HOW TO USE THIS BOOK

W0036007

STEP 1

Refer to the index at the back of the book. You can find any drug by any name in less than 5 seconds. All drugs are cross-indexed by generic and all known trade names. The index is easily distinguished by a printed blue bar at the edge of the pages. Drugs are also indexed by pharmacologic action. With one turn of the page, all drugs included in the text with similar pharmacologic actions and their page numbers are available to you. Everything is strictly alphabetized; you will never be required to refer to additional pages to locate a drug.

STEP 2

Turn to the single page number given after the name of the drug. All information about the drug is included as continuous reading. You will rarely be required to turn to another section of the book to be completely informed. Specific breakdowns of each drug (Usual Dose, Pediatric Dose, Dose Adjustments, Dilution, Compatibility, Rate of Administration, Actions, Indications and Uses, Precautions, Contraindications, Drug/Lab Interactions, Side Effects, and Antidote) are consistent in format and printed in boldface type. Subheadings under these categories are in boldface. Scan quickly for Usual Dose, Dose Adjustments, Drug/Lab Interactions, Side Effects, or Antidote or carefully read all included information. The choice is yours. A quick scan will take 5 to 10 seconds. Even the most complicated drugs will take less than 2 minutes to read completely. Read each monograph carefully and completely before administering a drug to a specific patient for the first time, and review it any time a new drug is added to the patient's drug profile.

That's it! This is a fast, complete, and accurate reference for anyone administering intravenous medications. The spiral binding is specifically designed to lie flat, leaving your hands free to secure needed supplies, prepare your medication, or even ventilate a patient while you read the needed information.

Develop the "look it up" habit. Clear, concise language and simplicity of form contribute to quick, easy use of this handbook. Before your first use, read the Preface, as it contains lots of helpful information. Check out the *Intravenous Medications* website for monographs no longer included in this text and for other useful IV medication information: **http://evolve.elsevier.com/IVMeds**

General Dilution Chart
General Dilution Chart (Gm to mg)

Amount of Drug Required in Grams	Amount of Diluent						
	1000 mL	500 mL	250 mL	125 mL	100 mL	50 mL	25 mL
	mg/mL	mg/mL	mg/mL	mg/mL	mg/mL	mg/mL	mg/mL
20 Gm	20	40	80	160	200	400	800
19 Gm	19	38	76	152	190	380	760
18 Gm	18	36	72	144	180	360	720
17 Gm	17	34	68	136	170	340	680
16 Gm	16	32	64	128	160	320	640
15 Gm	15	30	60	120	150	300	600
14 Gm	14	28	56	112	140	280	560
13 Gm	13	26	52	104	130	260	520
12 Gm	12	24	48	96	120	240	480
11 Gm	11	22	44	88	110	220	440
10 Gm	10	20	40	80	100	200	400
9 Gm	9	18	36	72	90	180	360
8 Gm	8	16	32	64	80	160	320
7 Gm	7	14	28	56	70	140	280
6 Gm	6	12	24	48	60	120	240
5 Gm	5	10	20	40	50	100	200
4.5 Gm	4.5	9	18	36	45	90	180
4 Gm	4	8	16	32	40	80	160
3.5 Gm	3.5	7	14	28	35	70	140
3 Gm	3	6	12	24	30	60	120
2.5 Gm	2.5	5	10	20	25	50	100
2 Gm	2	4	8	16	20	40	80
1.5 Gm	1.5	3	6	12	15	30	60
1 Gm	1	2	4	8	10	20	40
0.5 Gm	0.5	1	2	4	5	10	20
0.25 Gm	0.25	0.5	1	2	2.5	5	10

To use chart:
1. Find mg/mL desired, and track to the amount of diluent desired and amount of drug in Gm required.
2. Find the amount of drug in Gm required, and track to the diluent desired and/or mg/mL desired.
3. Find the amount of diluent required, and track to the amount of drug in Gm and/or mg/mL desired.

Formula: Substitute any number for x

x Gm diluted in 1000 mL = x mg/mL (1 Gm in 1000 mL = 1 mg/mL)
x Gm diluted in 500 mL = $2x$ mg/mL (1 Gm in 500 mL = 2 mg/mL)
x Gm diluted in 250 mL = $4x$ mg/mL (1 Gm in 250 mL = 4 mg/mL)
x Gm diluted in 125 mL = $8x$ mg/mL (1 Gm in 125 mL = 8 mg/mL)
x Gm diluted in 100 mL = $10x$ mg/mL (1 Gm in 100 mL = 10 mg/mL)
x Gm diluted in 50 mL = $20x$ mg/mL (1 Gm in 50 mL = 20 mg/mL)
x Gm diluted in 25 mL = $40x$ mg/mL (1 Gm in 25 mL = 40 mg/mL)

Some variation occurs from the manufacturer's overfill or if the drug is in liquid form. If absolute accuracy is required, these variations can be avoided by withdrawing an amount in mL from the diluent equal to the manufacturer's overfill and/or an amount equal to the amount in mL of the drug. Consult the pharmacist for specific information on the manufacturer's overfill of infusion fluids used in your facility.

See next page.

General Dilution Chart (mg to mcg)

Amount of Drug Required in Milligrams	Amount of Diluent						
	1000 mL	500 mL	250 mL	125 mL	100 mL	50 mL	25 mL
	mcg/mL	mcg/mL	mcg/mL	mcg/mL	mcg/mL	mcg/mL	mcg/mL
20 mg	20	40	80	160	200	400	800
19 mg	19	38	76	152	190	380	760
18 mg	18	36	72	144	180	360	720
17 mg	17	34	68	136	170	340	680
16 mg	16	32	64	128	160	320	640
15 mg	15	30	60	120	150	300	600
14 mg	14	28	56	112	140	280	560
13 mg	13	26	52	104	130	260	520
12 mg	12	24	48	96	120	240	480
11 mg	11	22	44	88	110	220	440
10 mg	10	20	40	80	100	200	400
9 mg	9	18	36	72	90	180	360
8 mg	8	16	32	64	80	160	320
7 mg	7	14	28	56	70	140	280
6 mg	6	12	24	48	60	120	240
5 mg	5	10	20	40	50	100	200
4.5 mg	4.5	9	18	36	45	90	180
4 mg	4	8	16	32	40	80	160
3.5 mg	3.5	7	14	28	35	70	140
3 mg	3	6	12	24	30	60	120
2.5 mg	2.5	5	10	20	25	50	100
2 mg	2	4	8	16	20	40	80
1.5 mg	1.5	3	6	12	15	30	60
1 mg	1	2	4	8	10	20	40
0.5 mg	0.5	1	2	4	5	10	20
0.25 mg	0.25	0.5	1	2	2.5	5	10

To use chart:
1. Find the mcg/mL desired, and track to the amount of diluent desired and the amount of drug in mg required.
2. Find the amount of drug in mg required, and track to diluent desired and/or mcg/mL desired.
3. Find the amount of diluent required, and track to the amount of drug in mg and/or mcg/mL desired.

Formula: Substitute any number for x

x mg diluted in 1000 mL = x mcg/mL (1 mg in 1000 mL = 1 mcg/mL)
x mg diluted in 500 mL = $2x$ mcg/mL (1 mg in 500 mL = 2 mcg/mL)
x mg diluted in 250 mL = $4x$ mcg/mL (1 mg in 250 mL = 4 mcg/mL)
x mg diluted in 125 mL = $8x$ mcg/mL (1 mg in 125 mL = 8 mcg/mL)
x mg diluted in 100 mL = $10x$ mcg/mL (1 mg in 100 mL = 10 mcg/mL)
x mg diluted in 50 mL = $20x$ mcg/mL (1 mg in 50 mL = 20 mcg/mL)
x mg diluted in 25 mL = $40x$ mcg/mL (1 mg in 25 mL = 40 mcg/mL)

Some variation occurs from the manufacturer's overfill or if the drug is in liquid form. If absolute accuracy is required, these variations can be avoided by withdrawing an amount in mL from the diluent equal to manufacturer's overfill and/or an amount equal to the amount in mL of the drug. Consult the pharmacist for specific information on the manufacturer's overfill of infusion fluids used in your facility.

Elsevier's 2026
INTRAVENOUS MEDICATIONS

A Handbook for Nurses and Health Professionals

Shelly Rainforth Collins, PharmD, BCGP

President
Drug Information Consultants
Chesapeake, Virginia

41ST EDITION

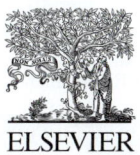

ELSEVIER

Elsevier
3251 Riverport Lane
St. Louis, Missouri 63043

ELSEVIER'S 2026 INTRAVENOUS MEDICATIONS, FORTYTWO EDITION

ISBN: 978-0-443-26959-2

Notice

Practitioners and researchers must always rely on their own experience and knowledge in evaluating and using any information, methods, compounds or experiments described herein. Because of rapid advances in the medical sciences, in particular, independent verification of diagnoses and drug dosages should be made. To the fullest extent of the law, no responsibility is assumed by Elsevier, authors, editors or contributors for any injury and/or damage to persons or property as a matter of products liability, negligence or otherwise, or from any use or operation of any methods, products, instructions, or ideas contained in the material herein.

Previous editions copyrighted 1973, 1977, 1981, 1984, 1988, 1989, 1990, 1991, 1993, 1994, 1995, 1996, 1997, 1998, 1999, 2000, 2001, 2002, 2003, 2004, 2005, 2006, 2007, 2008, 2009, 2010, 2011, 2012, 2013, 2014, 2015, 2016, 2017, 2018, 2019, 2020, 2021, 2022, 2023, 2024

International Standard Book Number: 978-0-443-12040-4

Content Strategist: Sonya Seigafuse
Content Development Specialist: Danielle M. Frazier
Publishing Services Manager: Deepthi Unni
Project Manager: Nayagi Anandan
Design Direction: Margaret Reid

Printed in United States of America

Last digit is the print number: 9 8 7 6 5 4 3 2 1

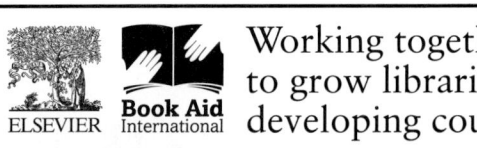

To my daughter,
Kristin Collins,
thank you for being such a joy.
I am so proud of the woman you have become.

To my father,
Charles Rainforth,
thank you for being the best dad
a girl could ever ask for.

This Year 2026 edition marks the 53rd year of publication of *Intravenous Medications*. All previous editions are considered out of date. We would like to welcome the expert contributions from the National Coalition for IV Push Safety in this new edition.

Intravenous Medications is designed for use anywhere intravenous medications are prepared and administered, such as in critical care areas, at the nursing station, in the office, in public health and home care settings, and by students and members of the armed services. Pertinent information can be found in a few seconds. Take advantage of its availability and quickly review every intravenous medication before administration.

When a medication is prescribed, the nurse must evaluate it for appropriateness and may need to prepare it, administer it, and observe the effects. If, after reviewing the information in *Intravenous Medications*, you have any questions about any order you are given, clarify it with the physician, consult the pharmacist, or consult your supervisor. The circumstances will determine whom you will approach first. If the physician thinks it is imperative to carry out an order even though you have unanswered questions, never hesitate to request that the physician administer the medication instead of you. In this era of constant change, the physician should be willing to provide you, your supervisor, and/or the pharmacist with current studies documenting the validity and appropriateness of orders.

All information presented in this handbook pertains only to the intravenous use of the drug and not necessarily to intramuscular, subcutaneous, oral, or other means of administration.

Several of the drugs in this text and on the Evolve website are biosimilars. Biosimilars are biological products that are licensed (approved) by the FDA because they are highly similar to an already FDA-approved biological product (known as the reference product (known as the reference product, such as trastuzumab [Herceptin]) but have allowable differences because they are made from living organisms. Biosimilars also have no clinically meaningful differences in terms of safety, purity, and potency from the reference product.

Many new uses have been approved for established drugs, and numerous safety issues have been identified by the FDA. All of these changes are incorporated so that our readers have the most current information available.

We continually strive to make the information in this handbook informative and easy to access. **We continue to identify drugs with a Black Box Warning BBW in the main heading of the monograph.** In addition, **Black Box Warning statements are shaded** in light gray, **and a different typeface is used** for instant identification wherever they appear in the text. *Blue-screened text* emphasizes a special circumstance not covered by a Black Box Warning. The FDA is now identifying **Limitations of Use** of drugs under Indications. Previously this information had been placed in Precautions. Common Toxicity Criteria (CTC) are available at https://ctep.cancer.gov/protocoldevelopment/electronic_applications/ctc.htm.

The Joint Commission and the **Institute for Safe Medication Practices (ISMP)** have strongly emphasized various ways to reduce errors in drug ordering and administration. *Intravenous Medications* uses both generic and trade names and spells out all symbols (except in charts where space is limited). The symbols are included in the Key to Abbreviations (p. xvii) if you need a refresher.

The Joint Commission, the ISMP, the American Pharmaceutical Association, and several other organizations have identified "High-Alert Medications" (a list of medications with the highest risk of injury when misused). The websites of these organizations contain considerable information and identify common risk factors and suggested strategies to reduce the risk of errors. All IV medications are considered high risk because they have an immediate effect, are irretrievable, and can cause life-threatening side effects with incorrect usage.

We advise the readers to consider several important sources for intravenous medication safety such the National Coalition for IV Push Safety, the Infusion Nurses Society, and the Institute for Safe Medication Practices.

Elsevier offers electronic versions of *Intravenous Medications* for handheld devices, tablets, laptops, and desktop computers. These electronic versions are convenient and portable alternatives or supplements to the printed book. In addition, all drugs currently on the Evolve IV Meds website **(http://evolve.elsevier.com/IVMeds)** for *Intravenous Medications* (because of space limitations for the print version) are **now all** incorporated in these electronic versions in alphabetical order to give you a complete package. Although the electronic versions are accessible wherever you have an electronic device, keep in mind that on some devices the entire monograph may not be visible at the same time. It is the user's responsibility to be familiar with the complete monograph and *all* aspects of each drug before administration.

Health care today is an intense environment. The speed of change is overwhelming, but the authors and publisher of *Intravenous Medications* have a commitment to provide all healthcare professionals who have the responsibility to administer IV medications with annual editions that incorporate complete, accurate, and current information in a clear, concise, accessible, and reliable tool. FDA websites are monitored throughout the year and provide many important updates, such as dose changes, new pediatric doses, additional disease-specific doses, refinements in dosing applications, new indications, new drug interactions, additional precautions, updates on post-marketing side effects, and new information on antidotes. Most drugs currently approved for intravenous use are included in the print version or are on the Evolve website: **http://evolve.elsevier.com/ IVMeds/**. (See pp. xiv and xv for a listing.) Helpful charts for dilution and/or rate of administration are incorporated in selected monographs. A General Dilution Chart to simplify calculations is found on the inside front cover. Front matter material provides a Key to Abbreviations and Important IV Therapy Facts.

Appreciation is extended to Sonya Seigafuse, Danielle M. Frazier, and Jodi M. Willard at Elsevier and to Joe Rekart at Graphic World.

And a thank you to the users of this reference. By seeking out this information, you serve your patients' needs and contribute to the safe administration of intravenous medications.

CONTENTS

Ado-Trastuzumab
Agalsidase Beta
Alfentanil Hydrochloride
Alglucerase
Alglucosidase Alfa
Alpha$_1$-Proteinase Inhibitor (Human)
Amifostine
Ammonium Chloride
Amobarbital Sodium
Anthrax Immune Globulin Intravenous (Human)
Antivenin (*Latrodectus mactans*)
Antivenin (*Micrurus fulvius*)

Antivenin Crotalidae Polyvalent Immune Fab (Ovine)
Arginine Hydrochloride
Ascorbic Acid
Asparaginase *Erwinia chrysanthemi*
Atracurium Besylate
Axicabtagene Ciloleucel
Azathioprine Sodium
Blinatumomab
Botulism Immune Globulin (Intravenous Human)
Brentuximab
Busulfan

Designed to facilitate quick reference, each entry begins with the generic name of the drug in boldface type. **Medications with a Black Box Warning are identified with a symbol BBW in the main heading**. Phonetic pronunciations appear just below the generic name. Drug categories follow. The primary category may be followed by additional ones representing the multiple uses of a medication. Associated trade names are under the generic name. Boldface type and alphabetical order enable the reader to verify correct drug names easily. The use of a Canadian maple leaf symbol (♣) after a trade name indicates availability in Canada only.

Headings within drug monographs are as follows.

USUAL ADULT DOSE: Doses recommended are the usual range for adults unless specifically stated otherwise. This information is presented first to enable the nurse to verify that the medication order is within acceptable parameters while checking the order and before preparation.

> **Pretreatment:** This subheading section alerts you to situations that must or should be completed before administering the medication. Many of the newer medications can cause fetal harm, so you will find the statement "Verify pregnancy status" here. You will also be alerted to premedication, baseline studies, pretesting, immunization, prehydration, and other requirements indicated before treatment and will be referred to the place in the monograph containing needed additional information.

PEDIATRIC DOSE: Pediatric doses are specifically stated when different from the adult dose. Not all medications are labeled for use in pediatric patients, and off-label use is common. See Maternal/Child for information on safety and effectiveness for use in pediatric patients. A ready-to-administer product should be used with caution if only administering a partial dose to prevent unintentional overdose.

INFANT AND/OR NEONATAL DOSE: This information is included if available and distinct from Pediatric Dose. See Maternal/Child for information on safety and effectiveness for use in pediatric patients, including infants and neonates. Medications for pediatric patients would likely be supplied by the pharmacy in a syringe or syringe pump administration or retrograde injection.

ALL AGE DOSE ADJUSTMENTS: Any situation that requires increasing or decreasing a dose is mentioned here. The range covers adjustments needed for elderly, debilitated, or hepatic or renal impairment patients; adjustments required by race or gender; or adjustments required in the presence of other medications or as physical conditions are monitored.

DILUTION: Medications given IV push may be available in ampules, vials, manufactured prefilled syringes, compounded prefilled syringes, and ready-to-assemble products such as Carpuject™. It is important to note that routine dilution of IV push medications is contraindicated unless required by the manufacturer, hospital policy, or other evidence-based guidelines. It is not appropriate to use prefilled saline flush syringes to dilute or reconstitute IV medications unless approved for this use by the U.S. Food and Drug Administration (FDA; see the label of the product you use).

> **Secondary Infusion Bags:** Certain medications may be available in more than one form (e.g., Mini-Bag Plus, ADD-Vantage™, Duplex®); follow the manufacturer's directions for reconstitution and stability. Appropriate diluents are listed, but refer to local protocols and standards. Standardization of concentrations is advised and guided by organizations such as the American Society of Health-System Pharmacists' Standardize 4 Safety initiative. Links to selected standards are listed here: National Adult Continuous Infusion Standards are available at https://www.ashp.org/-/media/assets/pharmacy-practice/s4s/docs/Adult-Infusion-Standards.pdf and pediatric standards are available at https://www.ashp.org/-/media/assets/pharmacy-practice/s4s/docs/Pediatric-Infusion-Standards.pdf.

The Solution Compatibility Chart on the inside back cover has been expanded and updated. For pediatric patients, most come diluted from the pharmacy, and standard concentrations for pediatric medications should be established locally. For any medication that must be diluted by the nurse prior to administering, please refer to the front pages entitled Preparation and Administration of Injectable Medications. Generic dilution charts for grams to milligrams and milligrams to micrograms are featured on the inside front cover and facing page.

Filters: A medication in a glass ampule should be filtered when drawn up to eliminate the possibility of glass shards being injected. A filter needle or filter straw is used to draw the solution from the ampule, and that device is replaced with a standard needle to inject into a bag or contents administered to a patient through a needleless port. Use of an in-line filter device for medications should be done according to local protocol or manufacturer guidance. Multiple in-line filters are available, and pore size should be matched to the product being administered. Consult your pharmacist if more information is needed than is provided in this book.

Storage: Medications prepared at the site of administration should be administered within 4 hours unless specifically noted on the label or in medication information sources and should be used only for a single patient. The product should be labeled completely (patient name, medication, concentration, date and time prepared, and initials of person doing the preparation) unless administered immediately. Aseptic intravenous compounding will generally be done in special clean rooms and the final product delivered to the location of the patient. Sterile compounded solutions should be properly labeled for an individual patient and stored under optimal conditions—generally refrigerated, although some medications should stay at room temperature. This detail should be on the product along with a label suggesting either "do not use" beyond a specific date (beyond use date, or BUD) and time or "do not hang" after a specific date and time (although these can generally hang for up to 24 additional hours). Consult local policies for specific terminology and standards.

COMPATIBILITIES The focus of this section is **compatibility** between two medications. **Any medication not listed as compatible should be considered incompatible**. Only the manufacturer's recommendations for **compatibility** or **incompatibility** are listed and may be specific to the concentration and/or solution. No third-party compatibilities or incompatibilities are listed. Multiple medications are sometimes administered through the same site, but that compatibility is often not studied or defined.

A manufacturer's listing may include detailed information on potential interaction with specific plastic tubing/containers or other medications or devices. If the manufacturer provides no information, that will be stated.

If there are other sources that list specific compatibilities dependent on concentration or manufacturer, a statement to this effect follows so you know other compatibilities may exist. An updated digital database (e.g., Lexicomp, Trissels, Micromedex, King Guide, Clinical Pharmacology) may be available in your location. Wall charts are not ideal for this purpose due to their rapidly becoming outdated. Always consult a pharmacist for clarification of compatibilities, specific concentrations, or doses.

Administration of IV Infusion: What steps should you consider before administering any medication? Please refer to the new section at the front of the book entitled Preparation and Administration of Injectable Medications. If the medication you wish to administer is not listed in the **Compatibility** section, *consider it to be incompatible*. If you are unable to discontinue the infusion of an incompatible drug, you must have another IV access.

RATE OF ADMINISTRATION: Accepted rates of administration are listed. Potential adverse effects from too rapid or slow injection rates are also listed but may not be complete. Suggested rates for infants, children, or the elderly are listed when available and are often administered with the aid of a controlled infusion device. Although the speed that a medication is given via IV push may be important, for small-volume doses it is the rate of flush following the medication that dictates delivery into the vasculature. The residual volume from the administration site (Y-site or needleless connector) and the vascular device fill volume must be factored into the rate of administration. Do not use running IV fluid to control the rate of administration. Charts are available in selected monographs.

MEDICATION ACTIONS: Clear, concise statements outline the origin of each medication, how it affects body systems, its length of action, and methods of excretion. If a medication crosses the placental barrier or is secreted in breast milk, it will be mentioned here if that information is available.

INDICATIONS AND USES: When a medication is reviewed by the FDA, it is labeled for specific indications. Once a medication is marketed, prescribers are allowed to use it for other indications, ideally with adequate supporting literature (known as "off-label" use) or under a specific protocol for the facility. However, specific contraindications, warnings, and precautions should be evaluated prior to use, including consideration of pregnancy, breastfeeding, extremes of age or weight, medication interactions, and potential adverse effects, and care setting. **Limitations of Use** are now being identified by the manufacturer in FDA-approved labeling to describe situations where the risk-to-benefit profile of a medication is uncertain and has implications for the safe and effective use of the medication.

CONTRAINDICATIONS: Contraindications are situations where the medication should not be used, and this book includes those specifically listed by the manufacturer in the approved label. Consult with the prescriber if an ordered medication is contraindicated for the patient.

PRECAUTIONS: The section on precautions covers many areas of information needed before injecting any medication, including Black Box Warnings from the prescribing information as previously defined. **Black Box Warning statements are shaded** in light gray, **and a different typeface is used** for instant identification wherever they appear in the text. The range of information in this category covers all facets not covered under specific headings. Additional subdivisions may be included.

Monitor: This subheading includes information such as required prerequisites for medication administration, parameters for evaluation, and patient assessments.

Patient Education: This subheading addresses only specific, important issues required for short-term IV use. It is expected that the health professional will review the major points in the medication profile with the patient, including name of medication, purpose, effects and side effects, special instructions, and duration of treatment. There are certain medications that require a Risk Evaluation and Mitigation Strategy (REMS), which is a medication safety program that the FDA can require for certain medications with serious safety concerns to help ensure that the benefits of the medication outweigh its risk. Medications with a REMS are noted in the patient education section.

Maternal/Child: This subheading addresses use in pregnancy, childbirth, and lactation; safety for use in pediatric patients; and any special impact on infants and neonates.

Elderly: This subheading is included whenever specific information impacting this patient group is available. The Beers Criteria for Potentially Inappropriate Medication Use in Older Adults recommendations are incorporated into the guidance regarding medications that should be avoided in most older patients or in certain situations. For more information on Beers criteria, see https://dcri.org/beers-criteria-medication-list. Always consider age-related organ impairment (e.g., cardiac, hepatic, renal, insufficient bone marrow reserve), history of previous or concomitant disease or medication therapy, and route of excretion when determining dose and evaluating side effects.

DRUG/LAB INTERACTIONS: Drug/drug or drug/lab interactions are listed here. To help identify these interactions more easily, **single medications, medication categories when there are multiple medications, and specific tests are in boldface type**. If a potential

interaction within the patient's medication profile is noted, consult a pharmacist immediately. Interactions may increase or decrease medication effectiveness or alter the likelihood of an adverse effect. Check with the lab first on drug/lab interactions; acceptable
monitoring alternatives may be available. After this consultation, notify the prescriber if
appropriate. To facilitate recognition, common trade names accompany generic names or
examples are presented.

SIDE EFFECTS: In some monographs, the most common side effects may be listed first,
followed by the most serious side effects. In all monographs, they are listed in alphabetical order. Specific symptoms of overdose are listed where available or distinct from
usual doses.

ANTIDOTE: Specific antidotes are listed in this section if available. In addition, specific
nursing actions to reverse undesirable side effects are listed.

Within a heading, there may be references to other sections within an individual
monograph (e.g., see Precautions, see Monitor, see Dose Adjustments, see Maternal/
Child). These references indicate additional requirements and should be consulted before
administering the medication.

<	less than	CVA	cerebrovascular accident
>	more than	CVP	central venous pressure
$^1/_4$NS	one-fourth normal saline (0.2%)	D10NS	10% dextrose in normal saline
$^1/_3$NS	one-third normal saline (0.33%)	D10W	10% dextrose in water
$^1/_2$NS	one-half normal saline (0.45%)	D5/$^1/_4$NS	5% dextrose in one-quarter normal saline (0.2%)
ABGs	arterial blood gases		
ACE	angiotensin-converting enzyme	D5/$^1/_3$NS	5% dextrose in one-third normal saline (0.33%)
ACT	activated coagulation time		
ACTH	adrenocorticotropic hormone	D5/$^1/_2$NS	5% dextrose in one-half normal saline (0.45%)
AF	atrial fibrillation		
A/G	albumin-to-globulin ratio	D5LR	5% dextrose in lactated Ringer's solution
AIDS	acquired immunodeficiency syndrome		
ALT	alanine aminotransferase (SGPT)	D5NS	5% dextrose in normal saline
AMI	acute myocardial infarction	D5R	5% dextrose in Ringer's solution
ANC	absolute neutrophil count	D5W	5% dextrose in water
aPTT	activated partial thromboplastin time	DC	discontinued
ARDS	adult respiratory distress syndrome/ acute respiratory distress syndrome	DEHP	diethylhexylphthalate
		DIC	disseminated intravascular coagulation
AST	aspartate aminotransferase (SGOT)		
AUC	area under the curve	dL	deciliter(s) (100 mL)
AV	atrioventricular	dMMR	deficient mismatch repair
BMD	bone mass density	DNA	deoxyribonucleic acid
BP	blood pressure	ECG	electrocardiogram
BSA	body surface area	EEG	electroencephalogram
BUN	blood urea nitrogen	eGFR	estimated glomerular filtration rate
BWFI	bacteriostatic water for injection	ESRD	end-stage renal disease
C	Celsius	F	Fahrenheit
Ca	calcium	FSH	follicle-stimulating hormone
CABG	coronary artery bypass graft	GI	gastrointestinal
CAD	coronary artery disease	GFR	glomerular filtration rate
CAPD	continuous ambulatory peritoneal dialysis	GGT	gamma-glutamyl transferase
		Gm	gram(s)
CBC	complete blood cell count	gr	grain(s)
CDAD	*Clostridium difficile*–associated diarrhea	gtt	drop(s)
		GU	genitourinary
CHF	congestive heart failure	Hb	hemoglobin
Cl	chloride	Hct	hematocrit
CMV	cytomegalovirus	HCV	hepatitis C virus
CNS	central nervous system	Hg	mercury
CO_2	carbon dioxide	HIV	human immunodeficiency virus
COPD	chronic obstructive pulmonary disease	hr	hour
CPK	creatine kinase	HR	heart rate
CrCl	creatinine clearance	HSCT	hematopoietic stem cell transplant
CRF	chronic renal failure	IBW	ideal body weight
CRT	controlled room temperature (20°C to 25°C; 68°F to 77°F)	ICU	intensive care unit
		IgA	immune globulin A
CSF	cerebrospinal fluid	IGIV	immune globulin intravenous
C/S	culture and sensitivity	ÍL	microliters, μL, mm^3
CTCAE	Common Terminology Criteria for Adverse Events	IM	intramuscular
		INR	international normalized ratio

IP	intrapleural	PRCA	pure red cell aplasia
IU	international unit(s)	PRES	posterior reversible encephalopathy syndrome
IV	intravenous		
IVIG	intravenous immunoglobulin	PSVT	paroxysmal supraventricular tachycardia
K	potassium		
KCl	potassium chloride	PT	prothrombin time
kg	kilogram(s)	PTT	partial thromboplastin time
L	liter(s)	PVC	polyvinyl chloride; premature ventricular contraction
lb	pound(s)		
LDH	lactic dehydrogenase	R	Ringer's injection or solution
LFT	liver function test	RBC	red blood cell
LH	luteinizing hormone	refrigerate	temperature at 2°C to 8°C (36°F to 46°F)
LR	lactated Ringer's injection or solution		
M	molar	RNA	ribonucleic acid
m²	meter squared	RPLS	reversible posterior leukoencephalopathy syndrome
MAO	monoamine oxidase		
MAP	mean arterial pressure	RT	room temperature
mcg	microgram(s)	RTS	room-temperature stable
mCi	millicurie(s)	SA	sinoatrial
mEq	milliequivalent	SC	subcutaneous
Mg	magnesium	SCr	serum creatinine
mg	milligram(s)	SIADH	syndrome of inappropriate antidiuretic hormone
MI	myocardial infarction		
min	minute	SOB	shortness of breath
mL	milliliter	S/S	signs and symptoms
mmol	millimole(s)	SW or SWI	sterile water for injection
mm³	cubic millimeters, μL, ÍL	TEN	toxic epidermal necrolysis
MDRSP	multidrug-resistant *Streptococcus pneumoniae*	TIA	transient ischemic attacks
		TLS	tumor lysis syndrome
MRI	magnetic resonance imaging	TNA	3-in-1 combination of amino acids, glucose, and fat emulsion
MSI-H	microsatellite instability-high		
Na	sodium	TPN	2-in-1 combination of amino acids and glucose; total parenteral nutrition
NaCl	sodium chloride		
NCI	National Cancer Institute; see CTCAE	TRALI	transfusion-related acute lung injury
ng	nanogram (millimicrogram)	TSH	thyroid-stimulating hormone
NS	normal saline (0.9%)	TT	thrombin time
NSAID	nonsteroidal anti-inflammatory drug	μL	microliters, mm³, ÍL
NSCLC	non–small-cell lung cancer	ULN	upper limits of normal
NSR	normal sinus rhythm	URI	upper respiratory infection
N/V	nausea and vomiting	UTI	urinary tract infection
OTC	over-the-counter	VEGF	vascular endothelial growth factor
PAC	premature atrial contraction	VF	ventricular fibrillation
PaO₂	arterial oxygen pressure	VS	vital signs
PCA	patient-controlled analgesia	VT	ventricular tachycardia
PCP	*Pneumocystis jiroveci* pneumonia	v/v	volume-to-volume ratio
pg	picogram	WBC	white blood cell
pH	hydrogen ion concentration	WBCT	whole blood clotting time
PML	progressive multifocal leukoencephalopathy	w/v	weight-to-volume ratio
		w/w	weight-to-weight ratio
PO	by mouth/orally		

IMPORTANT IV THERAPY FACTS

- Read the Preface and the Format and Content of *Intravenous Medications* sections at least once. They'll answer many of your questions and save you time.

USUAL DOSE

- Doses calculated on body weight are usually based on pretreatment weight and not on edematous weight.
- Normal renal or hepatic function is usually required for drugs metabolized by these routes.
- Formula to calculate creatinine clearance (CrCl) from serum creatinine value (Cockcroft–Gault equation):

$$\text{Males: } \frac{\text{Weight in kg} \times (140 - \text{Age in years})}{72 \times \text{Serum creatinine (mg/dL)}} = \text{CrCl}$$

Females: $0.85 \times$ Male CrCl value calculated from above formula.

- Children: $K \times \dfrac{\text{Linear length or height (cm)}}{\text{SCr (mg/100 mL)}}$

  K for children >1 year of age = 0.55
  K for infants = 0.45

- Lean body weight (LBW)
  Males: 50 kg + 2.3 kg for each inch over 5 feet
  Females: 45.5 kg + 2.3 kg for each inch over 5 feet
  Children weighing 15 kg or less: Use actual body weight in kg

- Formula to calculate body surface area (BSA):

$$\text{BSA (M}^2) = \sqrt{\frac{\text{Height (cm)} \times \text{Weight (kg)}}{3600}}$$

- To prevent unintentional overdose, a premixed solution such as DUPLEX or Galaxy containers available in a specific dose (e.g., 1 Gm, 2 Gm) should be used in pediatric patients *only when the individual dose is the entire contents of the container and not any fraction thereof.*

DILUTION

- Check all labels (drugs, diluents, and solutions) to confirm appropriateness for IV use.
- Sterile technique is imperative in all phases of preparation.
- Use a filter needle when withdrawing IV meds from ampules to eliminate possible pieces of glass.
- Pearls:
  1 Gm in 1 Liter yields 1 mg/mL.
  1 mg in 1 Liter yields 1 mcg/mL.
  % of a solution equals the number of grams/100 mL (5% = 5 Gm/100 mL).
- Pediatric dilution:
  If you dilute 6.0 mg/kg in 100 mL, 1 mL/hr equals 1.0 mcg/kg/min.
  If you dilute 0.6 mg/kg in 100 mL, 1 mL/hr equals 0.1 mcg/kg/min.
- To prevent unintentional overdose, a premixed solution such as DUPLEX or Galaxy containers available in a specific dose (e.g., 1 Gm, 2 Gm) should be used in pediatric patients *only when the individual dose is the entire contents of the container and not any fraction thereof.*
- See charts on inside front cover.

- Do not use bacteriostatic diluents containing benzyl alcohol for neonates, as doing so may cause a fatal toxic syndrome. Signs and symptoms (S/S) include CNS depression, hypotension, intracranial hemorrhage, metabolic acidosis, renal failure, respiratory problems, and seizures.
- Ensure adequate mixing of all drugs added to a solution.
- When combining drugs in a solution (additives), always consider the required rate adjustment of each drug.
- Examine solutions for clarity and any possible leakage.
- Frozen infusion solutions should be thawed at room temperature (25°C; 77°F) or under refrigeration. Do not force by immersion in water baths or in the microwave. All ice crystals must be melted before administration. Do not refreeze.
- Syringe prepackaging for use in specific pumps is now available for many drugs. Concentrations are often the strongest permissible, but length of delivery is accurate.
- Controlled room temperature (CRT) is considered to be 25°C (77°F). Most medications tolerate variations in temperature from 15°C to 30°C (59°F to 86°F).

INCOMPATIBILITIES

- Some manufacturers routinely suggest discontinuing the primary IV for intermittent infusion, which is usually done to avoid any possibility of incompatibility. Flushing the line before and after administration may be indicated and/or appropriate for some drugs.
- The brand of intravenous fluids or additives, concentrations, containers, rate and order of mixing, pH, and temperature all affect solubility and compatibility. Consult your pharmacist with any questions, and document appropriate instructions on the care plan.

TECHNIQUES

- **Do not hang** IV infusions in flexible plastic containers **in series connection, do not pressurize** IV infusions in flexible plastic containers **to increase flow rates without first fully evacuating residual air from the container, and do not use vented IV administration sets** with IV infusions in flexible plastic containers. **All may result in air embolism.**
- Confirm the patency of peripheral and/or central sites. Avoid extravasation.
- Avoid accidental arterial injection, as it can cause gangrene.

RATE OF ADMINISTRATION

- Life-threatening reactions (time-related overdose or allergy) are frequently precipitated by a too-rapid rate of injection.
- If a common IV line is used to administer other drugs through the same IV line, flush the IV line before and after each infusion with a compatible solution (e.g., NS, D5W). When flushing before administration, be sure to flush with an amount adequate to clear the previous drug (e.g., mL of drug or mL of lumen of catheter). When flushing after administration, be sure to flush with an amount at least equal to that of the drug administered (e.g., mL of drug or mL of lumen of catheter).

PATIENT EDUCATION

- A well-informed patient is a great asset; review all appropriate drug information with every conscious patient.

SIDE EFFECTS

- Reactions may be caused by a side effect of the drug itself, allergic response, overdose, or the underlying disease process.

RESOURCES

PUBLICATIONS

The following publications have been used as a resource to assemble the information found in *Intravenous Medications*. Additional and more detailed information on drugs may be found in these publications:

American Hospital Formulary Service Drug Information, 2020, Bethesda, MD, American Society of Health-System Pharmacists (updated via website).

Handbook on Injectable Drugs, 2021, Bethesda, MD, American Society of Health-System Pharmacists.

Lexi-CLINICAL SUITE, Wolters Kluwer Lexicomp mobile application software.

The Elsevier Guide to Oncology Drugs & Regimens, 2006, Huntington, NY, Elsevier.

Manufacturers' literature.

WEBSITE RESOURCES

http://www.accessdata.fda.gov/scripts/cder/drugsatfda—drug approvals and updates

http://www.fda.gov/safety/medwatch/default.htm—safety information

http://evolve.elsevier.com/IVMeds

http://www.cancer.gov—Common Terminology Criteria for Adverse Events (CTCAE)

http://www.blackboxrx.com—listing of all drugs with a Black Box Warning

PREPARATION AND ADMINISTRATION OF INJECTABLE DRUGS

Follow these steps after order verification and the appropriate steps for safe medication use.

GENERAL CONSIDERATIONS

Medications are prepared at the bedside when they are not provided in ready-to-administer form by the pharmacy or if the product stability requires preparation immediately before administration. Here is a simple list of **Do's and Don'ts**.

DO	DON'T
• Gather materials (drug, diluent, disinfecting swabs/devices, syringes, needles, label) onto a clean surface (general aseptic field) in a location without interruptions, away from sinks or other sources of contamination.	• Prepare hazardous drugs outside of approved areas (follow safe handling procedures).
• Perform hand hygiene.	• Re-use a single-use vial.
• Inspect materials for integrity (packaging clean, dry, and intact/undamaged) and expiration date.	• Use a multi-use vial on more than one patient unless local policies describe specific exceptions.
• Disinfect surfaces such as the vial, ampule neck, and injection site on a bag and let the product dry.	• Withdraw drug from a commercially available ready-to-use cartridge syringe.
• Keep key parts and key sites sterile.	• Dilute unless directed by the manufacturer.
• Add a tip cap to a syringe if not immediately administered.	• Use a saline flush solution from a pre-filled syringe to dilute or reconstitute a drug unless the flush syringe is labeled for that use.
• Label the product with the patient name, drug name, strength/dose, and time if not immediately administered.	• Recap used needles.
• Dispose of extra drug, used needles, and syringes in an approved device/location.	• Reuse a sterile saline flush syringe, even on the same patient.
• Obtain an independent double-check for high-alert medications according to local policies.	• Use the product more than 4 hours after preparation.
• Disinfect the injection port on IV tubing according to the device directions prior to administration.	

PROCEDURES

Preparing a Medication from an Ampule

1. Disinfect the neck of the ampule prior to entry and allow the disinfectant to dry.
2. Flick the ampule to ensure that all drug is in the body of the container.
3. Using a paper towel or gauze square, snap the neck of the ampule away from your body.
4. Use a syringe that is the appropriate size for the volume to be given to draw up the dose.
5. Take the cap off of the filter needle/straw, place your sterile needle/straw into the ampule, and draw up the needed amount of liquid.
6. Dispose of the ampule glass in a sharps container.
7. Remove the filter needle (do not inject through a filter needle); use a new sterile needle if injecting into a bag.
8. Refer to general considerations above.

Preparing a Medication from a Vial

1. Disinfect vial septum (the plastic cap on a vial is not a sterile barrier) and allow the disinfectant to dry.
2. Use a blunt needle to remove the contents of the vial.
3. To draw up the dose, use a syringe that is the appropriate size for the volume to be given.
4. Insert the needle into the vial, invert the vial, and withdraw the vial contents into the syringe.
5. Adjust the volume in the syringe according to the prescribed dose; some vials contain overfill, or the prescribed dose is less than the vial contents.
6. Dispose of the used syringe/needle safely after use.
7. Refer to general considerations above.

Reconstituting a Drug

Reconstitution is the process of adding a liquid diluent to a dry drug to make a specific concentration of liquid drug.

1. Disinfect the septum of the diluent and drug vials (the plastic cap on a vial is not a sterile barrier).
2. Attach a blunt needle to a syringe.
3. Pull the plunger back on the syringe to the volume of diluent you plan to withdraw (this will prevent a vacuum from forming) and inject air into the diluent vial.
4. Keeping the same needle and syringe in the vial, withdraw the amount of diluent needed.
5. Remove the syringe/needle from the diluent vial.
6. Inject the diluent into the powdered medication vial. Direct the solution toward the wall of the vial to minimize foaming.
7. Remove the syringe and needle from the vial.
   a. Swirl the vial to dissolve the drug.
   b. Inspect to ensure that the drug is dissolved and that no visible particles remain.
8. Withdraw the ordered dose of drug into a new sterile syringe of an appropriate size for the dose, using a new needle, and dispose of the used needle safely in a sharps container.
9. Refer to general considerations above.

Diluting a Drug

Dilution is the process of adding a liquid diluent to a liquid drug to make a specific concentration of the liquid drug.

1. Only dilute a liquid drug when recommended by manufacturer or local policy.
2. Using the steps above, draw the drug into the appropriately sized syringe.
3. Using the same needle and syringe, insert the needle into the diluent vial and withdraw the appropriate amount of diluent. **Do not inject the drug into the diluent vial**.
4. Remove the needle and syringe from the vial. Swirl gently to mix.
5. Remove the needle prior to attaching to needleless injection port or replace with tip cap.
   a. Do not use a saline flush solution from a prefilled syringe to dilute a medication.
   b. Do not inject a medication into another syringe through the syringe tip.

Preparing an Infusion Bag

1. Obtain or draw up the exact amount of drug to be added to the bag using the procedures described above.
   a. No more than two drugs may be added to an infusion bag when prepared outside the pharmacy.
2. Remove bag overwrap.
3. Disinfect the injection port on the bag and inject the drug.
4. Mix gently to ensure the drug is completely distributed.
5. Label and use within 4 hours as directed above.

IV Push Administration

1. Use barcode scanning if not already done or repeat the "rights" for safe medication use.
   a. Obtain an independent double check as appropriate for local policies.
2. Confirm vascular access patency with a flush/aspiration prior to each use and ensure appropriateness of that site for the drug and concentration to be administered.
   a. Use a 10-mL-diameter syringe to assess patency and give initial flush for central lines.
   b. Always use two sterile saline flush syringes, one before and one after medication administration. Do not reuse saline flush syringes.
3. Disinfect the needleless injection port of tubing, nearest the patient.
4. Stop the infusion.
5. Flush tubing with the first sterile saline flush syringe to clear IV fluids and injection port.
6. Attach medication syringe to the injection port and inject at the prescribed rate of administration.
7. Remove drug syringe.
8. Disinfect injection port.
9. Flush tubing with a second sterile saline flush syringe. Inject flush at the same rate as the medication rate of administration. (This is how the drug is administered completely at the desired rate).
   a. Never leave a syringe attached to an injection port.
10. Lock the vascular access device according to the device and local practice protocols or resume primary infusion.
11. Document drug administration if not already completed.

IVPB Administration

1. Use barcode scanning if not already done or repeat the "rights" for safe medication use.
   a. Obtain an independent double check as appropriate for local policies.
2. Confirm vascular access patency with a flush/aspiration prior to each use, and ensure appropriateness of that site for the drug and concentration to be administered.
   a. Use a 10-mL-diameter syringe to assess patency and give initial flush for central lines.
3. Disinfect the needleless injection port of tubing (per device directions) containing a compatible solution.
   a. Choose a port above the infusion device where it will control the IVPB rate.
   b. Do not interrupt a continuous therapeutic infusion for an IVPB drug.
4. If the drug and primary fluid are **not compatible**, stop the infusion and flush tubing with saline or dextrose as appropriate for the drug per the drug manufacturer's directions prior to drug administration.
   a. After the drug injection or infusion, repeat flush with saline/dextrose as compatible.
5. If the drug and primary fluid are **compatible**, you may continue the primary infusion or use the infusion pump/device to control which fluid infuses per local protocols.
6. Disinfect the port prior to each insertion including saline flush.
7. Lock the vascular access device according to the device and local practice protocols or resume primary infusion.
8. Document drug administration if not already completed.

Note that some drugs will be supplied with specific materials to facilitate preparation. Follow the manufacturer's guidelines for the use of those products.
Consult the Infusion Nurses Society Infusion Therapy Standards of Practice for detailed information, and always know the local practice policies and procedures.

ABATACEPT
(a-**BAY**-ta-sept)

Antirheumatic
Disease-modifying agent
Selective T-cell
costimulation blocker

Orencia

pH 7.2 to 7.8

USUAL DOSE
Pretreatment: Pretesting required; see Monitor. See Maternal/Child.

Dose is based on body weight in kilograms as shown in the following chart. After the initial dose, repeat administration at 2 and 4 weeks. Administer every 4 weeks thereafter. May be used as monotherapy or concomitantly with disease-modifying antirheumatic drugs (DMARDs) other than TNF antagonists; see Contraindications and Drug Interactions. May be given by SQ injection or as an IV infusion; formulation and dose are different; see Indications and prescribing information.

Abatacept Adult Dosing Guidelines		
Body Weight (kg)	**Dose (mg)**	**Number of Vials**
<60 kg	500 mg	2 vials
60 to 100 kg	750 mg	3 vials
>100 kg	1,000 mg	4 vials

Patients transitioning from IV therapy to subcutaneous administration should administer the first subcutaneous dose instead of the next scheduled IV dose. Abatacept is dosed weekly in the subcutaneous regimen. When administered for treatment of rheumatoid arthritis, it may be initiated with or without an IV loading dose. If the subcutaneous regimen is initiated with an IV loading dose, determine loading dose as outlined in the previous chart. The first subcutaneous injection should be administered within a day of the IV loading dose. A loading dose **is not** used when administered for treatment of psoriatic arthritis.

PEDIATRIC DOSE
May be given by SQ injection (2 years of age and older) or as an IV infusion (6 years of age and older) in pediatric patients. Formulation and dose are different; see Indications and prescribing information. When administered subcutaneously, **do not** administer an IV loading dose. May be used as monotherapy or concomitantly with methotrexate.

Pediatric patients 6 to 17 years of age who weigh less than 75 kg: 10 mg/kg/dose based on patient's body weight at each administration. After the initial dose, repeat administration at 2 and 4 weeks. Administer every 4 weeks thereafter.

Pediatric patients 6 to 17 years of age who weigh more than 75 kg: See Usual Dose and the Abatacept Adult Dosing Guidelines chart. Do not exceed a maximum dose of 1,000 mg.

DOSE ADJUSTMENTS
There is a trend toward a higher clearance with increasing body weight; see Usual Dose. No specific dose adjustments are required based on age or gender when corrected for body weight. ▪ The effects of renal or hepatic impairment have not been studied.

DILUTION
Using **ONLY the silicone-free disposable syringe provided** with each vial and an 18- to 21-gauge needle, reconstitute each 250-mg vial with 10 mL SWFI; final concentration is 25 mg/mL. (If reconstituted with a siliconized syringe, the solution must be discarded.) Direct stream of SWFI toward side of vial. Do not use vial if vacuum is not present. Rotate or swirl vial gently until contents have dissolved. Do not shake. After dissolution, vent vial with a needle to dissipate any foam that may be present. Solution should

be clear and colorless to pale yellow. Reconstituted solution must be further diluted to 100 mL as follows: From a 100-mL infusion bag or bottle, withdraw a volume of NS equal to the volume of reconstituted abatacept solution required for the patient's dose (for 2 vials, remove 20 mL; for 3 vials, remove 30 mL; for 4 vials, remove 40 mL). Using the *same silicone-free disposable syringe provided,* slowly add the reconstituted abatacept into the infusion bag or bottle. Mix gently.

Orencia prefilled syringes and Orencia ClickJet autoinjectors are intended for subcutaneous use only and are not intended for IV infusion.

Filter: Administration through a 0.2- to 1.2-micron, nonpyrogenic, low–protein binding filter is required.

Storage: Refrigerate unopened vials at 2° to 8°C (36° to 46°F). Do not use beyond expiration date. Protect from light by storing in original packaging. Before administration, the diluted solution may be stored at RT or refrigerated; however, infusion of the diluted solution should be completed within 24 hours of reconstitution. Discard diluted solution if not administered within 24 hours. Any unused portion in a vial must be discarded.

COMPATIBILITY

Manufacturer states, "Should not be infused concomitantly in the same intravenous line with other agents." **Compatibility** studies have not been performed.

RATE OF ADMINISTRATION

Administration through a 0.2- to 1.2-micron, nonpyrogenic, low–protein binding filter is required.

A single dose equally distributed over 30 minutes.

ACTIONS

A selective T-cell costimulation modulator. Acts as a selective biologic response modulator by inhibiting T-lymphocyte activation. Activated T-lymphocytes are implicated in the pathogenesis of rheumatoid arthritis and psoriatic arthritis. Abatacept reduces pain and joint inflammation and slows the progression of structural damage to bone and cartilage. Mean half-life is 13.1 days (range 8 to 25 days).

INDICATIONS AND USES

Reduce the S/S, induce a major clinical response, inhibit the progression of structural damage, and improve the physical function in adult patients with moderately to severely active rheumatoid arthritis. May be used as monotherapy or concomitantly with DMARDs other than TNF antagonists. May be given IV or SQ. Adult infusion patients may transition to SQ injection; see prescribing information. ▪ Reduce the S/S in pediatric patients 2 years of age and older with moderately to severely active polyarticular juvenile idiopathic arthritis. May be used as monotherapy or concomitantly with methotrexate. SQ injection may be used in pediatric patients 2 years of age and older. IV dosing has not been studied in patients younger than 6 years of age; see prescribing information. ▪ Treatment of adult patients with active psoriatic arthritis. May be used with or without nonbiologic DMARDs.

Limitation of use: Should not be administered concomitantly with TNF antagonists (e.g., adalimumab [Humira], etanercept [Enbrel]) or other biologic rheumatoid arthritis therapy, such as anakinra (Kineret).

CONTRAINDICATIONS

Manufacturer states, "None." Consider known hypersensitivity to abatacept or any of its components (maltose, monobasic sodium phosphate). See Limitation of Use and Drug/Lab Interactions.

PRECAUTIONS

Concurrent use with a TNF antagonist (e.g., adalimumab [Humira], etanercept [Enbrel]) is associated with an increased risk of infections with no associated increased efficacy when compared with use of the TNF antagonist alone. Concurrent use is not recommended; see Limitation of Use, Contraindications, and Drug/Lab Interactions. ▪ Hypersensitivity reactions, including anaphylaxis, have been reported and can occur after the first infusion. Emergency medical equipment and medications for treating these reactions must be readily available. ▪ Serious infections, including sepsis and pneumonia, have been reported; some have been fatal. Patients receiving concomitant immunosuppressive therapy may be at increased risk. ▪ Use caution in patients with a history of recurrent infections, underlying conditions that may predispose them to infections, or chronic, latent, or localized infections; see Monitor. ▪ Antirheumatic therapies have been associated with hepatitis B reactivation. ▪ Use with caution in patients with COPD. May be at increased risk for developing respiratory adverse events (e.g., COPD exacerbation, cough, dyspnea, rhonchi). ▪ As with all therapeutic proteins, there is a potential for immunogenicity. ▪ T-cells mediate cellular immune responses. Drugs that inhibit T-cell activation, including abatacept, may affect patient defenses against infection and malignancies. The impact of abatacept on the development and course of malignancies is not fully understood. ▪ See Maternal/Child.

Monitor: Evaluate patients for latent tuberculosis (TB) with a TB skin test. Patients testing positive in TB screening should be treated with a standard TB regimen before initiating therapy with abatacept. ▪ Screening for viral hepatitis should be performed before initiating therapy with abatacept. ▪ Monitor for S/S of infection, especially if transitioning patient from TNF antagonist therapy to therapy with abatacept. Discontinue therapy if a serious infection develops. ▪ Monitor COPD patients for worsening of respiratory status. ▪ Monitor for S/S of hypersensitivity or infusion-related reactions; see Side Effects. ▪ See Precautions and Drug/Lab Interactions.

Patient Education: Read manufacturer's patient information sheet before each infusion. ▪ Review disease states, medication list, and vaccination status with physician; see Precautions. ▪ Report S/S of allergic reaction (e.g., rash, itching, wheezing), infusion reaction (e.g., dizziness, headache), or infection promptly. Discuss previous infections, current infections, or exposure to TB. Educate patient of increased risk of infections and to consider wearing mask in indoor crowded situations.

Maternal/Child: Safety for use in pregnancy has not been established. Use caution. ▪ There is no information regarding the presence of abatacept in human milk, the effects on the breast-fed infant, or the effects on milk production. ▪ A pregnancy registry has been established; contact manufacturer. ▪ Safety and effectiveness for use in pediatric patients under 2 years of age not established. IV dosing has not been studied in patients younger than 6 years of age. ▪ Safety and effectiveness for uses other than juvenile idiopathic arthritis in pediatric patients have not been established. ▪ Patients with juvenile idiopathic arthritis should be brought up-to-date with all immunizations before initiating therapy with abatacept. ▪ Because it is unknown whether abatacept can cross the placenta and because it is an immunomodulatory agent, the safety of administering live vaccines to infants exposed to abatacept in utero is unknown. Consider risk versus benefit.

Elderly: Specific differences in safety and efficacy not noted. The frequency of serious infection and malignancy in patients over 65 years of age was greater than for those under age 65. However, there is a higher incidence of infection and malignancy in the elderly population in general. Use caution; see Precautions.

DRUG/LAB INTERACTIONS

Formal drug interaction studies have not been conducted. ▪ Methotrexate, NSAIDs, corticosteroids, and TNF antagonists do not appear to influence abatacept clearance. ▪ Concurrent use with a **TNF antagonist** (e.g., adalimumab, etanercept, infliximab) is associated with an increased risk of serious infections and no significant additional efficacy over use of the TNF antagonist alone. Concurrent use is not recommended. ▪ With the IV formulation, falsely elevated blood glucose readings may occur on the day of the infusion with **specific blood glucose monitoring systems** that react to drug products containing maltose. IV formulation contains maltose; SQ formulation does not contain maltose; see prescribing information. ▪ Safety and efficacy of concurrent use with **anakinra** has not been established. Concurrent use is not recommended. ▪ **Live virus vaccines** should not be given concurrently with or within 3 months of abatacept. ■ May blunt the effectiveness of some **vaccinations.**

SIDE EFFECTS

In adult and pediatric patients, side effects are similar in type and frequency. The most commonly reported side effects are headache, nasopharyngitis, nausea, and upper respiratory tract infections. The most serious adverse effects are infections and malignancies. Infections are the most likely adverse event to cause interruption or discontinuation of therapy. Acute infusion-related reactions (cough, dizziness, dyspnea, flushing, headache, hypertension, hypotension, nausea, pruritus, rash, urticaria, wheezing) have been reported and usually occur within 1 hour of the infusion. Hypersensitivity reactions (anaphylaxis [rare], dyspnea, hypotension, urticaria) have been reported, usually within 24 hours of infusion. Other reactions include back or extremity pain, COPD exacerbation, dyspepsia, immunogenicity (antibody formation), and rhonchi.

Post-Marketing: New or worsening psoriasis and vasculitis (including cutaneous vasculitis and leukocytoclastic vasculitis).

ANTIDOTE

Notify physician of any side effects; most will be treated symptomatically. During clinical studies, most infusion-related reactions were mild to moderate, and therapy was discontinued in very few patients. Discontinue abatacept for any serious reaction or infection. Therapy may need to be interrupted in patients who develop infections. Treat infusion and hypersensitivity reactions as indicated (e.g., oxygen, diphenhydramine, epinephrine, corticosteroids, vasopressors, and/or fluids). Resuscitate as necessary.

ACETAMINOPHEN BBW

(ah-**SEAT**-ah-**MIN**-oh-fen)

Ofirmev

Antipyretic
Analgesic

pH 5.5

USUAL DOSE

Pretreatment: Baseline studies may be indicated; see Monitor.

May be given as a single or repeated dose. Minimum dosing interval is 4 hours. No dose adjustment is necessary when converting from oral to IV dosing.

Care must be taken to avoid dosing errors, which could result in accidental overdose and death. In particular, be careful to ensure that:

- Dose in milligrams and milliliters is not confused
- Dosing is based on weight (using kg, not pounds) for patients under 50 kg
- Infusion pump is programmed properly
- Total daily dose of acetaminophen from all sources (i.e., all routes [IV, oral, and rectal]) and all acetaminophen-containing products does not exceed maximum daily limits.

Summary of Acetaminophen Dosing in Adults and Adolescents				
Age-Group	Dose Given q 4 hr	Dose Given q 6 hr	Maximum Single Dose	Maximum Total Daily Dose of Acetaminophen (By All Routes)
Adults and adolescents (13 years and older) weighing ≥50 kg	650 mg	1,000 mg	1,000 mg	4,000 mg in 24 hr
Adults and adolescents (13 years and older) weighing <50 kg	12.5 mg/kg	15 mg/kg	15 mg/kg (up to 750 mg)	75 mg/kg in 24 hr (up to 3,750 mg)

PEDIATRIC DOSE

See comments under Usual Dose.

Management of pain and reduction of fever in pediatric patients 2 to 12 years of age: 15 mg/kg every 6 hours or 12.5 mg/kg every 4 hours. Do not exceed a maximum single dose of 15 mg/kg or a maximum daily dose of 75 mg/kg/day. Minimum dosing interval is 4 hours.

Reduction of fever in infants 29 days to 2 years of age: 15 mg/kg every 6 hours to a maximum daily dose of acetaminophen 60 mg/kg/day, with a minimum dosing interval of 6 hours.

Reduction of fever in neonates, including premature neonates born at 32 weeks or more gestational age, up to 28 days chronologic age: 12.5 mg/kg every 6 hours to a maximum daily dose of acetaminophen of 50 mg/kg/day, with a minimum dosing interval of 6 hours.

DOSE ADJUSTMENTS

A reduced total daily dose of acetaminophen may be appropriate in patients with hepatic impairment or active liver disease. ▪ A reduced total daily dose and longer dosing intervals may be appropriate in patients with a CrCl less than or equal to 30 mL/min.

DILUTION

Available in a single-use vial or bag containing 1,000 mg/100 mL (10 mg/mL) of acetaminophen. For adults and adolescent patients weighing 50 kg or more requiring a 1,000-mg dose, administer the dose by inserting a vented IV set through the septum of the 100-mL vial or a nonvented IV set through the administration spike port of the 100-mL bag. Doses less than 1,000 mg should be withdrawn from the container and placed into a separate empty container before administration to avoid inadvertent administration of an overdose. Withdraw appropriate dose (650 mg or weight-based) from 100-mL vial or bag and place in an empty container (e.g., syringe, glass bottle, plastic IV container) for IV infusion.

Filter: Information not available.

Storage: Store unopened vial or bag at CRT. Do not refrigerate or freeze. Do not remove bag from overwrap until ready to use. After removing the outer wrap, check the container for minute leaks by squeezing the solution bag firmly. Discard 6 hours after entry into the container or transfer into an empty container. Single-use product. Discard any unused solution.

COMPATIBILITY

Manufacturer states, "Do not add other medications to solution. **Incompatible** with diazepam and chlorpromazine. Do not administer simultaneously."

Other sources suggest specific **compatibilities** dependent on concentration and manufacturer; consult a pharmacist.

RATE OF ADMINISTRATION

Administer as an infusion, equally distributed over 15 minutes. Pediatric doses up to 600 mg may be drawn up into a syringe and delivered via a syringe pump.

ACTIONS

A nonsalicylate antipyretic and a nonopioid analgesic agent. Exact mechanism of action is unknown but is thought to act through central actions. Widely distributed into most tissues except fat. Low protein binding (10% to 25%). Half-life is approximately 2 to 3 hours. Metabolized in the liver via three different pathways. Metabolites excreted in the urine.

INDICATIONS AND USES

Management of mild to moderate pain in adults and pediatric patients 2 years of age and older. ▪ Management of moderate to severe pain with adjunctive opioid analgesics in adults and pediatric patients 2 years of age and older. ▪ Reduction of fever in adults and pediatric patients.

CONTRAINDICATIONS

Known hypersensitivity to acetaminophen or to any components of the IV formulation. ▪ Patients with severe hepatic impairment or severe active liver disease.

PRECAUTIONS

Acetaminophen has been associated with cases of acute liver failure, at times resulting in liver transplant and death. Most cases of liver injury are associated with the use of acetaminophen at doses that exceed the maximum daily limits and often involve more than one acetaminophen-containing product. Do not exceed the maximum recommended daily dose. ▪ Use with caution in patients with hepatic impairment or active hepatic disease, alcoholism, chronic malnutrition, severe hypovolemia (e.g., due to dehydration or blood loss), or severe renal impairment (CrCl less than or equal to 30 mL/min). ▪ Serious, sometimes fatal, skin reactions such as acute generalized exanthematous pustulosis, Stevens-Johnson syndrome, and toxic epidermal necrolysis have been reported rarely. ▪ Hypersensitivity and anaphylactic reactions have been reported. ▪ Care must be taken when prescribing, preparing, or administering acetaminophen to avoid dosing errors, which could result in accidental overdose and death; see Usual Dose. ▪ Antipyretic effects may mask fever in patients treated for postsurgical pain.

Monitor: Baseline SCr and liver function tests may be indicated. ▪ Monitor for S/S of hypersensitivity reaction (e.g., pruritus; rash; respiratory distress; swelling of the face, mouth, and throat; urticaria). ▪ Monitor for S/S of serious skin reactions.

Maternal/Child: Epidemiologic studies on oral acetaminophen use in pregnant females have not reported a clear association between acetaminophen use and birth defects, miscarriage, or adverse maternal or fetal outcomes. Safety of IV formulation for use in pregnancy not established. Use only if clearly needed. ▪ Safety for use in breastfeeding not established. Acetaminophen is secreted in human milk in small quantities after oral administration. Use caution. ▪ The effectiveness for treatment of acute pain has not been established in pediatric patients less than 2 years of age. ▪ The safety and effectiveness for treatment of fever in pediatric patients, including premature neonates born at 32 weeks or more gestational age, is supported by adequate and well-controlled studies.

Elderly: No overall differences in safety and efficacy were observed between older and younger patients, but greater sensitivity of some older individuals cannot be ruled out.

DRUG/LAB INTERACTIONS

Substances that induce or regulate hepatic cytochrome enzyme CYP2E1 (e.g., ethanol, isoniazid) may alter the metabolism of acetaminophen and increase its hepatotoxic potential. Effects have not been studied. ▪ Chronic acetaminophen doses of 4,000 mg/day may cause an increase in INR in patients stabilized on **warfarin.** Effect of short-term use on INR has not been studied. Monitoring of INR recommended. ▪ **Many available analgesics contain acetaminophen in combination with another analgesic** (e.g., hydrocodone/acetaminophen oxycodone/acetaminophen). **Over-the-counter cold and allergy preparations and sleep aids** may also contain acetaminophen in combination with other active ingredients. Monitor total daily dose of acetaminophen coming from all possible sources.

SIDE EFFECTS

Adult patients: The most common adverse reactions were headache, insomnia, nausea, and vomiting. Less frequently reported side effects included anemia, anxiety, dyspnea, fatigue, fever, and hypersensitivity reactions, including anaphylaxis, hypertension, hypokalemia, hypotension, increased aspartate aminotransferase, infusion site pain, muscle spasms, peripheral edema, and trismus.

Pediatric patients: The most common adverse reactions were constipation, nausea, pruritus, and vomiting. Less commonly reported side effects included abdominal pain, agitation, anemia, atelectasis, diarrhea, fever, headache, hypersensitivity reaction, hypertension, hypervolemia, hypoalbuminemia, hypokalemia, hypomagnesemia, hypophosphatemia, hypotension, injection site pain, muscle spasm, oliguria, pleural effusion, pulmonary edema, stridor, and wheezing.

Overdose: Early symptoms may include diaphoresis, general malaise, nausea, and vomiting. More serious adverse effects include hepatic necrosis, renal tubular necrosis, hypoglycemic coma, and thrombocytopenia.

ANTIDOTE

Notify the physician of significant side effects. Discontinue immediately at the first appearance of skin rash or any other sign of hypersensitivity. Treat as indicated (e.g., diphenhydramine, epinephrine, albuterol). Resuscitate as necessary. If an acetaminophen overdose is suspected, obtain a serum acetaminophen level and baseline liver function studies. *N*-acetylcysteine antidote may be indicated. See acetylcysteine monograph. Contact a regional poison control center for additional information.

ACETAZOLAMIDE SODIUM

(ah-set-ah-**ZOE**-la-myd **SO**-dee-um)

Antiglaucoma
Anticonvulsant
Diuretic
Urinary alkalinizer

Diamox   pH 9.2

USUAL DOSE

Pretreatment: Baseline studies indicated; see Monitor.

Antiglaucoma agent: 250 mg to 1 Gm/24 hr. May be given as 250-mg doses at 4- to 6-hour intervals. In the treatment of secondary glaucoma and in the preoperative treatment of some cases of acute congestive (closed-angle) glaucoma, the preferred dose is 250 mg every 4 hours. In acute cases, to rapidly lower intraocular pressure, an initial single dose of 500 mg followed by 125 to 250 mg at 4-hour intervals may be given.

Edema of congestive heart failure or drug therapy: 250 to 375 mg or 5 mg/kg of body weight as a single dose daily; when loss of edematous fluid stops, reduce to every other day or give for 2 days followed by a day of rest.

Anticonvulsant: *Adults and pediatric patients:* Dose in epilepsy may range from 8 to 30 mg/kg/24 hr in divided doses every 6 to 12 hours (2 to 7.5 mg/kg every 6 hours or 4 to 15 mg/kg every 12 hours). Reduce initial daily dose when given with other anticonvulsants.

Urinary alkalinization: *Adults and pediatric patients:* 5 mg/kg/dose every 8 to 12 hours.

PEDIATRIC DOSE

See Maternal/Child.

Acute antiglaucoma agent: 5 to 10 mg/kg every 6 hours. Do not exceed 1,000 mg/24 hr.

Edema of congestive heart failure or drug therapy: 5 mg/kg as a single dose daily or every other day; see comment under Usual Dose. Do not exceed 1,000 mg/24 hr.

Slowly progressive hydrocephalus in infants 2 weeks to 10 months (unlabeled): 20 mg/kg/24 hr in equally divided doses every 8 hours (8.3 mg/kg every 8 hours). Up to 100 mg/kg/24 hr or a maximum dose of 2 Gm/24 hr has been used.

DOSE ADJUSTMENTS

Reduced dose required when introducing acetazolamide into a treatment regimen with other anticonvulsants. ▪ Administer every 12 hours in patients with a CrCl from 10 to 50 mL/min. Avoid use in patients with a CrCl less than 10 mL/min (ineffective).

DILUTION

Each 500 mg should be diluted in 5 mL SWFI. May then be given by IV injection or added to standard IV fluids. IM administration not recommended.

Storage: Reconstituted solution stable for 12 hours at RT or 3 days refrigerated.

COMPATIBILITY

Compatibility information not available from manufacturer.

Other sources suggest a few specific **compatibilities** dependent on concentration and manufacturer; consult a pharmacist.

RATE OF ADMINISTRATION

500 mg over at least 1 to 3 minutes or added to IV fluids to be given over 4 to 8 hours.

ACTIONS

A potent carbonic anhydrase inhibitor and nonbacteriostatic sulfonamide, acetazolamide depresses the tubular reabsorption of sodium, potassium, and bicarbonate. Excreted unchanged in the urine, producing diuresis, alkalinization of the urine, and a mild degree of metabolic acidosis.

INDICATIONS AND USES

Adjunctive treatment of edema due to congestive heart failure, drug-induced edema, centrencephalic epilepsies (petit mal, unlocalized seizures), chronic simple (open-angle) glaucoma, and secondary glaucoma, and preoperatively in acute angle-closure glaucoma when delay of surgery is desired to lower intraocular pressure. ▪ Used orally for acute mountain sickness.

Unlabeled uses: Metabolic alkalosis, urine alkalinization, and respiratory stimulant in COPD.

CONTRAINDICATIONS

Depressed sodium and potassium levels, hyperchloremic acidosis, marked kidney or liver disease, adrenocortical insufficiency, and hypersensitivity to acetazolamide or any of its components. Long-term use contraindicated in some glaucomas.

PRECAUTIONS

Chemically related to sulfonamides; may cause serious reactions in sensitive patients. ▪ May be alternated with other diuretics to achieve maximum effect. ▪ Greater diuretic action is achieved by skipping a day of treatment rather than increasing dose; failure in therapy may be due to overdose or too-frequent dosage. ▪ IM administration not recommended. Administration by IV injection is preferred. ▪ Use with caution in impaired respiratory function (e.g., pulmonary disease, edema, infection, obstruction); may cause severe respiratory acidosis. ▪ Potassium excretion is proportional to diuresis. Hypokalemia may result from diuresis or with severe cirrhosis. ▪ Introduce or withdraw gradually when used as an anticonvulsant.

Monitor: Obtain baseline CBC and platelet count before use and monitor during therapy. ▪ Periodic monitoring of electrolytes is recommended.

Patient Education: Consider birth control options.

Maternal/Child: Category C: has been shown to be teratogenic in animal studies. Use during pregnancy only if potential benefit justifies potential risks to the fetus. ▪ Discontinue breast-feeding or discontinue acetazolamide. ▪ Safety for use in pediatric patients not established, but no problems are documented.

Elderly: Use caution; no documented problems, but age-related renal impairment may be a factor.

DRUG/LAB INTERACTIONS

May cause hypokalemia with concurrent use of **steroids.** ▪ Hypokalemia may cause toxicity and fatal cardiac arrhythmias with **digoxin** or interfere with **insulin or oral antidiabetic agent** response, thus causing hyperglycemia. ▪ Alkalinization of urine by acetazolamide potentiates **amphetamines, ephedrine, flecainide, methenamine, procainamide, pseudoephedrine, quinidine, and tricyclic antidepressants** by decreasing rate of excretion. ▪ May decrease response to **lithium, methotrexate, some antidepressants, phenobarbital, salicylates, and urinary anti-infectives** by increasing rate of excretion. ▪ Metabolic acidosis induced by acetazolamide may potentiate **salicylate** toxicity (anorexia, tachypnea, lethargy, coma, and death can occur with high-dose aspirin). ▪ Alkalinity may cause **false-positive urinary protein** and possibly **urinary steroid tests.** ▪ May depress **iodine uptake** by the thyroid.

SIDE EFFECTS

Minimal with short-term therapy. Respond to symptomatic treatment or withdrawal of drug: acidosis, anorexia, bone marrow suppression, confusion, crystalluria, drowsiness, fever, hemolytic anemia, hypokalemia (ECG changes, fatigue, muscle weakness, vomiting), paresthesias, photosensitivity, polyuria, rash, renal calculus, and thrombocytopenic purpura.

ANTIDOTE

Notify physician of any adverse effects and discontinue drug if necessary. Treat hypersensitivity reactions as indicated; may require epinephrine, airway management, oxygen, IV fluids, antihistamines, corticosteroids, and pressor amines. Moderately dialyzable (20% to 40%).

ACETYLCYSTEINE INJECTION

(ah-see-till-**SIS**-tay-een in-**JEK**-shun)

Antidote

Acetadote

pH 6 to 7.5

USUAL DOSE (ADULT AND PEDIATRIC)

Recommended dosage in adults and pediatric patients with acute acetaminophen ingestion: Total dose is at least 300 mg/kg within first 24 hours as 3 separate, sequential doses (i.e., 3-bag method to administer the loading, second, and third doses). The total recommended infusion time for the 3 doses is 21 hours. Total volume administered for patients less than 40 kg and for those requiring fluid restriction can be adjusted as clinically needed; see the following dosage charts for patients who weigh from 5 to 20 kg, from 21 to 40 kg, and for patients weighing 41 kg or greater. Consider osmolarity; see Dilution and Precautions.

Distribute doses as indicated in the following guidelines:

Dosage for patients who weigh 5 to 20 kg:

Loading dose: 150 mg/kg diluted in 3 mL/kg of diluent administered at least over 1 hour.

Second dose: 50 mg/kg diluted in 7 mL/kg of diluent administered over 4 hours.

Third dose: 100 mg/kg diluted in 14 mL/kg of diluent administered over 16 hours. Continue NAC at 6.25 mg/kg/hr until stopping criteria are met: Drawn level, AST/ALT and INR every 12 to 24 hours. Stopping criteria: APAP level less than 10, INR less than 2, ALT/AST is normal for patient or if elevated, has decreased from peak (20% to 25%), and patient is clinically well.

Acetylcysteine Dosage Guide by Weight in Patients 5 to 20 kg						
Body Weight (kg)	Loading Dose: 150 mg/kg diluted in 3 mL/kg of diluent administered over at least 1 hour		Second Dose: 50 mg/kg diluted in 7 mL/kg of diluent administered over 4 hours		Third Dose: 100 mg/kg diluted in 14 mL/kg of diluent administered over 16 hours	
	Loading Dose (mg)	Diluent Volume (mL)	Second Dose (mg)	Diluent Volume (mL)	Third Dose (mg)	Diluent Volume (mL)
5 kg[a]	750 mg	15 mL	250 mg	35 mL	500 mg	70 mL
10 kg	1,500 mg	30 mL	500 mg	70 mL	1,000 mg	140 mL
15 kg	2,250 mg	45 mL	750 mg	105 mL	1,500 mg	210 mL
20 kg	3,000 mg	60 mL	1,000 mg	140 mL	2,000 mg	280 mL

[a]Recommended dosage for patients less than 5 kg has not been studied.

Dosage for patients who weigh 21 to 40 kg:

Loading dose: 150 mg/kg diluted in 100 mL of diluent administered over at least 1 hour.

Second dose: 50 mg/kg diluted in 250 mL of diluent administered over 4 hours.

Third dose: 100 mg/kg diluted in 500 mL of diluent administered over 16 hours.

Acetylcysteine Dosage Guide by Weight in Patients 21 to 40 kg		
Body Weight (kg)	Loading Dose: 150 mg/kg in 100 mL of diluent administered over at least 1 hour	Second Dose: 50 mg/kg in 250 mL of diluent administered over 4 hours	Third Dose: 100 mg/kg in 500 mL of diluent administered over 16 hours
	Total Acetylcysteine Dose (mg)	Total Acetylcysteine Dose (mg)	Total Acetylcysteine Dose (mg)
21 kg	3,150 mg	1,050 mg	2,100 mg
30 kg	4,500 mg	1,500 mg	3,000 mg
40 kg	6,000 mg	2,000 mg	4,000 mg

Dosage for patients who weigh 41 kg or greater:
Loading dose: 150 mg/kg diluted in 200 mL of diluent administered over at least 1 hour.
Second dose: 50 mg/kg diluted in 500 mL of diluent administered over 4 hours.
Third dose: 100 mg/kg diluted in 1,000 mL of diluent administered over 16 hours.

Acetylcysteine Dosage Guide by Weight in Patients 41 kg or Greater			
Body Weight (kg)	Loading Dose: 150 mg/kg in 200 mL of diluent administered over at least 1 hour	Second Dose: 50 mg/kg in 500 mL of diluent administered over 4 hours	Third Dose: 100 mg/kg in 1,000 mL of diluent administered over 16 hours
	Total Acetylcysteine Dose (mg)	Total Acetylcysteine Dose (mg)	Total Acetylcysteine Dose (mg)
41 kg	6,150 mg	2,050 mg	4,100 mg
50 kg	7,500 mg	2,500 mg	5,000 mg
60 kg	9,000 mg	3,000 mg	6,000 mg
70 kg	10,500 mg	3,500 mg	7,000 mg
80 kg	12,000 mg	4,000 mg	8,000 mg
90 kg	13,500 mg	4,500 mg	9,000 mg
≥100 kg	15,000 mg	5,000 mg	10,000 mg

DOSE ADJUSTMENTS
Therapy extending beyond 21 hours at 6.25 mg/kg/hr if stop criteria are not met, especially in suspected massive overdose, concomitant ingestion of other substances, or in patients with pre-existing liver disease. In these cases, absorption and/or half-life of acetaminophen may be prolonged. Obtain acetaminophen levels and ALT/AST and INR before the end of the 21-hour infusion. If acetaminophen levels are still above 10 mcg/ml, or in cases in which ALT/AST or INR remains greater than or equal to 2, continue the infusion and contact a regional poison control center. ▪ Specific information and/or recommendations are not available for patients with impaired hepatic or renal function.

DILUTION
Available in single-dose vials containing 6 Gm/30 mL. May be diluted in D5W, ½NS, or SWFI. See Usual Dose for dilution guidelines based on weight. Total volume administered should be adjusted for patients less than 40 kg or for those requiring fluid restriction. Hyponatremia and seizures may result from large volumes in small pediatric patients. ▪ A hyperosmolar solution. Caution is advised when the diluent volume is decreased; hyperosmolarity of the solution is increased as shown in the following chart.

Acetylcysteine Concentration and Osmolarity			
Acetylcysteine Concentration (mg/mL)	Osmolarity in ½NS (mOsmol/L)	Osmolarity in D5W (mOsmol/L)	Osmolarity in SWFI (mOsmol/L)
7 mg/mL	245 mOsmol/L	343 mOsmol/L	91 mOsmol/L[a]
24 mg/mL	466 mOsmol/L	564 mOsmol/L	312 mOsmol/L

[a]Osmolarity should be adjusted to a physiologically safe level (generally not less than 150 mOsmol/L in pediatric patients).

Color of acetylcysteine may change from colorless to a slight pink or purple once the stopper is punctured; quality is not affected.
Filters: Data not available, and use is not required by manufacturer.
Storage: Store unopened vials at CRT. Diluted solution is stable for 24 hours at CRT. Do not use previously opened vials for IV administration. Discard unused portions.

COMPATIBILITY
Manufacturer states, "**Compatible** with D5W, ½NS, and SWFI."

RATE OF ADMINISTRATION
Usual total infusion time of all 3 doses is 20 to 24 hours. Rate reduction may be required to manage S/S of infusion reactions; see Monitor and Antidote.

Loading dose: An infusion evenly distributed over 60 minutes.

Second dose: An infusion evenly distributed over 4 hours.

Third dose: An infusion evenly distributed over 16 hours.

ACTIONS
Acetaminophen doses of 150 mg/kg or greater have been associated with hepatotoxicity. Acetylcysteine is an antidote for acetaminophen overdose that protects the liver by maintaining or restoring the glutathione levels (metabolites formed after an overdose of acetaminophen may deplete the hepatic stores of glutathione and cause binding of the metabolite to protein molecules within the hepatocyte, resulting in cellular necrosis). It may also act by forming an alternate substrate and detoxifying the reactive metabolite of acetaminophen. Acetylcysteine is postulated to form cysteine and disulfides. Cysteine is further metabolized to form glutathione and other metabolites. Half-life is approximately 5.6 hours. Crosses the placental barrier. Some excretion in urine.

INDICATIONS AND USES
To prevent or lessen hepatic injury after ingestion of a potentially hepatotoxic quantity of acetaminophen in patients with acute ingestion or repeated supratherapeutic ingestion (RSI).

CONTRAINDICATIONS
Known hypersensitivity to acetylcysteine or any of its components. Many clinicals believe that a previous hypersenstivity reaction does not preclude use in subsequent overdose.

PRECAUTIONS
For IV administration only. ▪ Should be administered in a facility equipped to monitor the patient and respond to any medical emergency. ▪ Most effective against severe hepatic injury when administered within 8 hours of ingestion. Administration before 4 hours does not allow enough time to determine an actual need for treatment with acetylcysteine; serum levels drawn before 4 hours have passed may be misleading. Effectiveness diminishes gradually after 8 hours. Should be administered if 24 hours or less has passed since ingestion, because the reported time of ingestion may not be correct and it does not appear to worsen the patient's condition. ▪ Total volume administered should be adjusted for patients less than 40 kg and for patients requiring fluid restriction. If volume is not adjusted, fluid overload can occur, potentially resulting in hyponatremia, seizure, and death; see Usual Dose. ▪ Anaphylactoid reactions have been reported and usually occur soon after initiation of the infusion. Use caution in patients with asthma or a history of bronchospasm. Death occurred in a patient with asthma. ▪ Acute flushing and erythema of the skin may occur. These reactions usually occur within 30 to 60 minutes of beginning the infusion and often resolve spontaneously despite continued infusion or slowing infusion rate. ▪ Clearance decreased and half-life prolonged in patients with various stages of liver damage. ▪ The Rumack-Matthew nomogram does not apply to patients with repeated supratherapeutic ingestion (RSI), which is defined as ingestion of acetaminophen at doses higher than those recommended for extended periods of time. For treatment information, see prescribing information for a professional assistance line for acetaminophen overdose, or contact a regional poison control center. ▪ The Rumack-Matthew nomogram may underestimate the risk for hepatotoxicity in patients with chronic alcoholism, malnutrition, or CYP2E1 enzyme-inducing drugs (e.g., isoniazid). Consideration should be given to treating these patients even if the acetaminophen concentrations are in the nontoxic range. ▪ Vial stopper does not contain natural rubber latex. ▪ See Monitor and Antidote.

Monitor: Obtain baseline AST, ALT, bilirubin, INR, SCr, BUN, blood glucose, and electrolytes to monitor hepatic and renal function and electrolyte and fluid balance. Continue monitoring as indicated.

Preferred method of treatment: Estimate time of acetaminophen ingestion. If less than 24 hours since overdose, draw an acetaminophen level at 4 hours postingestion or as soon as possible thereafter to clarify the need for intervention with acetylcysteine. The serum acetaminophen level should be evaluated on the Rumack-Matthew nomogram to determine the probability of toxicity (see package insert for copy of nomogram). ▪ If serum acetaminophen level is below the treatment line on the nomogram, discontinue the acetylcysteine if initiated as a precaution. If the plasma level is above the treatment line on the nomogram, initiate or continue treatment.

Secondary options for treatment: If serum acetaminophen levels are not available within 8 hours, initiate treatment. Do not delay treatment more than 8 hours postingestion. ▪ If time of ingestion is unknown or if the patient is unreliable, consider empiric initiation of acetylcysteine treatment. ▪ If a serum acetaminophen level is not available or cannot be interpreted and less than 24 hours has elapsed since ingestion, administer acetylcysteine regardless of the quantity reported to have been ingested.

All treatment options: Monitor vital signs before, during, and after the infusion. ▪ Evaluate serum acetaminophen level on the Rumack-Matthew nomogram. ▪ Infusion reactions may begin with acute flushing and erythema of the skin. May resolve spontaneously despite continued infusion of acetylcysteine or may progress to an acute hypersensitivity reaction and/or anaphylaxis. Observe continuously for initial S/S of a hypersensitivity reaction (e.g., hypotension, rash, shortness of breath, wheezing). ▪ In suspected toxicity resulting from the extended-release acetaminophen preparation, an acetaminophen level drawn fewer than 8 hours postingestion may be misleading. Draw a second level at 8 to 10 hours after the acute ingestion. If either acetaminophen level falls above the toxicity line, acetylcysteine treatment should be initiated. ▪ See Precautions and Antidote.

Patient Education: Report S/S of hypersensitivity promptly (e.g., bronchospasm, hypotension, shortness of breath, wheezing).

Maternal/Child: Use during pregnancy only if clearly needed. Delaying treatment of acetaminophen overdose may increase the risk of maternal or fetal morbidity and mortality. ▪ Use caution; safety for use during breast-feeding not established; effects unknown. After 30 hours, acetylcysteine should be cleared from maternal blood, and breast-feeding can be resumed. ▪ No adequate or well-controlled studies in pediatric patients; use is based on clinical practice. Efficacy appears to be similar to that seen in adults; see Side Effects.

Elderly: Differences in response compared with younger adults not known.

DRUG/LAB INTERACTIONS

Drug-drug interaction studies have not been done.

SIDE EFFECTS

Adult and pediatric patients: Facial flushing, pruritus, rash, and urticaria have been reported most frequently and most commonly occur during the initial loading dose. Other reported side effects include edema, hypersensitivity reactions (including anaphylaxis), hypotension, nausea and vomiting, pharyngitis, respiratory symptoms (e.g., bronchospasm, chest tightness, cough, respiratory distress, shortness of breath, stridor, wheezing), rhinorrhea, rhonchi, tachycardia, and throat tightness.

Overdose: S/S of acute toxicity in animals included ataxia, convulsions, cyanosis, hypoactivity, labored respiration, and loss of righting reflex.

ANTIDOTE

Keep physician informed of all side effects. Flushing and erythema of the skin may occur and often resolve spontaneously. If other symptoms of a hypersensitivity reaction occur (e.g., bronchospasm, dyspnea, hypotension, wheezing), discontinue acetylcysteine and treat with diphenhydramine or epinephrine as indicated. After symptoms subside, the infusion may be carefully resumed. If S/S of hypersensitivity recur, discontinue infusion permanently and consider alternate treatments. Contact a regional poison control center for possible treatment alternatives. Hemodialysis may remove some acetylcysteine.

ACYCLOVIR
(ay-**SYE**-kloh-veer)

Antiviral

Zovirax

pH 11

USUAL DOSE
Pretreatment: See Precautions and Monitor.

In all situations for adults, adolescents, children, and neonates, do not exceed a maximum dose of 20 mg/kg every 8 hours.

Adults and adolescents (12 years of age and older):

Herpes simplex infections; mucosal and cutaneous HSV infections in immunocompromised patients: 5 mg/kg of body weight every 8 hours for 7 days.

Severe initial clinical episodes of herpes genitalis: 5 mg/kg every 8 hours for 5 days.

Herpes simplex encephalitis: 10 mg/kg every 8 hours for 10 days.

Herpes zoster infections (shingles) in immunocompromised patients: 10 mg/kg every 8 hours for 7 days.

PEDIATRIC DOSE
Herpes simplex infections; mucosal and cutaneous HSV infections in immunocompromised patients: *Pediatric patients 3 months to 12 years:* 10 mg/kg every 8 hours for 7 days.

Herpes simplex encephalitis: *Pediatric patients 3 months to 12 years:* 20 mg/kg every 8 hours for 10 days.

Herpes zoster infections (shingles) in immunocompromised patients: *Pediatric patients under 12 years:* 20 mg/kg every 8 hours for 7 days.

NEONATAL DOSE
Neonatal herpes simplex virus infections: *PMA of at least 34 weeks:* 20 mg/kg every 8 hours for 21 days.

PMA of less than 34 weeks: 20 mg/kg every 12 hours for 21 days.

Doses recommended should be used with caution in neonates with ongoing medical conditions affecting their renal function beyond the effect of prematurity.

DOSE ADJUSTMENTS
Calculate dose by ideal body weight in obese individuals. ■ Reduced dose may be indicated in the elderly based on the potential for decreased renal function and concomitant disease or drug therapy. ■ In adults and pediatric patients (older than 3 months) with impaired renal function, reduce dose and/or adjust dosing interval based on CrCl as indicated in the following chart.

Acyclovir Dosage Adjustments for Adults and Pediatric Patients With Renal Impairment		
Creatinine Clearance (mL/min per 1.73 M²)	Percent of Recommended Dose	Dosing Interval (hours)
>50 mL/min	100%	Every 8 hr
≥25-50 mL/min	100%	Every 12 hr
≥10-25 mL/min	100%	Every 24 hr
≤0-10 mL/min	50%	Every 24 hr

Plasma concentrations decrease with hemodialysis; adjustment of the dosing schedule is recommended so that an additional dose is administered after each dialysis. No supplemental dose is indicated in peritoneal dialysis after adjustment of the dosing interval.

DILUTION
Initially dissolve each 500 mg with 10 mL SWFI (1,000 mg with 20 mL). Concentration equals 50 mg/mL. Do not use bacteriostatic water for injection (BWFI); will cause precipitation. Shake well to dissolve completely. Also available in liquid vials. Withdraw the desired dose and further dilute in an amount of solution to provide a concentration less

than 7 mg/mL (70-kg adult at 5 mg/kg equals 350 mg dissolved in a total of 100 mL of solution equals 3.5 mg/mL). **Compatible** with most standard electrolyte and glucose infusion solutions.

Filters: No data available from manufacturer.

Storage: Store unopened vials at CRT. Use reconstituted solution within 12 hours; high pH may result in etching of glass vial surface after 12 hours. Use solution fully diluted for administration within 24 hours. Manufacturer will supply data showing stability for longer periods under specific conditions.

COMPATIBILITY

Manufacturer lists BWFI as **incompatible.** Dilution in biologic or colloidal fluids (e.g., blood products, protein solutions) is not recommended.

Other sources suggest specific **compatibilities** dependent on concentration and manufacturer; consult a pharmacist.

RATE OF ADMINISTRATION

A single dose must be administered at a constant rate over 1 hour as an infusion. Renal tubular damage will occur with too-rapid rate of injection. Acyclovir crystals will occlude renal tubules. Use of an infusion pump or microdrip (60 gtt/mL) recommended.

ACTIONS

An antiviral agent with activity against HSV types 1 (HSV-1) and 2 (HSV-2) and varicella-zoster virus (VZV). Inhibits replication of viral DNA. Widely distributed in tissues and body fluids. Metabolized to a small extent in the liver. Half-life is approximately 2.5 hours. Excreted mainly as unchanged drug in the urine. Crosses the placental and blood-brain barriers. Secreted in breast milk.

INDICATIONS AND USES

Treatment of initial and recurrent mucosal and cutaneous herpes simplex (HSV-1 and HSV-2) infections in immunosuppressed patients. ▪ Severe initial clinical episodes of herpes genitalis in immunocompetent patients. ▪ Herpes simplex encephalitis. ▪ Neonatal and infant herpes simplex virus infections. ▪ Herpes zoster infections (shingles) in immunocompromised patients. ▪ Oral acyclovir is used to treat varicella zoster (chickenpox).

Unlabeled uses: Prevention of HSV reactivation in HSCT, treatment of disseminated HSV or VZV, or empiric treatment of suspected encephalitis in immunocompromised patients with cancer.

CONTRAINDICATIONS

Hypersensitivity to acyclovir or valacyclovir (Valtrex). The ganciclovir monograph indicates a contraindication for ganciclovir with acyclovir.

PRECAUTIONS

Confirm diagnosis of HSV (HSV-1 or HSV-2) through laboratory culture. Initiate therapy as quickly as possible after symptoms are identified. ▪ For IV use only; avoid IM or SQ injection. ▪ Use caution in patients with underlying neurologic abnormalities; those with serious renal, hepatic, or electrolyte abnormalities; or significant hypoxia. ▪ Use caution in patients receiving interferon or intrathecal methotrexate, or with patients who have had previous neurologic reactions to cytotoxic drugs. ▪ Incidence of CNS adverse events may be more common in the elderly or in patients with decreased renal function. ▪ Isolates of HSV (HSV-1 or HSV-2) and VZV with reduced susceptibility to acyclovir have been identified. Consider the possibility of viral resistance to acyclovir in patients who show poor clinical response. ▪ Thrombotic thrombocytopenic purpura/hemolytic uremic syndrome (TTP/HUS) has been reported in immunocompromised patients receiving acyclovir. Deaths have occurred. ▪ See Contraindications.

Monitor: Maintain adequate hydration and urine flow before and during infusion. Encourage fluid intake of 2 to 3 L/day. ▪ Monitor CBC, liver function tests, and renal function;

abnormal renal function (decreased CrCl can occur), concomitant use of other nephrotoxic drugs, pre-existing renal disease, and dehydration make further renal impairment with acyclovir more likely. ▪ Confirm patency of vein; will cause thrombophlebitis. Rotate site of infusion.

Patient Education: Maintain adequate hydration. Virus remains dormant and can still spread to others. ▪ Avoid sexual intercourse when visible herpes lesions are present. Use condoms routinely.

Maternal/Child: Use during pregnancy only if benefits outweigh risk to fetus. ▪ Breast milk concentrations can be higher than maternal serum concentrations. Discontinue breast-feeding or evaluate very carefully. ▪ 10 mg/kg and 20 mg/kg doses in pediatric patients from 3 months to 16 years achieved concentrations similar to those in adults receiving 5 mg/kg to 10 mg/kg. ▪ Use with caution in neonates; they have an age-related decrease in clearance and an increase in half-life (3.8 hours).

Elderly: Effectiveness is similar to younger adults. ▪ Plasma concentrations are higher in the elderly compared to younger adults; may be due to age-related changes in renal function. ▪ Duration of pain after healing was longer in patients 65 years or older. ▪ Incidence of side effects (e.g., CNS adverse events [coma, confusion, hallucinations, somnolence], dizziness, nausea, renal adverse events, vomiting) was increased. ▪ See Dose Adjustments and Precautions.

DRUG/LAB INTERACTIONS

See Precautions. May cause neurotoxicity (e.g., severe drowsiness and lethargy) with **zidovudine.** ▪ Concurrent use with other **nephrotoxic agents** (e.g., aminoglycosides [gentamicin, tobramycin], cisplatin) may increase risk of nephrotoxicity, especially in patients with pre-existing renal impairment. ▪ Potentiated by **probenecid.** ▪ Synergistic effects with **ketoconazole and interferon** have been noted. Clinical importance not established.

SIDE EFFECTS

Acute renal failure, aggressive behavior, agitation, alopecia, angioedema, ataxia, coma, confusion, delirium, diaphoresis, disseminated intravascular coagulation (DIC), dizziness, dysarthria (difficulty articulating words), elevated transaminase levels, encephalopathy, gastrointestinal distress, hallucinations, headache, hematuria, hemolysis, hives, hyperbilirubinemia, hypersensitivity reactions (e.g., anaphylaxis), hypotension, inflammation at injection site, lethargy, leukocytoclastic vasculitis, leukopenia, lymphadenopathy, nausea, obtundation, peripheral edema, phlebitis, photosensitive rash, pruritus, rash, seizures, tissue necrosis, transient increased BUN or SCr levels, tremors, urticaria, and vomiting. Some patients (fewer than 1%) may have abdominal pain, anemia, anorexia, anuria, chest pain, diarrhea, edema, fatigue, fever, hemoglobinemia, hepatitis, hypokalemia, ischemia of digits, jaundice, leukocytosis, lightheadedness, myalgia, neutropenia, neutrophilia, paresthesia, psychosis, pulmonary edema with cardiac tamponade, rigors, skin reactions (e.g., erythema multiforme, Stevens-Johnson syndrome, toxic epidermal necrolysis), thirst, thrombocytosis, thrombocytopenia, and visual abnormalities.

ANTIDOTE

Notify physician of all side effects. Discontinue drug with onset of CNS side effects. Treatment will be symptomatic and supportive. Adequate hydration is indicated to prevent precipitation of acyclovir in the renal tubules. A 6-hour session of hemodialysis will reduce plasma acyclovir concentration by approximately 60%. Hemodialysis may be indicated in patients with acute renal failure and anuria. Treat anaphylaxis and resuscitate as necessary.

ADENOSINE
(ah-**DEN**-oh-seen)

Adenocard, Adenoscan

Antiarrhythmic
Diagnostic agent

pH 4.5 to 7.5

USUAL DOSE

Adenocard: Conversion of acute paroxysmal supraventricular tachycardia (PSVT): 6 mg initially as a rapid bolus by the peripheral IV route. If supraventricular tachycardia not eliminated in 1 to 2 minutes, give 12 mg. May repeat 12-mg dose in 1 to 2 minutes if needed. Do not exceed 12 mg in any single dose. Give undiluted directly into a vein. If given into an IV line, use the port closest to the insertion site and follow with a rapid NS flush to be certain the solution reaches the systemic circulation. For heart transplant patients: Initial dose should be reduced to 1 mg; may increase subsequent doses up to 3 mg, if needed.

Do not administer a repeat dose to patients who develop a high-level block on one dose of adenosine.

Adenoscan: Noninvasive diagnosis of coronary artery disease with thallium tomography: 140 mcg/kg/min (0.14 mg/kg/min) as a 6-minute continuous peripheral infusion (total dose of 0.84 mg/kg). Injection should be as close to the venous access as possible. Inject thallium at 3 minutes. May be injected directly into adenosine infusion set. Dose should be based on total body weight. There are no data on the safety or efficacy of alternative Adenoscan infusion protocols. Safety and efficacy of Adenoscan administered by the intracoronary route have not been established. ▪ See Drug/Lab Interactions.

PEDIATRIC DOSE

See Maternal/Child.

Adenocard: Conversion of acute paroxysmal supraventricular tachycardia (PSVT) in pediatric patients weighing less than 50 kg: 0.05 to 0.1 mg/kg. May increase dose by 0.05 to 0.1 mg/kg increments every 2 minutes until PSVT is terminated or maximum dose is reached (0.3 mg/kg or 12 mg). AHA guidelines recommend 0.1 mg/kg rapid IV push. Follow each dose with a 5- to 10-mL NS flush. Double to 0.2 mg/kg if a second dose is required. Maximum first dose is 6 mg. Maximum second dose and maximum single dose is 12 mg. ▪ See comments in Usual Dose.

Pediatric patients weighing more than 50 kg: Same as Usual Dose.

DOSE ADJUSTMENTS

Metabolism of adenosine is independent of hepatic or renal function. No dose adjustment indicated. ▪ See Drug/Lab Interactions; alternative therapy (e.g., calcium channel blockers) may be indicated.

DILUTION

Solution must be clear; do not use if discolored or particulate matter present. Give undiluted for both indications.

Storage: Store at CRT 15° to 30° C (59° to 86° F); refrigeration will cause crystallization. If crystals do form, dissolve by warming to room temperature. Discard unused portion.

COMPATIBILITY

Manufacturer states that thallium-201 is **compatible** with Adenoscan and may be injected directly into the Adenoscan infusion set.

Other sources suggest a few specific **compatibilities** dependent on concentration and manufacturer; consult a pharmacist.

RATE OF ADMINISTRATION

Adenocard: *Conversion of acute PSVT:* Must be given as a rapid bolus IV injection over 1 to 2 seconds. Follow each dose with NS flush; see Usual Dose.

Adenoscan: *Pharmacologic stress testing:* See Usual Dose.

ACTIONS

A naturally occurring nucleoside present in all cells of the body. Has many functions. When given as a rapid IV bolus of 6 or 12 mg, adenosine usually has no systemic hemodynamic effects. As a rapid IV bolus, it has antiarrhythmic properties, slowing cardiac conduction (particularly at the AV node), interrupting re-entry pathways through the AV node, and restoring sinus rhythm in patients with PSVT, including PSVT associated with Wolff-Parkinson-White syndrome. When used as a diagnostic aid and given as a continuous infusion, adenosine acts as a vasodilator. Dilates normal coronary vessels, increasing blood flow. Has little effect on stenotic arteries. When administered with thallium-201, helps differentiate between areas of heart supplied by normal blood flow and areas supplied by stenotic coronary arteries. When larger doses are given by infusion, adenosine decreases BP and produces a reflexive increase in HR. Adenocard and Adenoscan have the same molecular structure, solvent, diluent, and concentration. The difference in their actions is in the rate of administration; however, the FDA has approved Adenocard for converting PSVT and Adenoscan for pharmacologic stress testing. When used for treatment of PSVT, it is effective within 1 minute. When used for diagnostic purposes, maximum effect is reached within 2 to 3 minutes of starting the infusion. Coronary blood flow velocity returns to basal levels within 1 to 2 minutes after the infusion is discontinued. Half-life is estimated to be less than 10 seconds. Adenosine is salvaged immediately by erythrocytes and blood vessel endothelial cells and metabolized for natural uses throughout the body (regulation of coronary and systemic vascular tone, platelet function, lipolysis in fat cells, intracardiac conduction).

INDICATIONS AND USES

Adenocard: To convert acute PSVT to normal sinus rhythm; a first-line agent according to AHA. Includes PSVT associated with accessory bypass tracts (Wolff-Parkinson-White syndrome). Does not convert atrial flutter, atrial fibrillation, or ventricular tachycardia to normal sinus rhythm (NSR).

Adenoscan: Adjunct to thallium-201 myocardial perfusion scintigraphy in patients unable to exercise adequately. (Results are similar to exercise stress testing.)

CONTRAINDICATIONS

Known hypersensitivity to adenosine. ▪ Sinus node disease, such as symptomatic bradycardia or sick sinus syndrome, and second- or third-degree AV block unless a functioning artificial pacemaker is in place. ▪ Known or suspected bronchoconstrictive or bronchospastic lung disease (e.g., asthma).

PRECAUTIONS

Both preparations: Emergency resuscitation drugs and equipment must always be available. ▪ Initiate continuous ECG monitoring prior to starting therapy, if possbile, as there may be short-lasting first-, second-, or third-degree heart block or sinus bradycardia. Usually self-limiting due to short half-life. Patients who develop high-level block should not be given additional doses of adenosine. ▪ May cause dyspnea, bronchoconstriction, and respiratory compromise. Use with caution in patients with obstructive lung disease not associated with bronchoconstriction (e.g., emphysema, bronchitis). Avoid use in patients with bronchoconstrictive or bronchospastic disease (e.g., asthma); see Contraindications.

Adenocard: ▪ Transient or prolonged episodes of asystole and ventricular fibrillation have been reported. Deaths have occurred. In most instances, these cases were associated with the concomitant use of digoxin and, less frequently, with digoxin and verapamil. ▪ Some slowing of ventricular response may occur if atrial flutter or fibrillation is also present.

Adenoscan: Use with caution in patients with pre-existing first-degree AV block or bundle branch block. ▪ Fatal and nonfatal cardiac arrest, sustained ventricular tachycardia (requiring resuscitation), and MI have been reported. Avoid use in patients with S/S of myocardial ischemia (e.g., unstable angina) or cardiovascular instability; may be at increased risk for adverse cardiac events. ▪ Can cause significant hypotension. Use with caution in patients with autonomic dysfunction, stenotic valvular heart disease, pericarditis or pericardial effusion, stenotic carotid artery disease with cerebrovascular insufficiency, or uncorrected hypovolemia; may be at increased risk for hypotensive complications. ▪ Hemorrhagic and ischemic cerebrovascular accidents have occurred. ▪ New onset or recurrence of convulsive seizures has occurred following administration of Adenoscan. Some seizures are prolonged and require emergent anticonvulsive management. Aminophylline may increase the risk of seizures associated with Adenoscan; see Antidote. ▪ Hypersensitivity reactions (e.g., chest discomfort, dyspnea, erythema, flushing, throat tightness, and rash) have occurred. ▪ Hypertension has been reported; usually resolves spontaneously within several minutes but, in some cases, has lasted for several hours. ▪ Atrial fibrillation has been reported. In reported cases, it began 1.5 to 3 minutes into the infusion, lasted for 15 seconds to 6 hours, and spontaneously converted to NSR.

Monitor: *Adenocard: Conversion of acute PSVT:* Must reach systemic circulation; see Usual Dose. ▪ ECG monitoring during administration recommended. Monitor BP. At the time of conversion to normal sinus rhythm, PVCs, PACs, atrial fibrillation, sinus bradycardia, sinus tachycardia, skipped beats, and varying degrees of AV nodal block are seen on the ECG in many patients. Usually last only a few seconds and resolve without intervention. ▪ Less likely to precipitate hypotension if arrhythmia does not terminate.

Adenoscan: Pharmacologic stress testing: ECG monitoring during administration recommended. Monitor HR and BP at regular intervals during infusion. ▪ Obtain images when infusion complete and redistribution images 3 to 4 hours later. ▪ Monitor for S/S of hypersensitivity reactions.

Patient Education: Avoid consumption of any products containing methylxanthines, including caffeinated coffee, tea, or other caffeinated beverages; caffeine-containing drug products; aminophylline; and theophylline before the myocardial perfusion imaging study. Caution patient that they may experience a brief period of chest pressure/discomfort after administration. ▪ Review medical history (e.g., history of seizures or respiratory compromise). ▪ Promptly report any potential side effects.

Maternal/Child: Category C: Use in pregnancy only if clearly needed. Some references recommend avoiding early pregnancy. ▪ Safety for use in pediatric patients not established, but has been used for conversion of PSVT in neonates, infants, children, and adolescents. Safety for use in pharmacologic stress testing in patients under 18 years not established. ▪ Interrupt nursing after administration of Adenoscan.

Elderly: Response similar to that seen in younger patients; however, greater sensitivity of some older patients cannot be ruled out. May have diminished cardiac function, nodal dysfunction, concomitant disease, or drug therapy that may alter hemodynamic function and produce severe bradycardia or AV block.

DRUG/LAB INTERACTIONS

Both preparations: Effects antagonized by **methylxanthines** (e.g., caffeine, theophylline); larger doses may be required or adenosine may not be effective. ▪ Potentiated by **dipyridamole**; smaller doses of adenosine may be indicated. Safety and efficacy of adenosine in the presence of dipyridamole have not been systematically evaluated. ▪ Cardiovascular effects increased by **nicotine;** rapid injection may induce anginal pain. ▪ May produce a higher degree of heart block with **carbamazepine.** ▪ Concomitant use with **digoxin alone or digoxin in combination with verapamil** associated with rare cases of ventricular fibrillation; see Precautions. ▪ See Usual Dose. ▪ **Adenoscan:** Before using Adenoscan for pharmacologic stress testing, avoid (or withhold for at least 5 half-lives) **adenosine antagonists** (e.g., methylxanthines) **and/or potentiators** (e.g., dipyridamole). ▪ Has been used with other cardioactive agents such as **beta-adrenergic blockers, angiotensin-converting enzyme inhibitors, and calcium channel blockers** without apparent adverse interactions, but its effectiveness with these agents has not been fully evaluated.

SIDE EFFECTS

Both preparations: Generally predictable, short lived, and easily tolerated. Most will appear immediately and last less than 1 minute. Atrial fibrillation, bronchospasm, chest pressure or discomfort, dizziness, dyspnea and/or shortness of breath, facial flushing, GI discomfort, headache, hypertension, light-headedness, nausea, numbness, PACs, PVCs, sinus bradycardia, sinus tachycardia, skipped beats, and varying degrees of AV nodal block. Less than 1% of patients complain of apprehension; blurred vision; burning; chest pain; head pressure; heavy arms; hyperventilation; hypotension; metallic taste; neck and back pain; palpitations; pressure in groin; seizures; sweating; throat, neck, or jaw discomfort; tight throat; and tingling in arms. Serious side effects may include arrhythmias (persistent), including VT, VF, atrial fibrillation, and torsades de pointes; bronchospasm (severe); myocardial infarction; pulmonary edema; and third-degree AV block. Asystole with fatal outcome has been reported.

Post-Marketing: *Both preparations:* Seizure activity, including tonic-clonic (grand mal) seizures, and loss of consciousness. *Adenoscan:* Cardiac failure, cerebrovascular accident (including intracranial hemorrhage), fatal and nonfatal cardiac arrest, hypersensitivity reactions, injection site reactions, myocardial infarction, respiratory arrest, throat tightness, ventricular arrhythmia, and vomiting. *Adenocard:* Atrial fibrillation, bradycardia, prolonged asystole, torsades de pointes, transient increase in blood pressure, VF, and VT.

ANTIDOTE

Notify physician of any side effect that lasts more than 1 minute. If a side effect persists, decrease rate of infusion (Adenoscan [pharmacologic stress testing]). Discontinue in any patient who develops severe respiratory difficulties or in any patient who develops persistent or symptomatic high-grade AV block or hypotension. Treat side effects symptomatically if indicated. Bradycardia may be refractory to atropine. Short half-life generally precludes overdose problems, but aminophylline 50 to 125 mg as a slow infusion is a competitive antagonist. Methylxanthine use (e.g., theophylline) is not recommended in patients who experience seizures in association with Adenoscan. Resuscitate as necessary.

ADUCANUMAB
(a-due-**KAN**-eu-mab)

Aduhelm

Anti-amyloid
Monoclonal antibody
Immune globulin

USUAL DOSE

1 mg/kg once every 4 weeks for 2 infusions, then 3 mg/kg every 4 weeks for 2 infusions, then 6 mg/kg every 4 weeks for 2 infusions, then 10 mg/kg every 4 weeks thereafter.

PEDIATRIC DOSE

Safety and efficacy have not been established.

DOSE ADJUSTMENTS

Renal: No dosage adjustments provided by manufacturer.
Hepatic: No dosage adjustments provided by manufacturer.

DILUTION

Once patient-specific dose is calculated, withdraw the required volume and add to 100 mL of NS. Gently invert to mix *(do not shake).* Allow to warm to room temperature if refrigerated.

COMPATIBILITY

Do not administer simultaneously with any other medication or IV solutions other than NS.

RATE OF ADMINISTRATION

Administer as an IV infusion over 60 minutes using a 0.22-micron in-line filter.

ACTIONS

Aducanumab reduces amyloid beta plaques; the accumulation of such plaques is the defining characteristic of Alzheimer disease.

INDICATIONS AND USES

Alzheimer disease.

CONTRAINDICATIONS

No contraindications listed by manufacturer.

Continued

PRECAUTIONS

Amyloid-related imaging abnormalities–edema (ARIA-E) and/or ARIA-hemosiderin deposition may occur within the first 8 doses. If patients experience symptoms such as headache, altered mental status, dizziness, nausea, or visual disturbance, a clinical evaluation must be performed and MRI if indicated. Depending on severity, the drug may need to be discontinued, the dose reduced, or the patient carefully monitored as indicated by physician.

Monitor: MRI of brain before initiation and before infusion numbers 7 and 12.

Patient Education: Have patient report symptoms such as headache, altered mental status, dizziness, nausea, or visual disturbance to physician immediately.

Maternal/Child: No adverse events were observed in animal reproduction studies; however, aducanumab is known to cross the placenta. It is not known if aducanumab is present in breast milk.

Elderly: Refer to Usual Dose and Precautions.

DRUG/LAB INTERACTIONS

No known significant drug interactions.

SIDE EFFECTS

Hemosiderosis, microhemorrhage, brain edema, falling, headache, diarrhea, altered mental status, confusion, delirium, disorientation, urticaria, angioedema.

ANTIDOTE

Discontinue infusion and treat appropriately for severe hypersensitivity reactions.

ALBUMIN (HUMAN)
(al-**BYOO**-min **HU**-man)

Plasma volume expander
(plasma protein fraction)

Albumin (Human Preservative Free) 5%, 20%, & 25%, Albuminar 5% & 25%, AlbuRx 5% & 25%, Albutein 5% & 25%, Buminate 5% & 25%, Flexbumin 25%, Human Albumin Grifols 25%, Normal Serum Albumin, Plasbumin 5%, 20%, & 25%

pH 6.4 to 7.4

USUAL DOSE

Variable, depending on patient condition (e.g., presence of hemorrhage, hypovolemia, or shock, pulse, BP, hemoglobin and hematocrit, and amount of pulmonary or venous congestion present). Fluid and protein requirements and underlying condition determine the concentration of albumin used. 5% is usually indicated in hypovolemic or intravascularly depleted patients, and 20% or 25% is appropriate when fluid and sodium intake should be minimized (e.g., cerebral edema, hypoproteinemia, pediatric patients). The initial dose is usually 12.5 to 25 Gm. Amount of 5% given may be increased to 0.5 Gm/lb of body weight (10 mL/lb) with careful monitoring of the patient. Available as 5% solution (5 Gm/100 mL), 20% solution (20 Gm/100 mL), or 25% solution (25 Gm/100 mL). The maximum dose is 6 Gm/kg/24 hr or 250 Gm in 48 hours (250 Gm is equal to 5 L of 5% or 1 L of 25%). In the absence of active hemorrhage, the total dose usually does not exceed the normal circulating mass of albumin (e.g., 2 Gm/kg of body weight).

Hypoproteinemia (hypoalbuminemia): 50 to 75 Gm as a 5% or 25% solution. Repeat doses may be required in patients who continue to lose albumin.

Hypovolemia: 12 to 25 Gm as a 5%, 20%, or 25% solution. May be repeated in 15 to 30 minutes if response inadequate. If 25% solution is used, additional fluids may be needed.

Burns: Electrolyte replacement and crystalloids (e.g., IV fluids) to maintain plasma volume are required in the first 24 hours. Then begin with 25 Gm and adjust as necessary to maintain albumin level from 2 to 3 Gm/dL.

Acute nephrosis or acute nephrotic syndrome: 20 to 25 Gm of a 25% solution with a loop diuretic (e.g., furosemide [Lasix], torsemide [Demadex]) daily for 7 to 10 days.

Hemodialysis: 100 mL of a 20% or 25% solution.

Red blood cell resuspension: 20 to 25 Gm of a 20% or 25% solution/liter of RBCs.

Cardiopulmonary bypass: Achieve a plasma albumin of 2.5 Gm/dL and hematocrit concentration of 20% with either a 5% or 25% solution. Use crystalloids (IV fluids) as a pump prime.

PEDIATRIC DOSE

0.5 to 1 Gm/kg/dose. 25% solution is usually used in infants and other pediatric patients; *do not use in preterm infants.* Monitor hemodynamic response closely. Maximum dose 6 Gm/kg/24 hr or 250 Gm/48 hr.

Hypoproteinemia (hypoalbuminemia): 0.5 to 1 Gm/kg/dose. Repeat every 1 to 2 days as needed.

Hypovolemia: 0.5 to 1 Gm/kg/dose. May be repeated in 15 to 30 minutes if response inadequate.

Hemolytic disease of the newborn: 1 Gm/kg (4 mL/kg) of 25% albumin. One source recommends giving 1 hour before exchange transfusion. Another recommends 1 to 2 hours before blood transfusion or with transfusion (exchange 50 mL of albumin 25% for 50 mL plasma). *Do not use in preterm infants.*

Burns: See Usual Dose.

DILUTION

May be given undiluted or further diluted with NS or D5W for infusion. NS is the preferred diluent. When sodium restriction is required, D5W may be substituted. The use of SWFI as a diluent is not recommended. Life-threatening hemolysis and acute renal failure can result if a sufficient volume of SWFI is used as a diluent. The 5% product is isotonic and osmotically approximates human plasma. One volume of 25% to four volumes of diluent is isotonic. Use only clear solutions.

Storage: Store at CRT. Use within 4 hours after opening. Discard unused portions.

COMPATIBILITY

Do not use SWFI as a diluent; see Dilution. Manufacturers state, "Do not mix with protein hydrolysates, amino acid mixtures, or solutions containing alcohol." Manufacturers also state, "May be administered in conjunction with or combined with other parenterals such as whole blood, plasma, glucose, saline, or sodium lactate."

Other sources suggest a few specific **compatibilities** dependent on concentration and manufacturer; consult a pharmacist.

RATE OF ADMINISTRATION

Variable, depending on indication, present blood volume, patient response, and concentration of solution. A too-rapid rate, especially in the presence of normal blood volume, may cause circulatory overload and pulmonary edema. Averages are:

Normal blood volume: 1 to 2 mL/min.

Deficient blood volume (hypovolemia): A single dose as rapidly as tolerated. Repeat dose as rapidly as tolerated if indicated. As volume approaches normal, slow 5% to 1 to 2 mL/min and 25% to 1 mL/min to prevent circulatory overload and pulmonary edema.

Hypoproteinemia: 2 to 3 mL/min in adults; a single dose over 30 to 120 minutes in pediatric patients.

Infants and other pediatric patients: For uses other than hypovolemia and hypoproteinemia, the rate of administration should be about one-fourth to one-half the adult rate.

ACTIONS

A sterile natural plasma protein substance prepared by a specific process, which makes it free from the danger of serum hepatitis. A blood volume expander that accounts for 70% to 80% of the colloid oncotic pressure of plasma. Expands blood volume proportionately to amount of circulating blood, improves cardiac output, prevents marked hemoconcentration, aids in reduction of edema, and raises serum protein levels. Low sodium content helps to maintain electrolyte balance and should promote diuresis in presence of edema (contains 130 to 160 mEq sodium/L). Also acts as a transport protein that binds both endogenous and exogenous substances, including bilirubin and certain drugs.

INDICATIONS AND USES

Hypovolemia (with or without shock [actual or impending], with or without hemorrhage); 5% if hypovolemic, 25% if adequate hydration or edema is present. ▪ Hypoalbuminemia from inadequate production (e.g., burns, congenital analbuminemia, endocrine disorders, infection, liver disease, major injury, malignancy, malnutrition). ▪ Hypoalbuminemia from excessive catabolism (e.g., burns, major injury, nephrosis, pancreatitis, pemphigus [chronic relapsing skin disease], peritonitis, thyrotoxicosis). ▪ Hypoalbuminemia from loss from the body (e.g., hemorrhage, burn exudates, excessive renal excretion, exfoliative dermatoses, exudative enteropathy [e.g., inflammatory bowel disease]). ▪ Hypoalbuminemia from redistribution within the body (e.g., cirrhosis with ascites, inflammatory conditions, major surgery). ▪ Hypoalbuminemia secondary to pulmonary edema in adult respiratory distress syndrome (ARDS). ▪ Raising plasma oncotic pressure to treat edema of nephrosis. ▪ Cardiopulmonary bypass surgery. ▪ Hemolytic disease of the newborn (bilirubin binding activity) as adjunct to exchange transfusion. ▪ Provide adequate volume and prevent hypoproteinemia as an adjunct to RBC resuspension.

Unlabeled uses: Large-volume paracentesis, spontaneous bacterial peritonitis in patients with cirrhosis.

CONTRAINDICATIONS

Anemia (severe) or cardiac failure in the presence of normal or increased intravascular volume, hypersensitivity to albumin, pulmonary edema. ▪ Buminate 25% should not be used in patients with chronic renal impairment; contains aluminum.

PRECAUTIONS

Whole blood or packed cells probably indicated if more than 1,000 mL 5% albumin required in hemorrhage; are adjunctive to use of large amounts of serum albumin to prevent anemia. Is not a substitute for whole blood in situations in which both the oxygen-carrying capacity and plasma volume expansion provided by whole blood are required. ▪ May be given regardless of patient blood group. ▪ Use caution in hypertension, low cardiac reserve, hepatic or renal failure, or lack of albumin deficiency. ▪ Use caution in patients with normal or increased intravascular volume; however, patients with hypoproteinemia may have normal blood volume. ▪ Use caution in patients with burns, hypoproteinemia, or hypovolemia; an FDA-issued Dear Doctor letter identified concerns of an excess mortality rate when albumin administration was compared to NS administration in these critically ill patients. Trauma patients with concomitant traumatic brain injuries may also be at risk for increased mortality. ▪ Made from human plasma and may contain infectious agents (e.g., HIV, Creutzfeldt-Jakob disease, hepatitis B, hepatitis C). Numerous steps in the manufacturing process are used to make the potential for infection extremely remote. ▪ 25 Gm of albumin is the osmotic equivalent of 2 units of fresh frozen plasma. 25 Gm of albumin provides as much plasma protein as 500 mL of plasma or 2 units of whole blood. ▪ Albumin is not a source of nutrition.

Monitor: Monitor BP. ▪ Monitor for S/S of a hypersensitivity reaction (e.g., chest pain, dizziness, dyspnea, fever, flushing, hypotension, nausea, pruritus, rash, rigors, urticaria). ▪ Hemoglobin, hematocrit, electrolyte, and serum protein evaluations are mandatory during therapy. Alkaline phosphatase may be elevated. ▪ Hyponatremia may result from administration of large volumes of albumin diluted in D5W; additional monitoring of electrolytes may be required. ▪ Observe patient carefully for increased bleeding resulting from more normal BP, circulatory embarrassment, pulmonary edema, or lack of diuresis. Central venous and/or pulmonary wedge pressure readings are most helpful. ▪ Maintain hydration with additional fluids, especially in dehydrated patients. ▪ Normal plasma albumin is 3.5 to 6 Gm/dL.

Maternal/Child: Category C: safety for use during pregnancy not established. ▪ Do not use 25% solution in preterm infants.

Elderly: Monitor fluid intake carefully; more susceptible to circulatory overload and pulmonary edema. ▪ Plasma albumin levels may be more volatile.

DRUG/LAB INTERACTIONS
Specific information not available.

SIDE EFFECTS
Chills, fever, headache, hypotension, nausea, salivation, skin rash or hives, tachycardia, vomiting.

Major: Congestive heart failure, decreased myocardial contractility, hypersensitivity reactions including anaphylaxis (rare), precipitous hypotension, pulmonary edema, and salt and water retention.

ANTIDOTE
Notify the physician of all side effects. Minor side effects are generally tolerated and treated symptomatically. For major side effects, discontinue albumin and treat symptomatically. Resuscitate as necessary.

ALDESLEUKIN BBW
(al-des-**LOO**-kin)

Antineoplastic
Immunomodulator
Biologic response modifier
Recombinant interleukin-2

Interleukin-2 Recombinant, Proleukin

pH 7.2 to 7.8

USUAL DOSE
(International units [IU])

Pretreatment: Patient selection restricted. Prescreening and baseline studies required; see Precautions/Monitor.

Standard high-dose regimen: Intermittent IV: 600,000 International units (IU)/kg (0.037 mg/kg) every 8 hours for 14 doses. After 9 days of rest, repeat for up to 14 more doses; this constitutes one course (two 5-day [14 or fewer doses] treatment cycles separated by a rest period of 9 days). Treat with 28 doses or until dose-limiting toxicity requiring ICU-level support occurs. Dose is based on actual patient weight.

Retreatment: Evaluate for response 4 weeks after course completion and again before scheduling start of the next course. Additional courses are considered if there is some tumor shrinkage following the previous course and retreatment is not contraindicated. At least 7 weeks from hospital discharge should elapse before a subsequent course is administered.

Sometimes given in combination with other agents.

DOSE ADJUSTMENTS
Information on dosing in obese and underweight patients is not available; base dose on actual patient weight. ▪ Doses are frequently withheld for toxicity. Doses are actually withheld, not reduced in amount. Median number of doses actually administered in a first course is 20 for metastatic renal cell carcinoma patients and 18 for metastatic melanoma patients. Continuous infusions can be interrupted as indicated by patient symptoms. ▪ Hold doses and restart based on the following chart:

Guidelines for Holding Doses of Aldesleukin	
Hold Dose for	**May Give Next Dose if**
CARDIOVASCULAR	
Atrial fibrillation, supraventricular tachycardia, bradycardia that requires treatment or is recurrent or persistent.	Patient is asymptomatic with full recovery to normal sinus rhythm.
Systolic BP <90 mm Hg with increasing requirements for pressors.	Systolic BP ≥90 mm Hg and stable or improving requirements for pressors.
Any ECG change consistent with MI or ischemia with or without chest pain; suspicion of cardiac ischemia or myocarditis.	Patient is asymptomatic; MI and myocarditis have been ruled out; clinical suspicion of angina is low; there is no incidence of ventricular hypokinesia.
PULMONARY	
O$_2$ saturation <90%.	O$_2$ saturation >90%.
CENTRAL NERVOUS SYSTEM	
Mental status changes (e.g., agitation, confusion, lethargy, somnolence). May result in coma.	Mental status changes completely resolved.
BODY AS A WHOLE	
Sepsis syndrome; patient is clinically unstable.	Sepsis syndrome has resolved; patient is clinically stable; infection is under treatment.
UROGENITAL	
SCr >4.5 mg/dL or a SCr of ≥4 mg/dL in presence of severe volume overload, acidosis, or hyperkalemia.	SCr <4 mg/dL, and fluid and electrolyte status is stable.
Persistent oliguria, urine output of <10 mL/hr for 16 to 24 hr with rising SCr.	Urine output >10 mL/hr with a decrease of SCr >1.5 mg/dL or normalization of SCr.
DIGESTIVE	
Signs of hepatic failure, including encephalopathy, increasing ascites, liver pain, hypoglycemia.	Discontinue for remainder of current course. May consider a new course of treatment in 7 weeks if all signs of hepatic failure have resolved.
Stool guaiac repeatedly >3 to 4$^+$.	Stool guaiac negative.
SKIN	
Bullous dermatitis or marked worsening of pre-existing skin condition (avoid topical steroid therapy).	Resolution of all signs of bullous dermatitis.

- After withholding a dose, no dose should be given until patient is globally assessed and specific criteria for restarting aldesleukin are met.

DILUTION   (International units [IU])

Each 22,000,000 IU vial (1.3 mg) must be reconstituted with 1.2 mL of preservative-free SWFI (18,000,000 IU/mL [1.1 mg (1,100 mcg)/mL]). Sterile technique imperative. Direct diluent to side of vial and gently swirl to avoid excess foaming. Do not shake. Further dilute the calculated dose in 50 mL D5W. Desired final infusion concentration is 30 to 70 mcg/mL. If the total dose is 1.5 mg or less (patient weighs less than 40 kg), the dose of aldesleukin should be diluted in a smaller volume of D5W so the final concentration remains in the acceptable range. Plastic infusion containers are preferred over glass. Do not use any filters for dilution or administration. Do not use any other diluent or infusion solution; may cause increased aggregation. Bring to room temperature before administration.

Filters: Do not use any filters for dilution or administration.

Storage: Store in refrigerator before and after reconstitution and dilution. Do not freeze. Protect from light. No stability problems will occur at CRT for 48 hours after dilution but has no preservatives. Do not use beyond expiration date on vial.

COMPATIBILITY

Manufacturer recommends not mixing with other drugs in the same container. Bacteriostatic water for injection (BWFI) or NS will increase aggregation.

Other sources suggest a few specific **compatibilities** dependent on concentration and manufacturer; consult a pharmacist.

RATE OF ADMINISTRATION

Intermittent IV: A single dose as an intermittent infusion over 15 minutes. Flush main line IV with D5W before and after each use. Manufacturer recommends that any keep-open IV in place for intermittent administration be D5W.

ACTIONS

A genetically engineered recombinant protein that possesses the biologic activity of naturally occurring interleukin-2 (IL-2). Exact mechanism of action is unknown. Immunoregulatory properties include enhancement of lymphocyte mitogenesis and stimulation of long-term growth of human IL-2 dependent cell lines, enhancement of lymphocyte cytotoxicity, induction of killer cell (lymphokine-activated [LAK] and natural [NK]) activity, and induction of interferon-gamma production. Immunologic effects occur in a dose-dependent manner and include activation of cellular immunity with profound lymphocytosis, eosinophilia, and thrombocytopenia, as well as the production of cytokines, including tumor necrosis factor, IL-1, and gamma interferon. Half-life is approximately 85 minutes. Eliminated by metabolism in the kidney with little or no bioactive protein excreted in urine.

INDICATIONS AND USES

Prescreening mandatory. Eligibility requirements for treatment are specific; see Precautions and Contraindications. ▪ Treatment of metastatic renal cell carcinoma in adults. Patient selection should include assessment of performance status. See prescribing information for details. ▪ Treatment of adults with metastatic melanoma.

Unlabeled uses: Acute myelogenous leukemia after autologous BMT.

CONTRAINDICATIONS

Abnormal thallium stress test or pulmonary function tests. ▪ Known hypersensitivity to interleukin-2 or any component of aldesleukin. ▪ Patients with organ allografts. ▪ Exclude from treatment any patient with significant cardiac, pulmonary, renal, hepatic, or CNS impairment; any patient requiring treatment with steroidal agents; and any patient at higher risk for cardiovascular adverse events during periods of hypotension and fluid shifts.

Retreatment is permanently contraindicated in patients who experienced specific toxicities in a previous course of therapy (see the following chart).

Contraindications for Retreatment With Aldesleukin	
Organ System	**Symptom**
Cardiovascular	Sustained ventricular tachycardia $\geq$5 beats. Cardiac rhythm disturbances not controlled or unresponsive to management. Chest pain with ECG changes consistent with angina or myocardial infarction. Cardiac tamponade.
Pulmonary	Intubation required more than 72 hours.
Renal	Renal failure requiring dialysis for more than 72 hours.
Central nervous system	Coma or toxic psychosis lasting more than 48 hours. Repetitive or difficult-to-control seizures.
Gastrointestinal	Bowel ischemia or perforation. Bleeding requiring surgery.

PRECAUTIONS

Administered in the hospital under the supervision of a qualified physician (usually a medical oncologist and/or immunologist). Intensive care facilities and specialists in cardiopulmonary and/or intensive care medicine must be available. ■ Capillary leak syndrome (CLS [extravasation of plasma proteins and fluid into the extravascular space and loss of vascular tone]) can begin immediately after aldesleukin treatment starts and results in hypotension and reduced organ perfusion that can be severe enough to result in death. CLS may be associated with angina, arrhythmias (supraventricular and ventricular), edema, GI bleed or infarction, mental status changes, myocardial infarction, renal insufficiency, and respiratory insufficiency requiring intubation. Extravasation of protein and fluid into the extravascular space will lead to edema and the creation of new effusions. ■ Therapy should be restricted to patients with normal cardiac and pulmonary functions as defined by appropriate tests. ■ Use extreme caution in patients with normal thallium stress tests and pulmonary function tests who have a history of prior cardiac or pulmonary disease. ■ Patients who have had a nephrectomy are eligible for treatment if SCr is less than 1.5 mg/dL (85% of patients in one study). ■ Mental status changes (e.g., irritability, confusion, depression) may be indicators of bacteremia or early bacterial sepsis, hypoperfusion, occult CNS malignancy, or direct aldesleukin-induced CNS toxicity. Mental status changes due solely to aldesleukin may progress for several days before recovery begins. Permanent neurologic deficits have been reported. ■ Withhold administration in patients who develop moderate to severe lethargy or somnolence; continued administration may result in coma. ■ May exacerbate disease symptoms in clinically unrecognized or untreated CNS metastases. Thoroughly evaluate and treat CNS metastases before aldesleukin therapy. New neurologic signs, symptoms, and anatomic lesions have been reported in patients without evidence of CNS metastases. Clinical manifestations include agitation, ataxia, change in mental status, hallucinations, obtundation, speech difficulties, and coma. Cortical lesions and demyelination have been seen using MRI studies. Neurologic S/S usually resolve following discontinuation of therapy; however, there have been reports of permanent damage. ■ Use extreme caution in patients with a history of seizures (may cause seizures), patients with fixed requirements for large volumes of fluid (e.g., hypercalcemia), those with autoimmune disorders (e.g., Crohn disease, ulcerative colitis, psoriasis), previous cytotoxic drug therapy or radiation therapy, and patients sensitive to *Escherichia coli*–derived proteins. ■ May cause autoimmune disease and inflammatory disorders or exacerbate pre-existing conditions. ■ Serious manifestations of eosinophilia involving eosinophilic infiltration of cardiac and pulmonary tissues can occur following aldesleukin administration. ■ Associated with impaired neutrophil function and an increased risk of disseminated infection, including sepsis and bacterial endocarditis. Pre-existing bacterial infections should be adequately treated before beginning therapy. Patients with indwelling central lines are at increased risk for infection with gram-positive organisms. Antibiotic prophylaxis with ciprofloxacin, nafcillin, or vancomycin has been associated with a reduced incidence of staphylococcal infections. ■ Induces significant hypotension; discontinue antihypertensives during treatment. ■ Kidney and liver function are impaired during aldesleukin therapy. ■ May impair thyroid function; changes may suggest autoimmunity; thyroid replacement therapy has been required in a few patients. ■ May cause hyperglycemia and/or diabetes mellitus. ■ Anti-aldesleukin antibodies have been detected in some patients. Impact of antibody formation on efficacy and safety of aldesleukin is unknown. ■ See Drug/Lab Interactions.

Monitor: A central venous catheter (double or triple lumen) is frequently ordered on admission (required for continuous infusion). A minimum of two IV lines is usually required (one for the aldesleukin and its keep-open IV and one for other needed fluids and medications). Flushing of line with D5W before and after aldesleukin is imperative. Ability to record CVP and draw blood samples should be available. ■ Admission chest x-ray, ECG, CBC with differential and platelet count, blood chemistries including electrolytes and renal and liver function tests, T_3, T_4, PT, PTT, urinalysis, and body weight should be obtained. Adequate pulmonary function, normal arterial blood gases, and normal ejection fraction should be documented. ■ During drug administration obtain daily CBC with differential and platelet count, blood chemistries including electrolytes, renal and hepatic function tests, and chest x-rays. ▪ Continuous cardiac monitoring is indicated (required with BP below 90 mm Hg or any cardiac irregularity). ▪ Monitoring and flexibility in management of fluid balance and organ perfusion status are imperative. Requires constant management and balancing of effects of fluid shifts to prevent the consequences of hypovolemia (e.g., impaired organ perfusion) or fluid accumulation (e.g., edema, pulmonary edema, ascites, pulmonary effusion), which may exceed the patient's tolerance. ▪ Assess hypovolemia by central venous catheterization and frequent central venous pressure monitoring. Administer colloids (albumin, plasmanate) or crystalloids (IV fluids) as indicated for a BP drop of 20 mm Hg or greater or a systolic BP less than 90. ▪ Frequent neuro checks required (note agitation, blurred vision, confusion, depression, irritability, and persistent somnolence). ▪ Vital signs and strict I&O are required every 2 to 4 hours (much more frequently as side effects develop). ▪ Weigh daily. ▪ Assess thyroid function periodically. ▪ An ECG and cardiac enzymes are indicated for any S/S of chest pain, murmurs, gallops, irregular rhythm, or palpitations. A repeat thallium study is indicated for evidence of cardiac ischemia or CHF; may indicate ventricular hypokinesia due to MI or myocarditis. ▪ Obtain a urinalysis as indicated. ▪ Assess pulmonary function through examination, vital signs, and pulse oximetry. Arterial blood gases are indicated for any dyspnea or respiratory impairment. ▪ If fever occurs several days into treatment or recurs after subsiding, assume infection first, then drug. Confusion, depression, or irritability may also suggest infection. Draw cultures; administer appropriate antibiotics. ▪ Patients who have had nephrectomies may be more at risk for increases in serum BUN or creatinine, electrolyte shifts, and reduced urine output. Evaluate fluid, electrolyte, and acid-base status promptly if any of the above occur. Gradual increases without other complications (marked fluid overload, hyperkalemia, acidosis) are frequently tolerated (SCr must not exceed 4.5 mg/dL). ▪ Maintain pulmonary status as needed with O_2 and diuretics. Assess pulmonary status with chest x-rays. ▪ Monitor central and peripheral IV sites to reduce potential for infection. ▪ No restrictions on activity; use caution ambulating (orthostatic hypotension). ▪ No restrictions on diet. Encouragement may be required (anorexia and/or mouth sores). ▪ Monitor for thrombocytopenia (platelet count less than 50,000/mm³). Initiate precautions to prevent excessive bleeding (e.g., inspect IV sites, skin, and mucous membranes; use extreme care during invasive procedures; test urine, emesis, stool, and secretions for occult blood). ▪ Specific preparation required for discharge; refer to literature. ▪ Manufacturer supplies excellent brochures for nurses and physicians with detailed guidelines in chart form on all aspects of monitoring, toxicity, and treatment. ▪ Complete review and adequate preparation of all aspects of this therapy with the patient and family are imperative. Can reduce psychological stress of toxicity. ▪ Tumor regression has continued for up to 12 months after one or more courses of therapy. ▪ See Dose Adjustments, Contraindications, and Antidote.

Patient Education: Many side effects will occur; report any changes you perceive so they can be evaluated and treated if needed (e.g., changes in breathing, chest or other pain, temperature, mood, light-headedness, fatigue). ▪ Request assistance for ambulation and always sit on the side of the bed first. ▪ Take only prescribed medications. ▪ Avoid alcohol. ▪ Use of effective contraceptive measures recommended for fertile males and females. ▪ Use 15 SPF sunscreen in sunlight to protect against photosensitivity. ▪ See Appendix D, p. 1311, for additional information. ▪ Manufacturer supplies a patient education booklet; review thoroughly and discuss with your physician and nurse.

Maternal/Child: Category C: benefits must outweigh risks. Contraceptive measures required before initial administration and throughout treatment. ▪ Discontinue breast-feeding. ▪ Safety for use in pediatric patients under 18 years of age not established; studies show responsiveness and toxicity similar.

Elderly: Response rates and toxicity similar to that seen in younger adults; however, some increased incidence of severe urogenital toxicities and dyspnea was noted in the elderly. ▪ Use caution; consider age-related organ impairment.

DRUG/LAB INTERACTIONS

May cause interactions with **psychotropic drugs** (e.g., analgesics, antiemetics, narcotics, sedatives, tranquilizers) because aldesleukin also affects central nervous function. ▪ Concomitant use with **cardiotoxic agents** (e.g., doxorubicin [Adriamycin]), **hepatotoxic agents** (e.g., methotrexate, asparaginase), **myelotoxic agents** (e.g., cytotoxic chemotherapy, radiation therapy), **and nephrotoxic agents** (e.g., aminoglycosides, indomethacin) may increase toxicity in these organ systems and/or delay excretion of these agents, increasing their toxicity. ▪ Acute, atypical adverse reactions have been reported in patients treated with aldesleukin and subsequently administered **radiographic iodinated contrast media.** Reactions have included chills, diarrhea, edema, fever, hypotension, nausea, oliguria, pruritus, rash, and vomiting. Most reactions were reported when contrast media were given within 4 weeks after the last dose of aldesleukin. ▪ **Glucocorticoids** (e.g., dexamethasone) reduce aldesleukin-induced side effects but also reduce its antitumor effectiveness. ▪ Aldesleukin-induced hypotension may be potentiated by **beta-blockers and other antihypertensive agents** (e.g., ACE inhibitors, calcium channel blockers). ▪ Concurrent use with **interferon-alfa** may increase incidence of MI, myocarditis, ventricular hypokinesia, and severe rhabdomyolysis. ▪ May cause hypersensitivity reactions in patients receiving combination regimens **(high-dose aldesleukin and antineoplastics)**. ▪ Aldesleukin may decrease clearance and increase plasma levels of **indinavir.** ▪ Capable of altering numerous lab values; see literature.

SIDE EFFECTS

Frequent, predictable, often severe; are usually clinically manageable and frequently require intensive care management. Begin to occur shortly after therapy begins (chills, fatigue, fever, hypotension, nausea, vomiting). Frequency and severity are dose-related and schedule-dependent. Most are reversible within 2 or 3 days of discontinuation of therapy. Even with intensive management, side effects can progress to death.

Initially anorexia, arthralgia, chills, fatigue, fever, nausea, and vomiting occur. Initial symptoms of capillary leak syndrome are edema, electrolyte abnormalities, hypotension, oliguria, respiratory distress, significant weight gain, and tachycardia. Effects of CLS **successively** result in *hypovolemia,* which in turn leads to hypotension → hypoperfusion → sinus tachycardia → angina → myocardial ischemia and infarction → arrhythmias (supraventricular and ventricular) → decreased renal perfusion → prerenal azotemia → oliguria → anuria; *fluid retention/weight gain,* which in turn leads to rales → dyspnea → cough → tachypnea → hypoxia → pleural effusion → respiratory insufficiency requiring intubation → diarrhea → edema of the bowel → refractory acidosis → edema → ascites; and *breakdown of blood-brain barrier* (neuropsychiatric toxicity [e.g., agitation, combativeness, confusion, hallucinations, lethargy, psychosis, somnolence]). Abdominal pain and GI bleeding may be related to diarrhea, vomiting, stomatitis, duodenal ulcer formation, bowel ischemia, infarction, or perforation. Cerebral edema and concomitant medications may impact many side effects. Lethargy and/or somnolence may lead to coma. Anemia and thrombocytopenia may occur; coagulation abnormalities (PT, PTT) reflect liver dysfunction. Hemodynamic effects similar to septic shock may be caused by tumor necrosis factor. Erythematous rash and pruritus (can progress to dry desquamation) can occur in almost all patients and are extremely uncomfortable. See Precautions and Drug/Lab Interactions.

Post-Marketing: Anaphylaxis, angioedema, cardiac tamponade, cardiomyopathy, cellulitis, cerebral hemorrhage, cerebral lesions, cholecystitis, colitis, demyelinating neuropathy, encephalopathy, eosinophilia, extrapyramidal syndrome, fatal endocarditis, fatal subdural and subarachnoid hemorrhage, febrile neutropenia, gastritis, hepatitis, hepatosplenomegaly, hypertension, hyperthyroidism, injection site necrosis, insomnia, intestinal obstruction, lymphocytopenia, myopathy, myositis, neuralgia, neuritis, neutropenia, pneumonia (bacterial, fungal, viral), retroperitoneal hemorrhage, rhabdomyolysis, urticaria.

ANTIDOTE

Temporarily discontinue aldesleukin and notify physician immediately of arrhythmias or rhythm changes, chest pain, marked changes in HR, positive neuropsychiatric check (agitation, blurred vision, persistent extreme somnolence), systolic BP below 90 mm Hg, apical HR over 120, temperature over 38° C (100.4° F), respirations over 25/min, complaints of dyspnea, decreased breath sounds, increased sputum production, severe diarrhea associated with refractory acidosis, vomiting refractory to treatment, acute changes in GI status. May be restarted based on patient response. Hold any subsequent dose for failure to maintain organ perfusion; see Dose Adjustments. Fever is routinely treated with acetaminophen and indomethacin or Naprosyn; increased doses may be needed. Suggested treatments include slow IV meperidine for chills and rigidity; diphenoxylate or loperamide PO for diarrhea; diphenhydramine 25 mg PO q 6 hr, a soothing skin cream, and oatmeal baths for urticaria and pruritus; temazepam for insomnia; ondansetron for nausea. Treat edema with furosemide once BP has normalized. IV fluids, albumin or plasmanate, and Trendelenburg positioning are used to maintain fluid balance and BP. If organ perfusion and BP are not sustained by dopamine 1 to 5 mcg/kg/min as a continuous infusion, increase to 6 to 10 mcg/kg/min or add phenylephrine (1 to 5 mcg/kg/min). Prolonged use of pressors at relatively high doses may cause cardiac arrhythmias. Treat arrhythmias as indicated (usually sinus or supraventricular tachycardia [adenosine, verapamil]). Use O_2 for decreased Pao_2. Use packed RBCs for anemia and to ensure maximum oxygen-carrying capacity. Platelet transfusions are indicated for thrombocytopenia or to reduce risk of GI bleeding. Use of blood modifiers to treat bone marrow toxicity may be indicated. Special precautions may be required (e.g., avoid IM injections; test urine, emesis, stool, secretions for occult blood). All treatment is supportive; recovery should begin within a few hours of cessation of aldesleukin. With normalized BP, diuretics (furosemide) can hasten recovery. Low-dose haloperidol may help severe mental status changes.

More rapid onset of dose-limiting toxicities will occur with overdose. **Dexamethasone** is indicated to counteract life-threatening toxicities. May result in loss of therapeutic effect.

ALEMTUZUMAB BBW
(ah-lem-**TOOZ**-uh-mab)

Monoclonal Antibody
Antineoplastic
Immunomodulator

Campath ▪ Lemtrada

pH 6.8 to 7.4

USUAL DOSE
CAMPATH
Pretreatment: Verify pregnancy status; baseline studies indicated; see Monitor and Maternal/Child.

Premedication, dose escalation to the recommended maintenance dose, and anti-infective prophylaxis are required.

Premedication: Diphenhydramine 50 mg and acetaminophen 500 to 1,000 mg should be administered 30 minutes before the first dose, at dose escalations, and as clinically indicated. For cases in which severe infusion-related reactions have occurred, corticosteroids may be administered to help prevent or minimize subsequent reactions.

Dose escalation: Dose escalation is required at initiation of therapy or if dosing is held for 7 or more days during treatment. Initiate at a dose of 3 mg daily. When this dose is tolerated (infusion-related toxicities are Grade 2 or less), the daily dose should be increased to 10 mg. When the 10-mg dose is tolerated, the maintenance dose of 30 mg may be initiated. In most cases, dose escalation to the maintenance dose of 30 mg can be achieved in 3 to 7 days.

Maintenance dose: 30 mg/day administered three times a week on alternate days (e.g., Monday, Wednesday, Friday). Total duration of therapy, including dose escalation, is 12 weeks. Single doses greater than 30 mg or cumulative weekly doses greater than 90 mg have been associated with an increased incidence of pancytopenia and should **not** be administered.

Anti-infective prophylaxis: Administer sulfamethoxazole/trimethoprim DS twice daily three times a week (or equivalent) as *Pneumocystis jiroveci* pneumonia (PCP) prophylaxis and famciclovir (Famvir) 250 mg twice daily or equivalent as herpetic prophylaxis at the start of alemtuzumab therapy. Continue PCP and herpes viral prophylaxis for a minimum of 2 months after completion of therapy or until the CD4+ count is equal to or greater than 200 cells/mm^3, whichever occurs later.

LEMTRADA
Pretreatment: Verify pregnancy status. Pretesting required and baseline studies indicated; see Precautions and Monitor. Before starting treatment with Lemtrada:
• Complete any necessary immunizations at least 6 weeks before treatment with Lemtrada.
• Determine whether the patient has a history of varicella or has been vaccinated for varicella zoster virus (VZV). If not, test the patient for antibodies to VZV and consider vaccination if antibody-negative. Postpone treatment until 6 weeks after VZV vaccination.
• Perform tuberculosis screening according to local guidelines.
• Instruct patients to avoid potential sources of *Listeria monocytogenes*.

Premedication: *Corticosteroids:* Administer high-dose corticosteroids (1,000 mg methylprednisolone [Solu-Medrol] or equivalent) immediately before Lemtrada infusion for the first 3 days of each treatment course. Also consider pretreatment with antihistamines and/or antipyretics.

Herpes prophylaxis: Administer antiviral prophylaxis for herpetic viral infections starting on the first day of each treatment course and continue for a minimum of 2 months following treatment with Lemtrada or until the CD4+ lymphocyte count is at least 200 cells/mcL, whichever occurs later.

Lemtrada: Recommended dose is 12 mg/day administered by IV infusion for 2 treatment courses.

First treatment course: 12 mg/day as an infusion on 5 consecutive days (60 mg total dose).
Second treatment course: 12 mg/day as an infusion on 3 consecutive days (36 mg total dose) administered 12 months after the first treatment course.
Subsequent treatment courses: After the second treatment course, subsequent treatment courses of 12 mg/day on 3 consecutive days (36 mg total dose) may be administered as needed at least 12 months after the last dose of any prior treatment courses.

DOSE ADJUSTMENTS
CAMPATH AND LEMTRADA
Withhold alemtuzumab during serious infections or other serious adverse reactions until resolution.

CAMPATH
There are no dose modifications recommended for lymphopenia. ▪ Discontinue alemtuzumab for autoimmune anemia or autoimmune thrombocytopenia. ▪ Recommendations for dose modification for severe neutropenia or thrombocytopenia are listed in the following chart.

Alemtuzumab Dose Modification for Neutropenia or Thrombocytopenia	
Hematologic Values	**Dose Modification**[a]
ANC less than 250/mm^3 and/or platelet count equal to or less than 25,000/mm^3	
First occurrence	Withhold alemtuzumab therapy. Resume alemtuzumab at 30 mg when ANC is equal to or greater than 500/mm^3 and platelet count is equal to or greater than 50,000/mm^3.
Second occurrence	Withhold alemtuzumab therapy. Resume alemtuzumab at 10 mg when ANC is equal to or greater than 500/mm^3 and platelet count is equal to or greater than 50,000/mm^3.
Third occurrence	Discontinue alemtuzumab therapy.
Equal to or greater than 50% decrease from baseline in patients initiating therapy with a baseline ANC equal to or less than 250/mm^3 and/or a baseline platelet count equal to or less than 25,000/mm^3	
First occurrence	Withhold alemtuzumab therapy. Resume alemtuzumab at 30 mg upon return to baseline value(s).
Second occurrence	Withhold alemtuzumab therapy. Resume alemtuzumab at 10 mg upon return to baseline value(s).
Third occurrence	Discontinue alemtuzumab therapy.

[a]If the delay between dosing is equal to or more than 7 days, resume alemtuzumab therapy at 3 mg and escalate to 10 mg and then to 30 mg as tolerated; see Usual Dose and Rate of Administration.

DILUTION
CAMPATH
Available as a 30 mg/1 mL single-use vial. ***Do not shake*** vial before use. Contains no preservatives; sterile technique is imperative. Withdraw the necessary amount of Campath from the vial into a syringe:

- To prepare the 3-mg dose, withdraw 0.1 mL into a 1-mL syringe calibrated in increments of 0.01 mL.
- To prepare the 10-mg dose, withdraw 0.33 mL into a 1-mL syringe calibrated in increments of 0.01 mL.
- To prepare the 30-mg dose, withdraw 1 mL in either a 1-mL or 3-mL syringe calibrated in 0.1-mL increments.

Inject the appropriate dose into 100 mL of NS or D5W. Gently invert the bag to mix solution. Discard any unused drug.

LEMTRADA
Available as a 12 mg/1.2 mL single-use vial. ***Do not freeze or shake*** vial before use. Contains no preservatives; sterile technique is imperative. Withdraw 1.2 mL of Lemtrada

from the vial into a syringe and inject into 100 mL of NS or D5W. Gently invert the bag to mix solution.

Filters: Specific information not available.

Storage: *Campath:* Store vials in refrigerator at 2° to 8° C (36° to 46° F). ***Do not freeze or shake.*** If accidentally frozen, thaw at 2° to 8° C before administration. Protect from direct sunlight.

Lemtrada: Store vials in refrigerator at 2° to 8° C (36° to 46° F) in original carton to protect from light. ***Do not freeze or shake.***

Campath and Lemtrada: Prepared solution may be stored at RT (15° to 25° C [Lemtrada] or 15° to 30° C [Campath]) or refrigerated. Protect from light and use within 8 hours of dilution.

COMPATIBILITY

Campath and Lemtrada: Manufacturer states, "Do not add or simultaneously infuse other drug substances through the same intravenous line."

Campath: Compatible with PVC bags and PVC or polyethylene-lined PVC administration sets.

RATE OF ADMINISTRATION

Campath and Lemtrada: *Do not administer* as an IV push or bolus.

Campath: A single dose as an infusion over 2 hours. Subcutaneous administration is unlabeled but has been used.

Lemtrada: A single dose as an infusion over 4 hours starting within 8 hours of dilution. Extend duration of infusion if clinically indicated.

ACTIONS

A recombinant, DNA-derived, humanized monoclonal antibody (Campath-1H) that binds to the 21-28 kD cell surface glycoprotein, CD52. CD52 is expressed on the surface of both normal and malignant B- and T-lymphocytes, natural killer (NK) cells, most monocytes, macrophages, and a subpopulation of granulocytes. A proportion of bone marrow cells, including some CD34+ cells, also express variable levels of CD52. The proposed mechanism of action for **Campath** is antibody-dependent cellular-mediated lysis following cell surface binding of Campath to the leukemic cells. The precise mechanism of action by which **Lemtrada** exerts its therapeutic effects in multiple sclerosis is unknown but is presumed to involve binding to CD52. Following cell surface binding to T- and B-lymphocytes, **Lemtrada** results in antibody-dependent cellular cytolysis and complement-mediated lysis. Circulating T- and B-lymphocytes are depleted after each treatment course. Lymphocyte counts then increase slowly over time, with B-cell counts recovering within 6 months and T-cell counts recovering after 12 months. Alemtuzumab exhibits nonlinear kinetics. **Campath** AUC and half-life increase with repeated dosing. Mean half-life was 11 hours (range 2 to 32 hours) after the first 30-mg dose and was 6 days (range 1 to 14 days) after the last 30-mg dose. The half-life of **Lemtrada** was approximately 2 weeks and was comparable between courses.

INDICATIONS AND USES

CAMPATH

As a single agent for treatment of B-cell chronic lymphocytic leukemia (B-CLL).

LEMTRADA

Treatment of patients with relapsing forms of multiple sclerosis (MS). Because of its safety profile, use is generally reserved for patients who have had an inadequate response to two or more drugs indicated for the treatment of MS.

CONTRAINDICATIONS

CAMPATH

Manufacturer states, "None."

LEMTRADA

Contraindicated in patients who are infected with human immunodeficiency virus (HIV) because it causes prolonged reductions of CD4+ lymphocyte counts.

PRECAUTIONS
CAMPATH AND LEMTRADA
Administered by or under the direction of a physician specialist in a facility with adequate diagnostic and treatment facilities to monitor patient and respond to any medical emergency. ▪ As with all therapeutic proteins, there is a potential for immunogenicity.

CAMPATH
Serious and, in rare instances, fatal pancytopenia/marrow hypoplasia, autoimmune idiopathic thrombocytopenia, and autoimmune hemolytic anemia have been reported. Have occurred at recommended dose. Myelosuppression may be prolonged. Do not exceed maximum daily or weekly recommended dose. See Usual Dose, Dose Adjustments, and Antidote. ▪ Campath treatment results in severe and prolonged lymphopenia with a concomitant increased incidence of opportunistic infections. Serious and sometimes fatal bacterial, viral, fungal, and protozoan infections have been reported. Prophylaxis directed against PCP and herpes virus infections is recommended. Prophylaxis has been shown to decrease but not eliminate the occurrence of these infections. See Usual Dose, Dose Adjustments, Monitor, and Antidote. ▪ Serious and sometimes fatal infusion reactions can occur; see Monitor. ▪ Administer only irradiated blood products to avoid transfusion-associated graft-versus-host disease (TAGVHD) unless immediate transfusion is required.

LEMTRADA
Available only through the Lemtrada REMS program because of the risks of autoimmunity, infusion reactions, and malignancies; see prescribing information. ▪ Treatment with Lemtrada can result in the formation of autoantibodies and increase the risk of serious autoimmune-mediated conditions. May cause serious, sometimes fatal, autoimmune conditions such as immune thrombocytopenia and antiglomerular basement membrane disease. Several other autoimmune disorders have also been reported in a small number of patients. ▪ Immune thrombocytopenia (ITP) has occurred and has been diagnosed more than 3 years after the last Lemtrada dose. Antiplatelet antibodies did not precede ITP onset. ▪ Glomerular nephropathies (e.g., membranous glomerulonephritis, anti-glomerular basement membrane [anti-GBM] disease) have occurred, and some resulted in ESRD requiring dialysis or renal transplantation. May occur up to 40 months after the last dose of Lemtrada. ▪ Newly diagnosed autoimmune thyroid disorders (e.g., Graves disease, hyperthyroidism, hypothyroidism, autoimmune thyroiditis, goiter) have been reported and have occurred more than 7 years after the first Lemtrada dose. Thyroidectomy was required in some patients. In patients with ongoing thyroid disorder, consider benefit versus risk of Lemtrada administration. ▪ Autoimmune cytopenias (e.g., neutropenia, hemolytic anemia, pancytopenia) have occurred. Prompt medical attention is indicated if a cytopenia is confirmed. ▪ Causes cytokine release syndrome, which may result in serious and life-threatening infusion reactions. ▪ Cases of pulmonary alveolar hemorrhage with an onset of within 48 hours of the Lemtrada infusion have been reported in post-marketing use. ▪ May cause an increased risk of malignancies, including thyroid cancer, melanoma, and lymphoproliferative disorders. ▪ Cases of lymphoproliferative disorders and lymphoma have occurred in Lemtrada-treated patients with MS, including a MALT lymphoma, Castleman disease, and a fatality following treatment of non–Epstein Barr virus-associated Burkitt lymphoma. ▪ Because Lemtrada is an immunomodulatory therapy, caution should be exercised in initiating it in patients with pre-existing or ongoing malignancies. ▪ Serious and life-threatening stroke (including ischemic and hemorrhagic stroke) has been reported within 3 days of administration, with most cases occurring within 1 day. Cases of cervicocephalic (e.g., vertebral, carotid) arterial dissection involving multiple arteries have been reported within 3 days of Lemtrada administration. ▪ Autoimmune hepatitis causing clinically significant liver injury, including acute liver failure requiring transplant, has occurred. ▪ Serious infections, including appendicitis, gastroenteritis, herpes viral infections (genital herpes, herpes simplex, herpes zoster, oral herpes), human papillomavirus (HPV [including cervical dysplasia]), pneumonia, tooth infection, and tuberculosis, have occurred. Fungal infections (e.g., oral and vaginal candidiasis) and *Listeria monocytogenes* infections (e.g., meningitis, encephalitis, sepsis, and gastroenteritis), including fatal cases of *Listeria* meningoencephalitis, have

also been reported. ▪ Serious and sometimes fatal opportunistic infections (e.g., aspergillosis, coccidioidomycosis, cytomegalovirus, histoplasmosis, nocardiosis, and PCP) have occurred. ▪ Serious and sometimes fatal bacterial, protozoan, and viral infections, including those due to reactivation of latent infections reported with Campath, may occur in patients treated with Lemtrada. ▪ No data are available on reactivation of hepatitis B virus (HBV) or hepatitis C virus (HCV) because these patients were excluded from trials. Consider screening patients at high risk for HBV or HCV infections; may be at risk for irreversible liver damage. ▪ Lemtrada may increase the risk of acute acalculous cholecystitis. ▪ Progressive multifocal leukoencephalopathy has occurred in a patient with MS. ▪ Hypersensitivity pneumonitis and pneumonitis with fibrosis have occurred. ▪ Lymphopenia is common; total lymphocyte counts increased to reach the lower limit of normal 6 to 12 months after each course of Lemtrada. ▪ See Monitor and Drug/Lab Interactions.

Monitor: *Campath:* Obtain a baseline CBC, including differential and platelet count. Monitor weekly or more frequently if worsening anemia, neutropenia, or thrombocytopenia develops. ▪ Infusion reactions, including acute cardiac insufficiency, angioedema, anaphylactoid shock, ARDS, bronchospasm, cardiac arrhythmias and/or arrest, chills, dyspnea, fever, hypotension, MI, N/V, pulmonary infiltrates, rash, respiratory arrest, rigors, syncope, and/or urticaria may occur. Reactions may be severe. Acute infusion-related reactions were most common during the first week of therapy in clinical studies. Premedicate patient and monitor carefully during infusion. Withhold Campath for Grade 3 or 4 infusion reactions. Gradual escalation to the recommended maintenance dose is required at the initiation of therapy and after interruption of therapy for 7 or more days. See Usual Dose. ▪ Monitor for S/S of any infection. ▪ Monitor for CMV infection during therapy and for at least 2 months after completion of therapy. Treat confirmed infection or viremia as indicated with ganciclovir (Cytovene) or equivalent. ▪ Monitor for thrombocytopenia (platelet count less than 50,000/mm³). Initiate precautions to prevent excessive bleeding (e.g., inspect IV sites, skin, and mucous membranes; use extreme care during invasive procedures; test urine, emesis, stool, and secretions for occult blood). ▪ CD4+ counts should be followed after therapy until recovery to equal to or greater than 200 cells/mm³. See Usual Dose.

Lemtrada: Obtain baseline CBC with differential, serum creatinine levels, urinalysis with urine cell counts, a test of thyroid function (e.g., thyroid-stimulating hormone [TSH] level), and serum transaminases ALT, AST, and total bilirubin levels. Measure the urine protein-to-creatine ratio before initiating therapy. ▪ Repeat CBC, SCr, and urinalysis with urine cell counts at monthly intervals; repeat TSH every 3 months. Repeat serum transaminases and total bilirubin levels periodically. Continue for 48 months after the last dose. After 48 months, perform testing based on clinical findings that suggest autoimmunity (e.g., ITP, anti-GBM disease, thyroid disorders, cytopenias). Symptoms of autoimmune hemolytic anemia may include chest pain, dark urine, jaundice, tachycardia, and weakness. ▪ TB screening recommended before initiating therapy with Lemtrada. Treat appropriately if screening is positive. ▪ Monitor vital signs before the infusion and periodically during the infusion. ▪ Monitor for S/S of an infusion reaction (e.g., anaphylaxis, angioedema, bradycardia, bronchospasm, chest pain, fever, headache, hypertension, hypotension, rash, tachycardia [including atrial fibrillation], transient neurologic symptoms) during and for a minimum of 2 hours after each infusion. Serious infusion reactions have been reported more than 24 hours after an infusion. ▪ Additional monitoring may be indicated in patients predisposed to cardiovascular or pulmonary compromise. ▪ Monitor for symptoms of thyroid cancer (e.g., new lump or swelling in the neck, pain in the front of the neck, persistent hoarseness or other voice changes, trouble swallowing or breathing, a constant cough not due to an upper respiratory tract infection). ▪ Perform baseline and yearly skin examinations to monitor for melanoma. ▪ Monitor for thrombocytopenia (platelet count less than 50,000/mm³) and S/S of ITP (e.g., easy bruising, petechiae, spontaneous mucocutaneous bleeding, heavier than normal or irregular menstrual bleeding). Initiate precautions to prevent excessive bleeding (e.g., inspect IV sites, skin, and mucous membranes; use extreme care during invasive procedures; test urine, emesis, stool, and secretions for occult blood). Hemoptysis may also be indicative of anti-GBM disease, and an appropriate differential diagnosis must be undertaken. ▪ Monitor for S/S of nephropathy or anti-GBM disease (e.g., change in color of urine, decreased urine output, dyspnea, edema, elevated SCr levels, hematuria or proteinuria, hemoptysis [from alveolar hemorrhage]) during treatment and after treatment is completed. Anti-GBM disease can be life-threatening if left untreated. Early evaluation and treatment is required to improve outcomes, including preservation of renal function. For urine dipstick results of 1+ protein or greater, measure the urine protein-to-creatinine ratio. For ratios greater than 200 mg/g, increase in SCr greater than 30%, or unexplained hematuria, perform further evaluation for nephropathies. Increased SCr with hematuria or signs of pulmonary involvement of anti-GBM disease (e.g., hemoptysis, exertional dyspnea) warrant immediate evaluation. ▪ Monitor for unexplained liver enzyme elevations and symptoms suggestive of hepatic dysfunction (e.g., abdominal pain, anorexia, fatigue, jaundice and/or dark urine, unexplained nausea, and vomiting). If S/S of autoimmune hepatitis occur, promptly measure serum transaminases and total bilirubin and interrupt or discontinue treatment as appropriate. ▪ Monitor for S/S of infection and consider delaying administration in patients with active infection until the infection is fully controlled. Monitor for symptoms of *Listeria* infection (fever, chills, diarrhea, nausea, vomiting, headache, pain in joints and muscles, neck stiffness, difficulty walking, mental status changes, coma, and other neurologic changes). *Listeria* infection can lead to significant complications or death. ▪ Monitor for S/S of acute acalculous cholecystitis (e.g., abdominal pain, abdominal tenderness, fever, nausea, and vomiting). Leukocytosis and abnormal liver enzymes are also commonly observed. Acute acalculous cholecystitis is associated with high morbidity and mortality rates. If suspected, evaluate and treat promptly. ▪ Monitor for S/S suggestive of PML (e.g., changes in thinking; disturbance of vision, memory, or orientation leading to confusion; personality changes; and progressive weakness on one side of the body or clumsiness of limbs). Typical symptoms associated with PML are diverse and progress over days to weeks. MRI findings may be apparent before clinical S/S. Withhold treatment and perform appropriate diagnostic evaluation at the first S/S of PML. ▪ Annual HPV screening is recommended for female patients. ▪ See Drug/Lab Interactions.

Patient Education: *Campath and Lemtrada:* Promptly report any unusual side effects or signs of bleeding or bruising, infection (e.g., fever or swollen glands), or infusion reaction (e.g., difficulty breathing, rash). ▪ See Appendix D, p. 1311.

Campath: Females of childbearing potential and males of reproductive potential should use effective contraceptive methods during treatment and for a minimum of 6 months following therapy. ▪ Irradiation of blood products is required. ▪ Take prophylactic anti-infectives for PCP and herpes virus as prescribed.

Lemtrada: Review Medication Guide before each treatment course. ▪ Complete any necessary immunizations at least 6 weeks before treatment with Lemtrada. ▪ Inform healthcare provider of previous Campath use. ▪ To avoid in utero exposure to Lemtrada, females of childbearing potential should use effective contraceptive measures during treatment and for 4 months following therapy. ▪ Serious infusion reactions may occur after the infusion is complete. ▪ Seek immediate medical attention if symptoms of stroke or cervicocephalic arterial dissection occur (e.g., neck pain, weakness on one side of the body, facial droop, difficulty with speech, sudden severe headache). ▪ Seek immediate medical help for bruising, petechiae, spontaneous mucocutaneous bleeding (e.g., epistaxis, hemoptysis), or heavier than normal or irregular menstrual bleeding. ▪ Promptly report abdominal pain, anorexia, bleeding, chest pain or tightness, cough, dark urine, easy bruising, fatigue, hemoptysis, jaundice, shortness of breath, tachycardia, unexplained nausea or vomiting, and wheezing. ▪ May cause thyroid disorders. Promptly report symptoms (e.g., weight loss or gain, fast heartbeat or palpitations, eye swelling, constipation, or feeling cold). ▪ May increase the risk of malignancies, including thyroid cancer and melanoma. ▪ Baseline and yearly skin examinations recommended. ▪ Carry the LEMTRADA REMS Patient Safety Information Card in case of emergency. ▪ Take prescribed medication for herpes prophylaxis as directed by healthcare provider. ▪ Yearly HPV screening is recommended. ▪ May increase the risk of suicidal thoughts and behavior. Promptly report emergence or worsening of S/S of depression, any unusual changes in mood or behavior, or thoughts about self-harm. ▪ Seek prompt medical help for symptoms of *Listeria* infection. ▪ Avoid or adequately heat foods that are potential sources of *L. monocytogenes* (e.g., deli meat, dairy products made with unpasteurized milk, soft cheeses, or undercooked meat, seafood, or poultry) before starting treatment. The incubation period for *L. monocytogenes* ranges from 3 to 70 days; in most cases S/S of invasive listeriosis start within 1 month of exposure to *L. monocytogenes*. ▪ Report S/S of acute acalculous cholecystitis. ▪ Periodic laboratory monitoring required for prolonged period of time (48 months or longer). ▪ Encourage females exposed to Lemtrada during pregnancy to enroll in the pregnancy exposure registry; see Lemtrada prescribing information.

Maternal/Child: Campath and Lemtrada: May cause fetal harm. Effective contraception required; see Patient Education.

Campath: Discontinue breast-feeding during treatment. ▪ Safety and effectiveness for use in pediatric patients not established.

Lemtrada: Autoantibodies may be transferred from the mother to the fetus during pregnancy. Placental transfer of antithyroid antibodies resulting in neonatal Graves disease has been reported. ▪ May induce persistent thyroid disorders. Untreated hypothyroidism in pregnant females increases the risk of miscarriage and may have effects on the fetus, including mental retardation and dwarfism. ▪ There are no data on the presence of alemtuzumab in human milk, the effects on the breast-fed infant, or the effects of the drug on milk production. ▪ Safety and effectiveness for use in pediatric patients less than 17 years of age not established. Use is not recommended in pediatric patients due to the risks of autoimmunity, infusion reactions, and stroke and because it may increase the risk of malignancies (lymphoma, lymphoproliferative disorders, melanoma, and thyroid).

Elderly: ***Campath:*** Clinical studies did not include sufficient numbers of patients 65 years of age and older to determine whether they respond differently than younger patients. Other clinical experience has not identified differences in response.

Lemtrada: Clinical studies did not include sufficient numbers of patients age 65 and over. Differences in response compared with younger adults not known.

DRUG/LAB INTERACTIONS

Campath and Lemtrada

Do not administer **chloroquine or live virus vaccines** to patients receiving alemtuzumab. ▪ Campath and Lemtrada both contain the same active ingredient, **alemtuzumab**. Before use in a patient who has received **either Campath or Lemtrada** previously, consider the potential for additive and long-lasting effects on the immune system.

Campath

No formal drug interaction studies have been performed.

Lemtrada

Concomitant use with antineoplastic or immunosuppressive therapies could increase the risk of immunosuppression.

SIDE EFFECTS

Campath

The most common serious side effects are cytopenias (anemia, lymphopenia, neutropenia, thrombocytopenia), infections (CMV viremia, CMV infection, other infections), and infusion reactions (chills, dyspnea, fever, hypotension, nausea, rash, tachycardia, urticaria). GI symptoms (abdominal pain, diarrhea, N/V) and neurologic symptoms (insomnia, anxiety) are also commonly reported. Autoimmune hemolytic anemia or autoimmune idiopathic thrombocytopenia, headache, hypertension, tremor, and many other adverse reactions have been reported less frequently.

Lemtrada

The most common serious side effects include acute acalculous cholecystitis, autoimmunity, autoimmune hepatitis, cervicocephalic arterial dissection, glomerular nephropathies, immune thrombocytopenia, infections, infusion reactions, malignancies, other autoimmune cytopenias, PML, pneumonitis, stroke, and thyroid disorders. The most common side effects reported include abdominal pain, arthralgia, back pain, diarrhea, dizziness, fatigue, fever, flushing, fungal infections, headache, herpes viral infection, insomnia, nasopharyngitis, nausea and vomiting, oropharyngeal pain, pain in extremities, paresthesia, pruritus, rash, sinusitis, thyroid gland disorders, upper respiratory tract infection, urinary tract infection, urticaria. Lymphopenia and suicidal behavior have also been reported. All side effects listed under Campath may occur.

Post-Marketing: *Campath:* Acute acalculous cholecystitis, aplastic anemia, cardiotoxicity (e.g., cardiomyopathy, CHF, and decreased ejection fraction [some patients had been previously treated with cardiotoxic agents]), cerebrovascular disorders (cervicocephalic arterial dissection, stroke [including hemorrhagic and ischemic]), chronic inflammatory demyelinating polyradiculoneuropathy, EBV-associated lymphoproliferative disorder, fatal infusion reactions, fatal transfusion-associated graft-versus-host disease, Goodpasture's syndrome, Graves disease, Guillain-Barré syndrome, optic neuropathy, reactivation of latent viruses, serum sickness, and tumor lysis syndrome.

Lemtrada: Acalculous cholecystitis, autoimmune hepatitis, hemophagocytic lymphohistiocytosis, neutropenia, opportunistic infections, PML, pulmonary alveolar hemorrhage, thrombocytopenia, and vasculitis. Post-marketing symptoms under Campath may occur.

ANTIDOTE

CAMPATH AND LEMTRADA

Notify physician of all side effects. Treatment of most reactions will be supportive. Therapy should be temporarily discontinued during serious infection, serious hematologic toxicity (except lymphopenia), or other serious toxicity until the infection or adverse event resolves. Discontinue medication for severe reactions. Infusion reactions may be treated with acetaminophen, antihistamines (e.g., diphenhydramine), corticosteroids (e.g., hydrocortisone), epinephrine, and meperidine as indicated. Treat hypersensitivity reactions with epinephrine, antihistamines, and corticosteroids as needed. Resuscitate as indicated.

CAMPATH

Discontinue medication permanently for severe reactions, including autoimmune anemia or thrombocytopenia. Administration of irradiated blood products and/or blood modifiers (e.g., darbepoetin [Aranesp], epoetin alfa [Epogen], filgrastim [Neupogen, Zarxio], pegfilgrastim [Neulasta], sargramostim [Leukine]) may be indicated to treat bone marrow toxicity. Median durations of neutropenia were 28 to 37 days, and median durations of thrombocytopenia were 9 to 21 days. Median time to recovery of CD4+ counts to equal to or greater than 200/mm^3 is 2 to 6 months; however, full recovery of CD4+ and CD8+ counts may take more than 12 months. Discontinue alemtuzumab and provide supportive therapy in overdose.

LEMTRADA

Consider pretreatment with antihistamines and/or antipyretics. Epinephrine and atropine were administered to a number of patients who experienced an infusion reaction in clinical trials. If ITP is suspected, obtain a CBC. If ITP is confirmed, treat appropriately. If anti-GBM disease is suspected, urgent evaluation and treatment are required. Anti-GBM disease can lead to renal failure requiring dialysis or transplantation and can be life-threatening if left untreated. There is no known antidote for overdose.

ALLOPURINOL SODIUM
(al-oh-**PYOUR**-ih-nohl **SO**-dee-um)

Antigout
Antihyperuricemic
Antineoplastic adjunct

Aloprim

pH 11.1 to 11.8

USUAL DOSE

Pretreatment: Baseline studies indicated; see Monitor.

Allopurinol: IV and oral doses are therapeutically equivalent. Oral dose can replace an IV dose at any time. See Monitor.

200 to 400 mg/M^2/day as a single infusion or in equally divided doses at 6-, 8-, or 12-hour intervals (50 to 100 mg/M^2 every 6 hours, 67 to 133 mg/M^2 every 8 hours, or 100 to 200 mg/M^2 every 12 hours). Total dose should not exceed 600 mg/day.

PEDIATRIC DOSE

Recommended starting dose is 200 mg/M^2/day. Usually given in equally divided doses at 6- to 8-hour intervals (50 mg/M^2 every 6 hours or 67 mg/M^2 every 8 hours). Another source says the daily dose may be given at 6-, 8-, or 12-hour intervals or as a single daily infusion. Studies found no significant difference in dose response in pediatric patients. See comments in Usual Dose.

DOSE ADJUSTMENTS

In patients with impaired renal function not on dialysis, reduce dose based on CrCl according to the following chart.

Allopurinol Dosing in Impaired Renal Function	
CrCl (mL/min)	**Dose**
10-20 mL/min	200 mg daily
3-10 mL/min	100 mg daily
<3 mL/min	100 mg daily at extended intervals (more than 24 hr if necessary)

Treat with the lowest effective dose to minimize side effects. ▪ Dose with normal renal function may be increased or decreased based on electrolytes and serum uric acid levels. ▪ Lower doses and/or extended intervals may be required in the elderly; consider potential for decreased organ function, concomitant disease, or other drug therapy. ▪ See Drug/Lab Interactions.

DILUTION

Available as a single-dose vial containing 500 mg of allopurinol. Reconstitute with 25 mL of SWFI (yields 20 mg/mL). Swirl until completely dissolved. Must be further diluted with NS or D5W. Maximum concentration for administration is 6 mg/mL. 19 mL of additional diluent per 20 mg (1 mL) yields 1 mg/mL, 9 mL of additional diluent yields 2 mg/mL, and 2.3 mL of additional diluent yields 6 mg/mL.

Storage: Store unopened vials at CRT. Do not refrigerate the reconstituted and/or diluted product; begin infusion within 10 hours of reconstitution.

COMPATIBILITY

Manufacturer recommends administering sequentially and flushing before and after administration. Manufacturer lists the following drugs as **incompatible:** amikacin, amphotericin B (conventional), carmustine, cefotaxime, chlorpromazine, clindamycin, cytarabine, dacarbazine, daunorubicin, diphenhydramine, doxorubicin, doxycycline, floxuridine, gentamicin, idarubicin, imipenem-cilastatin, mechlorethamine, meperidine, methylprednisolone, metoclopramide, minocycline, nalbuphine, ondansetron, prochlorperazine, promethazine, sodium bicarbonate, streptozocin, tobramycin, and vinorelbine. *Do not use solutions containing sodium bicarbonate.*

Other sources suggest a few specific **compatibilities** dependent on concentration and manufacturer; consult a pharmacist.

RATE OF ADMINISTRATION

Manufacturer's recommendation not available. A maximum dose should take at least $\frac{1}{2}$ to 1 hour or more based on volume with diluent and patient comfort and/or requirements. Include in hydration fluids. See Compatibility.

ACTIONS

A xanthine oxidase inhibitor. Metabolized to oxypurinol. Acts on purine catabolism without disrupting the biosynthesis of purines. Reduces the production of uric acid by inhibiting the biochemical reactions immediately preceding its formation. Decreases uric acid concentrations in both serum and urine. Prevents or decreases urate deposition, decreasing the occurrence or progression of gout or urate nephropathy. Reduction of serum uric acid concentration occurs in 2 to 3 days. Peak concentrations are related to dose. Pharmacokinetic and plasma profiles of allopurinol and oxypurinol, as well as half-lives and systemic clearance, are similar with IV or oral administration. Systemic exposure to oxypurinol is also similar by both routes at each dose level. Cleared by glomerular filtration; some oxypurinol is reabsorbed in the kidney tubules. Secreted in breast milk.

INDICATIONS AND USES

Management of patients with leukemia, lymphoma, and solid tumor malignancies who are receiving cancer therapy that causes elevations of serum and urinary uric acid levels and who cannot tolerate oral therapy. Consider prophylactic use before initiation of and during chemotherapy in patients who are NPO, are nauseated and vomiting, or have malabsorption problems, dysphagia, or GI tract dysfunctions. Used prophylactically before the initiation of and during chemotherapy to prevent hyperuricemia caused by tumor lysis syndrome (TLS) and its sequela, acute uric acid nephropathy (AUAN).

Unlabeled uses: Preservation of cadaveric kidneys for transplantation.

CONTRAINDICATIONS

Any patient who has had a severe reaction to allopurinol (usually a hypersensitivity reaction).

PRECAUTIONS

For IV infusion only. ▪ A skin rash or other beginning signs of hypersensitivity may be followed by exfoliative, urticarial, and purpuric lesions; Stevens-Johnson syndrome; generalized vasculitis; irreversible hepatotoxicity; and/or rarely death. ▪ Incidence of hypersensitivity reactions may be increased in patients with decreased renal function who are receiving concurrent thiazides (e.g., chlorothiazide); use with caution. ▪ See Drug/Lab Interactions.

Monitor: Whenever possible, begin allopurinol therapy 24 to 48 hours before the start of chemotherapy known to cause tumor cell lysis (including adrenocorticosteroids). ▪ Monitor serum uric acid levels and electrolytes before and during therapy. Monitor serum uric acid levels to determine dose and frequency required to maintain uric acid levels within the normal range. ▪ Hydration with 3,000 mL/M^2/day (twice the level of maintenance fluid replacement) is recommended to promote a high volume of urine output (more than 2 L/day in adults) with low urate concentration. ▪ Maintain urine at neutral or slightly alkaline pH. To increase solubility of uric acid, alkalinity of urine may be increased with sodium bicarbonate. ▪ Monitor renal and hepatic systems before and during therapy. ▪ Monitoring of liver function suggested in patients with pre-existing liver disease, in patients with increases in liver function tests, and in patients who develop anorexia, pruritus, or weight loss. ▪ Observe for symptoms of TLS (e.g., hyperuricemia, hyperkalemia, hyperphosphatemia, and hypocalcemia). If untreated, may develop AUAN leading to renal failure requiring hemodialysis. ▪ Bone marrow suppression has been reported; monitor CBC periodically.

Patient Education: Maintain adequate hydration, avoid alcoholic drinks, and report nausea and vomiting and decreased urine production. ▪ Report promptly blood in the urine, painful urination, irritation of the eyes, skin rash, or swelling of the lips or mouth. ▪ Major acute toxicities may be allergic or renal. ▪ May cause drowsiness; use caution in activities that require alertness. Request assistance for ambulation.

Maternal/Child: Category C: potential benefits must justify potential risks to fetus. ▪ Use caution if required during breast-feeding.

Elderly: Lower-end initial doses or extended intervals may be appropriate in the elderly; see Dose Adjustments.

DRUG/LAB INTERACTIONS

May increase toxicity of **didanosine**; concurrent use not recommended. ▪ Inhibits metabolism and increases effects and toxicity of **thiopurines** (e.g., azathioprine, mercaptopurine). Reduce dose of thiopurine to one-third to one-fourth. ▪ **Uricosuric agents** (e.g., sulfinpyrazone, probenecid, colchicine) may increase elimination of active metabolites of allopurinol; may increase urinary excretions of uric acid. ▪ Prolongs half-life of **dicumarol;** monitor PT or PTT and adjust anticoagulant dose as indicated. ▪ Frequency of skin rash increased with **ampicillin/amoxicillin.** ▪ Bone marrow suppression may be increased when given concurrently with **cytotoxic agents** (e.g., cyclophosphamide); risk of bleeding or infection may be increased. ▪ May prolong half-life of **chlorpropamide.** ▪ Hypersensitivity reactions may be increased with **ACE inhibitors or thiazide diuretics**. ▪ Concurrent use with **cyclosporine** may increase cyclosporine serum levels. A reduced dose of cyclosporine may be indicated; monitoring of cyclosporine serum levels suggested. ▪ May decrease clearance and increase toxicity of **theophyllines**.

SIDE EFFECTS

Fewer than 1% of patients have had side effects directly attributable to allopurinol. Most were hypersensitivity reactions (e.g., nausea and vomiting, rash, and renal failure/insufficiency) and of mild to moderate severity. Xanthine crystalluria has been rarely reported in long-term therapy with oral allopurinol.

ANTIDOTE

Discontinue allopurinol at the first sign of skin rash or any other allergic reaction. Do not restart. Keep physician informed of all side effects. Symptoms of TLS require immediate intervention and correction of electrolyte abnormalities to avoid kidney damage. Treat hypersensitivity reactions as indicated; may require epinephrine, diphenhydramine, corticosteroids, and/or oxygen. Allopurinol is dialyzable, but effectiveness of hemodialysis or peritoneal dialysis in an overdose is not known.

ALPROSTADIL BBW
(al-**PROSS**-tah-dill)

Prostaglandin E$_1$, Prostin VR Pediatric

Prostaglandin
(ductus arteriosus
patency adjunct)

USUAL DOSE
Pediatric patients: Begin with 0.05 to 0.1 mcg/kg/min. When therapeutic response is achieved, reduce infusion rate in increments to the lowest dose that maintains the response (e.g., reduce from 0.1 to 0.05 or from 0.025 to 0.01 mcg/kg/min). If necessary, dose may be increased gradually to a maximum of 0.4 mcg/kg/min. Generally these higher rates do not produce greater effects. May be given through infusion in a large vein or, if necessary, through an umbilical artery catheter placed at the ductal opening.

DILUTION
Each 500 mcg (1 mL) must be further diluted with NS or D5W. When using a volumetric infusion chamber, the appropriate amount of IV infusion solution should be added to the chamber first. The undiluted alprostadil should then be added to the IV infusion solution, avoiding direct contact of the undiluted solution with the wall of the volumetric infusion chamber; see Compatibility. Various volumes of infusion solution may be used depending on infusion pump capabilities and desired infusion rate.

Guidelines for Dilution of 500 mcg (1 mL) of Alprostadil and Rate of Infusion for Desired Dose of Alprostadil			
Diluent (mL)	Concentration (mcg/mL)	Desired Dose (mcg/kg/min)	Rate of Infusion (mL/min/kg)
250 mL	2 mcg/mL	0.1 mcg/kg/min	0.05 mL/min/kg
100 mL	5 mcg/mL	0.1 mcg/kg/min	0.02 mL/min/kg
50 mL	10 mcg/mL	0.1 mcg/kg/min	0.01 mL/min/kg
25 mL	20 mcg/mL	0.1 mcg/kg/min	0.005 mL/min/kg

Storage: Refrigerate until dilution. Prepare fresh solution for administration every 24 hours.

COMPATIBILITY
Manufacturer states that undiluted alprostadil may interact with the plastic sidewalls of the volumetric infusion chamber, causing a change in the appearance of the chamber and creating a hazy solution. Should this occur, the solution and the volumetric infusion chamber should be replaced; see Dilution.

Other sources suggest specific **compatibilities** dependent on concentration and manufacturer; consult a pharmacist.

RATE OF ADMINISTRATION
See Usual Dose. Infusion pump capable of delivering 0.005, 0.01, 0.02, or 0.05 mL/min/kg required. Use for the shortest time possible at the lowest rate therapeutically effective. Decrease rate of infusion *stat* if a significant fall in arterial pressure occurs.

ACTIONS
A naturally occurring acidic lipid. A prostaglandin. Has various pharmacologic effects, including vasodilation, inhibition of platelet aggregation, and stimulation of the intestinal and uterine smooth muscle. Lowers blood pressure by decreasing peripheral resistance. A reflex increase in cardiac output and heart rate accompanies the reduction in blood pressure. Smooth muscle of the ductus arteriosus is susceptible to alprostadil's relaxing effect. Infants with congenital defects that restrict the pulmonary or systemic blood flow may benefit from alprostadil infusion. In some infants with restricted pulmonary blood flow, an increase in blood PO$_2$ was observed. In some infants with restricted systemic blood flow, an increase in pH in those who were acidotic, an increase in SBP, and a

decrease in the ratio of pulmonary artery pressure to aortic pressure were seen. Rapid metabolism by oxidation (80% in one pass through the lungs) necessitates administration by continuous infusion. Remainder excreted as metabolites in the urine.

INDICATIONS AND USES
Temporarily maintain the patency of the ductus arteriosus until corrective or palliative surgery can be performed on neonates who have congenital heart defects and who depend on the patent ductus for survival. Such congenital heart defects include pulmonary atresia, pulmonary stenosis, tricuspid atresia, tetralogy of Fallot, interruption of the aortic arch, coarctation of the aorta, or transposition of the great vessels. ■ Used by intercavernosal injection to treat impotence.

CONTRAINDICATIONS
None known.

PRECAUTIONS
Usually administered by trained personnel in pediatric intensive care facilities. ■ Establish a diagnosis of cyanotic heart disease (restricted pulmonary blood flow). Not indicated for infant respiratory distress syndrome (hyaline membrane disease). ■ Response is poor in infants with Po_2 values of 40 torr or more or those more than 4 days old. More effective with lower Po_2. ■ Apnea has been experienced in 10% to 12% of treated neonates; see Monitor. ■ Use caution in neonates with bleeding tendencies; inhibits platelet aggregation. ■ Administration of alprostadil to neonates may result in gastric outlet obstruction secondary to antral hyperplasia. Appears to be related to duration of therapy and cumulative dose. Risk of long-term infusion should be weighed against the possible benefits in a critically ill neonate; see Monitor. ■ Cortical proliferation of the long bones has been observed in infants during long-term infusions. May regress after withdrawal of drug.

Monitor: Monitor respiratory status continuously. Ventilatory assistance must be immediately available. May cause apnea, especially in infants under 2 kg. Apnea usually appears during the first hour of infusion. ■ Monitor arterial pressure intermittently by umbilical artery catheter, auscultation, or Doppler transducer. Decrease rate of infusion *stat* if a significant fall in arterial pressure occurs. ■ Decrease or stop infusion if infant develops increased respiratory distress; bleeding, bruising, or hematoma formation; or sudden changes in cardiac status (e.g., decreased BP, bradycardia, cardiac arrest, cyanosis). ■ Measure effectiveness with increase of Po_2 in infants with restricted pulmonary blood flow and increase of BP and blood pH in infants with restricted systemic blood flow. ■ Monitor for evidence of antral hyperplasia and gastric outlet obstruction in neonates receiving more than 120 hours of therapy at recommended doses.

DRUG/LAB INTERACTIONS
No drug interactions have been reported between alprostadil and the therapy that is standard in neonates with restricted pulmonary or systemic blood flow. Standard therapy includes **antibiotics** such as penicillin or gentamicin; **vasopressors** such as dopamine and isoproterenol; **cardiac glycosides**; and **diuretics** such as furosemide. ■ Inhibits **platelet aggregation.**

SIDE EFFECTS
Apnea, bradycardia, cardiac arrest, cerebral bleeding, cortical proliferation of long bones, diarrhea, DIC, edema, fever, flushing, hyperextension of the neck, hyperirritability, hypokalemia, hypotension, hypothermia, seizures, sepsis, tachycardia. Many other side effects have occurred in 1% or less of infants receiving alprostadil.

Overdose: Apnea, bradycardia, fever, flushing, hypotension.

ANTIDOTE
Notify physician of all side effects. Discontinue immediately if apnea occurs. Institute emergency measures. If infusion is restarted, use extreme caution. Decrease or stop infusion if infant develops increased respiratory distress; bleeding, bruising, or hematoma formation; or sudden changes in cardiac status (e.g., decreased BP, bradycardia, cardiac arrest, cyanosis). Decrease rate if pyrexia, hypotension, or fall in arterial pressure occurs.

ALTEPLASE

(**AL**-teh-playz)

Thrombolytic agent

Activase, rt-PA✦, Tissue Plasminogen Activator, tPA ▪ Cathflo Activase

pH 7.3

USUAL DOSE

Pretreatment: Baseline studies required; see Monitor.

Selected indications (e.g., acute ischemic stroke, acute myocardial infarction [AMI] in patients weighing less than 65 or 67 kg) require exact weight-adjusted dosing. To deliver an accurate dose without possibility of overdose, calculate desired dose and **withdraw** any amount ***NOT*** needed from a 50- or 100-mg vial and **discard**. In all situations follow total dose with at least 30 mL of NS or D5W through the IV tubing to ensure administration of total dose.

Acute Myocardial Infarction

Administer as soon as possible after onset of symptoms. Total dose is based on patient weight and should not exceed 100 mg regardless of selected administration regimen (accelerated infusion and 3-hour infusion are outlined in the following sections).

Accelerated infusion: Recommended accelerated infusion dose consists of an IV bolus over 1 to 2 minutes followed by an IV infusion as shown in the following chart.

Accelerated Infusion Weight-Based Doses for Patients With AMI			
Patient Weight (kg)	**IV Bolus**	**First 30 Minutes**	**Next 60 Minutes**
>67 kg	15 mg	50 mg	35 mg
≤67 kg	15 mg	0.75 mg/kg	0.5 mg/kg

The safety and efficacy of accelerated infusion of alteplase have only been investigated with concomitant administration of heparin and aspirin. See comments under Usual Dose.

3-hour infusion: For patients weighing 65 kg or more, administer a total dose of 100 mg titrated over 3 hours as an IV infusion. Initially, administer 60 mg over the first hour (with 6 to 10 mg of this administered as a bolus over 1 to 2 minutes). Follow with 20 mg/hr for 2 hours. For smaller patients (less than 65 kg), calculate total dose using 1.25 mg/kg of body weight administered over 3 hours (with 0.075 mg/kg administered as a bolus over 1 to 2 minutes). Follow with 0.675 mg/kg over the first hour and 0.25 mg/kg/hr for 2 hours. Weight-based doses are shown in the following chart. See comments under Usual Dose.

3-Hour Infusion Weight-Based Doses for Patients With AMI				
Patient Weight (kg)	**Bolus**	**Rest of 1st Hour**	**2nd Hour**	**3rd Hour**
≥65 kg	6 to 10 mg	50 to 54 mg	20 mg	20 mg
<65 kg	0.075 mg/kg	0.675 mg/kg	0.25 mg/kg	0.25 mg/kg

Acute Ischemic Stroke

Administer as soon as possible but within 3 hours after onset of symptoms. Perform non–contrast-enhanced CT or MRI before administration to rule out intracranial bleed. Recommended dose is 0.9 mg/kg. Do not exceed the maximum dose of 90 mg. See comments in Usual Dose. Give a bolus of 10% of the calculated dose over 1 minute followed by balance of calculated dose (90%) as an infusion evenly distributed over 60 minutes. Do not give aspirin, heparin, or warfarin for 24 hours; see Precautions.

PULMONARY EMBOLISM

100 mg administered over 2 hours as an IV infusion. Begin parenteral anticoagulation near the end of or immediately following the alteplase infusion when the partial thromboplastin time (PTT) or thrombin time (TT) returns to twice normal or less.

CENTRAL VENOUS ACCESS DEVICE (CVAD) OCCLUSIONS, CATHFLO ACTIVASE

See Rate of Administration, Precautions, Monitor, and Maternal/Child.

Patient weight 30 kg or greater: Instill 2 mg in 2 mL into the occluded catheter.

Patient weight less than 30 kg: Instill 110% of the internal lumen volume of the occluded catheter into the occluded catheter. Do not exceed 2 mg in 2 mL.

Attempt to aspirate blood from the catheter after 30 minutes of dwell time. If catheter function has been restored, aspirate 4 to 5 mL of blood in patients equal to or greater than 10 kg or 3 mL of blood in patients less than 10 kg to remove Cathflo Activase and residual clot, then gently irrigate the catheter with NS.

If catheter function has not been restored (unable to aspirate blood), allow the first dose to remain in the catheter for 90 additional minutes of dwell time and then attempt to aspirate again (total elapsed time is 120 minutes). If catheter function has been restored, aspirate and irrigate as above. If function has not been restored, a second dose may be instilled and the dwell time and aspiration process repeated.

DILUTION

Myocardial infarction, stroke, and pulmonary embolism: Must be reconstituted with SWFI without preservatives (provided by manufacturer). Available in 50- and 100-mg vials. May be administered as reconstituted solution at 1 mg/mL or further diluted immediately before administration in an equal volume of NS or D5W to yield a concentration of 0.5 mg/mL using either polyvinyl chloride bags or glass vials. Slight foaming is expected; let stand for several minutes to dissipate large bubbles. Do not shake. Mix by swirling or slow inversion; avoid agitation during dilution.

50-mg vial: Use a large-bore (18-gauge) needle and syringe to direct the stream of provided diluent (SWFI) into the lyophilized cake. A vacuum must be present when the diluent is added to the powder for injection. Do not use if vacuum is not present.

Bolus dose can be given when indicated by withdrawing the calculated dose from the infusion and injecting it through a med port. When obtaining the bolus dose, **do not** prime syringe with air; insert needle into the alteplase vial stopper to withdraw dose. Remove portion of dose that is not needed and waste prior to starting the infusion. An NS bag should be infused after alteplase is emptied to ensure complete delivery of the desired dose. Alternately, the IV pump can be programmed to deliver the appropriate volume as a bolus at the initiation of the infusion. Administer balance of dose, using either a polyvinyl chloride bag or glass vial and infusion set. Adjust pump rate as required. Complete by flushing tubing with IV solution.

100-mg vial: Does not contain a vacuum. Diluent and transfer device provided. Insert one end of transfer device into upright vial of diluent (do not invert diluent vial yet). Hold alteplase vial upside down and push center of vial down onto piercing pin. Now invert vials and allow diluent to flow into alteplase. Small amount (0.5 mL) of diluent will not transfer. Swirl gently to dissolve. Do not shake. Process takes several minutes. Remove any quantity of drug in excess of that specified for patient treatment; see Usual Dose.

Bolus dose can be given when indicated by direct IV injection by programming the IV pump to deliver the appropriate volume as a bolus at the initiation of the infusion as described previously. When withdrawing the bolus dose from a 100-mg vial, the needle should be inserted away from the puncture mark made by the transfer device. Administer the balance of dose by inserting an infusion set into puncture site created by piercing pin. Hang by plastic capping on bottom of vial. Prime tubing with alteplase and administer. Adjust pump rate of delivery as required. Complete by flushing tubing with IV solution.

Cathflo Activase for CVAD occlusion: Supplied as a sterile lyophilized powder in 2-mg vials. Must be reconstituted with 2.2 mL of SWFI without preservatives. Direct diluent stream into the powder. Allow to stand undisturbed until large bubbles dissipate; may foam slightly. Mix by swirling gently; do not shake. Should be completely dissolved within

3 minutes. Final concentration is 1 mg/mL. If the 2-mg vials are not available, some pharmacies dilute 50 mg of alteplase with 50 mL of SWFI without preservatives (1 mg/mL). Withdraw 2.2 mL (2.2 mg) into 2- or 5-mL sterile disposable syringes. In studies, these were transferred to sterile glass vials and frozen. Defrost and use as needed (22 prepared doses).

Filters: Specific information not available.

Storage: *Systemic alteplase:* Protect from light in cartons. May be stored at CRT or refrigerated before and/or after reconstitution. Manufacturer recommends reconstitution immediately before use. Must be used within 8 hours of reconstitution. Discard unused solution. Stable as a 0.5 mg/mL solution in NS or D5W for 8 hours at CRT.

Cathflo Activase: Refrigerate unopened vials; protect from light during extended storage. Reconstitution immediately before use is recommended, but solution may be used up to 8 hours after reconstitution if refrigerated at 2° to 30° C (36° to 46° F). Do not use beyond expiration date on vial. Discard unused solution.

COMPATIBILITY

Manufacturer states, "No other medication should be added to infusion solutions containing alteplase"; see Dilution.

Other sources suggest a few specific **compatibilities** dependent on concentration and manufacturer; consult a pharmacist.

RATE OF ADMINISTRATION

Systemic alteplase: See specific rates for each diagnosis under Usual Dose. In all situations use an infusion pump (preferred) or a metriset with microdrip (60 drop/mL) and IV tubing to facilitate accurate administration. Flushing of IV line required. NS preferred for flushing of IV line.

Cathflo Activase: Avoid excessive pressure or force while attempting to clear catheters; see Usual Dose, Precautions, and Monitor.

ACTIONS

A tissue plasminogen activator and enzyme produced by recombinant DNA technology. It binds to fibrin in a thrombus and converts plasminogen to plasmin. This initiates local fibrinolysis and dissolution of the clot. Onset of action is prompt. Cleared from the plasma by the liver within 5 (50%) to 10 (80%) minutes after the infusion is discontinued. Some fibrinolytic activity may persist for up to 1 hour after completion of the infusion.

Cathflo Activase: When Cathflo Activase is administered for restoration of function to central venous access devices according to the manufacturer's instructions, circulating plasma levels of alteplase are not expected to reach pharmacologic concentrations.

INDICATIONS AND USES

Systemic alteplase: Use in AMI for the reduction of the incidence of congestive heart failure and the reduction of mortality associated with AMI. ▪ Treatment of acute ischemic stroke. Exclude intracranial hemorrhage as the primary cause of stroke S/S before initiation of treatment. ▪ Lysis of acute massive pulmonary embolism defined as (1) acute pulmonary emboli obstructing blood flow to a lobe or to multiple lung segments, or (2) acute pulmonary emboli accompanied by unstable hemodynamics (e.g., failure to maintain BP without supportive measures).

Limitation of use: In patients with AMI, the risk of stroke may outweigh the benefit produced by thrombolytic therapy in patients whose AMI puts them at low risk for death or heart failure.

Cathflo Activase: Restoration of function to CVADs as assessed by the ability to withdraw blood.

Unlabeled uses: *Systemic alteplase:* Treatment of acute ischemic stroke 3 to 4.5 hours after symptom onset. Has been shown to restore blood flow to frostbitten limbs. Has been used in peripheral arterial occlusion, prosthetic valve thrombosis, and submassive pulmonary embolism.

CONTRAINDICATIONS

All indications: Known hypersensitivity to alteplase or its components.

Acute myocardial infarction/pulmonary embolism: Do not administer for the treatment of AMI or pulmonary embolism in the following situations in which the risk of bleeding is greater than the potential benefit: active internal bleeding, bleeding diathesis, history of recent cerebrovascular accident, recent (within 3 months) intracranial or intraspinal surgery or serious head trauma, current severe uncontrolled hypertension, presence of intracranial conditions that may increase the risk of bleeding (e.g., some neoplasms, arteriovenous malformation, or aneurysm).

Acute ischemic stroke: Do not administer to treat acute ischemic stroke in the following situations in which the risk of bleeding is greater than the potential benefit: current intracranial hemorrhage (on pretreatment evaluation), subarachnoid hemorrhage, active internal bleeding, presence of intracranial conditions that may increase the risk of bleeding (e.g., some neoplasms, arteriovenous malformation, or aneurysm), recent (within 3 months) intracranial or intraspinal surgery or serious head trauma, bleeding diathesis, or current severe uncontrolled hypertension.

PRECAUTIONS

All systemic indications: Administered under the direction of a physician knowledgeable in its use and with appropriate emergency drugs and diagnostic and laboratory facilities available. ▪ Alteplase can cause significant, sometimes fatal, internal or external bleeding. May be internal bleeding (involving intracranial or retroperitoneal sites or the GI, GU, or respiratory tracts) or external bleeding, especially at arterial and venous puncture sites. Use extreme care with the patient; avoid IM injections and any trauma to the patient who is receiving alteplase. Avoid invasive procedures (e.g., arterial puncture and venipuncture). If these procedures are absolutely necessary, use extreme precautionary methods. To minimize bleeding from noncompressible sites, avoid internal jugular and subclavian venous punctures. If an arterial puncture is necessary, use an upper extremity vessel that is accessible to manual compression, apply pressure for at least 30 minutes, and monitor the puncture site closely. ▪ Fatal cases of hemorrhage associated with traumatic intubation in patients receiving alteplase have been reported. ▪ Aspirin and heparin have been administered concomitantly with and following infusions of alteplase in the management of AMI and PE. However, the administration of heparin and aspirin concomitantly with and following infusions of alteplase for the treatment of acute ischemic stroke during the first 24 hours after symptom onset has not been investigated. Because heparin, aspirin, or alteplase may cause bleeding complications, carefully monitor for bleeding. Hemorrhage can occur 1 or more days after administration of alteplase while patients are still receiving anticoagulant therapy. ▪ The risk of bleeding with alteplase therapy for all systemic indications is increased and should be weighed against the anticipated benefit in any of the following conditions: recent major surgery or procedure (e.g., CABG, obstetric delivery, organ biopsy, previous puncture of noncompressible vessels), recent intracranial hemorrhage, recent GI or GU bleeding, cerebrovascular disease, hypertension (systolic above 175 mm Hg or diastolic above 110 mm Hg), recent trauma, acute pericarditis, subacute bacterial endocarditis, hemostatic defects (including those secondary to severe hepatic or renal disease), significant liver dysfunction, pregnancy, hemorrhagic ophthalmic conditions (e.g., diabetic hemorrhagic retinopathy), septic thrombophlebitis or occluded AV cannula at seriously infected site, patients taking anticoagulants, advanced age, or any situation in which bleeding might be hazardous or difficult to manage because of location. ▪ Cholesterol embolism has been reported rarely and is associated with invasive procedures (e.g., cardiac catheterization, angiography, vascular surgery) and/or anticoagulant therapy; see Side Effects. ▪ Hypersensitivity, including urticarial/anaphylactic reactions, have been reported. Fatalities have occurred. Angioedema has been observed during and up to 2 hours after infusion in patients treated for acute ischemic stroke and AMI. In many cases patients received concomitant angiotensin-converting enzyme inhibitors. See Drug/Lab Interactions and Antidote.

Myocardial infarction: Reperfusion arrhythmias can occur (e.g., sinus bradycardia, accelerated idioventricular rhythm, PVCs, ventricular tachycardia); have antiarrhythmic medications available.

Acute ischemic stroke: Because of the higher risk of intracranial hemorrhage in patients treated for acute ischemic stroke, treatment facility must be able to provide evaluation and management of intracranial hemorrhage. ▪ Risk of intracranial hemorrhage may be increased in patients with severe neurologic deficit at presentation. However, efficacy results suggest a reduced but still favorable clinical outcome for these patients. ▪ Treatment may begin before coagulation study results are known in patients without recent use of oral anticoagulants or heparin. Discontinue infusion if pretreatment INR is greater than 1.7 or if an elevated aPTT is identified.

Pulmonary emboli: Thrombolytics can increase the risk of thromboembolic events in patients with high likelihood of left heart thrombus, such as patients with mitral stenosis or atrial fibrillation. ▪ Treatment with alteplase does not constitute adequate treatment of underlying deep venous thrombosis. ▪ Risk of re-embolization due to lysis of underlying DVT should be considered.

Cathflo Activase: Consider causes of catheter dysfunction other than thrombus formation (e.g., catheter malposition, mechanical failure, constriction by a suture, lipid deposits or drug precipitates within the catheter lumen). ▪ Do not apply vigorous suction during attempts to determine catheter occlusion; may risk damage to the vascular wall or collapse of soft-walled catheters. ▪ Avoid excessive pressure during instillation of Cathflo Activase into the catheter; may cause rupture of the catheter or expulsion of the clot into the circulation. ▪ Use caution with patients who have active internal bleeding, thrombocytopenia, or other hemostatic defects (including those secondary to hepatic or renal disease). ▪ Use caution in patients who have conditions for which bleeding constitutes a significant hazard, who would be difficult to manage because of location of the bleeding, who are at high risk for embolic complications (e.g., venous thrombosis in the region of the catheter), or who have had any of the following within 48 hours: surgery, obstetric delivery, percutaneous biopsy of viscera or deep tissues, or puncture of noncompressible vessels. ▪ Use caution in the presence of known or suspected infection in the catheter; may release a localized infection into the systemic circulation. ▪ Hypersensitivity, including urticaria, angioedema, and anaphylaxis, has been reported. ▪ See Monitor. ▪ Safety and effectiveness of doses greater than 2 mg have not been established.

Monitor: ***All systemic indications:*** Establish a separate IV line for alteplase. ▪ Obtain appropriate laboratory studies (e.g., PT, TT, PTT, INR, aPTT, CBC, fibrinogen levels, platelets). ▪ Diagnosis-specific baseline studies (e.g., ECG, troponin in myocardial infarction, noncontrast CT brain scan, neurologic assessment in acute ischemic stroke, and CT or pulmonary angiography in pulmonary embolism) are indicated. ▪ Monitor the patient carefully and frequently for pain and signs of bleeding; observe catheter sites frequently and apply pressure dressings to any recently invaded site; watch for hematuria, hematemesis, bloody stool, petechiae, hematoma, flank pain, or muscle weakness; perform neuro checks. Continue until normal clotting function returns. ▪ Monitor BP and maintain within appropriate limits with antihypertensives or vasopressors as indicated. ▪ Monitor for signs of a hypersensitivity reaction (e.g., laryngeal edema, rash, shock) during and for several hours after infusion. ▪ Watch for extravasation; may cause ecchymosis and/or inflammation. Restart IV at another site and apply local therapy. ▪ See Precautions and Drug/Lab Interactions.

Myocardial infarction: Monitor ECG.

Acute ischemic stroke: Before the initiation of therapy, determine actual time of onset of stroke. ▪ During and following alteplase administration, frequently monitor and control BP. The 2013 AHA/ASA guidelines for early management of acute ischemic stroke recommend (1) monitoring BP every 15 minutes for 2 hours, every 30 minutes for 6 hours, then every 1 hour for 18 hours; and (2) performing neurologic assessments every 15 minutes during infusion, every 30 minutes thereafter for the next 6 hours, and then hourly until 24 hours after treatment. ▪ Hemorrhage in the brain occurs frequently during treatment with alteplase; monitor carefully. Acute neurologic deterioration, new headache, acute hypertension, or nausea and vomiting may indicate the occurrence of intracranial hemorrhage. If intracranial hemorrhage is suspected, discontinue alteplase and obtain a CT scan.

Cathflo Activase: Aseptic technique imperative. ▪ Avoid force while attempting to clear catheters; may rupture catheter or dislodge clot into the circulation. ▪ Monitor for S/S of a hypersensitivity reaction. ▪ See Precautions.

Patient Education: Compliance with all measures to minimize bleeding (e.g., strict bed rest) is very important. ▪ Avoid use of razors, toothbrushes, and other sharp items. Use caution while moving to avoid excessive bumping. ▪ Report all S/S of bleeding (e.g., unusual bruising, pink or brown urine, red or black or tarry stools, coughing up blood, vomiting blood or blood that looks like coffee grounds, headache or stroke symptoms). Apply local pressure if indicated. Expect oozing from IV sites.

Maternal/Child: *Systemic alteplase:* Safety for use in pregnancy and breast-feeding not established. ▪ Safety and effectiveness for use in pediatric patients not established.

Cathflo Activase: Use during pregnancy only if benefits justify potential risk to the fetus. ▪ Use caution during breast-feeding. ▪ Has been used in patients 2 weeks to 17 years of age. Rates of serious adverse events as well as restoration of catheter function similar to adults.

Elderly: *Systemic alteplase:* Possible increased risk of bleeding with advanced age (e.g., age greater than 77 years). In acute ischemic stroke, efficacy results suggest a reduced but still favorable clinical outcome for elderly patients treated with alteplase.

Cathflo Activase: No incidents of intracranial hemorrhage, embolic events, or major bleeding events were observed during studies. ▪ Use caution in the elderly with conditions known to increase the risk of bleeding; see Precautions.

DRUG/LAB INTERACTIONS

Risk of bleeding may be increased by any medicine that affects blood clotting, including **anticoagulants** (e.g., heparin, warfarin); **any medication that may cause hypoprothrombinemia, thrombocytopenia, or GI ulceration or bleeding** (e.g., selected antibiotics [e.g., cefotetan], aspirin, NSAIDs); **and/or any other medication that inhibits platelet aggregation** (e.g., clopidogrel, dipyridamole, glycoprotein GP IIb/IIIa receptor antagonists [e.g., eptifibatide, tirofiban]). ▪ Concomitant **angiotensin-converting enzyme inhibitors** increase the risk of angioedema. ▪ **Coagulation tests and measures of fibrinolytic activity** may be unreliable; specific procedures can be used; notify the lab of alteplase use.

SIDE EFFECTS

Systemic alteplase: Bleeding is most common: internal (GI tract, GU tract, retroperitoneal, or intracranial sites) and superficial or external bleeding (ecchymosis, epistaxis, gingival bleeding, venous cutdowns, arterial punctures, sites of recent surgical intervention). Mild to serious hypersensitivity reactions (e.g., anaphylactoid reaction, laryngeal edema, orolingual angioedema, rash, urticaria) have occurred. Cholesterol embolization can occur with thrombolytics but has been reported rarely. It may present with acute renal failure, bowel infarction, cerebral infarction, gangrenous digits, hypertension, livedo reticularis, myocardial infarction, pancreatitis, purple toe syndrome, retinal artery occlusion, rhabdomyolysis, or spinal cord infarction. Fatalities have been reported.

Post-Marketing: The following events may be life-threatening:

Acute ischemic stroke: Cerebral edema, cerebral herniation, embolism, new ischemic stroke, seizure.

Acute myocardial infarction: Arrhythmias, AV block, cardiac arrest, cardiac tamponade, cardiogenic shock, electromechanical dissociation, fever, heart failure, hypotension, mitral regurgitation, myocardial reinfarction, myocardial rupture, nausea and/or vomiting, pericardial effusion, pericarditis, pulmonary edema, recurrent ischemia, thromboembolism.

Pulmonary embolism: Hypotension, pleural effusion, pulmonary edema, pulmonary reembolization, thromboembolism.

Cathflo Activase: Gastrointestinal bleeding, hypersensitivity reactions (e.g., anaphylaxis, angioedema, urticaria), sepsis, and venous thrombosis have occurred. There were no reports of intracranial hemorrhage or pulmonary emboli during clinical trials.

ANTIDOTE

Systemic alteplase: Notify physician of all side effects. Note even the most minute bleeding tendency. Oozing at IV sites is expected. Control minor bleeding by local pressure. For severe bleeding in a critical location or suspected intracranial bleeding, discontinue alteplase and any heparin therapy immediately. Obtain PT, aPTT, platelet count, and fibrinogen. Draw blood for type and cross-match. Transfuse as indicated. Consider protamine if heparin has been used. Treat reperfusion arrhythmias with appropriate antiarrhythmic; VT or VF may require cardioversion. Treat minor hypersensitivity reactions symptomatically. If anaphylaxis or angioedema occur, discontinue infusion immediately and initiate appropriate treatment with antihistamines (e.g., diphenhydramine), IV corticosteroids, or epinephrine; resuscitate as necessary.

Cathflo Activase: Discontinue Cathflo Activase and withdraw it from the catheter if serious bleeding in a critical location (e.g., intracranial, gastrointestinal, retroperitoneal, pericardial) occurs. Discontinue drug and treat anaphylaxis as indicated; resuscitate as necessary. In the event of accidental administration of a 2-mg dose directly into the systemic circulation, the concentration of circulating levels of alteplase would be expected to return to exogenous levels of 5 to 10 ng/mL within 30 minutes.

AMIKACIN SULFATE BBW
(am-ih-**KAY**-sin **SUL**-fayt)

Antibacterial
(aminoglycoside)

pH 3.5 to 5.5

USUAL DOSE

Up to 15 mg/kg of body weight/24 hr equally divided into 2 or 3 doses at equally divided intervals (5 mg/kg every 8 hours or 7.5 mg/kg every 12 hours). Dosage based on ideal weight of lean body mass.

Studies suggest that in certain populations a single daily dose of 15 to 20 mg/kg (instead of divided into 2 or 3 doses) may provide higher peak levels and enhance drug effectiveness while actually reducing or having no adverse effects on risk of toxicity. Various procedures for monitoring blood levels are in use. Some health facilities are monitoring with trough levels; others may draw levels at predetermined times and plot the concentration on nomograms. Depending on the protocol in place, doses or intervals may be adjusted. See Dose Adjustments and Precautions.

PEDIATRIC DOSE

15 to 22.5 mg/kg/24 hr equally divided into 2 or 3 doses and given every 8 to 12 hours (5 to 7.5 mg/kg every 8 hours or 7.5 to 11.25 mg/kg every 12 hours). Do not exceed 1.5 Gm/24 hr. A single daily dose is also being used in pediatric patients. See comments under Usual Dose.

NEWBORN DOSE

See Maternal/Child.

10 mg/kg of body weight as a loading dose, then 7.5 mg/kg/dose. Intervals of 7.5 mg/kg dose adjusted based on age as follows:

Under 28 weeks' gestation and under 7 days of age: Give every 24 hours.

Under 28 weeks' gestation and over 7 days or 28 to 34 weeks' gestation and under 7 days of age: Give every 18 hours.

Continued

28 to 34 weeks' gestation and over 7 days of age or over 34 weeks' gestation and under 7 days of age: Give every 12 hours.

Over 34 weeks' gestation and over 7 days of age: Give every 8 hours.

DOSE ADJUSTMENTS

Reduce daily dose commensurate with amount of renal impairment and/or increase intervals between injections. ▪ Once-daily dosing is not usually used in patients with ascites, burns covering more than 20% of the total body surface area, CrCl less than 40 mL/min (including patients requiring dialysis), CrCl greater than 120 mL/min, cystic fibrosis, endocarditis, mycobacterium infections, or in infants or pregnancy. ▪ Reduced dose or extended intervals may be required in the elderly. ▪ See Drug/Lab Interactions.

DILUTION

Each 500 mg or fraction thereof is diluted with 100 to 200 mL D5W, D5NS, or NS. Amount of diluent may be decreased proportionately with dosage for infants and other pediatric patients. Available for pediatric injection as 50 mg/mL.

Storage: Stable for 24 hours at RT at concentrations of 0.25 and 5 mg/mL when diluted in specific solutions; see prescribing information.

COMPATIBILITY

Do not physically premix with other drugs; administer separately as recommended by manufacturer. Inactivated in solution with beta-lactam antibiotics (e.g., cephalosporins, penicillins) and vancomycin. Do not mix in the same solution. Appropriate spacing required because of physical **incompatibilities**. See Drug/Lab Interactions.

Solution: Manufacturer lists D5W, D5 in ¼NS, D5 in ½NS, NS, LR, D5 in Normosol M (Plasma-Lyte 56 in D5W), D5 in Normosol R (Plasma-Lyte 148 in D5W).

Other sources suggest specific **compatibilities** dependent on concentration and manufacturer; consult a pharmacist.

RATE OF ADMINISTRATION

A single dose over at least 30 to 60 minutes. Infants should receive a 1- to 2-hour infusion.

ACTIONS

An aminoglycoside antibiotic with neuromuscular blocking action. Bactericidal against many gram-negative organisms resistant to other antibiotics including other aminoglycosides such as gentamicin, kanamycin, and tobramycin. Well distributed through all body fluids. Usual half-life is 2 to 3 hours. Crosses the placental barrier. Excreted in the kidneys. Cross-allergenicity does occur between aminoglycosides.

INDICATIONS AND USES

Short-term treatment of serious infections caused by susceptible organisms (e.g., gram-negative bacteria) generally resistant to alternate drugs that have less potential toxicity. ▪ Effective in infections of the respiratory and urinary tracts, CNS (including meningitis), skin and soft tissue, intra-abdominal (including peritonitis), bacterial septicemia (including neonatal sepsis), burns, and postoperative infections. ▪ Considered initial therapy in suspected gram-negative infections after culture and sensitivity are drawn. ▪ In certain severe infections (e.g., neonatal sepsis), empiric concomitant treatment with an antibiotic effective against gram-positive organisms (e.g., penicillin) may be required until the results of C/S are obtained.

Unlabeled uses: Treatment of *Mycobacterium avium* complex, a common infection in AIDS (part of a multiple [3 to 5] drug regimen), tuberculosis.

CONTRAINDICATIONS

Known amikacin or aminoglycoside sensitivity. Sulfite sensitivity may be a contraindication.

PRECAUTIONS

Sensitivity studies indicated to determine susceptibility of causative organism to amikacin. ▪ Response should occur in 24 to 48 hours. Safety for use longer than 14 days not established. ▪ Superinfection may occur from overgrowth of nonsusceptible organisms. ▪ May contain sulfites; use caution in patients with asthma. ▪ Single daily dosing has been used effectively in abdominal, pelvic inflammatory, and GU infections in patients with normal renal function. Not recommended in bacteremia caused by *Pseudomonas aeruginosa,* endocarditis, meningitis, during pregnancy, or in patients less than 6 weeks postpartum. Limited data available for use in all other situations (e.g., burns, cystic fibrosis, elderly, pediatrics, renal impairment). ▪ Potentially nephrotoxic, ototoxic, and neurotoxic. Risk of nephrotoxicity and neurotoxicity (e.g., auditory and vestibular ototoxicity) increased in patients with pre-existing renal damage or in normal renal function with prolonged use. Partial or total irreversible deafness may continue to develop after amikacin is discontinued. ▪ Use with caution in patients with muscular disorders (e.g., myasthenia gravis, parkinsonism) because these drugs may aggravate muscle weakness. ▪ *Clostridium difficile*–associated diarrhea (CDAD) has been reported. May range from mild diarrhea to fatal colitis. Consider in patients who present with diarrhea during or after treatment with amikacin. ▪ See Monitor and Drug/Lab Interactions.

Monitor: Maintain good hydration. ▪ Narrow range between toxic and therapeutic levels. Periodically monitor peak and trough concentrations. Manufacturer recommends avoiding peak serum concentrations greater than 35 mcg/mL and trough serum concentrations above 10 mcg/mL. ▪ Monitor urine protein, presence of cells and casts, and decreased specific gravity. Watch for decreased urine output, rising BUN and SCr, and declining CrCl levels. Dose adjustment may be necessary. ▪ Closely monitor patients with impaired renal function for nephrotoxicity and neurotoxicity (e.g., auditory and vestibular ototoxicity); nephrotoxicity may be reversible. ▪ In extended treatment, monitor serum levels, electrolytes, and renal, auditory, and vestibular functions frequently. ▪ See Drug/Lab Interactions.

Patient Education: Report promptly any changes in balance, hearing loss, weakness, or dizziness. ▪ Consider birth control options. ▪ Promptly report diarrhea or bloody stools that occur during treatment or up to several months after an antibiotic has been discontinued; may indicate CDAD and require treatment.

Maternal/Child: Category D: avoid pregnancy. Potential hazard to fetus. ▪ Safety for use during breast-feeding not established; use extreme caution. ▪ Peak concentrations are generally lower in infants and young children. ▪ Use extreme caution in premature infants and neonates; immature kidney function will result in prolonged half-life.

Elderly: Consider less toxic alternatives. ▪ Longer intervals between doses may be more important than smaller doses. ▪ Monitor renal function and drug levels carefully. Measurement of CrCl more useful than BUN or SCr to assess renal function. ▪ Half-life prolonged.

DRUG/LAB INTERACTIONS
Synergistic when used in combination with **beta-lactam antibiotics** (e.g., cephalosporins, penicillins) **and vancomycin.** Synergism may be inconsistent; see Compatibility. ▪ Concurrent use topically or systemically with any other **ototoxic or nephrotoxic agents** should be avoided. May have dangerous additive effects with **anesthetics, other neuromuscular blocking antibiotics, diuretics, beta-lactam antibiotics** (e.g., cephalosporins), **vancomycin, and many others.** ▪ Neuromuscular blocking muscle relaxants (e.g., atracurium, succinylcholine) are potentiated by aminoglycosides. *Apnea can occur.* ▪ Aminoglycosides are potentiated by **anticholinesterases** and **antineoplastics.**

SIDE EFFECTS
Occur more frequently with impaired renal function, higher doses, prolonged administration, in dehydrated or elderly patients, and in patients receiving other ototoxic or nephrotoxic drugs. Fever, headache, hypotension, nausea, paresthesias, seizures, skin rash, tremor, and vomiting.

Major: Albuminuria, anemia, arthralgia, azotemia, CDAD, eosinophilia, loss of balance, neuromuscular blockade, oliguria, ototoxicity, RBCs and WBCs or casts in urine, respiratory depression or arrest, and rising SCr.

ANTIDOTE

Notify physician of all side effects. If minor side effects persist or any major symptom appears, discontinue drug and notify physician. Treatment is symptomatic, or a reduction in dose may be required. In overdose, hemodialysis may be indicated. Monitor fluid balance, CrCl, and plasma levels carefully. Complexation with ticarcillin may be as effective as hemodialysis. Consider exchange transfusion in the newborn. Calcium salts or neostigmine may reverse neuromuscular blockade. Treat CDAD with fluids, electrolytes, protein supplements, and appropriate antibiotics (e.g., oral vancomycin) as indicated. In severe cases, surgical evaluation may be indicated. Resuscitate as necessary.

AMINOCAPROIC ACID

(a-mee-noh-ka-**PROH**-ick **AS**-id)

Amicar

Antifibrinolytic
Antihemorrhagic

pH 6 to 7.6

USUAL DOSE

Pretreatment: Pretesting and baseline studies required; see Precautions and Monitor.

4 to 5 Gm initially over 1 hour. Follow with 1 Gm/hr for 8 hours or until bleeding is controlled. In acute bleeding syndromes, the 4- to 5-Gm dose may be given as a continuous infusion over the first hour, followed by a continuous infusion of 1 Gm/hr for 8 hours or until bleeding is controlled. Maximum dose is 30 Gm/24 hr.

Prevent recurrence of subarachnoid hemorrhage (unlabeled): 36 Gm/24 hr. One source suggests administering 18 Gm in 400 mL D5W every 12 hours for 10 days. Follow with oral therapy.

Prevention of perioperative bleeding during cardiac surgery (unlabeled): 10 Gm as an infusion over 20 to 30 minutes before skin incision. Follow with 1 to 2.5 Gm/hr (usually 2 Gm/hr) until the end of the operation. Infusion may be continued for 4 hours after protamine reversal of heparin. In addition, 10 Gm may be added to the cardiopulmonary bypass circuit priming solution. An alternate regimen is 10 Gm over 20 to 30 minutes before skin incision, followed by 10 Gm after heparin administration, then 10 Gm when cardiopulmonary bypass is discontinued and before protamine reversal of heparin. Another source suggests a loading dose of 80 mg/kg over 20 minutes followed by 30 mg/kg/hr, or a loading dose of 60 mg/kg over 20 minutes followed by 30 mg/kg/hr plus a 10-mg/kg dose in the priming solution of the cardiopulmonary bypass pump.

PEDIATRIC DOSE

Acute bleeding syndromes (unlabeled): See Maternal/Child. *Loading dose:* 100 to 200 mg/kg. Follow with a maintenance dose of 100 mg/kg/dose every 4 to 6 hours. Maximum dose is 30 Gm/24 hr.

DOSE ADJUSTMENTS

May accumulate in patients with renal impairment, and reduced doses are suggested; however, specific recommendations are not available from the manufacturer. Another source suggests decreasing dose to 15% to 25% of the normal dose in patients with renal impairment.

DILUTION

1 Gm equals 4 mL of prepared solution. Further dilute with **compatible** infusion solutions (NS, D5W, SWFI, or Ringer's solution). Up to 50 mL of diluent may be used for each 1 Gm.

Storage: Before use store at CRT. Do not freeze.

COMPATIBILITY

Compatible in D5W, Ringer's solution, and NS.

RATE OF ADMINISTRATION

5 Gm or fraction thereof over first hour in 250 mL of solution; then administer each succeeding 1 Gm over 1 hour in 50 to 100 mL of solution. Use of an infusion pump for accurate dose recommended. Rapid administration or insufficient dilution may cause hypotension, bradycardia, and/or arrhythmia.

ACTIONS

A 6-aminohexanoic acid that acts as an inhibitor of fibrinolysis. Inhibits plasminogen activator substances; to a lesser degree inhibits plasmin activity. Increases fibrinogen activity in clot formation by inhibiting the enzyme required for destruction of formed fibrin. Onset of action is prompt but will last less than 3 hours. Partially metabolized. Half-life is 2 hours. Excreted in urine. Easily penetrates RBCs and tissue cells after prolonged administration.

INDICATIONS AND USES

Useful in enhancing hemostasis when fibrinolysis contributes to bleeding. ▪ Treatment of fibrinolytic bleeding, which may be associated with surgical complications following heart surgery (with or without cardiac bypass procedures) and portacaval shunt, hematologic disorders such as aplastic anemia, acute and life-threatening abruptio placentae, hepatic cirrhosis, and neoplastic disease such as carcinoma of the prostate, lung, stomach, and cervix. ▪ Urinary fibrinolysis (normal physiologic phenomenon), which may result from severe trauma, anoxia, shock, surgical hematuria complications following prostatectomy and nephrectomy, or nonsurgical hematuria resulting from polycystic or neoplastic disease of the GU system.

Unlabeled uses: Prevent recurrence of subarachnoid hemorrhage. ▪ Control of bleeding in thrombocytopenia. ▪ Prevention of perioperative bleeding during cardiac surgery. ▪ Prophylaxis and treatment during dental surgical procedures (hemophilia and/or hemorrhage).

CONTRAINDICATIONS

Evidence of an active intravascular clotting process. ▪ Uncertainty as to whether the cause of bleeding is primary fibrinolysis (PF) or disseminated intravascular coagulation (DIC). This distinction must be made before administration; see Precautions. ▪ Do not use aminocaproic acid in the presence of DIC without concomitant heparin.

PRECAUTIONS

Should not be administered without a definite diagnosis and/or lab findings indicative of hyperfibrinolysis. ▪ The following tests are used to differentiate primary fibrinolysis (PF) from disseminated intravascular coagulation (DIC). Platelet count should be normal in PF but is usually decreased in DIC; protamine paracoagulation test is negative in PF and positive in DIC (a precipitate forms when protamine sulfate is dropped into citrated plasma); euglobulin clot lysis test is abnormal in PF but normal in DIC. ▪ In life-threatening situations, transfusion and other appropriate emergency measures may be required. ▪ Avoid use in patients with hematuria of upper urinary tract origin. Has caused glomerular capillary thrombosis in the renal pelvis and ureters, leading to intrarenal obstruction. ▪ Use with caution in patients with cardiac disease. May cause hypotension and bradycardia. Endocardial hemorrhage and fatty degeneration of the myocardium have been reported in animals. ▪ Use with caution in patients with hepatic disease. Etiology of bleeding may be multifactorial and difficult to diagnose. ▪ Use with caution in patients with renal impairment; see Dose Adjustments. Kidney stones have been reported in animal studies. ▪ Skeletal muscle weakness with necrosis of muscle fibers has been reported after prolonged use; see Monitor. ▪ An increased incidence of certain neurologic deficits (e.g., cerebral ischemia, cerebral vasospasm, hydrocephalus) associated with the use of antifibrinolytic agents in the treatment of subarachnoid hemorrhage has been reported. Relationship to drug therapy versus natural disease process or diagnostic procedures (e.g., angiography) is unclear.

Monitor: See Precautions and Contraindications. ▪ Use only in conjunction with general and specific tests to determine the amount of fibrinolysis present (e.g., fibrinogen, PT, aPTT). ▪ Monitor lab evaluations as appropriate for diagnosis (e.g., platelet count, clotting factors, CPK, AST). ▪ Vital signs, intake and output, any signs of bleeding, and neurologic assessment should be monitored based on patient condition. ▪ Observe for thromboembolic complications (e.g., chest pain, dyspnea, edema, hemoptysis, leg pain, or positive Homans' sign). ▪ Monitor for S/S of skeletal muscle damage. May range from mild myalgias with weakness to severe proximal myopathy with rhabdomyolysis, myoglobinuria, and acute renal failure. ▪ Monitor lab evaluations as appropriate for diagnosis (e.g., platelet count, clotting factors, CPK, AST).

Patient Education: Move slowly with help to avoid orthostatic hypotension.

Maternal/Child: Category C: safety for use in pregnancy and breast-feeding not established. ▪ Safety for use in pediatric patients not established but is used. ▪ Contains benzyl alcohol, which has been associated with "gasping syndrome" in neonates (sudden onset of gasping respirations, hypotension, bradycardia, and cardiovascular collapse).

Elderly: Consider age-related impaired organ function; reduced dose may be indicated.

DRUG/LAB INTERACTIONS

Potential for thrombus formation increased with concurrent use of **estrogens.** ▪ Frequently used with **clotting factor complexes** (e.g., factor IX complex, anti-inhibitor coagulant complex), but risk of thrombus formation may be increased. Delay administration for 8 or more hours after clotting factor complexes. ▪ Prolongation of template **bleeding time** has been reported during continuous infusions exceeding 24 Gm/day.

SIDE EFFECTS

Generally well tolerated. Abdominal pain, agranulocytosis, bradycardia, coagulation disorder, confusion, cramps, decreased vision, diarrhea, dizziness, dyspnea, edema, grand mal seizure, hallucinations, headache, hypersensitivity reactions (including anaphylaxis), hypotension, increased BUN and CPK, injection site reactions, intracranial hypertension, leukopenia, malaise, muscle weakness, myalgia, myopathy, myositis, nausea, peripheral ischemia, pruritus, pulmonary embolism, renal failure, rhabdomyolysis, rash, stuffy nose, stroke, syncope, tearing, thrombocytopenia, thrombophlebitis, thrombosis, tinnitus, or vomiting.

Overdose: Acute renal failure, convulsions, or death.

ANTIDOTE

Treat side effects symptomatically. Discontinue use of drug with any suspicion of thrombophlebitis, thromboembolic complications, or if CPK is elevated (myopathy). In life-threatening situations, fresh whole blood transfusions, fibrinogen infusions, and other emergency measures may be required. May be removed by hemodialysis or peritoneal dialysis.

AMINOPHYLLINE
(am-ih-**NOFF**-ih-lin)

Bronchodilator
Respiratory stimulant

pH 8.6 to 9

USUAL DOSE

To obtain maximum benefit with minimal risk of adverse effects, dosing must be individualized based on serum theophylline concentration and patient response. Monitor frequently to avoid toxicity. Only aminophylline premixed in solution or aminophylline containing 20 mg of theophylline for each 25 mg of aminophylline is intended for IV use (approximately 79% theophylline). *All doses are based on lean body weight;* theophylline does not distribute into fatty tissue. *All doses listed are milligrams of aminophylline to be administered.*

BRONCHODILATION IN ACUTE ASTHMA OR BRONCHOSPASM

With an average mean volume of distribution of 0.5 L/kg (range is 0.3 to 0.7 L/kg), each mg/kg of theophylline given over 30 minutes should result in an average 2 mcg/mL increase in serum theophylline concentration.

Adults, children, infants, and neonates who *have not* received a theophylline preparation in the previous 24 hours: An *initial loading dose* of 5 to 6 mg/kg of lean body weight (5.7 mg of aminophylline is equal to 4.6 mg/kg of theophylline) should produce a serum concentration of 10 mcg/mL (range 6 to 16 mcg/mL). Measure serum theophylline concentration in 30 minutes to determine if additional loading doses are indicated. Once a serum concentration of 10 to 15 mcg/mL is obtained with loading dose(s), it should be maintained with a continuous infusion. Rate of infusion is based on the pharmacokinetic parameters (e.g., volume of distribution, clearance, concomitant disease states) of the specific patient population and should achieve a target serum concentration of 10 mcg/mL. See Dose Adjustments and Monitor for recommendations of serum theophylline testing after an infusion is started.

Adults, children, infants, and neonates who *have* received a theophylline preparation in the previous 24 hours: *A serum theophylline concentration must be obtained before considering any loading dose.* For pediatric patients not receiving aminophylline or theophylline, give a loading dose of 5 to 7 mg/kg/dose. Maintenance dose is dependent on age. See the following chart for maintenance doses.

Once a serum concentration of 10 to 15 mcg/mL is obtained with or without loading dose(s), it should be maintained with a continuous infusion. Rate of infusion is based on the pharmacokinetic parameters (e.g., volume of distribution, clearance, concomitant disease states) of the specific patient population and should achieve a target serum concentration of 10 mcg/mL. See Dose Adjustments and Monitor for recommendations of serum theophylline testing after an infusion is started.

Maintenance infusion: Desired theophylline serum concentration is 10 mcg/mL. Most maintenance doses can be reduced within the first 12 hours based on serum theophylline levels and depending on patient condition and response; see Dose Adjustments. Because of a large interpatient variability in theophylline clearance, each patient may differ from the mean value used to calculate these infusion rates. Another serum concentration is recommended one expected half-life after starting the continuous infusion; see Dose Adjustments.

Aminophylline Infusion Rates Following an Appropriate Loading Dose	
Patient Population	**Aminophylline Infusion Rate in mg/kg/hr[a]** (Actual theophylline administered in mg/kg/hr is in parentheses)
Neonates up to 24 days of age	1.27 mg/kg *every 12 hours* (1 mg/kg *every 12 hours*)[b]
Neonates over 24 days of age	1.9 mg/kg *every 12 hours* (1.5 mg/kg *every 12 hours*)[b]
Infants 6 to 52 weeks of age	mg/kg/hr = [(0.008 × Age in weeks) + 0.21[c]] ÷ 0.79
Children 1 to 9 years	1 mg/kg/hr (0.8 mg/kg/hr)
Children 9 to 12 years	0.875 mg/kg/hr (0.7 mg/kg/hr)
Adolescent smokers 12 to 16 years	0.875 mg/kg/hr (0.7 mg/kg/hr)
Adolescent nonsmokers 12 to 16 years	0.625 mg/kg/hr (0.5 mg/kg/hr)[d]
Adults (healthy nonsmokers 16 to 60 years)	0.5 mg/kg/hr (0.4 mg/kg/hr)[d]
Elderly over 60 years	0.375 mg/kg/hr (0.3 mg/kg/hr)[e]
Cardiac decompensation, cor pulmonale, liver dysfunction, sepsis with multiorgan failure, or shock	0.25 mg/kg/hr (0.2 mg/kg/hr)[e]

[a]Lower initial dose may be required for patients receiving other drugs that decrease theophylline clearance (e.g., cimetidine [Tagamet]).
[b]To achieve a target concentration of 7.5 mcg/mL for neonatal apnea.
[c]The 0.21 factor was not adjusted from the theophylline formula because it may not have the same proportional value. See package insert or contact Abbott if additional information desired.
[d]Not to exceed 900 mg/day unless serum levels indicate need for a larger dose.
[e]Not to exceed 400 mg/day or 21 mg/hr (17 mg/hr as theophylline) unless serum levels indicate need for a larger dose.

Reverse Adenosine-Mediated Effects of Dipyridamole in Adults (Unlabeled)
50 to 100 mg over 30 to 60 seconds. Do not exceed a rate of 50 mg/30 sec. Maximum dose is 250 mg.

NEONATAL DOSE
Apnea and bradycardia of prematurity (unlabeled): *Loading dose:* 5 to 6 mg/kg given over 20 to 30 minutes. See all criteria under Usual Dose.

Maintenance dose: See Maintenance Infusion under Usual Dose. Manufacturer recommends keeping serum theophylline level at 7.5 mcg/mL. Another source recommends 1 to 2 mg/kg/dose every 6 to 8 hours.

DOSE ADJUSTMENTS
To determine if the concentration is accumulating or declining from the post–loading dose level, a serum concentration is recommended one expected half-life after starting the continuous infusion; see the following chart or see literature for a complete summary. If the level is declining (higher than average clearance), consider an additional loading dose or increasing the infusion rate. If the level is increasing, assume accumulation and decrease the infusion rate before the level exceeds 20 mcg/mL.

There are huge variances in patients with concurrent illness or altered physiologic states (e.g., acute pulmonary edema, COPD, cystic fibrosis, fever with acute viral respiratory illness in pediatric patients [9 to 15 years], liver disease, pregnancy, sepsis with multiorgan failure, thyroid disease); see package insert. ■ In patients with cor pulmonale, cardiac decompensation, liver dysfunction, or in those taking drugs that markedly reduce theophylline clearance (e.g., cimetidine), the initial aminophylline infusion rate should not exceed 21 mg/hr (17 mg/hr as theophylline) unless serum concentrations can be monitored every 24 hours. Up to 5 days may be required before steady state is reached in these patients; see Drug Interactions. ▪ To decrease the risk of side effects associated with unexpected large increases in serum theophylline concentration, dose adjustment recommendations should be considered as the upper limit.

Final Dose Adjustment Guided by Serum Theophylline Concentration[a]	
Peak Serum Concentration	**Dose Adjustment**
Less than 9.9 mcg/mL	If symptoms are not controlled and current dose is tolerated, increase infusion rate about 25%. Recheck serum concentration after 12 hours in pediatric patients and 24 hours in adults for further dose adjustment.
10 to 14.9 mcg/mL	If symptoms are controlled and current dose is tolerated, maintain infusion rate and recheck serum concentration at 24-hour intervals. If symptoms are not controlled and current dose is tolerated, consider adding additional medication(s) to treatment regimen.
15 to 19.9 mcg/mL	Consider 10% decrease in infusion rate to provide greater margin of safety, even if current dose is tolerated.[b]
20 to 24.9 mcg/mL	Decrease infusion rate by 25%, even if no side effects are present. Recheck serum concentration after 12 hours in pediatric patients and 24 hours in adults to guide further dose adjustment.
25 to 30 mcg/mL	Stop infusion for 12 hours in pediatric patients and 24 hours in adults and decrease subsequent infusion rate at least 25% even if no side effects are present. Recheck serum concentration after 12 hours in pediatric patients and 24 hours in adults to guide further dose adjustment. If symptomatic, stop infusion and consider need for overdose treatment; see Antidote.
Over 30 mcg/mL	Stop the infusion and treat overdose as indicated; see Antidote. If aminophylline is subsequently resumed, decrease infusion rate by at least 50% and recheck serum concentration after 12 hours in pediatric patients and 24 hours in adults to guide further dose adjustment.

[a]Dose increases should not be made in patients with an acute exacerbation of symptoms unless the steady-state serum theophylline concentration is less than 10 mcg/mL.

[b]Dose reduction and/or serum theophylline concentration measurement is indicated whenever side effects are present, physiologic abnormalities that can reduce theophylline clearance occur (e.g., sustained fever), or a drug that interacts with theophylline is added or discontinued; see Precautions and Drug/Lab Interactions.

DILUTION

Check vial carefully; must state, "For IV use." Warm to room temperature. Only the 25 mg/mL solution may be given by IV injection undiluted, but further dilution for infusion in at least 100 to 200 mL of D5W is preferred. NS or dextrose in saline solutions may be used. Available prediluted. Crystals will form if solution pH falls below 8.

Storage: Usually stored between 15° and 30° C (59° and 86° F). Protect from light and freezing.

COMPATIBILITY

Manufacturer states, "Should not be mixed in a syringe with other drugs but should be added separately to the IV solution," and recommends discontinuing other solutions infusing at the same site if there is a potential problem with admixture **incompatibility.** Manufacturer recommends avoiding admixtures with alkali labile drugs (e.g., epinephrine, norepinephrine, isoproterenol, penicillin G potassium). Precipitation in acidic media may occur with the undiluted solution but not to dilute solutions in IV infusions.

Other sources suggest specific **compatibilities** dependent on concentration and manufacturer; consult a pharmacist.

RATE OF ADMINISTRATION

A single dose over a minimum of 20 to 30 minutes. Most references suggest a minimum of 30 minutes. Do not exceed an average rate of 1 mL or 25 mg/min when giving by IV injection or as an infusion. Rapid administration may cause cardiac arrhythmias.

Discontinue primary infusion if theophylline administered by piggyback or additive tubing and a possible **incompatibility** problem exists.

Reverse adenosine-mediated effects of dipyridamole: See Usual Dose.

ACTIONS

An alkaloid xanthine derivative. It relaxes smooth muscle in the airways (bronchodilation) and suppresses the response of the airways to stimuli (nonbronchodilator prophylactic effects). Cardiac output, urinary output, and sodium excretion are increased. Skeletal and cardiac muscles are stimulated, as is the CNS to a lesser degree. There is peripheral vasodilation. It decreases pulmonary artery pressure and lowers the threshold of the respiratory center to CO_2. Well distributed throughout the body. In adults and pediatric patients over 1 year of age, 90% of a dose is metabolized in the liver. Because of a large interpatient variability in theophylline clearance, half-life varies extensively based on age, concurrent illness, or altered physiologic state; see Dose Adjustments, Precautions, Maternal/Child, and Elderly. Excreted in a changed form in the urine. Crosses the placental barrier. Secreted in breast milk.

INDICATIONS AND USES

Adjunct to inhaled beta-2 selective agonists (e.g., albuterol) and systemic corticosteroids for the treatment of acute exacerbations of the symptoms and reversible airflow obstruction associated with asthma and other chronic lung diseases (e.g., emphysema, chronic bronchitis). **Unlabeled uses:** Apnea and bradycardia of prematurity. ▪ Reduce bronchospasm in cystic fibrosis and acute descending respiratory infections. ▪ Relieve periodic apnea and increase arterial blood pH in patients with Cheyne-Stokes respirations. ▪ Reverse adenosine-mediated effects of dipyridamole- (Persantine), adenosine- (Adenoscan), or regadenoson- (Lexiscan) induced adverse reactions (e.g., angina pectoris, bronchospasm, severe hypotension, ventricular arrhythmias).

CONTRAINDICATIONS

Known hypersensitivity to theophylline or ethylenediamine.

PRECAUTIONS

Theophylline clearance may be reduced in neonates (term and premature); children less than 1 year; elderly (over 60 years); infants less than 3 months of age with reduced renal function; patients with acute pulmonary edema, congestive heart failure, cor pulmonale, hypothyroidism, liver disease (e.g., cirrhosis, acute hepatitis), sepsis with multiorgan failure, shock; or in patients with a fever of 102° F or more for 24 hours or more, or lesser temperature elevations for longer periods. Risk of severe toxicity increased in these patient populations; dose reduction and more frequent monitoring may be required. ▪ Use with extreme caution in patients with active peptic ulcer disease, cardiac arrhythmias (not including bradyarrhythmias), or seizures; may exacerbate these conditions. ▪ Initiate oral therapy as soon as symptoms are adequately improved. ▪ See Maternal/Child and Drug/Lab Interactions.

Monitor: Monitor serum levels as directed in Usual Dose and Dose Adjustments to achieve maximum benefit with minimum risk. Each 0.5 mg/kg will increase serum theophylline by 1 mcg/mL. 10 mcg/mL to less than 20 mcg/mL is considered therapeutic. Peak serum level is best measured 20 to 30 minutes after initial loading dose, a half-life after the initial infusion, or 12 to 14 hours into continuous infusion. ▪ Monitor vital signs, including lung sounds. ▪ Monitor for all signs of toxicity; see Side Effects. Serious toxicity may not be preceded by less severe side effects. ▪ Serum theophylline measurements are indicated before making a dose increase; whenever signs or symptoms of toxicity are present; whenever a new illness presents, an existing illness worsens, or a change in treatment regimen is initiated that may alter theophylline clearance (e.g., sustained fever, hepatitis [see Precautions], or drugs that may interact [see Drug/Lab Interactions]); and every 24 hours throughout the infusion. ▪ Stop the IV infusion and obtain a serum theophylline concentration immediately in any patient on aminophylline who develops nausea or vomiting (particularly repetitive vomiting) or if any other signs of toxicity occur, even if another cause is suspected. ▪ Dose increases should not be made in patients with an acute exacerbation of symptoms unless the steady-state serum theophylline concentration is less than

10 mcg/mL. ▪ Patients with a very high initial clearance rate (low steady-state serum theophylline concentrations at above-average doses) are likely to experience large changes in serum concentration in response to dose changes. ▪ Maintain hydration. ▪ See Precautions, Maternal/Child, Elderly, and Drug/Lab Interactions.

Patient Education: Do not take or discontinue any prescription or over-the-counter medication, including herbal products, without physician's approval. ▪ Promptly report S/S of toxicity (e.g., nausea and vomiting).

Maternal/Child: Category C: use in pregnancy only if clearly indicated. ▪ Neonates may have therapeutic blood levels and may develop apnea from theophylline withdrawal. ▪ Elimination of drug is prolonged in premature infants, neonates, and children up to 1 year. Use with extreme caution in pediatric patients. Has caused fatal reactions. Elimination reaches maximum values by 1 year of age, remains fairly constant to 9 years of age, and slowly decreases by approximately 50% to adult values at 16 years of age. ▪ Pediatric patients under the age of 1 year, as well as neonates with decreased renal function, require careful attention to dosing and frequent monitoring of serum theophylline concentrations. ▪ Secreted in breast milk; some sources recommend discontinuing breast-feeding. If the decision is made to breast-feed, monitor infant for evidence of side effects.

Elderly: Compared to healthy young adults, clearance of theophylline is decreased an average of 30% in healthy elderly. Monitor dosing carefully; frequent serum theophylline concentrations are recommended. See Dose Adjustments, Precautions, and Monitor.

DRUG/LAB INTERACTIONS

Review of patient drug profile by pharmacist is imperative at time of initiation of aminophylline and with any change in medication regimen. ▪ Do not use one **xanthine derivative** concurrently with another **xanthine derivative, ephedrine, or other sympathomimetic drugs.** ▪ Xanthines antagonize or potentiate or are themselves antagonized or potentiated by many drug groups. Monitor serum levels as indicated. **Theophylline clearance increased and serum levels decreased by aminoglutenide, barbiturates, carbamazepine, isoproterenol, phenytoin, rifampin, smoking, and sulfinpyrazone. Theophylline clearance decreased and serum levels increased by alcohol, allopurinol, beta-adrenergic blockers, cimetidine, ciprofloxacin, clarithromycin, disulfiram, erythromycin, estrogen-containing oral contraceptives, fluvoxamine, interferon alfa-A, methotrexate, mexiletine, pentoxifylline, propafenone, tacrine, thiabendazole, and verapamil.** ▪ Inhibits **pancuronium;** increased doses of pancuronium may be required to achieve neuromuscular blockade. ▪ **Carbamazepine and loop diuretics** (e.g., furosemide) may increase or decrease serum levels. ▪ Reduces sedative effect of **benzodiazepines** (e.g., diazepam, midazolam) **and of propofol**; increased doses of sedatives may be required. To avoid respiratory depression, reduce sedative dose if aminophylline is discontinued or if dose is significantly reduced. ▪ May decrease **lithium** levels. Dose adjustment and monitoring of lithium levels may be indicated. ▪ Concurrent use with **ketamine** may lower aminophylline seizure level. ▪ Concurrent use with **ephedrine** may increase nausea, nervousness, and insomnia. ▪ May increase **lab values** for free fatty acids, glucose, HDL, LDL, total cholesterol, uric acid, and urinary free cortisol excretion. ▪ Caffeine and xanthine metabolites in neonates or patients with renal dysfunction may cause readings from some **immunoassay techniques** to be higher than the actual serum theophylline concentration. ▪ Interferes with **dipyridamole-assisted MI perfusion studies.**

SIDE EFFECTS

Headache, insomnia, nausea, and vomiting most common when peak serum concentrations are less than 20 mcg/mL. Rarely a severe hypersensitivity reaction of the skin (e.g., exfoliative dermatitis) may occur. Toxicity resulting in death may occur suddenly at levels less than 20 mcg/mL, especially in certain populations (see Precautions); may occur more frequently with serum levels above 20 mcg/mL. Anxiety, arrhythmias (e.g., atrial fibrillation, ventricular fibrillation), cardiac arrest, convulsions, delirium, dizziness, flushing, hyperpyrexia, intractable seizures, nausea, peripheral vascular collapse, persistent vomiting, restlessness, temporary hypotension.

Overdose: *Acute:* Acid/base disturbances, arrhythmias (e.g., sinus tachycardia), hyperglycemia, hypokalemia, seizures (usually with serum concentrations over 100 mcg/mL), vomiting, and death have occurred.

Chronic: All of the above plus various arrhythmias, seizures (with serum concentration greater than 30 mcg/mL), and death.

ANTIDOTE

With onset of any side effect, discontinue drug and notify physician. ■ Stop the IV infusion and obtain a serum theophylline concentration immediately in any patient on aminophylline who develops nausea or vomiting (particularly repetitive vomiting) or if any other signs of toxicity occur, even if another cause is suspected. ■ For mild symptoms the physician may choose to continue the drug at a decreased dose and rate of administration. All side effects will be treated symptomatically. Maintain adequate ventilation and adequate hydration. Grand mal seizures may not respond to anticonvulsants. Diazepam may be most effective. Treat atrial arrhythmias with verapamil, and ventricular arrhythmias with lidocaine or procainamide. Use dopamine for hypotension. Do not use stimulants. Resuscitate as necessary.

MANUFACTURER'S SPECIFIC RECOMMENDATIONS FOR ACUTE AND CHRONIC OVERDOSE

Acute overdose (e.g., excessive loading dose or excessive infusion rate for less than 24 hours) or chronic overdose (e.g., excessive infusion rate for more than 24 hours): Serum concentration 20 to 30 mcg/mL:
Stop the infusion, monitor the patient, and obtain a serum theophylline concentration in 2 to 4 hours to ensure that the concentration is decreasing.

Acute overdose with a serum concentration of 30 to 100 mcg/mL or chronic overdose with serum concentrations greater than 30 mcg/mL in patients less than 60 years of age:
Stop the infusion. Administer multiple-dose, oral-activated charcoal and measures to control emesis. Monitor the patient and obtain serial theophylline concentrations every 2 to 4 hours to determine the effectiveness of therapy and to determine further treatment decisions. Institute extracorporeal removal if emesis, seizures, or cardiac arrhythmias cannot be adequately controlled.

Acute overdose with a serum concentration greater than 100 mcg/mL or chronic overdose with serum concentrations greater than 30 mcg/mL in patients 60 years or older:
Stop the infusion. Consider prophylactic anticonvulsant therapy. Administer multiple-dose oral-activated charcoal and measures to control emesis. Consider extracorporeal removal, even if the patient has not experienced a seizure. Monitor the patient and obtain serial theophylline concentrations every 2 to 4 hours to determine the effectiveness of therapy and to determine further treatment decisions.

Extracorporeal removal:
Weigh risk versus benefits. Charcoal hemoperfusion is the most effective and increases theophylline clearance up to sixfold, but hypotension, hypocalcemia, and platelet consumption and bleeding diatheses may occur. Hemodialysis is about as efficient as multiple-dose oral-activated charcoal and has a lower risk of serious complications. Consider hemodialysis when charcoal hemoperfusion is not feasible and multiple-dose oral-activated charcoal is ineffective because of intractable emesis. Serum theophylline concentrations may rebound 5 to 10 mcg/mL after either treatment is discontinued due to redistribution of theophylline from the tissue compartment. Peritoneal dialysis is ineffective, and exchange transfusions in neonates have been minimally effective.

AMIODARONE HYDROCHLORIDE

Antiarrhythmic

(am-ee-**OH**-dah-rohn hy-droh-**KLOR**-eyed)

Nexterone, Pacerone

pH 4.08

USUAL DOSE

Pretreatment: See Maternal/Child.

TREATMENT AND PROPHYLAXIS OF VENTRICULAR TACHYCARDIA (VT) AND VENTRICULAR FIBRILLATION (VF)

1,000 mg over the first 24 hours in 3 distinct segments; two loading infusions and a maintenance infusion. Use of a dedicated central venous catheter preferred.

Rapid loading infusion: 150 mg specifically diluted solution (1.5 mg/mL) over 10 minutes (15 mg/min). Follow immediately with the slow-loading infusion.

Slow loading infusion: 360 mg specifically diluted solution (1.8 mg/mL) at 1 mg/min over the next 6 hours.

Maintenance infusion: 540 mg of 1.8 mg/mL solution at 0.5 mg/min over 18 hours. Maintenance infusion is usually continued at 0.5 mg/min for 48 to 96 hours or until ventricular arrhythmias are stabilized; see Dose Adjustments. Transfer to oral therapy as soon as feasible (guidelines are in package insert).

TREATMENT OF BREAKTHROUGH VENTRICULAR FIBRILLATION (VF) OR HEMODYNAMICALLY UNSTABLE VENTRICULAR TACHYCARDIA (VT)

At any time that breakthrough VF or hemodynamically unstable VT occurs during administration, a supplemental rapid loading infusion (150 mg over 10 minutes) may be repeated. May be specifically diluted 1.5 mg/mL solution or rate of the maintenance infusion (1.8 mg/mL) may be temporarily increased to equal 150 mg (83.33 mL) over 10 minutes. In life-threatening arrhythmias, AHA guidelines state that this rapid loading infusion (150 mg over 10 minutes) may be repeated every 10 minutes as needed and recommend a maximum cumulative dose of 2.2 Gm/24 hr.

CARDIAC ARREST (UNLABELED)

300 mg (6 mL) or 5 mg/kg as a bolus injection. Flush with 10 mL D5W or NS. Should be given through a separate IV line immediately after the first dose of epinephrine (1 mg) and before the fourth electrical countershock. Supplemental doses of 150 mg (3 mL) may be given for recurrent bouts of VT/VF. AHA guidelines recommend a first dose of 300 mg IV push and a second dose, if needed, of 150 mg IV push.

SUPRAVENTRICULAR ARRHYTHMIAS (UNLABELED)

150 mg over 10 minutes as a loading dose (15 mg/min). Follow with an infusion of 360 mg over 6 hours (1 mg/min) followed by a maintenance infusion of 0.5 mg/min for 18 hours.

INTRAVENOUS TO ORAL TRANSITION

Guidelines for IV to oral transition are located in manufacturer's literature. See Prescribing Information or consult pharmacist.

PEDIATRIC DOSE

Safety for use in pediatric patients (particularly infants and neonates) not established and not recommended; see Maternal/Child.

Treatment of refractory pulseless VT, VF (unlabeled): AHA guidelines recommend 5 mg/kg by IV bolus (maximum single dose is 300 mg). May repeat to a maximum of 15 mg/kg/24 hr. Total dose in adolescents is 2.2 Gm/24 hr.

Treatment of perfusing supraventricular and ventricular arrhythmias (unlabeled): AHA guidelines recommend 5 mg/kg as an infusion over 20 to 60 minutes (maximum single dose 300 mg). May repeat to a maximum of 15 mg/kg/24 hr. Total dose in adolescents is 2.2 Gm/24 hr.

DOSE ADJUSTMENTS

The first 24-hour dose may be individualized for each patient; however, in controlled clinical trials mean daily doses above 2,100 mg were associated with an increased risk of hypotension. Do not exceed an initial infusion rate of 30 mg/min. ▪ Rate of maintenance infusion may be increased to achieve effective arrhythmia suppression. ▪ Based on experience from clinical studies, a maintenance infusion of up to 0.5 mg/min can be continued for 2 to 3 weeks regardless of the patient's age, renal function, or left ventricular function. ▪ One source suggests a reduced dose in hepatic failure. ▪ Dose selection should be cautious in the elderly. Reduced initial doses may be indicated based on the potential for decreased organ function and concomitant disease or drug therapy.

DILUTION

Available as a premixed solution in 1.5 mg/mL and 1.8 mg/mL concentrations or as a vial that must be further diluted. To further dilute vials, do not use evacuated glass intravenous bottles. Use only commercially available D5W solutions in polyolefin or glass containers in any prepared solution that will be given over more than 2 hours. PVC containers are suitable only for dilution of the rapid loading dose; see Compatibility and Precautions.

Rapid-loading infusion: Dilute 150 mg (3 mL) in 100 mL D5W; concentration is 1.5 mg/mL.

Slow-loading infusion and maintenance infusion: Dilute 900 mg (18 mL) in 500 mL D5W; concentration is 1.8 mg/mL. Dilutions from 1 to 6 mg/mL have been used for maintenance solutions after the first 24 hours. Use of a central venous catheter is recommended; however, concentrations over 2 mg/mL for longer than 1 hour must be administered through a central venous catheter. Higher concentrations (3 to 6 mg/mL) have caused peripheral vein phlebitis and hepatocellular necrosis; see Precautions.

Cardiac arrest (unlabeled): Loading dose (300 mg or 5 mg/kg) or supplemental boluses (150 mg) may be given undiluted.

Filters: Use of a 0.2-micron in-line filter recommended by manufacturer. States "filtering does not affect potency." Another source suggests no significant loss of drug potency with the use of a 0.22-micron cellulose ester membrane filter.

Storage: Store ampules and premixed solutions in their carton at CRT. Use solutions diluted in PVC containers within 2 hours; use those diluted in glass or polyolefin containers within 24 hours. Protect from light and freezing.

COMPATIBILITY

Manufacturer recommendations include: Do not use evacuated glass intravenous bottles. Administer through a dedicated IV line (central venous catheter preferred). Absorbs to PVC tubing but loss accounted for in specified dose; follow infusion regimen closely. Leaches out plasticizers, including DEHP, from IV tubing. The degree of leaching increases when the solution is infused at a higher concentration or a slower infusion rate than recommended. Manufacturer lists aminophylline, argatroban, bivalirudin, cefazolin, ceftazidime, digoxin, furosemide, heparin, imipenem-cilastatin, magnesium sulfate, nitroprusside sodium, piperacillin/tazobactam, potassium phosphates, sodium bicarbonate, and sodium phosphates as **incompatible** at the **Y-site** with amiodarone in D5W. Aminophylline, ampicillin/sulbactam, and micafungin in NS are also listed as **incompatible** at the **Y-site**.

Other sources suggest specific **compatibilities** dependent on concentration and manufacturer; consult a pharmacist.

RATE OF ADMINISTRATION

Volumetric pump required for administration. Surface properties of diluted solution reduce drop size; use of a drop counter infusion set causes underdosing. Use of a 0.2-micron in-line filter is also recommended. A central venous catheter is recommended for all concentrations and is required for concentrations greater than 2 mg/mL. Adhere to prescribed rates; risk of hypotension is increased in the first hours of treatment and with increased rates; may cause secondary renal or hepatic failure; see Precautions. Do not use plastic containers in a series; could result in air embolism.

Rapid-loading infusion or breakthrough treatment of VF/VT: 150 mg over 10 minutes (15 mg/min). Do not exceed a rate of 30 mg/min.

Slow-loading infusion: 1 mg/min or 33.3 mL/hr (0.556 mL/min) of 1.8 mg/mL solution for 6 hours.

Maintenance infusion: 0.5 mg/min or 16.6 mL/hr (0.278 mL/min) of 1.8 mg/mL solution for 18 hours. A continuing maintenance solution should deliver 720 mg/24 hr at 0.5 mg/min whether the concentration is 1.8 mg/mL or 6 mg/mL. May be continued at this rate for up to 2 to 3 weeks as described in Usual Dose.

Cardiac arrest (unlabeled): Loading or supplemental doses by IV bolus injection. Follow with 10 mL flush of D5W or NS through Y-tube or three-way stopcock. May be given through a free-flowing infusion of D5W (D5W or NS may be used for Nexterone). After return of spontaneous circulation (ROSC), initiate the slow loading and maintenance infusions as above.

ACTIONS

An antiarrhythmic agent. Generally considered a Class III antiarrhythmic drug, but possesses characteristics of all four antiarrhythmic classes. Decreases number of VT/VF events. It prolongs the duration of action potentials, depresses conduction velocity, slows conduction and prolongs refractoriness at the AV node, and exhibits some alpha and beta blockade activity. Raises the threshold for VF and may prevent its recurrence. Also has vasodilatory effects that decrease cardiac workload and myocardial oxygen consumption. Uptake by the myocardium is rapid; antiarrhythmic effect is prompt (clinically relevant within hours); however, full effect may take days. Has an exceptionally long half-life. Highly protein bound. Metabolized in the liver by cytochrome P_{450} enzymes (specifically CYP3A4 and CYP2C8). Terminal elimination half-life after a single IV dose ranged from 9 to 36 days. Primarily excreted in bile. Crosses placental barrier. Secreted in breast milk.

INDICATIONS AND USES

Initiation of treatment and prophylaxis of frequently recurring VF and hemodynamically unstable VT in patients refractory to other therapy. Used until ventricular arrhythmias are stabilized; usually 48 to 96 hours, but may be given for longer periods. ▪ Treatment of patients taking oral amiodarone who are unable to take oral medication.

Unlabeled uses: Conversion of atrial fibrillation to a normal sinus rhythm and maintenance of a normal sinus rhythm. ▪ Cardiac arrest with persistent VT or VF if defibrillation, CPR, and vasopressor administration have failed. ▪ Control of hemodynamically stable monomorphic VT, polymorphic VT with a normal baseline QT interval, or wide-complex tachycardia of uncertain origin. ▪ Control of rapid ventricular rate due to accessory pathway conduction in pre-excited atrial arrhythmias. ▪ Heart rate control in patients with atrial fibrillation and heart failure with no accessory pathway. ▪ Pharmacologic adjunct to ICD (implantable cardioverter defibrillator) therapy to suppress symptomatic ventricular tachyarrhythmias in otherwise optimally treated patients with heart failure.

CONTRAINDICATIONS

Cardiogenic shock; corneal refractive laser surgery; known hypersensitivity to amiodarone or any of its components, including iodine; marked sinus bradycardia; second- or third-degree AV block unless a functioning pacemaker is available; sinus node dysfunction. See Drug/Lab Interactions.

PRECAUTIONS

Usually administered by or under the direction of the physician specialist with facilities for monitoring the patient and responding to any medical emergency. ▪ Because of the long half-life of amiodarone and its metabolite, the potential for adverse reactions or interactions, as well as observed adverse effects, can persist following amiodarone withdrawal. ▪ May cause increases in liver enzymes and bilirubin levels. However, in the majority of patients, liver enzyme elevations either improved during therapy or remained at baseline levels. Abnormal baseline hepatic enzymes are not a contraindication to use. ▪ Use of higher than recommended loading dose concentrations and increased rates of administration have been associated with hepatocellular necrosis, hepatic coma, acute renal failure, and death. ■ May worsen existing arrhythmias or precipitate new ones, primarily torsades de pointes or new-onset VF. Deaths have occurred. ■ Correct hypokalemia, hypomagnesemia, and hypocalcemia before use; may exaggerate a prolonged QTc and cause arrhythmias (e.g., torsades de pointes). ■ Combination of amiodarone with other antiarrhythmics that can prolong the QTc interval should be reserved for patients with life-threatening ventricular arrhythmias who do not respond to single agent therapy; see Drug/Lab Interactions. ■ Risk of QTc prolongation is increased with other medications that can prolong the QTc; see Drug/Lab Interactions. ■ Hypotension is the most common side effect. Usually occurs within the first several hours of therapy and appears to be rate-related. Do not exceed initial rates recommended by manufacturer. In some cases, hypotension has been refractory to treatment. Deaths have occurred. See Monitor and Antidote. ■ Drug-related bradycardia that is not dose related can occur. Patients with a predisposition to bradycardia or AV block should be treated with amiodarone in a setting in which a temporary pacemaker is available. ■ May cause visual impairment (e.g., optic neuropathy or optic neuritis); has progressed to permanent blindness. ■ May cause pulmonary toxicity (e.g., ARDS, bronchospasm, cough, dyspnea, hemoptysis, hypoxemia, pulmonary fibrosis, wheezing). Usually seen with long-term oral use, but acute pulmonary toxicity has been reported after IV use. Has progressed to respiratory failure and death. Patients with pre-existing lung disease may be at increased risk. ■ Monitor patients undergoing general anesthesia closely; may increase sensitivity to myocardial depressant and conduction defects of halogenated inhalation anesthetics (hypotension). ■ Use caution in patients with cardiomyopathy, hepatic failure, left ventricular dysfunction, or thyroid dysfunction. ■ May cause hypothyroidism or hyperthyroidism. Amiodarone-induced hyperthyroidism may result in thyrotoxicosis and/or the possibility of arrhythmia breakthrough or aggravation. Deaths have occurred. Severe hypothyroidism and myxedema coma, sometimes fatal, have been reported. ■ Thyroid nodules and/or thyroid cancer have been reported in patients treated with amiodarone. ■ Anaphylactic/anaphylactoid reactions, some fatal, have been reported. ■ See Compatibility and Drug/Lab Interactions.

Monitor: Continuous ECG and HR monitoring is mandatory to observe for arrhythmias. Watch for QTc prolongation; may worsen existing arrhythmia or precipitate a new arrhythmia, including torsades de pointes. Consider the possibility of hyperthyroidism if new signs of arrhythmia appear. ■ Monitor for bradycardia and AV block. ■ Monitor BP closely to minimize hypotension (occurs frequently with initial rates); see Rate of Administration, Precautions, and Antidote. ■ Confirm patency of vein. Incidence of phlebitis markedly increased with concentrations above 2.5 mg/mL. For infusions longer than 1 hour, do not exceed a concentration of 2 mg/mL unless a central venous line is used. ■ Monitor serum electrolytes and acid-base balance, especially in patients with prolonged diarrhea and those receiving diuretics. ■ Monitor liver enzymes (AST, ALT, GGT) and bilirubin for elevations indicating progressive injury. ■ Monitor pulmonary status (e.g., FiO_2, SaO_2, PaO_2, chest x-ray); baseline pulmonary function tests recommended; repeat as indicated. ■ Monitor thyroid function tests before treatment and periodically thereafter. Patients with a history of thyroid nodules, goiter, or other thyroid dysfunction and the elderly should be monitored closely. Amiodarone is eliminated slowly, and abnormal function tests may persist for weeks or months after it is discontinued. ■ Regular ophthalmic exams, including funduscopy and slit lamp exams, are recommended. Prompt ophthalmic exams recommended at first sign of visual impairment. May require discontinuation of amiodarone therapy. ■ Monitor for S/S of anaphylaxis/anaphylactoid reactions (e.g., cardiac arrest, cold sweat, cyanosis, flushing, hyperhidrosis, hypotension, hypoxia, rash, shock, tachycardia). ■ See Precautions and Drug/Lab Interactions.

Patient Education: Most manufacturers of corneal refractive laser surgery devices contraindicate this procedure in patients receiving amiodarone. ■ Report promptly any feelings of faintness, difficulty breathing, or pain or stinging along injection site. Review side effect profile, including S/S of hypothyroidism or hyperthyroidism. ■ Effective birth control recommended. ▪ Numerous drug interactions. Review all medications, including OTC medications, with physician or pharmacist. ▪ Avoid grapefruit juice if transitioned to oral amiodarone.

Maternal/Child: Category D: can cause fetal harm; avoid pregnancy or use only if benefit to mother justifies risk to fetus. Fetal exposure may increase potential for adverse experiences, including cardiac, thyroid, neurodevelopmental, neurologic, and growth effects in neonates. ▪ Discontinue breast-feeding. ▪ Safety for use during labor and delivery not established. ▪ Safety and effectiveness for use in pediatric patients not established. Use in pediatric patients is not recommended by the manufacturer. ▪ Vials contain benzyl alcohol, which has been associated with "gasping syndrome" in neonates (sudden onset of gasping respirations, hypotension, bradycardia, and cardiovascular collapse).

Elderly: Differences in response between the elderly and younger patients have not been identified; however, clearance is slower and half-life may be doubled (up to 47 days). See Dose Adjustments.

DRUG/LAB INTERACTIONS

Amiodarone has a long half-life; drug interactions may persist long after it is discontinued. *Contraindicated with nelfinavir and ritonavir.* Should not be given concurrently with **ibutilide.** ▪ Concurrent use with other **antiarrhythmic agents** (e.g., flecainide, procainamide, quinidine) increases their serum concentrations and may result in additive increases in QT prolongation and serious arrhythmias. Manufacturer recommends reducing the dose of previously given antiarrhythmic agents by 30% to 50% several days after starting amiodarone and then evaluating the need for continued therapy with the other antiarrhythmic agent after the effects of amiodarone have been established. Monitor serum levels if possible. ▪ QT prolongation has been reported with concomitant administration of amiodarone and **fluoroquinolones, halogenated inhalation anesthetic agents, macrolide antibiotics, azole antifungals, lithium, loratadine, phenothiazines** (e.g., prochlorperazine, promethazine), **trazodone, tricyclic antidepressants, and grapefruit juice (oral therapy);** see Precautions. ▪ May decrease metabolism and increase serum levels of **digoxin.** Reduce digoxin dose by 50% or withdraw completely when amiodarone therapy is initiated. ▪ Use with **potassium-depleting diuretics** may lead to increased risk of arrhythmias due to hypokalemia. ▪ Inhibits metabolism and increases anticoagulant effect (e.g., increased PT and INR) of **warfarin.** Dose reduction of the anticoagulant and careful monitoring of PT or INR recommended. Effects may persist long after amiodarone is discontinued. ▪ Coadministration with dabigatran may result in an elevated serum concentration of dabigatran. ▪ May decrease metabolism and increase serum levels of **flecainide, phenytoin, lidocaine, procainamide, quinidine, and theophylline** (aminophylline). May cause toxicity; monitor serum levels. Reduced doses indicated. ▪ May decrease metabolism and increase serum levels of **cyclosporine.** Monitor cyclosporine levels and renal function. ▪ May increase serum concentration of **methotrexate.** Monitor levels and for S/S of toxicity. ▪ Concomitant use with **HMG-CoA reductase inhibitors** that are CYP3A4 substrates (e.g., lovastatin, simvastatin) has been associated with myopathy/rhabdomyolysis. In patients taking amiodarone, limit the dose of lovastatin to 40 mg daily and limit the dose of simvastatin to 20 mg daily. Lower starting and maintenance doses of other CYP3A4 substrates (e.g., atorvastatin) may also be required. ▪ Amiodarone clearance increased and plasma levels decreased with **cholestyramine, phenytoin, rifampin, and St. John's wort.** ▪ **Cimetidine and protease inhibitors** (e.g., indinavir) may decrease clearance and increase plasma levels of amiodarone. ▪ Concomitant use of **drugs with depressant effects on the sinus and AV node** (e.g., beta-blockers, calcium channel blockers) can potentiate the electrophysiologic and hemodynamic effects of amiodarone, resulting in bradycardia, sinus arrest, and AV block. Monitoring of heart rate required. ▪ May inhibit conversion of **clopidogrel** to its active metabolite, resulting in ineffective inhibition of platelet aggregation. ▪ May inhibit conversion of the prodrug **cyclophosphamide** to its active metabolite. ▪ Monitor patients undergoing **general anesthesia** closely. May increase sensitivity to myocardial depressant and conduction defects of **halogenated inhalation anesthetics.** ▪ PO use for longer than 2 weeks may decrease metabolism and increase serum levels of **dextromethorphan**. ▪ Serious symptomatic bradycardia has occurred with coadministration with **ledipasvir/sofosbuvir** (Harvoni) or with **sofosbuvir** (Sovaldi). Mechanism unknown. Monitor heart rate in patients taking or recently discontinuing amiodarone when starting antiviral treatment. ▪ See Precautions.

SIDE EFFECTS

The most important adverse reactions are asystole/cardiac arrest/pulseless electrical activity, AV block, bradycardia, cardiogenic shock, CHF, hypotension, liver function abnormalities, torsades de pointes, and VT. The most common adverse reactions leading to discontinuation of IV amiodarone therapy are asystole/cardiac arrest/pulseless electrical activity, cardiogenic shock, hypotension, and VT. Other adverse reactions that have been reported include abnormal kidney function, atrial fibrillation, atrioventricular block, diarrhea, increased ALT and AST, lung edema, nodal arrhythmia, prolonged QT interval, respiratory disorder, shock, sinus bradycardia, Stevens-Johnson syndrome, thrombocytopenia, VF, and vomiting.

Post-Marketing: Anemia (aplastic and/or hemolytic), ARDS, confusion, cough, delirium, disorientation, dizziness, dyspnea, erythema multiforme, exfoliative dermatitis, hallucinations, hemoptysis, hypoxia, muscle weakness, myopathy, neutropenia, pancreatitis, pancytopenia, organizing pneumonia (may be fatal), rhabdomyolysis, syndrome of inappropriate antidiuretic hormone secretion (SIADH), toxic epidermal necrolysis (may be fatal), and many other side effects have been reported.

Overdose: AV block, bradycardia, cardiogenic shock, death, hepatotoxicity, and hypotension.

ANTIDOTE

Keep physician informed of all side effects and treat promptly as appropriate; many are life-threatening. Monitor hepatic enzymes closely. Reduce rate or discontinue for progressive hepatic injury. Treat hypotension and cardiogenic shock by slowing the infusion rate. Vasopressors, inotropic agents, and volume expansion may be indicated. Slow infusion rate or discontinue if bradycardia and/or AV block occur; may require a temporary pacemaker. If torsades de pointes occurs, stop all cardioactive drugs (e.g., antiarrhythmics, digoxin, antidepressants, phenothiazines) and normalize electrolytes (e.g., potassium, magnesium). Treat as indicated. Dose reduction or discontinuation of amiodarone may be required if thyroid abnormalities develop. Thyroid hormone supplementation may be required in hypothyroidism. Initiation of antithyroid drugs (e.g., propylthiouracil), beta-blockers (e.g., propranolol), and/or temporary corticosteroid therapy may be necessary for treatment of hyperthyroidism. In severe thyrotoxicosis where amiodarone cannot be discontinued, thyroidectomy may be used as treatment. Experience with surgical intervention is limited; could induce thyroid storm. Amiodarone is not dialyzable. Resuscitate as necessary.

AMISULPRIDE

Dopamine antagonist

Barhemsys

pH 4.75 to 5.25

USUAL DOSE

Prevention of postoperative nausea and vomiting (PONV): 5 mg as a single IV injection infused over 1 to 2 minutes at the time of induction of anesthesia.

Treatment of PONV: 10 mg as a single IV injection infused over 1 to 2 minutes in the event of nausea and/or vomiting after a surgical procedure.

DOSE ADJUSTMENTS

No dose adjustment required based on age, sex, race, or in patients with mild to moderate renal impairment (eGFR 30 to 89 mL/min/1.73 M^2). The pharmacokinetics of amisulpride in patients with severe renal impairment (eGFR less than 30 mL/min/1.73 M^2) have not been adequately studied.

DILUTION

Available as a clear, colorless solution in a single-dose vial containing 5 mg/2 mL (2.5 mg/mL). May be administered undiluted.

Storage: Store unopened vials at CRT. Protect from light. Amisulpride is subject to photo-degradation. Administer within 12 hours after the vial is removed from the protective carton.

COMPATIBILITY

Manufacturer states, "Amisulpride is chemically and physically compatible with SWFI, D5W, and NS, which may be used to flush an IV line before or after administration of amisulpride."

RATE OF ADMINISTRATION

A single dose equally distributed over 1 to 2 minutes.

ACTIONS

Amisulpride is a selective dopamine-2 (D2) and dopamine-3 (D3) receptor antagonist. D2 receptors are located in the chemoreceptor trigger zone (CTZ) and respond to the dopamine released from the nerve endings. Activation of CTZ relays stimuli to the vomiting center, which is involved in emesis. Studies in multiple species indicate that D3 receptors in the area postrema also play a role in emesis. Amisulpride has no appreciable affinity for any other receptor types apart from low affinities for $5\text{-}HT_{2B}$ and $5\text{-}HT_7$ receptors. Plasma protein binding is 25% to 30%. The mean elimination half-life is 4 to 5 hours. Amisulpride is minimally metabolized and does not appear to be metabolized by cytochrome P450 enzymes. Excreted in urine and feces as unchanged drug and metabolites. Secreted in breast milk.

INDICATIONS AND USES

Indicated in adults for:

- Prevention of postoperative nausea and vomiting (PONV), either alone or in combination with an antiemetic of a different class.
- Treatment of PONV in patients who have received antiemetic prophylaxis with an agent of a different class or who have not received prophylaxis.

CONTRAINDICATIONS

Hypersensitivity to amisulpride.

PRECAUTIONS

Causes dose- and concentration-dependent prolongation of the QT interval. Avoid in patients with congenital long QT syndrome and in patients taking droperidol; see Monitor. ▪ Avoid use in patients with severe renal impairment (eGFR less than 30 mL/min/1.73 M^2). Amisulpride is substantially excreted by the kidneys, and patients with severe renal impairment may have increased systemic exposure and an increased risk of adverse reactions.

Monitor: ECG monitoring is recommended in patients with pre-existing arrhythmias/cardiac conduction disorders, electrolyte abnormalities (e.g., hypokalemia or hypomagnesemia), and CHF, and in patients taking other medications (e.g., ondansetron [Zofran]) or with other medical conditions known to prolong the QT interval.

Patient Education: May cause cardiac arrhythmias. Contact provider immediately for light-headedness, a syncopal episode, or a perceived change in heart rate. ▪ Review all prescription and nonprescription medications with a healthcare professional.

Maternal/Child: Data unavailable. Use in pregnancy only if potential benefit justifies potential risk. ▪ Amisulpride is present in breast milk. Consider pumping and discarding milk for 48 hours after amisulpride administration to reduce infant exposure. ▪ Safety and effectiveness for use in pediatric patients have not been established.

Elderly: No overall differences in safety or effectiveness were observed between patients 65 years of age and older and younger patients, but greater sensitivity of some older individuals cannot be ruled out. Amisulpride is substantially excreted by the kidneys, and the risk of adverse reactions may be greater in patients with impaired renal function.

DRUG/LAB INTERACTIONS

Reciprocal antagonism of effects occurs between **dopamine agonist** (e.g., levodopa) and amisulpride. Avoid concomitant use. ▪ Avoid concomitant use with **droperidol**. Dose- and concentration-dependent QT prolongation caused by both agents may be additive. ▪ ECG monitoring is recommended in patients taking **other drugs known to prolong the QT interval** (e.g., ondansetron).

SIDE EFFECTS

Prevention of PONV: The most common adverse reactions were abdominal distension, chills, hypokalemia, increased blood prolactin concentrations, and procedural hypotension.

Treatment of PONV: The most common adverse reaction was infusion site pain.

Post-Marketing: The following adverse reactions have been reported during postapproval chronic oral use of amisulpride outside of the United States. (Amisulpride is not approved for oral dosing or chronic use in the United States.) Reported adverse reactions included agitation, agranulocytosis, angioedema, anxiety, bradycardia, confusional state, dystonia, extrapyramidal disorder, hypersensitivity, hypotension, increased hepatic enzymes, insomnia, neuroleptic malignant syndrome, prolonged QT interval, seizures, somnolence, torsades de pointes, urticaria, and ventricular tachycardia.

ANTIDOTE

Most side effects will be treated symptomatically. Keep physician informed and treat side effects as indicated. There is no specific antidote for an amisulpride overdose. Management includes cardiac monitoring and treatment of severe extrapyramidal symptoms. Weakly dialyzed; hemodialysis should not be used to eliminate the drug.

AMPHOTERICIN B BBW* ■
AMPHOTERICIN B LIPID-BASED PRODUCTS
(am-foe-**TER**-ih-sin)

Abelcet, AmBisome

Antifungal
Antiprotozoal (AmBisome)

pH 5 to 7 ■ 5 to 6

*The Black Box Warning applies only to the generic formulation.

USUAL DOSE

Pretreatment: Pretesting and baseline studies required; see Precautions and Monitor.

Each product has different biochemical, pharmacokinetic, and pharmacodynamic properties. They are not interchangeable from dose to dose, in a given patient, between each other or conventional amphotericin.

ABELCET (AMPHOTERICIN B LIPID COMPLEX INJECTION)

Adults and pediatric patients: 5 mg/kg/24 hr as an infusion. Repeat daily until clinical response or mycologic cure.

AMBISOME (AMPHOTERICIN B LIPOSOME FOR INJECTION)

Adults, children, and infants over 1 month of age: All doses are by infusion.

Empirical therapy in febrile, neutropenic patients: 3 mg/kg/24 hr.

Systemic fungal infections (e.g., *Aspergillus, Candida, Cryptococcus*): 3 to 5 mg/kg/24 hr.

Treatment of cryptococcal meningitis in HIV-infected patients: 6 mg/kg/24 hr.

Visceral leishmaniasis in immunocompetent patients: 3 mg/kg/24 hr on Days 1 through 5. Repeat 3 mg/kg on Day 14 and on Day 21. A repeat course of therapy may be useful if parasitic clearance is not achieved.

Visceral leishmaniasis in immunocompromised patients: 4 mg/kg/24 hr on Days 1 through 5. Repeat 4 mg/kg on Days 10, 17, 24, 31, and 38. During clinical studies, parasitic clearance was not achieved or relapse within 6 months occurred in 88.2% of patients. Usefulness of repeat courses not determined.

GENERIC (CONVENTIONAL AMPHOTERICIN B)

Adults and pediatric patients: Begin with a test dose of 0.1 mg/kg up to 1 mg maximum dose in 20 mL D5W. Infuse over 20 to 30 minutes. Determine size of therapeutic dose by intensity of reaction over a 2- to 4-hour period. Usual starting dose is 0.25 mg/kg of body weight/24 hr. Gradually increase dose by 5 to 10 mg/day (0.125 to 0.25 mg/kg in pediatric patients) to a final dose of 0.5 to 0.7 mg/kg. Total daily dose may range up to 1 mg/kg/day, or up to 1.5 mg/kg/24 hr may be given on alternate-day therapy. Several months of therapy are usually required and recommended for cure. Dosage must be adjusted to each specific patient. In some instances, higher doses can be used. Do not exceed a total daily dose of 1.5 mg/kg under any circumstances.

DOSE ADJUSTMENTS

ABELCET: Full dose usually required; base on SCr and overall patient condition.

AMBISOME: No dose adjustments suggested.

GENERIC (CONVENTIONAL): In all situations, gradual dose increases are essential. Whenever medicine is not given for 7 days or longer, restart treatment at lowest dosage level.

Patients with impaired cardio-renal function or a severe reaction to the test dose: Initiate with smaller daily doses (i.e., 5 to 10 mg).

Patients who experience amphotericin-induced nephrotoxicity: One source recommends reducing the total daily dose by 50% or administering the dose every other day.

Severe and rapidly progressive fungal infection: Initiate treatment with a daily dose of 0.3 mg/kg.

DILUTION

ABELCET: Available in 100-mg (20-mL) vials. Shake vial until all yellow sediment is dissolved. Maintain aseptic technique. Withdraw an exact total daily dose from one or more vials using one or more syringes and 18-gauge needles. Replace needle(s) on syringe(s) with the 5-micron filter(s) supplied with each vial. A new filter must be used for each 400 mg (80 mL) of Abelcet. Empty syringe contents through filter into an infusion of D5W. 4 mL of diluent (D5W) is required for each 1 mL (5 mg) of Abelcet to achieve a final concentration of 1 mg/mL. For **pediatric** and/or fluid-restricted patients (e.g., patients with cardiovascular disease) reduce diluent by half (approximate concentration of 2 mg/mL).

AMBISOME: Reconstitute each 50-mg vial with 12 mL SWFI (without a bacteriostatic agent) to yield 4 mg/mL. Shake vial vigorously for 30 seconds; forms a yellow translucent suspension. Withdraw an exact total daily dose from one or more vials using one or more 20-mL syringes and needles. Replace needle(s) with the 5-micron filter(s) supplied with each vial. A new filter must be used for each 50-mg vial. Empty syringe contents through filter into an infusion of D5W. Use sufficient diluent to achieve a final concentration of 1 to 2 mg/mL, pH 5 to 6. For **pediatric patients:** may be further diluted to concentrations of 0.2 to 0.5 mg/mL for infants and small children to provide adequate volume for infusion.

GENERIC (CONVENTIONAL): A 50-mg vial is initially diluted with 10 mL of SWFI (without a bacteriostatic agent); 5 mg equals 1 mL. Shake well until solution is clear. Further dilute each 1 mg in at least 10 mL of D5W. Dextrose must have a pH above 4.2. Concentration of solution must not be greater than 0.1 mg/mL. Do not use any other diluent. Use a sterile 20-gauge or larger needle at each step of the dilution. Maintain aseptic technique. Larger pore 1-micron filters may be used. Use only fresh solutions without evidence of precipitate or foreign matter. Light sensitive; protect from light during administration.

Filters: Abelcet: 5-micron filter(s) supplied with each vial. A new filter must be used for each 400 mg (80 mL) of Abelcet. Empty syringe contents through filter into an infusion solution. Do not use an in-line filter.

AmBisome: 5-micron filter(s) supplied with each vial. A new filter must be used for each 50-mg vial. Empty syringe contents through filter into an infusion solution. Do not use an in-line filter smaller than 1 micron.

Generic (Conventional): Larger pore 1-micron filters may be used; see Dilution.

Storage: Abelcet: Before reconstitution, refrigerate in carton until time of use and protect from light. Do not freeze. Diluted solution is stable 48 hours if refrigerated and an additional 6 hours at room temperature. Discard unused drug.

AmBisome: Unopened vials may be stored at temperatures up to 25° C (77° F). Vials reconstituted with SWFI may be refrigerated for up to 24 hours. Do not freeze. Infusion of fully diluted solution must begin within 6 hours. Discard unused drug.

Generic (Conventional): Before reconstitution, refrigerate vials and protect from light. Do not freeze. Preserve concentrate in refrigerator up to 7 days or 24 hours at room temperature. Use diluted solution promptly.

COMPATIBILITY

ALL FORMULATIONS

In all situations, use a separate infusion line or flush an existing line with D5W before and after administration.

ABELCET

Do not mix with any other diluent, drug, or solution. Use only D5W. Manufacturer states that **compatibility** with any other diluent has not been established.

Other sources suggest a few specific **compatibilities** dependent on concentration and manufacturer; consult a pharmacist.

AMBISOME/GENERIC

Do not mix with any other diluent, drug, or solution. Use only SWFI for reconstitution and D5W for dilution for infusion. Use of any other solution or the presence of a bacteriostatic agent (e.g., benzyl alcohol) may cause precipitation.

GENERIC (CONVENTIONAL)

Compatibility information not available from manufacturer.

Other sources suggest a few specific **compatibilities** dependent on concentration and manufacturer; consult a pharmacist.

RATE OF ADMINISTRATION

ALL AMPHOTERICINS: Rapid infusion may cause hypotension, hypokalemia, arrhythmia, and shock. Infusion reactions can occur with all amphotericin B formulations. See Precautions, Side Effects, and Antidote. With all formulations, flush existing line with D5W before and after administration or use a separate IV line.

ABELCET: Total daily dose as an infusion at 2.5 mg/kg/hr. Contents of diluted solution must be mixed by shaking at least every 2 hours. Do not use an in-line filter.

AMBISOME: Total daily dose as an infusion over 2 hours. Use of a controlled infusion device is recommended. Infusion time may be shortened to a minimum of 1 hour for patients who show no evidence of intolerance or infusion-related reactions. Infusion time may be extended for patient discomfort or acute reactions or if infusion volume is not tolerated. Do not use any in-line filter less than 1 micron.

GENERIC (CONVENTIONAL): Daily dose over 2 to 6 hours by slow IV infusion. Expected reactions usually less severe with slower rate. A minimum 1-micron filter may be used.

ACTIONS

Antifungal antibiotic agents that bind to the sterol component of fungal cell membranes resulting in leakage of cellular contents. May be fungistatic or fungicidal according to body fluid concentration and susceptibility of the fungus. Abelcet is amphotericin B complexed with two phospholipids in a 1:1 drug-to-lipid ratio. AmBisome is amphotericin B intercalated into a liposomal membrane with several components. Assay tests cannot distinguish lipid-based amphotericin from conventional amphotericin B. Modification of amphotericin to the various lipid-based products alters the drug's functional properties. It allows for increased levels of drug at the site of action (usually areas where the fungi are). Overall effect is increased effectiveness with less toxicity. Not effective against bacteria, rickettsiae, or viruses. Long terminal half-life probably reflects a slow redistribution from tissues. Actual distribution to organs is somewhat selective and may help to decide which product is best to use in a given situation. Route of metabolism not known. Excreted very slowly in the urine.

INDICATIONS AND USES

ABELCET: Treatment of invasive fungal infections in patients who are refractory to or intolerant of conventional amphotericin B therapy.

AMBISOME: Empirical therapy for presumed fungal infection in febrile, neutropenic patients. ■ Treatment of patients with aspergillosis, candida, and/or cryptococcus infections refractory to conventional amphotericin B or in patients in whom renal impairment or unacceptable toxicity precludes the use of conventional amphotericin B. ■ Treatment of visceral leishmaniasis. ■ Treatment of cryptococcal meningitis in HIV-infected patients.

GENERIC (CONVENTIONAL): Treatment of fungal infections that are progressive and potentially fatal, such as aspergillosis, cryptococcosis, blastomycosis, and disseminated forms of candidiasis, coccidioidomycosis, and histoplasmosis, mucormycosis, and sporotrichosis. These infections must be caused by specific organisms. Not recommended for treatment of noninvasive forms of fungal disease in patients with normal neutrophil counts.

Unlabeled uses: AmBisome has been used to prevent fungal infections in bone marrow transplant patients.

CONTRAINDICATIONS

All amphotericin formulations: Known sensitivity to amphotericin B or any components of its formulations unless a life-threatening situation is present.

PRECAUTIONS

ALL AMPHOTERICIN FORMULATIONS: Diagnosis should be positively established by culture or histologic study. ▪ Close clinical observation is imperative. Anaphylaxis has occurred; emergency equipment and supplies must be available. ▪ Infusion reactions are common and usually occur 1 to 3 hours after the start of the infusion. Frequency and severity of reactions generally diminish with subsequent doses. Pretreatment with antipyretics, antihistamines (e.g., diphenhydramine), and/or selective use of corticosteroids may be indicated. ▪ Use caution in patients receiving leukocyte transfusions; may cause acute pulmonary toxicity. Separate times of administration as much as possible. ▪ Nephrotoxicity is the usual dose-limiting factor for use of conventional amphotericin B. Impairment may improve with dose reduction or alternate-day therapy, but some residual dysfunction is possible. Lipid-based formulations are associated with less nephrotoxicity. Most studies show equivalent or superior effectiveness compared with conventional amphotericin. Introduction of lipid-based products to patients with increased CrCl and BUN from conventional amphotericin has decreased the CrCl and BUN.

ABELCET: Renal toxicity is dose dependent but has been consistently less nephrotoxic than conventional amphotericin B.

AMBISOME: Incidence of renal toxicity significantly lower than with conventional amphotericin B.

GENERIC (CONVENTIONAL): Should be used primarily for treatment of patients with progressive and potentially life-threatening fungal infections. It should not be used to treat noninvasive forms of fungal disease such as oral thrush, vaginal candidiasis, and esophageal candidiasis in patients with normal neutrophil counts. ▪ To prevent overdose, verify product name and dose, especially if dose exceeds 1.5 mg/kg. ▪ Therapy is often initiated in infusion centers. ▪ A small amount of heparin added to the infusion may reduce the incidence of thrombophlebitis. ▪ Meperidine (Demerol), nonsteroidal anti-inflammatory agents (e.g., ibuprofen), or hydrocortisone before administration may prevent febrile reactions, including chills; corticosteroids not recommended for concomitant use in other situations because they exaggerate hypokalemia. ▪ Prophylactic antiemetics and antihistamines are also appropriate.

Monitor: *All amphotericin formulations:* Obtain baseline CBC, PT, serum electrolytes, renal (e.g., creatine kinase, BUN, SCr), and liver function (e.g., ALT, AST) tests. Repeat frequently during therapy; recommended weekly. Monitor PT as indicated during therapy. ▪ Discontinue or reduce dose until renal function improves if increase in BUN or SCr is clinically significant. Side effects (e.g., hypokalemia, hypomagnesemia, impaired renal function) may be life-threatening. ▪ Monitor vital signs and I&O. Record every 30 minutes for up to 4 hours after infusion is complete. ▪ Monitor for S/S of hypersensitivity or infusion reactions (e.g., chest pain, dizziness, dyspnea, fever, flushing, hypotension, nausea, pruritus, rash, rigors, urticaria). ▪ Encourage fluids to maintain hydration.

Patient Education: *All amphotericin formulations:* Review all medical conditions and medications before beginning treatment. ▪ Discomfort associated with infusion. ▪ Promptly report S/S of an acute reaction (e.g., anorexia, chills, fever, headache, hypotension, nausea or vomiting, shortness of breath). ▪ Long-term therapy required to effect a cure. ▪ Report diarrhea, fever, increased or decreased urination, loss of appetite, sore throat, stomach pain, and any unusual bleeding or bruising, tiredness, or weakness. ▪ Maintain adequate hydration.

Maternal/Child: *All amphotericin formulations:* Category B: has been used successfully during pregnancy but adequate studies not available. Use only if clearly needed. ▪ Safety for use in breast-feeding and pediatric patients not established. Discontinue nursing. ▪ Conventional amphotericin B has been used in pediatric patients. Lipid-based preparations have been used in pediatric patients without any unexpected side effects. Safety of use of AmBisome in infants under 1 month of age not established.

Elderly: Consider age-related impaired body functions. Lipid-based preparations have been used without unexpected side effects.

DRUG/LAB INTERACTIONS

Drug interaction studies have not been done for lipid-based preparations, but interactions similar to conventional amphotericin B are expected. ▪ **Corticosteroids** will increase hypokalemia and may cause arrhythmias. Use with caution only if indicated to control drug reactions or, if necessary, monitor serum electrolytes and cardiac function closely. ▪ Hypokalemic effect may be increased with **thiazides,** may potentiate **digoxin** toxicity, and/or may enhance the curariform effect of **neuromuscular blocking agents;** monitor serum potassium levels. ▪ Avoid use or use extreme caution with other **nephrotoxic drugs** (e.g., **aminoglycosides, selected antibiotics** [e.g., vancomycin], **anesthetics, antituberculars** [e.g., capreomycin], **diuretics, pentamidine**). Nephrotoxic effects are additive. Frequent monitoring of renal function indicated if any other nephrotoxic drug must be used. ▪ Nephrotoxicity and myelotoxicity are both increased when given concurrently with **zidovudine.** ▪ Potentiates nephrotoxicity of **cyclosporine;** alternate immunosuppressive therapy recommended. ▪ Concurrent use with **antineoplastic agents** (e.g., cisplatin, methotrexate) **or radiation therapy** may increase renal toxicity and incidence of bronchospasm and hypotension. ▪ Enhances antifungal effects of **flucytosine and other antiinfectives.** May increase toxicity. ▪ Antagonism between amphotericin B and **imidazole antifungals** (e.g., ketoconazole, miconazole, fluconazole) has been reported. ▪ Acute pulmonary toxicity occurred in patients receiving **leukocyte transfusion;** separate administration times as much as possible. ▪ **False elevations of serum phosphate** may occur if patient samples are analyzed using the PHOSm assay.   ·

SIDE EFFECTS

Lipid-Based Preparations: Most side effects similar to conventional amphotericin B but occur with less frequency and intensity. Acute reactions, including fever and chills, may occur within 1 to 3 hours of starting the infusion. Infusion-related cardiorespiratory reactions may include dyspnea, hypertension, hyperventilation, hypotension, hypoxia, tachycardia, and vasodilation. Arrhythmia, bronchospasm, and shock can occur. Anaphylaxis and cardiac arrest from overdose have been reported.

Generic (Conventional): Common even at doses below therapeutic; may begin to occur within 15 to 20 minutes: anorexia, chills, convulsions, diarrhea, fever, headache, phlebitis, vomiting. Anaphylactoid reactions, anemia, cardiac disturbances (including fibrillation and arrest), coagulation defects, hypertension, hypokalemia, hypotension, and numerous other side effects occur fairly frequently. Renal function impaired in 80% of patients. May reverse after treatment ends, but some permanent damage likely.

Post-Marketing: *AmBisome:* Agranulocytosis, angioedema, bronchospasm, cyanosis/hypoventilation, edema, erythema, hemorrhagic cystitis, pulmonary edema, rhabdomyolysis.

ANTIDOTE

All Amphotericin Formulations: Notify the physician of all side effects. Many are reversible if the drug is discontinued. Some will respond to symptomatic treatment. Acute reactions (e.g., fever, chills, hypotension, nausea, and vomiting) usually lessen with subsequent doses. These acute infusion-related reactions can be managed by pretreatment with antipyretics, antihistamines, and/or corticosteroids or reduction of the rate of infusion and prompt treatment with antihistamines and/or corticosteroids and meperidine (Demerol) for chills. If anaphylaxis or serious respiratory distress occurs, discontinue amphotericin and treat as necessary. Give no further infusions. Hemodialysis not effective in overdose. Discontinue if BUN and alkaline phosphatase are abnormal. Dantrolene has been used to prevent (50 mg PO) or treat (50 mg IV) severe, shaking chills.

Generic (Conventional): Administration of conventional amphotericin B on alternate days may decrease the incidence of some side effects. Urinary alkalinizers may minimize renal tubular acidosis.

Abelcet: Overdose has caused cardiac arrest. Discontinue drug and treat symptomatically.

AMPICILLIN SODIUM AND SULBACTAM SODIUM

(am-pih-**SILL**-in **SO**-dee-um and sull-**BACK**-tam **SO**-dee-um)

Unasyn

Antibacterial (penicillin and beta-lactamase inhibitor)

pH 8 to 10

USUAL DOSE

Adults and pediatric patients weighing 40 kg or more: 1.5 to 3 Gm every 6 hours (1 Gm ampicillin with 0.5 Gm sulbactam to 2 Gm ampicillin with 1 Gm sulbactam). All commercial preparations in the United States have a 2:1 ratio of ampicillin to sulbactam (e.g., 1.5 Gm = 1 Gm ampicillin plus 0.5 Gm sulbactam). Do not exceed 4 Gm *sulbactam*/24 hr. *All doses in this monograph include ampicillin and sulbactam within the recommended dose.*

PEDIATRIC DOSE

IV use for more than 14 days is not recommended. See comments under Usual Dose.

Skin and skin structure infections in pediatric patients over 1 year of age and less than 40 kg: 300 mg/kg/day (200 mg/kg ampicillin and 100 mg/kg sulbactam) in equally divided doses as an infusion every 6 hours (75 mg/kg every 6 hours).

DOSE ADJUSTMENTS

May be indicated in the elderly. ▪ Reduce total daily dose in impaired renal function according to the following chart.

Ampicillin/Sulbactam Dose Guidelines in Impaired Renal Function	
Creatinine Clearance (mL/min per 1.73 M²)	**Dose/Frequency**
30 mL/min or more	Usual recommended dose q 6 to 8 hr
15 to 29 mL/min	Usual recommended dose q 12 hr
5 to 14 mL/min	Usual recommended dose q 24 hr
Hemodialysis patients[a]	Usual recommended dose q 24 hr On day of dialysis, give immediately after dialysis

[a]One source recommends 1.5 to 3 Gm every 12 to 24 hours for hemodialysis patients, given after dialysis on dialysis days. A dose of 3 Gm/24 hr has been recommended for peritoneal dialysis patients.

DILUTION

Each 1.5 Gm or fraction thereof must be initially reconstituted with 4 mL of SWFI (375 mg/mL). Allow to stand to dissipate foaming. Solution should be clear and colorless to pale yellow. Must be further diluted to a final concentration of 3 to 45 mg/mL in one of the following solutions and given by slow IV injection or as an intermittent IV infusion: D5W, D5 in ½NS, LR, or NS. Also available in piggyback vials, pharmacy bulk packages, and ADD-Vantage vials for use with ADD-Vantage infusion containers.

Storage: Store at CRT before dilution. Stability of different concentrations in each solution varies (see literature).

COMPATIBILITY

May be inactivated in solution with aminoglycosides (e.g., amikacin, gentamicin). Do not mix in the same solution. Appropriate spacing and/or separate sites required. See Drug/Lab Interactions.

Other sources suggest specific **compatibilities** dependent on concentration and manufacturer; consult a pharmacist.

RATE OF ADMINISTRATION

IV injection: A single dose over a minimum of 10 to 15 minutes.

Intermittent IV: A single dose over 15 to 30 minutes or longer, depending on amount of solution. Too-rapid injection may cause seizures.

ACTIONS

An antibacterial combination consisting of the semi-synthetic penicillin, ampicillin so-dium, and the beta-lactamase inhibitor sulbactam sodium. The addition of sulbactam extends the antibacterial spectrum of ampicillin to include many bacteria normally resis-tant to it and to other beta-lactam antibacterials. The antibacterial combination has a broad spectrum of bactericidal activity against selected gram-positive, gram-negative, and anaerobic organisms (see literature). Inhibits bacterial cell wall synthesis. Peak se-rum levels achieved by end of infusion. Widely distributed into many body tissues and fluids. Half-life is 1 hour. Crosses the placental barrier. Excreted in the urine. Secreted in breast milk.

INDICATIONS AND USES

Treatment of skin and skin structure, intra-abdominal, and gynecologic infections due to susceptible strains of specific organisms.

CONTRAINDICATIONS

History of serious hypersensitivity reactions (e.g., anaphylaxis or Stevens-Johnson syn-drome) to ampicillin, sulbactam, or other beta-lactam antibacterial drugs (e.g., penicillins and cephalosporins). ■ Patients with a previous history of cholestatic jaundice/hepatic dysfunction associated with ampicillin/sulbactam. ■ Infectious mononucleosis because of increased incidence of rash.

PRECAUTIONS

Hypersensitivity reactions, including fatalities, have been reported in patients on penicil-lin therapy; most likely to occur in patients with a history of penicillin allergy or sensitiv-ity to multiple allergens. There have been reports of individuals with a history of penicil-lin hypersensitivity experiencing severe reactions when treated with cephalosporins. Check history of previous hypersensitivity reactions to penicillins, cephalosporins, or other allergens. Actual incidence of cross-allergenicity not established but may be more common with first-generation cephalosporins. ■ Hepatic dysfunction, including hepatitis and cholestatic jaundice, has been associated with the use of ampicillin/sulbactam. He-patic toxicity is usually reversible; however, deaths have been reported. ■ May cause severe skin reactions (e.g., acute generalized exanthematous pustulosis [AGEP], dermati-tis exfoliative, erythema multiforme, Stevens-Johnson syndrome [SJS], and toxic epider-mal necrolysis [TEN]). ■ Studies indicated to determine the causative organism and susceptibility to ampicillin/sulbactam. ■ To reduce the development of drug-resistant bacteria and maintain its effectiveness, ampicillin and sulbactam should be used to treat or prevent only those infections proven or strongly suspected to be caused by bacteria. ■ Avoid prolonged use of this drug; superinfection caused by overgrowth of nonsuscep-tible organisms may result. ■ *Clostridium difficile*–associated diarrhea (CDAD) has been reported. May range from mild diarrhea to fatal colitis. Consider in patients who present with diarrhea during or after treatment with ampicillin and sulbactam.

Monitor: Watch for early symptoms of hypersensitivity reactions, especially in indi-viduals with a history of allergic problems. ■ Monitor for possible skin reactions. If a skin rash develops, monitor closely and discontinue if lesions progress. ■ AST may be increased. Renal, hepatic, and hematopoietic function should be checked during pro-longed therapy. Hepatic function should be monitored at regular intervals in patients with hepatic impairment. ■ May cause thrombophlebitis. Observe carefully and rotate infusion sites.

Patient Education: Promptly report any S/S of a hypersensitivity reaction (e.g., itching, rash, wheezing), fever, sore throat, unusual bleeding or bruising, severe stomach cramps and/or diarrhea, or seizures. ■ Promptly report diarrhea or bloody stools that occur during treatment or up to several months after an antibiotic has been discontinued; may indicate CDAD and require treatment.

Maternal/Child: Animal studies have not shown adverse effects on fertility or in the fetus. Use only if clearly needed. ■ Use caution with breast-feeding. May cause diarrhea, candidiasis, or allergic response in nursing infants. ■ Safety for IV use in pediatric patients over 1 year of age has been established for skin and skin structure infections but not for other uses; however, it is in use. Elimination rate markedly reduced in neonates. ■ Safety and effectiveness of IM use in pediatric patients not established.

Elderly: Consider degree of age-related impaired renal function. ■ See Dose Adjustments.

DRUG/LAB INTERACTIONS

Concurrent use with probenecid may result in increased and prolonged ampicillin and sulbactam blood levels. ■ Frequently used concomitantly with **aminoglycosides** (e.g., gentamicin), but these drugs must never be mixed in the same infusion (mutual inactivation). If given concurrently, administer at separate sites. ■ May be antagonized by **bacteriostatic antibiotics** (e.g., chloramphenicol, erythromycin, tetracyclines); may interfere with bactericidal action. ■ May decrease clearance and increase toxicity of **methotrexate**. ■ Ampicillin-induced skin rash potentiated by **allopurinol**. ■ False-positive glucose reaction with **Clinitest and Benedict's or Fehling's solution.** ■ May cause **false values** in other lab tests; see literature.

SIDE EFFECTS

Full scope of hypersensitivity reactions, including anaphylaxis, is possible. Diarrhea and rash occur most frequently. Abdominal distension; burning, discomfort, and pain at injection site; candidiasis; chest pain; chills; decreased hemoglobin, hematocrit, RBC, WBC, lymphocytes, neutrophils, and platelets; decreased serum albumin and total protein; dysuria; edema; epistaxis; erythema; facial swelling; fatigue; flatulence; glossitis; headache; increased alkaline phosphatase, BUN, creatinine, LDH, AST, ALT; increased basophils, eosinophils, lymphocytes, monocytes, and platelets; itching; malaise; mucosal bleeding; nausea and vomiting; phlebitis; RBCs and hyaline casts in urine; substernal pain; thrombophlebitis; tightness in throat; and urine retention can occur. May cause CDAD. Higher than normal doses may cause neurologic adverse reactions, including convulsions, especially with impaired renal function.

Post-Marketing: Abdominal pain, abnormal hepatic function, acute generalized exanthematous pustulosis, agranulocytosis, angioedema, black "hairy" tongue, cholestasis, cholestatic hepatitis, convulsions, dizziness, dyspepsia, dyspnea, erythema multiforme, exfoliative dermatitis, gastritis, hemolytic anemia, hyperbilirubinemia, jaundice, melena, positive direct Coombs' test, Stevens-Johnson syndrome, stomatitis, thrombocytopenic purpura, toxic epidermal necrolysis, tubulointerstitial nephritis, and urticaria.

ANTIDOTE

Notify the physician of any side effect. For severe symptoms, discontinue the drug, treat hypersensitivity reactions as indicated (e.g., antihistamines, epinephrine, corticosteroids) and resuscitate as necessary. Treat CDAD with fluids, electrolytes, protein supplements, and appropriate antibiotics (e.g., oral vancomycin) as indicated. In severe cases, surgical evaluation may be indicated. Hemodialysis may be effective in overdose.

ANGIOTENSIN II INJECTION
(an-jee-oh-**TEN**-sin too)

Giapreza

Peptide hormone
Vasopressor

pH 5.5

USUAL DOSE
Titrate to effect for each individual patient. Recommended starting dose is 20 nanograms (ng)/kg/min via continuous IV infusion. Use of a central venous line is recommended. Monitor blood pressure response and titrate angiotensin II every 5 minutes by increments of up to 15 ng/kg/min as needed to achieve or maintain target blood pressure. Do not exceed 80 ng/kg/min during the first 3 hours of treatment.

Once the underlying shock has sufficiently improved, down-titrate every 5 to 15 minutes by increments of up to 15 ng/kg/min based on blood pressure. Maintenance doses should not exceed 40 ng/kg/min. Doses as low as 1.25 ng/kg/min may be used.

DOSE ADJUSTMENTS
See Usual Dose. ▪ No dose adjustments required based on age, sex, or impaired renal or hepatic function.

DILUTION
Available in sterile vials containing 2.5 mg/mL or 5 mg/2 mL. Must be diluted in NS. Dilute the contents of one vial in 250 to 500 mL of NS to achieve a final concentration of 5,000 ng/mL or 10,000 ng/mL according to the following chart.

Preparation of Diluted Solutions of Angiotensin II				
Fluid Restricted?	Vial Strength	Withdraw Amount (mL)	Infusion Bag Size (mL)	Final Concentration (ng/mL)
No	2.5 mg/mL	1 mL	500 mL	5,000 ng/mL
Yes	2.5 mg/mL	1 mL	250 mL	10,000 ng/mL
Yes	5 mg/2 mL	2 mL	500 mL	10,000 ng/mL

Filters: Specific information not available.
Storage: Before use, refrigerate vials at 2° to 8° C (36° to 46° F). Diluted solution may be stored at RT or under refrigeration. Discard prepared solution after 24 hours whether stored under refrigeration or at RT. After use, discard vial and any unused portion of the drug product.

COMPATIBILITY
Must be diluted in NS. Specific information on **compatibility** with other fluids or drugs is not available.

RATE OF ADMINISTRATION
See Usual Dose. For IV infusion only. Administration through a central venous line is recommended.

ACTIONS
A synthetic form of human angiotensin II. Angiotensin II is a naturally occurring peptide hormone of the renin-angiotensin-aldosterone system (RAAS). It raises blood pressure by vasoconstriction and increased aldosterone release. Direct action of angiotensin II on the vessel wall is mediated by binding to the G-protein–coupled angiotensin II receptor type 1 on vascular smooth muscle cells, which stimulates calcium/calmodulin-dependent phosphorylation of myosin and causes smooth muscle contraction. Median time to reach the target mean arterial pressure end point is approximately 5 minutes. Half-life is less than 1 minute. Metabolized by aminopeptidase A and angiotensin-converting enzyme 2 to angiotensin-(2-8) [angiotensin III] and angiotensin-(1-7), respectively in plasma, erythrocytes, and many of the major organs (i.e., intestine, kidney, liver, and lung).

INDICATIONS AND USES
Treatment of hypotension in adults with septic or other distributive shock.

CONTRAINDICATIONS
Manufacturer states, "None."

PRECAUTIONS
A higher incidence of arterial and venous thrombotic and thromboembolic events occurred in patients receiving angiotensin II compared with placebo-treated patients. Deep venous thromboses were the major occurrence. Concurrent venous thromboembolism (VTE) prophylaxis is recommended.

Monitor: Monitor vital signs. Continuous monitoring is indicated in these critically ill patients. ■ Monitor for S/S of potential thromboembolic events, and administer VTE prophylaxis. ■ See Drug/Lab Interactions.

Maternal/Child: Published data on use in pregnancy are not available. However, septic or other distributive shock is a medical emergency that can be fatal if left untreated. Delaying treatment in pregnant females with hypotension associated with septic or other distributive shock is likely to increase the risk of maternal and fetal morbidity and mortality. ■ No data available on the presence of angiotensin II in human milk, the effects on the breast-fed infant, or the effects on milk production. ■ Safety and effectiveness for use in pediatric patients have not been established.

Elderly: No significant difference in safety or effectiveness between patients 65 years of age or older and younger patients.

DRUG/LAB INTERACTIONS
Response to angiotensin II may be increased with concomitant use of **angiotensin-converting enzyme (ACE) inhibitors**. ■ Response to angiotensin II may be decreased with concomitant use of **angiotensin II receptor blockers (ARBs)**.

SIDE EFFECTS
Thromboembolic events, including arterial and venous thrombotic events and deep vein thrombosis, are the most common adverse reactions. Acidosis, delirium, fungal infection, hyperglycemia, peripheral ischemia, tachycardia, and thrombocytopenia have also been reported.

Overdose: Hypertension, necessitating close monitoring and supportive care.

ANTIDOTE
Notify the physician of all side effects or unexpected changes in vital signs. For accidental overdose with hypertension, reduce rate or temporarily discontinue until condition stabilizes. Monitor and provide supportive care as indicated. Effects are expected to be brief because the half-life of angiotensin II is less than 1 minute. Should a hypersensitivity reaction occur, treat as indicated (e.g., antihistamines, epinephrine, corticosteroids). Resuscitate if indicated.

ANIDULAFUNGIN
(a-**nid**-yoo-luh-**FUN**-jin)

Antifungal
(echinocandin)

Eraxis

USUAL DOSE
Pretreatment: Pretesting and baseline studies required; see Monitor and Maternal/Child.
Candidemia and other *Candida* infections (intra-abdominal abscess and peritonitis): Begin with a *loading dose* of 200 mg as an infusion on Day 1. Follow with a daily dose of 100 mg as an infusion beginning on Day 2. Base duration of treatment on patient's clinical response. In general, antifungal therapy should continue for at least 14 days after the last positive culture.
Esophageal candidiasis: Begin with a *loading dose* of 100 mg as an infusion on Day 1. Follow with a daily dose of 50 mg as an infusion beginning on Day 2. Treat for a minimum of 14 days and for at least 7 days following resolution of symptoms. Relapse of esophageal candidiasis has occurred in patients with HIV infections; suppressive antifungal therapy may be considered after a course of treatment.

DOSE ADJUSTMENTS
No dose adjustment is indicated based on age, gender, or race; in patients with any degree of renal or hepatic insufficiency; or in patients using concomitant medications that are known metabolic substrates, inhibitors, or inducers of cytochrome P_{450} (CYP450) isoenzymes; see Drug/Lab Interactions. ■ No dose adjustment is required in patients with HIV who are receiving concomitant antiretroviral therapy (e.g., HIV protease inhibitors [e.g., amprenavir (Agenerase), indinavir (Crixivan), nelfinavir (Viracept), ritonavir (Norvir), saquinavir (Invirase)]).

DILUTION
Each 50-mg vial must be reconstituted with 15 mL of SWFI, and each 100-mg vial must be reconstituted with 30 mL of SWFI. The resulting concentration is 3.33 mg/mL. Aseptically transfer the reconstituted dose (50, 100, or 200 mg) into the appropriately sized IV container of D5W or NS for infusion as shown in the following chart. The final concentration of infusion solution is 0.77 mg/mL.

Dilution Requirements for Administration of Anidulafungin				
Dose (mg)	Number of Unit Packs Required	Total Reconstituted Volume (mL)	Volume of NS or D5W for Infusion	Total Infusion Volume (mL)
50 mg	1-50 mg	15 mL	50 mL	65 mL
100 mg	2-50 mg or 1-100 mg	30 mL	100 mL	130 mL
200 mg	4-50 mg or 2-100 mg	60 mL	200 mL	260 mL

Filters: No data available from manufacturer.
Storage: Store unopened vials at 2° to 8° C (36° to 46° F). Do not freeze. Excursions for 96 hours up to 25° C (77° F) are permitted, and the vial can be returned to storage at 2° to 8° C. Reconstituted solution can be stored at up to 25° C (77° F) for up to 24 hours. Infusion solution can be stored at temperatures up to 25° C for up to 48 hours or stored frozen for at least 72 hours.

COMPATIBILITY
Manufacturer states, "Do not mix or co-infuse with other medications or electrolytes. **Compatibility** of anidulafungin with intravenous substances, additives, or medications other than D5W or NS has not been established."

Other sources suggest specific **compatibilities** dependent on concentration and manufacturer; consult a pharmacist.

RATE OF ADMINISTRATION

Flush IV line with D5W or NS before and after infusion.

Do not exceed an infusion rate of 1.1 mg/min (equivalent to 1.4 mL/min or 84 mL/hr when diluted as directed). Infusion at a rate greater than 1.1 mg/min may cause histamine-mediated reactions (e.g., bronchospasm, dyspnea, flushing, hypotension, pruritus, rash, urticaria).

ACTIONS

A semi-synthetic lipopeptide, anidulafungin is an echinocandin, the newest class of antifungal agents. Acts by inhibiting the synthesis of 1,3-beta-D-glucan, an integral component of the fungal cell wall not present in mammalian cells. Extensively protein bound. Steady state is achieved after a loading dose. Not metabolized, it undergoes slow chemical degradation. Hepatic metabolism has not been observed. Anidulafungin is not a clinically relevant substrate, inducer, or inhibitor of cytochrome P_{450} (CYP450) isoenzymes. Terminal half-life ranges from 40 to 50 hours. Some excretion in feces, with minimal excretion in urine.

INDICATIONS AND USES

Treatment of the following fungal infections: candidemia and other forms of *Candida* infections (intra-abdominal abscess and peritonitis) and esophageal candidiasis.

Limitations of use: Has not been studied in *Candida* infections associated with endocarditis, osteomyelitis, and meningitis. ▪ Has not been studied in sufficient numbers of neutropenic patients to determine effectiveness.

CONTRAINDICATIONS

Hypersensitivity to anidulafungin or any of its components (e.g., fructose, mannitol, polysorbate 80, tartaric acid, sodium hydroxide, and/or hydrochloric acid) or to other echinocandins (e.g., micafungin [Mycamine]).

PRECAUTIONS

Do not give as an IV bolus; for IV infusion only. ▪ Abnormal liver function tests have been reported. Isolated cases of significant hepatic dysfunction, hepatitis, or worsening hepatic failure have occurred. ▪ *Candida* isolates with reduced susceptibility to anidulafungin have been reported, which suggests a potential for development of drug resistance. Clinical significance unknown. Cross-resistance with other echinocandins (e.g., micafungin [Mycamine]) has not been studied. ▪ Has been shown to be active against *Candida albicans* resistant to fluconazole (Diflucan). ▪ See Monitor and Antidote.

Monitor: Specimens for fungal culture, serologic testing, and histopathologic testing should be obtained before therapy to isolate and identify causative organisms. Therapy may begin as soon as all specimens are obtained and before results are known. Reassess after test results are known. ▪ Baseline CBC with differential and platelet count, BUN, and liver function tests (e.g., ALT, AST) may be indicated. ▪ Monitor for evidence of impaired hepatic function (e.g., increased ALT, AST, serum alkaline phosphatase). ▪ Monitor for S/S of infusion-related, possibly histamine-related, adverse reactions (e.g., bronchospasm, dyspnea, flushing, hypotension, pruritus, rash, urticaria). ▪ Anaphylaxis, including shock, has been reported. Monitor for S/S of a hypersensitivity reaction (e.g., bronchospasm, dyspnea, hives, hypotension, pruritus, rash, swelling of eyelids, lips, or face); discontinue infusion if a hypersensitivity reaction occurs.

Patient Education: Promptly report any hypersensitivity or infusion-related reactions (e.g., bronchospasm, dyspnea, dizziness, flushing, itching, rash, urticaria). Report S/S of liver dysfunction (anorexia, fatigue, jaundice, nausea and vomiting, dark urine, or pale stools).

Maternal/Child: Use during pregnancy only if benefits justify risk to fetus. Based on animal studies, anidulafungin can cause fetal harm when administered to a pregnant woman. ▪ Use caution if required during breast-feeding. Secreted in milk of drug-treated rats; not known if anidulafungin is secreted in human milk. Effects on breast-fed infants or on milk production unknown. ▪ Safety and effectiveness for use in pediatric patients 16 years of age or younger have not been established; however, some immunocompromised pediatric (2 through 11 years) and adolescent (12 through 17 years) patients with neutro-penia were included in studies; see prescribing information.

Elderly: Differences in response compared to younger adults not identified.

DRUG/LAB INTERACTIONS

Anidulafungin is not a clinically relevant substrate, inducer, or inhibitor of cytochrome P_{450} (CYP450) isoenzymes. It is considered unlikely that it will have a clinically relevant effect on the metabolism of drugs metabolized by CYP450 isoenzymes and/or other drugs likely to be coadministered with it.

SIDE EFFECTS

Patients treated for candidemia and other *Candida* infections: Deep vein thrombosis; diarrhea; elevated ALT, AST, alkaline phosphatase; fever; hypokalemia; insomnia; nausea; vomiting.

Patients treated for esophageal candidiasis: Anemia; diarrhea; dyspepsia (aggravated); elevated ALT, AST, and gamma-glutamyl transferase; fever; headache; leukopenia; nausea; neutropenia; phlebitis; rash; and vomiting.

Histamine-mediated reactions (e.g., bronchospasm, dyspnea, flushing, hypotension, pruritus, rash, urticaria) or hypersensitivity reactions (including anaphylaxis) may occur. Significant hepatic dysfunction (e.g., hepatitis, hepatocellular damage, hyperbilirubine-mia, or hepatic failure) has occurred. Many other side effects have been reported in small numbers of patients.

Post-Marketing: Anaphylactic reaction, anaphylactic shock, bronchospasm.

ANTIDOTE

Notify physician of all side effects; most will be treated symptomatically. Reduce rate of infusion if a histamine-mediated reaction occurs. If a hypersensitivity reaction occurs, discontinue anidulafungin and treat as indicated. Appropriate treatment may include oxygen, epinephrine, antihistamines (e.g., diphenhydramine), vasopressors (e.g., dopa-mine), corticosteroids, IV fluids, and ventilation equipment. S/S indicative of hepatic side effects may require evaluation of benefits versus risk of continuing anidulafungin therapy. Not removed by hemodialysis. Resuscitate as indicated.

ANIFROLUMAB

(an-i-**FROL**-ue-mab)

Saphnelo

USUAL DOSE
Adult: 300 mg IV every 4 weeks.

PEDIATRIC DOSE
Safety and efficacy have not been established.

DOSE ADJUSTMENTS
Renal: No dosage adjustments provided by manufacturer.
Hepatic: No dosage adjustments provided by manufacturer.

DILUTION
Before use, inspect vial and do not use if solution is cloudy, discolored, or contains particulate matter. Allow to warm to room temperature. *Do not shake vial.* Withdraw and discard 2 mL of NS from a 100-mL bag; withdraw 2 mL from the vial and add to the NS bag. Invert bag and mix gently; *do not shake*.

COMPATIBILITY
Do not administer simultaneously with any other medication or IV solutions other than NS.

RATE OF ADMINISTRATION
Use a separate line with an in-line, low–protein binding, 0.2-micron filter and infuse over 30 minutes. Upon completion, flush infusion set with 25 mL of NS.

ACTIONS
Anifrolumab is an IgG1-kappa monoclonal antibody that blocks the activity of type 1 interferon receptors, which in turn reduces inflammatory and immunologic processes associated with systemic lupus erythematosus.

INDICATIONS AND USES
Systemic lupus erythematosus.

CONTRAINDICATIONS
Anaphylaxis to anifrolumab or any component of the formulation.

PRECAUTIONS
Infusion reactions: Consider premedication in patients with a history of infusion reactions. Stop infusion and start supportive treatment if patient develops infusion-related reactions.
Infections: Serious and potentially fatal infections may occur during treatment. Patients are at increased risk for respiratory infections and herpes zoster.
Malignancy: Immunosuppressant therapy may increase the risk of malignancy.
Immunizations: Patients should be brought up-to-date with immunizations before starting therapy. Do not give live or live attenuated vaccines.
Monitor: Monitor for signs and symptoms of hypersensitivity and infection.
Patient Education: Contact physician for infection (fever, chills, sore throat, ear, sinus pain, cough, increased sputum or change in color of sputum, painful urination, mouth sores or wounds that do not heal); stomach pain or diarrhea; warm, red, or painful skin or sores on body; muscle pain; sweating; shingles; dizziness; headache; vomiting; fatigue; weakness.

Maternal/Child: Anifrolumab is a humanized monoclonal antibody (IgG1), and human IgG is known to cross the placenta. Data collection to monitor pregnancy and infant outcomes is ongoing. It is unknown whether anifrolumab will pass in breast milk; the manufacturer states the decision to breast-feed during therapy should consider the risk of infant exposure.

Elderly: Refer to adult dosing and precautions.

DRUG/LAB INTERACTIONS

There are many drug interactions with anifrolumab, and the following drugs should be avoided: bacilli Calmette-Guérin (BCG), baricitinib, belimumab, biologic antipsoriasis agents, biologic disease-modifying antirheumatic drugs, cladribine, dengue tetravalent vaccine, MMR and varicella virus vaccine, natalizumab, pimecrolimus, poliovirus vaccine, ruxolitinib, tacrolimus topical, talimogene laherparepvec, tertomotide, tofacitinib, typhoid vaccine, upadacitinib, vaccines (live), and yellow fever vaccine.

SIDE EFFECTS

Infection, bronchitis, upper respiratory tract infection, malignant neoplasm of breast, squamous cell carcinoma, hypersensitivity reaction, antibody development, herpes zoster infection, cough, infusion-related reactions, anaphylaxis, and angioedema.

ANTIDOTE

Discontinue infusion and treat appropriately for severe hypersensitivity reactions.

ANTIHEMOPHILIC FACTOR (HUMAN ▪ RECOMBINANT ▪ RECOMBINANT [Fc FUSION PROTEIN] ▪ RECOMBINANT [PEGYLATED] ▪ RECOMBINANT [PEGYLATED-aucl] ▪ RECOMBINANT [SINGLE CHAIN] ▪ RECOMBINANT [PORCINE SEQUENCE][a])

Antihemophilic agent

(an-tie-hee-moe-**FIL**-ik **FAK**-tor)

AHF, Factor VIII ▪ Hemofil M, Koate DVI ▪ Advate, Helixate FS, Kogenate FS, Kogenate FS Bio-Set, Kovaltry, Kovaltry Bio-Set, Novoeight, Nuwiq, Recombinate, Xyntha, Xyntha Solofuse ▪ Eloctate ▪ Adynovate ▪ Jivi ▪ Afstyla ▪ Obizur[a]

Available factor VIII products and their origins include the following:

Hemofil M, Koate DVI (Human): Blood product derivatives. May contain trace amounts of mouse or hamster protein.

Advate, Helixate FS, Kogenate FS, Kogenate FS Bio-Set, Kovaltry, Kovaltry Bio-Set, Novoeight, Xyntha, Xyntha Solofuse (Recombinant): Stabilized without human albumin. No human or animal-derived proteins are used in the purification or formulation processes. May contain trace amounts of mouse or hamster protein.

Recombinate (Recombinant): Stabilized in human albumin. May contain bovine protein and trace amounts of mouse or hamster protein.

Eloctate (Recombinant): B-domain–deleted recombinant factor VIII Fc (BDD-rFVIIIFc) fusion protein is the active ingredient. No human or animal-derived proteins are used in the purification or formulation processes.

Nuwiq (Recombinant): B-domain–deleted recombinant factor VIII (BDD-rFVIII) is the active ingredient. No human or animal-derived proteins are used in the purification or formulation processes.

Adynovate (Recombinant) PEGylated: The cell culture, pegylation, purification process, and formulation do not use additives of human or animal origins. May contain trace amounts of hamster protein.

Jivi (Recombinant) PEGylated-aucl: The cell culture, pegylation, purification process, and formulation do not use additives of human or animal origins. May contain trace amounts of mouse and hamster protein.

Afstyla (Recombinant): A single polypeptide chain with a truncated B-domain. No human or animal-derived proteins are used in the purification or formulation processes.

Obizur* (Recombinant): Porcine sequence. May contain trace amounts of hamster protein.

Alphanate and Humate P (see AHF and von Willebrand Factor Complex monograph): From human plasma; intermediate and high purity.

USUAL DOSE
(International units [IU])

Pretreatment: Pretesting and baseline studies required; see Monitor.

Adults and pediatric patients: Dosing is completely individualized. Dose, frequency, and duration of treatment are based on severity of the factor VIII deficiency, location and extent of bleeding, clinical condition of the patient, desired antihemophilic factor level, body weight, and presence of factor VIII inhibitors. Measure factor VIII level before administration; see Monitor. In general, a dose of 1 IU/kg will raise the plasma factor VIII activity by 2 IU/dL. On average, a plasma antihemophilic factor level of 20% to

[a]Recombinant (Porcine Sequence [Obizur]) is indicated for use only in acquired hemophilia. Not indicated for use in congenital hemophilia A.

40% of normal is required to control minor hemorrhage. A level of 30% to 60% of normal may be required to control moderate bleeding; greater percentages are required for major bleeding or surgical procedures.

All products except Obizur use a variation of the following formula.

To calculate the dose needed based on a desired factor VIII increase (%):

$$\text{Dose (IU)} = \text{Body weight (kg)} \times \text{Desired factor VIII increase (IU/dL or \% of normal)} \times 0.5$$

To calculate the expected % factor VIII increase for a given dose:

$$\text{Expected \% factor VIII increase} = (\#\text{ Units administered} \times 2) \div \text{Body weight (kg)}$$

The following charts outline AHF dosing recommendations for the various AHF products. *Consult individual product labeling for more detailed information.*

Control and Prevention of Bleeding Episodes				
Degree of Bleeding	**AHF Product**	**Required Peak Postinfusion Factor VIII Activity (as % of Normal or IU/dL)**	**Dose (IU/kg)**	**Frequency and Duration of Therapy**
Minor Early hemarthrosis, mild muscle bleed, or mild oral bleed Superficial muscle or soft tissue and oral bleeds	Advate	20 to 40	10 to 20 IU/kg	Repeat every 12 to 24 hr (8 to 24 hr in patients under 6 years of age) for 1 to 3 days until bleeding is resolved or healing is achieved.
	Adynovate Jivi[a]	20 to 40	10 to 20 IU/kg	Adynovate: Repeat every 12 to 24 hr until bleeding is resolved. Jivi: Repeat every 24 to 48 hr until bleeding is resolved.
	Afstyla	20 to 40	See formula	Repeat every 12 to 24 hr until bleeding is resolved.
	Eloctate	40 to 60	20 to 30 IU/kg	Repeat every 24 to 48 hr (12 to 24 hr in patients under 6 years of age) until bleeding is resolved or healing is achieved.
	Helixate FS Kogenate FS	20 to 40	10 to 20 IU/kg	Repeat dose if there is evidence of further bleeding until bleeding is resolved.
	Koate DVI	20	10 IU/kg	May respond to a single dose. Repeat if there is evidence of further bleeding.
	Kovaltry Kovaltry Bio-Set	20 to 40	See formula	Repeat every 12 to 24 hr for at least 1 day until bleeding episode as indicated by pain is resolved or healing is achieved.
	Novoeight Recombinate Xyntha Hemofil M	20 to 40	See formula	Repeat every 12 to 24 hr for at least 1 day (usually 1 to 3 days) until bleeding is resolved or healing is achieved.
	Nuwiq	20 to 40	See formula	Repeat every 12 to 24 hr for at least 1 day until bleeding is resolved.

Continued

Control and Prevention of Bleeding Episodes—cont'd				
Degree of Bleeding	AHF Product	Required Peak Postinfusion Factor VIII Activity (as % of Normal or IU/dL)	Dose (IU/kg)	Frequency and Duration of Therapy
Moderate Moderate bleeding into muscle (except iliopsoas), bleeding into oral cavity, definite hemarthroses, and known trauma	Advate	30 to 60	15 to 30 IU/kg	Repeat every 12 to 24 hr (8 to 24 hr in patients under 6 years of age) for 3 days or more until bleeding is resolved or healing is achieved.
	Adynovate Jivi[a]	30 to 60	15 to 30 IU/kg	Adynovate: Repeat every 12 to 24 hr until bleeding is resolved. Jivi: Repeat every 24 to 48 hr until bleeding is resolved.
	Afstyla	30 to 60	See formula	Repeat every 12 to 24 hr until bleeding is resolved.
	Eloctate	40 to 60	20 to 30 IU/kg	Repeat every 24 to 48 hr (12 to 24 hr in patients under 6 years of age) until bleeding is resolved or healing is achieved.
	Helixate FS Kogenate FS	30 to 60	15 to 30 IU/kg	Repeat every 12 to 24 hr until bleeding is resolved.
	Koate DVI	30 to 50	Initial: 15 to 25 IU/kg Repeat: 10 to 15 IU/kg	Repeat with lower dose every 8 to 12 hr if needed until bleeding is resolved or healing is achieved.
	Kovaltry Kovaltry Bio-Set	30 to 60	See formula	Repeat every 12 to 24 hr for 3 to 4 days or more until pain and acute disability are resolved.
	Novoeight Recombinate Xyntha Hemofil M	30 to 60	See formula	Repeat every 12 to 24 hr until pain and acute disability are resolved and/or adequate local hemostasis is achieved (approximately 3 to 4 days).
	Nuwiq	30 to 60	See formula	Repeat every 12 to 24 hr for 3 to 4 days or more until bleeding is resolved.

Continued

Control and Prevention of Bleeding Episodes—cont'd				
Degree of Bleeding	AHF Product	Required Peak Postinfusion Factor VIII Activity (as % of Normal or IU/dL)	Dose (IU/kg)	Frequency and Duration of Therapy
Major/Life-Threatening Significant GI bleed; intracranial, intra-abdominal, or intrathoracic bleeding; CNS bleeding; limb-threatening hemorrhage; bleeding into retropharyngeal or retroperitoneal spaces or iliopsoas sheath or into eyes/retina; fractures; head trauma	Advate	60 to 100	30 to 50 IU/kg	Repeat every 8 to 24 hr (6 to 12 hr in patients under 6 years of age) for 3 days or more until bleeding is resolved or healing is achieved.
	Adynovate Jivi[a]	60 to 100	30 to 50 IU/kg	Every 8 to 12 hr until bleeding is resolved.
	Afstyla	60 to 100	See formula	Repeat every 8 to 24 hr until bleeding is resolved.
	Eloctate	80 to 100	40 to 50 IU/kg	Repeat every 12 to 24 hr (8 to 24 hr in patients under 6 years of age) until bleeding is resolved or healing is achieved (approximately 7 to 10 days).
	Helixate FS Kogenate FS	80 to 100	Initial: 40 to 50 IU/kg Repeat: 20 to 25 IU/kg	Every 8 to 12 hr until bleeding is resolved.
	Koate DVI	80 to 100	Initial: 40 to 50 IU/kg Repeat: 20 to 25 IU/kg	Every 8 to 12 hr until bleeding is resolved.
	Kovaltry Kovaltry Bio-Set	60 to 100	See formula	Repeat every 8 to 24 hr until bleeding is resolved.
	Novoeight Recombinate Xyntha Hemofil M	60 to 100	See formula	Repeat every 8 to 24 hr until bleeding is resolved (approximately 7 to 10 days).
	Nuwiq	60 to 100	See formula	Repeat every 8 to 24 hr until bleeding is resolved.

IU, International unit.

[a]Jivi: Total recommended maximum dose per infusion is approximately 6,000 IU (rounded to vial size).

Continued

Perioperative Management (Surgical Prophylaxis)			
Type of Surgery	AHF Product	Required Peak Postinfusion Factor VIII Activity (as % of Normal or IU/dL)	Dose, Frequency, and Duration of Therapy
Minor Including tooth extraction	Advate	60 to 100	A single bolus infusion (30 to 50 IU/kg) beginning within 1 hr of operation. Optional additional dosing every 12 to 24 hr as needed to control bleeding. For dental procedures, adjunctive therapy may be considered.
	Adynovate	60 to 100	A single bolus infusion (30 to 50 IU/kg) beginning within 1 hr of operation. Repeat after 24 hours if necessary. Single dose or repeat as needed until bleeding is resolved.
	Afstyla	30 to 60	See formula. Repeat every 24 hr for at least 1 day until healing is achieved.
	Eloctate	50 to 80	25 to 40 IU/kg. Repeat every 24 hr (12 to 24 hr in patients under 6 years of age). Continue for at least 1 day until healing is achieved.
	Jivi[a]	30 to 60 Preoperative and postoperative	15 to 30 IU/kg. Repeat every 24 hr for at least 1 day until healing is achieved.
	Helixate FS Kogenate FS	30 to 60	15 to 30 IU/kg. Repeat every 12 to 24 hr until bleeding is resolved.
	Koate DVI	Not listed	See Major. Less intensive treatment schedules may provide adequate hemostasis.
	Kovaltry Kovaltry Bio-Set	30 to 60 Preoperative and postoperative	See formula. Repeat every 24 hr for at least 1 day until healing is achieved.
	Novoeight	30 to 60	See formula. Repeat every 24 hr for at least 1 day until healing is achieved.
	Nuwiq	30 to 60 Preoperative and postoperative	See formula. Repeat dose every 24 hr. Continue at least 1 day until healing is achieved.
	Recombinate Hemofil M	60 to 80	See formula. A single infusion plus oral antifibrinolytic therapy within 1 hr is sufficient in approximately 70% of cases.
	Xyntha	30 to 60	See formula. Repeat every 12 to 24 hr for 3 to 4 days until adequate local hemostasis is achieved. For tooth extraction, a single infusion plus oral antifibrinolytic therapy within 1 hr may be sufficient.

Continued

	Perioperative Management (Surgical Prophylaxis)—cont'd		
Type of Surgery	AHF Product	Required Peak Postinfusion Factor VIII Activity (as % of Normal or IU/dL)	Dose, Frequency, and Duration of Therapy
Major Examples include intracranial, intraabdominal, or intrathoracic surgery, joint replacement surgery	Advate Adynovate	80 to 120 Preoperative and postoperative	Preoperative: 40 to 60 IU/kg. Verify 100% activity has been achieved before surgery. Maintenance: 40 to 60 IU/kg every 8 to 24 hr (6 to 24 hr in patients under 6 years of age [Advate] or under 12 years of age [Adynovate]) depending on desired level of factor VIII and state of wound healing.
	Afstyla	80 to 100	See formula. Repeat every 8 to 24 hr until adequate wound healing, then continue for at least another 7 days to maintain a factor VIII activity of 30% to 60% (IU/dL).
	Eloctate	80 to 120 Preoperative and postoperative	Preoperative: 40 to 60 IU/kg. Verify 100% activity has been achieved before surgery. Follow with a repeat dose of 40 to 50 IU/kg after 8 to 24 hr (6 to 24 hr in patients under 6 years of age) and then every 24 hr to maintain factor VIII activity within target range until adequate wound healing; then continue for at least 7 days to maintain factor VIII activity within target range.
	Jivi[a]	80 to 100 Preoperative and postoperative	40 to 50 IU/kg. Repeat every 12 to 24 hours until adequate wound healing is complete, then continue therapy for at least another 7 days to maintain a Factor VIII activity of 30% to 60% (IU/dL).
	Helixate FS Kogenate FS	100	50 IU/kg preoperatively to achieve 100% activity. Repeat every 6 to 12 hr to keep factor VIII activity in desired range. Continue until healing is achieved.
	Koate DVI	100	50 IU/kg. Verify 100% activity has been achieved before surgery. Repeat infusions every 6 to 12 hr initially and for a total of 10 to 14 days until healing is complete.
	Kovaltry Kovaltry Bio-Set	80 to 100 Preoperative and postoperative	See formula. Repeat every 8 to 24 hr until adequate wound healing is achieved, then continue for at least another 7 days to maintain factor VIII activity of 30% to 60% (IU/dL).
	Novoeight	80 to 100 Preoperative and postoperative	See formula. Continue every 8 to 24 hr until adequate wound healing. Continue at reduced dose for at least 7 days to maintain a factor VIII activity at 30% to 60% (IU/dL).

Continued

Perioperative Management (Surgical Prophylaxis)—cont'd			
Type of Surgery	AHF Product	Required Peak Postinfusion Factor VIII Activity (as % of Normal or IU/dL)	Dose, Frequency, and Duration of Therapy
Major Examples include intracranial, intraabdominal, or intrathoracic surgery, joint replacement surgery	Nuwiq	80 to 100 Preoperative and postoperative	See formula. Repeat dose every 8 to 24 hr until adequate wound healing, then continue therapy for at least another 7 days to maintain a factor VIII activity of 30% to 60% (IU/dL).
	Recombinate Hemofil M	80 to 100 Preoperative and postoperative	See formula. Continue every 8 to 24 hr depending on the state of wound healing.
	Xyntha	60 to 100	See formula. Continue every 8 to 24 hr until threat is resolved or, in the case of surgery, until adequate local hemostasis and wound healing are achieved.

IU, International unit.

[a]Jivi: Total recommended maximum dose per infusion is approximately 6,000 IU (rounded to vial size).

Obizur (porcine preparation): Obizur does not use a formula. **Indicated for use only in acquired hemophilia. Not indicated for use in congenital hemophilia A.** The recommended dose of Obizur for minor, moderate, and/or major bleeding is 200 IU/kg as an initial dose. Subsequent doses may be given every 4 to 12 hours and should be titrated to individual clinical response and to maintain recommended factor VIII trough levels (50% to 100% of normal for minor or moderate bleeding and 100% to 200% of normal for an acute bleed, decreasing to 50% to 100% of normal after acute bleed is controlled, if required). Maintain the factor VIII activity within the target range. Plasma levels of factor VIII should not exceed 200% of normal or 200 IU/dL.

Routine prophylaxis to prevent or reduce the frequency of bleeding (e.g., severe factor VIII deficiency with frequent hemorrhages):

Advate: 20 to 40 IU/kg every other day (3 to 4 times per week). Alternately, an everythird-day dosing regimen targeted to maintain factor VIII trough levels greater than or equal to 1% may be used. Adjust dose based on patient response.

Adynovate: *Adults and adolescents (12 years of age or older):* Administer 40 to 50 IU/kg 2 times per week. *Pediatric patients (under 12 years of age):* 55 IU/kg 2 times per week with a maximum of 70 IU/kg/dose. Adjust dose based on patient's clinical response.

Afstyla: *Adults and adolescents (12 years of age or older):* Recommended starting regimen is 20 to 50 IU/kg administered 2 to 3 times weekly. *Pediatric patients (under 12 years of age):* Recommended starting regimen is 30 to 50 IU/kg administered 2 to 3 times weekly. More frequent or higher doses may be required in pediatric patients under 12 years of age to account for the higher clearance in this age-group. Adjust dose based on patient's response.

Eloctate: Initiate therapy with a dose of 50 IU/kg every 4 days. Adjust dose based on patient response (range 25 to 65 IU/kg at 3- to 5-day intervals). More frequent or higher doses up to 80 IU/kg may be required in pediatric patients under 6 years of age.

Jivi: Initiate therapy at 30 to 40 IU/kg twice weekly. Based on bleeding episodes, the regimen may be adjusted to 45 to 60 IU/kg every 5 days. Regimen may be further individually adjusted to less or more frequent dosing. Total recommended maximum dose per infusion is approximately 6,000 IU (rounded to vial size).

Helixate FS and Kogenate FS: *Adults:* 25 IU/kg 3 times a week. *Pediatric patients:* 25 IU/kg every other day.

Kovaltry, Kovaltry Bio-Set: *Adults and adolescents:* 20 to 40 IU/kg 2 or 3 times a week. *Pediatric patients 12 years of age or younger:* 25 to 50 IU/kg twice weekly, 3 times weekly, or every other day according to individual requirements.

Novoeight: *Adults and adolescents (12 years of age or older):* 20 to 50 IU/kg 3 times a week or 20 to 40 IU/kg every other day. *Pediatric patients (under 12 years of age):* 25 to 60 IU/kg 3 times a week or 25 to 50 IU/kg every other day.

Nuwiq: *Adults and adolescents (12 to 17 years of age):* 30 to 40 IU/kg every other day. *Pediatric patients (2 to 11 years of age):* 30 to 50 IU/kg every other day or 3 times per week.

DOSE ADJUSTMENTS

Titrate the dose and frequency to the patient's clinical response. ▪ If factor VIII level fails to increase as expected or if bleeding is not controlled after administration of the calculated dose, factor VIII antibodies (inhibitors) are probable; may respond to an increased dose, especially if titer is less than 10 Bethesda units/mL. Frequent determinations of circulating AHF levels indicated. ▪ Higher or more frequent dosing may be required in pediatric patients.

DILUTION

Products are available in multiple strengths. Actual number of AHF units is shown on each vial. Consult package insert of product to obtain product-specific information on dilution. All preparations provide diluent, and most provide administration equipment that may include transfer devices, needles (single- or double-ended), filters or filter needles, syringes, vial adapters, and/or administration sets for each vial. Use only the diluent provided, and maintain strict aseptic technique. Warm to room temperature (25° C [77° F]) before dilution and maintain throughout administration to avoid precipitation of active ingredients. If more than one vial is required to achieve the desired dose, multiple vials may be drawn into the same container (e.g., syringe). Follow manufacturer's instructions. Products do not contain a preservative, and all products must be used within 3 hours of reconstitution (4 hours for Afstyla and Novoeight).

Filters: Supplied by manufacturer if required.

Storage: Consult package insert of product to obtain product-specific information on storage requirements after reconstitution. Before reconstitution, store all formulations in original packages to protect from light at 2° to 8° C (35° to 46° F). (Recombinate may be stored at RT or under refrigeration.) Do not freeze. **All formulations except Adynovate and Obizur** can be stored at RT for 2 months or longer before reconstitution. **Adynovate** can be stored at RT for up to 1 month. Do not return to the refrigerator after storage at RT. **Afstyla** can be stored at RT, not to exceed 25° C (77° F), for a single period of up to 3 months (within the expiration date on carton and vial labels). Do not return product to the refrigerator. **Jivi** can be stored at RT for up to 6 months. Do not return to the refrigerator after storage at RT. **Obizur** should be refrigerated until use. Do not use beyond expiration dates on vials (or revised expiration date if stored at RT, whichever is earlier).

COMPATIBILITY

Administration through a separate line without mixing with other IV fluids or medications is recommended.

RATE OF ADMINISTRATION

Use administration set supplied by manufacturer, if provided. Rate of administration is based on patient comfort. Reduce rate of infusion or temporarily discontinue if there is a significant increase in heart rate or if S/S of hypersensitivity occur.

Advate, Adynovate: A single dose over 5 minutes or less. Do not exceed a rate of 10 mL/min.

Afstyla, Eloctate, Hemofil M: A single dose administered at a rate not to exceed 10 mL/min.

Jivi: A single dose administered over 1 to 15 minutes. Maximum infusion rate is 2.5 mL/min.

Helixate FS, Kogenate FS, Kogenate FS Bio-Set, Kovaltry, Kovaltry Bio-Set: A single dose over 1 to 15 minutes is usually well tolerated.

Koate-DVI: A single dose over 5 to 10 minutes.

Novoeight: A single dose over 2 to 5 minutes.

Nuwiq: A single dose at a maximum rate of 4 mL/min.

Obizur: A single dose at a rate of 1 to 2 mL/min.

Recombinate (reconstituted with 5 mL of SWFI): Do not exceed a rate of 5 mL/min.
Recombinate (reconstituted with 10 mL SWFI): Do not exceed a rate of 10 mL/min.
Xyntha, Xyntha Solofuse: A single dose over several minutes, based on patient comfort.

ACTIONS

AHF is one of nine major factors in the blood that must act in sequence to produce co-agulation, or clotting. It is the specific clotting factor deficient in patients with hemo-philia A (classic hemophilia). Administration of AHF can temporarily correct the coagu-lation defect in these patients. One international unit (IU) of AHF is approximately equal to the level of factor VIII activity in 1 mL of fresh pooled human plasma. **Adynovate** and **Jivi** exhibit an extended terminal half-life through pegylation, which reduces binding to the physiologic factor VIII clearance receptor (LRP1). **Afstyla** is expressed as a single-chain factor VIII molecule with covalent linkage between heavy and light chains, keep-ing the molecule in the single-chain form and resulting in increased stability and in-creased von Willebrand factor (vWF) affinity. vWF stabilizes factor VIII and protects it from degradation.

Recombinant porcine sequence AHF (Obizur): Patients with acquired hemophilia have nor-mal factor VIII genes but develop autoantibodies against their own factor VIII (i.e., in-hibitors). These autoantibodies neutralize circulating human factor VIII and create a functional deficiency of factor VIII. Obizur temporarily replaces the inhibited endoge-nous factor VIII that is needed for effective hemostasis in patients with acquired hemo-philia A.

INDICATIONS AND USES

On-demand treatment and control of bleeding episodes in adults and pediatric patients with hemophilia A (congenital factor VIII deficiency) **(all products *except* Jivi and Obizur)**.
▪ Perioperative management (surgical prophylaxis) in adults and pediatric patients with hemophilia A **(all products *except* Jivi and Obizur).** ▪ Routine prophylaxis to prevent or reduce the frequency of bleeding in adults and pediatric patients with hemophilia A **(Advate, Adynovate, Afstyla, Eloctate, Helixate FS, Kogenate FS, Kovaltry, Kovaltry Bio-Set, No-voeight, Nuwiq).** ▪ Routine prophylaxis to prevent bleeding episodes and risk of joint damage in pediatric patients without pre-existing joint damage **(Helixate FS, Kogenate FS).**
▪ On-demand treatment and control of bleeding episodes, perioperative management of bleeding, and routine prophylaxis to reduce the frequency of bleeding episodes in ado-lescent and adult patients (12 years and older) with hemophilia A **(Jivi).** ▪ Treatment of bleeding episodes in adults with *acquired hemophilia A (Obizur).*

Limitations of use: *All products:* Not indicated for treatment of von Willebrand disease.
Jivi: Jivi is not indicated for use in pediatric patients under 12 years of age due to greater risk for hypersensitivity reactions. ▪ **Jivi** is not indicated for use in previously untreated patients.

Obizur: Safety and efficacy of **Obizur** have not been established in patients with a baseline anti-porcine factor VIII inhibitor titer of greater than 20 Bethesda units. ▪ **Obizur is not indicated for treatment of congenital hemophilia A.**

CONTRAINDICATIONS

All products: Hypersensitivity to the specific product or to any component of a product (e.g., mouse, hamster, or bovine protein [monoclonal antibody–derived factor VIII, por-cine sequence]; various stabilizers; polysorbate 80; polyethylene glycol [PEG]).

PRECAUTIONS

Should be administered under the direction of a physician specialist. ▪ Hypersensitivity reactions (including anaphylaxis) are possible. ▪ Formation of neutralizing antibodies (inhibitors) to factor VIII can occur; see Monitor. ▪ In patients receiving **Jivi,** a clinical immune response associated with IgM anti-PEG antibodies (manifested as symptoms of acute hypersensitivity and/or loss of drug effect) has been observed, primarily in patients under 6 years of age. Symptoms of the clinical immune response were transient, and anti-PEG IgM titers decreased over time to undetectable levels. In cases of clinical sus-picion of loss of drug effect, conduct testing for Factor VIII inhibitors. A low post-infusion Factor VIII level in the absence of detectable Factor VIII inhibitors indicates that loss of drug effect is likely due to anti-PEG antibodies. Discontinue **Jivi** and switch patient to a previously effective Factor VIII product. ▪ Plasma-derived products may contain infectious agents that can cause disease (e.g., viruses and, theoretically, the Creutzfeldt-Jakob disease agent). The risk that these products will transmit an infectious agent has been reduced by screening plasma donors, testing for the presence of viruses, and inactivating and/or removing certain viruses during manufacturing. Hepatitis A and parvovirus 19 have been reported infrequently with plasma-based products, usually in immunocompromised patients or pregnant females. ▪ Intravascular hemolysis can occur when large volumes of plasma-derived products are given to individuals with blood groups A, B, or AB. Monitor for progressive anemia. ▪ Components of some products may contain latex; use caution to avoid a hypersensitivity reaction. ▪ Hemophilic patients with cardiovascular risk factors or diseases may be at the same risk as nonhemophilic patients for developing cardiovascular events when clotting has been normalized by treatment with factor VIII. ▪ Treatment of choice when volume or RBC replacement is not needed; avoids hypervolemia and hyperproteinemia. ▪ Not useful to treat other coagulation factor deficiencies. ▪ Catheter-related infections may occur if antihemophilic factor is administered via central venous access devices (CVADs). These infections have not been associated with the actual AHF product. ▪ Desmopressin may be the preferred treatment for mild to moderate hemophilia A (AHF levels that are at least 5%).

Monitor: *All products:* Identification of factor VIII deficiency with determination of circulating AHF levels should be obtained before administration. Monitor plasma factor VIII activity by the one-stage clotting assay (except **Afstyla** and **Jivi** [see below]) to confirm that adequate factor VIII levels have been achieved and maintained. Adjust dose as indicated. ▪ Monitor heart rate and blood pressure before and during treatment. ▪ Monitor for the development of factor VIII inhibitors. Should be suspected if factor VIII plasma levels are not obtained or if bleeding is not controlled with an appropriate dose. The Bethesda inhibitor assay determines if factor VIII inhibitors are present. Bethesda Units (BU) are used to report inhibitor levels. ▪ Monitor patients with a known or suspected inhibitor to factor VIII more frequently. ▪ Monitor for S/S of a hypersensitivity reaction (e.g., anaphylaxis, angioedema, chest or throat tightness, dizziness, dyspnea, face swelling, fever, flushing, hypotension, laryngeal edema, nausea, paresthesia, pruritus, rash, tachycardia, urticaria, vomiting, wheezing). ▪ Monitor for signs of bleeding. ▪ Monitor hemoglobin and hematocrit. ▪ Monitor patients with CVADs for S/S of infection. ▪ See Precautions.

Afstyla: Monitoring of plasma factor VIII levels by a chromogenic assay is preferred over the one-stage clotting assay routinely used in U.S. clinical laboratories (most accurately reflects the clinical hemostatic potential of Afstyla). The one-stage clotting assay result underestimates the factor VIII activity level compared with the chromogenic assay result by approximately one-half. *If the one-stage clotting assay is used, multiply the result by a conversion factor of 2 to determine the patient's factor VIII activity level.*

Jivi: Monitor the Factor VIII activity of Jivi in plasma using either a validated chromogenic substrate assay or a validated one-stage clotting assay. Validation required to prevent underestimation or overestimation of Factor VIII activity; see manufacturer's prescribing information.

Obizur: Monitor factor VIII activity 30 minutes and 3 hours after initial dose and 30 minutes after subsequent doses. Use of the Nijmegen-Bethesda inhibitor assay is recommended.

Patient Education: *All products:* Read manufacturer-supplied patient product information. ▪ Instruction for self-administration and proper storage and preparation may be appropriate. ▪ Discontinue antihemophilic factor and immediately report S/S of a hypersensitivity reaction (e.g., hives, hypotension, itching, rash, tightness of the chest, wheezing). ▪ Review prescription and nonprescription medications with a healthcare provider. ▪ Contact provider for lack of clinical response. May indicate development of inhibitors. ▪ Consult with healthcare provider before travel. Bring an adequate supply of AHF based on current treatment regimen.

Plasma-derived products: Report S/S of hepatitis A (e.g., persistent poor appetite and tiredness, fever, dark urine, yellowing of the skin, nausea, vomiting, and abdominal pain). ▪ Report S/S of parvovirus B19 (e.g., chills, drowsiness, fever, and runny nose followed 2 weeks later by a rash and joint pain).

Maternal/Child: Use during pregnancy only if clearly needed. ▪ Use caution during breast-feeding. ▪ Advate, Afstyla, Helixate FS, Kogenate FS, Kovaltry, Kovaltry Bio-Set, and Recombinate have been used in pediatric patients of all ages, including infants. Other formulations are indicated for use in pediatric patients but did not include newborns in clinical trials. ▪ *All products:* Clearance (based on kg body weight) is higher in the pediatric population. Half-life is shorter; see Dose Adjustments. ▪ *Jivi:* Safety and effectiveness in pediatric patients under 12 years of age has not been established. Jivi is not indicated in this age-group. Adverse reactions due to immune response to PEG, including hypersensitivity reactions and/or loss of drug effect, have been observed; see Precautions. ▪ *Obizur:* Safety and efficacy for use in pediatric patients not established.

Elderly: Numbers in clinical studies insufficient to determine whether the elderly respond differently from younger subjects.

DRUG/LAB INTERACTIONS
Specific information not available.

SIDE EFFECTS
May respond to reduced rate of administration. Serious adverse reactions include hypersensitivity reactions and factor VIII inhibitors.

Plasma-based AHF: Abdominal pain, blurred vision, bradycardia, chills, clouding or loss of consciousness, diarrhea, dizziness, dysgeusia, factor VIII inhibition, fever, flushing, headache, hemolytic anemia, hyperfibrinogenemia, hypersensitivity reactions (anaphylaxis, backache, chills, erythema, fever, hives, hypotension, nausea, pruritus, rash, tightness of chest, urticaria, wheezing), lethargy, paresthesias, somnolence, stinging at infusion site, tachycardia, tingling, or vomiting may occur.

Recombinant products: The most commonly reported side effects included arthralgia, back pain, central venous access device–associated infections, chills, cough, dizziness, dry mouth, epistaxis, fever, flushing, headache, increased hepatic enzymes, infusion site reactions (e.g., inflammation, pain), inhibitor formation in previously untreated or minimally treated patients, limb injury, malaise, nasopharyngitis, nausea, nonneutralizing anti–factor VIII antibody formation, paresthesia, skin-associated hypersensitivity reactions (e.g., erythema, pruritus, rash, urticaria), and generalized hypersensitivity reactions, including anaphylaxis.

Obizur: In clinical trials, development of inhibitors to porcine factor VIII occurred in more than 5% of patients.

Jivi: Anti-PEG antibodies.

ANTIDOTE
Most side effects usually subside spontaneously in 15 to 20 minutes and are generally related to the rate of infusion. Keep the physician informed. Slow or discontinue infusion temporarily if heart rate increases or beginning S/S of a hypersensitivity reaction occur. Discontinue immediately and treat hypersensitivity reactions (antihistamines, epinephrine, corticosteroids). Premedication with antihistamines (e.g., diphenhydramine) may be considered for patients with previous hypersensitivity reactions. Resuscitate as necessary.

ANTIHEMOPHILIC FACTOR ▪ VON WILLEBRAND FACTOR COMPLEX (HUMAN)

(an-tie-hee-moe-**FIL**-ik **FAK**-tor)

Antihemorrhagic

Alphanate, Humate-P

USUAL DOSE

(International units [IU])

Pretreatment: See Precautions.

Completely individualized. Based on degree of deficiency, desired antihemophilic factor level, body weight, severity of bleeding, and presence of factor VIII inhibitors. One international unit (IU) of factor VIII or 1 IU of von Willebrand factor:Ristocetin Cofactor (vWF:RCof) is approximately equal to the level of factor VIII activity or vWF:RCof found in 1 mL of fresh pooled human plasma.

ALPHANATE

Treatment of hemophilia A (adults): Dose requirements and frequency are calculated on the basis of an expected initial response of 2% of normal FVIII:C IU/kg of body weight administered. Assess adequacy of treatment by clinical effects and monitoring of factor VIII activity. See Precautions. The following general dosages are recommended for adult patients:

Alphanate Dose Guidelines for the Treatment of Adults With Hemophilia A	
Hemorrhagic Event	**Dosage (AHF FVIII:C IU/kg body weight)**
Minor hemorrhage: Bruises, cuts, or scrapes or uncomplicated joint hemorrhage	FVIII:C levels should be brought to 30% of normal (15 FVIII IU/kg twice daily) until hemorrhage stops and healing has been achieved (1 to 2 days).
Moderate hemorrhage: Nose, mouth, and gum bleeds; dental extractions; hematuria	FVIII:C levels should be brought to 50% (25 FVIII IU/kg twice daily). Continue until healing has been achieved (2 to 7 days on average).
Major hemorrhage: Joint or muscle hemorrhage, major trauma, hematuria, intracranial and/or intraperitoneal bleeding	FVIII:C levels should be brought to 80% to 100% of normal for at least 3 to 5 days (40 to 50 FVIII IU/kg twice daily). Then maintain at 50% (25 FVIII IU/kg twice daily) until healing has been achieved. May require treatment for up to 10 days.
Surgery	Before surgery, FVIII:C levels should be brought to 80% to 100% of normal (40 to 50 FVIII IU/kg twice daily). For the next 7 to 10 days or until healing has been achieved, patient should be maintained at 60% to 100% FVIII levels (25 to 50 FVIII IU/kg twice daily).

IU, International unit.

Continued

Alphanate Dose Guidelines for Prophylaxis During Surgery and Invasive Procedures of Adult and Pediatric Patients With von Willebrand Disease (Except Type 3 Patients Undergoing Surgery)	
Bleeding Prophylaxis for Surgical or Invasive Procedures	Dosage (AHF vWF:RCof IU/kg body weight)
Adult	Preoperative dose: 60 vWF:RCof IU/kg body weight. Subsequent infusions: 40 to 60 vWF:RCof IU/kg body weight at 8- to 12-hour intervals as clinically needed. Dosing may be reduced after the third postoperative day. Continue treatment until healing is complete.
Adult	**Minor procedure:** vWF activity of 40% to 50% for at least 1 to 3 days postoperatively.
Adult	**Major procedure:** vWF activity of 40% to 50% for at least 3 to 7 days postoperatively.
Pediatric	Initial dose: 75 vWF:RCof IU/kg body weight. Subsequent infusions: 50 to 75 vWF:RCof IU/kg body weight at 8- to 12-hour intervals as clinically needed. Dosing may be reduced after the third postoperative day. Continue treatment until healing is complete.

IU, International unit.

♣HUMATE-P

Treatment of hemophilia A (adults): As a general rule, 1 IU of factor VIII activity per kg body weight will increase the circulating factor VIII level by approximately 2 IU/dL. Assess adequacy of treatment by clinical effects and monitoring of factor VIII activity. See Precautions. The following general dosages are recommended for adult patients:

Humate-P Dose Recommendations for the Treatment of Hemophilia A[a]	
Hemorrhage Event	Dosage (IU[b] FVIII:C/kg body weight)
Minor • Early joint or muscle bleed • Severe epistaxis	Loading dose 15 IU FVIII:C/kg to achieve FVIII:C plasma level of approximately 30% of normal; one infusion may be sufficient. If needed, half of the loading dose may be given once or twice daily for 1-2 days.
Moderate • Advanced joint or muscle bleed • Neck, tongue, or pharyngeal hematoma without airway compromise • Tooth extraction • Severe abdominal pain	Loading dose 25 IU FVIII:C/kg to achieve FVIII:C plasma level of approximately 50% of normal. Followed by 15 IU FVIII:C/kg every 8-12 hours for first 1-2 days to maintain FVIII:C plasma level at 30% of normal. Then same dose once or twice a day for up to 7 days or until adequate wound healing.
Life-threatening • Major operations • Gastrointestinal bleeding • Neck, tongue, or pharyngeal hematoma with potential for airway compromise • Intracranial, intra-abdominal, or intrathoracic bleeding • Fractures	Initially 40-50 IU FVIII:C/kg. Followed by 20-25 IU FVIII:C/kg every 8 hours to maintain FVIII:C plasma level at 80%-100% of normal for 7 days. Then continue the same dose once or twice a day for another 7 days to maintain the FVIII:C level at 30%-50% of normal.

[a]In all cases, the dose should be adjusted individually by clinical judgment of the potential for compromise of a vital structure and by frequent monitoring of factor VIII activity in the patient's plasma.
[b]*IU*, International unit.

Treatment of von Willebrand Disease (vWD) (adults and pediatric patients): As a rule, 40 to 80 IU vWF:RCof (corresponding to 16 to 32 IU factor VIII in Humate-P) per kg body weight given every 8 to 12 hours. Repeat doses are administered as needed based on monitoring of appropriate clinical and laboratory measures. Expected levels of vWF:RCof are based on an expected in vivo recovery of 1.5 IU/dL rise per IU/kg vWF:RCof administered. The administration of 1 IU of factor VIII per kg body weight can be expected to lead to a rise in circulating vWF:RCof of approximately 3.5 to 4 IU/dL. The following general dosages are recommended for adult and pediatric patients:

Humate-P Dose Recommendations for Treatment of von Willebrand Disease in Adult and Pediatric Patients		
Classification	**Hemorrhage**	**Dosage (IU[a] vWF:RCof/kg body weight)**
TYPE 1		
Mild *(Where use of desmopressin is known or suspected to be inadequate)* Baseline vWF:RCof activity typically >30% of normal (i.e., >30 IU/dL)	**Major (examples)** • Severe or refractory epistaxis • GI bleeding • CNS trauma • Traumatic hemorrhage	Loading dose 40 to 60 IU/kg. Then 40 to 50 IU/kg every 8 to 12 hours for 3 days to keep the nadir level of vWF:RCof >50% of normal (i.e., >50 IU/dL). Then 40 to 50 IU/kg daily for a total of up to 7 days of treatment.
Moderate or Severe Baseline vWF:RCof activity typically <30% of normal (i.e., <30 IU/dL)	**Minor (examples)** • Epistaxis • Oral bleeding • Menorrhagia	40 to 50 IU/kg (1 or 2 doses)
	Major (examples) • Severe or refractory epistaxis • GI bleeding • CNS trauma • Hemarthrosis • Traumatic hemorrhage	Loading dose of 50 to 75 IU/kg Then 40 to 60 IU/kg every 8 to 12 hours for 3 days to keep the nadir level of vWF:RCof >50% of normal (i.e., >50 IU/dL) Then 40 to 60 IU/kg daily for a total of up to 7 days of treatment *Factor VIII:C levels should be monitored and maintained according to the guidelines for hemophilia A therapy.*[b]
TYPE 2 (ALL VARIANTS) AND TYPE 3		
	Minor (clinical indications above)	40 to 50 IU/kg (1 or 2 doses)
	Major (clinical indications above)	Loading dose of 60 to 80 IU/kg Then 40 to 60 IU/kg every 8 to 12 hours for 3 days to keep the nadir level of vWF:RCof >50% of normal (i.e., >50 IU/dL) Then 40 to 60 IU/kg daily for a total of up to 7 days of treatment *Factor VIII:C levels should be monitored and maintained according to the guidelines for hemophilia A therapy.*[b]

[a]*IU,* International unit.
[b]In instances where both FVIII and vWF levels must be monitored.

Prevention of excessive bleeding during and after surgery in vWD: In the case of emergency surgery, administer a loading dose of 50 to 60 IU/kg Humate-P and closely monitor the patient's trough coagulation factor levels. Measurement of incremental in vivo recovery (IVR) and assessment of baseline plasma vWF:RCof and FVIII:C levels are recommended in all patients before surgery. As shown in the following charts, calculation of the loading dose requires four values: the target peak plasma vWF:RCof level, the baseline vWF:RCof level, body weight (BW) in kilograms, and IVR. If individual recovery values are not available, a standardized loading dose can be used based on an assumed vWF:RCof IVR of 2 IU/dL per IU/kg of vWF:RCof product administered.

Continued

vWF:RCof and FVIII:C Humate-P Loading Dose Recommendations for the Prevention of Excessive Bleeding During and After Surgery			
Type of Surgery	vWF:RCof Target Peak Plasma Level	FVIII:C Target Peak Plasma Level	Calculation of Loading Dose (to be administered 1 to 2 hours before surgery)
Major	100 IU/dL	80 to 100 IU/dL	Δ^a vWF:RCof × BW (kg)/IVR^b = IU vWF:RCof required. If incremental IVR is not available, assume an IVR of 2 IU/dL per IU/kg and calculate the loading dose as follows: (100 − Baseline plasma vWF:RCof) × BW (kg)/2. In the case of emergency surgery, administer a dose of 50 to 60 IU/kg.
Minor/oral ^{c}	50 to 60 IU/dL	40 to 50 IU/dL	Δ^a vWF:RCof × BW (kg)/IVR^b = IU vWF:RCof required.

IU, International unit.

$^a\Delta$ = Target peak plasma vWF:RCof − Baseline plasma vWF:RCof.

^{b}IVR = Incremental recovery as measured in the patient.

^{c}Oral surgery is defined as removal of fewer than three teeth, if the teeth are nonmolars and have no bony involvement. Removal of more than one impacted wisdom tooth is considered major surgery due to the expected difficulty of the surgery and the expected blood loss, particularly in subjects with type 2A or type 3 vWD. Removal of more than two teeth is considered major surgery in all patients.

vWF:RCof and FVIII:C Target Trough Plasma Level and Minimum Duration of Treatment Recommendations for Subsequent Maintenance Doses of Humate-P for the Prevention of Excessive Bleeding During and After Surgery					
Type of Surgery	vWF:RCof Target Trough Plasma Levels^a		FVIII:C Target Trough Plasma Levels^a		Minimum Duration of Treatment
	Up to 3 Days Following Surgery	After Day 3	Up to 3 Days Following Surgery	After Day 3	
Major	>50 IU/dL	>30 IU/dL	>50 IU/dL	>30 IU/dL	72 hours
Minor	≥30 IU/dL	—	—	>30 IU/dL	48 hours
Oral^b	≥30 IU/dL	—	—	>30 IU/dL	8 to 12 hours^c

IU, International unit.

^{a}Trough levels for either coagulation factor should not exceed 100 IU/dL.

^{b}See note on oral surgery in previous chart.

^{c}At least one maintenance dose following surgery based on individual pharmacokinetic values.

PEDIATRIC DOSE

Treatment of hemophilia A (unlabeled): For immediate control of bleeding, follow the general recommendations for dosing and administration for adults. See Usual Dose and Maternal/Child.

DOSE ADJUSTMENTS

Adjust subsequent doses based on FVIII:C plasma level achieved or as outlined in specific charts.

DILUTION

Consult individual product instructions in the package insert; each product has a specific process for dilution. Information may be updated frequently. **Alphanate** provides diluent, a double-ended transfer needle, and a microaggregate filter for use in administration. **Humate-P** provides diluent and a filter transfer set.

Alphanate and Humate-P: Actual number of AHF units is shown on each vial. Use only the diluent provided and maintain strict aseptic technique. Use a plastic syringe to prevent binding to glass surfaces. Warm to room temperature (25° C [77° F]) before dilution and maintain throughout administration to avoid precipitation of active ingredients.

Filters: Filters supplied by manufacturer; see Dilution.

Storage: *Alphanate:* Refrigerate before use. Avoid freezing. May be stored at CRT for up to 2 months. Label vial with date removed from refrigeration. *Humate-P:* Store up to 25° C (up to 77° F). Avoid freezing. *Alphanate and Humate-P:* Do not refrigerate after reconstitution. Confirm expiration date on vial. Administer within 3 hours of reconstitution to ensure sterility. Discard any unused solution.

COMPATIBILITY

Compatibility information not available from manufacturer. Administration through a separate line without mixing with other IV fluids or medications is generally recommended for these products; consult a pharmacist.

RATE OF ADMINISTRATION

Inject solution slowly. Rapid administration may result in vasomotor reactions.

Humate-P recommends a maximum rate of 4 mL/min.

Alphanate recommends a maximum rate not to exceed 10 mL/min.

ACTIONS

A purified, sterile, lyophilized concentrate of antihemophilic factor (factor VIII) and von Willebrand Factor (vWF). Factor VIII is an essential cofactor in the activation of factor X, leading ultimately to the formation of thrombin and fibrin. It is the specific clotting factor deficient in patients with hemophilia A (classic hemophilia). vWF is important for correcting the coagulation defect in patients with von Willebrand disease (vWD). It promotes platelet aggregation and platelet adhesion on damaged vascular endothelium and acts as a stabilizing carrier protein for the procoagulant protein factor VIII. vWF activity is measured with an assay that uses an agglutinating cofactor called Ristocetin (RCof). The vWF:RCof assay provides a quantitative measurement of vWF function by determining how well vWF helps platelets adhere to one another. Reduced vWF:RCof activity indicates a deficiency of vWF. Following administration of FVIII/vWF, there is a rapid increase of plasma factor VIII activity, followed by a rapid decrease in activity and then a slower rate of decrease in activity. The mean initial half-life in hemophilic patients is 8.3 to 27.5 hours with Alphanate and 12.2 hours (range: 8.4 to 17.4 hours) with Humate-P. In patients with vWD, bleeding time decreases. Antihemophilic factor/von Willebrand Factor Complex is obtained from pooled human fresh frozen plasma. Multiple methods of purification are used to inactivate infectious agents, including viruses.

INDICATIONS AND USES

ALPHANATE

Prevention and control of bleeding in patients with factor VIII deficiency due to hemophilia A or acquired factor VIII deficiency. ▪ Prophylaxis for surgical and/or invasive procedures in adult and pediatric patients with von Willebrand disease (vWD) (type 1 or 2) in which the use of desmopressin is either ineffective or contraindicated. ▪ Not indicated for patients with severe vWD (type 3).

HUMATE-P

Treatment and prevention of bleeding in adult patients with hemophilia A. ▪ Treatment of spontaneous and trauma-induced bleeding episodes and prevention of excessive bleeding during and after surgery in adult and pediatric patients with severe vWD or with mild or moderate vWD in which the use of desmopressin is known or suspected to be inadequate. ▪ Safety and efficacy of prophylactic dosing to prevent spontaneous bleeding and to prevent excessive bleeding related to surgery have not been established in patients with vWD.

CONTRAINDICATIONS

ALPHANATE: None known when used as indicated.

HUMATE-P: History of anaphylactic or severe systemic response to AHF-vWF preparations or known hypersensitivity to any of its components.

PRECAUTIONS

ALPHANATE AND HUMATE-P: For IV use only. ▪ Important to establish that coagulation disorder is caused by factor VIII or vWF deficiency. Not useful in treatment of other deficiencies. ▪ Healthcare professionals should use caution during administration; may have risk of exposure to viral infection. ▪ Manufactured from human plasma. Risk of transmitting infectious agents (e.g., HIV, hepatitis and, theoretically, Creutzfeldt-Jakob disease) has been greatly reduced by screening, testing, and manufacturing techniques. However, risk of transmission cannot be totally eliminated. ▪ Hepatitis A and B vaccines are recommended for patients receiving plasma derivatives. ▪ Thrombotic events have been reported. Use caution in patients with known risk factors for thrombosis. Incidence may be higher in females. ▪ Inhibitors may develop with large or frequent doses; see Monitor.

Monitor: Complex contains blood group isoagglutinins (anti-A and anti-B). When very large or frequently repeated doses are needed, as when inhibitors are present or when presurgical and postsurgical care is involved, patients of blood groups A, B, and AB should be monitored for signs of intravascular hemolysis and decreasing hematocrit values; see Antidote. ▪ Replacement therapy should be monitored by appropriate coagulation tests, especially in cases involving major surgery. Monitor factor VIII and vWF:RCof as indicated in dosing guidelines.

Patient Education: Prophylactic hepatitis A and hepatitis B vaccines recommended. ▪ Report symptoms of possibly transmitted viral infections immediately. Symptoms may include anorexia, arthralgias, fatigue, jaundice, low-grade fever, nausea, or vomiting. ▪ Report rash or any other sign of hypersensitivity reaction promptly.

Maternal/Child: Category C: use only if clearly needed. ▪ Adequate and well-controlled studies with long-term evaluation of joint damage have not been done in pediatric patients. Joint damage may result from suboptimal treatment of hemarthroses. ▪ Safety and effectiveness for use in neonates with vWD have not been established. Has been used safely in infants, children, and adolescents with vWD.

Elderly: Numbers insufficient to determine differences in response compared with younger adults. Consider overall status in dosing.

DRUG/LAB INTERACTIONS
Specific information not available.

SIDE EFFECTS
ALPHANATE AND HUMATE-P: Usually well tolerated. Rare cases of hypersensitivity reactions, including anaphylaxis, have been reported (symptoms may include chest tightness, edema, fever, pruritus, rash, throat tightness). Other reported side effects include chills, headache, lethargy, nausea and vomiting, paresthesia, phlebitis, somnolence, and vasodilation. Inhibitors of factor VIII may occur.

Post-Marketing: *Alphanate:* In addition to the above, cardiac arrest, femoral venous thrombosis, flushing, itching, joint pain, pulmonary embolus, seizure, shortness of breath, swelling of the parotid gland, urticaria. *Humate-P:* Hypersensitivity reactions (including anaphylaxis), development of inhibitors to factor VIII, hemolysis, hypervolemia, thromboembolic complications.

ANTIDOTE
Keep physician informed of all side effects. If mild reactions occur (mild allergic reaction, chills, nausea, or stinging at the infusion site) and additional treatment is indicated, a product from a different lot should be considered. Discontinue immediately at first sign of a moderate to severe hypersensitivity reaction. Treat as necessary (antihistamines, epinephrine, corticosteroids). Development of acute hemolytic anemia, increased bleeding tendency, or hyperfibrinogenemia may require transfusion with Type O red blood cells. Discontinue administration of Alphanate/Humate-P and consider alternative therapy. Resuscitate as necessary.

ANTITHROMBIN III (HUMAN)

(an-tie-**THROM**-bin)

Anticoagulant
Antithrombotic

AT-III, Thrombate III

pH 6.5 to 7.5

USUAL DOSE

Pretreatment: See Precautions.

Antithrombin III: Loading dose, maintenance dose, and dosing intervals are completely individualized based on confirmed diagnosis (see Precautions), patient weight, clinical condition, degree of deficiency, type of surgery or procedure involved, physician judgment, desired level of antithrombin III (AT-III), and actual plasma levels achieved as verified by appropriate lab tests. One unit/kg should raise the level of AT-III by 1.4%. The desired AT-III level after the first dose should be about 120% of normal (normal is 0.1 to 0.2 Gm/L). AT-III levels must be maintained at normal or at least above 80% of normal for 2 to 8 days depending on individual patient factors. Usually achieved by administration of a maintenance dose once daily. Concomitant administration of heparin usually indicated; see Drug/Lab Interactions.

Calculate the initial loading dose using the following formula (assumes a plasma volume of 40 mL/kg):

$$\text{Dosage units } = \frac{(\text{Desired AT-III level } [\%] - \text{Baseline AT-III } [\%]) \times \text{Body weight (kg)}}{\div 1.4\%}$$

For a 70-kg patient with a baseline AT-III level of 57% the initial dose of Thrombate III would be $(120\% - 57\%) \times 70 \div 1.4 = 3{,}150$ International units (IU). Measurement of plasma levels is suggested pre-infusion, 20 minutes postinfusion (peak), 12 hours postinfusion, and preceding next infusion (trough). If recovery differs from the anticipated rise of 1.4% for each IU/kg, modify the formula accordingly. If the above patient has a 20-minute AT-III level of 147%, the increase in AT-III measured for each 1 IU/kg administered is $(147\% - 57\%) \times 70 \text{ kg} \div 3{,}150 \text{ IU} = 2\%$ rise for each IU/kg administered. This in vivo recovery would be used to calculate future doses. A maintenance dose of approximately 60% of the loading dose every 24 hours is the average required to maintain plasma levels between 80% and 120%. Dose and interval based on plasma levels.

DOSE ADJUSTMENTS

See Drug/Lab Interactions.

DILUTION

Diluent, double-ended needles for dilution, and filter needle for aspiration into a syringe are provided. Warm unopened diluent and concentrate to room temperature. Enter diluent bottle with double-ended transfer needle first. Enter vacuum concentrate bottle with double-ended transfer needle at a 45-degree angle. Direct diluent from above to sides of vial to gently moisten all contents. Remove diluent bottle and transfer needle; swirl continuously until completely dissolved. Draw into a syringe through the filter needle. Remove filter needle; replace with an administration set (not provided). For larger doses, several bottles may be drawn into one syringe. Use a separate filter needle for each bottle.

Filters: Filter needle supplied by manufacturer; see Dilution. For larger doses, several bottles may be drawn into one syringe. Use a separate filter needle for each bottle.

Storage: Store in refrigerator before dilution; avoid freezing. Do not refrigerate after reconstitution. Use within 3 hours of reconstitution.

Continued

COMPATIBILITY

Administration through a separate line without mixing with other IV fluids or medications is recommended.

RATE OF ADMINISTRATION

Too-rapid injection may cause dyspnea.

A single dose over 10 to 20 minutes.

ACTIONS

Manufactured from human plasma, purified and heat treated through specific processes, AT-III is a plasma-based protein produced by the body to inactivate specific clotting proteins and control clot formation. Identical to heparin cofactor I, a factor in plasma necessary for heparin to exert its anticoagulant effect. It inactivates thrombin and the activated forms of factors IX, X, XI, and XII (all coagulation enzymes except factors VIIa and XIIIa). Increases AT-III levels within 30 minutes and has a half-life of up to 3 days.

INDICATIONS AND USES

Treatment of patients with hereditary AT-III deficiency to prevent thrombosis during surgical or obstetric procedures (replacement therapy) or during acute thrombotic episodes.

CONTRAINDICATIONS

None when used as indicated.

PRECAUTIONS

For IV use only. ■ Confirm diagnosis of hereditary AT-III deficiency based on a clear family history of venous thrombosis as well as decreased plasma AT-III levels and the exclusion of acquired deficiency. Present laboratory tests may not be able to identify all cases of congenital AT-III deficiency. ■ Every unit of plasma used to manufacture AT-III is tested and found nonreactive for HBsAg and negative for antibody to HIV by FDA-approved tests, then heat-treated by a special process. Even with these precautions, individuals who receive multiple infusions may develop viral infection, particularly non-A, non-B hepatitis. HIV infection remains a remote possibility. ■ May reverse heparin resistance.

Monitor: See varying methods for measuring AT-III levels under Usual Dose. Should be measured at least twice daily until the patient is stabilized and peak and trough levels established, then measured daily. All blood work should be drawn immediately before the next infusion of AT-III.

Patient Education: Inform of risks of thrombosis in connection with pregnancy and surgery and the fact that AT-III deficiency is hereditary.

Maternal/Child: Neonatal AT-III levels should be measured immediately after birth if parents are known to have AT-III deficiency (fatal neonatal thromboembolism [e.g., aortic thrombi] has occurred). Treatment of the neonate should be under the direction of a physician knowledgeable about coagulation disorders. Normal full-term and premature infants have lower than adult averages of AT-III plasma levels. ■ Category B: use only if clearly indicated. Fetal abnormalities not noted when administered in the third trimester. ■ Safety for use in pediatric patients not established.

DRUG/LAB INTERACTIONS

Half-life of AT-III decreases with concurrent **heparin** treatment. The anticoagulant effect of heparin is enhanced, and a reduced dose of heparin and low-molecular-weight heparins (LMWHs) is indicated to avoid bleeding.

SIDE EFFECTS

Bowel fullness, chest pain, chest tightness, chills, cramps, dizziness, fever, film over eye, foul taste in mouth, hives, light-headedness, oozing and hematoma formation, and shortness of breath have occurred with Thrombate III. Some patients with acquired AT-III deficiency diagnosed with disseminated intravascular coagulation (DIC) have had diuretic and vasodilatory effects. Rapid infusion may cause dyspnea.

ANTIDOTE

Levels of 150% to 210% found in a few patients have not caused any apparent complications. Observe for bleeding. Reduce rate of infusion immediately for dyspnea. Decrease rate or interrupt infusion as indicated until side effects subside. Keep physician informed of patient's lab values and condition.

ANTITHROMBIN RECOMBINANT
(an-tie-**THROM**-bin re-**KOM**-be-nant)

Atryn

Anticoagulant
Antithrombotic

pH 7

USUAL DOSE
(International units [IU])

Pretreatment: See Precautions. Baseline studies required; see Monitor.

Dose must be individualized for each patient and is based on the pretreatment level of functional antithrombin (AT) (expressed in percentage of normal) and on body weight in kilograms according to the following chart. Treatment goal is to restore and maintain functional AT activity levels between 80% and 120% (0.8 to 1.2 IU/mL) of normal. Treatment should be initiated before delivery or approximately 24 hours before surgery to ensure AT level is in the target range. Different dosing formulas are used for the treatment of surgical and pregnant patients. Pregnant females being treated with antithrombin recombinant for any peripartum or perioperative event, including a cesarean section, should be treated according to the dosing formula for pregnant females.

Antithrombin Recombinant Dosing Formula for Surgical Patients and Pregnant Females	
Loading Dose (IU)	**Maintenance Dose (IU/hr)**
Surgical Patients	
$\dfrac{(100 - \text{Baseline AT activity level})}{2.3} \times \text{Body weight (kg)}$	$\dfrac{(100 - \text{Baseline AT activity level})}{10.2} \times \text{Body weight (kg)}$
Pregnant Females	
$\dfrac{(100 - \text{Baseline AT activity level})}{1.3} \times \text{Body weight (kg)}$	$\dfrac{(100 - \text{Baseline AT activity level})}{5.4} \times \text{Body weight (kg)}$

IU, International unit.

Check AT level just after surgery or delivery; AT activity may be rapidly decreased by surgery or delivery. If AT activity level is below 80%, administer an additional bolus dose to rapidly restore decreased AT activity level. Then restart the maintenance dose at the same rate of infusion as before the bolus. Monitor AT activity at least once or twice daily and adjust doses according to the chart in Dose Adjustments. Continue treatment until adequate follow-up anticoagulation is established.

DOSE ADJUSTMENTS

Antithrombin Recombinant AT Activity Monitoring and Dose Adjustment			
Initial Monitor Time	**AT Level**	**Dose Adjustment**	**Recheck AT Level**
2 hr after initiation of treatment	<80%	Increase by 30%	2 hr after each dose adjustment
	80% to 100%	None	6 hr after initiation of treatment or dose adjustment
	>120%	Decrease by 30%	2 hr after each dose adjustment

DILUTION
Bring vials to RT no more than 3 hours before reconstitution. Each vial contains approximately 1,750 IU; exact potency is stated on the carton and label. Immediately before use, each vial **must** be reconstituted with 10 mL SWFI. **Do not shake.** Draw the reconstituted solution from one or more vials into a sterile syringe. May administer reconstituted solution directly or may further dilute in an infusion bag containing NS (e.g., dilute to obtain a final concentration of 100 IU/mL). Administer using an infusion set with a 0.22-micron in-line filter.

Filters: Use of a 0.22-micron in-line filter required during infusion.

Storage: Before use, refrigerate vials between 2° and 8° C (36° and 46° F). Use reconstituted or diluted solution within 8 to 12 hours of preparation. Do not use beyond expiration date on vial. Discard unused product.

COMPATIBILITY
Compatibility information not available from manufacturer; consult a pharmacist. Because of specific use and unique formulation, consider administering through a separate line without mixing with other IV fluids or medications.

RATE OF ADMINISTRATION
Loading dose: Administer as an infusion over 15 minutes. Follow immediately with the **maintenance dose** as a continuous infusion at the calculated IU/hr rate.

ACTIONS
A recombinant human antithrombin produced by DNA technology. A DNA coding sequence for human antithrombin and a mammary gland–specific DNA sequence are introduced into genetically engineered goats. The goats' milk contains the antithrombin. The amino acid sequence of antithrombin recombinant is identical to that of human plasma-derived antithrombin. Purified through numerous processes to eliminate potential viruses. AT is the principal inhibitor of thrombin and factor Xa. AT neutralizes the activity of thrombin and factor Xa by forming a complex that is rapidly removed from the circulation. When AT is bound to heparin, the ability of antithrombin to inhibit thrombin and factor Xa can be enhanced by greater than 300- to 1,000-fold. Half-life range based on IU/kg is 11.6 to 17.7 hours. This recombinant formulation has a shorter half-life and more rapid clearance compared with plasma-derived antithrombin (e.g., Thrombate III). Secreted in breast milk.

INDICATIONS AND USES
Prevention of perioperative and peripartum thromboembolic events in patients with hereditary antithrombin deficiency. ■ **Not indicated for treatment** of thromboembolic events in patients with hereditary antithrombin deficiency.

CONTRAINDICATIONS
Known hypersensitivity to goat and goat milk proteins.

PRECAUTIONS
For IV use only. ■ Confirm diagnosis of hereditary antithrombin deficiency. ■ Hypersensitivity reactions may occur at any time during the infusion, thus requiring discontinuation of the infusion. ■ The anticoagulant effect of drugs that use antithrombin to exert their anticoagulation (e.g., heparin, low-molecular-weight heparins such as enoxaparin [Lovenox]) may be altered when antithrombin recombinant is added or withdrawn. Avoid excessive or insufficient anticoagulation by monitoring coagulation tests suitable

for the anticoagulant used (e.g., aPTT and anti-factor Xa activity). To avoid bleeding or thrombosis, perform these tests regularly and at close intervals, especially during the first hours after the start or withdrawal of antithrombin recombinant. ▪ See Drug/Lab Interactions.

Monitor: Specific coagulation tests are required before administration and throughout the infusion process; see Usual Dose and Precautions. ▪ Monitor throughout the infusion for S/S of a hypersensitivity reaction (e.g., hives, hypotension, generalized urticaria, tightness of the chest, wheezing, and/or anaphylaxis). ▪ Monitor for S/S of bleeding or thrombosis.

Patient Education: Inform physician of a past or present allergy to goats or goat milk. ▪ Promptly report S/S of a hypersensitivity reaction (e.g., rash, shortness of breath, wheezing). ▪ Risk of bleeding increased when used with other anticoagulants. Report bleeding from any source.

Maternal/Child: Category C: use during pregnancy only if clearly needed. Studies have not shown that antithrombin recombinant increases the risk of fetal abnormalities if administered during the third trimester of pregnancy. Adverse reactions have not been reported in neonates born to females treated with antithrombin recombinant during clinical trials. ▪ Indicated for prevention of thromboembolic events in females with hereditary antithrombin deficiency during labor and delivery. ▪ Levels that appear in breast milk are estimated to be the same as in normal lactating females; however, use only if clearly needed and with caution during breast-feeding. ▪ Safety and effectiveness for use in pediatric patients not established.

Elderly: Numbers in clinical studies insufficient to determine whether elderly patients respond differently than younger subjects. Dosing should be cautious in the elderly. Reduced doses may be indicated based on the potential for decreased organ function and concomitant disease or drug therapy.

DRUG/LAB INTERACTIONS

The anticoagulant effect of **heparin and low-molecular-weight heparin** is enhanced by antithrombin. Concurrent use with these anticoagulants may alter the half-life of antithrombin. Concurrent use with **heparin, low-molecular-weight heparins** such as enoxaparin (Lovenox), **or other anticoagulants** that use antithrombin to exert their anticoagulant effect must be monitored clinically and biologically. To avoid excessive anticoagulation, perform regular coagulation tests (aPTT and, where appropriate, anti-factor Xa activity) at close intervals and adjust the dose of anticoagulant as indicated.

SIDE EFFECTS

Hemorrhage and infusion site reactions were most commonly reported. Hemorrhage may be serious (intra-abdominal, hemarthrosis, and postprocedural). Less common side effects include feeling hot, hematoma, hematuria, hepatic enzyme abnormalities, hypersensitivity reactions (including anaphylaxis), and noncardiac chest pain.

ANTIDOTE

Keep physician informed of patient's lab values and condition. Discontinue the infusion if a hypersensitivity reaction occurs. ▪ Treat anaphylaxis immediately with oxygen, epinephrine, antihistamines (e.g., diphenhydramine), vasopressors (e.g., dopamine), corticosteroids, albuterol, IV fluids, and ventilation equipment as indicated. Resuscitate as necessary.

ANTITHYMOCYTE GLOBULIN (RABBIT) BBW

Immunosuppressant

(an-tie-**THI**-mo-cite **GLOB**-you-lin)

Thymoglobulin, Atgam (equine)[a]

pH 7 to 7.4

USUAL DOSE

Pretreatment: Baseline studies indicated; see Monitor.

Premedication: To reduce the incidence and intensity of side effects during the infusion of anti-thymocyte globulin; premedication 1 hour before the infusion with corticosteroids (e.g., dexamethasone), acetaminophen, and/or an antihistamine (e.g., diphenhydramine) is recommended.

Anti-thymocyte globulin: 1.5 mg/kg of body weight daily for 7 to 14 days. Given as an infusion into a high-flow vein. Used in conjunction with maintenance immunosuppression (e.g., tacrolimus [Prograf], mycophenolate [Cell-Cept]); see Drug/Lab Interactions.

DOSE ADJUSTMENTS

Reduce dose by one-half if WBC count is between 2,000 and 3,000 cells/mm^3 or if platelet count is between 50,000 and 75,000 cells/mm^3. ▪ Consider withholding dose or stopping anti-thymocyte therapy if WBC count falls below 2,000 cells/mm^3 or platelets fall below 50,000 cells/mm^3.

DILUTION

Calculate the number of vials required (25 mg/vial); 5 mL of SWFI as diluent per vial is supplied. Drug and diluent must be warmed to room temperature before dilution. Absolute sterile technique required throughout dilution process. For each vial required use a new syringe and needle. Withdraw 5 mL of diluent and inject into lyophilized powder. Rotate vial gently until powder is completely dissolved. Do not shake. Each reconstituted vial contains 25 mg (5 mg/mL). Must be further diluted by transferring into 50 mL of infusion solution (saline or dextrose) for each 25 mg of anti-thymocyte globulin. Total volume is usually between 50 to 500 mL. Invert the infusion bag gently once or twice to mix the solution.

Filters: Use of a 0.22-micron in-line filter recommended.

Storage: Refrigerate and protect from light until removed to prepare for reconstitution. Do not freeze. Do not use after expiration date on vial. Use reconstituted vials within 4 hours. Use infusion solutions immediately. Discard unused drug.

COMPATIBILITY

Administration through a separate line without mixing with other IV fluids or medications is suggested because of specific use and potential for anaphylaxis.

Other sources suggest a few specific **compatibilities** dependent on concentration and manufacturer; consult a pharmacist.

RATE OF ADMINISTRATION

Use of a high-flow vein and a 0.22-micron filter recommended. Well-tolerated and less likely to produce side effects (e.g., chills and fever) when administered at the recommended rate and the patient is premedicated.

Initial dose: A total daily dose equally distributed over a minimum of 6 hours.

Subsequent doses: A total daily dose equally distributed over a minimum of 4 hours.

ACTIONS

A purified, pasteurized, gamma immune globulin, obtained by immunization of rabbits with human thymocytes. Mechanism of action not fully understood. May induce immunosuppression by T-cell depletion and immune modulation. Made up of a variety of antibodies that recognize key receptors on T-cells (those cells responsible for attacking and

---

[a]See Index for monograph of Lymphocyte Immune Globulin, the equine product of Anti-Thymocyte Globulin.

rejecting a foreign substance within the body). Anti-thymocyte globulin antibodies can inactivate and kill these T-cells, thus reversing the rejection process. May prevent organ loss and reduce the need for retransplantation. T-cell depletion is usually observed within a day of initiating thymoglobulin therapy. Half-life averages 2 to 3 days but the drug remains active, targeting the offending immune cells for days to weeks after treatment.

INDICATIONS AND USES
Treatment of kidney transplant acute rejection in conjunction with concomitant immunosuppression.
Unlabeled uses: Compassionate use in the treatment of acute rejection in bone marrow, heart, and liver transplants. Treatment of myelodysplastic syndrome (MDS).

CONTRAINDICATIONS
Patients with a known allergy to rabbit proteins, an acute viral illness, or a history of anaphylaxis during rabbit immunoglobulin administration.

PRECAUTIONS
Administered only under the direction of a physician experienced in immunosuppressive therapy and management of renal transplant patients in a facility with adequate laboratory and supportive medical resources. ■ Not considered effective for treating antibody-mediated (humoral) rejections. ■ Prolonged use or overdose in combination with other immunosuppressive agents may cause over-immunosuppression resulting in severe infections and may increase the incidence of lymphoma or posttransplant lymphoproliferative disease (PTLD) or other malignancies. Use of appropriate antiviral, antibacterial, antiprotozoal, and/or antifungal prophylaxis is recommended. In clinical trials, viral prophylaxis with ganciclovir infusion was used. ■ In clinical trials, anti-rabbit antibodies developed in 68% of patients. Controlled studies on repeat use of anti-thymocyte globulin in patients with anti-rabbit antibodies have not been conducted. Use caution if repeat courses are indicated; monitoring of lymphocyte count is recommended to ensure that T-cell depletion is achieved. ■ If anaphylaxis occurs during or after therapy, further administration of anti-thymocyte globulin is contraindicated.
Monitor: Obtain baseline and monitor WBC and platelet counts during therapy. Thrombocytopenia or neutropenia may occur and are reversible following dose adjustment; see Dose Adjustments. ■ Close clinical observation is imperative. Monitor for side effects during and after infusion. Anaphylaxis has occurred; emergency equipment, medications, and supplies must be available. ■ Monitoring of the lymphocyte count (i.e., total lymphocyte count and T-cell counts [absolute and/or subset]) may help assess the degree of T-cell depletion. ■ Monitor carefully for signs of infection. ■ Prophylactic antibiotics may be indicated pending results of C/S in a febrile neutropenic patient. ■ See Precautions and Drug/Lab Interactions.
Patient Education: Imperative that all medications (especially immunosuppressants) be reviewed with physician. ■ Report any previous hypersensitivity/anaphylactic reaction. ■ Report acute viral infections immediately. ■ Promptly report chest pain, irregular or rapid heartbeat, shortness of breath, swelling of the face or throat, or wheezing during infusion of medication. ■ See Appendix D, p. 1311. ■ May be associated with an increased risk of malignancy.
Maternal/Child: Category C: safety for use during pregnancy and breast-feeding not established. Safety and effectiveness for use in pediatric patients not established. Use only if clearly needed. ■ Has been used in pediatric patients in limited European studies and in the United States for compassionate use. Response similar to adults.
Elderly: Specific information not available.

DRUG/LAB INTERACTIONS
Concurrent use with **immunosuppressants** (e.g., azathioprine, cyclosporine, mycophenolate, tacrolimus) may potentiate the immunosuppressive action of these agents; many transplant centers decrease maintenance immunosuppression therapy during the period of antibody therapy. ■ May **stimulate the production of antibodies,** which cross-react with rabbit immune globulins. ■ May interfere with **rabbit antibody-base immunoassays** and with **cross-match or panel-reactive antibody cytotoxicity assays.**

SIDE EFFECTS

Are dose-limiting. Abdominal pain, asthenia, diarrhea, dizziness, dyspnea, fever, headache, hyperkalemia, hypertension, infection, infusion reaction (e.g., chills and fever), leukopenia, malaise, nausea, pain, peripheral edema, tachycardia, and thrombocytopenia were reported frequently. Anaphylaxis has been reported.

Overdose: Leukopenia or thrombocytopenia.

ANTIDOTE

Notify physician of all side effects. Most can be managed symptomatically. Manage leukopenia or thrombocytopenia during therapy or in overdose with dose reduction. Infusion reactions are managed with premedication and reduction in the rate of infusion. Treat infections aggressively; see Precautions. May require discontinuation of therapy. Discontinue infusion and/or therapy immediately if anaphylaxis occurs. Treat anaphylaxis immediately with epinephrine, diphenhydramine, oxygen, vasopressors (e.g., dopamine), corticosteroids, IV fluids, and ventilation equipment as indicated. Resuscitate as necessary.

APREPITANT

(ap-**RE**-pi-tant)

Cinvanti, Aponvie

Antiemetic
Substance P/NK$_1$
Receptor antagonist

USUAL DOSE

Pretreatment: See Maternal/Child.

Adult dose: *Highly emetogenic chemotherapy:* 130 mg IV approximately 30 minutes before chemotherapy on Day 1.

Moderately emetogenic chemotherapy: 100 mg IV 30 minutes before chemotherapy on Day 1.

DOSE ADJUSTMENTS

No dose adjustment indicated based on age, race, gender, renal status (including patients with ESRD undergoing dialysis), or mild to moderate hepatic insufficiency. Data in patients with severe hepatic insufficiency (Child-Pugh score >9) not available.

DILUTION

Supplied as an opaque, off-white to amber emulsion in a single-dose glass vial containing 130 mg/18 mL aprepitant.

Intravenous injection over 2 minutes: Withdraw **18 mL for the 130-mg dose** or **14 mL for the 100-mg dose**. Do not dilute.

Intravenous infusion over 30 minutes: Withdraw **18 mL for the 130-mg dose** or **14 mL for the 100-mg dose**. Transfer drug into a non-PVC infusion bag filled with 100 mL of NS or D5W. Gently invert the bag 4 to 5 times. Avoid shaking.

Filters: Specific information not available.

Storage: Before use, vials should be refrigerated at 2° to 8° C (36° to 46° F) or can remain at RT for up to 60 days. The diluted solution is stable at ambient RT for 6 hours in NS or for 12 hours in D5W or for up to 72 hours if stored under refrigeration in NS or D5W.

COMPATIBILITY

Manufacturer states, "Use only non-DEHP tubing and non-PVC infusion bags. Should not be mixed or reconstituted with solutions for which physical and chemical **compatibility** have not been established. Aprepitant for injection is **incompatible** with any solutions containing divalent cations (e.g., calcium or magnesium), including lactated Ringer's solution and Hartmann's solution."

RATE OF ADMINISTRATION

Injection: A single dose as an injection over 2 minutes. Flush infusion line with NS before and after administration of aprepitant.

Infusion: A single dose as an infusion equally distributed over 30 minutes. Use only non-DEHP tubing.

Complete the injection or infusion approximately 30 minutes before administration of chemotherapy.

ACTIONS

A selective high-affinity antagonist of human substance P/neurokinin$_1$ (NK$_1$) receptors. Has little or no affinity for 5-HT$_3$, dopamine, and corticosteroid receptors. Aprepitant inhibits emesis induced by cytotoxic chemotherapeutic agents, such as cisplatin, via central actions. Crosses the blood-brain barrier and occupies brain NK$_1$ receptors. Augments the antiemetic activity of the 5-HT$_3$-receptor antagonist ondansetron and the corticosteroid dexamethasone and inhibits both the acute and delayed phases of cisplatin-induced emesis. Highly protein bound. Undergoes extensive metabolism, primarily by CYP3A4 and to a lesser extent by CYP1A2 and CYP2C19. Eliminated primarily by metabolism; not renally excreted. Half-life is approximately 9 to 13 hours.

INDICATIONS AND USES

Used in combination with other antiemetic agents in adults for the prevention of acute and delayed nausea and vomiting associated with initial and repeat courses of highly emetogenic chemotherapy (HEC), including high-dose cisplatin, and for the prevention of nausea and vomiting associated with initial and repeat courses of moderately emetogenic chemotherapy (MEC).

Limitation of use: Aprepitant has not been studied for the treatment of established nausea and vomiting.

CONTRAINDICATIONS

Hypersensitivity to any component of the product. ▪ Concurrent use with pimozide (Orap); see Drug/Lab Interactions.

PRECAUTIONS

Aprepitant is a substrate, weak to moderate (dose-dependent) inhibitor, and inducer of CYP3A4. Use with caution in patients receiving concomitant medications that are substrates, strong or moderate CYP3A4 inhibitors, or strong CYP3A4 inducers; see Drug/Lab Interactions. ▪ Use with caution in patients with severe hepatic insufficiency (Child-Pugh score >9); see Dose Adjustments. ▪ Serious hypersensitivity reactions, including anaphylaxis, have been observed during or soon after administration; see Monitor.

Monitor: Monitor for S/S of a hypersensitivity reaction during and after the infusion (e.g., anaphylaxis, dyspnea, eye swelling, flushing, pruritus, wheezing). ▪ Monitor IV site. ▪ See Drug/Lab Interactions.

Patient Education: Read FDA-approved patient information before starting therapy. ▪ Discontinue use of aprepitant and promptly report S/S of a hypersensitivity reaction (e.g., difficulty breathing or swallowing, hives, itching, rash). ▪ Efficacy of hormonal contraceptives may be reduced during and for 28 days after administration of the last dose of aprepitant. Alternative or backup methods of nonhormonal effective contraception (such as condoms or spermicides) should be used during treatment and for 1 month after the last dose of aprepitant. ▪ Numerous drug interactions possible. A complete review of all prescription, nonprescription, and herbal products is required before each dose. ▪ Patients on chronic warfarin therapy should have their INR checked in the 2-week period, particularly at 7 to 10 days, following initiation of regimen. ▪ Report infusion site reactions.

Maternal/Child: Avoid pregnancy due to alcohol content; may cause fetal harm, including CNS abnormalities, behavioral disorders, and impaired intellectual development. ▪ Information on use during breast-feeding not available. Use caution. ▪ Safety and effectiveness for use in pediatric patients not established.

Elderly: Response similar to that seen in younger patients. Use caution when dosing; consider decreased hepatic, renal, or cardiac function and concomitant disease or other drug therapy.

DRUG/LAB INTERACTIONS

Aprepitant is a substrate, weak-to-moderate (dose-dependent) inhibitor, and inducer of CYP3A4. It is also an inducer of CYP2C9. ▪ Use of aprepitant with other drugs that are CYP3A4 substrates may result in increased plasma concentration of the concomitant drug. ▪ Concurrent use with **pimozide** is *contraindicated*. Inhibition of CYP3A4 could result in elevated plasma concentrations of pimozide, potentially causing serious or life-threatening reactions such as QT prolongation; see Contraindications. ▪ Efficacy of **hormonal contraceptives** may be reduced during and for 28 days after administration of the last dose of aprepitant (decreased estrogen and progestin exposure); see Patient Education. ▪ Patients on chronic **warfarin** therapy should be closely monitored over a 2-week period, particularly at 7 to 10 days after initiation of aprepitant with each chemotherapy cycle. Coadministration may result in a clinically significant decrease in INR. ▪ Aprepitant can increase plasma concentrations of **dexamethasone** and **methylprednisolone**. When given concurrently with aprepitant, reduce the dexamethasone and methylprednisolone PO doses by approximately 50% and the methylprednisolone IV dose by approximately 25%. (Dexamethasone doses listed in Usual Dose take the drug interaction into account.) ▪ Coadministration of aprepitant with **chemotherapy agents metabolized by CYP3A4** (e.g., ifosfamide, vinblastine, and vincristine) should be done with caution and careful monitoring. ▪ May increase plasma levels of **benzodiazepines**. Monitor for sedation. ▪ Aprepitant is a CYP2C9 inducer. Has been shown to induce the metabolism of **CYP2C9 substrates** (e.g., tolbutamide, warfarin), thus decreasing plasma concentrations. Monitor patients receiving CYP2C9 substrates as indicated (e.g., plasma drug concentrations, therapeutic effect/efficacy, blood sugar control). ▪ Avoid concomitant use with **moderate to strong CYP3A4 inhibitors** (e.g., clarithromycin, diltiazem, itraconazole, ketoconazole, nefazodone, nelfinavir, ritonavir, troleandomycin); may increase aprepitant plasma concentrations. ▪ Coadministration with **strong CYP3A4 inducers** (e.g., carbamazepine, phenytoin, rifampin) may decrease aprepitant plasma concentrations and decrease efficacy. Avoid concurrent use. ▪ Aprepitant is unlikely to interact with drugs that are **substrates for the P-glycoprotein transporter**. ▪ Aprepitant did not have clinically important effects on the pharmacokinetics of **5-HT$_3$antagonists** (e.g., dolasetron, granisetron, ondansetron).

SIDE EFFECTS

The most common side effects reported include eructation, fatigue, headache, and infusion site reactions. Other reported side effects include abdominal pain or distention, acid reflux, acne, anemia, anxiety, bradycardia, cardiovascular disorder, chest discomfort, chills, cognitive disorder, conjunctivitis, constipation, cough, decreased neutrophil count, disorientation, dizziness, dream abnormality, dry mouth, dysgeusia, dysuria, edema, epigastric discomfort, euphoria, febrile neutropenia, flatulence, flushing, gait disturbance, gastroesophageal reflux disease, hematuria (microscopic), hyperglycemia, hyperhidrosis, hyponatremia, increased alkaline phosphatase, infusion site reactions, lethargy, muscle cramps or weakness, myalgia, nausea, neutropenic colitis, oily skin, palpitations, perforating duodenal ulcer, pharyngitis, photosensitivity, polydipsia, polyuria, postnasal drip, pruritus, rash, skin lesions, sneezing, somnolence, stomatitis, thirst, throat irritation, tinnitus, vomiting, and weight gain and/or weight loss.

Post-Marketing: Hypersensitivity reactions (including anaphylaxis), pruritus, rash, Stevens-Johnson syndrome, toxic epidermal necrolysis, and urticaria have been reported. Ifosfamide-induced neurotoxicity after aprepitant and ifosfamide coadministration has also been reported.

ANTIDOTE

Keep physician informed of all side effects. Most minor side effects will be treated symptomatically. Discontinue aprepitant at the first sign of hypersensitivity. Treat hypersensitivity reactions as indicated; may require epinephrine, airway management, oxygen, IV fluids, antihistamines, corticosteroids, and pressor amines. Do not reinitiate aprepitant in patients who experience a severe hypersensitivity reaction. Aprepitant is not removed by hemodialysis.

ARGATROBAN
(ahr-**GAT**-troe-ban)

USUAL DOSE

Pretreatment: Discontinue all parenteral anticoagulants (e.g., heparin) and obtain baseline blood tests including an aPTT (prophylaxis or treatment) and ACT (PCI) before administration of argatroban; see Monitor.

Prophylaxis or treatment of thrombosis in patients with heparin-induced thrombocytopenia (HIT/ HITTS): Begin *argatroban* with an initial dose of 2 mcg/kg/min as a continuous infusion. Steady-state levels usually obtained within 1 to 3 hours. Check the aPTT in 2 hours and after any dose change. Adjust the mcg/kg/min dose (not to exceed 10 mcg/kg/min) as clinically indicated until the steady-state aPTT is 1.5 to 3 times the initial baseline value (not to exceed 100 seconds).

Anticoagulant in patients with or at risk for HIT/HITTS undergoing percutaneous coronary interventions (PCI): *Aspirin* 325 mg 2 to 24 hours before planned PCI was administered in studies. Begin *argatroban* with an initial infusion of 25 mcg/kg/min via a large-bore IV line. Next, administer a bolus of 350 mcg/kg over 3 to 5 minutes. 5 to 10 minutes after completion of bolus dose, check the ACT. The PCI may proceed if the ACT is greater than 300 seconds but less than 450 seconds. If ACT is less than 300 seconds, give an additional IV bolus of 150 mcg/kg, increase the infusion rate to 30 mcg/kg/min, and check the ACT in 5 to 10 minutes. If ACT is greater than 450 seconds, decrease the infusion rate to 15 mcg/kg/min and recheck the ACT in 5 to 10 minutes. When a therapeutic ACT has been achieved (between 300 and 450 seconds), the infusion dose in effect at the time the therapeutic ACT is achieved should be continued for the duration of the procedure. For situations outside these parameters, see Dose Adjustments. If anticoagulation is required after PCI, continue argatroban but lower infusion rate to 2 mcg/kg/min. Draw an aPTT in 2 hours and adjust the infusion rate as clinically indicated (not to exceed 10 mcg/kg/min) to reach an aPTT between 1.5 and 3 times baseline value (not to exceed 100 seconds); see All Situations in Monitor if transfer to oral anticoagulation is indicated.

DOSE ADJUSTMENTS

All situations: No dose adjustment indicated in patients with impaired renal function, or based on age or gender. ■ In patients with hepatic impairment, initiate therapy at a lower dose and carefully titrate until the desired level of anticoagulation is reached. Achievement of steady-state aPTT levels may take longer and require more dose adjustments of argatroban in patients with hepatic impairment compared with patients with normal hepatic function.

Prophylaxis or treatment of thrombosis in patients with heparin-induced thrombocytopenia (HIT/ HITTS): Reduce initial dose to 0.5 mcg/kg/min in patients with moderate or severe hepatic impairment. There is a fourfold decrease in argatroban clearance in these patients; titrate dose carefully and monitor aPTT closely.

Anticoagulant in patients with or at risk for HIT/HITTS undergoing percutaneous coronary interventions (PCI): In case of dissection, impending abrupt closure, thrombus formation during the procedure, or inability to achieve or maintain an ACT over 300 seconds, additional bolus doses of 150 mcg/kg may be given and the infusion rate increased to 40 mcg/kg/min. Check the ACT after each additional bolus or change in rate of infusion. ■ In patients with hepatic impairment undergoing PCI, carefully titrate argatroban until desired level of anticoagulation is achieved. See Precautions for patients with clinically significant liver disease.

DILUTION

Available premixed at a final concentration of 1 mg/mL or as a 250-mg vial that must be diluted in 250 mL of NS, D5W, or LR to a concentration of 1 mg/mL. Mix by repeated inversion of the diluent bag for a minimum of 1 minute. Solution may initially be briefly hazy. Use of diluent at RT is recommended. Colder temperatures can slow down the rate of dissolution of precipitates. The vial should be discarded if the solution is cloudy or if an insoluble precipitate is noted. Do not expose prepared solutions to direct sunlight.

Storage: Store vials in carton at CRT, protected from light and freezing. Diluted solution stable in ambient indoor light for 24 hours at 20° to 25° C (68° to 77° F). Light-resistant measures such as foil protection for IV lines are not necessary. Prepared solutions may be stable for up to 96 hours when protected from light and stored at 20° to 25° C (68° to 77° F) or refrigerated. Prepared solutions should not be exposed to direct sunlight. Store premixed bags in original carton at 20° to 25° C (68° to 77° F). Do not refrigerate or freeze. Protect from light.

COMPATIBILITY

Manufacturer states, "Should not be mixed with other drugs prior to dilution in a suitable IV fluid." Other sources suggest specific **compatibilities** dependent on concentration and manufacturer; consult a pharmacist.

RATE OF ADMINISTRATION

Prophylaxis or treatment of thrombosis in patients with heparin-induced thrombocytopenia (HIT/HITTS): 2 mcg/kg/min. See Usual Dose and/or Dose Adjustments as needed.

Anticoagulant in patients with or at risk for HIT/HITTS undergoing percutaneous coronary interventions (PCI): See Usual Dose and/or Dose Adjustments for specific rates and criteria.

ACTIONS

An anticoagulant that is a highly selective synthetic direct thrombin inhibitor. It reversibly binds to the thrombin active site and exerts its anticoagulant effects by inhibiting thrombin-catalyzed or induced reactions, including fibrin formation; activation of coagulation factors V, VIII, and XIII and protein C; and platelet aggregation. Highly selective for thrombin with little or no effect on related serine proteases (trypsin, factor Xa, plasmin, and kallikrein). Inhibits both free and clot-bound thrombin. Does not require the cofactor antithrombin III for antithrombic activity. Produces a dose-dependent increase in aPTT, ACT, INR, PT, and TT. Anticoagulant effects are immediate. Steady-state levels of both drug and anticoagulant effect are usually attained within 1 to 3 hours and are maintained until the infusion is discontinued or the dose adjusted. Distribution is primarily in the extracellular fluid. Metabolized in the liver. Half-life range is 39 to 51 minutes. Excreted primarily in feces with some excretion in urine.

INDICATIONS AND USES

An anticoagulant for prophylaxis or treatment of thrombosis in patients with heparin-induced thrombocytopenia (HIT). ■ An anticoagulant in adult patients with or at risk for heparin-induced thrombocytopenia undergoing percutaneous coronary intervention (PCI). May be used in combination with aspirin.

CONTRAINDICATIONS

Hypersensitivity to argatroban or any of its components and patients with overt major bleeding.

PRECAUTIONS

All situations: Hemorrhage can occur at any site. Intracranial and retroperitoneal hemorrhage has been reported. Use with extreme caution in disease states and other circumstances in which there is an increased danger of hemorrhage, including severe hypertension; immediately following lumbar puncture; spinal anesthesia; major surgery, especially involving the brain, spinal cord, or eye; hematologic conditions associated with increased bleeding tendencies such as congenital or acquired bleeding disorders and gastrointestinal lesions such as ulcerations. ■ Concomitant therapy with thrombolytic agents (e.g., alteplase [tPA], reteplase, streptokinase), antiplatelet agents, or other anticoagulants may increase the risk of bleeding, including life-threatening intracranial bleeding; see Drug/Lab Interactions. ■ Safety and effectiveness of argatroban for cardiac indications other than PCI in patients with HIT not established. ■ Use caution in patients with hepatic disease; argatroban clearance is decreased four-fold and elimination half-life is increased. Full reversal of anticoagulant effect may require longer than 4 hours. See Dose Adjustments.

PCI: Avoid use of argatroban in PCI patients with clinically significant hepatic disease or AST/ALT levels equal to or greater than 3 times the upper limit of normal. These patients were not included in clinical trials.

Monitor: *All situations:* Obtain baseline and monitor platelet count, hemoglobin, hematocrit, and occult blood in stool in addition to required aPTT or ACT; see Usual Dose and specific parameters as follows. ■ Other coagulation tests (e.g., PT, INR, and TT) are affected by argatroban, but therapeutic ranges for these tests have not been identified. ■ Observe carefully for symptoms of a hemorrhagic event (e.g., unexplained fall in hematocrit, fall in hemoglobin, fall in BP, or any other unexplained symptom). ■ HIT is a serious, immune-mediated complication of heparin therapy that may result in subsequent venous and arterial thrombosis. Initial treatment of HIT is to discontinue all heparin, but patients still require anticoagulation for prevention and treatment of thromboembolic events. ■ Initiate oral anticoagulation with warfarin (Coumadin) when appropriate. Do not use a loading dose of warfarin; use the expected daily dose. Monitor INR daily. Concurrent use with warfarin results in prolongation of the PT and INR beyond that produced by warfarin alone. With doses of argatroban up to 2 mcg/kg/min, argatroban can be discontinued when the INR is greater than 4 on combined therapy. After argatroban is discontinued, repeat the INR in 4 to 6 hours. If the INR is below the desired therapeutic range, resume the infusion of argatroban and repeat the procedure daily until the desired therapeutic range on warfarin alone is reached. See Drug/Lab Interactions. With doses of argatroban more than 2 mcg/kg/min the INR relationship is less predictable. Reduction of dose to 2 mcg/kg/min is recommended.

Prophylaxis or treatment of thrombosis: Obtain a baseline aPTT before treatment begins. Repeat aPTT in 2 hours, after any dose adjustment, and as indicated to achieve desired target aPTT of 1.5 to 3 times baseline. ■ Repeated administration has been tolerated with no loss of anticoagulant activity and no evidence of neutralizing antibodies. No change in dose is required.

PCI: Obtain baseline ACT before dosing; repeat ACT 5 to 10 minutes after bolus dosing, after a change in infusion rate, and at the end of the PCI procedure. Draw additional ACTs every 20 to 30 minutes during a prolonged procedure. ■ Follow standard procedures for maintenance and care of venous or arterial sheaths. In clinical studies, sheaths were removed no sooner than 2 hours after discontinuing argatroban and when ACT had decreased to less than 160 seconds. ■ See Dose Adjustments if anticoagulation is required after PCI.

Patient Education: Review medication and medical history with physician. ■ Report all episodes of bleeding. ■ Report tarry stools. ■ Compliance with all measures to minimize bleeding is very important (e.g., avoid use of razors, toothbrushes, other sharp items). ■ Use caution while moving to avoid excess bumping. ■ Promptly report any S/S of hypersensitivity reaction (e.g., airway reactions, rash, dizziness).

Maternal/Child: Use during pregnancy only if clearly needed. There are risks to the mother associated with untreated thrombosis in pregnancy and a risk of hemorrhage in the mother, fetus, and neonates associated with the use of anticoagulants. Monitor neonates for bleeding. ■ No data on the presence of argatroban in human milk or on its effects on milk production. ■ Safety and effectiveness for use in pediatric patients not established. ■ Has been used in a small number of pediatric patients with HIT or HITTS who require an alternative to heparin therapy. See package insert for dosing recommendations and monitoring parameters. Clearance was 50% lower in seriously ill pediatric patients compared with healthy adults.

Elderly: Response similar to that in younger patients; efficacy is not affected by age. Safety analysis suggests that older patients tend to have an increased risk of events compared with younger patients; however, older patients have increased underlying conditions that may predispose them to adverse reactions.

DRUG/LAB INTERACTIONS

If argatroban is to be initiated after cessation of **heparin** therapy, allow sufficient time for heparin's effect on the aPTT to decrease before initiating argatroban therapy. ▪ Drug interactions have not been demonstrated between argatroban and concomitantly administered **aspirin or acetaminophen.** ▪ The safety and effectiveness of argatroban with thrombolytic agents and glycoprotein IIb/IIIa antagonists (e.g., eptifibatide, tirofiban) have not been established. ▪ Risk of bleeding may be increased by any medicine that affects blood clotting, including **anticoagulants** (e.g., heparin, warfarin); **any medication that may cause hypoprothrombinemia, thrombocytopenia, or GI ulceration or bleeding** (e.g., selected antibiotics [e.g., cefotetan], aspirin, NSAIDs); **and/or any other medication that inhibits platelet aggregation** (e.g., clopidogrel, valproic acid). ▪ Concurrent use with **warfarin** results in prolongation of the PT and INR beyond that produced by warfarin alone; see Monitor. The combination causes no further reduction in vitamin K dependent factor Xa than that seen with warfarin alone. Relationship between INR obtained on combined therapy and INR obtained on warfarin alone is dependent on both the dose of argatroban and the thromboplastin reagent used.

SIDE EFFECTS

All situations: Bleeding is the most frequent adverse event. Hypersensitivity reactions (e.g., coughing, dyspnea, hypotension, rash) have been reported, most frequently in patients who also received streptokinase or contrast media.

Prophylaxis or treatment of thrombosis: The most common side effects are cardiac arrest, diarrhea, dyspnea, fever, hypotension, and sepsis. Hemorrhagic events included brachial bleed, a decreased hemoglobin and hematocrit, GI bleed, groin bleed, GU bleed, hematuria, hemoptysis, intracranial bleed, limb and below-knee amputation stump, and multisystem hemorrhage and DIC. Abdominal pain, abnormal renal function, arrhythmias (e.g., atrial fibrillation, ventricular tachycardia), cerebrovascular disorder, coughing, infection, nausea, pain, pneumonia, UTI, and vomiting have occurred.

PCI: The most common side effects are back pain, chest pain, headache, hypotension, nausea, and vomiting. Retroperitoneal and GI bleeding occurred in a few patients. Other minor bleeding included coronary arteries, a decreased hemoglobin and hematocrit, GI bleeding, GU bleeding, hematuria, groin, hemoptysis, and access site (venous or arterial). Abdominal pain, bradycardia, fever, and MI and other serious coronary events have occurred.

Overdose: Symptoms of acute toxicity in animals included clonic convulsions, coma, loss of righting reflex, paralysis of hind limbs, and tremors.

ANTIDOTE

No specific antidote is available. Obtain aPTT, ACT, and/or other coagulation tests. Overdose with or without bleeding may be controlled by discontinuing argatroban or by decreasing the infusion dose; aPTT should return to baseline within 2 to 4 hours after discontinuation. Reversal may take longer in patients with hepatic impairment. If life-threatening bleeding develops and excessive plasma levels of argatroban are suspected, immediately stop argatroban infusion. Determine aPTT and hemoglobin, and prepare for blood transfusion as appropriate. Follow current guidelines for treatment of shock as indicated (fluid, vasopressors [e.g., dopamine], Trendelenburg position, plasma expanders [e.g., albumin]). Approximately 20% of argatroban may be cleared through a 4-hour dialysis session.

ATEZOLIZUMAB BBW
(**A**-te-zoe-**LIZ**-ue-mab)

Monoclonal antibody (anti-PD-L1)
Antineoplastic agent

Tecentriq

pH 5.8

USUAL DOSE

Pretreatment: Verify pregnancy status. Pretesting required in selected patients and baseline studies indicated; see Precautions and Monitor.

Locally advanced or metastatic urothelial carcinoma or previously treated non–small-cell lung cancer (as a single agent): 840 mg every 2 weeks, 1,200 mg every 3 weeks, or 1,680 mg every 4 weeks. Administered as an intravenous infusion over 60 minutes until disease progression or unacceptable toxicity. For all dosages, if the first infusion is tolerated, all subsequent infusions may be delivered over 30 minutes.

First-line treatment of metastatic nonsquamous non–small-cell lung cancer: 1,200 mg every 3 weeks administered as an IV infusion over 60 minutes followed by bevacizumab, paclitaxel, and carboplatin on Day 1 of each 21-day cycle for a maximum of 4 to 6 cycles of chemotherapy. If the first infusion is tolerated, all subsequent infusions may be delivered over 30 minutes. Following completion of 4 to 6 cycles of paclitaxel and carboplatin, and if bevacizumab is discontinued, the recommended dose of atezolizumab is 840 mg every 2 weeks, 1,200 mg every 3 weeks, or 1,680 mg every 4 weeks administered as an intravenous infusion over 60 minutes (administer subsequent infusions over 30 minutes if 60 minutes was tolerated) until disease progression or unacceptable toxicity. Refer to prescribing information for bevacizumab, paclitaxel, and carboplatin for recommended dosing information.

Locally advanced or metastatic triple-negative breast cancer (TNBC): 840 mg administered as an IV infusion over 60 minutes, followed by 100 mg/M^2 paclitaxel protein-bound. For each 28-day cycle, atezolizumab is administered on Days 1 and 15, and paclitaxel protein-bound is administered on Days 1, 8, and 15 until disease progression or unacceptable toxicity. Atezolizumab and paclitaxel protein-bound may be discontinued for toxicity independently of each other. If the first infusion is tolerated, all subsequent infusions may be delivered over 30 minutes. Refer to prescribing information for paclitaxel protein-bound before initiation.

Small-cell lung cancer (SCLC): 1,200 mg administered intravenously over 60 minutes every 3 weeks until disease progression or unacceptable toxicity. When administered in combination with carboplatin and etoposide, administer atezolizumab before chemotherapy when given on the same day. Refer to the prescribing information for the chemotherapy agents administered in combination with atezolizumab for recommended dosing information. Following completion of 4 cycles of carboplatin and etoposide, the recommended dose of atezolizumab is 840 mg every 2 weeks, or 1,200 mg every 3 weeks, or 1,680 mg every 4 weeks. Administer until disease progression or unacceptable toxicity. If the first infusion is tolerated, all subsequent infusions may be delivered over 30 minutes

DOSE ADJUSTMENTS

No dose reductions are recommended. Recommended dose modifications for adverse reactions are provided in the following chart.

Atezolizumab Dose Modifications Recommended for Adverse Reactions		
Adverse Reaction	Severity of Adverse Reaction[a]	Dose Modifications
Pneumonitis[b]	Grade 2	Withhold dose until Grade 1 or resolved and corticosteroid dose is less than or equal to prednisone 10 mg/day (or equivalent).
	Grade 3 or 4	Permanently discontinue.[b]
Hepatitis[b]	AST or ALT more than 3 and up to 8 × ULN or total bilirubin more than 1.5 and up to 3 × ULN	Withhold dose until Grade 1 or resolved and corticosteroid dose is less than or equal to prednisone 10 mg/day (or equivalent).
	AST or ALT more than 8 × ULN or total bilirubin more than 3 × ULN	Permanently discontinue.[b]
Colitis or diarrhea[b]	Grade 2 or 3	Withhold dose until Grade 1 or resolved and corticosteroid dose is less than or equal to prednisone 10 mg/day (or equivalent).
	Grade 4	Permanently discontinue.[b]
Endocrinopathies (including but not limited to hypophysitis, adrenal insufficiency, hyperthyroidism, and type 1 diabetes mellitus)[b]	Grade 2, 3, or 4	Withhold dose until Grade 1 or resolved and clinically stable on hormone replacement therapy.
Other immune-mediated adverse reactions involving a major organ[b]	Grade 3	Withhold dose until Grade 1 or resolved and corticosteroid dose is less than or equal to prednisone 10 mg/day (or equivalent).
	Grade 4	Permanently discontinue.[b]
Infections[b]	Grade 3 or 4	Withhold dose until Grade 1 or resolved.
Infusion-related reactions[b]	Grade 1 or 2	Interrupt or slow the rate of infusion.
	Grade 3 or 4	Permanently discontinue.[b]
Persistent Grade 2 or 3 adverse reaction (excluding endocrinopathies)	Grade 2 or 3 adverse reaction that does not recover to Grade 0 or 1 within 12 weeks after last atezolizumab dose	Permanently discontinue.[b]
Inability to taper corticosteroid	Inability to reduce to less than or equal to prednisone 10 mg/day (or equivalent) within 12 weeks after last atezolizumab dose	Permanently discontinue.[b]
Recurrent Grade 3 or 4 adverse reaction	Recurrent Grade 3 or 4 (severe or life-threatening) adverse reaction	Permanently discontinue.[b]

[a]National Cancer Institute Common Terminology Criteria for Adverse Events (NCI CTCAE) version 4.
[b]See Precautions, Monitor, and Antidote.

- No dose adjustments are recommended for patients with mild or moderate renal impairment or mild hepatic impairment.

DILUTION

Atezolizumab is a colorless to slightly yellow solution available in a single-dose vial containing either 840 mg/14 mL or 1,200 mg/20 mL (60 mg/mL). Discard the vial if the solution is cloudy or discolored or if visible particles are observed. *Do not shake the vial.* Select the appropriate vial(s) based on the prescribed dose. Withdraw the required volume of atezolizumab from the vial(s) and transfer into a 250-mL polyvinyl chloride (PVC), polyethylene (PE), or polyolefin (PO) infusion bag containing NS. Dilute only with NS. Mix diluted solution by gentle inversion. *Do not shake.*

Filters: May use with or without a sterile, nonpyrogenic, low–protein-binding, in-line filter (pore size of 0.2-0.22 micron).

Storage: Store at 2° to 8° C (36° to 46° F) in original carton to protect from light. Does not contain a preservative. Do not freeze or shake. Administer immediately once prepared. If diluted solution is not used immediately, it can be stored at RT for up to 6 hours (from time of preparation and including infusion time) or refrigerated at 2° to 8° C (36° to 46° F) for no more than 24 hours. Discard empty vials of atezolizumab.

COMPATIBILITY

Manufacturer states, "Do not coadminister other drugs through the same intravenous line." **Compatible** only with NS.

RATE OF ADMINISTRATION

Do not administer as an intravenous push or bolus.

A single dose as an infusion equally distributed over 60 minutes through an IV line with or without a sterile, nonpyrogenic, low–protein binding, in-line filter (pore size of 0.2-0.22 micron). If the first infusion is tolerated, all subsequent infusions may be delivered over 30 minutes. Interrupt or slow the rate of infusion for mild or moderate infusion reactions. Permanently discontinue if a Grade 3 or 4 infusion reaction occurs.

ACTIONS

Atezolizumab is a programmed death ligand-1 (PD-L1) blocking antibody. PD-L1 may be expressed on tumor cells and/or tumor-infiltrating immune cells and can contribute to inhibition of the antitumor immune response in the tumor microenvironment. Binding of PD-L1 to the PD-1 and B7.1 receptors found on T-cells and antigen-presenting cells suppresses cytotoxic T-cell activity, T-cell proliferation, and cytokine production. Atezolizumab is a Fc-engineered, humanized, monoclonal antibody that binds to PD-L1 and blocks its interactions with the PD-1 and B7.1 receptors. This releases the PD-L1/PD-1–mediated inhibition of the immune response, including activation of the antitumor immune response without inducing antibody-dependent cellular cytotoxicity. In syngeneic mouse tumor models, blocking PD-L1 activity resulted in decreased tumor growth. Terminal half-life is approximately 27 days. The population PK analysis suggests a steady state is obtained after 6 to 9 weeks (2 to 3) cycles of repeated dosing.

INDICATIONS AND USES

Treatment of adult patients with locally advanced or metastatic urothelial carcinoma (MUC) who (1) are not eligible for cisplatin-containing chemotherapy and whose tumors express PD-L1 (PD-L1–stained tumor-infiltrating immune cells [IC] covering 5% or more of the tumor area) as determined by an FDA-approved test, or (2) are not eligible for any platinum-containing chemotherapy regardless of PD-L1 status, or (3) have disease progression during or following platinum-containing chemotherapy or within 12 months of neoadjuvant or adjuvant chemotherapy. This indication is approved under accelerated approval based on tumor response rate and durability of response. Continued approval may be contingent on verification and description of clinical benefit in confirmatory trial(s). ▪ Treatment of adult patients with metastatic NSCLC who have disease progression during or following platinum-containing chemotherapy. Given as a single agent. Patients with *EGFR* or *ALK* genomic tumor aberrations should have disease progression on FDA-approved therapy for NSCLC harboring these aberrations before receiving atezolizumab. ▪ First-line treatment of adult patients with metastatic nonsquamous non–small-cell lung cancer (Nsq NSCLC) with no EGFR or ALK genomic tumor aberrations. Given in combination with bevacizumab, paclitaxel, and carboplatin.

■ Treatment of adult patients with unresectable locally advanced or metastatic triple-negative breast cancer (TNBC) whose tumor expresses PD-L1 (PD-L1 stained tumor-infiltrating immune cells [IC] of any intensity covering ≥1% of the tumor area) as determined by an FDA-approved test. Given in combination with paclitaxel protein-bound. This indication is approved under accelerated approval based on progression-free survival. Continued approval may be contingent on verification and description of clinical benefit in confirmatory trial(s). ■ First-line treatment of adult patients with extensive-stage small-cell lung cancer (ES-SCLC). Given in combination with carboplatin and etoposide.

CONTRAINDICATIONS
Manufacturer states, "None."

PRECAUTIONS
Immune-mediated pneumonitis or interstitial lung disease (defined as requiring the use of systemic corticosteroids), including fatal cases, have occurred with atezolizumab. ■ Liver test abnormalities and immune-mediated hepatitis (defined as requiring the use of systemic corticosteroids), including fatal cases, has occurred with atezolizumab. ■ Immune-mediated colitis or diarrhea (defined as requiring the use of systemic corticosteroids) has occurred with atezolizumab. ■ Immune-related endocrinopathies, including adrenal insufficiency, hypophysitis/hypopituitarism, type 1 diabetes mellitus (including diabetic ketoacidosis), and thyroid disorders, have occurred with atezolizumab. ■ Atezolizumab can cause other severe and fatal immune-mediated adverse reactions that may involve any organ system (e.g., cardiac, dermatologic, gastrointestinal, hematologic, musculoskeletal, neurologic, ophthalmologic, renal, or vascular). May occur during or after treatment with atezolizumab; see Monitor. ■ Severe infections, including fatal cases, have been reported. Urinary tract infections were more common in patients with urothelial carcinoma; pneumonia was more common in patients with NSCLC. ■ Severe, sometimes life-threatening infusion-related reactions have been reported; see Rate of Administration. ■ See Dose Adjustments and Monitor for criteria to withhold or discontinue atezolizumab therapy and for medications for treatment of atezolizumab-related adverse reactions. ■ Effect of severe renal impairment or moderate or severe hepatic impairment on pharmacokinetics of atezolizumab is unknown. ■ A protein substance; has the potential for immunogenicity.

Monitor: Select cisplatin-ineligible patients with previously untreated locally advanced or metastatic urothelial carcinoma for treatment with atezolizumab based on the PD-L1 expression on tumor-infiltrating immune cells. Select patients with locally advanced or metastatic triple-negative breast cancer for treatment with atezolizumab in combination with paclitaxel protein-bound based on the PD-L1 expression of tumor-infiltrating immune cells. For information on FDA-approved tests, see http://www.fda.gov/companiondiagnostics. ■ Obtain baseline liver function studies and thyroid function tests and monitor periodically during treatment. ■ For any suspected immune-mediated adverse reaction, ensure adequate evaluation to confirm etiology or to exclude other causes. ■ Monitor for S/S of **pneumonitis** (e.g., chest pain, new or worsening cough, shortness of breath). Evaluate with radiographic imaging. Administer steroids (1 to 2 mg/kg/day prednisone equivalents, followed by corticosteroid taper) for Grade 2 or greater pneumonitis. Withhold or permanently discontinue atezolizumab based on the severity. See Dose Adjustments. ■ Monitor patients for S/S of **hepatitis** (e.g., easy bruising or bleeding, jaundice, lethargy, pain on right side of the abdomen, severe nausea or vomiting). Monitor AST, ALT, and bilirubin periodically during and after treatment with atezolizumab. Administer corticosteroids (1 to 2 mg/kg/day prednisone equivalents, followed by corticosteroid taper) for Grade 2 or higher elevations in AST, ALT, or bilirubin. Interrupt or permanently discontinue atezolizumab based on severity; see Dose Adjustments. ■ Monitor patients for S/S of **diarrhea or colitis**. Withhold atezolizumab treatment for Grade 2 or 3 diarrhea or colitis. If symptoms persist for longer than 5 days or recur, administer 1 to 2 mg/kg prednisone or equivalent per day followed by corticosteroid taper. Interrupt atezolizumab or permanently discontinue based on the severity. See Dose

Adjustments. ▪ Monitor for S/S of **hypophysitis** (e.g., fatigue, headache, dizziness or fainting, changes in vision, or low levels of hormones produced by the pituitary [ACTH], thyroid stimulating hormone [TSH], follicle-stimulating hormone [FSH], luteinizing hormone [LH], growth hormone [GH], or prolactin). For Grade 2 or higher hypophysitis, administer corticosteroids (1 to 2 mg/kg/day prednisone equivalents, followed by corticosteroid taper) and hormone replacement as clinically indicated. Interrupt therapy based on severity; see Dose Adjustments. ▪ Monitor for S/S of immune-mediated **thyroid disorders**. Monitor thyroid function tests periodically during treatment. Initiate hormone replacement therapy or medical management of hyperthyroidism as clinically indicated. Continue atezolizumab for hypothyroidism and interrupt for hyperthyroidism based on the severity; see Dose Adjustments. ▪ Monitor for S/S of **adrenal insufficiency** (e.g., fatigue, nausea, vomiting, hypotension, hyponatremia, hyperkalemia, low cortisol). For Grade 2 or higher adrenal insufficiency, administer prednisone 1 to 2 mg/kg/day or equivalent followed by a taper and hormone replacement as clinically indicated. Interrupt atezolizumab based on the severity; see Dose Adjustments. ▪ Monitor for S/S of **diabetes mellitus** (hyperglycemia, increased thirst, urination). Monitor serum glucose and, if indicated, initiate treatment with insulin for type 1 diabetes mellitus. Interrupt atezolizumab based on the severity; see Dose Adjustments. ▪ Monitor for S/S of **other immune-mediated adverse reactions** (e.g., cardiac [myocarditis], dermatologic [bullous dermatitis, pemphigoid, erythema multiforme, Stevens-Johnson syndrome (SJS)/toxic epidermal necrolysis (TEN)], gastrointestinal [pancreatitis, including increases in serum amylase or lipase levels], general [systemic inflammatory response syndrome, histiocytic necrotizing lymphadenitis], hematologic [autoimmune hemolytic anemia, immune thrombocytopenic purpura], musculoskeletal [myositis, rhabdomyolysis], neurologic [Guillain-Barré syndrome, myasthenia syndrome/myasthenia gravis, demyelination, immune-related meningoencephalitis, aseptic meningitis, encephalitis, facial and abducens nerve paresis, polymyalgia rheumatica, autoimmune neuropathy, and Vogt-Koyanagi-Harada syndrome], ophthalmologic [uveitis, iritis], renal [nephrotic syndrome, nephritis], vascular [vasculitis]). For suspected Grade 2 immune-mediated adverse reactions, exclude other causes and initiate corticosteroids as clinically indicated. For severe (Grade 3 or 4) adverse reactions, administer prednisone 1 to 2 mg/kg/day or equivalents, followed by a taper. Interrupt or permanently discontinue atezolizumab based on the severity of the reaction; see Dose Adjustments. If uveitis occurs in combination with other immune-mediated adverse reactions, evaluate for Vogt-Koyanagi-Harada syndrome, which has been observed with other products in this class and may require treatment with systemic steroids to reduce the risk of permanent vision loss. ▪ Monitor for S/S of **infection**. Initiate antibiotic therapy in patients with suspected or confirmed bacterial infections; see Dose Adjustments. ▪ Monitor for S/S of **infusion-related reactions** (e.g., chills, fever, flushing, hypotension, hypoxemia, pruritus, rash, rigors, wheezing). Interrupt, slow the rate of infusion, or permanently discontinue based on the severity. For Grade 1 or 2 infusion-related reactions, consider using premedications with subsequent doses.

Patient Education: Review FDA-approved Medication Guide. ▪ Verify pregnancy status in females of reproductive potential before initiating atezolizumab. ▪ Effective contraception required during treatment and for at least 5 months after the last dose of atezolizumab. ▪ Advise patients to contact their healthcare provider immediately for S/S of infusion-related reactions (e.g., chills, feeling faint, fever, flushing, hypoxemia, pruritus, rigors, wheezing). ▪ Some side effects may require corticosteroid treatment and interruption or discontinuation of atezolizumab. ▪ Promptly report S/S of pneumonitis (e.g., new or worsening cough, chest pain, shortness of breath). ▪ Promptly report S/S of hepatitis (e.g., easy bruising or bleeding, jaundice, lethargy, pain on right side of abdomen, severe nausea or vomiting). ▪ Promptly report S/S of colitis (e.g., blood or mucus in stools, diarrhea, severe abdominal pain). ▪ Promptly report S/S of hypophysitis, hyperthyroidism, hypothyroidism, adrenal insufficiency, or type 1 diabetes mellitus, including diabetic ketoacidosis. S/S may include constipation, dizziness or fainting, extreme tiredness, feeling cold, hair loss, headaches that will not go away, increased thirst or urination, and weight gain or weight loss. ■ Numerous side effects are possible. Report any side effect or change in condition to healthcare provider. ■ Keeping scheduled appointments for blood work or other laboratory tests is imperative. ■ May impair fertility in females of reproductive potential.

Maternal/Child: Based on its mechanism of action, atezolizumab can cause fetal harm when administered to a pregnant woman. ■ Do not breast-feed while taking atezolizumab and for at least 5 months after receiving the last dose. ■ Safety and effectiveness for use in pediatric patients have not been established.

Elderly: No overall difference in safety or efficacy has been observed between younger patients and patients 65 years of age and older.

DRUG/LAB INTERACTIONS
The drug interaction potential of atezolizumab is unknown.

SIDE EFFECTS
The most common adverse reactions with atezolizumab as a single agent are cough, decreased appetite, dyspnea, fatigue/asthenia, and nausea. The most common adverse reactions when used in combination with other antineoplastic drugs in patients with NSCLC and SCLC were alopecia, constipation, decreased appetite, diarrhea, fatigue/asthenia, and nausea. The most common adverse reactions when used in combination with paclitaxel protein-bound were alopecia, anemia, constipation, cough, decreased appetite, diarrhea, fatigue, headache, nausea, neutropenia, peripheral neuropathies, and vomiting.

Urothelial carcinoma: The most common Grade 3 or 4 adverse reactions reported include ALT increase, anemia, blood creatinine increase, decreased appetite, diarrhea, fatigue, hyponatremia, hypotension, intestinal obstruction, pain (back/neck), renal failure, sepsis, and urinary tract infection. Serious adverse reactions included acute kidney injury, diarrhea, intestinal obstruction, renal failure, and sepsis. Other adverse reactions included cough, peripheral edema, infusion reactions, pruritus, rash, respiratory tract infection, upper respiratory tract infection, venous thromboembolism, and vomiting. Diarrhea/colitis, dyspnea, fatigue, hypersensitivity, and sepsis led to discontinuation. Deaths resulted from cardiac arrest, intestinal obstruction, myocardial infarction, pneumonitis, respiratory distress or failure, and sepsis.

NSCLC: The most common adverse reactions reported include cough, decreased appetite, dyspnea, and fatigue. The most common Grade 3 or 4 adverse reactions include diarrhea, decreased appetite, dehydration, fatigue/asthenia, hypertension, febrile neutropenia, nausea, pneumonia, and pulmonary embolism. Deaths resulted from aortic dissection, aspiration pneumonia, cardiac arrest, cerebrovascular accident, chronic obstructive pulmonary disease, febrile neutropenia, hemoptysis, intestinal ischemia, intestinal obstruction, intracranial hemorrhage, pneumonia, pulmonary embolism, and pulmonary hemorrhage.

TNBC: The most common Grade 3 or 4 adverse reactions included anemia, decreased neutrophil count, fatigue, hypokalemia, increased AST, neutropenia, peripheral neuropathies, and pneumonia. The most frequent serious adverse reactions were dyspnea, fever, pneumonia, and urinary tract infection. The most common adverse reaction leading to discontinuation was peripheral neuropathy. Fatal adverse reactions included aspiration, autoimmune hepatitis, mucosal inflammation, pneumonia, pulmonary embolism, and septic shock. Numerous laboratory abnormalities occurred. See prescribing information for complete list.

SCLC: The most common Grade 3 or 4 adverse reactions were asthenia, diarrhea, fatigue/asthenia, febrile neutropenia, infusion-related reactions, and pneumonia. Fatal adverse reactions included neutropenia, pneumonia, and respiratory failure. Other adverse reactions included alopecia, anemia, constipation, decreased appetite, increased ALT, nausea, leukopenia, lymphopenia, thrombocytopenia, and vomiting.

See prescribing information for complete list of adverse reactions based on diagnosis.

See Precautions for additional serious adverse reactions that have been reported with the administration of atezolizumab.

ANTIDOTE

Keep physician informed of all side effects. May constitute a medical emergency or will be treated symptomatically as indicated. Interrupt or slow the rate of administration in patients with mild or moderate infusion reactions. See Dose Adjustments and Monitor for when to interrupt or permanently discontinue atezolizumab and for treatment specifics for immune-mediated adverse reactions. Treat hypersensitivity/infusion reactions as needed (e.g., oxygen, antihistamines, epinephrine, corticosteroids, vasopressors, and/or fluids). There is no information on overdose with atezolizumab.

ATROPINE SULFATE
(**AH**-troh-peen **SUL**-fayt)

Atropine

Anticholinergic
Antiarrhythmic
Antidote

pH 3 to 6.5

USUAL DOSE

IV administration is usually preferred, but subcutaneous, intramuscular, and endotracheal administration are possible. For administration via an endotracheal tube, dilute 1 to 2 mg in no more than 10 mL of SW or NS.

Titrate dose based on HR, PR interval, BP, and symptoms. Manufacturer-recommended adult doses are outlined in the following chart.

Manufacturer-Recommended Adult Dosage		
Use	**Dose**	**Repeat**
Antisialagogue or other antivagal	0.5 to 1 mg	1 to 2 hours
Organophosphorus[a] or muscarinic mushroom poisoning	2 to 3 mg[b]	20 to 30 minutes
Bradyasystolic cardiac arrest	1 mg	3 to 5 minutes; 3 mg maximum total dose

[a]Atropine is given in conjunction with pralidoxime for organophosphate insecticide and nerve agent poisoning.
[b]Higher doses have been used in severe poisoning. Consult a regional poison control center.

Other sources recommend the following doses:

Inhibition of salivation and secretions (preanesthesia): 0.4 to 0.6 mg 30 to 60 minutes preoperatively and repeat every 4 to 6 hours as needed.

Bradycardia: 0.5 mg every 3 to 5 minutes, not to exceed a total dose of 3 mg or 0.04 mg/kg.

Reversal of neuromuscular blockade: 15 to 30 mcg/kg administered with neostigmine or 7 to 10 mcg/kg administered with edrophonium. Administer in a separate syringe either concurrently or a few minutes before administering the anticholinesterase agent. If bradycardia is present, administer atropine first.

Cardiac asystole or pulseless electrical activity: AHA guidelines state, "Routine use during pulseless electrical activity or asystole is unlikely to have a therapeutic benefit."

PEDIATRIC DOSE

Fatal dose of atropine in pediatric patients may be as low as 10 mg. See Maternal/Child.

Dosing in pediatric patients has not been well studied. The manufacturer lists a usual initial dose of 0.01 to 0.03 mg/kg. Doses less than 0.1 mg have been associated with a paradoxical bradycardia.

Other sources recommend the following doses:

Inhibition of salivation and secretions (preanesthesia): Administer 30 to 60 minutes preoperatively and repeat every 4 to 6 hours as needed. *Infants; weight less than 5 kg:* 0.02 mg/kg/dose. There is no documented minimum dose for patients in this age/weight range. *Infants and children; weight equal to or more than 5 kg:* 0.01 to 0.02 mg/kg/dose; maximum single dose should not exceed 0.4 mg. Minimum recommended dose is 0.1 mg.

Bradycardia: *Infants; weight less than 5 kg:* 0.02 mg/kg/dose. There is no documented minimum dose for patients in this age/weight range. *Infants and children; weight equal to or more than 5 kg:* 0.02 mg/kg/dose; maximum single dose should not exceed 0.5 mg. May repeat one time in 3 to 5 minutes; maximum total dose should not exceed 1 mg. Minimum recommended dose is 0.1 mg.

Antidote for acute poisoning from exposure to anticholinesterase compounds (e.g., organophosphate compounds, nerve gases, mushroom poisoning): 0.05 to 0.1 mg/kg; repeat every 5 to 10 minutes until muscarinic S/S subside. Administer repeat doses as needed based on recurrence of symptoms.

Reversal of neuromuscular blockade: 0.01 to 0.02 mg/kg of atropine concomitantly with 0.04 mg/kg of neostigmine. See Usual Dose for additional information.

DOSE ADJUSTMENTS

Reduced dose may be indicated in the elderly based on decreased organ function and/or concomitant disease or other drug therapy. ▪ See Precautions, Drug/Lab Interactions, and Pediatric Dose.

DILUTION

May be given undiluted. Do not add to IV solutions. Inject through Y-tube or three-way stopcock of infusion set.

Storage: Store at CRT.

COMPATIBILITY

Compatibility information not available from manufacturer.

Other sources suggest specific **compatibilities** dependent on concentration and manufacturer; consult a pharmacist.

RATE OF ADMINISTRATION

Administer undiluted by rapid IV injection. Slow injection may cause a paradoxical bradycardia.

ACTIONS

Atropine is an anticholinergic drug and a potent belladonna alkaloid. An antimuscarinic agent that competitively antagonizes the muscarine-like actions of acetylcholine and other choline esters. Produces local, central, and peripheral effects on the body. Main therapeutic uses are peripheral, affecting smooth muscle, cardiac muscle, and exocrine gland cells. Increases heart rate and cardiac output and dries secretions. Widely distributed, metabolized by the liver via enzymatic hydrolysis, and excreted in urine. Half-life in adults is approximately 3 hours. Half-life in pediatric patients and adults over 65 years of age may be more than doubled. Crosses placental barrier. Secreted in breast milk.

INDICATIONS AND USES

Temporary blockade of severe or life-threatening muscarinic effects (e.g., as an antisialagogue, an antivagal agent, an antidote for organophosphorus or muscarinic mushroom poisoning, and for treatment of bradyasystolic cardiac arrest).

CONTRAINDICATIONS

Manufacturer states, "None." Other sources list hypersensitivity to atropine. No contraindications exist in the treatment of life-threatening organophosphorus or carbamate insecticide or nerve agent poisoning.

PRECAUTIONS

Use with caution in patients with coronary artery disease. When recurrent use is essential, the total dose should be restricted to 2 to 3 mg (0.03 to 0.04 mg/kg) to avoid the detrimental effects of atropine-induced tachycardia on myocardial oxygen demand. ▪ May precipitate acute glaucoma. ▪ May convert partial organic pyloric stenosis into complete obstruction. ▪ May cause complete urinary retention in patients with prostatic hypertrophy. ▪ May cause thickening of bronchial secretions and the formation of viscid mucous plugs in patients with chronic lung disease. ▪ Use with caution in patients with cardiovascular disease, pulmonary disease, autonomic neuropathy, GI disease (e.g., paralytic ileus, intestinal atony, severe ulcerative colitis, toxic megacolon), hyperthyroidism, myasthenia gravis, and renal or hepatic impairment.

Monitor: Vital signs and/or ECG based on specific situation. ▪ Monitor for resolution or return of symptoms in episodes of poisoning. ▪ Monitor for S/S of atropine toxicity (e.g., blurred vision, delirium, fever, muscle fasciculations, hot, dry skin).

Patient Education: Use caution if task requires alertness; may cause blurred vision, dizziness, or drowsiness. ▪ Report eye pain, flushing, or skin rash promptly. ▪ Report dry mouth, difficulty urinating, constipation, or increased light sensitivity.

Maternal/Child: Category C: safety for use in pregnancy, breast-feeding, and pediatric patients not established. ▪ Pediatric patients may be more sensitive to anticholinergic effects.

Elderly: May be more sensitive to adverse effects. ▪ Potential for constipation and urinary retention increased. ▪ See Dose Adjustments.

DRUG/LAB INTERACTIONS

May have additive effects when used in combination with **other agents with anticholinergic properties** (e.g., glycopyrrolate, phenothiazines, tricyclic antidepressants). ▪ May potentiate effects of many oral drugs by delaying gastric emptying and increasing absorption (e.g., **atenolol, digoxin, nitrofurantoin, thiazide diuretics**). ▪ Decreases the rate of **mexiletine** absorption without altering the relative oral bioavailability. ▪ Antagonizes **anticholinesterase inhibitors** (e.g., edrophonium, pyridostigmine).

SIDE EFFECTS

Most side effects of atropine are directly related to its antimuscarinic action. Blurred vision, dryness of the mouth, photophobia, and tachycardia commonly occur. Other possible reactions include anhidrosis (leading to heat intolerance), constipation, dilation of the pupils, flushing, heat prostration from decreased sweating, hypersensitivity reactions (e.g., skin rashes that in some cases progressed to exfoliation), nausea, paralytic ileus, tachycardia, urinary hesitancy and retention (especially in males), and vomiting.

Overdose: *Excessive doses* may cause ataxia; difficulty swallowing; dilated pupils; dizziness; fatigue; hot, dry skin; palpitations; restlessness; thirst; and tremor. *Toxic doses* may lead to restlessness and excitation, hallucinations, delirium, and coma. *Severe intoxication* may lead to depression and circulatory collapse, paralysis, coma, respiratory failure, and death.

ANTIDOTE

Discontinue if side effects increase or are severe. Notify physician. Use standard treatments to manage cardiac arrhythmias. Physostigmine salicylate (1 to 4 mg [0.5 to 1 mg in pediatric patients]) reverses most cardiovascular and CNS effects. Repeat doses as needed. Diazepam or a short-acting barbiturate may be administered as needed to control marked excitement and convulsions. Large doses should be avoided because central depressant action may coincide with the depression that occurs late in atropine poisoning. Central stimulants are not recommended. Artificial respiration with oxygen may be necessary. Ice bags and alcohol sponges help to reduce fever, especially in pediatric patients. Atropine is not removed by dialysis.

AVELUMAB
(a-**VEL**-ue-mab)

Bavencio

Antineoplastic agent
Monoclonal antibody (Anti-PD-L1)

pH 5 to 5.6

USUAL DOSE

Pretreatment: Verify pregnancy status. Baseline studies required; see Monitor.

Premedication: Premedicate with an antihistamine (e.g., diphenhydramine) and acetaminophen before the first 4 infusions of avelumab. Administer for subsequent avelumab doses based on clinical judgment and the presence/severity of prior infusion reactions. See Monitor.

Metastatic Merkel cell carcinoma and urothelial carcinoma: 800 mg as an IV infusion over 60 minutes every 2 weeks until disease progression or unacceptable toxicity.

Renal cell carcinoma: 800 mg as an IV infusion over 60 minutes every 2 weeks in combination with axitinib 5 mg orally taken twice daily (12 hours apart) with or without food until disease progression or unacceptable toxicity. When axitinib is used in combination with avelumab, dose escalation of axitinib above the initial 5-mg dose may be considered at intervals of 2 weeks or longer. Review the full prescribing information for axitinib before initiation.

DOSE ADJUSTMENTS

Recommended Dose Modifications for Avelumab		
Treatment-Related Adverse Reaction	**Severity of Adverse Reactions**[a]	**Dose Modification**
Pneumonitis	Grade 2 pneumonitis	Withhold avelumab. Resume avelumab in patients with complete or partial resolution (Grade 0 to 1) of pneumonitis after corticosteroid taper.
	Grade 3 or 4 pneumonitis or recurrent Grade 2 pneumonitis	Permanently discontinue avelumab.
Hepatitis For avelumab in combination with axitinib, see the following chart.	AST or ALT more than 3 and up to 5 × ULN or total bilirubin more than 1.5 and up to 3 × ULN	Withhold avelumab. Resume avelumab in patients with complete or partial resolution (Grade 0 to 1) of hepatitis after corticosteroid taper.
	AST or ALT more than 5 × ULN or total bilirubin more than 3 × ULN	Permanently discontinue avelumab.
Colitis	Grade 2 or 3 diarrhea or colitis	Withhold avelumab. Resume avelumab in patients with complete or partial resolution (Grade 0 to 1) of colitis or diarrhea after corticosteroid taper.
	Grade 4 diarrhea or colitis or recurrent Grade 3 diarrhea or colitis	Permanently discontinue avelumab.
Endocrinopathies (including but not limited to hypothyroidism, hyperthyroidism, adrenal insufficiency, hyperglycemia)	Grade 3 or 4 endocrinopathies	Withhold avelumab. Resume avelumab in patients with complete or partial resolution (Grade 0 to 1) of endocrinopathies after corticosteroid taper.

Continued

Recommended Dose Modifications for Avelumab—cont'd		
Treatment-Related Adverse Reaction	**Severity of Adverse Reactions[a]**	**Dose Modification**
Nephritis and renal dysfunction	Serum creatinine more than 1.5 and up to 6 × ULN	Withhold avelumab. Resume avelumab in patients with complete or partial resolution (Grade 0 to 1) of nephritis and renal dysfunction after corticosteroid taper.
	Serum creatinine more than 6 × ULN	Permanently discontinue avelumab.
Other immune-mediated adverse reactions, including but not limited to anemia, arthritis, bullous dermatitis, demyelination, encephalitis, erythema multiforme, exfoliative dermatitis, Guillain-Barré syndrome, hemolytic anemia, histiocytic necrotizing lymphadenitis, hypophysitis, hypopituitarism, iritis, myasthenia gravis, myocarditis, myositis, pancreatitis, pemphigoid, psoriasis, rhabdomyolysis, Stevens-Johnson syndrome (SJS)/toxic epidermal necrolysis (TEN), uveitis, and vasculitis[b]	For any of the following: • Moderate or severe clinical signs or symptoms of an immune-mediated adverse reaction not described above • Grade 3 or 4 endocrinopathies	Withhold avelumab pending clinical evaluation. Resume avelumab in patients with complete or partial resolution (Grade 0 to 1) of other immune-mediated adverse reactions after corticosteroid taper.
	For any of the following: • Life-threatening adverse reaction (excluding endocrinopathies) • Recurrent severe immune-mediated adverse reaction • Requirement for 10 mg/day or greater prednisone or equivalent for more than 12 weeks • Persistent Grade 2 or 3 immune-mediated adverse reactions lasting 12 weeks or longer	Permanently discontinue avelumab.
Infusion-related reaction	Grade 1 or 2	Interrupt or slow the rate of infusion.
	Grade 3 or 4	Permanently discontinue avelumab.

[a]Toxicity was graded per National Cancer Institute Common Terminology Criteria for Adverse Events (CTCAE), Version 4.

[b]Observed with avelumab or with other anti-PD-1/PD-L1 monoclonal antibodies.

Recommended Dose Modifications for Avelumab in Combination With Axitinib		
Treatment-Related Adverse Reaction	**Severity of Adverse Reactions[a]**	**Dose Modification**
Hepatitis	AST or ALT >3 and ≤5 × ULN or total bilirubin >1.5 and ≤3 × ULN	Withhold both avelumab and axitinib until these adverse reactions recover to Grades 0-1. If persistent (>5 days) consider corticosteroid therapy (initial dose of 0.5 to 1 mg/kg/day prednisone or equivalent followed by a taper). Consider rechallenge with a single drug or sequential rechallenge with both drugs after recovery. Reduce dose per the axitinib full prescribing information if rechallenging with axitinib.
	AST or ALT ≥5 × ULN or >3 × ULN with concurrent total bilirubin ≥2 × ULN or total bilirubin ≥3 × ULN	Permanently discontinue avelumab and axitinib and consider corticosteroid therapy (initial dose of 0.5 to 1 mg/kg/day prednisone or equivalent followed by a taper).
Cardiovascular events	Grade 3-4	Permanently discontinue avelumab and axitinib.

[a]Toxicity was graded per National Cancer Institute Common Terminology Criteria for Adverse Events (CTCAE), Version 4.

No pharmacokinetic differences were observed in patient subgroups defined by age, gender, race, PD-L1 status, tumor burden, and hepatic and renal function (mild, moderate, or severe renal insufficiency; mild to moderate impaired hepatic function). The pharmacokinetics of avelumab is unknown in patients with severe hepatic impairment. ■ In patients with advanced RCC, avelumab clearance in patients who tested positive for treatment-emergent antidrug antibodies (ADA) was 15% higher as compared with clearance in patients who tested negative. ■ See Monitor and Precautions.

DILUTION

Available as a 200 mg/10 mL (20 mg/mL) clear, colorless to slightly yellow solution in a single-dose vial. Withdraw the required volume of avelumab from the vial(s) and inject it into a 250-mL infusion bag containing either NS or ½NS. Gently invert the bag to mix the diluted solution, and avoid foaming or excessive shearing. ***Do not shake***. Inspect the solution to ensure it is clear, colorless, and free of visible particles.

Filters: Use of sterile, nonpyrogenic, low–protein-binding in-line filter (pore size of 0.2 micron) required.

Storage: Before use, refrigerate vials at 2° to 8° C (36° to 46° F) in original carton to protect from light. Do not freeze or shake. Store diluted avelumab at RT up to 25° C (77° F) for no more than 4 hours from the time of dilution **OR** under refrigeration at 2° to 8° C (36° to 46° F) for no more than 24 hours from the time of dilution. Do not freeze. If refrigerated, allow the diluted solution to come to RT before administration. Protect diluted solution from light. Discard any partially used or empty vials.

COMPATIBILITY

Manufacturer states, "Do not coadminister other drugs through the same intravenous line."

RATE OF ADMINISTRATION

A single dose equally distributed over 60 minutes through an IV line containing a sterile, nonpyrogenic, low–protein-binding in-line filter (pore size of 0.2 micron). Interrupt or slow the rate of infusion for mild or moderate infusion-related reactions; see Dose Adjustments.

ACTIONS

A human IgG1 lambda monoclonal antibody. Avelumab is a programmed death ligand-1 (PD-L1) blocking antibody. Avelumab binds PD-L1 and blocks the interaction between PD-L1 and its receptors PD-1 and B7.1. This interaction releases the inhibitory effects of PD-L1 on the immune response, resulting in the restoration of immune responses, including antitumor immune responses. Shown to induce antibody-dependent cell-mediated cytotoxicity (ADCC) in vitro. Primary elimination mechanism is proteolytic degradation. Terminal half-life was 6.1 days in patients receiving 10 mg/kg. When avelumab 10 mg/kg was administered in combination with axitinib 5 mg, the respective exposures of avelumab and axitinib were comparable to the single agents.

INDICATIONS AND USES

Treatment of adults and pediatric patients 12 years and older with metastatic Merkel cell carcinoma (MCC). ▪ Treatment of patients with locally advanced or metastatic urothelial carcinoma (UC) who have disease progression during or following platinum-containing chemotherapy or who have disease progression within 12 months of neoadjuvant or adjuvant treatment with platinum-containing therapy. These indications are approved under accelerated approval based on tumor response and duration of response. Continued approval may be contingent on verification and description of clinical benefit in confirmatory trials. ▪ Treatment of patients with advanced renal cell carcinoma (RCC) in combination with axitinib.

CONTRAINDICATIONS

Manufacturer states, "None."

PRECAUTIONS

Avelumab can cause immune-mediated pneumonitis, including fatal cases. ▪ Avelumab can cause immune-mediated hepatitis, including fatal cases. ▪ Avelumab can cause immune-mediated colitis. ▪ Avelumab can cause immune-mediated endocrinopathies (e.g., adrenal insufficiency, thyroid disorders [hypothyroidism/hyperthyroidism], Type 1 diabetes mellitus, including diabetic ketoacidosis). ▪ Avelumab can cause immune-mediated thyroid disorders. Thyroid disorders can occur at any time during treatment. Manage hypothyroidism with hormone-replacement therapy. Initiate medical management for control of hyperthyroidism. ▪ Avelumab can cause type 1 diabetes mellitus, including diabetic ketoacidosis. Withhold avelumab and administer antihyperglycemics or insulin in patients with severe or life-threatening hyperglycemia. ▪ Avelumab can cause immune-mediated nephritis. ▪ Avelumab can result in other severe and fatal immune-mediated adverse reactions; see Dose Adjustments. These immune-mediated reactions may involve any organ system. Most immune-mediated reactions initially manifest during avelumab treatment but may occur after discontinuation. ▪ Avelumab can cause severe or life-threatening infusion-related reactions. These reactions may occur after completion of the infusion. Premedicate with an antihistamine and acetaminophen before the first 4 infusions; see Usual Dose. ▪ Avelumab in combination with axitinib can cause severe and fatal cardiovascular events. Optimize management of cardiovascular risk factors such as diabetes, dyslipidemia, or hypertension. ▪ A protein substance; has a potential for immunogenicity. **Monitor:** Obtain baseline serum creatinine, serum glucose, liver function tests, and thyroid function tests before initiating treatment, and monitor periodically during treatment and as indicated based on clinical evaluation. ▪ When using avelumab in combination with axitinib, consider baseline and periodic evaluations of left ventricular ejection fraction and more frequent monitoring of liver enzymes. ▪ Monitor for S/S of pneumonitis, and evaluate patients with suspected pneumonitis with radiographic imaging. ▪ Monitor for S/S of colitis. ▪ Monitor for S/S of adrenal insufficiency during and after treatment. Administer corticosteroids as appropriate for adrenal insufficiency. ▪ Monitor for hyperglycemia or other S/S of diabetes. For patients with severe or life-threatening hyperglycemia, resume treatment with avelumab when metabolic control is achieved with insulin replacement or antihyperglycemics. ▪ Monitor for other possible immune-mediated adverse reactions. Evaluate to confirm or rule out an immune-mediated adverse reaction and to exclude other causes. Use of high-dose corticosteroids and/or hormone replacement therapy may be indicated. ▪ Monitor for S/S of infusion-related reactions, including abdominal pain, back pain, chills, dyspnea, fever, flushing, hypotension, urticaria, and wheezing. ▪ Administer corticosteroids (initial dose of 1 to 2 mg/kg/day prednisone or equivalent, followed by a corticosteroid taper) for Grade 2 or greater colitis, hepatitis, nephritis, pneumonitis, or other immune-mediated reactions. ▪ Monitor for S/S of cardiovascular events. ▪ See Precautions and Dose Adjustments.

Patient Education: Review manufacturer's medication guide. ▪ Review medical conditions and medications with healthcare provider. ▪ Avoid pregnancy; females of child-bearing potential should use effective contraception during treatment with avelumab and for at least 1 month after the last dose. ▪ Promptly report S/S of pneumonitis (e.g., chest pain, new or worsening cough, or shortness of breath). ▪ Promptly report S/S of hepatitis (e.g., easy bruising or bleeding, jaundice, lethargy, pain on the right side of abdomen, or severe nausea or vomiting). ▪ Promptly report S/S of colitis (e.g., diarrhea or severe abdominal pain). ▪ Promptly report S/S of endocrinopathies (e.g., adrenal insufficiency, diabetes mellitus, hyperthyroidism, or hypothyroidism). ▪ Promptly report S/S of nephritis and renal dysfunction (e.g., blood in urine, decreased urine output, loss of appetite, swelling in ankles, or any other symptoms of renal dysfunction). ▪ Promptly report S/S of infusion-related reactions (e.g., chills, fever, hives, and shortness of breath or wheezing). ▪ Promptly report S/S of cardiovascular events (e.g., dyspnea, new or worsening chest discomfort, or peripheral edema).

Maternal/Child: Based on its mechanism of action, avelumab can cause fetal harm. Females of reproductive potential should use effective contraception during treatment with avelumab and for at least 1 month after the last dose. ▪ Discontinue breast-feeding during therapy with avelumab and for at least 1 month after final dose. ▪ Safety and effectiveness for use in pediatric patients under 12 years of age not established.

Elderly: Studies with MCC did not include sufficient numbers of patients 65 years of age and older to determine whether they respond differently than younger patients. No overall differences in safety or efficacy were reported between elderly patients and younger patients in UC or RCC studies.

DRUG/LAB INTERACTIONS
Formal drug interaction studies have not been conducted.

SIDE EFFECTS
The most common side effects reported were abdominal pain, cough, decreased appetite, diarrhea, dysphonia, dyspnea, fatigue, headache, hepatoxicity, hypertension, hypothyroidism, infusion-related reactions, mucositis, musculoskeletal pain, nausea, palmar-plantar erythrodysesthesia, peripheral edema, rash, and urinary tract infections. Other side effects reported were arthralgia, constipation, decreased weight, dizziness, fever, pruritus, and vomiting. Laboratory abnormalities included anemia; decreased hemoglobin and platelet count; hyperglycemia; hyperkalemia; hyponatremia; increased alkaline phosphatase, ALT, amylase, AST, bilirubin, cholesterol, creatinine, GGT, lipase, and triglycerides; lymphopenia; neutropenia; and thrombocytopenia. Serious immune-mediated colitis, immune-mediated endocrinopathies, immune-mediated hepatitis (as a single agent and in combination with axitinib) and hepatoxicity, immune-mediated nephritis and renal dysfunction, immune-mediated pneumonitis, and other immune-mediated reactions have occurred. Major adverse cardiovascular events have also occurred. For complete list of adverse reactions, see full prescribing information.

ANTIDOTE
Keep physician informed of all side effects. May constitute a medical emergency or will be treated symptomatically as indicated. Withhold or permanently discontinue avelumab as outlined in the chart in Dose Adjustments. Discontinue avelumab and axitinib for Grade 3 or 4 cardiovascular events. For life-threatening infusion reactions, immediately and permanently stop avelumab and administer appropriate supportive treatment. For less severe infusion reactions, management may involve temporarily stopping the infusion, reducing the infusion rate, and/or administering symptomatic treatment (e.g., IV saline, diphenhydramine, bronchodilators such as albuterol and acetaminophen). Resuscitate if indicated.

Axatilimab
(AX a TIL I mab)

Monoclonal Antibody

Niktimvo

USUAL DOSE

The recommended dosage of NIKTIMVO is 0.3 mg/kg (maximum 35 mg) every 2 weeks in adult and pediatric patients weighing ≥40 kg.

PEDIATRIC DOSE

The recommended dosage of NIKTIMVO is 0.3 mg/kg (maximum 35 mg) every 2 weeks in adult and pediatric patients weighing ≥40 kg.

DOSE ADJUSTMENTS

Renal: No dosage adjustments provided by manufacturer

Hepatic: No dosage adjustments provided by manufacturer

Dosage adjustments based on adverse reactions:

Adverse Reaction Grade 1 or 2 ■ Temporarily interrupt the infusion until resolution or decrease infusion rate by 50% ■ Initiate symptomatic treatment (eg, antihistamines and antipyretics) ■ For subsequent infusions, premedicate and resume the infusion at 50% of the prior infusion rate.

Grade 3 or 4 Permanently discontinue. Elevation of aspartate aminotransferase (AST) or alanine aminotransferase (ALT; on day of dosing) Grade 3 with total bilirubin ≤ Grade 1 withhold NIKTIMVO until recovery to Grade 2, then resume at 0.2 mg/kg (maximum 23 mg) every 2 weeks.

Elevation of AST or ALT (regardless of time of the reaction): AST or ALT ≥3 times upper limit of normal (ULN) with total bilirubin ≥2 times ULN and alkaline phosphatase (ALP) <2 times ULN, withhold and investigate for drug-induced liver injury. If confirmed, permanently discontinue. Grade 4, permanently discontinue.

Elevation of CPK, amylase, or lipase ≥ Grade 3 ■ If diagnostic evaluation results show no evidence of end-organ damage, continue without dose reduction ■ If diagnostic evaluation results show evidence of end-organ damage, permanently discontinue. Symptomatic ≥ Grade 3 Permanently discontinue.

Other nonhematologic adverse reactions Grade 3, withhold until recovery to Grade 2 ■ If delayed by ≤4 weeks from the planned infusion, resume at 0.2 mg/kg (maximum 23 mg) every 2 weeks ■ If delayed by >4 weeks from the planned infusion, permanently discontinue. Grade 4 Permanently discontinue.

DILUTION

■ Withdraw the calculated volume of solution from the vial and add it into an intravenous infusion bag containing 0.9% Sodium Chloride Injection to achieve a final concentration between the range of 0.24 mg/mL and 0.75 mg/mL. Discard vial with any unused portion. Mix diluted solution by gentle inversion. Do not shake. Discard if the solution is cloudy, discolored, or contains extraneous particulate matter other than trace amounts of translucent to white particles.

Administration

Administer diluted solution by intravenous infusion over 30 minutes through a dedicated infusion line that includes a sterile, low-protein binding 0.2-micron in-line or add-on polyethersulfone (PES) filter • Do not coadminister other drugs through the same infusion line • After administration, flush the infusion line with 0.9% Sodium Chloride Injection.

ACTIONS

Axatilimab-csfr is a monoclonal antibody that binds to colony-stimulating factor-1 receptors (CSF-1R) expressed on monocytes and macrophages. Blocking CSF-1R with axatilimab-csfr reduces the levels of these circulating proinflammatory and profibrotic monocytes and monocyte-derived macrophages, as demonstrated by a reduction of nonclassical monocyte counts in nonclinical studies with axatilimab-csfr, and inhibits the activity of pathogenic macrophages in tissues.

INDICATIONS AND USES
Treatment of chronic graft-versus-host disease

CONTRAINDICATIONS
No contraindications are listed by manufacturer.

PRECAUTIONS
Infusion-Related Reactions: Interrupt or slow the rate of infusion or permanently discontinue NIKTIMVO based on severity of reaction.

Monitoring Parameters: Monitor AST, ALT, ALP, creatine phosphokinase (CPK), amylase, and lipase before the start of NIKTIMVO therapy, every 2 weeks for the first month, and every 1 to 2 months thereafter until abnormalities are resolved.

Patient Education: Advise patients and caregivers that infusion-related reactions may occur during NIKTIMVO treatment. Inform patients and caregivers of the signs and symptoms of infusion-related reactions and to seek medical care should signs and symptoms occur.

Maternal/Child: Pregnancy considerations: May cause fetal harm. Advise females of reproductive potential of the potential risk to a fetus and to use effective contraception.

Breastfeeding considerations: It is not known if axatilimab is present in breast milk.

Elderly: No specific recommendations; refer to adult dosing.

DRUG/LAB INTERACTIONS
No drug interaction information is listed in prescribing information.

SIDE EFFECTS
The most common ($\geq$15%) adverse reactions, including laboratory abnormalities, are increased AST, infection (pathogen unspecified), increased ALT, decreased phosphate, decreased hemoglobin, viral infection, increased GGT, musculoskeletal pain, increased lipase, fatigue, increased amylase, increased calcium, increased CPK, increased ALP, nausea, headache, diarrhea, cough, bacterial infection, pyrexia, and dyspnea.

ANTIDOTE
There is no antidote; stop infusion for hypersensitivity reactions and treat appropriately.

AZACITIDINE

(ay-za-**SYE**-ti-deen)

Vidaza

Antineoplastic
Antimetabolite

USUAL DOSE

Pretreatment: Verify pregnancy status. Baseline studies indicated; see Monitor.

Premedication: Prophylactic administration of antiemetics (e.g., granisetron, ondansetron [Zofran]) is indicated before each dose.

First treatment cycle: An initial dose of 75 mg/M^2 as an IV infusion or as a SQ injection once daily for 7 days is recommended for all patients regardless of baseline hematology.

Subsequent treatment cycles: Cycles should be repeated every 4 weeks. Dose may be increased to 100 mg/M^2 if no beneficial effect is seen after 2 treatment cycles and if no toxicity other than nausea and vomiting has occurred. Treatment is recommended for a minimum of 4 to 6 cycles; however, a complete or partial response may require additional treatment cycles. Repeat cycles may be administered as long as the patient continues to benefit. See Dose Adjustments for dose delay or reduction recommendations for hematologic response, renal toxicities, and/or electrolyte disturbances.

DOSE ADJUSTMENTS

After administration of the recommended dosage for the first cycle, adjust dosage for subsequent cycles based on nadir counts and hematologic response as outlined in the following chart.

Dose Adjustments of Azacitidine Based on Baseline Hematologic Responses		
In any given subsequent cycle for patients with a baseline (start of treatment) WBC equal to or greater than 3 × 10⁹/L (3,000 cells/mm³), ANC equal to or greater than 1.5 × 10⁹/L (1,500 cells/mm³), and platelets equal to or greater than 75 × 10⁹/L (75,000 cells/mm³): Adjust the dose based on nadir counts according to the following chart.		

Nadir Counts		% Dose in the Next Cycle
ANC (cells/mm³)	**Platelets (cells/mm³)**	
<500 cells/mm³	<25,000 cells/mm³	50%
500 to 1,500 cells/mm³	25,000 to 50,000 cells/mm³	67%
>1,500 cells/mm³	≥50,000 cells/mm³	100%

In any given subsequent cycle for patients with a baseline (start of treatment) WBC less than 3 × 10⁹/L (3,000 cells/mm³), ANC less than 1.5 × 10⁹/L (1,500 cells/mm³), or platelets less than 75 × 10⁹/L (75,000 cells/mm³): Adjust the dose based on nadir counts and bone marrow biopsy cellularity at the time of the nadir according to the following chart. *The exception is the presence of clear improvement in differentiation (% of mature granulocytes is higher and ANC is higher than at the onset of that course) at the time of the next cycle. If this improvement occurs, the dose of the current treatment should be continued.*

WBC or Platelet Nadir (% Decrease in Counts from Baseline)	Bone Marrow Biopsy Cellularity at Time of Nadir (%)		
	30% to 60%	15% to 30%	<15%
	% Dose in the Next Course		
50% to 75%	100%	50%	33%
>75%	75%	50%	33%

If a nadir as defined in this chart has occurred, give the next course 28 days after the start of the preceding course, provided that both the WBC and the platelet count are greater than 25% above the nadir and are rising. If a greater than 25% increase above the nadir is not seen by Day 28, counts should be reassessed every 7 days. If a 25% increase is not seen by Day 42, reduce the scheduled dose by 50%.

Dose adjustments of azacitidine based on renal toxicity and serum electrolytes: If unexplained reductions in serum bicarbonate levels to less than 20 mEq/L occur, reduce the dose by 50% on the next course. ▪ If unexplained elevations of BUN or SCr occur, delay the next cycle until values return to baseline and then reduce the dose by 50% on the next course. Severe renal impairment (CrCl less than 30 mL/min) has no major effect on exposure of azacitidine after multiple SQ administrations. Therefore azacitidine can be administered to patients with renal impairment without Cycle 1 dose adjustment. (IV route was not studied.) ▪ Use care in dose selection for the elderly; reduced doses may be indicated based on overall renal function.

DILUTION
Specific techniques required; see Precautions. Available as a lyophilized powder in single-use vials containing 100 mg. More than one vial may be required for a single dose. Reconstitute each vial with 10 mL SWFI. Vigorously shake or roll each vial until all solids are dissolved. Solution equals 10 mg/mL. Withdraw the required amount of azacitidine to deliver the desired dose and inject into a 50- or 100-mL infusion bag of NS or LR. Administration must be complete within 1 hour of reconstitution. Discard unused portions appropriately.

Filters: Specific information not available.

Storage: Store in cartons at CRT. Reconstituted solutions may be held at 25° C (77° F), but administration must be complete within 1 hour of reconstitution.

COMPATIBILITY
Manufacturer lists azacitidine as **incompatible** with D5W, hetastarch, or any solution that contains bicarbonate. These solutions have the potential to increase the rate of degradation of azacitidine.

RATE OF ADMINISTRATION
A single dose equally distributed over 10 to 40 minutes. Administration must be complete within 1 hour of reconstitution.

ACTIONS
A pyrimidine nucleoside analog of cytidine. Azacitidine is believed to exert its antineoplastic effects by causing hypomethylation of DNA and direct cytotoxicity on abnormal hematopoietic cells in the bone marrow. Cytotoxic effects cause the death of rapidly dividing cells, including cancer cells that are no longer responsive to normal growth-control mechanisms. Nonproliferating cells are relatively insensitive to azacitidine. This hypomethylation of DNA may restore normal function to genes that are critical for cellular differentiation and proliferation. May be metabolized by the liver. Half-life is 4 hours. Primarily excreted in urine with minimal excretion in feces.

INDICATIONS AND USES
Treatment of patients with the following French-American-British (FAB) myelodysplastic syndrome (MDS) subtypes such as refractory anemia (RA), refractory anemia with ringed sideroblasts (if accompanied by neutropenia or thrombocytopenia or requiring transfusions), refractory anemia with excess blasts (RAEB), refractory anemia with excess blasts in transformation (RAEB-T), and chronic myelomonocytic leukemia (CMMoL).

CONTRAINDICATIONS
Known hypersensitivity to azacitidine. ▪ Patients with advanced malignant hepatic tumors.

PRECAUTIONS

Follow guidelines for handling cytotoxic agents; see Appendix A, p. 1308. ■ If azacitidine comes into contact with skin, immediately wash with soap and water. If it comes into contact with mucous membranes, flush thoroughly with water. ■ Administer by or under the direction of a physician specialist in a facility with adequate diagnostic and treatment facilities to monitor the patient and respond to any medical emergency. ■ Use caution in patients with liver disease; potentially hepatotoxic in patients with severe pre-existing hepatic impairment; see Contraindications. Cases of progressive hepatic coma and death have been reported in patients with extensive tumor burden due to metastatic disease, especially when baseline albumin is less than 3 Gm/dL. ■ Reports of renal abnormalities (e.g., elevated serum creatinine, renal failure, and death) have occurred in patients treated with azacitidine in combination with other chemotherapeutic agents for non-MDS conditions. Patients with renal impairment may be at increased risk for renal toxicity. ■ Renal tubular acidosis (a fall in serum bicarbonate to less than 20 mEq/L in association with an alkaline urine and hypokalemia [serum potassium less than 3 mEq/L]) developed in 5 patients with chronic myelogenous leukemia (CML) (an unapproved use) treated with azacitidine and etoposide. ■ May cause fatal or serious tumor lysis syndrome (TLS), including in patients with MDS; may occur despite concomitant use of uric acid–lowering drugs (e.g., allopurinol [Aloprim]). ■ The effects of age, race, gender, or hepatic impairment on the pharmacokinetics of azacitidine have not been studied. ■ Anemia, neutropenia, and thrombocytopenia may be dose-limiting toxicities.

Monitor: Verify pregnancy status of females of reproductive potential before initiating azacitidine. ■ Obtain a baseline CBC with platelets, and monitor before each dosing cycle and as indicated to monitor response and toxicity between cycles. ■ Obtain baseline renal and hepatic function (BUN, SCr, LFT, bilirubin) studies and electrolytes; monitor with each cycle and during treatment as indicated. ■ Monitor for tumor lysis syndrome. Monitor uric acid levels and maintain hydration. Uric acid–lowering drugs (e.g., allopurinol [Aloprim]) may be indicated. ■ Use prophylactic antiemetics to reduce nausea and vomiting and to increase patient comfort. ■ Monitor for S/S of infection. Prophylactic antibiotics may be indicated pending results of C/S in a febrile neutropenic patient. ■ Monitor for thrombocytopenia (platelet count less than 50,000/mm³). Initiate precautions to prevent excessive bleeding (e.g., inspect IV sites, skin, and mucous membranes; use extreme care during invasive procedures; test urine, emesis, stool, and secretions for occult blood). ■ Avoid administration of live virus vaccine to immunocompromised patients. ■ See Precautions and Antidote.

Patient Education: Avoid pregnancy; effective contraception required for females of reproductive potential during treatment and for 6 months after the final dose. Effective contraception required for males with female partners of reproductive potential during treatment and for 3 months after the final dose. ■ Patients should report a suspected pregnancy immediately. ■ Azacitidine may have an effect on male or female fertility. ■ Inform physician about any underlying liver or renal disease.

Maternal/Child: Avoid pregnancy; may cause fetal harm. ■ Discontinue breast-feeding during treatment and for 1 week after the final dose. ■ Safety and effectiveness for use in pediatric patients not established.

Elderly: Safety and effectiveness similar to younger adults. ■ Consider age-related renal impairment; dosing should be cautious; see Dose Adjustments. Monitor renal function.

DRUG/LAB INTERACTIONS

Formal drug interaction studies have not been completed. ■ Effect on metabolism by some known microsomal enzyme inhibitors or inducers has been studied in vitro. Does not appear to inhibit CYP2B6 or CYP2C8. Potential to inhibit other CYP enzymes is not known. Does not appear to induce CYP1A2, CYP2C19, or CYP3A4/5. ■ Do not administer **live virus vaccines** to patients receiving antineoplastic agents.

SIDE EFFECTS

Hypokalemia, petechiae, rigors, and weakness are the most common side effects. Other common side effects include anemia; constipation; diarrhea; ecchymosis; fever; injection site bruising, erythema, and pain; leukopenia; nausea; neutropenia; thrombocytopenia; and vomiting. Febrile neutropenia, fever, leukopenia, neutropenia, pneumonia, and thrombocytopenia were the most frequent causes of dose reduction, delay, and discontinuation. Infusion site erythema or pain and catheter site reactions such as infection, erythema, or hemorrhage were reported with IV administration. Elevated SCr, hepatic coma, hypokalemia, renal failure, renal tubular acidosis, and tumor lysis syndrome have also been reported. Numerous other side effects may be associated with azacitidine.

Post-Marketing: Injection site necrosis, interstitial lung disease, necrotizing fasciitis (including fatal cases), Sweet's syndrome (acute febrile neutrophilic dermatosis), tumor lysis syndrome.

ANTIDOTE

Notify physician of any side effects. Most will be treated symptomatically. Dose may be reduced or delayed for hematologic toxicity, renal toxicity, or electrolyte disturbances. See Dose Adjustments for specific criteria. Blood and blood products, antibiotics, and other adjunctive therapies must be available. No known antidote; monitor blood counts and provide supportive care in overdose. Resuscitate as necessary.

AZITHROMYCIN

Antibacterial (macrolide)

(az-**zith**-roh-**MY**-sin)

Zithromax

USUAL DOSE

Community-acquired pneumonia: 500 mg as a single daily dose for a minimum of 2 days. Follow with 500 mg of oral azithromycin as a single daily dose. Total course of therapy (IV + oral) should be 7 to 10 days.

Pelvic inflammatory disease: 500 mg as a single daily dose for 1 to 2 days. Follow with 250 mg of oral azithromycin as a single daily dose. Total course of therapy (IV + oral) should be 7 days. If anaerobic microorganisms are also suspected, concurrent administration of an antibacterial agent with anaerobic activity is recommended (e.g., metronidazole [Flagyl]).

DOSE ADJUSTMENTS

No dose adjustment provided by manufacturer for patients with impaired liver or renal function; see Precautions. ■ See Drug/Lab Interactions.

DILUTION

Each 500-mg vial must be reconstituted with 4.8 mL SWFI. Shake well to ensure dilution (100 mg/mL). Further dilute each 500 mg of reconstituted solution with 250 to 500 mL of one of the following solutions: 5% dextrose in water (D5W), normal saline (NS), ½NS, D5 in ⅓NS, D5 in ½NS, D5 in ½NS with 20 mEq KCl, Ringer's lactate (LR), D5LR, D5 in Normosol M, D5 in Normosol R. 500 mL diluent yields 1 mg/mL, 250 mL yields 2 mg/mL. Concentrations greater than 2 mg/mL have caused local IV site reactions and should be avoided.

Storage: Store vials at or below 30°C (86°F). Reconstituted or diluted solution stable at CRT for 24 hours. Diluted solution stable for up to 7 days if refrigerated.

COMPATIBILITY

Manufacturer states, "Other IV substances, additives, or medications should not be added to azithromycin, or infused simultaneously through the same IV line." Flush IV line with a **compatible** IV fluid before and after administration.

Other sources suggest specific **compatibilities** dependent on concentration and manufacturer; consult a pharmacist.

RATE OF ADMINISTRATION
Do not give by IV bolus; must be infused over at least 1 hour.
1 mg/mL dilution: A single dose equally distributed over 3 hours.
2 mg/mL dilution: A single dose equally distributed over 1 hour.

ACTIONS
A macrolide antibiotic. Active against selected organisms, including aerobic gram-positive and gram-negative organisms and other organisms, including *Chlamydia* and *Mycoplasma pneumoniae*. Interferes with microbial protein synthesis by binding a ribosomal subunit of a susceptible microorganism. Terminal half-life of 68 hours allows for once-daily dosing. Prolonged half-life is thought to result from extensive uptake and subsequent release of drug from tissues. Studies to assess the metabolism of azithromycin have not been performed. Excreted primarily as unchanged drug in bile. Up to 14% excreted in urine within 24 hours. Excreted in breast milk in small amounts.

INDICATIONS AND USES
Treatment of community-acquired pneumonia and pelvic inflammatory disease caused by susceptible strains of specific organisms (e.g., *Staphylococcus aureus, Streptococcus pneumoniae, Haemophilus influenzae, Legionella pneumophila, Neisseria gonorrhoeae, Chlamydia trachomatis.* See product insert for complete list of organisms). Administered to patients who require initial IV therapy. Many other indications for oral use.

CONTRAINDICATIONS
Hypersensitivity to any macrolide antibiotic. ▪ Patients with a history of cholestatic jaundice/hepatic dysfunction associated with prior use of azithromycin.

PRECAUTIONS
For IV use only. ▪ Specific sensitivity studies are indicated to determine susceptibility of the causative organism to azithromycin. ▪ To reduce the development of drug-resistant bacteria and maintain its effectiveness, azithromycin should be used only to treat infections proven or strongly suspected to be caused by susceptible bacteria. ▪ Has demonstrated cross-resistance with erythromycin. ▪ Serious hypersensitivity reactions, including angioedema, anaphylaxis, dermatologic reactions (e.g., acute generalized exanthematous pustulosis [AGEP], Stevens-Johnson syndrome, toxic epidermal necrolysis), and cases of drug reaction with eosinophilia and systemic symptoms (DRESS), have been reported. Use extreme caution; hypersensitivity reactions have recurred even after azithromycin was discontinued and hypersensitivity reactions treated. Fatalities have been reported. ▪ Hepatotoxicity, including abnormal liver function, hepatitis, cholestatic jaundice, hepatic necrosis, and hepatic failure, have been reported; deaths have occurred. The pharmacokinetics of azithromycin in patients with hepatic impairment have not been established. ▪ Use caution in patients with impaired renal function. Data unavailable. ▪ Macrolide antibiotics (including azithromycin) have caused prolonged cardiac repolarization and QT intervals, imparting a risk of developing cardiac arrhythmia and torsades de pointes, which can be fatal. Consider risk/benefit of azithromycin use in at-risk patients, such as patients with known prolonged QT intervals; a history of torsades de pointes, congenital long QT syndrome, bradyarrhythmias, or uncompensated heart failure; patients taking drugs known to prolong the QT interval; patients with ongoing proarrhythmic conditions (e.g., uncorrected hypokalemia or hypomagnesemia) or clinically significant bradycardia; and patients receiving Class Ia (quinidine, procainamide) or Class III (amiodarone, dofetilide, sotalol) antiarrhythmic agents. ▪ Timing of transfer to oral therapy should be based on clinical response. ▪ Avoid prolonged use; superinfection caused by overgrowth of nonsusceptible organisms may result. ▪ *Clostridium difficile*–associated diarrhea (CDAD) has been reported. May range from mild diarrhea to fatal colitis. Consider in patients who present with diarrhea during or after treatment with azithromycin. ▪ May cause exacerbations of symptoms of myasthenia gravis or new onset of myasthenia syndrome.
Monitor: Monitor vital signs. ▪ Observe closely for signs of a hypersensitivity reaction; see Antidote. ▪ Monitoring of liver function may be indicated; see Precautions. ▪ ECG monitoring for QT prolongation may be indicated; see Precautions. ▪ Monitor infusion

site for inflammation and/or extravasation. ■ Contains 4.96 mEq of sodium/vial. Observe for electrolyte imbalance and cardiac irregularities. May aggravate CHF. ■ See Drug/Lab Interactions and Antidote.

Patient Education: Discontinue azithromycin and report any signs of an allergic reaction immediately (difficulty breathing, itching, rash, swelling). ■ Discontinue azithromycin and report S/S of hepatitis (e.g., dark urine, jaundice, loss of appetite, malaise, nausea and vomiting). ■ Promptly report diarrhea or bloody stools that occur during treatment or up to several months after an antibiotic has been discontinued; may indicate CDAD and require treatment. ■ Parents or caregivers of neonates who have received azithromycin should report vomiting or irritability with feedings. ■ Review all prescription and nonprescription medications with your healthcare provider.

Maternal/Child: Safety for use during pregnancy not established; use with caution and only if clearly needed. Available data do not suggest an increased risk for major birth defects, miscarriage, or adverse maternal or fetal outcomes with azithromycin use in pregnant females. ■ Azithromycin is present in human milk. Monitor breast-fed infant for diarrhea, vomiting, or rash. ■ Safety and effectiveness of IV formulation for use in pediatric patients under 16 years of age not established. ■ Infantile hypertrophic pyloric stenosis (IHPS) has been reported after the use of azithromycin in neonates (treatment up to 42 days of life). Caregivers should contact their physician if vomiting or irritability with feeding occurs. ■ Has been administered to pediatric patients age 6 months to 16 years by the oral route. The most common side effects in this age-group included abdominal pain, diarrhea, headache, nausea, rash, and vomiting.

Elderly: Response similar to that seen in younger adults. ■ May be more susceptible to development of drug-associated effects on the QT interval and torsades de pointes than younger patients. ■ May respond with a blunted natriuresis to salt loading; see Monitor. ■ Consider age-related organ impairment.

DRUG/LAB INTERACTIONS

May increase the anticoagulant effects of **warfarin**; monitoring of PT is indicated. ■ Coadministration with **nelfinavir** results in increased azithromycin levels. Dose adjustment is not recommended, but close monitoring for known side effects (e.g., liver enzyme abnormalities, hearing impairment) is suggested. ■ May have a modest effect on the pharmacokinetics of **atorvastatin, carbamazepine, cetirizine, didanosine, efavirenz, fluconazole, indinavir, midazolam, nelfinavir, sildenafil, sulfamethoxazole/trimethoprim, theophylline, triazolam,** or **zidovudine**. No dose adjustment required with coadministration of these drugs. ■ **Efavirenz and fluconazole** may have a modest effect on the pharmacokinetics of azithromycin. No dose adjustment is necessary with coadministration of these drugs. Use caution when coadministered with **digoxin, colchicine,** or **phenytoin**. Interactions have not been reported in clinical trials with azithromycin, but studies have not been performed to evaluate potential drug-drug interactions. Drug interactions have been observed with these drugs and other macrolide antibiotics.

SIDE EFFECTS

Usually mild to moderate in severity and reversible after azithromycin discontinued. The most commonly reported side effects are abdominal pain, diarrhea, nausea and vomiting. Less frequently reported side effects include anorexia; dizziness; dyspnea; injection site pain or local inflammation; pruritus; rashes; stomatitis; and vaginitis. Reported laboratory abnormalities include decreased platelet count; elevated AST, ALT, alkaline phosphatase, bilirubin, creatinine, LDH; leukopenia; and neutropenia.

Post-Marketing: Arrhythmias (e.g., ventricular tachycardia, hypotension, QT prolongation, and torsades de pointes), asthenia, CDAD, CNS toxicity (e.g., agitation, convulsions, headache, hyperactivity, somnolence, syncope), constipation, dermatologic reactions (including acute generalized exanthematous pustulosis [AGEP], pruritus, Stevens-Johnson syndrome, toxic epidermal necrolysis, and urticaria), DRESS, dyspepsia, fatigue, hearing disturbances (including hearing loss, deafness, and/or tinnitus), hepatotoxicity (e.g., hepatitis and cholestatic jaundice, cases of hepatic necrosis, and hepatic failure [some resulting in death]), hypersensitivity reactions (e.g., anaphylaxis, angioedema), interstitial nephritis, malaise, oral candidiasis, pancreatitis, paresthesia, pyloric stenosis, acute renal failure, and taste/smell perversion and/or loss.

ANTIDOTE

Notify physician of any side effects. Discontinue azithromycin for hypersensitivity reactions and S/S of hepatotoxicity. Treat hypersensitivity reactions as indicated and resuscitate as necessary. Hypersensitivity reactions have recurred after azithromycin has been discontinued and initial treatment completed. Prolonged observation is required. Mild cases of CDAD may respond to discontinuation of azithromycin. Treat CDAD with fluids, electrolytes, protein supplements, and appropriate antibiotics (e.g., oral vancomycin) as indicated. In severe cases, surgical evaluation may be indicated.

AZTREONAM
(az-**TREE**-oh-nam)

Azactam

Antibacterial
(monobactam)

pH 4.5 to 7.5

USUAL DOSE

Pretreatment: See Precautions.

Dose and route determined by susceptibility of the causative organism(s), severity and site of infection, and condition of the patient. IV route recommended for patients requiring single doses greater than 1 Gm or those with bacterial septicemia, localized parenchymal abscess (e.g., intra-abdominal abscess), peritonitis, or other severe systemic or life-threatening infections.

Urinary tract infection: 500 mg to 1 Gm every 8 or 12 hours.

Moderately severe systemic infections: 1 or 2 Gm every 8 or 12 hours.

Severe systemic or life-threatening infections: 2 Gm every 6 or 8 hours. Use the full suggested dose. Do not exceed 8 Gm/24 hr.

Normal renal function required. Duration of therapy depends on the severity of the infection. Continue for at least 2 days after all symptoms of infection subside. Can produce therapeutic serum levels given intraperitoneally in dialysis fluid.

PEDIATRIC DOSE

See Maternal/Child.

Mild to moderate infections: 30 mg/kg every 8 hours.

Moderate to severe infections: 30 mg/kg every 6 or 8 hours. Maximum recommended dose is 120 mg/kg/24 hr.

Cystic fibrosis: 50 mg/kg every 6 to 8 hours. Maximum dose is 200 mg/kg/day not to exceed 8 Gm/24 hr. Higher doses have been used.

NEONATAL DOSE

Neonatal doses are **unlabeled;** see Maternal/Child.

30 mg/kg/dose. Interval between doses based on age and weight as follows:

Less than 1,200 Gm and 0 to 4 weeks of age: Give every 12 hours.

1,200 to 2,000 Gm and 0 to 7 days of age: Give every 12 hours.

1,200 to 2,000 Gm and over 7 days of age: Give every 8 hours.

More than 2,000 Gm and 0 to 7 days of age: Give every 8 hours.

More than 2,000 Gm and over 7 days of age: Give every 6 hours.

DOSE ADJUSTMENTS

Dosing in the elderly should be cautious and reduced based on CrCl; consider potential for decreased organ function and concomitant disease or drug therapy. ▪ Prolonged serum levels may occur in patients with transient or persistent renal insufficiency. After an initial loading dose of 1 or 2 Gm, reduce succeeding doses by 50% in patients with CrCl between 10 and 30 mL/min/1.73 M^2. ▪ After an initial loading dose of 500 mg,

1 Gm, or 2 Gm, reduce succeeding doses by 75% in patients with CrCl less than 10 mL/min/1.73 M^2 or in patients supported by dialysis. For serious or life-threatening infections, in addition to the maintenance doses, give 12.5% of the initial dose after each dialysis session.

DILUTION

Usually light yellow, may become slightly pink on standing; does not affect potency.

IV injection: Reconstitute a single dose with 6 to 10 mL of SWFI. Shake immediately and vigorously. Use immediately and discard any unused solution.

Intermittent IV: Initially reconstitute each single dose with a minimum of 3 mL of SWFI. Shake immediately and vigorously. Must be further diluted in at least 50 mL of D5W, NS, or other **compatible** infusion solutions for each 1 Gm of aztreonam (see chart on inside back cover or literature). Concentration should not exceed 20 mg/mL or 2% w/v. Available in vials and premixed Galaxy infusion bags.

Storage: Store vials at RT before use. Concentrations exceeding 2% should be used promptly unless prepared with SWFI or NS. Other reconstituted or diluted solutions are stable for 48 hours at CRT or up to 7 days if refrigerated. Vials are for single use only; discard unused amounts. Store aztreonam in Galaxy plastic containers at or below −20° C (−4° F). Thaw frozen container at RT or in a refrigerator. **Do not** force thaw by immersion in a water bath or by microwave irradiation. Thawed solutions are stable for 14 days refrigerated or for 48 hours at RT. Do not refreeze.

COMPATIBILITY

Manufacturer lists as **incompatible** with metronidazole (Flagyl IV) and nafcillin (Nallpen).

Other sources suggest specific **compatibilities** dependent on concentration and manufacturer; consult a pharmacist.

RATE OF ADMINISTRATION

IV injection: A single dose equally distributed over 3 to 5 minutes.

Intermittent IV: A single dose over 20 to 60 minutes. May be given through Y-site. Do not infuse simultaneously with other drugs or solutions except in proven **compatibility**. Flush common IV tubing before and after administration.

ACTIONS

A synthetic monobactam antibiotic. Bactericidal through inhibition of bacterial cell wall synthesis to a wide spectrum of specific gram-negative aerobic organisms, including *Pseudomonas aeruginosa*. Has activity in the presence of some beta-lactamases (both penicillinases and cephalosporinases) of gram-negative and gram-positive bacteria. Widely distributed into many body fluids and tissues. Serum half-life averages 1.7 hours; range is 1.5 to 2 hours. Primarily excreted in the urine with some excretion through feces. Crosses placental barrier. Secreted in breast milk.

INDICATIONS AND USES

Treatment of serious lower respiratory tract, urinary tract, skin and skin structure, gynecologic, and intra-abdominal infections and bacterial septicemia. Most effective against specific gram-negative organisms (see literature). ▪ Adjunctive therapy to surgery for the management of infections caused by susceptible organisms, including abscesses, infections complicating hollow viscus perforations, cutaneous infections, and infections of serous surfaces.

CONTRAINDICATIONS

Known hypersensitivity to aztreonam or its components.

PRECAUTIONS

Specific studies are indicated to identify the causative organism and susceptibility to aztreonam. ▪ To reduce the development of drug-resistant bacteria and maintain its effectiveness, aztreonam should be used to treat or prevent only those infections proven or strongly suspected to be caused by bacteria. ▪ Before C/S data are available, concurrent initial antimicrobial therapy with agents to cover gram-positive and/or anaerobic microorganisms may be indicated in seriously ill patients. ▪ Avoid prolonged use of drug; superinfection caused by overgrowth of nonsusceptible organisms may result. ▪ Can result in hypersensitivity reactions with or without prior exposure. ▪ Cross-reactivity with other beta-lactam antibiotics (e.g., penicillins, cephalosporins, and/or carbapenems) is rare but can occur. Use with caution in patients with a history of hypersensitivity reactions to beta-lactam antibiotics. ▪ *Clostridium difficile*–associated diarrhea (CDAD) has been reported. May range from mild diarrhea to fatal colitis. Consider in patients who present with diarrhea during or after treatment with aztreonam. ▪ Toxic epidermal necrolysis has been reported rarely in patients receiving aztreonam who have undergone BMT and have other risk factors (e.g., radiation therapy, sepsis).

Monitor: Watch for early symptoms of a hypersensitivity reaction. Use caution in patients with known sensitivity to penicillins, cephalosporins, or carbapenems. ▪ Monitor renal and hepatic function, especially in the elderly. ▪ Monitor renal function with concurrent administration of higher doses or prolonged administration of aminoglycosides (e.g., gentamicin). ▪ May cause thrombophlebitis. Use small needles and large veins and rotate infusion sites.

Patient Education: Report pain or burning at injection site or S/S of a hypersensitivity reaction (e.g., difficulty breathing, flushing, itching, rash). ▪ Promptly report diarrhea or bloody stools that occur during treatment or up to several months after an antibiotic has been discontinued; may indicate CDAD and require treatment.

Maternal/Child: Category B: use in pregnancy only if clearly needed. ▪ Consider discontinuing breast-feeding. ▪ Safety and effectiveness for use in pediatric patients between 9 months and 16 years of age has been established. ▪ Safety and effectiveness for use in infants under 9 months of age and for treatment of pediatric patients with septicemia and skin and skin-structure infections (where the skin infection is believed or known to result from *H. influenzae* type b) not established. ▪ Higher doses of aztreonam may be indicated in pediatric patients with cystic fibrosis. ▪ IV route is suggested for pediatric patients; data are limited for IM injection and impaired renal function.

Elderly: Reduced doses may be indicated. Monitor renal function; see Dose Adjustments. ▪ Response is similar to that seen in younger patients; however, clearance is decreased and half-life is prolonged.

DRUG/LAB INTERACTIONS

Antagonism may occur with **beta-lactamase–inducing antibiotics** (e.g., cefoxitin, imipenem); do not use concurrently. ▪ Aztreonam and **aminoglycosides** have been shown to be synergistic against many gram-negative aerobic bacilli. May be used concomitantly in severe infections. Nephrotoxicity and ototoxicity can be markedly increased when both drugs are utilized. ▪ See Side Effects.

SIDE EFFECTS

Diarrhea, nausea and vomiting, phlebitis/thrombophlebitis, and rash occur most frequently. Less frequently reported reactions include abdominal cramps; altered taste; breast tenderness; CDAD (including pseudomembranous colitis); chest pain; confusion; diaphoresis; diplopia; dizziness; dyspnea; elevated alkaline phosphatase, AST, ALT, platelets, and SCr; encephalopathy; eosinophilia; erythema multiforme; exfoliative dermatitis; fever; flushing; GI bleeding; halitosis; headache; hematologic changes (e.g., anemia, leukocytosis, neutropenia, pancytopenia, thrombocytopenia, thrombocytosis); hepatitis; hypersensitivity reactions (e.g., anaphylaxis, angioedema, bronchospasm); hypotension; insomnia; jaundice; malaise; mouth ulcer; muscular aches; nasal congestion; numb tongue; paresthesia; petechiae; positive Coombs' test; prolonged PT and PTT; pruritus; purpura; seizures; sneezing; tinnitus; toxic epidermal necrolysis; transient ECG changes (ventricular bigeminy and PVCs); urticaria; vaginal candidiasis; vaginitis; vertigo; weakness; wheezing.

ANTIDOTE

Notify physician of any side effects. Discontinue the drug if indicated. Treat hypersensitivity reactions as indicated and resuscitate as necessary. Mild cases of CDAD may respond to discontinuation of drug. Treat CDAD with fluids, electrolytes, protein supplements, and appropriate antibiotics (e.g., oral vancomycin) as indicated. In severe cases, surgical evaluation may be indicated. Hemodialysis or peritoneal dialysis may be useful in overdose.

BASILIXIMAB BBW
(**bah**-zih-**LIX**-ih-mab)

Simulect

Recombinant monoclonal antibody
Immunosuppressant

USUAL DOSE
Pretreatment: Baseline studies indicated; see Monitor.

Basiliximab should only be administered once it has been determined that the patient will receive the graft and concomitant immunosuppression. Patients who have received a previous course of basiliximab should only be re-exposed to a subsequent course of therapy with extreme caution. Used concurrently with cyclosporine (Sandimmune) and corticosteroids.

Organ rejection prophylaxis in renal transplant: 2 doses of 20 mg each as an infusion. Administer the first dose within 2 hours before transplantation. Give the second dose 4 days after transplantation. Withhold the second dose if complications such as severe hypersensitivity reactions to basiliximab or graft loss occur.

PEDIATRIC DOSE
Less than 35 kg: 2 doses of 10 mg each (discard remaining product after each dose).
35 kg or more: 2 doses of 20 mg each.

In all pediatric patients, administer the first dose within 2 hours before transplantation. Give the second dose 4 days after transplantation. See Actions and Maternal/Child. Withhold second dose if complications occur (e.g., hypersensitivity reactions or graft loss).

DOSE ADJUSTMENTS
No dose adjustments indicated.

DILUTION
Reconstitute each single 20-mg vial with 5 mL of SWFI. Reconstitute each 10-mg vial with 2.5 mL SWFI. Shake gently to dissolve powder. After reconstitution, may be given as an IV injection or may be further diluted to 50 mL with NS or D5W. When mixing, gently invert to avoid foaming; do not shake.

Storage: Store unopened vials in the refrigerator (2° to 8° C [36° to 46° F]). Should be used within 4 hours of reconstitution. If necessary, may be refrigerated for up to 24 hours. Discard prepared solution after 24 hours.

COMPATIBILITY
Manufacturer states, "Other drug substances should not be added or infused simultaneously through the same IV line." No **incompatibilities** observed with polyvinyl chloride bags and administration sets.

RATE OF ADMINISTRATION
May be given through a peripheral or central vein.

IV injection: May be given as a bolus injection over 30 to 60 seconds. Incidence of N/V and local reaction including pain increased.

Infusion: A single dose properly diluted over 20 to 30 minutes.

ACTIONS
A chimeric (murine/human) monoclonal antibody produced by recombinant DNA technology. Functions as an immunosuppressant. Specifically binds to and blocks the interleukin-2 receptor alpha chain (IL-2Rα, also known as CD25 antigen), thereby inhibiting IL-2 driven proliferation of activated T-cells, which play a key role in organ rejection. Reduces/minimizes acute rejection. IL-2Rα is expressed selectively on activated, but not resting, T-cells. This selectivity prevents the profound generalized immunosuppression seen with other immunosuppressants used in organ transplantation and may decrease the risk of infection and development of lymphoproliferative disorders. Two 20-mg doses block the receptor for 4 to 6 weeks posttransplantation, the critical risk period for acute organ rejection. Has reduced the incidence of biopsy-confirmed acute rejections while minimizing side effects seen with other immunosuppressants. Clinical benefit

demonstrated in a broad range of patients, regardless of age, gender, race, donor type, or history of diabetes mellitus as long as serum levels exceed 0.2 mg/mL (by ELISA). Mean half-life is 4 to 10.4 days. Half-life is increased (5.2 to 17.8 days) and distribution volume and clearance are decreased by approximately 50% in pediatric patients 2 to 11 years of age. Crosses the placental barrier. May be secreted in breast milk.

INDICATIONS AND USES

Prophylaxis of acute organ rejection in patients receiving renal transplants. Used as part of an immunosuppressive regimen that includes cyclosporine and corticosteroids. Dosing regimen may also include either azathioprine or mycophenolate (CellCept IV).

CONTRAINDICATIONS

Known hypersensitivity to basiliximab or any of its components (composite of human and murine antibodies).

PRECAUTIONS

Usually administered by or under the direction of a physician experienced in immunosuppressive therapy and management of organ transplant patients. Adequate laboratory and supportive medical resources must be available. ■ Severe acute (onset within 24 hours) hypersensitivity reactions including anaphylaxis have been reported both with initial exposure and/or following re-exposure after several months. Emergency equipment and drugs for the treatment of severe hypersensitivity reactions must be readily available. Withhold the second dose of basiliximab if a hypersensitivity reaction occurs. ■ Readministration after an initial course of therapy has not been studied in humans, but other monoclonal antibodies have precipitated anaphylactoid reactions. ■ Potential for causing lymphoproliferative disorders, cytomegalovirus (CMV), and other opportunistic infections is unknown. ■ Use with caution in patients with infections or malignancies. ■ It is not known whether basiliximab use will have a long-term effect on the ability of the immune system to respond to antigens first encountered during induced immunosuppression. ■ Low titers of anti-idiotype antibodies and human antimurine antibodies (HAMA) to basiliximab have been detected in some patients during treatment; no adverse effects have been noted.

Monitor: Obtain baseline CBC with differential and platelets and baseline renal and liver tests if not already completed for other immunosuppressant agents. ■ Monitor vital signs. ■ Observe closely for signs of infection (fever, sore throat, tiredness) or unusual bleeding or bruising. ■ Prophylactic antibiotics may be indicated pending results of C/S in a febrile immunosuppressed patient. ■ Symptoms of cytokine release syndrome (e.g., chills, fever, dyspnea, and malaise) have not been reported but may occur; observe carefully. ■ See Drug/Lab Interactions.

Patient Education: Immediately report difficulty in breathing or swallowing, rapid heartbeat, rash, or itching. ■ Report swelling of lower extremities and weakness. ■ Avoid pregnancy; females with childbearing potential should use effective contraception before beginning basiliximab therapy, during therapy, and for 2 months after completion. ▪ See Appendix D.

Maternal/Child: Category B: use during pregnancy only if benefits justify the potential risk to the fetus. Avoid pregnancy; effective contraception required; see Patient Education. ▪ Discontinue breast-feeding. ▪ Has been used in pediatric patients from 2 to 15 years of age. No adequate or well-controlled studies completed. See differences in Actions. Most frequent side effects were fever and urinary infections.

Elderly: Age-related dosing not required. Adverse events similar to younger adults. Use caution when giving immunosuppressive drugs to the elderly.

DRUG/LAB INTERACTIONS

Has been administered concurrently with **anti-lymphocyte globulin** (ALG), **anti-thymocyte globulin, azathioprine, corticosteroids, cyclosporine, muromonab CD3, and mycophenolate**; no additional adverse reactions noted. ▪ **May increase or decrease numerous lab values,** including serum calcium and potassium and fasting blood glucose.

SIDE EFFECTS

Basiliximab did not appear to alter the pattern, frequency, or severity of known side effects associated with the use of immunosuppressive drugs. Abdominal pain, anemia, constipation, diarrhea, edema, fever, headache, hyperkalemia, hypersensitivity reactions (including anaphylaxis, bronchospasm, capillary leak syndrome, cardiac failure, cytokine release syndrome, dyspnea, hypotension, pruritus, pulmonary edema, rash, respiratory failure, sneezing, tachycardia, urticaria, wheezing), hypertension, hypokalemia, insomnia, nausea, pain, peripheral edema, upper respiratory infections, urinary tract infections. Incidence of N/V and local reaction including pain increased with bolus injection. Severe hypersensitivity reactions (including anaphylaxis), capillary leak syndrome, and cytokine release syndrome have been reported. Incidence of infections, lymphomas, or other malignancies similar to placebo groups in studies.

ANTIDOTE

Notify physician of all side effects. Most will be treated symptomatically. Basiliximab may be discontinued or alternate immunosuppressive agents substituted. Discontinue immediately if anaphylaxis occurs, and treat with oxygen, epinephrine, corticosteroids, and/or antihistamines. Resuscitate as necessary.

BELATACEPT `BBW`

(bel-**AT**-a-sept)

**Immunosuppressant
(selective T-cell
costimulation blocker)**

Nulojix

pH 7.2 to 7.8

USUAL DOSE

Pretreatment: Ascertain Epstein-Barr virus (EBV) serology before treatment. Testing for latent TB indicated; see Contraindications and Monitor.

Administration of higher-than-recommended doses or more frequent dosing of belatacept is not recommended because of an increased risk of posttransplant lymphoproliferative disorder (PTLD), progressive multifocal leukoencephalopathy (PML), and serious CNS infections.

Premedication is not required. Base the total infusion dose on actual body weight at the time of transplantation.

Dosing of Belatacept for Kidney Transplant Recipients[a]	
Dosing for Initial Phase	**Dose**
Day 1 (day of transplantation, before implantation) and Day 5 (approximately 96 hours after Day 1 dose)	10 mg/kg
End of Week 2 and Week 4 after transplantation	10 mg/kg
End of Week 8 and Week 12 after transplantation	10 mg/kg
Dosing for Maintenance Phase	**Dose**
End of Week 16 after transplantation and every 4 weeks (plus or minus 3 days) thereafter	5 mg/kg

[a]The dose prescribed must be evenly divisible by 12.5 mg (evenly divisible increments are 0, 12.5, 25, 37.5, 50, 62.5, 75, 87.5, and 100). For example: At 10 mg/kg/dose, a patient weighing 64 kg would receive 640 mg. The closest doses evenly divisible by 12.5 below and above 640 mg are 637.5 mg and 650 mg. The nearest dose is 637.5 mg, and this would be the actual prescribed dose.

Regimen includes basiliximab (Simulect) induction, mycophenolate mofetil (MMF, CellCept), and corticosteroids.
Basiliximab: 20 mg IV on the day of transplantation and 4 days later.
Mycophenolate mofetil: 1 Gm twice daily as an initial dose. Adjust dose based on clinical signs of adverse events or efficacy failure.
Corticosteroid doses should be consistent with those used in clinical trials. In Studies 1 and 2, methylprednisolone 500 mg IV was given on arrival to the OR on Day 1. Methylprednisolone 250 mg IV was given on Day 2, and prednisone 100 mg PO was given on Day 3. In clinical trials, the median corticosteroid doses were tapered to approximately 15 mg (10 to 20 mg) per day by the first 6 weeks and remained at approximately 10 mg (5 to 10 mg) per day for the first 6 months posttransplant; see Precautions. Actual corticosteroid dosing in clinical trials is summarized in the following chart.

Actual Corticosteroid[a] Dosing in Studies 1 and 2		
	Median (Q1-Q3) Daily Dose[b,c]	
Day of Dosing	Study 1	Study 2
Week 1	31.7 mg (26.7 to 50 mg)	30 mg (26.7 to 50 mg)
Week 2	25 mg (20 to 30 mg)	25 mg (20 to 30 mg)
Week 4	20 mg (15 to 20 mg)	20 mg (15 to 22.5 mg)
Week 6	15 mg (10 to 20 mg)	16.7 mg (12.5 to 20 mg)
Month 6	10 mg (5 to 10 mg)	10 mg (5 to 12.5 mg)

[a]Corticosteroid = Prednisone or prednisolone.
[b]Protocols allowed for flexibility in determining corticosteroid dose and rapidity of taper after Day 15. It is not possible to distinguish corticosteroid doses used to treat acute rejection versus doses used in a maintenance regimen.
[c]Q1 and Q3 are the 25th and 75th percentiles of daily corticosteroid doses, respectively.

DOSE ADJUSTMENTS
Do not modify the dose during the course of therapy unless there is a change in body weight of greater than 10%. ■ Age, gender, race, renal function, hepatic function, diabetes, and concomitant dialysis do not affect the clearance of belatacept.

DILUTION
Belatacept is for IV infusion only. *Must be reconstituted/prepared using only the silicone-free disposable syringe provided with each vial. This syringe will be required for both reconstitution and the preparation of the final infusion. Maintain sterility. Any solution prepared with other than the provided silicone-free syringe must be discarded.*

Each vial contains 250 mg of belatacept lyophilized powder. Calculate the number of vials needed to provide the total infusion dose. Reconstitute the contents of each vial with 10.5 mL of SWFI, NS, or D5W using the silicone-free disposable syringe and an 18- to 21-gauge needle. Direct the stream of diluent to the glass wall of the vial. To avoid foaming, rotate the vial and swirl gently until contents are completely dissolved. *Avoid prolonged or vigorous agitation. Do not shake.* Reconstituted solution yields 25 mg/mL and should be clear to slightly opalescent and colorless to pale yellow. Calculate the total volume of reconstituted solution required to provide the prescribed dose:

Volume of 25 mg/mL belatacept solution (in mL) = Prescribed dose (in mg) ÷ 25 mg/mL

The reconstituted solution must be further diluted in infusion fluid. If reconstituted with SWFI, dilute with either NS or D5W. If reconstituted with NS, further dilute with NS. If reconstituted with D5W, further dilute with D5W. From the appropriate-size infusion bag or bottle (typically an infusion volume of 100 mL is appropriate, but volumes from 50 to 250 mL may be used), withdraw a volume of infusion fluid equal to the total volume of reconstituted belatacept required to provide the prescribed dose. Using the same silicone-free disposable syringe used for reconstitution, withdraw the required amount of belatacept and inject it into the infusion bag or bottle. Gently rotate to ensure mixing. Concentration should range from 2 mg/mL to 10 mg/mL.

Filters: Must be administered with a nonpyrogenic, low–protein-binding, 0.2- to 1.2-micron filter.

Storage: Refrigerate vials of lyophilized powder at 2° to 8° C (36° to 46° F) in carton to protect from light. The reconstituted solution should be further diluted in infusion fluid immediately. The infusion must be completed within 24 hours. Infusion solution can be refrigerated protected from light for up to 24 hours. A maximum of 4 hours of those 24 hours can be at RT 20° to 25° C (68° to 77° F) and room light. Discard any unused solution remaining in vials.

COMPATIBILITY

Manufacturer states, "Must be reconstituted/prepared using only the silicone-free disposable syringe provided with each vial. Any solution prepared with other than the provided silicone-free syringe must be discarded" and "Infuse in a separate line; should not be infused concomitantly in the same IV line with other agents."

RATE OF ADMINISTRATION

A single dose evenly distributed over 30 minutes.

ACTIONS

A selective T-cell costimulation blocker. Produced by recombinant DNA technology. Binds to CD80 and CD86 on antigen-presenting cells, thereby blocking CD28-mediated costimulation of T-lymphocytes. Belatacept-mediated costimulation blockade results in the inhibition of cytokine production by T-cells required for antigen-specific antibody production by B-cells and inhibits T-lymphocyte proliferation. Activated T-lymphocytes are the predominant mediators of immunologic rejection. Half-life ranges from 6.1 to 15.1 days.

INDICATIONS AND USES

Prophylaxis of organ rejection in adult patients receiving a kidney transplant. Used in combination with basiliximab induction, mycophenolate mofetil, and corticosteroids.

Limitations of use: Use only in patients who are Epstein-Barr virus (EBV) seropositive.

- Use for prophylaxis of organ rejection in transplanted organs other than the kidney not established.

CONTRAINDICATIONS

Transplant recipients who are Epstein-Barr virus (EBV) seronegative or who have unknown EBV serostatus because of risk of posttransplant lymphoproliferative disorder (PTLD) predominantly involving the CNS.

PRECAUTIONS

For IV infusion only. ▪ Usually administered by or under the direction of a physician experienced in immunosuppressive therapy and management of kidney transplant patients. Adequate laboratory and supportive medical resources must be available. ▪ Increased risk for developing posttransplant lymphoproliferative disorder (PTLD), predominantly involving the CNS, compared with patients on a cyclosporine-based regimen. Recipients without immunity to Epstein-Barr virus (EBV) are at a particularly increased risk; therefore use in EBV-seropositive patients only. Do not use belatacept in transplant recipients who are EBV-seronegative or who have unknown EBV serostatus. ▪ Other known risk factors for PTLD include cytomegalovirus (CMV) infection and T-cell–depleting therapy. Use T-cell–depleting therapies to treat acute rejection with caution. CMV prophylaxis is recommended for at least 3 months after transplantation. Patients who are EBV seropositive and CMV seronegative may be at increased risk for PTLD compared with patients who are EBV seropositive and CMV seropositive. ▪ Minimization of the corticosteroid dose to 5 mg/day between Day 3 and Week 6 posttransplantation has been associated with an increased rate and grade of acute rejection, particularly Grade III rejection. Graft loss occurred in some patients. Corticosteroid use should be consistent with clinical trial experience; see Usual Dose. ▪ Increased susceptibility to infection and possible development of malignancies may result from immunosuppression. Increased risk of developing other malignancies, including malignancies of the skin, appears related to intensity and duration of use. Avoid prolonged exposure to UV light and sunlight. Risk of developing bacterial, viral (e.g., CMV and herpes), fungal, and protozoal infections, including opportunistic infections such as tuberculosis (TB) or polyoma virus–associated nephropathy (PVAN), is increased and may lead to serious (including fatal) outcomes. Prophylaxis for *Pneumocystis jiroveci* is recommended after transplantation. ▪ The coadministration (at the same or nearly the same time) of anti-thymocyte globulin and belatacept may pose a risk for venous thrombosis of the renal allograft; see Drug/Lab Interactions. ▪ PML (a rapidly progressive and fatal opportunistic infection of the CNS that is caused by the JC virus) has been reported. ▪ Infusion-related reactions have occurred within 1 hour of infusion; however, no serious reactions or anaphylaxis were reported in studies. ■ Use in liver transplant patients is not recommended because of an increased risk of graft loss and death. ■ Anti-belatacept antibody development was not associated with an altered clearance of belatacept. The clinical impact of anti-belatacept antibodies has not been determined. ■ Do not administer live virus vaccines; see Drug/Lab Interactions.

Monitor: Ascertain EBV serology before starting therapy with belatacept. ■ Monitor for new or worsening neurologic, cognitive, or behavioral signs and symptoms. May indicate PTLD or PML. ■ PML is usually diagnosed by brain imaging, CSF testing for JC viral DNA, and/or brain biopsy. Consultation with a specialist (e.g., neurologist and/or infectious disease specialist) should be considered. ■ Evaluate patients for latent tuberculosis (TB). Patients testing positive in TB screening should be treated with a standard TB regimen before initiating belatacept therapy. ■ Monitor for S/S of infection; see Antidote. ■ Monitor renal function closely and consider PVAN if renal function is deteriorating. ■ New-onset diabetes, dyslipidemia, and hypertension may occur; monitor blood sugar, lipid panel, and BP. ■ Monitor for infusion reactions (primarily hypertension and hypotension). ■ See Precautions.

Patient Education: Read manufacturer's patient information sheet before each infusion. ■ Risk of other malignancies, especially skin cancer, is increased. Report S/S of skin cancer, such as suspicious moles or lesions. Limit exposure to sunlight and UV light. Wear protective clothing and use a sunscreen with a high protection factor. ■ Promptly report confusion, thinking problems, and loss of memory; decreased strength or weakness on one side of the body; and changes in mood or behavior, walking or talking, and vision. ■ Promptly report S/S of infection (e.g., fever, malaise). Adherence to prescribed antimicrobial prophylaxis is imperative. ■ Information on use in pregnant females is not available. Pregnancy registry available to monitor maternal-fetal outcomes. ■ Live vaccines should be avoided.

Maternal/Child: Insufficient data to inform on drug-associated risk in pregnant females. ■ There are no data on the presence of belatacept in human milk or on the effects on breastfed infants or human milk production; consider risk versus benefit. ■ Safety and effectiveness for use in pediatric patients under 18 years of age not established.

Elderly: Safety and effectiveness similar to that seen in younger adults.

DRUG/LAB INTERACTIONS

A change of **mycophenolic acid (MPA)** exposure may occur with a crossover from **cyclosporine to belatacept** or from **belatacept to cyclosporine** in patients concomitantly receiving **MMF**. Cyclosporine decreases MPA exposure by preventing enterohepatic recirculation of MPA, whereas belatacept does not. A higher MMF dosage may be needed after switching from belatacept to cyclosporine because cyclosporine may cause lower MPA concentrations and increase the risk of graft rejection. A lower MMF dosage may be needed after switching from cyclosporine to belatacept because this switch may result in higher MPA concentrations and increase the risk for adverse reactions related to MPA. ■ If **anti-thymocyte globulin** (or any other cell-depleting immunosuppressive induction treatment) and belatacept will be administered concomitantly, a 12-hour interval between the two administrations is suggested to reduce the risk of venous thrombosis of the renal allograft. ■ Avoid the use of **live vaccines** during treatment with belatacept, including but not limited to intranasal influenza, measles, mumps, rubella, oral polio, BCG, yellow fever, varicella, and Ty21a typhoid vaccines.

SIDE EFFECTS

Anemia, constipation, cough, diarrhea, fever, graft dysfunction, headache, hyperkalemia, hypertension, hypokalemia, leukopenia, nausea, peripheral edema, urinary tract infection, and vomiting are most common. Posttransplant lymphoproliferative disorder (PTLD), predominantly CNS PTLD; other malignancies; and serious infections, including JC virus–associated progressive multifocal leukoencephalopathy (PML) and polyoma virus–associated nephropathy (PVAN), are the most serious potential side effects and may be life threatening. Abdominal pain, acne, anxiety, arthralgia, back pain, bronchitis, cytomegalovirus (CMV) and herpes infections, dizziness, dyslipidemia, dyspnea, dysuria, hematuria, hypercholesterolemia, hyperglycemia, hyperuricemia, hypocalcemia, hypomagnesemia, hypophosphatemia, hypotension, increased creatinine, influenza, infusion reactions, insomnia, nasopharyngitis, new-onset diabetes, proteinuria, renal tubular necrosis, tremor, tuberculosis, and upper respiratory infections may occur.

Post-Marketing: Anaphylaxis and venous thrombosis of the renal allograft (with coadministration of anti-thymocyte globulin).

ANTIDOTE

Notify physician of all side effects. Most will be treated symptomatically. In case of overdose, it is recommended that the patient be monitored for any S/S of adverse reactions and appropriate symptomatic treatment instituted. If PML is confirmed or if patient develops evidence of PVAN, consider reducing or discontinuing immunosuppression, taking into account the risk to the allograft. Therapy may need to be interrupted in patients who develop infections. Treat infusion reactions as indicated. Resuscitate as necessary.

BELIMUMAB
(be-**LIM**-ue-mab)

Benlysta

Monoclonal antibody

pH 6.5

USUAL DOSE

Pretreatment: Baseline studies indicated; see Monitor.

Premedication: Consider premedication (e.g., antihistamines, H_2 antagonists, and/or corticosteroids) to help prevent or minimize hypersensitivity/infusion reactions.

Belimumab: 10 mg/kg as an infusion at 2-week intervals for the first 3 doses. Administer at 4-week intervals thereafter.

DOSE ADJUSTMENTS

No dose adjustment is recommended for patients with renal or hepatic impairment.

DILUTION

Provided as a lyophilized powder in a single-dose vial for reconstitution and dilution before IV infusion. Available in two strengths (120 mg or 400 mg). Allow vial to reach RT before reconstitution (approximately 10 to 15 minutes). Using a 21- to 25-gauge needle, reconstitute the 120-mg vial with 1.5 mL SWFI and the 400-mg vial with 4.8 mL SWFI. Concentration for both will equal 80 mg/mL. Direct the SWFI toward the side of the vial to minimize foaming. Gently swirl for 60 seconds. Allow to sit at RT and gently swirl for 60 seconds every 5 minutes until completely dissolved. *Do not shake.* Reconstitution may take up to 30 minutes. If reconstituted with a mechanical swirler, do not exceed 500 rpm and/or a duration of 30 minutes. Protect from sunlight. Solution should be opalescent and colorless to pale yellow. Small air bubbles are expected and are acceptable.

Patients weighing more than 40 kg: The desired dose of the reconstituted solution must be further diluted to 250 mL with NS, ½NS, or LR by withdrawing and discarding a volume equal to the desired dose from a 250-mL infusion bag or bottle of NS, ½NS, or LR.

Patients weighing less than or equal to 40 kg: Withdraw and discard a volume equal to the desired dose from a 100-mL infusion bag or bottle of NS, ½NS, or LR so that the resulting belimumab concentration in the infusion bag does not exceed 4 mg/mL. Add the desired dose of belimumab to the infusion bag or bottle and invert to mix the solution; see Storage.

Filters: No data available from manufacturer.

Storage: Before use, refrigerate vials (2° to 8° C [36° to 46° F]) in original carton, protected from light. Do not freeze. Avoid exposure to heat. Do not use beyond expiration date. Reconstituted solution, if not used immediately, should be refrigerated and protected from direct sunlight. Solution diluted in NS, ½NS, or LR may be refrigerated or kept at RT. Total time from reconstitution to completion of the infusion should not exceed 8 hours. Discard any unused product.

COMPATIBILITY

Manufacturer states, "**Incompatible** with dextrose solutions," "No **incompatibilities** with polyvinylchloride or polyolefin bags observed," and "Should not be infused concomitantly in the same IV line with other agents."

RATE OF ADMINISTRATION

A single dose, properly diluted, as an infusion equally distributed over 1 hour. Slow or interrupt infusion rate if an infusion reaction develops. Do not administer as an IV push or bolus.

ACTIONS

A recombinant, DNA-derived, humanized monoclonal antibody. It is a B-lymphocyte stimulator (BLyS)–specific inhibitor that blocks the binding of soluble BLyS (a B-cell survival factor) to its receptors on B-cells. Does not bind with B-cells directly. However, by binding BLyS, it inhibits the survival of B-cells (including auto-reactive B-cells) and reduces the differentiation of B-cells into immunoglobulin-producing plasma cells. Significantly reduces circulating CD19+, CD20+, naïve, and activated B-cells, and the SLE B-cell subset. Reductions in IgG and anti–double-strand DNA antibodies and increases in complement (C3 and C4) were observed as early as Week 8 and sustained through Week 52. In pediatric dosing, the pharmacodynamic response was consistent with the adult data. Terminal half-life is 19.4 days.

INDICATIONS AND USES

As an IV infusion in the treatment of patients 5 years of age and older or as a subcutaneous injection in patients 18 years of age and older with active, autoantibody-positive, systemic lupus erythematosus (SLE) who are receiving standard therapy.

Limitations of use: Efficacy has not been evaluated in patients with severe active lupus nephritis or severe active central nervous system lupus. Has not been studied in combination with other biologics or IV cyclophosphamide. Use of belimumab is not recommended in these situations.

CONTRAINDICATIONS

Patients who have experienced an anaphylactic hypersensitivity reaction with belimumab.

PRECAUTIONS

120-mg and 400-mg single-dose vials are for IV infusion only. Also available for SQ injection in a prefilled autoinjector or a single-dose (200 mg/mL) prefilled glass syringe. ▪ Administered under the direction of a physician knowledgeable in its use in a facility with adequate diagnostic and treatment facilities to monitor the patient and respond to any medical emergency. ▪ Serious hypersensitivity/infusion reactions, including anaphylaxis and death, have occurred. Acute hypersensitivity reactions usually occur within hours of the infusion. Nonacute reactions, including rash, nausea, fatigue, myalgia, headache, and facial edema, may occur up to a week following the infusion. Hypersensitivity, including serious reactions, has occurred in patients who have previously tolerated an infusion of belimumab. Patients with a history of multiple drug allergies or significant hypersensitivity may be at increased risk. Administration of premedications (which can mask or mitigate a reaction) and the overlap in S/S may make it difficult to distinguish between a hypersensitivity reaction and an infusion reaction. ▪ Serious and sometimes fatal infections have been reported. Use with caution in patients with severe or chronic infections. ▪ Cases of JC virus–associated progressive multifocal leukoencephalopathy (PML) resulting in neurologic deficits, including fatal cases, have been reported. Risk factors for PML include treatment with immunosuppressant therapies and impairment of immune function. ▪ Psychiatric events, including depression, suicidal ideation and behavior, insomnia, and anxiety, have been reported. Most patients had a history of depression or other serious psychiatric disorders and were receiving psychoactive medications. ▪ More deaths were reported with belimumab than with placebo during the controlled period of clinical trials. Etiologies included cardiovascular disease, infection, and suicide. No single cause of death predominated. ▪ The impact of treatment with belimumab on the development of malignancies is not known. The mechanism of action of belimumab could increase the risk for the development of malignancies. ▪ Anti-belimumab antibodies developed in a small percentage of patients. Clinical relevance is unknown. ▪ Response rates were lower in Black/African-American patients; use with caution.

Monitor: Obtain a baseline CBC, including a differential and platelet count. Monitor as indicated. ▪ Monitor for hypersensitivity reactions carefully during and for an appropriate period of time after administration; delayed onset of severe hypersensitivity reactions has been reported. S/S reported include anaphylaxis, angioedema, dyspnea, hypotension, pruritus, rash, and urticaria. ▪ On the day of the infusion, monitor for S/S of an infusion reaction (e.g., bradycardia, headache, hypotension, myalgia, nausea, rash, urticaria). ▪ Monitor for S/S of PML, such as new-onset or deteriorating neurologic signs and symptoms. Consultation with a neurologist is recommended. ▪ Consider interrupting therapy if a new infection develops during treatment with belimumab, and monitor patient closely. ▪ Monitor for S/S of psychiatric events (e.g., depression, and suicidal ideation and behavior).

Patient Education: Read FDA-approved medication guide. ▪ Females of childbearing potential should use effective contraceptive methods during treatment and for a minimum of 4 months after the final treatment. ▪ Manufacturer has established a pregnancy registry, and patients who are or who become pregnant are encouraged to register. ▪ Tell your healthcare provider if you are allergic to any medications. ▪ Promptly report anxiousness, difficulty breathing; dizziness or fainting; headache; itching; low blood pressure; nausea; skin rash, redness, or swelling; swelling of the face, lips, mouth, tongue, or throat; may indicate a hypersensitivity/infusion reaction. ▪ Promptly report diarrhea, chest discomfort or pain, chills, cold sweats, coughing up mucus, dizziness, fever, nausea, new or worsening depression or suicidal thoughts, pain or burning with urination, unusual changes in behavior or mood, frequent urination, warm, red, or painful skin or sores on your body. ▪ Promptly report new or worsening neurologic symptoms (e.g., confusion, difficulty talking or walking, dizziness, loss of balance, memory loss, or vision problems). ▪ Do not receive live vaccines while taking belimumab.

Maternal/Child: Monoclonal antibodies, including belimumab, are actively transported across the placenta during the third trimester of pregnancy and may affect immune response in infants exposed to belimumab in utero. However, there are risks to both the mother and the fetus associated with SLE. Use during pregnancy only if the potential benefit justifies the potential risk to the fetus. ▪ Clinical data are lacking regarding safety during breast-feeding. Consider risk versus benefit. ▪ Safety and effectiveness of IV administration has been established in pediatric patients 5 years of age and older. The safety and effectiveness for use in pediatric patients under 5 years of age has not been established. ▪ Risks and benefits should be considered before administering live or live-attenuated vaccines to infants exposed to belimumab in utero. Monitor the infant of a treated mother for B-cell reduction and other immune dysfunction.

Elderly: Numbers in clinical studies are insufficient to determine if the elderly respond differently than younger subjects; use with caution.

DRUG/LAB INTERACTIONS

Formal drug interaction studies have not been performed. ▪ Has not been studied in combination with other **biologics, including B-cell–targeted therapies or IV cyclophosphamide;** concurrent use is not recommended. ▪ Do not administer **live virus vaccines** for 30 days before or concurrently with belimumab. ▪ Risks and benefits should be considered before administering live or live-attenuated vaccines to infants exposed to belimumab in utero.

SIDE EFFECTS

Bronchitis, depression, diarrhea, fever, insomnia, migraine, nasopharyngitis, nausea, pain in extremities, and pharyngitis were most commonly reported. Cystitis, leukopenia, and viral gastroenteritis have also been reported. Serious side effects include depression and suicidality, hypersensitivity reactions (including anaphylaxis), infusion reactions, malignancy, serious infections, and death.

Post-Marketing: Fatal anaphylaxis.

ANTIDOTE

Notify physician of all side effects. Treatment of most side effects will be supportive. Consider interrupting therapy if a new infection develops during treatment with belimumab. If PML is confirmed, consider discontinuing immunosuppressant therapy, including belimumab. Slow or interrupt infusion rate if an infusion reaction develops. Infusion reactions may be treated with acetaminophen, antiemetics, H_2 antagonists, or corticosteroids as indicated. Discontinue if a serious hypersensitivity reaction occurs. Treat hypersensitivity reactions as indicated; may require epinephrine, airway management, oxygen, IV fluids, antihistamines, corticosteroids, and pressor amines.

BELINOSTAT   Antineoplastic
(be-**LIN**-oh-stat)

Beleodaq

USUAL DOSE

Pretreatment: Verify pregnancy status. Baseline studies indicated; see Monitor.

Belinostat: 1,000 mg/M² administered over 30 minutes by IV infusion once each day on Days 1 through 5 of a 21-day cycle. Cycles can be repeated every 21 days until disease progression or unacceptable toxicity.

DOSE ADJUSTMENTS

Before the start of each cycle and before resuming treatment following toxicity, the absolute neutrophil count (ANC) should be greater than or equal to 1×10^9/L (1,000/mm³), and the platelet count should be greater than or equal to 50×10^9/L (50,000/mm³). ▪ Other toxicities must be CTCAE Grade 2 or less before retreatment. ▪ Reduce the starting dose of belinostat to 750 mg/M² in patients known to be homozygous for the UGTIA1*28 allele. ▪ See the following chart for dose modifications for hematologic and nonhematologic toxicities. Base the dose adjustments for thrombocytopenia and neutropenia on platelet and absolute neutrophil nadir (lowest value) counts in the preceding cycle of therapy.

Dose Modifications for Hematologic and Nonhematologic Toxicities	
Hematologic Toxicities	**Dose Modification**
Platelet count $\geq 25 \times 10^9$/L and nadir ANC $\geq 0.5 \times 10^9$/L	No change
Nadir ANC $<0.5 \times 10^9$/L (any platelet count)	Decrease dose by 25% (750 mg/M²)
Platelet count $<25 \times 10^9$/L (any nadir ANC)	
Nonhematologic Toxicities	**Dose Modification**
Any CTCAE Grade 3 or 4 adverse reactionª	Decrease dose by 25% (750 mg/M²)
Recurrence of CTCAE Grade 3 or 4 adverse reaction after two dose reductions	Discontinue Beleodaq

ªFor nausea, vomiting, and diarrhea, dose modify only if the duration is greater than 7 days with supportive management.

▪ Data insufficient to recommend dosing in patients with moderate to severe hepatic impairment (bilirubin greater than 1.5 times the ULN) or in patients with a CrCl 39 mL/min or less.

DILUTION

Specific techniques required; see Precautions. Available in single-use vials containing lyophilized powder equivalent to 500 mg belinostat. Reconstitute each vial with 9 mL of SWFI (concentration is 50 mg/mL). Swirl contents until no visible particles remain. Withdraw the required dose and transfer to an infusion bag containing 250 mL of NS. Do not use if cloudiness or particulates are observed.

Filters: Use of an infusion set with a 0.22-micron in-line filter is required for administration.

Storage: Store in original packaging at CRT until use. Reconstituted vials may be stored for up to 12 hours at 15° to 25° C (59° to 77° F). Fully diluted solution may be stored at 15° to 25° C (59° to 77° F) for up to 36 hours, including infusion time.

COMPATIBILITY

Compatibility information not available from manufacturer; consult a pharmacist.

RATE OF ADMINISTRATION

A single dose as an IV infusion equally distributed over 30 minutes through an infusion set with a 0.22-micron in-line filter. Infusion time may be extended to 45 minutes for infusion site pain or other symptoms potentially attributable to the infusion.

ACTIONS

A histone deacetylase (HDAC) inhibitor. HDACs catalyze the removal of acetyl groups from the lysine residues of histones and some non-histone proteins. In vitro, belinostat caused the accumulation of acetylated histones and other proteins, inducing cell-cycle arrest and/or apoptosis of some transformed cells. It shows preferential cytotoxicity toward tumor cells compared with normal cells. Highly bound to protein. Primarily metabolized by UGT1A1. Also undergoes some metabolism by selected cytochrome P_{450} isoenzymes. Elimination half-life is 1.1 hours. Excreted primarily in urine and to a lesser extent in feces.

INDICATIONS AND USES

Treatment of patients with relapsed or refractory peripheral T-cell lymphoma. This indication is approved under accelerated approval based on tumor response rate and duration of response. An improvement in survival or disease-related symptoms has not been established. Continued approval may be contingent on verification and description of clinical benefit in confirmatory trials.

CONTRAINDICATIONS

Manufacturer states, "None."

PRECAUTIONS

Follow guidelines for handling cytotoxic agents. See Appendix A. ▪ Usually administered by or under the direction of a physician specialist with adequate diagnostic and treatment facilities to monitor the patient and respond to any medical emergency. ▪ Can cause thrombocytopenia, leukopenia (neutropenia and lymphopenia), and/or anemia. See Monitor and Dose Adjustments. ▪ Serious and sometimes fatal infections, including pneumonia and sepsis, have occurred. Do not administer belinostat to patients with an active infection. Patients with a history of extensive or intensive chemotherapy may be at higher risk for life-threatening infections. ▪ Can cause fatal hepatotoxicity and liver function test abnormalities. Interrupt or adjust dose until recovery, or permanently discontinue belinostat based on the severity of the hepatic toxicity; see Monitor and Dose Adjustments. ▪ Tumor lysis syndrome (TLS) has occurred. May cause acute renal failure requiring dialysis and can be fatal. ▪ Gastrointestinal toxicity has been reported. ▪ Belinostat is metabolized in the liver. Use caution in patients with hepatic impairment. Patients with moderate and severe hepatic impairment (total bilirubin greater than 1.5 times the ULN) were excluded from clinical trials. ▪ See Monitor.

Monitor: Obtain baseline CBC, including platelets, and monitor weekly. ▪ Obtain baseline serum chemistry tests, including renal and hepatic function, before the start of the first dose of each cycle. ▪ Observe closely for signs of infection. Prophylactic antibiotics may be indicated pending results of C/S in a febrile neutropenic patient. ▪ Monitor for S/S of TLS; early signs are flank pain and hematuria. May progress to renal failure, hyperkalemia, hypocalcemia, hyperuricemia, or hyperphosphatemia. Monitoring of serum electrolytes, uric acid, urine output, and renal function indicated. ▪ Prevention and treatment of hyperuricemia due to TLS may be accomplished with adequate hydration and, if necessary, with uric acid–lowering drugs (e.g., allopurinol). ▪ Monitor for thrombocytopenia (platelet count less than 50,000 mm^3). Initiate precautions to prevent excessive bleeding (e.g., inspect IV sites, skin, and mucous membranes; use extreme care during invasive procedures; test urine, emesis, stool, and secretions for occult blood). ▪ Nausea, vomiting, and diarrhea may require the use of antiemetic and/or antidiarrheal medications. Use prophylactically to increase patient comfort.

Patient Education: Review manufacturer's patient information leaflet. ▪ Avoid pregnancy. Effective birth control recommended for females of reproductive potential during treatment and for 6 months after the last dose and for males with female partners of reproductive potential during treatment and for 3 months after the last dose. ▪ May impair male fertility. ▪ Promptly report nausea, vomiting, and diarrhea; antiemetics and/or antidiarrheals may be indicated. ▪ Promptly report symptoms of infection (e.g., fever). ▪ Report bloody stools, bruising, fatigue. ▪ Laboratory monitoring is imperative. ▪ See Appendix D, p. 1311.

Maternal/Child: Based on its mechanism of action and findings of genotoxicity, belinostat can cause fetal harm. ▪ Discontinue breast-feeding. ▪ Safety and effectiveness for use in pediatric patients not established.

Elderly: Patients 65 years of age and older had a higher response rate to belinostat than did younger adults. ▪ No clinically meaningful differences in serious side effects were observed in patients based on age.

DRUG/LAB INTERACTIONS

Avoid concomitant administration of belinostat with **strong inhibitors of UGT1A1** (e.g., atazanavir). ▪ Belinostat did not increase the AUC or C_{max} of **warfarin** (Coumadin). Dose adjustment of warfarin is not required when coadministered with belinostat. ▪ Likely a glycoprotein (P-gp) substrate but not likely to inhibit P-gp.

SIDE EFFECTS

The most common side effects reported are anemia, fatigue, fever, nausea, and vomiting. Serious side effects reported include hematologic toxicity (anemia, lymphopenia, neutropenia, thrombocytopenia), hepatotoxicity and liver function abnormalities, increased SCr, infections (pneumonia, sepsis), multiorgan failure, and tumor lysis syndrome. Anemia, fatigue, febrile neutropenia, and multiorgan failure were reported as the reason for discontinuation of treatment. Other side effects reported include abdominal pain, chills, constipation, cough, decreased appetite, diarrhea, dizziness, dyspnea, headache, hypokalemia, hypotension, increased blood lactate dehydrogenase, infusion site pain, peripheral edema, phlebitis, prolonged QT, pruritus, and rash. Treatment-related deaths have occurred.

ANTIDOTE

Notify physician of all side effects. Minor side effects may be treated symptomatically. Supportive therapy as indicated will help sustain the patient in toxicity. Interrupt or adjust dose until recovery, or permanently discontinue belinostat based on the severity of the hematologic or hepatic toxicity. Hematologic toxicity may require dose adjustment. Neutropenia may be treated with filgrastim. Severe thrombocytopenia or anemia may require transfusion. Should a hypersensitivity reaction occur, treat as indicated.

BENDAMUSTINE HYDROCHLORIDE

(ben-deh-**MUS**-teen)

Antineoplastic
Alkylating agent

Bendeka, Treanda, Belrapzo, Vivimusta

pH 2.5 to 3.5

USUAL DOSE

Pretreatment: Verify pregnancy status. Baseline studies indicated; see Monitor.

Premedication: Premedication with antihistamines (e.g., diphenhydramine), antipyretics (e.g., acetaminophen), and corticosteroids may be indicated; see Monitor and Antidote.

Chronic lymphocytic leukemia (CLL): 100 mg/M^2 as an IV infusion on Days 1 and 2 of a 28-day cycle. May be repeated for up to 6 cycles.

Non-Hodgkin lymphoma (NHL): 120 mg/M^2 as an IV infusion on Days 1 and 2 of a 21-day cycle. May be repeated for up to 8 cycles.

DOSE ADJUSTMENTS

Chronic lymphocytic leukemia (CLL) and non-Hodgkin lymphoma (NHL): Delay treatment for Grade 4 hematologic toxicity or clinically significant nonhematologic toxicity equal to or greater than Grade 2. In addition, dose reduction may be indicated; see specific indication. Re-initiate treatment, if indicated, when nonhematologic toxicity has recovered to equal to or less than Grade 1 and/or the ANC has recovered to equal to or greater than 1,000 cells/mm^3 and platelets have recovered to equal to or greater than 75,000 cells/mm^3. ■ No dose adjustment indicated based on age or gender; see Precautions.

Chronic lymphocytic leukemia (CLL): Reduce dose to 50 mg/M^2 on Days 1 and 2 of each cycle for Grade 3 or greater hematologic toxicity. If Grade 3 or greater toxicity recurs, reduce dose to 25 mg/M^2 on Days 1 and 2 of each cycle. ■ Reduce dose to 50 mg/M^2 on Days 1 and 2 of each cycle for clinically significant Grade 3 or greater nonhematologic toxicity. ■ Dose re-escalation in subsequent cycles may be considered by the treating physician.

Non-Hodgkin lymphoma (NHL): Reduce dose to 90 mg/M^2 on Days 1 and 2 of each cycle for Grade 4 hematologic toxicity. If Grade 4 toxicity recurs, reduce the dose to 60 mg/M^2 on Days 1 and 2 of each cycle. ■ Reduce dose to 90 mg/M^2 on Days 1 and 2 of each cycle for Grade 3 or greater nonhematologic toxicity. If Grade 3 or greater toxicity recurs, reduce the dose to 60 mg/M^2 on Days 1 and 2 of each cycle.

DILUTION

Specific techniques required; see Precautions. Treanda is available in **two formulations:** a solution **(Treanda Injection)** and a lyophilized powder **(Treanda for Injection).** Formulations have different concentrations. **Do not mix or combine the two formulations.**

Treanda Injection is available as a solution in 45 mg/0.5 mL and 180 mg/2 mL single-use vials. **Do not use with devices containing polycarbonate or acrylonitrile-butadiene-styrene (ABS), including closed-system transfer devices (CSTDs), adapters, and syringes when preparing the infusion bag.** Must be diluted in a biosafety cabinet or a containment isolator. Aseptically withdraw the volume needed for the required dose and transfer to a 500-mL infusion bag of NS or D2.5/½NS using a polypropylene syringe with a metal needle and polypropylene hub. (Polypropylene syringes are translucent in appearance.) Final concentration of infusion solution should be 0.2 to 0.7 mg/mL. Mix thoroughly; solution should be clear and colorless to slightly yellow; see Compatibility. After dilution of **Treanda Injection** in the infusion bag, devices that contain ABS or polycarbonate, including infusion sets, may be used.

Treanda for Injection and **generic products** are available as a lyophilized powder in 25- and 100-mg single-use vials. **If a CSTD or adapter that contains polycarbonate or ABS is to be used as supplemental protection during preparation, use only this formulation (lyophilized powder for injection).** Reconstitute each 25-mg vial with 5 mL SWFI and each 100-mg vial with 20 mL SWFI; concentration is 5 mg/mL. Shake well. Should completely dissolve in 5 minutes. Within 30 minutes of reconstitution, withdraw the desired dose from the vial(s) and further dilute in 500 mL of NS or D2.5/½NS. Final concentration should be 0.2 to 0.6 mg/mL. Mix thoroughly; solution should be clear and colorless to slightly yellow.

Bendeka is available as a ready-to-dilute solution in 100 mg/4 mL multiple-dose vials. Withdraw the volume needed for the required dose and immediately transfer into a 50-mL infusion bag of NS, D5W, or D2.5/½NS. The final concentration should be 1.85 to 5.6 mg/mL. The final admixture should be a clear and colorless to yellow solution.

Filters: Specific information not available.

Storage: *All formulations:* Retain in original package to protect from light. **Bendeka** must be stored in the refrigerator at 2° to 8° C (36° to 46° F) in original carton to protect from light. When refrigerated, the contents may partially freeze. Allow the vial to reach room temperature (RT) (15° to 30° C [59° to 86° F]) before use. If particulate matter is observed after achieving RT, the product should be discarded. Solution diluted in NS or D2.5/½NS is stable for 6 hours at RT and in room light or for 24 hours refrigerated. Solution diluted in D5W is stable for 3 hours at RT and in room light or for 24 hours refrigerated. Administration must be completed within these times (e.g., 3, 6, or 24 hours based on type of storage and solution used). **Bendeka** is supplied as a multiple-dose vial that is stable for up to 28 days after initial vial entry when stored in its original carton under refrigeration. Manufacturer recommends no more than 6 dose withdrawals from each vial. **Treanda Injection** must be stored in the refrigerator. Solution diluted in NS or D2.5/½NS is stable for 2 hours at RT and in room light or for 24 hours refrigerated. Administration must be completed within these times (e.g., 2 or 24 hours based on type of storage). **Treanda for Injection and generic products** may be stored at CRT. Solution diluted in NS or D2.5/½NS is stable for 3 hours at RT and in room light or for 24 hours refrigerated. Administration must be completed within these times. Discard any unused solution.

COMPATIBILITY

Manufacturer states, "Use SWFI for reconstitution (for **Treanda for Injection**) and then (for **both formulations**) either NS or D2.5/½NS for dilution. No other diluents have been shown to be **compatible**."

Treanda Injection: Contains N,N-dimethylacetamide (DMA), which is **incompatible** with devices that contain polycarbonate or ABS. Devices, including CSTDs, adapters, and syringes that contain polycarbonate or ABS, have been shown to dissolve when they come into contact with DMA. This **incompatibility** leads to device failure (e.g., leaking, breaking, or operational failure of CSTD components), possible product contamination, and potential serious adverse health consequences to the practitioner or patient.

RATE OF ADMINISTRATION

Bendeka: *All indications:* Total daily dose as an infusion equally distributed over 10 minutes.

Treanda and generic products: *Chronic lymphocytic leukemia (CLL):* Total daily dose as an infusion equally distributed over 30 minutes.

Non-Hodgkin lymphoma (NHL): Total daily dose as an infusion equally distributed over 60 minutes.

ACTIONS

A bifunctional mechlorethamine derivative. An alkylating agent. Active against both quiescent and dividing cells. Exact mode of action unknown. May lead to cell death by damaging the DNA in cancer cells as well as by disrupting normal cell division. Highly protein bound. Distributes freely in human red blood cells. Extensively metabolized via hydrolytic, oxidative, and conjugative pathways. Half-life of the parent compound is approximately 40 minutes. Half-life of the two active metabolites, M3 and M4, are approximately 3 hours and 30 minutes, respectively. Excreted in urine and feces.

INDICATIONS AND USES

Treatment of patients with chronic lymphocytic leukemia (CLL). Study demonstrated a higher rate of overall response and a longer progression-free survival for bendamustine compared with chlorambucil (Leukeran). Effectiveness compared with first-line therapies other than chlorambucil has not been studied. ▪ Treatment of patients with indolent B-cell non-Hodgkin lymphoma that has progressed during or within 6 months of treatment with rituximab (Rituxan) or a rituximab-containing regimen.

CONTRAINDICATIONS

Bendeka: Known hypersensitivity to bendamustine, polyethylene glycol 400, propylene glycol, or monothioglycerol.

Treanda: Known hypersensitivity to bendamustine.

PRECAUTIONS

Follow guidelines for handling cytotoxic agents. See Appendix A, p. 1308. ▪ Administered by or under the direction of the physician specialist in a facility equipped to monitor the patient and respond to any medical emergency. ▪ Do not use in patients with a CrCl less than 40 mL/min (Bendeka) or less than 30 mL/min (Treanda). Use with caution in patients with mild or moderate renal impairment; no formal studies conducted. ▪ Use with caution in patients with mild hepatic impairment. Do not use in patients with moderate hepatic impairment (AST or ALT 2.5 to 10 times the ULN and total bilirubin 1.5 to 3 times the ULN) or severe hepatic impairment (total bilirubin greater than 3 times the ULN). No formal studies conducted. ▪ Myelosuppression may be severe and require dose delays and/or subsequent dose reductions. Deaths from myelosuppression-related adverse reactions have occurred; see Dose Adjustments. ▪ Infections, including hepatitis, pneumonia, and sepsis, have been reported. Has been associated with septic shock and death. ▪ Patients treated with bendamustine are at risk for reactivation of infections, including (but not limited to) hepatitis B, cytomegalovirus, *Mycobacterium tuberculosis,* and herpes zoster; see Monitor. ▪ Infusion reactions are common. In rare instances anaphylaxis or anaphylactoid reactions have occurred. Usually occur in the second and/or subsequent cycles of therapy. ▪ Tumor lysis syndrome (TLS) has been reported and may occur in the first treatment cycle. S/S are renal insufficiency, hyperkalemia, hypocalcemia, hyperuricemia, or hyperphosphatemia. May lead to acute renal failure and death. ▪ Fatal and serious skin reactions, including toxic skin reactions (Stevens-Johnson syndrome [SJS], toxic epidermal necrolysis [TEN], and drug reaction with eosinophilia and systemic syndrome [DRESS]), rash, and bullous exanthema, have been reported. Reactions have occurred when bendamustine was given as a single agent and in combination with other anticancer agents or allopurinol; see Drug/Lab Interactions and Antidote. ▪ Fatal and serious cases of liver injury have been reported. Combination therapy, progressive disease, or reactivation of hepatitis B were confounding factors in some patients. Most cases were reported within the first 3 months of therapy. ▪ Premalignant and malignant diseases, including myelodysplastic syndrome, myeloproliferative disorders, acute myeloid leukemia, and bronchial carcinoma have been reported. Causal relationship has not been determined.

Monitor: Patients should undergo appropriate measures (including clinical and laboratory monitoring, prophylaxis, and treatment) for infection and/or infection reactivation before treatment. ▪ Obtain baseline CBC with differential and platelet count. Monitor CBC with differential weekly, and monitor platelet count each cycle. Hematologic nadir usually occurs in the third week. If recovery to recommended values does not occur by the first day of the next scheduled cycle, delay dose until recovery occurs; see Dose Adjustments. ▪ Obtain baseline CrCl, AST, ALT, and total bilirubin; repeat as indicated. ▪ Monitor closely for S/S of infusion or hypersensitivity reactions (e.g., chills, fever, pruritus, rash). Discontinue bendamustine if a severe reaction occurs. Inquire about possible symptoms that suggest a minor reaction after the first infusion. Consider premedication with antihistamines (e.g., diphenhydramine), antipyretics (e.g., acetaminophen), and corticosteroids in patients who have experienced a Grade 1 or 2 infusion reaction; see Antidote. ▪ Monitor for S/S of TLS. In patients at risk for TLS, prevention and treatment of hyperuricemia may be accomplished with vigorous hydration. Allopurinol has been used during the beginning of bendamustine therapy. However, there may be an increased risk of severe skin toxicity with concomitant use of allopurinol and bendamustine; see Drug/Lab Interactions. Monitor uric acid levels. Monitor electrolytes, particularly potassium, and treat as indicated. ▪ Monitor patients with skin reactions closely. Withhold or discontinue bendamustine if skin reactions are severe or progressive. ▪ Use prophylactic antiemetics to reduce nausea and vomiting and increase patient comfort. ▪ Observe for S/S of infection (e.g., fever) or reactivation of infection. Prophylactic antibiotics may be indicated pending results of C/S in a febrile neutropenic patient. ▪ Monitor for thrombocytopenia (platelet count less than 50,000 cells/mm^3). Initiate precautions to prevent excessive bleeding (e.g., inspect IV sites, skin, and mucous membranes; use extreme care during invasive procedures; test urine, emesis, stool, and secretions for occult blood). ▪ Monitor IV site for signs of extravasation during and after administration (e.g., infection, pain, redness, swelling, necrosis); extravasation has resulted in hospitalization.

Patient Education: Avoid pregnancy; effective birth control is recommended for both men and females throughout treatment and for 3 months (for men) and 6 months (for females) after treatment is complete; report a suspected pregnancy immediately. ▪ May pose a risk to reproductive capacity in both males and females. May cause impaired spermatogenesis, azoospermia, and total germinal aplasia in males. ▪ Promptly report signs of infection (e.g., chills, fever) or allergic reaction (e.g., dyspnea, itching, rash) and severe or worsening skin reactions, including itching or rash. ▪ Promptly report signs of liver toxicity (e.g., anorexia, bleeding or bruising, jaundice). ▪ Frequent laboratory monitoring required. ▪ Promptly report IV site burning or stinging. ▪ Report other side effects such as nausea, vomiting, or diarrhea. Symptomatic treatment can be provided. ▪ May cause fatigue. Avoid driving or operating any dangerous tools or machinery if this side effect is experienced. ▪ See Appendix D, p. 1311.

Maternal/Child: Avoid pregnancy; can cause fetal harm. Males and females of childbearing age must use effective birth control. ▪ If the drug is used during pregnancy or if the patient becomes pregnant during therapy, inform the patient of the potential hazard to the fetus. ▪ Has the potential for serious side effects; breast-feeding is not recommended during treatment and for at least 1 week after the last dose. ▪ Effectiveness for use in pediatric patients not established. Evaluation of one small Phase 1/2 trial suggests that the safety profile in pediatric patients is similar to that seen in adults; see prescribing information.

Elderly: Side effect profile similar for all age-groups studied. Patients over age 65 years with CLL had a lower overall response rate and a shorter progression-free survival than CLL patients under age 65. In NHL patients, efficacy (overall response rate and duration of response) was similar for all age-groups.

DRUG/LAB INTERACTIONS

No formal drug interaction studies have been conducted. ▪ Active metabolites of bendamustine are formed via cytochrome P$_{450}$ CYP1A2. **Inhibitors of CYP1A2** (e.g., ciprofloxacin, fluvoxamine) may increase plasma concentrations of bendamustine and decrease plasma concentrations of active metabolites. **Inducers of CYP1A2** (e.g., omeprazole, smoking) may decrease plasma concentrations of bendamustine and increase plasma concentrations of its active metabolites. Use caution or consider alternative treatments if concomitant treatment with CYP1A2 inhibitors or inducers is indicated. ▪ Not likely to inhibit metabolism via other selected CYP isoenzymes or to induce the metabolism of substrates of cytochrome P$_{450}$ enzymes. ▪ Incidence of severe skin reactions (e.g., SJS, TEN, and DRESS) may be increased when bendamustine is given concomitantly with **allopurinol and other medications known to cause these syndromes** (e.g., rituximab). ▪ In vitro data suggest that P-glycoprotein, breast cancer resistance protein (BCRP), and/or other efflux transporters may have a role in bendamustine transport.

SIDE EFFECTS

Anorexia, constipation, cough, diarrhea, dyspnea, fatigue, fever, headache, myelosuppression (anemia, febrile neutropenia, leukopenia, lymphopenia, neutropenia, thrombocytopenia), nausea, rash, stomatitis, vomiting, and weight loss were most common. Other side effects reported include abdominal pain; anxiety; arthralgia; asthenia; back pain; bone pain; chest pain; chills; decreased CrCl; dehydration; depression; dizziness; dry mouth; dry skin; dysgeusia; dyspepsia; elevated AST, ALT, and bilirubin levels; gastro-esophageal reflux disease; herpes simplex and herpes zoster; hypersensitivity and/or infusion reactions (e.g., anaphylaxis [rare], pruritus, rash); hypertension; hyperuricemia; hypokalemia; infections; infusion site reactions; insomnia; malignancies; nasal congestion; nasopharyngitis; night sweats; oral candidiasis; pain; peripheral edema; pharyngolaryngeal pain; pneumonia; sepsis; stomatitis; tachycardia; TLS; and wheezing. Hypersensitivity reactions and fever required study withdrawal in some patients.

Post-Marketing: Anaphylaxis, cardiac disorders (atrial fibrillation, CHF [some fatal], MI [some fatal], palpitation), DRESS, extravasation resulting in hospitalization, infusion site reactions (irritation, pain, phlebitis, pruritus, swelling), pancytopenia, *Pneumocystis jiroveci* pneumonia, pneumonitis, Stevens-Johnson syndrome, and toxic epidermal necrolysis.

Overdose: Ataxia, cardiac arrhythmias, convulsions, respiratory distress, sedation, tremor.

ANTIDOTE

Keep physician informed of all side effects and hematologic parameters. Side effects may decrease in severity with reduced dose. Bone marrow depression may require withholding bendamustine until recovery occurs. Administration of whole blood products (e.g., packed RBCs, platelets, leukocytes) may be required. Selected blood modifiers (e.g., erythropoiesis-stimulating agents, filgrastim, pegfilgrastim, sargramostim) may be indicated to treat bone marrow toxicity. Discontinue the infusion immediately for any life-threatening side effect (e.g., clinically significant bronchospasm, cardiac arrhythmias, severe hypotension). Consider premedication with antihistamines (e.g., diphenhydramine), antipyretics (e.g., acetaminophen), and corticosteroids in subsequent cycles in patients who have experienced a Grade 1 or 2 hypersensitivity and/or infusion reaction. Grade 3 or 4 reactions have not typically been rechallenged; consider discontinuing bendamustine. Withhold or discontinue bendamustine if skin reactions are severe or progressive. There is no specific antidote. Supportive therapy as indicated will help sustain the patient in toxicity. ECG monitoring may be indicated to evaluate cardiac side effects.

BENZTROPINE MESYLATE
(**BENS**-troh-peen **MES**-sih-layt)

Antidyskinetic
Antiparkinson
Anticholinergic

Cogentin   pH 5 to 8

USUAL DOSE

Individualized based on age, weight, and type of parkinsonism. One dose daily, usually at bedtime, provides relief for most patients; however, divided doses (two or four times daily) may be beneficial in selected patients. Has a cumulative action. Initiate treatment with lower doses. Increase in increments of 0.5 mg at 5- to 6-day intervals until optimal results are obtained without excessive side effects or a maximum dose of 6 mg is reached.

Idiopathic parkinsonism: 0.5 to 1 mg/day at bedtime. Up to 4 to 6 mg/day may be required.

Postencephalitic parkinsonism: 2 mg/day. May be given in 1 or more doses. In highly sensitive patients, begin with a 0.5-mg dose at bedtime and increase as indicated.

Drug-induced extrapyramidal disorders: 1 to 4 mg given once or twice daily. Most effective with extrapyramidal disorders that develop soon after beginning treatment with neuroleptic agents (e.g., phenothiazines, haloperidol). Withhold after 1 to 2 weeks. If still needed, may be restarted. Drug-induced extrapyramidal disorders that develop slowly may not respond to benztropine.

Acute dystonic reactions: 1 to 2 mg usually provides quick relief.

PEDIATRIC DOSE

Has atropine-like side effects but may be used with caution in pediatric patients over 3 years of age. See Usual Dose and begin at low end of dosing range. See Contraindications.

DOSE ADJUSTMENTS

Begin with the lower end of the dosing range and increase gradually, especially in thin or elderly patients. In the elderly, consider potential for age-related impaired organ function and concomitant disease or drug therapy. ■ Reduced doses may be indicated if weakness and/or inability to move a particular muscle group occurs (may be more frequent with larger doses). ■ Reduced doses may be indicated during hot weather, especially with concomitant use of other atropine-like drugs; in patients with alcoholism, CNS disease, or other chronic illnesses; and in patients who do manual labor in a hot environment. ■ Reduce dose or temporarily discontinue for severe dry mouth that results in difficulty swallowing or speaking or for loss of appetite and weight.

DILUTION

1 mL of prepared solution equals 1 mg. May be given undiluted.

Storage: Store at CRT. Do not freeze.

COMPATIBILITY

Compatibility information not available from manufacturer.

Other sources suggest a few specific **compatibilities** dependent on concentration and manufacturer; consult a pharmacist.

RATE OF ADMINISTRATION

A single dose equally distributed over 1 minute.

ACTIONS

Has both anticholinergic and antihistaminic effects. Onset of action occurs within minutes by IV or IM route. Undergoes hepatic metabolism.

INDICATIONS AND USES

Adjunct in therapy of all forms of parkinsonism. ■ Control of extrapyramidal disorders (except tardive dyskinesia) due to neuroleptic drugs (e.g., haloperidol, phenothiazines [e.g., chlorpromazine, prochlorperazine]).

CONTRAINDICATIONS

Pediatric patients under 3 years of age. ■ Known hypersensitivity to benztropine or its components.

PRECAUTIONS

IV route seldom used except in acute drug reactions or psychotic episodes. ■ Use caution in patients with tachycardia and/or prostatic hypertrophy; monitor closely. ■ Use with caution in patients with glaucoma. May be used in patients with simple glaucoma; however, benztropine is not recommended for use in patients with angle-closure glaucoma. ■ Mental and/or physical abilities required for performance of hazardous tasks may be impaired. ■ Concomitant use with phenothiazines and/or tricyclic antidepressants may cause fever, GI upset, heat intolerance, heat stroke, hyperthermia, and paralytic ileus. Fatalities have occurred. ■ May produce anhidrosis (deficient or absent sweating). ■ May aggravate the symptoms of tardive dyskinesia; see Contraindications. ■ May intensify symptoms (e.g., mental confusion and excitement, visual hallucinations) and may precipitate a toxic psychosis in patients with mental disorders, especially with larger doses.

Monitor: Has a cumulative action; close observation is required. ■ Monitor for S/S of paralytic ileus (e.g., abdominal pain, constipation, distention), especially in patients receiving other anticholinergic or neuroleptic agents. ■ May cause dysuria and/or urinary retention; monitor urine output. ■ Observe for weakness and inability to move particular muscle groups; see Dose Adjustments. ■ See Precautions and Drug/Lab Interactions.

Patient Education: Promptly report abdominal pain or distention, constipation, fever, GI upset, heat intolerance, inability to sweat, and pain or difficulty urinating. ■ Ability to perform hazardous tasks may be impaired.

Maternal/Child: Safety for use during pregnancy and breast-feeding not established. ■ May inhibit lactation. ■ Has atropine-like effects; do not use in pediatric patients under

3 years of age, and use caution in pediatric patients over 3 years of age. See Pediatric Dose and Contraindications.

Elderly: See Dose Adjustments and Precautions. ■ May produce agitation, confusion, disorientation, hallucinations, or psychotic-like symptoms. ■ Has the potential to increase memory impairment. ■ Chronic use may precipitate glaucoma.

DRUG/LAB INTERACTIONS

Concomitant use with **phenothiazines and/or tricyclic antidepressants** may cause fever, GI upset, heat intolerance, heat stroke, hyperthermia, and paralytic ileus. ■ Use with **other anticholinergic agents** may increase the risk of adverse anticholinergic effects (e.g., blurred vision, delirium, dry mouth, hyperpyrexia). ■ May reduce effectiveness of **neuroleptic drugs** (e.g., haloperidol) and increase the risk of adverse anticholinergic effects. Use with haloperidol may worsen schizophrenic symptoms and may precipitate tardive dyskinesia. ■ May reduce the effectiveness of levodopa by reducing the amount of levodopa absorbed in the GI tract. Monitor pharmacologic response to levodopa closely with concomitant use.

SIDE EFFECTS

Blurred vision, constipation, depression, dilated pupils, dry mouth, dysuria, exacerbation of pre-existing psychotic symptoms, fever, heat stroke, hypersensitivity reaction (e.g., skin rash), hyperthermia, listlessness, nausea, nervousness, numbness of fingers, paralytic ileus, tachycardia, toxic psychosis (e.g., confusion, disorientation, memory impairment, visual hallucinations), urinary retention, vomiting.

Overdose: In addition to the above side effects, anhidrosis; ataxia; CNS depression; coma; convulsions; delirium; dizziness; dysphagia; glaucoma; headache; hot, dry, flushed skin; hypertension; muscle weakness; mydriasis; palpitations; respiratory arrest; and shock may occur.

ANTIDOTE

Notify the physician of all side effects. If a hypersensitivity reaction (e.g., skin rash) is not controlled by dose reduction, discontinue benztropine. Treat overdose with physostigmine salicylate 1 to 2 mg SQ or IV to reverse symptoms of anticholinergic intoxication. May be repeated in 2 hours if indicated. Observe for relapses up to 12 hours. Treat symptoms of overdose symptomatically. Respiratory support, diazepam for CNS excitement (use with caution to avoid subsequent depression), local miotics (e.g., pilocarpine ophthalmic) for mydriasis (pupil dilation) or cycloplegia (paralysis of the ciliary muscle of the eye), cold applications (e.g., ice bags, alcohol sponges) for hyperpyrexia, a vasopressor (e.g., dopamine) and IV fluids for circulatory collapse, and darkening of the room for photophobia may all be indicated. Resuscitate as necessary.

BEVACIZUMAB ■
BEVACIZUMAB-awwb[a] ■
BEVACIZUMAB-bvzr[a]
(beh-vah-**SIZZ**-ih-mab)

Recombinant monoclonal antibody
Vascular Endothelial Growth
Factor (VEGF) Inhibitor
Antineoplastic

Avastin, Mvasi[a], Zirabev[a], Vegzemla, Alymsys   pH 6.2

USUAL DOSE

Bevacizumab-awwb[a] (Mvasi), bevacizumab-maly (Alymsys) and bevacizumab-adcd (Vegzelma) and bevacizumab-bvzr[a] (Zirabev) and bevacizumab-adcd (Vegzemla) are biosimilar drugs of bevacizumab (Avastin). Unless specifically stated otherwise, the use of the name *bevacizumab* or *bevacizumab products* applies to all formulations.

Pretreatment: Do not begin therapy until at least 28 days following surgery and the wound is fully healed. Verify pregnancy status. Baseline studies indicated; see Monitor.

BEVACIZUMAB PRODUCTS

May be used in combination with other antineoplastic agents or as a single agent. See Dose Adjustments, Monitor, and Precautions.

Metastatic colorectal cancer (mCRC): Recommended doses are either 5 mg/kg or 10 mg/kg IV every 2 weeks when used in combination with intravenous 5-FU–based chemotherapy. Administer 5 mg/kg IV every 2 weeks when used in combination with bolus IFL (irinotecan, fluorouracil, leucovorin calcium). Administer 10 mg/kg IV every 2 weeks when used in combination with FOLFOX4 (fluorouracil, leucovorin calcium, and oxaliplatin).

Administer 5 mg/kg IV every 2 weeks or 7.5 mg/kg IV every 3 weeks when used in combination with a fluoropyrimidine-irinotecan–based or a fluoropyrimidine-oxaliplatin–based chemotherapy in patients who have progressed on a first-line bevacizumab-containing regimen.

First-line non-squamous, non–small-cell lung cancer (NSCLC): 15 mg/kg IV every 3 weeks in combination with carboplatin and paclitaxel.

Recurrent glioblastoma: 10 mg/kg IV every 2 weeks.

Metastatic renal cell carcinoma (mRCC): 10 mg/kg IV every 2 weeks in combination with interferon alfa.

Persistent, recurrent, or metastatic cervical cancer: 15 mg/kg IV every 3 weeks administered in combination with paclitaxel and cisplatin, or in combination with paclitaxel and topotecan.

BEVACIZUMAB (AVASTIN)

Stage III or IV epithelial ovarian, fallopian tube, or primary peritoneal cancer after initial surgical resection: 15 mg/kg IV every 3 weeks in combination with carboplatin and paclitaxel for up to 6 cycles, followed by bevacizumab 15 mg/kg IV every 3 weeks as a single agent for a total of up to 22 cycles or until disease progression, whichever occurs earlier.

Platinum-resistant recurrent epithelial ovarian, fallopian tube, or primary peritoneal cancer: 10 mg/kg IV every 2 weeks in combination with paclitaxel, pegylated liposomal doxorubicin, or topotecan (weekly); or 15 mg/kg IV every 3 weeks in combination with topotecan (every 3 weeks).

Platinum-sensitive recurrent epithelial ovarian, fallopian tube, or primary peritoneal cancer: 15 mg/kg IV every 3 weeks when administered in combination with carboplatin and paclitaxel for 6 to 8 cycles, followed by bevacizumab 15 mg/kg IV every 3 weeks as a single agent until disease progression. Alternatively, 15 mg/kg IV every 3 weeks when administered

---

[a]Please see p. xi for more information on biosimilars.

in combination with carboplatin and gemcitabine for 6 to 10 cycles, followed by bevacizumab 15 mg/kg IV every 3 weeks as a single agent until disease progression.

DOSE ADJUSTMENTS

No dose reduction for bevacizumab products is recommended. ▪ Modify doses for adverse reactions based on the following chart.

Dose Modifications for Adverse Reactions		
Adverse Reaction	**Severity**	**Dose Modification**
Gastrointestinal perforation and fistulae	• Gastrointestinal perforation, any grade • Tracheoesophageal fistula, any grade • Fistula, Grade 4 • Fistula formation involving any internal organ	Discontinue bevacizumab
Wound healing complications	• Wound healing complications requiring medical intervention • Necrotizing fasciitis	Discontinue bevacizumab
Hemorrhage	• Grade 3 or 4	Discontinue bevacizumab
	• Recent history of hemoptysis of ½ teaspoon (2.5 mL) or more	Withhold bevacizumab
Thromboembolic events	• Arterial thromboembolism, severe	Discontinue bevacizumab
	• Venous thromboembolism, Grade 4	Discontinue bevacizumab
Hypertension	• Hypertensive crisis • Hypertensive encephalopathy	Discontinue bevacizumab
	• Hypertension, severe	Withhold bevacizumab if not controlled with medical management; resume once controlled
Posterior reversible encephalopathy syndrome (PRES)	• Any	Discontinue bevacizumab
Renal injury and proteinuria	• Nephrotic syndrome	Discontinue bevacizumab
	• Proteinuria greater than or equal to 2 Gm/24 hr in absence of nephrotic syndrome	Withhold bevacizumab until proteinuria less than 2 grams/24 hr
Infusion reaction	• Severe infusion reaction	Discontinue bevacizumab
	• Clinically significant	Interrupt infusion; resume at a decreased rate of infusion after symptoms resolve
	• Mild, clinically insignificant	Decrease infusion rate
Congestive heart failure	• Any	Discontinue bevacizumab

▪ See Monitor and Precautions.

DILUTION

Available in single-use vials containing 100 mg in 4 mL or 400 mg in 16 mL (25 mg/mL). Calculate desired dose and choose the appropriate vial or combination of vials. Withdraw the required volume of the bevacizumab product and dilute in a total volume of 100 mL of NS.

Filters: Not required by manufacturer; however, studies with *Avastin* using a 0.2-micron in-line filter were done, and drug potency appeared to be maintained.

Storage: Store in original carton in refrigerator at 2° to 8° C (36° to 46° F) until time of use. Protect from light. ***Do not shake or freeze.*** Diluted solutions may be refrigerated for up to 8 hours. Contains no preservatives; unused portions must be discarded.

COMPATIBILITY

Manufacturer states, "Do not administer or mix with dextrose solutions." **Incompatibilities** with polyvinylchloride or polyolefin bags have not been observed with *Avastin.*

RATE OF ADMINISTRATION

Must be given as an IV infusion.

Initial infusion: A single dose equally distributed over 90 minutes.

Second infusion: If the initial infusion is well tolerated, the second infusion may be administered equally distributed over 60 minutes.

Subsequent infusions: If the 60-minute infusion is well tolerated, subsequent infusions may be administered equally distributed over 30 minutes.

ACTIONS

A humanized IgG_1 monoclonal antibody produced by recombinant DNA technology. Has antiangiogenesis properties. The interaction of human vascular endothelial growth factor (VEGF) with its receptors leads to endothelial cell proliferation and new blood vessel formation. By binding VEGF, bevacizumab prevents the interaction of VEGF with its receptors on the surface of endothelial cells, thus inhibiting the development of new blood vessels around tumors (a tumor-starving mechanism) and resulting in a reduction of microvascular growth and an inhibition of metastatic disease progression. Predicted time to steady-state was 84 days. Half-life is approximately 20 days (range is 11 to 50 days). IgG antibodies may cross the placental barrier and be secreted in breast milk.

INDICATIONS AND USES

BEVACIZUMAB PRODUCTS

First- or second-line treatment of metastatic colorectal cancer. Used in combination with intravenous 5-fluorouracil–based chemotherapy (e.g., IFL, FOLFOX4). ▪ Second-line treatment of metastatic colorectal cancer in patients who have progressed on a first-line bevacizumab-containing regimen. Used in combination with fluoropyrimidine-irinotecan–based or fluoropyrimidine-oxaliplatin–based chemotherapy. ▪ First-line treatment of patients with unresectable, locally advanced, recurrent, or metastatic non-squamous, non–small-cell lung cancer. Given in combination with carboplatin and paclitaxel. ▪ Treatment of recurrent glioblastoma in adults. ▪ Treatment of metastatic renal cell cancer. Given in combination with interferon alfa. ▪ Treatment of persistent, recurrent, or metastatic cervical cancer. Given in combination with paclitaxel and cisplatin or paclitaxel and topotecan.

BEVACIZUMAB (AVASTIN)

Treatment of patients with platinum-resistant recurrent epithelial ovarian, fallopian tube, or primary peritoneal cancer who received no more than 2 prior chemotherapy regimens. Given in combination with paclitaxel, pegylated liposomal doxorubicin, or topotecan. ▪ Treatment of patients with platinum-sensitive recurrent epithelial ovarian, fallopian tube, or primary peritoneal cancer. Given in combination with carboplatin and paclitaxel or with carboplatin and gemcitabine, followed by bevacizumab as a single agent. ▪ Treatment of patients with Stage III or IV epithelial ovarian, fallopian tube, or primary peritoneal cancer following initial surgical resection. Given in combination with carboplatin and paclitaxel, followed by bevacizumab as a single agent.

Limitation of use: Bevacizumab products are not indicated for adjuvant treatment of colon cancer.

CONTRAINDICATIONS

Manufacturer states, "No known contraindications"; see Precautions and Antidote. ▪ Avoid use in patients with ovarian cancer who have evidence of rectosigmoid involvement by pelvic examination or bowel involvement on CT scan or clinical symptoms of bowel obstruction.

PRECAUTIONS
Must be given as an infusion. ■ Should be administered by or under the direction of a physician specialist in a facility equipped to monitor the patient and respond to any medical emergency. ■ Incidence of wound healing and surgical complications, including serious and fatal complications, is increased in patients receiving bevacizumab. Withhold bevacizumab for a minimum of 28 days after major surgery; surgical incision must be fully healed. Withhold at least 28 days before elective surgery (half-life is approximately 20 days but has a wide range). ■ GI perforation with or without fistula formation and/or intra-abdominal abscesses has occurred; deaths have been reported. The majority of cases occurred within the first 50 days of initiation of bevacizumab. Consider GI perforation in any patient with complaints of abdominal pain associated with constipation, fever, nausea, and vomiting. ■ Nongastrointestinal fistula formation has been reported, in some cases with a fatal outcome. Serious fistula formations involving tracheoesophageal, bronchopleural, biliary, vaginal, renal, and bladder areas have been reported. Most events occurred within the first 6 months of bevacizumab therapy. ■ Necrotizing fasciitis (including fatal cases) has been reported, usually secondary to wound healing complications, gastrointestinal perforation, or fistula formation. ■ Severe or fatal hemorrhage, including CNS hemorrhage, epistaxis, GI bleed, hematemesis, hemoptysis, and vaginal bleeding, occurred up to five times more frequently in patients receiving bevacizumab compared with patients receiving chemotherapy alone. Do not administer bevacizumab to patients with serious bleeding or a recent history of hemoptysis of 1/2 teaspoon or more of red blood. ■ May cause severe hypertension that may be persistent. Treatment is required; see Monitor and Antidote. ■ Posterior reversible encephalopathy syndrome (PRES) has been reported. Onset of symptoms occurred from 16 hours to 1 year after initiation of therapy. May present with blindness and other visual and neurologic disturbances, confusion, headache, lethargy, and seizures. Mild to severe hypertension may be present. MRI is required to confirm diagnosis. Symptoms usually resolve gradually with discontinuation of bevacizumab and treatment of hypertension. ■ Proteinuria occurred during studies and progressed to nephrotic syndrome in some patients. Findings consistent with thrombotic microangiopathy have been found on kidney biopsy in some patients. In some but not all patients, proteinuria decreased within several months after therapy was discontinued. Increased serum creatinine levels have occurred and may not return to baseline. ■ CHF has been reported. Incidence is higher in patients receiving chemotherapy plus bevacizumab compared with patients receiving chemotherapy alone. ■ Infusion reactions are infrequent but have occurred. ■ Serious and sometimes fatal arterial thromboembolic events (ATEs) (e.g., CVA [stroke], MI, TIA, angina) have been reported. The risk of developing an ATE was increased in patients with a history of arterial thromboembolism or diabetes and in patients greater than 65 years of age. ■ Venous thromboembolic events (e.g., deep vein thrombosis, intra-abdominal thrombosis, and pulmonary embolism) have been reported. ■ Increases the risk of ovarian failure in premenopausal females receiving bevacizumab (Avastin) with chemotherapy for adjuvant treatment of a solid tumor. Recovery of ovarian function is defined as resumption of menses, a positive serum β-HCG pregnancy test, or an FSH level less than 30 mIU/mL. Recovery of ovarian function occurred in some but not all females following discontinuation of therapy. Long-term effects of bevacizumab on fertility are unknown. ■ A protein substance, it has the potential for producing an immune response. Neutralizing antibodies against bevacizumab have been found using a specific immunosorbent assay; clinical significance is not known. ■ See Drug/Lab Interactions, Maternal/Child, and Antidote.
Monitor: Obtain baseline BP, CBC with differential and platelets, and urinalysis. ■ Monitor for S/S of an infusion reaction (e.g., chest pain, chills, diaphoresis, headache, hypertension, hypertensive crisis associated with neurologic S/S, oxygen desaturation, rigors, wheezing). ■ Monitor BP at least every 2 to 3 weeks; monitor more frequently in patients with hypertension. Treat hypertension with appropriate antihypertensive therapy. Continue to monitor BP at regular intervals after bevacizumab therapy is discontinued. ■ Repeat CBC with differential and platelets as indicated. ■ Monitor for the

development or worsening of proteinuria by serial dipstick urinalysis. Patients with a 2+ or greater urine dipstick reading should undergo further assessment with a 24-hour urine collection. Monitor patients with moderate to severe proteinuria until improvement and/ or resolution is observed. Repeat urinalyses and/or 24-hour urine collections as indicated. ▪ Monitor for S/S of CHF (e.g., cyanosis, dyspnea on exertion, edema, fatigue on exertion, hypoxemia, jugular venous distension, orthopnea, pulmonary rales, tachycardia, third heart sound). ▪ Check surgical wounds for wound dehiscence. ▪ Monitor for S/S of any type of bleeding. ▪ Monitor for GI perforation or fistula formulation (e.g., abdominal pain, constipation, fever, hypotension, nausea and vomiting). ▪ Monitor for S/S of thromboembolic events. ▪ Monitor for S/S of PRES. Obtain MRI to confirm diagnosis if indicated. ▪ See Dose Adjustments (Dose Modifications for Adverse Reactions), Rate of Administration, Precautions, and Antidote.

Patient Education: May cause fetal harm; avoid pregnancy. Females of reproductive potential should use effective contraception during treatment with and for 6 months after the last dose of bevacizumab; see Maternal/Child. Females should report a suspected pregnancy immediately. ▪ Increases risk of ovarian failure and may impair fertility. ▪ Full disclosure of health history is imperative. ▪ Promptly report any S/S of CHF. ▪ Promptly report any S/S of an infusion reaction. ▪ Promptly report any unusual or unexpected symptoms or side effects (e.g., abdominal pain, bleeding from any source, constipation, dyspnea, fever, persistent cough, rigors, sudden onset of worsening neurologic function, vomiting, wound separation). ▪ Increased risk of arterial and venous thromboembolic events and wound healing complications. ▪ Routine monitoring of BP and renal function required. ▪ See Appendix D, p. 1311.

Maternal/Child: May cause fetal harm based on findings from animal studies and the drug's mechanism of action. Animal models link angiogenesis and VEFG and VEFG Receptor 2 to critical aspects of female reproduction, embryofetal development, and postnatal development. ▪ Discontinue breast-feeding during treatment with bevacizumab and for 6 months after the final dose. ▪ Safety and effectiveness for use in pediatric patients not established. Nonmandibular osteonecrosis has been reported in pediatric patients under 18 years of age who have received bevacizumab. Bevacizumab is not approved for this patient population.

Elderly: Overall survival was similar compared to younger adults; however, the incidence of some side effects was increased (e.g., arterial thromboembolic events).

DRUG/LAB INTERACTIONS

Drug interaction studies have not been completed. ▪ Has been administered with **carboplatin, paclitaxel, and interferon alfa.** May decrease paclitaxel exposure. ▪ Several cases of microangiopathic hemolytic anemia (MAHA) have been reported in patients with solid tumors who are receiving concomitant therapy with bevacizumab and **sunitinib malate** (Sutent). This combination therapy is not approved and not recommended.

SIDE EFFECTS

The most common side effects include back pain, dry skin, epistaxis, exfoliative dermatitis, headache, hypertension, lacrimation (excess), proteinuria, rectal hemorrhage, rhinitis, and taste alteration. Major, dose-limiting, and potentially life-threatening side effects include arterial thromboembolic events (e.g., angina, cerebral infarction, MI, TIA), bleeding episodes (e.g., CNS hemorrhage, epistaxis [severe], GI hemorrhage, hemoptysis, vaginal bleeding), CHF, GI perforations (with or without fistula formation [may be complicated by intra-abdominal abscess]), hypertensive crises, infusion reactions, nongastrointestinal fistula formation, ovarian failure, posterior reversible encephalopathy syndrome (PRES), proteinuria with or without nephrotic syndrome, surgery and wound healing complications, and venous thromboembolic events (e.g., deep vein thrombosis, intra-abdominal thrombosis, pulmonary embolism). Other side effects have been reported depending on chemotherapy regimen and include abdominal pain, anal fistula, anorexia, anxiety, arthralgia, asthenia, chest pain, confusion, constipation, cough, diarrhea, dizziness, dysarthria, dysphonia, dyspnea, fatigue, gingival bleeding, hematologic toxicity (e.g., leukopenia, lymphopenia, neutropenia, thrombocytopenia), hemorrhoids, hyperglycemia, hyperkalemia, hypoalbuminemia, hypocalcemia, hypomagnesemia, hyponatremia, increased serum creatinine, infection, insomnia, mucosal inflammation, muscular weakness, myalgia, nail disorder, nasal mucosal disorder, nausea, pain (extremity, neck, pelvic), palmar-plantar erythrodysesthesia syndrome, peripheral edema, peripheral sensory neuropathy, pneumonitis/pulmonary infiltrates, proctalgia, rhinitis, sinusitis, stomatitis, syncope, urinary tract infection, vomiting, weight loss. Additional side effects may occur.

Post-Marketing: Anastomotic ulceration, gallbladder perforation, GI ulcer, intestinal necrosis, mesenteric venous occlusion, nasal septum perforation, osteonecrosis of the jaw, pancytopenia, polyserositis, pulmonary hypertension, renal thrombotic microangiopathy (manifested as severe proteinuria).

ANTIDOTE

Keep physician informed of all side effects. May constitute a medical emergency or will be treated symptomatically as indicated. Patients who develop gastrointestinal vaginal fistula may also have a bowel obstruction and require surgical intervention, as well as a diverting ostomy. Discontinue if any of the following develop: GI perforation (any grade), fistula formation involving any internal organ, formation of any grade tracheo-esophageal fistula or any Grade 4 fistula, wound dehiscence or wound healing complications requiring medical intervention, necrotizing fasciitis, Grade 3 or 4 hemorrhage, nephrotic syndrome, a severe arterial thromboembolic event, life-threatening (Grade 4) venous thromboembolic events (including pulmonary embolism), PRES, hypertensive crisis, hypertensive encephalopathy, or CHF. Treat these side effects aggressively; see Dose Adjustments (Dose Modifications for Adverse Reactions), Precautions and Monitor. Discontinue bevacizumab for severe infusion reactions and treat as indicated (e.g., epinephrine, diphenhydramine, IV fluids, oxygen). Temporarily withhold for recent history of hemoptysis, severe hypertension, proteinuria, or less severe infusion reactions as outlined in Dose Adjustments (Dose Modifications for Adverse Reactions). Withhold bevacizumab for at least 28 days before elective surgery (half-life is approximately 20 days but has a wide range). Incision must be fully healed before therapy is resumed.

BEZLOTOXUMAB
(bez-loe-**TOX**-ue-mab)

Monoclonal Antibody

Zinplava   pH 6

USUAL DOSE

A single dose of 10 mg/kg administered as an IV infusion over 60 minutes. The safety and efficacy of repeat administration in patients with *Clostridium difficile* infection (CDI) has not been studied. Administer in conjunction with antibacterial drug treatment for CDI.

DOSE ADJUSTMENTS

None noted. Exposure of bezlotoxumab was not influenced by age, gender, race, comorbid conditions, or renal or hepatic impairment.

DILUTION

Available in a 1,000 mg/40 mL (25 mg/mL) clear to moderately opalescent, colorless to pale yellow solution in a single-dose vial. Withdraw the calculated dose based on the patient's weight, and transfer into an IV bag containing either NS or D5W to prepare a diluted solution with a final concentration of 1 mg/mL to 10 mg/mL. Mix diluted solution by gentle inversion. ***Do not shake.***

For example, a 70-kg patient would require a dose of 700 mg (10 mg/kg $\times$ 70 kg). Withdraw 700 mg (28 mL) and transfer to a 100-mL bag of IV solution to prepare a diluted solution with a final concentration of 5.4 mg/mL (700 mg $\div$ 128 mL = 5.4 mg/mL).

Filter: Infuse through a sterile, nonpyrogenic, low–protein binding, 0.2- to 5-micron in-line or add-on filter.

Storage: Store vials in refrigerator at 2° to 8° C (36° to 46° F). Keep in original carton to protect from light. *Do not freeze or shake vials or diluted solution.* Vials may be stored at RT protected from light for no more than 24 hours. Diluted solution may be stored either at RT for up to 16 hours or refrigerated for up to 24 hours. These time limits include storage of the infusion solution in the IV bag through the duration of the infusion. If refrigerated, allow the diluted solution to come to RT before administration. Discard any unused portion left in the vial.

COMPATIBILITY

Manufacturer states, "Do not coadminister other drugs simultaneously through the same infusion."

RATE OF ADMINISTRATION

A single dose as an infusion equally distributed over 60 minutes. Infuse through a sterile, nonpyrogenic, low–protein binding, 0.2- to 5-micron in-line or add-on filter. May be infused through a peripheral or central line. If diluted solution has been refrigerated, bring to RT before administration.

ACTIONS

A human monoclonal antibody that binds to *C. difficile* toxin B and neutralizes its effects. It does not bind to *C. difficile* toxin A. Bezlotoxumab is eliminated by catabolism and has an elimination half-life of approximately 19 days.

INDICATIONS

To reduce the recurrence of *Clostridium difficile* infection (CDI) in patients 18 years of age or older who are receiving antibacterial drug treatment for CDI and are at a high risk for CDI recurrence.

Limitation of use: Bezlotoxumab is not indicated for the treatment of CDI. It is not an antibacterial drug and should be used only in conjunction with antibacterial drug treatment of CDI.

CONTRAINDICATIONS

Manufacturer states, "None."

PRECAUTIONS

Do not administer as an IV push or bolus. ▪ Heart failure has been reported. In clinical trials it occurred primarily in patients with underlying congestive heart failure (CHF). In this population there were more deaths in the bezlotoxumab-treated patients than in the placebo-treated patients. In patients with a history of CHF, bezlotoxumab should be reserved for use when benefit outweighs the risk. ▪ A protein product; has the potential for immunogenicity.

Monitor: Monitor for S/S of infusion-related reactions (e.g., dizziness, dyspnea, fatigue, fever, headache, hypertension, and nausea). In clinical trials most reactions were rated as mild to moderate in severity. ▪ Monitor for S/S of heart failure.

Patient Education: Read FDA-approved Patient Information. ▪ Use of bezlotoxumab does not take the place of antibacterial treatment for CDI. Antibacterial treatment must be continued as directed.

Maternal/Child: Information is not available for use during pregnancy or breast-feeding. Use with caution and only if benefit justifies risk. ▪ Safety and effectiveness have not been established for use in pediatric patients.

Elderly: No overall differences in safety and effectiveness have been observed between elderly patients and younger patients.

DRUG/LAB INTERACTIONS

Because bezlotoxumab is eliminated by catabolism, no metabolic drug-drug interactions are expected.

SIDE EFFECTS

The most common side effects reported include fever, headache, and nausea. The most common serious side effect was heart failure. Infusion-related reactions occurring on the day of or on the day after the infusion were reported and included dizziness, dyspnea, fatigue, fever, headache, hypertension, and nausea.

ANTIDOTE

Keep physician informed of all side effects. Most will be treated symptomatically as indicated. Treat infusion-related reactions as indicated (e.g., oxygen, diphenhydramine, epinephrine, corticosteroids, vasopressors, and/or fluids). There is no clinical experience with overdose.

BIVALIRUDIN

(**by**-val-ih-**ROO**-din)

Angiomax

Anticoagulant
(direct thrombin inhibitor)

pH 5 to 6

USUAL DOSE

Pretreatment: Baseline studies indicated; see Monitor.

Initiate just before percutaneous coronary intervention (PCI). Given in combination with aspirin.

Aspirin: 300 to 325 mg before PCI and daily thereafter.

Bivalirudin: Begin with an IV bolus dose of 0.75 mg/kg. Follow immediately with an infusion at 1.75 mg/kg/hr for the duration of the PCI procedure. Perform an ACT 5 minutes after the bolus dose has been administered. An additional bolus dose of 0.3 mg/kg should be given if needed. See chart in Rate of Administration. Extended duration of infusion following PCI at 1.75 mg/kg/hr for up to 4 hours postprocedure should be considered in patients with ST segment elevation MI (STEMI). May be administered in combination with a glycoprotein IIb/IIIa inhibitor (e.g., eptifibatide, tirofiban) when clinically indicated. Combined use may increase the risk of bleeding.

DOSE ADJUSTMENTS

Reduce infusion rate in impaired renal function as indicated in the following chart. No reduction in the bolus dose is needed.

Guidelines for Bivalirudin Dose Adjustments in Impaired Renal Function[a]	
Renal Function (GFR)	**Infusion Rate (mg/kg/hr)**
GFR ≥30 mL/min	1.75 mg/kg/hr
GFR <30 mL/min	1 mg/kg/hr
Patients on hemodialysis	0.25 mg/kg/hr

[a]The ACT should be monitored in renally impaired patients.

DILUTION

Available in two formulations: (1) a vial containing 250 mg of lyophilized powder, and (2) a refrigerated, ready-to-use premixed vial containing 250 mg/50 mL or 500 mg/100 mL (5 mg/mL).

Vial (lyophilized powder): *Bolus and initial infusion:* Reconstitute each 250-mg vial with 5 mL SWFI. Gently swirl to dissolve. Reconstituted solution is clear to opalescent and colorless to slightly yellow. Each 250-mg vial must be further diluted in 50 mL of D5W or NS. Withdraw and discard 5 mL from a 50-mL infusion bag containing D5W or NS. Add the contents of the reconstituted vial to the infusion bag to yield a final concentration of 5 mg/mL.

Premixed ready-to-use vials: Once removed from refrigerator, use immediately.

Storage: *Vial (lyophilized powder):* Store unopened vials at CRT. Do not freeze reconstituted or diluted solution. Reconstituted solution stable for 24 hours refrigerated. Concentrations between 0.5 mg/mL and 5 mg/mL are stable at RT for up to 24 hours. Discard unused portion of reconstituted solution.

Premixed ready-to-use vials: Store in refrigerator between 2° and 8° C (36° and 46° F). Excursions are permitted to 20° to 25° C (68° to 77° F). Avoid excess heat.

COMPATIBILITY

Manufacturer states, "**Do not** administer the following drugs in the same IV line with bivalirudin: Alteplase, amiodarone, amphotericin B (conventional), chlorpromazine, diazepam, dobutamine, prochlorperazine, reteplase, streptokinase, and vancomycin. All are **incompatible** through the same IV line (**Y-site** or piggyback)."

No **incompatibilities** have been observed with administration sets.

Other sources suggest specific **compatibilities** dependent on concentration and manufacturer; consult a pharmacist.

RATE OF ADMINISTRATION

The following chart details, by patient weight in kilograms, the amount of the bolus dose, and the rate in mL/hr of the infusion.

Bivalirudin Dosing Guidelines		
	Using 5 mg/mL Concentration	
Weight (kg)	Bolus (0.75 mg/kg) (mL)	Infusion (1.75 mg/kg/hr) (mL/hr)
43–47	7 mL	16 mL/hr
48–52	7.5 mL	17.5 mL/hr
53–57	8 mL	19 mL/hr
58–62	9 mL	21 mL/hr
63–67	10 mL	23 mL/hr
68–72	10.5 mL	24.5 mL/hr
73–77	11 mL	26 mL/hr
78–82	12 mL	28 mL/hr
83–87	13 mL	30 mL/hr
88–92	13.5 mL	31.5 mL/hr
93–97	14 mL	33 mL/hr
98–102	15 mL	35 mL/hr
103–107	16 mL	37 mL/hr
108–112	16.5 mL	38.5 mL/hr
113–117	17 mL	40 mL/hr
118–122	18 mL	42 mL/hr
123–127	19 mL	44 mL/hr
128–132	19.5 mL	45.5 mL/hr
133–137	20 mL	47 mL/hr
138–142	21 mL	49 mL/hr
143–147	22 mL	51 mL/hr
148–152	22.5 mL	52.5 mL/hr

ACTIONS

An anticoagulant that is a specific and reversible direct thrombin inhibitor. It directly inhibits thrombin by specifically binding both to the catalytic site and to the anion-binding exosite of circulating and clot-bound thrombin. It inhibits coagulant effects by preventing thrombin-mediated cleavage of fibrinogen to fibrin; activation of factors V, VIII, and XIII; and activation of platelets. Exhibits dose- and concentration-dependent anticoagulant activity as evidenced by prolongation of ACT, aPPT, PT and TT. Anticoagulant effect is immediate. Cleared from plasma by a combination of renal mechanisms and proteolytic cleavage. The binding of bivalirudin to thrombin is reversible, resulting in recovery of thrombin active site functions. Coagulation times return to baseline approximately 1 hour after completion of infusion. Half-life averages 25 minutes. 20% of unchanged drug excreted in urine.

INDICATIONS AND USES

An anticoagulant for use in patients undergoing percutaneous coronary intervention (PCI), including patients with heparin-induced thrombocytopenia and heparin-induced thrombocytopenia and thrombosis syndrome. Used concurrently with aspirin.
Unlabeled uses: Heparin-induced thrombocytopenia (HIT) complicated by thrombosis.
■ Used as a substitute for heparin in patients with acute HIT who require cardiac surgery (e.g., coronary artery bypass graft [CABG]).

CONTRAINDICATIONS

Hypersensitivity to bivalirudin or its components; active major bleeding.

PRECAUTIONS

For IV use only. ■ Most bleeding associated with the use of bivalirudin in PCI occurs at the site of arterial puncture; however, hemorrhage can occur at any site. Consider a hemorrhagic event if there is an unexplained fall in BP or hematocrit and discontinue bivalirudin. ■ Use with caution in disease states and other circumstances in which there is an increased risk of bleeding, including severe hypertension; immediately following lumbar puncture; spinal anesthesia; major surgery, especially involving the brain, spinal cord, or eye; hematologic conditions associated with increased bleeding tendencies such as congenital or acquired bleeding disorders and gastrointestinal lesions such as ulcerations. ■ Has been associated with an increased risk of thrombus formation when used in gamma brachytherapy (percutaneous intracoronary brachytherapy). Fatalities have occurred. Imperative to maintain meticulous catheter technique, with frequent aspiration and flushing to minimize conditions of stasis within the catheter and vessels. ■ Acute stent thrombosis (fewer than 4 hours) has been observed at a greater frequency in bivalirudin-treated patients compared with heparin-treated patients with STEMI undergoing primary PCI. Patients should remain for at least 24 hours in a facility capable of managing ischemic complications and should be carefully monitored following primary PCI for S/S consistent with myocardial ischemia. ■ Half-life extended in patients with impaired renal function; see Dose Adjustments. ■ As with all therapeutic proteins, there is the potential for immunogenicity. ■ See Drug/Lab Interactions.
Monitor: Before therapy, obtain platelet count, hemoglobin and hematocrit, SCr, ACT, and aPTT. ■ Dose is not titrated to ACT; however, the ACT was checked at 5 minutes and again in 45 minutes during original clinical studies. ■ Monitor anticoagulation status in patients with impaired renal function receiving reduced doses. ■ Observe carefully for symptoms of a hemorrhagic event (e.g., unexplained fall in hematocrit or fall in BP). ■ Monitor patients with disease states associated with an increased risk of bleeding more frequently for bleeding. ■ Monitor STEMI patients undergoing primary PCI for S/S consistent with myocardial ischemia for a minimum of 24 hours following the procedure.
Patient Education: Risk of bleeding may be increased; discuss medical history and list of all medications (prescription and over-the-counter) with your healthcare provider; see Drug Interactions. ■ Report all episodes of bleeding. ■ Report tarry stools. ■ Compliance with all measures to minimize bleeding is very important (e.g., avoid use of razors, toothbrushes, other sharp items). ■ Use caution while moving to avoid excess bumping.

Maternal/Child: Safety for use during pregnancy not established. ▪ Not known if bivalirudin is secreted in human milk; use caution if required during breast-feeding. ▪ Safety and effectiveness for use in pediatric patients not established.

Elderly: Response similar to younger adults. ▪ See Dose Adjustments for the elderly with impaired renal function. ▪ Bleeding events are more common in the elderly.

DRUG/LAB INTERACTIONS

Coadministration with **heparin, warfarin, thrombolytics, or glycoprotein IIb/IIIa inhibitors** is associated with an increased risk of major bleeding events. ▪ Concomitant use with **other agents that alter hemostasis** such as **other anticoagulants** (e.g., enoxaparin, apixaban, rivaroxaban), **nonsteroidal anti-inflammatory drugs, and platelet aggregation inhibitors** (e.g., clopidogrel, prasugrel) may increase the risk of bleeding. ▪ Bivalirudin affects INR; therefore INR measurements made in patients who have been treated with bivalirudin may not be useful for determining the appropriate dose of warfarin.

SIDE EFFECTS

Bleeding is the most frequent adverse event; incidence in clinical studies was less than with heparin. Other reported side effects include abdominal pain, angina pectoris, anxiety, back pain, bradycardia, dyspepsia, fever, headache, hypertension, hypotension, injection site pain, insomnia, nausea, nervousness, pain, pelvic pain, thrombocytopenia, urinary retention, and vomiting.

Post-Marketing: Cardiac tamponade, elevated INR, fatal hemorrhage, hypersensitivity reactions (including anaphylaxis), pulmonary hemorrhage, and thrombus formation during PCI with and without intracoronary brachytherapy, including reports of fatal outcomes.

Overdose: Bleeding, death due to hemorrhage.

ANTIDOTE

No specific antidote is available. Overdose with or without bleeding may be controlled by discontinuing bivalirudin. Discontinuation leads to a gradual reduction in anticoagulant effects due to metabolism of the drug depending on dose/overdose and concentration achieved. ACT or aPTT should return to normal within 1 to 4 hours after discontinuation. Reversal may take longer in patients with renal impairment. If life-threatening bleeding develops and excessive plasma levels of bivalirudin are suspected, immediately stop infusion. Determine aPTT, ACT, and hemoglobin and prepare for blood transfusion as appropriate. Follow current guidelines for treatment of shock as indicated (fluid, vasopressors [e.g., dopamine], Trendelenburg position, plasma expanders [e.g., albumin, hetastarch]). Treat hypersensitivity reactions as indicated; may require epinephrine, airway management, oxygen, IV fluids, antihistamines, corticosteroids, and pressor amines. Bivalirudin is removed by hemodialysis.

BLEOMYCIN SULFATE BBW
(blee-oh-**MY**-sin **SUL**-fayt)

Antineoplastic
(antibiotic)

Blenoxane

pH 4.5 to 6

USUAL DOSE
Pretreatment: Verify pregnancy status. Baseline studies indicated; see Monitor.

Squamous cell carcinoma, non-Hodgkin lymphoma, testicular carcinoma: 0.25 to 0.5 units/kg of body weight/dose (10 to 20 units/M^2), once or twice weekly (1 unit equals 1 mg). The first two doses in lymphoma patients should not exceed 2 units in order to rule out hypersensitivity.

Hodgkin disease: Dosage as above. After a 50% response, a maintenance dose of 1 unit daily or 5 units weekly is recommended.

DOSE ADJUSTMENTS
Unit/kg dose based on average weight in presence of edema or ascites. ▪ Dose selection in the elderly should be cautious; consider decreased renal function and concomitant disease or drug therapy. ▪ Reduce dose in impaired renal function as indicated in the following chart.

CrCl (mL/min)	Bleomycin Dose
50 mL/min and above	100%
40–50 mL/min	70%
30–40 mL/min	60%
20–30 mL/min	55%
10–20 mL/min	45%
5–10 mL/min	40%

DILUTION
Specific techniques required; see Precautions. Each 15 units or fraction thereof must be reconstituted with 5 mL or more of NS. For IV injection, further dilution is not necessary, but has been further diluted in 50 to 100 mL NS and given as an intermittent infusion. May be given through Y-tube of a free-flowing IV.

Filters: No data available from manufacturer. Another source indicates no significant drug loss with the use of a 0.22-micron filter.

Storage: Refrigerate powder. Diluted solution stable at room temperature for 24 hours.

COMPATIBILITY
Manufacturer states, "Should not be reconstituted or diluted with D5W or other dextrose-containing diluents."

Other sources suggest specific **compatibilities** dependent on concentration and manufacturer; consult a pharmacist.

RATE OF ADMINISTRATION
IV injection: Each 15- to 30-unit dose over 10 minutes.

Intermittent infusion: A single dose over 15 to 30 minutes or 1 unit/minute.

ACTIONS
An antibiotic antineoplastic agent, cell cycle phase-specific, that seems to act by splitting and fragmentation of double-stranded DNA. Inhibits DNA synthesis and, to a lesser extent, RNA and protein synthesis. It localizes in tumors. Improvement usually noted within 2 to 3 weeks. Widely distributed throughout the body. Inactivated by an enzyme that is widely distributed in normal tissue with the exception of the skin and lungs. Half-life is approximately 2 hours. About 60% to 70% excreted in urine.

INDICATIONS AND USES

Testicular carcinoma; may induce complete remission with vinblastine and cisplatin. ▪ Palliative treatment, adjunct to surgery or radiation, in patients not responsive to other chemotherapeutic agents or those with squamous cell carcinoma of the skin, head, esophagus, neck, or GU tract, including the cervix, vulva, scrotum, and penis; in Hodgkin disease and other lymphomas. ▪ Injected into pleural cavity to treat malignant pleural effusion.

CONTRAINDICATIONS

Patients who have demonstrated a hypersensitive or idiosyncratic reaction to it.

PRECAUTIONS

Follow guidelines for handling cytotoxic agents. See Appendix A, p. 1308. ▪ May be given by the IM, IV, SQ, or IP routes. ▪ Administered by or under the direction of the physician specialist. ▪ Administer in a facility with adequate diagnostic and treatment facilities to monitor the patient and respond to any medical emergency. ▪ May be used with other antineoplastic drugs to achieve tumor remission. ▪ Pulmonary toxicity may progress from nonspecific pneumonitis to pulmonary fibrosis and death. Pulmonary toxicity increases markedly with advancing age or with total doses greater than 400 units but has been seen in younger patients and in patients treated with lower doses. It may occur at lower doses when bleomycin is used in combination with other antineoplastic agents. Risk of developing pulmonary toxicity is greater when O_2 is administered in surgery. To prevent this side effect, it has been recommended that the FiO_2 be maintained at concentrations approximating that of room air during surgery and in the postoperative period. Additionally, fluid replacement should be closely monitored and focus more on colloid (e.g., albumin) administration rather than on crystalloid (e.g., NS, LR) administration. ▪ A severe idiosyncratic reaction (similar to anaphylaxis) has been reported in approximately 1% of lymphoma patients. S/S include hypotension, mental confusion, fever, chills, and wheezing; may be immediate or delayed for several hours. More common after the first or second doses. ▪ Use with extreme caution in patients with significant renal impairment or compromised pulmonary function.

Monitor: Obtain a baseline chest x-ray, and recheck every 1 to 2 weeks to detect pulmonary changes. ▪ To identify subclinical pulmonary toxicity, monitor pulmonary diffusion capacity for carbon monoxide monthly. Should remain 30% to 35% above pretreatment value. Earliest signs of pulmonary toxicity are rales and dyspnea. ▪ Monitor renal, hepatic, and central nervous systems and skin for symptoms of toxicity. ▪ Determine patency of vein; avoid extravasation. ▪ Maintain adequate hydration. ▪ Prophylactic antiemetics may reduce nausea and vomiting and increase patient comfort. ▪ Observe closely for all signs of infection. Prophylactic antibiotics may be indicated pending results of C/S in a febrile neutropenic patient. ▪ Acetaminophen, diphenhydramine, and steroids (e.g., hydrocortisone) may be used prophylactically to reduce incidence of fever and anaphylaxis. ▪ See Precautions.

Patient Education: Use effective contraception. ▪ Report any possible side effects promptly. ▪ Report stinging or burning at IV site promptly. ▪ See Appendix D, p. 1311. ▪ Pulmonary toxicity more likely in smokers.

Maternal/Child: Category D: avoid pregnancy. ▪ Not recommended during breastfeeding. ▪ Safety and effectiveness for use in pediatric patients not established. Volume of distribution and half-life is comparable to that in adults.

Elderly: Response similar to that seen in younger adults; however, pulmonary toxicity is more common in patients older than 70 years of age. ▪ See Dose Adjustments; monitoring of renal function suggested.

DRUG/LAB INTERACTIONS

See Precautions. ▪ Vascular toxicities (e.g., myocardial infarction, CVA, thrombotic microangiopathy, cerebral arteritis) or Raynaud's phenomenon have occurred rarely when bleomycin is used in combination with **other antineoplastic agents.** ▪ May decrease GI absorption of **digoxin and hydantoins** (e.g., phenytoin). ▪ Do not administer **live virus vaccines** to patients receiving antineoplastic drugs. ▪ Causes sensitization of lung tissue to O_2; increases risk of pulmonary toxicity with **O_2 and general anesthetics.** ■ **Cisplatin** may inhibit renal elimination and increase toxicity.

SIDE EFFECTS

Alopecia, anorexia, chills, dyspnea, fever, hypotension, malaise, nausea, phlebitis (infrequent), rales, scleroderma-like skin changes, stomatitis, tenderness of the skin, tumor site pain, vomiting, weight loss.

Major: Severe idiosyncratic reaction similar to anaphylaxis (up to 6 hours after test dose), chest pain (acute with sudden onset suggestive of pleuropericarditis), pneumonitis, pulmonary fibrosis, skin toxicity (including nodules on hands, desquamation of skin, hyperpigmentation, and gangrene).

ANTIDOTE

Notify the physician of all side effects. Minor side effects will be treated symptomatically. Discontinue the drug immediately and notify the physician of any symptom of major side effects. Provide immediate treatment (epinephrine and diphenhydramine for anaphylaxis, antibiotics and steroids for pneumonitis) or supportive therapy as indicated.

BORTEZOMIB

Antineoplastic

(bore-**TEH**-zo-mib)

Velcade

pH 2 to 6.5

USUAL DOSE

Pretreatment: Verify pregnancy status. Baseline studies indicated; see Monitor.

Previously untreated multiple myeloma: 1.3 mg/M^2/dose as an IV bolus. Given in combination with oral melphalan and oral prednisone for nine 6-week cycles as outlined in the following chart. For Cycles 1 to 4, administer twice weekly (Days 1, 4, 8, 11, 22, 25, 29, 32). For Cycles 5 to 9, administer once weekly (Days 1, 8, 22, 29). At least 72 hours should elapse between consecutive doses of bortezomib.

Dosage Regimen for Patients With Previously Untreated Multiple Myeloma Twice-Weekly Bortezomib (Cycles 1-4 When Used in Combination with Melphalan and Prednisone)											
Week	**1**				**2**		**3**	**4**		**5**		**6**
Bortezomib (1.3 mg/M^2)	Day 1	—	—	Day 4	Day 8	Day 11	Rest period	Day 22	Day 25	Day 29	Day 32	Rest period
Melphalan (9 mg/M^2) Prednisone (60 mg/M^2)	Day 1	Day 2	Day 3	Day 4	—	—	Rest period	—	—	—	—	Rest period
Once-Weekly Bortezomib (Cycles 5-9 When Used in Combination With Melphalan and Prednisone)											
Week	**1**				**2**		**3**	**4**		**5**		**6**
Bortezomib (1.3 mg/M^2)	Day 1	—	—	—	Day 8	—	Rest period	Day 22	—	Day 29	—	Rest period
Melphalan (9 mg/M^2) Prednisone (60 mg/M^2)	Day 1	Day 2	Day 3	Day 4	—	—	Rest period	—	—	—	—	Rest period

Previously untreated mantle cell lymphoma: 1.3 mg/M^2/dose as an IV bolus. Given in combination with intravenous rituximab, cyclophosphamide, doxorubicin, and oral prednisone (VcR-CAP) for six 3-week cycles as outlined in the following chart. Bortezomib is administered first, followed by rituximab. Bortezomib is administered twice weekly for 2 weeks (Days 1, 4, 8, 11), followed by a 10-day rest period on Days 12 to 21. For patients with a response first documented at Cycle 6, two additional VcR-CAP cycles are recommended. At least 72 hours should elapse between consecutive doses of bortezomib.

Dosage Regimen for Patients With Previously Untreated Mantle Cell Lymphoma								
Twice Weekly Bortezomib (Six 3-week Cycles)[a]								
Week	1					2		3
Bortezomib (1.3 mg/M²)	Day 1	—	—	Day 4	—	Day 8	Day 11	Rest period
Rituximab (375 mg/M²) Cyclophosphamide (750 mg/M²) Doxorubicin (50 mg/M²)	Day 1	—	—	—	—	—	—	Rest period
Prednisone (100 mg/M²)	Day 1	Day 2	Day 3	Day 4	Day 5	—	—	Rest period

[a]Dosing may continue for 2 more cycles (for a total of 8 cycles) if response is first seen at Cycle 6.

Relapsed multiple myeloma and relapsed mantle cell lymphoma: 1.3 mg/M²/dose as an IV bolus 2 times a week for 2 weeks (Days 1, 4, 8, and 11). Follow with a 10-day rest period (Days 12 through 21). At least 72 hours should elapse between doses of bortezomib (e.g., Days 1, 4, 8, and 11). A treatment cycle is 21 days. See Dose Adjustments. For extended therapy of more than 8 cycles, bortezomib may be administered on the above standard schedule or, for relapsed multiple myeloma, on a maintenance schedule of once weekly for 4 weeks (Days 1, 8, 15, and 22), followed by a 13-day rest period (Days 23 to 35).

Patients with multiple myeloma who have previously responded to treatment with bortezomib (either alone or in combination) and who have relapsed at least 6 months after their prior therapy may be started on bortezomib at the last tolerated dose. Retreated patients are administered bortezomib twice weekly (Days 1, 4, 8, and 11) every 3 weeks for a maximum of 8 cycles. At least 72 hours should elapse between consecutive doses of bortezomib. Bortezomib may be administered either alone or in combination with dexamethasone.

Combination therapy in multiple myeloma (unlabeled in bortezomib prescribing information): *Bortezomib:* Administer 1.3 mg/M² as an IV bolus on Days 1, 4, 8, and 11 every 3 weeks. *Doxil:* Administer 30 mg/M² on Day 4 following bortezomib. Continue for up to 8 cycles until disease progression or the occurrence of unacceptable toxicity.

DOSE ADJUSTMENTS

Dose adjustments are based on clinical toxicities. ■ Starting dose adjustments are not required for patients with renal insufficiency, including those requiring dialysis. Bortezomib may be partially removed by dialysis. Administer after dialysis. ■ No significant difference in the pharmacokinetics of bortezomib based on age, sex, or renal impairment; see Precautions. ■ See the following charts for recommended starting dose modifications for patients with moderate to severe hepatic impairment; dose adjustments in combination therapy with melphalan and prednisone; dose adjustments in combination therapy with rituximab, cyclophosphamide, doxorubicin, and prednisone; dose adjustments in relapsed multiple myeloma and mantle cell lymphoma; and dose modifications for bortezomib-related neuropathic pain and/or peripheral sensory or motor neuropathy.

	Bilirubin Level	SGOT (AST) Levels	Modification of Starting Dose
Recommended Starting Dose Modification for Bortezomib in Patients With Hepatic Impairment			
Mild	≤1 × ULN	>ULN	None
Mild	>1 to 1.5 × ULN	Any	None
Moderate	>1.5 to 3 × ULN	Any	Reduce bortezomib to 0.7 mg/M² in the first cycle. Consider dose escalation to 1 mg/M² or further dose reduction to 0.5 mg/M² in subsequent cycles based on patient tolerance.
Severe	>3 × ULN	Any	

Combination therapy with melphalan and prednisone in previously untreated multiple myeloma: Before each treatment cycle, platelet count should be equal to or greater than 70×10^9/L, and ANC should be equal to or greater than 1×10^9/L. Nonhematologic toxicities should have resolved to Grade 1 or baseline. Dose modifications for subsequent cycles are outlined in the following chart.

Toxicity	Dose Modification or Delay
Dose Modifications During Cycles of Combination Bortezomib, Melphalan, and Prednisone Therapy[a]	
Hematologic toxicity during a cycle: If prolonged Grade 4 neutropenia or thrombocytopenia, or thrombocytopenia with bleeding, is observed in the previous cycle	Consider reducing the melphalan dose by 25% in the next cycle.
If platelet count is ≤30 × 10⁹/L or ANC is not above 0.75 × 10⁹/L on a bortezomib-dosing day (other than Day 1)	Withhold bortezomib dose.
If several bortezomib doses in consecutive cycles are withheld due to toxicity	Reduce bortezomib dose by 1 dose level (from 1.3 mg/M² to 1 mg/M², or from 1 mg/M² to 0.7 mg/M²).
Grade ≥3 nonhematologic toxicities	Withhold bortezomib therapy until symptoms of the toxicity have resolved to Grade 1 or baseline. Bortezomib may then be re-initiated with 1 dose-level reduction (from 1.3 mg/M² to 1 mg/M², or from 1 mg/M² to 0.7 mg/M²). For bortezomib-related neuropathic pain and/or peripheral neuropathy, hold or modify bortezomib as outlined in the chart for dose modification for bortezomib-related neuropathic pain and/or peripheral neuropathy.

[a]Graded according to Common Terminology Criteria for Adverse Events (CTCAE).

Combination therapy with IV rituximab, cyclophosphamide, doxorubicin, and oral prednisone in previously untreated mantle cell lymphoma: Before the first day of each cycle (other than Cycle 1), platelet count should be equal to or greater than 100×10^9/L, and ANC should be equal to or greater than 1.5×10^9/L. Hemoglobin should be equal to or greater than 8 g/dL, and nonhematologic toxicities should have resolved to Grade 1 or baseline. Dose modifications for Days 4, 8, and 11 are outlined in the following chart.

Dose Modifications on Days 4, 8, and 11 During Cycles of Combination Bortezomib, Rituximab, Cyclophosphamide, Doxorubicin, and Prednisone Therapy	
Toxicity	**Dose Modification or Delay**
Hematologic Toxicity	
Grade 3 or higher neutropenia or a platelet count below 25×10^9/L	Withhold bortezomib therapy for up to 2 weeks until the patient has an ANC at or above 0.75×10^9/L and a platelet count at or above 25×10^9/L. • If the toxicity does not resolve after bortezomib has been withheld, discontinue bortezomib. • If toxicity resolves such that the patient has an ANC at or above 0.75×10^9/L and a platelet count at or above 25×10^9/L, bortezomib dose should be reduced by 1 dose level (from 1.3 mg/M^2 to 1 mg/M^2, or from 1 mg/M^2 to 0.7 mg/M^2).
Grade 3 or higher nonhematologic toxicities	Withhold bortezomib therapy until symptoms of the toxicity have resolved to Grade 2 or better. Bortezomib may then be re-initiated with 1 dose-level reduction (from 1.3 mg/M^2 to 1 mg/M^2, or from 1 mg/M^2 to 0.7 mg/M^2). For bortezomib-related neuropathic pain and/or peripheral neuropathy, hold or modify bortezomib as outlined in the chart for dose modification for bortezomib-related neuropathic pain and/or peripheral neuropathy.

For information concerning rituximab, cyclophosphamide, doxorubicin, and prednisone, see manufacturer's prescribing information.

Relapsed multiple myeloma and relapsed mantle cell lymphoma: Withhold dose if a Grade 3 nonhematologic toxicity (e.g., 6 to 10 emeses/24 hr, severe infection) or a Grade 4 hematologic toxicity (e.g., thrombocytopenia less than 25,000/mm³) occurs. When symptoms have resolved, resume treatment with a dose reduced by 25% (1.3 mg/M^2/dose reduced to 1 mg/M^2/dose, 1 mg/M^2/dose reduced to 0.7 mg/M^2/dose). ■ See doxorubicin monograph for additional dose adjustments required in Doxil and bortezomib combination therapy for treatment of multiple myeloma. ■ Reduce dose in patients who develop bortezomib-related neuropathic pain and/or peripheral sensory or motor neuropathy according to the following chart.

Recommended Dose Modification for Bortezomib-Related Neuropathic Pain and/or Peripheral Sensory or Motor Neuropathy	
Severity of Peripheral Neuropathy Signs and Symptoms[a]	**Modification of Dose and Regimen**
Grade 1 (asymptomatic; loss of deep tendon reflexes or paresthesias) without pain or loss of function	No action.
Grade 1 with pain or Grade 2 (moderate symptoms; limiting instrumental Activities of Daily Living [ADL])[b]	Reduce dose to 1 mg/M^2.
Grade 2 with pain or Grade 3 (severe toxicity symptoms; limiting self-care ADL[c])	Withhold therapy until toxicity resolves. When toxicity resolves, re-initiate with a reduced dose of 0.7 mg/M^2 and change treatment schedule to once per week.
Grade 4 (life-threatening consequences; urgent intervention indicated)	Discontinue bortezomib.

[a]Graded according to Common Terminology Criteria for Adverse Events (CTCAE), v. 4.0.
[b]Instrumental ADL (e.g., preparing meals, shopping for groceries or clothes, using telephone, managing money).
[c]Self-care ADL (e.g., bathing, dressing and undressing, feeding self, using the toilet, taking medications, and not bedridden).

DILUTION
Specific techniques required; see Precautions. For IV use, reconstitute each 3.5-mg vial **only with 3.5 mL NS.** Concentration equals 1 mg/mL. *The SQ route uses less diluent and results in a different concentration (2.5 mg/mL).* To prevent overdosage, use caution when diluting and calculating volume to administer. Manufacturer supplies a sticker that specifies indicated route of administration. Place sticker on syringe of prepared bortezomib.

Storage: Stable until expiration date when stored at CRT in original package and protected from light. Reconstituted solution stable at 25° C (77° F) for up to 8 hours in a syringe or in original vial when exposed to normal indoor lighting. Must be given within 8 hours.

COMPATIBILITY
Compatibility information not available from manufacturer; consult a pharmacist.

RATE OF ADMINISTRATION
A single dose as an IV bolus injection over 3 to 5 seconds. May be given into a peripheral vein. To ensure the full dose is administered, flush with NS after injection.

May also be given through an IV port if the primary IV is temporarily discontinued. Flush with NS before and after administration.

ACTIONS
A reversible inhibitor of the 26S proteasome, which is a large protein complex that degrades ubiquitinated proteins. The blocking of this proteasome disrupts numerous biologic pathways related to the growth and survival of cancer cells and can lead to cell death. Distributes widely to peripheral tissues. Over 80% is bound to plasma proteins. Mean elimination half-life after multiple doses ranges from 76 to 108 hours after the 1.3 mg/M^2 dose. Metabolized in the liver via selected cytochrome P_{450} enzymes. Pathways of elimination in humans have not been determined.

INDICATIONS
Treatment of patients with multiple myeloma. ▪ Treatment of patients with mantle cell lymphoma.

Unlabeled use: Treatment of multiple myeloma in combination with doxorubicin liposomal injection in patients who have received one prior therapy but have not previously received bortezomib.

CONTRAINDICATIONS
Hypersensitivity to bortezomib or any component of the formulation (e.g., boron or mannitol), not including local reactions. ▪ Intrathecal administration.

PRECAUTIONS
Follow guidelines for handling cytotoxic agents. See Appendix A, p. 1308. ▪ Velcade may be given IV or SQ depending on dilution. Generic formulations of bortezomib are for IV use only. ▪ Administered by or under the supervision of a physician experienced in the use of antineoplastic therapy in a facility equipped to monitor the patient and respond to any medical emergency. ▪ Bortezomib therapy causes peripheral neuropathy. Both sensory and motor peripheral neuropathy have been reported. Use caution in patients with pre-existing peripheral neuropathy; symptoms may worsen. Many have been treated previously with neurotoxic agents. Incidence of peripheral neuropathy may be less with SQ administration. Use of the SQ route may be considered for patients who have pre-existing or are at high risk for peripheral neuropathy. ▪ May cause orthostatic/postural hypotension. Use with caution in patients with a history of syncope, in patients receiving concomitant medications that may cause hypotension, and in patients who are dehydrated. ▪ Hypersensitivity reactions (including anaphylactic reactions) have been reported. ▪ Thrombocytopenia and neutropenia have been reported; see Monitor. ▪ Gastrointestinal and intracerebral hemorrhages have occurred during thrombocytopenia in association with bortezomib. ▪ Acute development or exacerbation of CHF and/or new onset of decreased left ventricular ejection fraction has been reported. ▪ Acute respiratory distress syndrome (ARDS) and acute diffuse infiltrative pulmonary disease of unknown etiology such as pneumonitis, interstitial pneumonia, lung infiltration have occurred. ▪ Pulmonary hypertension in the absence of left heart failure or significant

pulmonary disease has been reported. ▪ Posterior reversible encephalopathy syndrome (PRES), formerly termed reversible posterior leukoencephalopathy syndrome (RPLS), has occurred. Patients may present with visual or neurologic disturbances. MRI may be used to confirm diagnosis. ▪ Use caution in patients with moderate to severe liver impairment. Clearance decreased; see Monitor and Dose Adjustments. ▪ Use caution in patients who are receiving multiple concomitant medications and/or who have serious underlying medical conditions; asymptomatic increases in liver enzymes, hyperbilirubinemia, hepatitis, and rare cases of acute liver failure have been reported. May be reversible if bortezomib is discontinued. Information on rechallenging these patients is limited. ▪ Tumor lysis syndrome has been reported; patients with a high tumor burden are at increased risk. ▪ Cases, sometimes fatal, of thrombotic microangiopathy, including thrombotic thrombocytopenic purpura/hemolytic uremic syndrome (TTP/HUS), have been reported. ▪ GI adverse events, including constipation, diarrhea, ileus, nausea, and vomiting, have been reported and may require treatment. ▪ Consider antiviral prophylaxis. Herpes simplex and herpes zoster reactivation have been reported.

Monitor: Obtain baseline CBC with differential and platelet count; repeat before each cycle and monitor as needed during treatment. Monitor platelet count before each dose. ▪ Obtain baseline electrolytes, including serum calcium and potassium. Monitor fluid and electrolyte balance and replace as indicated. Prevent dehydration. ▪ Obtain baseline bilirubin and AST and repeat as indicated; see Dose Adjustments. Monitor patients with impaired liver function closely for S/S of bortezomib toxicity. ▪ Monitor BP closely. Dehydration and/or concomitant medications may contribute to hypotension. Assist with ambulation. ▪ Monitor patients at risk for or with existing heart disease closely for S/S of CHF (e.g., exertional dyspnea, orthopnea, edema, tachycardia, pulmonary rales, a third heart sound, jugular venous distention) and/or for new onset of decreased left ventricular ejection fraction. ▪ Use prophylactic antiemetics to reduce nausea and vomiting and increase patient comfort. ▪ Antidiarrheal medication (e.g., loperamide [Imodium]) may be indicated. ▪ Monitor for S/S of peripheral neuropathy (e.g., burning sensation, discomfort, hyperesthesia [sensitivity of skin], hypoesthesia [impairment of any sense, especially touch], neuropathic pain or weakness, paresthesia [abnormal sensation such as burning, prickling]). Incidence may be increased in patients treated previously with neurotoxic agents (e.g., cisplatin, thalidomide [Thalomid], vinca alkaloids [e.g., vincristine]). See Dose Adjustments; may require change of dose or schedule. Improvement in or a resolution of peripheral neuropathy has been reported following dose adjustment or discontinuation of bortezomib. ▪ Monitor for neutropenia and thrombocytopenia (platelet count less than 50,000/mm^3). Occurs in a cyclical pattern with nadirs occurring after the last dose of each cycle and typically recovering before initiation of the next cycle. Initiate precautions to prevent excessive bleeding (e.g., inspect IV sites, skin, and mucous membranes; use extreme care during invasive procedures; test urine, emesis, stool, and secretions for occult blood). ▪ Monitor uric acid levels before and during therapy. Hydration and uric acid–lowering drugs (e.g., allopurinol [Aloprim]) may be indicated for serious tumor lysis syndrome. ▪ Monitor for S/S of TTP/HUS (e.g., fever, microangiopathic hemolytic anemia [see schistocytes in a blood smear], renal failure, thrombocytopenia, and neurologic manifestations). ▪ Hypoglycemia and hyperglycemia have been reported in patients taking oral diabetic agents. Monitor blood glucose levels and adjust antidiabetic medications as indicated; see Drug/Lab Interactions. ▪ Monitor respiratory status closely. Any change in condition should be evaluated promptly and treated as indicated. ▪ Monitor for S/S associated with development of PRES (e.g., blindness, confusion, headache, hypertension, lethargy, seizures, and other visual and neurologic disturbances).

Patient Education: Verify pregnancy status of females of reproductive potential before initiating therapy. ▪ Avoid pregnancy. Females of reproductive potential should use effective contraception during treatment with bortezomib and for 7 months after treatment. Males with female sexual partners of reproductive potential should use effective contraception during treatment with bortezomib and for 4 months after treatment. Should pregnancy occur, notify physician immediately and discuss potential hazards. ▪ May have an effect on male and female fertility. ▪ May cause dizziness, fatigue, hypotension, or syncope; use caution when driving or operating machinery. ▪ Review all medications with your physician and/or pharmacist; effects of medications for high blood pressure and other medications that may lower blood pressure may increase hypotension. Other agents may increase peripheral neuropathy. May interfere with medications for diabetes. ▪ Promptly report bleeding, constipation, decreased appetite, fever, or an increase in blood pressure ▪ Review of monitoring requirements and adverse events before therapy is imperative. ▪ Avoid dehydration; promptly report diarrhea, dizziness, fainting spells, light-headedness, muscle cramps, and vomiting. ▪ Promptly report any signs of infection (e.g., chills, fever, night sweats) or signs of bleeding (e.g., bruising, tarry stools, blood in urine, pinpoint red spots on skin). ▪ Promptly report symptoms of peripheral neuropathy (e.g., burning sensation [feet or hands], numbness, pain, tingling, or weakness in the arms or legs). If these symptoms pre-existed, report if they seem to be worse. ▪ Promptly report shortness of breath, cough, or other lung problems. ▪ Promptly report swelling of the ankles, feet, or legs. ▪ Report any visual or neurologic disturbances. ▪ Promptly report jaundice or right upper quadrant pain. ▪ Promptly report rash, severe injection site reactions, or skin pain. ▪ See Appendix D, p. 1311.

Maternal/Child: Based on the mechanism of action and findings in animals, bortezomib can cause fetal harm. Use of effective contraception required. ▪ Discontinue breast-feeding during treatment and for up to 2 months after treatment. ▪ Safety and effectiveness for use in pediatric patients not established.

Elderly: Safety and effectiveness similar to other age-groups; however, greater sensitivity in the elderly cannot be ruled out. In clinical trials, patients over 65 years of age had a slightly increased incidence of Grade 3 or 4 toxicity.

DRUG/LAB INTERACTIONS

Drug interaction studies are limited. ▪ Bortezomib is a substrate of CYP3A4, 2C19, and 1A2; concomitant administration of **inhibitors or inducers of selected cytochrome P$_{450}$ enzymes** may cause toxicity or reduce effectiveness of bortezomib. Consult pharmacist. **Inhibitors** may reduce metabolism and increase serum levels of bortezomib. ▪ Coadministration with **ketoconazole**, an inhibitor, increases bortezomib exposure. Monitor for toxicity. Other examples of **inhibitors** include cimetidine, erythromycins, grapefruit juice, antifungal agents (e.g., itraconazole), nefazodone, and ritonavir. Patients receiving bortezomib in conjunction with a strong CYP3A4 inhibitor should be closely monitored. ▪ **Inducers** may increase metabolism and decrease serum levels and effectiveness of bortezomib. Examples of **inducers** may include carbamazepine, phenobarbital, phenytoin, and rifampin. Concomitant use of **strong CYP3A4 inducers** (e.g., rifampin) is not recommended. ▪ Hypotension may be increased by **agents that induce hypotension** (e.g., alcohol, antihypertensives [e.g., ACE inhibitors (e.g., lisinopril)], beta-blockers [e.g., atenolol]). ▪ May increase or decrease the effects of **oral antidiabetic agents** (e.g., glyburide, glipizide). Monitor blood glucose levels and adjust dose of antidiabetic medication as indicated.

SIDE EFFECTS

Diarrhea, fatigue, peripheral neuropathy, excessive vomiting, and thrombocytopenia may be dose limiting. Most common side effects reported include anemia, anorexia, constipation, diarrhea, fatigue, fever, leukopenia, lymphopenia, nausea and vomiting, neuralgia, neutropenia, peripheral neuropathy, rash, and thrombocytopenia. Abdominal distention, abdominal pain, alopecia, arthralgia, asthenia, bronchitis, cardiac failure, chills, cough, decreased appetite, dehydration, dizziness, dysesthesia, edema, febrile neutropenia, headache, hypertension, hypoesthesia, hypotension, hyperglycemia, malaise, nasopharyngitis, paresthesia, peripheral edema, pneumonia, psychotic disorders (e.g., anxiety, agitation, confusion, insomnia, mental status change, suicidal ideation), reactivation of herpesvirus infections (zoster and simplex), respiratory tract infections, stomatitis, upper abdominal pain, weakness, and weight loss have also been reported. Numerous other side effects have been reported that may or may not be related to bortezomib and include hypersensitivity reactions (including anaphylaxis and immune complex–mediated hypersensitivity), ARDS and other pulmonary disorders, bleeding (e.g., GI, intracerebral), CVA, GI disorders (serious [e.g., acute pancreatitis, ischemic colitis, paralytic ileus]), hepatic disorders (e.g., cholestasis, liver failure, portal vein thrombosis), hyperbilirubinemia, hypernatremia, hyperuricemia, hypocalcemia, hypokalemia, hyponatremia, infections (e.g., aspergillosis, bacteremia, herpes, listeriosis, oral candidiasis, septic shock, toxoplasmosis, URI), MI, pleural effusion, PRES, pulmonary embolism, pulmonary hypertension, renal disorders (e.g., acute or chronic renal failure, calculus, hemorrhagic cystitis, hydronephrosis), respiratory distress, and tumor lysis syndrome. See prescribing information for additional side effects.

Post-Marketing: Acute diffuse infiltrative pulmonary disease, acute febrile neutrophilic dermatosis (Sweet's syndrome), blindness, cardiac tamponade, chalazion/blepharitis, deafness (bilateral), herpes meningoencephalitis, ischemic colitis, ophthalmic herpes, optic neuropathy, PRES, progressive multifocal leukoencephalopathy (PML), and Stevens-Johnson syndrome/toxic epidermal necrolysis.

Overdose: Profound progressive hypotension, tachycardia, and decreased cardiac contractility. Symptomatic hypotension and thrombocytopenia with fatal outcomes have been reported in patients who received more than twice the recommended dose.

ANTIDOTE

Keep physician informed of all side effects. Most will be treated symptomatically as indicated. See Dose Adjustments for dosing modifications based on toxicity. Temporarily discontinue bortezomib if severe thrombocytopenia occurs (less than 25,000 or 30,000/mm^3, depending on indication); may be resumed at a reduced dose after thrombocytopenia is resolved. Severe thrombocytopenia may require platelet transfusions. Reduce dose, withhold dose, or discontinue based on S/S of peripheral neuropathy. Symptoms of peripheral neuropathy may improve or return to baseline if bortezomib is discontinued. Hypotension may respond to adjustment of antihypertensive medications, hydration, or administration of mineralocorticoids and/or sympathomimetics. Withhold bortezomib for Grade 3 neutropenia. Recovery from neutropenia may be spontaneous or may be treated with filgrastim or pegfilgrastim. Treat anemia as indicated with whole blood products (e.g., packed RBCs) or blood modifiers (e.g., darbepoetin alfa [Aranesp], epoetin alfa). For new or worsening cardiopulmonary symptoms, consider interrupting bortezomib until a prompt and comprehensive diagnostic evaluation is conducted. For symptoms of serious liver dysfunction, interrupt bortezomib to assess reversibility. Discontinue bortezomib in patients who develop PRES. In overdose, monitor V/S continuously and provide supportive care. Maintain BP with dopamine, epinephrine, or norepinephrine as needed. Maintain body temperature. If diagnosis of TTP/HUS is suspected, stop treatment and evaluate. If diagnosis is excluded, consider restarting. There is no specific antidote; supportive therapy will help sustain the patient in toxicity. Resuscitate as indicated.

BREXANOLONE BBW

(brex-**AN**-oh-lone)

Zulresso

Gamma-aminobutyric acid (GABA)
A receptor-positive modulator

USUAL DOSE

Initiate brexanolone treatment early enough in the day to allow for recognition of excessive sedation.

Brexanolone is administered as a 60-hour IV infusion as outlined below:

- 0 to 4 hours: Initiate with a dosage of 30 mcg/kg/hr
- 4 to 24 hours: Increase dosage to 60 mcg/kg/hr
- 24 to 52 hours: Increase dosage to 90 mcg/kg/hr (a reduction in dosage to 60 mcg/kg/hr may be considered during this time period for patients who do not tolerate 90 mcg/kg/hr)
- 52 to 56 hours: Decrease dosage to 60 mcg/kg/hr
- 56 to 60 hours: Decrease dosage to 30 mcg/kg/hr

DOSE ADJUSTMENTS

If excessive sedation occurs at any time during the infusion, stop the infusion until the symptoms resolve. The infusion may be resumed at the same or lower dose as clinically indicated. ▪ Dosage adjustment in patients with any degree of hepatic impairment is unnecessary. ▪ No dosage adjustment is recommended in patients with mild, moderate, or severe renal impairment. ▪ Avoid use in patients with end-stage renal disease (ESRD) with an eGFR of less than 15 mL/min/1.73 M^2 because of the potential accumulation of the solubilizing agent, betadex sulfobutyl ether sodium.

DILUTION

Available as a 100 mg/20 mL (5 mg/1 mL) single-dose vial containing a preservative-free, clear colorless solution. To compound a single infusion bag, withdraw 20 mL of brexanolone from the vial and place in a polyolefin, non-DEHP, nonlatex infusion bag. Immediately dilute with 40 mL of SWFI, and further dilute with 40 mL of NS (total volume of 100 mL) to achieve a final concentration of 1 mg/mL. Administer immediately or refrigerate for later use. The 60-hour infusion will generally require the preparation of five infusion bags. Additional bags will be needed for patients weighing 90 kg or more.

Filters: Manufacturer states, "Do not use in-line filter infusion sets."

Storage: Store unopened vials at 2° to 8° C (36° to 46° F) protected from light. *Do not freeze.* If the diluted solution is not used immediately, store refrigerated for up to 96 hours. The diluted solution can be used for up to 12 hours of infusion time at RT. Discard any unused solution after 12 hours of infusion.

COMPATIBILITY

Manufacturer states, "Prepare and store in a polyolefin, non-DEHP, nonlatex infusion bag," "Use a PVC, non-DEHP, nonlatex infusion set," and "Administer via a dedicated line. Do not inject other medications into the infusion bag or mix with brexanolone."

RATE OF ADMINISTRATION

Administer via a dedicated line using a PVC, non-DEHP, nonlatex infusion set. Use a programmable peristaltic infusion pump to ensure accurate delivery. Fully prime infusion administration sets with admixture before inserting into the pump and connecting to the venous catheter.

ACTIONS

A neuroactive steroid gamma-aminobutyric acid (GABA) A receptor-positive modulator. The mechanism of action of brexanolone in the treatment of postpartum depression (PPD) is not fully understood but is thought to be related to its positive allosteric modulation of GABA A receptors. Exhibits extensive distribution into tissues. Plasma protein binding is greater than 99%. The terminal half-life is approximately 9 hours. Extensively metabolized by non–CYP-based pathways. Metabolites are pharmacologically inactive.

Excreted in feces (primarily as metabolites) and in urine (with less than 1% as unchanged brexanolone). Secreted in breast milk.

INDICATIONS AND USES

Treatment of postpartum depression (PPD) in adults.

CONTRAINDICATIONS

Manufacturer states, "None."

PRECAUTIONS

A healthcare provider must be available on site to continuously monitor the patient, and intervene as necessary, for the duration for the brexanolone infusion. ▪ Patients treated with brexanolone are at risk of somnolence, excessive sedation, sudden loss of consciousness, or an altered state of consciousness during administration; see Dose Adjustments. Time to full recovery from loss or altered state of consciousness after dose interruption ranged from 15 to 60 minutes. There was no clear association between loss or alteration of consciousness and pattern or timing of dose. Not all patients who experienced a loss or alteration of consciousness reported sedation or somnolence before the episode. ▪ In pooled analyses of placebo-controlled trials of chronically administered antidepressant drugs (SSRIs and other antidepressant classes), the incidence of suicidal thoughts and behaviors in antidepressant-treated patients 24 years of age and younger was greater than in placebo-treated patients. There was considerable variation in the risk of suicidal thoughts and behaviors among drugs, but an increased risk was identified in young patients for most drugs studied. Consider changing the therapeutic regimen, including discontinuing brexanolone, in patients whose depression becomes worse or in patients who experience emergent suicidal thoughts and behaviors. ▪ Brexanolone is a Schedule IV controlled substance, with the potential for abuse and dependence. In PPD trials, end of treatment occurred through tapering, so it was not possible to assess whether abrupt discontinuation produced withdrawal symptoms indicative of physical dependence. It is recommended that brexanolone be tapered according to the dosage recommendations unless symptoms warrant immediate discontinuation; see Usual Dose and Dose Adjustments. ▪ Brexanolone is available only through a restricted program under a Risk Evaluation and Mitigation Strategy (REMS) called the ZULRESSO REMS; see manufacturer's prescribing information for requirements.

Monitor: Monitor for excessive sedation and sudden loss of consciousness. ▪ Assess for excessive sedation every 2 hours during planned, nonsleep periods. Immediately stop the infusion if there are S/S of excessive sedation. After symptoms resolve, the infusion may be resumed at the same rate or at a reduced rate as clinically appropriate. ▪ Patients must be accompanied during interactions with their child(ren) because of the potential for excessive sedation and sudden loss of consciousness. ▪ Monitor for hypoxia using continuous pulse oximetry equipped with an alarm. Immediately stop the infusion if pulse oximetry indicates hypoxia. The infusion should not be resumed. ▪ Monitor for worsening depression or suicidal ideation.

Patient Education: Read the FDA-approved patient labeling (Medication Guide). ▪ Avoid pregnancy. In the event of a pregnancy, enrollment in the National Pregnancy Registry for Antidepressants is encouraged. ▪ After the infusion, avoid potentially hazardous activities requiring mental alertness, such as driving, until any sedative effects have dissipated. ▪ Request assistance during interactions with child(ren) because of the potential for excessive sedation and sudden loss of consciousness. Must not be the primary caregiver. ▪ Review all medications with a healthcare provider; drug interactions are possible. ▪ Brexanolone can be abused or lead to dependence. ▪ Report signs of excessive sedation that may occur during the infusion (patient and caregiver). ▪ Report worsening depression or the emergence of suicidal thoughts and behavior (patient and caregiver). ▪ Brexanolone is available only through a restricted program called the ZULRESSO REMS. Patient enrollment and monitoring is required.

Maternal/Child: Based on animal studies of other drugs that enhance GABAergic inhibition, brexanolone may cause fetal harm when administered to a pregnant woman. Patients exposed to brexanolone during pregnancy are encouraged to enroll in the National

Pregnancy Registry for Antidepressants. ■ Present in breast milk, but infant exposure is expected to be low. Consider risk versus benefit for mother and infant. ■ Safety and effectiveness in pediatric patients have not been established.

Elderly: PPD is a condition associated with pregnancy; there is no geriatric experience with brexanolone.

DRUG/LAB INTERACTIONS

Drug interactions studies have not been conducted. ■ Concomitant use with other CNS depressants (e.g., alcohol, antidepressants, benzodiazepines, opioids) may increase the likelihood or severity of adverse reactions related to sedation. ■ No clinically significant differences in the pharmacokinetics of phenytoin (CYP2C9 substrate) were observed when used concomitantly with brexanolone.

SIDE EFFECTS

The most commonly reported adverse reactions were dry mouth, flushing/hot flush, loss of consciousness, and sedation/somnolence. Adverse reactions leading to treatment discontinuation were sedation-related effects (loss of consciousness, presyncope, syncope, and vertigo) or infusion site pain. Adverse reactions leading to dose reduction or interruption were sedation-related effects (dizziness, fatigue, loss of consciousness, somnolence, syncope), changes in blood pressure, and infusion site events. Other reported adverse events include diarrhea, dyspepsia, oropharyngeal pain, and tachycardia.

Overdose: May result in excessive sedation, including loss of consciousness and the potential for accompanying respiratory changes.

ANTIDOTE

Notify physician of all side effects. Most will be treated symptomatically. Immediately stop the infusion for S/S of excessive sedation. After symptoms resolve, the infusion may be resumed at the same or reduced rate as clinically appropriate. Immediately stop the infusion for hypoxia. The infusion should not be resumed. In case of overdose, stop the infusion immediately and initiate supportive measures as necessary. Brexanolone is rapidly cleared from plasma.

BRIVARACETAM

(**BRIV**-a-**RA**-se-tam)

Anticonvulsant

Briviact

pH 5.5

USUAL DOSE

Pretreatment: Baseline studies indicated; see Monitor. See Maternal/Child.

Brivaracetam may be initiated with either IV or oral administration. When initiating treatment, gradual dose escalation is not required. Dose should be based on clinical response and tolerability. IV injection may also be used when oral administration is temporarily not feasible and should be administered at the same dose and frequency as oral brivaracetam. Use of the IV formulation beyond 4 consecutive days of treatment has not been studied.

Patients 16 years of age and older (monotherapy or adjunctive therapy): 50 mg twice daily (100 mg/day) is the recommended starting dose. Based on individual patient tolerability and therapeutic response, the maintenance dose may be adjusted down to a minimum of 25 mg twice daily (50 mg/day) or up to a maximum of 100 mg twice daily (200 mg/day).

DOSE ADJUSTMENTS

See Usual Dose. ■ Recommended starting dose for all stages of hepatic impairment (for patients 16 years of age and older) is 25 mg twice daily (50 mg/day), with a recommended maximum dose of 75 mg twice daily (150 mg/day). ■ For patients receiving concomitant rifampin, increase the dose by up to 100% (i.e., double the dose); see Drug/Lab Interactions. ■ No dose adjustment required for patients with impaired renal function; see Precautions.

DILUTION

A clear, colorless solution available as 50 mg/5 mL (10 mg/mL) in a single-use vial. Withdraw the desired dose. May be administered without further dilution or may be further diluted with NS, D5W, or LR and given as an infusion.

Filters: Specific information not available.

Storage: Store at CRT before use. Do not freeze. Diluted solution should not be stored for more than 4 hours at RT; may be stored in polyvinyl chloride (PVC) bags. Discard any unused portion of vial.

COMPATIBILITY

Compatibility information not available from manufacturer. Consider specific use; consult pharmacist.

RATE OF ADMINISTRATION

A single dose as an IV injection or infusion over 2 to 15 minutes. Flush IV line before and after injection.

ACTIONS

An antiepileptic (anticonvulsant) drug. The precise mechanism of action is unknown. Displays a high and selective affinity for synaptic vesicle protein 2A (SV2A) in the brain, which may contribute to the anticonvulsant effect. Weakly bound to plasma proteins. Primarily metabolized by hydrolysis and secondarily by hydroxylation. The hydrolysis reaction is mediated by hepatic and extrahepatic amidase. The hydroxylation pathway is mediated primarily by CYP2C19. Terminal plasma half-life is approximately 9 hours. May cross the placental barrier. Eliminated primarily by metabolism and by excretion in urine.

INDICATIONS AND USES

Treatment of partial-onset seizures in patients 16 years of age and older. IV injection may be used when oral administration is temporarily not feasible; see Maternal/Child.

CONTRAINDICATIONS

Known hypersensitivity to brivaracetam or any of its inactive ingredients.

PRECAUTIONS

For IV use only. ■ Antiepileptic drugs (AEDs) increase the risk of suicidal thoughts or behavior in patients taking these drugs for any indication. Patients treated with any AED for any indication should be monitored for the emergence or worsening of depression, suicidal thoughts or behavior, and/or any unusual changes in mood or behavior. Some behavioral changes may resolve without intervention. Others may require dose reduction or discontinuation of brivaracetam. ■ Associated with CNS side effects (somnolence, fatigue, dizziness, coordination difficulties [abnormal gait, ataxia, balance disorder, incoordination]). The risk is greatest early in treatment but can occur at any time; see Monitor and Patient Education. ■ Has been associated with behavioral and psychiatric abnormalities (e.g., aggression, agitation, altered mood, anger, anxiety, apathy, belligerence, depression, emotional lability, irritability, mood swings, nervousness, psychomotor hyperactivity, restlessness, tearfulness, and psychotic symptoms, including hallucinations, paranoia, acute psychosis, and suicidal ideation). ■ Hypersensitivity reactions have been reported. ■ Avoid abrupt withdrawal to minimize the risk of increased seizure frequency and status epilepticus. ■ Not recommended for use in patients with end-stage renal disease who are undergoing dialysis; data not available.

Monitor: Obtain baseline and periodic liver function tests. ■ Monitor for the emergence or worsening of depression, suicidal thoughts or behavior, and/or any unusual changes in mood or behavior. ■ Observe for seizure activity. ■ Observe closely for signs of CNS side effects; see Precautions. ■ Monitor for S/S of a hypersensitivity reaction; angioedema and bronchospasm have been reported. If a reaction occurs, discontinue brivaracetam.

Patient Education: Review manufacturer's medication guide. ■ May cause dizziness, coordination difficulties, and somnolence; use caution when performing tasks that require alertness or coordination (e.g., operating machinery, driving). ■ May increase the risk of suicidal thoughts and behavior. Promptly report the emergence or worsening of S/S of depression, any unusual changes in mood or behavior, or thoughts of self-harm. ▪ Promptly report S/S of a hypersensitivity reaction (e.g., hypotension, rash, tightness of the chest, urticaria, wheezing). ▪ Females who are pregnant or who become pregnant should be encouraged to enroll in the North American Antiepileptic Drug (NAAED) Pregnancy Registry. ▪ Do not discontinue without consulting a healthcare provider. Must be gradually withdrawn to reduce the potential for increased seizure frequency and status epilepticus.

Maternal/Child: Use during pregnancy only if the potential benefit justifies the potential risk to the fetus. Based on animal studies, may cause fetal harm. ▪ Insufficient data on effects during breast-feeding; consider risk versus benefit. ▪ The safety of brivaracetam injection in pediatric patients has not been established; however, *oral* brivaracetam can be used and is indicated for the treatment of partial-onset seizures in patients 4 years of age and older. See prescribing information. ▪ Safety and effectiveness for use in patients 16 years of age and older have been established.

Elderly: Numbers in clinical studies insufficient to determine if elderly patients respond differently than younger patients. Dose selection should usually start at the low end. Consider decreased hepatic, renal, or cardiac function and concomitant disease or other drug therapy.

DRUG/LAB INTERACTIONS

Coadministration with rifampin decreases brivaracetam plasma concentrations. Brivaracetam dose should be increased by up to 100% while patients are receiving concomitant treatment with rifampin. ▪ Coadministration with carbamazepine may increase exposure to the active metabolite of carbamazepine. Consider carbamazepine dose reduction if tolerability issues arise. ▪ Increases plasma concentrations of phenytoin. Monitor phenytoin levels when concomitant brivaracetam is added to or discontinued from ongoing phenytoin therapy. ▪ Coadministration of brivaracetam with levetiracetam provided no added therapeutic benefit.

SIDE EFFECTS

Dizziness, fatigue, nausea, sedation, somnolence, and vomiting are most common. Cerebellar coordination and balance disturbances, constipation, decreased neutrophil count, decreased white blood cell count, dysgeusia, euphoric mood, feeling drunk, and infusion site pain and irritability have also been reported. See Precautions.

Overdose: Anxiety, balance disorder, bradycardia, diplopia, dizziness, fatigue, nausea, somnolence, and vertigo.

ANTIDOTE

Keep physician informed of all side effects. Some may not require intervention, and others may improve with a reduced dose or discontinuation of brivaracetam. Treat hypersensitivity reactions immediately with oxygen, epinephrine, antihistamines, vasopressors, corticosteroids, albuterol, IV fluids, and ventilation equipment as indicated. Support patient as required in overdose. There is no specific antidote. Ensure adequate airway, oxygenation, and ventilation and monitor vital signs, cardiac rate, and rhythm. Hemodialysis is not expected to enhance clearance. Resuscitate as necessary.

BUMETANIDE BBW

(byou-**MET**-ah-nyd)

Diuretic (loop)

pH 6.8 to 7.8

Bumex

USUAL DOSE
0.5 to 1 mg. May be repeated at 2- to 3-hour intervals. Do not exceed 10 mg/24 hr. Can be used for patients allergic to furosemide. 1:40 mg ratio (bumetanide to furosemide) is used to determine dose. Individualize dose and schedule; see Precautions/Monitor.

DOSE ADJUSTMENTS
Start at lower end of dosing range in the elderly. Consider decreased cardiac, hepatic, or renal function; concomitant disease; and other drug therapy.

DILUTION
May be given undiluted. Not usually added to IV solutions but **compatible** with D5W, NS, and LR. Usually given through Y-tube of infusion set. Use only freshly prepared solutions for infusion. Discard after 24 hours.

COMPATIBILITY
Compatibility information not available from manufacturer.

Other sources suggest specific **compatibilities** dependent on concentration and manufacturer; consult a pharmacist.

RATE OF ADMINISTRATION
A single dose by IV injection over 1 to 2 minutes. Give infusion at prescribed rate.

ACTIONS
A sulfonamide diuretic, antihypertensive, and antihypercalcemic agent related to the thiazides. A loop diuretic agent. Extremely potent. Onset of action is within minutes and duration of action may last 4 to 6 hours. Apparently acts on the proximal and distal ends of the tubule and the ascending limb of the loop of Henle to excrete water, sodium, chloride, and potassium. Will produce diuresis in alkalosis or acidosis. Rapidly distributed, it is excreted primarily in the urine.

INDICATIONS AND USES
Edema associated with congestive heart failure, cirrhosis of the liver with ascites, renal diseases including nephrotic syndrome. ▪ Acute pulmonary edema. ▪ Edema unresponsive to other diuretic agents. ▪ Diuresis in patients allergic to furosemide. ▪ Adjunct in combination with other antihypertensive agents in the treatment of hypertensive crisis.
Unlabeled uses: Treatment of hypercalcemia.

CONTRAINDICATIONS
Anuria, known hypersensitivity to bumetanide. Use caution in patients with hepatic coma or in states of severe electrolyte depletion. Do not use until condition is improved or corrected. See Precautions.

PRECAUTIONS
May be used concurrently with aldosterone antagonists (e.g., spironolactone [Aldactone]) for more effective diuresis and to prevent excessive potassium loss. ▪ May increase blood glucose; has precipitated diabetes mellitus. ▪ May lower serum calcium level, causing tetany. ▪ In rare instances may precipitate an acute attack of gout. ▪ Risk of ototoxicity increased with higher doses, rapid injection, decreased renal function, or concurrent use with other ototoxic drugs; see Drug/Lab Interactions. ▪ Patients allergic to sulfonamides may have an allergic reaction to bumetanide. ▪ Excessive doses can lead to profound diuresis with water and electrolyte depletion.
Monitor: Monitor for excessive diuresis with water and electrolyte depletion. Routine checks on electrolyte panel, CO_2, serum glucose, uric acid, and BUN are necessary during therapy. Potassium chloride replacement may be required.
Patient Education: Hypotension may cause dizziness; move slowly, and request assistance to sit on edge of bed or ambulate. ▪ May decrease potassium levels and require a supplement.

Maternal/Child: Category C: use in pregnancy only if clearly needed. ▪ Consider discontinuing breast-feeding. ▪ Safety and effectiveness for use in pediatric patients not established. ▪ Has been used in infants age 4 days to 6 months at doses ranging from 0.005 mg/kg to 0.1 mg/kg. Maximal diuretic effect seen at doses of 0.035 to 0.04 mg/kg. Elimination half-life decreases during the first month of life from approximately 6 hours at birth to 2.4 hours at 1 month.

Elderly: Response similar to that seen in younger patients; however, dose selection should be cautious; see Dose Adjustments. Consider increased sensitivity to hypotensive and electrolyte effects and increased risk of circulatory collapse or thromboembolic episodes. ▪ Monitoring of renal function suggested.

DRUG/LAB INTERACTIONS

Causes excessive potassium depletion with **corticosteroids, thiazide diuretics, amphotericin B**. ▪ Potentiates **antihypertensive drugs**; reduced dose of the antihypertensive agent or both drugs may be indicated. ▪ May cause transient or permanent deafness with doses exceeding the usual or when given in conjunction with **other ototoxic drugs** (e.g., aminoglycosides, cisplatin). ▪ **Amphotericin B** may increase potential for ototoxicity and nephrotoxicity; avoid concurrent use. ▪ Nephrotoxicity increased by other **nephrotoxic agents** (e.g., acyclovir, aminoglycosides, cyclosporine, vancomycin); avoid concurrent use. ▪ May increase serum levels of **lithium** (may cause toxicity). ▪ May cause cardiac arrhythmias with **amiodarone or digoxin** (potassium depletion). ▪ Risk of cardiotoxicity increased with **pimozide**; concurrent use not recommended. ▪ May enhance or inhibit actions of **nondepolarizing muscle relaxants or theophyllines.** ▪ May cause hyperglycemia with **insulin or sulfonylureas** by decreasing glucose tolerance. ▪ Effects may be inhibited by **ACE inhibitors, NSAIDs, probenecid, or** in patients with cirrhosis and ascites who are taking **salicylates.** ▪ May cause profound diuresis and serious electrolyte abnormalities with **thiazide diuretics** because of synergistic effects. ▪ Do not use concomitantly with **ethacrynic acid**; risk of ototoxicity markedly increased. ▪ Smoking may increase secretion of ADH-decreasing diuretic effects and cardiac output. ▪ See Precautions.

SIDE EFFECTS

Usually occur in prolonged therapy, seriously ill patients, or following large doses.

Abdominal pain, arthritic pain, azotemia, dizziness, ECG changes, elevated SCr, encephalopathy, headache, hyperglycemia, hyperuricemia, hypocalcemia, hypochloremia, hypomagnesemia, hyponatremia, hypotension, impaired hearing, muscle cramps, nausea, pruritus, rash.

Major: Anaphylactic shock, blood volume reduction, circulatory collapse, dehydration, excessive diuresis, hypokalemia, metabolic acidosis, thrombocytopenia, vascular thrombosis, and embolism.

ANTIDOTE

If minor side effects are noted, discontinue the drug and notify the physician, who may treat the side effects symptomatically and continue the drug. If side effects are progressive or any major side effect occurs, discontinue the drug immediately and notify the physician. Treatment of major side effects is symptomatic and aggressive and includes fluid and electrolyte replacement. Resuscitate as necessary.

BUPRENORPHINE HYDROCHLORIDE BBW
(byou-pren-**OR**-feen hy-droh-**KLOR**-eyed)

Narcotic analgesic
(agonist-antagonist)
Anesthesia adjunct

Buprenex

pH 3.5 to 5.5

USUAL DOSE
Individualize dose, taking into account the patient's severity of pain, response, prior analgesic treatment experience, and risk factors for addiction, abuse, and misuse. Use lowest effective dose for the shortest duration consistent with the patient's treatment goals.

Pain control (adults and pediatric patients over 12 years of age): 0.3 mg (1 mL). Repeat every 6 hours as necessary. May be repeated in 30 to 60 minutes, if indicated.

PEDIATRIC DOSE
Pain control (2 to 12 years of age): 2 to 6 mcg/kg of body weight/dose every 4 to 6 hours as needed. A repeat dose in 30 to 60 minutes is **not** recommended. Longer intervals (6 to 8 hours) may be sufficient for some patients. Determine appropriate interval through clinical assessment. See Maternal/Child.

DOSE ADJUSTMENTS
Reduce dose in high-risk patients (e.g., elderly or debilitated, respiratory disease), when other CNS depressants have been given, and in the immediate postoperative period; see Drug/Lab Interactions. ▪ Reduced dose may be required in impaired liver function.

DILUTION
May be given undiluted.

Filters: Not required by manufacturer; however, 0.2-micron filters were used during manufacturing. No loss of drug potency expected.

Storage: Before use, store at CRT. Avoid freezing and/or prolonged exposure to light.

COMPATIBILITY
Compatibility information not available from manufacturer.

Other sources suggest specific **compatibilities** dependent on concentration and manufacturer; consult a pharmacist.

RATE OF ADMINISTRATION
A single dose over at least 2 minutes.

ACTIONS
A synthetic narcotic agonist-antagonist analgesic. Buprenorphine is a partial agonist at the mu-opioid receptor and an antagonist at the kappa-opioid receptor. 0.3 mg buprenorphine is approximately equivalent to 10 mg morphine in analgesic and respiratory depressant effects. It demonstrates narcotic antagonist activity and has been shown to be equipotent with naloxone as an antagonist of morphine. Pain relief is effected within minutes and lasts up to 6 hours. Metabolized in the liver. Primarily excreted through feces and to a lesser extent in the urine. Crosses the placental barrier. Secreted in breast milk.

INDICATIONS AND USES
Management of pain severe enough to require an opioid analgesic and for which alternate treatments are inadequate.

Limitations of use: Because of the risk of addiction, abuse, and misuse, even at recommended doses, reserve buprenorphine for use in patients for whom alternative treatment options (e.g., nonopioid analgesics or opioid combination products):

• Have not been tolerated or are not expected to be tolerated.
• Have not provided adequate analgesia or are not expected to provide adequate analgesia.

CONTRAINDICATIONS

Hypersensitivity to buprenorphine (e.g., anaphylaxis) or any other ingredient in the formulation. ▪ Significant respiratory depression. ▪ Acute or severe bronchial asthma in an unmonitored setting or in the absence of resuscitative equipment. ▪ Known or suspected GI obstruction, including paralytic ileus.

PRECAUTIONS

Buprenorphine exposes patients and other users to the risks of opioid addiction, abuse, and misuse, which can lead to overdose and death. Assess each patient's risk before prescribing buprenorphine, and monitor all patients regularly for the development of these behaviors and conditions. The potential for these risks should not, however, prevent the prescribing of buprenorphine for the proper management of pain in any given patient. ▪ Strategies to reduce the risk of diversion or misuse should be employed by healthcare facilities that use this and other controlled substances. ▪ See prescribing information for further discussion regarding abuse, addiction, physical dependence, and tolerance. ▪ Serious, life-threatening, or fatal respiratory depression may occur. Respiratory depression may occur at any time, but risk is greatest during initiation of therapy or after a dose increase. To reduce the risk of respiratory depression, proper dosing and titration are essential. Overestimating the buprenorphine dose when converting patients from another opioid product can result in a fatal overdose with the first dose. ▪ CO_2 retention from respiratory depression can exacerbate the sedating effects of opioids. ▪ Use caution with asthma, COPD, or other chronic pulmonary diseases or with respiratory depression or difficulty from any source; patients are at increased risk for decreased respiratory drive, including apnea, even at recommended doses. ▪ Use caution in elderly, cachectic, or debilitated patients; respiratory depression is more likely to occur. Use caution in pediatric patients, elderly or debilitated patients, or patients with severe impairment of renal, hepatic, or pulmonary function; myxedema or hypothyroidism; adrenocortical insufficiency; CNS depression or coma; toxic psychoses; prostatic hypertrophy or urethral stricture; acute alcoholism; delirium tremens; or kyphoscoliosis. ▪ Cases of adrenal insufficiency have been reported with opioid use. If adrenal insufficiency is diagnosed, treat with physiologic replacement doses of corticosteroids and wean the patient off the opioid to allow adrenal function to recover. Another opioid may be tried; some cases reported use of a different opioid without recurrence of adrenal insufficiency. ▪ Cases of serotonin syndrome have been reported during concomitant use of opioids with serotonergic drugs. ▪ Prolongation of the QTc interval has been reported in some patients. Avoid buprenorphine in patients who have a history of long-QT syndrome or an immediate family member with this condition or in patients receiving concurrent treatment with Class IA antiarrhythmic agents (e.g., quinidine, procainamide), Class III antiarrhythmic agents (e.g., amiodarone, sotalol), or other medications that prolong the QT interval. Consider risk in patients with hypokalemia, hypomagnesemia, or clinically unstable cardiac disease (e.g., heart failure, MI, and significant bradycardia). Periodic ECG monitoring is recommended in these patients. ▪ May cause severe hypotension, including orthostatic hypotension and syncope, in ambulatory patients. Patients whose ability to maintain BP has already been compromised by a reduced blood volume or concurrent administration of certain CNS depressant drugs (e.g., phenothiazines or general anesthetics) are at increased risk. ▪ In patients with circulatory shock, buprenorphine may cause vasodilation and can further reduce cardiac output and BP. Avoid buprenorphine in patients with circulatory shock. ▪ Use caution in patients with head injury, brain tumors, or increased intracranial pressure. Respiratory depression may cause increased P_{CO_2}, cerebral vasodilation, and increased intracranial pressure. Clinical course of head injury may be obscured. ▪ Cases of acute and chronic hypersensitivity to buprenorphine have been reported. ▪ Use caution in patients with biliary tract disease, including acute pancreatitis. May cause spasm of the sphincter of Oddi. Opioids may cause increases in amylase. ▪ Buprenorphine may increase the frequency of seizures in patients with seizure disorders. ▪ May precipitate withdrawal symptoms if stopped too quickly after prolonged use or if patient has been taking opiates. ▪ Tolerance (the need for increasing doses to maintain a defined effect such as analgesia [in the absence of disease progression or other external factors]) can develop with chronic use. ▪ See Maternal/Child and Drug/Lab Interactions.

Monitor: Naloxone, oxygen, and controlled respiratory equipment must be available. ▪ Observe patient frequently and monitor vital signs. Monitor for respiratory depression, especially during initiation of therapy (within the first 24 to 72 hours) or after a dose increase. ▪ Keep patient supine to minimize side effects; orthostatic hypotension and fainting may occur. Observe closely when initiating or titrating therapy and during ambulation. ▪ Monitor patients who may be susceptible to the intracranial effects of CO_2 retention for signs of sedation and respiratory depression. ▪ Monitor for S/S of hypersensitivity reactions (e.g., anaphylactic shock, angioneurotic edema, bronchospasm, hives, pruritus, rash). ▪ Monitor patients with biliary tract disease for worsening of symptoms. ▪ Monitor patients with a history of seizure disorders for worsening seizure control. ▪ Pain control usually more effective with routinely administered doses. Determine appropriate interval through clinical assessment. ▪ Periodic ECG monitoring may be indicated in patients at risk for QT prolongation. ▪ Monitor for S/S of serotonin syndrome (e.g., mental status changes [e.g., agitation, coma, hallucinations], autonomic instability [e.g., hyperthermia, labile blood pressure, tachycardia], neuromuscular aberrations [e.g., hyperreflexia, incoordination, rigidity], and/or GI symptoms [e.g., diarrhea, nausea, vomiting]). Onset of symptoms may occur within hours to days of concomitant use of opioids with serotonergic drugs. ▪ Monitor patients regularly for the development of opioid addiction, abuse, and misuse.

Patient Education: Review medications with provider. ▪ Avoid use of alcohol or other CNS depressants. ▪ Promptly report S/S of serotonin syndrome. ▪ Use caution performing any task requiring alertness; may cause dizziness, euphoria, and sedation. ▪ Request assistance for ambulation. ▪ May result in severe constipation. Scheduled bowel regimen recommended. ▪ May result in addiction, abuse, and misuse, even when taken as recommended.

Maternal/Child: Safety for use during pregnancy and labor and delivery not established. Use only when clearly needed. Closely monitor neonates exposed to buprenorphine during labor and delivery for signs of respiratory depression. ▪ Prolonged use of buprenorphine during pregnancy can result in neonatal opioid withdrawal syndrome, which may be life-threatening if not recognized and treated. Infants born to mothers receiving buprenorphine during pregnancy should be monitored closely and treated for neonatal opioid withdrawal syndrome if indicated. See literature for treatment protocols. ▪ Discontinue breast-feeding. ▪ Not recommended in pediatric patients under 2 years of age.

Elderly: See Dose Adjustments. ▪ May be more sensitive to effects (e.g., respiratory depression, urinary retention, constipation, dizziness). ▪ Analgesia should be effective with lower doses. ▪ Consider possibility of decreased organ function.

DRUG/LAB INTERACTIONS

Concomitant use with benzodiazepines or other CNS depressants (e.g., nonbenzodiazepine sedative/hypnotics, anxiolytics, tranquilizers, muscle relaxants, general anesthetics, antipsychotics, other opioids, alcohol) may result in profound sedation, respiratory depression, coma, and death. Reserve concomitant use for patients for whom alternative treatment options are inadequate. Use minimum effective dose for the shortest duration possible, and monitor for S/S of respiratory depression and sedation. ▪ May decrease analgesic effects of **other narcotics;** avoid concurrent use. ▪ Clearance decreased and serum levels increased by **cytochrome P$_{450}$ inhibitors** (e.g., azole antifungal agents, macrolide antibiotics, protease inhibitors). Monitor with concurrent use; dose adjustment may be indicated. ▪ Clearance increased and serum levels decreased by **cytochrome P$_{450}$ inducers** (e.g., carbamazepine, phenytoin, rifampin). Use caution; dose adjustments may be indicated. ▪ Serotonin syndrome has been reported with the concomitant use of opioids, including buprenorphine, and other **drugs that affect the serotonergic neurotransmitter system** (e.g., selective serotonin reuptake inhibitors [SSRIs], serotonin and norepinephrine reuptake inhibitors [SNRIs], tricyclic antidepressants [TCAs], triptans, 5-HT3 receptor antagonists, mirtazapine, trazodone, tramadol, MAO inhibitors, linezolid, and intravenous methylene blue). Careful observation, particularly during treatment initiation and dose adjustment, is required with concomitant use. ▪ Severe and unpredictable potentiation of **MAO inhibitors** (e.g., selegiline, phenelzine, tranylcypromine, linezolid) has been reported. MAO inhibitor interactions may manifest as serotonin syndrome or opioid toxicity (e.g., respiratory depression, coma). Use of buprenorphine is not recommended for patients taking MAOIs or within 14 days of stopping such treatment. ▪ **Mixed agonist/antagonist analgesics** (e.g., butorphanol, nalbuphine) may reduce the analgesic effect of buprenorphine and/or precipitate withdrawal symptoms. Avoid concomitant use. ▪ Buprenorphine may enhance the neuromuscular blocking action of **skeletal muscle relaxants** (e.g., cyclobenzaprine, orphenadrine), increasing the degree of respiratory depression. Monitor patient and decrease dose if indicated. ▪ Opioids can reduce the efficacy of **diuretics** by inducing the release of antidiuretic hormone. Increase dose of diuretic if needed. ▪ Concomitant use with **anticholinergic drugs** may increase the risk of urinary retention and/or severe constipation, which may lead to paralytic ileus. ▪ **Nucleoside reverse transcriptase inhibitors (NRTIs)** do not appear to induce or inhibit the P450 enzyme pathway, thus no interactions with buprenorphine are expected. ▪ **Non-nucleoside reverse transcriptase inhibitors (NNRTIs)** are metabolized principally by CYP3A4. Efavirenz, nevirapine, and etravirine are known CYP3A inducers, whereas delavirdine is a CYP3A inhibitor. Significant pharmacokinetic interactions between NNRTIs (e.g., efavirenz and delavirdine) and buprenorphine have been shown in clinical studies, but these pharmacokinetic interactions did not result in any significant pharmacodynamic effects. Monitor patients and adjust buprenorphine dose if indicated. ▪ Some **protease inhibitors** (PIs) with CYP3A4 inhibitory activity (atazanavir and atazanavir/ritonavir) resulted in elevated levels of buprenorphine and norbuprenorphine. Symptoms of opioid excess and sedation have been reported. Monitor patient and reduce dose if indicated.

SIDE EFFECTS

Sedation is the most common side effect. Other commonly reported side effects include constipation, dizziness, headache, hypotension, hypoventilation, miosis, nausea, sweating, vertigo, and vomiting. Serious side effects include acute and chronic hypersensitivity reactions (e.g., anaphylaxis, angioneurotic edema, bronchospasm, hives, pruritus, rash), addiction, adrenal insufficiency, increased intracranial pressure, life-threatening respiratory depression, neonatal opioid withdrawal syndrome, QTc prolongation, seizure, and severe hypotension. Numerous other reactions have been reported in fewer than 1% of patients.

Overdose: Airway obstruction (partial or complete), atypical snoring, bradycardia, cold and clammy skin, constricted pupils, death, hypotension, pulmonary edema, respiratory depression, skeletal muscle flaccidity, and somnolence progressing to stupor and coma. Marked mydriasis rather than miosis may be seen with hypoxia in overdose situations.

Post-Marketing: Cases of serotonin syndrome have been reported with concomitant use of opioids and serotonergic drugs.

ANTIDOTE

With increasing severity of any side effect or onset of symptoms of overdose, discontinue the drug and notify the physician. An opioid antagonist (e.g., naloxone hydrochloride) will help to reverse respiratory depression but should be reserved for clinically significant respiratory or circulatory depression. Repeat dosing of the antagonist may be needed due to the long-acting depressant effects of buprenorphine (36 to 48 hours). Carefully monitor the patient until spontaneous respiration is reliably re-established. A patent airway, artificial ventilation, oxygen therapy, and other symptomatic treatment must be instituted promptly. Treat anaphylaxis and resuscitate as necessary.

BUTORPHANOL TARTRATE BBW
(byou-**TOR**-fah-nohl **TAHR**-trayt)

Narcotic analgesic
(agonist-antagonist)
Anesthesia adjunct

Butorphanol Tartrate PF, Stadol, Stadol PF

pH 3 to 5.5

USUAL DOSE
Pain control: 1 mg. Repeat every 3 to 4 hours as necessary. Range is 0.5 to 2 mg.

Preoperative or preanesthetic: 2 mg 60 to 90 minutes before surgery. Individualize dose. Usually given IM.

Labor: 1 to 2 mg at full term in early labor; may be repeated after 4 hours. Use alternate analgesia if delivery is expected to occur within 4 hours.

Adjunct to balanced anesthesia: 2 mg just before induction or 0.5 to 1 mg in increments during anesthesia. Increments may be up to 0.06 mg/kg and should be based on previous sedative, analgesic, and hypnotic drugs. Patients seldom require less than 4 mg or more than 12.5 mg. Administered only under the direction of the anesthesiologist.

DOSE ADJUSTMENTS
Reduce dose to half of the recommended dose and increase the interval between doses to at least 6 hours for impaired liver or renal function and in the elderly; adjust as indicated by patient response. ▪ Another source suggests that patients with a glomerular filtration rate (GFR) of 10 to 50 mL/min receive 75% of the usual dose given at the normal dosage interval and that patients with a GFR less than 10 mL/min receive 50% of the usual dose given at the normal dosage interval. No dose adjustment is necessary for patients with a GFR greater than 50 mL/min. ▪ Reduce dose when other CNS depressants have been given and in the immediate postoperative period. Use the smallest effective dose and extend intervals between doses. ▪ See Drug/Lab Interactions.

DILUTION
May be given undiluted. Avoid aerosol spray while preparing a syringe for use. Rinse with cool water following skin contact. Available preservative free.

Storage: Store at CRT. Protect from light and freezing.

COMPATIBILITY
Compatibility information not available from manufacturer.

Other sources suggest specific **compatibilities** dependent on concentration and manufacturer; consult a pharmacist.

RATE OF ADMINISTRATION
Each 2 mg or fraction thereof over 3 to 5 minutes. Frequently titrated according to symptom relief and respiratory rate.

ACTIONS
A potent narcotic analgesic with some narcotic agonist-antagonist effects. Exact mechanism of action is unknown. Analgesia similar to morphine is produced. Does produce respiratory depression, but this does not increase markedly with larger doses. Pain relief is effected almost immediately, peaks at 30 minutes, and lasts about 2 to 4 hours. Causes some hemodynamic changes that increase the workload of the heart. Metabolized in the liver. Excreted in urine and feces. Crosses the blood-brain barrier and placental barrier. Secreted in breast milk.

INDICATIONS AND USES
Relief of moderate to severe pain. ▪ Preoperative or preanesthetic medication, as a supplement to anesthesia. ▪ Relief of pain during early labor.

CONTRAINDICATIONS
Hypersensitivity to butorphanol or its components (some products contain benzethonium chloride).

PRECAUTIONS

Butorphanol exposes patients and other users to the risks of opioid addiction, abuse, and misuse, which can lead to overdose and death. Assess each patient's risk before prescribing butorphanol, and monitor all patients regularly for the development of these behaviors and conditions. Strategies to reduce the risk of diversion or misuse should be used by healthcare facilities that use this and other controlled substances. ▪ See prescribing information for further discussion regarding abuse, addiction, physical dependence, and tolerance. ▪ Not used for narcotic-dependent patients because of antagonist activity. ▪ May increase cardiac workload; use in myocardial infarction, ventricular dysfunction, and coronary insufficiency only if benefits outweigh risks. ▪ Use caution in respiratory depression or difficulty from any source, obstructive respiratory conditions, head injury, and impaired liver or kidney function. ▪ May elevate cerebrospinal pressure. ▪ In overdose situations, always consider the possibility of multiple drug ingestion. ▪ Cases of serotonin syndrome have been reported during concomitant use of butorphanol with serotonergic drugs.

Monitor: Naloxone, oxygen, and controlled respiratory equipment must be available. Duration of action of butorphanol usually exceeds that of naloxone; repeated dosing may be necessary. ▪ Observe patient frequently and monitor vital signs. ▪ Monitor for respiratory depression, especially during initiation of therapy (within the first 24 to 72 hours) or after a dose increase. ▪ Keep patient supine to minimize side effects; orthostatic hypotension and fainting may occur. Observe closely during ambulation. ▪ Monitor for S/S of serotonin syndrome (e.g., mental status changes [e.g., agitation, coma, hallucinations], autonomic instability [e.g., hyperthermia, labile blood pressure, tachycardia], neuromuscular aberrations [e.g., hyperreflexia, incoordination, rigidity], and/or GI symptoms [e.g., diarrhea, nausea, vomiting]). Onset of symptoms may occur within hours to days of concomitant use of opioids with serotonergic drugs. ▪ Pain control usually more effective with routinely administered doses. Determine appropriate interval through clinical assessment.

Patient Education: Avoid use of alcohol or other CNS depressants (e.g., antihistamines, diazepam). ▪ Promptly report S/S of serotonin syndrome. ▪ Use caution performing any task requiring alertness; may cause dizziness, euphoria, and sedation. ▪ Request assistance for ambulation. ▪ May be habit forming.

Maternal/Child: Category C: safety for use in pregnant females before 37 weeks' gestation not established; use only if benefit justifies potential risk to fetus. ▪ Prolonged use of butorphanol during pregnancy can result in neonatal opioid withdrawal syndrome, which may be life threatening if not recognized and treated. Infants born to mothers receiving butorphanol during pregnancy should be monitored closely and treated for neonatal opioid withdrawal syndrome, if indicated. See literature for treatment protocols. ▪ Has been associated with transient (10 to 90 minutes) sinusoidal fetal heart rate patterns. Use caution if abnormal fetal heart rate is present. Alternative analgesia suggested if delivery is expected to occur within 4 hours. ▪ Use caution in breast-feeding; an estimated 4 mcg/L has been found in breast milk; monitor for excess sedation and/or respiratory depression. ▪ Safety and effectiveness for use in pediatric patients under 18 years of age not established.

Elderly: Mean half-life may be extended by 25%, may be more sensitive to effects (e.g., respiratory depression, constipation, dizziness, urinary retention). ▪ Analgesia should be effective with lower doses; see Dose Adjustments. ▪ Consider decreased organ function, concomitant disease, or other drug therapy.

DRUG/LAB INTERACTIONS

Concomitant use of butorphanol with **benzodiazepines** and other **CNS depressants** (e.g., sedative/hypnotics, anxiolytics, tranquilizers, muscle relaxants, general anesthetics, antipsychotics, other opioids, alcohol) may result in profound sedation, respiratory depression, coma, and death. Hypotension can also occur. Reserve concomitant use for patients for whom alternative treatment options are inadequate. Limit dose and duration of treatment to the minimum required and monitor patients carefully for S/S of respiratory depression and sedation. ▪ Serotonin syndrome has been reported with the concomitant use of opioids, including butorphanol, and other **drugs that affect the serotonergic neurotransmitter system** (e.g., selective serotonin reuptake inhibitors [SSRIs], serotonin and norepinephrine reuptake inhibitors [SNRIs], tricyclic antidepressants

[TCAs], triptans, 5-HT3 receptor antagonists, mirtazapine, trazodone, tramadol, MAO inhibitors, linezolid, and intravenous methylene blue). Careful observation, particularly during treatment initiation and dose adjustment, is required with concomitant use. ▪ **Medications that affect hepatic metabolism of drugs** (e.g., aminophylline, cimetidine, erythromycin) may interfere with the metabolism of butorphanol. Reduced doses of butorphanol and/or longer intervals between doses may be indicated. ▪ May decrease analgesic effects of **other narcotics;** avoid concurrent use. ▪ May cause an increase in conjunctival changes with **pancuronium.**

SIDE EFFECTS

Dizziness, nausea and/or vomiting, and somnolence occur most frequently. Abdominal pain, anorexia, anxiety, asthenia, bronchitis, clammy skin, confusion, constipation, cough, diplopia, dizziness, drug dependence, dry mouth, dyspnea, euphoria, floating feeling, flushing, hallucinations, headache, hypersensitivity reactions (e.g., pruritus), hypotension, insomnia, lethargy, nervousness, palpitations, paresthesia, respiratory depression, sweating, tremor, unusual dreams, vasodilation, vertigo, warmth. May cause increased pulmonary artery pressure, pulmonary wedge pressure, left ventricular end-diastolic pressure, systemic arterial pressure, pulmonary vascular resistance, and cardiac workload.

Overdose: Cardiovascular insufficiency, hypoventilation, coma, and death. May be associated with ingestion of multiple drugs.

ANTIDOTE

With increasing severity of any side effect or onset of symptoms of overdose, discontinue the drug and notify the physician. Most side effects will be treated symptomatically. Treat hypertension with antihypertensives (e.g., nitroglycerin, nitroprusside sodium). Naloxone hydrochloride will reverse respiratory depression. Duration of action of butorphanol usually exceeds that of naloxone; repeated dosing may be necessary. A patent airway, adequate ventilation, oxygen therapy, and other symptomatic treatment must be instituted promptly. Vasodilation may cause hypotension.

C1 ESTERASE INHIBITOR (HUMAN OR RECOMBINANT)

Protein C1 Inhibitors

(C 1 **ES**-ter-ase in-**HIB**-it-or)

Berinert, Cinryze, Ruconest

Available C1 esterase inhibitor products include:

Berinert: Plasma-derived C1 esterase inhibitor (human) pH 4.5 to 8.5

Cinryze: Plasma-derived C1 esterase inhibitor (human) pH 6.6 to 7.4

Ruconest: (Recombinant) C1 esterase inhibitor pH 6.8

USUAL DOSE
(International units [IU])

BERINERT

Treatment of an acute attack: 20 international units/kg (IU/kg) as an IV injection. Doses lower than 20 international units/kg (IU/kg) should not be administered.

CINRYZE

Routine prophylaxis dosing: 1,000 units as an IV injection over 10 minutes (1 mL/min). May be repeated every 3 or 4 days as necessary for routine prophylaxis against angioedema attacks in patients with hereditary angioedema (HAE).

RUCONEST

Treatment of an acute attack: 50 international units/kg (IU/kg) with a maximum of 4,200 international units (IU) administered as a slow IV injection over approximately 5 minutes. If symptoms persist, a second dose may be administered. Do not exceed 4,200 international units/dose (IU/dose).

DILUTION
(International units [IU])

BERINERT

Available in a kit containing one 500–international unit (IU) vial of Berinert, one 10-mL vial of SWFI, one Mix2Vial filtered transfer set, and one alcohol swab. Bring components to room temperature (RT). Berinert is a lyophilized concentrate and requires reconstitution. The Mix2Vial transfer set provided requires a specific technique to accomplish reconstitution; see manufacturer's literature for instructions. Alternately, for each vial of Berinert and provided diluent, place all components on a flat surface, remove the flip caps from the drug and diluent vials, swab the vials with alcohol, and allow them to dry. Insert one end of a double-ended transfer needle into the diluent. Invert the diluent bottle and insert the other end of the transfer needle into the drug vial. Diluent will be drawn into the drug vial by a vacuum. Remove the transfer device and diluent vial. Gently swirl the drug vial to fully dissolve. Solution should be colorless, clear, and free from visible particles. Do not use if solution is cloudy, discolored, or contains particulates. Concentration equals 50 units/mL. Calculate volume required to supply the calculated dose. Attach a vented filter spike to a 10-mL (or larger) syringe and withdraw the contents. Contents of multiple vials may be pooled in a single administration device (e.g., syringe). Use a new double-ended transfer needle and a new vented filter spike or a new unused Mix2Vial for each vial requiring reconstitution.

CINRYZE

If refrigerated, bring components to RT (two 500-unit vials of Cinryze and two 5-mL vials of SWFI [not supplied by manufacturer]). Use of a silicone-free syringe is recommended for reconstitution and administration. Access the diluent vial before the Cinryze vial to prevent loss of vacuum. For each 500-unit vial, insert one end of a double-ended transfer needle into the SWFI diluent. Invert the bottle of diluent and rapidly insert the other end of the transfer needle into the slightly angled Cinryze vial. Diluent will be drawn into the Cinryze vial by a vacuum. Do not use if there is no vacuum. Remove the transfer device and diluent vial. Gently swirl the Cinryze vial until the powder is completely dissolved. Do not use if solution is turbid or discolored (should be colorless to slightly blue and clear). Attach a filter needle to a 10-mL syringe and withdraw 500 units (5 mL) from each vial (total dose 1,000 units in 10 mL [100 units/mL]).

Rᴜᴄᴏɴᴇꜱᴛ

Bring components to room temperature (vials of Ruconest and SWFI as diluent [not supplied by manufacturer]). Remove the flip caps from the drug and diluent vials, swab the vials with alcohol, and allow them to dry. Using the syringe/needle or syringe/vial adapter, withdraw 14 mL of SWFI from the diluent vial. Remove the syringe and transfer the diluent to the Ruconest vial. Add the diluent slowly to avoid forceful impact on the powder. Swirl the vial slowly to mix and avoid foaming. If indicated, repeat this procedure using another 14 mL of diluent using a new vial adapter and a second vial of Ruconest. Concentration equals 150 international units/mL (IU/mL). Calculate volume required to supply the calculated dose and draw up into a syringe. Contents of both vials may be pooled into a single administration syringe. Do not use if solution is cloudy, discolored, or contains particulates.

Filters: Bᴇʀɪɴᴇʀᴛ: A Mix2Vial filtered transfer set is provided for each single-use dose or, alternately, a double-ended needle and a vented filter spike are required.

Cɪɴʀʏᴢᴇ ᴀɴᴅ Rᴜᴄᴏɴᴇꜱᴛ: Specific information not available.

Sᴛᴏʀᴀɢᴇ: All Formulations: Store in carton at 2° to 25° C (36° to 77° F) until ready for use. Do not freeze. Protect from light. Do not use beyond expiration date. For single use only. Discard unused drug.

Bᴇʀɪɴᴇʀᴛ: Reconstituted solution must be used within 8 hours; do not refrigerate or freeze.

Cɪɴʀʏᴢᴇ: Reconstituted solution must be administered at RT within 3 hours of preparation.

Rᴜᴄᴏɴᴇꜱᴛ: Use reconstituted solution immediately, or refrigerate and use within 8 hours. Do not freeze.

COMPATIBILITY

Bᴇʀɪɴᴇʀᴛ: Manufacturer states, "Do not mix Berinert with other medicinal products, and administer by a separate infusion line."

Cɪɴʀʏᴢᴇ: Manufacturer states, "Do not mix with other materials."

Rᴜᴄᴏɴᴇꜱᴛ: Manufacturer states, "Do not mix with other medicinal products or solutions. Administer by a separate infusion line."

RATE OF ADMINISTRATION

Bᴇʀɪɴᴇʀᴛ: A single dose at a rate of approximately 4 mL/min.

Cɪɴʀʏᴢᴇ: A single dose equally distributed over 10 minutes (1 mL/min).

Rᴜᴄᴏɴᴇꜱᴛ: A single dose equally distributed over approximately 5 minutes.

ACTIONS

C1 esterase inhibitor is a normal constituent of human blood and is a serine proteinase inhibitor. It has an important inhibiting potential on several of the major cascade systems, including the complement system, the intrinsic coagulation (contact) system, the fibrinolytic system, and the coagulation cascade. Hereditary angioedema (HAE) patients have low levels of endogenous or functional C1 esterase inhibitor. Although the events that induce attacks of angioedema in HAE patients are not well defined, it is thought that increased vascular permeability and the clinical manifestation of HAE attacks (e.g., local tissue swelling of hands, feet, limbs, face, intestinal tract, and airway [larynx or trachea]) are primarily mediated through contact system activation. Suppression of contact system activation by C1 esterase inhibitor through the inactivation of plasma kallikrein and factor XIIa is thought to modulate vascular permeability by preventing the generation of bradykinin. Supplying additional C1 esterase inhibitor activity by IV injection facilitates the normal process. Plasma levels of C1 inhibitor increase within 1 hour or less of IV administration of Cinryze. The mean half-life is 22 hours for **Berinert,** 56 hours for **Cinryze,** and 2.5 hours for **Ruconest.**

INDICATIONS AND USES

Bᴇʀɪɴᴇʀᴛ: Treatment of acute abdominal, facial, or laryngeal attacks of hereditary angioedema (HAE) in adult and adolescent patients. ▪ Safety and effectiveness for use as prophylactic therapy not established.

Cɪɴʀʏᴢᴇ: Routine prophylaxis against angioedema attacks in adolescent and adult patients with HAE.

Ruconest: Treatment of acute attacks in adult and adolescent patients with HAE.

Limitation of use: Ruconest: Effectiveness not established in HAE patients with laryngeal attacks.

CONTRAINDICATIONS

All Formulations: Known life-threatening hypersensitivity reactions, including anaphylaxis to C1 esterase inhibitor preparations.

Ruconest: Is contraindicated in patients with a history of allergy to rabbits or rabbit-derived products.

PRECAUTIONS

All Formulations: For intravenous use only. ▪ Initiate treatment under the supervision of a qualified health care professional experienced in the treatment of HAE. ▪ Severe hypersensitivity reactions, including anaphylaxis, may occur. Epinephrine should be immediately available. See Antidote. ▪ Serious arterial and venous thromboembolic (TE) events (e.g., basilar artery thrombosis, multiple pulmonary microemboli, and thrombosis) have been reported at recommended doses of C1 esterase inhibitor products, and other TE events (e.g., myocardial infarction, pulmonary embolism, arterial thrombosis, deep vein thrombosis) have been reported in patients receiving off-label high-dose C1 esterase inhibitor therapy. Risk factors may include the presence of an indwelling venous catheter/access device, prior history of thrombosis, underlying atherosclerosis, use of oral contraceptives or certain androgens, morbid obesity, and immobility. Weigh benefits of treatment versus risk.

Berinert and Cinryze: Made from human plasma and may contain infectious agents (e.g., HIV, Creutzfeldt-Jakob disease, hepatitis B, or hepatitis C). Numerous steps in the manufacturing process are used to reduce the potential for infection.

Monitor: All Formulations: Observe for symptoms of a hypersensitivity reaction (e.g., anaphylaxis, generalized urticaria, hives, hypotension, tightness in the chest, wheezing). Reaction may occur during injection or after injection is complete. ▪ Symptoms of an HAE attack may be similar to S/S of hypersensitivity reactions. Evaluate carefully to initiate the correct treatment. There is usually no itching or hives with an HAE attack. ▪ Monitor patients with known risk factors for thrombotic events during and after administration; see Precautions.

Patient Education: All Formulations: Inform patients of the risks for infectious agent transmission and of safety precautions taken during the manufacturing process. ▪ Promptly report symptoms of a hypersensitivity reaction (e.g., difficulty breathing, feeling faint, hives, itching, tightness in the chest, wheezing). ▪ Promptly report symptoms of a possible thrombosis (e.g., altered consciousness or speech; loss of sensation or motor power; new-onset swelling and pain in the abdomen, chest, or limbs; shortness of breath). ▪ Appropriately trained patients may self-administer upon recognition of an HAE attack. However, given the potential for airway obstruction during an acute laryngeal HAE attack, patients experiencing such an attack should be advised to seek immediate medical attention after self-administration of **Berinert**. ▪ Discuss all medications used (e.g., prescription, nonprescription, over-the-counter, herbal, supplements) with the physician. ▪ Consult a health care professional before travel.

Maternal/Child: Berinert and Cinryze: Category C: Safety and effectiveness for use during pregnancy, labor, and delivery have not been established; use only if clearly needed.

Ruconest: Category B: Safety and effectiveness during pregnancy, labor, and delivery have not been established; use only if clearly needed.

All Formulations: Not known if C1 esterase inhibitor is secreted in human milk; use only if clearly needed during breast-feeding. ▪ *Berinert:* Safety and effectiveness for use in pediatric patients under 12 years of age not established. ▪ *Cinryze:* Safety and effectiveness for use in neonates, infants, or other pediatric patients not established. Clinical studies included patients 9, 14, and 16 years of age. ▪ *Ruconest:* Safety and effectiveness were evaluated in 17 adolescent patients (13 to 17 years of age) treated for 52 HAE attacks with no serious adverse reactions. Abdominal pain, headache, and oropharyngeal pain did occur.

Elderly: All Formulations: Numbers in clinical studies insufficient to determine if the elderly respond differently than do younger subjects.

DRUG/LAB INTERACTIONS
ALL FORMULATIONS: No drug interaction studies have been conducted.

SIDE EFFECTS
BERINERT: The most common side effect observed was dysgeusia (an altered sense of taste). An increase in the severity of pain associated with HAE was the most serious side effect during clinical trials. Other reported side effects include abdominal pain, back pain, diarrhea, facial pain, headache, muscle spasm, nausea, and vomiting.

CINRYZE: The most common side effects reported include headache, nausea, rash, and vomiting. The most serious reaction observed in clinical studies was a cerebrovascular accident. Hypersensitivity reactions, including anaphylaxis, hives, hypotension, tightness of the chest, urticaria, and wheezing, have occurred.

RUCONEST: The most common side effects reported include diarrhea, headache, and nausea. Hypersensitivity with anaphylaxis was the most serious reaction reported.

POST-MARKETING: Berinert: Reported side effects from use outside the United States include hypersensitivity/anaphylactic reactions, viral transmission (e.g., acute hepatitis C), chills, fever, and injection site pain or redness.

CINRYZE: Local infusion site reactions (including inflammation or hematoma) and thromboembolic events (including catheter-related and deep venous thrombosis, transient ischemic attack, and stroke).

RUCONEST: Abdominal pain and rash.

ANTIDOTE
ALL FORMULATIONS: Keep the physician informed of side effects. Interrupt or discontinue injection if indicated (e.g., hypersensitivity reaction, thrombotic event). If appropriate and if symptoms subside, infusion may be resumed at a tolerated rate. ▪ Discontinue C1 esterase inhibitor and treat anaphylaxis immediately with oxygen, epinephrine, antihistamines (e.g., diphenhydramine), vasopressors (e.g., dopamine), corticosteroids, albuterol, IV fluids, and ventilation equipment as indicated. Resuscitate as necessary.

CAFFEINE CITRATE
(**KAF**-feen **SIT**-rayt)

Cafcit

CNS stimulant
Respiratory stimulant adjunct

pH 4.7

PEDIATRIC DOSE
Pretreatment: Baseline studies may be indicated; see Precautions and Monitor.

The dose expressed as caffeine base is one-half the dose when expressed as caffeine citrate. The recommended loading dose and maintenance dose are listed in the following chart.

Guidelines for Loading and Maintenance Doses of Caffeine Citrate		
	Dose of Cafcit (volume)	**Dose Expressed as Caffeine Citrate**
Loading dose	1 mL/kg	20 mg/kg for 1 dose
Maintenance dose	0.25 mL/kg	5 mg/kg every 24 hours

Begin maintenance dose 24 hours after loading dose. Maintenance dose may be given IV or orally. Duration of treatment beyond 10 to 12 days has not been studied. See Precautions.

DOSE ADJUSTMENTS
May adjust maintenance dose using serum concentrations of caffeine. ▪ To avoid toxicity in neonates with impaired renal or hepatic function, use with caution and monitor serum concentrations.

DILUTION

Both the IV and the oral doses are supplied in vials containing 60 mg/3 mL of caffeine citrate (30 mg/3 mL of caffeine base). Confirm that vial is for IV use. Withdraw calculated dose and dilute with sufficient D5W to administer at the recommended rate of administration.

Storage: Store at CRT. Single-use vial. Discard any unused solution. Stable for 24 hours at room temperature when mixed with any of the solutions listed by the manufacturer in Compatibility.

COMPATIBILITY

Solution: Manufacturer lists D5W; another source adds D5/¼NS, D5/¼NS with 20 mEq KCl/L.

Additive: Manufacturer lists amino acid solution 8.5%, calcium gluconate 10%, D5W, dextrose 50%, dopamine 40 mg/mL diluted to 0.6 mg/mL with D5W, fentanyl 50 mcg/mL diluted to 10 mcg/mL with D5W, heparin sodium 1,000 units/mL diluted to 1 unit/mL with D5W, IV fat emulsion 20%.

Other sources suggest a few specific **compatibilities** dependent on concentration and manufacturer; consult a pharmacist.

RATE OF ADMINISTRATION

Use of a syringe pump infuser is recommended.

Loading dose: Infuse over 30 minutes.

Maintenance dose: Infuse over 10 minutes.

ACTIONS

A bronchial smooth muscle relaxant, a CNS and cardiac stimulant, and a diuretic. Structurally related to other methylxanthines (e.g., theophylline and theobromine). Exact mechanism of action in apnea of prematurity is not known. Postulated mechanisms include stimulation of the respiratory center, increased minute ventilation, decreased threshold to hypercapnia, increased response to hypercapnia, increased skeletal muscle tone, decreased diaphragmatic fatigue, increased metabolic rate, increased oxygen consumption, blood vessel dilatation, central vessel vasoconstriction, and smooth muscle relaxation. Readily distributes into the brain. Caffeine levels in the CSF of preterm neonates approximate plasma levels. Metabolized in the liver by the cytochrome P_{450} system. Metabolism and elimination in the preterm neonate are much slower than in adults due to immature hepatic and/or renal function. Mean half-life and fraction excreted unchanged in the urine is inversely related to gestational/postconceptual age. In neonates, the half-life is approximately 3 to 4 days and the fraction excreted unchanged in the urine is approximately 86% (within 6 days). By 9 months of age, the metabolism of caffeine approximates that seen in adults (half-life is 5 hours and amount excreted unchanged is 1%). Interconversion between caffeine and theophylline has been reported in preterm neonates. After theophylline administration, caffeine levels are approximately 25% of theophylline levels. After caffeine administration, 3% to 5% of caffeine administered converts to theophylline.

INDICATIONS AND USES

Short-term treatment of apnea of prematurity in infants more than 28 but less than 33 weeks' gestational age. In one study apnea of prematurity was defined as having at least 6 apnea episodes of more than 20 seconds' duration in a 24-hour period with no other identifiable cause of apnea.

Unlabeled uses: Prevention of postoperative apnea in former preterm infants.

CONTRAINDICATIONS

Hypersensitivity to any of its components.

PRECAUTIONS

Apnea of prematurity is a diagnosis of exclusion. Other causes of apnea (e.g., CNS disorders, primary lung disease, anemia, sepsis, metabolic disturbances, cardiovascular abnormalities, or obstructive apnea) should be ruled out or properly treated before initiating therapy with caffeine citrate. ■ Reports in the literature suggest a possible association between the use of methylxanthines and the development of necrotizing enterocolitis.

Necrotizing enterocolitis, resulting in death in some cases, has been reported in neonates receiving caffeine citrate. ▪ Is a CNS stimulant. Use with caution in infants with seizure disorders. ▪ May increase heart rate, left ventricular output, and stroke volume. Use with caution in infants with cardiovascular disease. ▪ Duration of treatment of apnea of prematurity in trials has been limited to 10 to 12 days. Safety and efficacy of therapy beyond this time have not been established. ▪ Safety and efficacy for use in prophylactic treatment of sudden infant death syndrome (SIDS) or before extubation in mechanically ventilated infants have not been established. ▪ Use with caution in infants with impaired renal or hepatic function; see Dose Adjustments and Monitor. ▪ Patients sensitive to other xanthines (e.g., aminophylline) may also be sensitive to caffeine.

Monitor: Obtain baseline serum caffeine levels in infants previously treated with theophylline because preterm infants metabolize theophylline to caffeine; see Actions. Levels should also be obtained in infants born to mothers who ingested caffeine before delivery, as caffeine readily crosses the placenta. Caffeine levels ranged from 8 to 40 mg/L in clinical trials. A therapeutic plasma concentration range has not been determined, but one source suggests 5 to 25 mcg/mL. Serious toxicity has been reported at levels exceeding 50 mg/L. Monitor levels periodically during treatment to avoid toxicity. Monitoring is especially important in infants with impaired renal or hepatic function; see Dose Adjustments. ▪ Monitor serum glucose periodically. Hypoglycemia and hyperglycemia have been reported. ▪ Monitor for S/S of necrotizing enterocolitis (e.g., gastric distension, vomiting, bloody stools). Screening stools for occult blood may be helpful in identifying early-onset necrotizing enterocolitis.

Patient Education: Caregivers should be instructed to consult physician if infant continues to have apnea events and to not increase the dose of caffeine citrate without consulting a physician. ▪ Contact physician at the first sign of lethargy or GI intolerance (e.g., abdominal distension, vomiting, or bloody stools). ▪ Dose must be accurately measured, and any unused solution must be discarded.

Maternal/Child: Category C: no controlled studies; benefits should outweigh risks. ▪ Half-life is increased in pregnant women. ▪ Half-life may be in excess of 100 hours in infants under 6 months of age due to immature liver function.

DRUG/LAB INTERACTIONS
Metabolized by the cytochrome P_{450} system. Lower caffeine doses may be required with coadministration of medications that **inhibit the P_{450} system,** decreasing the elimination of caffeine (e.g., cimetidine and ketoconazole]). Higher caffeine doses may be needed with coadministration of medications that **induce the P_{450} system,** increasing the elimination of caffeine (e.g., phenobarbital and phenytoin). ▪ Interconversion between caffeine and **theophylline** has been reported. Concurrent use of these drugs is not recommended; see Actions.

SIDE EFFECTS
Cardiovascular effects (e.g., tachycardia, increased left ventricular output, and increased stroke volume), CNS stimulation (e.g., irritability, jitteriness, restlessness), GI effects (e.g., feeding intolerance, gastritis, increased gastric aspirate, and necrotizing enterocolitis), hyperglycemia, hypoglycemia, renal effects (e.g., increased urine output, increased CrCl, and increased sodium and calcium excretion).

Overdose: Signs and symptoms of caffeine overdose in the preterm infant may include elevated BUN, elevated total leukocyte concentration, fever, fine tremor of extremities, hyperglycemia, hypertonia, insomnia, jitteriness, nonpurposeful jaw and lip movements, opisthotonos, seizures, tachypnea, tonic-clonic movements, or vomiting.

ANTIDOTE
Notify the physician of any side effects. Treatment of overdose is primarily symptomatic and supportive. Seizures may be treated with intravenous administration of diazepam or a barbiturate such as pentobarbital. Caffeine levels have been shown to decrease after exchange transfusions. Resuscitate as necessary.

CALASPARGASE PEGOL-mknl
(kal-**AS**-par-jase **PEG**-ol)

Asparlas

Antineoplastic agent
Enzyme

pH 7.3

USUAL DOSE
Pretreatment: Verify pregnancy status in females of reproductive potential before starting treatment with calaspargase pegol-mknl.
Adult and pediatric patients (1 month to 21 years of age): 2,500 units/M^2 IV. Do not administer more frequently than every 21 days.

DOSE ADJUSTMENTS
See Monitor. If adverse reactions occur, modify treatment according to the following chart.

Calaspargase-Pegol-mknl Dose Modifications for Adverse Reactions		
Adverse Reaction	**Severity[a]**	**Action**
Infusion reaction or hypersensitivity reaction	Grade 1	Reduce the infusion rate by 50%.
	Grade 2	Interrupt the infusion of calaspargase pegol-mknl. Treat the symptoms. When symptoms resolve, resume the infusion and reduce the infusion rate by 50%.
	Grade 3 to 4	Discontinue calaspargase pegol-mknl permanently.
Hemorrhage	Grade 3 to 4	Hold calaspargase pegol-mknl. Evaluate for coagulopathy and consider clotting factor replacement as needed. Resume calaspargase pegol-mknl with the next scheduled dose if bleeding is controlled.
Pancreatitis	Grade 3 to 4	Hold calaspargase pegol-mknl for elevations of lipase or amylase >3 × ULN until enzyme levels stabilize or are declining. Discontinue calaspargase pegol-mknl permanently if clinical pancreatitis is confirmed.
Thromboembolism	Uncomplicated deep vein thrombosis	Hold calaspargase pegol-mknl. Treat with appropriate antithrombotic therapy. Upon resolution of symptoms, consider resuming calaspargase pegol-mknl while continuing antithrombotic therapy.
	Severe or life-threatening thrombosis	Discontinue calaspargase pegol-mknl permanently. Treat with appropriate antithrombotic therapy.
Hepatoxicity	Total bilirubin >3 to ≤10 × ULN	Hold calaspargase pegol-mknl until total bilirubin levels go down to ≤1.5 × ULN.
	Total bilirubin >10 × ULN	Discontinue calaspargase pegol-mknl and do not make up for missed doses.

[a]Grade 1 is mild, Grade 2 is moderate, Grade 3 is severe, and Grade 4 is life-threatening.

DILUTION
Available as a clear, colorless solution in a single-dose vial containing 3,750 units/5 mL (750 units/mL). Dilute calaspargase pegol-mknl in 100 mL of NS or D5W using aseptic technique. ***Do not shake or vigorously agitate***. Discard any unused portion left in vials.
Storage: Store unopened vials refrigerated at 2° to 8° C (36° to 46° F) in carton to protect from light. Do not shake or freeze. Unopened vials may be stored at RT for no more than

48 hours. The diluted solution may be stored up to 4 hours at RT or refrigerated at 2° to 8° C (36° to 46° F) for up to 24 hours. Protect from light. Discard the vial for any particulate matter, cloudiness, or discoloration. **Do not administer** if calaspargase pegol-mknl has been shaken or vigorously agitated, frozen, or stored at RT for more than 48 hours.

COMPATIBILITY
Manufacturer states, "Do not infuse other drugs through the same intravenous line during administration of calaspargase pegol-mknl."

RATE OF ADMINISTRATION
A single dose as an infusion over 1 hour. After dilution, administer immediately into a running infusion of NS or D5W.

ACTIONS
Calaspargase pegol-mknl contains an asparagine-specific, enzyme-derived *Escherichia coli* as a conjugate of L-asparaginase and monomethoxypolyethylene glycol with a succinimidyl carbonate linker. L-asparaginase is an enzyme that catalyzes the conversion of the amino acid L-asparagine into aspartic acid and ammonia. The pharmacologic effect of calaspargase pegol-mknl is thought to be based on selective killing of leukemic cells due to depletion of plasma L-asparagine. Leukemic cells with low expression of asparagine synthetase have a reduced ability to synthesize L-asparagine and therefore depend on an exogenous source of L-asparagine for survival. The half-life is 16.1 days.

INDICATIONS AND USES
Treatment of acute lymphoblastic leukemia (ALL) in pediatric and young adult patients 1 month to 21 years of age. Administered as a component of a multiagent chemotherapeutic regimen.

CONTRAINDICATIONS
Patients with a history of any of the following: serious hypersensitivity reactions, including anaphylaxis, to pegylated L-asparaginase therapy; serious thrombosis during previous L-asparaginase therapy; serious pancreatitis during previous L-asparaginase therapy; serious hemorrhagic events during previous L-asparaginase therapy. ▪ Patients with severe hepatic impairment.

PRECAUTIONS
Administered by or under the direction of a physician specialist in a facility with adequate diagnostic and treatment facilities to monitor the patient and respond to any medical emergency. ▪ Hypersensitivity reactions, including anaphylaxis, can occur. ▪ Pancreatitis has been reported. ▪ Serious thrombotic events, including sagittal sinus thrombosis, have been reported. ▪ Hemorrhage associated with increased PT, PTT, and hypofibrinogenemia has occurred. ▪ Hepatoxicity and abnormal liver function, including elevations of transaminase, elevations of bilirubin (direct and indirect), reduced serum albumin, and reduced plasma fibrinogen can occur. ▪ As with all therapeutic proteins, there is the potential for immunogenicity.

Monitor: Monitor patients at least weekly, with bilirubin, transaminases, glucose, and clinical examinations until recovery from cycle of therapy. ▪ Monitor for S/S of hemorrhage or thrombosis. Obtain coagulation parameters, including PT, PTT, and fibrinogen, as indicated. ▪ Evaluate patients with abdominal pain for evidence of pancreatitis. Assess serum amylase and/or lipase levels to confirm early signs of pancreatic inflammation. ▪ Monitor patients for S/S of hypersensitivity reactions (e.g., angioedema, bronchospasm, dyspnea, erythema, eye swelling, hypotension, lip swelling, pruritus, and rash). Observe patient during and for at least 1 hour after infusion. ▪ Evaluate bilirubin and transaminases at least weekly during cycles of treatment that include calaspargase pegol-mknl through at least 6 weeks after the last dose. ▪ See Antidote.

Patient Education: Promptly report all side effects, especially unusual bleeding or bruising, excessive thirst, frequent urination, hypersensitivity reactions (e.g., dizziness, feeling faint, flushing, hives, itching, nausea, pruritus, shortness of breath), jaundice, S/S of thrombosis (e.g., arm or leg swelling, chest pain, headache, shortness of breath), severe abdominal pain, or severe nausea or vomiting. ▪ Advise females of reproductive potential to avoid becoming pregnant while receiving calaspargase pegol-mknl. Females should use effective contraceptive methods, including a barrier method, during treatment and for at least 3 months after the last dose. Use of oral contraceptives is not recommended.

Maternal/Child: Based on animal studies, calaspargase pegol-mknl can cause fetal harm when administered to a pregnant woman. ▪ Do not breast-feed while receiving calaspargase pegol-mknl and for 3 months after the last dose. ▪ Safety and effectiveness of calaspargase pegol-mknl has been established in pediatric patients between 1 month and 17 years of age (no data for the age-group under 1 month of age).

DRUG/LAB INTERACTIONS
Specific information not available.

SIDE EFFECTS
The most common adverse reactions were abnormal clotting studies, increased bilirubin, elevated transaminase, and pancreatitis. Other side effects include arrhythmia, cardiac failure, diarrhea, dyspnea, embolic and thrombotic events, fungal infection, hemorrhages, hypersensitivity, pneumonia, and sepsis.

ANTIDOTE
Notify physician of all side effects. Symptomatic and supportive treatment may be indicated. Discontinue in patients who experience a serious hypersensitivity reaction or a serious thrombotic event. Discontinue in patients if pancreatitis is suspected. If pancreatitis is confirmed, do not resume. If serious liver toxicity occurs, discontinue treatment and provide supportive care. Treat hypersensitivity reactions as indicated; may require epinephrine, airway management, oxygen, IV fluids, antihistamines (e.g., diphenhydramine), corticosteroids (e.g., hydrocortisone sodium succinate), and pressor amines (e.g., dopamine). Consider appropriate replacement therapy in patients with severe or symptomatic coagulopathy.

CALCITRIOL
(**kal**-si-**TRYE**-ole)

Calcijex

Vitamin D

pH 5.9 to 7

USUAL DOSE
Pretreatment: Baseline studies indicated; see Monitor.

Effectiveness of calcitriol therapy is dependent on adequate daily intake of calcium. The RDA of calcium in adults is 800 mg. Calcium supplementation or proper dietary measures must be initiated and maintained.

Hypocalcemia and/or secondary hyperparathyroidism: Recommended initial dose, depending on the severity of hypocalcemia and/or secondary hyperparathyroidism, is 1 mcg (0.02 mcg/kg) to 2 mcg administered at each hemodialysis treatment (three times weekly, approximately every other day). Initial doses have ranged from 0.5 to 4 mcg three times weekly.

Information supplied by the manufacturer suggests that the relative dosing of paricalcitol to calcitriol is 4:1. When converting a patient from calcitriol to paricalcitol, the initial dose of paricalcitol should be four times greater than the patient's dose of calcitriol.

PEDIATRIC DOSE
Hypocalcemia in end-stage renal disease (ESRD) (unlabeled): 0.01 to 0.05 mcg/kg/dose given 3 times a week; see Maternal/Child. See all comments under Usual Dose.

DOSE ADJUSTMENTS
Adjust dosing based on patient response. Begin dosing at lower end of dose range in the elderly; see Elderly. If a satisfactory response is not observed, dose may be increased by

0.5 to 1 mcg at 2- to 4-week intervals. Monitor serum calcium, phosphorus, and calcium × phosphorus product (Ca × P) frequently during any dose adjustment period; see Monitor. ▪ Discontinue therapy if elevated calcium level or a Ca × P product of greater than 70 is noted. Re-initiate therapy at a lower dose when parameters normalize. ▪ Calcitriol dose may need to be reduced as the parathyroid hormone (PTH) levels decrease in response to therapy. The currently accepted target range for intact parathyroid hormone (iPTH) in chronic renal failure (CRF) patients is no more than 1.5 to 3 times the nonuremic upper limit of normal. Incremental dosing must be individualized and commensurate with PTH, serum calcium, and phosphorus levels. The following chart is a suggested approach to dose titration.

Calcitriol Suggested Dosing Guidelines	
PTH Levels	**Calcitriol Dose**
The same or increasing	Increase
Decreasing by <30%	Increase
Decreasing by >30% but <60%	Maintain
Decreasing by >60%	Decrease
1.5–3 times the upper limit of normal	Maintain

DILUTION
May be given undiluted. Available in 1-mcg/mL ampules.
Storage: Store ampules at CRT. Protect from light. Calcitriol may be drawn up into a syringe up to 8 hours before administration but must be protected from direct sunlight.
COMPATIBILITY
Y-site: D5W, NS, SWFI.
RATE OF ADMINISTRATION
Administer as a bolus dose into the venous line at the end of hemodialysis.
ACTIONS
The active form of vitamin D_3 (cholecalciferol). Must be metabolically activated in liver and kidney before it is fully active on its target tissues. In bone, acts with PTH to stimulate resorption of calcium. In kidneys, increases tubular reabsorption of calcium. Stimulates intestinal calcium transport and directly suppresses synthesis and release of PTH from the parathyroid gland. A vitamin D–resistant state may exist in uremic patients because of the failure of the kidney to adequately convert precursors to the active compound, calcitriol. Duration of action is 3 to 5 days.
INDICATIONS AND USES
Management of hypocalcemia in patients undergoing chronic renal dialysis. Has been shown to significantly reduce elevated PTH levels, which results in improvement in renal osteodystrophy.
CONTRAINDICATIONS
Patients with hypercalcemia or evidence of vitamin D toxicity.
PRECAUTIONS
Because calcitriol is the most potent form of vitamin D available, oral vitamin D supplements should be discontinued during treatment. ▪ Dietary phosphorus should be restricted and a non–aluminum phosphate–binding compound (e.g., calcium acetate, sevelamer) should be administered to control serum phosphorus levels in patients undergoing dialysis.
Monitor: Obtain baseline serum calcium, phosphorus, aluminum, albumin, and PTH assays. ▪ Serum calcium levels should be corrected for serum albumin using the following equation: Corrected Ca = observed Ca + 0.8 × (normal albumin − observed albumin).

For example: If serum calcium is 7 mg/dL and observed albumin is 2.5 Gm/dL, Corrected Ca = 7 + 0.8 × (4 − 2.5) = 8.2 mg/dL. All decisions regarding therapy should be based on corrected calcium values. ■ Monitor magnesium, alkaline phosphatase, and 24-hour urinary calcium and phosphorus periodically. ■ Criteria used to determine if calcitriol should be administered include serum calcium less than 11.5 mg/dL, Ca × P less than 70, serum albumin less than 60 mcg/L (within normal limits), and PTH more than 3 times the upper limit of normal. ■ Serum calcium, phosphorus, and the Ca × P product should be monitored twice weekly during dose titration. Once stable, decrease monitoring to once monthly. See Dose Adjustments. ■ PTH levels, once stable, should be monitored every 3 months. Adynamic bone lesions may develop if PTH levels are suppressed to abnormal levels. If PTH levels fall below the target range (1.5 to 3 times the upper limit of normal), the calcitriol dose should be reduced. Discontinuation may result in rebound effect. Therefore gradual titration downward to a new maintenance dose is recommended; see Dose Adjustments. ■ Overdosage of vitamin D is dangerous. May induce hypercalcemia and/or hypercalciuria. If clinically significant hypercalcemia develops, dose should be reduced or held. Chronic hypercalcemia can lead to generalized vascular calcification, nephrocalcinosis, and other soft-tissue calcification. The serum Ca × P product should not be allowed to exceed 70. Radiographic evaluation of suspect anatomic regions may be useful in early detection of this condition; see Side Effects and Antidote. ■ Use with caution in patients receiving digoxin. Hypercalcemia may precipitate cardiac arrhythmias; see Drug/Lab Interactions.

Patient Education: Report symptoms of hypercalcemia promptly. Dose adjustment or treatment may be required. Strict adherence to dietary supplementation of calcium and restriction of phosphorus is required to ensure optimal effectiveness of therapy. Phosphate-binding compounds (e.g., calcium acetate [PhosLo]) may be needed to control serum phosphorus levels in patients with CRF, but excessive use of aluminum-containing products (e.g., aluminum hydroxide gel [Alternagel]) should be avoided. ■ Avoid use of unapproved nonprescription medications, including magnesium-containing antacids.

Maternal/Child: Category C: safety for use in pregnancy not established. Benefits must outweigh risks. ■ Safety for use in breast-feeding not established. A decision should be made whether to discontinue nursing or to discontinue the drug. ■ Safety and effectiveness have been studied in a small number of pediatric patients, ages 13 to 18 years, with ESRD on hemodialysis. The mean weekly dose ranged from 1 to 1.4 mcg. Use in this study program appeared to be safe and effective. See package insert for study information.

Elderly: Begin dosing at lower end of dose range. Consider age-related organ impairment, concomitant disease, and/or drug therapy; see Dose Adjustments.

DRUG/LAB INTERACTIONS

Specific interaction studies have not been performed. ■ **Digoxin** toxicity is potentiated by hypercalcemia. Use caution when calcitriol is prescribed concomitantly with digoxin compounds. ■ **Phosphate or vitamin D–related compounds** should not be taken concomitantly with calcitriol. ■ **Magnesium-containing antacids** and calcitriol should not be used concomitantly. Hypermagnesemia may result.

SIDE EFFECTS

Overdose or chronic administration may lead to hypercalcemia, hypercalciuria, and hyperphosphatemia. High intake of calcium and phosphate concomitant with calcitriol therapy may lead to similar abnormalities. Signs and symptoms of vitamin D intoxication associated with hypercalcemia include *Early:* bone pain, constipation, dry mouth, headache, metallic taste, muscle pain, nausea, somnolence, vomiting, and weakness. *Late:* albuminuria, anorexia, cardiac arrhythmias, conjunctivitis (calcific), decreased libido, ectopic calcification, elevated AST and ALT, elevated BUN, hypercholesterolemia, hypertension, hyperthermia, nocturia, overt psychosis (rare), pain at injection site, pancreatitis, photophobia, polydipsia, polyuria, pruritus, rhinorrhea, and weight loss. Rare cases of hypersensitivity reactions, including anaphylaxis, have been reported.

ANTIDOTE

Notify physician of any side effects. Treatment of patients with clinically significant hypercalcemia (more than 1 mg/dL above the upper limit of normal range) consists of supportive measures, immediate dose reduction or interruption of therapy, initiation of a low-calcium diet, withdrawal of calcium supplements, patient mobilization, attention to fluid and electrolyte imbalances, assessment of electrocardiographic abnormalities (critical in patients receiving digoxin), and hemodialysis or peritoneal dialysis against a calcium-free dialysate, as warranted. Hypercalcemia usually resolves in 2 to 7 days. Monitor serum calcium levels frequently until calcium levels return to within normal limits. May re-initiate calcitriol therapy at a dose 0.5 mcg less than prior dose. See Dose Adjustments.

CALCIUM CHLORIDE
(**KAL**-see-um **KLOR**-eyed)

Electrolyte replenisher
Antihypocalcemic
Cardiotonic
Antihyperkalemic
Antihypermagnesemic

pH 5.5 to 7.5

USUAL DOSE

In a 10% solution, 10 mL (1 Gm) contains 13.6 mEq (272 mg) of calcium; 1 mL (100 mg), 1.36 mEq (27.2 mg). **All doses based on a 10% solution.**

Hypocalcemic disorders (prophylaxis, treatment, electrolyte replacement, maintenance): 500 mg to 1 Gm at intervals of 1 to 3 days. Repeat doses may be required and are based on patient response or serum calcium levels. May be given as part of a TPN program.

Magnesium intoxication: 500 mg. Observe for signs of recovery before giving any additional calcium.

Hyperkalemia ECG disturbances of cardiac function: 100 mg to 1 Gm; titrate dose by monitoring ECG changes. American Heart Association guidelines recommend 500 mg to 1 Gm as a dose. Repeat as needed.

Cardiac arrest or cardiotoxicity in the presence of hypocalcemia or hypermagnesemia. Note: routine use of calcium is not recommended due to lack of improved survival. 500-1000 mg as a rapid bolus.

Overdose of calcium channel blockers or beta-adrenergic blockers (unlabeled): AHA guidelines recommend 500 mg to 1 Gm. May repeat as needed.

PEDIATRIC DOSE

Do not administer into a scalp vein in pediatric patients; see Precautions, Monitor, and Maternal/Child.

Hypocalcemic disorders: 0.027 to 0.05 mL/kg of body weight (2.7 to 5 mg/kg) of a 10% solution. Up to 10 mL (1 Gm)/day may be required. No data from clinical trials are available regarding repeat doses. Sources suggest repeat doses every 4 to 6 hours based on patient response or serum calcium levels.

Cardiac arrest in the presence of hyperkalemia or hypocalcemia, hypermagnesemia or calcium channel antagonist toxicitiy: 20 mg/kg/dose (maximum dose 2000 mg).

DILUTION

For intermittent IV infusion, dilute to a maximum concentration of 20 mg/ml.

COMPATIBILITY

Calcium salts not generally mixed with carbonates, phosphates, sulfates, or tartrates. *Extreme caution and a specific multistep process are required when calcium and phosphates are combined in parenteral nutrition solutions. Consult pharmacist.*

Other sources suggest specific **compatibilities** dependent on concentration and manufacturer; consult a pharmacist.

RATE OF ADMINISTRATION

For IV administration only. Avoid rapid administration (do not exceed 100 mg/min, except in cardiac arrest). For intermittent IV infusion, infuse diluted solution over 1 hour or no greater than 45-90 mg/kg/hours (0.6 to 1.2 mEq/kg/hr). Administer via a central or deep vein is preferred; do not use small hand or foot veins as severe necrosis and sloughing may occur.

ACTIONS

Calcium is a basic element prevalent in the human body. It affects bones, nerves, muscles, glands, cardiac and vascular tone, and normal coagulation of the blood. It is excreted in the urine and feces.

INDICATIONS AND USES

Calcium preparations other than calcium chloride are often preferred except in cardiac resuscitation or calcium channel blocker toxicity. ▪ Increase plasma calcium levels in hypocalcemic disorders (e.g., tetany [neonatal, parathyroid deficiency], vitamin D deficiency, alkalosis, conditions associated with intestinal malabsorption). ▪ Treat ECG disturbances caused by hyperkalemia. ▪ Adjunctive therapy in sensitivity reactions (especially with urticaria), insect bites or stings (relieve muscle cramping), acute symptoms of lead colic, rickets, or osteomalacia. ▪ Cardiac resuscitation only to treat hypocalcemia, hyperkalemia, hypermagnesemia or calcium-channel–blocker toxicity (verapamil, diltiazem), or after open heart surgery if epinephrine does not produce effective myocardial contractions. ▪ Antidote for cardiac and respiratory depression of magnesium sulfate toxicity.

Unlabeled uses: Treatment of arrhythmias and/or hypotension caused by an overdose of calcium channel blockers or beta-adrenergic blockers. ▪ Prevention of hypotension caused by calcium channel blockers.

CONTRAINDICATIONS

Digitalized patients, hypercalcemia, ventricular fibrillation. Not recommended in the treatment of asystole and electromechanical dissociation.

PRECAUTIONS

Three times more potent than calcium gluconate. ▪ For IV use only. ▪ See Drug/Lab Interactions.

Monitor: Confirm patency of vein; select a large vein and use a small needle to reduce vein irritation. Administration into a central or deep vein is preferred. Necrosis and sloughing will occur with IM or SC injection or extravasation. ▪ Keep patient recumbent after injection to prevent postural hypotension. ▪ Monitor vital signs carefully. ▪ Monitor serum calcium levels as indicated. May cause hyperchloremic acidosis.

Maternal/Child: Category C: safety for use in pregnancy and breast-feeding not established. Use only when clearly needed. ▪ Rarely used IV in pediatric patients. Use of a less irritating salt preferred because of small vein size.

DRUG/LAB INTERACTIONS

Will increase **digoxin** toxicity and may cause arrhythmias. If necessary, give small amounts very slowly. ▪ Potentiated by **thiazide diuretics**; may cause hypercalcemia or calcium toxicity. ▪ May reduce plasma levels of **atenolol**. ▪ Can reduce neuromuscular paralysis and respiratory depression produced by **antibiotics such as kanamycin.** ▪ Antagonizes **verapamil;** can reverse clinical effects. ▪ May cause metabolic alkalosis and inhibit binding of potassium with **sodium polystyrene sulfonate.**

SIDE EFFECTS

Usual doses will produce a local burning sensation, moderate drop in BP, and peripheral vasodilation. May cause bradycardia; cardiac arrest; heat waves; metallic, calcium, or chalky taste; prolonged state of cardiac contraction; sense of oppression; or tingling sensation, especially with a too-rapid rate of administration.

Overdose: Coma, intractable nausea and vomiting, lethargy, markedly elevated plasma calcium level, weakness, and sudden death.

ANTIDOTE

If extravasation occurs, immediately stop infusion and disconnect; gently aspirate extravasated solution. Do NOT flush the line. Initiate hyaluronidase antidote; remove needle/cannula; apply cold compresses; elevate extremity. Hyaluronidase: inject 1-1.7 mL intradermally or subcutaneously as 5 separate 0.2-0.3 mL injections into area of extravasation (using 25 -guage needle) at the leading edge in a clockwise manner. May also inject hyaluronidase through the catheter that caused the infiltration.

CALCIUM GLUCONATE
(**KAL**-see-um **GLOO**-koh-nayt)

Electrolyte replenisher

pH 6 to 8.2

USUAL DOSE

Individualize dose within the recommended ranges listed in the following chart based on severity of symptoms of hypocalcemia, the serum calcium level, and the acuity of onset of hypocalcemia.

All doses based on a 10% solution, which yields 10 Gm/100 mL or 100 mg/mL. (1 mL of calcium gluconate contains 9.3 mg [0.465 mEq] of elemental calcium.)

Dosing Recommendations in mg of Calcium Gluconate for Neonate, Pediatric, and Adult Patients			
Patient Population	Initial Dose	Subsequent Doses (if needed)	
		Bolus	Continuous Infusion
Adult	1,000 mg-2,000 mg	1,000 mg-2,000 mg every 6 hr	Initiate at 5.4-21.5 mg/kg/hr
Pediatric (>1 month to <17 years)	29-60 mg/kg	29-60 mg/kg every 6 hr	Initiate at 8-13 mg/kg/hr
Neonate (≤1 month)	100-200 mg/kg	100-200 mg/kg every 6 hr	Initiate at 17-33 mg/kg/hr

For bolus administration, DO NOT exceed a rate of:
- 200 mg/min in adult patients.
- 100 mg/min in pediatric patients.

For continuous infusions, adjust rate as needed based on serum calcium levels.

Calcium channel blocker overdose (unlabeled): 60 mg/kg/dose over 5 to 10 minutes (not to exceed 3,000 to 6,000 mg/dose); may repeat every 10 to 20 minutes for 3 to 4 additional doses. Alternatively, may initiate an infusion at 60 to 150 mg/kg/hr. Titrate to maintain adequate hemodynamic response.

Beta-blocker overdose (unlabeled): 60 mg/kg over 5 to 10 minutes followed by an infusion at 60 to 150 mg/kg/hr. Titrate to maintain adequate hemodynamic response.

PEDIATRIC AND NEONATAL DOSE

See Usual Dose, Precautions/Monitor, and Maternal/Child. ▪ Do not administer into a scalp vein.

DOSE ADJUSTMENTS

For patients with renal impairment, initiate therapy at the lowest dose of the recommended dose range for all age-groups and monitor serum calcium every 4 hours. Accumulation may occur. ▪ Dose selection for the elderly should start at the lowest dose of the recommended dose range, reflecting the potential for decreased organ function and concomitant disease or drug therapy.

DILUTION

Supplied as a 10% solution in single-dose vials or pharmacy bulk packages. May be given by bolus IV administration or as a continuous IV infusion.

Bolus: Dilute required dose in D5W or NS to a final concentration of 10 to 50 mg/mL before administration.

Continuous Infusion: Dilute required dose in D5W or NS to a final concentration of 5.8 to 10 mg/mL before administration. Solution should appear clear and colorless to slightly yellow.

Storage: Store at CRT. Do not freeze. Manufacturer recommends immediate administration of diluted solution. Discard unused portion in singe-dose vial immediately. Discard any unused portion of the pharmacy bulk package within 4 hours of initial entry into the vial. Supersaturated solutions may precipitate. If a precipitate is present, dissolve by warming the vial to 60° to 80° C (140° to 176° F) with occasional agitation until the solution becomes clear. Shake vigorously. Allow to cool to RT before administration.

COMPATIBILITY

Do not mix calcium gluconate with ceftriaxone. Concurrent use can lead to formation of ceftriaxone-calcium precipitates. Calcium-containing solutions and ceftriaxone may be administered sequentially in patients older than 28 days of age provided the infusion lines are thoroughly flushed between infusions with a **compatible** solution. *Do not* administer calcium gluconate and ceftriaxone simultaneously via a Y-site in any age group. Calcium salts should not be mixed with phosphates, bicarbonates, or minocycline. *Extreme caution and a specific multistep process are required when calcium and phosphates are combined in parenteral nutrition solutions. Consult pharmacist.*

Other sources suggest specific **compatibilities** dependent on concentration and manufacturer; consult a pharmacist.

RATE OF ADMINISTRATION

Administer via a secure IV line to avoid calcinosis cutis and tissue necrosis; see Precautions. ▪ Rapid administration may cause vasodilation, decreased BP, bradycardia, cardiac arrhythmias, syncope, and cardiac arrest. May be administered by slow bolus administration or continuous infusion.

Bolus: Administer slowly. *Adult:* DO NOT exceed a rate of 200 mg/min.

Pediatric patients (including neonates): DO NOT exceed a rate of 100 mg/min.

Infusion: Adjust rate as needed based on serum calcium levels. Bolus rates should not be exceeded.

In all situations, stop or slow infusion rate if patient complains of discomfort.

ACTIONS

IV administration of calcium gluconate increases serum ionized calcium level. Ionized calcium and gluconate are normal constituents of body fluids. Calcium in the body is distributed mainly in the skeleton (99%). Only 1% of the total body calcium is distributed within the extracellular fluids and soft tissues. About 50% of total serum calcium is in the ionized form and represents the biologically active part. Calcium plays a role in cardiac, neuromuscular, structural, and blood coagulation systems within the body. It crosses the placental barrier and is secreted in breast milk. It is excreted in the feces and urine.

INDICATIONS AND USES

Treatment of acute symptomatic hypocalcemia in pediatric and adult patients.

Unlabeled uses: Treatment of calcium-channel–blocker overdose (e.g., diltiazem, verapamil).
- Treatment of beta-blocker overdose (e.g., atenolol, metoprolol).

Limitation of Use: Safety for long-term use has not been established.

CONTRAINDICATIONS

Hypercalcemia. ■ Neonates (28 days of age or younger) receiving ceftriaxone.

PRECAUTIONS

Has only one-third the potency of calcium chloride. ■ For IV use only. ■ Cardiac arrhythmias may occur if calcium and cardiac glycosides (e.g., digoxin) are administered together. Hypercalcemia increases the risk of digoxin toxicity. ■ Concomitant use of ceftriaxone and calcium gluconate is contraindicated in neonates due to cases of fatal outcomes in which a crystalline material was observed in the lungs and kidneys at autopsy after ceftriaxone and calcium were administered simultaneously through the same IV line. Concomitant administration can lead to the formation of ceftriaxone-calcium precipitates that may act as emboli, resulting in vascular spasm or infarction; see Contraindications and Compatibility. ■ IV administration and local trauma may result in calcinosis cutis. May occur with or without extravasation and is characterized by abnormal dermal deposits of calcium salts. Serious complications may include tissue necrosis, ulceration, and secondary infection. ■ Rapid administration may cause vasodilation, decreased BP, bradycardia, cardiac arrhythmias, syncope, and cardiac arrest. ■ Calcium gluconate contains aluminum (up to 400 mcg/L). In impaired kidney function, aluminum may reach toxic levels. Premature neonates are particularly at risk because of their immature kidneys and requirement for calcium and phosphate, which also contain aluminum. Research indicates that patients with impaired renal function who receive more than 4 to 5 mcg/kg/day of parenteral aluminum are at risk for developing CNS or bone toxicity associated with aluminum accumulation.

Monitor: Confirm patency of vein; select a large vein and use a small needle to reduce vein irritation. ■ Monitor patient, vital signs, and ECG during administration. ■ Monitor serum calcium every 4 to 6 hours during intermittent (bolus) infusions and every 1 to 4 hours during continuous infusion. More frequent monitoring may be required in patients with renal impairment; see Dose Adjustments. ■ Monitor for calcinosis cutis; may clinically manifest as papules, plaques, or nodules that may be associated with erythema, swelling, or induration ■ Keep patient recumbent after injection to prevent postural hypotension.

Patient Education: Promptly report pain or discomfort at injection site.

Maternal/Child: Safety for use in pregnancy not established; benefits must outweigh risk. There are risks to the mother and the fetus associated with hypocalcemia in pregnancy. ■ Maternal hypocalcemia can result in an increased rate of spontaneous abortion, premature and dysfunctional labor, and possibly pre-eclampsia. ■ Infants born to mothers with hypocalcemia can have associated fetal and neonatal hyperparathyroidism, which in turn can cause fetal and neonatal skeletal demineralization, subperiosteal bone resorption, osteitis fibrosa cystica, and neonatal seizures. Infants born to mothers with hypocalcemia should be carefully monitored for signs of hypocalcemia or hypercalcemia, including neuromuscular irritability, apnea, cyanosis, and cardiac rhythm disorders. ■ Calcium is present in breast milk. There are no data on the effects of calcium gluconate administration on the breast-fed infant or milk production. Consider risk of infant exposure, benefits of breast-feeding to the infant, and benefits of treatment to the mother. ■ Safety and effectiveness of calcium gluconate have been established in pediatric patients for the treatment of acute, symptomatic hypocalcemia. ■ See Precautions and Contraindications.

Elderly: Dose selection should start at the lowest dose of the recommended dose range; see Dose Adjustments.

DRUG/LAB INTERACTIONS

Hypercalcemia increases the risk of **digoxin** toxicity and may cause arrhythmias. If necessary, give small amounts of calcium very slowly. ■ **Calcipotriene, estrogen, teriparatide, thiazide diuretics, vitamin A, and vitamin D** may cause hypercalcemia. Monitor calcium concentration in patients taking these drugs concurrently. ■ Administration of calcium may reduce the response to **calcium channel blockers**.

SIDE EFFECTS

The most common adverse reactions are calcification, calcinosis cutis, local soft tissue inflammation, and necrosis due to extravasation. Bradycardia, cardiac arrest, cardiac arrhythmias, hypotension, syncope, and vasodilation can occur with too-rapid rate of administration. Serious adverse reactions are described in Precautions.

Overdose: Coma, confusion, depression, diminished ability to concentrate urine and diuresis, disorientation, fatigue, hallucinations, hypercalcemia, hypotonicity, seizures, weakness, and sudden death.

ANTIDOTE

If side effects occur, further dilution and decrease in the rate of administration may be necessary. If side effects persist, discontinue the drug and notify the physician. In an overdose situation, immediately discontinue administration and provide supportive treatments to restore intravascular volume and promote calcium excretion in the urine if necessary. Monitoring of fluid, electrolytes, and cardiac and respiratory status is imperative. If extravasation occurs or clinical manifestations of calcinosis cutis are noted, immediately discontinue IV administration at that site. For extravasation, inject affected area with hyaluronidase, using a 25-gauge needle. Apply dry, cold compresses and elevate extremity. Resuscitate as necessary.

CANGRELOR

(**KAN**-grel-or)

Antiplatelet agent

Kengreal

USUAL DOSE

Cangrelor: 30 mcg/kg as an IV **bolus** followed immediately by a 4 mcg/kg/min IV infusion. Initiate the bolus infusion prior to percutaneous coronary intervention (PCI). The maintenance infusion should ordinarily be continued for at least 2 hours or for the duration of PCI, whichever is longer.

Transitioning to oral P2Y$_{12}$ therapy: To maintain platelet inhibition after discontinuation of cangrelor infusion, an oral P2Y$_{12}$ platelet inhibitor should be administered. Administer one as described below:

Ticagrelor (Brilinta): 180 mg at any time during cangrelor infusion or immediately after discontinuation.

Prasugrel (Effient): 60 mg immediately after discontinuation of cangrelor. Do not administer prasugrel before discontinuation of cangrelor.

Clopidogrel (Plavix): 600 mg immediately after discontinuation of cangrelor. Do not administer clopidogrel before discontinuation of cangrelor.

DOSE ADJUSTMENTS

No dose adjustments needed based on sex, age, renal status, or hepatic function. ■ The impact of weight on drug exposure is accounted for by the use of weight-based dosing.

DILUTION

Available as a sterile lyophilized powder in single-use 10-mL vials containing 50 mg cangrelor. Reconstitute each 50-mg vial with 5 mL of SWFI. Swirl gently until all material is dissolved. Avoid vigorous mixing. Allow any foam to settle. Ensure that the contents of the vial are fully dissolved and the reconstituted material is a clear, colorless to pale yellow solution. Before administration, each reconstituted vial must be further diluted with NS or D5W. Withdraw the contents from the reconstituted vial and add to a 250-mL bag of NS or D5W. Mix the bag thoroughly. Final concentration is 200 mcg/mL and should be sufficient for at least 2 hours of dosing. Patients 100 kg and over will require a minimum of 2 bags.

Storage: Store vials of cangrelor at CRT (20° to 25° C [68° to 77° F]), with excursions between 15° and 30° C (59° and 86° F) permitted. Reconstituted cangrelor should be further diluted immediately. Cangrelor is stable at RT for 12 hours diluted in D5W and for 24 hours diluted in NS. Discard any unused portion of reconstituted solution remaining in the vial.

COMPATIBILITY
Manufacturer states, "Administer cangrelor via a dedicated IV line."

RATE OF ADMINISTRATION
Administer cangrelor via a dedicated IV line.

Bolus: Administer the bolus volume rapidly (less than 1 minute) from the diluted bag via manual IV push or pump. Ensure the bolus is completely administered before the start of PCI. Start the infusion immediately after administration of the bolus.

Infusion: Administer at 4 mcg/kg/min. Continue for at least 2 hours or for the duration of PCI, whichever is longer.

ACTIONS
A direct $P2Y_{12}$ platelet receptor inhibitor that blocks adenosine diphosphate (ADP)–induced platelet activation and aggregation. It binds selectively and reversibly to the $P2Y_{12}$ receptor to prevent further signaling and platelet activation. When given according to the recommended regimen, platelet inhibition occurs within 2 minutes. Metabolism of cangrelor is independent of hepatic function and does not interfere with other drugs metabolized by hepatic enzymes. It is deactivated rapidly in the circulation by dephosphorylation to its primary metabolite, a nucleoside that has negligible antiplatelet activity. After discontinuation of the infusion, the antiplatelet effect decreases rapidly and platelet function returns to normal within 1 hour. The average elimination half-life is about 3 to 6 minutes. Excreted in urine and feces.

INDICATIONS AND USES
An adjunct to percutaneous coronary intervention (PCI) to reduce the risk of periprocedural myocardial infarction (MI), repeat coronary revascularization, and stent thrombosis (ST) in patients who have not been treated with a $P2Y_{12}$ platelet inhibitor and are not being given a glycoprotein IIb/IIIa inhibitor.

CONTRAINDICATIONS
Patients with significant active bleeding. ▪ Known hypersensitivity (e.g., anaphylaxis) to cangrelor or any component of the product.

PRECAUTIONS
For IV use only. ▪ Bleeding is the most common complication encountered during therapy. ▪ Drugs that inhibit platelet $P2Y_{12}$ function, including cangrelor, increase the risk of bleeding. ▪ Once cangrelor is discontinued, there is no antiplatelet effect after 1 hour. ▪ Serious hypersensitivity reactions have been reported.

Monitor: Monitor for S/S of bleeding. ▪ Monitor for S/S of hypersensitivity reactions (e.g., anaphylaxis, hypotension, pruritus, rash, urticaria, or wheezing).

Patient Education: Promptly report S/S of a hypersensitivity reaction (e.g., hives, rash, shortness of breath or troubled breathing, swelling of eyelids, lips, or face).

Maternal/Child: Use during pregnancy only if clearly needed. Life-sustaining therapy should not be withheld due to potential concerns regarding effects on the fetus. Use during labor and delivery may increase the risk for maternal bleeding and hemorrhage. Performance of neuraxial blockade procedures is not advised during use of cangrelor due to potential risk of spinal hematoma. When possible, discontinue cangrelor 1 hour before labor, delivery, or neuraxial blockade. ▪ Data not available. Due to its short half life, cangrelor exposure is expected to be very low in the breast-fed infant. ▪ Safety and effectiveness for use in pediatric patients not established.

Elderly: No overall difference in safety or effectiveness between older and younger patients has been observed.

DRUG/LAB INTERACTIONS

If **clopidogrel** or **prasugrel** is administered during cangrelor infusion, it will have no antiplatelet effect until the next dose is administered. Therefore **clopidogrel** and **prasugrel** should not be administered until cangrelor infusion is discontinued. ▪ Administration of **ticagrelor** during cangrelor infusion does not attenuate the antiplatelet effect of ticagrelor. ▪ Coadministration of cangrelor with unfractionated **heparin**, **aspirin**, and **nitroglycerin** was formally studied in healthy subjects, with no evidence of an effect on the pharmacokinetics and pharmacodynamics of cangrelor. ▪ Cangrelor has been coadministered with bivalirudin, low-molecular-weight heparin, clopidogrel, prasugrel, and ticagrelor without clinically detectable interactions.

SIDE EFFECTS

The most common adverse reaction is bleeding.

Coronary artery dissection, coronary artery perforation, and dyspnea were the most frequent events leading to discontinuation of cangrelor. Serious cases of hypersensitivity, including angioedema, anaphylactic reactions, anaphylactic shock, bronchospasm, and stridor, have occurred. Decreased renal function was reported in a small number of patients with severe renal impairment (creatinine clearance less than 30 mL/min).

ANTIDOTE

There is no specific treatment to reverse the antiplatelet effect of cangrelor, but the effect is gone within 1 hour after discontinuation of the drug. Treat anaphylaxis immediately with oxygen, epinephrine, antihistamines, vasopressors, corticosteroids, albuterol, IV fluids, and ventilation equipment as indicated. Resuscitate as necessary.

CARBOPLATIN BBW
(**KAR**-boh-plah-tin)

Antineoplastic
(alkylating agent)

pH 5 to 7

USUAL DOSE

Pretreatment: Baseline studies indicated; see Monitor. See Maternal/Child.

Before giving a dose in a cycle, it is recommended that platelets be above 100,000/mm³ and neutrophils above 2,000/mm³; see Dose Adjustments. The Calvert formula for carboplatin dosing based on pre-existing renal function and/or desired platelet nadir determines the patient's dose.

$$\text{Total dose (mg)} = (\text{Target AUC}) \times (\text{GFR} + 25)$$

Dose is calculated in milligrams, not mg/M². The ordering physician determines the target AUC (area under the curve) and supplies the required information on the GFR (glomerular filtration rate) or CrCl, as well as the desired response. The pharmacist calculates the correct dose. See package insert for additional information.

Initial treatment of advanced ovarian cancer in combination with cyclophosphamide: Carboplatin 300 mg/M² plus cyclophosphamide 600 mg/M² on Day 1 every 4 weeks for 6 cycles or carboplatin dose targeted by Calvert equation to an AUC of 6 to 7 plus cyclophosphamide 600 mg/M² on Day 1 every 4 weeks.

Palliative treatment of recurrent ovarian cancer after prior chemotherapy: *As a single agent:* With normal renal function (CrCl greater than 60 mL/min), give 360 mg/M² on Day 1 every 4 weeks or, alternately, a dose targeted by Calvert equation to an AUC of 4 to 6 appears to provide an appropriate dose range in these patients.

DOSE ADJUSTMENTS

Single agent or combination therapy. Dose adjustment is based on nadir after prior dose according to the following chart.

Carboplatin Dose Based on Bone Marrow Suppression		
Platelets/mm^3	Neutrophils/mm^3	Adjusted Dose (from Prior Course)[a]
>100,000	>2,000	Increase to 125%
50,000-100,000	500-2,000	No adjustment
<50,000	<500	Decrease to 75%

[a]Percentages apply to carboplatin as a single agent or to both carboplatin and cyclophosphamide in combination.

Once the dose has been increased to 125% of the starting dose, no further dose increases are indicated. ▪ With impaired renal function (CrCl 16 to 40 mL/min), give 200 mg/M^2; CrCl 41 to 59 mL/min, give 250 mg/M^2. Dose recommendation not available for patients with a CrCl less than 16 mL/min. ▪ Bone marrow suppression is more severe in patients who have had prior therapy, especially with cisplatin and when carboplatin is used with other bone marrow–suppressing therapies or radiation, and may be more severe in the elderly. Reduced dose may be indicated. Monitor carefully and manage dose and timing to reduce additive effects.

DILUTION

Specific techniques required; see Precautions. Available as a premixed solution (10 mg/mL) and as a lyophilized powder. Immediately before use, reconstitute each 10 mg of carboplatin lyophilized powder with 1 mL of SWFI, D5W, or NS (50 mg with 5 mL, 150 mg with 15 mL, 450 mg with 45 mL). All yield 10 mg/mL. Both preparations may be further diluted with NS or D5W to concentrations as low as 0.5 mg/mL. Do not use needles or IV tubing with aluminum parts to mix or administer; a precipitate will form and decrease potency. Best to mix lyophilized preparation immediately before use.

Storage: *Premixed solutions:* Stable to the date indicated on the package stored at CRT and protected from light. Multidose vials maintain microbial, chemical, and physical stability for up to 14 days at RT (25° C [77° F]) following multiple-needle entries. *Lyophilized powder:* Store unopened vials at CRT. Protect from light. Reconstituted solutions are stable for 8 hours at RT (25° C [77° F]). Discard 8 hours after dilution.

COMPATIBILITY

Forms a precipitate if in contact with aluminum (e.g., needles, syringes, catheters).

Other sources suggest specific **compatibilities** dependent on concentration and manufacturer; consult a pharmacist.

RATE OF ADMINISTRATION

A single dose as an infusion over a minimum of 15 minutes. Extend administration time based on amount of diluent and patient condition.

ACTIONS

An alkylating agent. Better tolerated by patients, carboplatin causes less nausea and vomiting, less neurotoxicity, and less nephrotoxicity than cisplatin. Myelosuppression is generally reversible and manageable with antibiotics and transfusions. Produces interstrand DNA cross-links and is cell-cycle nonspecific. Not bound to plasma proteins. Half-life is 2.6 to 5.9 hours. Majority of carboplatin is excreted in the urine within 24 hours.

INDICATIONS AND USES

Initial treatment of advanced ovarian cancer in combination with other approved chemotherapeutic agents (e.g., cyclophosphamide). ▪ Palliative treatment of recurrent ovarian cancer after prior chemotherapy, including patients treated with cisplatin.

Unlabeled uses: Treatment of bladder cancer, non–small-cell lung cancer, and small-cell lung cancer.

CONTRAINDICATIONS
Hypersensitivity to cisplatin or other platinum-containing compounds or mannitol; severe bone marrow suppression; significant bleeding.

PRECAUTIONS
Follow guidelines for handling cytotoxic agents. See Appendix A. ▪ Usually administered by or under the direction of the physician specialist in a facility with adequate diagnostic and treatment facilities to monitor the patient and respond to any medical emergency. ▪ Bone marrow suppression is dose related and may be severe, resulting in infection and/or bleeding. Anemia may be cumulative and may require transfusion support. Bone marrow suppression increased in patients who have received prior therapy, especially regimens including cisplatin, and in patients with impaired kidney function. ▪ Anaphylaxis has been reported and may occur within minutes of administration. ▪ Risk of hypersensitivity increased in patients previously exposed to platinum therapy. Patients sensitive to other platinum compounds (e.g., cisplatin) may be sensitive to carboplatin; see Contraindications. ▪ Peripheral neurotoxicity is uncommon, but risk may be increased in patients over 65 years of age and in patients previously treated with cisplatin. ▪ Secondary malignancies, including acute nonlymphocytic leukemia, myeloproliferation syndrome, and carcinoma, have been reported in patients treated with alkylating agents. ▪ See Drug/Lab Interactions.

Monitor: BUN and SCr should be done before each dose. CrCl, WBC, platelet count, and hemoglobin are recommended before each dose and weekly thereafter. Platelet count recommended to be 100,000/mm^3 and neutrophils 2,000/mm^3 before a dose can be repeated; see Dose Adjustments. Anemia is frequent and cumulative. Transfusion is often indicated. ▪ Excessive hydration or forced diuresis not required, but maintain adequate hydration and urinary output. ▪ Nausea and vomiting are frequently severe but less than with cisplatin; generally last 24 hours. Prophylactic administration of antiemetics is indicated. Various protocols are used. ▪ Observe for symptoms of hypersensitivity reactions during administration; epinephrine, corticosteroids, and antihistamines should be available. ▪ Observe closely for symptoms of infection. Prophylactic antibiotics may be indicated pending results of C/S in a febrile neutropenic patient. ▪ Monitor for thrombocytopenia (platelet count less than 50,000/mm^3). Initiate precautions to prevent excessive bleeding (e.g., inspect IV sites, skin, and mucous membranes; use extreme care during invasive procedures; test urine, emesis, stool, and secretions for occult blood).

Patient Education: Effective birth control recommended. Manufacturer provides a patient information booklet. ▪ See Appendix D.

Maternal/Child: Category D: avoid pregnancy. ▪ Discontinue breast-feeding. ▪ Safety and effectiveness for use in pediatric patients not established. ▪ Significant hearing loss has been reported in pediatric patients; occurred with higher-than-recommended doses of carboplatin in combination with other ototoxic agents.

Elderly: Neurotoxicity and myelotoxicity may be more severe. ▪ Consider possibility of decreased renal function. ▪ See Dose Adjustments and Precautions.

DRUG/LAB INTERACTIONS
Nephrotoxicity and ototoxicity are additive when used with other **ototoxic or nephrotoxic agents** (e.g., acyclovir, aminoglycosides [e.g., gentamicin], cisplatin, rifampin, quinidine). Use with caution. ▪ Bone marrow toxicity increased with other **antineoplastic agents, radiation therapy, and/or other agents that may cause blood dyscrasias** (e.g., anticonvulsants [e.g., phenytoin], cephalosporins, mycophenolate, rituximab). Dose adjustment of either or both drugs may be indicated. ▪ Do not administer **live virus vaccines** to patients receiving antineoplastic drugs. ▪ See Dose Adjustments.

SIDE EFFECTS
Allergic reactions, including anaphylaxis, can occur during administration. Alopecia (rare), anemia, anorexia, bleeding, bone marrow suppression (usually reversible), bronchospasm, bruising, changes in taste, constipation, death, decreased serum electrolytes, decreased urine output, dehydration, diarrhea, erythema, fatigue, fever, hemolytic uremic

syndrome (rare, cancer-associated), hypotension, infection, laboratory test abnormalities (alkaline phosphatase, aspartate aminotransferase [AST], BUN, SCr, total bilirubin), nausea and vomiting (severe), neutropenia, ototoxicity, peripheral neuropathies, pruritus, rash, stomatitis, thrombocytopenia, urticaria, visual disturbances, weakness.

ANTIDOTE

Notify physician of all side effects. Symptomatic and supportive treatment is indicated. Withhold carboplatin until myelosuppression has resolved. Administration of whole blood products (e.g., packed RBCs, platelets, leukocytes) may be required. Blood modifiers (e.g., darbepoetin alfa, epoetin alfa, filgrastim, pegfilgrastim, sargramostim) may be indicated to treat bone marrow toxicity. Treat anaphylaxis with epinephrine, corticosteroids, oxygen, and antihistamines. There is no specific antidote.

CARMUSTINE (BCNU) BBW

(kar-**MUS**-teen)

BiCNU

Antineoplastic
(alkylating agent/
nitrosourea)

pH 5.6 to 6

USUAL DOSE

Pretreatment: Verify nonpregnancy status. Baseline testing and studies required; see Monitor.

Premedication: Administration of antiemetics is recommended.

Carmustine: Initial dose as a single agent in previously untreated patients is 150 to 200 mg/M^2. May be given as a single dose, or one-half of the calculated dose may be given initially and repeated the next day. Repeat every 6 weeks if bone marrow is sufficiently recovered. Repeat course should not be administered until leukocytes are above 4,000/mm³, platelets are above 100,000/mm³, and ANC is above 1,000/mm³. Subsequent doses should be adjusted according to hematologic response of previous dose (see Dose Adjustments).

DOSE ADJUSTMENTS

Bone marrow toxicity can be delayed and cumulative. Dose adjustments must be considered *based on the nadir blood counts from the prior dose* according to the following chart. Do not administer a repeat course of carmustine until blood counts recover.

Carmustine Dose Adjustment Based on Bone Marrow Suppression		
Nadir After Prior Dose		**Percentage of Prior Dose to Be Given**
Leukocytes/mm³	Platelets/mm³	%
≥4,000	≥100,000	100%
3,000-3,999	75,000-99,999	100%
2,000-2,999	25,000-74,999	70%
<2,000	<25,000	50%

Lower doses accordingly when carmustine is used in combination with other myelosuppressive drugs or in patients with depleted bone marrow reserve. ■ Do not administer carmustine to patients with compromised renal function. Carmustine should be discontinued in patients with a CrCl less than 10 mL/min. ▪ Dosing should be cautious in the elderly. Lower-end initial doses may be indicated. Consider decrease in cardiac, hepatic, and renal function; concomitant disease; or other drug therapy; see Elderly.

DILUTION

Specific techniques required; see Precautions. Initially dilute 100-mg vial with supplied sterile diluent (3 mL of dehydrated alcohol injection). Further dilute with 27 mL of SWFI. Each mL will contain 3.3 mg carmustine. The reconstituted solution should be a clear, colorless to yellowish solution. Withdraw desired dose and further dilute in up to 500 mL of NS or D5W and give as an infusion. A concentration of 0.2 mg/mL is desired. Use glass or polypropylene containers.

Filters: No significant loss of potency with any size cellular ester membrane filter when reconstituted or diluted as recommended.

Storage: Must be protected from light in all forms. Store unopened vials of the dry drug (carmustine) and supplied diluent in refrigerator (2° to 8° C [36° to 46° F]). After reconstitution as directed, carmustine is stable for 24 hours under refrigeration. Reconstituted vials should be examined for crystal formation before use. If crystals have formed, they may be redissolved by warming the vial to RT with agitation. After reconstitution and after further dilution to a concentration of 0.2 mg/mL in NS or D5W, may be stored at RT but must be used within 8 hours. Fully diluted solution may also be stored under refrigeration for 24 hours and an additional 6 hours at RT. Temperatures above 30.5° C (86.9° F) will cause liquefaction of the drug powder; discard immediately. Product is intended for single use. Discard any unused solution.

COMPATIBILITY

Manufacturer lists as **incompatible** with polyvinyl chloride infusion bags; use only glass or polypropylene containers. Ensure polypropylene containers are PVC-free and DEHP-free.

Other sources suggest a few specific **compatibilities** dependent on concentration and manufacturer; consult a pharmacist.

RATE OF ADMINISTRATION

Each single dose must be given as a slow IV infusion over at least 2 hours. Administration over fewer than 2 hours can lead to pain and burning at the injection site. The rate of administration should not exceed 1.66 mg/M^2/min. Reduce rate for pain or burning at injection site, flushing of the skin, or suffusion of the conjunctiva.

ACTIONS

An alkylating agent of the nitrosourea group with antitumor activity, cell-cycle phase nonspecific. Exact mechanism of action is unknown. Alkylates DNA and RNA and may inhibit several key enzymatic processes. Metabolites may contribute to antineoplastic and toxic activities. Effectively crosses the blood-brain barrier. Elimination half-life ranges from 15 to 75 minutes. Excreted in changed form in urine. Small amounts excreted as respiratory CO_2.

INDICATIONS AND USES

Palliative therapy as a single agent or in established combination therapies in the treatment of brain tumors, multiple myeloma, Hodgkin lymphoma, and some non-Hodgkin lymphomas.

CONTRAINDICATIONS

Hypersensitivity to carmustine or its components.

PRECAUTIONS

Follow guidelines for handling cytotoxic agents. See Appendix A. ▪ Administered by or under the direction of the physician specialist. ▪ Delayed bone marrow suppression, notably thrombocytopenia and leukopenia, is a dose-limiting, common, and severe toxic effect of carmustine. May contribute to bleeding and overwhelming infection. ▪ Pulmonary toxicity is dose related. Risk is increased with a cumulative dose greater than 1,400 mg/M^2. Other risk factors include a past history of lung disease and duration of treatment. Toxicity is characterized by pulmonary infiltrates and/or fibrosis. Delayed-onset pulmonary toxicity has occurred years after treatment and can result in death, particularly in patients who received it in childhood or early adolescence. ▪ Secondary malignancies, including acute leukemia and bone marrow dysplasias, have been reported in patients treated with alkylating agents.

Monitor: Determine absolute patency and quality of vein and adequate circulation of extremity. Severe cellulitis may result from extravasation. ▪ Obtain baseline CBC, including leukocyte and platelet counts. Monitor weekly for at least 6 weeks after each dose. Wait at least 6 weeks between doses. Thrombocytopenia occurs at about 4 weeks postadministration, and leukopenia occurs at about 5 to 6 weeks. Each persists for 1 to 2 weeks. ▪ Obtain baseline pulmonary function studies and monitor pulmonary function frequently during treatment. Risk of pulmonary toxicity is increased in patients with a baseline below 70% of the predicted forced vital capacity (FVC) or carbon monoxide diffusing capacity (DLco). ▪ Obtain baseline and periodic SCr. Monitor patients with compromised renal function closely for toxicity; see Dose Adjustments. ▪ Periodic monitoring of liver function tests is recommended. ▪ Nausea and vomiting can be severe. Prophylactic administration of antiemetics recommended. ▪ Avoid contact of carmustine solution with the skin. Immediately wash the skin or mucosa with soap and water if contact occurs. ▪ Observe for any signs of infection. Prophylactic antibiotics may be indicated pending results of C/S in a febrile neutropenic patient. ▪ Maintain hydration. ▪ Monitor for thrombocytopenia (platelet count less than 50,000/mm^3). Initiate precautions to prevent excessive bleeding (e.g., inspect IV sites, skin, and mucous membranes; use extreme care during invasive procedures; test urine, emesis, stool, and secretions for occult blood). ▪ Long-term monitoring for the development of secondary malignancies is recommended.

Patient Education: Avoid pregnancy. Females of reproductive potential should use highly effective contraception during treatment and for at least 6 months after completion of therapy. Males of reproductive potential should use effective contraception during treatment and for at least 3 months after completion of therapy. ▪ Male fertility may be compromised. ▪ Promptly report stinging or burning at IV site. ▪ Weekly laboratory monitoring required. ▪ Promptly report shortness of breath, cough, or other S/S of pulmonary toxicity. ▪ Seek medical attention in the event of a seizure. ▪ See Appendix D.

Maternal/Child: Avoid pregnancy. Can cause fetal harm based on mechanism of action and findings in animals. ▪ Discontinue breast-feeding. ▪ Safety and effectiveness for use in pediatric patients not established. Risk versus benefit must be carefully considered due to a high risk of pulmonary toxicity occurring years after treatment and resulting in death.

Elderly: Dose selection should be cautious; see Dose Adjustments. ▪ Toxicity may be increased. ▪ Monitoring of renal function is suggested.

DRUG/LAB INTERACTIONS

Potentiated by **cimetidine**; increased myelosuppression (e.g., leukopenia and neutropenia) have been reported with concurrent use. ▪ Phenobarbital induces the metabolism of carmustine and may compromise its antitumor activity. ▪ Inhibits **digoxin and phenytoin;**

may reduce serum levels. ▪ Do not administer **vaccines** to patients receiving antineoplastic drugs. ▪ See Dose Adjustments.

SIDE EFFECTS

The most common adverse reactions are myelosuppression, nausea, pneumonitis, pulmonary toxicity, renal toxicity, and vomiting. Many reactions are dose related and can be reversed. Bone marrow toxicity (especially leukopenia and thrombocytopenia) is most pronounced at 4 to 6 weeks; can be severe and cumulative with repeated dosage. Other reported reactions include acute leukemia and bone marrow dysplasias (following long-term therapy), anemia, anorexia, blurred vision, chest pain, conjunctival edema and hemorrhage, diarrhea, elevated liver function test, encephalopathy, flushing of skin and suffusion of conjunctiva from too-rapid infusion rate, gynecomastia, headache, hyperpigmentation and burning of skin (from actual contact with solution), hypersensitivity reactions, hypotension, loss of depth perception, nausea and vomiting, neuroretinitis, opportunistic infections, pulmonary infiltrates or fibrosis, renal abnormalities, seizures, tachycardia, and veno-occlusive disease.

ANTIDOTE

Notify physician of all side effects. Most will decrease in severity with reduced dosage, increased time span between doses, or symptomatic treatment. May reduce therapeutic effectiveness. Bone marrow suppression may require withholding carmustine until recovery occurs. Administration of whole blood products (e.g., packed RBCs, platelets, leukocytes) may be required. Blood modifiers (e.g., darbepoetin alfa, epoetin alfa, filgrastim, pegfilgrastim, sargramostim) may be indicated to treat bone marrow toxicity. There is no specific antidote. Supportive therapy as indicated will help sustain the patient in toxicity.

CASIMERSEN
Antisense oligonucleotide
(**KAS**-i-**MER**-sen)

Amondys 45   pH 7.5

USUAL DOSE

30 mg/kg once a week.

PEDIATRIC DOSE

30 mg/kg/dose once a week.

DOSE ADJUSTMENTS

Renal: No dosage adjustments provided by manufacturer.
Hepatic: No dosage adjustments provided by manufacturer.

DILUTION

Allow vials to reach room temperature before dilution. Inspect for particulate matter before and after dilution; do not use if small particles are observed. Mix contents of each vial by inverting 2 or 3 times; *do not shake*. Use a 21-gauge or smaller needle to withdraw calculated volume, and dilute with NS to a total volume of 100 to 150 mL. Gently invert 2 or 3 times to mix.

COMPATIBILITY

Do not administer simultaneously with any other medication or IV solutions other than NS.

RATE OF ADMINISTRATION

Administer as an IV infusion over 35 to 60 minutes immediately after dilution. Use a 0.2-micron filter attached to primary IV tubing. Complete infusion within 4 hours.

ACTIONS

Casimersen binds exon 45 of dystrophin premessenger RNA. This results in exclusion of this exon during mRNA procession, which allows for production of internally truncated dystrophin protein in patients with genetic mutations that are amenable to exon 45 skipping.

INDICATIONS AND USES

Duchenne muscular dystrophy (DMD) in patients who have a confirmed mutation of the DMD gene that is amenable to exon 45 skipping.

CONTRAINDICATIONS

None listed.

PRECAUTIONS

Kidney toxicity: Nephrotoxicity, including potentially fatal glomerulonephritis, has been reported; monitor kidney function. Serum creatinine may not be a reliable measure of renal function in patients with DMD; refer to a nephrologist.

Monitor: Monitor for signs/symptoms of renal disfunction. Monitor proteinuria by dipstick urinalysis (baseline and monthly), and monitor serum cystatin C and urine protein-to-creatinine ratio (baseline and every 3 months). Monitor for hypersensitivity reactions during infusion.

Patient Education: Notify physician of signs of cold; cough; fever; dizziness; headache; joint pain; mouth, ear, or throat pain; stomach upset; or signs of allergic reaction (hives; rash; chest tightness; trouble breathing or swallowing; swelling of mouth, face, lips, tongue, or throat; unusual hoarseness).

Maternal/Child: DMD usually affects males, so no pregnancy information is available. The risk versus benefit of breast-feeding should be considered.

Elderly: No specific problems documented.

DRUG/LAB INTERACTIONS

No known significant interactions.

SIDE EFFECTS

Nausea, dizziness, headache, arthralgia, otalgia, otitis media, cough, oropharyngeal pain, upper respiratory infection, fever.

ANTIDOTE

Discontinue infusion and treat appropriately for severe hypersensitivity reactions or severe renal toxicity.

CASPOFUNGIN ACETATE

(**kas**-po-**FUN**-jin **AS**-ah-tayt)

Cancidas

Antifungal
(echinocandin)

pH 6.6

USUAL DOSE

Pretreatment: Verify pregnancy status. Baseline studies indicated; see Monitor.

Empirical therapy: 70 mg as an infusion on Day 1. Beginning on Day 2, reduce subsequent doses to 50 mg/day. Duration of empiric therapy is based on clinical response and should continue at least until resolution of neutropenia. Patients found to have a fungal infection should be treated for a minimum of 14 days after the last positive culture; treatment should continue for at least 7 days after both neutropenia and clinical symptoms have resolved.

Candidemia and other *Candida* infections: 70 mg as an infusion on Day 1. Beginning on Day 2, reduce subsequent doses to 50 mg/day. Duration of treatment is based on clinical and microbiologic response. Usually continued for at least 14 days after the last positive culture. Persistently neutropenic patients may require a longer course of therapy pending resolution of the neutropenia.

Esophageal candidiasis: 50 mg daily as an infusion. Continue for 7 to 14 days after symptom resolution. A 70-mg loading dose has not been studied for this indication. Suppressive oral therapy following treatment with caspofungin may be considered to decrease the risk of relapse of oropharyngeal candidiasis in patients with HIV infections.

Invasive aspergillosis: 70 mg as an infusion on Day 1. Beginning on Day 2, reduce subsequent doses to 50 mg/day. Duration of treatment is based on severity of the underlying disease, recovery from immunosuppression, and clinical response.

PEDIATRIC DOSE

Pediatric patients 3 months to 17 years of age (for all indications): 70 mg/M^2 as an infusion on Day 1. Beginning on Day 2, reduce subsequent doses to 50 mg/M^2/day. Regardless of the patient's calculated dose, the loading dose and/or the daily maintenance dose should not exceed a maximum of 70 mg. Duration of therapy for each indication should be individualized as outlined in Usual Dose.

DOSE ADJUSTMENTS

All diagnoses: *Adult and pediatric patients:* Dose adjustment is not indicated based on age, gender, or race. ▪ See Drug/Lab Interactions.

Adults: Dose adjustment is not indicated in patients with impaired renal function or in patients with mild impaired hepatic function (Child-Pugh score 5 to 6). ▪ In patients with moderate hepatic insufficiency (Child-Pugh score 7 to 9), reduce daily doses to 35 mg with a 70-mg loading dose administered on Day 1 where appropriate. ▪ Dose may be increased from 50 to 70 mg daily in empirically treated febrile neutropenic patients who are not clinically responding to the 50-mg dose; experience is limited. ▪ In patients receiving concurrent administration of rifampin, increase the daily dose to 70 mg. An increase in the daily dose to 70 mg/day should be considered in patients who are not clinically responding and are taking other inducers and/or mixed inducers/inhibitors of caspofungin clearance, specifically carbamazepine, dexamethasone, efavirenz, nevirapine, and phenytoin.

Pediatric patients: If the 50-mg/M^2 daily dose is well tolerated but does not provide adequate clinical response, it may be increased to 70 mg/M^2 (not to exceed a total dose of 70 mg). ▪ There is no experience in pediatric patients with any degree of hepatic insufficiency. ▪ In pediatric patients receiving concurrent administration of rifampin (Rifadin), increase the daily dose to 70 mg/M^2 (not to exceed an actual daily dose of 70 mg). Consider a daily dose of 70 mg/M^2 (not to exceed a total dose of 70 mg) in pediatric patients receiving other inducers of caspofungin clearance, specifically carbamazepine, dexamethasone, efavirenz, nevirapine, and phenytoin.

DILUTION

Available in 70-mg and 50-mg single-dose vials. Select appropriate vial size. If refrigerated product is used, allow vial to come to room temperature. Reconstitute selected dose with 10.8 mL of NS, SWFI, or BWFI. Mix gently to achieve a clear solution; should dissolve completely. The 70-mg vial will yield 7 mg/mL, and the 50-mg vial will yield 5 mg/mL.

Adults: Based on the concentrations noted above, withdraw the appropriate volume required to provide the correct dose and add to an IV bag or bottle containing 250 mL of NS, ½NS, ¼NS, or LR for infusion. In fluid-restricted or pediatric patients, the appropriate volume of caspofungin may be added to reduced volumes of the above solutions, not to exceed a final concentration of 0.5 mg/mL.

Pediatric patients: The choice of vial used should be based on the total dose to be administered. Pediatric doses less than 50 mg should be withdrawn from a 50-mg vial, if available, to ensure accuracy. After reconstitution, withdraw the volume required to provide the correct dose, and add to a volume of NS, ½NS, ¼NS, or LR for infusion to achieve a final concentration not to exceed 0.5 mg/mL.

Storage: *Cancidas:* Refrigerate unopened vials. *Generic:* Store at CRT.

Reconstituted vials of either product may be stored at or below 25° C (77° F) for 1 hour before preparing as an infusion solution. Discard any unused reconstituted solution. Fully diluted solutions may be stored at or below 25° C (77° F) for 24 hours or refrigerated for 48 hours.

COMPATIBILITY

Manufacturer states, "Do not mix or co-infuse caspofungin with other medications. Do not use diluents containing dextrose."

Other sources suggest specific **compatibilities** dependent on concentration and manufacturer; consult a pharmacist.

RATE OF ADMINISTRATION

A single dose as an infusion evenly distributed over 1 hour. **Do not** administer by IV bolus administration.

ACTIONS

An echinocandin antifungal. A glucan synthesis inhibitor. It inhibits the synthesis of beta (1,3)-D-glucan, an essential component of the cell wall of susceptible *Aspergillus* and *Candida* species. Beta (1,3)-D-glucan is not found in human cells. Extensively bound to albumin (97%). After completion of an IV infusion, plasma concentrations decline in several phases, each with its own half-life (e.g., β-phase: 9 to 11 hours; γ-phase: 40 to 50 hours). Distribution, rather than excretion or biotransformation, is the primary mechanism influencing plasma clearance. Slowly metabolized by hydrolysis and *N*-acetylation. Excreted in urine and feces.

INDICATIONS AND USES

The following indications apply to adult and pediatric patients 3 months of age and older.

Empirical therapy for presumed fungal infections in febrile, neutropenic patients. ▪ Treatment of invasive aspergillosis in patients who are refractory to or intolerant of other therapies (i.e., amphotericin B and/or itraconazole). *Limitation of use:* Has not been studied for initial therapy for invasive aspergillosis. ▪ Treatment of esophageal candidiasis. *Limitation of use:* Has not been approved for the treatment of oropharyngeal candidiasis. ▪ Treatment of candidemia and the following *Candida* infections: intra-abdominal abscesses, peritonitis, and pleural space infections. *Limitation of use:* Has not been studied in endocarditis, osteomyelitis, and meningitis due to *Candida*.

CONTRAINDICATIONS

Known hypersensitivity to caspofungin or any of its components.

PRECAUTIONS

Concomitant use with cyclosporine is not recommended unless the potential benefit outweighs the risk; see Monitor and Drug/Lab Interactions. ▪ Abnormal LFTs have been seen in healthy volunteers and in adult and pediatric patients treated with caspofungin. In some patients with serious underlying conditions who were receiving multiple concomitant medications with caspofungin, isolated cases of clinically significant hepatic dysfunction, hepatitis, and hepatic failure have been reported. A causal relationship to caspofungin has not been established. ▪ There is no clinical experience in adult patients with severe hepatic insufficiency (Child-Pugh score greater than 9) or in pediatric patients with any degree of hepatic impairment. ▪ Hypersensitivity reactions, including anaphylaxis, have been reported. ▪ Histamine-mediated reactions, including angioedema, bronchospasm, facial swelling, pruritus, rash, and sensation of warmth, have also been reported. ▪ Cases of Stevens-Johnson syndrome (SJS) and toxic epidermal necrolysis (TEN), some with a fatal outcome, have been reported. Use caution in patients with a history of allergic skin reactions. ▪ Clinical failures due to drug resistance in patients receiving caspofungin therapy have been reported.

Monitor: Most patients have serious underlying medical conditions (e.g., bone marrow transplant, HIV, malignancies) requiring multiple concomitant medications. Obtain baseline studies as required and repeat as indicated. ▪ Monitor vital signs. ▪ Observe for S/S of a hypersensitivity/histamine-mediated reaction (e.g., angioedema, bronchospasm, facial swelling, pruritus, rash, sensation of warmth). ▪ Monitor liver function tests (e.g., AST, ALT). Evaluate risk versus benefit of continuing therapy in patients with evidence of worsening hepatic function. ▪ Monitor liver function in patients receiving therapy with both caspofungin and cyclosporine. Risk/benefit of continued concomitant therapy should be evaluated in patients who develop abnormal liver function tests. ▪ See Drug/Lab Interactions.

Patient Education: Review all medical conditions and medications before beginning treatment. ▪ Promptly report pain at infusion site, symptoms of hypersensitivity reactions (e.g., angioedema, bronchospasm, facial swelling, pruritus, rash, sensation of warmth), or hepatic toxicity (e.g., jaundice). ▪ Advise of the potential risk to a fetus. Inform health care provider if pregnant, become pregnant, or are thinking about becoming pregnant. ▪ Inform health care provider if plan to breast-feed infant.

Maternal/Child: Based on animal studies, may cause fetal harm. ▪ There are no data on the presence of caspofungin in human milk, the effects on the breast-fed child, or the effects on milk production. Has been found in the milk of lactating, drug-treated rats. ▪ Safety and effectiveness for use in neonates and infants under 3 months of age has not been established.

Elderly: Response similar to that in younger patients. Dose adjustment is not required; however, greater sensitivity of some older individuals cannot be ruled out.

DRUG/LAB INTERACTIONS

Concomitant use with **cyclosporine** is not recommended unless benefit outweighs risk. An increase in the AUC of caspofungin and increases in liver function tests have been reported. ▪ Pharmacokinetics of caspofungin are not altered by **amphotericin B, itraconazole, mycophenolate, nelfinavir, or tacrolimus**. ▪ Serum concentrations of tacrolimus may be somewhat decreased with concomitant administration; monitor tacrolimus concentrations and adjust dose as indicated. ▪ **Inducers of caspofungin clearance** (e.g., carbamazepine, dexamethasone, efavirenz, nevirapine, phenytoin, rifampin) may significantly increase caspofungin clearance and necessitate an increase in caspofungin dose; see Dose Adjustments.

SIDE EFFECTS

Side effect profile is similar in both adult and pediatric patients. Incidence difficult to assess because of multiple medical conditions and multiple medications. The most commonly reported side effects include chills, diarrhea, elevated liver function tests (e.g., alkaline phosphatase, ALT, AST), fever, hypokalemia, hypotension, and rash. Other side effects reported include abdominal pain; anemia; ARDS; central line infection; cough; decreased hematocrit, hemoglobin, and WBC; diaphoresis; dyspnea; erythema; flushing; headache; hyperbilirubinemia; hypercalcemia; hyperglycemia; hyperkalemia; hypertension; hypomagnesemia; increased BUN/SCr; increased RBCs and protein in urine; infusion-related reactions; injection site reactions; mucosal inflammation; nausea; peripheral edema; phlebitis; pneumonia; pulmonary edema; radiographic infiltrates; respiratory failure; tachycardia; tachypnea; and vomiting. Possible histamine-mediated/hypersensitivity reactions (e.g., angioedema, bronchospasm, facial swelling, pruritus, rash, sensation of warmth) and anaphylaxis have been reported.

Post-Marketing: Erythema multiforme, hepatic necrosis, hepatobiliary adverse reactions (e.g., clinically significant hepatic dysfunction, hepatitis, hepatic failure) in adult and pediatric patients with serious underlying medical conditions, increased gamma-glutamyl transferase, pancreatitis, peripheral edema, renal dysfunction (clinically significant), skin exfoliation, Stevens-Johnson syndrome, swelling, and toxic epidermal necrolysis.

ANTIDOTE

Notify physician of all side effects; most will be treated symptomatically. Discontinue caspofungin and notify physician of abnormal liver function tests progressing to clinical S/S of liver disease. Rash may be the first sign of an exfoliative skin disorder in immunocompromised patients; discontinue caspofungin and notify physician. Histamine-mediated reactions may require discontinuation of caspofungin and/or appropriate treatment. Discontinue caspofungin at the first S/S of a serious hypersensitivity reaction. Treat anaphylaxis as indicated. Resuscitate as necessary. Not removed by hemodialysis.

CEFAZOLIN SODIUM
(sef-**AYZ**-oh-lin **SO**-dee-um)

Antibacterial
(cephalosporin)

Ancef, Kefzol

pH 4.5 to 7

USUAL DOSE

Pretreatment: Baseline studies indicated; see Monitor.

Cefazolin: 250 mg to 2 Gm every 8 hours. Up to 6 Gm is usual, but 12 Gm in 24 hours has been used, depending on severity of infection.

Mild infections: 250 to 500 mg every 8 hours.

Moderate to severe infections: 500 mg to 1 Gm every 8 hours.

Life-threatening infections (e.g., endocarditis, septicemia): 2 Gm every 8 hours.

Pneumococcal pneumonia: 500 mg every 12 hours.

Acute, uncomplicated urinary tract infections: 1 Gm every 12 hours.

Perioperative prophylaxis: 1 to 2 Gm 30 minutes to 1 hour before incision. For lengthy procedures (e.g., 2 hours or more), 0.5 to 1 Gm may be repeated in the OR. Administer every 6 to 8 hours for 24 hours postoperatively.

Endocarditis prophylaxis (unlabeled): 1 Gm 30 minutes before surgery.

PEDIATRIC DOSE

Mild to moderate infections: 25 to 100 mg/kg/day, divided every 8 hours. Maximum daily dose is 6 gm/day.

Severe infections: 100-150 mg/kg/day divided every 6-8 hours; maximum daily dose 12 gm/day.

Perioperative prophylaxis: The manufacturer does not provide dosage recommendations in pediatric patients. However, one source recommends 30 mg/kg (not to exceed 2 Gm) administered within 60 minutes of the surgical incision.

Endocarditis prophylaxis (unlabeled): 50 mg/kg 30 minutes before the start of surgery. Do not exceed 1 Gm.

NEONATAL DOSE

See Maternal/Child. American Academy of Pediatrics (AAP) recommends:

7 days of age or younger regardless of weight: 25 mg/kg every 12 hours.

8 to 28 days of age; weight 2 kg or less: 25 mg/kg every 12 hours.

8 to 28 days of age; weight more than 2 kg: 25 mg/kg every 8 hours.

DOSE ADJUSTMENTS

Reduced doses or extended intervals may be indicated in the elderly; consider age-related impaired organ function, nutritional status, and concomitant disease or drug therapy. In impaired renal function, the initial dose in adults and pediatric patients should be as above. Reduce all subsequent doses according to the following charts.

Cefazolin Dose Guidelines in Impaired Renal Function for Adults		
CrCl	**Dose**	**Frequency**
CrCl >55 mL/min	Full	Normal
CrCl 35–54 mL/min	Full	q 8 hr or less frequently
CrCl 11–34 mL/min	½ Usual dose	q 12 hr
CrCl 10 mL/min	½ Usual dose	q 18–24 hr

Cefazolin Dose Guidelines in Impaired Renal Function for Pediatric Patients		
Creatinine Clearance (mL/min)	Dose	Frequency
>70 mL/min	Full	Normal
41–70 mL/min	60% of normal daily dose[a]	q 12 hr
21–40 mL/min	25% of normal daily dose[a]	q 12 hr
5–20 mL/min	10% of normal daily dose[a]	q 24 hr

[a]In equally divided doses.

DILUTION

Each 1 Gm or fraction thereof of the lyophilized powder must be reconstituted with at least 2.5 mL of SWFI. Shake well. To reduce the incidence of thrombophlebitis, may be further diluted in 50 to 100 mL of D5W, NS, or other **compatible** infusion solutions (see chart on inside back cover or literature) and given as an intermittent infusion. Available in several forms (other than vials of lyophilized powder), including dual-chamber DUPLEX containers with dextrose, premixed with dextrose in a frozen Galaxy container, Add-Vantage vials, and pharmacy bulk vials. Refer to manufacturer's prescribing information for specific preparation and storage requirements.

Storage: Before reconstitution of the lyophilized powder, protect from light and store at CRT. Give within 24 hours of preparation if stored at CRT or within 10 days if under refrigeration. Discard pharmacy bulk vials within 4 hours after initial entry.

COMPATIBILITY

May be used concomitantly with aminoglycosides (e.g., amikacin, gentamicin), but these drugs must never be mixed in the same infusion (mutual inactivation). If given concurrently, administer separately and flush IV line before and after administration.

Other sources suggest specific **compatibilities** dependent on concentration and manufacturer; consult a pharmacist.

RATE OF ADMINISTRATION

IV injection: Over 3 to 5 minutes.

Intermittent infusion: Extend administration time as indicated by amount of solution and condition of patient. Usually administered over 30 to 60 minutes.

ACTIONS

A semi-synthetic, first-generation cephalosporin antibiotic that is bactericidal through inhibition of cell wall synthesis to some gram-positive and gram-negative organisms, including staphylococci and streptococci. Peak serum levels achieved by end of infusion. Widely distributed in most tissues and body fluids (CSF minimal), including bone, gallbladder, myocardium, and skin and soft tissue. Serum half-life is 1.8 hours. Excreted rapidly in the urine. Crosses the placental barrier. Secreted in breast milk.

INDICATIONS AND USES

Treatment of serious infections of the bone, joints, skin, soft tissue, respiratory tract, biliary tract, and GU tract; septicemia; and endocarditis. Effective only if the causative organism is susceptible. ▪ Perioperative prophylaxis.

Unlabeled uses: Prophylaxis of bacterial endocarditis.

CONTRAINDICATIONS

Previous immediate hypersensitivity reaction (e.g., anaphylaxis, serious skin reactions) to cefazolin or the cephalosporin class of antibiotics, penicillins, or other beta-lactams; see Precautions. ▪ Premixed solutions containing dextrose may be contraindicated in patients with known allergies to corn or corn products.

PRECAUTIONS

Hypersensitivity reactions, including fatalities, have been reported and include reports of individuals with a history of penicillin hypersensitivity or sensitivity to multiple allergens experiencing severe reactions when treated with cephalosporins. Check history of previous hypersensitivity reactions to penicillins, cephalosporins, or other allergens. Actual incidence of cross-allergenicity not established but may be more common with first-generation cephalosporins. ■ Hypersensitivity reactions have been reported with administration of corn-derived, dextrose-containing products to patients with or without a history of hypersensitivity to corn products. Cefazolin in the DUPLEX and Galaxy containers contains dextrose. ■ Sensitivity studies indicated to determine susceptibility of the causative organisms to cefazolin. ■ To reduce the development of drug-resistant bacteria and maintain its effectiveness, cefazolin should be used to treat or prevent only those infections proven or strongly suspected to be caused by bacteria. ■ Continue antibiotic therapy for at least 2 to 3 days after all symptoms of infection subside. ■ Avoid prolonged use of drug; superinfection caused by overgrowth of nonsusceptible organisms may result. ■ Use caution in patients with impaired renal function, allergies, or a history of GI disease (especially colitis). ■ With inappropriately high doses, seizures may occur in patients with impaired renal function. ■ May be associated with an elevated INR, especially in patients with impaired renal or hepatic function, those with a poor nutritional state, and those receiving extended courses of antimicrobial therapy. ■ *Clostridium difficile*–associated diarrhea (CDAD) has been reported. May range from mild diarrhea to fatal colitis. Consider in patients who present with diarrhea during or after treatment with cefazolin.

Monitor: Obtain baseline PT/INR and monitor, especially in at-risk patients (see Precautions); vitamin K may be indicated. ■ Watch for early symptoms of hypersensitivity reactions. ■ See Drug/Lab Interactions; additional monitoring may be indicated (e.g., renal function, drug serum levels, PT/INR).

Patient Education: Report promptly any bleeding or bruising, diarrhea, or symptoms of hypersensitivity (e.g., difficulty breathing, hives, itching, rash). ■ Promptly report diarrhea or bloody stools that occur during treatment or up to several months after an antibiotic has been discontinued; may indicate CDAD and require treatment.

Maternal/Child: Category B: safety for use during pregnancy and breast-feeding not established. No problems documented. ■ Safety for use in premature infants and neonates under 1 month of age not established; immature renal function will increase blood levels. See Pediatric Dose.

Elderly: No specific problems documented. ■ See Usual Dose and Dose Adjustments.

DRUG/LAB INTERACTIONS

Risk of nephrotoxicity may be increased with **aminoglycosides and other nephrotoxic agents** (e.g., loop diuretics). ■ **Probenecid** inhibits excretion, resulting in elevated cefazolin levels. Dose reduction of cefazolin may be necessary. ■ May be antagonized by **bacteriostatic antibiotics** (e.g., chloramphenicol, erythromycin, tetracyclines); may interfere with bactericidal action. ■ May result in false-positive reaction for **urine glucose** except with enzyme-based tests (e.g., Clinistix). ■ Positive direct Coombs' tests have been reported. ■ See Compatibility and Side Effects.

SIDE EFFECTS

Anorexia; CDAD; diarrhea; elevated BUN and creatinine levels; elevated PT/INR; hypersensitivity reactions, including anaphylaxis; leukopenia; local site pain; nausea and vomiting; neutropenia; oral thrush; phlebitis; positive direct and indirect Coombs' test; pruritis; transient elevation of AST, ALT, and alkaline phosphatase; seizures (large doses); thrombophlebitis; vaginal itching or discharge. Hypoprothrombinemia (rare) and hemolytic anemia may occur. Hepatitis and renal failure have been reported. Aplastic anemia, erythema multiforme, hemolytic anemia, hemorrhage, hepatic impairment (including cholestasis), pancytopenia, renal impairment, Stevens-Johnson syndrome, toxic epidermal necrolysis, and toxic nephropathy have been reported with cephalosporin-class antibiotics.

ANTIDOTE

Notify the physician of any side effects. Discontinue the drug if indicated. Mild cases of CDAD may respond to discontinuation of cefazolin. Treat CDAD with fluids, electrolytes, protein supplements, and appropriate antibiotics (e.g., oral vancomycin) as indicated. In severe cases, surgical evaluation may be indicated. Discontinue cefazolin and treat hypersensitivity reaction as indicated (airway, oxygen, IV fluids, antihistamines [e.g., diphenhydramine], corticosteroids [e.g., hydrocortisone sodium succinate], epinephrine, pressor amines [e.g., dopamine]) and resuscitate as necessary. Hemodialysis may be useful in overdose.

CEFEPIME AND ENMETAZOBACTAM

(seh fuh **peem** and En MET azo bactam)

Cephalosporin Combination

Exblifep

USUAL DOSE
2.5 Gm (cefepime 2 Gm and enmetazobactam 500 mg) IV every 8 hours.

PEDIATRIC DOSE:
Safety and effectiveness have not been established.

DOSE ADJUSTMENTS
Renal: *Estimated glomerular filtration rate (eGFR) 30 to 59 mL/min:* 1.25 Gm (cefepime 1 g and enmetazobactam 250 mg) IV every 8 hours.[Ref]

eGFR 15 to 29 mL/min: 1.25 Gm (cefepime 1 Gm and enmetazobactam 250 mg) IV every 12 hours.

eGFR <15 mL/min: 1.25 Gm (cefepime 1 Gm and enmetazobactam 250 mg) IV as a loading dose on day 1 of treatment, followed by 625 mg (cefepime 500 mg and enmetazobactam 125 mg) IV every 24 hours thereafter.[Ref]

Hemodialysis, intermittent (thrice weekly) Dialyzable (cefepime: 30%; enmetazobactam: 35%): 1.25 g (cefepime 1 Gm and enmetazobactam 250 mg) IV as a loading dose on day 1 of treatment, followed by 625 mg (cefepime 500 mg and enmetazobactam 125 mg) IV every 24 hours thereafter. On dialysis days, administer after dialysis.

Hepatic: No dosage adjustments are provided in the manufacturer's labeling.

RECONSTITUTION AND DILUTION
Reconstitution: Reconstitute vial with 10 mL of normal saline (NS), dextrose 5% in water (D5W), or D2.5W and 1/2NS from a 250-mL infusion bag. Mix gently to dissolve. Reconstituted solution will have a concentration of 200 mg/mL (cefepime 160 mg/mL and enmetazobactam 40 mg/mL) and a final volume of ~13 mL. Immediately withdraw the required amount of reconstituted solution and further dilute in the 250-mL infusion bag used for reconstitution. The same injection solution should be used for both reconstitution and dilution.

Cefepime and Enmetazobactam Dose Preparation[Ref]			
Cefepime and enmetazobactam dose	Number of vials to reconstitute for further dilution	Volume to withdraw from reconstituted vial for further dilution	Volume of infusion bag
2.5 Gm (cefepime 2 Gm and enmetazobactam 500 mg)	1 vial	Entire contents of vial (~13 mL)	250 mL
1.25 Gm (cefepime 1 Gm and enmetazobactam 250 mg)	1 vial	6.5 mL	250 mL
625 mg (cefepime 500 mg and enmetazobactam 125 mg)	1 vial	3.3 mL	250 mL

Dilution for infusion Immediately withdraw the required amount of reconstituted solution and further dilute in the 250-mL infusion bag used for reconstitution. The same injection solution should be used for both reconstitution and dilution.

COMPATIBILITY
Compatible with D5W, NS, ½ NS—consult with hospital pharmacist for other compatibility questions.

RATE OF ADMINISTRATION
Administer by IV infusion over 2 hours. If patient has eGFR >130 mL/min, give over 4 hours.

ACTIONS

Cefepime binds to penicillin-binding proteins, which inhibits the final transpeptidation step of peptidoglycan synthesis in bacterial cell walls, inhibiting cell wall synthesis.

Enmetazobactam is a beta-lactamase inhibitor that protects cefepime from degradation by certain serine beta-lactamases (e.g., extended spectrum beta-lactamases).

INDICATIONS AND USES

Urinary tract infection, complicated (pyelonephritis or urinary tract infection with systemic signs/symptoms).

CONTRAINDICATIONS

Hypersensitivity to cefepime, enmetazobactam, any component of the formulation, or other beta-lactam drugs.

PRECAUTIONS

May be associated with increased International Normalized Ratio.

Hypersensitivity: Hypersensitivity reactions have been reported. Serious, occasionally fatal hypersensitivity reactions (including anaphylaxis), and serious skin reactions have been reported in patients receiving beta-lactams.

Neurotoxicity: Severe neurologic reactions (some fatal) have been reported, including encephalopathy, aphasia, myoclonus, seizures, and nonconvulsive status epilepticus. Risk may be increased in the presence of kidney impairment; ensure dose is adjusted for kidney function and discontinue therapy if patient develops neurotoxicity; effects are often reversible upon discontinuation of cefepime. Use with caution in patients with history of seizure disorder.

Superinfection: Prolonged use may result in fungal or bacterial superinfection, including *Clostridioides difficile*-associated diarrhea and pseudomembranous colitis.

Kidney impairment: Use with caution in patients with kidney impairment (creatinine clearance ≤60 mL/min).

Monitoring parameters Kidney function: In patients with changing kidney function, monitor serum creatinine and eGFR at least daily.

PATIENT EDUCATION

Notify nurse and physician of any itching, swelling, redness (signs of allergic reaction). Notify physician of any watery diarrhea.

MATERNAL/CHILD

Pregnancy considerations: Adverse events were not observed in animal reproduction studies.

Breastfeeding considerations: Cefepime is present in breast milk; excretion of enmetazobactam is not known.

According to the manufacturer, the decision to breastfeed during therapy should take into consideration the risk of infant exposure, the benefits of breastfeeding to the infant, and the benefits of treatment to the mother.

Elderly: No specific recommendations; refer to adult dosing.

DRUG/LAB INTERACTIONS

Avoid the following drugs: BCG (Intravesical), cholera vaccine, and fecal microbiota. Other drug interactions include aminoglycosides, furosemide, mycohenolate, and warfarin.

SIDE EFFECTS

Most common side effects include elevated liver tests (serum transaminases), diarrhea, increased bilirubin, injection site reaction, headache, and nausea.

ANTIDOTE

There is no antidote; stop infusion for hypersensitivity reactions and treat appropriately.

CEFEPIME HYDROCHLORIDE
(seh-fuh-**peem** hy-droh-**KLOR**-eyed)

Antibacterial
(cephalosporin)

Maxipime

pH 4 to 6

USUAL DOSE
Pretreatment: Baseline studies indicated; see Monitor.

Adults: Range is from 1-2 Gm every 8-12 hours. Dose and frequency based on severity of disease and/or specific susceptibility of the causative organism according.

PEDIATRIC DOSE
Pediatric patients 2 months to 16 years; weight up to 40 kg: 50 mg/kg every 12 hours with the duration of therapy as outlined under Usual Dose. Increase frequency to every 8 hours for empiric monotherapy in febrile neutropenia and for treatment of pneumonia due to *Pseudomonas aeruginosa.* Do not exceed adult dose.

DOSE ADJUSTMENTS
In impaired renal function, the initial dose should be as stated earlier (except in patients undergoing hemodialysis). All remaining doses should be reduced based on CrCl according to the following chart (e.g., if the normal dose is 1 Gm every 12 hours with a CrCl greater than 60, the maintenance dose would be reduced to 1 Gm every 24 hours with a CrCl between 30 and 60 mL/min). Dose reductions should be comparable in *pediatric patients.*

Cefepime Dose Guidelines in Impaired Renal Function				
Creatinine Clearance (mL/min)	Recommended Maintenance Schedule (relative to normal dosing schedule)			
Normal Recommended Dosing Schedule (>60 mL/min)	500 mg q 12 hr	1 Gm q 12 hr	2 Gm q 12 hr	2 Gm q 8 hr
30-60 mL/min	500 mg q 24 hr	1 Gm q 24 hr	2 Gm q 24 hr	2 Gm q 12 hr
11-29 mL/min	500 mg q 24 hr	500 mg q 24 hr	1 Gm q 24 hr	2 Gm q 24 hr
<11 mL/min	250 mg q 24 hr	250 mg q 24 hr	500 mg q 24 hr	1 Gm q 24 hr
CAPD	500 mg q 48 hr	1 Gm q 48 hr	2 Gm q 48 hr	2 Gm q 48 hr
Hemodialysis[a]	1 Gm on Day 1, then 500 mg q 24 hr.			1 Gm q 24 hr

[a]On hemodialysis days, cefepime should be administered following hemodialysis. Whenever possible, administer at the same time each day.

Consult literature for conversion formula if dose is to be based on SCr. ▪ Reduced dose may be required in the elderly based on renal function. ▪ Dose adjustment not required in impaired hepatic function.

DILUTION
Vials of the lyophilized powder for IM/IV use may be reconstituted with D5W, NS, SWFI, (see the following chart) and then further diluted with NS, D5W, D10W, D5NS, D5LR. Concentrations between 1 mg/mL and 40 mg/mL are acceptable. (500 mg reconstituted with 5 mL = 100 mg/mL, further diluted with 95 mL = 5 mg/mL, with 45 mL = 10 mg/mL.) Available in several forms (other than vials of lyophilized powder), including Add-Vantage vials, dual-chamber DUPLEX containers with dextrose, and premixed with dextrose in a frozen Galaxy container. Refer to manufacturer's prescribing information for specific preparation and storage requirements.

Cefepime Dilution Guidelines			
Single-Dose Vials for Intravenous Administration	Amount of Diluent to Be Added (mL)	Approximate Available Volume (mL)	Approximate Cefepime Concentration (mg/mL)
CEFEPIME VIAL CONTENT			
500 mg (IV)	5 mL	5 mL	100 mg/mL
1 Gm (IV)	10 mL	10.5 mL	100 mg/mL
2 Gm (IV)	10 mL	12.5 mL	160 mg/mL
ADD-VANTAGE			
1-Gm vial	50 mL	50 mL	20 mg/mL
1-Gm vial	100 mL	100 mL	10 mg/mL
2-Gm vial	50 mL	50 mL	40 mg/mL
2-Gm vial	100 mL	100 mL	20 mg/mL

Filters: Specific information from studies not available; contact manufacturer for further information.

Storage: See manufacturer's directions. Recommendations for storing vary from CRT (20° to 25° C [68° to 77° F]) to 2° to 25° C (36° to 77° F) in the dry state; protect from light. Most reconstituted or diluted solutions are stable for 24 hours at CRT and 7 days if refrigerated (recommendations may vary with diluent). As with other cephalosporins, the color of cefepime tends to darken depending on storage conditions; however, the product potency is not adversely affected when stored as recommended.

COMPATIBILITY

Manufacturer recommends temporarily discontinuing other solutions infusing at the same site during intermittent infusion. May be used concomitantly with aminoglycosides (e.g., gentamicin, tobramycin), aminophylline, metronidazole, and vancomycin, but these drugs must never be mixed in the same infusion (mutual inactivation or other potential interactions). If concurrent therapy with cefepime is indicated, each of these antibiotics can be administered separately. Flush IV line before and after administration.

Other sources suggest specific **compatibilities** dependent on concentration and manufacturer; consult a pharmacist.

RATE OF ADMINISTRATION

Do not use plastic containers in a series connection; could result in air embolism. May be given (off label) as extended infusion: IV 2 Gm infused over 3–4 hours or Continuous infusion: 4–6 Gm infused over 24 hours. May give a first does of 2 Gm over 30 minutes followed by infusion.

Intermittent infusion: A single dose equally distributed over 30 minutes.

ACTIONS

A semi-synthetic, broad-spectrum, fourth-generation cephalosporin antibiotic. Bactericidal to a wide range of both gram-positive and gram-negative organisms. Cefepime is highly resistant to hydrolysis by most beta-lactamases and exhibits rapid penetration into gram-negative bacterial cells. Acts by inhibition of bacterial wall synthesis. Peak serum levels achieved by end of infusion; half-life is 1.7 to 2.3 hours. Well distributed into many body fluids and tissues. Partially metabolized; 85% excreted unchanged in urine. Secreted in breast milk.

INDICATIONS AND USES

Treatment of moderate to severe pneumonia caused by susceptible organisms, including cases associated with concurrent bacteremia. ▪ Treatment of uncomplicated and complicated urinary tract infections caused by susceptible organisms, including pyelonephritis and cases associated with concurrent bacteremia. ▪ Treatment of uncomplicated skin and skin structure infections caused by susceptible organisms. ▪ Empiric monotherapy in the treatment of febrile neutropenic patients; see Precautions. ▪ Treatment of complicated intra-abdominal infections in adults; used in combination with metronidazole (Flagyl). ▪ See literature for list of susceptible organisms.

CONTRAINDICATIONS
Patients who have shown immediate hypersensitivity reactions to cefepime, any cephalosporin, penicillin, or other beta-lactam antibiotic; see Precautions. ▪ Premixed solutions containing dextrose may be contraindicated in patients with known allergies to corn or corn products.

PRECAUTIONS
Hypersensitivity reactions, including anaphylaxis, have been reported. Check history of previous hypersensitivity reactions to penicillins, cephalosporins, or other allergens. Cross-sensitivity among beta-lactam antibacterial agents has been documented; however, the actual incidence of cross-allergenicity is not established. ▪ Specific sensitivity studies are indicated to determine susceptibility of the causative organism to cefepime. ▪ To reduce the development of drug-resistant bacteria and maintain its effectiveness, cefepime should be used to treat or prevent only those infections proven or strongly suspected to be caused by bacteria. ▪ IM injection is used only for mild to moderate urinary tract infections due to *E. coli*. ▪ Avoid prolonged use of drug; superinfection caused by overgrowth of nonsusceptible organisms may result. ▪ May decrease prothrombin activity, especially in patients with impaired renal or hepatic function, those in a poor nutritional state, and those receiving extended courses of antimicrobial therapy. ▪ Serious neurologic adverse events, including aphasia, encephalopathy (changes in consciousness, including coma, confusion, hallucinations, and stupor), myoclonus, nonconvulsive status epilepticus, and seizures, have occurred; life-threatening or fatal events have been reported. Patients with impaired renal function may be at greater risk, especially if doses are not properly adjusted; see Dose Adjustments and monitor closely. In most cases, neurotoxicity was reversible and resolved after cefepime was discontinued and/or after hemodialysis. ▪ *Clostridium difficile*–associated diarrhea (CDAD) has been reported. May range from mild diarrhea to fatal colitis. Consider in patients who present with diarrhea during or after treatment with cefepime. ▪ Higher-end doses may increase incidence and severity of rash and require cefepime to be discontinued. ▪ Insufficient data exist for monotherapy of febrile neutropenia in patients at high risk for severe infection (e.g., history of recent bone marrow transplant, hypotension on presentation, underlying hematologic malignancy, severe or prolonged neutropenia). ▪ Positive direct Coombs' tests have been reported during treatment with cefepime. Discontinue drug and institute appropriate therapy in patients who develop hemolytic anemia.

Monitor: Obtain baseline CBC with differential and platelets and SCr. ▪ Obtain baseline PT and monitor, especially in at-risk patients (see Precautions); vitamin K may be indicated. ▪ Watch for early symptoms of a hypersensitivity reaction. ▪ Monitor for neurotoxicity (e.g., aphasia, encephalopathy, myoclonus, nonconvulsive status epilepticus, seizures). ▪ May cause thrombophlebitis. ▪ Monitor and re-evaluate frequently the need for continued antimicrobial treatment in patients whose fever resolves but who remain neutropenic for more than 7 days. ▪ See Drug/Lab Interactions.

Patient Education: Promptly report any bleeding or bruising or symptoms of hypersensitivity (e.g., difficulty breathing, hives, itching, rash). ▪ Promptly report diarrhea or bloody stools that occur during treatment or up to several months after an antibiotic has been discontinued; may indicate CDAD and require treatment. ▪ Promptly report neurologic S/S (e.g., aphasia, change in consciousness, confusion, hallucinations, seizures, stupor).

Maternal/Child: Category B: safety for use during pregnancy, labor and delivery, and breast-feeding not established; use only if clearly needed. ▪ Safety and effectiveness have not been established for use in infants under 2 months of age, in pediatric patients for treatment of complicated intra-abdominal infections, or for treatment of serious infections in pediatric patients in whom the suspected or proven pathogen is *Haemophilus influenzae* type b. ■ An alternate agent with demonstrated clinical effectiveness should be used in pediatric patients in whom meningitis or meningeal seeding from a distant infection site is suspected or documented. ■ Pharmacokinetics in pediatric patients and adults is similar. Dose modification similar to adults is indicated in impaired renal function; see Dose Adjustments. ■ Immature renal function of infants and small children will increase blood levels of all cephalosporins. ■ Positive Coombs' test may be observed in newborns whose mothers have received cephalosporin antibiotics before parturition.

Elderly: Consider age-related impaired organ function, nutritional status, and concomitant disease or drug therapy; reduced dose or extended intervals may be indicated. Serious adverse reactions (e.g., aphasia, encephalopathy, myoclonus, nonconvulsive status epilepticus, seizures) have occurred in elderly patients with renal impairment given unadjusted doses of cefepime; see Dose Adjustments. Monitor for hypocalcemia.

DRUG/LAB INTERACTIONS

Risk of nephrotoxicity may be increased with **aminoglycosides and other nephrotoxic agents** (e.g., loop diuretics); monitor renal function closely. ■ Risk of ototoxicity may be increased when administered with aminoglycosides (e.g., gentamicin). ■ May have a false-positive reaction for **urine glucose** except with enzyme-based tests (e.g., Clinistix). ■ See Compatibility and Side Effects.

SIDE EFFECTS

Decreased phosphorus, increased ALT and AST, increased PT and PTT, local reactions (including phlebitis), pain and/or inflammation, positive Coombs' test, and rash are the most common adverse reactions. At the highest doses (2 Gm every 8 hours), the most common adverse reactions are diarrhea, fever, headache, nausea, pruritis, rash, and vomiting. Other reported adverse reactions include the full scope of hypersensitivity reactions (e.g., anaphylaxis, itching, rash, shock, urticaria); bone marrow suppression (e.g., agranulocytosis, anemia, leukopenia, neutropenia, thrombocytopenia); CDAD; colitis; decreased calcium (more common in elderly); elevated alkaline phosphatase, BUN, calcium, creatinine, eosinophils, phosphorus, potassium, and total bilirubin; erythema; neurotoxicity (e.g., seizures [large doses, or standard doses in renally impaired patients]); oral moniliasis; and vaginitis. Aplastic anemia, erythema multiforme, hemolytic anemia, hemorrhage, hepatic dysfunction (including cholestasis), pancytopenia, renal dysfunction, Stevens-Johnson syndrome, toxic epidermal necrolysis, and toxic nephropathy have been reported with cephalosporin-class antibiotics.

Overdose: Encephalopathy (disturbances of consciousness, including confusion, hallucinations, stupor, and coma), myoclonus, neuromuscular excitability, nonconvulsive status epilepticus, seizures.

Post-Marketing: Agranulocytosis, anaphylaxis, aphasia, encephalopathy, myoclonus, seizures, nonconvulsive status epilepticus.

ANTIDOTE

Notify physician of any side effects. Discontinue cefepime and treat hypersensitivity reactions as indicated (airway, oxygen, IV fluids, epinephrine, corticosteroids, pressor amines [e.g., dopamine], antihistamines [e.g., diphenhydramine]). Resuscitate as necessary. Discontinue cefepime if neurotoxicity develops, and institute supportive measures as indicated. Mild cases of CDAD may respond to discontinuation of cefepime. Treat CDAD with fluids, electrolytes, protein supplements, and appropriate antibiotics (e.g., oral vancomycin) as indicated. In severe cases, surgical evaluation may be indicated. Hemodialysis may be useful in overdose.

CEFIDEROCOL
(**SEF**-i-**DER**-oh-kol)

Fetroja

Antibacterial
(cephalosporin)

pH 5.2 to 5.8

USUAL DOSE

Pretreatment: Baseline studies indicated; see Monitor.

Cefiderocol: 2 Gm every 8 hours administered as an IV infusion over 3 hours; see Dose Adjustments. Duration of therapy is 7 to 14 days. Duration guided by the severity of infection and the patient's clinical status.

DOSE ADJUSTMENTS

Adjust dose in patients with CrCl less than 60 mL/min as outlined in the following chart.

Recommended Dosage of Cefiderocol for Patients With CrCl Less Than 60 mL/min			
Estimated Creatinine Clearance (CrCl)[a]	Dose	Frequency	Infusion Time
Patients with CrCl 30 to 59 mL/min	1.5 Gm	q 8 hr	3 hr
Patients with CrCl 15 to 29 mL/min	1 Gm	q 8 hr	3 hr
ESRD patients (CrCl <15 mL/min) with or without intermittent HD[b]	0.75 Gm	q 12 hr	3 hr

[a]CrCl, Creatinine clearance estimated by Cockcroft-Gault equation.
[b]Cefiderocol is removed by hemodialysis (HD); thus complete hemodialysis (HD) at the latest possible time before the start of cefiderocol dosing.
ESRD, End-stage renal disease; *HD*, hemodialysis.

■ Increase dosage to 2 Gm IV every 6 hours in patients with a CrCl 120 mL/min or greater. ■ Reduced dose or extended intervals may be indicated in elderly patients; consider age-related impaired renal function and concomitant disease states. ■ No clinically significant differences in pharmacokinetics of cefiderocol were observed based on age, sex, or race. ■ Dose reduction is not required in impaired hepatic function.

DILUTION

Available as a sterile, lyophilized powder in a 1-Gm vial. Reconstitute each 1-Gm vial with 10 mL of either NS or D5W. Shake gently to dissolve. Allow vial(s) to stand until foam dissipates (typically within 2 minutes). The final volume of reconstituted solution will be approximately 11.2 mL. To prepare the required dose, withdraw the appropriate volume of reconstituted solution from the vial as indicated in the following chart and add to an infusion bag containing 100 mL of NS or D5W. Resulting solution should be clear and colorless.

Preparation of Cefiderocol Doses			
Cefiderocol Dose	Number of 1-g Cefiderocol Vials to Be Reconstituted	Volume to Withdraw From Reconstituted Vial(s)	Total Volume of Cefiderocol Reconstituted Solution for Further Dilution Into at Least 100 mL
2 Gm	2 vials	11.2 mL (entire contents) of each vial	22.4 mL
1.5 Gm	2 vials	11.2 mL (entire contents) of first vial AND 5.6 mL from second vial	16.8 mL
1 Gm	1 vial	11.2 mL (entire contents)	11.2 mL
0.75 Gm	1 vial	8.4 mL	8.4 mL

Filter: Data not available.

Storage: Refrigerate vials at 2° to 8° C (36° to 46° F) in original carton to protect from light. Reconstituted solution is stable for 1 hour at RT. Diluted solution in the infusion bag is stable for 4 hours at RT. Discard any unused solution in the vial.

COMPATIBILITY

Compatible with NS and D5W. The manufacturer states that, "The compatibility of cefiderocol solution for administration with solutions containing other drugs or other diluents has not been established."

RATE OF ADMINISTRATION

A single dose as an infusion equally distributed over 3 hours.

ACTIONS

A cephalosporin antibacterial drug with activity against gram-negative aerobic bacteria. Cefiderocol functions as a siderophore and binds to extracellular free ferric iron. In addition to passive diffusion via porin channels, cefiderocol is actively transported across the outer cell membrane of bacteria into the periplasmic space using a siderophore iron uptake mechanism. Cefiderocol exerts bactericidal action by inhibiting cell wall biosynthesis through binding to penicillin-binding proteins. Cefiderocol has no clinically relevant *in vitro* activity against most gram-positive bacteria and anaerobic bacteria. Plasma protein binding (primarily to albumin) is 40% to 60%. Minimally metabolized. Terminal elimination half-life is 2 to 3 hours. Primarily excreted by the kidneys.

INDICATIONS AND USES

Treatment of complicated urinary tract infections (cUTIs), including pyelonephritis caused by susceptible gram-negative microorganisms (*Escherichia coli, Klebsiella pneumoniae, Proteus mirabilis, Pseudomonas aeruginosa,* and *Enterobacter cloacae* complex), in patients 18 years of age or older who have limited or no alternative treatment options. Approval of this indication is based on limited clinical safety and efficacy data.

CONTRAINDICATIONS

Known history of severe hypersensitivity to cefiderocol or other beta-lactam antibacterial drugs or to any other component of cefiderocol.

PRECAUTIONS

In a multinational, randomized open-label trial in critically ill patients with carbapenem-resistant gram-negative bacterial infections, an increase in all-cause mortality was observed in patients treated with cefiderocol compared with patients treated with best available therapy (BAT). Patients with nosocomial pneumonia, bloodstream infections, sepsis, or cUTIs were included in the trial. The increase in all-cause mortality occurred in patients treated for nosocomial pneumonia, bloodstream infections, or sepsis. The safety and efficacy of cefiderocol has not been established for the treatment of nosocomial pneumonia, bloodstream infections, or sepsis. Reserve cefiderocol for use in patients who have limited or no alternative treatment options for the treatment of cUTIs.
■ Serious and occasionally fatal hypersensitivity (anaphylactic) reactions and serious skin reactions have been reported in patients receiving beta-lactam antibacterial drugs. These reactions are more likely to occur in patients with a history of a beta-lactam hypersensitivity and/or a history of sensitivity to multiple allergens. Hypersensitivity reactions have been reported with cefiderocol. Check history of previous hypersensitivity reactions to other cephalosporins, penicillins, or carbapenems. Cross-sensitivity among beta-lactam antibacterial drugs has been established. ■ Specific sensitivity studies indicated to determine susceptibility of causative organism to cefiderocol. ■ Cross-resistance with other classes of antibacterial drugs has not been identified; therefore isolates resistant to other antibacterial drugs may be susceptible to cefiderocol. ■ To reduce the development of drug-resistant bacteria and maintain its effectiveness, cefiderocol should be used to treat or prevent only those infections proven or strongly suspected to be caused by bacteria. ■ *Clostridium difficile*–associated diarrhea (CDAD) has been reported. May range from mild diarrhea to fatal colitis. Consider in patients who present with diarrhea during or after treatment with cefiderocol. ■ Cephalosporins, including cefiderocol, have been implicated in triggering seizures. Nonconvulsive status epilepticus (NCSE),

encephalopathy, coma, asterixis, neuromuscular excitability, and myoclonia have been reported with cephalosporins, particularly in patients with a history of epilepsy and/or when recommended dosages of cephalosporins were exceeded due to renal impairment; see Dose Adjustments. Anticonvulsant therapy should be continued in patients with known seizure disorders.

Monitor: Obtain baseline and periodic CBC and SCr. ▪ Monitor CrCl in all patients with fluctuating renal function and adjust dosage accordingly; see Dose Adjustments. ▪ CrCl 120 mL/min or greater may be seen in seriously ill patients who are receiving IV fluid resuscitation. ▪ Monitor for S/S of a hypersensitivity reaction. ▪ Monitor for S/S of CNS adverse reactions. If CNS adverse reactions (including seizures) occur, patients should undergo a neurologic evaluation to determine whether cefiderocol should be discontinued. ▪ Closely monitor the clinical response to therapy in patients with a cUTI.

Patient Education: Review list of allergies and medical conditions with provider. Report promptly any symptoms of hypersensitivity (e.g., difficulty breathing, hives, itching, rash) or neurologic symptoms (e.g., confusion, myoclonus, seizures). ▪ Promptly report diarrhea or bloody stools that occur during treatment or up to several months after an antibiotic has been discontinued; may indicate CDAD and require treatment.

Maternal/Child: Safety for use during pregnancy and breast-feeding not established. No problems documented. Use caution. ▪ Safety and efficacy for use in pediatric patients younger than 18 years of age not established.

Elderly: No specific differences in safety or effectiveness were observed between elderly and younger patients. ▪ See Dose Adjustments.

DRUG/LAB INTERACTIONS

Cefiderocol may result in **false-positive dipstick tests** (urine protein, ketones, or occult blood). Use alternate clinical laboratory methods of testing to confirm positive tests.

SIDE EFFECTS

The most common adverse reactions include candidiasis, constipation, cough, diarrhea, elevations in liver tests, headache, hypokalemia, infusion site reactions, nausea, rash, and vomiting. Adverse reactions leading to discontinuation of therapy include diarrhea, hypersensitivity reactions, and increased hepatic enzymes. Less commonly reported adverse reactions include abdominal pain, atrial fibrillation, bradycardia, CHF, cholecystitis, cholelithiasis, *C. difficile* infection, decreased appetite, dry mouth, dyspnea, dysgeusia, fever, fluid overload, gallbladder pain, hypersensitivity reactions, hypocalcemia, increased creatine phosphokinase, insomnia, peripheral edema, pleural effusion, prolonged INR and PT, pruritus, restlessness, seizures, stomatitis, and thrombocytosis.

ANTIDOTE

Notify physician of any side effects. Discontinue the drug if indicated. Treat hypersensitivity reactions as indicated and resuscitate as necessary. Mild cases of CDAD may respond to discontinuation of cefiderocol. Treat CDAD with fluids, electrolytes, protein supplements, and appropriate antibiotics (e.g., oral vancomycin) as indicated. In severe cases, surgical evaluation may be indicated. Approximately 60% of cefiderocol is removed by a 3- to 4-hour hemodialysis session.

CEFOTAXIME SODIUM
(sef-oh-**TAX**-eem **SO**-dee-um)

Antibacterial
(cephalosporin)

Claforan

pH 5 to 7.5

USUAL DOSE

Range is 2 to 12 Gm/24 hr. Depends on seriousness of infection. Maximum daily dose is 12 Gm. Duration of treatment depends on the organism and infection being treated. A minimum of 10 days is recommended for infections caused by *group A beta-hemolytic streptococci* to guard against the risk of rheumatic fever or glomerulonephritis.

Uncomplicated infections: 1 Gm every 12 hours.

Moderate to severe infections: 1 to 2 Gm every 8 hours.

Serious infections and septicemia: 2 Gm every 6 to 8 hours.

Life-threatening infections: 2 Gm every 4 hours.

For moderate to life-threatening infections, higher doses are often reduced after a positive clinical response.

Disseminated gonococcal infections: 1 Gm every 8 hours; continue for 24 to 48 hours after symptoms improve. Transfer to oral cefixime to complete a minimum of 1 week of treatment.

Perioperative prophylaxis: 1 Gm 30 to 90 minutes before incision. Equal to or less than 60 minutes is recommended. May be repeated in a lengthy procedure. In *cesarean section* give initial dose after cord is clamped, then 1 Gm at 6 and 12 hours postoperatively.

PEDIATRIC DOSE

Maximum daily dose 12 Gm/24 hr. Differentiation between premature and normal gestational age is not necessary.

0 to 1 week of age: 50 mg/kg/dose every 12 hours.

1 to 4 weeks of age: 50 mg/kg/dose every 8 hours. One source increases the interval to every 12 hours in infants weighing less than 1,200 Gm.

1 month to 12 years, weight less than 50 kg: 50 to 180 mg/kg/24 hr equally divided into 4 to 6 doses (8.3 to 30 mg/kg/dose every 4 hours or 12.5 to 45 mg/kg/dose every 6 hours). Use higher-end doses for serious infections, including meningitis.

Weight 50 kg or more: See Usual Dose.

DOSE ADJUSTMENTS

In impaired renal function with a CrCl less than 20 mL/min/1.73 M^2, reduce dose by one-half and maintain same dosing interval. ■ Reduced doses or extended intervals may be indicated in the elderly. Consider age-related impaired organ function, nutritional status, and concomitant disease or drug therapy. ■ See Usual Dose and Drug/Lab Interactions.

DILUTION

Each dose of the lyophilized powder (500 mg, 1 Gm, 2 Gm) must be reconstituted with 10 mL SWFI, D5W, NS, or other **compatible** infusion solution (see chart on inside back cover or literature). Do not prepare with diluents having a pH above 7.5; see Compatibility. Solution color ranges from pale yellow to light amber. May be further diluted with 50 to 100 mL of **compatible** solutions and given as an intermittent infusion or added to larger volumes and given as a continuous infusion. (1 Gm in 14 mL of SWFI is isotonic.)

Available in several forms (other than vials of lyophilized powder), including premixed with dextrose in a frozen Galaxy container, in ADD-Vantage vials for use with ADD-Vantage infusion containers, and in pharmacy bulk vials. Refer to manufacturer's prescribing information for specific preparation and storage requirements.

Storage: Store unopened cartons at CRT. Protect from excessive light. Stability of reconstituted solutions ranges from 12 hours at RT to 10 days refrigerated depending on concentration, diluent, and infusion container; see prescribing information.

COMPATIBILITY

May be used concomitantly with aminoglycosides (e.g., amikacin, gentamicin), but these drugs must never be mixed in the same infusion (mutual inactivation). If given concurrently, administer separately and flush the IV line before and after administration. Manufacturer recommends temporarily discontinuing other solutions infusing at the same site during intermittent infusion and states, "Do not add supplementary medications to premixed plastic IV containers." Manufacturer also states, "Should not be prepared with solutions having a pH above 7.5, such as sodium bicarbonate."

Other sources suggest specific **compatibilities** dependent on concentration and manufacturer; consult a pharmacist.

RATE OF ADMINISTRATION

See Compatibility. Injection and intermittent infusion may be given through Y-tube of infusion set.

IV injection: A single dose equally distributed over a minimum of 3 to 5 minutes. Rapid bolus injections (less than 60 seconds) have caused life-threatening arrhythmias.

Intermittent IV: A single dose over 30 minutes.

Continuous infusion: 500 to 1,000 mL over 6 to 24 hours, depending on total dose and concentration.

ACTIONS

A broad-spectrum, third-generation cephalosporin antibiotic. Bactericidal to many gram-negative, gram-positive, and anaerobic organisms. Effective against many otherwise resistant organisms. Inhibits bacterial cell wall synthesis. Distributed into most body tissues and fluids, including inflamed meninges. Some metabolites formed. Half-life is approximately 1 hour. Excreted in the urine. Crosses placental barrier. Secreted in breast milk.

INDICATIONS AND USES

Treatment of serious lower respiratory tract, urinary tract, skin and skin structure, intra-abdominal, bone and joint, CNS, gynecologic infections, and bacteremia/septicemia. Most effective against specific organisms (see literature). ▪ Perioperative prophylaxis.

Unlabeled uses: Treatment of disseminated gonococcal infections and Lyme disease.

CONTRAINDICATIONS

Previous hypersensitivity reaction to cephalosporins; see Precautions. ▪ Premixed solutions containing dextrose may be contraindicated in patients with known allergies to corn or corn products.

PRECAUTIONS

Hypersensitivity reactions, including fatalities, have been reported and include reports of individuals with a history of penicillin hypersensitivity or sensitivity to multiple allergens experiencing severe reactions when treated with cephalosporins. Check history of previous hypersensitivity reactions to penicillins, cephalosporins, or other allergens. Actual incidence of cross-allergenicity not established but may be more common with first-generation cephalosporins. ▪ Sensitivity studies indicated to determine susceptibility of the causative organism to cefotaxime. ▪ To reduce the development of drug-resistant bacteria and maintain its effectiveness, cefotaxime should be used to treat or prevent only those infections proven or strongly suspected to be caused by bacteria. ▪ Continue for 2 to 3 days after all symptoms of infection subside. ▪ Avoid prolonged use of drug; superinfection caused by overgrowth of nonsusceptible organisms may result. ▪ Use caution in patients with impaired renal function, allergies, or a history of GI disease (especially colitis). ▪ *Clostridium difficile*–associated diarrhea (CDAD) has been reported. May range from mild diarrhea to fatal colitis. Consider in patients who present with diarrhea during or after treatment with cefotaxime. ▪ Granulocytopenia and, rarely, agranulocytosis can occur, especially during prolonged therapy; see Monitor.

Monitor: Watch for early symptoms of a hypersensitivity reaction. ▪ Monitor CBC if duration of treatment is more than 10 days. ▪ May cause thrombophlebitis. Use small needles and large veins, and rotate infusion sites. ▪ See Drug/Lab Interactions; additional monitoring may be indicated (e.g., renal function, drug serum levels, PT).

Patient Education: Report promptly any bleeding or bruising or symptoms of hypersensitivity (e.g., difficulty breathing, hives, itching, rash). ▪ Promptly report diarrhea or bloody stools that occur during treatment or up to several months after an antibiotic has been discontinued; may indicate CDAD and require treatment.

Maternal/Child: Category B: safety for use during pregnancy and breast-feeding not established. No problems documented. ▪ Immature renal function of infants and small children will increase blood levels of all cephalosporins.

Elderly: No specific problems documented; see Dose Adjustments.

DRUG/LAB INTERACTIONS

Risk of nephrotoxicity may be increased with **aminoglycosides and other nephrotoxic agents** (e.g., loop diuretics [e.g., furosemide], NSAIDs [e.g., ibuprofen, naproxen]). ▪ **Probenecid** inhibits excretion of cefotaxime, decreasing clearance by approximately 50%. Limit administration of cefotaxime to no more than 6 Gm/day when given concurrently with probenecid. ▪ May be antagonized by **bacteriostatic antibiotics** (e.g., chloramphenicol, erythromycin, tetracyclines); may interfere with bactericidal action. ▪ See Compatibility and Side Effects. ▪ May cause a positive direct **Coombs' test.** ▪ May produce a false-positive reaction for **urine glucose** except with enzyme-based tests (e.g., Clinistix).

SIDE EFFECTS

Generally well tolerated. The most common side effect is a local reaction at the injection site. Less frequent reactions include a full scope of hypersensitivity reactions, including anaphylaxis; CDAD; colitis; decreased hemoglobin or decreased hematocrit; decreased platelet functions; diarrhea; dyspnea; elevation of AST, ALT, total bilirubin, alkaline phosphatase, LDH, and BUN (transient); eosinophilia; fever; leukopenia; local site pain; nausea; oral thrush; positive direct Coombs' test; prolonged PT; seizures (large doses); thrombophlebitis; transient neutropenia; vaginitis; vomiting. Generally resolve after cephalosporins are discontinued. Aplastic anemia, erythema multiforme, hemolytic anemia, hemorrhage, hepatic dysfunction (including cholestasis), pancytopenia, renal dysfunction, Stevens-Johnson syndrome, toxic epidermal necrolysis, and toxic nephropathy have been reported with cephalosporin-class antibiotics.

Post-Marketing: Arrhythmia (with rapid injection), cutaneous reactions (e.g., isolated cases of erythema multiforme, Stevens-Johnson syndrome, toxic epidermal necrolysis), encephalopathy (e.g., impairment of consciousness, abnormal movements and seizures), hematologic reactions (e.g., agranulocytosis, hemolytic anemia, thrombocytopenia), hepatic reactions (e.g., cholestasis, elevated gamma-glutamyl transferase [GGT] and bilirubin, hepatitis, jaundice), renal reactions (e.g., interstitial nephritis and transient elevations in SCr).

ANTIDOTE

Notify the physician of any side effects. Discontinue the drug if indicated. Mild cases of CDAD may respond to discontinuation of cefotaxime. Treat CDAD with fluids, electrolytes, protein supplements, and appropriate antibiotics (e.g., oral vancomycin) as indicated. In severe cases, surgical evaluation may be indicated. Treat hypersensitivity reactions as indicated and resuscitate as necessary. Hemodialysis may be useful in overdose.

CEFOTETAN DISODIUM
(sef-oh-**TEE**-tan dye-**SO**-dee-um)

Antibacterial
(cephalosporin)

pH 4.5 to 6.5

USUAL DOSE

Range is 1 to 6 Gm/24 hr for 5 to 10 days. Do not exceed 6 Gm/24 hr.

Urinary tract infections: 500 mg to 2 Gm every 12 hours or 1 to 2 Gm every 12 to 24 hours.

Moderate infections: 1 or 2 Gm every 12 hours.

Moderate infections of skin and skin structure: 2 Gm every 24 hours or 1 Gm every 12 hours. Give 1 or 2 Gm every 12 hours if *Klebsiella pneumoniae* is the causative organism.

Serious infections: 2 Gm every 12 hours.

Life-threatening infections: 3 Gm every 12 hours.

Pelvic inflammatory disease: 2 Gm every 12 hours for 14 days. Transfer to oral therapy at any time it is clinically appropriate, usually 48 hours after clinical improvement.

Perioperative prophylaxis: 1 to 2 Gm IV 30 to 60 minutes before incision except during cesarean section. Given only after clamping the umbilical cord in *cesarean section.*

PEDIATRIC DOSE

Unlabeled: 20 to 40 mg/kg of body weight every 12 hours; see Maternal/Child.

DOSE ADJUSTMENTS

Reduced doses or extended intervals may be indicated in the elderly; consider age-related impaired organ function, nutritional status, and concomitant disease or drug therapy.

■ Reduce total daily dose if renal function impaired according to the following chart.

Cefotetan Dose Guidelines in Impaired Renal Function	
Creatinine Clearance (mL/min)	**Dose/Frequency**
>30 mL/min	Usual recommended dose q 12 hr
10-30 mL/min	Usual recommended dose q 24 hr or $^1/_2$ usual recommended dose q 12 hr
<10 mL/min	Usual recommended dose q 48 hr or $^1/_4$ usual recommended dose q 12 hr
Hemodialysis patients	$^1/_4$ usual adult dose q 24 hr on days between dialysis sessions $^1/_2$ usual adult dose on the day of dialysis

DILUTION

IV injection: Reconstitute each 1 Gm of the lyophilized powder with 10 mL of SWFI (2 Gm with 20 mL). Shake well and let stand until clear.

Intermittent IV: *Vials:* A single dose may be further diluted or initially diluted with 50 to 100 mL of D5W or NS. Also available in dual-chamber DUPLEX containers and pharmacy bulk packaging. Refer to manufacturer's prescribing information for specific preparation and storage requirements.

Filters: No data available from manufacturer.

Storage: Store vials below 22° C (72° F); protect from light. Administer within 24 hours of preparation or within 96 hours if refrigerated. Stable after dilution for 1 week if frozen; thaw at room temperature before use; discard remaining solution; do not refreeze. Slight yellowing does not affect potency.

COMPATIBILITY

May be used concomitantly with aminoglycosides (e.g., amikacin, gentamicin), but these drugs must never be mixed in the same infusion (mutual inactivation). If given concurrently, administer separately and flush the IV line before and after administration. Manufacturer recommends temporarily discontinuing other solutions infusing at the same site during intermittent infusion and states, "Do not add supplementary medications to premixed plastic IV containers" (e.g., Galaxy).

Other sources suggest specific **compatibilities** dependent on concentration and manufacturer; consult a pharmacist.

RATE OF ADMINISTRATION
See Compatibility. May be given through Y-tube of infusion set.
IV injection: A single dose equally distributed over 3 to 5 minutes.
Intermittent IV: A single dose equally distributed over 30 minutes.

ACTIONS
A broad-spectrum, second-generation cephalosporin antibiotic. Bactericidal to selected gram-negative, gram-positive, and anaerobic organisms. Inhibits bacterial cell wall synthesis. Effective against many otherwise resistant organisms. Peak serum levels achieved at end of infusion. Widely distributed in most tissues, body fluids (CSF minimal), bone, gallbladder, myocardium, and skin and soft tissue. Half-life is from 3 to 4.6 hours. Primarily excreted in the urine. Crosses placental barrier. Secreted in breast milk.

INDICATIONS AND USES
Treatment of serious lower respiratory tract, urinary tract, skin and skin structure, gynecologic, intra-abdominal, and bone and joint infections. Most effective against specific organisms (see literature). ▪ Perioperative prophylaxis.

CONTRAINDICATIONS
Previous hypersensitivity reaction to cephalosporins or related antibiotics (penicillins). Absolute only if reaction was serious and in patients who have experienced a cephalosporin-associated hemolytic anemia. ▪ Premixed solutions containing dextrose may be contraindicated in patients with known allergies to corn or corn products.

PRECAUTIONS
Specific sensitivity studies are indicated to determine susceptibility of the causative organism to cefotetan. ▪ To reduce the development of drug-resistant bacteria and maintain its effectiveness, cefotetan should be used to treat or prevent only those infections proven or strongly suspected to be caused by bacteria. ▪ Continue for at least 2 or 3 days after all symptoms of infection subside. ▪ Avoid prolonged use of drug; superinfection caused by overgrowth of nonsusceptible organisms may result. ▪ Use caution in patients with impaired renal function, a history of GI disease (especially colitis), bleeding disorders or allergies, and those receiving an extended course of cephalosporins. ▪ *Clostridium difficile*–associated diarrhea (CDAD) has been reported. May range from mild diarrhea to fatal colitis. Consider in patients who present with diarrhea during or after treatment with cefotetan. ▪ Hemolytic anemia, including fatalities, has been reported. Discontinue cefotetan immediately if anemia develops during the course of therapy. May present during treatment or up to 2 to 3 weeks following therapy completion.
Monitor: Watch for early symptoms of a hypersensitivity reaction. ▪ Use extreme caution in the penicillin-sensitive patient; incidence of cross-sensitivity may be up to 10%. ▪ May cause hypoprothrombinemia (deficiency of prothrombin [factor II]); 10 mg/week of prophylactic vitamin K may be indicated in elderly, debilitated, or other patients with vitamin K deficiency. Monitor PT. ▪ May cause thrombophlebitis. Use small needles and large veins, and rotate infusion sites. ▪ Observe for electrolyte imbalance and cardiac irregularities. Contains 3.5 mEq sodium per Gm. ▪ Monitor for S/S of hemolytic anemia, including CBC if indicated. ▪ See Drug/Lab Interactions; additional monitoring may be indicated (e.g., renal function, drug serum levels, PT).
Patient Education: Avoid alcohol or alcohol-containing preparations; may cause abdominal cramps, flushing, headache, nausea and vomiting, shortness of breath, sweating, and tachycardia. ▪ Report promptly any bleeding or bruising or symptoms of hypersensitivity (e.g., difficulty breathing, hives, itching, rash). ▪ Promptly report diarrhea or bloody stools that occur during treatment or up to several months after an antibiotic has been discontinued; may indicate CDAD and require treatment.

Maternal/Child: Category B: safety for use during pregnancy not established. Use only if clearly needed. ▪ Use caution if breast-feeding. ▪ Safety for use in pediatric patients not established. Immature renal function of infants and small children will increase blood levels of all cephalosporins.

Elderly: See Dose Adjustments. ▪ Safety and effectiveness similar to younger adults; however, greater sensitivity of some older individuals cannot be ruled out. ▪ Monitoring of renal function suggested.

DRUG/LAB INTERACTIONS

May produce symptoms of acute intolerance with **alcohol** (a disulfiram-like reaction with abdominal cramps, headache, flushing, nausea and vomiting, shortness of breath, sweating, tachycardia). Patient must abstain from alcohol during treatment and until at least 72 hours after discontinuation. ▪ Risk of nephrotoxicity may be increased with **aminoglycosides and other nephrotoxic agents** (e.g., loop diuretics). ▪ Sources differ on inhibition of excretion by **probenecid.** ▪ May be antagonized by **bacteriostatic antibiotics** (e.g., chloramphenicol, erythromycin, tetracyclines); may interfere with bactericidal action. ▪ Bleeding tendency increased with **any medicine that affects blood clotting** (e.g., heparin and oral anticoagulants [warfarin], thrombolytic agents [e.g., alteplase (tPA)], salicylates, NSAIDs, sulfinpyrazone). ▪ Large amounts of cephalosporins and/or salicylates may induce **hypoprothrombinemia. ▪ False increases in creatinine levels** with Jaffe method. ▪ **False-positive for urine glucose** except with enzyme-based tests (e.g., Clinistix). ▪ **Positive direct Coombs' test.** ▪ See Compatibility and Side Effects.

SIDE EFFECTS

Full scope of hypersensitivity reactions, including anaphylaxis. Bleeding episodes; burning, discomfort, and pain at injection site; CDAD; diarrhea; elevated alkaline phosphatase, AST, ALT, and LDH; eosinophilia; nausea; prolonged PT; seizures (large doses); thrombocytosis. Hypoprothrombinemia (rare) and hemolytic anemia may occur.

ANTIDOTE

Notify physician of any side effects. Discontinue the drug if indicated. Treat hypersensitivity reactions as indicated and resuscitate as necessary. Mild cases of CDAD may respond to discontinuation of cefotetan. Treat CDAD with fluids, electrolytes, protein supplements, and appropriate antibiotics (e.g., oral vancomycin) as indicated. In severe cases, surgical evaluation may be indicated. Bleeding episodes may respond to vitamin K or require discontinuation of drug. Fresh frozen plasma, packed red cells, or platelet concentrates may be indicated in abnormal bleeding tendencies confirmed by lab evaluations. If bleeding is due to platelet dysfunction, discontinue and use an alternate antibiotic. Blood transfusions (e.g., packed red cells) may be indicated if hemolytic anemia develops. Hemodialysis is only slightly useful in overdose.

CEFOXITIN SODIUM
(seh-**FOX**-ih-tin **SO**-dee-um)

Antibacterial
(cephalosporin)

Mefoxin

pH 4.2 to 7

USUAL DOSE

Range is 1 to 2 Gm every 6 to 8 hours. Dose based on severity of disease, susceptibility of pathogens, and condition of patient.

Cefoxitin Dosing Guidelines		
Type of Infection	**Dose and Frequency**	**Total Daily Dose**
Uncomplicated forms[a] of infections such as pneumonia, urinary tract infection, cutaneous infection	1 Gm every 6 to 8 hr	3 to 4 Gm
Moderately severe or severe infections	1 Gm every 4 hr or 2 Gm every 6 to 8 hr	6 to 8 Gm
Infections commonly needing antibiotics in higher doses (e.g., gas gangrene)	2 Gm every 4 hr or 3 Gm every 6 hr	12 Gm

[a]Including patients in whom bacteremia is absent or unlikely.

Perioperative prophylaxis: 2 Gm 30 minutes to 1 hour before incision. Follow with 2 Gm every 6 hours for no more than 24 hours.

Prophylaxis during cesarean section: Either a single 2-Gm dose after clamping the umbilical cord or a 3-dose regimen consisting of 2 Gm given as soon as the umbilical cord is clamped followed by 2 Gm in 4 hours and again in 8 hours.

PEDIATRIC DOSE

Pediatric patients over 3 months of age: Manufacturer recommends 80 to 160 mg/kg/24 hr divided into 4 to 6 equal doses (20 to 40 mg/kg every 6 hours or 13.3 to 26.7 mg/kg every 4 hours), with higher doses being used for more severe or serious infections. Other sources recommend: *Mild to moderate infections:* 80 mg/kg/24 hr in equally divided doses every 6 to 8 hours (20 mg/kg every 6 hours or 26.66 mg/kg every 8 hours). *Severe infections:* 160 mg/kg/24 hr in equally divided doses every 6 hours (40 mg/kg every 6 hours). Do not exceed adult dose and/or 12 Gm.

Perioperative prophylaxis in pediatric patients over 3 months of age: 30 to 40 mg/kg 30 minutes to 1 hour before incision and every 6 hours for no more than 24 hours.

NEONATAL DOSE (unlabeled)

Use sterile cefoxitin sodium USP only. Other formulations may contain benzyl alcohol.

90 to 100 mg/kg/24 hr in equally divided doses every 8 hours (30 to 33.3 mg/kg every 8 hours).

DOSE ADJUSTMENTS

Reduced dose or extended intervals may be indicated in the elderly; consider age-related impaired organ function, nutritional status, and concomitant disease or drug therapy. ■ In impaired renal function, the initial dose should be as previously listed, but all remaining maintenance doses should be based on CrCl according to the following chart. See Drug/Lab Interactions.

Cefoxitin Maintenance Dose in Adults With Impaired Renal Function		
Creatinine Clearance (mL/min)	Dose (Gm)	Frequency
30-50 mL/min	1-2 Gm	q 8-12 hr
10-29 mL/min	1-2 Gm	q 12-24 hr
5-9 mL/min	0.5-1 Gm	q 12-24 hr
<5 mL/min	0.5-1 Gm	q 24-48 hr

Hemodialysis patients should receive a loading dose of 1 to 2 Gm after each dialysis in addition to the maintenance dose listed in the previous chart.

In pediatric patients, **the manufacturer recommends reducing the dose and frequency consistent with the recommendations for adults.**

DILUTION

1 Gm of the lyophilized powder must be reconstituted with at least 10 mL, and 2 Gm with 10 or 20 mL, of SWFI, BWFI, D5W, or NS. May be given as an intermittent injection, or a single dose may be further diluted in 50 to 1,000 mL of most common infusion solutions (see chart on inside back cover and literature). The use of butterfly needles and dilution in up to 1,000 mL of D5W, D5NS, or NS are preferred when administering larger doses as a continuous infusion. Also available in dual-chamber DUPLEX containers and as a frozen, premixed solution. Refer to manufacturer's prescribing information for specific preparation and storage requirements. May be given through a Y-tube, additive infusion set, or as a continuous infusion.

Storage: Storage before use is dependent on product. Reconstituted solutions are stable at RT for 6 hours, and 7 days if refrigerated. Solutions diluted in 50 to 1,000 mL diluent are stable for an additional 18 hours at RT and an additional 48 hours if refrigerated.

COMPATIBILITY

May be used concomitantly with aminoglycosides (e.g., amikacin, gentamicin), but these drugs must never be mixed in the same infusion (mutual inactivation). If given concurrently, administer separately and flush the IV line before and after administration. Manufacturer recommends temporarily discontinuing other solutions infusing at the same site during intermittent infusion. Do not introduce additives to the DUPLEX® container.

Other sources suggest specific **compatibilities** dependent on concentration and manufacturer; consult a pharmacist.

RATE OF ADMINISTRATION

See Dilution. Each 1 Gm or fraction thereof over 3 to 5 minutes or longer as indicated by amount of solution and condition of the patient. Intermittent infusions are commonly given over 30 minutes. Rate of continuous infusion should be by physician order.

ACTIONS

A semi-synthetic, second-generation cephalosporin antibiotic that is bactericidal to many gram-positive, gram-negative, and anaerobic organisms. Inhibits bacterial cell wall synthesis. Has activity in the presence of some beta-lactamases, both penicillinases and cephalosporinases, of gram-negative and gram-positive bacteria. Peak serum levels achieved by end of infusion. Widely distributed into many body tissues and fluids (CSF minimal). Passes into pleural and joint fluids and is detectable in antibacterial concentrations in bile. Half-life is 41 to 59 minutes. Excreted rapidly in the urine. Crosses the placental barrier. Secreted in breast milk.

INDICATIONS AND USES

Treatment of serious lower respiratory, urinary, intra-abdominal, gynecologic, bone and joint, skin and skin structure infections, and septicemia. Effective only if the causative organism is susceptible. If *C. trachomatis* is a suspected pathogen, antichlamydial coverage should be added. ▪ Perioperative prophylaxis in patients undergoing uncontaminated gastrointestinal surgery, vaginal or abdominal hysterectomy, or cesarean section.

CONTRAINDICATIONS

Previous hypersensitivity reaction to cefoxitin or other cephalosporins; see Precautions. ▪ Premixed solutions containing dextrose may be contraindicated in patients with known allergies to corn or corn products.

PRECAUTIONS

Hypersensitivity reactions, including fatalities, have been reported and include reports of individuals with a history of penicillin hypersensitivity or sensitivity to multiple allergens experiencing severe reactions when treated with cephalosporins. Check history of previous hypersensitivity reactions to penicillins, cephalosporins, or other allergens. Actual incidence of cross-allergenicity not established but may be more common with first-generation cephalosporins. ▪ Sensitivity studies indicated to determine susceptibility of the causative organism to cefoxitin. ▪ To reduce the development of drug-resistant bacteria and maintain its effectiveness, cefoxitin should be used to treat or prevent only those infections proven or strongly suspected to be caused by bacteria. ▪ Avoid prolonged use of drug; superinfection caused by overgrowth of nonsusceptible organisms may result. ▪ Use caution in patients with impaired renal function, allergies, or a history of GI disease (especially colitis). ▪ *Clostridium difficile*–associated diarrhea (CDAD) has been reported. May range from mild diarrhea to fatal colitis. Consider in patients who present with diarrhea during or after treatment with cefoxitin. ▪ Continue treatment for group A beta-hemolytic streptococcal infections for 10 days or more to decrease the risk of rheumatic fever or glomerulonephritis.

Monitor: Watch for early symptoms of a hypersensitivity reaction. ▪ Use extreme caution in the penicillin-sensitive patient; cross-sensitivity has been reported. ▪ Thrombophlebitis may result from prolonged or high dosage; use small needles and larger veins, and rotate infusion sites. ▪ Periodic monitoring of CBC, SCr, and liver function tests is recommended during prolonged therapy. ▪ See Drug/Lab Interactions; additional monitoring may be indicated (e.g., renal function, drug serum levels, PT).

Patient Education: Report promptly any bleeding or bruising or symptoms of hypersensitivity (e.g., difficulty breathing, hives, itching, rash). ▪ Promptly report diarrhea or bloody stools that occur during treatment or up to several months after an antibiotic has been discontinued; may indicate CDAD and require treatment.

Maternal/Child: Safety for use during pregnancy and breast-feeding not established. No problems documented. ▪ Safety and effectiveness for use in pediatric patients from birth to 3 months of age not established. ▪ Do not use formulations containing benzyl alcohol in infants and children under 3 months of age. ▪ Immature renal function will increase blood levels. ▪ Eosinophilia and elevated AST associated with higher doses in infants and children.

Elderly: Response similar to that seen in younger adults. Dose selection should be cautious; see Dose Adjustments. Monitoring of renal function suggested.

DRUG/LAB INTERACTIONS

Risk of nephrotoxicity may be increased with **aminoglycosides and other nephrotoxic agents** (e.g., loop diuretics such as furosemide). ▪ **Probenecid** inhibits excretion. Reduced dose of cefoxitin may be required with concomitant use. ▪ May be antagonized by **bacteriostatic antibiotics** (e.g., chloramphenicol, erythromycin, tetracyclines); may interfere with bactericidal action. ▪ Cephalosporins may enhance the anticoagulant effects of **vitamin K antagonists** (e.g., warfarin). ▪ False-positive reaction for **urine glucose** has been reported with Clinitest reagent tablets. Glucose tests based on enzymatic glucose oxidase reactions (e.g., Clinistix) is recommended. ▪ False increases in **creatinine levels** with Jaffe method. ▪ False increases in **urinary 17-hydroxy-corticosteroids levels** have been reported with high concentrations of cefoxitin in the urine. ▪ See Compatibility and Side Effects.

SIDE EFFECTS

Local site reactions (e.g., thrombophlebitis) are most common. Acute renal failure; anemia; CDAD; colitis; hypersensitivity reactions (including anaphylaxis, angioedema, dyspnea, eosinophilia, fever, flushing, interstitial nephritis, pruritus, rash [including exfoliative dermatitis and toxic epidermal necrolysis], urticaria); elevations in SCr and BUN; hypotension; jaundice; leukopenia; nausea and vomiting; neutropenia; oral thrush; phlebitis; positive direct Coombs' test; possible exacerbation of myasthenia gravis prolonged PT; proteinuria; seizures (large doses); thrombocytopenia; and transient elevation of AST, ALT, and alkaline phosphatase have occurred. Hypoprothrombinemia (rare) and hemolytic anemia may occur. Abdominal pain, agranulocytosis, aplastic anemia, erythema multiforme, hemolytic anemia, hemorrhage, hepatic dysfunction (including cholestasis), pancytopenia, renal dysfunction, Stevens-Johnson syndrome, superinfection, toxic epidermal necrolysis, toxic nephropathy, and vaginitis have been reported with cephalosporin-class antibiotics.

ANTIDOTE

Notify physician of any side effects. Discontinue the drug if indicated. Treat CDAD with fluids, electrolytes, protein supplements, and appropriate antibiotics (e.g., oral vancomycin) as indicated. In severe cases, surgical evaluation may be indicated. Treat hypersensitivity reactions as indicated and resuscitate as necessary. Hemodialysis may be useful in overdose.

CEFTAROLINE FOSAMIL
(cef-**TAR**-oh-leen **FOS**-a-mil)

Teflaro

Antibacterial
(cephalosporin)

pH 4.8 to 6.5

USUAL DOSE

Pretreatment: Baseline studies indicated; see Monitor.

Ceftaroline: 600 mg every 8-12 hours as an IV infusion over 5-60 minutes. Duration of therapy should be guided by the severity and the site of infection and the patient's clinical and bacteriologic progress.

PEDIATRIC DOSE

Dosage is based on the age and weight of the child as outlined in the following charts. Duration of therapy should be guided by the severity and site of infection and the patient's clinical and bacteriologic progress.

Dosage of Ceftaroline by Indication in Pediatric Patients 2 Months of Age and Older				
Indication	**Age Range**	**Dosage and Frequency**	**Infusion Time**	**Recommended Duration of Therapy**
Acute bacterial skin and skin structure infection (ABSSSI) **OR** Community-acquired bacterial pneumonia (CABP)	2 months to <2 years	8 mg/kg q 8 hr	5-60 minutes	5-14 days
	≥2 years to <18 years (≤33 kg)	12 mg/kg q 8 hr		
	≥2 years to <18 years (>33 kg)	400 mg/kg q 8 hr **OR** 600 mg q 12 hr		

Dosage of Ceftaroline in Pediatric Patients Under 2 Months of Age (Gestational Age 34 Weeks and Older and Postnatal Age 12 Days and Older[a])				
Indication	**Age Range**	**Dosage and Frequency**	**Infusion Time**	**Recommended Duration of Treatment**
Acute bacterial skin and skin structure infection (ABSSSI)	0[a] to less than 2 months	6 mg/kg q 8 hr	30-60 minutes	5-14 days

[a]Gestational age 34 weeks and older and postnatal age 12 days and older.

DOSE ADJUSTMENTS

Dose adjustment required with renal impairment as outlined in the following chart.

Dosage of Ceftaroline in Adult Patients With Renal Impairment	
Estimated CrCl[a] (mL/min)	Recommended Dosage Regimen
>50 mL/min	600 mg q 12 hr
>30 to ≤50 mL/min	400 mg q 12 hr
≥15 to ≤30 mL/min	300 mg q 12 hr
End-stage renal disease, including hemodialysis[b]	200 mg q 12 hr[c]

[a]CrCl as calculated by Cockcroft-Gault formula.
[b]End-stage renal disease is defined as CrCl <15 mL/min.
[c]Ceftaroline is hemodialyzable; administer after hemodialysis on hemodialysis days.

- No dose adjustment is required in pediatric patients with CrCl >50 mL/min/1.73 M^2, estimated using the Schwartz equation. There is insufficient information to recommend a dosage regimen for pediatric patients with a CrCl <50 mL/min/1.73 M^2. - Dose adjustment is not indicated based on gender, race, or hepatic function. - Reduced dose may be indicated in the elderly based on age-related renal impairment.

DILUTION
Available in single-dose glass vials containing 600 mg or 400 mg. Reconstitute with 20 mL of SWFI, NS, D5W, or LR as shown in the following chart. Mix gently. Time to dissolution is less than 2 minutes.

Preparation of Ceftaroline for Intravenous Use			
Dosage Strength (mg)	Volume of Diluent to Be Added (mL)	Approximate Ceftaroline Concentration (mg/mL)	Amount to Be Withdrawn
400 mg	20 mL	20 mg/mL	**Adult:** Total volume **Pediatric**[a]: Volume based on age and weight
600 mg	20 mL	30 mg/mL	**Adult:** Total volume **Pediatric**[a]: Volume based on age and weight

[a]The recommended dosage of ceftaroline is based on the age and weight of the child.

Further dilute the reconstituted solution in 50 to 250 mL. Use the same diluent for further dilution unless SWFI was used. If SWFI was used as the initial diluent, further dilute the reconstituted solution in NS, D5W, D2.5/0.45NS, or LR.

Adults: When preparing a 600-mg ceftaroline dose in a 50-mL infusion bag, withdraw 20 mL of the infusion solution before injecting the reconstituted drug into the bag. Resultant concentration approximately 12 mg/mL.

Adult or pediatric patients weighing more than 33 kg: When preparing a 400-mg ceftaroline dose in a 50-mL infusion bag, withdraw 20 mL of the infusion solution before injecting the reconstituted drug into the bag. Resultant concentration approximately 8 mg/mL.

Pediatric patients weighing 33 kg or less: When preparing a ceftaroline dose in a 50-mL infusion bag, the amount of solution withdrawn from the reconstituted ceftaroline vial will vary according to the weight and age of the child.

The final solution concentration should not exceed 12 mg/mL. Infusion solution ranges from clear light yellow to dark yellow depending on the concentration and the storage conditions.

Filter: Data not available.

Storage: Store unopened vials at CRT. Diluted solution should be used within 6 hours when stored at RT or within 24 hours when refrigerated.

COMPATIBILITY
Manufacturer states, "Should not be mixed with or physically added to solutions containing other drugs." **Compatibility** with other drugs has not been established.

Other sources suggest specific **compatibilities** dependent on concentration and manufacturer; consult a pharmacist.

RATE OF ADMINISTRATION

Adults and pediatric patients 2 months of age and older: A single dose equally distributed over 5 to 60 minutes.

Pediatric patients under 2 months of age: A single dose equally distributed over 30 to 60 minutes.

ACTIONS

A semi-synthetic, broad-spectrum cephalosporin. Ceftaroline fosamil, a prodrug, is converted into the bioactive ceftaroline in plasma by a phosphatase enzyme. Bactericidal to many gram-negative and gram-positive organisms. Inhibits bacterial cell wall synthesis. Protein binding is minimal (20%). Ceftaroline undergoes hydrolysis, forming an inactive metabolite. Half-life is approximately 2.2 to 3 hours. Both ceftaroline and its metabolites are primarily eliminated by the kidneys.

INDICATIONS AND USES

Treatment of adults and pediatric patients (at least 34 weeks gestational age and 12 days postnatal age) with acute bacterial skin and skin structure infection (ABSSSI) caused by susceptible strains of microorganisms. ▪ Treatment of adults and pediatric patients 2 months of age and older with community-acquired bacterial pneumonia (CABP) caused by susceptible strains of microorganisms.

CONTRAINDICATIONS

Known serious hypersensitivity to ceftaroline or other members of the cephalosporin class.

PRECAUTIONS

Hypersensitivity reactions, some fatal, and serious skin reactions have been reported in patients receiving beta-lactam antibiotics. Check history of previous hypersensitivity reactions to penicillins, cephalosporins, carbapenems, or other allergens. Cross-sensitivity among beta-lactam antibacterial agents has been established; however, the actual incidence of cross-allergenicity is not established. ▪ Specific sensitivity studies are indicated to determine susceptibility of the causative organism to ceftaroline. ▪ To reduce the development of drug-resistant bacteria and maintain its effectiveness, ceftaroline should be used to treat or prevent only those infections proven or strongly suspected to be caused by susceptible bacteria. ▪ Although cross-resistance may occur, some isolates resistant to other cephalosporins may be susceptible to ceftaroline. ▪ *Clostridium difficile*–associated diarrhea (CDAD) has been reported. May range from mild diarrhea to fatal colitis. Consider in patients who present with diarrhea during or after treatment with ceftaroline. ▪ Seroconversion from a negative to a positive direct Coombs' test occurred in approximately 10% of adult patients and in approximately 18% of pediatric patients in clinical trials. No adverse reactions representing hemolytic anemia were reported. If anemia develops during or after treatment with ceftaroline, drug-induced hemolytic anemia should be considered and diagnostic studies, including a direct Coombs' test, should be performed.

Monitor: Watch for early symptoms of a hypersensitivity reaction. ▪ Obtain baseline CBC with differential and platelet count and SCr.

Patient Education: Promptly report S/S of a hypersensitivity reaction (e.g., rash, hives, wheezing, shortness of breath). ▪ Promptly report diarrhea or bloody stools that occur during treatment or up to several months after an antibiotic has been discontinued; may indicate CDAD and require treatment.

Maternal/Child: Safety for use during pregnancy not established; use only if clearly needed. ▪ No data are available regarding the presence of ceftaroline in human milk, the effects of ceftaroline on breast-fed infants, or the effects on milk production; use caution. ▪ Safety and effectiveness for use in pediatric patients at least 34 weeks gestational age and 12 days postnatal age for treatment of ABSSSI have been established. ▪ Safety and effectiveness for use in pediatric patients less than 34 weeks gestational age and 12 days postnatal age for treatment of ABSSSI have not been established. ▪ Safety and effectiveness for use in pediatric patients under 2 months of age for treatment of CABP have not been established.

Elderly: No specific problems documented. Efficacy and safety appear similar to that seen in younger patients. Consider age-related renal impairment; see Dose Adjustments.

DRUG/LAB INTERACTIONS

No clinical drug-drug interaction studies have been conducted. There is minimal potential for drug-drug interactions between ceftaroline and CYP450 substrates, inhibitors, or inducers; drugs known to undergo active renal secretion; and drugs that may alter renal blood flow.

SIDE EFFECTS

The most common side effects occurring in both adult and pediatric patients were diarrhea, nausea, and rash. Additional side effects more commonly reported in pediatric patients included fever and vomiting. Hypersensitivity reactions were the most frequently reported serious side effects leading to discontinuation of therapy. Other less frequently reported side effects included CDAD, constipation, hypokalemia, increased transaminases (ALT, AST), phlebitis, seroconversion from a negative to a positive direct Coombs' test, and vomiting. Several other side effects were reported in less than 2% of the population studied.

Post-Marketing: Agranulocytosis, eosinophilic pneumonia, leukopenia.

ANTIDOTE

Notify physician of any side effects. Discontinue the drug if indicated. Treat hypersensitivity reactions as indicated (e.g., diphenhydramine, epinephrine, albuterol) and resuscitate as necessary. Discontinue ceftaroline for suspected drug-induced hemolytic anemia and initiate supportive therapy as indicated (e.g., transfusion). Mild cases of CDAD may respond to discontinuation of ceftaroline. Treat CDAD with fluids, electrolytes, protein supplements, and appropriate antibiotics (e.g., oral vancomycin) as indicated. In severe cases, surgical evaluation may be indicated. Ceftaroline is partially removed by hemodialysis.

CEFTAZIDIME	Antibacterial
(sef-**TAY**-zih-deem)	(cephalosporin)
Fortaz, Tazicef	pH 5 to 8

USUAL DOSE

Pretreatment: Baseline studies indicated; see Monitor.

Range is from 250 mg to 2 Gm every 8 to 12 hours. Dosage based on severity of infection, condition and renal function of the patient, and susceptibility of the causative organism.

Uncomplicated urinary tract infections: 250 mg every 12 hours.

Complicated urinary tract infections: 500 mg every 8 to 12 hours.

Uncomplicated pneumonia; mild skin and skin structure infections: 500 mg to 1 Gm every 8 hours.

Bone and joint infections: 2 Gm every 12 hours.

Severe or life-threatening infections (especially in immunocompromised patients), meningitis, serious gynecologic and intra-abdominal infections: 2 Gm every 8 hours.

Pseudomonal lung infections in cystic fibrosis patients (must have normal renal function): 30 to 50 mg/kg of body weight every 8 hours. Do not exceed 6 Gm/24 hr.

PEDIATRIC DOSE

Pediatric patients 1 month to 12 years of age: 30 to 50 mg/kg of body weight every 8 hours. Reserve higher doses for immunocompromised pediatric patients or for those with cystic fibrosis or meningitis. Do not exceed 6 Gm/24 hr.

NEONATAL DOSE

Neonates up to 4 weeks of age: 30 mg/kg every 12 hours. Other dosing regimens based on age and weight are available in the pediatric literature.

DOSE ADJUSTMENTS

Reduced dose or extended intervals may be indicated in the elderly; consider age-related impaired organ function, nutritional status, and concomitant disease or drug therapy. ■ In impaired renal function, an initial loading dose of 1 Gm may be given, but all remaining doses should be based on CrCl according to the following chart. Adjustment for pediatric patients is similar to adults; consider body surface area or lean body mass and reduce dosing frequency.

Ceftazidime Maintenance Dose in Impaired Renal Function		
Creatinine Clearance (mL/min)	**Dose[a]**	**Frequency**
31-50 mL/min	1 Gm	q 12 hr
16-30 mL/min	1 Gm	q 24 hr
6-15 mL/min	500 mg	q 24 hr
<5 mL/min	500 mg	q 48 hr
Hemodialysis patients	1 Gm	After each dialysis session
Peritoneal dialysis patients	500 mg	q 24 hr

[a]If the normal dose would be lower than the doses in the chart, use the lower dose.

In patients with impaired renal function who have severe infection (normally requiring a 6 Gm/24 hr dose), the dose in the previous chart may be increased by 50% or the dosing frequency may be increased. In patients undergoing hemodialysis, give a loading dose of 1 Gm followed by 1 Gm after each dialysis. ■ In peritoneal dialysis patients (CAPD), give a loading dose of 1 Gm followed by 500 mg every 24 hours. In addition to IV use, ceftazidime can be incorporated in the dialysis fluid at a concentration of 250 mg for 2 L of dialysis fluid. ▪ Dose reduction not required in impaired hepatic function.

DILUTION

IV injection: Directions for the initial preparation of ceftazidime solutions are outlined in the following chart.

Preparation of Ceftazidime Solutions[a]			
Size	Amount of Diluent to Be Added (mL)	Approximate Available Volume (mL)	Approximate Ceftazidime Concentration (mg/mL)
500-mg vial	5.3	5.7[b]	100
1-Gm vial	10	10.8[c]	100
2-Gm vial	10	11.5[d]	170

[a]Directions may vary slightly depending on manufacturer. Consult prescribing information for product-specific reconstitution and dilution instructions.
[b]To obtain a dose of 500 mg, withdraw 5 mL from vial after reconstitution.
[c]To obtain a dose of 1 Gm, withdraw 10 mL from vial after reconstitution.
[d]To obtain a dose of 2 Gm, withdraw 11.5 mL from vial after reconstitution.

Reconstitute with SWFI as outlined in the chart. Shake well. Dilution generates CO_2. Invert vial and completely depress plunger of syringe. Insert needle through stopper and keep it within the solution. Expel bubbles from solution in syringe before injection.

Intermittent IV infusion: A single dose may be further diluted in 50 to 100 mL of D5W, NS, or other **compatible** infusion solutions for injection (see literature or chart on inside back cover).

Storage: Store unopened vials in carton at CRT. Protect from light. Stability of reconstituted and diluted solution is product specific; consult manufacturer's prescribing information. Selected products may be frozen for up to 3 months after initial dilution; thaw at room temperature (see instructions); do not refreeze. Will be light yellow to amber in color depending on concentration and diluent.

COMPATIBILITY

May be used concomitantly with aminoglycosides (e.g., amikacin, gentamicin, and tobramycin), but these drugs must never be mixed in the same infusion (mutual inactivation). May exhibit a physical **incompatibility** with vancomycin depending on concentration. If aminoglycosides or vancomycin are given concurrently, administer separately and flush IV line before and after administration. Manufacturer recommends temporarily discontinuing other solutions infusing at the same site during intermittent infusion and states, "Do not add supplementary medications to premixed plastic IV containers."

Other sources suggest specific **compatibilities** dependent on concentration and manufacturer; consult a pharmacist.

RATE OF ADMINISTRATION

See Compatibility. May be given through Y-tube of infusion set.

IV injection: A single dose equally distributed over 3 to 5 minutes.

Intermittent IV infusion: A single dose over 15 to 30 minutes. May also be given (off label) as extended infusion: IV 2 gm every 8 hours over 3-4 hours or my continuous infusion: 6 gm infused over 24 hours. May give first 2 gm dose over 30 minutes before starting infusion.

ACTIONS

A broad-spectrum, third-generation cephalosporin antibiotic. Bactericidal to selected gram-negative, gram-positive, and anaerobic organisms. Effective against many otherwise resistant organisms, including *Pseudomonas aeruginosa*. Inhibits bacterial cell wall synthesis and has activity in the presence of some beta-lactamases of gram-negative and gram-positive bacteria. Peak serum levels achieved by end of infusion. Therapeutic levels distributed into many body fluids and tissues, including CSF and aqueous humor.

Half-life is 1.9 hours. Excreted unchanged in the urine. Crosses placental barrier. Secreted in breast milk.

INDICATIONS AND USES

Treatment of the following infections caused by susceptible isolates of the designated microorganisms (see prescribing information): lower respiratory tract, urinary tract, skin and skin structure, bone and joint, gynecologic, intra-abdominal, CNS infections (including meningitis), and bacterial septicemia. Has been used alone in cases of confirmed or suspected sepsis and in combination with other antibacterial drugs such as aminoglycosides, vancomycin, and clindamycin in severe and life-threatening infections and in immunocompromised patients.

CONTRAINDICATIONS

History of hypersensitivity reaction to ceftazidime or the cephalosporin class of antibiotics; see Precautions. ▪ Premixed solutions containing dextrose may be contraindicated in patients with known allergies to corn or corn products.

PRECAUTIONS

Hypersensitivity reactions, including fatalities, have been reported and include reports of individuals with a history of penicillin hypersensitivity or sensitivity to multiple allergens experiencing severe reactions when treated with cephalosporins. Check history of previous hypersensitivity reactions to penicillins, cephalosporins, or other allergens. Actual incidence of cross-allergenicity not established but may be more common with first-generation cephalosporins. ▪ Hypersensitivity reactions have been reported with administration of corn-derived, dextrose-containing products in patients with or without a history of hypersensitivity to corn products. Ceftazidime in the DUPLEX container contains dextrose. ▪ Specific sensitivity studies indicated to determine susceptibility of causative organism to ceftazidime. Inducible type I beta-lactamase resistance has been noted with some organisms and can develop during therapy, leading to clinical failure. Periodic susceptibility testing may be indicated. ▪ To reduce the development of drug-resistant bacteria and maintain its effectiveness, ceftazidime should be used to treat only those infections proven or strongly suspected to be caused by bacteria. ▪ Use with caution in patients with renal impairment. Elevated levels of ceftazidime in these patients can lead to asterixis, coma, encephalopathy, myoclonus, neuromuscular excitability, and seizures; see Dose Adjustments. ▪ May be associated with a fall in prothrombin activity. Patients at risk include those with renal or hepatic impairment, those with poor nutritional status, and those receiving a protracted course of antimicrobial therapy. See Monitor. ▪ Avoid prolonged use of drug; superinfection caused by overgrowth of nonsusceptible organisms may result. ▪ Use caution in patients with a history of GI disease (especially colitis). ▪ An immune-mediated hemolytic anemia has been reported in patients receiving cephalosporin class antibiotics, including ceftazidime. ▪ *Clostridium difficile*–associated diarrhea (CDAD) has been reported. May range from mild diarrhea to fatal colitis. Consider in patients who present with diarrhea during or after treatment with ceftazidime. ▪ Continue for at least 2 days after all symptoms of infection subside.

Monitor: Obtain baseline and periodic CBC and SCr. ▪ Watch for early symptoms of a hypersensitivity reaction. ▪ Monitor PT and administer vitamin K as indicated; see Precautions. ▪ See Drug/Lab Interactions; additional monitoring may be indicated (e.g., renal function, drug serum levels, PT).

Patient Education: Report promptly any bleeding or bruising, symptoms of hypersensitivity (e.g., difficulty breathing, hives, itching, rash), or neurologic symptoms (e.g., confusion, myoclonus, seizures). ▪ Promptly report diarrhea or bloody stools that occur during treatment or up to several months after an antibiotic has been discontinued; may indicate CDAD and require treatment.

Maternal/Child: Category B: safety for use during pregnancy and breast-feeding not established. No problems documented. Use caution. ▪ Immature renal function of infants and small children will increase blood levels of all cephalosporins. ▪ Only specific solutions can be used in pediatric patients.

Elderly: No specific differences in safety or effectiveness were observed between elderly and younger patients. ▪ See Usual Dose and Dose Adjustments.

DRUG/LAB INTERACTIONS

Risk of nephrotoxicity and ototoxicity may be increased with **aminoglycosides and other nephrotoxic and/or ototoxic agents** (e.g., loop diuretics such as furosemide). ▪ May be antagonized by **bacteriostatic antibiotics** (e.g., chloramphenicol, erythromycin, tetracyclines); may interfere with bactericidal action. ▪ **Probenecid** inhibits excretion of ceftazidime and may increase serum concentrations. ▪ Cephalosporins may enhance the anticoagulant effects of **vitamin K antagonists** (e.g., warfarin). ▪ May reduce the effectiveness of **oral estrogen/progesterone contraceptives.** ▪ May have a false-positive reaction for **urine glucose** except with enzyme-based tests (e.g., Clinistix). ▪ See Compatibility and Side Effects.

SIDE EFFECTS

The most common adverse reactions occurring in fewer than 2% of patients include hypersensitivity reactions, GI symptoms, and CNS reactions. Full scope of hypersensitivity reactions (including anaphylaxis, bronchospasm, cardiopulmonary arrest, hypotension); abdominal pain; angioedema; burning, discomfort, and pain at injection site; candidiasis; CDAD; colitis; diarrhea; dizziness; elevated alkaline phosphatase, AST, ALT, GGT, and BUN/SCr; erythema multiforme; fever; headache; nausea and vomiting; paresthesia; phlebitis; prolonged PT; pruritus; rash; renal impairment; seizures (large doses or in patients with renal impairment); Stevens-Johnson syndrome; toxic epidermal necrolysis; toxic nephropathy; urticaria; vaginitis. Hypoprothrombinemia (rare) and hemolytic anemia may occur. Aplastic anemia, erythema multiforme, hemolytic anemia, hemorrhage, hepatic dysfunction (including cholestasis), pancytopenia, renal dysfunction, Stevens-Johnson syndrome, toxic epidermal necrolysis, and toxic nephropathy have been reported with cephalosporin-class antibiotics.

Overdose: Asterixis, coma, encephalopathy, neuromuscular excitability, and seizures may occur in patients with renal impairment; see Precautions.

Post-Marketing: Hyperbilirubinemia, jaundice.

ANTIDOTE

Notify physician of any side effects. Discontinue the drug if indicated. Treat hypersensitivity reaction as indicated and resuscitate as necessary. Mild cases of CDAD may respond to discontinuation of ceftazidime. Treat CDAD with fluids, electrolytes, protein supplements, and appropriate antibiotics (e.g., oral vancomycin) as indicated. In severe cases, surgical evaluation may be indicated. Hemodialysis may be useful in overdose.

CEFTAZIDIME/AVIBACTAM

(sef-**TAY**-zih-deem a-vih-**BAK**-tam)

Antibacterial
(cephalosporin/beta-lactamase inhibitor)

Avycaz

USUAL DOSE

Pretreatment: Baseline studies indicated; see Monitor.

18 years of age or older: 2.5 Gm (2 Gm ceftazidime/0.5 Gm avibactam) every 8 hours as an infusion over 2 hours.

PEDIATRIC DOSE

Dose of Ceftazidime/Avibactam in Patients 3 Months to Less Than 18 Years of Age					
Infection	Age Range	Dose	Frequency	Infusion Time (hours)	Duration of Treatment
cIAI[a] and cUTI including Pyelonephritis	2 years to less than 18 years[b]	62.5 mg/kg to a maximum of 2.5 Gm (Ceftazidime 50 mg/kg and avibactam 12.5 mg/kg to a maximum dose of ceftazidime 2 Gm and avibactam 0.5 Gm)	Every 8 hours	2	cIAI: 5 to 14 days cUTI: 7 to 14 days
	6 months to less than 2 years	62.5 mg/kg (Ceftazidime 50 mg/kg and avibactam 12.5 mg/kg)			
	3 months to less than 6 months	50 mg/kg (Ceftazidime 40 mg/kg and avibactam 10 mg/kg)			

[a]Ceftazidime/avibactam was used in combination with metronidazole in cIAI pediatric patients in clinical studies (metronidazole dose used was 10 mg/kg q 8 hr).

[b]For pediatric patients (2 years or older) with eGFR ≤50 mL/min/1.73 M^2, dosage adjustments are recommended; see Dose Adjustments.

DOSE ADJUSTMENTS

No dose adjustment is recommended based on age, gender, or hepatic impairment.

- Reduced dose may be indicated in the elderly based on age-related renal impairment.
- Dose adjustment required for patients with moderate and severe renal impairment and end-stage renal disease according to the following charts.

Ceftazidime-Avibactam Dosing in Adult Patients With Renal Impairment	
Estimated CrCl (mL/min)	Recommended Dose Regimen
>50 mL/min	2.5 Gm (2 Gm/0.5 Gm) IV every 8 hours.
31 to 50 mL/min	1.25 Gm (1 Gm/0.25 Gm) IV every 8 hours.
16 to 30 mL/min	0.94 Gm (0.75 Gm/0.19 Gm) IV every 12 hours.
6 to 15 mL/min[a]	0.94 Gm (0.75 Gm/0.19 Gm) IV every 24 hours.
≤5 mL/min[a]	0.94 Gm (0.75 Gm/0.19 Gm) IV every 48 hours.

[a]Both ceftazidime and avibactam are hemodialyzable; administer after hemodialysis on hemodialysis days.

Ceftazidime-Avibactam Dosing in Pediatric Patients 2 Years and Older With Renal Impairment[a]		
Estimated eGFR[b] (mL/min/1.73M²)	Dose	Frequency
31 to 50 mL/min	31.25 mg/kg to a maximum of 1.25 Gm (ceftazidime 25 mg/kg and avibactam 6.25 mg/kg to a maximum dose of ceftazidime 1 Gm and avibactam 0.25 Gm)	Every 8 hours
16 to 30 mL/min	23.75 mg/kg to a maximum of 0.94 Gm (ceftazidime 19 mg/kg and avibactam 4.75 mg/kg to a maximum dose of ceftazidime 0.75 Gm and avibactam 0.19 Gm)	Every 12 hours
6 to 15 mL/min	23.75 mg/kg to a maximum of 0.94 Gm (ceftazidime 19 mg/kg and avibactam 4.75 mg/kg to a maximum dose of ceftazidime 0.75 Gm and avibactam 0.19 Gm)	Every 24 hours
≤5 mL/min[c]	23.75 mg/kg to a maximum of 0.94 Gm (ceftazidime 19 mg/kg and avibactam 4.75 mg/kg to a maximum dose of ceftazidime 0.75 Gm and avibactam 0.19 Gm)	Every 48 hours

[a]Dosing was derived based on the population PK modeling, which assumed similar proportional effects of renal impairment in adults and pediatric patients 2 years of age and older.
[b]As calculated using the Schwartz bedside formula.
[c]Both ceftazidime and avibactam are hemodialyzable; administer after hemodialysis on hemodialysis days.

DILUTION

Available as single-use vials containing 2 Gm ceftazidime and 0.5 Gm avibactam. Reconstitute each vial with 10 mL of SWFI, NS, D5W, all combinations of dextrose and sodium chloride injection containing up to 2.5% dextrose and 0.45% NS, or LR injection. Mix gently. Reconstituted solution will have an approximate final volume of 12 mL, an approximate ceftazidime concentration of 167 mg/mL, and an approximate avibactam concentration of 42 mg/mL. Must be further diluted before infusion. Withdraw the required dose from the vial according to the following chart and transfer into an infusion bag containing the same diluent used for reconstitution of the powder (except SWFI) to achieve a final ceftazidime concentration of 8 to 40 mg/mL and a final avibactam concentration of 2 to 10 mg/mL. If SWFI was used for reconstitution, use any of the other appropriate diluents listed previously for dilution.

Preparation of Ceftazidime-Avibactam to Achieve Required Doses in Adult and Pediatric Patients (Weighing 40 kg or More)	
Ceftazidime-Avibactam Dose	Volume to Withdraw From Reconstituted Vial for Further Dilution to 50 to 250[a] mL
2.5 Gm (2 Gm/0.5 Gm)	Entire contents (12 mL)
1.25 Gm (1 Gm/0.25 Gm)	½ of vial contents (6 mL)
0.94 Gm (0.75 Gm/0.19 Gm)	4.5 mL

[a]Dilution to 250 mL should be used only for the 2.5-Gm dose.

To prepare doses for pediatric patients weighing less than 40 kg, follow the constitution instruction in the previous chart to yield a solution with a final ceftazidime-avibactam concentration of approximately 209 mg/mL (ceftazidime concentration of 167 mg/mL and avibactam concentration of 42 mg/mL). Use these concentrations to calculate the volume of ceftazidime-avibactam required to prepare the prescribed dose. Ensure that contents are completely dissolved. Infusion solution ranges from clear to light yellow.
Filters: Specific information not available.
Storage: Before use, store at CRT in original carton to protect from light. The reconstituted solution may be held for no longer than 30 minutes before dilution in a suitable

infusion solution. Fully diluted solutions may be stored for 12 hours at room temperature or for 24 hours refrigerated at 2° to 8° C (36° to 46° F). Use refrigerated solution within 12 hours of subsequent storage at RT.

COMPATIBILITY

Manufacturer states **compatible** with the more commonly used IV infusion fluids in infusion bags (including Baxter Mini-Bag Plus); see Dilution. Simulated **Y-site compatibility** studies using a solution of ceftazidime and avibactam at concentrations of 20 mg/mL and 5 mg/mL, respectively, were performed. **Compatible** drugs with the corresponding **compatible** diluent (D5W, NS, or LR) include amikacin, azithromycin, aztreonam, ceftaroline, colistimethate, daptomycin, dexmedetomidine, dopamine, furosemide, gentamicin, imipenem-cilastatin, levofloxacin, magnesium sulfate, metronidazole, norepinephrine, phenylephrine, vasopressin, and vecuronium. Depending on the diluent, the following drugs may also be **compatible** at the **Y-site** (see prescribing information for specific information): ertapenem, heparin, linezolid, meropenem, potassium chloride, potassium phosphates, sodium bicarbonate, tedizolid, and tobramycin.

RATE OF ADMINISTRATION

A single dose as an infusion equally distributed over 2 hours.

ACTIONS

Ceftazidime-avibactam is an antibacterial combination product consisting of the cephalosporin ceftazidime pentahydrate and the beta-lactamase inhibitor avibactam sodium. Ceftazidime is a cephalosporin antibacterial drug with in vitro activity against certain gram-negative and gram-positive bacteria. Active against several gram-negative bacteria in clinical infections. Its bactericidal action results from inhibition of cell wall biosynthesis and is mediated through binding to penicillin-binding proteins (PBPs). Avibactam is a non–beta-lactam beta-lactamase inhibitor that inactivates certain beta-lactamases that degrade ceftazidime. Less than 10% of ceftazidime is protein bound. Both ceftazidime and avibactam are excreted mainly by the kidneys, primarily as unchanged drug. Terminal half-life is approximately 2.8 hours. Ceftazidime is excreted in human milk in low concentrations.

INDICATIONS AND USES

Treatment of infections caused by susceptible isolates of designated organisms in the conditions and patient populations listed below. ▪ Used in combination with metronidazole for the treatment of complicated intra-abdominal infections (cIAI) in adult and pediatric patients 3 months of age or older. ▪ Treatment of complicated urinary tract infections (cUTI), including pyelonephritis, in adult and pediatric patients 3 months of age or older. ▪ Treatment of hospital-acquired bacterial pneumonia and ventilator-associated bacterial pneumonia (HABP/VABP) in patients 18 years of age or older.

CONTRAINDICATIONS

Known serious hypersensitivity to ceftazidime-avibactam, ceftazidime, avibactam-containing products, or other members of the cephalosporin class.

PRECAUTIONS

For IV infusion only; do not administer as an IV bolus. ▪ In a cIAI trial, clinical cure rates were lower in a subgroup of patients with a baseline CrCl of 30 mL/min to less than or equal to 50 mL/min compared with patients with a CrCl of greater than 50 mL/min. Reduction in clinical cure rates was more marked in patients treated with ceftazidime-avibactam plus metronidazole compared with meropenem-treated patients. Within this subgroup, patients treated with ceftazidime/avibactam received a 33% lower daily dose than is currently recommended for patients with a CrCl of 30 mL/min to less than or equal to 50 mL/min; see Monitor. ▪ Serious and occasionally fatal hypersensitivity (anaphylactic) reactions and serious skin reactions have been reported in patients receiving beta-lactam antibacterial drugs. Check history of previous hypersensitivity reactions to other cephalosporins, penicillins, or carbapenems. Cross-sensitivity among beta-lactam antibacterial drugs has been established. ▪ Specific sensitivity studies are indicated to determine susceptibility of the causative organism to ceftazidime-avibactam. ▪ To reduce the development of drug-resistant bacteria and maintain its effectiveness, ceftazidime-avibactam should be used to treat only those infections proven or strongly suspected to be caused by susceptible bacteria. ▪ No cross-resistance with other classes of antimicrobials has been identified. Some isolates resistant to other cephalosporins (including ceftazidime) and to carbapenems may be susceptible to ceftazidime-avibactam. ▪ *Clostridium difficile* –associated diarrhea (CDAD) has been reported for nearly all systemic antibacterial agents and may range in severity from mild diarrhea to fatal colitis. Consider in patients who present with diarrhea during or after treatment with ceftazidime-avibactam. ▪ Central nervous system reactions (e.g., asterixis, coma, encephalopathy, myoclonia, neuromuscular excitability, nonconvulsive status epilepticus, and seizures) have been reported in patients treated with ceftazidime, particularly in patients with renal impairment. Adjust dose based on CrCl.

Monitor: Obtain baseline and periodic SCr. Monitor CrCl at least daily in patients with changing renal function. Adjust dose of ceftazidime-avibactam accordingly; see Dose Adjustments. ▪ Monitor for S/S of a hypersensitivity reaction (e.g., hypotension, rash, urticaria, tightness of the chest, wheezing).

Patient Education: Promptly report S/S of a hypersensitivity reaction (e.g., hives, rash, shortness of breath, wheezing). ▪ Promptly report diarrhea or bloody stools that occur during treatment or up to several months after an antibiotic has been discontinued; may indicate CDAD and require treatment. ▪ Promptly report neurologic S/S (e.g., encephalopathy [disturbance of consciousness including confusion, hallucinations, stupor, and coma], myoclonus, and seizures). ▪ Full course of therapy must be completed.

Maternal/Child: Use during pregnancy only if clearly needed. ▪ No information is available on the effects of ceftazidime and avibactam on breast-fed pediatric patients or on milk production; use caution during breast-feeding. ▪ Safety and effectiveness in the treatment of cIAI and cUTI have been established in pediatric patients 3 months to less than 18 years of age. Safety and effectiveness in pediatric patients under 3 months of age with cIAI or cUTI have not been established. Safety and effectiveness in patients under 18 years of age with HABP/VABP have not been established.

Elderly: Incidence of side effects may be higher in elderly patients being treated for cIAI. This finding was not identified in the cUTI or HABP/VABP trials. ▪ Consider age-related renal impairment, monitoring of renal function, and dose with caution; see Dose Adjustments.

DRUG/LAB INTERACTIONS

Formal drug interaction studies have not been conducted. ▪ In vitro, avibactam is a substrate of OAT1 and OAT3. Coadministration with **probenecid** prolongs the half-life of avibactam and is not recommended. ▪ In vitro studies have not demonstrated antagonism between ceftazidime-avibactam and colistin, levofloxacin (Levaquin), linezolid (Zyvox), metronidazole (Flagyl), tigecycline (Tygacil), tobramycin, or vancomycin. ▪ May have a false-positive reaction for **urine glucose** except with enzyme-based tests (e.g., Clinistix).

SIDE EFFECTS

The most common side effects reported in adults are diarrhea, nausea, and vomiting. The most common side effects reported in pediatric patients are diarrhea, infusion site phlebitis, rash, and vomiting. The safety profile of ceftazidime-avibactam in pediatric patients is similar to adults with cIAI and cUTI. Hypersensitivity reactions, skin reactions, central nervous system reactions, and CDAD may be severe. Other reported side effects include abdominal pain, constipation, dizziness, headache, pruritus, and upper abdominal pain. Other side effects have been reported in fewer than 1% of patients.

ANTIDOTE

Notify physician of any side effects. Discontinue the drug if indicated. Treat hypersensitivity reactions as indicated (e.g., diphenhydramine, epinephrine, albuterol) and resuscitate as necessary. Mild cases of CDAD may respond to discontinuation of ceftazidime-avibactam. Treat CDAD with fluids, electrolytes, protein supplements, and appropriate antibiotics (e.g., oral vancomycin) as indicated. In severe cases, surgical evaluation may be indicated. Both ceftazidime and avibactam can be removed from the circulation by hemodialysis.

CEFTOBIPROLE MEDOCARIL
(sef toe BYE prole)

Cephalosporin 5th generation

Zevtera

USUAL DOSE
Note: In the US, doses are expressed as amount of ceftobiprole medocaril. Ceftobiprole medocaril (prodrug) 667 mg is equivalent to ceftobiprole 500 mg (active drug).

Therapy for *Staphylococcus aureus*, including methicillin-resistant S. aureus (MRSA): 667 mg IV every 6 hours for 8 days, followed by 667 mg IV every 8 hours for ≤14 days starting from day of first negative blood culture. Longer courses are need for endocarditis or metastatic sites of infection.

Community-acquired pneumonia: 667 mg IV every 8 hours for minimum of 5 days (or 7 days if MRSA is isolated). *Not recommended for hospital-acquired pneumonia.

Skin and soft tissue infection: 667 mg IV every 8 hours for ≤5 days; may extend up to 14 days depending on severity and clinical response

PEDIATRIC DOSE
Community-acquired pneumonia: Infants ≥3 months of age and children <12 years of age: 20 mg/kg/dose IV every 8 hours; maximum dose is 667 mg/dose.

Children ≥12 years of age and adolescents <18 years of age: 13.3 mg/kg/dose IV every 8 hours; maximum dose: 667 mg/dose.

DOSE ADJUSTMENTS
Renal: *If recommended dose is ceftobiprole medocaril 667 mg IV every 6 hours:*

Creatinine clearance (CrCl) 30 to <50 mL/min: 667 mg IV every 8 hours.

CrCl 15 to <30 mL/min: 333 mg IV every 8 hours.

CrCl <15 mL/min: 333 mg IV every 24 hours.

If recommended dose is ceftobiprole medocaril 667 mg IV every 8 hours:

CrCl 30 to <50 mL/min: 667 mg IV every 12 hours.

CrCl 15 to <30 mL/min: 333 mg IV every 12 hours.

CrCl <15 mL/min: 333 mg IV every 24 hours.

Hemodialysis, intermittent (thrice weekly): 333 mg IV every 24 hours; administer after hemodialysis on dialysis days.

Peritoneal dialysis: 333 mg IV every 24 hours.

PEDIATRIC PATIENTS WITH ALTERED RENAL FUNCTION
Adolescents <18 years of age and children ≥12 years of age

Estimated glomerular filtration rate (eGFR) 30 to <50 mL/min/1.73 m^2: 10 mg/kg/dose IV every 12 hours; maximum dose: 667 mg

eGFR 15 to <30 mL/min/1.73 m^2: 10 mg/kg/dose IV every 12 hours; maximum dose: 333 mg

eGFR <15 mL/min/1.73 m^2 data are not sufficient to recommend specific dosage adjustments; however, dosage adjustments are probably necessary.

Children 6 to <12 years of age

eGFR 30 to <50 mL/min/1.73 m^2: 10 mg /kg/dose IV every 12 hours; maximum dose: 667 mg/dose.

eGFR 15 to <30 mL/min/1.73 m^2: 10 mg /kg/dose IV every 24 hours; maximum dose: 333 mg/dose.

eGFR <15 mL/min/1.73 m^2: Data are not sufficient to recommend specific dosage adjustments; however, dosage adjustments are probably necessary.

Children 2 to <6 years of age

eGFR 30 to <50 mL/min/1.73 m^2: 13.3 mg /kg/dose IV every 12 hours; maximum dose: 667 mg/dose.

eGFR 15 to <30 mL/min/1.73 m^2: 3.3 mg /kg/dose IV every 24 hours; maximum dose: 333 mg/dose.

eGFR <15 mL/min/1.73 m²: Data are not sufficient to recommend specific dosage adjustments, however, dosage adjustments are probably necessary.

Children <2 years of age and infants ≥3 months of age

No dosage adjustments are provided in the manufacturer's labeling; dosage adjustment likely necessary.

Hepatic: No dosage adjustments are provided in the manufacturer's labeling.

RECONSTITUTION AND DILUTION

Reconstitution: *Adults:* Reconstitute powder with 10 mL sterile water for injection (SWFI) or dextrose 5% in water (D5W) to make a final concentration of 66.7 mg/mL. Shake vigorously until dissolved completely; may take up to 10 minutes. Resulting volume of reconstituted solution is 10.6 mL.

Dilution for infusion

667 mg dose: Withdraw 10 mL of reconstituted solution and inject into 250 mL normal saline (NS) or D5W. Invert bag gently 5 to 10 times until mixed.

333 mg dose: Withdraw 5 mL of reconstituted solution and inject into 125 mL NS or D5W. Invert bag gently 5 to 10 times until mixed.

Pediatric Patients: Adolescents <18 years of age and children ≥12 years of age

Reconstitute 667-mg vial with 10 mL of D5W or SWFI. Shake vigorously until dissolution is completed; may take up to 10 minutes; Resultant concentration: 66.7 mg/mL; volume after reconstitution: ~10.6 mL. Further dilute in NS or D5W to a final concentration of 2.67 mg/mL. After dilution, gently invert 5 to 10 times.

Children <12 years of age and infants ≥3 months of age

Reconstitute 667-mg vial with 10 mL of D5W. Shake vigorously until dissolution is completed; may take up to 10 minutes. Resultant concentration: 66.7 mg ceftobiprole medocaril/mL; volume after reconstitution: ~10.6 mL. Further dilute dose in D5W to a final concentration of 5.33 mg ceftobiprole medocaril/mL. After dilution, gently invert 5 to 10 times.

COMPATIBILITY

Incompatible with calcium-containing IV solutions; Precipitation may occur when mixed with calcium-containing solutions. Do not mix or simultaneously administer ceftobiprole and calcium-containing solutions in the same IV line.

RATE OF ADMINISTRATION

Administer by IV infusion over 2 hours.

ACTIONS

Prodrug converted in vivo to active drug with bactericidal activity by inhibiting bacterial cell wall synthesis through binding to one or more of the penicillin-binding proteins (PBPs), including PBP2a in MRSA and PBP2b and PBP2x in penicillin-resistant *S. pneumoniae.*

INDICATIONS AND USES

Bloodstream infection, community-acquired pneumonia, skin and soft tissue infection.

CONTRAINDICATIONS

Severe hypersensitivity to ceftobiprole medocaril, other members of the cephalosporins class, or any component of the formulation.

PRECAUTIONS

Seizures and other adverse CNS reactions have been reported, particularly in patients with a history of epilepsy or when recommended doses were exceeded due to kidney impairment.

Serious hypersensitivity reactions, including anaphylaxis. Question patients about previous hypersensitivity reactions to other cephalosporins, penicillins, and other beta-lactam antibiotics. Cross-sensitivity has been established. If given to a patient with penicillin or other beta-lactam allergy, use with caution; if a hypersensitivity reaction occurs, discontinue and institute supportive therapy.

Use may result in bacterial or fungal superinfection. *Clostridium difficile*–associated diarrhea (CDAD) and pseudomembranous colitis have been reported with use.

Use with caution in patients with renal impairment. Dosage adjustment is required with CrCl <50 mL/min.

Patient Education: Notify provider of extended diarrhea, stomach pain, vomiting. May cause low sodium and potassium levels; contact provider with headache, confusion, seizures, muscle pain, weakness or cramping or abnormal heartbeat. Notify provider if dark urine or yellow eyes or skin occur. Notify provider immediately with any signs of allergic reaction (rash; hives; itching; red, swollen, blistered, or peeling skin with or without fever; wheezing; tightness in the chest or throat; trouble breathing, swallowing, or talking; unusual hoarseness; or swelling of the mouth, face, lips, tongue, or throat).

Maternal/Child

Pregnancy considerations: Adverse events were not observed in animal reproduction studies.

Breastfeeding considerations: It is not known if ceftobiprole is present in breast milk.

Elderly: No specific recommendations; refer to adult dosing.

DRUG/LAB INTERACTIONS

Avoid the following drugs: Bacilus Guérin (BCG) vaccine (Intravesical), cholera vaccine, fecal microbiota.

SIDE EFFECTS

Most common side effects include nausea and anemia.

ANTIDOTE

There is no antidote; stop infusion for hypersensitivity reactions and treat appropriately.

CEFTOLOZANE/TAZOBACTAM

(sef-**TOL**-oh-zane/**TAZ**-oh-**BAK**-tam)

Antibacterial
(cephalosporin/
beta-lactamase inhibitor)

Zerbaxa

USUAL DOSE

Pretreatment: Baseline studies indicated; see Monitor.

1.5 Gm (ceftolozane 1 Gm and tazobactam 0.5 Gm) to 3 Gm (ceftolozane 2 Gm and tazobactam 1 Gm) every 8 hours as an infusion over 1 hour. Guide duration of treatment by the severity and site of the infection and the patient's clinical and bacteriologic progress.

DOSE ADJUSTMENTS

No dose adjustment is recommended based on age, gender, hepatic impairment, or race.

■ Dose adjustment is required for patients with a CrCl of 50 mL/min or less according to the following chart.

Ceftolozane/Tazobactam Dosing in Patients With Renal Impairment		
Estimated CrCl (mL/min)	**Complicated Intra-abdominal Infections and Complicated Urinary Tract Infections, Including Pyelonephritis**	**Hospital-Acquired Bacterial Pneumonia and Ventilator-Associated Bacterial Pneumonia**
30 to 50 mL/min	750 mg (500 mg and 250 mg) IV every 8 hours	1.5 Gm (1 Gm and 0.5 Gm) IV every 8 hours
15 to 29 mL/min	375 mg (250 mg and 125 mg) IV every 8 hours	750 mg (500 mg and 250 mg) IV every 8 hours
End-stage renal disease (ESRD) on hemodialysis (HD)	A single loading dose of 750 mg (500 mg and 250 mg) followed by a 150 mg (100 mg and 50 mg) maintenance dose administered every 8 hours for the remainder of the treatment period (on hemodialysis days, administer the dose at the earliest possible time following completion of dialysis)	A single loading dose of 2.25 Gm (1.5 Gm and 0.75 Gm) followed by a 450 mg (300 mg and 150 mg) maintenance dose administered every 8 hours for the remainder of the treatment period (on hemodialysis days, administer the dose at the earliest possible time following completion of dialysis)

DILUTION

Available as single-dose vials containing 1 Gm ceftolozane and 0.5 Gm tazobactam. Reconstitute each vial with 10 mL of SWFI or NS and gently shake to dissolve. Final volume is approximately 11.4 mL. Reconstituted solution is *NOT* for direct injection.

Withdraw the required dose from the vial(s) according to the following chart and transfer to an infusion bag containing 100 mL of NS or D5W.

Preparation of Ceftolozane/Tazobactam to Achieve Required Doses	
Ceftolozane/Tazobactam Dose	**Volume to Withdraw From Reconstituted Vial(s)**
3 Gm (2 Gm and 1 Gm)	Two vials of 11.4 mL each (entire contents from 2 vials)
2.25 Gm (1.5 Gm and 0.75 Gm)	11.4 mL for one vial (entire contents) and 5.7 mL from a second vial
1.5 Gm (1 Gm and 0.5 Gm)	11.4 mL (entire contents)
750 mg (500 mg and 250 mg)	5.7 mL
450 mg (300 mg and 150 mg)	3.5 mL
375 mg (250 mg and 125 mg)	2.9 mL
150 mg (100 mg and 50 mg)	1.2 mL

Infusion solutions range from clear, colorless solutions to clear and slightly yellow.
Filters: Specific information not available.
Storage: Refrigerate vials at 2° to 8° C (36° to 46° F) in original carton to protect from light. Solutions reconstituted with SWFI or NS may be held for 1 hour before transfer and dilution. Fully diluted solutions may be stored for 24 hours at room temperature or for 7 days if refrigerated. Do not freeze reconstituted or diluted solutions.

COMPATIBILITY

Compatibility with other drugs not established. Manufacturer states, "Ceftolozane/ tazobactam should not be mixed with other drugs or physically added to solutions containing other drugs."

Other sources suggest a few specific **compatibilities** dependent on concentration and manufacturer; consult a pharmacist.

RATE OF ADMINISTRATION

A single dose as an infusion equally distributed over 1 hour (per manufacturer); some reference suggest the 3-Gm dose be administerd over 3 hours.

ACTIONS

Ceftolozane/tazobactam is an antibacterial combination product consisting of the cephalosporin antibacterial drug ceftolozane sulfate and the beta-lactamase inhibitor tazobactam sodium. Its bactericidal action results from inhibition of cell wall biosynthesis and is mediated through binding to penicillin-binding proteins (PBPs). Tazobactam sodium is an irreversible inhibitor of some beta-lactamases (enzymes [e.g., certain penicillinases and cephalosporinases] produced by bacteria and capable of hydrolyzing/inactivating penicillins and cephalosporins). Active against a variety of gram-negative, gram-positive, and anaerobic bacteria. Protein binding of ceftolozane and tazobactam is approximately 16% to 21% and 30%, respectively. Ceftolozane does not appear to be metabolized to an appreciable extent. Tazobactam is hydrolyzed to an inactive metabolite. Half-life of ceftolozane is approximately 3 to 4 hours. Half-life of tazobactam is approximately 2 to 3 hours. Both ceftolozane and tazobactam are eliminated by the kidneys—ceftolozane as the unchanged parent drug and tazobactam as the unchanged parent drug and its inactive metabolite.

INDICATIONS AND USES

Treatment of patients 18 years of age or older with infections caused by susceptible isolates of designated organisms in the conditions listed below. ■ Used in combination with metronidazole for the treatment of complicated intra-abdominal infections (cIAI). ■ Treatment of complicated urinary tract infections (cUTI), including pyelonephritis. ■ Treatment of hospital-acquired bacterial pneumonia and ventilator-associated bacterial pneumonia (HABP/VABP).

CONTRAINDICATIONS

Known serious hypersensitivity to ceftolozane/tazobactam, piperacillin/tazobactam, or other members of the beta-lactam class.

PRECAUTIONS

For IV infusion only; do not administer as an IV bolus. ▪ Decreased efficacy was seen in cIAI and cUTI trials in patients with a baseline CrCl of 30 to 50 mL/min; see Monitor. ▪ Serious and occasionally fatal hypersensitivity (anaphylactic) reactions have been reported in patients receiving beta-lactam antibacterial drugs. Check the history of previous hypersensitivity reactions to penicillins, cephalosporins, or other beta-lactam antibacterial drugs. Cross-sensitivity has been established. ▪ Specific sensitivity studies are indicated to determine susceptibility of the causative organism to ceftolozane/tazobactam. ▪ Bacteria resistant to other cephalosporins may be susceptible to ceftolozane/tazobactam, although cross-resistance may occur. ▪ To reduce the development of drug-resistant bacteria and maintain its effectiveness, ceftolozane/tazobactam should be used to treat only those infections proven or strongly suspected to be caused by bacteria. ▪ *Clostridium difficile*–associated diarrhea (CDAD) has been reported for nearly all systemic antibacterial agents and may range in severity from mild diarrhea to fatal colitis. Consider in patients who present with diarrhea during or after treatment with ceftolozane/tazobactam.

Monitor: Monitor the CrCl at least daily in patients with changing renal function. Adjust dose of ceftolozane/tazobactam accordingly. ▪ Monitor for S/S of a hypersensitivity reaction (e.g., hypotension, rash, urticaria, tightness of the chest, wheezing).

Patient Education: Promptly report S/S of a hypersensitivity reaction (e.g., hives, rash, shortness of breath, wheezing). ▪ Promptly report diarrhea or bloody stools that occur during treatment or up to several months after an antibiotic has been discontinued; may indicate CDAD and require treatment.

Maternal/Child: Use during pregnancy only if the potential benefit outweighs the possible risk. ▪ Use caution during breast-feeding. ▪ Safety and effectiveness for use in pediatric patients not established.

Elderly: A higher incidence of adverse reactions occurs in patients 65 years of age and older. ▪ In the complicated intra-abdominal infection clinical trial, cure rates were lower in patients 65 years of age or older in the ceftolozane/tazobactam group compared with the comparator group. This finding in the elderly population was not seen in the complicated UTI trial. ▪ Consider age-related renal impairment, monitoring of renal function, and dose with caution; see Dose Adjustments.

DRUG/LAB INTERACTIONS

Ceftolozane/tazobactam is not metabolized in the liver. No significant drug-drug interactions are anticipated between ceftolozane/tazobactam and substrates, inhibitors, and inducers of cytochrome P_{450} enzymes. ▪ It is not a substrate for P-glycoprotein (P-gp). ▪ Tazobactam is a known substrate for OAT1 and OAT3. Coadministration with the OAT1/OAT3 inhibitor **probenecid** prolongs the half-life of tazobactam by 71%.

SIDE EFFECTS

The most common side effects reported in either cIAI or cUTI are diarrhea, fever, headache, and nausea. The most common side effects reported in HABP/VABP are diarrhea, increase in hepatic transaminases, and renal impairment/renal failure. Hypersensitivity reactions and CDAD may be severe. Other reported side effects include abdominal pain, anemia, anxiety, atrial fibrillation, constipation, dizziness, hypokalemia, hypotension, increased ALT and AST, insomnia, intracranial hemorrhage, rash, thrombocytosis, and vomiting. Other side effects have been reported in fewer than 1% of patients.

ANTIDOTE

Notify physician of any side effects. Discontinue the drug if indicated. Treat hypersensitivity reactions as indicated (e.g., diphenhydramine, epinephrine, albuterol) and resuscitate as necessary. Mild cases of CDAD may respond to discontinuation of ceftolozane/tazobactam. Treat CDAD with fluids, electrolytes, protein supplements, and appropriate antibiotics (e.g., oral vancomycin) as indicated. In severe cases, surgical evaluation may be indicated. Both ceftolozane and tazobactam are partially removed by hemodialysis.

CEFTRIAXONE SODIUM
(sef-try-**AX**-ohn **SO**-dee-um)

Rocephin

Antibacterial
(cephalosporin)

pH 6.6 to 6.7

USUAL DOSE

Adults and pediatric patients over 12 years: 1 to 2 Gm/24 hr. May be given as a single dose every 24 hours or equally divided into 2 doses and given every 12 hours depending on the type and severity of the infection. Do not exceed a total dose of 4 Gm/24 hr.
Meningitis: 2 Gm every 12 hours.
Disseminated gonococcal infections (unlabeled): 1 Gm daily for 24 to 48 hours. Transfer to oral dosing after improvement is noted, and continue for a total of 7 days of therapy.
Perioperative prophylaxis: 1 Gm IV 30 minutes to 2 hours before incision. Used primarily in patients undergoing coronary artery bypass surgery and in contaminated or potentially contaminated surgeries.
Lyme disease (unlabeled): 2 Gm daily for 14 days (range 14 to 28 days).

PEDIATRIC DOSE

See Maternal/Child.
Pediatric patients 1 month to 12 years of age: *Skin and soft tissue:* 50 to 75 mg/kg of body weight/24 hr as a single dose or in equally divided doses every 12 hours (25 to 37.5 mg/kg every 12 hours). Do not exceed a total dose of 2 Gm/24 hr.
Other serious infections (other than meningitis): 50 to 75 mg/kg of body weight/24 hr in equally divided doses every 12 hours (25 to 37.5 mg/kg every 12 hours). Do not exceed a total dose of 2 Gm/24 hr.
Bacterial meningitis: Begin with a loading dose of 100 mg/kg on day 1 (do not exceed a total dose of 4 Gm), follow with 100 mg/kg/day (not to exceed 4 Gm) as a single dose or in equally divided doses every 12 hours (50 mg/kg every 12 hours). Continue for 7 to 14 days depending on the causative organism.
Lyme disease (unlabeled): 50 to 75 mg/kg/day for 14 days (range 10 to 28 days). Maximum dose is 2 Gm.

NEONATAL DOSE

See Contraindications, Rate of Administration, and Maternal/Child before administration to neonates.
Neonatal doses may also be given IM.
The American Academy of Pediatrics (AAP) recommends the following:
28 days of age or younger regardless of weight: 50 mg/kg/day as a single daily dose.
Bacterial meningitis: Same as Pediatric Dose.
Infants born to mothers with gonococcal infections: 25 to 50 mg/kg one time only (do not exceed 125 mg).

DOSE ADJUSTMENTS

In adults with both hepatic and renal impairment, dose should not exceed 2 Gm daily.
■ Dose adjustment not required for elderly patients with doses up to 2 Gm/day provided there is no severe renal and hepatic impairment. ■ See Drug/Lab Interactions.

DILUTION

Initially reconstitute each 250 mg of sterile powder with 2.4 mL (500 mg with 4.8 mL, 1 Gm with 9.6 mL, 2 Gm with 19.2 mL) of SWFI, NS, D5W, D10W, D5NS, or D5/½NS for injection (see chart on inside back cover or literature for additional diluents). Each mL will contain 100 mg. A single dose must be further diluted to the desired concentration with the same solution and given as an intermittent infusion. Shake well. Concentrations of 10 mg/mL to 40 mg/mL are recommended for intermittent infusion. Color of solution ranges from light yellow to amber depending on length of storage, concentration, and diluent used. Should not be reconstituted, further diluted, or simultaneously administered with calcium-containing IV solutions. A precipitate can form; see Compatibility.

Also available in a premixed frozen Galaxy container, in dual-chamber DUPLEX containers, in ADD-Vantage vials for use with ADD-Vantage infusion containers, and in pharmacy bulk packages. Refer to manufacturer's prescribing information for specific preparation and storage requirements.

Storage: See manufacturer's directions. Recommendations for storing vary from CRT (20° to 25° C [68° to 77° F]) to RT (25° C [77° F]) or below and protect from light. Stable at RT for at least 24 hours in stated solutions or selected solutions up to 10 days if refrigerated (see prescribing information). D5NS and D5/½NS should not be refrigerated. Stability and color (light yellow to amber) depend on concentration and diluent. Solutions reconstituted in D5W or NS in concentrations between 10 and 40 mg/mL and then frozen at −20° C in PVC or polyolefin containers remain stable for 26 weeks.

COMPATIBILITY

Manufacturer states, "Do not use diluents containing calcium, such as Ringer's solution or Hartmann's solution, to reconstitute or further dilute ceftriaxone. Particulate formation can result. Ceftriaxone and calcium-containing solutions, including continuous calcium-containing infusions such as parenteral nutrition, should not be mixed or coadministered simultaneously via a **Y-site**." However, in patients other than neonates, ceftriaxone and calcium-containing solutions may be administered sequentially if the infusion lines are thoroughly flushed between infusions with a **compatible** fluid; see Contraindications and Precautions. Manufacturer lists as **compatible** with metronidazole as an **additive** in NS or D5W if the concentration of metronidazole does not exceed 5 to 7.5 mg/mL with ceftriaxone 10 mg/mL as an admixture. Mixture is stable at RT for 24 hours. Precipitation will occur if refrigerated or if concentration of metronidazole exceeds 8 mg/mL. No studies have been done with Flagyl IV RTU. Manufacturer lists aminoglycosides (e.g., gentamicin), amsacrine, fluconazole, and vancomycin as **incompatible** and states, "May be given sequentially with thorough flushing of the IV line with **compatible** solution between the administrations."

Other sources suggest specific **compatibilities** dependent on concentration and manufacturer; consult a pharmacist.

RATE OF ADMINISTRATION

Intermittent IV: A single dose over 30 minutes.

Neonates: Intravenous doses should be given over 60 minutes to reduce the risk of bilirubin encephalopathy.

ACTIONS

A broad-spectrum, third-generation cephalosporin antibiotic. Bactericidal to selected gram-negative, gram-positive, and anaerobic organisms. Effective against many otherwise resistant organisms. Inhibits bacterial cell wall synthesis. Therapeutic concentrations achieved in many body fluids and tissues, including CSF. Highly protein bound. Has a long half-life (range is 5.8 to 8.7 hours), allowing once-a-day dosing for many indications. Peak serum levels achieved by end of infusion. Excreted through urine, bile, and feces. Crosses placental barrier. Secreted in breast milk.

INDICATIONS AND USES

Treatment of serious lower respiratory tract, urinary tract, skin and skin structure, bone and joint, and intra-abdominal infections. ■ Bacterial septicemia. ■ Meningitis. ■ Most effective against specific organisms (see literature). ■ Perioperative prophylaxis. ■ Given IM for additional indications (e.g., acute bacterial otitis, uncomplicated gonorrhea, and pelvic inflammatory disease).

Unlabeled uses: Treatment of Lyme disease and numerous other infections. ■ Disseminated gonococcal infections. ■ IM for CDC recommendation for chancroid.

CONTRAINDICATIONS

Known hypersensitivity to ceftriaxone, any of its excipients, or other cephalosporins; see Precautions. ■ Premature neonates up to a postmenstrual age of 41 weeks (gestational age + chronologic age). ■ Hyperbilirubinemic neonates; see Maternal/Child. ■ Co-administration with calcium-containing IV solutions, including parenteral nutrition, in infants up to 28 days of age is contraindicated because of the risk of precipitation of ceftriaxone-calcium salt. Cases of fatal outcomes in which a crystalline material was observed in the lungs and kidneys on autopsy have been reported in neonates receiving ceftriaxone and calcium-containing fluids; see Precautions and Compatibility. ▪ Intravenous administration of ceftriaxone solutions containing lidocaine is contraindicated. When lidocaine solution is used as a solvent with ceftriaxone for intramuscular injection, these contraindications do not apply; see IM prescribing information. ▪ Solutions containing dextrose may be contraindicated in patients with hypersensitivity to corn products.

PRECAUTIONS

Hypersensitivity reactions, including fatalities, have been reported. Obtain history of previous hypersensitivity reactions to penicillins, cephalosporins, other beta-lactam agents, or other allergens. Ceftriaxone should be administered with caution to any patient with such a history. Actual incidence of cross-allergenicity not established but may be more common with first-generation cephalosporins. ▪ Sensitivity studies are indicated to determine susceptibility of the causative organism to ceftriaxone. ▪ To reduce the development of drug-resistant bacteria and maintain its effectiveness, ceftriaxone should be used to treat or prevent only those infections proven or strongly suspected to be caused by bacteria. ▪ Continue for at least 2 days after all symptoms of infection subside. Usual course of therapy is 4 to 14 days; *S. pyogenes* requires treatment for 10 days. ▪ Should not be reconstituted, further diluted, or simultaneously administered with calcium-containing IV solutions. A precipitate can form; see Compatibility. There have been no reports of an interaction between ceftriaxone and oral calcium-containing products or between IM ceftriaxone and oral or IV calcium-containing products. ▪ May be associated with an alteration in prothrombin time. Patients at risk include those with impaired vitamin K synthesis or low vitamin K stores (e.g., chronic hepatic disease and malnutrition). Vitamin K administration (10 mg weekly) may be necessary if the prothrombin time is prolonged before or during therapy. ▪ Avoid prolonged use of drug; superinfection caused by overgrowth of nonsusceptible organisms may result. ▪ Use caution in patients with both impaired renal and hepatic function, allergies, or a history of GI disease (especially colitis). ▪ *Clostridium difficile*–associated diarrhea (CDAD) has been reported. May range from mild diarrhea to fatal colitis. Consider in patients who present with diarrhea during or after treatment with ceftriaxone. ▪ Immune-mediated hemolytic anemia has been reported in both adults and pediatric patients. Fatalities have occurred. ▪ Ceftriaxone-calcium precipitates in the gallbladder have been observed in patients receiving ceftriaxone. These precipitates appear on sonogram and may be misinterpreted as gallstones. Patients may be asymptomatic or may develop symptoms of gallbladder disease. The abnormalities appear to be transient and reversible with the discontinuation of ceftriaxone; see Antidote. ▪ Ceftriaxone-calcium precipitates in the urinary tract have been observed in patients receiving ceftriaxone and may be detected as sonographic abnormalities. Patients may be asymptomatic or may develop symptoms of urolithiasis, ureteral obstruction, and postrenal acute renal failure. The condition appears to be reversible with discontinuation of ceftriaxone and institution of appropriate management; see Antidote. ▪ Pancreatitis, possibly secondary to biliary obstruction, has been reported.

Monitor: Watch for early symptoms of a hypersensitivity reaction. ▪ Monitor PT/INR and administer vitamin K as indicated; see Precautions. ▪ Monitor CBC for development of cephalosporin-induced anemia. ▪ Ensure adequate hydration and monitor renal function. ▪ See Dose Adjustments and Drug/Lab Interactions; additional monitoring may be indicated (e.g., renal function, drug serum levels, PT).

Patient Education: Report promptly any bleeding or bruising or symptoms of hypersensitivity (e.g., difficulty breathing, hives, itching, rash). ▪ Promptly report diarrhea or bloody stools that occur during treatment or up to several months after an antibiotic has been discontinued; may indicate CDAD and require treatment.

Maternal/Child: Category B: safety for use during pregnancy not established. No problems documented. ▪ Use caution during breast-feeding. Low concentrations of ceftriaxone are excreted in human milk. ▪ Safety and effectiveness of ceftriaxone in neonates, infants, and pediatric patients have been established. Immature renal function of infants and small children will increase blood levels of all cephalosporins. ▪ Use is contraindicated in hyperbilirubinemic neonates. Ceftriaxone can displace bilirubin from its binding sites on albumin. Risk of bilirubin encephalopathy exists; see Contraindications and Precautions. ▪ Ceftriaxone is also contraindicated in premature neonates up to a postmenstrual age of 41 weeks and in neonates 28 days of age or younger if they require calcium-containing IV solutions; see Contraindications. ▪ The probability of ceftriaxone-calcium precipitates in the gallbladder or urinary tract appears to be greatest in pediatric patients.

Elderly: Response similar to other age-groups; however, greater sensitivity of the elderly cannot be ruled out; see Dose Adjustments.

DRUG/LAB INTERACTIONS

Risk of nephrotoxicity may be increased with **aminoglycosides and other nephrotoxic agents** (e.g., loop diuretics such as furosemide). ▪ May be antagonized by **bacteriostatic antibiotics** (e.g., chloramphenicol, erythromycin, tetracyclines); may interfere with bactericidal action. ▪ Concomitant use with **vitamin K antagonists** (e.g., warfarin) may increase the risk of bleeding. Monitor coagulation parameters frequently, and adjust anticoagulant dose accordingly. ▪ May cause false-positive **Coombs' test.** ▪ The presence of ceftriaxone may falsely lower estimated blood glucose values obtained with some **blood glucose monitoring systems.** Consult manufacturer's instructions and use alternative testing methods if necessary. ▪ May produce false-positive reaction for **urine glucose** except with enzyme-based tests (e.g., Clinistix). ▪ See Compatibility and Side Effects.

SIDE EFFECTS

Full scope of hypersensitivity reactions (e.g., anaphylaxis with fatal outcome, chills, fever, and pruritus) has been reported. Agranulocytosis; allergic pneumonitis; "biliary sludge" or pseudolithiasis; bleeding episodes; burning, discomfort, and pain at injection site; casts in urine; CDAD; colitis; diarrhea; dizziness; dysgeusia; elevated alkaline phosphatase, bilirubin, BUN, creatinine, AST, and ALT; headache; leukopenia; nausea and vomiting; nephrolithiasis; pancreatitis; prolonged PT; renal precipitations; seizures; thrombophlebitis. Other hematologic reactions (e.g., anemia, eosinophilia, hemolytic anemia, leukopenia, lymphopenia, neutropenia, thrombocytopenia, thrombocytosis) may occur. Aplastic anemia, erythema multiforme, hemolytic anemia, hemorrhage, hepatic dysfunction (including cholestasis), pancytopenia, renal dysfunction, Stevens-Johnson syndrome, toxic epidermal necrolysis, and toxic nephropathy have been reported with cephalosporin-class antibiotics.

Post-Marketing: Dermatologic reactions (e.g., acute generalized exanthematous pustulosis, allergic dermatitis, exanthema, and isolated cases of Stevens-Johnson syndrome and toxic epidermal necrolysis), genitourinary reactions (e.g., oliguria, postrenal acute renal failure, ureteric obstruction), kernicterus, stomatitis, symptomatic precipitation of ceftriaxone-calcium salt in the gallbladder. Fatal cases of ceftriaxone-calcium precipitates in lungs and kidneys of neonates have been reported; see Contraindications, Precautions, and Maternal/Child.

ANTIDOTE

Notify physician of any side effects. Discontinue the drug if indicated (e.g., CDAD, hypersensitivity reactions, seizures, S/S of gallbladder disease, or S/S suggestive of urolithiasis, oliguria, or renal failure). Treat hypersensitivity reactions as indicated and resuscitate as necessary. Mild cases of CDAD may respond to discontinuation of ceftriaxone. Treat CDAD with fluids, electrolytes, protein supplements, and appropriate antibiotics (e.g., oral vancomycin) as indicated. In severe cases, surgical evaluation may be indicated. Vitamin K may be useful in bleeding episodes, or drug may need to be discontinued. Not removed by hemodialysis.

CEFUROXIME SODIUM
(sef-your-**OX**-eem **SO**-dee-um)

Zinacef

Antibacterial
(cephalosporin)

pH 5 to 8.5

USUAL DOSE

Cefuroxime: Dependent on seriousness of infection. Usual dose is 750 mg to 1.5 Gm every 8 hours for 5 to 10 days. Maximum dose is 3 Gm every 8 hours.

Uncomplicated infections (gonococcal, pneumonia, skin and soft tissue, urinary tract): 750 mg every 8 hours.

PEDIATRIC DOSE

Do not exceed adult dose.

Pediatric patients 3 months of age or older: 50 to 100 mg/kg/day in equally divided doses every 6 to 8 hours (12.5 to 25 mg/kg every 6 hours or 16.7 to 33.3 mg/kg every 8 hours). Higher-end dosing used for more serious infections.

Bone and joint infections: 50 mg/kg every 8 hours. Up to 1.5 Gm/dose has been given.

Bacterial meningitis: 200 to 240 mg/kg/day in equally divided doses every 6 to 8 hours (50 to 60 mg/kg every 6 hours or 66.7 to 80 mg/kg every 8 hours); see Precautions.

NEONATAL DOSE

Neonatal doses are unlabeled; see Precautions and Maternal/Child.

The American Academy of Pediatrics suggests the following doses:

Neonates: 7 days of age or younger regardless of weight: 50 mg/kg every 12 hours.

Neonates from 8 to 28 days of age weighing 2 kg or less: 50 mg/kg every 8 to 12 hours.

Neonates from 8 to 28 days of age weighing more than 2 kg: 50 mg/kg every 8 hours.

DOSE ADJUSTMENTS

Reduced doses or extended intervals may be indicated in the elderly; consider age-related impaired organ function, nutritional status, and concomitant disease or drug therapy.

Adults: Reduce total daily dose if renal function impaired according to the following chart. ■ See Drug/Lab Interactions.

Cefuroxime Dose Guidelines in Impaired Renal Function in Adults		
Creatinine Clearance (mL/min)	**Dose**	**Frequency**
>20 mL/min	750 mg-1.5 Gm	q 8 hr
10-20 mL/min	750 mg	q 12 hr
<10 mL/min	750 mg	q 24 hr
Hemodialysis patients	An additional dose of 750 mg at end of each dialysis session	

Pediatric patients: In pediatric patients with impaired renal function, reduce frequency as indicated in the chart for adults.

DILUTION

Reconstitute 750 mg with 8.3 mL SWFI. Reconstitute 1.5 Gm with 16 mL SWFI. Shake well. May be further diluted to 50 or 100 mL with D5W, NS, or other **compatible** infusion solution (see chart on inside back cover or literature) and given as an intermittent infusion, or added to 500 to 1,000 mL and given as a continuous infusion. Also available in dual-chamber DUPLEX containers, ADD-Vantage vials, Twist vials, premixed frozen Galaxy bags, and pharmacy bulk packaging. Refer to manufacturer's prescribing information for specific preparation and storage requirements.

Storage: In dry state, store between 15° and 30° C (59° to 86° F); protect from light. Reconstituted vials are stable for 24 hours at CRT or 48 hours if refrigerated. Diluted solutions may be stable for up to 7 days if refrigerated.

COMPATIBILITY

May be used concomitantly with aminoglycosides (e.g., amikacin, gentamicin), but these drugs must never be mixed in the same infusion (mutual inactivation). If given concurrently, administer separately and flush the IV line before and after administration. Manufacturer recommends temporarily discontinuing other solutions infusing at the same site during intermittent infusion and lists sodium bicarbonate **incompatible** as a diluent.

Other sources suggest specific **compatibilities** dependent on concentration and manufacturer; consult a pharmacist.

RATE OF ADMINISTRATION

See Compatibility. Injection or intermittent infusion may be given through Y-tube of infusion set.

IV injection: A single dose equally distributed over 3 to 5 minutes.

Intermittent IV: A single dose over 15 to 30 minutes.

Continuous infusion: 500 to 1,000 mL over 6 to 24 hours, depending on total dose and concentration.

ACTIONS

A broad-spectrum, second-generation cephalosporin antibiotic. Bactericidal to selected gram-negative and gram-positive organisms. Effective against many otherwise resistant organisms. Inhibits bacterial cell wall synthesis. Peak serum levels achieved by end of infusion. Widely distributed. 50% bound to serum proteins. Therapeutic concentrations found in pleural fluid, joint fluid, bile, sputum, bone, aqueous humor, and CSF. Half-life is 80 minutes. Excreted in the urine. Crosses placental barrier. Secreted in breast milk.

INDICATIONS AND USES

Treatment of patients with infections caused by susceptible strains of designated organisms in the following diseases: serious lower respiratory tract, urinary tract, bone and joint, skin and skin structure infections, septicemia, and meningitis. ■ Perioperative prophylaxis. ■ Used IM to treat gonorrhea.

CONTRAINDICATIONS

Previous hypersensitivity reaction to cephalosporins; see Precautions. ■ Premixed solutions containing dextrose may be contraindicated in patients with known allergies to corn or corn products.

PRECAUTIONS

Hypersensitivity reactions, including fatalities, have been reported and include reports of individuals with a history of penicillin hypersensitivity or sensitivity to multiple allergens experiencing severe reactions when treated with cephalosporins. Check history of previous hypersensitivity reactions to penicillins, cephalosporins, or other allergens. Actual incidence of cross-allergenicity not established but may be more common with first-generation cephalosporins. ■ Sensitivity studies indicated to determine susceptibility of the causative organism to cefuroxime. ■ To reduce the development of drug-resistant bacteria and maintain its effectiveness, cefuroxime should be used to treat or prevent only those infections proven or strongly suspected to be caused by bacteria. ■ Continue for at least 2 to 3 days after all symptoms of infection subside. ■ Continue treatment of *Streptococcus pyogenes* infections for a minimum of 10 days to decrease the risk of rheumatic fever or glomerulonephritis. ■ Avoid prolonged use of drug; superinfection caused by overgrowth of nonsusceptible organisms may result. ■ Use caution in patients with impaired renal function, allergies, or a history of GI disease (especially colitis). ■ *Clostridium difficile*–associated diarrhea (CDAD) has been reported. May range from mild diarrhea to fatal colitis. Consider in patients who present with diarrhea during or after treatment with cefuroxime. ▪ May be associated with a fall in prothrombin activity. Patients at risk include those with renal or hepatic impairment, patients with poor nutritional status, patients receiving a protracted course of antimicrobial therapy, and patients previously stabilized on anticoagulant therapy; see Monitor. ▪ Mild to moderate hearing loss has been reported in a few pediatric patients treated for meningitis.

Monitor: Obtain baseline SCr and monitor renal function periodically during therapy. ▪ Watch for early symptoms of a hypersensitivity reaction. ▪ May cause thrombophlebitis. Use small needles and large veins, and rotate infusion sites. ▪ Monitor PT and administer vitamin K as indicated. ▪ See Drug/Lab Interactions; additional monitoring may be indicated (e.g., renal function, drug serum levels).

Patient Education: Report promptly any bleeding or bruising or symptoms of hypersensitivity (e.g., difficulty breathing, hives, itching, rash). ▪ Promptly report diarrhea or bloody stools that occur during treatment or up to several months after an antibiotic has been discontinued; may indicate CDAD and require treatment.

Maternal/Child: Category B: safety for use during pregnancy and breast-feeding not established. No problems documented. ▪ Is used in infants under 3 months of age, but safety not established; immature renal function will increase blood levels.

Elderly: See Dose Adjustments. ▪ Response similar to other age groups; however, greater sensitivity of the elderly cannot be ruled out.

DRUG/LAB INTERACTIONS

Risk of nephrotoxicity may be increased with **aminoglycosides and other nephrotoxic agents** (e.g., loop diuretics such as furosemide). ▪ **Probenecid** inhibits excretion. Reduced dose of cefuroxime may be required with concomitant use. ▪ May be antagonized by **bacteriostatic antibiotics** (e.g., chloramphenicol, erythromycin, tetracyclines); bactericidal action may be negated. ▪ May cause a false-negative reaction in specific **blood glucose** tests (ferricyanide). ▪ False-positive reaction for **urine glucose** except with enzyme-based tests (e.g., Clinistix). ▪ False-positive **Coombs' test.** ▪ See Compatibility and Side Effects.

SIDE EFFECTS

Full scope of hypersensitivity reactions, including anaphylaxis, drug fever, erythema multiforme, interstitial nephritis, positive Coombs' test, pruritus, rash, Stevens-Johnson syndrome, toxic epidermal necrolysis, and urticaria. CDAD; decreased hemoglobin, hematocrit, or platelet functions; diarrhea; elevation of AST, ALT, total bilirubin, alkaline phosphatase, LDH, and BUN/SCr (transient); eosinophilia; fever; leukopenia; local site pain; nausea; oral thrush; seizures (large doses and decreased renal function); transient neutropenia; thrombocytopenia; and thrombophlebitis have occurred. Abdominal pain, agranulocytosis, aplastic anemia, colitis, hemolytic anemia, hemorrhage, hepatic dysfunction (including cholestasis), pancytopenia, prolonged prothrombin time, renal dysfunction, toxic nephropathy, and vaginitis, including vaginal candidiasis, have been reported with cephalosporin-class antibiotics.

Post-Marketing: Angioedema, cutaneous vasculitis, seizures.

ANTIDOTE

Notify physician of any side effects. Discontinue the drug if indicated. Mild cases of CDAD may respond to discontinuation of drug. Treat CDAD with fluids, electrolytes, protein supplements, and appropriate antibiotics (e.g., oral vancomycin) as indicated. In severe cases, surgical evaluation may be indicated. Treat hypersensitivity reactions and resuscitate as necessary. Hemodialysis or peritoneal dialysis may be somewhat useful in overdose.

CEMIPLIMAB-rwlc
(se-**MIP**-li-mab-rwlc)

Libtayo

Antineoplastic
Monoclonal antibody (Anti-PD-1)

pH 6

USUAL DOSE
Pretreatment: Verify pregnancy status, baseline studies indicated; see Monitor.
Cemiplimab-rwlc: 350 mg administered as an IV infusion over 30 minutes every 3 weeks until disease progression or unacceptable toxicity.

DOSE ADJUSTMENTS
Withhold or discontinue cemiplimab-rwlc to manage adverse reactions as outlined in the following chart. No dose reduction of cemiplimab-rwlc is recommended.

Recommended Dose Modifications for Cemiplimab-rwlc Adverse Reactions		
Adverse Reaction	**Severity**[a]	**Cemiplimab-rwlc Dosage Modifications**
Severe and Fatal Immune-Mediated Adverse Reactions		
Pneumonitis	Grade 2	Withhold[b]
	Grade 3 or 4	Permanently discontinue
Colitis	Grade 2 or 3	Withhold[b]
	Grade 4	Permanently discontinue
Hepatitis	If AST or ALT increases to more than 3 and up to 10 × ULN or if total bilirubin increases up to 3 × ULN	Withhold[b]
	If AST or ALT increases to more than 10 × ULN or total bilirubin increases to more than 3 × ULN	Permanently discontinue
Endocrinopathies	Grade 2, 3, or 4	Withhold if clinically necessary
Other immune-mediated adverse reactions involving a major organ	Grade 3	Withhold[b]
	Grade 4	Permanently discontinue
Recurrent or persistent immune mediated adverse reactions	Recurrent Grade 3 or 4 Grade 2 or 3 persistent for 12 weeks or longer after last cemiplimab-rwlc dose Requirement for 10 mg per day or greater prednisone or equivalent lasting 12 weeks or longer after last cemiplimab-rwlc dose	Permanently discontinue
Other Adverse Reactions		
Infusion-related reactions	Grade 1 or 2	Interrupt or slow the rate of the infusion
	Grade 3 or 4	Permanently discontinue

[a] Toxicity graded per National Cancer Institute Common Terminology Criteria for Adverse Events, v4.0 (NCI CTCAE v4).
[b] Resume in patients with complete or partial resolution (Grade 0 or 1) after corticosteroid taper.

DILUTION
Available as a clear to slightly opalescent, colorless to pale-yellow solution in a single-use vial containing 350 mg/7 mL (50 mg/mL). Discard the vial if the solution is cloudy, discolored, or contains extraneous particulate matter other than trace amounts of translucent-to-white particles. Withdraw 7 mL and dilute with NS or D5W to a final

concentration between 1 and 20 mg/mL (e.g., mix 350 mg in 100 mL to obtain a final concentration of 3.5 mg/mL). Mix the diluted solution by gentle inversion. ***Do not shake***. **Filters:** Must be administered through an IV line containing a sterile, in-line, or add-on 0.2- to 5-micron filter.

Storage: Before use, refrigerate at 2° to 8° C (36° to 46° F) in original carton to protect from light. Do not freeze or shake. After preparation, store the prepared infusion at room temperature for no more than 8 hours from the time of preparation to the end of the infusion, or refrigerate for no more than 24 hours from the time of preparation to the end of the infusion. Administration time is included in storage time. If refrigerated, allow the diluted solution to come to room temperature before administration. Do not freeze. Discard partially used vials.

COMPATIBILITY

Compatibility information not available from manufacturer; consult a pharmacist.

RATE OF ADMINISTRATION

A single dose as an infusion equally distributed over 30 minutes through an IV line containing a sterile, in-line, or add-on 0.2- to 5-micron filter. Interrupt, slow the rate of infusion, or permanently discontinue based on severity of any infusion-related reaction; see Dose Adjustments and Antidote.

ACTIONS

An antineoplastic agent. Cemiplimab-rwlc is a programmed death receptor-1 (PD-1) blocking antibody; a recombinant human immunoglobulin G4 (IgG4) monoclonal antibody that binds to the PD-1 receptor and blocks its interaction with PD-L1 and PD-L2. Binding of the PD-1 ligands PD-L1 and PD-L2 to the PD-1 receptor found on T-cells inhibits T-cell proliferation and cytokine production. Upregulation of the PD-1 ligands occurs in some tumors, and signaling through this pathway can contribute to inhibition of active T-cell immune surveillance of tumors. Blocking the interaction between PD-1 and the PD-1 ligands releases the PD-1 pathway–mediated inhibition of the immune response, including the antitumor immune response. In syngeneic mouse tumor models, blocking PD-1 activity resulted in decreased tumor growth. Mean elimination half-life is 19 days. Steady-state concentrations were reached after approximately 4 months of treatment when cemiplimab-rwlc was administered at a dose of 350 mg every 3 weeks.

INDICATIONS AND USES

Treatment of patients with metastatic cutaneous squamous cell carcinoma (CSCC) or locally advanced CSCC who are not candidates for curative surgery or curative radiation therapy.

CONTRAINDICATIONS

Manufacturer states, "None."

PRECAUTIONS

Immune-mediated adverse reactions, which may be severe or fatal, can occur in any organ system or tissue. These reactions usually occur during treatment but can also manifest after discontinuation of therapy. Early identification and management are essential to ensure safe use. ▪ Severe immune-mediated pneumonitis, including fatal cases, have occurred with cemiplimab-rwlc treatment. ▪ Severe immune-mediated colitis has been reported. ▪ Immune-mediated hepatitis, including fatal cases, has occurred with cemiplimab-rwlc treatment. ▪ Immune-mediated nephritis has occurred with cemiplimab-rwlc treatment. ▪ Immune-mediated skin adverse reactions, including erythema multiforme and pemphigoid, have been reported. Rare cases of Stevens-Johnson syndrome (SJS) and toxic epidermal necrolysis (TEN) have also been reported. ▪ Systemic corticosteroids were required in all patients with pneumonitis, colitis, hepatitis, nephritis, and dermatologic adverse reactions during clinical trials. ▪ Immune-mediated endocrinopathies, including adrenal insufficiency, hypophysitis (which can result in hypopituitarism), hypothyroidism, hyperthyroidism, and Type 1 diabetes mellitus (with possible diabetic ketoacidosis), have been reported. ▪ Numerous other immune-mediated adverse reactions, some with fatal outcome, were reported in fewer than 1% of patients who received cemiplimab-rwlc or other PD-1/PD-L1 blocking antibodies.

- Severe infusion reactions have been reported. ■ See Dose Adjustments, Monitor, and Antidote for required dose adjustments, indicated criteria and medications for treatment, and criteria for withholding or discontinuation of cemiplimab-rwlc. ■ A protein substance; has a potential for immunogenicity.

Monitor: Obtain clinical chemistries, including liver and thyroid function tests, at baseline and periodically during treatment. ■ Monitor for S/S of immune-mediated adverse reactions, and institute medical management promptly. Include specialty consultation as appropriate; see Dose Adjustments. ■ For Grade 3 or 4 and certain Grade 2 immune-mediated adverse reactions, administer corticosteroids (1 to 2 mg/kg/day prednisone or equivalent) or other appropriate therapy until improvement to Grade 1 or less followed by a corticosteroid taper over 1 month. Consider administration of other systemic immunosuppressants in patients whose immune-mediated adverse reaction is not controlled with corticosteroids. Institute hormone replacement therapy for endocrinopathies as warranted. ■ Monitor for infusion reactions; see Dose Adjustments and Rate of Administration. ■ Monitor patients for S/S of pneumonitis (e.g., abnormal chest x-ray, chest pain, new or worsening cough, or shortness of breath). ■ Monitor patients for colitis. ■ Monitor for S/S of hepatitis (e.g., easy bruising or bleeding, jaundice, lethargy, pain on the right side of the abdomen, severe nausea or vomiting, abnormal LFTs). ■ Monitor renal function periodically. ■ Monitor for S/S of hypophysitis (e.g., fatigue, headache, low levels of the hormones produced by the pituitary [adrenocorticotropic hormone (ACTH), thyroid-stimulating hormone (TSH), follicle-stimulating hormone (FSH), luteinizing hormone (LH), growth hormone (GH), prolactin]). Administer hormone replacement therapy and corticosteroids as clinically indicated. ■ Monitor for S/S of adrenal insufficiency (e.g., fatigue, nausea, vomiting, hypotension, hyponatremia, hyperkalemia, low cortisol concentrations). Administer corticosteroids as clinically indicated. ■ Monitor for changes in thyroid function. Administer hormone replacement therapy for hypothyroidism. Initiate medical management for control of hyperthyroidism (e.g., methimazole, propylthiouracil). ■ Monitor for hyperglycemia. Administer insulin when clinically indicated. ■ Monitor for development of a rash. ■ Monitor patient for any other clinically significant immune-mediated adverse reactions. Examples of other immune-mediated adverse reactions that have occurred include aplastic anemia, autoimmune neuropathy, duodenitis, encephalitis, gastritis, Guillain-Barré syndrome, hemolytic anemia, hemophagocytic lymphohistiocytosis, histiocytic necrotizing lymphadenitis, immune thrombocytopenic purpura, iritis, meningitis, myasthenic syndrome/myasthenia gravis, myelitis and demyelination, myocarditis, myositis, nerve paresis, pancreatitis, pericarditis, polymyalgia rheumatica, rhabdomyolysis, sarcoidosis, solid organ transplant rejection, systemic inflammatory response syndrome, uveitis, and vasculitides. If uveitis occurs in combination with other immune-mediated adverse reactions, consider a Vogt-Koyanagi-Harada–like syndrome, which may require treatment with systemic steroids to reduce the risk of permanent vison loss. For any suspected immune-mediated adverse reactions, exclude other causes. Based on the severity of the adverse reaction, withhold or discontinue cemiplimab-rwlc, administer high-dose corticosteroids and, if appropriate, initiate hormone replacement therapy.

Patient Education: Review manufacturer's medication guide. ■ Effective contraception required during treatment with cemiplimab-rwlc and for at least 4 months following the last dose of cemiplimab-rwlc. ■ Promptly report a known or suspected pregnancy. ■ Some side effects may require corticosteroid treatment and interruption or discontinuation of cemiplimab-rwlc. ■ Promptly report any S/S of an infusion-related reaction. ■ Promptly report S/S of pneumonitis (e.g., chest pain, new or worsening cough, or shortness of breath). ■ Promptly report S/S of colitis (e.g., diarrhea, blood or mucus in stools, or severe abdominal pain). ■ Promptly report S/S of hepatitis (e.g., easy bruising or bleeding, jaundice, lethargy, pain on the right side of the abdomen, severe nausea or vomiting). ■ Promptly report S/S of kidney dysfunction (e.g., blood in urine, decreased urine output, loss of appetite, swelling in ankles). ■ Promptly report S/S of hypophysitis, adrenal insufficiency, hypothyroidism, hyperthyroidism, or diabetes mellitus; see

Monitor. ■ Promptly report development of a rash. ■ Keeping scheduled appointments for blood work or other laboratory tests is imperative.

Maternal/Child: Avoid pregnancy. Based on mechanism of action and data from animal studies, cemiplimab-rwlc can cause fetal harm when administered to a pregnant woman. Animal studies have shown that inhibition of the PD-1/PD-L1 pathway can lead to increased risk of immune-mediated rejection of the developing fetus, resulting in fetal death. Human IgG4 is known to cross the placental barrier, and cemiplimab-rwlc is an IgG4 immunoglobin. ■ Discontinue breast-feeding. ■ Safety and effectiveness have not been established for use in pediatric patients.

Elderly: No overall differences in safety or efficacy were reported between elderly patients and younger patients.

DRUG/LAB INTERACTIONS
No formal pharmacokinetic drug-drug interaction studies conducted with cemiplimab-rwlc.

SIDE EFFECTS
The most common adverse reactions were diarrhea, fatigue, and rash. The most common Grade 3 to 4 adverse reactions were cellulitis, fatigue, hypertension, musculoskeletal pain, pneumonia, sepsis, skin infection, and urinary tract infection. Several immune-mediated reactions have been reported, including colitis, dermatologic adverse reactions/rash, endocrinopathies, hepatitis, nephritis and renal dysfunction, pneumonitis; see Precautions, Monitor, and Antidote. Other reported reactions include constipation, decreased appetite, nausea, and pruritus. Laboratory abnormalities include anemia, hypercalcemia, hypoalbuminemia, hyponatremia, hypophosphatemia, increased AST and INR, and lymphopenia.

ANTIDOTE
Keep physician informed of all side effects. May constitute a medical emergency or will be treated symptomatically as indicated. Treat side effects aggressively; see Monitor. Follow guidelines for withholding or discontinuing therapy as outlined in Dose Adjustments. Interrupt or slow the rate of administration in patients with mild or moderate infusion reactions. Discontinue in patients with a severe or life-threatening infusion reaction and treat as indicated. Initiate corticosteroid therapy as outlined in Monitor for immune-mediated reactions (e.g., pneumonitis, colitis, hepatitis, renal dysfunction, hypophysitis, adrenal insufficiency, hyperthyroidism or hypothyroidism, rash, and other clinically significant immune-mediated adverse reactions). Hormone replacement may also be indicated; see Monitor. Resuscitate if indicated.

CETIRIZINE HYDROCHLORIDE
(se-**TIR**-a-zeen)

Histamine H$_1$ antagonist

Quzyttir

pH 4.5 to 6.5

USUAL DOSE
Adults and adolescents 12 years of age and older: 10 mg as an IV injection over 1 to 2 minutes once every 24 hours.

PEDIATRIC DOSE
Pediatric patients 6 to 11 years of age: 5 mg or 10 mg depending on symptom severity as an IV injection over 1 to 2 minutes once every 24 hours.

Pediatric patients 6 months to 5 years of age: 2.5 mg as an IV injection over 1 to 2 minutes once every 24 hours.

DOSE ADJUSTMENTS

Not recommended in pediatric patients under 6 years of age with impaired renal or hepatic function. ■ No dose adjustment required in other patients with hepatic impairment or in renal impairment, including patients on dialysis; see Monitor.

DILUTION

Available as a ready-to-use, clear, colorless solution in a single-dose vial containing 10 mg/mL.

Filters: Specific information not available.

Storage: Store at CRT. Discard any unused portion.

COMPATIBILITY

Compatibility information not available from manufacturer; consult a pharmacist.

RATE OF ADMINISTRATION

A single dose as an IV push over 1 to 2 minutes.

ACTIONS

A selective histamine-1 (H_1) receptor antagonist. Its principal effects are mediated via selective inhibition of peripheral H_1 receptors. It has negligible anticholinergic and antiserotonergic activity. Activity persists for at least 24 hours. Peak concentrations achieved in 0.03 hours (range 0.03 to 2 hours). Mean plasma protein binding is 93%. Metabolized to a limited extent by oxidative O-dealkylation to a metabolite with negligible antihistaminic activity. Mean elimination half-life is 8.3 hours. Excreted primarily in urine. Secreted in breast milk.

INDICATIONS AND USES

Treatment of acute urticaria in adults and pediatric patients 6 months of age and older.

Limitation of use: Not recommended in pediatric patients under 6 years of age with impaired renal or hepatic function.

CONTRAINDICATIONS

Known hypersensitivity to cetirizine hydrochloride or any of its ingredients, levocetirizine, or hydroxyzine.

PRECAUTIONS

Somnolence/sedation have been reported.

Monitor: Observe for effectiveness. ■ Monitor for somnolence/sedative effects. ■ Monitor for antihistamine side effects in patients with renal or hepatic impairment.

Patient Education: May cause somnolence/sedation. Exercise caution when driving a car or operating potentially dangerous machinery. ■ Avoid concurrent use with alcohol or other CNS depressants. May cause additional reduction in alertness and additional impairment of CNS performance.

Maternal/Child: No adequate and well-controlled studies in pregnant women. No evidence to date of fetal harm in animal studies. ■ Present in breast milk. Consider risk versus benefits. ■ Safety and effectiveness have been established in pediatric patients 6 months to 17 years of age. ■ Safety and effectiveness in pediatric patients under 6 months of age have not been established.

Elderly: Response similar to that seen in younger adults, but greater sensitivity of some older individuals cannot be ruled out.

DRUG/LAB INTERACTIONS

Formal drug interaction studies are not available. ■ **Alcohol and/or other CNS depressants** may increase somnolence/sedation effects. ■ A small decrease in the clearance of cetirizine may occur with larger **theophylline** doses.

SIDE EFFECTS

The most common adverse reactions (incidence less than 1%) are dysgeusia, dyspepsia, feeling hot, headache, hyperhidrosis, paresthesia, and presyncope. Somnolence/sedation have also been reported.

ANTIDOTE

Notify physician of all side effects. Minor side effects may be tolerated or treated symptomatically. Not removed by dialysis.

CETUXIMAB BBW
(seh-**TUX**-ih-mab)

Recombinant monoclonal antibody
Antineoplastic
Epidermal growth factor receptor (EGFR) inhibitor

Erbitux

pH 7 to 7.4

USUAL DOSE

Pretreatment: Verify pregnancy status. Preassessment required to determine appropriate patient selection for patients with colorectal cancer; baseline studies indicated; see Monitor.

Premedication: To prevent or attenuate severe infusion reactions, premedicate with an H_1 antagonist (e.g., diphenhydramine 50 mg) IV 30 to 60 minutes before the first dose. Premedication for subsequent infusions should be based on clinical judgment and the presence/severity of previous infusion reactions.

Squamous cell carcinoma of the head and neck (SCCHN) in combination with radiation therapy or in combination with platinum-based therapy with 5-FU: *First infusion:* 400 mg/M² as an initial loading dose 1 week **before the initiation** of a course of radiation therapy or on the day of initiation of platinum-based therapy with 5-FU. Complete cetuximab administration 1 hour before beginning platinum-based therapy with 5-FU.

Subsequent infusions: 250 mg/M² once each week for the duration of radiation therapy (6 to 7 weeks) or until disease progression or unacceptable toxicity when administered with platinum-based therapy with 5-FU. Complete infusion 1 hour before radiation therapy or platinum-based therapy with 5-FU.

Squamous cell carcinoma of the head and neck as monotherapy:

First infusion: 400 mg/M² as an initial loading dose.

Subsequent infusions: 250 mg/M² once each week as a maintenance dose. Continue until disease progression or unacceptable toxicity.

Colorectal cancer in combination with irinotecan, FOLFIRI, or as monotherapy: Determine epidermal growth factor receptor (EGFR)-expression status and absence of a *Ras* mutation before initiating treatment; see Indications.

First infusion: 400 mg/M² as an initial loading dose. Complete infusion 1 hour before irinotecan or FOLFIRI (irinotecan, 5-FU, leucovorin) when given as combination therapy.

Subsequent infusions: 250 mg/M² once each week as a maintenance dose. Complete infusion 1 hour before irinotecan or FOLFIRI when given as combination therapy. Continue until disease progression or unacceptable toxicity.

DOSE ADJUSTMENTS

No dose adjustment required based on age, gender, race, or hepatic or renal function. ▪ No dose adjustment indicated for mild to moderate skin toxicity. ▪ Reduce, delay, or discontinue cetuximab to manage adverse reactions as described in the following chart.

Recommended Cetuximab Dosage Modifications for Adverse Reactions		
Adverse Reaction	**Severity[a]**	**Dosage Modification**
Infusion reactions	Grade 1 or 2	Reduce infusion rate by 50%.
	Grade 3 or 4	Discontinue cetuximab immediately and permanently.
Dermatologic toxicities and infectious sequelae (e.g., acneiform rash, mucocutaneous disease)	1st occurrence; Grade 3 or 4	Delay infusion 1 to 2 weeks; if condition improves, continue at 250 mg/M². If no improvement, discontinue cetuximab.
	2nd occurrence; Grade 3 or 4	Delay infusion 1 to 2 weeks; if condition improves, continue at 200 mg/M². If no improvement, discontinue cetuximab.
	3rd occurrence; Grade 3 or 4	Delay infusion 1 to 2 weeks; if condition improves, continue at 150 mg/M². If no improvement, discontinue cetuximab.
	4th occurrence; Grade 3 or 4	Discontinue cetuximab.
Pulmonary toxicity	Acute onset or worsening pulmonary symptoms	Delay infusion 1 to 2 weeks; if condition improves, continue at the dose that was being administered at the time of occurrence. If no improvement in 2 weeks or interstitial lung disease (ILD) is confirmed, discontinue cetuximab.

[a]National Cancer Institute (NCI) Common Toxicity Criteria (CTC), version 2.0.

DILUTION
Available in 100 mg/50 mL and 200 mg/100 mL single-use vials (2 mg/mL). Multiple vials may be needed for each dose. May pool volume required to provide calculated dose into an empty evacuated container. Solution is clear and may contain small amounts of easily visible white particulates. *Do not shake or dilute.*

Filters: Use of a low–protein binding, 0.22-micron in-line filter is required; see Rate of Administration.

Storage: Refrigerate vials at 2° to 8° C (36° to 46° F). Do not freeze. Preparations in infusion containers are chemically and physically stable for 12 hours if refrigerated or 8 hours at CRT (20° to 25° C [68° to 77° F]). Discard remaining solution in the infusion container after 8 hours at CRT. Discard any unused portion of the vial.

COMPATIBILITY
Compatibility information not available from manufacturer; consult a pharmacist.

RATE OF ADMINISTRATION
Do not administer as an IV push or bolus. Must be given as an infusion via an infusion pump or a syringe pump. Must be administered through a low–protein binding, 0.22-micron in-line filter.

First infusion: The initial loading dose should be infused evenly distributed over 2 hours (120 minutes). Do not exceed a rate of 10 mg/min (5 mL/min). In patients who have Grade 1 or 2 infusion reactions, decrease the rate of administration by 50%; see Dose Adjustments.

Subsequent infusions: Weekly maintenance doses should be infused evenly distributed over 1 hour (60 minutes). Do not exceed a rate of 10 mg/min (5 mL/min). In patients who have Grade 1 or 2 infusion reactions, decrease the rate of administration by 50%; see Dose Adjustments.

ACTIONS
An antineoplastic agent. A human/mouse monoclonal antibody produced by recombinant DNA technology that acts as an epidermal growth factor receptor (EGFR) antagonist. Cetuximab is composed of the Fv regions of a murine anti-EGFR antibody with human IgG1 heavy and kappa light-chain constant regions. Designed to bind to the EGFR found on the surface of both normal cells and tumor cells, resulting in inhibition of cell growth, induction of apoptosis, and decreased matrix metalloproteinase and vascular endothelial

growth factor production. Antitumor effects were not observed in tumor cells that did not express the EGFR. With the recommended dose regimen, cetuximab concentrations reached steady-state levels by the third weekly infusion with a mean half-life of 112 hours (range 63 to 230 hours). IgG antibodies may cross the placental barrier and may be secreted in breast milk.

INDICATIONS AND USES

Initial treatment of locally or regionally advanced SCCHN in combination with radiation therapy. ▪ First-line treatment of patients with recurrent locoregional disease or metastatic SCCHN in combination with platinum-based therapy with 5-FU. ▪ Used as a single agent for the treatment of patients with recurrent or metastatic SCCHN in whom platinum-based chemotherapy has failed. ▪ Treatment of K-*Ras* wild type, EGFR–expressing metastatic colorectal cancer (mCRC) as determined by FDA-approved tests for this use. Used in combination with FOLFIRI (irinotecan, 5-fluorouracil, leucovorin) for first-line treatment. Used in combination with irinotecan (Camptosar) in patients who are refractory to irinotecan-based chemotherapy. Used as a single agent in patients who cannot tolerate irinotecan or in those who have failed treatment with irinotecan (Camptosar)– and oxaliplatin (Eloxatin)–based regimens.

Limitation of use: Not indicated for treatment of *Ras*-mutant colorectal cancer or when the results of the *Ras* mutation tests are unknown.

CONTRAINDICATIONS

Manufacturer states, "None." However, a repeat dose is contraindicated in any patient who has a severe infusion reaction. ▪ Use with caution in patients with known hypersensitivity to murine proteins, cetuximab, or any of its components.

PRECAUTIONS

Do not administer as an IV push or bolus. Must be given as an infusion via an infusion pump or a syringe pump. ▪ Should be administered by or under the direction of the physician specialist in a facility equipped to monitor the patient and respond to any medical emergency. ▪ Severe infusion reactions have occurred, and some have been fatal. Most severe reactions occur with the first infusion and have occurred even with the use of prophylactic antihistamines. Risk of anaphylactic reactions may be increased in patients with a history of tick bites, red meat allergy, or in the presence of IgE antibodies directed against galactose-α-1,3-galactose (alpha-gal). ▪ Cardiopulmonary arrest and/or sudden death has been reported in patients with SCCHN treated with cetuximab and radiation and in patients with SCCHN treated with cetuximab and a combination of platinum-based therapy with 5-FU. Carefully consider the use of cetuximab in combination with radiation therapy or platinum-based therapy with 5-FU in patients with head and neck cancer who have a history of arrhythmias, coronary artery disease, or congestive heart failure. ▪ Pulmonary toxicity, including interstitial lung disease (ILD), has been reported. ▪ Severe dermatologic toxicities, including acneiform rash, skin drying and fissuring, and inflammatory and infectious sequelae (e.g., blepharitis [inflammation of the eyelids], cellulitis [diffuse subcutaneous inflammation of connective tissues], cheilitis [inflammation of the lip], conjunctivitis, hypertrichosis, and keratitis/ulcerative keratitis with decreased visual acuity), have occurred and may be dose limiting. Complications involving *S. aureus* sepsis and abscesses requiring incision and drainage have been reported. Life-threatening and fatal bullous mucocutaneous disease with blisters, erosions, and skin sloughing has been observed. ▪ In a controlled study, the addition of cetuximab to radiation and cisplatin led to an increased incidence of serious toxicity and death without any improvement in progression-free survival. Cetuximab is not indicated for the treatment of SCCHN in combination with radiation and cisplatin. ▪ May cause electrolyte abnormalities. ▪ A protein substance, it has the potential for producing immunogenicity. However, there does not appear to be a relationship between the appearance of antibodies to cetuximab and the safety or antitumor activity of the molecule. ▪ See Monitor and Antidote.

Monitor: Determine EGFR-expression status and the absence of a *Ras* mutation in patients with metastatic colorectal cancer (mCRC) using FDA-approved tests before initiating treatment. See prescribing information for access to FDA-approved tests. Use of cetuximab in patients with *Ras* mutant mCRC resulted in no clinical benefit and increased tumor progression, toxicity, and mortality. Expression of EGFR has been detected in nearly all patients with SCCHN, so determination of EGFR-expression status is not required in this patient population. ▪ Monitor VS frequently. ▪ Observe patient closely during every infusion and for at least 1 hour after each infusion. Monitor longer to confirm resolution of the event in patients requiring treatment for infusion reactions. Infusion reactions can occur during or several hours after completion of the infusion, even in patients who are premedicated with diphenhydramine and/or who have not had infusion reactions with previous doses; see Precautions. S/S of severe reactions may include hypotension, rapid onset of airway obstruction (e.g., bronchospasm, hoarseness, stridor), loss of consciousness, MI, shock, and/or cardiac arrest. ▪ Monitor serum electrolytes, including magnesium, calcium, and potassium, weekly during therapy and for 8 weeks following completion. Electrolyte loss may occur from days to months after initiating cetuximab. Oral or parenteral electrolyte replacement may be indicated. ▪ Monitor for S/S of dermatologic toxicity such as acneiform rash (e.g., multiple follicular-pustular–appearing lesions on the face, upper chest, back, and extremities), skin drying, and fissuring. Dose adjustments or termination of therapy may be indicated; see Dose Adjustments and Precautions. The first onset of acneiform rash may occur within the first 2 weeks, may subside when treatment is discontinued, or may persist for longer periods. The rash lasted more than 28 days after stopping cetuximab in most patients. Inflammatory or infectious sequelae (e.g., blepharitis, cellulitis, cheilitis) may develop and should be treated promptly. ▪ Monitor for S/S of interstitial lung disease (e.g., dyspnea on exertion, nonproductive cough, inspiratory crackles on chest examination). Acute onset or worsening symptoms may require interruption or discontinuation of cetuximab therapy. ▪ See Dose Adjustments, Rate of Administration, Precautions, and Antidote.

Patient Education: Verify pregnancy status in females of reproductive potential before initiating therapy. Avoid pregnancy; use of effective birth control recommended for females during therapy and for 2 months after the last dose. See Maternal/Child. Women should report a suspected pregnancy immediately. ▪ Review potential side effects before therapy. ▪ Report any unusual or unexpected symptoms or side effects promptly, including infusion-related reactions (e.g., dyspnea, feeling of faintness, hives, wheezing), respiratory reactions (e.g., cough, shortness of breath), or dermatologic toxicities. ▪ Review medical history with provider before initiating therapy. ▪ Sunlight can worsen the skin reactions that may occur. Limit exposure to the sun (use sunscreen, wear hat and protective clothing) while receiving and for 2 months following the last dose of cetuximab. ▪ See Appendix D.

Maternal/Child: Can cause fetal harm when administered to a pregnant woman. ▪ Discontinue breast-feeding during treatment with cetuximab and for 60 days following the last dose. ▪ Safety and effectiveness for use in pediatric patients not established.

Elderly: Safety and effectiveness similar to younger adults in CRC trials. SCCHN studies did not include sufficient numbers of patients over age 65 years to determine any differences in efficacy or toxicity.

DRUG/LAB INTERACTIONS

No drug interaction studies have been completed. ▪ No pharmacokinetic interaction was observed between cetuximab and irinotecan, cetuximab and cisplatin, and cetuximab and carboplatin. ▪ Increased incidence of death and serious toxicity have been observed when **cetuximab, cisplatin, and radiation therapy** have been used concomitantly.

SIDE EFFECTS

The most common side effects are cutaneous adverse reactions (e.g., nail changes, pruritus, rash), diarrhea, headache, and infection. The most serious side effects are cardiopulmonary arrest, dermatologic toxicity, infusion reactions, and interstitial lung disease. **SCCHN:** Anorexia; elevated ALT, AST, and alkaline phosphatase; mucositis/stomatitis/pharyngitis; and radiation dermatitis/toxicities.

Colorectal cancer: Anxiety, arthralgia, confusion, constipation, cough, depression, dyspnea, fatigue, insomnia, malaise, mouth dryness, neuropathy, neutropenia, pain, stomatitis, and taste disturbance.

All diagnoses: Acneiform rash, asthenia, chills, conjunctivitis, dehydration, dyspepsia, electrolyte abnormalities (e.g., hypocalcemia, hypokalemia, hypomagnesemia), fever, nausea and vomiting, and weight loss.

Post-Marketing: Aseptic meningitis, Stevens-Johnson syndrome, toxic epidermal necrolysis, life-threatening and fatal bullous mucocutaneous disease.

ANTIDOTE

Keep physician informed of all side effects. May constitute a medical emergency or will be treated symptomatically as indicated. Hypersensitivity or infusion-related side effects may resolve with reduction in the rate of infusion by 50% and by continued use of premedication with diphenhydramine. Discontinue cetuximab immediately for severe infusion reactions requiring medical intervention and/or hospitalization; *do not rechallenge.* Treat hypersensitivity or infusion reactions as indicated; may require use of epinephrine, corticosteroids, diphenhydramine, bronchodilators (e.g., albuterol, aminophylline), IV saline, oxygen, and/or acetaminophen. Dermatologic toxicities may be dose limiting (see Dose Adjustments) or may be treated with topical and/or oral antibiotics as appropriate. Use of topical corticosteroids is not recommended. Interrupt cetuximab for acute onset or worsening of pulmonary symptoms. Treat as indicated; permanently discontinue cetuximab for confirmed interstitial lung disease. Replace electrolytes as indicated. Resuscitate if indicated.

CHLOROTHIAZIDE SODIUM

(klor-oh-**THIGH**-ah-zyd **SO**-dee-um)

Diuretic (thiazide)
Antidiuretic (diabetes insipidus)

Diuril

pH 9.2 to 10

USUAL DOSE

Pretreatment: Baseline studies indicated; see Monitor.

IV and oral doses are therapeutically equivalent. Oral dose can replace an IV dose at any time. 0.5 to 1 Gm once or twice daily. Individualize based on patient response. Use of the smallest dose necessary to achieve desired response is indicated. Some patients respond to intermittent therapy (e.g., every other day or 3 to 5 days out of a week). Intermittent therapy may decrease the incidence of excessive response and the resulting undesirable electrolyte imbalance. Another source suggests the following:

Diuretic: 250 mg every 6 to 12 hours. Up to 2 Gm/24 hr may be indicated.

PEDIATRIC DOSE

Safety and effectiveness in pediatric patients not established; all pediatric doses are **unlabeled;** experience has been limited; see Maternal/Child.

Under 6 months of age (unlabeled): Begin with 1 to 4 mg/kg every 12 hours. May increase to 10 to 20 mg/kg every 12 hours if needed.

6 months of age or older (unlabeled): Begin with 2 mg/kg every 12 hours or 4 mg/kg every 24 hours. May increase to 10 mg/kg every 12 hours if needed.

DOSE ADJUSTMENTS

See Drug/Lab Interactions. ▪ If progressive renal impairment occurs, consider withholding or discontinuing diuretic therapy. ▪ Caution and lower-end dosing suggested in the elderly. Consider potential for age-related impaired organ function and concomitant disease or drug therapy.

DILUTION

Each 0.5 Gm must be reconstituted with at least 18 mL of SW (yields 28 mg/mL). Never use less than 18 mL of SW. Prepare immediately before use. May be given as an IV injection or may be further diluted in dextrose or NS solutions and given as an infusion.

Storage: Store in powder form at CRT. Contains no preservatives; use reconstituted solution immediately and discard unused portion.

COMPATIBILITY

Manufacturer lists as **incompatible** with whole blood or its derivatives.

Other sources suggest a few specific **compatibilities** dependent on concentration and manufacturer; consult a pharmacist.

RATE OF ADMINISTRATION

0.5 Gm or fraction thereof as a slow IV injection (e.g., over 2 to 3 minutes) or as an infusion (rate dependent on volume of diluent and patient condition).

ACTIONS

A diuretic and antihypertensive agent. It affects the distal renal tubular mechanism of electrolyte reabsorption. Excretion of sodium and chloride occurs in approximately equal amounts. There is some loss of potassium and bicarbonate. The specific mechanism of its antihypertensive effect is not known; however, it does not affect normal blood pressure. Effectiveness is noted within 15 to 30 minutes. Half-life is approximately 1 to 2 hours; duration of action is 6 to 12 hours. Not metabolized but rapidly excreted unchanged in the urine. Crosses the placental barrier but not the blood-brain barrier. Secreted in breast milk.

INDICATIONS AND USES

Adjunctive therapy in edema associated with congestive heart failure, hepatic cirrhosis, and corticosteroid and estrogen therapy. ▪ May be useful in edema due to various forms of renal dysfunction (e.g., nephrotic syndrome, acute glomerulonephritis, chronic renal failure). ▪ Edema of pregnancy when edema results from the above conditions (e.g., pathologic causes). ▪ Used rarely during a normal pregnancy (in the absence of cardiovascular disease) for edema that causes extreme discomfort not relieved by rest. ▪ Adjunctive therapy in the treatment of hypertension.

CONTRAINDICATIONS

Anuria. ▪ Hypersensitivity to chlorothiazide, any of its components, or other sulfonamide-derived drugs.

PRECAUTIONS

IV use indicated in patients unable to take oral medication or in emergency situations. For IV use only; do not use IM or SC. ▪ Use with caution in severe renal disease; thiazides may precipitate azotemia. ▪ Use with caution in patients with impaired renal function; cumulative effects may develop. ▪ Use with caution in patients with impaired hepatic function or progressive liver disease; minor alterations of fluid and electrolyte balance may precipitate hepatic coma. ▪ Sensitivity reactions may occur in patients with or without a history of allergy or bronchial asthma. ▪ Exacerbation and/or activation of systemic lupus erythematosus has been reported. ▪ May increase glucose levels, uric acid levels, total cholesterol, HDL, triglycerides, and urine output of magnesium. ▪ May decrease calcium excretion. Marked hypercalcemia may indicate hidden hyperparathyroidism; discontinue thiazides before testing for parathyroid function. ▪ Antihypertensive effects may be increased in postsympathectomy patients. ▪ See Monitor and Drug/Lab Interactions.

Monitor: Determine absolute patency of vein. Avoid extravasation. ▪ Obtain baseline and perform repeat checks routinely of electrolyte panel, CO_2, BUN, uric acid, and glucose. ▪ May precipitate excessive diuresis with water and electrolyte depletion. Monitor for S/S of fluid or electrolyte imbalance (e.g., confusion, drowsiness, dryness of mouth, hypochloremic alkalosis, hypokalemia, hyponatremia, hypotension, lethargy, muscle fatigue, muscle pain or cramps, nausea and vomiting, oliguria, restlessness, seizures, tachycardia, thirst, weakness) and replace electrolytes as necessary. Monitor serum and urine electrolytes more closely in patients who are vomiting or receiving parenteral fluids. Monitor VS closely. ▪ Monitor closely for hypokalemia (especially during brisk diuresis) in patients with severe cirrhosis or during prolonged treatment. May cause cardiac arrhythmias and/or increase the potential for toxic effects of digoxin. Potassium supplements or the use of potassium-sparing diuretics may be indicated. ▪ See Precautions and Drug/Lab Interactions.

Patient Education: Take only prescribed medications. ▪ Promptly report dizziness, diarrhea, muscle weakness or cramps, nausea, or vomiting. ▪ May cause hypokalemia and require a potassium supplement.

Maternal/Child: Category C: use only if clearly needed. Crosses the placental barrier; has been found in cord blood and may harm the fetus. ▪ Discontinue breast-feeding. ▪ Use in infants and pediatric patients has been limited and is not generally recommended; see Pediatric Dose.

Elderly: Differences in response compared to younger adults not identified. ▪ Dose selection should be cautious; see Dose Adjustments. May have increased sensitivity to hypotensive and electrolyte effects. Monitoring of renal function suggested.

DRUG/LAB INTERACTIONS

Do not give simultaneously with **whole blood or its derivatives.** ▪ Has antihypertensive actions. May have an additive effect used concurrently with **other antihypertensive agents;** reduced doses of both agents may be indicated. ▪ Potential for orthostatic hypotension is increased with concurrent use of **alcohol, barbiturates, or narcotics.** ▪ May cause hyperglycemia. Monitor **blood glucose levels** and adjust doses of insulin and oral antidiabetic agents as indicated. ▪ Electrolyte depletion (especially hypokalemia) may increase with concurrent administration of **other drugs that cause potassium loss,** such as amphotericin B or corticosteroids. ▪ May have a decreased response to **pressor amines** (e.g., norepinephrine); monitor carefully. ▪ Concurrent use with **lithium** not recommended; renal excretion of lithium is decreased and potential for lithium toxicity is increased. ▪ **NSAIDs** may decrease the effects of diuretics; monitor carefully. ▪ Raises blood uric acid; dose adjustment of **antigout agents** (e.g., allopurinol, colchicine) may be indicated. ▪ Synergistic effects with **loop diuretics** (e.g., furosemide, torsemide) may cause profound diuresis and serious electrolyte abnormalities. ▪ Hypokalemia and hypomagnesemia may cause **digoxin-induced arrhythmias;** monitor potassium levels. ▪ Hypersensitivity reactions to **allopurinol** may be increased. ▪ May prolong **antineoplastic** (e.g., methotrexate) induced leukopenia. ▪ **May cause hypercalcemia** through decreased calcium excretion or increased bone release or by enhancing action of vitamin D. ▪ May decrease effects of **anticoagulants.** ▪ Discontinue thiazides before **testing for parathyroid function;** see Precautions.

SIDE EFFECTS

Agranulocytosis, alopecia, anorexia, aplastic anemia, blurred vision (transient), constipation, cramping, diarrhea, dizziness, electrolyte imbalance, erythema multiforme (including Stevens-Johnson syndrome, exfoliative dermatitis, and toxic epidermal necrolysis), GI upset, glycosuria, headache, hematuria, hemolytic anemia, hyperglycemia, hypersensitivity reactions, hypotension, jaundice, leukopenia, muscle spasm, nausea and vomiting, orthostatic hypotension, pancreatitis, paresthesias, renal dysfunction, renal failure, restlessness, sialadenitis (inflammation of a salivary gland), thrombocytopenia, vertigo, weakness, yellow vision.

Overdose: Most common S/S are those caused by electrolyte depletion (e.g., hypokalemia, hyponatremia, hypochloremic alkalosis) and dehydration resulting from excessive diuresis. Cardiac arrhythmias may occur if digoxin is used concurrently.

ANTIDOTE

Notify physician of all side effects. Minor side effects may be treated symptomatically. Reduce chlorothiazide dose or discontinue if side effects are moderate or severe. Treatment of moderate to severe side effects is symptomatic and aggressive. If progressive renal impairment or S/S of hepatic coma occur, consider withholding or discontinuing diuretic therapy. Treatment of overdose is symptomatic and supportive. Correct dehydration, electrolyte imbalance, hepatic coma, and hypotension. Maintain an adequate airway and use oxygen or artificial ventilation for respiratory distress as indicated. Amount of chlorothiazide removed by hemodialysis has not been established. Resuscitate as necessary.

CHLORPROMAZINE HYDROCHLORIDE BBW

(klor-**PROH**-mah-zeen hy-droh-**KLOR**-eyed)

**Phenothiazine
Antipsychotic
Antiemetic**

Thorazine

pH 3 to 5

USUAL DOSE

Use of the IV route is reserved for the treatment of acute nausea and vomiting in surgery, intractable hiccups, and tetanus.

Acute nausea and vomiting in surgery: 2 mg. May repeat at 2-minute intervals as indicated. Do not exceed 25 mg. Usually given as an infusion.

Intractable hiccups: 25 to 50 mg diluted in 500 to 1,000 mL of NS. Given as a slow IV infusion with patient flat in bed. Monitor BP closely.

Tetanus: 25 to 50 mg as an infusion of at least 1 mg/mL. Individualize dose to patient response and tolerance. Repeat every 6 to 8 hours. Usually given in conjunction with barbiturates.

PEDIATRIC DOSE

See Maternal/Child. IV route rarely used for pediatric patients. Not recommended for use in infants under 6 months of age.

Acute nausea and vomiting in surgery, pediatric patients 6 months of age or older: 1 mg. May repeat at 2-minute intervals as indicated. Monitor for hypotension. Another source suggests 2.5 to 4 mg/kg/24 hr in equally divided doses every 6 to 8 hours (0.625 to 1 mg/kg every 6 hours or 0.83 to 1.33 mg/kg every 8 hours). Usual IV/IM dose does not exceed 2.5 to 4 mg/kg/24 hr or 40 mg/24 hr (whichever is less) in pediatric patients 6 months to 5 years of age or up to 23 kg (50 lb), and 75 mg/24 hr in pediatric patients 5 to 12 years of age.

Tetanus: 0.55 mg/kg of body weight (0.25 mg/lb) every 6 to 8 hours. Do not exceed 40 mg/24 hr for up to 23 kg (50 lb) and 75 mg/24 hr for up to 50 kg (50 to 100 lb), except in severe cases.

DOSE ADJUSTMENTS

Adjust dose to the individual and severity of condition. Reduce dose of any medication potentiated by phenothiazines by one-fourth to one-half. See Drug/Lab Interactions. ▪ Reduce dose by one-fourth to one-half in the elderly, debilitated patients, or emaciated patients, and increase very gradually by response.

DILUTION

Each 25 mg (1 mL) must be diluted with 24 mL of NS for injection. 1 mL will equal 1 mg. May be further diluted in 500 to 1,000 mL of NS and given as an infusion. Handle carefully; may cause contact dermatitis. Sensitive to light. Slightly yellow color does not alter potency. Discard if markedly discolored.

Storage: Store at CRT. Protect from light and freezing.

COMPATIBILITY

Compatibility information not available from manufacturer. Other sources suggest specific **compatibilities** dependent on concentration and manufacturer; consult a pharmacist.

RATE OF ADMINISTRATION

Titrate to symptoms and vital signs. See Precautions.

IV injection: Each 1 mg or fraction thereof over 1 minute.

Infusion: Given very slowly. Do not exceed 1 mg/min.

Pediatric rate: Do not exceed 1 mg or fraction thereof over 2 minutes.

ACTIONS

A phenothiazine derivative with effects on the central, autonomic, and peripheral nervous systems. A psychotropic agent. Decreases anxiety and tension, relaxes muscles, produces sedation, and tranquilizes. Has an antiemetic effect and potentiates CNS depressants. Has strong antiadrenergic and anticholinergic activity. Also possesses slight antihistaminic and antiserotonin activity. Onset of action is prompt and of short duration in small IV doses. Extensively metabolized in liver and kidney and excreted primarily in urine. Crosses the placental barrier. Secreted in breast milk.

INDICATIONS AND USES

The IV route is used only for the treatment of acute nausea and vomiting in surgery, the treatment of intractable hiccups, and as an adjunct in the treatment of tetanus. ▪ Used IM or PO for the treatment of schizophrenia and the management of psychotic disorders. ▪ Also indicated IM, PO, or rectally to relieve restlessness and apprehension before surgery, to manage acute intermittent porphyria, to control manic episodes in manic-depressive illness, and to treat severe behavioral problems in pediatric patients.

Unlabeled uses: Treatment of phencyclidine (PCP) psychosis. ▪ Treatment of migraine headaches (IV or IM). ▪ To reduce choreiform movements of Huntington's disease.

CONTRAINDICATIONS

Hypersensitivity to phenothiazines, comatose or severely depressed states, or the presence of large amounts of CNS depressants (e.g., alcohol, barbiturates, narcotics).

PRECAUTIONS

Not approved for dementia-related psychosis; mortality risk in elderly dementia patients taking conventional or atypical antipsychotics is increased; most deaths are due to cardiovascular or infectious events. ▪ Use of the IV route is reserved for the treatment of acute nausea and vomiting in surgery, intractable hiccups, and tetanus. IM injection preferred. ▪ Use caution in patients with bone marrow suppression; glaucoma; cardiovascular, liver, renal, and chronic respiratory diseases; and acute respiratory diseases of pediatric patients. ▪ Re-exposure of patients who have experienced jaundice, skin reactions, or blood dyscrasias with a phenothiazine is not recommended. Cross-sensitivity may occur. ▪ May produce ECG changes (e.g., prolonged QT interval, changes in T waves). ▪ Use with caution in patients with a history of seizure disorders; may lower seizure threshold. ▪ Extrapyramidal symptoms caused by chlorpromazine may be confused with CNS signs of an undiagnosed disease (e.g., Reye's syndrome or encephalopathy). ▪ May mask diagnosis of brain tumor, drug intoxication, and intestinal obstruction. ▪ Tardive dyskinesia (potentially irreversible involuntary dyskinetic movements) may develop. Use smallest doses and shortest duration of therapy to minimize risk. ▪ Neuroleptic malignant syndrome (NMS) characterized by hyperpyrexia, muscle rigidity, altered mental status, and autonomic instability has been reported; see Antidote. ▪ May cause paradoxical excitation in pediatric patients and the elderly. ▪ Use phenothiazines with extreme caution in pediatric patients with a history of sleep apnea, a family history of SIDS, or in the presence of Reye's syndrome. ▪ May contain sulfites; use caution in patients with asthma. ▪ Taper dose gradually following high dose or extended therapy to prevent possible occurrence of withdrawal symptoms (e.g., dizziness, gastritis, nausea, tremors, and vomiting).

Monitor: Keep patient in supine position throughout treatment and for at least 30 minutes after treatment. Ambulate slowly and carefully; may cause postural hypotension. ▪ Monitor BP and pulse before and during administration and between doses. ▪ Cough reflex is often depressed; monitor closely if nauseated or vomiting to prevent aspiration. ▪ Anticholinergic and cardiac effects may be troublesome during anesthesia. For patients receiving phenothiazines, taper and discontinue preoperatively if they will not be continued after surgery. ▪ May discolor urine pink to reddish brown. ▪ Photosensitivity of skin is possible. ▪ See Drug/Lab Interactions.

Patient Education: Request assistance for ambulation; may cause dizziness or fainting. ▪ Observe caution when performing tasks that require alertness. ▪ Avoid use of alcohol and other CNS depressants (e.g., diazepam, narcotics). ▪ Possible eye and skin photosensitivity. Avoid unprotected exposure to sun. ▪ Urine may discolor to pink or reddish brown.

Maternal/Child: See Precautions and Contraindications. ▪ Category C: use during pregnancy only when clearly needed. Use near term may cause maternal hypotension and adverse neonatal effects (e.g., extrapyramidal syndrome, hyperreflexia, hyporeflexia, jaundice). ▪ Fetuses and infants have a reduced capacity to metabolize and eliminate; may cause embryo toxicity, increase neonatal mortality, or cause permanent neurologic damage. May contain benzyl alcohol; use not recommended in neonates. ▪ Not recommended during breast-feeding. Increases risk of dystonia and tardive dyskinesia. ▪ Pediatric patients metabolize antipsychotic agents more rapidly than adults and are at increased risk to develop extrapyramidal actions, especially during acute illness (e.g., chickenpox, CNS infections, dehydration, gastroenteritis, measles); monitor closely.

Elderly: See Dose Adjustments and Precautions. ▪ Have a reduced capacity to metabolize and eliminate. May have increased sensitivity to postural hypotension, anticholinergic and sedative effects. ▪ Increased risk of extrapyramidal side effects (e.g., tardive dyskinesia, parkinsonism).

DRUG/LAB INTERACTIONS

Use with **epinephrine** not recommended; may cause precipitous hypotension. ▪ Use with **agents that produce hypotension** (e.g., antihypertensives, benzodiazepines, diuretics, lidocaine, paclitaxel) may produce severe hypotension. ▪ Increased CNS, respiratory depression, and hypotensive effects with **CNS depressants** (e.g., narcotics, alcohol, anesthetics, and barbiturates); reduced doses of these agents usually indicated. ▪ Chlorpromazine does not potentiate the anticonvulsant actions of **barbiturates.** Doses of **anticonvulsant barbiturates** should not be decreased if chlorpromazine is introduced. Instead begin chlorpromazine at a lower dose and titrate to effect. ▪ Chlorpromazine may lower the seizure threshold. It may also interfere with **phenytoin and valproic acid** clearance, increasing potential for toxicity. Dose adjustment of anticonvulsants may be necessary. ▪ Additive effects with **MAO inhibitors** (e.g., selegiline), **anticholinergics, antihistamines, antihypertensives, hypnotics, muscle relaxants, rauwolfia alkaloids, and thiazide diuretics;** dose adjustment may be necessary. ▪ **Barbiturates** may also increase metabolism of chlorpromazine and reduce its effects. ▪ Risk of cardiotoxicity increased with **pimozide;** concurrent use not recommended. ▪ Risk of additive QT interval prolongation, cardiac depressant effects, and cardiac arrhythmias increased with **disopyramide, erythromycin, probucol, procainamide, and quinidine.** ▪ Concurrent use with **antidepressants, tricyclic antidepressants, or MAO inhibitors** (e.g., selegiline) may increase effects of both drugs; risk of NMS may be increased. ▪ Use with **antithyroid drugs** may increase risk of agranulocytosis. ▪ May inhibit antiparkinson effects of **levodopa.** ▪ May decrease pressor response to **ephedrine.** ▪ May increase anticholinergic effect of **orphenadrine.** ▪ May decrease effects of **oral anticoagulants.** ▪ Concurrent use with **haloperidol, droperidol, or metoclopramide** may cause increased extrapyramidal effects. ▪ Use with **metrizamide** (Amipaque) may lower seizure threshold; discontinue chlorpromazine 48 hours before myelography and do not resume for 24 hours after test is completed. ▪ Metabolism and clearance of chlorpromazine is increased in cigarette **smokers;** decreased plasma levels and effectiveness may occur; dose adjustment of chlorpromazine may be indicated. ▪ Decreased drowsiness may occur in cigarette **smokers.** May be offset by increased doses of chlorpromazine. ▪ Use caution during anesthesia with **barbiturates** (e.g., methohexital, thiopental); may increase frequency and severity of hypotension and neuromuscular excitation. ▪ Encephalopathic syndrome has been reported with concurrent use of **lithium;** monitor for S/S of neurologic toxicity. ▪ Capable of innumerable other interactions. ▪ May cause false-positive **pregnancy test** and false-positive **amylase, PKU, and other urine tests.**

SIDE EFFECTS

Usually transient if drug is discontinued, but may require treatment if severe. Anaphylaxis, cardiac arrest, distorted Q and T waves, drowsiness, excitement, extrapyramidal symptoms (e.g., abnormal positioning, extreme restlessness, pseudoparkinsonism, weakness of extremities), fever, hematologic toxicities (e.g., agranulocytosis, aplastic anemia, leukopenia, thrombocytopenia), hypersensitivity reactions, hypertension, hypotension (occurs less frequently in smokers), melanosis, photosensitivity, tachycardia, tardive dyskinesia, and many others.

Overdose: Can cause convulsions, hallucinations, and death.

ANTIDOTE

Discontinue the drug at onset of any side effect and notify the physician. Discontinue chlorpromazine and all drugs not essential to concurrent therapy immediately if NMS occurs. Will require intensive symptomatic treatment, medical monitoring, and management of concomitant medical problems. Counteract hypotension with norepinephrine or phenylephrine and IV fluids. Counteract extrapyramidal symptoms with benztropine or diphenhydramine. Use diazepam followed by phenytoin for convulsions or hyperactivity. Maintain a clear airway and adequate hydration. Epinephrine is contraindicated for hypotension; further hypotension will occur. Phenytoin may be helpful in ventricular arrhythmias. Avoid analeptics such as caffeine and sodium benzoate in treating respiratory depression and unconsciousness; they may cause convulsions. Resuscitate as necessary. Not removed by dialysis.

CIPROFLOXACIN BBW

(sip-row-**FLOX**-ah-sin)

Cipro IV

Antibacterial
(fluoroquinolone)

pH 3.5 to 4.6

USUAL DOSE
Pretreatment: Baseline studies indicated; see Monitor.
Dose and duration based on severity and nature of the infection, susceptibility of the causative organsim. Usual dose is 200 to 400 mg every 8 to 12 hours.

PEDIATRIC DOSE
Used only when alternate therapy cannot be used; see Precautions and Maternal/Child.
In all situations, do not exceed an IV dose of 400 mg.
Inhalation anthrax (postexposure): 10 mg/kg every 12 hours IV. Do not exceed 400 mg/dose IV. Begin administration as soon as possible after suspected or confirmed exposure. May transfer to oral therapy when appropriate with a dose of 15 mg/kg PO every 12 hours. Do not exceed a 500-mg dose PO. Administer for 60 days.
Complicated UTIs or pyelonephritis in patients from 1 to 17 years of age: Dosing and initial route (IV or PO) should be determined by severity of infection. 6 to 10 mg/kg IV every 8 hours. Do not exceed 400 mg/dose IV. May transfer to oral therapy with a dose of 10 to 20 mg/kg PO every 12 hours at discretion of physician. Do not exceed a 750-mg dose PO. Total duration of treatment is 10 to 21 days.
Plague: 10 mg/kg every 8 to 12 hours IV. Do not exceed 400 mg/dose IV. Begin administration as soon as possible after suspected or confirmed exposure. May transfer to oral therapy when appropriate with a dose of 15 mg/kg PO every 8 to 12 hours. Do not exceed a 500-mg dose PO. Administer for 10 to 21 days.
Pulmonary exacerbations of cystic fibrosis in patients from 5 to 17 years of age (unlabeled): 10 mg/kg/dose IV every 8 hours. Do not exceed 400 mg/dose. May transfer to oral therapy when appropriate at a dose of 20 mg/kg/dose PO every 12 hours; see Monitor.

DOSE ADJUSTMENTS
Increase interval between doses (200 to 400 mg every 18 to 24 hours) if CrCl is less than 30 mL/min (see literature for additional information). ■ Information on dosing adjustments for pediatric patients with renal insufficiency is not available. ■ Dose reduction not required based on age; see Elderly. ■ See Drug/Lab Interactions.

DILUTION
Available prediluted in D5W in latex-free plastic infusion containers ready for use. A clear, colorless to slightly yellow solution. Do not hang plastic containers in series; may cause air embolism. Also available in 20- and 40-mL vials containing 10 mg/mL (1% solution), which must be diluted with NS, D5W, SWFI, D10W, D5/¼NS, D5/½NS, or LR to a final concentration of 1 to 2 mg/mL.
Filters: No recommendations available from manufacturer.
Storage: Store vials between 5° and 30° C (41° and 86° F). Store flexible containers and vials between 5° and 25° C (41° and 77° F); protect from light, excessive heat, and freezing. Vials diluted in recommended solutions are stable for up to 14 days refrigerated or at room temperature if the final diluted concentration is between 0.5 and 2 mg/mL.

COMPATIBILITY

Manufacturer recommends temporarily discontinuing other solutions infusing at the same site during intermittent infusion through a **Y-site** or volume control and that ciprofloxacin be administered separately and the IV line be flushed before and after administration of any other drug.

Other sources suggest specific **compatibilities** dependent on concentration and manufacturer; consult a pharmacist.

RATE OF ADMINISTRATION

A single dose must be equally distributed over 60 minutes as an infusion. Too-rapid administration and/or the use of a small vein may increase incidence of local site inflammation and other side effects. May be given through a Y-tube of infusion set. Temporarily discontinue other solutions infusing at the same site.

ACTIONS

A synthetic, broad-spectrum antimicrobial agent, a fluoroquinolone. Bactericidal to a wide range of aerobic gram-negative and gram-positive organisms through interference with the enzymes needed for bacterial DNA replication, transcription, repair, and recombination. Onset of action is prompt, and serum levels are dose related. Half-life averages 5 to 6 hours. Readily distributed to body fluids (saliva, nasal and bronchial secretions, sputum, skin blister fluid, lymph, peritoneal fluid, bile and prostatic secretions). Found in lung, skin, fat, muscle, cartilage, and bone. Levels in cerebrospinal fluid and eye fluids are lower than plasma levels. Limited metabolism. Excreted primarily as unchanged drug in the urine, usually within 24 hours. A small amount is excreted in the bile and feces. Crosses placental barrier. Secreted in breast milk.

INDICATIONS AND USES

Treatment of infections caused by susceptible isolates of designated organisms in the conditions and patient populations listed below. ▪ Treatment of skin and skin structure infections in adults. ▪ Treatment of bone and joint infections in adults. ▪ Treatment of complicated intra-abdominal infections in adults (used in combination with metronidazole). ▪ Treatment of nosocomial pneumonia in adults. ▪ Empiric treatment of febrile neutropenia in adults (used in combination with piperacillin sodium). ▪ Treatment of inhalational anthrax (postexposure) to reduce the incidence or progression of disease in adults or pediatric patients following exposure to aerosolized *Bacillus anthracis* (Anthrax). ▪ Treatment of plague (including pneumonic and septicemic plague) due to *Yersinia pestis*, and prophylaxis for plague in adults and pediatric patients from birth to 17 years of age. ▪ Treatment of chronic bacterial prostatitis in adults. ▪ Treatment of lower respiratory infections in adults (*not* the drug of first choice in treatment of presumed or confirmed pneumonia secondary to *Streptococcus pneumoniae*). ▪ Treatment of acute exacerbations of chronic bronchitis (AECB) in adults. Because ciprofloxacin has been associated with serious adverse reactions and because for some patients AECB is self-limiting, reserve ciprofloxacin for treatment of AECB in patients who have no alternative treatment options. ▪ Treatment of urinary tract infections (UTIs) in adults. ▪ Treatment of complicated UTI and pyelonephritis due to *Escherichia coli* in pediatric patients 1 to 17 years of age. Although effective, ciprofloxacin is not the drug of first choice because of an increased incidence of adverse reactions compared with controls; see Maternal/Child. ▪ Treatment of acute sinusitis in adults. Because ciprofloxacin has been associated with serious adverse reactions and because for some patients acute sinusitis is self-limiting, reserve ciprofloxacin for treatment of acute sinusitis in patients who have no alternative treatment options. ▪ Oral route of administration indicated for treatment of other infections (e.g., infectious diarrhea, typhoid fever, urethral and cervical gonococcal infections).

Unlabeled uses: Cystic fibrosis. ▪ Infective endocarditis. ▪ Surgical prophylaxis. ▪ Tularemia.

CONTRAINDICATIONS

Known hypersensitivity to ciprofloxacin or any other quinolone antimicrobial agent (e.g., levofloxacin) or any of the product components. ▪ Concomitant administration with tizanidine is contraindicated.

PRECAUTIONS

To reduce the development of drug-resistant bacteria and maintain its effectiveness, ciprofloxacin should be used to treat or prevent only those infections proven or strongly suspected to be caused by bacteria. ▪ Specific culture and sensitivity studies indicated to determine susceptibility of the causative organism to ciprofloxacin. ▪ The emergence of bacterial resistance to fluoroquinolones and the occurrence of cross-resistance with other fluoroquinolones have been observed and are of concern. Proper use of fluoroquinolones and other classes of antibiotics is encouraged to avoid the emergence of resistant bacteria from overuse. ▪ *Pseudomonas aeruginosa* may develop resistance during treatment. Ongoing culture and sensitivity studies indicated. ▪ If anaerobic organisms are suspected of contributing to the infection, appropriate therapy should be administered. ▪ Prolonged use may cause superinfection because of overgrowth of nonsusceptible organisms. Monitor carefully. ▪ Fluoroquinolones, including ciprofloxacin, have been associated with disabling and potentially irreversible serious adverse reactions that have occurred together in the same patient. Commonly seen adverse reactions include tendinitis and tendon rupture, arthralgia, myalgia, peripheral neuropathy, changes in blood glucose levels, and CNS effects (e.g., anxiety, confusion, depression, hallucinations, insomnia, severe headaches). These reactions can occur within hours to weeks after starting ciprofloxacin and have been seen in patients of any age and in patients without any pre-existing risk factors. Discontinue ciprofloxacin immediately and avoid the use of fluoroquinolones, including ciprofloxacin, in patients who experience any of these serious adverse reactions. ▪ Fluoroquinolones, including ciprofloxacin, have been associated with an increased risk of seizures (convulsions), increased intracranial pressure (pseudotumor cerebri), dizziness, and tremors. May trigger seizures or lower the seizure threshold. Use caution in patients with epilepsy or known or suspected CNS disorders that may predispose them to seizures or lower the seizure threshold (e.g., severe cerebral arteriosclerosis, previous history of convulsion, reduced cerebral blood flow, altered brain structure, or stroke) or in the presence of other risk factors that may predispose them to seizures (e.g., drugs that may lower the seizure threshold, renal dysfunction). ▪ Fluoroquinolones, including ciprofloxacin, have been associated with an increased risk of psychiatric adverse reactions that include toxic psychosis, psychotic reactions progressing to suicidal ideations/thoughts, hallucinations, or paranoia; depression; self-injurious behavior such as attempted or completed suicide; anxiety, agitation, or nervousness; confusion, delirium, disorientation, or disturbances in attention; insomnia or nightmares; and memory impairment. These reactions may occur following the first dose. ▪ Tendinitis and tendon rupture that required surgical repair or resulted in prolonged disability have been reported in patients of all ages receiving quinolones. Most frequently involves the Achilles tendon but has also been reported with the shoulder, hand, biceps, thumb, and other tendon sites. ▪ Inflammation and tendon rupture may occur during or up to months after fluoroquinolone therapy and may occur bilaterally. Risk may be increased in patients over 60 years of age; in patients taking corticosteroids; in patients with heart, kidney, or lung transplants; with strenuous physical activity; and in patients with renal failure or previous tendon disorders such as rheumatoid arthritis. Avoid ciprofloxacin in patients who have a history of tendon disorders or have experienced tendinitis or tendon rupture. Discontinue ciprofloxacin immediately if patient experiences pain, swelling, inflammation, or rupture of a tendon. ▪ Fluoroquinolones have neuromuscular blocking activity and may exacerbate muscle weakness in patients with myasthenia gravis. Serious adverse events, including requirement for ventilatory support and deaths, have been reported in patients with myasthenia gravis. Avoid use in patients with a known history of myasthenia gravis. ▪ Fluoroquinolones, including ciprofloxacin, have been associated with an increased risk of peripheral neuropathy. Cases of sensory or sensorimotor axonal polyneuropathy resulting in paresthesias, hypoesthesias, dysesthesias (impairment of sensitivity or touch), or weakness have been reported. Symptoms may occur soon after initiation of therapy and may be irreversible. Avoid ciprofloxacin in patients who have previously experienced peripheral neuropathy. ■ Serious and occasionally fatal hypersensitivity (anaphylactic) reactions have been reported. ■ Prolongation of the QT interval on ECG and infrequent cases of arrhythmia (including torsades de pointes) have been reported with the use of some fluoroquinolones, including ciprofloxacin. Avoid ciprofloxacin in patients with known prolongation of the QT interval, in patients with risk factors for QT prolongation or torsades de pointes (e.g., congenital long QT syndrome, uncorrected electrolyte imbalances [e.g., hypokalemia, hypomagnesemia], and cardiac disease [e.g., heart failure, MI, and significant bradycardia]), and in patients receiving concurrent treatment with Class 1A antiarrhythmic agents (e.g., quinidine, procainamide), Class III antiarrhythmic agents (e.g., amiodarone, sotalol), tricyclic antidepressants, macrolides, or antipsychotics. ■ Other serious events (sometimes fatal) due to hypersensitivity or uncertain etiology have been reported with fluoroquinolones, including ciprofloxacin. Manifestations may include allergic pneumonitis, renal or hepatic impairment/failure, hematologic toxicity, and dermatologic toxicity; see Side Effects, Post-Marketing. These reactions usually occur following administration of multiple doses. Discontinue ciprofloxacin at the first appearance of a skin rash, jaundice, or other signs of hypersensitivity. Cases of severe hepatic toxicity, including necrosis, life-threatening hepatic failure, and fatal events, have been reported. Acute liver injury is rapid in onset (range 1 to 39 days) and is often associated with hypersensitivity. Temporary increase in transaminases, alkaline phosphatase, or cholestatic jaundice, especially in patients with previous liver damage, has also been reported. ■ Epidemiologic studies report an increased rate of aortic aneurysm and dissection within 2 months after use of fluoroquinolones, particularly in elderly patients. In patients with a known aortic aneurysm or who are at greater risk for aortic aneurysms, ciprofloxacin use should be limited to cases in which no alternative antibacterial treatments are available. ■ *Clostridium difficile*–associated diarrhea (CDAD) has been reported. May range from mild diarrhea to fatal colitis. Consider in patients who present with diarrhea during or after treatment with ciprofloxacin. ■ Moderate to severe photosensitivity/phototoxicity reactions have been reported in patients receiving quinolones; see Patient Education. ■ Fluroquinolones, including ciprofloxacin, have been associated with disturbances of blood glucose, including symptomatic hyperglycemia and hypoglycemia, usually in diabetic patients receiving concomitant treatment with an oral hypoglycemic agent (e.g., glyburide) or with insulin. In these patients, careful monitoring of blood glucose is recommended. Severe cases of hypoglycemia resulting in coma or death have been reported. Ciprofloxacin and other quinolones should be reserved for cases in which no other drugs are available.

Monitor: Monitor for S/S of hypersensitivity reaction (e.g., cardiovascular collapse, dyspnea, itching, loss of consciousness, pharyngeal or facial edema, tingling, urticaria). May cause anaphylaxis with the first or succeeding doses, even in patients without known hypersensitivity. Emergency equipment must always be available. ■ Monitor for S/S of peripheral neuropathy. Discontinue ciprofloxacin at the first symptoms of neuropathy (e.g., pain, burning, tingling, numbness, and/or weakness) or if patient is found to have deficits in light touch, pain, temperature, position sense, vibratory sensation, and/or motor strength. ■ Monitor for CNS adverse effects, including altered mental status, seizures, and changes in mood or behavior. ■ Monitor for S/S of tendinitis or tendon rupture. ■ ECG monitoring for QT prolongation may be indicated in selected patients. ■ Maintain adequate hydration and acidity of urine throughout treatment. Can form crystals in concentrated alkaline urine. ■ Monitor hematopoietic, hepatic, and renal systems during prolonged treatment. Patients with severe infections and severe renal impairment and hepatic insufficiency require careful monitoring. ■ Monitor blood glucose, especially in diabetic patients. ■ Use of large veins recommended to reduce incidence of local irritation. Symptoms of local irritation do not preclude further administration of ciprofloxacin unless they recur or worsen. Generally resolve when infusion complete. ■ Concomitant use with theophylline may cause serious and fatal reactions, including cardiac arrest, respiratory failure, seizures, and/or status epilepticus. If concomitant use cannot be avoided, monitor serum levels of theophylline and adjust dose as indicated. ■ Doses will increase slightly with transfer to oral ciprofloxacin (e.g., 200 mg IV every 12 hours equals 250 mg PO every 12 hours; 400 mg IV every 12 hours equals 500 mg PO every 12 hours; 400 mg IV every 8 hours equals 750 mg PO every 12 hours). ■ See Drug/Lab Interactions.

Patient Education: A patient medication guide is available from the manufacturer. ■ Discontinue ciprofloxacin and promptly report the development of any severe adverse reaction. ■ Capable of numerous drug interactions. Review all prescription and nonprescription medications with your health care provider. ■ Inform physician of any history of myasthenia gravis. Patients with a history of myasthenia gravis should avoid using ciprofloxacin. ■ Photosensitivity has been reported. Avoid excessive sunlight or artificial ultraviolet light. May cause severe sunburn; wear protective clothing, use sunscreen, and wear dark glasses outdoors. Report a sunburn-like reaction or skin eruption promptly. ■ Effects of caffeine- or theophylline-containing preparations may be increased; promptly report difficulty breathing, palpitations, and/or seizures. Limit or eliminate concurrent use. Monitor if concurrent use is necessary. ■ Promptly report tendon pain or inflammation, weakness, or the inability to use a joint; rest and refrain from exercise. Symptoms may be irreversible. ■ Promptly report skin rash or any other hypersensitivity reaction. ■ Promptly report pain, burning, tingling, numbness, and/or weakness. Nerve damage can be permanent. ■ Promptly report development of any CNS side effects (e.g., convulsions, dizziness, light-headedness, change in mood or behavior). ■ Inform physician of any history of seizures. ■ Request assistance with ambulation; may cause dizziness and light-headedness. Use caution in tasks that require alertness. ■ Parents should inform physician of any history of joint-related problems and should promptly report any joint-related problems that develop during or after therapy. ■ Promptly report diarrhea or bloody stools that occur during treatment or up to several months after an antibiotic has been discontinued; may indicate CDAD and require treatment. ■ Promptly report any S/S of hepatic toxicity (e.g., dark-colored urine, fever, itching, light-colored bowel movement, loss of appetite, nausea, right upper quadrant tenderness, tiredness, weakness, yellowing of skin). ■ May prolong QT interval. Review medications and medical history. ■ Drink fluids liberally to avoid formation of highly concentrated urine and crystal formation. ■ Seek emergency medical care if sudden chest, stomach, or back pain is experienced. ■ Diabetic patients taking oral hypoglycemic agents or insulin should discontinue ciprofloxacin and contact their provider if they experience a hypoglycemic reaction.

Maternal/Child: Category C: use during pregnancy only if benefits justify potential risk to fetus and mother. ■ Discontinue breast-feeding. ■ May erode cartilage of weight-bearing joints or cause other signs of arthropathy (arthralgia, arthritis) in infants and children. Indicated for treatment of complicated UTIs or pyelonephritis. Although effective, it is not the drug of first choice for this indication due to adverse reactions. Also indicated for inhalation anthrax (postexposure) and for treatment of and prophylaxis for the plague. The risk-benefit assessment indicates that administration of ciprofloxacin for these indications is appropriate. ■ Has been used in infants and children to treat serious infections unresponsive to other antibiotic regimens.

Elderly: Safety and effectiveness similar to younger adults. ■ May be at increased risk of experiencing side effects (e.g., aortic aneurysm and dissection, CNS effects, drug-associated effects on the QT interval, tendinitis, tendon rupture); see Precautions. Half-life may be slightly extended because of age-related renal impairment; see Dose Adjustments. Monitoring of renal function may be useful.

DRUG/LAB INTERACTIONS

Review of patient medication profile required. ■ Ciprofloxacin is an inhibitor of the hepatic CYP1A2 enzyme pathway. Coadministration with other drugs metabolized by this route, such as **clozapine, methylxanthines** (e.g., theophylline), **olanzapine, ropinirole, tizanidine,** or **zolpidem,** results in increased plasma concentrations of these drugs, which may cause significant toxicity. ■ **Concomitant administration with tizanidine is contraindicated** (hypotensive and sedative effects potentiated). ■ Concurrent use with **zolpidem** is not recommended. ■ May cause serious or fatal reactions with **theophylline** (e.g., cardiac arrhythmias or arrest, respiratory failure, or seizures). If must be used concomitantly, monitor serum levels of theophylline and decrease dose as appropriate. Observe closely with **caffeine** intake; has caused similar problems. Elevated serum levels of other xanthine derivatives (e.g., pentoxifylline-containing products) have also been seen with concurrent use. ■ Use with **cyclosporine** may cause an increase in SCr and nephrotoxic effects. Monitor SCr if concurrent use required. ■ May potentiate **oral anticoagulants** (e.g., warfarin); monitor PT/INR. ■ Potentiated by **probenecid.** Use with caution and monitor for possible ciprofloxacin toxicity. ■ Severe hypoglycemia has been reported with concomitant use of **oral antidiabetic agents** (e.g., glyburide, glimepiride); monitor serum glucose levels. ■ May increase or decrease serum **phenytoin** levels; monitor phenytoin levels with concomitant use and repeat phenytoin levels shortly after completion of ciprofloxacin therapy. ■ Risk of CNS stimulation and seizures may be increased with concurrent use of **NSAIDs** with high doses of quinolones. ■ Concurrent use with **methotrexate** requires close monitoring. May inhibit renal tubular transport of methotrexate, thereby increasing methotrexate serum levels and the risk of toxicity. ■ Coadministration with **drugs that prolong the QT interval,** such as **Class IA or III antiarrhythmic agents** (e.g., amiodarone, disopyramide, procainamide, quinidine), **tricyclic antidepressants, macrolide antibiotics,** and **antipsychotics,** may increase the risk of QT prolongation and life-threatening arrhythmias. Concurrent use is not recommended. ■ Fivefold increase in **duloxetine** exposure with concurrent use. Avoid use if possible. If must be given concurrently, monitor for duloxetine toxicity. ■ Twofold increase in **sildenafil** exposure. Use with caution. ■ May cause a false-positive when **testing urine for opiates;** more specific testing methods may be indicated. ■ See Side Effects.

SIDE EFFECTS

Central nervous system disturbances, diarrhea, eosinophilia, headache, hepatic enzyme abnormalities (elevation of alkaline phosphatase, AST, ALT, LDH, serum bilirubin), local IV site reactions, nausea and vomiting, rash, and restlessness are reported most frequently. Other less frequent reactions include abdominal pain; allergic reactions (e.g., anaphylaxis, cardiovascular collapse, death, dyspnea, edema [facial, pharyngeal, or pulmonary], fever, itching, loss of consciousness, urticaria); cardiovascular effects (e.g., cardiac arrest, QT interval prolongation, tachycardia, torsades de pointes, vasodilation); CDAD; CNS effects (e.g., confusion, depression, hallucinations, light-headedness, seizures, tingling, toxic psychosis, tremors); crystalluria; elevated platelet counts, BUN, serum amylase, serum creatinine, serum creatine phosphokinase, serum potassium, uric acid, and triglycerides; hyperglycemia; hypoglycemia; increased intracranial pressure; peripheral neuropathy (e.g., pain, burning, tingling, numbness and/or weakness [see Precautions, Monitor]); photosensitivity/phototoxicity and vision changes; respiratory arrest; status epilepticus; tendinitis; and tendon rupture. Capable of numerous other reactions in fewer than 1% of patients.

Post-Marketing: Acute generalized exanthematous pustulosis (AGEP), allergic pneumonitis, arthralgia, exacerbation of myasthenia gravis, hematologic abnormalities (agranulocytosis, anemia [hemolytic and aplastic], leukopenia, pancytopenia, thrombocytopenia, thrombotic thrombocytopenic purpura), increased INR in patients treated with vitamin K antagonists, interstitial nephritis, liver abnormalities (e.g., acute hepatic necrosis or failure, hepatitis, jaundice), myalgia, polyneuropathy, serum sickness, severe dermatologic reactions (e.g., toxic epidermal necrolysis [Lyell's syndrome], Stevens-Johnson syndrome), vasculitis.

ANTIDOTE

Keep physician informed of all side effects. Many will require symptomatic treatment; monitor closely. Death may result from some of these side effects. Discontinue ciprofloxacin at the first appearance of a skin rash or major side effect (hypersensitivity, CDAD, CNS symptoms, dermatologic reactions, hepatoxicity, hypoglycemia, peripheral neuropathy, phototoxicity, or tendinitis or tendon rupture). Treat hypersensitivity reactions with epinephrine, airway management, oxygen, IV fluids, antihistamines (diphenhydramine), corticosteroids (hydrocortisone sodium succinate), and pressor amines (dopamine) as indicated. Treat CNS symptoms as indicated. Mild cases of CDAD may respond to discontinuation of ciprofloxacin. Treat CDAD with fluids, electrolytes, protein supplements, and appropriate antibiotics (e.g., oral vancomycin) as indicated. In severe cases, surgical evaluation may be indicated. In overdose, observe carefully, provide supportive treatment, maintain hydration, and monitor renal function and urinary pH and acidify, if required, to prevent crystalluria. No specific antidote; up to 10% may be removed by hemodialysis or peritoneal dialysis. Maintain patient until drug excreted.

CISPLATIN BBW
(sis-**PLAH**-tin)

CDDP

Antineoplastic
(alkylating agent)

pH 3.5 to 4.5

USUAL DOSE

Pretreatment: Verify nonpregnancy status. Baseline studies indicated; see Monitor.

Prehydration required; see Precautions and Monitor. See Dose Adjustments. May be given in combination with amifostine to reduce nephrotoxicity and neurotoxicity of cisplatin. See amifostine monograph. Administration as a 6- to 8-hour infusion with intravenous hydration and mannitol has been used to reduce nephrotoxicity. Doses greater than 100 mg/M^2 once every 3 to 4 weeks are rarely used.

Metastatic testicular tumors: Used in combination with other approved chemotherapeutic agents. 20 mg/M^2 daily for 5 days per cycle.

Metastatic ovarian tumors: 75 to 100 mg/M^2 on Day 1 every 4 weeks. Used in combination with cyclophosphamide (Cytoxan) 600 mg/M^2 IV on Day 1 every 4 weeks. Another regimen (unlabeled in cisplatin prescribing information) uses paclitaxel 135 mg/M^2 (as a 24-hour infusion) followed by cisplatin 75 mg/M^2. Both agents are given once every 3 weeks for 6 courses. See paclitaxel monograph; premedication required. Used as a *single agent,* the dose of cisplatin is 100 mg/M^2 every 4 weeks.

First-line treatment of ovarian cancer (unlabeled in cisplatin prescribing information): Given in combination with paclitaxel as follows: Give paclitaxel 135 mg/M^2 as an infusion over 24 hours. Follow with cisplatin 75 mg/M^2 as an infusion over 6 to 8 hours. Repeat every

3 weeks. See paclitaxel monograph; premedication required. Other dose combinations and infusion times are being used.

Advanced bladder cancer: 50 to 70 mg/M^2 once every 3 to 4 weeks. 50 mg/M^2 is recommended once every 4 weeks for patients heavily pretreated with radiation or chemotherapy. Numerous other doses and combinations are used.

Non–small-cell lung cancer (unlabeled in cisplatin prescribing information): Given in combination with gemcitabine as follows: gemcitabine 1,000 mg/M^2 as an infusion on Days 1, 8, and 15 of each 28-day cycle. Follow the gemcitabine infusion on Day 1 with cisplatin 100 mg/M^2. See gemcitabine monograph; other dosing schedules are in use. Another regimen uses a combination of paclitaxel and cisplatin as follows: paclitaxel 135 mg/M^2 as an infusion over 24 hours followed by cisplatin 75 mg/M^2 over 6 to 8 hours. Repeat every 3 weeks. See paclitaxel monograph; premedication required. Also used with docetaxel 75 mg/M^2 infused over 1 hour followed immediately by an infusion of cisplatin 75 mg/M^2 over 30 to 60 minutes. Repeat every 3 weeks. See docetaxel monograph; premedication required.

DOSE ADJUSTMENTS

All doses adjusted based on prior radiation therapy or chemotherapy. ▪ Repeat doses may not be given unless SCr is below 1.5 mg/100 mL and/or BUN is below 25 mg/100 mL. Renal toxicity becomes more prolonged and severe with repeated courses. Renal function must return to normal before next dose is given. ▪ Platelets should be 100,000/mm^3 and leukocytes 4,000/mm^3; verify auditory acuity as within normal limits. ▪ Dosing should be cautious in the elderly. Lower-end initial doses may be indicated. Consider decrease in cardiac, hepatic, and renal function; concomitant disease; or other drug therapy; see Elderly.

DILUTION

Specific techniques required; see Precautions. Available in liquid form, 1 mg/mL. Withdraw desired dose. Immediately before use, manufacturer recommends diluting a single dose in 2 liters of D5⅟2NS or D5⅟3NS containing 37.5 Gm of mannitol. Do not use D5W. Will decompose if adequate chloride ion not available. Is also diluted in smaller amounts of NS (100 to 500 mL). Do not use needles or IV tubing with aluminum parts to administer; a precipitate will form, and potency will decrease. See Monitor for additional optional additives.

Storage: Cisplatin remaining in multidose vial is stable at CRT for 28 days protected from light or 7 days under fluorescent light. Do not refrigerate. Protect from light if it will not be used within 6 hours.

COMPATIBILITY

Manufacturer states, "Do not use needles, IV sets, or equipment containing aluminum." Aluminum reacts with cisplatin, causing precipitate formation and loss of potency. A precipitate will form if reconstituted solutions are refrigerated.

Other sources suggest specific **compatibilities** dependent on concentration and manufacturer; consult a pharmacist.

RATE OF ADMINISTRATION

Administer as a slow IV infusion; *should not be given as a rapid IV injection.* Rates vary based on protocol. Manufacturer suggests administering each 1 liter of infusion solution over 3 to 4 hours. Give total dose (2 liters) over 6 to 8 hours. Rate must be sufficient to maintain hydration and diuresis. Infusion times of 30 to 120 minutes are common, but infusion time has also been extended to 24 hours/dose. One source recommends a maximum rate not to exceed 1 mg/min. Too-rapid administration increases nephrotoxicity and ototoxicity.

ACTIONS

A heavy metal complex (platinum and chloride atoms). Has properties similar to alkylating agents and is cell-cycle nonspecific. Inhibits DNA synthesis by formation of DNA cross-links. Concentration is highest in liver, prostate, and kidney; somewhat lower in bladder, muscle, testicle, pancreas, and spleen. Heavily protein bound. Only one-fourth to one-half of the drug is excreted in the urine by the end of 5 days. Platinum may be present in tissues for as long as 180 days after the last administration. Secreted in breast milk.

INDICATIONS AND USES

Treatment of metastatic testicular tumors; used in combination therapy with other approved chemotherapy agents in patients who have already received appropriate surgical and/or radiotherapeutic procedures. ▪ Treatment of metastatic ovarian tumors; used in combination therapy with other approved chemotherapy agents in patients who have already received appropriate surgical and/or radiotherapeutic procedures. ▪ Used as a single agent as secondary treatment in patients with metastatic ovarian tumors refractory to standard chemotherapy who have not previously received cisplatin therapy. ▪ Used as a single agent for treatment of patients with transitional cell bladder cancer that is no longer amenable to local treatment such as surgery and/or radiotherapy. ▪ Is used in specific combinations with other chemotherapeutic drugs.

Unlabeled uses: First-line therapy for treatment of advanced cancer of the ovary in combination with paclitaxel. ▪ First-line treatment of patients with inoperable, locally advanced, or metastatic non–small-cell lung cancer (NSCLC) in combination with gemcitabine, paclitaxel, or docetaxel. ▪ Treatment of cancers of the brain, adrenal cortex, breast, cervix, uterus, endometrium, head and neck, esophagus, lung, and liver; osteogenic sarcomas; and numerous other malignancies.

CONTRAINDICATIONS

Hypersensitivity to cisplatin or other platinum-containing compounds, myelosuppressed patients, pre-existing impaired renal function, or hearing deficit.

PRECAUTIONS

Follow guidelines for handling cytotoxic agents. See Appendix A. ▪ Administered by or under the direction of the physician specialist. ▪ Adequate facilities and emergency resuscitation equipment and supplies must always be available. ▪ Renal toxicity can be cumulative and may be severe. ▪ Other major dose-related toxicities include myelosuppression, nausea, and vomiting. ▪ Ototoxicity (tinnitus, loss of high-frequency hearing, and/or deafness) can be significant and may be more pronounced in pediatric patients. ▪ Anaphylaxis has been reported and may occur within minutes of cisplatin administration. ▪ Labeling changed to read, "Doses greater than 100 mg/M^2/cycle once every 3 to 4 weeks are rarely used." This is an effort to eliminate serious errors resulting from confusion with carboplatin. Flip-off seal on vial now says, "Call Dr. if dose greater than 100 mg/M^2/cycle." ▪ Neuropathies may occur with higher doses, greater frequency of average doses, or prolonged therapy. Usually occur after prolonged therapy but have been reported after a single dose. If symptoms of neuropathy are observed, discontinue cisplatin. ▪ See Elderly.

Monitor: Obtain baseline CBC, SCr, BUN, CrCl and calcium, magnesium, potassium, and sodium levels. Repeat CBC weekly and other listed labs before each subsequent cycle. ▪ Hydrate patient with 1 to 2 L of infusion fluid for 8 to 12 hours before cisplatin administration. Urine output should exceed 100 to 150 mL/hr. ▪ Maintain adequate hydration and urine output of at least 100 to 200 mL/hr for 24 hours after each dose. ▪ Nausea and vomiting are frequently severe and prolonged (up to a week). May begin within 1 to 4 hours of administration or may be delayed. Prophylactic administration of antiemetics recommended. Fosaprepitant (Emend), ondansetron (Zofran), metoclopramide (Reglan), or dexamethasone are effective in most patients. ▪ Ototoxicity is cumulative; test hearing before administration and regularly during treatment. Ototoxicity increased in pediatric patients. ▪ Monitor uric acid levels before and during treatment and maintain hydration. Allopurinol and alkalinization of urine may be indicated. ▪ Monitor for anaphylactic-like reactions (e.g., bronchoconstriction, facial edema, hypotension, tachycardia). ▪ Monitor liver function periodically. ▪ Perform neurologic exams on a regular basis. Neuropathy may present as paresthesias, areflexia, and loss of proprioception and vibratory sensation. ▪ Replace depleted electrolytes as necessary. ▪ Observe closely for signs of infection. Prophylactic antibiotics may be indicated pending results of C/S in a febrile neutropenic patient. ▪ Monitor infusion site carefully during infusion; local soft tissue toxicity has been reported with extravasation. ▪ Monitor for thrombocytopenia (platelet count less than 50,000/mm^3). Initiate precautions to prevent excessive bleeding (e.g., inspect IV sites, skin, and mucous membranes; use extreme care during invasive procedures; test urine, emesis, stool, and secretions for occult blood).

Patient Education: Effective birth control recommended. ▪ See Appendix D.

Maternal/Child: Category D: avoid pregnancy; can cause fetal harm. Has a mutagenic potential. ▪ Discontinue breast-feeding. ▪ Safety and effectiveness for use in pediatric patients not established. ▪ Ototoxicity increased in pediatric patients. All pediatric patients should have audiometric monitoring performed before initiation of therapy, before each dose, and for several years after therapy.

Elderly: Dose selection should be cautious; see Dose Adjustments. ▪ Response (e.g., effectiveness) is similar to younger adults, but length of survival may be shorter. ▪ Incidence of myelosuppression (e.g., severe leukopenia, neutropenia, thrombocytopenia), infectious complications, nephrotoxicity, and peripheral neuropathy may be increased.

DRUG/LAB INTERACTIONS

Ototoxicity and nephrotoxicity are potentiated with other **ototoxic or nephrotoxic agents** (e.g., aminoglycosides and loop diuretics). Concurrent use not recommended. ▪ Serum levels of **anticonvulsant agents** (e.g., phenytoin) may become subtherapeutic when used concurrently with cisplatin. Monitor anticonvulsant levels; increased doses may be indicated. ▪ Bone marrow toxicity increased with **other antineoplastic agents and/or radiation therapy.** ▪ Synergistic with **etoposide**; may be beneficial. ▪ May affect renal excretion and increase toxicity of many drugs **(e.g., bleomycin, methotrexate).** ▪ Response duration may be shortened with concurrent use of **pyridoxine (vitamin B$_6$) and altretamine.** ▪ Do not administer **live virus vaccines** to patients receiving antineoplastic agents.

SIDE EFFECTS

Are frequent; can occur with the initial dose and will become more severe with succeeding doses. Dose-related and cumulative renal insufficiency, including renal failure, is the major dose-limiting toxicity (often noted during the second week following a dose). Acute leukemia, alopecia, anaphylaxis (facial edema, hypotension, tachycardia, and wheezing within minutes of administration), asthenia, cardiac abnormalities, dehydration, diarrhea, electrolyte disturbances (hypocalcemia, hypokalemia, hypomagnesemia, hyponatremia, hypophosphatemia), elevated serum amylase, hemolytic anemia, hepatotoxicity, hyperuricemia, malaise, myelosuppression, nausea and vomiting (acute or delayed), syndrome of inappropriate antidiuretic hormone secretion (SIADH), neurotoxicity (including peripheral neuropathy that may be reversible, leukoencephalopathy, and reversible posterior leukoencephalopathy syndrome [RPLS]), ocular toxicity (e.g., blurred vision, cerebral blindness, optic neuritis, papilledema), ototoxicity including tinnitus and hearing loss in the high-frequency range, peripheral neuropathy (may be irreversible), vascular toxicities (e.g., cerebral arteritis, CVA, MI, or thrombotic microangiopathy [hemolytic-uremic syndrome (HUS)]), and vestibular toxicity.

Overdose: Deafness, intractable nausea and vomiting, kidney failure, liver failure, neuritis, ocular toxicity, significant myelosuppression, and death.

ANTIDOTE

Notify physician of all side effects. Cisplatin may have to be discontinued permanently or until recovery. Symptomatic and supportive treatment is indicated. Administration of whole blood products (e.g., packed RBCs, platelets, leukocytes) and/or blood modifiers (e.g., darbepoetin alfa [Aranesp], epoetin alfa [Epogen], filgrastim [Neupogen, Zarxio], pegfilgrastim [Neulasta], sargramostim [Leukine]) may be indicated to treat bone marrow toxicity. Pretreatment with amifostine may reduce nephrotoxic, neurotoxic, and hematologic effects. Treat anaphylaxis with epinephrine, corticosteroids, oxygen, and antihistamines. There is no specific antidote. Hemodialysis appears to have little effect on removing platinum from the body because of the rapid and high degree of protein binding.

CLADRIBINE BBW
(**KLAD**-rih-bean)

Leustatin

Antineoplastic
(antimetabolite)

pH 5.5 to 8

USUAL DOSE

Pretreatment: Verify pregnancy status. Baseline studies indicated; see Monitor.

In all situations, may be administered on an outpatient basis with an appropriate pump and a central venous line in place. Administer any subsequent course with extreme caution. Hematologic recovery must be considered.

Hairy cell leukemia: 0.09 mg/kg/day equally distributed as a continuous infusion over 24 hours. Repeat daily for 7 consecutive days.

Chronic lymphocytic leukemia and Waldenström's macroglobulinemia (unlabeled): 0.1 mg/kg/day equally distributed as a continuous infusion over 24 hours for 7 consecutive days.

Acute myeloid leukemia and mantle cell lymphoma (unlabeled): 5 mg/M^2/day over 2 hours for 5 days.

DOSE ADJUSTMENTS

May be required with severe bone marrow impairment, with prior radiation or myelosuppressive agents. ■ May be required in severe renal insufficiency; effects of renal or hepatic impairment on excretion of cladribine not yet clarified for humans. ■ See Drug/Lab Interactions.

DILUTION

Specific techniques required; see Precautions. Available in single-use 10-mL vials containing 10 mg (1 mg/mL). Contains no preservatives; aseptic technique imperative. May develop a precipitate at low temperatures. Warm naturally to RT and shake vigorously. Do not heat or microwave.

Inpatient continuous infusion: Add the calculated daily dose of cladribine through a sterile 0.22-micron disposable hydrophilic syringe filter to an infusion bag containing 500 mL of NS.

Outpatient continuous infusion: A total 7-day dose is added to a calculated amount of bacteriostatic NS to make a total volume of 100 mL. Add the calculated dose of cladribine (7 days × 0.09 mg/kg or 0.09 mL/kg) to the infusion reservoir through the sterile 0.22-micron disposable hydrophilic syringe filter, then add the calculated amount of bacteriostatic NS to the reservoir through the filter. Total volume in the reservoir should equal 100 mL. Specific equipment (i.e., a sterile medication reservoir and pump capable of delivering accurate minute amounts into a central venous line [presently using SIMS Deltec medication cassette with SIMS Deltec pump]) and a specific process, including the use of a 0.22-micron syringe filter, are required. Preparation of cassette usually done by pharmacist. Line of cassette remains clamped until attached to central venous line and pump is functional. See literature for details, and follow all specific instructions for medication pump.

Filters: To minimize the risk of microbial contamination, a 0.22-micron hydrophilic syringe filter is required in the preparation of the outpatient continuous infusion.

Storage: Protect from light. Refrigerate before reconstitution. Never refreeze. Discard any unused concentrate. *500 mL dilution* is stable for at least 24 hours at RT under normal fluorescent light; may be refrigerated for up to 8 hours after dilution. Immediate use preferred. *100 mL dilution* is stable in reservoir of medication cassette for 7 days if correctly diluted.

COMPATIBILITY

D5W will cause degradation of cladribine. Manufacturer states, "Adherence to the recommended diluents and infusion systems is advised."

Other sources suggest specific **compatibilities** dependent on concentration and manufacturer; consult a pharmacist.

RATE OF ADMINISTRATION

Inpatient continuous infusion: A single dose properly diluted evenly distributed as an infusion over 24 hours.

Outpatient continuous infusion: Administered through a central venous line (very concentrated solution). Medication reservoir and pump required (presently using Pharmacia Deltec medication cassette and pump worn as a portable pack). Set rate for equal distribution of 100 mL over 7 days. Follow all specific instructions for pump.

ACTIONS

A chlorinated purine nucleoside analog and synthetic antineoplastic agent. Mechanism of action is not known, but it is believed to be cytotoxic by inhibiting both DNA synthesis and repair. Affects both dividing and resting cells. The 7-day course for hairy cell leukemia has resulted in complete response in a majority of patients with no evidence of persistent bone marrow disease. Crosses the blood-brain barrier. Average half-life is 4.2 to 9.2 hours. Specific methods of metabolism and routes of excretion are not known. Some drug does appear in urine.

INDICATIONS AND USES

Treatment of active hairy cell leukemia (HCL) as defined by clinically significant anemia, neutropenia, thrombocytopenia, or disease-related symptoms.

Unlabeled uses: Treatment of acute myeloid leukemia, chronic lymphocytic leukemia, mantle cell lymphoma, and Waldenström's macroglobulinemia.

CONTRAINDICATIONS

Hypersensitivity to cladribine or any of its components; neonates (7-day dilution contains benzyl alcohol).

PRECAUTIONS

Follow guidelines for handling cytotoxic agents. See Appendix A. ▪ Administered by or under the direction of the physician specialist. ▪ Anticipate severe suppression of bone marrow function, including neutropenia, anemia, and thrombocytopenia; usually reversible and appears to be dose dependent. ▪ Myelosuppressive effects are most notable during the first month after therapy. ▪ Serious, sometimes fatal, infections have been reported (e.g., respiratory tract infections, pneumonia, viral skin infections, sepsis). ▪ Neurologic toxicity, including paraparesis and quadriparesis, has been reported. Usually occurs with higher doses but has been seen with standard dosing regimens. ▪ Because of the possibility of increased toxicity, use caution in known or suspected renal or hepatic insufficiency, or any severe bone marrow impairment, or prior cytotoxic or radiation therapy. ▪ Acute nephrotoxicity has been observed with high doses (4 to 9 times the recommended dose for HCL). Risk of toxicity increased when given concurrently with other nephrotoxic agents and/or therapies. ▪ Rare cases of tumor lysis syndrome have been reported. ▪ Appears to be no relationship between serum concentrations and ultimate clinical outcome. ▪ Additional courses did not improve overall response. ▪ Current studies suggest that overall response rate may be decreased in patients previously treated with splenectomy, deoxycoformycin (pentostatin), and in patients refractory to alpha-interferon. ▪ May cause prolonged bone marrow hypocellularity; clinical significance not known.

Monitor: Obtain baseline CBC with differential and platelets before therapy. May be repeated as indicated, but usually not required again until 7 or 8 days after treatment begins; then monitor as indicated for at least 4 to 8 weeks (anemia, neutropenia, thrombocytopenia, infection [bacterial, fungal, or viral], and bleeding are common and must be treated promptly). Monitoring schedule facilitates outpatient treatment; keep in close contact with patient. ▪ Consider possibility of infection if fever occurs; appropriate lab tests, x-rays, and broad-spectrum antibiotics may be indicated, especially in a febrile neutropenic patient. ▪ Monitor uric acid levels before and during treatment; maintain hydration; allopurinol may be indicated (preferred agent). ▪ Monitor renal and hepatic function periodically. ▪ Platelet count usually returns to normal in 12 days (may be delayed if severe baseline thrombocytopenia was present), absolute neutrophil count (ANC) usually returns to normal in 5 weeks, and hemoglobin in 8 weeks. All should be normal by 9 weeks. ▪ Complete response is indicated by an absence of hairy cells in bone marrow and peripheral blood and normalization of peripheral blood parameters. Confirm response with bone marrow aspiration and biopsy between 9 weeks and 4 months. ▪ Prophylactic antiemetics may improve patient comfort. ▪ Monitor for thrombocytopenia (platelet count less than 50,000/mm^3). Initiate precautions to prevent excessive bleeding (e.g., inspect IV sites, skin, and mucous membranes; use extreme care during invasive procedures; test urine, emesis, stool, and secretions for occult blood). Avoid constipation and avoid alcohol and aspirin (risk of GI bleeding).

Patient Education: Avoid pregnancy; consider birth control options and future fertility. ▪ Report fever, bleeding, cough, edema, injection site reactions, malaise, mouth sores, rashes, shortness of breath, stomach pain, and tachycardia promptly. Maintain hydration. ▪ Manufacturer supplies a patient education booklet; review thoroughly and discuss with physician and nurse. ▪ Review all literature provided with pump to deliver outpatient dosing. ▪ See Appendix D.

Maternal/Child: Category D: avoid pregnancy; has potential to cause fetal harm. Has caused suppression of testicular cells in monkeys; effect on human fertility unknown. ▪ Discontinue breast-feeding. ▪ Safety for use in pediatric patients not established. Investigationally used in higher doses to treat relapsed acute leukemia. Dose-limiting toxicity occurred.

Elderly: Geriatric-specific problems not encountered in studies to date. Consider age-related organ impairment.

DRUG/LAB INTERACTIONS

Increased toxicity with other **myelosuppressive agents** (e.g., methotrexate). ▪ May raise concentration of blood uric acid; increased doses of **antigout agents** (e.g., allopurinol) may be indicated; **avoid uricosurics** (e.g., probenecid, sulfinpyrazone). ▪ Do not administer **live attenuated vaccines** to patients receiving antineoplastic agents.

SIDE EFFECTS

Fever occurs first. Onset of thrombocytopenia begins in 7 to 10 days followed by anemia (severe) and neutropenia (severe). Fatigue, headache, injection site reactions, infection, nausea, and rash are common. Many other side effects may or may not be related to cladribine: abdominal pain, abnormal breath sounds, abnormal chest sounds, anorexia, arthralgia, asthenia, chills, constipation, cough, diaphoresis, diarrhea, dizziness, edema, epistaxis, erythema, insomnia, malaise, myalgia, pain, petechiae, pruritus, purpura, shortness of breath, tachycardia, trunk pain, weakness, vomiting.

Post-Marketing: Most of these additional side effects occurred in patients who received multiple courses of cladribine and include altered level of consciousness, aplastic anemia, conjunctivitis, elevated bilirubin and transaminases, hemolytic anemia, hypereosinophilia, hypersensitivity, myelodysplastic syndrome, neurologic toxicity, opportunistic infections, pulmonary interstitial infiltrates (usually with an infectious etiology), renal impairment, Stevens-Johnson syndrome, toxic epidermal necrolysis, and tumor lysis syndrome.

Overdose: Acute nephrotoxicity, irreversible neurologic toxicity (paraparesis/quadriparesis), severe bone marrow suppression (anemia, neutropenia, and thrombocytopenia).

ANTIDOTE

Keep physician informed of all side effects; many will be treated symptomatically as indicated. Platelet or RBC transfusions are frequently required to treat anemia or thrombocytopenia, especially during the first month. Filgrastim (Neupogen, Zarxio) or pegfilgrastim (Neulasta) may be used to increase neutrophil count, although recovery is usually spontaneous. Use specific antibiotics to combat infection. Discontinue cladribine if renal toxicity, neurotoxicity, or overdose occurs. No specific antidote for overdose. Supportive therapy as indicated will help sustain the patient in toxicity. Resuscitate if indicated.

CLEVIDIPINE BUTYRATE
(klev-**ID**-i-peen **BUE**-tih-rate)

Calcium channel blocker
Antihypertensive

Cleviprex

pH 6 to 8

USUAL DOSE
Must be individualized to achieve the desired BP reduction. Titrate to patient response and BP goal.

Initial dose: 1 to 2 mg/hr (2 to 4 mL/hr) as a continuous infusion.

Dose titration: Initially, double the dose at 90-second intervals. As the BP approaches goal, increase the dose by less than doubling and lengthen the time between dose adjustments to every 5 to 10 minutes. In general, a 1- to 2-mg/hr increase in dose will produce an additional 2- to 4-mm Hg decrease in systolic pressure. The maximum dose used for most patients in studies was 16 mg/hr.

Maintenance dose: The desired therapeutic response for most patients occurs at 4 to 6 mg/hr (8 to 12 mL/hr). Doses as high as 32 mg/hr (64 mL/hr) have been administered. Data are limited. Because of lipid-load restrictions, no more than 1,000 mL or an average of 21 mg/hr (42 mL/hr) is recommended per 24-hour period. In studies, most infusions were administered for less than 24 hours. There is little experience with infusions lasting more than 72 hours at any dose.

Transition to oral therapy: Discontinue or titrate the infusion downward while establishing appropriate oral therapy. Consider the lag time of onset of oral agent's effect. See Monitor.

DOSE ADJUSTMENTS
Lower-end initial doses may be indicated in the elderly. Consider the potential for decreased organ function and concomitant disease or drug therapy. ▪ Patients with abnormal hepatic or renal function may receive the initial dose listed under Usual Dose.

DILUTION
Strict aseptic technique is imperative. Available as a single-dose, ready-to-use vial containing a 0.5-mg/mL phospholipid emulsion that can support microbial growth. Invert vial gently several times before use to ensure uniformity of emulsion.

Filter: No data available from manufacturer.

Storage: Refrigerate unopened vials at 2° to 8° C (36° to 46° F) or store at 25° C (77° F) for up to 2 months. Vials stored at RT should not be returned to the refrigerator. Do not freeze. Protect from light until administration. Once vial is punctured, use within 4 hours and discard any unused portion, including that which is currently being infused.

COMPATIBILITY
Manufacturer states, "Should not be administered in the same line as other medications. Should not be diluted, but can be administered via a Y-tube or medication port with SWFI, NS, D5W, D5NS, D5LR, LR, and 10% amino acid."

RATE OF ADMINISTRATION
Administer as a continuous infusion as outlined in Usual Dose. Use of an infusion device required. May be given through a central or peripheral line.

ACTIONS
A dihydropyridine calcium channel blocker. Mediates the influx of calcium during depolarization in arterial smooth muscle. Reduces mean arterial BP by decreasing systemic vascular resistance in a dose-dependent manner. Does not reduce cardiac filling pressure (preload), confirming the lack of effect on venous capacitance vessels. Vasodilation and the resulting decrease in BP may produce a reflex increase in heart rate. Onset of effects begins within 2 to 4 minutes. Evidence of tolerance or hysteresis has not been observed in patients receiving infusions of up to 72 hours' duration. Full recovery of BP is achieved 5 to 15 minutes after the infusion is stopped. Rapidly distributed. Highly protein bound. Metabolized by hydrolysis in the blood and extravascular tissues, making its

elimination unlikely to be affected by hepatic or renal dysfunction. Half-life is approximately 15 minutes. Excreted primarily in urine and, to a lesser extent, in feces.

INDICATIONS AND USES
Reduction of BP when oral therapy is not feasible or not desirable.

CONTRAINDICATIONS
Allergies to soybeans, soy products, eggs, or egg products. ■ Defective lipid metabolism such as pathologic hyperlipidemia, lipoid nephrosis, or acute pancreatitis if accompanied by hyperlipidemia. ■ Severe aortic stenosis (afterload reduction can be expected to reduce myocardial oxygen delivery).

PRECAUTIONS
For IV use only. ■ Strict aseptic technique required; see Dilution. ■ May produce systemic hypotension and reflex tachycardia. Dose reduction may be indicated. ■ Use caution in patients with lipid metabolism disorders. Contains approximately 0.2 Gm of lipid per mL. Lipid intake restrictions may be necessary in these patients. A reduction in the quantity of concurrently administered lipids (e.g., propofol, IV fat) may be necessary to compensate for the amount of lipid infused as part of the clevidipine formulation. See Usual Dose. ■ May produce a negative inotropic effect and exacerbate heart failure. ■ Rebound hypertension may occur in patients undergoing prolonged therapy; see Monitor. ■ Has not been studied for the treatment of hypertension associated with pheochromocytoma.

Monitor: Monitor BP and HR during infusion and until vital signs are stable. ■ Rebound hypertension may occur in patients who receive a prolonged infusion and are not transitioned to other antihypertensive therapies. Monitor BP for at least 8 hours after the infusion is discontinued. ■ During transition to oral therapy, continue BP monitoring until patient is stabilized. ■ Monitor heart failure patients closely.

Patient Education: Promptly report signs of a hypertensive emergency (e.g., neurologic symptoms, vision changes, evidence of CHF). ■ Continued follow-up and treatment of pre-existing hypertension required.

Maternal/Child: Category C: use during pregnancy only if potential benefit justifies potential risk to the fetus. ■ Safety in labor and delivery not established. Other calcium channel blockers suppress uterine contractions in humans. ■ Safety for use in breast-feeding not established; effects unknown. ■ Safety and effectiveness for use in pediatric patients not established.

Elderly: Response similar to that seen in younger adults; however, greater sensitivity in the elderly cannot be ruled out. ■ See Dose Adjustments.

DRUG/LAB INTERACTIONS
Formal studies have not been conducted. ■ Does not have the potential for inducing or inhibiting the cytochrome P_{450} system. ■ Use of **beta-blockers** as treatment for clevidipine-induced reflex tachycardia is not recommended. Experience is limited. ■ If used concomitantly with **beta-blockers** and beta-blockers are to be discontinued, withdraw beta-blocker therapy gradually. Clevidipine will not protect against the effects of abrupt beta-blocker withdrawal.

SIDE EFFECTS
Acute renal failure, atrial fibrillation, cardiac arrest, dyspnea, flushing, headache, hypotension, myocardial infarction, nausea, peripheral edema, rebound hypertension, reflex tachycardia, syncope, and vomiting.

Post-Marketing: Decreased oxygen saturation (possible pulmonary shunting), hypersensitivity reactions, increased blood triglycerides, ileus.

ANTIDOTE
Notify physician of any side effects; most will be treated symptomatically. Reduce dose for systemic hypotension or reflex tachycardia. Discontinue for suspected overdose. Reduction in antihypertensive effects should be seen within 5 to 15 minutes. Monitor BP and support if needed. Resuscitate as necessary.

CLINDAMYCIN PHOSPHATE BBW
(klin-dah-**MY**-cin **FOS**-fayt)

Antibacterial
Antiprotozoal
(lincosamide)

Cleocin Phosphate

pH 5.5 to 7

USUAL DOSE
Doses based on susceptibility of specific organisms; see literature.

Serious infections: 600 to 1,200 mg/24 hr in 2, 3, or 4 equally divided doses (300 to 600 mg every 12 hours, 200 to 400 mg every 8 hours, or 150 to 300 mg every 6 hours).

More severe infections: 1,200 to 2,700 mg/24 hr in 2, 3, or 4 equally divided doses (600 to 1,350 mg every 12 hours, 400 to 900 mg every 8 hours, or 300 to 675 mg every 6 hours).

Life-threatening infections: Up to 4,800 mg/24 hr has been given.

Acute pelvic inflammatory disease (unlabeled): 900 mg every 8 hours. Used in combination with gentamicin. Continue both drugs for at least 24 hours after patient improves. Complete 14-day treatment program with oral doxycycline or clindamycin.

CNS toxoplasmosis in AIDS (unlabeled): 600 mg every 6 hours. Used in combination with pyrimethamine (Daraprim) and leucovorin.

***Pneumocystis jiroveci* pneumonia (unlabeled):** 600 mg every 6 hours or 900 mg every 8 hours. Used in combination with primaquine.

Babesiosis (unlabeled): 1,200 to 2,400 mg/24 hr in 4 equally divided doses (300 to 600 mg every 6 hours). Continue for 7 to 10 days. Used in combination with quinine.

Prophylaxis of bacterial endocarditis: 600 mg IV or PO 30 minutes before procedure.

PEDIATRIC DOSE
Pediatric patients over 1 month to 16 years of age: 20 to 40 mg/kg of body weight/24 hr in 3 or 4 equally divided doses based on the seriousness of the infection (5 to 10 mg/kg every 6 hours or 6.66 to 13.3 mg/kg every 8 hours). Alternately 350 mg/M^2/24 hr may be used (87.5 mg/M^2 every 6 hours or 116.6 mg/M^2 every 8 hours). 450 mg/M^2/24 hr may be used for more serious infections if necessary (112.5 mg/M^2 every 6 hours or 150 mg/M^2 every 8 hours).

Prophylaxis of bacterial endocarditis: 20 mg/kg IV or PO 30 minutes before procedure. Do not exceed adult dose.

NEONATAL DOSE
See Maternal/Child.

Under 1 month of age, full term: 15 to 20 mg/kg/day in 3 to 4 equally divided doses (3.75 to 5 mg/kg every 6 hours or 5 to 6.7 mg/kg every 8 hours).

DOSE ADJUSTMENTS
Dose adjustments are not required in the presence of mild to moderate renal or hepatic disease and should not be required in severe disease; see Monitor.

DILUTION
Available prediluted in 300-, 600-, and 900-mg doses, in ADD-Vantage vials for use with ADD-Vantage infusion containers, as a 150 mg/mL solution in flip-top vials, in ready-to-use Galaxy bags, and in pharmacy bulk packages (for use only by the pharmacy). Dilute ADD-Vantage vials with 50 to 100 mL of D5W or NS. Doses prepared using the 150 mg/mL solutions are most commonly diluted in 50 to 100 mL of D5W, NS, or other **compatible** infusion solution. Concentration of clindamycin in diluent should not exceed 18 mg/mL. See chart on inside back cover or product insert for additional diluents. May be further diluted in larger amounts of **compatible** infusion solutions and given as a continuous infusion after the initial dose.

Storage: Store vials at CRT before use. Administration as soon as possible after dilution is recommended. Stable at CRT for at least 24 hours in **compatible** infusion solutions. See manufacturer's literature for additional stability data if diluted solutions are kept at RT, refrigerated, or frozen. Frozen solutions should be thawed at room temperature and not refrozen.

COMPATIBILITY

Manufacturer lists as **compatible** for 24 hours at RT with IV solutions containing sodium chloride, glucose, calcium, or potassium and with solutions containing vitamin B complex in concentrations usually used clinically. Manufacturer states, "No **incompatibility** has been demonstrated with the antibiotics carbenicillin, cephalothin, gentamicin, kanamycin, or penicillin."

Manufacturer lists as **incompatible** with aminophylline, ampicillin, barbiturates, calcium gluconate, magnesium sulfate, phenytoin.

Other sources suggest specific **compatibilities** dependent on concentration and manufacturer; consult a pharmacist.

RATE OF ADMINISTRATION

Should not be administered intravenously undiluted as a bolus. Severe hypotension and cardiac arrest can occur with too-rapid injection.

Intermittent infusion: 30 mg or fraction thereof over at least 1 minute (each 300 mg over a minimum of 10 minutes/1,200 mg over a minimum of 40 to 60 minutes). Do not give more than 1,200 mg in single 1-hour infusion.

Continuous infusion: Administer initial dose at 10 (15 or 20) mg/min over 30 minutes (rapid infusion rate). Will result in serum levels above 4 (5 or 6) mcg/mL. To maintain these serum levels, continue infusion at 0.75 (1 or 1.25) mg/min.

ACTIONS

A semi-synthetic antibiotic that quickly converts to active clindamycin. Bacteriostatic with activity against gram-positive aerobes and anaerobes, as well as some gram-negative anaerobes. It inhibits bacterial protein synthesis by binding to the 50S subunit of the ribosome. Widely distributed in most body fluids and tissues. There is no clinically effective distribution to cerebrospinal fluid. Predominantly metabolized by cytochrome P_{450} CYP3A4. Half-life is approximately 3 hours. Excreted in urine and feces in small amounts. Crosses placental barrier. Secreted in breast milk.

INDICATIONS AND USES

Treatment of serious infections caused by susceptible anaerobic bacteria. ■ Treatment of serious infections due to susceptible strains of streptococcal, pneumococcal, and staphylococcal bacteria in penicillin-allergic patients. ■ Conditions for which clindamycin is indicated include septicemia, lower respiratory tract infections (including pneumonia, empyema, and lung abscess), skin and skin structure, gynecologic (including endometritis, nongonococcal tubo-ovarian abscess, pelvic cellulitis, and postsurgical vaginal cuff infection), intra-abdominal (including peritonitis and intra-abdominal abscess), and bone and joint infections (including acute hematogenous osteomyelitis).

Unlabeled uses: Alternative to sulfonamides with pyrimethamine to treat CNS toxoplasmosis in AIDS patients. ■ Treat *Pneumocystis jiroveci* pneumonia in combination with primaquine. ■ Treatment of babesiosis. ■ Prophylaxis of bacterial endocarditis. ■ Treatment of acute pelvic inflammatory disease.

CONTRAINDICATIONS

Known hypersensitivity to clindamycin or lincomycin.

PRECAUTIONS

To reduce the development of drug-resistant bacteria and maintain its effectiveness, clindamycin should be used to treat or prevent only those infections proven or strongly suspected to be caused by bacteria. ■ Sensitivity studies are indicated to determine susceptibility of the causative organism to clindamycin. ■ Cross-resistance is sometimes observed among lincosamides, macrolides, and streptogramin B. Macrolide-inducible resistance to clindamycin occurs in some isolates of macrolide-resistant bacteria. Macrolide-resistant isolates of staphylococci and beta-hemolytic streptococci should be screened for induction of clindamycin resistance. ■ Avoid prolonged use; superinfection caused by overgrowth of nonsusceptible organisms may result. ■ Because its use has been associated with severe colitis, it should be reserved for serious infections in which less toxic antimicrobial agents are inappropriate. ▪ *Clostridium difficile*–associated diarrhea (CDAD) has been reported. May range from mild diarrhea to fatal colitis. Consider in patients who present with diarrhea during or after treatment with clindamycin. ▪ Use caution with a history of GI, severe renal, or liver disease, and in patients with a history of asthma or significant allergies. ▪ Severe hypersensitivity reactions, including severe skin reactions such as toxic epidermal necrolysis, drug reaction with eosinophilia and systemic symptoms (DRESS), and Stevens-Johnson syndrome (SJS), some with fatal outcomes, have been reported. ▪ Serious anaphylactic reactions have been reported. ▪ Certain infections may require incision and drainage or other indicated surgical procedures in addition to antibiotic therapy. ▪ Not appropriate to treat meningitis.

Monitor: Capable of causing severe, even fatal, colitis; observe for symptoms of diarrhea. ▪ Periodic blood cell counts and liver and kidney studies are indicated in prolonged therapy. ▪ Monitor liver enzymes periodically in patients with severe liver disease. ▪ Monitor for S/S of hypersensitivity reactions, including severe skin and anaphylactic reactions.

Patient Education: Promptly report diarrhea or bloody stools that occur during treatment or up to several months after an antibiotic has been discontinued; may indicate CDAD and require treatment. ▪ Do not treat diarrhea without notifying physician.

Maternal/Child: In clinical trials with pregnant women, the systemic administration of clindamycin during the second or third trimesters has not been associated with an increased frequency of congenital abnormalities. Should be used during the first trimester only if clearly needed. ▪ Has the potential to cause adverse effects on the GI flora of a breast-fed infant. Consider risk versus benefit and the possibility of alternate therapy. Monitor the infant for S/S of adverse reactions (diarrhea, candidiasis or, rarely, CDAD) if administered to a breast-feeding mother. ▪ Some dosage forms contain benzyl alcohol, which has been associated with a fatal "gasping syndrome" in neonates. ▪ Benzyl alcohol can cross the placenta. ▪ Monitor organ system functions if used in pediatric patients. ▪ In cases of beta-hemolytic streptococcal infections, treatment should be continued for at least 10 days.

Elderly: CDAD may occur more frequently in elderly patients (over 60 years of age) and may be more severe. Monitor carefully for changes in bowel frequency; may not tolerate diarrhea well.

DRUG/LAB INTERACTIONS
May potentiate **neuromuscular blocking agents**. ▪ May decrease **cyclosporine** levels. Monitor and adjust dose if necessary. ▪ Clindamycin is predominantly metabolized by CYP3A4 and to a lesser extent by CYP3A5. **Inhibitors of CYP3A4 and CYP3A5** (e.g., protease inhibitors, azole antifungals) may increase clindamycin concentrations. Monitor for possible adverse reactions. **Inducers of CYP3A4 and CYP3A5** (e.g., rifampin) may reduce clindamycin concentrations, decreasing effectiveness.

SIDE EFFECTS
Abdominal pain, abnormal liver function tests, agranulocytosis, anaphylaxis, angioedema, azotemia, cardiac arrest, CDAD, diarrhea, drug reaction with eosinophilia and systemic symptoms (DRESS), eosinophilia (transient), exfoliative dermatitis, hypersensitivity reactions, hypotension, injection site reactions, jaundice, leukopenia, metallic taste, nausea, neutropenia (transient), oliguria, polyarthritis (rare), proteinuria, pruritus, pseudomembranous colitis, severe skin reactions (e.g., toxic epidermal necrolysis, acute generalized exanthematous pustulosis [AGEP], erythema multiforme), skin rashes, thrombophlebitis, urticaria, vaginitis, vomiting.

ANTIDOTE
Notify the physician of any side effects. Discontinue the drug if indicated (e.g., CDAD, diarrhea, hypersensitivity reactions, severe skin reaction), treat hypersensitivity reactions as indicated, and resuscitate as necessary. Mild cases of CDAD may respond to discontinuation of drug. Treat CDAD with fluids, electrolytes, protein supplements, and appropriate antibiotics (e.g., oral vancomycin) as indicated. In severe cases, surgical evaluation may be indicated. Hemodialysis or CAPD will not decrease blood levels in toxicity.

CLOFARABINE
(kloh-**FARE**-ah-bean)

Clolar

Antineoplastic
(metabolic inhibitor)

pH 4.5 to 7.5

PEDIATRIC DOSE

Pretreatment: Verify pregnancy status. Baseline studies required; see Monitor.

Premedication: Consider prophylactic antiemetic medications. Consider use of prophylactic steroids (e.g., hydrocortisone 100 mg/M^2 on Days 1 through 3) to mitigate or prevent the development of systemic inflammatory response syndrome (SIRS) or capillary leak syndrome (e.g., hypotension, pulmonary edema, tachycardia, tachypnea). See Drug/Lab Interactions.

Clofarabine: 52 mg/M^2 as an infusion each day for 5 consecutive days. Dose is based on body surface area (BSA), which is calculated using the actual height and weight before the start of each cycle. Repeat every 2 to 6 weeks; see Dose Adjustments. Frequency is based on recovery or return to baseline organ function. Median time between cycles during clinical studies was 28 days (range 12 to 55 days).

DOSE ADJUSTMENTS

Administer subsequent cycles no sooner than 14 days from the starting day of the previous cycle provided the patient's ANC is greater than or equal to 0.75×10^9/L. ■ Reduce dose by 50% in patients with a CrCl between 30 and 60 mL/min. Information is insufficient to make a dose recommendation in patients with a CrCl less than 30 mL/min or in patients on dialysis. ■ Reduce the dose of the next cycle by 25% in patients experiencing a Grade 4 neutropenia (ANC less than 0.5×10^9/L) that lasts 4 or more weeks. ■ Withhold clofarabine if a clinically significant infection develops. When the infection is clinically controlled, restart therapy at full dose. ■ Discontinue if hypotension develops at any time during the 5 days of administration. ■ Discontinue drug immediately if Grade 3 or higher increases in SCr, liver enzymes, or bilirubin occur; see Monitor and Antidote. May be restarted (generally with a 25% dose reduction) when the patient is stable and organ function has returned to baseline. ■ Discontinue drug immediately if S/S of SIRS or capillary leak syndrome occur; see Monitor and Antidote. May be restarted (generally with a 25% dose reduction) when the patient is stable. ■ Withhold clofarabine if a Grade 3 noninfectious nonhematologic toxicity occurs (excluding transient elevations in serum transaminases and/or serum bilirubin and/or nausea and vomiting that is controlled by antiemetics). With resolution or a return to baseline, restart clofarabine at a 25% dose reduction. ■ Discontinue therapy if a Grade 4 noninfectious nonhematologic toxicity occurs.

DILUTION

Specific techniques required; see Precautions. Available in single-use 20-mL vials containing 20 mg (1 mg/mL). Contains no preservatives; aseptic technique is imperative.

Calculate the exact number of vials needed to achieve the total dosing volume required.

$$\text{Total number of vials required} = \text{Total dose (mg)} \div 20 \text{ mg}$$

$$\text{Dosing volume (mL)} = \text{Total dose (mg)}$$

For example, a child with a body surface area (BSA) of 0.75 M^2 would need a dose of 39 mg of clofarabine (39 ÷ 20 mg = 1.95 vials, so 2 vials of clofarabine would be needed; 39 mg equals a dosing volume of 39 mL).

Withdraw the calculated dose from the vial(s). Using a 0.2-micron syringe filter, add the calculated dose to a sufficient volume of D5W or NS to provide a final concentration between 0.15 mg/mL and 0.4 mg/mL (e.g., 39 mg [39 mL in the example above] added to 100 mL of D5W or NS will provide a final concentration of approximately 0.28 mg/mL).

Filters: Use of a 0.2-micron syringe filter is recommended for use during dilution in D5W or NS.

Storage: Store unopened vials at CRT. Diluted solutions may be stored at CRT but must be used within 24 hours.

COMPATIBILITY

Manufacturer states, "To prevent drug **incompatibilities,** no other medications should be administered through the same IV line."

RATE OF ADMINISTRATION

A single dose properly diluted and evenly distributed as an infusion over 2 hours.

ACTIONS

A purine nucleoside metabolic inhibitor. Acts by inhibiting DNA synthesis. Also disrupts the mitochondrial membrane, causing the release of mitochondrial proteins, cytochrome C, and apoptosis-inducing factor, which leads to cell death. Is cytotoxic to rapidly proliferating and quiescent cancer cell types in vitro. Results in a rapid reduction of peripheral leukemia cells. Metabolism in the liver is very limited. Pathways of nonhepatic elimination not known. Estimated half-life is 5.2 hours. Excreted primarily in the urine.

INDICATIONS AND USES

Treatment of pediatric patients 1 to 21 years of age with relapsed or refractory acute lymphoblastic leukemia (ALL) after treatment with at least two prior regimens. This indication is based on response rate. There are no trials verifying an improvement in disease-related symptoms or increased survival with clofarabine.

Unlabeled uses: Treatment of other relapsed or refractory leukemias, including acute myelocytic leukemia (AML), myelodysplastic syndrome (MDS), and chronic myeloid leukemia in blast phase.

CONTRAINDICATIONS

Manufacturer states, "None."

PRECAUTIONS

Follow guidelines for handling cytotoxic agents. See Appendix A. ▪ Administered by or under the direction of the physician specialist in a facility with adequate diagnostic and treatment facilities to monitor the patient and respond to any medical emergency. ▪ At the initiation of treatment, most patients have hematologic impairment as a manifestation of the leukemia. Clofarabine causes myelosuppression, which may be severe and prolonged. Treatment may result in prolonged and severe neutropenia, including febrile neutropenia. Patients may be at an increased risk for infection, including severe and fatal sepsis and opportunistic infections. ▪ Use with great caution in patients with impaired hepatic or renal function. ▪ May develop tumor lysis syndrome, cytokine release syndrome, systemic inflammatory response syndrome, capillary leak syndrome, and organ dysfunction; deaths have been reported; see Monitor. ▪ Serious and fatal hemorrhage, including cerebral, GI, and pulmonary hemorrhage, has occurred. Most cases were associated with thrombocytopenia; see Monitor. ▪ Patients who have previously received a hematopoietic stem cell transplant (HSCT) are at higher risk for hepatotoxicity suggestive of veno-occlusive disease (VOD) following treatment with clofarabine (40 mg/M^2) used in combination with etoposide (VePesid 100 mg/M^2) and cyclophosphamide (Cytoxan 440 mg/M^2); has also been reported with monotherapy. ▪ Severe and fatal hepatotoxic events, including hepatitis and hepatic failure, have been reported; see Monitor. ▪ Renal toxicity, including Grade 3 or 4 elevated creatinine, acute renal failure, and hematuria, have been reported; see Monitor and Dose Adjustments. ▪ Fatal and serious cases of enterocolitis (neutropenic colitis, cecitis, and *C. difficile* colitis) have been reported. Occurs more frequently within 30 days of treatment and in the setting of combination chemotherapy. May lead to necrosis, perforation, hemorrhage, or sepsis complications. ▪ Serious and fatal skin reactions (Stevens-Johnson syndrome [SJS] and toxic epidermal necrolysis [TEN]) have been reported. ▪ Safety and effectiveness in adults not established. In a Phase 1 study of adults with refractory and/or relapsed hematologic malignancies, the pediatric dose of 52 mg/M² was not tolerated.

Monitor: Obtain baseline CBC with differential and platelets and serum electrolytes. Bone marrow suppression is expected. Appears to be dose-dependent and is usually reversible (with interruption of clofarabine treatment) but can be severe; monitor regularly and more frequently in patients who develop cytopenias. Monitoring of CBC and platelets is recommended daily during the 5 days of clofarabine administration, then 1 to 2 times weekly or as clinically indicated. ▪ Obtain baseline renal and hepatic function studies (e.g., SCr, bilirubin, ALT, AST), and uric acid levels. Monitor renal and hepatic function closely during the 5 days of clofarabine administration. Monitor for S/S of hepatitis and hepatic failure. Discontinue drug immediately if Grade 3 or higher increases in SCr, liver enzymes, or bilirubin occur; see Antidote. ▪ Monitor HR, BP, and respiratory status closely during infusion. Hypotension should be reported immediately; see Antidote. ▪ Monitor for S/S of tumor lysis syndrome (e.g., hyperkalemia, hyperphosphatemia, hyperuricemia, hypocalcemia, metabolic acidosis, urate crystalluria, and renal failure). Adequate hydration and antihyperuricemics (e.g., allopurinol) are indicated to prevent and/or treat hyperuricemia due to tumor lysis syndrome. ▪ Monitor for S/S of cytokine release syndrome (e.g., hypotension, pulmonary edema, tachycardia, tachypnea); may develop into systemic inflammatory response syndrome (SIRS)/capillary leak syndrome (rapid onset of respiratory distress, hypotension, pleural and pericardial effusion, and multiorgan failure). Close monitoring and early intervention may reduce risk; see Pediatric Dose and Antidote. To reduce the effects of tumor lysis and other adverse events (e.g., SIRS), the continuous administration of IV fluids throughout the 5 days of clofarabine treatment is recommended. ▪ Observe closely for signs of infection. Prophylactic antibiotics may be indicated pending the result of C/S in a febrile neutropenic patient. ▪ Use prophylactic antiemetics to reduce nausea and vomiting and increase patient comfort. ▪ Monitor for thrombocytopenia (platelet count less than 50,000/mm³). Initiate precautions to prevent excessive bleeding (e.g., inspect IV sites, skin, and mucous membranes; use extreme care during invasive procedures; test urine, emesis, stool, and secretions for occult blood). ▪ Monitor patients for S/S of enterocolitis and treat promptly. ▪ Monitor for development of skin reactions.

Patient Education: Avoid pregnancy; effective birth control recommended for men and women. Report a suspected pregnancy immediately. ▪ Drink plenty of fluids and avoid dehydration that may be caused by diarrhea and vomiting; report promptly if significant. ▪ Laboratory monitoring required. ▪ Promptly report bleeding, decreased urine output, dizziness, fainting spells, infection, jaundice, light-headedness, rapid respiratory rate, or a rapid heart rate. ▪ Review medications with pharmacist or physician. Avoid medications that may be hepatotoxic or nephrotoxic, including OTC or herbal medications. ▪ Skin rash may occur; report promptly if significant. ▪ See Appendix D.

Maternal/Child: Category D: avoid pregnancy; may cause fetal harm. Also has dose-related effects on male reproductive organs in animals. ▪ Discontinue breast-feeding.

Elderly: Not indicated in this patient population.

DRUG/LAB INTERACTIONS

Clinical drug-drug interactions have not been studied; however, the following cautions should be considered. ▪ Primarily excreted by the kidneys; minimize exposure to drugs with known renal toxicity during the 5 days of clofarabine administration (e.g., **aminoglycosides, amphotericin B, NSAIDs** [e.g., ibuprofen, naproxen], **rifampin**). Risk of renal toxicity may be increased. ▪ The liver is a known target organ for toxicity; consider avoiding drugs known to induce hepatic toxicity (e.g., **amiodarone, NSAIDs** [e.g., ibuprofen, naproxen], **phenothiazines** [e.g., prochlorperazine], **zidovudine**). ▪ Close monitoring is required with concomitant administration of medications affecting blood pressure or cardiac function (e.g., **diuretics** [furosemide], **calcium channel blockers** [diltiazem], **and other antihypertensives**). ▪ Cytochrome P$_{450}$ inhibitors (e.g., cimetidine, erythromycins, antifungal agents [e.g., itraconazole], ritonavir, verapamil) and cytochrome P_{450} inducers (e.g., carbamazepine, phenobarbital, phenytoin, rifampin) are unlikely to affect the metabolism of clofarabine. The effect on cytochrome P_{450} substrates has not been studied.

SIDE EFFECTS

Bone marrow suppression (e.g., anemia, leukopenia, neutropenia, thrombocytopenia) is anticipated, appears to be dose dependent, and is usually reversible. Anxiety, diarrhea, fatigue, febrile neutropenia, fever, flushing, headache, mucosal inflammation, nausea and vomiting, palmar-plantar erythrodysesthesia syndrome, pruritus, and rash occur most frequently. SIRS/capillary leak syndrome (e.g., rapid onset of respiratory distress, hypotension, pleural and pericardial effusion, and multiorgan failure) has occurred and can be fatal. Hepatotoxicity (elevated AST, ALT, bilirubin), renal toxicity (elevated SCr, acute renal failure), and veno-occlusive disease of the liver have occurred. Serious and fatal hemorrhage (cerebral, GI, and pulmonary), enterocolitis (neutropenic colitis, cecitis, and *C. difficile* colitis), and skin reactions (SJS and TEN) have been reported. Numerous additional side effects may occur and include abdominal pain, anorexia, arthralgia, back pain, cardiac toxicity (e.g., pericardial effusion, tachycardia), confusion, constipation, cough, depression, dermatitis, dizziness, dyspnea, edema, elevated creatinine, epistaxis, erythema, gingival bleeding, hematuria, hepatobiliary toxicity (e.g., elevated AST, ALT, bilirubin), hepatomegaly, hypertension, hypotension, infections (e.g., bacteremia, cellulitis, herpes simplex, oral candidiasis, pneumonia, sepsis, staphylococcal), injection site pain, irritability, jaundice, lethargy, myalgia, pain, petechiae, pleural effusion, renal toxicity, respiratory distress, rigors, somnolence, sore throat, transfusion reaction, tremor, weight loss.

Post-Marketing: Bone marrow failure, GI hemorrhage (including fatalities), hepatic failure, hepatitis, hyponatremia, Stevens-Johnson syndrome, toxic epidermal necrolysis, and veno-occlusive disease.

ANTIDOTE

Keep physician informed of all side effects; most will be treated symptomatically as indicated. Discontinue if hypotension develops at any time during the 5 days of administration. Discontinue clofarabine immediately if early S/S of SIRS or capillary leak (e.g., hypotension) appear. Use of albumin, diuretics, and steroids may be indicated. May consider restarting (usually at a lower dose) after the patient is stabilized and organ function has returned to baseline. Discontinue clofarabine immediately if substantial increases in SCr, liver enzymes, or bilirubin occur. May be restarted (possibly at a lower dose) when the patient is stable and organ function has returned to baseline. Discontinue clofarabine for exfoliative or bullous rash or if SJS or TEN is suspected. Bone marrow suppression must be resolved before additional doses can be given. Administration of whole blood products (e.g., packed RBCs, platelets, or leukocytes) and/or blood modifiers (e.g., darbepoetin alfa [Aranesp], epoetin alfa [Epogen], filgrastim [Neupogen, Zarxio], pegfilgrastim [Neulasta], sargramostim [Leukine]) may be indicated to treat bone marrow toxicity. Use specific antibiotics to combat infection. No specific antidote for overdose. Supportive therapy as indicated will help sustain the patient in toxicity. Should a hypersensitivity reaction occur, treat with antihistamines, corticosteroids, epinephrine, and oxygen as indicated. Resuscitate if indicated.

COAGULATION FACTOR VIIa (RECOMBINANT) RTS BBW

Antihemorrhagic

(ko-ag-yew-**LA**-shun **FAK**-ter 7a [re-**KOM**-be-nant])

NovoSeven RT

pH 5.5

USUAL DOSE

HEMOPHILIA A OR B PATIENTS WITH INHIBITORS

Bleeding episodes: 90 mcg/kg every 2 hours until hemostasis is achieved or until the treatment has been judged to be ineffective. Doses between 35 and 120 mcg/kg have been used successfully. Minimum effective dose has not been established. The dose and dosing interval may be adjusted based on the severity of the bleeding and the degree of homeostasis achieved. In clinical studies, a decision on outcome was reached for a majority of patients with joint or muscle bleeds within 8 doses, although more doses were required for severe bleeds. For severe bleeds, dosing should continue at 3- to 6-hour intervals after hemostasis is achieved to maintain the hemostatic plug. The appropriate duration of posthemostatic dosing has not been studied and should be minimized; see Precautions. If a new bleeding episode or rebleeding occurs, return to 2-hour dosing intervals.

Surgical intervention: 90 mcg/kg immediately before the intervention. Repeat every 2 hours during intervention. *For minor surgery,* postsurgical dosing should be administered every 2 hours for 48 hours and then every 2 to 6 hours until healing has occurred. *For major surgery,* postsurgical dosing should be administered every 2 hours for 5 days and then every 4 hours until healing has occurred. Additional doses may be given if required.

CONGENITAL FACTOR VII DEFICIENCY PATIENTS

Bleeding episodes and surgical intervention: 15 to 30 mcg/kg every 4 to 6 hours until hemostasis is achieved. Doses as low as 10 mcg/kg have been effective. Dose and dosing interval should be adjusted to each individual based on the severity of bleeding and the degree of hemostasis achieved. Minimal effective dose has not been determined.

ACQUIRED HEMOPHILIA

70 to 90 mcg/kg every 2 to 3 hours until hemostasis is achieved. Minimum effective dose has not been determined.

PEDIATRIC DOSE

See Usual Dose. Clinical studies were conducted with dosing determined according to body weight and not according to age. See Maternal/Child.

DOSE ADJUSTMENTS

Dose and administration interval may be adjusted based on the severity of the bleeding and the degree of hemostasis achieved. If patient develops intravascular coagulation or thrombosis, dosage should be reduced or treatment stopped; see Monitor.

DILUTION

NovoSeven RT is room temperature stable (RTS); aseptic technique is imperative. Available in packages that contain 1-, 2-, or 5-mg vials with a specified volume of histidine diluent. Select the appropriate vial package based on the calculated dose. Bring vial and diluent to RT. Do not exceed 37° C (98.6° F). Reconstitute powder with provided diluent, aiming the needle (20- to 26-gauge needle recommended) and the stream of diluent against the side of the vial. Do not inject the diluent directly on the powder. Do not use SWFI or other diluents. Gently swirl vial until powder is completely dissolved. Final concentration of reconstituted solution is 1 mg/mL (1,000 mcg/mL).

Storage: Before reconstitution, refrigerate or store between 2° and 25° C (36° and 77° F). Avoid exposure to direct sunlight. Do not freeze. After reconstitution, store at RT or refrigerate. Should be used within 3 hours. Do not freeze reconstituted product or store in syringe. Discard unused product.

COMPATIBILITY

Manufacturer states, "Intended for IV injection only and should not be mixed with infusion solutions. Do not store reconstituted solution in syringes." If line needs to be flushed before or after NovoSeven RT administration, use NS.

RATE OF ADMINISTRATION

A single dose as a slow IV injection over 2 to 5 minutes, depending on dose administered.

ACTIONS

A vitamin K–dependent glycoprotein structurally similar to human plasma–derived factor VIIa. Produced by recombinant DNA technology. Promotes hemostasis by activating the extrinsic pathway of the coagulation cascade. When complexed with tissue factor, can activate coagulation factor X to factor Xa, and coagulation factor IX to factor IXa. Factor Xa, in complex with other factors, then converts prothrombin to thrombin. This leads to the formation of a hemostatic plug by converting fibrinogen to fibrin. Half-life is 2.3 hours. Duration of action is 3 hours.

INDICATIONS AND USES

Treatment of bleeding episodes or prevention of bleeding in surgical interventions or invasive procedures in hemophilia A or B patients with inhibitors to factor VIII or factor IX and in patients with acquired hemophilia. ■ Treatment of bleeding episodes or prevention of bleeding in surgical interventions or invasive procedures in patients with congenital FVII deficiency.

CONTRAINDICATIONS

Manufacturer states, "None." Use with caution in patients with known hypersensitivity to coagulation factor VIIa (recombinant), any of its components, and in patients with known hypersensitivity to mouse, hamster, or bovine proteins.

PRECAUTIONS

For intravenous bolus administration only. ■ Should be administered to patients only under the direct supervision of a physician experienced in the treatment of bleeding disorders. ■ Thrombotic events have been reported in clinical trials as well as through post-marketing surveillance following coagulation factor VIIa (recombinant) RTS use for each of the approved indications. Patients with disseminated intravascular coagulation (DIC), advanced atherosclerotic disease, crush injury, septicemia, or concomitant treatment with aPCCs/PCCs (activated or nonactivated prothrombin complex concentrates) may have an increased risk of developing thrombotic events due to circulating tissue factor or predisposing coagulopathy. Use caution in patients with an increased risk of thromboembolic complications. These include, but are not limited to, patients with a history of coronary artery disease (CAD), liver disease, DIC, or postoperative immobilization; elderly patients; and neonates. ■ Coagulation factor VIIa has been studied in placebo-controlled trials outside the approved indications to control bleeding in intracranial hemorrhage, advanced liver disease, trauma, cardiac surgery, spinal surgery, and other therapeutic areas. Safety and effectiveness have not been established in these settings, and the use is not approved by the FDA. Arterial and venous thrombotic and thromboembolic events have been reported during post-marketing surveillance. Studies have shown an increased risk of arterial thromboembolic adverse events (e.g., MI, myocardial ischemia, cerebral infarction, and cerebral ischemia) with coagulation factor VIIa when administered outside the current approved guidelines. ■ Biologic and clinical effects of prolonged elevated levels of factor VIIa have not been studied; therefore, the duration of posthemostatic dosing should be minimized, and patients should be appropriately monitored by a physician experienced in the treatment of hemophilia during this time period.

Monitor: Evaluation of hemostasis should be used to determine the effectiveness of therapy and to provide a basis for modification of the treatment schedule; coagulation parameters do not necessarily correlate with or predict the effectiveness of therapy. Coagulation parameters (e.g., PT, aPTT, plasma FVII clotting activity [FVII:C]) may be used as an adjunct to the clinical evaluation of hemostasis in monitoring the effectiveness and treatment schedule, although these parameters have shown no direct correlation to achieving hemostasis. ■ Patients with factor VII deficiency should be monitored for PT and factor

VII coagulant activity before and after treatment. If the factor VIIa activity fails to reach the expected level, if PT is not corrected, or if bleeding is not controlled after treatment with the recommended doses, antibody formation should be suspected and analysis for antibodies should be performed. ■ The normal factor VII plasma concentration is 0.5 mcg/mL. Factor VIIa levels of 15% to 25% (0.075 to 0.125 mcg/mL) are generally sufficient to achieve normal hemostasis. ■ Monitor patients for the development of signs or symptoms of activation of the coagulation system or thrombosis. When there is laboratory confirmation of intravascular coagulation or presence of clinical thrombosis, dosage should be reduced or the treatment stopped, depending on the patient's symptoms; see Dose Adjustments.

Patient Education: Discuss benefits versus risk of therapy and signs of hypersensitivity reactions including hives, urticaria, chest tightness, wheezing, hypotension, and anaphylaxis. ■ Signs of bleeding may be similar to signs of thrombosis and can include new-onset swelling and pain in the limbs or abdomen, new-onset chest pain, shortness of breath, loss of sensation or motor power, or altered consciousness or speech.

Maternal/Child: Category C: safety for use during pregnancy not established. Use only if clearly indicated and benefit justifies potential risk to the fetus. ■ Discontinue breast-feeding. ■ Thrombotic events have been reported in women without a prior diagnosis of bleeding disorders who have received coagulation factor VIIa for uncontrolled post-partum hemorrhage. ■ A decision should be made whether to discontinue nursing or to discontinue the drug. ■ The safety and effectiveness have not been studied to determine if there are differences among various age groups from infants to adolescents (0 to 16 years of age); see Pediatric Dose.

Elderly: Numbers in clinical studies insufficient to determine if the elderly respond differently than younger subjects.

DRUG/LAB INTERACTIONS
The risk of potential interaction between factor VIIa and coagulation factor concentrates has not been adequately evaluated. Simultaneous use of **activated prothrombin complex concentrates** (e.g., anti-inhibitor coagulant complex [Feiba]) **or prothrombin complex concentrates** (e.g., factor IX [AlphaNine SD, BeneFIX]) should be avoided.

SIDE EFFECTS
Generally well tolerated. The majority of patients reporting side effects received more than 12 doses. The most common side effects are arthralgia, edema, fever, headache, hemorrhage, hypertension, hypotension, injection site reaction, nausea, pain, rash, and vomiting. Most serious adverse reactions are thrombotic events; however, the risk in patients with hemophilia and inhibitors is considered to be low. Fatal and nonfatal thrombotic events have been reported when used for both labeled and off-label indications. Other side effects include arthrosis, bradycardia, coagulation disorder, decreased fibrinogen plasma, decreased prothrombin, decreased therapeutic response, DIC, hemarthrosis, hypersensitivity reactions, increased fibrinolysis, pneumonia, pruritus, purpura, renal function abnormalities, shock, subdural hematoma, thrombosis, urticaria.

Post-Marketing: High D-dimer levels and consumptive coagulopathy; thromboembolic events, including myocardial ischemia and/or infarction, cerebral ischemia and/or infarction, thrombophlebitis, arterial thrombosis, deep vein thrombosis, and related pulmonary embolism; and isolated cases of hypersensitivity reactions (including anaphylaxis) have occurred following use in both labeled and unlabeled indications.

ANTIDOTE
Discontinue drug and notify physician of any major side effects. Treat hypersensitivity reactions as indicated. For thrombosis or DIC, anticoagulation with heparin may be indicated.

COAGULATION FACTOR X (HUMAN)

(ko-ag-yew-**LA**-shun **FAK**-ter X)

Coagadex

USUAL DOSE

Dose, frequency, and duration must be individualized based on the severity of the factor X deficiency, location and extent of bleeding, patient's clinical condition, and individual clinical response. Each vial is labeled with the actual factor X potency/content in International units (IU). The dose to achieve a desired in vivo peak increase in factor X level can be calculated with the following formula.

$$\text{Dose (IU)} = \text{Body weight (kg)} \times \text{Desired factor X rise (IU/dL)} \times 0.5$$

The desired factor X rise is the difference between the patient's plasma factor X level and the desired level. The dosing formula is based on the observed recovery of 2 IU/dL per IU/kg (i.e., for each 1 IU/kg of factor X administered, the circulating factor X level increases by approximately 2 IU/dL).

On-demand treatment and control of bleeding episodes: 25 IU/kg at the first sign of bleeding. Repeat every 24 hours until the bleed stops. Do not administer more than 60 IU/kg daily.

Perioperative management of bleeding: Do not administer more than 60 IU/kg daily.

Presurgery: Calculate the dose of coagulation factor X required to raise plasma factor X levels to 70 to 90 IU/dL using the following formula.

$$\text{Required dose (IU)} = \text{Body weight (kg)} \times \text{Desired factor X rise (IU/dL)} \times 0.5$$

Postsurgery: Repeat dose as necessary to maintain plasma factor X levels at a minimum of 50 IU/dL until there is no longer a risk of bleeding due to surgery.

DOSE ADJUSTMENTS

Adjust dose and duration based on factor X levels, location and extent of bleeding, patient's clinical condition, and clinical response to therapy.

DILUTION

Supplied in single-use glass vials containing approximately 250 or 500 IU (approximately 100 IU/mL after reconstitution) of factor X activity, packaged with 2.5 or 5 mL of SWFI, respectively, and a Mix2Vial transfer device. The total number of IUs available is clearly marked on each vial. Record the batch number of each vial. Consult instructions for reconstitution and administration in the package insert. If stored in the refrigerator, warm to room temperature (25° C [77° F]) before reconstitution. If more than 1 vial is required, use a new Mix2Vial transfer set for each vial of drug. Solution from multiple vials can be pooled into a single syringe. Do not shake. Do not use if the reconstituted solution is cloudy or contains any particles. The reconstituted solution should be clear or slightly pearl-like in appearance.

Filters: Incorporated into the Mix2Vial.

Storage: Store in refrigerator or at RT (2° to 30° C [36° to 86° F]) in original carton to protect from light until ready to use. Do not freeze. Do not use beyond the expiration date on the product vial. Should be used immediately but must be used within 1 hour of reconstitution.

COMPATIBILITY

Compatibility information not available from manufacturer; consult a pharmacist.

RATE OF ADMINISTRATION

A single dose may be administered as an infusion at a rate of 10 mL/min up to a maximum rate of 20 mL/min; consider patient comfort. Reduce rate of administration or interrupt the infusion if a marked increase in pulse occurs.

ACTIONS

Coagulation factor X is a plasma-derived, purified concentrate of human coagulation factor X. It temporarily replaces the missing factor X needed for effective hemostasis. After conversion to its active form (factor Xa), it associates with factor Va to form the prothrombinase complex, which activates prothrombin to thrombin. Thrombin then acts on soluble fibrinogen and factor XIII to generate a cross-linked fibrin clot. Mean half-life is approximately 30.3 hours.

INDICATIONS AND USES

Treatment of adults and pediatric patients (12 years of age and above) with hereditary factor X deficiency for on-demand treatment and control of bleeding episodes and perioperative management of bleeding in patients with mild hereditary factor X deficiency. **Limitation of use:** Perioperative management of bleeding in major surgery in patients with moderate and severe hereditary factor X deficiency has not been studied.

CONTRAINDICATIONS

Life-threatening hypersensitivity reactions to coagulation factor X or any of the product components.

PRECAUTIONS

For IV use only. ■ Administered under the direction of a physician knowledgeable in the treatment of coagulation disorders in a facility with adequate diagnostic and treatment facilities to monitor the patient and respond to any medical emergency. ■ Hypersensitivity reactions, including anaphylaxis, have occurred; see Monitor. ■ Manufactured from human plasma. Risk of transmitting infectious agents (e.g., HIV, hepatitis and, theoretically, Creutzfeldt-Jakob disease) has been greatly reduced by screening, testing, and manufacturing techniques. However, risk of transmission cannot be totally eliminated. Health care professionals should use caution during administration; may have risk of exposure to viral infection. ■ Contains trace human proteins other than factor X. ■ Neutralizing antibodies (inhibitors) to factor X may occur; see Monitor.

Monitor: Monitor BP and pulse during infusion. If a marked increase in pulse occurs, either reduce rate of infusion or interrupt the infusion. ■ Throughout the infusion, monitor for S/S of a hypersensitivity reaction (e.g., angioedema, chest tightness, chills, fever, headache, hypotension, lethargy, nausea, pruritus, rash, restlessness, tachycardia, urticaria, wheezing). ■ Monitor plasma factor X activity by performing a validated test (e.g., one-stage clotting assay) to confirm that adequate factor X levels have been achieved and maintained. ■ In surgery patients, monitor postinfusion plasma factor X levels before and after surgery to ensure that hemostatic levels are obtained and maintained. ■ Monitor for the development of factor X inhibitors. Perform a Nijmegen-Bethesda inhibitor assay if expected factor X plasma levels are not attained or if bleeding is not controlled with the expected dose of coagulation factor X.

Patient Education: Review manufacturer's medication guide. ■ Promptly report S/S of a hypersensitivity reaction (e.g., dizziness, hives, itching, rash, tightness of the chest, wheezing). ■ Report a lack of clinical response to therapy; may be a manifestation of an inhibitor. ■ Report symptoms of possibly transmitted viral infections immediately. Symptoms may include anorexia, arthralgias, fatigue, jaundice, low-grade fever, nausea, or vomiting. ■ If traveling, bring an adequate supply of medication based on current treatment regimen.

Maternal/Child: Use during pregnancy or labor and delivery only if clearly needed. ■ Safety for use during breast-feeding not known; consider benefit versus risk. ■ Safety and effectiveness for use in pediatric patients under 12 years of age not established.

Elderly: Numbers insufficient to determine differences in response between older and younger patients.

DRUG/LAB INTERACTIONS

Drug interaction studies have not been performed. ■ Use with caution in patients who are receiving other plasma products that may contain factor X (e.g., fresh frozen plasma, prothrombin complex concentrates [e.g., Kcentra]). ■ Based on its mechanism of action, coagulation factor X is likely to be counteracted by direct and indirect factor Xa inhibitors (e.g., apixaban, edoxaban, rivaroxaban).

SIDE EFFECTS

The most common side effects observed are back pain, fatigue, infusion site erythema, and infusion site pain. Hypersensitivity reactions have occurred.

ANTIDOTE

Keep the physician informed of side effects. Slow or interrupt infusion for a marked increase in pulse rate or a mild hypersensitivity reaction. Discontinue the infusion immediately if a severe hypersensitivity reaction occurs. Treat hypersensitivity as necessary (e.g., antihistamines, epinephrine, corticosteroids). Resuscitate as necessary.

COAGULATION FACTOR Xa (RECOMBINANT), INACTIVATED-zhzo BBW

Antidote

(ko-ag-yew-**LA**-shun **FAK**-ter Xa)

Andexxa

pH 7.8

USUAL DOSE

There are two dosing regimens.

Coagulation Factor Xa (recombinant) Dosing Regimens		
Dose[a]	Initial IV Bolus	Follow-on IV Infusion
Low dose	400 mg at a target rate of 30 mg/min	4 mg/min for up to 120 minutes
High dose	800 mg at a target rate of 30 mg/min	8 mg/min for up to 120 minutes

[a]The safety and effectiveness of more than one dose have not been evaluated.

The recommended dosing regimen is based on the specific FXa inhibitor, dose of FXa inhibitor, and time since the patient's last dose of the FXa inhibitor as outlined in the following chart.

Coagulation Factor Xa (Recombinant) Dose Based on Rivaroxaban or Apixaban Dose			
FXa Inhibitor	FXa Inhibitor Last Dose	Timing of FXa Inhibitor Last Dose Before Coagulation Factor Xa (Recombinant) Initiation	
		<8 Hours or Unknown	≥8 Hours
Rivaroxaban	≤10 mg	Low dose	Low dose
Rivaroxaban	>10 mg/Unknown	High dose	Low dose
Apixaban	≤5 mg	Low dose	Low dose
Apixaban	>5 mg/Unknown	High dose	Low dose

DILUTION

Available as a lyophilized powder in single-use vials of 100 mg of coagulation factor Xa (recombinant), inactivated-zhzo. To reduce the total reconstitution time needed during preparation, reconstitute all required vials in succession. The low-dose regimen will require 4 vials for the bolus and 5 vials for the infusion. The high-dose regimen will require 8 vials for the bolus and 10 vials for the infusion.

IV bolus preparation: Reconstitute each 100-mg vial with 10 mL of SWFI using a 10-mL syringe and a 20-gauge (or higher) needle. Direct the solution onto the inside wall of the vial to minimize foam (final concentration 10 mg/mL). Gently swirl each vial until completely dissolved. **Do not shake.** Typical dissolution time for each vial is approximately

3 minutes. If dissolution is incomplete, discard the vial and do not use the product. Using a 60-mL or larger syringe with a 20-gauge (or higher) needle, withdraw the reconstituted solution from each of the vials until the required dosing volume is achieved. Transfer the solution into an empty polyolefin or polyvinyl chloride IV bag with a volume of 250 mL or less.

Continuous IV infusion preparation: Follow the same procedure outlined for the IV bolus preparation. Reconstitute the number of vials needed based on the dose regimen. More than one 40- to 60-mL syringe, or an equivalent 100-mL syringe, may be used for transfer of the reconstituted solution to the IV bag.

Filters: Must be administered through an IV line containing a sterile 0.2- or 0.22-micron in-line polyethersulfone or equivalent low–protein-binding filter.

Storage: Store unopened vials at 2° to 8° C (36° to 46° F). Do not freeze. Reconstituted solution in vials is stable at RT for up to 8 hours or may be stored for up to 24 hours at 2° to 8° C (36° to 46° F). Reconstituted solution in IV bags is stable at RT for up to 8 hours or may be stored for up to 16 hours at 2° to 8° C (36° to 46° F). Discard partially used vials.

COMPATIBILITY
Compatibility information not available from manufacturer; consult a pharmacist.

RATE OF ADMINISTRATION
Administered through an IV line containing a sterile 0.2- or 0.22-micron in-line polyethersulfone or equivalent low–protein-binding filter.

IV bolus: Administer at a target rate of 30 mg/min.

IV continuous infusion: Within 2 minutes after the bolus dose, administer the continuous IV infusion as outlined in Usual Dose for up to 120 minutes.

ACTIONS
The active ingredient in coagulation factor Xa (recombinant), inactivated-zhzo is a genetically modified variant of human factor Xa. It exerts its procoagulant effect by binding and sequestering the FXa inhibitors rivaroxaban and apixaban. A second procoagulant effect is its ability to bind and inhibit the activity of tissue factor pathway inhibitor (TFPI). Inhibition of TFPI activity can increase tissue factor-initiated thrombin generation. In dose-ranging studies, dosing as a bolus followed by a 2-hour continuous infusion resulted in a rapid decrease in anti-FXa activity (within 2 minutes after the completion of the bolus administration) followed by reduced anti-FXa activity that was maintained throughout the duration of the continuous infusion. The anti-Xa activity returned to placebo levels approximately 2 hours after completion of a bolus or continuous infusion. TFPI activity in plasma was sustained for at least 22 hours following coagulation factor Xa (recombinant) administration. Half-life ranges from 5 to 7 hours.

INDICATIONS AND USES
Indicated for patients treated with rivaroxaban and apixaban when reversal of anticoagulation is needed due to life-threatening or uncontrolled bleeding.

This indication is approved under accelerated approval based on the change from baseline in anti-FXa activity in healthy volunteers. An improvement in hemostasis has not been established. Continued approval for this indication may be contingent on the results of studies to demonstrate an improvement in hemostasis in patients.

Limitation of use: Coagulation factor Xa (recombinant) has not been shown to be effective for, and is not indicated for, the treatment of bleeding related to any FXa inhibitors other than apixaban and rivaroxaban.

CONTRAINDICATIONS
Manufacturer states, "None."

PRECAUTIONS
For IV use only. ■ Treatment with coagulation factor Xa (recombinant) has been associated with serious and life-threatening adverse events, including arterial and venous thromboembolic events, ischemic events (including myocardial infarction and ischemic stroke), cardiac arrest, and sudden deaths. Thromboembolic events have been observed within 30 days after administration of coagulation factor Xa (recombinant). The median time to the first event was 6 days.

■ Patients being treated with FXa inhibitor therapy have underlying disease states that predispose them to thromboembolic events. Reversing FXa inhibitor therapy exposes patients to the thrombotic risk of their underlying disease. To reduce the risk of thrombosis, resume anticoagulant therapy as soon as medically appropriate following treatment with coagulation factor Xa (recombinant). ■ The safety of coagulation factor Xa (recombinant) has not been evaluated in patients who experienced thromboembolic events or disseminated intravascular coagulation within 2 weeks before the life-threatening bleeding event requiring treatment with coagulation factor Xa (recombinant). ■ Safety of coagulation factor Xa (recombinant) also has not been evaluated in patients who received prothrombin complex concentrates, recombinant factor VIIa, or whole blood products within 7 days before the bleeding event. ■ Re-elevation or incomplete reversal of anticoagulant activity can occur. In studies, there was a rapid and substantial decrease in anti-FXa activity corresponding to the coagulation factor Xa (recombinant) bolus that was sustained through the end of the continuous infusion. After the infusion, there was an increase in anti-FXa activity that peaked 4 hours after infusion. ■ As with all therapeutic proteins, there is a potential for immunogenicity.

Monitor: Monitor for thromboembolic events and initiate anticoagulation when medically appropriate. ■ Monitor for symptoms and signs that precede cardiac arrest and provide treatment as needed. ■ Monitor for S/S of ischemic events. ■ Standard clinical assessments (e.g., VS, hemoglobin measurements, CT assessments relevant to the type of bleeding [e.g., GI, cerebral]) may be used to evaluate effective hemostasis. ■ An anti-Xa activity assay that is calibrated to each specific factor Xa inhibitor may be available at some facilities and can be used to rule out clinically significant serum concentrations and quantify the anticoagulant effect of the given anti-Xa inhibitor.

Patient Education: Reversing FXa inhibitor therapy increases the risk of thromboembolic events. Arterial and venous thromboembolic events, ischemic events, cardiac events, and sudden death were observed within 30 days after administration of coagulation factor Xa (recombinant). Report S/S of thrombosis (e.g., limb or abdominal swelling and/or pain, chest pain or pressure, shortness of breath, loss of sensation or motor power, altered consciousness, vision, or speech).

Maternal/Child: Safety for use during pregnancy, labor and delivery, and during breast-feeding not established; use with caution and only if clearly indicated. ■ Safety and effectiveness for use in pediatric patients not established.

Elderly: No overall differences in safety or efficacy were observed between the elderly and younger patients, but greater sensitivity of some older individuals cannot be ruled out.

DRUG/LAB INTERACTIONS

There are no known significant interactions.

SIDE EFFECTS

The most common side effects observed were infusion-related reactions, pneumonia, and urinary tract infections. Infusion-related reactions included cough, dysgeusia, dyspnea, feeling hot, and flushing. Thromboembolic events reported after administration of coagulation factor Xa (recombinant) included acute myocardial infarction, acute respiratory failure, cardiac arrest, cardiac thrombus, cardiogenic shock, congestive heart failure, deep venous thrombosis, embolic stroke, iliac artery thrombosis, ischemic stroke, nonsustained ventricular tachycardia, pulmonary embolism, and sudden death. No thromboembolic events were observed in healthy volunteers who received FXa inhibitors and were treated with coagulation factor Xa (recombinant).

ANTIDOTE

Notify physician of any side effect and treat as appropriate.

COLISTIMETHATE SODIUM

(koh-lis-tih-**METH**-ayt **SO**-dee-um)

Coly-Mycin M

USUAL DOSE
Pretreatment: Baseline studies indicated; see Monitor and Precautions.

Adult and pediatric dose: Based on severity of the infection. Dosage expressed in terms of colistin base. Range is 2.5 to 5 mg/kg/24 hr of colistin base equally divided into 1-2 doses. Can be given via nebulization as 150 mg every 8 hours over 60 minutes. Do not exceed the maximum dose of 5 mg/kg/24 hr.

PEDIATRIC DOSE
See Usual Dose.

DOSE ADJUSTMENTS
In obese patients, base dose on ideal body weight. ▪ Caution and lower-end dosing suggested in the elderly. Consider age-related impaired organ function and concomitant disease or drug therapy. ▪ Dose reduction may alleviate neurologic adverse reactions. ▪ Reduce dose or increase time interval in patients with impaired renal function based on the following chart.

Suggested Modification of Dosage Schedules of Colistimethate Sodium for Adults With Impaired Renal Function				
	Normal	**Mild**	**Moderate**	**Severe**
CrCl (mL/min)	≥80	50-79	30-49	10-29
Dosage Schedule	2.5-5 mg/kg divided into 2 to 4 doses per day	2.5-3.8 mg/kg divided into 2 doses per day	2.5 mg/kg once daily or divided into 2 doses per day	1.5 mg/kg every 36 hours

Note: The suggested total daily dose is calculated from colistin base activity.

DILUTION
Reconstitute a 150-mg vial with 2 mL SWFI. Swirl gently to avoid frothing. Concentration equals 75 mg/mL colistin base. May be further diluted in a desired amount (e.g., 100 to 1,000 mL) of D5W, D5NS, D5/½NS, NS, D5/¼NS, or LR for infusion.

Filters: No significant loss of drug potency noted with filtration through a 0.22-micron cellulose ester membrane filter.

Storage: Store at CRT before use. Reconstituted solutions are stable for up to 7 days at RT or refrigerated. Freshly prepare fully diluted solutions and complete administration within 24 hours.

COMPATIBILITY
Compatibility information not available from manufacturer. Other sources suggest a few specific **compatibilities** dependent on concentration and manufacturer; consult a pharmacist.

RATE OF ADMINISTRATION
IV over 30-60 minutes.

ACTIONS
A polypeptide antibiotic. A surface-active agent that penetrates into and disrupts the bacterial cell membrane. Has bactericidal activity against selected aerobic gram-negative organisms. Serum half-life is 2 to 3 hours. Excreted in urine. Crosses placental barrier.

INDICATIONS AND USES

Treatment of acute or chronic infections due to sensitive strains of gram-negative bacilli (e.g., *Enterobacter aerogenes*, *Escherichia coli*, *Klebsiella pneumoniae*, and *Pseudomonas aeruginosa*).

CONTRAINDICATIONS

Hypersensitivity to colistimethate or its components. ▪ Not indicated for infections due to *Proteus* or *Neisseria*.

PRECAUTIONS

To reduce the development of drug-resistant bacteria and maintain its effectiveness, colistimethate sodium should be used only to treat those infections that are proven or strongly suspected to be caused by susceptible bacteria. ▪ May cause nephrotoxicity, which is thought to be a dose-dependent effect; use caution in patients with impaired renal function, including the elderly; see Dose Adjustments. ▪ Usual doses in patients with impaired renal function will lead to high serum levels, which may lead to acute renal insufficiency, renal shutdown, and neurotoxicity, including muscle weakness and apnea. ▪ Avoid prolonged use of drug; superinfection caused by overgrowth of nonsusceptible organisms may result. ▪ *Clostridium difficile*–associated diarrhea (CDAD) has been reported. ▪ Has caused transient neurologic disturbances (e.g., circumoral paresthesia or numbness, tingling or formication [feeling of something crawling on the skin] of extremities, generalized pruritus, dizziness, vertigo, and slurring of speech).

Monitor: Obtain baseline BUN and serum creatinine. ▪ Monitor for diminishing urine output, rising BUN and SCr, and decreased CrCl as indicated during therapy; dose reduction may be required. Nephrotoxicity may be reversible with discontinuation of colistimethate. ▪ Monitor for S/S of neuromuscular disturbances. ▪ Motor coordination may be impaired; supervise ambulation. ▪ See Drug/Lab Interactions.

Patient Education: May cause dizziness and vertigo. Request assistance with ambulation and do not drive vehicles or use hazardous machinery while on therapy. ▪ Promptly report sensations of numbness or tingling, generalized itching, severe dizziness or vertigo, and slurring of speech. ▪ Promptly report diarrhea or bloody stools that occur during treatment or up to several months after an antibiotic has been discontinued; may indicate CDAD and require treatment.

Maternal/Child: Category C: use during pregnancy only if the potential benefit justifies the potential risk to the fetus. ▪ Use caution during breast-feeding; similar drugs (e.g., colistin sulfate) are secreted in breast milk. ▪ Use caution and monitor pediatric patients closely. Side effects are similar to adults; however, neonates, infants, and children either cannot or may not report them.

Elderly: Dose selection should be cautious; see Dose Adjustments and Precautions. ▪ Differences in response compared to younger adults not identified. ▪ Monitoring of renal function is suggested.

DRUG/LAB INTERACTIONS

Risk of respiratory paralysis and renal dysfunction is increased with **certain other antibiotics** (e.g., aminoglycosides). Concurrent use is not recommended; if necessary, use extreme caution. *Apnea can occur.*

SIDE EFFECTS

Apnea; CDAD; decreased CrCl; decreased urine output; dizziness; fever; generalized itching, urticaria, and rash; GI upset; hypersensitivity reactions, including anaphylaxis; increased BUN and SCr; nephrotoxicity; paresthesia; respiratory distress; seizures; slurred speech; tingling of extremities and tongue; vertigo.

Overdose: Neuromuscular blockade (e.g., ataxia, confusion, disorders of speech, dizziness, lethargy, nystagmus, paresthesia). Respiratory muscle paralysis may lead to apnea, respiratory arrest, and death. May also cause acute renal failure (e.g., decreased urine output and increases in BUN and SCr and decreased CrCl).

ANTIDOTE

Notify the physician of all side effects. Reduction in dose may alleviate symptoms. If symptoms of impaired renal function or overdose occur, discontinue the drug immediately and notify the physician. Nephrotoxicity may be reversible. Maintain an adequate airway and artificial ventilation as indicated. After drug plasma levels have fallen, colistimethate may be restarted in reduced doses if indicated. Treat allergic reactions symptomatically with antihistamines, pressor amines, and corticosteroids. Mild cases of CDAD may respond to discontinuation of colistimethate. Information not available on ability of hemodialysis or peritoneal dialysis to remove colistimethate in overdose. Resuscitate as indicated.

CONIVAPTAN HYDROCHLORIDE

Arginine vasopressin antagonist

(kon-ih-**VAP**-tan hy-droh-**KLOR**-eyed)

Vaprisol

pH 3.4 to 3.8

USUAL DOSE

Loading dose: 20 mg as an IV infusion over 30 minutes. Follow with 20 mg administered as a **continuous infusion** evenly distributed over 24 hours. May be administered for an additional 1 to 3 days as a continuous infusion of 20 mg/day. The total duration of infusion (after the loading dose) should not exceed 4 days.

DOSE ADJUSTMENTS

If the serum sodium does not rise at the desired rate, the dose may be titrated up to 40 mg as a continuous infusion over 24 hours. 40 mg is the maximum daily dose. ▪ A reduced dose may be required if the patient experiences an undesirably rapid rate of rise of serum sodium; see Precautions. ▪ If hyponatremia persists or recurs (after initial interruption of therapy) and the patient has no evidence of neurologic sequelae, conivaptan may be resumed at a reduced dose; see Monitor. ▪ A reduced dose may also be required in patients who develop hypotension or hypovolemia; see Monitor. ▪ No dose adjustment indicated in patients with mild hepatic impairment. ▪ Reduced dose required in patients with moderate (Child-Pugh Class B) and severe (Child-Pugh Class C) hepatic impairment. Initiate with a loading dose of 10 mg. Follow with a continuous infusion of 10 mg over 24 hours for 2 days to a maximum of 4 days. If sodium is not rising at the desired rate, the conivaptan dose may be titrated up to 20 mg/day. ▪ Use in patients with severe renal impairment (CrCl less than 30 mL/min) is not recommended; see Contraindications.

DILUTION

Available in a single-use, ready-to-use (RTU) plastic container containing 20 mg conivaptan in 100 mL D5W. If the RTU container is being administered as a 40-mg dose, administer two consecutive 20 mg/100 mL containers over 24 hours.

Storage: Store at 25° C (77° F); however, brief exposure up to 40° C (104° F) does not adversely affect the product. Avoid excessive heat. Protect from light and freezing. Do not remove container from overwrap until ready to use. Overwrap is a moisture and light barrier.

COMPATIBILITY

Manufacturer states, "Should not be mixed or administered with lactated Ringer's or furosemide. Should not be combined with any other product in the same intravenous line or bag. **Compatible** at the Y-site with NS at a flow rate for conivaptan of 4.2 mL/hr and NS at either 2.1 mL/hr or 6.3 mL/hr."

RATE OF ADMINISTRATION

Loading dose: A single dose equally distributed over 30 minutes as an infusion.
Continuous infusion: A single dose equally distributed over 24 hours.

ACTIONS

A nonpeptide, dual arginine vasopressin (AVP) antagonist of V_{1A} and V_2 receptors. The level of AVP in the blood is critical for the regulation of water and electrolyte balance and is usually elevated in both euvolemic and hypervolemic hyponatremia. (In euvolemic hyponatremia there is an increase in total body water, but the sodium content remains the same; in hypervolemic hyponatremia both sodium and water content in the body increase, but the water gain is greater). AVP excess is associated with hyponatremia without edema. The AVP effect is mediated through V_2 receptors that help maintain plasma osmolality within the normal range. Conivaptan blocks V_2 receptors in the renal collecting ducts, resulting in aquaresis (excretion of free water). This is generally accompanied by increased net fluid loss, increased urine output, and decreased urine osmolality within the normal range. Conivaptan is highly protein bound. It is metabolized in the liver by the cytochrome P_{450} isoenzyme, CYP3A. Its half-life is 5.3 to 8.1 hours, depending on dose. Primarily excreted in the feces and, to a lesser extent, in urine. Crosses the placenta in animals.

INDICATIONS AND USES

To raise serum sodium in the hospitalized patient with euvolemic and hypervolemic hyponatremia. Euvolemic hyponatremia may occur in the syndrome of inappropriate antidiuretic hormone secretion (SIADH, an inability of the body to excrete dilute urine) or in the setting of certain conditions, including hypothyroidism, adrenal insufficiency, and pulmonary disorders.

Limitations of use: Conivaptan has not been shown to be effective for treatment of the S/S of heart failure. ▪ It has not been established that raising serum sodium with conivaptan provides a symptomatic benefit.

CONTRAINDICATIONS

Patients with hypovolemic hyponatremia. ▪ Coadministration with potent CYP3A inhibitors, such as clarithromycin, indinavir, itraconazole, ketoconazole, and ritonavir; see Drug Interactions. ▪ Anuria (no benefit expected).

PRECAUTIONS

For IV use only. ▪ Use only in hospitalized patients. ▪ Safety for use in hypervolemic hyponatremic patients with underlying CHF has not been established. Should be used to raise sodium in these patients only after other treatment options have been considered. Incidence of adverse cardiac events may be increased. ▪ An overly rapid increase in serum sodium concentration (more than 12 mEq/L/24 hr) may result in serious sequelae. Although not observed in clinical trials, osmotic demyelination syndrome has been reported following rapid correction of low serum sodium concentration. Osmotic demyelination results in dysarthria, mutism, dysphagia, lethargy, affective changes, spastic quadriparesis, seizures, coma, or death. Patients with severe malnutrition, alcoholism, or advanced liver disease may be at increased risk; use slower rates of correction; see Monitor. ▪ Reduced doses required in patients with moderate or severe hepatic impairment; see Dose Adjustments. ▪ May cause significant infusion site reaction; see Monitor.

Monitor: Administer via a large vein. Monitor infusion site and rotate every 24 hours. ▪ Monitor serum sodium concentration and neurologic status closely during therapy. If an overly rapid increase in serum sodium concentration occurs (greater than 12 mEq/L/24 hr), administration should be discontinued. If the sodium continues to rise, administration should not be resumed. If hyponatremia persists or recurs (after initial interruption of therapy) and the patient has no evidence of neurologic sequelae, conivaptan may be resumed at a reduced dose. ▪ Monitor vital signs, urine output and osmolality, and volume status of patient. Discontinue therapy in patients who develop hypotension or hypovolemia. Once the patient is again euvolemic and is no longer hypotensive, therapy may be resumed at a reduced dose; see Dose Adjustments.

Patient Education: Promptly report any burning at the infusion site or other side effects. ▪ Request assistance for ambulation. ▪ Review list of allergies and medications with physician or pharmacist.

Maternal/Child: Use during pregnancy only if benefits justify risk to the fetus. Has been shown to cause fetal harm in animals. ▪ Discontinue breast-feeding. ▪ Safety and effectiveness for use in pediatric patients have not been studied.

Elderly: Response similar to that seen in the general study population.

DRUG/LAB INTERACTIONS

A substrate of CYP3A. Concomitant use with **potent CYP3A4** inhibitors such as clarithromycin, indinavir, itraconazole, ketoconazole, and ritonavir increases conivaptan exposure and is contraindicated. ▪ A potent inhibitor of CYP3A. Coadministration with **CYP3A4 substrates** (e.g., amlodipine, midazolam, and simvastatin) results in increased exposure of the other drug. Avoid concomitant use with drugs eliminated primarily by CYP3A-mediated metabolism. Subsequent treatment with CYP3A substrates may be initiated no sooner than 1 week after the infusion of conivaptan is complete. ▪ May decrease clearance and increase serum concentration of **digoxin.** Monitor digoxin levels.

SIDE EFFECTS

The most common adverse reactions are infusion site reactions (e.g., erythema, pain, phlebitis), fever, headache, hypokalemia, and orthostatic hypotension. Other reactions that occurred in more than 2% of patients include anemia, atrial fibrillation, confusion, constipation, diarrhea, hypertension, hypomagnesemia, hyponatremia, hypotension, insomnia, nausea, peripheral edema, pharyngolaryngeal pain, pneumonia, pruritus, pyrexia, ST segment depression on ECG, thirst, urinary tract infection, and vomiting.

ANTIDOTE

Notify physician of any side effects. Most will be treated symptomatically. Discontinue therapy if there is an overly rapid increase in serum sodium concentration or if the patient experiences hypotension or hypovolemia. Discontinue therapy permanently if neurologic sequelae are present; see Precautions, Monitor, and Dose Adjustments. Resuscitate as necessary.

COSYNTROPIN

(koh-**SIN**-troh-pin)

Cortrosyn

Diagnostic agent
(adrenocorticotropic)

pH 5.5 to 7.5

USUAL DOSE

Pretreatment: See Drug/Lab Interactions. Baseline blood draw indicated.

Cosyntropin: 250 mcg (0.25 mg). The liquid formulation of cosyntropin is for IV use only. Cortrosyn may be used IV or IM.

PEDIATRIC DOSE

Pediatric patients over 2 years of age: See Usual Dose.

Pediatric patients 2 years of age or less: 125 mcg (0.125 mg).

DILUTION

Available as a lyophilized powder or as a solution. Reconstitute powder with 1 mL NS. For IV use, both formulations should be diluted with 2 to 5 mL of NS. May be given directly IV after this initial dilution or further diluted in D5W or NS and given as an infusion (250 mcg in 250 mL equals 1 mcg/mL).

Storage: *Lyophilized powder:* Store at CRT. *Liquid formulation:* Store at 2° to 8° C (36° to 46° F); protect from light and freezing. Discard any unused drug.

COMPATIBILITY

Manufacturer states, "Should not be added to blood or plasma; may be inactivated by enzymes." Consider specific use.

RATE OF ADMINISTRATION

IV injection: A single dose over 2 minutes.

Infusion: A single dose at a rate of approximately 40 mcg/hr over 6 hours. Used to provide a greater stimulus to the adrenal gland. Infusions over 4 to 8 hours have been used.

ACTIONS

A synthetic subunit of adrenocorticotropic hormone (ACTH). Stimulates the adrenal cortex to secrete adrenocortical steroids (17-OH corticosteroids, 17-ketosteroids, and/or 17-ketogenic steroids). Does not increase cortisol secretion in patients with primary adrenocortical insufficiency. Peak plasma cortisol levels occur in 1 to 2 hours depending on formulation used.

INDICATIONS AND USES

Diagnostic aid for screening patients presumed to have adrenocortical insufficiency.

CONTRAINDICATIONS

Hypersensitivity to cosyntropin, synthetic ACTH, or any of the excipients.

PRECAUTIONS

Hypersensitivity reactions, including anaphylaxis, have been reported. Administer in a facility equipped to monitor the patient and respond to any medical emergency. ▪ Cosyntropin is preferable to ACTH because it is less likely to cause hypersensitivity reactions. May be used in patients who have had a hypersensitivity reaction to natural ACTH. ▪ Accuracy of diagnosis can be complicated by concomitant medications; see Drug/Lab Interactions. ▪ Any condition that elevates or lowers cortisol binding globulin levels can increase or decrease plasma total cortisol levels, respectively. For example, cortisol binding globulin levels can be low in cirrhosis or nephrotic syndrome.

Monitor: Collect a baseline blood sample of 6 to 7 mL before administration of cosyntropin. Collect a second blood sample 30 minutes and/or 60 minutes after administration; see prescribing information for sampling and blood storage requirements. Stimulated plasma cortisol levels of less than 18 to 20 mcg/dL at 30 or 60 minutes after cosyntropin administration are suggestive of adrenocortical insufficiency. ▪ Measurement of cortisol binding globulin levels may be recommended to ensure accuracy of interpretation of plasma total cortisol levels. ▪ Monitor for S/S of hypersensitivity reactions. ▪ Check BP frequently; may cause elevated BP and salt and water retention. ▪ See Drug/Lab Interactions and Precautions.

Patient Education: Promptly report S/S of a hypersensitivity reaction (e.g., hives, rash, shortness of breath or troubled breathing, swelling of eyelids, lips, or face).

Maternal/Child: Category C: use during pregnancy only if benefits outweigh risks. ▪ Use with caution during breast-feeding.

DRUG/LAB INTERACTIONS

Cortisone or hydrocortisone use may falsely elevate or, in a paradoxical response, lower plasma cortisol levels. **Spironolactone** use may also result in a falsely elevated cortisol level. Patients receiving cortisone, hydrocortisone, or spironolactone should omit their pretest doses on the day of testing. ▪ Use of **synthetic glucocorticoid preparations** (oral, inhaled, or injectable) might suppress plasma cortisol levels. ▪ Use of **estrogen-containing products** increases cortisol binding globulin levels, which can elevate plasma total cortisol levels. Discontinue estrogen-containing products 4 to 6 weeks before testing. Alternatively, concomitant measurement of cortisol binding globulin at the time of testing can be done; if cortisol binding globulin levels are elevated, plasma total cortisol levels are considered inaccurate. ▪ May accentuate electrolyte loss associated with **diuretic therapy.**

SIDE EFFECTS

Bradycardia, hypertension, peripheral edema, rash, and tachycardia have been reported. Hypersensitivity reactions, including anaphylaxis (rare), have occurred.

ANTIDOTE

Notify the physician of any side effect. Keep epinephrine and diphenhydramine available to treat anaphylaxis. Resuscitate as necessary.

CYCLOPHOSPHAMIDE
(sye-kloh-**FOS**-fah-myd)

Antineoplastic
(alkylating agent/
nitrogen mustard)

Lyophilized Cytoxan, ✦Procytox

pH 3 to 7.5

USUAL DOSE
Pretreatment: Verify pregnancy status.

Although effective alone in susceptible malignancies, cyclophosphamide is more frequently used concurrently or sequentially with other antineoplastic agents. **Doses may be expressed in mg/kg or mg/M².** During or immediately after administration, adequate amounts of fluid should be ingested or infused to force diuresis and thus reduce the risk of urinary toxicity. Cyclophosphamide should be administered in the morning; see Monitor.

Malignant diseases (adult and pediatric patients): *As a single agent:* The initial dose may be 40 to 50 mg/kg of body weight, usually given in divided doses over 2 to 5 days. Alternate dosing schedules are 3 to 5 mg/kg twice weekly or 10 to 15 mg/kg every 7 to 10 days. Higher doses have been used with some protocols based on the condition being treated. Adequate hydration is indicated, and the use of mesna can be considered to attenuate or reduce the incidence of hemorrhagic cystitis. **Combination protocols:** Numerous combination therapies are in use. Has been used with bleomycin, bortezomib, carboplatin, cisplatin, dacarbazine, dexamethasone, docetaxel, doxorubicin, epirubicin, etoposide, fludarabine, fluorouracil, methotrexate, prednisone, procarbazine, rituximab, topotecan, vinblastine, and vincristine. See literature for various regimens.

Adjuvant treatment of operable node-positive breast cancer: Treatment protocol includes cyclophosphamide, doxorubicin, and docetaxel. Administer cyclophosphamide 500 mg/M² and doxorubicin 50 mg/M². One hour later, give docetaxel 75 mg/M². Repeat every 3 weeks for 6 cycles. See docetaxel (Taxotere) and doxorubicin (Adriamycin) monographs.

PEDIATRIC DOSE
Malignant diseases: See Usual Dose.

DOSE ADJUSTMENTS
Dosages must be adjusted based on antitumor activity and/or leukopenia. Total leukocyte count is a good, objective guide for regulating dosage. Withhold therapy in patients with neutrophils less than or equal to 1,500/mm³ and platelets less than 50,000/mm³. ▪ When used as a component of a multidrug regimen, it may be necessary to reduce the dose of cyclophosphamide as well as the doses of the other drugs. ▪ Dosing should be cautious in the elderly. Lower-end initial doses may be indicated. Consider decrease in cardiac, hepatic, and renal function; concomitant disease; or other drug therapy; see Elderly.

DILUTION
Specific techniques required; see Precautions. Contains no preservatives; aseptic technique imperative. Each 100 mg must be diluted with 5 mL of NS or SWFI; yields 20 mg/mL (a 2% solution). Shake solution gently and allow to stand until clear. A 2% solution reconstituted with NS may be injected directly or further diluted to a minimum concentration of 0.2% (2 mg/mL) for infusion. A 2% solution reconstituted with SWFI is hypotonic and should not be injected directly. It **must** be further diluted to a minimum concentration of 0.2% (2 mg/mL). D5W, ½NS, and D5NS are **compatible** diluents. Do not use heat to facilitate dilution. See Monitor.

Filters: May be filtered through available micron sizes of cellulose ester membrane filters.
Storage: Store unopened vials at or below 25° C (77° F). Cyclophosphamide that is reconstituted in SWFI must be used immediately. Do not store. If reconstituted in NS or further diluted, it must be used within 24 hours when stored at RT. Solutions reconstituted in NS or further diluted in ½NS are stable up to 6 days if refrigerated. Solutions

further diluted in D5W or D5NS are stable for 36 hours if refrigerated. Do not use cyclophosphamide vials if there are signs of melting (clear or yellowish viscous liquid or droplets).

COMPATIBILITY

Compatibility information not available from manufacturer. Other sources suggest specific **compatibilities** dependent on concentration and manufacturer; consult a pharmacist.

RATE OF ADMINISTRATION

Rate may vary depending on protocol. May be given by IV push or as an intermittent or continuous infusion. Inject or infuse very slowly to reduce the likelihood of adverse reactions that may be administration rate–dependent (e.g., facial swelling, headache, nasal congestion, scalp burning). Duration of infusion should be appropriate for the volume to be infused.

ACTIONS

An alkylating agent of the nitrogen mustard group with antitumor activity; cell cycle phase nonspecific, but most effective in S phase. Cyclophosphamide is a prodrug that is activated by hepatic microsomal enzymes. It is thought to prevent cell division by cross-linking DNA strands and preventing DNA synthesis. Elimination half-life is 3 to 12 hours. Metabolized in the liver, it or its metabolites are excreted in the urine. Secreted in breast milk.

INDICATIONS AND USES

Although effective alone in susceptible malignancies, cyclophosphamide is more frequently used concurrently or sequentially with other antineoplastic agents. Cyclophosphamide has been used in the treatment of the following malignancies: malignant lymphomas (e.g., Hodgkin disease, lymphocytic lymphoma, mixed-cell–type lymphomas, histiocytic lymphoma, Burkitt's lymphoma), multiple myeloma, leukemias (e.g., chronic lymphocytic leukemia, chronic granulocytic leukemia, acute myelogenous and monocytic leukemia, acute lymphoblastic [stem cell] leukemia in children), mycosis fungoides, neuroblastoma, adenocarcinoma of the ovary, retinoblastoma, and carcinoma of the breast. ▪ Adjuvant treatment of operable node-positive breast cancer in combination with doxorubicin and docetaxel. ▪ Used orally to treat many other indications, including biopsy-proven nephrotic syndrome, in pediatric patients when disease fails to respond to primary therapy or when primary therapy causes intolerable side effects.

Limitation of use: Safety and effectiveness for the treatment of nephrotic syndrome in adults or of other renal disease have not been established.

Unlabeled uses: Ewing's sarcoma, granulomatosis with polyangiitis (GPA, Wegener's granulomatosis), lupus nephritis, non-Hodgkin lymphoma, severe rheumatologic conditions. ▪ Transplant conditioning and many others; see literature.

CONTRAINDICATIONS

Hypersensitivity to cyclophosphamide, any of its metabolites, or to other components of the product. ▪ Urinary outflow obstruction.

PRECAUTIONS

Follow guidelines for handling cytotoxic agents. See Appendix A. ▪ Administered by or under the direction of the physician specialist. ▪ Myelosuppression (leukopenia, neutropenia, thrombocytopenia, and anemia), bone marrow failure, and severe immunosuppression may lead to serious and sometimes fatal infections. Sepsis and septic shock can occur. Latent infections (e.g., tuberculosis, viral hepatitis) can be reactivated. ▪ Hemorrhagic cystitis, pyelitis, ureteritis, and hematuria have been reported. Urotoxicity can be fatal. ▪ Exclude or correct any urinary tract obstructions before starting treatment; see Contraindications. ▪ Use with caution, if at all, in patients with active urinary tract infections. ▪ Myocarditis, myopericarditis, pericardial effusions including cardiac tamponade, and congestive heart failure have been reported and may be fatal. Supraventricular and ventricular arrhythmias (including severe QT prolongation) have been reported. Risk of cardiotoxicity may be increased with high doses, in the elderly, in patients with pre-existing cardiac disease, and in patients with previous radiation treatment to the cardiac region and/or previous or concomitant treatment with other cardiotoxic drugs (e.g., bleomycin, doxorubicin). ▪ Pneumonitis, pulmonary fibrosis, pulmonary veno-occlusive disease, and other forms of pulmonary toxicity leading to respiratory failure have been reported during and after treatment with cyclophosphamide. Late-onset pneumonitis (greater than 6 months after the start of therapy) appears to be associated with increased mortality. Pneumonitis may develop years after treatment. ▪ Development of secondary malignancies has been reported in patients treated with cyclophosphamide used alone or in association with other antineoplastic agents. May develop several years after treatment has been discontinued. ▪ Risk of bladder cancer may be reduced by prevention of hemorrhagic cystitis. ▪ Veno-occlusive disease (VOD) has been reported. Fatalities have occurred. A cytoreductive regimen in preparation for bone marrow transplantation that consists of cyclophosphamide in combination with whole-body irradiation, busulfan, or other agents has been identified as a major risk factor. VOD has also been reported to develop gradually in patients receiving long-term, low-dose, immunosuppressive doses of cyclophosphamide; in patients with pre-existing hepatic impairment; in patients who have received abdominal radiation; and in patients with low performance status. ▪ Hyponatremia associated with increased total body water, acute water intoxication, and a condition that resembles syndrome of inappropriate antidiuretic hormone secretion (SIADH) has been reported. ▪ Use caution in patients with impaired renal function. ▪ Use with caution in patients with impaired hepatic function. Reduced conversion to active metabolite may cause decreased efficacy. ▪ May interfere with normal wound healing. ▪ Do not administer any live virus vaccine to patients receiving antineoplastic drugs. ▪ Anaphylaxis resulting in death has been reported.

Monitor: Monitor CBC and platelets and SCr frequently; see Dose Adjustments. ▪ Check urinary sediment regularly for presence of erythrocytes and other signs of urotoxicity and/or nephrotoxicity. ▪ Aggressive hydration with forced diuresis and frequent bladder emptying can reduce the frequency and severity of bladder toxicity. Mesna has been used to prevent severe bladder toxicity. ▪ Monitor patients with severe renal impairment (CrCl 10 to 24 mL/min) for signs and symptoms of toxicity. ▪ Observe continuously for infection. Prophylactic antibiotics may be indicated pending results of C/S in a febrile neutropenic patient. Antimycotics and/or antivirals may also be indicated. ▪ Monitor patients with risk factors for cardiotoxicity. ▪ Monitor patients for signs and symptoms of pulmonary toxicity. ▪ Use antiemetics for patient comfort. ▪ Monitor for thrombocytopenia (platelet count less than 50,000/mm^3). Initiate precautions to prevent excessive bleeding (e.g., inspect IV sites, skin, and mucous membranes; use extreme care during invasive procedures; test urine, emesis, stool, and secretions for occult blood).

Patient Education: Effective birth control recommended. Female patients should use highly effective contraception during and for up to 1 year after completion of treatment. Male patients with a female partner who is or may become pregnant should use a condom during and for at least 4 months after treatment. ▪ Male and female reproductive function and fertility may be impaired. ▪ Interferes with oogenesis and spermatogenesis. May cause sterility in both sexes. ▪ Increase fluid intake and void frequently. ▪ Promptly report any signs or symptoms of infection, any urinary symptoms, new or worsening shortness of breath, cough, swelling of the ankles/legs, palpitations, weight gain, dizziness, loss of consciousness, or other side effects. ▪ See Appendix D.

Maternal/Child: Category D: may produce fetal harm. ▪ Discontinue breast-feeding. ▪ Safety profile in pediatric patients similar to that of adults. ▪ See Patient Education.

Elderly: Consider age-related organ impairment. Dose selection should be cautious; see Dose Adjustments. Toxicity may be increased. Monitoring of renal function is suggested.

DRUG/LAB INTERACTIONS

Severe myelosuppression may be expected in patients pretreated with and/or receiving concomitant chemotherapy and/or radiation therapy. ▪ Concomitant use of **protease inhibitors** (e.g., atazanavir, indinavir, nelfinavir, ritonavir, saquinavir) may increase the concentration of cytotoxic metabolites. Use of protease inhibitor–based regimens was found to be associated with a higher incidence of infections and neutropenia in patients receiving cyclophosphamide, doxorubicin, and etoposide (CDE) than in patients receiving a nonnucleoside reverse transcriptase inhibitor–based regimen (e.g., delavirdine [Rescriptor], nevirapine [Viramune]). ▪ Increased hematotoxicity and/or immunosuppression may result from the combined effect of cyclophosphamide and **ACE inhibitors** (e.g., enalapril, lisinopril), **allopurinol, natalizumab, paclitaxel, thiazide diuretics** (e.g., hydrochlorothiazide), and **zidovudine**. ▪ Cardiotoxicity may result from a combined effect of cyclophosphamide and **anthracyclines** (e.g., doxorubicin, liposomal doxorubicin, epirubicin), **cytarabine, pentostatin** (Nipent), **radiation therapy** of the cardiac region, and **trastuzumab**. ▪ Increased pulmonary toxicity may result from a combined effect of cyclophosphamide and **amiodarone, filgrastim**, and **sargramostim**. ▪ Increased nephrotoxicity may result from the combined effect of cyclophosphamide and **amphotericin B and indomethacin**. ▪ Risk of hepatotoxicity is increased when administered with **azathioprine**. ▪ Increased incidence of hepatic VOD and mucositis when administered with **busulfan**. ▪ Increased incidence of mucositis when administered with **protease inhibitors** (e.g., atazanavir, indinavir, nelfinavir, ritonavir, saquinavir). ▪ Increased risk of hemorrhagic cystitis may result from a combined effect of cyclophosphamide and past or concomitant **radiation treatment**. ▪ Higher incidence of noncutaneous malignant solid tumors in patients with Wegener's granulomatosis when administered with **etanercept**. ▪ Acute encephalopathy has been reported in patients receiving **metronidazole** and cyclophosphamide. ▪ Concomitant use with **tamoxifen** may increase the risk of thromboembolic complications. ▪ May increase or decrease activity of **anticoagulants** (e.g., warfarin); monitor INR and adjust dose as indicated. ▪ May reduce serum **digoxin** and **cyclosporine** levels. ▪ May prolong neuromuscular blockade and prolonged respiratory depression caused by **succinylcholine**. These effects are dose dependent and may occur up to several days after cyclophosphamide is discontinued. Alert the anesthesiologist. ▪ May decrease effectiveness of oral **quinolone antibiotics** (e.g., ciprofloxacin, levofloxacin). ▪ Capable of many other interactions.

SIDE EFFECTS

The most commonly reported side effects are alopecia (regrowth may be slightly darker), diarrhea, febrile neutropenia, fever, nausea, neutropenia, and vomiting. Other side effects include abdominal pain, amenorrhea, anorexia, gonadal suppression, impaired wound healing, leukopenia (see Precautions), malaise, mucosal ulcerations, darkening of skin and fingernails, susceptibility to infection, including opportunistic infections.

Major: Anaphylaxis, bone marrow suppression (anemia, leukopenia, thrombocytopenia) or failure, hemorrhagic cystitis or ureteritis (reversible), infection, pneumonitis, pulmonary fibrosis, rash, renal tubular necrosis (reversible), secondary neoplasia, SIADH, urinary tract and renal toxicity (e.g., bladder fibrosis, hemorrhagic cystitis, ureteritis), veno-occlusive disease.

Post-Marketing: Numerous side effects have been identified from post-marketing surveillance. These include acute respiratory distress syndrome, arthralgia, ascites, asthenia, bronchospasm, cardiotoxicity (e.g., arrhythmias, cardiac arrest, cardiac failure, cardiogenic shock, cardiomyopathy, myocardial infarction, myocarditis, pericarditis), chest pain, chills, cholestasis, colitis, convulsions, disseminated intravascular coagulation, dizziness, dyspnea, edema, encephalopathy, fatigue, fever, fluid retention, headache, hemolytic-uremic syndrome, hepatic encephalopathy, hepatitis, hepatotoxicity with hepatic failure, hyperglycemia, hypertension, hypoglycemia, hyponatremia, hypotension, increased liver function tests, infusion site reactions, interstitial pneumonitis, malaise, muscle spasms, myalgia, pancreatitis, paresthesia, peripheral neuropathy, pruritus, pulmonary edema, radiation recall dermatitis, reversible posterior leukoencephalopathy syndrome, rhabdomyolysis, Stevens-Johnson syndrome, stomatitis, toxic epidermal necrolysis, visual impairment, and many others.

ANTIDOTE

No specific antidote available. Minor side effects will be treated symptomatically if necessary. Discontinue the drug in cases of severe hemorrhagic cystitis. Urotoxicity may require interruption of treatment or cystectomy. Mesna has been used to decrease the incidence of cystitis. Interrupt therapy, reduce dose, or discontinue in patients who have or who develop potentially serious infections. Administration of whole blood products (e.g., packed RBCs, platelets, leukocytes) and/or blood modifiers (e.g., darbepoetin alfa [Aranesp], epoetin alfa [Epogen], filgrastim [Neupogen, Zarxio], pegfilgrastim [Neulasta], sargramostim [Leukine]) may be indicated to treat bone marrow toxicity. Leukocyte and thrombocyte nadirs are usually reached in the first or second week of treatment. Peripheral blood cell counts are expected to normalize after approximately 20 days. Supportive therapy as indicated will help sustain the patient in toxicity. Cyclophosphamide and its metabolites are dialyzable.

CYCLOSPORINE BBW
(sye-kloh-**SPOR**-een)

Immunosuppressant

Sandimmune

USUAL DOSE
Pretreatment: Baseline studies may be indicated; see Monitor.

Cyclosporine: 5 to 6 mg/kg of body weight as a single dose 4 to 12 hours before transplantation. Repeat once each day until oral dosage form can be tolerated. Individualized adjustment is imperative and may be required on a daily basis. Administered at one-third of the oral dose in patients temporarily unable to take oral cyclosporine. Administered in conjunction with adrenal corticosteroids; different regimens used; see prescribing information.

PEDIATRIC DOSE
Same as adult dose; however, higher doses may be required. See Maternal/Child.

DOSE ADJUSTMENTS
Reduced dose may be required in impaired renal function and in patients with severe hepatic impairment. ▪ Higher doses may be required in pediatric patients. ▪ Lower-end doses may be indicated in the elderly. Consider impaired organ function and concomitant disease or other drug therapy. ▪ Cyclosporine (Sandimmune) is not bioequivalent to Neoral (a brand of cyclosporine oral solution). Conversion from Neoral dosing to Sandimmune may result in lower cyclosporine blood concentrations. Blood concentration monitoring is indicated to avoid potential underdosing. ▪ See Monitor and Drug/Lab Interactions.

DILUTION
Each 50 mg should be diluted immediately before use with 20 to 100 mL of NS or D5W and given as an infusion. May leach phthalate from polyvinylchloride containers; use diluents in glass infusion bottles. Dilute immediately before use and discard unused portion.

Filters: Filtered through a 0.45-micron polypropylene filter during manufacturing. Has a high ethanol content, which the filter must accommodate. A large-bore needle filter may be used when withdrawing cyclosporine from an ampule. Adsorption should be negligible, but if there is concern, draw diluent through the same filter. In-line filtering is acceptable. Manufacturer indicates that cyclosporine molecules are small enough to pass through an in-line filter as small as 0.22 microns. Loss of potency is not expected. Another source used 0.22- and 0.45-micron filters and indicates an initial loss of potency that recovered to full concentration.

Storage: Before use, store ampules at CRT. Protect from light. Discard diluted solution after 24 hours.

COMPATIBILITY
Leaches out plasticizers, including DEHP from PVC infusion bags and IV tubing; use of non-PVC containers and IV tubing recommended.

Other sources suggest a few specific **compatibilities** dependent on concentration and manufacturer; consult a pharmacist.

RATE OF ADMINISTRATION

A single dose properly diluted as a slow IV infusion equally distributed over 2 to 6 hours.

ACTIONS

A potent immunosuppressive agent. Interferes with IL-2 production and blocks T-cell proliferative signals during early T-cell activation. Prolongs survival of kidney, liver, and heart allogeneic transplants in the human. Measured by specific or nonspecific assays. Extensively metabolized by the cytochrome P_{450} hepatic enzyme system. Half-life is 19 hours (range 10 to 27 hours). Primarily excreted in bile and to a small extent in urine. Crosses the placental barrier. Secreted in breast milk.

INDICATIONS AND USES

Prophylaxis of organ rejection in kidney, liver, and heart allogeneic transplants in conjunction with adrenocortical steroids. ▪ Treatment of chronic rejection in patients previously treated with other immunosuppressive agents. Reserve parenteral formulation for when oral administration not feasible.

Unlabeled uses: Decrease frequency of pancreatic or corneal allograft rejection. ▪ Prevention of acute graft-versus-host disease. ▪ Crohn's disease.

CONTRAINDICATIONS

Hypersensitivity to cyclosporine or to Cremophor EL (polyoxyethylated castor oil).

PRECAUTIONS

Anaphylactic reactions have been reported with the IV formulation. These reactions may be related to the IV vehicle Cremophor EL; patients who experienced these reactions have subsequently been treated with the oral formulation of cyclosporine without incident. Because of the risk of anaphylaxis, IV cyclosporine should be reserved for patients who are unable to take oral therapy. ▪ Usually administered in the hospital by or under the direction of a physician experienced in immunosuppressive therapy and management of organ transplant patients. ▪ Adequate laboratory and supportive medical resources must be available. ▪ All formulations may be given concomitantly with adrenocortical steroids. Manufacturer has a Black Box Warning. *Do not administer cyclosporine with any other immunosuppressive agent except adrenocortical steroids.* ▪ Can cause hepatotoxicity and nephrotoxicity; see Monitor. In impaired renal function, if rejection is severe, try other immunosuppressive therapy or allow rejection and removal of the kidney rather than increase dose of cyclosporine. ▪ May cause lymphomas and other malignancies, particularly those of the skin. Increased risk of developing a malignancy appears to be related to the intensity and duration of immunosuppression. Some malignancies may be fatal. ▪ Patients receiving immunosuppressive therapies, including cyclosporine and cyclosporine-containing regimens, are at increased risk for infections (viral, bacterial, fungal, protozoal). Both generalized and localized infections can occur. Opportunistic infections include polyomavirus infections (e.g., JC virus–associated progressive multifocal leukoencephalopathy [PML]; polyoma virus–associated nephropathy [PVAN], especially due to BK virus infection). Pre-existing infections may be aggravated. Latent infections may be reactivated. Fatal outcomes have been reported. ▪ Encephalopathy has been reported, including posterior reversible encephalopathy syndrome (PRES). May manifest as impaired consciousness, convulsions, visual disturbances (including blindness), loss of motor function, movement disorders, and psychiatric disturbances. Predisposing factors may include hypertension, hypomagnesemia, hypocholesterolemia, high-dose corticosteroids, high cyclosporine blood levels, and graft-versus-host disease. Patients receiving liver transplants may be more susceptible to encephalopathy than patients receiving kidney transplants. Reversal of encephalopathy has occurred after discontinuation or dose reduction of cyclosporine. ▪ Convulsions have been reported, particularly in patients receiving concomitant therapy with high-dose methylprednisolone. ▪ Significant hyperkalemia (sometimes associated with hyperchloremic acidosis) and hyperuricemia have been reported. ▪ A syndrome of thrombocytopenia and microangiopathic hemolytic anemia that may result in graft failure has been reported. ▪ Optic disc edema, including papilledema, with possible visual impairment secondary to benign intracranial hypertension has been reported. ▪ See Drug/Lab Interactions.

Monitor: Observe for S/S of an anaphylactic reaction (e.g., blood pressure changes; bronchospasm; dyspnea; edema of face, tongue, or throat; itching; rash; tachycardia; wheezing). Monitor continuously for the first 30 minutes of the infusion and frequently thereafter. ▪ Can cause hepatotoxicity and nephrotoxicity. Monitor BUN, SCr, serum bilirubin, and liver enzymes frequently. Timing and amount of rise in BUN and creatinine and degree of nephrotoxicity or hepatotoxicity distinguish between need for dose reduction or symptoms of organ rejection. ▪ May be difficult to distinguish between nephrotoxicity and rejection. Up to 20% of patients may have simultaneous nephrotoxicity and rejection. See package insert for a chart discussing differential diagnoses for each. ▪ Monitor cyclosporine blood levels. Measured by specific or nonspecific assay. 24-hour specific trough values of 100 to 200 ng/mL of whole blood or 24-hour nonspecific trough values of 250 to 800 ng/mL of whole blood minimize side effects and rejection events. Nonspecific assays trough values are higher because they include metabolites. Plasma levels may range from $\frac{1}{2}$ to $\frac{1}{5}$ of whole blood levels. Consistent use of one assay is recommended. Confirm assay method to evaluate appropriately. ▪ Observe constantly for signs of infection (fever, sore throat, tiredness) or unusual bleeding or bruising. ▪ Prophylactic antibiotics may be indicated pending results of C/S. ▪ Monitor for development of PVAN and BK virus–associated nephropathy (e.g., deteriorating renal function and renal graft loss). Dose reduction may be indicated. ▪ Monitor for development of PML (e.g., apathy, ataxia, cognitive deficiencies, confusion, hemiparesis). If symptoms appear, consultation with a neurologist may be indicated. ▪ Monitor BP. Hypertension is a common side effect. Initiation or modification of antihypertensive therapy may be indicated; do not use potassium-sparing diuretics (e.g., spironolactone [Aldactone]); may increase risk of hyperkalemia. ▪ Monitor for S/S of encephalopathy and/or PRES. ▪ See Precautions and Drug/Lab Interactions.

Patient Education: Use effective birth control. Do not use oral contraceptives. See Appendix D. ▪ Do not make any changes in formulation (e.g., IV, capsules, oral solution) without physician direction; products are not equivalent. May require dose adjustment. ▪ Review side effects with a health care professional and report all side effects promptly. ▪ Capable of multiple drug-drug interactions; obtain physician approval before adding or stopping medications. ▪ Compliance with frequent laboratory tests is imperative.

Maternal/Child: Category C: safety for use in pregnancy not established. Should not be used unless benefit to the mother justifies potential risk to the fetus. Use in men and women capable of conception not established. Reported outcomes of pregnancies in women who received cyclosporine are difficult to evaluate. It is not possible to separate the effects of cyclosporine from the effects of other medications, underlying maternal disorders, or other aspects of the transplantation process. Negative outcomes included prematurity, low birth weight, fetal loss, and various malformations. ▪ Discontinue breast-feeding. ▪ Safety for use in pediatric patients not established but has been used in patients as young as 6 months of age. Accidental parenteral overdose in premature neonates has caused serious symptoms of intoxication.

Elderly: Dose selection should be cautious; see Dose Adjustments. ▪ Differences in response compared to younger adults not identified.

DRUG/LAB INTERACTIONS

Interactions are numerous and potentially life threatening. Review of drug profile by pharmacist imperative. ▪ Risk of nephrotoxicity increased when given with other drugs that may potentiate renal dysfunction. Use extreme caution and monitor renal function closely. If impairment of renal function is significant, either reduce the dose of cyclosporine and/or the coadministered drug, or consider an alternative treatment. Manufacturer lists **antibiotics** (e.g., ciprofloxacin, gentamicin, tobramycin, sulfamethoxazole/trimethoprim, vancomycin), **antifungals** (e.g., amphotericin B, ketoconazole), **anti-inflammatory drugs** (e.g., azapropazone, colchicine, diclofenac, naproxen, sulindac), **H_2 antagonists** (e.g., cimetidine, famotidine), **immunosuppressives** (e.g., tacrolimus), **antineoplastics, and fibric acid derivatives** (e.g., fenofibrate). Other sources list **acyclovir, foscarnet** (Foscavir), **selected quinolones, and numerous other nephrotoxic drugs**. ▪ Concurrent administration with **colchicine** may cause cyclosporine toxicity (e.g., GI, hepatic, renal, and neuromuscular toxicity). Cyclosporine may decrease the clearance and increase the toxic effects of colchicine (e.g., myopathy, neuropathy), especially in patients with renal impairment. With concurrent use, close clinical observation is required. Reduce colchicine dose or discontinue as indicated. ▪ May increase **diclofenac** (Voltaren) serum levels with concomitant administration; initiate diclofenac dose at the lower end of the therapeutic range. ▪ Cyclosporine is extensively metabolized by CYP3A4 and is a substrate of the multidrug efflux transporter P-glycoprotein. **Drugs that inhibit or induce CYP3A4, P-glycoprotein transporter, or organic anion transporter proteins** will result in an alteration of cyclosporine concentrations. Toxicity or allograft rejection may occur. Compounds that decrease cyclosporine absorption, such as **orlistat**, should be avoided. ▪ Cyclosporine plasma levels may be increased with concurrent use of **protease inhibitors** (e.g., boceprevir, indinavir, nelfinavir, ritonavir, saquinavir, telaprevir), which are metabolized by cytochrome P_{450} 3A; use caution. ▪ Drugs that inhibit the cytochrome P_{450} system may decrease the metabolism of cyclosporine and increase its serum concentrations. Manufacturer lists **allopurinol, amiodarone, antibiotics** (e.g., azithromycin, clarithromycin, erythromycin, quinupristin/dalfopristin), **antifungals** (e.g., fluconazole, voriconazole), **bromocriptine, calcium channel blockers, danazol, glucocorticoids, imatinib, metoclopramide, nefazodone, and oral contraceptives.** Monitor blood levels with concurrent use to avoid cyclosporine toxicity. ▪ Drugs that decrease cyclosporine concentrations should be avoided. Manufacturer lists **antibiotics, anticonvulsants, bosentan, octreotide, orlistat, terbinafine, St. John's wort, and sulfinpyrazone.** Other sources list **sulfamethoxazole/trimethoprim;** monitor levels and adjust cyclosporine dose as indicated to avoid transplant rejection. ▪ **Rifabutin** (Mycobutin) may increase metabolism of cyclosporine; use care with concomitant use. ▪ Cyclosporine inhibits CYP3A4 and the multidrug efflux transporter P-glycoprotein and may increase plasma concentrations of co-medications that are substrates of CYP3A4, P-glycoprotein, or organic anion transporter proteins. Cyclosporine reduces clearance and may increase blood levels of **ambrisentan, bosentan, dabigatran, digoxin, etoposide, methotrexate, NSAIDs, prednisolone, repaglinide, sirolimus, and other drugs.** May decrease the volume distribution of **digoxin** and cause toxicity rather quickly. With concurrent use, monitor digoxin levels, reduce digoxin dose, or discontinue as indicated. ▪ Concomitant use with **NSAIDs**, particularly in dehydrated patients, may potentiate renal dysfunction. ▪ Avoid concurrent use with **bosentan**. ▪ When coadministering **ambrisentan** with cyclosporine, the ambrisentan dose should *not* be titrated to the recommended maximum daily dose. ▪ Cyclosporine may decrease the clearance of **HMG-CoA reductase inhibitors (statins)**. Cases of myotoxicity (including muscle pain and weakness, myositis, and rhabdomyolysis) have been reported with concomitant use. Dose reduction of statins is indicated. Statins may be temporarily withheld or discontinued in patients with S/S of myopathy or potential for renal injury, including renal failure, secondary to rhabdomyolysis. ▪ Coadministration with **aliskiren** (Tekturna) is not recommended. ▪ May decrease **mycophenolate** levels. Monitor levels closely when cyclosporine is added or removed from a drug regimen containing mycophenolate. ▪ Concurrent use of cyclosporine with **imipenem-cilastatin** may increase CNS toxicity of both agents. ▪ Potentiates **nondepolarizing muscle relaxants**; will prolong neuromuscular blockade. ▪ Do not use **potassium-sparing diuretics**; may increase risk of hyperkalemia. Use caution when coadministered with **other potassium-sparing drugs, potassium-containing drugs**, and/or in patients on a **potassium-rich diet.** Hyperkalemia can occur. ▪ May cause convulsions with high doses of **methylprednisolone**. ▪ May be given in combination with **steroids** but has additive effects with other **immunosuppressive agents**; may increase risk of lymphoma. ▪ Concurrent administration with **sirolimus** increases blood levels of sirolimus. To minimize the effect on blood levels, administer sirolimus 4 hours after cyclosporine dose. ▪ Elevations in SCr have been reported with coadministration of **sirolimus** and cyclosporine. Effect is usually reversible with cyclosporine dose reduction. ▪ Serum levels may increase with **chloroquine** (Aralen). ▪ Avoid use in psoriasis patients receiving **other immunosuppressive agents or radiation therapy, including PUVA and UVB.** Immunosuppression may be excessive. ▪ May increase the plasma concentrations of **repaglinide**, which increases the risk for hypoglycemia. Monitor blood glucose levels closely. ▪ Concurrent use with **nifedipine** has caused gingival hyperplasia; avoid use in patients who develop gingival hyperplasia. ▪ High doses of cyclosporine (e.g., IV doses of 16 mg/kg/day) may increase the exposure to **anthracycline antibiotics** in cancer patients. ▪ Monitor serum creatinine when used with **NSAIDs** in rheumatoid arthritis patients. ▪ Vaccinations may be less effective. Avoid use of **live virus vaccines** in patients receiving cyclosporine. ▪ **Grapefruit juice** may affect certain enzymes of the P_{450} enzyme system and should be avoided.

SIDE EFFECTS

The most common side effects include gum hyperplasia, hirsutism, hypertension, renal dysfunction, and tremor. Other side effects include acne, convulsions, cramps, diarrhea, encephalopathy, glomerular capillary thrombosis, headache, hepatotoxicity, hyperkalemia, hyperuricemia, hypomagnesemia, infection, leukopenia, lymphoma, microangiopathic hemolytic anemia, nausea and vomiting, paresthesia, skin rash, and thrombocytopenia. Hypersensitivity reactions including anaphylaxis have occurred. Stevens-Johnson syndrome and toxic epidermal necrolysis have occurred rarely.

Post-Marketing: Headache, including migraine; hepatotoxicity and liver injury, including cholestasis, hepatitis, jaundice, and liver failure with serious and/or fatal outcomes; isolated cases of pain in the lower extremities; JC virus–associated PML, sometimes fatal; and PVAN, especially due to BK virus infection, resulting in graft loss.

ANTIDOTE

Notify physician of all side effects. Most can be treated symptomatically. Drug may be decreased or discontinued or other immunosuppressive agents utilized. Consider reducing total immunosuppression in transplant patients who develop PML or PVAN; may place graft at risk. Discontinue infusion at the first sign of a severe hypersensitivity reaction. Treat hypersensitivity as indicated; may require oxygen, epinephrine, antihistamines (e.g., diphenhydramine), vasopressors, corticosteroids, albuterol, IV fluids, and/or ventilation equipment. Nephrotoxicity, hepatotoxicity, encephalopathy (including PRES), or hematopoietic depression may require temporary reduction of dosage or permanent withholding of treatment. Dialysis is not effective in overdose.

CYSTEINE HYDROCHLORIDE
(**SIS**-te-een)

Amino acid

Elcys, Nouress

pH 1 to 2.5

USUAL DOSE

Pretreatment: Baseline studies indicated; see Monitor.

Cysteine: Dose should be individualized based on the patient's clinical condition (ability to adequately metabolize amino acids), body weight, and nutritional/fluid requirements, as well as additional energy given orally/enterally to the patient. Before initiating parenteral nutrition, review all medications, gastrointestinal function, and laboratory data (e.g., electrolytes [including magnesium, calcium, and phosphorus], glucose, urea/creatinine, liver panel, complete blood count, and triglyceride level [if adding lipid emulsion]). Recommended daily doses for Elcys and Nouress are based on recommended daily protein (amino acid) requirement and are included in the following charts.

Recommended Daily Dose of Elcys in Pediatric Patients and Adults			
Age	Recommended Protein[a] Requirement (Gm AA/kg/day)[b]	Recommended Dosage (mg Elcys/Gm AA)	Recommended Volume (mL Elcys/Gm AA)
Preterm and term infants under 1 month of age	3 to 4 Gm/kg/day	22 mg	0.44 mL
Pediatric patients 1 month to under 1 year of age	2 to 3 Gm/kg/day	22 mg	0.44 mL
Pediatric patients 1 to 11 years of age	1 to 2 Gm/kg/day	22 mg	0.44 mL
Pediatric patients 12 to 17 years of age	0.8 to 1.5 Gm/kg/day	7 mg	0.14 mL
Adults: Stable patients	0.8 to 1 Gm/kg/day	7 mg	0.14 mL
Adults: Critically ill patients[b]	1.5 to 2 Gm/kg/day	7 mg	0.14 mL

[a]Protein is provided as amino acids (AA).
[b]Includes patients requiring more than 2 to 3 days in the ICU with organ failure, sepsis, or postoperative major surgery. Do not use in patients with conditions that are contraindicated.
AA, Amino acid.

Recommended Daily Dose of Nouress in Neonates (Preterm and Term Infants Under 1 Month of Age)			
Dosage	Protein[a] Requirement (Gm AA/kg/day)	Dosage (mg Nouress/Gm AA)	Volume (mL Nouress/Gm AA
Neonates	3 to 4 Gm/kg/day	22 mg	0.44 mL

[a]Protein is provided as amino acids (AA).

DILUTION

Available as a clear, colorless solution in 10-mL single-dose vials containing 500 mg/ 10 mL (50 mg/mL). **Must be diluted and used as an admixture in the parenteral nutrition (PN) solution.** Strict aseptic techniques must be used throughout the mixing process. Review manufacturer's specific instructions in prescribing information. Initially transfer the desired amount of cysteine into the amino acid solution (this will be used later in the mixing process). Amino acid solution containing cysteine may be mixed with dextrose injection. A specific mixing sequence must be followed to minimize pH-related problems.

- *First,* transfer dextrose injection into the parenteral nutrition pooling container;
- *Second,* transfer phosphate salt;
- *Third,* transfer the cysteine-containing amino acid solution;
- *Fourth,* transfer electrolytes; and

- *Fifth,* transfer trace elements into the pooling container. Use gentle agitation during admixing to minimize localized concentration effects; shake containers gently after each addition. Evaluate all additions for compatibility and stability; consult a pharmacist. If an automated compounder is to be used, refer to its instructions for use. Inspect the final PN solution to ensure that precipitates have not formed. Discard if any precipitates are observed.

Filters: Elcys: Use a 0.22-micron in-line filter for administration without lipid emulsion. *Nouress*: Use a 0.22-micron in-line filter for administration.

Storage: *Both formulations:* Store unopened vials at CRT. Avoid excessive heat. Protect from freezing. If accidentally frozen, discard the vial. Promptly use mixed solutions. Any storage of the admixture should be under refrigeration at 2° to 8° C (36° to 46° F) and limited to no longer than 24 hours. After removal from the refrigerator, inspect for precipitates, use promptly, and complete the infusion within 24 hours. Discard if precipitates are observed. Discard any remaining admixture. *Nouress*: Protect from light. Vial stoppers are not made with natural rubber latex.

COMPATIBILITY

Calcium and phosphate ratios must be considered. Excess addition of calcium and phosphate, especially in the form of mineral salts, may result in the formation of calcium phosphate precipitates. *Elcys:* If infused with lipid emulsion, do not use administration sets and lines that contain di-2-ethylhexyl phthalate (DEHP). Administration sets that contain polyvinyl chloride (PVC) components have DEHP as a plasticizer.

RATE OF ADMINISTRATION

Use a dedicated line for PN solutions. Infuse into a central or peripheral line. Choice of venous route depends on osmolarity of the final infusate. Solutions with osmolarity of 900 mOsm/L or greater must be infused through a central catheter. Use a nonvented infusion set to prevent air embolism. Infuse at the prescribed rate. IV lipid emulsions can be infused concurrently into the same vein as the prepared PN solution by a Y-connector located near the infusion site. Flow rates of each solution should be controlled by separate infusion pumps.

ACTIONS

Endogenous cysteine is synthesized from methionine by the enzyme cystathionase via the trans-sulfuration pathway and serves as a precursor substrate for both glutathione and taurine. Provides cysteine to the systemic circulation of patients who require PN and cannot synthesize adequate quantities of cysteine due to insufficient or deficient cystathionase activity

INDICATIONS AND USES

Elcys: Indicated for use as an additive to amino acid solutions to meet the nutritional requirements of newborn infants requiring total parenteral nutrition (TPN) and of adult and pediatric patients with severe liver disease who may have impaired enzymatic processes and require TPN. It can also be added to amino acid solutions to provide a more complete profile of amino acids for protein synthesis.

Nouress: Indicated for use as an additive to amino acids solutions to meet nutritional requirements of neonates (preterm and term infants under 1 month of age) requiring TPN.

CONTRAINDICATIONS

Known hypersensitivity to one or more amino acids. ▪ Patients with inborn errors of amino acid metabolism due to risk of severe metabolic or neurologic complications. ▪ Patients with pulmonary edema or acidosis due to low cardiac output.

PRECAUTIONS

Must be diluted and used as an admixture in PN solutions; ***NOT for direct IV infusion.*** ▪ Before administration of PN solutions, correct severe fluid, electrolyte, and acid-base disorders. ▪ Pulmonary vascular precipitates causing pulmonary vascular emboli and pulmonary distress have been reported in patients receiving PN. In some fatal cases, pulmonary embolism occurred as a result of calcium phosphate precipitates. Precipitation following passage through an in-line filter and suspected in vivo precipitate formation have also been reported. ▪ The infusion of hypertonic nutrient injections into a peripheral vein may result in vein irritation, vein damage, and/or thrombosis. Cysteine must be diluted, and solutions with an osmolarity of 900 mOsm/L or greater must be infused through a central catheter. ■ IV infusion of amino acids may induce a rise in blood urea nitrogen (BUN), especially in patients with impaired hepatic or renal function. ■ Administration may result in metabolic acidosis in preterm infants, and serum amino acid imbalances, metabolic alkalosis, prerenal azotemia, hyperammonemia, stupor, and coma in patients with hepatic impairment. ■ Hepatobiliary disorders are known to develop in some patients without pre-existing liver disease who receive PN, including cholecystitis, cholelithiasis, cholestasis, hepatic steatosis, fibrosis, and cirrhosis, possibly leading to hepatic failure. ■ Contains aluminum that may be toxic. Aluminum may reach toxic levels with prolonged parenteral administration in patients with renal impairment. Preterm infants are particularly at risk for aluminum toxicity because their kidneys are immature and because they require large amounts of calcium and phosphate solutions, which also contain aluminum. Amounts greater than 4 to 5 mcg/kg/day of parenteral aluminum can accumulate aluminum to levels associated with CNS and bone toxicity. These toxicities may occur at lower rates of administration.

Monitor: Obtain baseline CBC, electrolytes (including calcium, magnesium, and phosphorus), glucose, liver panel, urea/creatinine, and triglyceride level (if adding lipid emulsion). ■ Monitor fluid and electrolyte status, serum osmolarity, blood glucose, liver and kidney function, blood count, and coagulation parameters throughout treatment. ■ Monitor patients with hepatic or renal impairment frequently to assess function and fluid balance. ■ Monitor acid-base balance. Significant deviations from normal concentrations may require the use of additional electrolyte supplements. ■ Monitor for S/S of pulmonary distress. ■ Monitor the infusion site and catheter periodically for precipitates and signs of vein irritation. Venous thrombophlebitis is the primary complication of peripheral access. Remove catheter as soon as possible if thrombophlebitis develops. ■ Monitor for hepatobiliary disorders (acid-base balance, liver function parameters, and ammonia levels). A clinician knowledgeable in liver disease should assess patients developing signs of hepatobiliary disorders early to identify possible causative and contributory factors and possible therapeutic and prophylactic interventions. ■ Hyperammonemia in infants can result in neurocognitive delays. Monitor blood ammonia levels frequently in infants. ■ Monitor for aluminum toxicity. Elcys aluminum exposure is not more than 0.21 mcg/kg/day at recommended doses. Nouress exposure is not more than 0.25 mcg/kg/day at recommended doses.

Patient Education: Frequent laboratory monitoring required. ■ Promptly report any irritation at the infusion site, shortness of breath, or other unexpected side effects.

Maternal/Child: Neither formulation is expected to cause major birth defects, miscarriage, or adverse maternal or fetal outcomes. Nouress is not approved for use in adults. ■ Data available on the effects of cysteine on infants, either directly or through breast milk, do not suggest a significant risk of adverse reactions from exposure. ■ Safety and efficacy established for use in pediatric patients; see Indications. ■ Hyperammonemia in infants can result in neurocognitive delays. Monitor blood ammonia levels frequently in infants.

Elderly: Clinical studies with Elcys have not been performed to determine whether patients 65 years of age and older respond differently from younger patients.

DRUG/LAB INTERACTIONS
Specific information not available.

SIDE EFFECTS
Most common adverse reactions are fever, generalized flushing, local reactions (erythema, phlebitis, thrombosis at the infusion site, and warm sensation), and nausea. *Nouress* adds metabolic acidosis. Serious adverse reactions include acid-base imbalance, aluminum toxicity, hepatobiliary disorders, hyperammonemia, increased BUN, pulmonary embolism due to pulmonary vascular precipitates, and vein damage and thrombosis.

Overdose: Overhydration or solute overload may occur.

ANTIDOTE

Notify the physician of all side effects. Adverse reactions related to PN may respond to an adjustment in amino acids, dextrose, or other additives and/or an adjustment in rate. Treat symptomatically and resuscitate as necessary. Stop infusion immediately for any signs of pulmonary distress, and initiate a medical evaluation. In the event of overhydration or solute overload from overdosage, re-evaluate the patient and institute appropriate corrective measures.

CYTARABINE BBW
(sye-**TAIR**-ah-bean)

ARA-C, Cytosar♣, Cytosar-U♣

Antineoplastic
(antimetabolite)

pH 7.4 to 7.7

USUAL DOSE

Pretreatment: Verify pregnancy status. Baseline studies indicated; see Monitor.

Dose is variable depending on specific regimen or protocol. Consult guidelines for current treatment regimens.

Acute nonlymphocytic leukemia in adult and pediatric patients: *Combination chemotherapy:* Manufacturer lists a dose of 100 mg/M^2/24 hr as a continuous infusion or 100 mg/M^2 as an IV injection every 12 hours. Repeat daily on Days 1 through 7.

Acute myelocytic leukemia or erythroleukemia in adult and pediatric patients: Manufacturer lists a dose of 100 mg/M^2/24 hr as a continuous infusion or 200 mg/M^2/day continuous infusion (as 100 mg/M^2 over 12 hours every 12 hours) for 7 days.

DOSE ADJUSTMENTS

Dose reduction may be indicated in impaired hepatic or renal function. ▪ See Precautions/Monitor. ▪ Usually used with other antineoplastic drugs in specific doses to achieve tumor remission. ▪ Withhold or modify dose based on degree of bone marrow suppression; see Monitor.

DILUTION

Specific techniques required; see Precautions. Available in multiple concentrations. Read label carefully. May be given by IV injection as is or further diluted in NS or D5W and given as an infusion. Use only clear solutions.

Storage: Store unused vials at CRT in carton to protect from light. When infusion solutions are prepared in D5W or NS, 94% to 96% of cytarabine remains present after 8 days. Immediate use preferred.

COMPATIBILITY

Compatibility information not available from manufacturer. Other sources suggest specific **compatibilities** dependent on concentration and manufacturer; consult a pharmacist.

RATE OF ADMINISTRATION

IV injection: Each 100 mg or fraction thereof over 15 to 30 minutes. When large IV doses are given too quickly, patients are frequently nauseated and may vomit for several hours postinjection. This problem tends to be less severe when the drug is infused.

IV infusion: Single daily dose properly diluted over 30 minutes to 24 hours, depending on amount of infusion solution and dosage regimen.

ACTIONS

An antimetabolite that inhibits synthesis of DNA. Cell-cycle specific for S phase. It is a pyrimidine analog that is incorporated into DNA. It inhibits DNA polymerase, resulting in decreased DNA synthesis and repair. Through various chemical processes this deprivation acts more quickly on rapidly growing cells and causes their death. A potent bone marrow suppressant. Crosses the blood-brain barrier. Serum half-life averages 1 to 3 hours. Metabolized in the liver and excreted in the urine.

INDICATIONS AND USES

Used in combination with other approved anticancer drugs for remission induction in acute nonlymphocytic leukemia in adults and pediatric patients. Also used for treatment of acute lymphocytic leukemia (ALL), the blast phase of chronic myelocytic leukemia, and acute myelocytic leukemia (AML). ▪ Is used intrathecally in the treatment of meningeal leukemia. A liposomal formulation (DepoCyt) is available for intrathecal use only; lipofoam molecules contained in this product are much too large for IV use.

CONTRAINDICATIONS

Hypersensitivity to cytarabine, pre-existing drug-induced bone marrow suppression.

PRECAUTIONS

Follow guidelines for handling cytotoxic agents. See Appendix A. ▪ Administered by or under the direction of a physician specialist in a facility with adequate diagnostic and treatment facilities to monitor the patient and respond to any medical emergency. Must be able to monitor drug tolerance and protect and maintain a patient compromised by drug toxicity. The main toxic effect of cytarabine is bone marrow suppression with leukopenia, thrombocytopenia, and anemia. Complications of bone marrow suppression include infection resulting from granulocytopenia and hemorrhage secondary to thrombocytopenia. Use with caution in patients with pre-existing drug-induced bone marrow suppression. Less serious toxicity includes nausea, vomiting, diarrhea and abdominal pain, oral ulceration, and hepatic dysfunction. Weigh benefit versus risk of known toxic effects before initiating therapy. ▪ Remissions induced by cytarabine are brief unless followed by maintenance therapy. ▪ Severe, and sometimes fatal, GI, pulmonary, cardiac, or CNS toxicity has occurred with experimental cytarabine regimens. Toxicities are different (e.g., reversible corneal toxicity, hemorrhagic conjunctivitis, cerebral and cerebellar dysfunction, severe GI ulceration) from those seen with conventional therapy. Deaths have been reported. ▪ Cases of cardiomyopathy and a syndrome of sudden respiratory distress rapidly progressing to pulmonary edema and radiographically pronounced cardiomegaly have been reported following experimental high-dose therapy. ▪ Do not use product containing benzyl alcohol if experimental high-dose therapy is administered. ▪ Use with caution and possibly at reduced doses in patients with renal or hepatic impairment. ▪ May induce hyperuricemia (tumor lysis syndrome) secondary to rapid lysis of neoplastic cells. ▪ Acute pancreatitis has been reported in patients receiving cytarabine by continuous infusion and in patients being treated with cytarabine who have had prior treatment with L-asparaginase.

Monitor: Leukocyte and platelet counts should be monitored daily. ▪ During induction therapy, WBC depression is biphasic with the first nadir occurring at Days 7 to 9 and a deeper fall at Days 15 to 24. Platelet depression begins around Day 5 and reaches a nadir at Days 12 to 15. ▪ Hold or modify therapy for platelet count less than 50,000 or polymorphonuclear granulocytes less than 1,000 cells/mm^3. Counts may continue to fall after the drug is stopped and may reach lowest values after drug-free intervals of 12 to 14 days. Restart therapy when bone marrow recovery is confirmed. Patients whose drug is withheld until "normal" peripheral blood values are attained may escape from control. ▪ Monitor hepatic and renal function at regular intervals during therapy. ▪ Perform bone marrow examinations frequently after blasts have disappeared from the peripheral blood. ▪ Higher total doses tolerated by IV injection compared with IV infusion, but the incidence and intensity of nausea and vomiting are increased. ▪ Prophylactic administration of antiemetics recommended. ▪ Be alert for signs of bone marrow suppression, bleeding, infection, or neurotoxicity. These side effects are dose- and schedule-dependent. ▪ Monitor for thrombocytopenia (platelet count less than 50,000/mm^3). Initiate precautions to prevent excessive bleeding (e.g., inspect IV sites, skin, and mucous membranes; use extreme care during invasive procedures; test urine, emesis, stool, and secretions for occult blood). ▪ Prophylactic antibiotics may be indicated pending results of C/S in a febrile neutropenic patient. ▪ Monitor uric acid levels and maintain hydration; allopurinol may be indicated. ▪ Monitor for S/S of pancreatitis (e.g., elevated amylase, nausea, vomiting, upper abdominal pain).

Patient Education: Effective birth control recommended. ▪ See Appendix D. ▪ Promptly report early signs of neurotoxicity (e.g., ataxia, confusion, lethargy) or bone marrow suppression (e.g., infection, bleeding).

Maternal/Child: Avoid pregnancy. Can cause fetal harm when administered to a pregnant woman, especially during the first trimester. ▪ Discontinue breast-feeding. ▪ Benzyl alcohol may cause a fatal "gasping syndrome" in premature infants. ▪ See Drug/Lab Interactions.

Elderly: Consider age-related organ impairment; toxicity may be increased.

DRUG/LAB INTERACTIONS

May inhibit **digoxin** absorption. ▪ Do not administer any **live virus vaccines** to patients receiving antineoplastic drugs. ▪ May cause acute pancreatitis in patients who previously received **L-asparaginase.** ▪ May antagonize action of **gentamicin** against *Klebsiella.* ▪ May antagonize antifungal actions of **flucytosine**.

SIDE EFFECTS

Abdominal pain, anorexia, bleeding, bone marrow suppression (e.g., anemia, leukopenia, thrombocytopenia), bone pain, cardiomyopathy, chest pain, conjunctivitis, diarrhea, esophagitis, fever, hepatic dysfunction, hypersensitivity reactions, hyperuricemia, malaise, megaloblastosis, mucosal bleeding, myalgia, nausea, oral and anal ulceration, pancreatitis, peripheral motor and sensory neuropathies, rash, stomatitis, thrombophlebitis, vomiting. Higher than usual dose regimens may cause severe coma, GI ulcerations and peritonitis, personality changes, pulmonary toxicity, somnolence, or death.

ANTIDOTE

Notify the physician of all side effects. Most will be treated symptomatically. Some toxicity is necessary to produce remission. Discontinue or withhold the drug for serious bone marrow suppression. Administration of whole blood products (e.g., packed RBCs, platelets, leukocytes) and/or blood modifiers (e.g., darbepoetin alfa [Aranesp], epoetin alfa [Epogen], filgrastim [Neupogen, Zarxio], pegfilgrastim [Neulasta], sargramostim [Leukine]) may be indicated to treat bone marrow toxicity. Drug must be restarted as soon as signs of bone marrow recovery occur, or its effectiveness will be lost. Use corticosteroids for cytarabine syndrome (fever, myalgia, bone pain, occasional chest pain, maculopapular rash, conjunctivitis, malaise). Usually occurs in 6 to 12 hours after administration. Continue cytarabine if patient responds to corticosteroids. There is no specific antidote; supportive therapy as indicated will help to sustain the patient in toxicity.

CYTOMEGALOVIRUS IMMUNE GLOBULIN INTRAVENOUS (HUMAN) BBW*

Passive immunizing agent
Antibacterial
Antiviral

(**sigh**-toh-**meg**-ah-lo-**VIGH**-rus ih-**MUNE** GLAW-byoo-lin)

CMV-IGIV, CytoGam

*This drug is on the Black Box Warning list; however, a BBW is not provided in the parenteral prescribing information.

USUAL DOSE

150 mg/kg is the maximum recommended dose per infusion.

Kidney transplant: 150 mg/kg of body weight as an IV infusion. This initial dose must be given within 72 hours of transplant. Additional infusions of 100 mg/kg are given at 2, 4, 6, and 8 weeks posttransplant, then reduced to 50 mg/kg at 12 and 16 weeks posttransplant.

Heart, liver, lung, and pancreas transplants: 150 mg/kg of body weight as an IV infusion. This initial dose must be given within 72 hours of transplant. Consider use in combination with ganciclovir (Cytovene) 10 mg/kg/day for 14 days. Additional infusions of cytomegalovirus IGIV containing 150 mg/kg are given at 2, 4, 6, and 8 weeks posttransplant, then reduced to 100 mg/kg at 12 and 16 weeks posttransplant.

DILUTION

Absolute sterile technique required; contains no preservatives. Available in 20- and 50-mL vials (50 mg/mL); multiple vials may be required. Use only if clear and colorless. Enter vial only once and initiate infusion within 6 hours. Must be completely infused within 12 hours of dilution. See Rate of Administration.

Filters: Use of an in-line filter (pore size 15 microns [0.2 microns acceptable]) is required; see Rate of Administration.

Storage: Store dry powder in refrigerator between 2° and 8° C (36° to 46° F).

COMPATIBILITY

Administration through a separate infusion line recommended. If absolutely necessary, may be piggybacked in a pre-existing line containing NS, ½NS, dextrose 2.5%, 5%, 10%, or 20% in water or saline. Do not dilute CMV-IGIV more than one part to two parts of any of these solutions.

RATE OF ADMINISTRATION

Use of an in-line filter (pore size 15 microns [0.2 microns acceptable]) and a constant infusion pump (e.g., IVAC) is required. Begin with a rate of 15 mg/kg/hr. May be increased to 30 mg/kg/hr in 30 minutes if no discomfort or adverse effects. May be increased in another 30 minutes to 60 mg/kg/hr if no discomfort or adverse effects. Do not exceed the 60 mg/kg/hr rate or allow the volume infused to exceed 75 mL/hr regardless of mg/kg/hr dose. Slow rate of infusion at onset of patient discomfort or any adverse reactions. Infusion must be complete within 12 hours of dilution. Subsequent doses may be increased at 15-minute intervals using the same mg/kg/hr rates and adhering to the volume maximum of 75 mL/hr.

ACTIONS

A sterile solution of immunoglobulin G (IgG). Derived from pooled adult human plasma selected for high titers of antibody for cytomegalovirus (CMV). Purified by a specific process. Can raise the relevant antibody levels sufficiently to attenuate or reduce the incidence of serious CMV disease. Antibody levels will last 2 to 3 weeks. Recent studies of combined prophylaxis with CMV-IGIV and ganciclovir have shown reductions in the incidence of serious CMV-associated disease in CMV-seronegative recipients of CMV-seropositive organs below that expected from one drug alone.

INDICATIONS AND USES

Prophylaxis of CMV disease associated with transplantation of kidney, heart, liver, lung, and pancreas. In transplants of these organs other than kidney from CMV-seropositive donors to seronegative recipients, prophylactic CMV-IGIV should be considered in combination with ganciclovir.

CONTRAINDICATIONS
History of a prior severe reaction associated with any human immunoglobulin preparations. Individuals with selective immunoglobulin A deficiency may develop antibodies to IgA and are at risk for anaphylaxis.

PRECAUTIONS
75% of untreated recipients would be expected to develop CMV disease. Use of CMV-IGIV has effected a 50% reduction in this disease rate. Effective results have been obtained with a variety of immunosuppressive regimens (e.g., combinations of azathioprine, cyclosporine, prednisone). ▪ A fatal CMV infection occurred even with ganciclovir treatment in one patient, who inadvertently missed a single injection.

Monitor: Continuous monitoring of vital signs is preferred. Must be monitored before infusion, at every rate change, at the midpoint, at the conclusion, and several times after completion. ▪ All supplies for emergency treatment of acute anaphylactic reaction must be available; see Antidote.

Patient Education: Adherence to the prescribed regimen is imperative.

Maternal/Child: Category C: safety for use during pregnancy or breast-feeding not established. Use only if clearly needed.

DRUG/LAB INTERACTIONS
Defer vaccination with any **live virus vaccine** (e.g., measles, mumps, rubella) until 3 months after CMV-IGIV administration.

SIDE EFFECTS
Incidence related to rate of administration; back pain, chills, fever, flushing, hypotension, muscle cramps, nausea, vomiting, wheezing. Hypersensitivity reactions, including anaphylaxis, are possible.

ANTIDOTE
With onset of any minor side effect, reduce rate of infusion immediately or discontinue temporarily. Discontinue CMV-IGIV if symptoms persist, and notify the physician. May be treated symptomatically and infusion resumed at a slower rate if symptoms subside. Discontinue CMV-IGIV if hypotension or anaphylaxis occur and treat immediately. Epinephrine, diphenhydramine, oxygen, vasopressors, corticosteroids, and ventilation equipment must always be available. Resuscitate as necessary.

DACARBAZINE BBW
(dah-**KAR**-bah-zeen)

Antineoplastic
(alkylating agent)

DTIC, DTIC-Dome

pH 3 to 4

USUAL DOSE
Pretreatment: See Maternal/Child.

Malignant melanoma: 2 to 4.5 mg/kg of body weight/24 hr for 10 days. May be repeated at 4-week intervals. May administer 250 mg/M^2 daily for 5 days. Repeat in 3 weeks. Has proved as effective in lesser doses as in larger doses. Individualized response determines dosage of subsequent treatments.

Hodgkin disease: 150 mg/M^2/24 hr for 5 days. Repeat every 4 weeks. Used in combination with other drugs in a specific regimen. An alternate regimen is 375 mg/M^2 on Days 1 and 15 every 4 weeks or 100 mg/M^2/day for 5 days. Given as part of a specific protocol.

DOSE ADJUSTMENTS
Dose (mg/kg) based on average weight in presence of edema or ascites. ■ Used with other antineoplastic drugs and radiation therapy in reduced doses to achieve tumor remission. ■ Dose reduction may be required in impaired liver and renal function.

DILUTION
Specific techniques required; see Precautions. Each 100-mg vial is diluted with 9.9 mL (200 mg with 19.7 mL) of SWFI (10 mg/mL). Further dilution in 50 to 250 mL of D5W or NS for infusion is preferred. May be given through Y-tube of infusion set through a free-flowing IV.

Storage: Discard in 6 to 8 hours if kept at room temperature. Reconstituted solution stable for 72 hours, diluted solution for 24 hours if refrigerated at 4° C (39° F).

COMPATIBILITY
Compatibility information not available from manufacturer; consult a pharmacist.

RATE OF ADMINISTRATION
Total dose over 30 to 60 minutes. More rapid rate may cause severe venous irritation.

ACTIONS
An antineoplastic agent. Exact mechanism of action is not known; may inhibit DNA and RNA synthesis. It is an alkylating agent, cell cycle phase nonspecific. Probably localizes in the liver and is excreted in the urine.

INDICATIONS AND USES
Metastatic malignant melanoma. ■ Hodgkin disease. ■ Soft-tissue sarcomas.

Unlabeled uses: Treatment of malignant pheochromocytoma with cyclophosphamide and vincristine. ■ Treatment of metastatic malignant melanoma with tamoxifen.

CONTRAINDICATIONS
Known hypersensitivity to dacarbazine.

PRECAUTIONS
Follow guidelines for handling cytotoxic agents. See Appendix A. ■ Administered by or under the direction of the physician specialist. ■ Bone marrow suppression is the most common toxicity. ■ Hepatic necrosis has been reported. ■ Consider potential for therapeutic benefit versus risk for toxicity. ■ Use caution in impaired liver and renal function.

Monitor: Determine absolute patency of vein; a stinging or burning sensation indicates extravasation; severe cellulitis and tissue necrosis will result. Discontinue injection; use another vein. ■ Monitor bone marrow function, white and RBC count, and platelet count frequently. ■ Nausea and vomiting may be reduced by restricting oral intake of fluid and foods for 4 to 6 hours before administration. Use prophylactic antiemetics. ■ Be alert for signs of bone marrow suppression, bleeding, or infection. ■ Monitor for thrombocytopenia (platelet count less than 50,000/mm^3). Initiate precautions to prevent excessive bleeding (e.g., inspect IV sites, skin, and mucous membranes; use extreme care during invasive procedures; test urine, emesis, stool, and secretions for occult blood). ▪ Prophylactic antibiotics may be indicated pending results of C/S in a febrile neutropenic patient.

Patient Education: Protect skin surfaces; may cause photosensitive skin reactions. ▪ Effective birth control recommended. ▪ Report burning or stinging at IV site promptly. ▪ See Appendix D, p. 1311.

Maternal/Child: Category C: safety for use in pregnancy or breast-feeding and in males and females capable of conception not established. ▪ Carcinogenic and teratogenic in animals. ▪ Discontinue breast-feeding.

Elderly: Consider age-related organ impairment; toxicity may be increased.

DRUG/LAB INTERACTIONS

Do not administer any **live virus vaccines** to patients receiving antineoplastic drugs. ▪ Inhibited by **phenobarbital and phenytoin.** ▪ Potentiates **allopurinol.** ▪ Effects of dacarbazine may be increased with **ciprofloxacin, isoniazid, fluvoxamine, ketoconazole, miconazole, and norfloxacin.** Effects may be decreased with **carbamazepine, phenobarbital, and rifampin.**

SIDE EFFECTS

Leukopenia and thrombocytopenia may be serious enough to cause death. Alopecia, anaphylaxis, anorexia, facial flushing, facial paresthesias, fever, hepatotoxicity, malaise, myalgia, nausea, skin necrosis, vomiting.

ANTIDOTE

Notify physician of all side effects. Most will be treated symptomatically. Bone marrow suppression may require temporary or permanent withholding of treatment. Administration of whole blood products (e.g., packed RBCs, platelets, leukocytes) and/or blood modifiers (e.g., darbepoetin alfa, epoetin alfa, filgrastim, pegfilgrastim, sargramostim) may be indicated to treat bone marrow toxicity. There is no specific antidote. Supportive therapy as indicated will help sustain the patient in toxicity. For extravasation, elevate extremity; consider injection of long-acting dexamethasone throughout extravasated tissue. Use a 27- or 25-gauge needle. Apply moist, warm compresses.

DALBAVANCIN
(**DAL**-ba-**VAN**-sin)

Dalvance

Antibacterial
(lipoglycopeptide)

USUAL DOSE

Pretreatment: Baseline studies indicated; see Precautions and Monitor.

1,500 mg. May be administered as a single dose or as a two-dose regimen with an initial dose of 1,000 mg followed 1 week later by 500 mg. Administer as an infusion over 30 minutes.

DOSE ADJUSTMENTS

Dosage should be adjusted in patients with renal impairment as outlined in the following chart.

Dosage of Dalbavancin in Patients With Renal Impairment		
Estimated CrCl[a]	Dalbavancin Single-Dose Regimen[b]	Dalbavancin Two-Dose Regimen[b]
≥30 mL/min or on regular hemodialysis	1,500 mg	1,000 mg followed 1 week later by 500 mg
<30 mL/min and not on regular hemodialysis	1,125 mg	750 mg followed 1 week later by 375 mg

[a]As calculated using the Cockcroft-Gault formula.
[b]Administered IV over 30 minutes.

- No dose adjustment is recommended for patients receiving regularly scheduled hemodialysis, and dalbavancin can be administered without regard to the timing of hemodialysis. ■ No dose adjustment is recommended for patients with mild hepatic impairment (Child-Pugh Class A). ■ Use caution when prescribed for patients with moderate or severe hepatic impairment (Child-Pugh Class B or C). No data are available to determine appropriate dosing in these patients. ■ No dose adjustment based on age or gender; see Elderly.

DILUTION

Available in single-use vials containing 500 mg of dalbavancin as a lyophilized powder. Reconstitute each 500-mg vial with 25 mL of SWFI or D5W. To avoid foaming, alternate between gentle swirling and inversion of the vial until contents are completely dissolved. *Do not shake.* Concentration is 20 mg/mL. Solution should be clear and colorless to yellow. Do not use if particulate matter remains. Transfer the required dose to an IV bag or bottle containing D5W. Diluted solution must have a final concentration of 1 mg/mL to 5 mg/mL.

Filters: Specific information not available.

Storage: Vials may be stored at CRT. Reconstituted vials and/or fully diluted solutions may be stored at RT or refrigerated at 2° to 8° C (36° to 46° F). Do not freeze. Total time from reconstitution to dilution to administration should not exceed 48 hours.

COMPATIBILITY

Manufacturer states, "Do not co-infuse dalbavancin with other medications or electrolytes. Saline-based infusion solutions may cause precipitation and should not be used. The **compatibility** of reconstituted dalbavancin with IV medications, additives, or substances other than D5W has not been established."

RATE OF ADMINISTRATION

A single dose as an infusion equally distributed over 30 minutes. If a common IV line is used to administer other drugs in addition to dalbavancin, flush the IV line before and after each dalbavancin infusion with D5W. Too-rapid infusion may cause "red-man syndrome," including back pain, flushing of the upper body, pruritus, rash, and/or urticaria. Temporarily stop or slow the infusion as indicated.

ACTIONS

Dalbavancin is a semi-synthetic lipoglycopeptide antibacterial drug. It interferes with cell wall synthesis by binding to the D-alanyl-D-alanine terminus of the stem pentapeptide in nascent cell wall peptidoglycan, thus preventing cross-linking. In vitro, dalbavancin is bactericidal against *Staphylococcus aureus* and *Streptococcus pyogenes* at concentrations similar to those sustained throughout treatment; see Indications. 93% bound to plasma proteins, primarily to albumin. Mean concentrations achieved in skin blister fluid remain above 30 mg/L up to 7 days after dosing. Effective half-life is approximately 346 hours. Excreted in feces and urine as unchanged drug and as a metabolite.

INDICATIONS AND USES

Treatment of adult patients with acute bacterial skin and skin structure infections (ABSSSI) caused by susceptible isolates of designated gram-positive microorganisms, including *Staphylococcus aureus* (both methicillin-susceptible [MSSA] and methicillin-resistant [MRSA] strains).

CONTRAINDICATIONS

Known hypersensitivity to dalbavancin. No data available on cross-reactivity between dalbavancin and other glycopeptides, including vancomycin.

PRECAUTIONS

Serious hypersensitivity (anaphylactic) and skin reactions have been reported. Check history of previous hypersensitivity reactions to glycopeptides (e.g., oritavancin, telavancin, vancomycin). Exercise caution in patients with a history of glycopeptide allergy; cross-sensitivity is possible. ■ Infusion-related reactions have been reported; see Rate of Administration. ■ Specific sensitivity studies are indicated to determine susceptibility of the causative organism to dalbavancin. ■ To reduce the development of drug-resistant bacteria and maintain its effectiveness, dalbavancin should be used to treat only those infections proven or strongly suspected to be caused by bacteria. ▪ *Clostridium difficile*–associated diarrhea (CDAD) has been reported for nearly all systemic antibacterial agents and may range in severity from mild diarrhea to fatal colitis. Consider in patients who present with diarrhea during or after treatment with dalbavancin. ▪ ALT elevations greater than 3 times the ULN occurred in some patients with normal baseline transaminase levels before treatment.

Monitor: Obtain baseline SCr. ▪ Monitor for S/S of hypersensitivity (e.g., hypotension, rash, urticaria, tightness of the chest, wheezing). ▪ Monitor for S/S of an infusion reaction; see Rate of Administration. ▪ See Precautions; baseline liver function studies may be indicated.

Patient Education: Promptly report S/S of a hypersensitivity reaction (e.g., hives, rash, shortness of breath, wheezing) or an infusion reaction (e.g., back pain, flushing of the upper body, pruritus, rash, and/or urticaria). ▪ Promptly report diarrhea or bloody stools that occur during treatment or up to several months after an antibiotic has been discontinued; may indicate CDAD and require treatment.

Maternal/Child: Use during pregnancy only if the potential benefit outweighs the possible risk to the fetus. ▪ Use caution during breast-feeding. ▪ Safety and effectiveness for use in pediatric patients not established.

Elderly: Consider age-related renal impairment, monitoring of renal function, and dose with caution; see Dose Adjustments.

DRUG/LAB INTERACTIONS

Clinical drug-drug interaction studies have not been conducted. ▪ There is minimal potential for drug-drug interactions between dalbavancin and substrates, inhibitors, and inducers of cytochrome P_{450} enzymes.

SIDE EFFECTS

The most common side effects reported are diarrhea, headache, and nausea. Hypersensitivity and/or infusion reactions may be severe. Increased ALT levels (reversible), pruritus, rash, and vomiting were also reported. Many other side effects occurred in fewer than 2% of patients.

Post-Marketing: Back pain as an infusion-related reaction.

ANTIDOTE

Notify physician of any side effects. Discontinue the drug if indicated. Treat hypersensitivity reactions as indicated (e.g., diphenhydramine, epinephrine, albuterol) and resuscitate as necessary. Temporarily discontinue or slow infusion for infusion-related reactions. Mild cases of CDAD may respond to discontinuation of dalbavancin. Treat CDAD with fluids, electrolytes, protein supplements, and appropriate antibiotics (e.g., oral vancomycin) as indicated. In severe cases, surgical evaluation may be indicated. Less than 6% of the recommended dose of dalbavancin is removed by hemodialysis.

DANTROLENE SODIUM
(**DAN**-troh-leen **SO**-dee-um)

Dantrium, Revonto ▪ Ryanodex

**Skeletal muscle relaxant
(direct acting)**

pH 9.5 ▪ 10.3

USUAL DOSE

In patients known to be susceptible to malignant hyperthermia (MH), oral dantrolene may be used prophylactically preoperatively. Oral or IV therapy should be used post-operatively for 1 to 3 days following IV treatment for MH crisis. Postoperative dosing is indicated after emergency treatment to prevent recurrence of the manifestations of MH.

Prophylactic dose: DANTRIUM, REVONTO: 2.5 mg/kg as an infusion. Begin administration 1¼ hours before anesthesia, and administer over 1 hour. Oral dantrolene may be used.

RYANODEX: 2.5 mg/kg as an IV injection over at least 1 minute. Begin administration 1¼ hours before surgery. If surgery is prolonged, administer additional individualized doses during anesthesia and surgery as needed.

ALL FORMULATIONS: Avoid agents that trigger MH (e.g., general anesthetics and depolarizing neuromuscular blocking agents [succinylcholine]).

Therapeutic or emergency dose: ALL FORMULATIONS: Discontinue all anesthetic agents at the first sign of a malignant hyperthermia reaction. Administration of 100% oxygen is recommended.

1 mg/kg of body weight as an initial dose as a rapid IV push. Repeat as necessary until symptoms subside or a cumulative dose of 10 mg/kg is reached. Entire regimen may be repeated if symptoms reappear. Dose required depends on degree of susceptibility to malignant hyperthermia, length of time of exposure to triggering agent, and time lapse between onset of crisis and beginning of treatment.

Post-crisis follow-up: An oral dose of 4 to 8 mg/kg/day for 1 to 3 days to prevent recurrences. If oral dosing not feasible, begin IV dose at 1 mg/kg and individualize by increasing based on patient response.

PEDIATRIC DOSE

Prophylactic, therapeutic, and post-crisis follow-up doses are the same as for adults; see Maternal/Child.

DOSE ADJUSTMENTS

Dose selection should be cautious in the elderly. Reduced doses may be indicated based on the potential for decreased organ function and concomitant disease or drug therapy.

DILUTION

DANTRIUM, REVONTO: Each 20 mg must be diluted with 60 mL SWFI without a bacteriostatic agent. Shake until solution is clear. May be administered through a Y-tube of infusion tubing. If large volumes will be used, transfer to plastic infusion bags; do not use glass bottles; see Compatibility.

RYANODEX: Reconstitute each 250-mg vial with 5 mL of SWFI without a bacteriostatic agent. Shake the vial to ensure an orange-colored uniform suspension. Do not reconstitute with D5W or NS; see Compatibility. May be administered directly into an indwelling catheter or through a Y-tube of a free-flowing infusion of D5W or NS.

Storage: ALL FORMULATIONS: Store undiluted vials at CRT and protect from light. Store diluted solution at CRT and protect from direct light. Discard after 6 hours.

COMPATIBILITY

DANTRIUM, REVONTO: Manufacturer states, "D5W, NS, and acidic solutions are **not compatible** and should not be used." May form a precipitate with glass bottles; use of plastic IV bags recommended.

RYANODEX: Do not dilute or transfer the reconstituted suspension to another container to infuse the product.

RATE OF ADMINISTRATION

Prophylactic dose: DANTRIUM, REVONTO: A single dose as an infusion distributed over 1 hour. RYANODEX: A single dose as an IV injection over at least 1 minute. If administering into an indwelling catheter without a free-flowing IV, flush line after administration of **Ryanodex** to ensure there is no residual drug left in the catheter.

Therapeutic or emergency dose: ALL FORMULATIONS: Each single dose should be given by rapid continuous IV push. Follow immediately with subsequent doses as indicated.

ACTIONS

A direct-acting skeletal muscle relaxant. Inhibits excitation-contraction coupling by interfering with the release of the calcium ion from the sarcoplasmic reticulum to reverse the physiologic cause of malignant hyperthermia and produce relaxation. The addition of dantrolene to the "triggered" malignant hyperthermic muscle cell may re-establish a normal level of ionized calcium in the myoplasm. Physiologic, metabolic, and biochemical changes associated with the malignant hyperthermia crisis may be reversed or attenuated. Has no appreciable effect on cardiovascular or respiratory function. Onset of action is prompt. Half-life of **Dantrium** and **Revonto** is 4 to 8 hours. Half-life of **Ryanodex** is 8.5 to 11.4 hours. Metabolized in the liver and excreted in urine. Readily crosses the placental barrier. Secreted in breast milk.

INDICATIONS AND USES

Treatment of malignant hyperthermia in conjunction with appropriate supportive measures. ▪ Prevention of malignant hyperthermia in patients at high risk.

CONTRAINDICATIONS

None.

PRECAUTIONS

Use caution in patients with impaired pulmonary or cardiac function or history of liver disease. ▪ Discontinue all anesthetic agents immediately when onset of malignant hyperthermia is recognized. Administration of 100% oxygen is recommended. ▪ Hepatotoxicity has been reported with oral dantrolene. ▪ Not indicated for use in patients with neuroleptic malignant syndrome (NMS).

Monitor: S/S of malignant hyperthermia crises include central venous desaturation, cyanosis and mottling of the skin, hypercarbia, increased utilization of anesthesia circuit carbon dioxide absorber, metabolic acidosis, skeletal muscle rigidity, tachycardia, tachypnea and, in many cases, fever. ▪ Monitor ECG, vital signs, electrolytes, and urine output continuously. ▪ Oxygen needs are increased. ▪ Manage metabolic acidosis. ▪ Institute cooling measures. ▪ Diuretics may be required to prevent or treat late kidney injury due to myoglobinuria. Consider amount of mannitol present in **Dantrium** or **Revonto** formulations. (**Ryanodex** does not contain a sufficient amount of mannitol to maintain diuresis.) ▪ Confirm absolute patency of vein; avoid extravasation. High pH may cause tissue necrosis. ▪ Associated with skeletal muscle weakness; see Patient Education.

- Ensure adequate ventilation; has been associated with dyspnea, respiratory muscle weakness, and decreased inspiratory capacity. ▪ Assess patients for difficulty swallowing and choking. ▪ Monitor hepatic function, including ALT, AST. ▪ Somnolence and dizziness may persist for up to 48 hours postdose. Ambulate with assistance.

Patient Education: May experience decreased grip strength, weakness in leg muscles, and light-headedness postoperatively. May persist for 48 hours. ▪ Request assistance for ambulation. ▪ Use caution when eating; choking and difficulty swallowing have been reported on day of administration. ▪ Avoid alcohol and other CNS depressants (e.g., diazepam [Valium]). ▪ Avoid tasks that require alertness. ▪ Promptly report bloody or tarry stools, itching, jaundice (yellow color) of eyes and skin, or skin rash.

Maternal/Child: Category C: embryocidal in animal studies. Use during pregnancy only if potential benefit justifies potential risk to the fetus. ▪ Discontinue breast-feeding. ▪ Safety and effectiveness for use in pediatric patients have been established. Dose is the same as for adults.

Elderly: Differences in responses between the elderly and younger patients have not been identified. Dose selection should be cautious; see Dose Adjustments.

DRUG/LAB INTERACTIONS

ALL FORMULATIONS: Avoid concurrent use of **calcium channel blockers and dantrolene**. Cardiovascular collapse, arrhythmias, and hyperkalemia have been reported. ▪ Ability to bind to plasma proteins inhibited by **warfarin**; increased by **tolbutamide**.

DANTRIUM AND REVONTO: May potentiate **vecuronium**-induced neuromuscular blockade.

RYANODEX: May potentiate the neuromuscular block when given with **muscle relaxants**. ▪ May potentiate the effects of **antipsychotic agents** (e.g., pimozide, clozapine) and **antianxiety agents** (e.g., diazepam) on the central nervous system. ▪ Concomitant use of **sedative agents** may increase the risk of somnolence and dizziness.

SIDE EFFECTS

Dizziness, drowsiness, loss of grip strength, and weakness in the legs are most common. Other reported side effects include erythema, hypersensitivity reactions (including anaphylaxis), injection site reactions, nausea, pulmonary edema, thrombophlebitis, tissue necrosis secondary to extravasation, urticaria.

ANTIDOTE

No specific antidote is available or needed when used correctly. Notify physician and initiate supportive measures (ensure adequate airway and ventilation, monitor ECG) in overdosage. Large amounts of IV fluids may be needed to prevent crystalluria. Treat anaphylaxis and resuscitate as necessary. Value of dialysis in overdose is not known.

DAPTOMYCIN
(**dap**-toe-**MY**-sin)

**Antibacterial
(cyclic lipopeptide)**

Cubicin, Cubicin RF

USUAL DOSE
Pretreatment: Baseline studies indicated; see Precautions and Monitor.

ALL FORMULATIONS

Dosages range between 4-10 mg/kg/day, depending on site of infection. Safety data for use more than 28 days is limited.

PEDIATRIC DOSE
CUBICIN AND CUBICIN RF: Merck & Co., Inc. has exclusive marketing rights. Cubicin and Cubicin RF are the only formulations approved for pediatric indications.

Complicated skin and skin structure infections (cSSSI): Dose is based on age according to the following chart.

Recommended Dose of Cubicin and Cubicin RF in Pediatric Patients (1 to 17 Years of Age) With cSSSI (Based on Age)		
Age Range	**Dose Regimen[a]**	**Duration of Therapy**
12 to 17 years	5 mg/kg once every 24 hours infused over 30 minutes	Up to 14 days
7 to 11 years	7 mg/kg once every 24 hours infused over 30 minutes	Up to 14 days
2 to 6 years	9 mg/kg once every 24 hours infused over 60 minutes	Up to 14 days
1 to <2 years	10 mg/kg once every 24 hours infused over 60 minutes	Up to 14 days

[a]Recommended dose regimen is for pediatric patients with normal renal function. Dose adjustment for pediatric patients with renal impairment not established.

CUBICIN RF: *Staphylococcus aureus bloodstream infections (bacteremia) in pediatric patients (1 to 17 years of age):* Dose is based on age according to the following chart.

Recommended Dosage of Cubicin RF in Pediatric Patients (1 to 17 Years of Age) With *S. aureus* Bacteremia (Based on Age)		
Age-Group	**Dosage[a]**	**Duration of Therapy**
12 to 17 years	7 mg/kg once every 24 hours infused over 30 minutes	Up to 42 days
7 to 11 years	9 mg/kg once every 24 hours infused over 30 minutes	Up to 42 days
1 to 6 years	12 mg/kg once every 24 hours infused over 60 minutes	Up to 42 days

[a]Recommended dosage is for pediatric patients (1 to 17 years of age) with normal renal function. Dosage adjustment for pediatric patients with renal impairment has not been established.

DOSE ADJUSTMENTS
ALL FORMULATIONS: No dose adjustment is required in adult patients with creatinine clearance 30 mL/min or higher. ▪ In patients with CrCl less than 30 mL/min, including patients undergoing hemodialysis or CAPD, administer a single dose (4 or 6 mg/kg) every 48 hours. If possible, administer dose following completion of hemodialysis on hemodialysis days. ▪ Dose adjustment for pediatric patients with renal impairment not established. ▪ No specific dose adjustments required based on age, gender, obesity, or mild to moderate hepatic impairment. Has not been studied in patients with severe hepatic impairment.

DILUTION

ALL FORMULATIONS EXCEPT CUBICIN RF

Available in 350-mg and 500-mg single-dose vials. Reconstitute each 350-mg vial with 7 mL of NS and each 500-mg vial with 10 mL of NS. Slowly direct NS to vial sides (50 mg/mL). Use of a transfer needle that is 21 gauge or smaller in diameter or a needleless device is recommended. Ensure wetting of entire daptomycin product. Allow vial to stand for 10 minutes, then gently rotate to ensure complete dilution. *To minimize foaming, avoid vigorous agitation or shaking during or after reconstitution.* Freshly reconstituted solutions range in color from pale yellow to light brown. Slowly remove the appropriate amount of the 50 mg/mL solution from the vial using a needle that is 21 gauge or smaller in diameter.

Adults: May be administered as a 50 mg/mL reconstituted solution or may be further diluted with 50 mL of NS before administration and given as an infusion.

Pediatric patients (30-minute infusion): Further dilute each dose to be administered over 30 minutes in 50 mL NS.

Pediatric patients (60-minute infusion): Further dilute each dose to be administered over 60 minutes in 25 mL NS.

CUBICIN RF

Reconstitute each single-dose 500-mg vial by directing 10 mL of *SWFI or BWFI* to vial sides (50 mg/mL). Use of a transfer needle that is 21 gauge or smaller in diameter is recommended. *DO NOT* use saline-based diluents for reconstitution, because this will result in a hyperosmotic solution that may result in infusion site reactions if the reconstituted product is administered as an IV injection over a period of 2 minutes. Slowly remove the appropriate amount of 50 mg/mL solution from the vial using a needle that is 21 gauge or smaller in diameter.

Adults: May be administered as a 50 mg/mL reconstituted solution or may be further diluted with 50 mL of NS before administration and given as an infusion.

Pediatric patients 7 to 17 years of age (30-minute infusion): Further dilute each dose to be administered over 30 minutes in 50 mL NS.

Pediatric patients 1 to 6 years of age (60-minute infusion): Further dilute each dose to be administered over 60 minutes in 25 mL NS.

Filters: No data available from manufacturer.

Storage: *Cubicin and generics:* Refrigerate unopened vials at 2° to 8° C (36° to 46° F). Both reconstituted and diluted solutions are stable for 12 hours at RT or up to 48 hours refrigerated. The combined time (vial and infusion bag) at RT should not exceed 12 hours. Combined refrigeration time (vial and infusion bag) should not exceed 48 hours.

Cubicin RF: In-use storage conditions for Cubicin RF are outlined in the following chart.

In-Use Storage Conditions for Cubicin RF Once Reconstituted in Acceptable IV Diluents				
			In-Use Shelf Life	
Container	**Diluent**		**RT**	**Refrigerated**
Vial	SWFI		1 day	3 days
	BWFI		2 days	3 days
Syringe	SWFI		1 day	3 days
	BWFI		2 days	5 days
IV bag	Reconstitution: SWFI for immediate dilution with NS		19 hours	3 days
	Reconstitution: BWFI for immediate dilution with NS		2 days	5 days

All formulations: Discard unused portion of vial.

COMPATIBILITY

ALL FORMULATIONS: Additives or other medications should not be added to daptomycin single-use vials or infusion bags, or infused simultaneously through the same intravenous line. If the same intravenous line is used for sequential infusion of several different drugs, the line should be flushed with a **compatible** infusion solution before and after infusion with daptomycin. ■ **Cubicin and generics** in the vial are **compatible** with NS, but **Cubicin RF in the vial** is **incompatible** and should **not** be reconstituted with NS because this will result in a hyperosmotic solution that may result in infusion site reactions if administered as the 2-minute IV injection. **All formulations** are **incompatible** with dextrose-containing diluents. ■ **All formulations:** Do not use in conjunction with ReadyMED® elastomeric infusion pumps; an **incompatibility** occurs because of an impurity leaching from this pump system into the daptomycin solution.

RECONSTITUTED CUBICIN: Compatible with NS and LR.

RECONSTITUTED CUBICIN RF: Compatible with NS, SWFI, and BWFI.

Other sources suggest a few specific **compatibilities** dependent on concentration and manufacturer for **Cubicin and generics**; consult a pharmacist.

RATE OF ADMINISTRATION

ALL FORMULATIONS

See Compatibility. Flushing of the IV line before and after infusion may be indicated.

Injection: *Adults:* A single dose properly reconstituted and administered over 2 minutes.

Infusion: *Adults:* A single dose properly diluted and administered over 30 minutes.

Pediatric patients 7 to 17 years of age: A single dose properly diluted and administered as an IV infusion over 30 minutes. Maintain infusion rate at 1.67 mL/min.

Pediatric patients 1 to 6 years of age: A single dose properly diluted and administered as an IV infusion over 60 minutes. Maintain infusion rate at 0.42 mL/min.

Do not administer as an injection in pediatric patients.

ACTIONS

Daptomycin is a cyclic lipopeptide antibacterial agent. Binds to bacterial cell membranes and causes a rapid depolarization of the membrane potential. Loss of the membrane potential leads to inhibition of protein, DNA, and RNA synthesis, which results in bacterial cell death. Exhibits bactericidal activity against aerobic gram-positive bacteria and has been shown to retain potency against antibiotic-resistant, gram-positive bacteria, including isolates resistant to methicillin. Cross-resistance between daptomycin and other antibacterial agents has not been reported. Highly protein bound, primarily to albumin. Site of metabolism has not been identified. Half-life is approximately 7 to 9 hours. Is excreted primarily by the kidney. A small fraction is excreted through the feces. Secreted in breast milk.

INDICATIONS AND USES

ALL FORMULATIONS: Treatment of adult patients with complicated skin and skin structure infections caused by susceptible strains of several aerobic gram-positive microorganisms. ■ Treatment of adults with *Staphylococcus aureus* bloodstream infections (bacteremia), including adult patients with right-sided infective endocarditis caused by methicillin-susceptible and methicillin-resistant isolates.

CUBICIN AND CUBICIN RF: Treatment of pediatric patients (1 to 17 years of age) with complicated skin and skin structure infections caused by susceptible strains of several aerobic gram-positive microorganisms. ■ Treatment of pediatric patients (1 to 17 years of age) with *Staphylococcus aureus* bloodstream infections (bacteremia).

Limitations of use: *All formulations:* Daptomycin is not indicated for treatment of left-sided infective endocarditis due to *S. aureus* and has not been studied in patients with prosthetic valve endocarditis. ■ **Not** indicated for treatment of pneumonia. ■ Not recommended in pediatric patients under 1 year of age; see Maternal/Child.

CONTRAINDICATIONS

Known hypersensitivity to daptomycin.

PRECAUTIONS

ALL FORMULATIONS: C/S indicated to determine susceptibility of causative organism to daptomycin. ■ To reduce the development of drug-resistant bacteria and maintain its effectiveness, daptomycin should be used to treat only those infections that are proven or strongly suspected to be caused by susceptible bacteria. ■ Combination therapy may be clinically indicated if the documented or presumed pathogens include gram-negative or anaerobic organisms. ▪ Eosinophilic pneumonia has been reported. Onset is usually 2 to 4 weeks after initiation of daptomycin and improves when therapy is discontinued. Patient may present with fever, dyspnea with hypoxic respiratory insufficiency, and diffuse pulmonary infiltrates or organizing pneumonia. ▪ Superinfection caused by the overgrowth of nonsusceptible organisms may occur with antibiotic use. Treat as indicated. ▪ *Clostridium difficile*–associated diarrhea (CDAD) has been reported. May range from mild diarrhea to fatal colitis. Consider in patients who present with diarrhea during or after treatment with daptomycin. ▪ Myopathy (defined as muscle aching or muscle weakness in conjunction with increases in creatine phosphokinase [CPK] values to greater than 10 times the ULN) has been reported. Rhabdomyolysis with or without acute renal failure has been reported. ▪ Cases of peripheral neuropathy have been reported. ▪ Hypersensitivity reactions, including anaphylaxis, have been reported. ▪ In clinical trials, decreased efficacy was observed in patients with moderate baseline renal impairment (CrCl less than 50 mL/min).

Monitor: *All formulations:* Obtain baseline and weekly SCr, BUN, and CPK levels. Patients who received recent prior or concomitant therapy with an HMG-CoA reductase inhibitor, patients with renal insufficiency, and patients who develop unexplained elevations in CPK while receiving daptomycin should be monitored more frequently. See Precautions and Antidote. ▪ Monitor for S/S of hypersensitivity reactions (e.g., dyspnea, fever, flushing, hypotension, nausea, pruritus, rash, urticaria). ▪ Monitor for the development of muscle pain or weakness, particularly in the distal extremities. ▪ Monitor for S/S of neuropathy and consider discontinuation. ▪ Repeat blood cultures indicated in patients with persisting or relapsing *S. aureus* infection or poor clinical response. MIC (minimum inhibitory concentration) susceptibility testing and diagnostic evaluation to rule out sequestered foci of infection may be indicated. Surgical intervention (e.g., débridement, removal of prosthetic device) and/or consideration of a change in antibacterial regimen may be required. ▪ Monitor for S/S of eosinophilic pneumonia (e.g., cough, fever, difficulty breathing, shortness of breath, diffuse pulmonary infiltrates or organizing pneumonia). Treatment with systemic steroids is recommended.

Patient Education: *All formulations:* Review side effects with physician. Promptly report muscle pain or weakness, S/S of a hypersensitivity reaction (e.g., hives, rash, shortness of breath or troubled breathing, swelling of eyelids, lips, or face), S/S of neuropathy (e.g., tingling or numbness, especially in the forearm or lower leg), or new or worsening cough, breathlessness, or fever. ▪ Review medications (prescription and nonprescription) with healthcare provider. ▪ Promptly report diarrhea or bloody stools that occur during treatment or up to several months after an antibiotic has been discontinued; may indicate CDAD and require treatment.

Maternal/Child: *All formulations:* Use during pregnancy only if clearly needed. ▪ Use caution during breastfeeding. Is present in breast milk. ▪ Safety and effectiveness of **Cubicin and Cubicin RF** in pediatric patients from 1 to 17 years of age for treatment of cSSSI and of **Cubicin RF** in pediatric patients from 1 to 17 years of age for treatment of *S. aureus* bloodstream infections (bacteremia) have been established. Avoid use of daptomycin in pediatric patients younger than 1 year of age. Animal studies suggest risk of potential effects on muscular, neuromuscular, and/or nervous systems (either peripheral and/or central). **Cubicin RF** has not been studied in pediatric patients with other bacterial infections.

Elderly: *All formulations:* Lower clinical success rates were seen in patients 65 years of age or older. In addition, adverse events were more common in this age-group. Consider age-related renal impairment. See Dose Adjustment.

DRUG/LAB INTERACTIONS

ALL FORMULATIONS: In vitro synergistic interactions occurred with **aminoglycosides, beta-lactam antibiotics, and rifampin** against some isolates of staphylococci and enterococci, including some methicillin-resistant *Staphylococcus aureus* (MRSA) isolates and some vancomycin-resistant enterococci isolates. ▪ Has been administered with **warfarin.** Does not appear to affect the pharmacokinetics of either drug. However, daptomycin can cause a significant concentration-dependent false prolongation of PT and elevation of INR when certain recombinant thromboplastin reagents are used for the assay. This drug-lab interaction can be minimized by drawing specimens for PT/INR near the time of trough plasma concentrations of daptomycin. Evaluation of PT/INR using an alternative method may be required. Evaluate for other causes of abnormally elevated PT/INR results. ▪ **HMG-CoA reductase inhibitors** may cause myopathy, which is manifested as muscle pain or weakness associated with elevated levels of CPK and possible rhabdomyolysis. Consider temporarily suspending the use of HMG-CoA reductase inhibitors in patients receiving daptomycin.

SIDE EFFECTS

Adult cSSSI patients: The most frequently reported side effects were abnormal liver function tests, diarrhea, dizziness, dyspnea, elevated CPK, headache, hypotension, rash, and urinary tract infections.

Pediatric cSSSI patients: The most frequently reported side effects included abdominal pain, diarrhea, elevated CPK, fever, headache, pruritus, and vomiting.

Adult *S. aureus* bacteremia/endocarditis patients: The most frequently reported side effects were abdominal pain, bacteremia, chest pain, edema, elevated CPK, hypertension, insomnia, pharyngolaryngeal pain, pruritus, sepsis, and sweating.

Pediatric *S. aureus* bacteremia patients: Elevated CPK and vomiting were the most frequently reported side effects.

All patients: Muscle pain or weakness, rhabdomyolysis (with or without renal failure), and peripheral neuropathy have been reported rarely. See Precautions. Hypersensitivity reactions including anaphylaxis, difficulty swallowing, hives, pruritus, shortness of breath, and truncal erythema have been reported. Other reactions have been reported in fewer than 1% of study patients. See manufacturer's literature.

Post-Marketing: Anaphylaxis; anemia; angioedema; CDAD; cough; difficulty swallowing; drug rash with eosinophilia and systemic symptoms (DRESS); eosinophilic pneumonia; fever; hives; nausea and vomiting; organizing pneumonia; peripheral neuropathy; platelet count decreased; pulmonary eosinophilia; pruritus; serious skin reactions, including Stevens-Johnson syndrome, vesiculobullous rash, and acute generalized exanthematous pustulosis; renal disorders, including acute kidney injury, renal insufficiency, and renal failure; rhabdomyolysis; shortness of breath; thrombocytopenia; truncal erythema; and visual disturbances.

ANTIDOTE

Notify physician of any side effects. Discontinue drug in patients with unexplained S/S of myopathy in conjunction with CPK elevation greater than 1,000 units/L (approximately 5 times the upper limit of normal) or in patients without reported symptoms who have marked elevation in CPK, with levels of greater than 2,000 units/L (equal to or greater than 10 times the ULN). Discontinue daptomycin at the first sign of eosinophilic pneumonia. Treatment with systemic steroids is recommended. Treat CDAD with fluids, electrolytes, protein supplements, and appropriate antibiotics (e.g., oral vancomycin) as indicated. In severe cases, surgical evaluation may be indicated. Discontinue daptomycin and treat hypersensitivity reactions as indicated (e.g., oxygen, diphenhydramine, epinephrine, corticosteroids, vasopressors, and/or fluids). Approximately 15% of daptomycin is removed during a 4-hour hemodialysis run. Approximately 11% is recovered over 48 hours with peritoneal dialysis. Use of a high-flux dialysis membrane may increase the amount of drug removal. Resuscitate as necessary.

DARBEPOETIN ALFA BBW
(DAR-beh-**poh**-eh-tin **AL**-fah)

Erythropoiesis-stimulating
agent (ESA)

Aranesp

pH 6 to 6.4

USUAL DOSE
Pretreatment: Baseline studies indicated; see Monitor.

Adult and pediatric patients: Rate of hemoglobin increase is dose dependent and varies among patients. Availability of iron stores, baseline hemoglobin, and concurrent medical problems affect the rate and extent of response. In controlled clinical trials, patients experienced greater risks for death, serious adverse cardiovascular reactions, and stroke when administered erythropoiesis-stimulating agents (ESAs) to target a hemoglobin level of greater than 11 Gm/dL. Use the lowest dose for each patient that will gradually increase the hemoglobin concentration to avoid the need for RBC transfusion. If a patient fails to respond or maintain a response, other etiologies should be considered and evaluated. See Monitor, Precautions, and Maternal/Child.

Anemia due to chemotherapy in cancer patients: Start only if Hgb is less than 10 g/dl and anticipated duration of myelosuppressive chemo is at least 2 additional months. 2.25 mcg/kg once weekly or 500 mcg once every 3 weeks until chemo is completed.

Anemia associated with chronic kidney disease (CKD) for patients on dialysis: Initiate darbepoetin when the hemoglobin level is less than 10 Gm/dL: *Starting dose:* 0.45 mcg/kg of body weight once per week or 0.75 mcg/kg once every 2 weeks as appropriate. May be given by IV or SQ injection. The IV route is recommended for patients on hemodialysis; see Precautions. See Dose Adjustments and Maternal/Child.

Anemia associated with chronic kidney disease (CKD) for patients NOT on dialysis: Consider initiating darbepoetin only when the hemoglobin level is less than 10 Gm/dL and the following two considerations apply: (1) the rate of hemoglobin decline indicates the likelihood of requiring a RBC transfusion, and (2) reducing the risk of alloimmunization and/or other RBC transfusion-related risks is a goal. *Starting dose:* 0.45 mcg/kg of body weight IV or SQ given once every 4 weeks as appropriate.

Conversion from epoetin alfa to darbepoetin alfa in patients with CKD on dialysis: Estimate starting weekly dose of darbepoetin for adult and pediatric patients based on the weekly dose of epoetin alfa at the time of substitution as shown in the following chart. Administer darbepoetin once per week in patients who were receiving epoetin alfa 2 to 3 times a week and once every 2 weeks in patients who were receiving epoetin alfa once per week. The route of administration (IV or SQ) should remain the same.

Estimated Darbepoetin Alfa Starting Dose Based on Previous Epoetin Alfa Dose for Patients With CKD on Dialysis		
Previous Weekly Epoetin Alfa Dose (units/week)	Darbepoetin Alfa Dose (mcg/week)	
	Adult	Pediatric
<1,500 units/week	6.25 mcg/week	See [a]
1,500 to 2,499 units/week	6.25 mcg/week	6.25 mcg/week
2,500 to 4,999 units/week	12.5 mcg/week	10 mcg/week
5,000 to 10,999 units/week	25 mcg/week	20 mcg/week
11,000 to 17,999 units/week	40 mcg/week	40 mcg/week
18,000 to 33,999 units/week	60 mcg/week	60 mcg/week
34,000 to 89,999 units/week	100 mcg/week	100 mcg/week
≥90,000 units/week	200 mcg/week	200 mcg/week

[a]Data insufficient to determine a darbepoetin alfa conversion dose in pediatric patients receiving a weekly epoetin alfa dose of less than 1,500 units/week.

Conversion from epoetin alfa to darbepoetin alfa in patients with CKD NOT on dialysis: The dose conversion shown in the previous chart (for patients with CKD on dialysis) does not accurately estimate the once-monthly dose of darbepoetin.

Anemia associated with chemotherapy in cancer patients: ESAs shortened overall survival and/or increased the risk of tumor progression or recurrence in clinical studies of patients with certain types of cancer; see Precautions. Initiate darbepoetin in patients undergoing cancer chemotherapy only if the hemoglobin is less than 10 Gm/dL and there is a minimum of 2 additional months of planned chemotherapy. Use the lowest dose necessary to avoid RBC transfusions. *Starting dose:* 2.25 mcg/kg of body weight SQ every week until completion of chemo-therapy course. An alternative schedule is 500 mcg SQ every 3 weeks until completion of chemotherapy course.

PEDIATRIC DOSE

Pediatric patients with CKD (under 18 years of age): Initiate darbepoetin when the hemo-globin level is less than 10 Gm/dL. *Starting dose:* 0.45 mcg/kg of body weight once per week as an IV or SQ injection. Patients not receiving dialysis may also be initiated at a dose of 0.75 mcg/kg once every 2 weeks. If the hemoglobin level approaches or exceeds 12 Gm/dL, reduce or interrupt the dose of darbepoetin.

DOSE ADJUSTMENTS

All patients with CKD: When adjusting therapy, consider hemoglobin rate of rise, hemoglo-bin rate of decline, ESA responsiveness, and hemoglobin variability. A single hemoglo-bin excursion may not require a dose adjustment. Dose should be started slowly and adjusted for each patient to achieve and maintain the lowest hemoglobin level sufficient to avoid the need for RBC transfusion. Allow sufficient time before adjusting a dose; increased hemoglobin levels may not be observed for 2 to 6 weeks. ▪ Do not increase the dose more frequently than once every 4 weeks. Decreases in dose can occur more frequently. Avoid frequent dose adjustments. ▪ If the hemoglobin rises rapidly (e.g., more than 1 Gm/dL in any 2-week period), reduce the dose by 25% or more as needed to reduce rapid responses. ▪ For patients who do not respond adequately (e.g., the he-moglobin has not increased by more than 1 Gm/dL) after 4 weeks of therapy, increase the dose by 25%. ▪ For patients who do not respond adequately over a 12-week escala-tion period, increasing the dose further is unlikely to improve response and may increase risks. Discontinue darbepoetin if responsiveness does not improve.

Adult patients with CKD on dialysis: If the hemoglobin level approaches or exceeds 11 Gm/dL, reduce or interrupt the dose of darbepoetin.

Adult patients with CKD NOT on dialysis: If the hemoglobin level exceeds 10 Gm/dL, reduce or interrupt the dose of darbepoetin and use the lowest dose sufficient to reduce the need for RBC transfusions.

Pediatric patients with CKD: See Pediatric Dose.

Anemia associated with chemotherapy in cancer patients:

Dose Adjustment in Patients Undergoing Cancer Chemotherapy		
Dose Adjustment	**Weekly Schedule**	**Every-3-Week Schedule**
If hemoglobin increases more than 1 Gm/dL in any 2-week period **or** If hemoglobin reaches a level needed to avoid RBC transfusion	Reduce dose by 40%	Reduce dose by 40%
If hemoglobin exceeds a level needed to avoid RBC transfusion	Withhold dose until hemoglobin approaches level at which RBC transfusions may be required Reinitiate at a dose 40% below the previous dose	Withhold dose until hemoglobin approaches level at which RBC transfusions may be required Reinitiate at a dose 40% below the previous dose
If hemoglobin increases by less than 1 Gm/dL **and** remains below 10 Gm/dL after 6 weeks of therapy	Increase dose to 4.5 mcg/kg/week	No dose adjustment
If there is no response as measured by hemoglobin levels **or** if RBC transfusions are still required after 8 weeks of therapy Following completion of a chemotherapy course	Discontinue darbepoetin	Discontinue darbepoetin

DILUTION
Available in numerous concentrations. Supplied in vials or prefilled syringes with needle guards (needle cover contains a derivative of latex). Must be given undiluted as an IV injection. Do not administer in conjunction with other drug solutions. **Do not shake** and keep covered to protect from room light until administration. Vigorous shaking or exposure to light will render solution biologically inactive. Single-dose vial contains no preservatives. Use only 1 dose per vial, then discard.
Filters: Not required; however, it was filtered during manufacturing with 0.2-micron filters. No significant loss of potency expected with use of non–protein binding filters of a similar size or larger.
Storage: Store in carton at 2° to 8° C (36° to 46° F). Do not freeze or shake. Protect from light.

COMPATIBILITY
Manufacturer states, "Do not administer in conjunction with other drug solutions."

RATE OF ADMINISTRATION
A single dose over at least 1 minute.

ACTIONS
An erythropoiesis-stimulating protein produced by recombinant DNA technology. Closely related to human erythropoietin. Production of endogenous erythropoietin is impaired in patients with chronic renal failure, and erythropoietin deficiency is the primary cause of their anemia. Darbepoetin has the same biologic effects as erythropoietin produced naturally by the kidneys. Stimulates bone marrow to produce RBCs, increasing the reticulocyte count within 10 days and the red cell count, hemoglobin, and hematocrit within 2 to 6 weeks. Normal iron stores are necessary because it steps up RBC production to a rate above what the body usually makes. New cells need iron, which is quickly depleted. Distribution is confined to the vascular space. Half-life is approximately 21 hours. Continued therapy will maintain improved RBC levels and decrease the need for transfusions.

INDICATIONS AND USES
Treatment of anemia associated with chronic kidney disease, including patients receiving dialysis and patients not receiving dialysis. ▪ As an SQ injection to treat chemotherapy-induced anemia in adult cancer patients who have nonmyeloid malignancies in which anemia is a result of the effect of concomitant myelosuppressive chemotherapy and who,

upon initiation of therapy, have a minimum of 2 additional months of planned chemotherapy.

Limitations of use: Not indicated for use in patients with cancer receiving hormonal agents, therapeutic biologic products, or radiotherapy unless receiving concomitant myelosuppressive chemotherapy. ▪ Not indicated for patients receiving myelosuppressive chemotherapy when the anticipated outcome is cure; see Precautions. ▪ Not indicated in patients with cancer receiving myelosuppressive chemotherapy in whom the anemia can be managed by transfusion. ▪ Has not been shown to improve quality of life, fatigue, or patient well-being; see Precautions. ▪ Not indicated as a substitute for an RBC transfusion in patients who require immediate correction of anemia.

CONTRAINDICATIONS

Known hypersensitivity to darbepoetin. ▪ Uncontrolled hypertension. ▪ Pure red cell aplasia (PRCA) that begins after treatment with darbepoetin or other erythropoietin agents.

PRECAUTIONS

May be given IV or SQ to patients not receiving dialysis. ▪ Erythropoiesis-stimulating agents (ESAs) increase the risk of death, MI, stroke, congestive heart failure, venous thromboembolism, thrombosis of hemodialysis vascular access, other thromboembolic events, and tumor progression or recurrence. Patients experienced greater risks of these adverse events when ESAs were administered to target a hemoglobin of greater than 11 Gm/dL. No trial has identified a hemoglobin target level, a darbepoetin dose, or a dosing strategy that does not increase these risks. Use the lowest darbepoetin dose sufficient to reduce the need for RBC transfusions. ▪ Use with caution in patients with coexistent cardiovascular disease and stroke. Patients with CKD and an insufficient hemoglobin response to ESA therapy may be at even greater risk for cardiovascular reactions and mortality than other patients. ▪ In clinical trials, ESAs increased the risk of death in patients undergoing CABG surgery and the risk of deep venous thrombosis in patients undergoing orthopedic procedures. ▪ Increases in hemoglobin of greater than 1 Gm/dL during any 2-week period have been associated with an increased incidence of cardiac arrest, neurologic events (e.g., seizures, stroke), exacerbations of hypertension, congestive heart failure (CHF), vascular thrombosis/ischemia/infarction, acute MI, deep vein thrombosis (DVT), pulmonary embolus, hemodialysis graft occlusion, and fluid overload/edema. See Dose Adjustments. ▪ Administration of ESAs to cancer patients shortened the overall survival time and/or increased the risk of tumor progression or recurrence in clinical studies of some patients with breast, cervical, head and neck, lymphoid, and non–small-cell lung malignancies. To minimize these risks, as well as the risks of serious cardiovascular and thrombovascular events, use the lowest dose needed to avoid a red blood cell transfusion. Use only to treat anemia due to concomitant myelosuppressive chemotherapy, and discontinue after completion of a chemotherapy course. ▪ BP may increase during therapy with darbepoetin. Hypertensive encephalopathy and seizures have been observed. ▪ Patients with uncontrolled hypertension should not be treated with darbepoetin until BP has been adequately controlled. ▪ In addition to low baseline hemoglobin and inadequate iron stores, delayed or diminished response may result from concurrent medical problems (e.g., infections, inflammatory or malignant processes, occult blood loss, underlying hematologic disease, folic acid or vitamin B_{12} deficiency, hemolysis, aluminum intoxication, osteofibrosis cystica, bone marrow fibrosis, pure red cell aplasia [PRCA], or anti-erythropoietin antibody–associated anemia). Correct or exclude other causes of anemia before initiating therapy. Not intended for use in anemia caused by iron or folate deficiencies, hemolysis, or GI bleeding or for use in treating symptoms of anemia, including dizziness, fatigue, low energy, poor quality of life, or shortness of breath. ▪ Safety and efficacy have not been established in patients with underlying hematologic diseases (e.g., hemolytic anemia, sickle cell anemia, thalassemia, porphyria). ▪ Therapy results in an increase in RBCs and a decrease in plasma volume, which could reduce dialysis efficiency; adjustment of dialysis prescription may be necessary. ▪ Darbepoetin increases the risk of seizures in patients with CKD. Use with caution in patients with epilepsy. ▪ As with all proteins, there is a potential for immunogenicity. The incidence of antibody development in patients receiving darbepoetin has not been determined. Use caution; hypersensitivity reactions and/or anaphylaxis can occur. ▪ Pure red cell aplasia (PRCA) and severe anemia, with or without other cytopenias, in association with neutralizing antibodies to erythropoietin have been observed. Most often reported in CKD patients receiving epoetin alfa by SQ injection. Evaluate any patient who develops a sudden loss of response to darbepoetin alfa accompanied by severe anemia and low reticulocyte count. Physicians may contact the manufacturer (Amgen) for help with evaluation of these patients. ▪ Blistering and skin exfoliation reactions, including erythema multiforme and Stevens-Johnson syndrome (SJS)/toxic epidermal necrolysis (TEN), have been reported. Discontinue therapy immediately if a severe cutaneous reaction is suspected. ▪ Darbepoetin is a growth factor that stimulates RBC production. Erythropoietin receptors are also found on the surfaces of normal, nonhematopoietic tissue and some malignant cell lines. The possibility that darbepoetin can act as a growth factor for any tumor type cannot be ruled out.

Monitor: Normal iron stores required to support epoetin-stimulated erythropoiesis. Transferrin saturation should be at least 20% and ferritin at least 100 ng/mL (100 mcg/L). Monitor before and during therapy. ▪ Monitor hemoglobin weekly in patients who are initiating therapy. Continue until stable and the maintenance dose has been established, then monitor at regular intervals (at least monthly). ▪ Monitor hemoglobin weekly for at least 4 weeks following adjustment of therapy. Once stabilized, continue to monitor at regular intervals (at least monthly). ▪ Monitor BP routinely. Initiation or intensification of antihypertensive therapy and dietary restrictions may be necessary. If BP is difficult to control by pharmacologic or dietary measures, the dose of darbepoetin should be reduced or withheld. ▪ Monitor for the presence of premonitory neurologic symptoms during the first several months after initiation of therapy. Seizures have been reported; see Precautions. ▪ Monitor for S/S of hypersensitivity reactions (e.g., anaphylaxis, angioedema, bronchospasm, rash, urticaria). ▪ Supplemental iron is usually required to increase and maintain iron stores. Administration of parenteral iron may be necessary in some patients.

Patient Education: Risk of seizures, especially for first several months of therapy. Do not drive or operate heavy equipment. Promptly report new-onset neurologic symptoms or change in seizure frequency. ▪ Stress the importance of compliance with diet, iron and vitamin (e.g., folic acid, B_{12}) supplementation, BP control, and dialysis regimen. ▪ Close monitoring of BP and hemoglobin is imperative. ▪ Promptly report S/S of a hypersensitivity reaction, pain or swelling in the legs, shortness of breath (SOB), increase in BP, dizziness, or loss of consciousness. ▪ Menses may resume; possibility of pregnancy. Contraception may be indicated. ▪ Additional instruction (e.g., equipment, techniques) will be required in patients who will self-administer (manufacturer supplies brochure). ▪ Increased risk of mortality, serious cardiovascular events, thromboembolic events, and tumor progression or recurrence. ▪ Read medication guide and instructions for use carefully. All patients should discuss the risks of using an ESA with a healthcare professional.

Maternal/Child: Use caution. Consider the benefits and risks of darbepoetin for the mother and possible risks to the fetus. ▪ Use caution in nursing mothers. ▪ Safety and effectiveness of darbepoetin alfa in pediatric patients with CKD receiving dialysis or not receiving dialysis have been established in the age-groups 1 month to 16 years. ▪ Safety and effectiveness were similar between adult and pediatric patients with CKD when darbepoetin was used for the initial treatment of anemia or when patients were transitioned from another erythropoietin to darbepoetin. ▪ Safety and effectiveness for use in pediatric cancer patients not established. ▪ Half-life and plasma concentrations in pediatric patients 3 years of age and older are similar to those seen in adults. See package insert.

Elderly: No differences in safety or efficacy were observed between older and younger patients.

DRUG/LAB INTERACTIONS

Specific information not available.

SIDE EFFECTS

Adult chronic kidney disease patients: Commonly reported adverse reactions include cough, dyspnea, hypertension, peripheral edema, and procedural hypotension. *Serious* adverse reactions include hypertension, increased mortality, MI, PRCA, seizures, serious hypersensitivity reactions, stroke, and thromboembolism. Other reported adverse reactions include angina, arteriovenous graft thrombosis, fluid overload, rash, and vascular access complications.

Pediatric chronic kidney disease patients: Commonly reported adverse reactions include convulsions, hypertension, injection site pain, and rash. *Serious* adverse reactions include convulsions and hypertension.

Cancer patients receiving chemotherapy: Commonly reported adverse reactions include abdominal pain, edema, and thrombovascular events. *Serious* adverse reactions include hypertension, increased mortality, increased risk of tumor progression or recurrence, MI, PRCA, seizures, serious hypersensitivity reactions, stroke, and thromboembolism.

Post-Marketing: PRCA and severe anemia, with or without other cytopenias, in association with neutralizing antibodies have been reported; see Precautions. Seizures, severe cutaneous reactions, and serious hypersensitivity reactions have also been reported.

ANTIDOTE

Notify physician of all side effects; most will be treated symptomatically. Excessive hypertension may require discontinuation of darbepoetin until BP is controlled or may respond to a reduction in dose of darbepoetin or to an increase in antihypertensive therapy. Reduce dose of darbepoetin in patients with an increase in hemoglobin of more than 1 Gm/dL in 2 weeks. May need to withhold darbepoetin until hemoglobin falls to desired goal. Consider phlebotomy in the event of overdose or polycythemia. If overdose or polycythemia does occur, monitor closely for cardiovascular events and hematologic abnormalities. When resuming therapy, monitor closely for evidence of rapid increases in hemoglobin concentration (greater than 1 Gm/dL within 14 days) and reduce dose as indicated. Adjustments in dialysis prescription may be required during dialysis to prevent clotting. Permanently discontinue therapy in patients with antibody-mediated anemia (PRCA). Patients should not be switched to other erythropoietic proteins, because antibodies may cross-react. Treat minor hypersensitivity reactions symptomatically. Discontinue drug and treat anaphylaxis as indicated; resuscitate as necessary.

DAUNORUBICIN AND CYTARABINE LIPOSOME FOR INJECTION BBW

Antineoplastic
(Anthracycline)

(DAW-noe-**ROO**-bi-sin and sye-**TAR**-a-been **LYE**-poe-sohm)

Vyxeos

USUAL DOSE

Do not interchange with other products containing daunorubicin and/or cytarabine. Vyxeos has different dose recommendations than daunorubicin hydrochloride, cytarabine, daunorubicin citrate liposome injection, and cytarabine liposome injection. Verify drug name and dose before preparation and administration to avoid dosing errors.

Pretreatment Requirements: Verify pregnancy status. Before initiating each cycle of Vyxeos, calculate the prior cumulative anthracycline exposure for the patient; see Precautions. Before initiating induction and each consolidation cycle, obtain an ECG and assess cardiac function by multigated radionuclide angiography (MUGA) scan or echocardiography (ECHO). Obtain CBC and liver and renal function studies before each consolidation cycle and as indicated; see Monitor.

Premedication: Administer prophylactic antiemetics before each treatment.

A full Vyxeos course consists of 1 to 2 cycles of induction and up to 2 cycles of consolidation. Do not start consolidation cycles until the absolute neutrophil count recovers to greater than 500/mm^3 and the platelet count recovers to greater than 50,000/mm^3 in the absence of unacceptable toxicity.

First cycle of induction: Daunorubicin 44 mg/M^2 and cytarabine 100 mg/M^2 as an IV infusion over 90 minutes on Days 1, 3, and 5.

Second induction cycle: If remission is not achieved with the first induction cycle, a second induction cycle may be administered 2 to 5 weeks after the first cycle if no unacceptable toxicity occurred. Administer daunorubicin 44 mg/M^2 and cytarabine 100 mg/M^2 as an IV infusion over 90 minutes on Days 1 and 3.

Consolidation: Administer the first consolidation cycle 5 to 8 weeks after the start of the last induction. Dose for consolidation is daunorubicin 29 mg/M^2 and cytarabine 65 mg/M^2 as an IV infusion over 90 minutes on Days 1 and 3. Administer the second consolidation cycle 5 to 8 weeks after the first in patients who do not show disease progression or unacceptable toxicity.

DOSE ADJUSTMENTS

Dose adjustment is not required for patients with mild or moderate renal impairment or in patients with hepatic impairment with a bilirubin level 3 mg/dL or less. ▪ No dose adjustment required based on age, body mass index, body weight, race, sex, and white blood cell count after adjusting dose by body surface area. ▪ Discontinue Vyxeos in patients who exhibit impaired cardiac function unless the benefit of continuing treatment outweighs the risk. ▪ If a planned dose is missed, administer the dose as soon as possible and adjust the dosing schedule accordingly to maintain the treatment interval. ▪ For hypersensitivity reactions of any grade/severity, interrupt the infusion immediately and manage symptoms. Reduce the rate of infusion or discontinue treatment as outlined in the following chart.

Management of Hypersensitivity Reactions to Vyxeos	
Mild symptoms	Once symptoms resolve, reinitiate infusion at half the previous rate of infusion. Consider premedication with antihistamines and/or corticosteroids for subsequent doses.
Moderate symptoms	Do not reinitiate infusion. For subsequent doses, premedicate with antihistamines and/or corticosteroids before initiating infusion at the same rate.
Severe/life-threatening symptoms	Permanently discontinue treatment. Treat according to the standard of care to manage symptoms, and monitor the patient until symptoms resolve.

DILUTION

Specific techniques required; see Precautions. Available as a lyophilized cake in a single-dose vial. Calculate the dose based on daunorubicin and individual patient's BSA. Calculate the number of vials required based on the daunorubicin dose. Remove required vials from refrigeration and equilibrate to RT for 30 minutes. Reconstitute each vial with 19 mL of SWFI. Immediately start a 5-minute timer and *carefully swirl the contents of the vial for 5 minutes* while gently inverting the vial every 30 seconds. Do not heat, vortex, or shake vigorously. After reconstitution, allow to rest for 15 minutes. Should be an opaque, purple, homogeneous dispersion. Each mL contains 2.2 mg of daunorubicin and 5 mg of cytarabine. Calculate the volume of reconstituted solution required using the following formula:

$$\text{Volume required (mL)} = \text{Dose of daunorubicin (mg/M}^2) \times \text{Patient's BSA (M}^2) \div 2.2 \text{ (mg/mL)}$$

Gently invert each vial 5 times before withdrawing the reconstituted product for further dilution. Withdraw the calculated volume and transfer to a 500-mL infusion bag of NS or D5W. Gently invert bag to mix the solution.

Filters: Manufacturer states, "An in-line membrane filter may be used for the IV infusion provided the minimum pore diameter of the filter is greater than or equal to 15 micrometers."

Storage: Refrigerate unreconstituted vials at 2° to 8° C (36° to 46° F) in original carton to protect from light. Should be stored in an upright position. Reconstituted product in the vial and fully diluted solutions may be refrigerated for up to 4 hours if not used immediately. Discard unused product.

COMPATIBILITY

Manufacturer states, "Do not mix Vyxeos with or administer as an infusion with other drugs."

RATE OF ADMINISTRATION

Use an infusion pump to administer by constant IV infusion over 90 minutes through a central venous catheter or a peripherally inserted central catheter. Flush the line before and after administration with NS or D5W.

ACTIONS

Vyxeos is a combination of daunorubicin and cytarabine in a 1:5 molar ratio encapsulated in liposomes. Daunorubicin is an anthracycline topoisomerase inhibitor, and cytarabine is a nucleoside metabolic inhibitor. The combination has been shown to have synergistic effects at killing leukemia cells in vitro and in murine models. Daunorubicin has antimitotic and cytotoxic activity. Cytarabine is a cell-cycle phase–specific antineoplastic agent, affecting cells only during the S-phase of cell division. Based on animal data, the liposomes enter and persist in the bone marrow and are taken up by leukemia cells to a greater extent than by normal bone marrow cells. After cellular internalization, liposomes undergo degradation, releasing cytarabine and daunorubicin within the intracellular environment. Half-life is 31.5 hours for daunorubicin and 40.4 hours for cytarabine. Metabolized to active and inactive metabolites with some excretion in urine.

INDICATIONS AND USES

Treatment of adults with newly diagnosed therapy-related acute myeloid leukemia (t-AML) or AML with myelodysplasia-related changes (AML-MRC).

CONTRAINDICATIONS

History of serious hypersensitivity reaction to cytarabine, daunorubicin, or any component of the formulation.

PRECAUTIONS

Follow guidelines for handling cytotoxic agents. See Appendix A, p. 1308. ▪ For IV use only. **Do not interchange with other products containing daunorubicin and/or cytarabine.** Vyxeos has different dose recommendations than daunorubicin hydrochloride, cytarabine, daunorubicin citrate liposome injection, and cytarabine liposome injection. Verify drug name and dose before preparation and administration to avoid dosing errors. ▪ Daunorubicin has been associated with severe local tissue necrosis at the site of drug extravasation. ▪ Serious or fatal hemorrhagic events associated with prolonged severe thrombocytopenia, including fatal CNS hemorrhages, have occurred. ▪ Contains the anthracycline daunorubicin, which has a known risk of cardiotoxicity. Prior therapy with anthracyclines, pre-existing cardiac disease, previous radiotherapy to the mediastinum, or concomitant use of cardiotoxic drugs may increase the risk of daunorubicin-induced cardiac toxicity. Assessment of cardiac function is required before initiating therapy; see Usual Dose. Discontinue therapy in patients with impaired cardiac function unless the benefit of initiating or continuing treatment outweighs the risk. Vyxeos treatment is not recommended in patients with an LVEF that is less than normal. ▪ Incidence of drug-induced CHF has been associated with cumulative doses of nonliposomal daunorubicin greater than 550 mg/M^2. Tolerable limit appears lower (400 mg/M^2) in patients who received radiation therapy to the mediastinum. Vyxeos treatment is not recommended in patients whose lifetime anthracycline exposure has reached the maximum cumulative limit. ▪ Serious or fatal hypersensitivity reactions, including anaphylaxis, have been reported with daunorubicin and cytarabine. ▪ Reconstituted Vyxeos contains copper gluconate (14% elemental copper). No clinical experience in patients with Wilson's disease or other copper-related metabolic disorders. The maximum theoretical total exposure of copper with the recommended dosing regimen is 106 mg/M^2. Use in patients with Wilson's disease only if the benefits outweigh the risks. ▪ Has not been studied in patients with severe renal impairment (CrCl 15 to 29 mL/min), ERSD, or a bilirubin level greater than 3 mg/dL.

Monitor: Pretreatment assessment required before initiating each cycle; see Usual Dose. ▪ Monitor blood counts regularly until recovery, and administer platelet transfusion support as required. ▪ Repeat MUGA scan or ECHO determinations of LVEF before consolidation and as clinically required. ▪ Monitor for S/S of a hypersensitivity reaction (e.g., chest pain, chills, dizziness, dyspnea, fever, flushing, hypotension, nausea, pruritus, rash, urticaria). ▪ In patients with Wilson's disease, risk of copper overload may require consultation with a hepatologist and nephrologist with expertise in managing acute copper toxicity. Monitor total serum copper, serum non-ceruloplasmin bound copper, 24-hour urine copper levels, and serial neuropsychological examinations in these patients. ▪ Determine absolute patency of vein. A stinging or burning sensation indicates extravasation; discontinue injection. Severe cellulitis and tissue necrosis will result from extravasation with conventional daunorubicin. ▪ Monitor for thrombocytopenia (platelet count less than 50,000/mm^3). Initiate precautions to prevent excessive bleeding (e.g., inspect IV sites, skin, and mucous membranes; use extreme care during invasive procedures; test urine, emesis, stool, and secretions for occult blood).

Patient Education: Review all current medications with provider. ▪ Promptly report IV site burning or stinging, S/S of a hypersensitivity reaction (e.g., light-headedness, rash, urticaria, tightness of the chest, wheezing), bleeding or bruising, dizziness, fever, infection, lack of coordination, loss of balance, numbness, severe headache, shortness of breath, sudden confusion, and swelling of extremities. ▪ Effective contraception required during treatment and for 6 months after the last dose of Vyxeos in females of reproductive potential and in males with female partners of reproductive potential. Verify pregnancy status before initiating treatment. Notify provider of known or suspected pregnancy. ▪ Periodic monitoring of blood counts imperative; transfusions may be required. ▪ See Appendix D, p. 1311.

Maternal/Child: Avoid pregnancy. Based on its mechanism of action, can cause fetal harm. Effective contraception required; see Patient Education. ▪ Has potential for serious adverse reactions in breast-fed infants; breast-feeding is not recommended during treatment and for at least 2 weeks after the last dose. ▪ Safety and effectiveness for use in pediatric patients not established.

Elderly: No overall differences in safety observed except for bleeding events, which occurred more frequently in elderly patients compared with younger patients.

DRUG/LAB INTERACTIONS

Risk of cardiotoxicity may increase with concomitant use of Vyxeos and **cardiotoxic agents** such as other anthracyclines (e.g., doxorubicin, idarubicin) or alkylating agents (e.g., cyclophosphamide, ifosfamide, cisplatin, carmustine, busulfan, chlormethine, and mitomycin) and/or radiation encompassing the heart. Assess cardiac function more frequently. ▪ Concomitant use with **hepatotoxic agents** (e.g., azathioprine, isoniazid, methotrexate, retinoids, sulfasalazine) may impair liver function and increase the toxicity of Vyxeos. Monitor hepatic function more frequently.

SIDE EFFECTS

Abdominal pain, arrhythmia, bacteremia, chills, constipation, cough, decreased appetite, diarrhea, dyspnea, edema, fatigue, febrile neutropenia, headache, hemorrhagic events, mucositis, musculoskeletal pain, nausea, pneumonia, rash, sleep disorders, and vomiting are most common. The most common serious adverse reactions are bacteremia, dyspnea, febrile neutropenia, hemorrhage, myocardial toxicity, pneumonia, and sepsis. Anxiety, catheter device/ injection site reaction, chest pain, delirium, dizziness, fungal infection, hemorrhoids, hypertension, hypotension, hypoxia, nonconduction cardiotoxicity, petechiae, pleural effusion, pruritus, renal insufficiency, sepsis, transfusion reactions, and visual impairment have also been reported. Laboratory abnormalities include prolonged cytopenias (neutropenia and thrombocytopenia) and chemistry abnormalities (alanine aminotransferase, hyperbilirubinemia, hypoalbuminemia, hypokalemia, and hyponatremia). Other serious side effects may include cardiotoxicity, copper overload, hypersensitivity reactions, and tissue necrosis.

ANTIDOTE
Most side effects will be treated symptomatically. Keep physician informed. Close monitoring of cumulative dosage of daunorubicin, CBC, ECG, and LVEF may prevent most serious and potentially fatal side effects. Supportive therapy as indicated will help sustain the patient in toxicity. See Dose Adjustments for management of hypersensitivity reactions and treat as appropriate (e.g., oxygen, antihistamines, epinephrine, corticosteroids, vasopressors, and/or fluids). Discontinue in patients with S/S of acute copper toxicity. Administration of whole blood products (e.g., packed RBCs, platelets, leukocytes) and/or blood modifiers (e.g., darbepoetin alfa, epoetin alfa, filgrastim, pegfilgrastim, sargramostim) may be indicated to treat bone marrow toxicity. See daunorubicin hydrochloride monograph for extravasation. Resuscitate as necessary.

DAUNORUBICIN HYDROCHLORIDE BBW
DAUNORUBICIN CITRATE
LIPOSOMAL INJECTION BBW

Antineoplastic
(anthracycline)

(daw-noh-**ROO**-bih-sin hy-droh-**KLOR**-eyed)
(daw-noh-**ROO**-bih-sin **SIH**-trate **LIP**-oh-sohm-ul)

Cerubidine ▪ DaunoXome

pH 4.5 to 6.5 ▪ 4.9 to 6

USUAL DOSE
ALL DAUNORUBICINS
Pretreatment: Verify pregnancy status. Baseline studies indicated; see Monitor.
CONVENTIONAL DAUNORUBICIN
Adult acute nonlymphocytic leukemia: 45 mg/M²/day on Days 1, 2, and 3 in adults under age 60 (adults over age 60 may require reduction to 30 mg/M²/day). Used in specific protocol combination therapy (e.g., cytarabine 100 mg/M²/day for 7 days). Regimen repeated every 3 to 4 weeks. In these subsequent courses, repeat daunorubicin, 30 to 45 mg/M²/day (depending on age) for only 2 days and cytarabine for only 5 days. To obtain a normal-appearing bone marrow may require up to 3 courses.
Adult acute lymphocytic leukemia: 45 mg/M²/day on Days 1, 2, and 3. Used in combination therapy (e.g., vincristine, prednisone, and L-asparaginase). In all situations, when remission is complete, an individual maintenance program should be established.
DAUNOXOME (LIPOSOMAL INJECTION)
Advanced, HIV-associated Kaposi's sarcoma: 40 mg/M² as an IV infusion. Repeat every 2 weeks. Continue treatment until there is evidence of disease progression (specifics outlined in package insert).
PEDIATRIC DOSE
CONVENTIONAL DAUNORUBICIN
See Maternal/Child.
Acute lymphocytic leukemia in pediatric patients 2 years of age and older: 25 mg/M²/day on Day 1 each week, vincristine 1.5 mg/M² on Day 1 each week, and prednisone 40 mg/M² PO daily. Remission should be obtained in 4 weeks. If a partial remission is obtained after 4 weeks, 1 or 2 more weeks of treatment may produce a complete remission.
Acute lymphocytic leukemia in infants and children under 2 years of age or less than 0.5 M² body surface: Calculate dose based on weight instead of body surface area: 1 mg/kg.
DAUNOXOME: Safety for use in pediatric patients not established.

DOSE ADJUSTMENTS
ALL DAUNORUBICINS: See Precautions/Monitor.

CONVENTIONAL DAUNORUBICIN: Profound bone marrow suppression is usually required to eradicate the leukemic cells and induce a complete remission. Evaluate bone marrow and peripheral blood to determine need for additional courses. ▪ See Usual Dose for adults over 60 years of age. ▪ Reduce dose in impaired hepatic or renal function according to the following chart.

Daunorubicin Dosing in Impaired Hepatic or Renal Function		
Serum Bilirubin	**Serum Creatinine**	**Dose Reduction**
1.2 to 3.0 mg	—	25%
>3 mg	—	50%
—	>3 mg	50%

DaunoXome: Reduce dose to 75% of normal (30 mg/M^2) if serum bilirubin is 1.2 to 3 mg/dL. Reduce dose to 50% of normal (20 mg/M^2) if serum bilirubin or creatinine is greater than 3 mg/dL. ▪ Withhold dose if absolute granulocyte count is less than 750 cells/mm^3.

DILUTION
Specific techniques required; see Precautions.

Conventional daunorubicin: Each 20 mg must be diluted with 4 mL of SWFI (5 mg/mL). Agitate gently to dissolve completely. Further dilute each dose with 10 to 15 mL of NS. Must be given through Y-tube of a free-flowing infusion of D5W or NS. May be added to 100 mL NS and given as an infusion. Use extreme caution.

DaunoXome: Dilute each single dose with an equal amount of D5W. Available as a 2 mg/mL preservative-free solution. Withdraw calculated volume (dose of DaunoXome) from vial; transfer to a sterile infusion bag that contains an equal volume of D5W. Desired concentration is 1 mg/mL. Do not use any other diluent. A translucent red liposomal dispersion; do not use if opaque. Do not use in-line filters for infusion. See Compatibility.

Filters: *DaunoXome:* Manufacturer states, "Do not use in-line filters for infusion."

Storage: *Conventional daunorubicin:* Protect from sunlight. Diluted solution stable 24 hours at room temperature, 48 hours if refrigerated; then discard.

DaunoXome: Refrigerate unopened vials; avoid freezing. Protect from light. Discard unused drug. Reconstituted solutions may be refrigerated for a maximum of 6 hours.

COMPATIBILITY
CONVENTIONAL DAUNORUBICIN

Manufacturer states, "Should not be administered mixed with other drugs or heparin."

Other sources suggest a few specific **compatibilities** dependent on concentration and manufacturer; consult a pharmacist.

DAUNOXOME

Manufacturer states, "The only fluid that may be mixed with DaunoXome is D5W. Must not be mixed with saline, bacteriostatic agents such as benzyl alcohol, or any other solution."

RATE OF ADMINISTRATION
CONVENTIONAL DAUNORUBICIN

IV injection: A single dose of properly diluted medication over 3 to 5 minutes.

IV infusion: A single dose evenly distributed over 30 to 45 minutes.

DAUNOXOME

A single dose as an infusion evenly distributed over 60 minutes. Do not use an in-line filter. Back pain, flushing, and chest tightness may occur. Usually subsides if infusion is stopped and usually does not recur if infusion is restarted at a slower rate after symptoms subside.

ACTIONS
CONVENTIONAL DAUNORUBICIN: A highly toxic antibiotic antineoplastic agent. Rapidly cleared from plasma, it inhibits synthesis of DNA. Cell-cycle specific for S phase; exact method

of action is unknown; antimitotic, cytotoxic, and immunosuppressive. Widely distributed in tissues, with the highest concentrations occurring in the spleen, kidneys, liver, lungs, and heart. Does not cross blood-brain barrier. Metabolized in the liver and other tissues. Elimination half-life is 18 to 30 hours. Slowly excreted in bile and urine.

DAUNOXOME: A liposomal preparation of daunorubicin formulated to maximize selectivity for solid tumors. In the circulation, the liposomal preparation protects the entrapped daunorubicin from chemical and enzymatic degradation, minimizes protein binding, and generally decreases uptake by normal (non–reticuloendothelial system) tissues. The mechanism of delivery is not known, but may be through the often altered and/or compromised vasculature of tumors. In animals, it has been shown to accumulate in tumors to a greater extent than conventional daunorubicin. Released over time within the cells of the solid tumor. Persists at high levels within tumor tissue for several days. It differs from conventional daunorubicin because it mostly confines itself to vascular fluid volume. Plasma clearance is slower and the AUC (area under the curve) is larger.

INDICATIONS AND USES

CONVENTIONAL DAUNORUBICIN: Treatment of acute nonlymphocytic leukemia in adults (myelogenous, monocytic, erythroid). ▪ Combination therapy for induction of remission in acute lymphocytic leukemia in adults and pediatric patients.

DAUNOXOME: Currently approved only for first-line cytotoxic therapy for advanced HIV-associated Kaposi's sarcoma.

CONTRAINDICATIONS

CONVENTIONAL DAUNORUBICIN: Hypersensitivity to daunorubicin or any of its components. *Not absolute:* Pre-existing bone marrow suppression, impaired cardiac function, pre-existing infection; see Precautions.

DAUNOXOME: History of hypersensitivity reaction to previous treatment with DaunoXome or any of its components (includes conventional daunorubicin). Not recommended in patients with less than advanced HIV-related Kaposi's sarcoma.

PRECAUTIONS

ALL DAUNORUBICINS: Follow guidelines for handling cytotoxic agents. See Appendix A, p. 1308. ▪ Administered by or under the direction of the physician specialist with facilities for monitoring the patient and responding to any medical emergency. ▪ For IV use only; do not give IM or SQ. ▪ Severe myelosuppression may occur and may lead to infection or hemorrhage. ▪ Use extreme caution in pre-existing drug-induced bone marrow suppression, existing heart disease, previous treatment with other anthracyclines (e.g., doxorubicin), or radiation therapy encompassing the heart. ▪ Incidence of myocardial toxicity increases after a total cumulative dose that exceeds 400 to 550 mg/M^2 in adults, 300 mg/M^2 in pediatric patients over 2 years of age, or 10 mg/kg in pediatric patients under 2 years of age. Potentially fatal congestive heart failure may occur either during therapy or months to years after therapy is complete. ▪ Urine may be reddish color (from dye, not hematuria).

Monitor: ALL DAUNORUBICINS: Monitor CBC including differential and platelet count before each dose. ▪ Monitoring of liver function, kidney function, ECG, chest x-ray, echocardiography, and systolic ejection fraction indicated before and during therapy; recommended before each course. ▪ Evaluation of cardiac function by medical history and physical exam is recommended before each dose; see Precautions. ▪ Monitor closely for S/S of hemorrhage or infection; may be life threatening. ▪ Prophylactic antibiotics may be indicated pending results of C/S in a febrile neutropenic patient. ▪ Determine absolute patency of vein. A stinging or burning sensation indicates extravasation; discontinue injection and use another vein. Severe cellulitis and tissue necrosis will result from extravasation with conventional daunorubicins; has not been observed with DaunoXome. ▪ Prophylactic antiemetics may reduce nausea and vomiting and increase patient comfort. ▪ Monitor uric acid levels; maintain hydration; uric acid–lowering drugs (e.g., allopurinol) may be indicated. ▪ Monitor for thrombocytopenia (platelet count less than 50,000/mm^3). Initiate precautions to prevent excessive bleeding (e.g., inspect IV sites, skin, and mucous membranes; use extreme care during invasive procedures; test urine, emesis, stool, and secretions for occult blood).

CONVENTIONAL DAUNORUBICIN: May cause acute congestive heart failure with total cumulative doses over 550 mg/M^2 in adults (400 mg/M^2 if previous treatment with doxorubicin or radiation therapy in area of heart), 300 mg/M^2 in pediatric patients over 2 years of age, and 10 mg/kg in pediatric patients under 2 years of age.

DaunoXome: May also cause cardiomyopathy. Monitoring of LVEF recommended at total cumulative doses of 320 mg/M^2, 480 mg/M^2, and every 240 mg/M^2 thereafter.

Patient Education: Effective birth control recommended. ▪ Report IV site burning or stinging promptly. ▪ Secondary leukemias have been reported. ▪ See Appendix D, p. 1311.

Maternal/Child: ALL DAUNORUBICINS: Category D: can cause fetal harm. Avoid pregnancy. ▪ Safety for use in breast-feeding not established; discontinue breast-feeding. ▪ Cardiotoxicity may be more frequent and occur at lower cumulative doses in pediatric patients. ▪ See Monitor.

DaunoXome: Safety for use in pediatric patients not established.

Elderly: Cardiotoxicity and myelotoxicity may be more severe. Consider age-related renal impairment. Safety of DaunoXome for use in the elderly has not been established.

DRUG/LAB INTERACTIONS

Concurrent use with **cyclophosphamide** may increase cardiotoxicity. ▪ Dose reduction may be required with concurrent use of **other myelosuppressive agents.** ▪ Concurrent use with **hepatotoxic agents** (e.g., high-dose methotrexate) may increase risk of toxicity. ▪ Risk of cardiotoxicity increased in patients previously treated with maximum cumulative doses of **other anthracyclines** (e.g., doxorubicin, idarubicin) **and/or radiation encompassing the heart.** ▪ Do not administer **vaccines or chloroquine** to patients receiving antineoplastic drugs. ▪ See Precautions.

SIDE EFFECTS

ALL DAUNORUBICINS: Bone marrow suppression and cardiotoxicity are dose related and dose limiting.

CONVENTIONAL DAUNORUBICIN: Acute congestive heart failure, alopecia (reversible), bone marrow suppression (marked with average doses), chills, decrease in systolic ejection fraction, depressed QRS voltage, diarrhea, fever, gonadal suppression, mucositis, myocarditis, nausea, pericarditis, skin rash, vomiting.

DaunoXome: Granulocytopenia is most common. Symptoms common to conventional daunorubicin may also occur. Infusion-related back pain, chest tightness, and flushing may be related to liposomal formulation.

Overdose: Will cause increased severity of myelosuppression, fatigue, nausea, and vomiting.

ANTIDOTE

Most side effects will be tolerated or treated symptomatically. Keep physician informed. Close monitoring of cumulative dosage, bone marrow, ECG, chest x-ray, echocardiography, and systolic ejection fraction may prevent most serious and potentially fatal side effects. There is no specific antidote. Supportive therapy as indicated will help sustain the patient in toxicity. Administration of whole blood products (e.g., packed RBCs, platelets, leukocytes) and/or blood modifiers (e.g., darbepoetin alfa, epoetin alfa, filgrastim, pegfilgrastim, sargramostim) may be indicated to treat bone marrow toxicity. For extravasation, aspirate as much infiltrated drug as possible, flood site with normal saline, and inject hydrocortisone sodium succinate or hyaluronidase throughout extravasated tissue. Use a 27- or 25-gauge needle. Cold, moist compresses may be helpful; elevate extremity. Site should be observed promptly by a reconstructive surgeon.

DECITABINE FOR INJECTION
(deh-**SIGHT**-ah-been for in-**JEK**-shun)

**Antineoplastic
(miscellaneous)**

Dacogen

pH 6.7 to 7.3

USUAL DOSE

Pretreatment: Verify pregnancy status. Baseline studies indicated; see Monitor.

There are two treatment options (a 3-day regimen and a 5-day regimen). With either regimen, treatment for a minimum of 4 cycles is recommended. A complete or partial response may take longer than 4 cycles.

Premedication: Standard antiemetic therapy is indicated.

Decitabine: *Option 1 (3-day regimen):* 15 mg/M^2 as an infusion over 3 hours. Repeat every 8 hours for 3 days. Repeat this complete cycle every 6 weeks. See Dose Adjustments and Monitor.

Option 2 (5-day regimen): 20 mg/M^2 as an infusion over 1 hour. Repeat once each day for 5 days. Repeat this complete cycle every 4 weeks. See Dose Adjustments and Monitor.

DOSE ADJUSTMENTS

Option 1 and Option 2: Hematologic recovery to at least an ANC equal to or greater than 1,000 cells/mm^3 and platelets equal to or greater than 50,000 cells/mm^3 is required before subsequent cycles are administered. ▪ If an SCr equal to or greater than 2 mg/dL, an ALT or a total bilirubin equal to or greater than 2 times the ULN, and/or an active or uncontrolled infection occur, do not restart decitabine therapy until the toxicity is resolved. ▪ No additional dose reductions are indicated based on age, gender, or race; see Precautions and Elderly. ▪ If hematologic recovery from a previous decitabine cycle requires more than 6 weeks but less than 8 weeks, delay repeat cycle of decitabine for up to 2 weeks. When therapy is restarted, reduce dose for that cycle to 11 mg/M^2 every 8 hours (33 mg/M^2/day, 99 mg/M^2/cycle). ▪ If hematologic recovery from a previous decitabine cycle requires more than 8 weeks but less than 10 weeks, assess the patient for disease progression (by bone marrow aspirates). If disease progression has not occurred, delay repeat cycle of decitabine for up to 2 more weeks to allow for hematologic recovery. When therapy is restarted, reduce dose for that cycle to 11 mg/M^2 every 8 hours (33 mg/M^2/day, 99 mg/M^2/cycle). In subsequent cycles, maintain or increase dose based on hematologic recovery.

DILUTION

Specific techniques required; see Precautions. Temperature of the diluent (NS or D5W) depends on time of administration and preparation.

If decitabine will be used within 15 minutes of preparation: Reconstitute a single vial (50 mg) with 10 mL of room temperature SWFI (each mL contains 5 mg of decitabine at a pH of 6.7 to 7.3). Further dilute immediately with room temperature NS or D5W to a final concentration of 0.1 to 1 mg/mL (further dilute each mL with 4 mL additional diluent for a 1 mg/mL concentration or 49 mL for a 0.1 mg/mL concentration). Must be used within 15 minutes of reconstitution.

If decitabine will not be used within 15 minutes of reconstitution: Decitabine must be reconstituted with room temperature SWFI and further diluted using cold (2° to 8° C) infusion fluids (NS or D5W) to a final concentration as above and stored at 2° to 8° C (36° to 46° F) for up to a maximum of 4 hours.

Filters: Specific information not available.

Storage: Store unopened vials at 25° C (77° F); excursions permitted to 15° to 30° C (59° to 86° F). Use of reconstituted and/or diluted solution within 15 minutes of reconstitution is preferred, or a specific process is required; see Dilution. Use the diluted, refrigerated solution within 4 hours from the time of preparation or discard.

COMPATIBILITY

Compatibility information not available from manufacturer; consult a pharmacist.

RATE OF ADMINISTRATION
Option 1: A single dose as an infusion equally distributed over 3 hours.
Option 2: A single dose as an infusion equally distributed over 1 hour.

ACTIONS
A hypomethylating antineoplastic agent. Cytotoxic to proliferating cells through a process that incorporates it into DNA, inhibits the enzyme DNA methyltransferase, and causes hypomethylation of DNA, leading to cell disintegration and/or death. This hypomethylation in neoplastic cells may restore normal function to genes that are critical for the control of cellular differentiation and proliferation and allow the formation of normal RBCs and platelets. Patients with myelodysplastic syndromes who have responded to decitabine have become transfusion independent. Terminal half-life range is 0.21 to 0.82 hours. Extensively metabolized by an unknown route(s). Protein binding is negligible.

INDICATIONS AND USES
Treatment of patients with myelodysplastic syndromes (MDS), including previously treated and untreated *de novo* and secondary MDS of all French-American-British subtypes (refractory anemia, refractory anemia with ringed sideroblasts, refractory anemia with excess blasts, refractory anemia with excess blasts in transformation, and chronic myelomonocytic leukemia) and intermediate-1, intermediate-2, and high-risk International Prognostic Scoring System groups.

CONTRAINDICATIONS
Manufacturer states, "None."

PRECAUTIONS
Follow guidelines for handling cytotoxic agents. See Appendix A, p. 1308. ▪ Administered by or under the direction of a physician specialist in a facility with adequate diagnostic and treatment facilities to monitor the patient and respond to any medical emergency. ▪ The effects of age, gender, race, or renal or hepatic impairment on the pharmacokinetics of decitabine have not been studied. ▪ Fatal and serious myelosuppression occurs in decitabine-treated patients. ▪ Myelosuppression and worsening neutropenia may occur more frequently in the first or second treatment cycles and may not indicate progression of underlying MDS. Neutropenia and thrombocytopenia may be dose-limiting toxicities. ▪ Patients with MDS produce poorly functioning and immature blood cells and experience anemia, bleeding, fatigue, infection, and weakness. High-risk MDS patients may experience bone marrow failure, which may lead to death from bleeding and infection. ▪ MDS can progress to acute leukemia (AML). ▪ Use caution in patients with renal or hepatic impairment; monitor more frequently for excessive toxicity. Use has not been studied.

Monitor: Obtain a baseline CBC with platelets and monitor before each dosing cycle and as indicated between cycles. ▪ Mange toxicity using dose-delay, dose-reduction, growth factors, and anti-infective therapies as needed. ▪ Obtain a baseline and monitor renal and hepatic function (BUN, SCr, bilirubin) as indicated. ▪ Use prophylactic antiemetics to reduce nausea and vomiting and increase patient comfort. ▪ Monitor for S/S of infection. Prophylactic antibiotics may be indicated pending results of C/S in a febrile neutropenic patient. ▪ Monitor for thrombocytopenia (platelet count less than $50,000/mm^3$). Initiate precautions to prevent excessive bleeding (e.g., inspect IV sites, skin, and mucous membranes; use extreme care during invasive procedures; test urine, emesis, stool, and secretions for occult blood). ▪ Avoid administration of live virus vaccine to immunocompromised patients. ▪ Observe for S/S of a hypersensitivity reaction; specific information not available. ▪ See Precautions and Antidote.

Patient Education: Avoid pregnancy; effective birth control recommended for both males and females; see Maternal/Child. Females should report a suspected pregnancy immediately. ▪ Discuss possible liver or kidney disease with a healthcare professional. ▪ Report S/S of infection (e.g., fever, sore throat), bruising, bleeding, or other suspected side effects.

Maternal/Child: Avoid pregnancy; may cause fetal harm. Females of childbearing potential should avoid becoming pregnant and use effective contraception while receiving decitabine and for 6 months after the last dose. Males with female partners of reproductive potential should use effective contraception while receiving treatment with decitabine and for 3 months after the last dose. ▪ Avoid breast-feeding during treatment with decitabine and for at least 1 week after the last dose. ▪ Safety and effectiveness for use in pediatric patients not established.

Elderly: The majority of patients in clinical trials were over 65 years of age. Safety and effectiveness similar to younger adults; however, greater sensitivity of some older individuals should be considered.

DRUG/LAB INTERACTIONS

Formal drug interactions studies have not been completed. In vitro studies suggest that decitabine is unlikely to inhibit or induce the activities of cytochrome P_{450} isoenzymes. ▪ Plasma protein binding is negligible; interactions due to displacement of more highly protein bound drugs from plasma proteins are not expected. ▪ Do not administer **live virus vaccines** to immunocompromised patients who are receiving antineoplastic agents.

SIDE EFFECTS

Cough, constipation, diarrhea, fatigue, fever, hyperglycemia, nausea, and petechiae have been reported most commonly. Bone marrow suppression (anemia, neutropenia, thrombocytopenia) was the most frequent cause of dose reduction, delay, and discontinuation. Grade 3 or 4 adverse events included febrile neutropenia, leukopenia, neutropenia, and thrombocytopenia. During clinical trials, therapy was also discontinued because of abnormal liver function tests, cardiopulmonary arrest, intracranial hemorrhage, *Mycobacterium avium* complex infection, and pneumonia. Atrial fibrillation, central line infection, febrile neutropenia, neutropenia, and pulmonary edema also resulted in delayed doses; bone marrow suppression (anemia, neutropenia, thrombocytopenia), depression, edema, lethargy, pharyngitis, and tachycardia resulted in reduced doses. Numerous other side effects may occur.

Post-Marketing: Acute febrile neutrophilic dermatosis (Sweet's syndrome) has been reported.

Overdose: Increased myelosuppression, including prolonged neutropenia and thrombocytopenia.

ANTIDOTE

Notify physician of any side effects. Most will be treated symptomatically. Dosage may be delayed for hematologic toxicity. Hematologic recovery to at least an ANC equal to or greater than 1,000 cells/mm³ and platelets equal to or greater than 50,000 cells/mm³ between cycles is required; see Dose Adjustments. If an SCr equal to or greater than 2 mg/dL, an ALT or a total bilirubin equal to or greater than 2 times the ULN, and/or an uncontrolled infection occur, discontinue decitabine therapy until the toxicity is resolved. Blood and blood products, antibiotics, and other adjunctive therapies must be available. Blood modifiers (e.g., darbepoetin alfa, epoetin alfa, filgrastim, pegfilgrastim, sargramostim) may be indicated to treat bone marrow toxicity. No known antidote; provide supportive care in overdose. ▪ Resuscitate as necessary.

DELAFLOXACIN BBW

(del-a-**FLOXS**-a-sin)

Antibacterial
(Fluoroquinolone)

Baxdela

USUAL DOSE

Pretreatment: Baseline studies indicated; see Precautions and Monitor.

Acute bacterial skin and skin structure infections (ABSSSI): 300 mg as an IV infusion over 60 minutes every 12 hours for 5 to 14 days.

Community-acquired bacterial pneumonia (CABP): 300 mg as an IV infusion over 60 minutes every 12 hours for 5 to 10 days. A 300-mg IV dose is equivalent to a 450-mg oral dose. Transfer to oral therapy at the discretion of the physician.

DOSE ADJUSTMENTS

No dose adjustment required in mild to moderate renal impairment (estimated glomerular filtration rate [eGFR] 30 to 89 mL/min/1.73 M^2). ▪ Reduce dose to 200 mg IV every 12 hours in severe renal impairment (eGFR 15 to 29 mL/min/1.73 M^2), and transfer to a 450-mg tablet orally every 12 hours at the discretion of the physician. ▪ Not recommended for use in end-stage renal disease (ESRD) (eGFR less than 15 mL/min/1.73 M^2), including patients on hemodialysis (information is insufficient to provide dosing recommendations). ▪ No dose adjustment required in patients with hepatic impairment.

DILUTION

Available in single-use vials. Reconstitute each 300-mg vial with 10.5 mL of D5W or NS. Shake vial vigorously until contents dissolve completely. Reconstituted vial contains 300 mg per 12 mL (25 mg/mL) as a clear yellow to amber-colored solution. Withdraw the desired dose (12 mL for a 300-mg dose and 8 mL for a 200-mg dose) from the reconstituted solution. Must be further diluted to a total volume of 250 mL with NS or D5W to achieve a concentration of 1.2 mg/mL for administration.

Filters: Specific information not available.

Storage: Before use, store vials at CRT. Reconstituted vials and diluted solution may be refrigerated at 2° to 8° C (36° to 46° F) or stored at 20° to 25° C (68° to 77° F) for up to 24 hours. Do not freeze. Discard unused solution.

COMPATIBILITY

Manufacturer states, "Do NOT administer delafloxacin for injection through the same IV line with any solution containing multivalent cations (e.g., calcium and magnesium). Do NOT co-infuse delafloxacin with other medications."

RATE OF ADMINISTRATION

Administer each 300- or 200-mg dose as an IV infusion equally distributed over 60 minutes. May be given through a Y-tube of infusion set. Temporarily discontinue other solutions infusing at the same site, and flush tubing with D5W or NS before and after delafloxacin; see Compatibility.

ACTIONS

A fluoroquinolone antibacterial drug. Antibacterial activity is due to the inhibition of both bacterial topoisomerase IV and DNA gyrase (topoisomerase II), enzymes that are required for bacterial DNA replication, transcription, repair, and recombination. Exhibits a concentration-dependent bactericidal activity against gram-positive and gram-negative bacteria in vitro. AUC comparable for IV and oral doses. 84% protein bound, primarily to albumin. Metabolized predominantly by glucuronidation. Mean half-life is 3.7 hours. Excreted as unchanged drug and glucuronide metabolites in urine and feces.

INDICATIONS AND USES

Treatment of adults with infections caused by susceptible strains of designated microorganisms in conditions listed in this section.

Treatment of acute bacterial skin and skin structure infections (ABSSSI). ▪ Treatment of adults with community-acquired bacterial pneumonia (CABP).

CONTRAINDICATIONS

Known hypersensitivity to delafloxacin, any of its components, or any of the fluoroquinolone class of antibacterial drugs.

PRECAUTIONS

For IV use only. ■ To reduce the development of drug-resistant bacteria and maintain its effectiveness, delafloxacin should be used to treat only those infections proven or strongly suspected to be caused by bacteria. Prescribing delafloxacin in the absence of a proven or strongly suspected bacterial infection is unlikely to provide benefit to the patient and increases the risk of development of drug-resistant bacteria. ■ Culture and sensitivity studies indicated to determine susceptibility of the causative organism to delafloxacin. ■ Cross-resistance between delafloxacin and other fluoroquinolone-class antibacterial agents has been observed; however, some isolates resistant to other fluoroquinolones may be susceptible to delafloxacin. ■ Prolonged use may cause superinfection because of overgrowth of nonsusceptible organisms. ■ Fluoroquinolones have been associated with disabling and potentially irreversible serious adverse reactions that have occurred together in the same patient. Commonly seen adverse reactions include tendinitis and tendon rupture, arthralgia, myalgia, peripheral neuropathy, and CNS effects (e.g., anxiety, confusion, depression, hallucinations, insomnia, severe headaches). These reactions can occur within hours to weeks after starting delafloxacin and have been seen in patients of any age and in patients without any pre-existing risk factors. Discontinue delafloxacin immediately and avoid the use of fluoroquinolones in patients who experience any of these serious adverse reactions. ■ Fluoroquinolones have been associated with an increased risk of tendinitis and tendon rupture in all ages. Most frequently involves the Achilles tendon but has also been reported with the shoulder, hand, biceps, thumb, and other tendon sites. ■ Tendon rupture or tendinitis may occur within hours of starting a fluoroquinolone or as long as several months after completion of fluoroquinolone therapy and may occur bilaterally. Risk may be increased in patients over 60 years of age, in patients taking corticosteroids, and in patients with heart, kidney, or lung transplants. Other risk factors include strenuous physical activity, renal failure, and previous tendon disorders such as rheumatoid arthritis. Avoid delafloxacin in patients who have a history of tendon disorders or have experienced tendinitis or tendon rupture. Discontinue delafloxacin immediately if patient experiences pain, swelling, inflammation, or rupture of a tendon. ■ Fluoroquinolones have been associated with an increased risk of peripheral neuropathy. Cases of sensory or sensorimotor axonal polyneuropathy resulting in paresthesias, hypoesthesias, dysesthesias (impairment of sensitivity or touch), or weakness have been reported. Symptoms may occur soon after initiation of therapy and may be irreversible. To minimize the development of an irreversible condition, discontinue delafloxacin if the patient experiences symptoms of peripheral neuropathy, including pain, burning, tingling, numbness, and/or weakness or other alterations of sensation, including light touch, pain, temperature, position sense, and vibratory sensation and/or motor strength. Avoid delafloxacin in patients who have previously experienced peripheral neuropathy. ■ Fluoroquinolones, including delafloxacin, have been associated with an increased risk of seizures (convulsions), increased intracranial pressure (pseudotumor cerebri), tremors, and light-headedness. May trigger seizures or lower the seizure threshold. Use caution in patients with epilepsy or known or suspected CNS disorders that may predispose patients to seizures or lower the seizure threshold (e.g., severe cerebral arteriosclerosis, previous history of convulsions, reduced cerebral blood flow, altered brain structure, or stroke) or in the presence of other risk factors that may predispose patients to seizures (e.g., drugs that may lower the seizure threshold, renal dysfunction). ■ Fluoroquinolones, including delafloxacin, have been associated with an increased risk of psychiatric adverse reactions, including toxic psychosis; psychotic reactions progressing to suicidal ideations/thoughts, hallucinations, paranoia; depression; or self-injurious behavior such as attempted or completed suicide; anxiety, agitation, restlessness or nervousness; confusion, delirium, disorientation, or disturbances in attention; insomnia or nightmares; and memory impairment. These reactions may occur after the first dose. ■ Fluoroquinolones have neuromuscular blocking activity and may exacerbate muscle weakness in persons with myasthenia gravis. Serious adverse events, including a requirement for ventilatory support and deaths, have been reported in these patients. Avoid use in patients with a known history of myasthenia gravis. ▪ Serious and occasionally fatal hypersensitivity and/or anaphylactic reactions have been reported and may occur after the first dose. ▪ *Clostridium difficile*–associated diarrhea (CDAD) has been reported. May range from mild diarrhea to fatal colitis. Consider in patients who present with diarrhea during or after treatment with delafloxacin. ▪ Epidemiologic studies report an increased rate of aortic aneurysm and dissection within 2 months after use of fluoroquinolones, particularly in elderly patients. In patients with a known aortic aneurysm or in patients who are at greater risk for aortic aneurysms, delafloxacin use should be limited to cases in which there are no alternative antibacterial treatments available. ▪ Fluoroquinolones, including delafloxacin, have been associated with disturbances of blood glucose, including symptomatic hyperglycemia and hypoglycemia, usually in diabetic patients receiving concomitant treatment with an oral hypoglycemic agent (e.g., glyburide) or with insulin. In these patients, careful monitoring of blood glucose is recommended. Severe cases of hypoglycemia resulting in coma or death have been reported. ▪ Use caution in patients with impaired renal function; see Dose Adjustments.

Monitor: Obtain baseline CBC with differential, SCr, and blood glucose. Monitor SCr and eGFR, especially in patients with severe renal impairment. If SCr increases, consider switching to delafloxacin tablets, if possible. ▪ Monitor for S/S of a hypersensitivity reaction (e.g., airway obstruction, angioedema, cardiovascular collapse, dyspnea, hypotension/shock, itching, loss of consciousness, tingling, urticaria, and other serious skin reactions). May cause anaphylaxis with the first or succeeding doses. Emergency equipment must always be available; see Precautions. ▪ Monitor for S/S of peripheral neuropathy. Discontinue delafloxacin at the first symptoms of neuropathy (e.g., pain, burning, tingling, numbness, and/or weakness) or if patient is found to have deficits in light touch, pain, temperature, position sense, vibratory sensation, and/or motor strength. ▪ Monitor for S/S of tendinitis or tendon rupture (e.g., tendon pain, swelling, or inflammation). ▪ Monitor for S/S of CNS effects (e.g., anxiety, confusion, depression, hallucinations, insomnia, paranoia, seizures). ▪ Monitor blood glucose, especially in diabetic patients. ▪ Monitor infusion site for inflammation and/or extravasation. ▪ See Precautions, Drug/Lab Interactions, and Antidote.

Patient Education: A patient medication guide is available from the manufacturer. ▪ Discontinue delafloxacin and promptly report the development of any severe adverse reaction. ▪ Review all medicines and disease history with pharmacist or physician before initiating treatment. ▪ Inform physician of any history of myasthenia gravis. ▪ Promptly report skin rash or any other hypersensitivity reaction. ▪ Discontinue delafloxacin and promptly report tendon pain, swelling or inflammation, weakness, or inability to use a joint. Avoid exercise and use of the affected area. ▪ Promptly report pain, burning, tingling, numbness, and/or weakness in extremities. Nerve damage can be permanent. ▪ Promptly report development of any CNS side effects (e.g., convulsions, dizziness, lightheadedness, change in mood or behavior). ▪ Inform physician of any history of seizures. ▪ Request assistance with ambulation; may cause dizziness and light-headedness. Use caution in tasks that require alertness. ▪ Promptly report diarrhea or bloody stools that occur during treatment or up to several months after an antibiotic has been discontinued; may indicate CDAD and require treatment. ▪ Seek emergency medical care if sudden chest, stomach, or back pain is experienced. ▪ Diabetic patients taking oral hypoglycemic agents or insulin should discontinue delafloxacin and contact their provider if they experience a hypoglycemic reaction. ▪ See Precautions, Monitor, and Antidote.

Maternal/Child: Safety for use in pregnancy not established; benefits must outweigh risks. ▪ Human data on safety during breast-feeding not available. Use caution if breast feeding; consider the mother's clinical need for delafloxacin and the health benefits to and potential adverse effects on the breast-fed infant. ▪ Not recommended for use in pediatric patients under 18 years of age; safety and effectiveness not established.

Elderly: Safety and effectiveness in elderly patients is similar to that in younger adults; however, they may experience an increased risk of side effects (e.g., aortic aneurysm and dissection, CNS effects, tendinitis, tendon rupture). Monitoring of renal function may be useful. ■ See Dose Adjustments and Precautions.

DRUG/LAB INTERACTIONS

Specific information not available. ■ Should not be coadministered with any solution containing multivalent cations (e.g., magnesium) through the same IV line. ■ In vitro drug combination studies with delafloxacin and aztreonam, ceftazidime, colistin, daptomycin, linezolid, meropenem, tigecycline, trimethoprim/sulfamethoxazole, and vancomycin demonstrated neither synergy nor antagonism.

SIDE EFFECTS

The most common side effects are diarrhea, elevated liver function tests (transaminases), headache, nausea, and vomiting. Serious side effects include CDAD, CNS effects, hypersensitivity reactions, peripheral neuropathy, and tendinitis and tendon rupture. Abdominal pain; abnormal dreams; anxiety; blurred vision; bradycardia; cardiac palpitations; dermatitis; dizziness; dysgeusia; dyspepsia; flushing; fungal infections; hyperglycemia; hypertension; hypoesthesia; hypoglycemia; hypotension; increased alkaline phosphatase, creatinine, creatine phosphokinase; infusion site bruising, discomfort, edema, erythema, extravasation, irritation, pain, phlebitis, swelling, and thrombosis; insomnia; myalgia; oral candidiasis; paresthesia; phlebitis; presyncope; pruritus; rash; renal impairment; renal failure; sinus tachycardia; syncope; tinnitus; urticaria; vertigo; and vulvovaginal candidiasis have been reported in fewer than 2% of patients.

ANTIDOTE

Keep physician informed of all side effects. Most minor side effects will be treated symptomatically; monitor closely. Discontinue delafloxacin at the first sign of any major side effect (CDAD, CNS symptoms, hypersensitivity reactions, symptoms of peripheral neuropathy, or tendon rupture). Treat hypersensitivity reactions as indicated with epinephrine, airway management, oxygen, IV fluids, antihistamines (e.g., diphenhydramine), corticosteroids (e.g., hydrocortisone sodium succinate), and pressor amines (e.g., dopamine). Treat CNS symptoms as indicated. Mild cases of CDAD may respond to discontinuation of delafloxacin. Treat CDAD with fluids, electrolytes, protein supplements, and appropriate antibiotics (e.g., oral vancomycin) as indicated. In severe cases, surgical evaluation may be indicated. Complete rest is indicated for an affected tendon until treatment is available. Treat overdose with observation and general supportive measures; about 19% of delafloxacin is removed by hemodialysis.

DESMOPRESSIN ACETATE

(des-moh-**PRESS**-in **AS**-ah-tayt)

DDAVP, 1-Deamino-8-D-Arginine Vasopressin

Hormone
Antidiuretic
Antihemorrhagic

pH 3.5 to 4

USUAL DOSE

Preassessment required based on diagnosis; see Monitor.

Diabetes insipidus: 2 to 4 mcg daily in 2 divided doses. Adjust each dose individually for an adequate diurnal rhythm of water turnover. IV dose has 10 times the antidiuretic effect of intranasal desmopressin.

Hemophilia A and von Willebrand's disease (Type 1): 0.3 mcg/kg of body weight. If used preoperatively, administer 30 minutes before the scheduled procedure. The necessity for repeat administration of desmopressin or the use of any blood products for hemostasis should be determined by laboratory response and the clinical condition of the patient; see Monitor.

DOSE ADJUSTMENTS

Many specific requirements depending on diagnosis; see Limitations of Use, Precautions, and Monitor. ▪ Dosing should be cautious in the elderly. Consider potential for decreased organ function and concomitant disease or drug therapy. See Elderly and Contraindications. ▪ Reduce dose accordingly (to $^1/_{10}$ of the intranasal dose) when transferring from intranasal to IV administration.

DILUTION

Diabetes insipidus: May be given undiluted.

Hemophilia A and von Willebrand's disease (Type 1): Dilute a single dose in 10 mL of NS for pediatric patients under 10 kg; 50 mL for adults and pediatric patients over 10 kg. Must be given as an infusion.

Storage: Refrigerate at 2° to 8° C (36° to 46° F). Use diluted product promptly.

COMPATIBILITY

Compatibility information not available from manufacturer; consult a pharmacist.

RATE OF ADMINISTRATION

Diabetes insipidus: A single dose by IV injection over 1 minute.

Hemophilia A and von Willebrand's disease (Type 1): A single dose as an infusion over 15 to 30 minutes.

ACTIONS

A synthetic analog of the natural hormone arginine vasopressin, an antidiuretic hormone affecting renal water conservation (human antidiuretic hormone—ADH). Has been shown to be more potent than arginine vasopressin in increasing plasma levels of factor VIII activity in patients with hemophilia A and von Willebrand's disease (Type 1). Produces dose-related increase in factor VIII levels within 30 minutes and peaks in 90 to 120 minutes. Onset of action as an antidiuretic is prompt. When administered by IV injection, desmopressin has an antidiuretic effect about 10 times that of an equivalent dose administered intranasally. Half-life is biphasic (7.8 minutes for fast phase and 75.5 minutes for slow phase). Increases water resorption in the kidney, increases urine osmolality, and decreases urine output. Increases plasma levels of von Willebrand factor, factor VIII, and t-PA, thereby contributing to a shortened activated partial thromboplastin time (aPTT) and bleeding time. Clinically effective antidiuretic doses are usually below the threshold levels for effects on vascular or visceral smooth muscle. Excreted in urine.

INDICATIONS AND USES

Diabetes insipidus: Antidiuretic replacement therapy in the management of central (cranial) diabetes insipidus and for the management of temporary polyuria and polydipsia following head trauma or surgery in the pituitary region.

Hemophilia A and von Willebrand's disease (Type 1): Indicated in patients with hemophilia A and in patients with mild to moderate classic von Willebrand's disease (Type I) who have factor VIII coagulant activity levels greater than 5%. In both indications, desmopressin will often maintain hemostasis during surgical procedures and postoperatively when administered 30 minutes before a scheduled procedure and will also stop bleeding in episodes of spontaneous or trauma-induced injuries such as hemarthroses, intramuscular hematomas, or mucosal bleeding.

Limitations of use: Ineffective for the treatment of nephrogenic diabetes insipidus. ▪ Not indicated for the treatment of hemophilia A or von Willebrand's disease (Type I) with factor VIII coagulant activity levels equal to or less than 5%; see Monitor. ▪ Not indicated for the treatment of hemophilia B. ▪ Not indicated in patients who have factor VIII antibodies. ▪ Not indicated for the treatment of severe classic von Willebrand's disease (Type I) and when there is evidence of an abnormal molecular form of factor VIII antigen.

CONTRAINDICATIONS

Infants under 3 months of age with hemophilia A or von Willebrand's disease, known hypersensitivity to desmopressin or any of the components of DDAVP injection, patients with moderate to severe renal impairment (CrCl less than 50 mL/min), and patients with hyponatremia or a history of hyponatremia.

PRECAUTIONS

A potent antidiuretic. Administration may lead to water intoxication and/or hyponatremia, which can be fatal. Fluid restriction is recommended. ▪ When administered to patients who do not have a need for the antidiuretic effect, fluid intake should be adjusted downward to decrease the potential occurrence of water intoxication and hyponatremia. Pediatric and elderly patients may be at increased risk. ▪ Should not be used to treat Type IIB von Willebrand's disease; platelet aggregation may be induced. ▪ Use with caution in patients with habitual or psychogenic polydipsia. May be more likely to drink excessive amounts of water, increasing their risk of hyponatremia. ▪ Use caution in patients with coronary artery insufficiency or hypertensive cardiovascular disease; has infrequently produced hypertension or hypotension, with a reflex increase in heart rate. ▪ Use with caution in patients predisposed to thrombus formation. There have been rare reports of thrombotic events following administration of desmopressin. ▪ Patients with conditions associated with fluid and electrolyte imbalance (e.g., cystic fibrosis, CHF, renal disorders) are prone to hyponatremia; use with caution. ▪ Severe hypersensitivity reactions, including anaphylaxis, have been reported. ▪ See Drug Interactions.

Monitor: *All diagnoses:* Monitor BP and pulse during infusion. ▪ Monitor fluid intake and urine volume. Monitor for S/S of hyponatremia, especially in high-risk patient populations (pediatric patients, the elderly, and patients with CHF). S/S may include headache, nausea and vomiting, decreased serum sodium, weight gain, restlessness, fatigue, lethargy, disorientation, depressed reflexes, loss of appetite, irritability, muscle weakness, muscle spasms, and abnormal mental status (e.g., confusion, decreased consciousness, hallucinations). Severe symptoms may include seizure, coma, and respiratory arrest caused by an extreme decrease in plasma osmolality.

Diabetes insipidus: Confirm diagnosis of diabetes insipidus with urinalysis, the water deprivation test, or the hypertonic saline infusion test. ▪ Fluid restriction indicated; see Precautions. ▪ Monitor continued response by measuring urine output and osmolality. Monitoring of plasma osmolality may be indicated. ▪ Monitor urine specific gravity and serum electrolytes. ▪ Monitor continued response by measuring urine output and osmolality. ▪ Monitoring of plasma osmolality may be indicated. ▪ Accuracy and effectiveness of dose measured by duration of sleep and adequate, not excessive, water turnover.

Hemophilia A: Determine factor VIII coagulant activity before administration for hemostasis. ▪ Monitor factor VIII coagulant activity, factor VIII antigen, factor VIII ristocetin cofactor (von Willebrand factor), and aPTT to assess patient status during treatment. ▪ Do not rely on desmopressin, but it may be considered for use in patients with factor VIII activity levels from 2% to 5% with careful monitoring. Generally used only when the factor VIII activity level is above 5%.

von Willebrand's disease (Type 1): Most effective when factor VIII activity level above 5%. ▪ Monitor bleeding time, factor VIII coagulant activity, factor VIII ristocetin cofactor activity, and factor VIII von Willebrand factor antigen during therapy to assess patient status. Patients with severe homozygous von Willebrand's disease with factor VIII coagulant activity and factor VIII von Willebrand factor antigen levels less than 1% are least likely to respond to treatment with desmopressin.

Hemophilia and von Willebrand's disease: Determine need for repeat administration of desmopressin or use of blood products by laboratory response as well as the clinical condition of the patient. Tachyphylaxis (lessening of response; i.e., a gradual diminution of the factor VIII activity increase) has been seen when given more frequently than every 48 hours.

Patient Education: Careful monitoring of fluid intake indicated in patients with diabetes insipidus. ■ When antidiuretic effect is not needed, caution patients (especially the young and the elderly) to limit fluid intake to satisfy thirst needs only; this decreases potential occurrence of water intoxication and hyponatremia.

Maternal/Child: Category B: use only when clearly indicated in pregnancy and breast-feeding. ■ Risk of hyponatremia and water intoxication increased in pediatric patients. Restrict fluid intake. ■ Safety for use in pediatric patients under 12 years of age with diabetes insipidus not established. ■ See Contraindications.

Elderly: Risk of hyponatremia and water intoxication increased. Use caution and restrict fluid intake. ■ Response similar to that seen in younger adults. Dosing should be cautious in the elderly. Monitor renal function; see Dose Adjustments.

DRUG/LAB INTERACTIONS

Has been used with aminocaproic acid without adverse effects. ■ May produce hypertension with other **vasopressors** (e.g., dopamine). ■ Use caution when administered concurrently with other medications that can increase the risk of water intoxication with hyponatremia (e.g., **carbamazepine, chlorpromazine, lamotrigine, NSAIDs, opiate analgesics, selective serotonin reuptake inhibitors, tricyclic antidepressants**).

SIDE EFFECTS

Mild abdominal cramps, nausea, transient headache, and vulval pain are most common and may disappear with reduced doses. Facial flushing, hypertension (slight), and/or hypotension with a compensatory tachycardia have occurred. May cause burning, local erythema, and swelling at site of injection. Most serious side effects include hyponatremia with resultant sequelae (see Precautions), water intoxication, and thrombotic events (cerebrovascular thrombosis, MI). Anaphylaxis has been reported.

Overdose: Confusion, continuing headache, drowsiness, problems passing urine, rapid weight gain due to fluid retention.

Post-Marketing: Hyponatremia (can be fatal), hyponatremic convulsions associated with concomitant use of oxybutynin (Ditropan) and imipramine (Tofranil-PM), thrombotic events (e.g., acute MI, acute cerebrovascular thrombosis).

ANTIDOTE

Notify physician of all side effects. Most will respond to reduction of dose or rate of administration, or symptomatic treatment. May need to discontinue drug. If overdose occurs, treat by reducing dose or frequency of administration, or discontinue drug if indicated. There is no known specific antidote for desmopressin acetate. Treat hypersensitivity with oxygen, epinephrine, antihistamines (e.g., diphenhydramine), vasopressors, corticosteroids, albuterol, IV fluids, and ventilation equipment as indicated. Resuscitate as necessary.

DEXAMETHASONE SODIUM PHOSPHATE

(dex-ah-**METH**-ah-zohn **SO**-dee-um **FOS**-fayt)

Hormone (corticosteroid)
Anti-inflammatory
Antiemetic
Immunosuppressant
Diagnostic agent (oral)

Decadron, Decadron Phosphate

pH 7 to 8.5

USUAL DOSE

The **usual initial dose** may vary from 0.5 to 9 mg/day depending on patient condition and response. Dosage must be individualized. IV dexamethasone is usually given in an emergency situation or when oral dosing is not feasible, and the parenteral dosage ranges are usually one-third to one-half the oral doses given every 12 hours. However, administration of dosages exceeding the usual dosages may be justified in certain overwhelming, acute, life-threatening situations. Repeat until adequate response, then decrease dose as indicated using the lowest dose that will maintain an adequate clinical response.

Anti-inflammatory: See average dose range above. Some sources recommend administering total daily dose divided every 6 to 12 hours.

Unresponsive shock: Several regimens have been suggested:

1 to 6 mg/kg as a single injection; *or*

40 mg. Repeat every 2 to 6 hours as needed; *or*

20 mg as a *loading dose,* followed by a continuous infusion of 3 mg/kg equally distributed over 24 hours. High-dose treatment is used until patient condition stabilizes, usually no longer than 48 to 72 hours.

Cerebral edema: *Loading dose:* 10 mg. *Maintenance dose:* 4 mg every 6 hours until maximum response has been noted (usually given IM). May be continued for several days postoperatively in patients requiring brain surgery. Switch to oral dexamethasone (1 to 3 mg three times daily) as soon as possible and taper over 5 to 7 days. Nonoperative cases may require continuous therapy to remain free of symptoms of increased intracranial pressure.

Cerebral edema in recurrent or inoperable brain tumors: 2 mg every 8 to 12 hours (usually given IM) to relieve symptoms of increased intracranial pressure. Adjust based on patient response.

Antiemetic in management of chemotherapy-associated nausea and vomiting (prevention): Several regimens are in use. Optimum dose has not been established.

Usual dose is 8 to 20 mg before chemotherapy. Lower doses (IV or PO) may be given over the next 24 to 72 hours if necessary. May be used alone or in combination with aprepitant or fosaprepitant and a 5-HT$_3$ antagonist (e.g., ondansetron) depending on emetogenic potential of chemotherapeutic agents.

Airway edema: *Adult and pediatric patients:* 0.5 to 2 mg/kg/24 hr in equally divided doses every 6 hours (0.125 to 0.5 mg/kg every 6 hours) beginning 24 hours before elective extubation. Continue for 4 to 6 doses after extubation.

Allergic conditions: (Usually given IM or PO) 4 to 8 mg on the first day, then PO in decreasing doses (1.5 mg every 12 hours on Days 2 and 3; 0.75 mg every 12 hours on Day 4; and 0.75 mg on Days 5 and 6).

Meningitis: *Adult and pediatric patients:* 0.15 mg/kg/dose every 6 hours for 2 to 4 days. Administer 10 to 20 minutes before or concurrently with the first dose of antibiotic.

Primary or secondary adrenocortical insufficiency (physiologic replacement): 0.03 to 0.15 mg/kg/24 hr or 0.6 to 0.75 mg/M^2/24 hr given in divided doses every 6 to 12 hours (0.015 to 0.075 mg/kg every 12 hours, or 0.0075 to 0.0375 mg/kg every 6 hours, or 0.3 to 0.375 mg/M^2 every 12 hours, or 0.15 to 0.1875 mg/M^2 every 6 hours). Usually given IM. Dexamethasone has minimal mineralocorticoid properties; may require a concomitant mineralocorticoid (e.g., fludrocortisone). Hydrocortisone is the drug of choice for this indication.

PEDIATRIC DOSE

See Maternal/Child. Dose should be based on the severity of the disease and the patient response rather than on strict adherence to a dose indicated by age, weight, or body surface area.

Cerebral edema: Use smallest effective dose (oral route preferred). Manufacturer recommends 0.2 mg/kg/24 hr in divided doses. An alternate source recommends: *Loading dose:* 1 to 2 mg/kg of body weight for 1 dose. *Maintenance dose:* 1 to 1.5 mg/kg/24 hr in equally divided doses every 4 to 6 hours (0.17 to 0.25 mg/kg every 4 hours or 0.25 to 0.375 mg/kg every 6 hours) for 5 days, then gradually decrease. Maximum dose is 16 mg/24 hr.

Airway edema: See Usual Dose.

Croup: 0.6 mg/kg/dose $\times$ 1 dose.

Antiemetic in management of chemotherapy-associated nausea and vomiting (prevention): Several regimens are in use. Optimum dose has not been established. Doses may range from 5 to 10 mg/M^2/dose. May be used alone or in combination with other antiemetics depending on emetogenic potential of chemotherapeutic agents.

Anti-inflammatory: 0.08 to 0.3 mg/kg/24 hr in equally divided doses every 6 to 12 hours (0.04 to 0.15 mg/kg every 12 hours or 0.02 to 0.075 mg/kg every 6 hours).

Meningitis: See Usual Dose.

DOSE ADJUSTMENTS

Use lowest possible dose required to control condition being treated. When dose reduction is possible, decrease dose gradually while monitoring for S/S of disease exacerbation. ■ Because complications of treatment with glucocorticoids depend on dose and duration of therapy, a risk/benefit decision must be made for each patient regarding dose and duration of treatment and whether daily or intermittent therapy should be used. ■ Clearance of corticosteroids is decreased in patients with hypothyroidism and increased in patients with hyperthyroidism. Dose adjustment may be required. ■ See Drug/Lab Interactions.

DILUTION

May be given undiluted or added to IV dextrose or saline solutions and given as an infusion.

Storage: Store at CRT. Avoid freezing. Protect from light. Use diluted solutions within 24 hours. Sensitive to heat; do not autoclave. Protect from freezing.

COMPATIBILITY

Compatibility information not available from manufacturer. Other sources suggest specific **compatibilities** dependent on concentration and manufacturer; consult a pharmacist.

RATE OF ADMINISTRATION

A single dose over at least 1 minute. Rapid administration may be associated with perineal burning or tingling. As an IV infusion, give at prescribed rate.

ACTIONS

An anti-inflammatory glucocorticoid. A synthetic adrenocortical steroid with minimal mineralocorticoid properties. Causes minimal sodium retention. Glucocorticoids cause profound and varied metabolic effects. They are primarily used for their potent anti-inflammatory effects on different organ systems and their ability to modify the body's immune response. The mechanism of antiemetic activity of dexamethasone has not been established. Approximately seven times as potent as prednisolone and 27 times as potent as hydrocortisone. Onset of action is prompt. Metabolized primarily in the liver and excreted as inactive metabolites in urine. Crosses the placental barrier. Excreted in breast milk.

INDICATIONS AND USES

May be used primarily as an anti-inflammatory or immunosuppressive agent for the treatment of various diseases, including endocrine, rheumatic, collagen, dermatologic, ophthalmic, gastrointestinal, respiratory, hematologic, and neoplastic diseases or disorders (see manufacturer's prescribing information). ■ Supplementary therapy for severe allergic/hypersensitivity reactions. ■ Reduction of acute edematous states (cerebral edema, airway edema). ▪ Shock unresponsive to conventional therapy. ▪ Acute exacerbations of disease for patients receiving steroid therapy. ▪ Adrenocortical insufficiency; total, relative, and operative. ▪ Has numerous other uses by other routes of administration (e.g., IM, intra-articular, intralesional, intrasynovial, soft-tissue injection, oral inhalant).

Unlabeled uses: Antiemetic for chemotherapy-induced nausea and vomiting (prevention). ▪ Adjunct to treatment of meningitis with antibiotics (to reduce incidence of ototoxicity). ▪ Dexamethasone or betamethasone is given IM to the mother to accelerate the production of lung surfactant in utero in the prevention of respiratory distress syndrome of premature infants.

CONTRAINDICATIONS

Systemic fungal infections. Another source lists hypersensitivity to any product component, including sulfites, and cerebral malaria.

PRECAUTIONS

Corticosteroids can produce reversible hypothalamic-pituitary-adrenal (HPA) axis suppression with the potential for glucocorticosteroid insufficiency after withdrawal of treatment. Adrenocortical insufficiency may result from too-rapid withdrawal of corticosteroids and may be minimized by gradual reduction of dosage. This type of relative insufficiency may persist for months after discontinuation of therapy; therefore hormone therapy should be reinstituted in any situation of stress occurring during that period (e.g., surgery, trauma, infection). If the patient is already receiving steroids, the dosage may need to be increased. Because mineralocorticoid secretion may be impaired, salt and/or a mineralocorticoid should be administered concurrently. ▪ Prolonged use of corticosteroids may increase susceptibility to infection, reactivate latent infectious diseases, or mask signs of infection. ▪ Pediatric patients who are on immunosuppressant corticosteroids are more susceptible to infection than healthy children. Infections such as chickenpox and measles can have a more serious or even fatal course. Adults and pediatric patients who have not had these diseases should take care to avoid exposure. If exposed, therapy with varicella zoster immune globulin (VZIG) or IVIG may be indicated. If chickenpox develops, treatment with antiviral agents should be considered. ▪ Corticosteroids should be used with great caution in patients with known or suspected *Strongyloides* (threadworm) infestation. Corticosteroid-induced immunosuppression may lead to *Strongyloides* hyperinfection and dissemination with widespread larval migration, often accompanied by severe enterocolitis and potentially fatal gram-negative sepsis. ▪ The use of dexamethasone in patients with active tuberculosis should be restricted to cases of fulminating or disseminated tuberculosis in which the corticosteroid is being used for management of disease in conjunction with an appropriate antituberculosis regimen. ▪ If corticosteroids are indicated in patients with latent tuberculosis or tuberculin reactivity, reactivation of the disease may occur. Chemoprophylaxis is indicated during prolonged corticosteroid therapy. ▪ Prolonged use of corticosteroids may produce posterior subcapsular cataracts or glaucoma with possible damage to the optic nerves and may enhance the establishment of secondary ocular infections due to fungi or viruses. ▪ Use with caution in patients with ocular herpes simplex; corneal perforation can occur. ▪ Use with caution in hypothyroidism and cirrhosis; effect of corticosteroids may be enhanced. ▪ Hypertension, sodium and water retention, and potassium and calcium excretion can occur with large doses of dexamethasone. Dietary sodium restriction and potassium supplementation may be necessary. Caution and close monitoring is required in patients with existing cardiovascular disease. ▪ Use with caution in patients with nonspecific ulcerative colitis (if there is a probability of impending perforation, abscess, or other pyogenic infection), diverticulitis, fresh intestinal anastomoses, active or latent peptic ulcer disease, renal insufficiency, hypertension, osteoporosis, and myasthenia gravis. ▪ Psychic derangements (e.g., euphoria, insomnia, mood swings, personality changes, severe depression, frank psychotic manifestations) can occur in patients receiving corticosteroids. Pre-existing emotional instability or psychotic tendencies may be aggravated. ▪ Rare instances of anaphylactoid reactions have been reported. ▪ Use with caution in patients who have had a recent MI. Ventricular free wall rupture has been reported. ▪ Use with caution in patients at risk for osteoporosis. Corticosteroids decrease bone formation, increase bone resorption, and decrease the protein matrix of the bone. May lead to inhibition of bone growth in pediatric patients and the development of osteoporosis at any age. ▪ An acute myopathy has been reported with the use of high doses of corticosteroids. Most often seen in patients with disorders of neuromuscular transmission (e.g., myasthenia gravis) or in patients receiving concomitant therapy with neuromuscular blocking drugs. Myopathy is generalized, may involve ocular and respiratory muscles, and may result in quadriparesis. Clinical improvement following discontinuation of corticosteroids may take weeks to years. ▪ Kaposi's sarcoma has been reported in patients receiving corticosteroid therapy, most often for chronic conditions. Clinical improvement may occur if therapy is discontinued. ▪ Some products may contain sulfites; use caution in patients with allergies.

Monitor: May increase insulin needs in diabetes; monitor blood glucose. ▪ Monitor electrolytes periodically. May cause sodium retention and potassium and calcium excretion. ▪ Monitoring of BP may be indicated; may cause hypertension secondary to fluid and electrolyte disturbances. ▪ Monitor for S/S of infection; S/S may be masked. ▪ Patients with latent tuberculosis should be monitored for reactivation of the disease. ▪ Periodic ophthalmic exams may be necessary with prolonged treatment. ▪ Monitor for S/S of a hypersensitivity reaction. ▪ Elevation of creatine kinase may occur with acute myopathy. Monitor if indicated. ▪ See Drug/Lab Interactions.

Patient Education: Promptly report edema, tarry stools, or weight gain. Promptly report anorexia, diarrhea, dizziness, fatigue, low blood sugar, nausea, weakness, weight loss, and vomiting. May indicate adrenal insufficiency after dose reduction or discontinuing therapy. ▪ May mask signs of infection and/or decrease resistance. ▪ Patients with diabetes may have an increased requirement for insulin or oral hypoglycemics. ▪ Avoid immunization with live virus vaccines. ▪ Carry ID stating steroid dependent if receiving prolonged therapy.

Maternal/Child: Category C: use with caution; benefits must outweigh risks. ▪ Discontinue breast-feeding. ▪ Observe newborn for hypoadrenalism if mother has received large doses. ▪ Monitor growth and development of pediatric patients receiving prolonged treatment. ▪ Use of a preservative-free solution recommended for neonates.

Elderly: Use cautiously in the smallest possible dose. Monitor BP, blood glucose, and electrolytes carefully. ▪ Increased risk of hypertension. ▪ Higher risk of glucocorticoid-induced osteoporosis.

DRUG/LAB INTERACTIONS

Some sources list additional interactions; review drug profile with pharmacist.

Aminoglutethimide and mitotane suppress adrenal function and increase metabolism of dexamethasone. Not recommended for concurrent use, or dexamethasone dose may need to be increased to be effective. Use of hydrocortisone suggested. ▪ Metabolism increased and effects reduced by **hepatic enzyme–inducing agents** (e.g., alcohol, barbiturates [e.g., phenobarbital], hydantoins [e.g., phenytoin], rifampin); dose adjustments may be required when adding or deleting from drug profile. ▪ Risk of hypokalemia increased with **amphotericin B or potassium-depleting diuretics** (e.g., thiazides, furosemide, ethacrynic acid). Monitor potassium levels and cardiac function. ▪ Increased risk of **digoxin** toxicity secondary to hypokalemia. ▪ May also decrease effectiveness of **potassium supplements;** monitor serum potassium. ▪ **Diuretics** decrease sodium and fluid retention effects of corticosteroids; corticosteroids decrease sodium excretion and diuretic effects of diuretics. ▪ Concurrent use with **NSAIDs** may increase the risk of GI toxicity. ▪ Aspirin should be used cautiously in conjunction with corticosteroids in hypoprothrombinemia. ▪ Increased activity of both cyclosporine and corticosteroids may occur when used concurrently. Convulsions have been reported with concurrent use. ▪ Clearance increased and effects decreased with **ephedrine.** ▪ May enhance the adverse/toxic effects of **anticholinesterases** (e.g., neostigmine); increased muscle weakness may occur. ▪ May decrease the effectiveness of **isoniazid, salicylates, and somatrem**; dose adjustments may be required. ■ Clearance decreased and effects increased with **estrogens, macrolide antibiotics** (e.g., azithromycin), **oral contraceptives, and ketoconazole.** ■ May interact with **anticoagulants, nondepolarizing muscle relaxants** (e.g., atracurium), **or theophyllines;** may inhibit or potentiate action; monitor carefully. ■ Monitor patients receiving **insulin** carefully; dose adjustments may be required. ■ Do not vaccinate with **live or live-attenuated virus vaccines** (e.g., smallpox) during therapy. Killed or inactivated vaccines may be administered. However, patients on corticosteroid therapy may exhibit a diminished response. ■ Toxic epidermal necrolysis has been reported with concomitant use of thalidomide and corticosteroids; use caution. ■ See Precautions. ■ Decreases uptake of **radioactive material** in cerebral edema; will alter brain scan.

SIDE EFFECTS
Do occur but are usually reversible: burning, itching, and tingling in the anogenital region; Cushing's syndrome; electrolyte imbalance; euphoria; fluid retention; glycosuria; headache; hyperglycemia; hypersensitivity reactions including anaphylaxis; hypertension; impaired wound healing; insomnia; leukocytosis; menstrual irregularities; mood swings; peptic ulcer; perforation and hemorrhage; protein catabolism; sweating; thromboembolism; tumor lysis syndrome; weakness; and many others.

ANTIDOTE
Notify the physician of any side effect. Treat side effects as indicated. Resuscitate as necessary for anaphylaxis and notify physician. Keep epinephrine immediately available.

DEXRAZOXANE
(dex-rah-**ZOX**-ayn)

Totect, Zinecard

Antidote
Extravasation antidote
Chemoprotective agent

pH 3.5 to 5.5

USUAL DOSE
Pretreatment: Verify pregnancy status and baseline studies required; see Monitor.
TOTECT
Administer once daily for 3 consecutive days. Initiate the first infusion as soon as possible and within 6 hours of extravasation. Doses should be given 24 hours apart (+ or − 3 hours); see Precautions. Recommended regimen is:
Day 1 and Day 2: 1,000 mg/M² not to exceed 2,000 mg.
Day 3: 500 mg/M² not to exceed 1,000 mg.
ZINECARD
Administered in conjunction with doxorubicin. Dose ratio of dexrazoxane to doxorubicin (Adriamycin) is 10:1 (e.g., 500 mg/M² dexrazoxane to 50 mg/M² doxorubicin). Do not administer doxorubicin before dexrazoxane. Doxorubicin dose must be given within 30 minutes after completion of the dexrazoxane injection.

DOSE ADJUSTMENTS
TOTECT AND ZINECARD
Decrease the recommended dose of dexrazoxane by 50% in patients with moderate to severe renal impairment (CrCl less than 40 mL/min). ■ Ratio of Zinecard to doxorubicin will be 5:1 (e.g., 250 mg/M² dexrazoxane to 50 mg/M² doxorubicin). ■ Consider age-related impaired organ function and concomitant disease or drug therapy in the elderly; see Elderly. ■ See Antidote. ■ Has not been evaluated in hepatic insufficiency.
ZINECARD
When administering Zinecard, the dose of dexrazoxane is dependent on the dose of doxorubicin. When the dose of doxorubicin is reduced (e.g., patients with hyperbilirubinemia), adjust the dexrazoxane dose accordingly. Maintain a 10:1 ratio (dexrazoxane to doxorubicin) except in patients with CrCl less than 40 mL/min; see above paragraph.

DILUTION

Specific techniques required; see Precautions.

TOTECT

Totect can be prepared with *either* SWFI and LR *or* 0.167 M sodium lactate injection and NS. More than 1 vial of Totect may be needed to prepare the calculated dose.

Preparation of Totect using SWFI and LR: Reconstitute each 500-mg vial of lyophilized Totect powder with 50 mL of SWFI (10 mg/mL). Withdraw the calculated dose and further dilute in 1,000 mL of LR. Reconstituted solution must be further diluted within 30 minutes of preparation.

Preparation of Totect using 0.167 M sodium lactate injection and NS: Reconstitute each 500-mg vial of lyophilized Totect powder with 50 mL of 0.167 M sodium lactate injection solution (10 mg/mL). (To prepare 50 mL of 0.167 M sodium lactate injection solution, add 1.67 mL of 5 mEq/mL sodium lactate injection to 50 mL SWFI.) Withdraw the calculated dose and further dilute in 1,000 mL of NS. Reconstituted solution must be further diluted within 30 minutes of preparation.

ZINECARD

Initially reconstitute each 250 mg (500 mg) with 25 mL (50 mL) of SWFI (10 mg/mL). Must be further diluted with LR. Concentration should range from 1.3 to 3 mg/mL. Further dilution of each 250-mg (500-mg) vial with 75 mL (150 mL) of LR would yield 2.5 mg/mL. Fully diluted solution has a pH of 3.5 to 5.5.

Storage: *Totect and Zinecard:* Store unopened vials at CRT. ***Totect:*** Store unopened vials in original carton to protect from light. Reconstituted solution should be further diluted within 30 minutes. Diluted product stable for 4 hours from time of reconstitution and dilution when stored below 25° C (77° F) or for up to 12 hours when stored refrigerated between 2° and 8° C (36° and 46° F). ***Zinecard:*** Reconstituted solution stable for 30 minutes at RT or, if necessary, up to 3 hours from the time of reconstitution under refrigeration at 2° to 8° C (36° to 46° F). Fully diluted solutions in LR are stable for 1 hour at RT or up to 4 hours if refrigerated at 2° to 8° C (36° to 46° F). Discard unused solutions.

COMPATIBILITY

Manufacturer states, "Should not be mixed or administered with other drugs"; degrades rapidly at a pH above 7.

Other sources suggest a few specific **compatibilities** dependent on concentration and manufacturer; consult a pharmacist.

RATE OF ADMINISTRATION

TOTECT

Administer a single dose as an IV infusion equally distributed over 1 to 2 hours. Infuse at RT with normal lighting in a large vein in an extremity/area other than the one affected by the extravasation.

ZINECARD

A single dose as an infusion over 15 minutes. Do not administer by IV push. Administer doxorubicin within 30 minutes after completion of Zinecard infusion.

ACTIONS

DEXRAZOXANE

Distributes throughout total body water. At least partly metabolized. Elimination half-life is 2.1 to 2.5 hours. Primarily excreted in urine. See Drug/Lab Interactions.

TOTECT

Diminishes tissue damage resulting from extravasation of anthracycline drugs. Exact mode of action unknown. May inhibit topoisomerase II reversibly.

ZINECARD

A cardioprotective agent. A potent intracellular chelating agent that readily penetrates cell membranes and interferes with iron-mediated free radical generation thought to be, in part, responsible for anthracycline-induced cardiomyopathy. Reduces the incidence of doxorubicin cardiomyopathy.

INDICATIONS AND USES

TOTECT

Treatment of extravasation resulting from IV anthracycline chemotherapy.

ZINECARD

Reduce the incidence and severity of cardiomyopathy associated with doxorubicin administration in females with metastatic breast cancer who have received a cumulative doxorubicin dose of 300 mg/M^2 and who will continue to receive doxorubicin therapy to maintain tumor control. ▪ *Do not use with the initiation of doxorubicin therapy.*

CONTRAINDICATIONS

TOTECT

None.

ZINECARD

Do not use with chemotherapy regimens that do not contain an anthracycline.

PRECAUTIONS

TOTECT AND ZINECARD

Follow guidelines for handling cytotoxic agents. See Appendix A, p. 1308. ▪ Usually administered by or under the direction of the physician specialist. ▪ For IV infusion only; do not administer IV push. ▪ May add to myelosuppression caused by chemotherapeutic agents. Febrile neutropenia has been reported when used with cytotoxic chemotherapy for management of anthracycline extravasation. ▪ Use with caution in patients with renal impairment; see Dose Adjustments. ▪ Has not been evaluated in hepatic impairment. ▪ Hypersensitivity reactions, including anaphylaxis, have been reported. Previous history of allergy to dexrazoxane products should be carefully considered before administration. Consider permanent discontinuation in patients with severe hypersensitivity reactions.

TOTECT

For IV administration; **not** for local infiltration into extravasation site. Remove cooling procedures such as ice packs, if used, from the extravasation area at least 15 minutes before administration to allow sufficient blood flow to the extravasated area. ▪ Use in patients with hepatic impairment is not recommended. Hepatic dysfunction (increases in transaminases and bilirubin) may occur (especially after doses of above 1,000 mg/M^2).

ZINECARD

Evidence indicates that the use of dexrazoxane with the initiation of fluorouracil, doxorubicin, and cyclophosphamide (FAC) therapy interferes with the antitumor efficacy of the regimen. In one breast cancer trial, a lower response rate and a shorter time to progression were seen in patients who received dexrazoxane with their first cycle of FAC therapy. This use is not recommended; see Indications. ▪ Secondary malignancies (e.g., acute myeloid leukemia [AML] and myelodysplastic syndrome [MDS]) have been reported in pediatric patients and adults who have received dexrazoxane in combination with chemotherapy (not indicated for use in pediatric patients).

Monitor: TOTECT AND ZINECARD: Pregnancy testing should be performed before the initiation of chemotherapy; if extravasation occurs, repeat pregnancy testing is not recommended before administration of dexrazoxane because treatment of extravasation of anthracycline chemotherapy should not be delayed. ▪ Obtain baseline and periodic renal and liver function tests as indicated. ▪ Monitor patients with impaired renal function for signs of hematologic toxicity. ▪ Monitor for S/S of hypersensitivity reaction (anaphylaxis, angioedema, bronchospasm, hypotension, loss of consciousness, respiratory distress, and skin reactions). ▪ Use of prophylactic antiemetics may be indicated.

TOTECT: Monitor CBC and differential and platelet count for increased bone marrow suppression during treatment with dexrazoxane and cytotoxic chemotherapy. ▪ Perform local examination for extravasation on a regular basis after treatment and until resolution. ▪ If vesicant compounds other than anthracyclines are being used through the same IV access (e.g., vincristine, mitomycin, and vinorelbine), consider treatments for these other vesicant compounds. Totect is not effective against the effects of vesicants other than anthracyclines.

ZINECARD: Obtain baseline CBC and repeat before each course of therapy. Administer Zinecard and chemotherapy only when adequate hematologic parameters are met. ■ Monitor cardiac function before and periodically during therapy to assess left ventricular ejection fraction (LVEF). ■ Reduces but does not eliminate the risk of doxorubicin-induced cardiotoxicity. Monitor for signs of congestive heart failure (e.g., basilar rales, S_3 gallop, paroxysmal nocturnal dyspnea, significant dyspnea on exertion, cardiomegaly by x-ray, or progressive decline from baseline of LVEF).

Patient Education: Myelosuppression, immunosuppression, and infections may occur. Monitor temperature frequently and report any fevers. Routine blood cell counts required. ■ Promptly report S/S of a hypersensitivity reaction (e.g., dizziness; fainting; hives; swelling of face, lips, tongue, or throat; trouble breathing). ■ Use of effective contraception required in females of reproductive potential during treatment and for 6 months after the last dose of dexrazoxane. Males with female partners of reproductive potential must use effective contraception during treatment and for 3 months after the last dose. Report a suspected pregnancy; see Maternal/Child. ■ May impair fertility in males of reproductive potential. Not known whether these effects on fertility are reversible. ■ Report pain at injection site promptly.

Maternal/Child: *Totect and Zinecard:* Avoid pregnancy. Can cause fetal harm. ■ *Totect:* Do not breast-feed during treatment and for 2 weeks after final dose. *Zinecard:* Discontinue breast-feeding. *Totect and Zinecard:* Safety for use in pediatric patients not established.

Elderly: Response similar to that seen in younger patients. ■ Monitor renal and hepatic function; see Dose Adjustments.

DRUG/LAB INTERACTIONS

TOTECT AND ZINECARD

May have additive bone marrow suppressant effects with **other bone marrow suppressants** (e.g., fluorouracil, cyclophosphamide). ■ Does not affect pharmacokinetics of **doxorubicin** or **epirubicin**. ■ Dexrazoxane is not an inhibitor for CYP1A, CYP2C9, CYP2C19, CYP2D6, or CYP3A.

TOTECT

Dimethylsulfoxide (DMSO) should not be used in patients who are receiving dexrazoxane for treatment of anthracycline-induced extravasation. Efficacy of Totect may be reduced.

ZINECARD

Not indicated for use in initiation of doxorubicin therapy; may interfere with antitumor effects of combination regimens.

SIDE EFFECTS

Administered to patients receiving chemotherapeutic agents; side effect profile reflects a combination of dexrazoxane, underlying disease, and chemotherapy. The most common side effects are fever, injection site pain, nausea, postoperative infection, and vomiting. Laboratory abnormalities may include decreased hemoglobin, neutrophils, platelets, WBCs, and sodium and increased AST, ALT, alkaline phosphatase, bilirubin, creatinine, LDH, and total calcium. Alopecia, anorexia, constipation, cough, depression, diarrhea, dizziness, dysphagia, dyspnea, fatigue, headache, infection, insomnia, peripheral edema, stomatitis, and urticaria have been reported.

ANTIDOTE

Keep physician informed of side effects; most will be treated symptomatically. Recovery from myelosuppression similar with or without dexrazoxane. Treat hypersensitivity reactions as needed (e.g., oxygen, antihistamines, epinephrine, corticosteroids, vasopressors, and/or fluids). There is no known antidote for dexrazoxane. Overdose with dexrazoxane can lead to signs of bone marrow failure. Treatment should be symptomatic. Hemodialysis or peritoneal dialysis may be useful.

DEXTRAN HIGH MOLECULAR WEIGHT

Plasma volume expander

(**DEX**-tran hi mo-**LEK**-u-ler)

Dextran 70, Dextran 75, Gentran 75

pH 3 to 7

USUAL DOSE

Variable, depending on amount of fluid loss and resultant hemoconcentration. Initially 30 Gm (500 mL). Total dose should not exceed 1.2 Gm/kg (20 mL/kg) of body weight in the first 24 hours for adult and pediatric patients. May give 0.6 Gm/kg (10 mL/kg) every 24 hours thereafter if indicated. *Use of Dextran 1 is indicated for prophylaxis of serious anaphylactic reactions in select patients; however, Dextran 1 is very limited in the United States.*

DILUTION

Available as a 6% solution in 500-mL bottles properly diluted in NS or D5W and ready for use. Dextran 70 (Cutter) is available in a 250-mL bottle. Use only clear solution. Crystallization of dextran can occur at low temperatures. Submerge in warm water and dissolve all crystals before administration.

Storage: Store at constant temperature not above 25° C (76° F). Discard partially used solution; no preservative added.

COMPATIBILITY

Compatibility information not available from manufacturer; consult a pharmacist. However, one source suggests that drugs should not be added to a dextran solution.

RATE OF ADMINISTRATION

Variable, depending on indication, present blood volume, and patient response. Initial 500 mL may be given at 20 to 40 mL/min if hypovolemic. If additional high molecular weight dextran is required, reduce flow to lowest rate possible to maintain hemodynamic status desired. In normovolemic patients, rate should not exceed 4 mL/min.

ACTIONS

A glucose polymer that approximates colloidal properties of human albumin. Provides hemodynamically significant plasma volume expansion in excess of the amount infused for about 24 hours. Dilutes total serum proteins and hematocrit values. Smaller dextran molecules are eliminated in urine; larger molecules are degraded to glucose.

INDICATIONS AND USES

Adjunct in treatment of shock or impending shock caused by burns, hemorrhage, surgery, or trauma.

Unlabeled uses: Treatment of nephrosis, toxemia of late pregnancy, and prevention of postoperative deep vein thrombosis.

CONTRAINDICATIONS

Severe bleeding disorders; marked hemostatic defects (e.g., thrombocytopenia, hypofibrinogenemia), even if drug-induced (e.g., heparin, warfarin); known hypersensitivity to dextran; breast-feeding and pregnancy unless a lifesaving measure; severe congestive cardiac failure; renal failure.

PRECAUTIONS

For IV use only. ■ Used when whole blood or blood products are not available. Not a substitute for whole blood or plasma proteins. ■ Use extreme caution in heart disease, impaired hepatic or renal function, congestive heart failure, pulmonary edema, in patients with edema and sodium retention of pathologic abdominal conditions, and in patients receiving anticoagulants or corticosteroids.

Monitor: Monitor pulse, BP, central venous pressure, and urine output every 5 to 15 minutes for the first hour and hourly thereafter while indicated. ■ Maintain hydration of patient with additional IV fluids; dextran promotes tissue dehydration. Avoid overhydration with dilution of electrolyte balance. ■ Change IV tubing or flush well with normal saline before infusing blood. Dextran will promote coagulation of blood in the tubing (glucose content). ▪ May reduce coagulability of the circulating blood. Observe patient for increased bleeding; maintain hematocrit above 30%. ▪ Hemoglobin, hematocrit, electrolyte, and serum protein evaluations are necessary during therapy. ▪ 500 mL contains 77 mEq of sodium and chloride. ▪ See Drug/Lab Interactions.

Maternal/Child: Category C: safety for use in pregnancy and breast-feeding not established.

DRUG/LAB INTERACTIONS

Draw blood for **laboratory tests and type and cross-match** before giving dextran, or notify laboratory of its use. May alter type and cross-match, blood sugar, total protein, and total bilirubin evaluation. ▪ May produce elevated **urine specific gravity** (also symptom of dehydration) and increase **AST and ALT.** ▪ See Monitor for interaction with blood.

SIDE EFFECTS

Bleeding, dehydration, fever, hypotension, joint pain, nausea, overhydration, tightness of the chest, urticaria, vomiting, wheezing. Severe anaphylaxis and death have occurred. Excessive doses have caused wound hematoma, seroma, and bleeding; distant bleeding (hematuria, melena); and pulmonary edema.

ANTIDOTE

Notify physician of any side effect. Discontinue the drug immediately at the first sign of a hypersensitivity reaction, provided other means of sustaining the circulation are available. Use epinephrine and/or antihistamines (diphenhydramine) as indicated. Factor VIII infusion may reverse excessive bleeding. Resuscitate as necessary.

DEXTRAN LOW MOLECULAR WEIGHT

Plasma volume expander

(**DEX**-tran lo mo-**LEK**-u-ler)

Dextran 40, Gentran 40, L.M.D. 10%, Rheomacrodex　　　**pH 3 to 7**

USUAL DOSE

Adjunct in shock: Variable, depending on amount of fluid loss and resultant hemoconcentration. Do not exceed 2 Gm/kg (20 mL/kg) of body weight total over first 24 hours and 1 Gm/kg (10 mL/kg) total over each succeeding 24 hours. Discontinue infusion after 5 days of therapy. *Dextran 1 is indicated for prophylaxis of serious anaphylactic reactions in select patients; however, its availability is limited in the United States.*

Prophylaxis of venous thrombosis and/or pulmonary embolism: 10 mL/kg of body weight on day of surgery. 500 mL daily for 2 to 3 days, then 500 mL every 2 to 3 days up to 2 weeks. Length of treatment based on risk of thromboembolic complication. *Note previous comment on use of dextran 1.*

As priming fluid: 10 to 20 mL/kg of body weight. Do not exceed this dose. May be used in conjunction with other priming fluids.

DILUTION

Available as a 10% solution in 500-mL bottles properly diluted in NS or D5W and ready for use. Use only clear solution. Crystallization of dextran can occur at low temperatures. Submerge in warm water and dissolve all crystals before administration.

Storage: Store at constant temperature not above 25° C (76° F). Discard partially used solution; no preservative added.

COMPATIBILITY

Compatibility information not available from manufacturer; consult a pharmacist. However, one source suggests that drugs should not be added to a dextran solution.

RATE OF ADMINISTRATION

Initial 500 mL may be given rapidly. Remainder of any desired daily dose should be evenly distributed over 8 to 24 hours depending on use. Slow rate or discontinue dextran for rapid increase of central venous pressure.

ACTIONS

A low-molecular-weight, rapid, but short-acting plasma volume expander. A colloid hypertonic solution, it increases plasma volume by once or twice its own volume. Helps to restore normal circulatory dynamics, increasing arterial and pulse pressure, central venous pressure, and cardiac output. Improves microcirculatory flow and prevents sludging in venous channels. Mobilizes water from body tissues and increases urine output.

INDICATIONS AND USES

Adjunctive therapy in the treatment of shock caused by hemorrhage, burns, trauma, or surgery. ■ Prophylaxis during surgical procedures with a high incidence of venous thrombosis and pulmonary embolism. ■ Pump priming during extracorporeal circulation.

CONTRAINDICATIONS

Severe bleeding disorders; marked hemostatic defects (e.g., thrombocytopenia, hypofibrinogenemia), even if drug-induced (e.g., heparin, warfarin); known hypersensitivity to dextran; breast-feeding and pregnancy unless a lifesaving measure; severe congestive cardiac failure; renal failure.

PRECAUTIONS

For IV use only. ■ Use caution in heart disease, renal shutdown, congestive heart failure, pulmonary edema, patients with edema and sodium retention, and patients taking corticosteroids.

Monitor: Monitor pulse, BP, central venous pressure (if possible), and urine output every 5 to 15 minutes for the first hour and hourly thereafter while indicated. ■ Slow rate or discontinue dextran for rapid increase of central venous pressure (normal 7 to 14 mm H_2O pressure). ■ If anuric or oliguric after 500 mL of dextran, discontinue the dextran. Mannitol may help increase urine flow. ■ Maintain hydration of patient with additional IV fluids; dextran promotes tissue dehydration. Avoid overhydration and dilution of serum electrolytes. ■ Change IV tubing or flush well with normal saline before superimposing blood. Dextran will promote coagulation of blood in the tubing (glucose content). ■ May reduce coagulability of the circulating blood slightly. Observe for bleeding complications, particularly following surgery or if patient is being anticoagulated. Maintain hematocrit above 30%. ■ 500 mL contains 77 mEq of sodium and chloride. ■ See Drug/Lab Interactions.

Maternal/Child: Category C: safety for use in pregnancy and breast-feeding not established.

DRUG/LAB INTERACTIONS

Draw blood for **laboratory tests and type and cross-match** before giving dextran, or notify laboratory of its use. May alter type and cross-match, blood sugar, total protein, and total bilirubin evaluation. ■ May produce elevated **urine specific gravity** (also a symptom of dehydration) and increase **AST and ALT.** ■ See Monitor for interaction with blood.

SIDE EFFECTS

Bleeding, dehydration, fever, hypotension, joint pain, nausea, overhydration, tightness of chest, urticaria, vomiting, wheezing. Severe anaphylaxis and death can occur. Excessive doses have caused wound hematoma, wound seroma, wound bleeding, distant bleeding (hematuria, melena), and pulmonary edema.

ANTIDOTE

Notify the physician of any side effect. Discontinue the drug immediately at the first sign of a hypersensitivity reaction, provided other means of sustaining the circulation are available. Use epinephrine and/or antihistamines (diphenhydramine) as indicated. Factor VIII infusion may reverse excessive bleeding. Resuscitate as necessary.

DEXTROSE
(**DEX**-trohs)

Glucose

Nutritional (carbohydrate)
Antidote

pH 3.2 to 6.5

USUAL DOSE

Depends on indication for use; age, weight, clinical condition of the patient; and laboratory determinants. The average normal adult requires 2 to 3 L of fluid daily to replace water loss through perspiration and urine.

Treatment of hypoglycemia: 10 to 25 Gm (20 to 50 mL of 50% dextrose or 40 to 100 mL of 25% dextrose). Repeat as needed.

Nutritional support: As part of a parenteral nutritional regimen that also includes amino acids, electrolytes, and possibly lipid emulsion. Dextrose dose is individualized to meet patient requirements.

Treatment of hyperkalemia (unlabeled): 25 Gm (50 mL of 50% dextrose) administered with 10 units of regular insulin over 5 to 30 minutes. Repeat as needed.

PEDIATRIC DOSE

Dose is dependent on indication for use, weight, clinical condition, and laboratory results.

Treatment of hypoglycemia: 0.5 to 1 Gm/kg/dose (2 to 4 mL/kg/dose of 25% dextrose). Do not exceed 25 Gm/dose. Repeat as needed. Subsequent continuous IV infusion of 10% dextrose may be needed to stabilize blood glucose levels. Further treatment should be guided by evaluation of the underlying disorder.

Nutritional support: See Usual Dose.

Treatment of hyperkalemia (unlabeled): 0.5 to 1 Gm/kg (2 mL/kg of 25% dextrose) administered with regular insulin. Usual ratio is 1 unit of insulin for every 4 to 5 Gm dextrose. Repeat as needed.

See Rate of Administration, Precautions, Monitor, and Maternal/Child.

NEONATAL DOSE

Dose is dependent on indication for use, weight, clinical condition, and laboratory results.

Treatment of hypoglycemia in neonates and low-birth-weight infants: 0.25 to 0.5 Gm/kg/dose (1 to 2 mL/kg/dose of 25% dextrose); do not exceed 25 Gm/dose. Larger or repeated single doses may be required in severe cases or older infants. Subsequent continuous IV infusion of 10% dextrose may be needed to stabilize blood glucose levels. Further treatment should be guided by evaluation of the underlying disorder.

Nutritional support: See Usual Dose.

See Rate of Administration, Precautions, Monitor, and Maternal/Child.

DOSE ADJUSTMENTS

Dosing should be cautious in newborns, especially premature infants with low birth weight, and in the elderly. Lower-end initial doses may be indicated. Consider decrease in organ function, concomitant disease, or other drug therapy. See Rate of Administration, Precautions, and Maternal/Child.

DILUTION

Available in several concentrations. Final concentration for administration will depend on indication for use. Depending on indication, may be given undiluted or further diluted to achieve desired concentration. Check label for aluminum content; see Precautions. Dextrose solutions are excellent media for bacterial growth. Do not use unless the solution is entirely clear.

Filters: One manufacturer states, "Use of a final filter is recommended during administration of all parenteral solutions, where possible."

Storage: Store at 20° to 25° C (68° to 77° F). Protect from freezing.

COMPATIBILITY
Will cause pseudoagglutination of red blood cells if administered simultaneously with whole blood. Consult pharmacist or refer to individual drug monograph before admixing with other drugs or solutions. Mix thoroughly.

RATE OF ADMINISTRATION
Rate dependent on concentration and indication for use. The maximum rate at which glucose can be infused without producing glycosuria is 0.5 Gm/kg/hr. At 0.8 Gm/kg/hr, 95% is retained and will cause glycosuria. For continuous infusions of concentrated dextrose, the administration rate should be governed by the patient's tolerance to dextrose, especially during the first few days of therapy. Increase rate gradually to the maximum required dose as indicated by frequent determinations of blood glucose levels. When discontinuing therapy, consideration should be given to gradually decreasing the infusion rate in the last hour to reduce the risk of hypoglycemia. Excessively rapid administration may cause hyperosmolar syndrome.

Excessive or rapid administration in very-low-birth-weight infants may cause hyperglycemia, increased serum osmolality, and possible intracerebral hemorrhage. Infusion rate and volume depend on the age, weight, and clinical and metabolic conditions of the patient and on concomitant therapy and should be determined by a consulting physician experienced in pediatric IV fluid therapy.

When higher concentrations are given peripherally, administer slowly (preferably through a small-bore needle into a large vein) to minimize venous irritation; see Precautions.

Do not hang flexible plastic containers in series connection, do not pressurize to increase flow rates without first fully evacuating residual air from the container, and do not use vented IV administration sets. All may result in air embolism.

ACTIONS
A parenteral fluid and nutrient replenisher. A monosaccharide, it provides glucose calories for metabolic needs. Metabolized to CO_2 and water. Its oxidation provides water to sustain volume and may help lower excess ketone production. Restores blood glucose levels. May help minimize liver glycogen depletion and may exert a protein-sparing action. Hypertonic solutions (20% to 50%) act as diuretics. When given in conjunction with insulin for the treatment of hyperkalemia, dextrose stimulates the uptake of potassium into cells, lowering serum potassium levels. Readily excreted by the kidneys, producing diuresis.

INDICATIONS AND USES
Parenteral replenishment of fluid and minimal carbohydrate calories ($2^{1}/2$%, 5%, 10%).
■ Source of calories and fluid replenishment when mixed with amino acids or other **compatible** IV fluids for patients requiring parenteral nutrition when oral or enteral nutrition is not possible or is insufficient or contraindicated (10% to 70%). ■ Treatment of acute symptomatic hypoglycemia in the neonate or older infant (25%). ■ Treatment of acute symptomatic hypoglycemia or insulin hypoglycemia (hyperinsulinemia or insulin shock). ■ As a diluent for IV administration of medications (usually $2^{1}/2$% to 10% solutions).
Unlabeled uses: Adjunctive treatment of hyperkalemia when administered concomitantly with insulin (25% or 50% solution).

CONTRAINDICATIONS
Known hypersensitivity to dextrose. Solutions containing dextrose may be contraindicated in patients with known allergies to corn or corn products. ■ Concentrated dextrose should not be used in severely dehydrated patients (may worsen hyperosmolar state) or in patients with intracranial or intraspinal hemorrhage, diabetic coma, or delirium tremens, especially if the patient is already dehydrated.

PRECAUTIONS
Administration of these solutions can cause fluid and/or solute overload, resulting in dilution of serum electrolyte concentrations, overhydration, congested states, or pulmonary edema. ■ If administered too rapidly, concentrated dextrose solutions may result in

significant hyperglycemia and possible hyperosmolar syndrome characterized by mental confusion and loss of consciousness. Hyperglycemia is associated with an increase in serum osmolality, resulting in osmotic diuresis, dehydration, and electrolyte losses. Patients with underlying CNS disease and renal impairment who receive dextrose infusions may be at greater risk for developing a hyperosmolar hyperglycemic state. ▪ Excessive administration of dextrose may result in significant hypokalemia and hypophosphatemia. ▪ Use with caution in patients with subclinical or overt diabetes and in patients receiving corticosteroids. ▪ Pulmonary embolism and pulmonary distress due to pulmonary vascular precipitates have been reported. Patients requiring calcium and phosphate supplementation may be at increased risk. However, precipitates have been reported even in the absence of phosphate salt in the parenteral solution. Precipitation after passage through an in-line filter and suspected in vivo precipitate formation have also been reported. ▪ Use dextrose with extreme caution in newborns, especially premature or low-birth-weight infants. Risk of developing hypoglycemia or hyperglycemia is increased; see Monitor. Hypoglycemia in the newborn can cause prolonged seizures, coma, and brain damage. Excessive or rapid administration of dextrose may result in increased serum osmolality and possible intracerebral hemorrhage. Hyperglycemia has also been associated with late-onset bacterial and fungal infections, retinopathy of prematurity, necrotizing enterocolitis, bronchopulmonary dysplasia, prolonged length of hospital stay, and death. ▪ Some solutions may contain aluminum. In impaired kidney function, aluminum may reach toxic levels. Premature neonates are particularly at risk because of their immature kidneys and requirement for calcium and phosphate, which also contain aluminum. Research indicates that patients with impaired renal function who receive greater than 4 to 5 mcg/kg/day of parenteral aluminum are at risk for developing CNS or bone toxicity associated with aluminum accumulation. ▪ The development of hepatobiliary disorders in some patients without pre-existing liver disease who receive parenteral nutrition has been reported. Disorders may include cholecystitis, cholelithiasis, cholestasis, hepatic steatosis, fibrosis, and cirrhosis, possibly leading to hepatic failure. ▪ Parenteral nutrition–associated liver disease (PNALD) has been reported in patients who receive parenteral nutrition for extended periods, especially preterm infants. May present as cholestasis or steatohepatitis. Exact etiology is unclear and may be multifactorial. ▪ Concentrated dextrose solutions should not be withdrawn abruptly. May cause rebound hypoglycemia. Reduce rate of administration gradually and then follow with administration of 5% or 10% dextrose solution. ▪ Patients who require parenteral nutrition are at high risk for infections. Risk is increased in patients with malnutrition-associated immunosuppression, hyperglycemia exacerbated by dextrose infusion, long-term use and poor maintenance of IV catheters, or immunosuppressive effects of other concomitant conditions, drugs, or other components of the parenteral formulation (e.g., lipid emulsion). ▪ Refeeding severely undernourished patients may result in refeeding syndrome characterized by the intracellular shift of potassium, phosphorus, and magnesium as the patient becomes anabolic. Thiamine deficiency and fluid retention may also develop. To prevent these complications, slowly increase nutrient intake, including dextrose solution. ▪ Hypersensitivity and infusion reactions, including anaphylaxis, have been reported. ▪ Infusion of hypertonic solutions into a peripheral vein may result in vein irritation, vein damage, and/or thrombosis.

Monitor: Type of laboratory monitoring depends on indication and may include baseline and periodic monitoring of CBC, renal and liver function tests, ammonia levels, serum glucose, and electrolytes. ▪ Monitor changes in fluid balance, electrolyte concentrations, and acid-base balance during prolonged therapy or as indicated by patient condition. ▪ Electrolytes, vitamins, and minerals are readily depleted. Watch for any signs of beginning deficiency and replace as needed. ▪ A vesicant at concentrations greater than 10%. Ensure proper catheter or needle position, confirm patency of vein, and avoid extravasation. Administration through a central line is required for prolonged infusions of concentrations over 10% to 12.5% or for solutions with an osmolarity of approximately 900 mOsm/L or more. Routine monitoring of infusion site required. ▪ Monitor blood glucose. Supplemental insulin may be required. ▪ Monitor for S/S of hypersensitivity reactions (angioedema, bronchospasm, chills, cyanosis, fever, hypotension, pruritus, and rash). ▪ Monitor for S/S of pulmonary distress. ▪ Inspect the solution, infusion set, and catheter periodically for formation of precipitates. ▪ Monitor for S/S of infection. ▪ Monitor for S/S that may indicate refeeding syndrome (hypokalemia, hypophosphatemia, hypomagnesemia, CHF, edema). ▪ See Rate of Administration and Precautions.

Pediatric patients: Monitor fluid intake, urine output, and serum electrolytes closely. Small volumes of fluid may affect fluid and electrolyte balance in very small infants and neonates. Renal function may be immature and the ability to excrete fluid and solute loads limited. ▪ Monitor serum glucose frequently in all pediatric patients but especially in infants, neonates, and low-birth-weight infants. Adequate glycemic control is imperative to avoid potential long-term adverse effects; see Precautions.

Pediatric Education: Promptly report development of any adverse event, including but not limited to S/S of infection, pulmonary distress, hypersensitivity reactions, or pain at injection site.

Maternal/Child: Category C: safety for use in pregnancy and breast-feeding not established. Malnutrition in pregnant females is associated with adverse maternal and fetal outcomes. Parenteral nutrition should be considered if a pregnant woman's nutritional requirements cannot be met by oral or enteral intake. Intrapartum maternal IV infusions of glucose-containing solutions may produce maternal hyperglycemia with subsequent fetal hyperglycemia and fetal metabolic acidosis. Fetal hyperglycemia can result in increased fetal insulin levels, which may result in neonatal hypoglycemia after delivery. Benefits must outweigh risks. Use caution and monitor fluid balance, glucose and electrolyte concentrations, and acid-base balance of both mother and child. ▪ See Precautions and Monitor.

Elderly: At increased risk for developing hyponatremia and hyponatremic encephalopathy. Lower-end initial doses may be indicated; see Dose Adjustments. Monitoring of renal function may be useful. Specific age-related differences in response have not been identified.

DRUG/LAB INTERACTIONS
See Monitor.

SIDE EFFECTS
Rare in small doses and at lower concentrations when administered at the appropriate rate. Side effects may include acidosis, alkalosis, aluminum toxicity, febrile reactions, fluid overload (congested states, pulmonary edema, overhydration, dilution of serum electrolyte concentrations), hepatobiliary disorders, hyperglycemia (during infusion), hyperosmolar syndrome (mental confusion, loss of consciousness), hypersensitivity reactions (e.g., anaphylaxis; coughing; difficulty breathing; periorbital, facial, and/or laryngeal edema; pruritus; sneezing; and urticaria), hypokalemia, hypophosphatemia, hypovitaminosis, infection, parenteral nutrition–associated liver disease, pulmonary embolism, rebound hypoglycemia (after infusion), refeeding syndrome, venous thrombosis or phlebitis.

ANTIDOTE
Discontinue the drug and notify the physician of the side effect. Provide symptomatic treatment as required. Dose reduction may be sufficient for management of some side effects. If signs of pulmonary distress occur, stop the infusion and initiate a medical evaluation. Patients developing signs of hepatobiliary disorders should be assessed by a clinician knowledgeable in liver disease. Treat hypersensitivity reactions as indicated (e.g., antihistamines, epinephrine, corticosteroids) and resuscitate as necessary.

DIAZEPAM BBW

(dye-**AYZ**-eh-pam)

Benzodiazepine
Sedative-hypnotic
Antianxiety agent
Anticonvulsant

Valium

pH 6.2 to 6.9

USUAL DOSE

Dose should be individualized. The usual recommended dose in older pediatric patients and adults is 2 to 20 mg IM or IV depending on the indication and its severity. In some conditions (e.g., tetanus), larger doses may be required. In acute conditions, the injection may be repeated within 1 hour, although an interval of 3 to 4 hours is usually satisfactory. Consider transition to oral therapy, if appropriate, once the acute symptomatology has been controlled.

Moderate anxiety disorders and symptoms of anxiety: 2 to 5 mg IV. Repeat in 3 to 4 hours if necessary.

Severe anxiety disorders and symptoms of anxiety: 5 to 10 mg IV. Repeat in 3 to 4 hours if necessary.

Acute alcohol withdrawal: 10 mg initially, then 5 to 10 mg in 3 to 4 hours if necessary.

Endoscopic procedures: 10 mg or less is usually effective given immediately before procedure begins; titrate to desired sedation (e.g., slurred speech). Up to 20 mg may be indicated if a narcotic is not used.

Muscle spasm: 5 to 10 mg. Repeat in 3 to 4 hours if necessary. Larger doses may be required in tetanus.

Status epilepticus and severe recurrent convulsive seizures: 5 to 10 mg. May be repeated at intervals of 10 to 15 minutes up to a total dose of 30 mg. May repeat in 2 to 4 hours. Another source suggests 0.15 to 0.2 mg/kg (maximum dose of 10 mg). May repeat one time.

Cardioversion: 5 to 15 mg 5 to 10 minutes before procedure begins.

PEDIATRIC DOSE

Safety for use in neonates not established but is used. Neonates and young infants have reduced or immature organ function; may be susceptible to prolonged CNS depression. Avoid small veins (e.g., dorsum of hand or wrist); see Monitor. Use in infants and children is most frequent in tetany and status epilepticus. Use of longer-acting anticonvulsants (e.g., phenobarbital, phenytoin) following diazepam may be indicated.

Tetanus in pediatric patients from 30 days of age to 5 years of age: 1 to 2 mg every 3 to 4 hours as necessary. Another source recommends a dose of 0.1 to 0.2 mg/kg/dose every 2 to 6 hours in infants and children, titrating as needed.
Respiratory assistance must be available.

Tetanus in pediatric patients 5 years of age or older: 5 to 10 mg every 3 to 4 hours as necessary. Respiratory assistance must be available.

Status epilepticus in neonates (unlabeled): 0.1 to 0.3 mg/kg/dose given over 3 to 5 minutes, every 15 to 30 minutes, to a maximum total dose of 2 mg (not recommended as first-line agent).

Status epilepticus in pediatric patients from 30 days of age to 5 years of age: 0.2 to 0.5 mg every 2 to 5 minutes to a maximum 5-mg dose. Another source suggests 0.1 to 0.3 mg/kg/dose given over 3 to 5 minutes every 5 to 10 minutes with a maximum dose of 10 mg for pediatric patients over 30 days of age.

Status epilepticus in pediatric patients 5 years of age or older: 1 mg every 2 to 5 minutes to a maximum 10-mg dose. May repeat in 2 to 4 hours if necessary.

DOSE ADJUSTMENTS

Lower doses (usually 2 to 5 mg) with slow titration should be used in elderly or debilitated patients and when other sedative medications are coadministered. ▪ See Drug/Lab Interactions.

DILUTION

Do not dilute or mix with any other drug. Should be given directly into the vein. Inject into IV tubing close to vein site only when direct IV injection is not feasible. Consider heparin lock for frequent injection.

Storage: Store at CRT in cartons to protect from light. Do not freeze.

COMPATIBILITY

Manufacturers recommend not mixing with any other drug or solution in syringe or solution. Precipitation can occur.

Other sources suggest a few specific **compatibilities** dependent on concentration and manufacturer; consult a pharmacist.

RATE OF ADMINISTRATION

Adults: 5 mg (1 mL) or fraction thereof over 1 minute. Maximum rate is 5 mg/min.

Infants and other pediatric patients: Give total dose over a minimum of 3 minutes in a dosage not to exceed 0.25 mg/kg.

ACTIONS

A benzodiazepine that binds to benzodiazepine receptors on the postsynaptic GABA neuron. Acts on parts of the limbic system, the thalamus and the hypothalamus, and induces calming effects. Exerts antianxiety, sedative/hypnotic, amnesic, anticonvulsant, skeletal muscle relaxant, and antitremor effects. Diminishes patient recall. Metabolized in the liver; stays in the body in appreciable amounts for several days and is excreted very slowly in the urine. Crosses the placental barrier. Secreted in breast milk.

INDICATIONS AND USES

Relief of acute anxiety when rapid action is required. ▪ Acute alcohol withdrawal (as an aid in symptomatic relief of acute agitation, tremor, impending or acute delirium tremens, and hallucinosis). ▪ As an adjunct in (1) endoscopic procedures; (2) skeletal muscle spasms associated with local pathology, cerebral palsy, athetosis, stiff-man syndrome, and tetanus; and (3) status epilepticus and severe recurrent convulsive seizures. ▪ As a premedication in patients undergoing surgical procedures (IM preferred) and cardioversion.

CONTRAINDICATIONS

Known hypersensitivity, acute narrow-angle glaucoma, and open-angle glaucoma unless receiving appropriate therapy.

PRECAUTIONS

Concomitant use of benzodiazepines and opioids (e.g., morphine, hydromorphone [Dilaudid], fentanyl) may result in profound sedation, respiratory depression, coma, and death; see Drug/Lab Interactions. ▪ Not recommended for treatment of petit mal or petit mal variant seizures; may precipitate tonic status epilepticus. ▪ Patients may experience a return to seizure activity after initial control; re-administration of diazepam may be needed. Once seizures are controlled, consideration should be given to the administration of agents useful in longer-term control of seizures. ▪ Avoid use in patients in shock, coma, or in acute alcoholic intoxication with depression of vital signs. ▪ Use caution in the elderly, those who are very ill, and those with limited pulmonary reserve (e.g., chronic lung disease) or unstable cardiac status; may be at increased risk of apnea and/or cardiac arrest. ▪ Withdrawal symptoms will occur after extended use. Gradual tapering of dose may be indicated. ▪ Use caution in patients with impaired renal or hepatic function. ▪ Intended for short-term use only. ▪ Available PO and as a rectal gel.

Monitor: See Dilution. ▪ To reduce the incidence of venous thrombosis, phlebitis, or local irritation, avoid smaller veins (such as the dorsum of the hand or wrist) and administer injection slowly. Extravasation or arterial administration hazardous. ▪ Oxygen, respiratory assistance, and flumazenil must always be available. ▪ Monitor vital signs. ▪ Monitor patients for respiratory depression and sedation, especially when used concomitantly with opioids and other CNS depressants; see Drug/Lab Interactions. ▪ EEG monitoring may be useful for monitoring seizure activity. ▪ Periodic CBC and liver function tests may be indicated with long-term use.

Patient Education: May produce drowsiness or dizziness. Request assistance with ambulation and use caution performing tasks that require alertness. Do not drive or operate hazardous machinery until all effects have subsided. ▪ Avoid use of alcohol or other CNS depressants (e.g., antihistamines, barbiturates). ▪ May be habit-forming with long-term use or high-dose therapy. ▪ Has amnesic potential; may impair memory. ▪ Consider birth control options.

Maternal/Child: Studies suggest an increased risk of birth deformities with use during pregnancy, especially in the first trimester. ▪ Not recommended during pregnancy, childbirth, or while breast-feeding. ▪ Efficacy and safety have not been established in neonates (30 days or less of age). ▪ May contain benzyl alcohol, which has been associated with fatal gasping syndrome in premature infants.

Elderly: See Dose Adjustments. Start with a small dose and increase gradually based on response. ▪ More sensitive to therapeutic and adverse effects (e.g., ataxia, dizziness, oversedation). ▪ IV injection may be more likely to cause apnea, bradycardia, hypotension, and cardiac arrest. ▪ See Precautions and Drug/Lab Interactions.

DRUG/LAB INTERACTIONS

Concomitant use of **benzodiazepines and opioids** (e.g., morphine, hydromorphone, fentanyl) may result in profound sedation, respiratory depression, coma, and death. Reserve concomitant prescribing of these drugs for use in patients for whom alternative treatment options are inadequate. Limit dosages and durations to the minimum required, and monitor for S/S of respiratory depression and sedation.

▪ When given concomitantly with a narcotic, the dosage of the narcotic should be reduced by at least one-third and administered in small increments. ▪ Concurrent use with other **CNS depressants** (e.g., alcohol, antihistamines, barbiturates, MAO inhibitors, phenothiazines, tricyclic antidepressants) may result in additive effects. Reduced dose may be indicated. Monitor for S/S of respiratory depression and sedation. ▪ May increase serum concentrations of **digoxin and phenytoin**; monitor serum levels. ▪ **Ritonavir** may increase risk of prolonged sedation and respiratory depression. ▪ Concurrent use with **beta-blockers, cimetidine, disulfiram, fluoxetine, isoniazid, itraconazole, ketoconazole, omeprazole**, and **probenecid** may inhibit hepatic metabolism, resulting in increased plasma concentrations of benzodiazepines. ▪ May decrease effectiveness of **levodopa**. ▪ Hypotensive effects of benzodiazepines may be increased by **any agent that induces hypotension** (e.g., antihypertensives, CNS depressants, diuretics, lidocaine, paclitaxel). ▪ Use with **rifampin** increases clearance and reduces effects of diazepam. ▪ **Theophyllines** (e.g., aminophylline) antagonize sedative effects of benzodiazepines. ▪ **Smoking** increases metabolism and clearance of diazepam, decreasing plasma levels and sedative effects. ▪ **Clozapine** has caused respiratory distress or cardiac arrest in a few patients; use concurrently with extreme caution. ▪ **Grapefruit juice** may affect certain enzymes of the P$_{450}$ enzyme system and should be avoided.

SIDE EFFECTS

Ataxia, drowsiness, fatigue, phlebitis, and venous thrombosis are the most commonly reported adverse reactions. Other reported reactions include apnea, blurred vision, bradycardia, cardiovascular collapse, changes in salivation, confusion, constipation, coughing, depressed respiration, depression, diplopia, dysarthria, dyspnea, headache, hiccups, hyperexcited states, hyperventilation, hypoactivity, hypotension, incontinence, jaundice, laryngospasm, nausea, neutropenia, nystagmus, rash, slurred speech, syncope, tremor, urinary retention, urticaria, and vertigo.

Overdose: Diminished reflexes, coma, confusion, and somnolence.

ANTIDOTE

Notify the physician of all side effects. Reduction of dosage may be required. Discontinue the drug for major side effects or paradoxical reactions, including hyperexcitability, hallucinations, and acute rage. Flumazenil will reverse all sedative effects of benzodiazepines. A patent airway, artificial ventilation, oxygen therapy, and other symptomatic treatment must be instituted promptly. Monitor respiration, heart rate, and BP. May cause emesis; observe closely. Treat hypersensitivity reaction, or resuscitate as necessary.

DIFELIKEFALIN
(dye-**FEL**-i-**KEF**-a-lin)

Korsuva

USUAL DOSE
0.5 mcg/kg IV into the venous line of the dialysis circuit at the end of each hemodialysis session.

PEDIATRIC DOSE
Not established.

DOSE ADJUSTMENTS
Renal: No dosage adjustments are provided by the manufacturer.
Hepatic: No dosage adjustments are provided by the manufacturer, although they should be avoided in severe hepatic impairment.

DILUTION
IV Bolus: Withdraw required volume from vial(s) into syringe. No further dilution is required. Discard any unused portion.

COMPATIBILITY
Do not administer simultaneously with any other medication or IV solutions other than normal saline.

RATE OF ADMINISTRATION
Give via IV bolus into the venous line of the hemodialysis circuit at the end of hemodialysis. Blood should not be circulating through the dialyzer. Give during or after the rinse back of circuit. If given after rinse back, flush with at least 10 mL of normal saline.

ACTIONS
Difelikefalin is a kappa opioid receptor agonist; the mechanism of action for pruritus has not been established.

INDICATIONS AND USES
Treatment of moderate to severe pruritus associated with chronic kidney disease in adults undergoing hemodialysis; has not been studied for peritoneal dialysis.

CONTRAINDICATIONS
None is listed by the manufacturer.

PRECAUTIONS
CNS effects include dizziness, mental status changes, gait disturbances, somnolence, and falls. Dizziness and somnolence are most likely to occur during the first few weeks of therapy and may diminish with continued dosing. Patients must be cautioned about driving or operating machinery. Risk of CNS sedative effects may be increased with use of concomitant CNS depressants.
Monitor: Mental status and relief of itching.
Patient Education: May cause CNS depression; advise patient to take fall precautions and avoid driving or operating machinery while taking. Notify provider of signs of allergic reaction.
Maternal/Child: There are no adequate data on developmental risks associated with the use in pregnant or lactating females.
Elderly: Somnolence is increased in patients greater than 65 years of age.

DRUG/LAB INTERACTIONS
Difelikefalin may enhance CNS depressant effects of other CNS depressant drugs.

SIDE EFFECTS
Hyperkalemia, diarrhea, nausea, falling, altered mental status

ANTIDOTE
There is no antidote.

DIGOXIN
(dih-**JOX**-in)

Cardiac glycoside
Antiarrhythmic
Inotropic agent

Digoxin Pediatric, Lanoxin, Lanoxin Pediatric

pH 6.8 to 7.2

USUAL DOSE

Individualize dosing, taking into account factors that affect digoxin blood levels (e.g., lean body weight [LBW], CrCl, age, concomitant disease states, concurrent medications). In general, the dose of digoxin used should be determined on clinical grounds. Dosing can be either initiated with a loading dose followed by maintenance dosing (if rapid titration is desired) or initiated with maintenance dosing without a loading dose. Parenteral administration of digoxin should be reserved for when rapid digitalization is medically necessary or when the drug cannot be taken orally. When changing from IV to oral dosing, increase oral dose by 20% to 25% to allow for reduced bioavailability of the oral product.

Loading dosing regimen in adults and pediatric patients:

Recommended Digoxin Injection Loading Dose for Adult and Pediatric Patients	
Age	**Total IV Loading Dose (mcg/kg)** Administer half of the total loading dose initially, then $1/4$ of the loading dose every 6–8 hours twice
Premature	15 to 25 mcg/kg
Full-term	20 to 30 mcg/kg
1 to 24 months	30 to 50 mcg/kg
2 to 5 years	25 to 35 mcg/kg
5 to 10 years	15 to 30 mcg/kg
Adults and pediatric patients over 10 years	8 to 12 mcg/kg

Maintenance dosing in adults and pediatric patients over 10 years of age: 2.4 to 3.6 mcg/kg/day given once daily. Doses may be adjusted every 2 weeks according to clinical response, serum drug levels, and toxicity.

PEDIATRIC DOSE

Use 0.1 mg/mL pediatric injection (100 mcg/mL). If using a tuberculin syringe to measure a pediatric dose, do not flush syringe with parenteral solution after contents are injected; may result in an overdose. The recommended starting maintenance dose in pediatric patients under 10 years of age is listed in the following chart. These recommendations assume the presence of normal renal function.

Recommended Starting Digoxin Maintenance Dosage in Pediatric Patients Under 10 Years of Age	
Age	**Dose Regimen (mcg/kg/dose)** **Given twice daily**
Premature	1.9 to 3.1 mcg/kg/dose
Full-term	3 to 4.5 mcg/kg/dose
1 to 24 months	4.5 to 7.5 mcg/kg/dose
2 to 5 years	3.8 to 5.3 mcg/kg/dose
5 to 10 years	2.3 to 4.5 mcg/kg/dose

DOSE ADJUSTMENTS

The following two charts provide recommended maintenance doses for specific patient populations based on lean body weight and renal function.

Corrected Creatinine Clearance[a]	Lean Body Weight (kg)[b]							Number of Days Before Steady State Achieved[c]
	40	**50**	**60**	**70**	**80**	**90**	**100**	
10 mL/min	64	80	96	112	128	144	160	19
20 mL/min	72	90	108	126	144	162	180	16
30 mL/min	80	100	120	140	160	180	200	14
40 mL/min	88	110	132	154	176	198	220	13
50 mL/min	96	120	144	168	192	216	240	12
60 mL/min	104	130	156	182	208	234	260	11
70 mL/min	112	140	168	196	224	252	280	10
80 mL/min	120	150	180	210	240	270	300	9
90 mL/min	128	160	192	224	256	288	320	8
100 mL/min	136	170	204	238	272	306	340	7

Digoxin Maintenance Dose (in mcg given ONCE daily) in Adults and Pediatric Patients Over 10 Years of Age Based on Lean Body Weight and Renal Function

[a]For adults, CrCl was corrected to a 70-kg body weight or 1.73 M² body surface area. For pediatric patients, the modified Schwartz equation may be used. The formula is based on height in cm and SCr in mg/dL where k is a constant and CCr is corrected to 1.73 M² body surface area. During the first year of life, the value of k is 0.33 for preterm infants and 0.45 for term infants. The k is 0.55 for pediatric patients and adolescent girls and 0.7 for adolescent boys:

$$GRF\ mL/min/1.73\ M^2 = (k \times Height)/SCr$$

[b]The doses listed assume average body composition.
[c]If no loading dose administered.

- Alternatively, the maintenance dose for adults and pediatric patients over 10 years of age may be estimated using the following formula:

$$Total\ maintenance\ dose\ (mcg) = Loading\ dose\ (mcg) \times \%\ Daily\ loss \div 100$$
$$Where\ \%\ daily\ loss = 14 + CrCl \div 5.$$

Corrected Creatinine Clearance[b]	Lean Body Weight (kg)[c]							Number of Days Before Steady State Achieved[d]
	5	**10**	**20**	**30**	**40**	**50**	**60**	
10 mL/min	8	16	32	48	64	80	96	19
20 mL/min	9	18	36	54	72	90	108	16
30 mL/min	10	20	40	60	80	100	120	14
40 mL/min	11	22	44	66	88	110	132	13
50 mL/min	12	24	48	72	96	120	144	12
60 mL/min	13	26	52	78	104	130	156	11
70 mL/min	14	28	56	84	112	140	168	10
80 mL/min	15	30	60	90	120	150	180	9
90 mL/min	16	32	64	96	128	160	192	8
100 mL/min	17	34	68	102	136	170	204	7

Digoxin Maintenance Dose[a] (in mcg given TWICE daily) in Pediatric Patients Under 10 Years of Age Based on Lean Body Weight and Renal Function

[a]Recommended doses are to be given twice daily.
[b]The modified Schwartz equation may be used to estimate creatinine clearance. See preceding chart.
[c]The doses listed assume average body composition.
[d]If no loading dose is administered.

■ Reduce dose in patients whose lean weight is an abnormally small fraction of their total body mass because of obesity or edema. ■ Monitor for S/S of digoxin toxicity and clinical response. Adjust dose based on toxicity, efficacy, and blood levels. ■ Reduce dose in partially digitalized patients, in patients with impaired renal function, and in the elderly. ■ Dose reduction may be required before cardioversion. ■ See Drug/Lab Interactions; adjustments may be required with numerous drugs. ■ Renal clearance diminished in neonates, including premature infants; adjust dose as indicated. ■ See Precautions.

DILUTION

Available as a 500 mcg (0.5 mg) in 2 mL injection (250 mcg [0.25 mg] per mL) and as a 100 mcg (0.1 mg) in 1 mL (pediatric) injection. May be given undiluted or each 1 mL may be diluted in 4 mL SWFI, NS, or D5W. Less diluent may cause precipitation. Use diluted solution immediately. Give through Y-tube of IV infusion set. See Pediatric Dose.

Storage: Store unopened vials at CRT protected from light.

COMPATIBILITY

Manufacturer recommends not mixing with other drugs in the same container and not administering simultaneously via the same IV line.

Other sources suggest specific **compatibilities** dependent on concentration and manufacturer; consult a pharmacist.

RATE OF ADMINISTRATION

Each single dose over a minimum of 5 minutes. Avoid bolus administration. Rapid administration may cause systemic and coronary arteriolar constriction.

ACTIONS

A cardiac glycoside obtained from *Digitalis lanata*. Inhibits Na-K ATPase, the "sodium pump" responsible for moving sodium ions out of cells and potassium ions into cells. The cardiologic consequences of this action are an increase in the force and velocity of myocardial systolic contraction (positive inotropic action), a slowing of the heart rate (negative chronotropic effect), decreased conduction velocity through the AV node, and a decrease in the degree of activation of the sympathetic nervous system and renin-angiotensin system (neurohormonal deactivating effect). Increases cardiac output and left ventricular ejection fraction and lowers pulmonary artery pressure, pulmonary capillary wedge pressure, and systemic vascular resistance. Widely distributed throughout the body. Onset of action is 5 to 30 minutes. Time to peak effect is 1 to 4 hours. Half-life is 1.5 to 2 days. Minimal metabolism. Rapidly excreted in urine, primarily as unchanged drug. Crosses the placenta and is secreted in breast milk.

INDICATIONS AND USES

Treatment of mild to moderate heart failure in adults. ■ To increase myocardial contractility in pediatric patients with heart failure. ■ Control of ventricular response rates in adult patients with chronic atrial fibrillation; see Precautions.

CONTRAINDICATIONS

Ventricular fibrillation and known hypersensitivity to digoxin or other digitalis preparations.

PRECAUTIONS

IV administration is the preferred parenteral route. Used only when oral therapy is not feasible or rapid therapeutic effect is necessary. ■ Commonly prolongs the PR interval; may cause severe sinus bradycardia or sinoatrial block in patients with pre-existing sinus node disease and may cause advanced or complete heart block in patients with pre-existing incomplete AV block. Consider insertion of a pacemaker before treatment with digoxin in these patients. ■ Use in patients with an accessory AV pathway (Wolff-Parkinson-White syndrome) increases risk of ventricular fibrillation and is not recommended. ■ Avoid use in patients with heart failure associated with preserved left ventricular systolic function (e.g., acute cor pulmonale, amyloid heart disease, constrictive pericarditis, idiopathic hypertrophic subaortic stenosis, restrictive cardiomyopathy). Patients with these conditions may experience a decreased cardiac output. Has been used for ventricular rate control in a subgroup of these patients with atrial fibrillation. ▪ Avoid use in patients with myocarditis; may precipitate vasoconstriction and promote production of pro-inflammatory cytokines. ▪ Use with caution in patients with impaired renal function; risk of toxicity increased; see Dose Adjustments. ▪ Use caution in patients with electrolyte disorders because potassium or magnesium depletion sensitizes the myocardium to digoxin; toxicity may occur with serum digoxin concentrations below 2 ng/mL. ▪ Use with caution in patients with hypercalcemia. May increase risk of digoxin toxicity. Maintain normocalcemia. ▪ Hypocalcemia may nullify effect of digoxin. If calcium levels need to be restored to normal, give calcium slowly and in small amounts. Serious arrhythmias have occurred in digitalized patients receiving calcium. ▪ Hypothyroidism may reduce requirements for digoxin. ▪ Addressing the underlying condition is suggested in patients with heart failure and/or atrial arrhythmias resulting from hypermetabolic or hyperdynamic states (e.g., hyperthyroidism, hypoxia, or arteriovenous shunt). Atrial arrhythmias associated with hypermetabolic states are particularly resistant to digoxin treatment. ▪ Patients with beriberi heart disease may fail to respond adequately to digoxin if the underlying thiamine deficiency is not treated concomitantly. ▪ Use is not recommended in patients with myocardial infarction. May cause an increase in myocardial oxygen demand and ischemia. ▪ Some clinicians suggest reducing or discontinuing the dose of digoxin for 1 to 2 days before an elective cardioversion of atrial fibrillation to avoid the induction of ventricular arrhythmias, but physicians must consider the consequences of increasing the ventricular response if digoxin is decreased or withdrawn. If digoxin toxicity is suspected, elective cardioversion should be delayed. If it is not prudent to delay cardioversion, the lowest possible energy level should be selected to avoid provoking ventricular arrhythmias. ▪ See Drug/Lab Interactions.

Monitor: Monitor for S/S of digoxin toxicity (anorexia, nausea, vomiting, vision changes, cardiac arrhythmias). ▪ Low body weight, advanced age, impaired renal function, hypomagnesemia, hypokalemia, and hypercalcemia may predispose patient to digoxin toxicity. Monitor electrolytes frequently during therapy. Avoid rapid changes. Supplements indicated to maintain normal serum electrolyte levels. ▪ Monitor renal function. ▪ Monitor digoxin levels. Draw at least 6 hours after the last dose, preferably just before the next dose. Serum digoxin levels less than 0.5 ng/mL have been associated with diminished efficacy, whereas levels above 2 ng/mL have been associated with increased toxicity without increased benefit. ▪ Monitor HR and BP. ▪ Baseline and periodic ECG monitoring suggested. May prolong the PR interval and cause depression of the ST segment on ECG. ▪ The earliest and most frequent manifestation of digoxin toxicity in infants and children is the appearance of cardiac arrhythmias, including sinus bradycardia. ECG monitoring recommended in pediatric patients to avoid intoxication. ▪ See Dose Adjustments, Precautions, and Drug/Lab Interactions.

Patient Education: Review all medications with pharmacist or physician. Capable of numerous drug interactions. ▪ Laboratory monitoring of digoxin levels and renal function required. ▪ Report any nausea, vomiting, persistent diarrhea, confusion, weakness, or vision disturbances.

Maternal/Child: Category C: use during pregnancy, labor, and delivery only if clearly needed. ▪ Use caution during breast-feeding. Digoxin does distribute into breast milk, but the estimated exposure of the nursing infant to digoxin via breast-feeding is far below the usual infant maintenance dose. ▪ Safety and effectiveness of digoxin in the control of ventricular rate in pediatric patients with atrial fibrillation have not been established. ▪ Safety and effectiveness in the treatment of heart failure in pediatric patients have not been established in well-controlled studies. However, in published literature of pediatric patients with heart failure of various etiologies, treatment with digoxin has been associated with improvements in hemodynamic parameters and in clinical S/S. ▪ Newborn infants display considerable variability in their tolerance to digoxin. Premature and immature infants are particularly sensitive. Dose must be reduced and individualized according to degree of maturity. ▪ Carefully titrate dose based on clinical response in pediatric patients with renal disease; see Dose Adjustments. ▪ See Monitor.

Elderly: Monitor carefully. Reduced dose may be indicated. Consider reduced body mass and reduced kidney function.

DRUG/LAB INTERACTIONS

Interactions are numerous. Careful monitoring required when initiating, adjusting, or discontinuing drugs that may interact with digoxin. Monitor serum levels carefully and adjust doses as indicated. ▪ Digoxin is a substrate for P-glycoprotein at the level of intestinal absorption, renal tubular secretion, and biliary-intestinal secretion. **Drugs that induce or inhibit P-glycoprotein** have the potential to alter digoxin pharmacokinetics. ▪ **Potassium-depleting diuretics** are a major contributing factor to digitalis toxicity. ▪ **Calcium** may produce serious arrhythmias in digitalized patients, particularly with too-rapid IV administration. ▪ **Amiodarone, propafenone, quinine, spironolactone**, and **verapamil** may increase serum digoxin concentration. Reduce digoxin dose by 15% to 30% and monitor levels. ▪ **Quinidine** and **ritonavir** may increase serum levels. Decrease digoxin dose by 30% to 50% and monitor levels. ▪ Synergistic with **beta-blockers** and **calcium channel blockers**. Additive effects on AV node conduction may result in bradycardia and/or advanced or complete heart block. ▪ **Ivabradine** can increase the risk of bradycardia. ▪ **ACE inhibitors, angiotensin receptor blockers, NSAIDs**, and **COX-2 inhibitors** (e.g., celecoxib) may impair excretion of digoxin. ▪ Coadministration with **dofetilide** has been associated with a higher incidence of torsades de pointes. ▪ Coadministration with **sotalol** has been associated with more proarrhythmic events than when either drug was administered alone. ▪ Sudden death was more common in patients receiving digoxin with **dronedarone** than when either drug was given alone. ▪ **Teriparatide** transiently increases serum calcium, which may predispose patients to digoxin toxicity. ▪ **Succinylcholine** may cause a sudden extrusion of potassium from muscle cells; may cause arrhythmias in digitalized patients. ▪ Increased risk of arrhythmias with **sympathomimetic amines** (e.g., dopamine, epinephrine, norepinephrine). ▪ Initiation of **thyroid treatment** may require an increase in digoxin dose. ▪ Endogenous substances of unknown composition (**digoxin-like immunoreactive substances [DLIS]**) can interfere with standard radioimmunoassays for digoxin. This interference usually results in a falsely elevated level but sometimes causes results to be falsely reduced. DLIS are present in up to half of all neonates and in varying percentages of pregnant females, patients with hypertrophic cardiomyopathy, patients with renal or hepatic dysfunction, and other patients who are volume expanded for any reason. **Spironolactone and some traditional Chinese and Ayurvedic medicines** may also interfere with different assays; see manufacturer's prescribing information for further information. ▪ See Precautions and Monitor.

SIDE EFFECTS

The overall incidence of adverse reactions with digoxin has been reported as 5% to 20%, with 15% to 20% of adverse reactions considered serious. Cardiac toxicity accounts for about one-half, GI disturbances for about one-fourth, and CNS and other toxicity for about one-fourth of these adverse reactions. ***Cardiac:*** Arrhythmias (e.g., first-degree, second-degree, or third-degree heart block [including asystole]; atrial tachycardia with block; AV dissociation; accelerated junctional [nodal] rhythm; unifocal or multiform ventricular premature contractions [especially bigeminy or trigeminy]; ventricular tachycardia; and ventricular fibrillation). ***GI:*** Abdominal pain, hemorrhagic necrosis of the intestines, intestinal ischemia, nausea and vomiting. ***CNS:*** Apathy, confusion, dizziness, headache, mental disturbances (e.g., anxiety, delirium, depression, hallucinations), and weakness. ***Other:*** Anorexia, gynecomastia, rash, thrombocytopenia, and visual changes.

Toxicity can cause death. The ***most common manifestation of excessive dosing in pediatric patients*** is the appearance of cardiac arrhythmias. Conduction disturbances or supraventricular tachyarrhythmias are the most common type of arrhythmia. Ventricular arrhythmias are less common.

Overdose: Anorexia, arrhythmias, CNS disturbances, fatigue, hyperkalemia, nausea and vomiting.

ANTIDOTE

Discontinue the drug at the first sign of toxicity, notify the physician, and place the patient on a cardiac monitor. Dosage may be decreased or discontinued. For severe toxicity, digoxin immune Fab is a specific antidote. Consider causes of toxicity (electrolyte disturbances, thyroid, concurrent medications) and correct/treat as indicated. Serum potassium must be obtained before administering potassium salts. See Precautions. Bradycardia and heart block caused by digoxin toxicity may respond to atropine. Ventricular arrhythmias may respond to lidocaine or phenytoin. A temporary pacemaker may also be used. With severe digoxin toxicity, potassium may be released from skeletal muscles, resulting in hyperkalemia. Hyperkalemia, if life-threatening, may be treated with D5W and insulin. Peritoneal dialysis or hemodialysis not effective in overdose.

DIGOXIN IMMUNE FAB (OVINE)   Antidote
(dih-**JOX**-in im-**MYOUN** fab)   **(digoxin intoxication)**

Digibind, DigiFab   pH 6 to 8

USUAL DOSE

Pretreatment: Testing for sensitivity to sheep serum and/or premedication may be indicated; see Contraindications and Monitor.

Acute toxicity in adults and pediatric patients: Determine dose by symptoms and clinical findings. Serum concentration may not reflect actual toxicity for 6 to 12 hours. Symptoms of life-threatening toxicity due to digoxin overdose include severe arrhythmias (e.g., VT, VF), progressive bradycardia, second- or third-degree heart block not responsive to atropine, and/or serum potassium levels exceeding 5 to 5.5 mEq/L in adults and 6 mEq/L in pediatric patients.

Dose in numbers of vials based on ingested dose is calculated by dividing the body load of digoxin in milligrams by 0.5. Each vial of **Digibind** contains 38 mg/vial and will bind 0.5 mg digoxin. Each vial of **DigiFab** contains 40 mg/vial and will bind 0.5 mg of digoxin. Dose may also be based on serum digoxin levels (see package insert; has charts for adults and pediatric patients).

An initial dose of up to 20 vials has been used. 20 vials will bind approximately 50 (0.25 mg) tablets of Lanoxin and should provide adequate treatment of most life-threatening ingestions in adult and pediatric patients. If ingested substance is unknown, if serum digoxin level is not available, or if there is concern about sensitivity to the serum, consider giving 10 vials. Observe clinical response and repeat if indicated. In clinical trials of Digibind the average dose was 10 vials. A single dose may be repeated in several hours if toxicity has not reversed or appears to recur. Febrile reactions are dose related.

Toxicity in chronic therapy: *Adults:* 6 vials should be adequate to reverse most cases of toxicity in adults in acute distress or if a serum digoxin concentration is not available.

Pediatric patients: less than 20 kg: 1 vial should be adequate if signs of toxicity are present.

DILUTION

Each vial must be diluted with 4 mL of SWFI (results in 9.5 mg/mL for Digibind and 10 mg/mL for DigiFab). Mix gently. May be given in this initial dilution or may be further diluted with any desired amount of NS (with **Digibind,** 34 mL NS/vial yields 1 mg/mL; with **DigiFab,** 36 mL NS/vial yields 1 mg/mL). Consider volume overload in pediatric patients when further diluting in NS. Administer to infants after initial dilution using a tuberculin syringe to deliver an accurate dose with less volume; for extremely small doses, dilute to 1 mg/mL before administration.

Filters: *Digibind:* Must be given through a 0.22-micron membrane filter.

Storage: Refrigerate unreconstituted vials. Use reconstituted solution promptly or store in refrigerator for up to 4 hours.

COMPATIBILITY

Compatibility information not available from manufacturer; consult a pharmacist.

RATE OF ADMINISTRATION

Decrease the rate of infusion or discontinue temporarily if an infusion reaction occurs. Do not give as an IV bolus injection unless cardiac arrest is imminent. Be prepared to treat anaphylaxis.

Digibind: Must be given through a 0.22-micron membrane filter. A single dose as an IV infusion equally distributed over 15 to 30 minutes.

DigiFab: A single dose as an infusion over 30 minutes.

ACTIONS

Antigen-binding fragments (Fab) prepared from specific antidigoxin antibodies produced in sheep are isolated and purified. Fab fragments bind molecules of digoxin and make them unavailable for binding at their site of action. Freely distributed in extracellular space. Reduces the level of free digoxin in the serum. Onset of action is prompt, with improvement in symptoms of toxicity within 30 minutes. Fab-digoxin complexes are cleared by the kidney. DigiFab is also cleared in the reticuloendothelial system.

INDICATIONS AND USES

Digibind: Treatment of patients with life-threatening digoxin intoxication or overdose (digoxin).

DigiFab: Treatment of patients with life-threatening or potentially life-threatening digoxin toxicity or overdose. Not indicated for milder cases of digoxin toxicity.

All formulations: Indicated for known suicidal or accidental consumption of fatal doses of digoxin, including ingestion of 10 mg or more of digoxin in previously healthy adults, 4 mg (or more than 0.1 mg/kg) in previously healthy pediatric patients, or ingestion causing steady-state serum concentrations greater than 10 ng/mL. ▪ Indicated for chronic ingestions causing steady-state serum digoxin concentrations exceeding 6 ng/mL in adults or 4 ng/mL in pediatric patients. ▪ Indicated for manifestations of life-threatening toxicity due to digoxin overdose, including severe ventricular arrhythmias (such as VT or VF), progressive bradycardia, or third-degree heart block not responsive to atropine. ▪ Also indicated when potassium concentrations are above 5 to 5.5 mEq/L in adults or 6 mEq/L in pediatric patients with rapidly progressive S/S of digoxin toxicity. ▪ See Precautions and Maternal/Child.

CONTRAINDICATIONS

None known when used for specific indications. If hypersensitivity exists and treatment is necessary, premedicate with corticosteroids and diphenhydramine and prepare to treat anaphylaxis.

PRECAUTIONS

Administered under the direction of the physician specialist with facilities for monitoring the patient and responding to any medical emergency. Cardiac arrest can result from ingestion of more than 10 mg digoxin by healthy adults, 4 mg digoxin by healthy pediatric patients, or serum digoxin levels above 10 ng/mL. ▪ Larger doses of digoxin immune Fab act more quickly but increase the possibility of febrile or hypersensitivity reactions. ▪ Use caution in impaired cardiac function. Inability to use cardiac glycosides may endanger patient. Support with dopamine or vasodilators. ▪ The clinical problem may not be caused by digoxin toxicity if the patient fails to respond to digoxin immune Fab. ▪ Consider that multiple drugs may have been used and are producing toxicity in suicide attempts. ▪ See Monitor and Drug/Lab Interactions.

Monitor: Although allergy testing is not required before treating life-threatening digoxin toxicity, patients allergic to ovine proteins or those who have previously received antibodies or Fab fragments produced from sheep are at risk. Determine patient response to any previous injections of serum of any type and history of any allergic-type reactions. In addition, **DigiFab** considers that patients with allergies to papain, chymopapain, other papaya extracts, or the pineapple enzyme bromelain may be at risk. *Digibind* provides the information below on sensitivity testing; that information is not included in the package insert for *DigiFab*. ▪ Test for sensitivity if indicated. Make a 1:100 solution by diluting 0.1 mL of reconstituted solution (10 mg/mL) with 9.9 mL sterile NS (100 mcg/mL).

Scratch test: Make a ¼-inch skin scratch through a drop of 1:100 dilution in NS. Inspect the site in 20 minutes. An urticarial wheal surrounded by a zone of erythema is a positive reaction.

Skin test: Inject 0.1 mL (10 mcg) of 1:100 dilution intradermally. Inspect the site in 20 minutes. An urticarial wheal surrounded by a zone of erythema is a positive reaction. Concomitant use of antihistamines may interfere with sensitivity tests. If skin testing causes a systemic reaction, place a tourniquet above the testing site and treat anaphylaxis.

▪ Serum digoxin or digitoxin concentration should be obtained before administration if at all possible. These measurements may be difficult to interpret if drawn soon after the last digitalis dose because at least 6 to 8 hours are required for equilibration of digoxin between serum and tissue. ▪ Standard treatment of digoxin intoxication includes withdrawal of the intoxicating agent; correction of electrolyte disturbances (especially hyperkalemia), acid-base imbalances, and hypoxia; and treatment of cardiac arrhythmias. ▪ Monitor VS, ECG, and potassium concentration frequently during and after drug administration. ▪ Monitor for S/S of an acute hypersensitivity reaction (e.g., angioedema, bronchospasm with wheezing or cough, erythema, hypotension, laryngeal edema, pruritus, stridor, tachycardia, urticaria). ▪ Potassium may be shifted from inside to outside the cell, causing increased renal excretion. May appear to have hyperkalemia while there is a total body deficit of potassium. When the digoxin effect is reversed, hypokalemia may develop rapidly. ▪ Do not redigitalize until all Fab fragments have been eliminated from the body. May take several days. May take longer in severe renal impairment, and reintoxication may occur by release of newly unbound digoxin into the blood. ▪ See Precautions and Drug/Lab Interactions.

Maternal/Child: Category C: use only when clearly indicated and benefits outweigh risks in pregnancy, breast-feeding, and infants. ▪ *Digibind* indicates that it should be used in infants and children if more than 0.3 mg of digoxin is ingested, if serum digoxin levels are equal to or greater than 6.4 nmol/L, or if there is underlying heart disease.

Patient Education: Contact the physician immediately if S/S of a delayed hypersensitivity reaction or serum sickness occur (e.g., rash, pruritus, urticaria).

Elderly: Consider age-related impaired renal function; monitor closely for recurrent toxicity; see Monitor.

DRUG/LAB INTERACTIONS

Will cause a precipitous rise in **total serum digoxin,** but most will be bound to the Fab fragment. Will interfere with digoxin immunoassay measurements until Fab fragment is completely eliminated. ▪ **Catecholamines** (e.g., epinephrine) may aggravate digoxin arrhythmias. ▪ See skin test in Monitor.

SIDE EFFECTS

Acute anaphylaxis with urticaria, respiratory distress, and vascular collapse is possible. Exacerbation of congestive heart failure and low cardiac output states and increased ventricular response in atrial fibrillation may occur due to withdrawal of digoxin effects. Hypokalemia may be life threatening.

ANTIDOTE

Notify the physician of all side effects. Discontinue the drug and treat anaphylaxis immediately. Corticosteroids, epinephrine, diphenhydramine, oxygen, IV fluids, vasopressors (dopamine), and ventilation equipment must always be available. Resuscitate as necessary. Treat hypokalemia cautiously when necessary. Support exacerbated cardiac conditions as necessary.

DIHYDROERGOTAMINE MESYLATE BBW

(dye-hy-droh-er-**GOT**-ah-meen **MES**-ih-layt)

D.H.E. 45

Ergot alkaloid
Migraine agent

pH 3.2 to 4

USUAL DOSE

Pretreatment: Verify pregnancy status; see Contraindications.

Abort or prevent headaches: 1 mg (1 mL). May be repeated in 1 hour. No more than 2 doses (2 mg total) may be given IV in 24 hours. Do not exceed 6 mg in 1 week; see Precautions. Administration of an antiemetic (e.g., metoclopramide [Reglan] 10 mg) PO 1 hour before dihydroergotamine is recommended.

Chronic intractable headache: 0.5 mg (0.5 mL). Administer an antiemetic IV (e.g., metoclopramide) about 10 minutes before injection.

Prevention of orthostatic hypotension associated with spinal or epidural anesthesia (unlabeled): 0.5 mg (0.5 mL). Give a few minutes before anesthetic.

PEDIATRIC DOSE

See Maternal/Child. Administration of an antiemetic (e.g., metoclopramide, prochlorperazine), usually PO, 1 hour before dihydroergotamine is recommended.

Pediatric patients 6 to 9 years of age: 100 to 150 mcg (0.1 to 0.15 mg).

Pediatric patients 9 to 12 years of age: 200 mcg (0.2 mg).

Pediatric patients 12 to 16 years of age: 250 to 500 mcg (0.25 to 0.5 mg).

For all age ranges, repeat up to 2 doses at 20-minute intervals if necessary. Another source suggests 250 mcg (0.25 mg) at the start of the attack. Repeat in 1 hour if necessary.

DILUTION

May be given undiluted.

Storage: Protect ampules from light and heat.

COMPATIBILITY

Compatibility information not available from manufacturer; consult a pharmacist.

RATE OF ADMINISTRATION

Administer slowly over 2-3 minutes, or can be given as a continuous infusion.

ACTIONS

An alpha-adrenergic blocking agent that causes constriction of both peripheral and cerebral blood vessels and produces depression of central vasomotor centers. Metabolized by the liver. Metabolites eliminated primarily in feces. Secreted in breast milk.

INDICATIONS AND USES

To abort or prevent vascular headaches (migraine, histamine cephalalgia). Used when rapid control is desired or other routes not feasible. ▪ Treatment of chronic intractable headache.

Unlabeled uses: To prevent orthostatic hypotension associated with spinal or epidural anesthesia. Use SQ to enhance heparin effects in preventing postoperative deep vein thrombosis after abdominal, thoracic, or pelvic surgeries or total hip replacement and IM or SQ to treat orthostatic hypotension.

CONTRAINDICATIONS

Breast-feeding, coronary artery disease, hepatic or renal disease, hypersensitivity, uncontrolled hypertension, peripheral vascular disease, pregnancy or females who may become pregnant, sepsis. ▪ Coadministration with potent CYP3A4 inhibitors, including protease inhibitors and macrolide antibiotics, is contraindicated; see Drug/Lab Interactions.

PRECAUTIONS

IM or SQ use is preferred but may be given IV to obtain a more rapid effect. ▪ Coadministration with potent CYP3A4 inhibitors, including protease inhibitors and macrolide antibiotics, increases the risk of vasospasm, leading to cerebral ischemia and/or ischemia of the extremities (peripheral). May be serious and/or life threatening; see Contraindications and Drug/Lab Interactions.

- Use only when a clear diagnosis of migraine has been established. Do not exceed dosing guidelines or use for chronic daily administration; see Usual Dose.

Monitor: Monitor vital signs; observe closely. ▪ See Drug/Lab Interactions.

Patient Education: Consider birth control options. ▪ Take only as directed. ▪ Report ineffectiveness or an increase in frequency or severity of headaches. ▪ Report chest pain, increased HR, itching, muscle pain or weakness of arms or legs, numbness or tingling of extremities, or swelling.

Maternal/Child: Category X: avoid pregnancy. See Contraindications. ▪ Safety for use in pediatric patients not established. Severe side effects (e.g., extrapyramidal reactions may occur). Pretreatment with an antiemetic may be helpful. Limit pediatric use to patients who have not responded to less toxic treatment.

Elderly: Increased risk of hypothermia and ischemic complications (e.g., cardiac, peripheral). ▪ Consider age-related renal impairment.

DRUG/LAB INTERACTIONS

Contraindicated with potent CYP3A4 inhibitors, including **antifungals**, **protease inhibitors** (e.g., ritonavir, nelfinavir, and indinavir), **and macrolide antibiotics**; see Contraindications and Precautions. ▪ Administer less potent CYP3A4 inhibitors with caution as vasospasm may occur. **Less potent inhibitors** include, but are not limited to, saquinavir, nefazodone, fluconazole, grapefruit juice, fluoxetine, fluvoxamine, zileuton, and clotrimazole. ▪ Opposes vasodilating effects of **nitrates**, decreasing their effectiveness. ▪ May cause hypertensive crisis in combination with other **vasopressors** (e.g., epinephrine). ▪ May cause peripheral vasoconstriction with ischemia and/or cyanosis with **beta-adrenergic blockers** and **nicotine.**

SIDE EFFECTS

Rare in therapeutic doses, but may include angina pectoris, blindness, gangrene, muscle pains, muscle weakness, nausea, numbness and tingling of the fingers and toes, pleural and retroperitoneal fibrosis, thirst, uterine bleeding, and vomiting.

ANTIDOTE

Discontinue the drug and notify the physician of any side effects. Another drug will probably be chosen if further treatment is indicated. Vasodilators (nitroprusside sodium) and CNS stimulants (e.g., caffeine and sodium benzoate) are indicated as an antidote. Heparin and low-molecular-weight dextran may be used to reduce thrombosis due to excessive vasoconstriction. Hemodialysis may be indicated. Resuscitate as necessary.

DILTIAZEM HYDROCHLORIDE
(dill-**TYE**-a-zem hy-droh-**KLOR**-eyed)

Calcium channel blocker
Antiarrhythmic

Cardizem

pH 3.7 to 4.1

USUAL DOSE
Pretreatment: Confirmation of diagnosis required; see Monitor.

Bolus: 0.25 mg/kg of body weight initially (20 mg for the average patient). Some patients may respond to an initial dose of 0.15 mg/kg. A second dose of 0.35 mg/kg may be given in 15 minutes if needed to achieve HR reduction (25 mg for the average patient). Any additional bolus doses used to achieve an appropriate response must be individualized to each patient.

Infusion: Patients with PSVT may respond to bolus doses and may not require an infusion, but to maintain reduction in HR in patients with atrial fibrillation or atrial flutter, immediately follow with an intravenous infusion at an initial rate of 10 mg/hr. Some patients may maintain response with an initial rate of 5 mg/hr. Infusion may be increased by 5 mg/hr increments to a maximum dose of 15 mg/hr. Discontinue infusion within 24 hours. Duration of infusion longer than 24 hours and infusion rates greater than 15 mg/hr have not been studied.

Transition to other antiarrhythmic agents as appropriate. In clinical trials, therapy with agents to maintain reduced heart rate in atrial fibrillation or atrial flutter or for prophylaxis of PSVT was generally started within 3 hours. Medications that were used included digoxin, quinidine, procainamide, calcium channel blockers (e.g., diltiazem, verapamil), beta-blockers (e.g., atenolol, metoprolol, propranolol). See prescribing information for individual agents.

DOSE ADJUSTMENTS
Specific mg/kg dose must be used for patients with low body weights. ▪ Reduced dose may be indicated in impaired hepatic or renal function. ▪ Dose selection should be cautious in the elderly. Reduced doses may be indicated based on potential for decreased organ function and concomitant disease or drug therapy. ▪ See Drug/Lab Interactions.

DILUTION
Available as a solution in 25-, 50-, or 125-mg vials (5 mg/mL) and, as a 100-mg ADD-Vantage vial. Dilute according to the following chart.

Dilution of Diltiazem Injection				
Diluent Volume	Quantity of Diltiazem Injection	Final Concentration	Administration	
			Dose	Infusion Rate
100 mL	125 mg (25 mL) (final volume 125 mL)	1 mg/mL	5 mg/hr 10 mg/hr 15 mg/hr	5 mL/hr 10 mL/hr 15 mL/hr
250 mL	250 mg (50 mL) (final volume 300 mL)	0.83 mg/mL	5 mg/hr 10 mg/hr 15 mg/hr	6 mL/hr 12 mL/hr 18 mL/hr
500 mL	250 mg (50 mL) (final volume 550 mL)	0.45 mg/mL	5 mg/hr 10 mg/hr 15 mg/hr	11 mL/hr 22 mL/hr 33 mL/hr
100 mL	100 mg (1 ADD-Vantage vial)	1 mg/mL	5 mg/hr 10 mg/hr 15 mg/hr	5 mL/hr 10 mL/hr 15 mL/hr

IV injection: May be given undiluted through Y-site of tubing containing NS, D5W, or D5/½NS.

Infusion: May be further diluted for infusion in any of the above solutions; see Dilution Chart above.

Filters: No data available from manufacturer.

Storage: Store vials containing solution under refrigeration at 2 to 8° C (36 to 46° F). Do not freeze. Some vials may be stored at room temperature for up to 1 month, then discarded. ADD-vantage vials may be stored at CRT. Do not freeze. Following dilution, infusion may be stored at RT or under refrigeration. Use within 24 hours. Discard unused medication and/or solution.

COMPATIBILITY

Consider any drug NOT listed as compatible to be INCOMPATIBLE until consulting a pharmacist; specific conditions may apply.

Manufacturer recommends that **all formulations** not be mixed with any other drugs in the same container and, if possible, that they not be co-infused in the same IV line.

Manufacturer lists **Diltiazem for Injection (ADD-Vantage)** in NS as **compatible** at the **Y-site** with aminophylline, ampicillin, ampicillin/sulbactam, hydrocortisone sodium succinate, insulin (regular U-100), methylprednisolone, nafcillin, and sodium bicarbonate.

Other sources suggest specific **compatibilities** dependent on concentration and manufacturer; consult a pharmacist.

RATE OF ADMINISTRATION

IV injection: Each single dose equally distributed over 2 minutes.

Infusion: 5 mg to 15 mg/hr based on patient response. See charts under Dilution for diluent, dose, and infusion rate information. Administer using an infusion pump.

ACTIONS

Directly inhibits the influx of calcium ions through slow channels during membrane depolarization of cardiac and vascular smooth muscle. Effective in supraventricular tachycardias because it slows conduction through the AV node and prolongs the effective refractory period. Has little or no effect on normal AV nodal conduction at normal heart rates. Slows ventricular rate in patients with a rapid ventricular response during atrial fibrillation or atrial flutter. Converts paroxysmal supraventricular tachycardia (PSVT) to normal sinus rhythm by interrupting the re-entry circuit in AV nodal re-entrant tachycardias and reciprocating tachycardias (e.g. Wolff-Parkinson-White syndrome [WPW]). Because of its effect on vascular smooth muscle, diltiazem decreases total peripheral resistance, resulting in a decrease in both diastolic and systolic BP. In patients with cardiovascular disease, diltiazem reduces BP, systemic vascular resistance, and coronary vascular resistance and increases coronary blood flow. In studies of patients with compromised myocardium (severe CHF, AMI, hypertrophic cardiomyopathy), administration of diltiazem did not produce a significant effect on contractility, left ventricular end diastolic pressure, or pulmonary capillary wedge pressure. The mean ejection fraction and cardiac output/index remained unchanged or increased. Produces less myocardial depression than verapamil. Effective within 3 minutes; maximum effect should occur within 2 to 5 minutes and last for 1 to 3 hours. 70% to 80% bound to plasma proteins. Metabolized in the liver. Half-life is approximately 3.4 hours following a bolus injection and increases to 4.1 to 4.9 hours with continuous infusion. Excreted in urine and feces. Secreted in breast milk.

INDICATIONS AND USES

Temporary control of rapid ventricular rate in atrial fibrillation or atrial flutter unless associated with an accessory bypass tract (e.g., Wolff-Parkinson-White syndrome or short PR syndrome). ■ Rapid conversion of paroxysmal supraventricular tachycardia (PSVT) to normal sinus rhythm including AV nodal re-entrant tachycardias and reciprocating tachycardias associated with an extranodal accessory pathway (e.g., Wolff-Parkinson-White syndrome or short PR syndrome).

CONTRAINDICATIONS

Atrial fibrillation or flutter when associated with an accessory bypass tract (e.g., Wolff-Parkinson-White or short PR syndrome), cardiogenic shock, known hypersensitivity to diltiazem, second- or third-degree AV block or sick sinus syndrome (unless functioning ventricular pacemaker in place), severe hypotension, patients receiving IV beta-adrenergic blocking agents (e.g., atenolol [Tenormin], propranolol [Inderal]) within a few hours, ventricular tachycardia. Not recommended for wide QRS tachycardias of uncertain origin.

PRECAUTIONS

For short-term use only. ■ Administration of IV diltiazem should take place in a facility with adequate personnel and emergency drugs and equipment (including a defibrillator) to monitor the patient and respond to any medical emergency. ■ While diltiazem will effectively decrease HR, cardioversion will probably be required to convert atrial fibrillation or atrial flutter to a normal sinus rhythm. ■ Appropriate vagal maneuvers (e.g., Valsalva maneuver) recommended before use of diltiazem in patients with paroxysmal supraventricular tachycardia if clinically appropriate. ■ Use IV diltiazem with caution in patients with pre-existing impaired ventricular function (e.g., congestive heart failure, acute myocardial infarction, or pulmonary congestion documented by x-ray); may exacerbate disease. Use of oral diltiazem in these patients is contraindicated. ■ May cause second- or third-degree AV block in sinus rhythm; discontinue diltiazem if high degree AV block occurs. ■ Can cause life-threatening tachycardia with severe hypotension in atrial fibrillation or flutter in patients with an accessory bypass tract and periods of asystole in patients with sick sinus syndrome; see Contraindications. ■ Use with caution in patients with PSVT who are hemodynamically compromised or are taking other drugs that decrease any or all of the following: peripheral resistance, intravascular volume, myocardial contractility or conduction. Symptomatic hypotension is possible. ■ Use with caution in impaired renal or hepatic function. ■ Ventricular premature beats (VPBs) may occur on conversion of PSVT to sinus rhythm; considered to have no clinical significance. ■ Rare instances of significant liver enzymes and other phenomena consistent with acute hepatic injury have been reported with use of oral diltiazem. ■ Rare cases of dermatologic toxicity progressing to erythema multiforme and/or exfoliative dermatitis has been reported with oral diltiazem.

Monitor: Accurate pretreatment diagnosis differentiating wide-complex QRS tachycardia of supraventricular origin from ventricular origin is imperative. ■ Continuous ECG monitoring required. ■ Monitor BP and HR closely. ■ See Drug/Lab Interactions.

Maternal/Child: Use during pregnancy only if potential benefit justifies the potential risk to the fetus. ■ Discontinue breast-feeding. ■ Safety and effectiveness for use in pediatric patients not established.

Elderly: Overall difference in response between the elderly and younger patients has not been identified, but greater sensitivity of some older individuals cannot be ruled out; see Dose Adjustments.

DRUG/LAB INTERACTIONS

Diltiazem is both a substrate and inhibitor of CYP3A4. Other **drugs that are substrates, inhibitors, or inducers of CYP3A4** may have a significant impact on the efficacy or toxicity of diltiazem. Patients taking drugs that are substrates of CYP3A4 may require dose adjustment when starting or stopping concomitantly administered diltiazem. ■ Do not give concomitantly (within a few hours) with **IV beta-adrenergic blocking agents**; see Contraindications. May result in bradycardia, AV block, and/or depression of contractility. Use extreme caution if these drugs are administered orally or if patient has received before admission; usually tolerated. ■ May result in additive effects with **any agent known to affect cardiac contractility and/or SA or AV node conduction** (e.g., digoxin, beta-blockers). ■ Is used with **digoxin,** but monitor for excessive slowing of HR and/or AV block.

- Coadministration with **amiodarone** or **clonidine** may result in bradycardia. Monitor closely. ■ May increase effects of certain **benzodiazepines** (e.g., midazolam), **buspirone**, and **methylprednisolone**. ■ May increase serum concentrations of **carbamazepine, cyclosporine, digoxin**, some **HMG-CoA reductase inhibitors** (e.g., atorvastatin, lovastatin, simvastatin), **nifedipine, quinidine, sirolimus, and tacrolimus**. Monitor serum levels and/or monitor for S/S of toxicity. ■ May potentiate cardiac effects of **anesthetics** (e.g., depression of cardiac contractility, conductivity, automaticity, and vascular dilation); titrate both drugs carefully. ■ Metabolism may be decreased and serum concentrations increased by **cimetidine** and some **azole antifungal agents** (e.g., itraconazole). ■ Metabolism may be increased and serum concentrations decreased by **CYP3A4 inducers** (e.g., rifampin). Avoid use if possible and consider alternative therapy. ■ May increase exposure to **ivabradine** and exacerbate bradycardia and conduction disturbances. Avoid concomitant use. ■ May enhance neurotoxicity of lithium. Variable effects on lithium concentrations have been reported.

SIDE EFFECTS

Arrhythmia (junctional rhythm or isorhythmic dissociation), flushing, hypotension (asymptomatic and symptomatic), and injection site reactions (burning, itching) occurred most frequently and were most often mild and transient but could have serious potential. Amblyopia, asthenia, asystole, atrial flutter, AV block (first- or second-degree), bradycardia, chest pain, congestive heart failure, constipation, dizziness, dry mouth, dyspnea, edema, elevated alkaline phosphatase and AST, headache, hyperuricemia, nausea, paresthesia, pruritus, sinus node dysfunction, sinus pause, sweating, syncope, ventricular arrhythmias, ventricular fibrillation, ventricular tachycardia, and vomiting have occurred. Additional side effects have been reported with oral diltiazem.

ANTIDOTE

Notify physician promptly of all side effects. Treatment will depend on clinical situation. IV fluids or the Trendelenburg position may be required for BP support. Vasopressors (e.g., dopamine or norepinephrine) may be used, if needed. Administer atropine (0.6 to 1 mg) for bradycardia. If no response, administer isoproterenol cautiously. Discontinue diltiazem if a high-degree AV block occurs. Treat with atropine as above. Fixed-high-degree AV block should be treated with cardiac pacing. Treat cardiac failure with inotropic agents (isoproterenol, dopamine, or dobutamine) and diuretics. Calcium chloride or calcium gluconate have been used to reverse the pharmacologic effects of diltiazem overdose with variable results. Treat hypersensitivity reactions or resuscitate as necessary. Not removed by hemodialysis.

DINUTUXIMAB BBW

(dye-new-**TUX**-ih-mab)

Antineoplastic
(monoclonal antibody)

Unituxin

pH 6.8

USUAL DOSE

Pretreatment: Verify pregnancy status. Verify adequate hematologic, respiratory, hepatic, and renal function *before initiating each course of dinutuximab*; see Monitor.

Administer required premedication and hydration *before initiation of each dinutuximab infusion.*

Hydration: Administer NS 10 mL/kg as an IV infusion over 1 hour just before initiating each dinutuximab infusion.

Premedication: *Analgesics:* Immediately before initiating dinutuximab infusion, administer morphine sulfate 50 mcg/kg IV. Follow with a morphine sulfate drip at an infusion rate of 20 to 50 mcg/kg/hr during and for 2 hours after completion of dinutuximab. Additional 25 to 50 mcg/kg IV doses of morphine may be administered as needed for pain up to once every 2 hours followed by an increase in the morphine infusion rate in clinically stable patients. Consider using fentanyl or hydromorphone (Dilaudid) if morphine is not tolerated. If pain is not managed adequately with opioids, consider use of gabapentin (Neurontin) or lidocaine in conjunction with IV morphine.

Antihistamines: 20 minutes before initiating dinutuximab infusion, administer an antihistamine such as diphenhydramine 0.5 to 1 mg/kg (maximum dose of 50 mg) IV over 10 to 15 minutes. Repeat every 4 to 6 hours as tolerated during the dinutuximab infusion.

Antipyretics: 20 minutes before initiating dinutuximab infusion, administer acetaminophen 10 to 15 mg/kg (maximum dose 650 mg). Repeat every 4 to 6 hours as needed for fever or pain. Administer ibuprofen 5 to 10 mg/kg every 6 hours as needed for control of persistent fever or pain.

Dinutuximab: 17.5 mg/M^2/day as an IV infusion over 10 to 20 hours for 4 consecutive days for a maximum of 5 cycles. See Rate of Administration.

Schedule of Dinutuximab Administration for Cycles 1, 3, and 5						
Cycle Day	**1 Through 3**	**4**	**5**	**6**	**7**	**8 Through 24[a]**
Dinutuximab		X	X	X	X	

[a]Cycles 1, 3, and 5 are 24 days in duration.

Schedule of Dinutuximab Administration for Cycles 2 and 4						
Cycle Day	**1 Through 7**	**8**	**9**	**10**	**11**	**12 Through 32[a]**
Dinutuximab		X	X	X	X	

[a]Cycles 2 and 4 are 32 days in duration.

DOSE ADJUSTMENTS

Manage adverse reactions by infusion interruption, infusion rate reduction, dose reduction, or permanent discontinuation of dinutuximab as outlined in the following charts; see Rate of Administration, Monitor, and Antidote.

Dinutuximab Dose Modification for Infusion-Related Reactions

Mild to moderate adverse reactions (e.g., transient rash, fever, chills, localized urticaria) that respond promptly to symptomatic treatment	Onset of reaction	Reduce dinutuximab infusion rate to 50% of the previous rate and monitor closely.
	After resolution	Gradually increase infusion rate up to a maximum rate of 1.75 mg/M^2/hr.
Prolonged or severe adverse reactions (e.g., mild bronchospasm without other symptoms, angioedema that does not affect the airway)	Onset of reaction	Immediately interrupt dinutuximab.
	After resolution	If S/S resolve rapidly, resume dinutuximab infusion at 50% of the previous rate and monitor closely.
	First recurrence	Discontinue dinutuximab until the following day. If symptoms resolve and continued treatment is warranted, premedicate with hydrocortisone 1 mg/kg IV (maximum dose 50 mg) and administer dinutuximab at a rate of 0.875 mg/M^2/hr in an intensive care unit.
	Second recurrence	Permanently discontinue dinutuximab.

Dinutuximab Dose Modification for Capillary Leak Syndrome

Moderate to severe but not life-threatening capillary leak syndrome	Onset of reaction	Immediately interrupt dinutuximab.
	After resolution	Resume dinutuximab infusion at 50% of the previous rate.
Life-threatening capillary leak syndrome	Onset of reaction	Discontinue dinutuximab for the current cycle.
	After resolution	In subsequent cycles, administer dinutuximab at 50% of the previous rate.
	First recurrence	Permanently discontinue dinutuximab.

Dinutuximab Dose Modification for Hypotension Requiring Medical Intervention

Symptomatic hypotension, systolic blood pressure (SBP) less than lower limit of normal for age, or SBP decreased by more than 15% compared to baseline	Onset of reaction	Interrupt dinutuximab infusion.
	After resolution	Resume dinutuximab infusion at 50% of the previous rate. If blood pressure remains stable for at least 2 hours, increase the infusion rate as tolerated up to a maximum rate of 1.75 mg/M^2/hr.

Dinutuximab Dose Modification for Severe Systemic Infection or Sepsis

Infections such as severe Grade 3 or 4 bacteremia requiring IV antibiotics or other urgent intervention	Onset of reaction	Discontinue dinutuximab until resolution of infection, and then proceed with subsequent cycles of therapy.

Dinutuximab Dose Modification for Neurologic Disorders of the Eye

Disorders such as blurred vision, dilated pupil with sluggish light reflex, eyelid ptosis, fixed or unequal pupils, mydriasis, papilledema, optic nerve disorder, or other visual disturbances that do not cause vision loss	Onset of reaction	Discontinue dinutuximab infusion until resolution.
	After resolution	Reduce dinutuximab dose by 50%.
	First recurrence or if accompanied by visual impairment	Permanently discontinue dinutuximab.

Continued

Dinutuximab Dose Modification for Severe Pain	
Severe pain	Decrease dinutuximab infusion rate to 0.875 mg/M^2/hr. Discontinue dinutuximab if pain is not adequately controlled despite infusion rate reduction and institution of maximum supportive measures. See Premedication, Analgesics.

DILUTION

Available in a single-use vial containing 17.5 mg/5 mL (3.5 mg/mL). Do not use if solution is cloudy, has pronounced discoloration, or contains particulate matter. Aseptically withdraw the required volume of dinutuximab and inject into a 100-mL bag of NS. Mix by gentle inversion. **Do not shake.**

Filters: Specific information not available.

Storage: Before use, store in refrigerator at 2° to 8° C (36° to 46° F) in outer carton to protect from light. Do not freeze or shake vials. Diluted solution may be refrigerated, but the infusion must begin within 4 hours of preparation. Discard diluted solution 24 hours after preparation. Discard unused contents of vial.

COMPATIBILITY

Compatibility information not available from manufacturer; consult a pharmacist.

RATE OF ADMINISTRATION

For use as a diluted IV infusion only. Do not administer as an IV push or bolus. Initiate at an infusion rate of 0.875 mg/M^2/hr for 30 minutes. Gradually increase as tolerated to a maximum rate of 1.75 mg/M^2/hr. Manage adverse reactions by infusion interruption, infusion rate reduction, dose reduction, or permanent discontinuation of dinutuximab; see Dose Adjustments.

ACTIONS

Dinutuximab is a chimeric monoclonal antibody produced in the murine myeloma cell line SP2/0. It binds to the glycolipid GD2. This glycolipid is expressed on neuroblastoma cells and on normal cells of neuroectodermal origin, including the central nervous system and peripheral nerves. Dinutuximab binds to cell surface GD2 and induces cell lysis of GD2-expressing cells through antibody-dependent, cell-mediated cytotoxicity (ADCC) and complement-dependent cytotoxicity (CDC). Terminal half-life is approximately 10 days.

INDICATIONS AND USES

Treatment of pediatric patients with high-risk neuroblastoma who achieve at least a partial response to prior first-line, multiagent, multimodality therapy. Used in combination with granulocyte-macrophage colony-stimulating factor (GM-CSF), interleukin-2 (IL-2), and 13-*cis*-retinoic acid (RA).

CONTRAINDICATIONS

History of anaphylaxis with dinutuximab.

PRECAUTIONS

For use as a diluted IV infusion only. Do not administer as an IV push or bolus. ▪ Administered under the direction of a physician knowledgeable in its use in a facility with adequate diagnostic and treatment facilities to monitor the patient and respond to any medical emergency. ▪ Serious and potentially life-threatening infusion reactions requiring urgent intervention, including blood pressure support, bronchodilator therapy, corticosteroids, infusion rate reduction, infusion interruption, or permanent discontinuation of dinutuximab, have occurred. ▪ Pain was reported in the majority of patients despite pretreatment with analgesics. Pain was most commonly described as abdominal, back, extremity, or musculoskeletal pain; chest pain; generalized pain; neuralgia; and arthralgia. ▪ Dinutuximab causes serious neurologic adverse reactions, including severe neuropathic pain and peripheral neuropathy. Severe neuropathic pain occurs in the majority of patients. Administer IV opioids before, during, and for 2 hours after completion of the infusion. Severe motor neuropathy has occurred; resolution did not occur in all cases. ▪ Urinary retention that persists for weeks to months after discontinuation of opioids has occurred. ▪ Transverse myelitis has occurred. ▪ Reversible posterior leukoencephalopathy syndrome (RPLS) has occurred. ▪ Capillary leak syndrome was reported. ▪ Severe hypotension was reported. Prehydration is required; see Usual Dose. ▪ Severe bacteremia requiring IV antibiotics or other urgent intervention has occurred. ▪ Neurologic disorders of the eye have been reported. ▪ Bone marrow suppression (e.g., severe anemia, febrile neutropenia, neutropenia, and thrombocytopenia) was reported. ▪ Electrolyte abnormalities (e.g., hypocalcemia, hypokalemia, and hyponatremia) occur in at least 25% of patients, and some developed inappropriate antidiuretic hormone secretion resulting in severe hyponatremia. ▪ Hemolytic-uremic syndrome has been reported. ▪ Has not been studied in patients with hepatic or renal impairment. ▪ A protein substance; has a potential for immunogenicity. ▪ See Dose Adjustments, Monitor, Maternal/Child, and Antidote.

Monitor: Verify that patients have adequate hematologic, respiratory, hepatic, and renal function before initiating each course of dinutuximab therapy. ▪ Administer required IV hydration and premedication with antihistamines, analgesics, and antipyretics before each dose. ▪ Obtain baseline CBC and platelets and monitor closely during therapy. ▪ Obtain baseline serum electrolytes and monitor daily during therapy. ▪ Monitor for S/S of an infusion reaction during and for at least 4 hours after completion of each infusion (e.g., bronchospasm, dyspnea, facial and upper airway edema, hypotension, stridor, urticaria). Infusion reaction generally occurred during or within 24 hours of completing an infusion. Because of an overlap in S/S, it is difficult to distinguish between infusion reactions and hypersensitivity reactions. ▪ Assess pain frequently; see Usual Dose, Dose Adjustments, and Antidote. ▪ Monitor for S/S of peripheral sensory or motor neuropathy (e.g., burning, numbness, tingling, or weakness). ▪ Monitor for S/S of prolonged urinary retention. ▪ Promptly evaluate any patient with S/S of transverse myelitis (e.g., incontinence, paresthesia, sensory loss, or weakness). Permanently discontinue if patient develops transverse myelitis. ▪ Monitor for S/S of RPLS (e.g., hypertension, lethargy, seizures, severe headache, or vision changes). If S/S of RPLS occur, institute appropriate medical treatment and permanently discontinue. ▪ Monitor for S/S of capillary leak syndrome (e.g., edema, fatigue, hemoconcentration, hypotension, light-headedness, nausea, weakness). Interrupt or discontinue dinutuximab. ▪ Monitor blood pressure closely. For symptomatic hypotension, interrupt or discontinue dinutuximab and provide supportive management. ▪ Monitor for S/S of infection and temporarily discontinue dinutuximab until resolution of the infection. ▪ Monitor for S/S of eye disorders (e.g., dilated pupil with sluggish light reflex or other visual disturbances that do not cause vision loss). Interrupt dinutuximab infusion until resolution. ▪ Monitor for S/S of hemolytic-uremic syndrome (e.g., anemia, decreased urine output, dizziness, edema, fatigue, hematuria, pallor, renal insufficiency). If symptoms appear, discontinue dinutuximab. ▪ See Dose Adjustments, Precautions, Maternal/Child, and Antidote.

Patient Education: Review manufacturer's medication guide. ▪ Effective contraception required during treatment with dinutuximab and for at least 2 months following the last dose of dinutuximab. ▪ Promptly report a known or suspected pregnancy. ▪ Some side effects may require extensive supportive treatment and interruption or discontinuation of dinutuximab. ▪ Promptly report S/S of an infusion reaction (e.g., difficulty breathing, dizziness, facial or lip swelling, light-headedness, urticaria) that occur during or within 24 hours following the infusion. ▪ Promptly report severe or worsening pain and S/S of neuropathy such as burning, numbness, tingling, or weakness. ▪ Promptly report edema, fatigue, light-headedness, or nausea. ▪ Promptly report blurred vision, diplopia, photophobia, ptosis, or unequal pupil size. ▪ Promptly report bruising or fatigue. ▪ Promptly report heart palpitations, muscle cramping, or seizures. ▪ Promptly report decreased urine output, edema, fainting, hematuria, inability to urinate, or pallor. ▪ Promptly report S/S of RPLS (e.g., hypertension, lethargy, seizures, severe headache, or vision changes).

Maternal/Child: Avoid pregnancy. Based on its mechanism of action, dinutuximab can cause fetal harm when administered to a pregnant woman. ▪ Discontinue breastfeeding. ▪ Safety and effectiveness for use in pediatric patients as part of a multiagent, multimodality therapy have been established; see Indications.

Elderly: Safety and effectiveness for use in the elderly have not been established.

DRUG/LAB INTERACTIONS

No drug-drug interaction studies have been reported with dinutuximab.

SIDE EFFECTS

The most common side effects reported in 25% or more of patients are anemia, capillary leak syndrome, diarrhea, fever, hypoalbuminemia, hypocalcemia, hypokalemia, hyponatremia, hypotension, increased ALT and AST, infusion reactions, lymphopenia, neutropenia, pain, thrombocytopenia, urticaria, and vomiting. The most common serious side effects reported in 5% or more of patients include capillary leak syndrome, fever, hypokalemia, hypotension, infections, infusion reactions, and pain. Decreased appetite, device-related infections, edema, hemorrhage, hyperglycemia, hypertension, hypertriglyceridemia, hypomagnesemia, hypophosphatemia, hypoxia, increased serum creatinine, nausea, neurologic disorders of the eye (e.g., blurred vision, eyelid ptosis, fixed or unequal pupils, mydriasis, optic nerve disorder, papilledema, photophobia), peripheral neuropathy, proteinuria, tachycardia, and weight increase have also been reported.

Post-Marketing: Neurotoxicity: prolonged urinary retention, transverse myelitis, and reversible posterior leukoencephalopathy syndrome (RPLS).

ANTIDOTE

Keep physician informed of all side effects. May constitute a medical emergency or will be treated symptomatically as indicated. Permanently discontinue dinutuximab in patients with any of the following: (1) Grade 3 or 4 anaphylaxis (life-threatening infusion reactions), (2) Grade 3 or 4 serum sickness, (3) Grade 3 pain unresponsive to maximum supportive measures, (4) Grade 4 sensory neuropathy or Grade 3 sensory neuropathy that interferes with daily activities for more than 2 weeks, (5) Grade 2 or greater peripheral motor neuropathy, (6) urinary retention that persists after discontinuation of opioids, (7) transverse myelitis, (8) reversible posterior leukoencephalopathy syndrome (RPLS), (9) subtotal or total vision loss, or (10) Grade 4 hyponatremia despite appropriate fluid management. Interrupt or discontinue dinutuximab and provide supportive management in (1) severe or prolonged infusion reactions, (2) symptomatic or severe capillary leak syndrome, (3) systemic infection, (4) symptomatic hypotension, and (5) patients with a dilated pupil and a sluggish light reflex or other visual disturbances that do not cause vision loss. Permanently discontinue dinutuximab and provide supportive management for signs of hemolytic-uremic syndrome. Treat these side effects aggressively; see Dose Adjustments, Precautions, and Monitor.

DIPHENHYDRAMINE HYDROCHLORIDE
(dye-fen-**HY**-drah-meen hy-droh-**KLOR**-eyed)

Antihistamine
Antidyskinetic/antiparkinsonism
Antiemetic
Antivertigo agent
Sedative-hypnotic

Benadryl, Benadryl PF, Diphenhydramine PF

pH 4 to 6.5

USUAL DOSE
10 to 50 mg. Up to 100 mg may be given. Individualize dose based on patient symptoms and response. Total dosage should not exceed 400 mg/24 hr.

PEDIATRIC DOSE
See Contraindications and Maternal/Child.

Pediatric patients after neonatal period: 1.25 mg/kg/dose every 6 hours as needed or 150 mg/M^2/24 hr in equally divided doses given every 6 hours (37.5 mg/M^2 every 6 hours). Never exceed a total dosage of 300 mg/24 hr.

Anaphylaxis or phenothiazine overdose: 1 to 2 mg/kg IV slowly.

DOSE ADJUSTMENTS
Reduce dose for the elderly or debilitated. ▪ See Drug/Lab Interactions.

DILUTION
May be given undiluted.

Filters: No data available from manufacturer.

Storage: Store below 40° C (104° F), preferably between 15° and 30° C (59° and 86° F). Protect from light and freezing.

COMPATIBILITY
Compatibility information not available from manufacturer; consult a pharmacist.

RATE OF ADMINISTRATION
25 mg or fraction thereof over 1 minute. Extend injection time in nonemergency situations and pediatric patients. See Maternal/Child.

ACTIONS
A potent antihistamine, it is capable of blocking the effects of histamine at various receptor sites, either eliminating a hypersensitivity reaction or greatly modifying it. It also has anticholinergic (antispasmodic), antiemetic, antivertigo, and sedative effects. It has rapid onset of action and is widely distributed throughout the body, including the CNS. A portion of this drug is metabolized in the liver; the rest is excreted unchanged in the urine. Half-life is 1 to 4 hours. Some secretion may occur in breast milk.

INDICATIONS AND USES
Allergic reactions to blood or plasma. ▪ Supplemental therapy to epinephrine in anaphylaxis and other uncomplicated allergic/hypersensitivity reactions requiring prompt treatment (e.g., angioedema, pruritus, urticaria). ▪ Preoperative or generalized sedation. ▪ Management of parkinsonism, including drug-induced (e.g., phenothiazines). ▪ Severe nausea and vomiting. ▪ Motion sickness. ▪ To replace oral therapy when it is impractical or contraindicated.

CONTRAINDICATIONS
Breast-feeding, hypersensitivity to antihistamines, newborn or premature infants.

PRECAUTIONS
IV route used only in emergency situations. ▪ Avoid SQ or perivascular injection. ▪ Use with extreme caution in infants, children, elderly or debilitated individuals, asthmatic attack, bladder neck obstruction, narrow-angle glaucoma, lower respiratory tract infections, prostatic hypertrophy, pyloroduodenal obstruction, and stenosing peptic ulcer.

Monitor: Will induce drowsiness. ▪ Monitor vital signs; observe closely. ▪ See Drug/Lab Interactions.

Patient Education: Do not drive or operate hazardous equipment until effects wear off. ▪ May cause drowsiness and dizziness; request help to ambulate. ▪ Avoid alcohol and other CNS depressants.

Maternal/Child: See Contraindications, Precautions, Monitor, and Side Effects. ▪ Category B: use only when clearly needed. May increase risk of abnormalities during the first trimester. ▪ Not recommended during breast-feeding. Small amounts may be distributed into breast milk, causing irritability or excitement in infants. ▪ Use extreme caution in infants and children; may cause hallucinations, convulsions, or death. May also reduce mental alertness and cause paradoxical excitation.

Elderly: See Dose Adjustments, Precautions, Monitor, and Side Effects. ▪ May cause confusion, dizziness, hyperexcitability, hypotension, and/or sedation. ▪ Sensitivity to anticholinergic effects is increased (e.g., blurred vision, constipation, dry mouth, urinary retention).

DRUG/LAB INTERACTIONS

Increases effectiveness of **epinephrine** and is often used in conjunction with it. ▪ Additive central nervous system effects with **alcohol, other CNS depressants** (e.g., hypnotics, sedatives, and tranquilizers), and **procarbazine**. Reduced dose of potentiated drug may be indicated. ▪ **MAO inhibitors** (e.g., selegiline) prolong and intensify the anticholinergic (drying) effects of antihistamines. Concurrent use not recommended. ▪ Effectiveness of many drugs is reduced in combination with diphenhydramine because of increased metabolism. ▪ May inhibit the wheal and flare reaction to **antigen skin tests.**

SIDE EFFECTS

Rare when used as indicated: anaphylaxis; blurring of vision; confusion; constipation; diarrhea; difficulty in urination; diplopia; drowsiness; drug rash; dryness of mouth, nose, and throat; epigastric distress; headache; hemolytic anemia; hypotension; insomnia; nasal stuffiness; nausea; nervousness; palpitations; photosensitivity; rapid pulse; restlessness; thickening of bronchial secretions; tightness of the chest and wheezing; tingling, heaviness, weakness of hands; urticaria; vertigo; vomiting. Overdose may cause convulsions, hallucinations, and death in pediatric patients.

ANTIDOTE

For exaggerated drowsiness or other disturbing side effects, discontinue the drug and notify the physician. Side effects will usually subside within a few hours or may be treated symptomatically. Treat hypotension promptly; may lead to cardiovascular collapse. Use dopamine, norepinephrine, or phenylephrine. Epinephrine is contraindicated for hypotension; further hypotension will occur. Propranolol is the drug of choice for ventricular arrhythmias. Treat convulsions with diazepam 0.1 mg/kg IV slowly. Some central anticholinergic effects may require physostigmine. Avoid analeptics (e.g., caffeine); may cause convulsions. Epinephrine must be available to treat anaphylaxis. Resuscitate as necessary.

DIPYRIDAMOLE
(dye-peer-**ID**-ah-mohl)

Coronary vasodilator
Diagnostic agent
Antiplatelet agent

Persantine

pH 2.2 to 3.2

USUAL DOSE
Pretreatment: See Monitor.

Myocardial perfusion imaging: 0.57 mg/kg of body weight equally distributed over 4 minutes (0.142 mg/kg/min). A 70-kg adult would receive a total dose of 39.9 mg (10 mg/min). Maximum dose is 60 mg. Thallium should be injected within 5 minutes following the 4-minute infusion of dipyridamole.

Antiplatelet agent (unlabeled): 250 mg/24 hr as an infusion.

DILUTION
Each 1 mL (5 mg) must be diluted with a minimum of 2 mL D5W, D5/½NS, or D5NS. Total volume should range from a minimum of 20 mL to 50 mL (39.9 mg [8 mL] would be diluted in a minimum of 16 mL for a total infusion of 24 mL; additional diluent can be used to facilitate titration). May not be given undiluted; will cause local irritation.

Antiplatelet agent: Each 250-mg dose should be diluted with 250 mL D5W (1 mg/mL). Concentration may be increased if larger doses required.

Storage: Undiluted drug should be stored at CRT and protected from direct light; avoid freezing.

COMPATIBILITY
Compatibility information not available from manufacturer; consult a pharmacist.

RATE OF ADMINISTRATION
A single dose must be equally distributed over 4 minutes (0.142 mg/kg/min).

Antiplatelet agent: 10 mg/hr as a continuous infusion. Use of a microdrip (60 drops/mL) or infusion pump recommended.

ACTIONS
A coronary vasodilator that will cause an increase in coronary blood flow velocity of from 3.8 to 7 times greater than resting velocity. Action may result from the inhibition of adenosine uptake. Peak velocity is reached in 2.5 to 8.7 minutes. Will cause a 20% increase in HR and a mild but significant decrease in systolic and diastolic BP in the supine position. Vital signs may take up to 30 minutes to return to baseline measurements. Used in combination with thallium, visualization shows dilation with sustained enhanced flow of intact vessels, leaving reduced pressure and flow across areas of hemodynamically important coronary vascular constriction. Results achieved are comparable to exercise-induced thallium imaging. Metabolized in the liver. Excreted in bile. Secreted in breast milk.

INDICATIONS AND USES
An alternative to exercise in thallium myocardial perfusion imaging for the evaluation of coronary artery disease in patients who cannot exercise adequately.

Unlabeled uses: Prophylactic inhibition of platelet aggregation in thromboembolism and myocardial infarction.

CONTRAINDICATIONS
Hypersensitivity to dipyridamole.

PRECAUTIONS
Administered by or under the direction of the cardiologist. ▪ Full facilities for treatment of any airway problem, cardiac emergency, or hypersensitivity, including laboratory analysis, must be available. ▪ Theophylline (aminophylline) and other emergency drugs must be immediately available. ▪ Patients with a history of unstable angina or a history of asthma may be at greater risk; use extreme caution. ▪ This drug has caused two fatal

myocardial infarctions as well as other serious side effects in a small percentage of patients; clinical information to be gained must be weighed against risk to the patient.

Monitor: An IV line with a Y-tube must be in place. ▪ Monitor vital signs continuously during infusion and for at least 15 minutes after or until return to baseline. ▪ ECG monitoring using at least 1 chest lead should be continuous. ▪ Patient is usually in a supine position, but tests have been conducted in a sitting position. Lower to supine with head tilted down (Trendelenburg) if hypotension occurs.

Maternal/Child: Category B: safety for use during pregnancy not established. Use only if clearly needed. ▪ Temporarily discontinue breast-feeding. ▪ Safety for use in pediatric patients not established.

DRUG/LAB INTERACTIONS

Theophylline bronchodilators reverse the effect of dipyridamole on myocardial blood flow. Interferes with dipyridamole-assisted **myocardial perfusion studies.** Withhold bronchodilators for 36 hours before testing.

SIDE EFFECTS

BP lability, chest pain/angina pectoris, dizziness, dyspnea, ECG abnormalities (e.g., extrasystoles, ST-T changes, tachycardia), fatigue, flushing, headache, hypertension, hypotension, nausea, pain (unspecified), paresthesia. Numerous other side effects occur in less than 1% of patients.

Major: Bronchospasm, cerebral ischemia (transient), fatal and nonfatal myocardial infarction, ventricular fibrillation, ventricular tachycardia (symptomatic) occurred in 0.3% of patients.

ANTIDOTE

Physician will be present throughout test administration. Theophylline (aminophylline) is an adenosine receptor antagonist and will reverse the adenosine-mediated effects of dipyridamole (e.g., angina pectoris, bronchospasm, severe hypotension, ventricular arrhythmias). If bronchospasm or chest pain occurs, administer 50 to 250 mg of theophylline at a rate not to exceed 50 mg over 30 seconds. If symptoms are not relieved by 250 mg of theophylline, sublingual nitroglycerin may be helpful. Persistent chest pain may indicate impending potentially fatal myocardial infarction. If patient condition permits, thallium may be injected and allowed to circulate for 1 minute before injection of theophylline; this will permit initial thallium perfusion imaging before reversal of vasodilatory effects of dipyridamole on coronary circulation. Use head-down supine position for hypotension before administering theophylline. After reversal of vasodilatory action, treat arrhythmias as indicated. Resuscitate as necessary.

DOBUTAMINE HYDROCHLORIDE
(doh-**BYOU**-tah-meen hy-droh-**KLOR**-eyed)

Adrenergic agonist
Inotropic agent

pH 2.5 to 5.5

USUAL DOSE
Pretreatment: See Monitor.
Dobutamine: 0.5 to 1 mcg/kg/min initially in patients likely to respond to minimum treatment. The usual effective initial dose ranges from 2.5 to 15 mcg/kg of body weight/min. AHA guidelines suggest 2 to 20 mcg/kg/min. Gradually adjust rate at 2- to 10-minute intervals to effect desired response. AHA guidelines recommend titrating so HR does not increase by more than 10% of baseline. Up to 40 mcg/kg/min has been used in some instances; increases potential for toxicity (e.g., myocardial ischemia). U.S. experience in controlled trials does not extend beyond 48 hours of therapy.

PEDIATRIC DOSE
AHA guidelines suggest 2 to 20 mcg/kg/min. Adjust rate to effect desired response; see Maternal/Child.

DOSE ADJUSTMENTS
Lower-end initial doses may be appropriate in the elderly based on potential for decreased organ function, concomitant disease, or other drug therapy. See Drug/Lab Interactions.

DILUTION
Available prediluted in D5W, or each 250-mg (20-mL) vial must be further diluted in at least 50 mL. Any amount of infusion solution desired above 50 mL may be used (250 mg in 1 L equals 250 mcg/mL; 250 mg in 500 mL equals 500 mcg/mL; 250 mg in 250 mL equals 1,000 mcg/mL). Adjust to fluid requirements of the patient. **Compatible** with D5W, D10W, D5/½NS, D5NS, D5/Isolyte M, LR, D5LR, Normosol-M in D5W, 20% Osmitrol in water, NS, or sodium lactate.
Filters: No data available from manufacturer. Another source suggests no significant drug loss through a 0.22-micron cellulose ester membrane filter.
Storage: Store premixed bags and vials at CRT; do not freeze. When mixed in infusion solution, use within 24 hours. Pink coloring of solution does not affect potency; will crystallize if frozen.

COMPATIBILITY
Manufacturer states, "Do not administer simultaneously with solutions containing sodium bicarbonate or any other strongly alkaline solution" (e.g., aminophylline, barbiturates). Manufacturer recommends not using other drugs as additives, not using in conjunction with other agents, and not using with diluents containing both sodium bisulfate and ethanol.

Other sources suggest a few specific **compatibilities** dependent on concentration and manufacturer; consult a pharmacist.

RATE OF ADMINISTRATION
Use of an infusion pump is recommended. Rate of infusion in mL/hr may be calculated using the following formula:

Rate (mL/hr) = [Dose (mcg/kg/min) $\times$ Weight (kg) $\times$ 60 min/hr] $\div$ Final concentration (mcg/mL)

Slowly titrate to desired response. May take up to 10 minutes to achieve peak effect of a specific dose. Half-life of dobutamine is only about 2 minutes. See Maternal/Child.

ACTIONS
A synthetic catecholamine chemically related to dopamine, it is a direct-acting inotropic agent whose primary activity results from stimulation of the beta-receptors. Induces short-term increases in cardiac output by improving stroke volume with minimum increases in rate and BP, minimum rhythm disturbances, and some decrease in systemic

vascular resistance. Effectiveness may decrease over time. Most use is short-term. Onset of action is 1 to 2 minutes; however, as much as 10 minutes may be required to obtain the peak effect. Has a very short duration of action. Half-life is 2 minutes; may be up to 5 minutes in preterm infants. Metabolized in the liver and other tissues. Metabolites are primarily excreted in the urine.

INDICATIONS AND USES
Short-term inotropic support in cardiac decompensation due to depressed contractility resulting from either organic heart disease or cardiac surgical procedures.

CONTRAINDICATIONS
Hypersensitivity to any components (contains sulfites), idiopathic hypertrophic subaortic stenosis, shock without adequate fluid replacement. ▪ Solutions containing dextrose may be contraindicated in patients with known allergy to corn or corn products.

PRECAUTIONS
Use extreme caution in myocardial infarction; increases in contractile force and HR may increase myocardial ischemia and size of infarction. ▪ Precipitous hypotension occurs rarely; usually reverses with a decrease in rate of administration; see Antidote. ▪ Use with caution in patients with atrial fibrillation; facilitates atrioventricular conduction, placing patients at risk for developing rapid ventricular response. Use digoxin preparation before starting dobutamine in patients with atrial fibrillation with rapid ventricular response. ▪ May precipitate or exacerbate ventricular ectopic activity but has rarely caused ventricular tachycardia. ▪ Reactions suggestive of hypersensitivity have been reported. ▪ Contains sulfites; use caution in patients with allergies. ▪ Ineffective if marked mechanical obstruction (e.g., severe valvular aortic stenosis) is present. ▪ Use for long-term treatment of CHF has been associated with increased risks of hospitalization and death. ▪ Solutions containing dextrose should be used with caution in patients with known or subclinical or overt diabetes mellitus.

Monitor: Correct hypovolemia and electrolyte disturbances (e.g., hypokalemia, hypomagnesemia) before initiating treatment. ▪ Continuous monitoring of ECG, BP, and HR required. Measure pulmonary wedge pressure, central venous pressure, and cardiac output if possible. ▪ May cause significant increase in BP or HR, especially systolic pressure. Patients with pre-existing hypertension may be at increased risk of developing an increased pressor response. ▪ Monitor for changes in fluid balance (input/output), electrolytes, and acid-base balance. ▪ Monitor for S/S of possible hypersensitivity reactions (e.g., bronchospasm, eosinophilia, fever, rash). ▪ See Drug/Lab Interactions.

Maternal/Child: Use only if benefits outweigh risks. ▪ Use caution in breast-feeding. ▪ Increases cardiac output and systemic BP in pediatric patients of every age-group, usually at infusion rates that are lower than those that cause significant tachycardia. Less effective than dopamine in premature neonates.

Elderly: Lower-end initial doses may be indicated; see Dose Adjustments. ▪ Differences in response compared to younger adults not identified, but greater sensitivity of some elderly cannot be ruled out.

DRUG/LAB INTERACTIONS
May be ineffective if **beta-blocking drugs** have been given. ▪ Produces higher cardiac output and lower pulmonary wedge pressure when given concomitantly with **nitroprusside sodium** than when either drug is used alone. ▪ May cause severe hypertension with **oxytocic drugs or guanethidine**. ▪ Pressor response increased with **tricyclic antidepressants** and **rauwolfia alkaloids** (e.g., reserpine); may cause hypertension. ▪ Use with caution in patients taking **MAO inhibitors**; prolonged hypertension may result from concurrent use.

SIDE EFFECTS
Anginal pain, chest pain, headache, hypertension, hypokalemia, hypotension, increased ventricular ectopic activity, myocardial ischemia, nausea, palpitations, phlebitis, shortness of breath, stress cardiomyopathy, tachycardia. Hypersensitivity reactions (e.g., bronchospasm, eosinophilia, fever, skin rash) have been reported. Local inflammatory changes may occur with infiltration.

Overdose: In addition to all of the above, overdose may cause anorexia, anxiety, excessive hypertension or hypotension, myocardial ischemia, tremor, ventricular tachycardia, and/or fibrillation, vomiting.

ANTIDOTE

Notify physician of all side effects. Many will resolve with a reduction in rate of administration. Decrease infusion rate and notify physician immediately if number of PVCs increases or there is a marked increase in pulse rate or BP. For accidental overdose, reduce rate or temporarily discontinue until condition stabilizes. Maintain a patent airway with adequate oxygenation and ventilation. Meticulously monitor and maintain patient's VS, blood gases, serum electrolytes, etc. Forced diuresis, peritoneal dialysis, hemodialysis, or charcoal hemoperfusion have not been established as beneficial for overdosage. Treat ventricular tachyarrhythmias with propranolol (Inderal) or lidocaine. Hypertension usually responds to a reduced rate or temporarily discontinuing dobutamine. Reduce rate or discontinue dobutamine if hypotension occurs. May require treatment with vasopressors (e.g., dopamine, norepinephrine). See Precautions.

DOCETAXEL BBW
(doh-seh-**TAX**-ell)

Taxotere

Antineoplastic agent
(taxane)

USUAL DOSE

Pretreatment: Verify pregnancy status. Baseline studies indicated; see Monitor.

Premedication for all patients except those with castration-resistant prostate cancer: Must be pretreated with oral corticosteroids to reduce the incidence and severity of fluid retention and hypersensitivity reactions. Usual regimen is dexamethasone 8 mg PO twice a day for 3 days. Begin 1 day before each docetaxel infusion.

Premedication for hormone-refractory prostate cancer: Administer oral dexamethasone 8 mg at 12 hours, 3 hours, and 1 hour before each docetaxel infusion (another steroid, prednisone, is part of the combination therapy).

Breast cancer: 60 to 100 mg/M^2 as an infusion. Repeat every 3 weeks.

Combination therapy for adjuvant treatment of operable node-positive breast cancer: 75 mg/M^2 as an infusion. Administer 1 hour after doxorubicin 50 mg/M^2 and cyclophosphamide 500 mg/M^2. Repeat every 3 weeks for 6 cycles. Prophylactic G-CSF (e.g., filgrastim) may be used to mitigate the risk of hematologic toxicity. See doxorubicin and cyclophosphamide monographs.

Prostate cancer (castration-resistant): 75 mg/M^2 as an infusion. Repeat every 3 weeks. Prednisone 5 mg PO twice daily is administered continuously throughout treatment. See Premedication.

Non–small-cell lung cancer (NSCLC) in chemotherapy-naïve patients: 75 mg/M^2 as an infusion over 1 hour. Follow immediately with cisplatin 75 mg/M^2 as an infusion over 30 to 60 minutes. Repeat regimen every 3 weeks. *Premedicate* with antiemetics and hydration as required for cisplatin administration; see cisplatin monograph.

NSCLC after failure of prior chemotherapy: 75 mg/M^2 as an infusion. Repeat every 3 weeks. Larger doses increased toxicity, infection, and treatment-related mortality.

Gastric adenocarcinoma: 75 mg/M^2 as an infusion over 1 hour. Follow immediately with cisplatin 75 mg/M^2 as an infusion over 1 to 3 hours (both on Day 1 only). *Premedicate* with antiemetics and hydration as required for cisplatin administration; see cisplatin and fluorouracil monographs. Follow the cisplatin infusion with fluorouracil 750 mg/M^2 as an infusion equally distributed over 24 hours. Repeat fluorouracil dose for 4 more 24-hour infusions (total of 5 days). Repeat regimen every 3 weeks. In the study, G-CSF (filgrastim) was recommended during the second and/or subsequent cycles to prevent or attenuate febrile neutropenia, documented infection with neutropenia, or neutropenia lasting more than 7 days.

Induction chemotherapy followed by radiotherapy for treatment of inoperable, locally advanced squamous cell cancer of the head and neck (SCCHN): 75 mg/M^2 as an infusion over 1 hour. Follow immediately with cisplatin 75 mg/M^2 as an infusion over 1 hour (both on Day 1 only). *Premedicate* with antiemetics and hydration as required for cisplatin administration; see cisplatin monograph. Follow the cisplatin infusion with fluorouracil 750 mg/M^2 as an infusion equally distributed over 24 hours. Repeat fluorouracil for four more 24-hour infusions (total of 5 days). See fluorouracil monograph. Repeat regimen every 3 weeks for a total of four cycles. Prophylactic antibiotics were used in clinical studies. In the study, G-CSF (filgrastim) was recommended during the second and/or subsequent cycles to prevent or attenuate febrile neutropenia, documented infection with neutropenia, or neutropenia lasting more than 7 days. Following chemotherapy, patients should receive radiotherapy.

Induction chemotherapy followed by chemoradiotherapy for treatment of locally advanced (unresectable, low surgical cure, or organ preservation) SCCHN: 75 mg/M^2 as an infusion over 1 hour. Follow with cisplatin 100 mg/M^2 as a 30-minute to 3-hour infusion (both on Day

1 only). **Premedicate** with antiemetics and hydration as required for cisplatin administration; see cisplatin monograph. Follow the cisplatin infusion with fluorouracil 1,000 mg/M^2 as an infusion equally distributed over 24 hours. Repeat fluorouracil for three more 24-hour infusions (total of 4 days). See fluorouracil monograph. Repeat regimen every 3 weeks for 3 cycles. Prophylactic antibiotics were used in clinical studies. In the study, G-CSF (filgrastim) was recommended during the second and/or subsequent cycles to prevent or attenuate febrile neutropenia, documented infection with neutropenia, or neutropenia lasting more than 7 days. Following chemotherapy, patients should receive chemoradiotherapy.

Treatment of ovarian cancer (unlabeled): 60 to 75 mg/M^2 as an infusion in combination with carboplatin. Repeat every 3 weeks.

Metastatic bladder cancer (unlabeled): 100 mg/M^2 every 3 weeks as a single agent or 35 mg/M^2 on Days 1 and 8 of a 21-day cycle in combination with gemcitabine and cisplatin. Administer for at least 6 cycles or until disease progression or unacceptable toxicity.

Treatment of esophageal cancer (unlabeled): 75 mg/M^2 as a 1-hour infusion every 21 days used in combination with fluorouracil and cisplatin.

DOSE ADJUSTMENTS

All diagnoses: Withhold therapy if neutrophils below 1,500/mm^3 or platelets below 100,000 cells/mm^3. A 25% reduction in the dose of docetaxel is recommended during subsequent cycles following severe neutropenia (less than 500/mm^3) lasting 7 days or more, febrile neutropenia, or a Grade 4 infection. ▪ Withhold therapy if bilirubin is greater than the ULN or if AST and/or ALT is greater than 1.5 times the ULN concomitant with alkaline phosphatase greater than 2.5 times the ULN. ▪ Discontinue therapy in patients who develop Grade 3 or higher peripheral neuropathy. ▪ Dose selection should be cautious in the elderly. Reduced doses may be indicated based on the potential for decreased organ function and concomitant disease or drug therapy. ▪ Consider additional dose adjustments when docetaxel is given in combination with other chemotherapeutic agents. ▪ See Precautions and Drug/Lab Interactions.

Breast cancer: Reduce dose to 75 mg/M^2 for patients initially dosed at 100 mg/M^2 who experience febrile neutropenia, severe neutropenia (neutrophils below 500/mm^3 for more than 1 week), severe or cumulative cutaneous reaction, or severe peripheral neuropathy. Further reduce to 55 mg/M^2 or discontinue docetaxel if any of the previously listed reactions persist. ▪ Patients receiving the lower dose of docetaxel (60 mg/M^2) may have the dose increased gradually if lower dose was well tolerated. ▪ Discontinue therapy in patients who develop Grade 3 or greater peripheral neuropathy.

Combination therapy for adjuvant treatment of operable node-positive breast cancer: Patients who experience febrile neutropenia should receive G-CSF (e.g., filgrastim) in all subsequent cycles. Patients who continue to experience this reaction should remain on G-CSF and have their docetaxel dose decreased to 60 mg/M^2. ▪ Reduce docetaxel dose to 60 mg/M^2 in patients who experience Grade 3 or 4 stomatitis. ▪ Reduce docetaxel dose from 75 to 60 mg/M^2 in patients who experience severe or cumulative cutaneous reactions or moderate neurosensory signs and/or symptoms. If side effects persist at the lower dose, discontinue therapy.

Prostate cancer: Reduce docetaxel dose from 75 to 60 mg/M^2 in patients who experience dose-limiting toxicities (e.g., febrile neutropenia, neutrophils less than 500 cells/mm^3 for more than 1 week, severe or cumulative cutaneous reactions, or moderate neurosensory signs and/or symptoms). If side effects persist at the lower dose, discontinue therapy.

Non–small-cell lung cancer after failure of prior chemotherapy: In NSCLC patients who experience either febrile neutropenia, neutrophils less than 500 cells/mm^3 for more than 1 week, severe or cumulative cutaneous reactions, or other Grade 3 or 4 nonhematologic toxicities, withhold docetaxel until resolution of toxicity, then resume at 55 mg/M^2. ▪ Discontinue therapy in patients who develop Grade 3 or greater peripheral neuropathy.

Non–small-cell lung cancer (NSCLC) in chemotherapy-naïve patients: Reduce dose to 65 mg/M^2 in patients whose nadir of platelet count during the previous course of therapy

Continued

was less than 25,000 cells/mm^3, in patients who experienced febrile neutropenia, and in patients with serious nonhematologic toxicities. Dose may be further reduced to 50 mg/M^2 as indicated. See cisplatin monograph for cisplatin dose adjustments.

Gastric adenocarcinoma and head and neck cancer: Patients who experience febrile neutropenia, documented infection with neutropenia, or neutropenia lasting more than 7 days should receive G-CSF (e.g., filgrastim) in all subsequent cycles. Patients who continue to experience this reaction should remain on G-CSF and have their docetaxel dose decreased to 60 mg/M^2. Reduce dose further to 45 mg/M^2 if subsequent episodes of complicated neutropenia occur. ■ Reduce docetaxel dose from 75 to 60 mg/M^2 in patients who experience Grade 4 thrombocytopenia. ■ Hold subsequent cycles of docetaxel until neutrophils recover to a level of greater than 1,500 cells/mm^3 and platelets recover to a level greater than 100,000 cells/mm^3. ■ If the previously mentioned toxicities persist, discontinue therapy. ■ Additional dose adjustments are outlined in the following chart.

Additional Recommended Dose Adjustments for Toxicities in Gastric Adenocarcinoma or Head and Neck Cancer Patients Treated With Docetaxel in Combination With Cisplatin and Fluorouracil	
Toxicity	**Dose Adjustment**
Diarrhea Grade 3	**First episode:** Reduce 5-FU dose by 20%. **Second episode:** Reduce docetaxel dose by 20%.
Diarrhea Grade 4	**First episode:** Reduce docetaxel and 5-FU doses by 20%. **Second episode:** Discontinue treatment.
Stomatitis/mucositis Grade 3	**First episode:** Reduce 5-FU dose by 20%. **Second episode:** Stop 5-FU only at all subsequent cycles. **Third episode:** Reduce docetaxel dose by 20%.
Stomatitis/mucositis Grade 4	**First episode:** Stop 5-FU only at all subsequent cycles. **Second episode:** Reduce docetaxel dose by 20%.
AST/ALT >2.5 to ≤5 × ULN and AP ≤2.5 × ULN, or AST/ALT >1.5 to ≤5 × ULN and AP >2.5 to ≤5 × ULN	Reduce docetaxel dose by 20%.
AST/ALT >5 × ULN and/or AP >5 × ULN	Discontinue docetaxel.
Peripheral neuropathy Grade 2	Reduce cisplatin dose by 20%.
Peripheral neuropathy Grade 3	Discontinue cisplatin treatment.
Ototoxicity Grade 3	Discontinue cisplatin treatment.
Rise in SCr ≥ Grade 2 (>1.5 × normal value) despite adequate rehydration	Determine CrCl before each subsequent cycle and consider the following dose reductions as outlined below.
CrCl ≥60 mL/min	Full dose of cisplatin given. Repeat CrCl before each treatment cycle.
CrCl >40 and <60 mL/min	Reduce dose of cisplatin by 50% at subsequent cycle. If CrCl was >60 mL/min at end of cycle, give full dose at the next cycle. If no recovery observed, omit cisplatin from the next treatment cycle.
CrCl <40 mL/min	Omit dose of cisplatin for **that treatment cycle only.** Discontinue cisplatin if CrCl remains at <40 mL/min. Reduce cisplatin dose by 50% if CrCl was >40 and <60 mL/min at end of cycle. Give full cisplatin dose if CrCl is >60 mL/min at end of cycle.
Plantar-palmar toxicity Grade 2 or greater	Discontinue fluorouracil until recovery, then reduce fluorouracil dose by 20%.
Other greater than Grade 3 toxicities except alopecia (can be permanent) and anemia	Delay 5-FU chemotherapy (for a maximum of 2 weeks from the planned date of infusion) until resolution to ≤Grade 1. If medically appropriate, resume treatment.

DILUTION

Specific techniques required; see Precautions. If docetaxel or diluted solution comes into contact with skin, immediately and thoroughly wash with soap and water. If docetaxel or diluted solution comes into contact with mucosa, immediately and thoroughly wash with water.

Available in multiple formulations, in **several concentrations, and as both single-use and multiple-use products; read label carefully.** Formulations are **NOT** interchangeable in a dose. **Do not use the two-vial formulation (injection concentrate and diluent [contains 13% ethanol in water for injection]) with the one-vial formulation. Read prescribing information carefully for product-specific dilution, storage, and stability information.**

Single-bottle formulations (generic and Taxotere): Available in 10 mg/mL and 20 mg/mL concentrations in multiple sizes. Manually rotate to mix thoroughly. Requires no initial dilution and is ready to add to an infusion solution; **read label carefully** to avoid overdose. Allow required number of vials to stand at room temperature for 5 minutes if refrigerated. Using a 21-gauge needle (product specific), withdraw required amount of docetaxel and inject via a single injection into a 250-mL infusion bag or bottle of NS or D5W; **see all formulations below.** Manually rotate to mix thoroughly.

Two-vial formulation (generic): Available in 20 mg/0.5 mL or in 80 mg/2 mL vials **(concentration is 2 times greater than the single-bottle formulation; read label carefully).** Allow required number of vials to stand at room temperature for 5 minutes if refrigerated. Reconstitute the appropriate vial (20 or 80 mg) with the entire contents of the diluent vial. Resulting concentration is 10 mg/mL. Mix well by repeated inversions for at least 45 seconds. **Do not shake.** Allow to stand until most of the foam dissipates. After this initial reconstitution, withdraw the required amount of 10 mg/mL concentrate and inject into a 250-mL bag or bottle of NS or D5W; **see all formulations below.**

All formulations: Final dilution should be in glass or polypropylene bottles or polypropylene or polyolefin plastic bags for infusion. Thoroughly mix the infusion by manual rotation. Should be administered through polyethylene-lined administration sets. Desired concentration should be between 0.3 and 0.74 mg/mL (100 mg in 250 mL = 0.4 mg/mL). If a dose greater than 200 mg is required, use a larger volume of NS or D5W so that a final concentration of 0.74 mg/mL is not exceeded. Solution should be clear.

Filters: Not required.

Storage: Storage requirements and stability are brand specific; check prescribing information. Some products may be stored at RT. Others require refrigeration. Docetaxel injection infusion solution is supersaturated and may therefore crystallize over time. If crystals appear, the solution must no longer be used and should be discarded.

Most formulations: Most formulations when fully diluted in NS or D5W should be used within 4 hours (including the 1-hour infusion time). **Taxotere** (one-vial formulation) is stable for 6 hours (including the 1-hour infusion time). At least one generic product is available as a multiple-dose vial that is stable for 28 days when refrigerated.

COMPATIBILITY

Leaches out plasticizers, including DEHP, from PVC infusion bags and administration sets. Use glass or polypropylene bottles or plastic (polypropylene or polyolefin) bags and polyethylene-lined administration sets to minimize patient exposure to leached DEHP. Do not allow concentrate to come into contact with plasticized PVC equipment or devices used to prepare and administer solutions.

Other sources suggest specific **compatibilities** dependent on concentration and manufacturer; consult a pharmacist.

RATE OF ADMINISTRATION

A single dose, properly diluted, equally distributed over 1 hour. Room temperature should be cool, and lighting should be low.

ACTIONS

An antineoplastic. A novel, semisynthetic, antimicrotubule agent derived from the needles of the yew plant. It inhibits cancer cell division. Microtubules assemble and disassemble during the cell cycle. Docetaxel promotes assembly and blocks disassembly of microtubules, preventing the cancer cells from dividing. The end result is cancer cell death. Highly protein bound. Metabolized in the liver by CYP3A4, an isoenzyme of the P_{450} family. Half-life is 11.1 hours. Eliminated primarily through feces and, to a lesser extent, urine and bile.

INDICATIONS AND USES

Treatment of locally advanced or metastatic breast cancer after failure of prior chemotherapy. ▪ In combination with doxorubicin and cyclophosphamide for adjuvant treatment of operable node-positive breast cancer. ▪ As a single agent in the treatment of locally advanced or metastatic NSCLC after failure of platinum-based chemotherapy (e.g., cisplatin). ▪ In combination with cisplatin for treatment of patients with unresectable, locally advanced, or metastatic NSCLC who have not previously received chemotherapy for this condition. ▪ In combination with prednisone for the treatment of castration-resistant metastatic prostate cancer. ▪ In combination with cisplatin and fluorouracil for the treatment of advanced gastric adenocarcinoma, including adenocarcinoma of the gastroesophageal junction, in patients who have not received prior chemotherapy for advanced disease. ▪ In combination with cisplatin and fluorouracil for induction therapy of locally advanced SCCHN. Following chemotherapy, patients should receive radiotherapy.

Unlabeled uses: Treatment of metastatic bladder cancer, esophageal cancer, ovarian cancer, soft tissue sarcomas, and adenocarcinomas of unknown primary site; consult literature.

CONTRAINDICATIONS

Baseline neutropenia less than 1,500 cells/mm^3. ▪ History of hypersensitivity reactions to docetaxel or other drugs formulated with polysorbate 80. ▪ Severe impaired liver function. In the United States, docetaxel is not recommended for patients with a bilirubin above the ULN or in patients with ALT and/or AST greater than 1.5 times the ULN range and increases in alkaline phosphatase greater than 2.5 times the ULN range; see Precautions.

PRECAUTIONS

Follow guidelines for handling cytotoxic agents. See Appendix A, p. 1308. ▪ Usually administered by or under the direction of the physician specialist. ▪ Adequate diagnostic and treatment facilities must be readily available. ▪ Incidence of treatment-related mortality increased in patients with abnormal liver function, in patients receiving higher doses, and in patients with NSCLC and a history of prior treatment with platinum-based chemotherapy who receive docetaxel as a single agent at a dose of 100 mg/M^2. ▪ Patients with elevations of bilirubin or abnormalities of transaminase concurrent with alkaline phosphatase are at increased risk for the development of Grade 4 neutropenia, febrile neutropenia, infections, severe thrombocytopenia, severe stomatitis, severe skin toxicity, and toxic death. ▪ Not recommended for patients with hepatic impairment; see Contraindications. Risk of toxicity and death is significant. Patients with isolated elevations of transaminases greater than 1.5 times the ULN have a higher rate of neutropenia Grade 4 but not of toxic death. Alcohol content of some products should be considered if given to patients with hepatic impairment. ▪ Reversible myelosuppression is the major dose-limiting toxicity of docetaxel. The median time to nadir was 7 days, and the median duration of severe neutropenia (fewer than 500 cells/mm^3) was 7 days. ▪ Febrile neutropenia occurred in patients dosed at 100 mg/M^2 but was uncommon in patients dosed at 60 mg/M^2. Hematologic responses, febrile reactions and infections, and rates of septic death for different regimens are dose related. ▪ Enterocolitis and neutropenic colitis (typhlitis) have occurred despite the coadministration of G-CSF. Use caution in patients with neutropenia, particularly in patients at risk for developing GI complications. ▪ Severe hypersensitivity reactions characterized by generalized rash/erythema, hypotension and/or bronchospasm or, rarely, fatal anaphylaxis have been reported. ▪ Patients who have previously experienced a hypersensitivity reaction to paclitaxel may develop a hypersensitivity reaction to docetaxel that may include severe or fatal reactions such as anaphylaxis. ▪ In addition to myelosuppression and hypersensitivity reactions, localized erythema of the extremities with edema followed by desquamation, severe fluid retention, severe neurosensory symptoms (e.g., dysesthesia, pain, paresthesia), and severe asthenia (usually in metastatic breast cancer patients) has been reported. ▪ Severe fluid retention may occur despite premedication with dexamethasone. ▪ Use with caution in patients with pleural effusion; may be exacerbated by docetaxel-induced fluid retention. ▪ Second primary malignancies, notably acute myeloid leukemia (AML), myelodysplastic syndrome (MDS), non-Hodgkin lymphoma (NHL), and renal cancer have been reported in patients treated with docetaxel-containing regimens. May occur months to years after docetaxel-containing therapy. ▪ Cystoid macular edema (CME) has been reported; see Monitor. ▪ Cases of intoxication have been reported with some formulations of docetaxel due to the alcohol content. Alcohol content may affect the CNS and should be considered in patients in whom alcohol intake should be avoided or minimized. May affect ability to drive or use machinery immediately after the infusion. ▪ When administering combination therapy, consult all appropriate drug monographs for relevant information. ▪ See Drug/Lab Interactions.

Monitor: Obtain baseline CBC with differential and platelets; monitor frequently during therapy and before each dose. See Dose Adjustments. ▪ Obtain baseline bilirubin, AST, ALT, and alkaline phosphatase; monitor as indicated during therapy (recommended before each dose). ▪ Obtain baseline and periodic renal function, if indicated. ▪ Determine absolute patency of vein. A stinging or burning sensation indicates extravasation; discontinue injection; use another vein. ▪ Obtain baseline vital signs; monitor during and after infusion. ▪ Monitor for hypersensitivity reactions, especially during the first and second infusions; may occur within minutes. Discontinue docetaxel if reaction is severe. Hypersensitivity reactions may occur even in patients premedicated with dexamethasone. ▪ Closely monitor patients with a previous history of hypersensitivity to paclitaxel during initiation of docetaxel therapy. ▪ Monitor for localized erythema of the palms of the hands and soles of the feet with or without desquamation. Skin eruptions generally occur within 1 week after docetaxel infusion, resolve before the next infusion, and are not disabling. However, severe reactions have been reported. A reduced dose may be indicated if severe. ▪ Monitor for fluid retention. Salt restriction and treatment with oral diuretics may be indicated. S/S of severe fluid retention include abdominal distension (severe), cardiac tamponade, dyspnea at rest, peripheral or generalized edema, pleural effusion. ▪ Observe for signs of peripheral neurotoxicity (e.g., neurosensory symptoms such as dysesthesia, pain, paresthesia, and peripheral motor neuropathy manifested primarily as distal extremity weakness); docetaxel may need to be discontinued; see Dose Adjustments. In patients with gastric adenocarcinoma or SCCHN, a baseline neurologic exam is recommended. Repeat every 2 cycles and at the end of treatment; see Dose Adjustments. ▪ Monitor patients for the onset of any GI toxicity. Enterocolitis and neutropenic enterocolitis may develop at any time and can lead to death as early as the first day of symptom onset. ▪ Observe for signs of infection. Use of prophylactic antibiotics may be indicated pending C/S in a febrile, neutropenic patient. Monitor patients receiving docetaxel (Taxotere), cisplatin, fluorouracil (5-FU) combination therapy closely for febrile neutropenia and/or neutropenic infection. ▪ Monitor for thrombocytopenia (platelet count less than 50,000/mm^3); see Dose Adjustments. Initiate precautions to prevent excessive bleeding (e.g., inspect IV sites, skin, and mucous membranes; use extreme care during invasive procedures; test urine, emesis, stool, and secretions for occult blood). ▪ Monitor for signs of existing or developing impaired vision. A prompt comprehensive ophthalmologic exam is indicated. If CME is diagnosed, discontinue docetaxel. ▪ Hematologic follow-up required due to risk of delayed second primary malignancies.

Patient Education: Avoid pregnancy. Females of reproductive potential should use effective contraception during treatment and for 6 months after the last dose of docetaxel. Male patients with female partners of reproductive potential should use effective contraception during treatment and for 3 months after the last dose. ▪ May impair fertility in males of reproductive potential. ▪ Review of monitoring requirements (e.g., CBCs, liver function tests) and adverse events before therapy imperative. ▪ Pretreatment with dexamethasone as prescribed is imperative. ▪ Report pain or burning at injection site and any unusual or unexpected symptoms or side effects as soon as possible (e.g., constipation, diarrhea, excessive tearing, fatigue, fever, hair loss [cases of permanent hair loss have been reported], hypersensitivity reaction [e.g., difficulty breathing, itching, rash], infusion site reaction, irregular and/or rapid heartbeat, nausea and vomiting, shortness of breath, swelling of feet and legs, weight gain, change in vision). ▪ Promptly report new or worsening symptoms of GI toxicity. ▪ Immediately report myalgia or cutaneous or neurologic reactions. ▪ Review all medications (prescription and nonprescription) and allergies with nurse and/or physician. ▪ Medication may contain alcohol. May affect ability to drive or operate machinery immediately after infusion. ▪ See Appendix D, p. 1311. ▪ Obtain name and telephone number of a contact person for emergencies, questions, or problems. ▪ Seek resources for counseling or supportive therapy. ▪ Risk of second primary malignancies requires hematologic follow-up. Changes in blood counts due to leukemia and other blood disorders may occur years after treatment.

Maternal/Child: Avoid pregnancy; may cause fetal harm. ▪ Avoid breast-feeding during treatment and for 1 week after the last dose of docetaxel. ▪ Effectiveness in pediatric patients as monotherapy or in combination have not been established. The overall safety profile of docetaxel in pediatric patients receiving monotherapy or combination treatment with cisplatin and 5-fluorouracil was consistent with the known safety profile in adults. Has been used in a small number of pediatric patients; see manufacturer's prescribing information. ▪ The alcohol content of docetaxel should be taken into account when given to pediatric patients.

Elderly: Dose selection should be cautious; see Dose Adjustments. ▪ May be at increased risk for developing side effects such as anemia, anorexia, diarrhea, dizziness, febrile neutropenia, infections, lethargy, nail changes, peripheral edema, stomatitis, and weight loss. ▪ Monitor hepatic function carefully.

DRUG/LAB INTERACTIONS

A substrate of CYP3A4. Metabolism may be modified by concomitant administration of other medications that induce, inhibit, or are metabolized by CYP3A4 (e.g., cyclosporine, phenytoin, phenobarbital, tacrolimus, and many others). ▪ Metabolism inhibited and serum levels increased with **strong CYP3A4 inhibitors** (e.g., imidazole antifungals [e.g., itraconazole, voriconazole], protease inhibitors [e.g., atazanavir, indinavir, nelfinavir, ritonavir, saquinavir], clarithromycin, and nefazodone). Avoid use. A pharmacokinetic study suggests considering a 50% dose reduction of docetaxel if coadministration of a strong CYP3A4 inhibitor is required; monitor closely for toxicity. ▪ Docetaxel clearance is not affected by coadministration of **prednisone, dexamethasone, fluorouracil, cyclophosphamide, doxorubicin,** or **cisplatin.** ▪ Do not administer **live virus vaccines** to patients receiving antineoplastic agents.

SIDE EFFECTS

Generally reversible but can be fatal. The most common side effects across all indications are alopecia, anemia, anorexia, asthenia, constipation, diarrhea, dysgeusia, dyspnea, febrile neutropenia, fluid retention (e.g., ascites, edema, pericardial effusion, pleural effusion), hypersensitivity reactions (e.g., back pain, chest tightness, chills, drug fever, dyspnea, flushing, hypotension, pruritus, rash), infection, mucositis, myalgia, nail disorders, nausea, neuropathy, neutropenia, pain, skin reactions, thrombocytopenia, and vomiting. Increased incidence of bone marrow suppression (anemia, leukopenia, neutropenia, thrombocytopenia) and/or severity of side effects is dose dependent and can be dose limiting. The most serious adverse reactions are alcohol intoxication, asthenia, cutaneous reactions, enterocolitis and neutropenic colitis, eye disorders, fluid retention, hematologic toxicity, hepatotoxicity, hypersensitivity, neurologic reactions, second primary malignancies, and toxic deaths. Abdominal pain; acute myeloid leukemia and myelodysplastic syndrome; acute pulmonary edema; acute respiratory distress syndrome; alcohol intoxication; altered hearing; amenorrhea; arthralgia; bleeding episodes; cardiac arrhythmias; CHF; colitis; confusion; conjunctivitis; cough; cutaneous reactions (e.g., localized rash on hands, feet, arms, face, thorax; erythema multiforme; severe hand and foot syndrome; Stevens-Johnson syndrome; toxic epidermal necrolysis); diarrhea; DIC (often in association with sepsis or multiorgan failure); dizziness; enteritis; esophagitis/dysphagia/odynophagia; eye disorders (e.g., CME); fatigue; fever with or without infection; gastrointestinal pain and cramping; heartburn; hepatitis (sometimes fatal, primarily in patients with pre-existing liver disease); hypotension; increased ALT, AST, and bilirubin; infusion site reactions; interstitial pneumonia; lethargy; lymphedema; myocardial ischemia; neurosensory symptoms (e.g., dysesthesia, pain, paresthesia); neutropenic infection; paresthesias (e.g., pain, burning sensation); perforation of the large intestine; renal insufficiency; seizures or transient loss of consciousness; stomatitis; taste perversion; tearing; vasodilation.

Overdose: Bone marrow suppression, mucositis, peripheral neurotoxicity.

Post-Marketing: Acute pulmonary edema, acute respiratory distress syndrome/pneumonitis, alopecia (permanent), anaphylactic shock, atrial fibrillation, bullous eruptions, chest pain, cutaneous lupus erythematosus, cystoid macular edema, deep vein thrombosis, dehydration, diffuse pain, disseminated intravascular coagulation (DIC) (often in association with sepsis or multiorgan failure), duodenal ulcer, dyspnea, ECG abnormalities, esophagitis, gastrointestinal perforation, GI hemorrhage, hearing disorders/loss, hepatitis, hyponatremia, ileus, interstitial lung disease, interstitial pneumonia, intestinal obstruction, ischemic colitis, lacrimation with or without conjunctivitis, MI, myelodysplastic syndrome, neutropenic enterocolitis, ototoxicity, pulmonary embolism, pulmonary fibrosis, radiation pneumonitis, radiation recall phenomenon, renal failure (most commonly associated with concomitant nephrotoxic drugs), renal insufficiency, respiratory failure, scleroderma-like changes (usually preceded by peripheral lymphedema), seizures, syncopy, tachycardia, thrombophlebitis, transient loss of consciousness, transient visual disturbances.

ANTIDOTE

Keep physician informed of all side effects. Most will be treated symptomatically as indicated. Most hypersensitivity reactions will subside with temporary discontinuation of docetaxel, and incidence seems to decrease with subsequent doses. Discontinue docetaxel if a severe hypersensitivity reaction occurs. Severe reactions may require epinephrine, antihistamines (e.g., diphenhydramine), corticosteroids (e.g., dexamethasone), or bronchodilators (e.g., albuterol). Patients with a history of a severe hypersensitivity reaction should not be rechallenged. If CME is diagnosed, discontinue docetaxel and initiate appropriate treatment. Consider alternative non-taxane cancer treatment. Neutropenia can be profound. Recovery is generally rapid and spontaneous but may be treated with filgrastim or pegfilgrastim. Severe thrombocytopenia may require platelet transfusions. Severe anemia (less than 8 Gm/dL) may require packed cell transfusions. Serious cutaneous reactions with desquamation (rare), serious fluid retention, persistent febrile neutropenia, severe peripheral neuropathy, or severe liver impairment may require discontinuation of docetaxel. There is no specific antidote for overdose. Supportive therapy will help sustain the patient in toxicity. Resuscitate if indicated.

DONANEMAB
(doe NAN e mab)

Kisunla

Anti-Amyloid Monoclonal
Antibody; Immunoglobulin;
Monoclonal Antibody

USUAL DOSE

700 mg IV every 4 weeks for 3 doses followed by 1400 mg IV every 4 weeks until amyloid plaques are reduced to minimal levels on amyloid positron emission tomography (PET) imaging.

PEDIATRIC DOSE

Efficacy and safety have not been established.

DOSE ADJUSTMENTS

Renal: No dosage adjustments provided by manufacturer.
Hepatic: No dosage adjustments provided by manufacturer.
Other dosage adjustments:

Amyloid-Related Imaging Abnormalities With Edema (ARIA-E)			
Clinical Symptom Severity	**ARIA-E severity on MRI**[Ref]		
	Mild	**Moderate**	**Severe**
Asymptomatic	May continue current dose and schedule.	Withhold donanemab until MRI displays radiographic resolution; use clinical judgment with resumption of dosing. Consider an MRI 2 to 4 months after initial identification to evaluate for resolution.	
Mild (e.g., discomfort with no change of normal daily activity)	May continue current dose and schedule.	Withhold donanemab until MRI displays radiographic resolution and symptoms resolve; use clinical judgment with resumption of dosing. Consider an MRI 2 to 4 months after initial identification to evaluate for resolution.	
Moderate or severe (e.g., symptoms ranging from discomfort that reduces or changes normal daily activity to incapacitating and not able to work or perform normal daily activity)	Withhold donanemab until MRI displays radiographic resolution and symptoms resolve; use clinical judgment with resumption of dosing. Consider an MRI 2 to 4 months after initial identification to evaluate for resolution.		

MRI, magnetic resonance image.

Amyloid-Related Imaging Abnormalities With Hemosiderin Deposition (ARIA-H)			
Clinical Symptom Severity	**ARIA-H severity on MRI(Ref)**		
	Mild	**Moderate**	**Severe**
Asymptomatic	May continue current dose and schedule.	Withhold donanemab until MRI displays radiographic resolution; use clinical judgment with resumption of dosing. Consider an MRI 2 to 4 months after initial identification to evaluate for resolution.	Withhold donanemab until MRI demonstrates radiographic stabilization; use clinical judgment when considering whether to continue or permanently discontinue therapy.
Symptomatic	Withhold donanemab until MRI displays radiographic resolution and symptoms resolve; use clinical judgment with resumption of dosing. Consider an MRI 2 to 4 months after initial identification to evaluate for resolution.		Withhold donanemab until MRI demonstrates radiographic stabilization and symptoms resolve; use clinical judgment when considering whether to continue or permanently discontinue therapy.

MRI, magnetic resonance image.

Hypersensitivity reaction signs/symptoms (eg, angioedema, anaphylaxis): Immediately discontinue infusion at first sign/symptom of hypersensitivity and initiate appropriate treatment.

Intracerebral hemorrhage (>1 cm in diameter)

Withhold donanemab until magnetic resonance image (MRI) displays radiographic stabilization and symptoms (if present) resolve.

Infusion reaction signs/symptoms (e.g., chills, nausea, vomiting, difficulty breathing, blood pressure changes)

Consider premedication with antihistamines, acetaminophen, nonsteroidal anti-inflammatory drugs, or corticosteroids before future infusions.[Ref]

DILUTION

Allow undiluted solution to come to room temperature before preparation. Withdraw required volume of donanemab and dilute with normal saline injection to a final concentration of 4 to 10 mg/mL. Gently invert diluted solution to mix; do not shake. Discard any unused portion left in the vial.[Ref]

Donanemab Dilution(Ref)		
Dose (volume)	**Volume of Normal Saline Injection Diluent**	**Final Concentration of Diluted Solution**
700 mg (40 mL)	30 to 135 mL	700 mg/70 mL (10 mg/mL) to 700 mg/175 mL (4 mg/mL)
1400 mg (80 mL)	60 to 270 mL	1400 mg/140 mL (10 mg/mL) to 1400 mg/350 mL (4 mg/mL)

Administration

Before IV infusion, allow the diluted solution to warm to room temperature if stored under refrigeration. Infuse over 30 minutes and flush line with NS after infusion is complete. Observe for infusion and hypersensitivity reactions during infusion and for at least 30 minutes after infusion. Discontinue infusion if hypersensitivity reaction.

ACTIONS

Donanemab is a humanized immunoglobulin gamma 1 (IgG_1) monoclonal antibody directed against insoluble N-truncated pyroglutamate amyloid beta. Donanemab reduces amyloid beta plaques, the accumulation of which is a defining pathophysiologic feature of Alzheimer's disease.

INDICATIONS AND USES

Treatment of Alzheimer disease; to be started in patients with mild cognitive impairment or mild dementia.

CONTRAINDICATIONS

Serious hypersensitivity (e.g., anaphylaxis) to donanemab or any component of the formulation.

PRECAUTIONS

Donanemab has a black box warning regarding amyloid-related imaging abnormalities (ARIA), characterized as ARIA with edema (ARIA-E) and ARIA with hemosiderin deposition (ARIA-H). Incidence and timing of ARIA vary among treatments. ARIA usually occurs early in treatment and is usually asymptomatic, although serious and life-threatening events rarely occur. Serious intracerebral hemorrhages >1 cm, some of which have been fatal, have been observed in patients treated with this class of medications. Ischemic stroke can occur and clinicians should consider whether such symptoms could be due to ARIA-E before giving thrombolytic therapy.

- Infusion reaction: Donanemab may cause infusion reactions, typically during infusion or within 30 minutes after infusion. Symptoms include chills, erythema, nausea, vomiting, difficulty breathing, dyspnea, sweating, blood pressure changes, headache, and chest pain. The highest incidence of infusion reactions occurs within the first 4 infusions.
- Polysorbate 80: Some dosage forms may contain polysorbate 80 (also known as Tweens). Hypersensitivity reactions, usually a delayed reaction, have been reported after exposure to pharmaceutical products containing polysorbate 80 in certain individuals

Monitor: PET or lumbar puncture to confirm presence of amyloid beta pathology (before initiation); apolipoprotein E $\epsilon4$ (ApoE $\epsilon4$) status testing (before initiation); brain MRI (before initiation [recent]; before infusions 2, 3,4, and 7; periodically, as appropriate in the setting of ARIA; e.g., 2 to 4 months after identification of ARIA) or if symptoms of ARIA develop; monitor closely for clinical and MRI changes; monitor for symptoms suggestive of ARIA (e.g., headache, altered mental status, visual changes, dizziness, nausea, gait difficulty, focal neurologic deficits, and seizure)

Patient Education: Contact physician with any of the following adverse effects:

- Headache, dizziness, upset stomach, change in eyesight, seizures, trouble walking, or confusion.
- Weakness on one side of the body, trouble speaking or thinking, changes in balance, drooping on one side of the face, or blurred eyesight.
- Infusion reactions such as chills; skin irritation; sweating; headache; chest pain; upset stomach or vomiting; signs of high or low blood pressure such as severe dizziness or headache, fainting, or changes in eyesight; or trouble breathing.
- Signs of an allergic reaction, such as rash; hives; itching; red, swollen, blistered, or peeling skin with or without fever; wheezing; tightness in the chest or throat; trouble breathing, swallowing, or talking; unusual hoarseness; or swelling of the mouth, face, lips, tongue, or throat.

Maternal/Child: Animal reproduction studies have not been conducted.

Breastfeeding considerations: It is not known if donanemab is present in breast milk.

Elderly: No specific recommendations; refer to adult dosing.

DRUG/LAB INTERACTIONS

Monitor therapy with the following drugs: efgartigimod alfa, rozanolixizumab, anticoagulants, thrombolytic agents, antiplatelet agents.

SIDE EFFECTS

Significant adverse reactions: ARIA, including ARIA consistent with vasogenic edema and/or sulcal effusions (ARIA-E) [Ref] and ARIA-H characterized by superficial siderosis, microhemorrhages, and macrohemorrhages [Ref] have been reported with donanemab therapy. Patients may develop ARIA-H with concomitant ARIA-E. In patients who developed ARIA (-E and/or -H) during donanemab clinical trials, most cases were asymptomatic with mild to moderate radiographic severity; however, serious and/or fatal symptoms have been reported [Ref]. Recurrent episodes of ARIA-E have also been described. Clinical symptoms suggesting ARIA may include abnormal gait, confusion, dizziness, focal neurologic deficits, headache, nausea, visual disturbance, and seizures. Resolution of ARIA-E occurred by 12 to 20 weeks in the majority of cases in clinical trials.

ARIA-E: Dose-related; related to the pharmacologic action. Increased cerebrovascular permeability due to antibody binding to deposited amyloid-beta results in an increase in extracellular fluid volume and vasogenic edema [Ref].

ARIA-H: Dose-related; related to the pharmacologic action. Leakage of blood from a vessel into adjacent tissue parenchyma or subarachnoid space/periadventitial compartments leaves residual deposits of iron in the form of hemosiderin, resulting in superficial siderosis and/or radiographic evidence of hemorrhage.

Other adverse reactions: Hemosiderosis, superficial siderosis: 15% to 25%.

Immunologic: Antibody development (87%; neutralizing: 100%).

Nervous system: Brain edema (ARIA-E: 24%; higher in apolipoprotein E ϵ4 carriers; Table 2), headache (13%; Table 3)

1% to 10%: *Hypersensitivity:* Hypersensitivity reaction (3%; including anaphylaxis, angioedema), infusion-related reaction (9%)

ANTIDOTE

There is no antidote; stop infusion for hypersensitivity reactions and treat appropriately.

DOPAMINE HYDROCHLORIDE BBW

(**DOH**-pah-meen hy-droh-**KLOR**-eyed)

Inotropic agent
Cardiac stimulant
Vasopressor

pH 2.5 to 5

USUAL DOSE

Where appropriate, restoration of blood volume with a suitable plasma expander or whole blood should be instituted or completed before administration of dopamine; the goal is a central venous pressure of 10 to 15 cm H_2O or a pulmonary wedge pressure of 14 to 18 mm Hg.

Adults: 2 to 5 mcg/kg of body weight/min initially in patients likely to respond to minimum treatment. 5 to 10 mcg/kg/min may be required initially to correct hypotension in the seriously ill patient. Gradually increase by 5 to 10 mcg/kg/min at 10- to 30-minute intervals until optimum response occurs. Average dose is 20 mcg/kg/min; over 50 mcg/kg/min has been required in some instances but is not recommended. If more than 20 mcg/kg/min is required to maintain BP, consider use of norepinephrine (Levophed) in addition. Doses over 20 mcg/kg/min decrease renal perfusion.

Bradycardia: AHA guidelines recommend dopamine infusion 2 to 20 mcg/kg/min. Titrate to desired effect; taper slowly. Indicated if atropine is ineffective. Alternately, transcutaneous pacing or epinephrine infusion 2 to 10 mcg/min may be used.

PEDIATRIC DOSE

See Maternal/Child. Note comments in Usual Dose. Usual starting dose is 1 to 5 mcg/kg/min. Dose increments range from 2.5 to 5 mcg/kg/min. Usual maximum dose is 15 to 20 mcg/kg/min. Doses up to 50 mcg/kg/min have been administered. Titrate dose gradually to desired effect.

DOSE ADJUSTMENTS

Reduce dose to one-tenth of the calculated amount for individuals who have been treated with MAO inhibitors (e.g., selegiline) within 2 to 3 weeks of administration of dopamine. ▪ Lower-end initial doses may be appropriate in the elderly based on potential for decreased organ function and concomitant disease or drug therapy. ▪ Reduce dose if possible if increased number of ectopic beats is observed. ▪ See Drug/Lab Interactions.

DILUTION

Each 200-mg, 400-mg, or 800-mg ampule must be diluted in 250 to 500 mL of the following IV solutions and given as an infusion: NS, D5W, D5NS, D5/½NS, D5LR, ⅙ M sodium lactate, or LR injection. See the following chart.

Final Dopamine Concentration (mcg/mL) When Dopamine 40 mg/mL or 80 mg/mL Is Mixed With Various Volumes of Infusion Solution			
Concentration of Dopamine	40 mg/mL		80 mg/mL
Volume of Dopamine	5 mL (200 mg)	10 mL (400 mg)	10 mL (800 mg)
250 mL diluent	800 mcg/mL	1,600 mcg/mL	3,200 mcg/mL
500 mL diluent	400 mcg/mL	800 mcg/mL	1,600 mcg/mL
1,000 mL diluent	200 mcg/mL	400 mcg/mL	800 mcg/mL

Also available prediluted in 250 mL or 500 mL of D5W. Dopamine concentration varies. More concentrated solutions may be used if absolutely necessary to reduce fluid volume. **Storage:** Store at CRT. Protect from freezing. Discard diluted solution after 24 hours. Do not use if solution is darker than slightly yellow.

COMPATIBILITY

Manufacturer states, "Do not add to sodium bicarbonate or any other strongly alkaline solution (e.g., aminophylline, barbiturates [e.g., phenobarbital]), oxidizing agents, or iron salts. Dopamine is inactivated in alkaline solution." Do not mix with alteplase or amphotericin B. Do not administer solutions containing dextrose through the same administration set as blood; may result in pseudoagglutination or hemolysis.

Other sources suggest specific **compatibilities** dependent on concentration and manufacturer; consult a pharmacist.

RATE OF ADMINISTRATION

Begin with recommended dose for body weight and seriousness of condition. Gradually increase by 5 to 10 mcg/kg/min to produce desired response. Titrate to desired hemodynamic or renal response. When titrating to the desired increase in systolic BP, the optimum dosage rate for renal response may be exceeded and may necessitate a rate reduction after the hemodynamic condition is stabilized. Use of a volumetric infusion pump is recommended for accuracy. Optimum urine flow determines correct evaluation of dosage. Decrease dose gradually; may cause marked hypotension if discontinued suddenly. Expansion of blood volume with IV fluids may be indicated. If hypotension occurs at lower infusion rate, the infusion rate should be rapidly increased until adequate blood pressure is obtained. If hypotension continues, dopamine should be discontinued, and a more potent vasoconstrictor agent (e.g., norepinephrine) should be administered. If a disproportionate rise in diastolic pressure is observed, the infusion rate should be decreased and the patient observed for further evidence of predominant vasoconstrictor activity unless such an effect is desired.

Dopamine Infusion Rate (mL/hr): 400 mcg/mL Concentration						
Desired Dose	**Weight in Kilograms**					
	50 kg	**60 kg**	**70 kg**	**80 kg**	**90 kg**	**100 kg**
	(mL/hr)	**(mL/hr)**	**(mL/hr)**	**(mL/hr)**	**(mL/hr)**	**(mL/hr)**
5 mcg/kg/min	37.5	45	52.5	60	67.5	75
10 mcg/kg/min	75	90	105	120	135	150
20 mcg/kg/min	150	180	210	240	270	300
30 mcg/kg/min	225	270	315	360	405	450
40 mcg/kg/min	300	360	420	480	540	600

Dopamine Infusion Rate (mL/hr): 800 mcg/mL Concentration						
Desired Dose	**Weight in Kilograms**					
	50 kg	**60 kg**	**70 kg**	**80 kg**	**90 kg**	**100 kg**
	(mL/hr)	**(mL/hr)**	**(mL/hr)**	**(mL/hr)**	**(mL/hr)**	**(mL/hr)**
5 mcg/kg/min	18.75	22.5	26.25	30	33.75	37.5
10 mcg/kg/min	37.5	45	52.5	60	67.5	75
20 mcg/kg/min	75	90	105	120	135	150
30 mcg/kg/min	112.5	135	157.5	180	202.5	225
40 mcg/kg/min	150	180	210	240	270	300

ACTIONS

Dopamine is a naturally occurring catecholamine that possesses alpha, beta, and dopaminergic receptor–stimulating actions. The effects of dopamine are dose-related. At low doses (0.5 to 2 mcg/kg/min), dopamine causes vasodilation in the renal, mesenteric, coronary, and intracerebral vascular beds, thereby increasing glomerular filtration rate, renal blood flow, sodium excretion, and urine flow. At medium doses (2 to 10 mcg/kg/min), beta-adrenoceptors are stimulated, resulting in improved myocardial contractility, increased sinoatrial rate, and enhanced impulse conduction in the heart. Systolic and pulse pressure may increase, but there is little, if any, effect on diastolic pressure at these doses. At higher doses (10 to 20 mcg/kg/min), alpha-adrenoceptors are stimulated, resulting in vasoconstriction and an increase in blood pressure. At doses above 20 mcg/kg/min, alpha effects predominate and vasoconstriction may compromise circulation in the limbs and override the dopaminergic effects of dopamine, reversing renal dilation and natriuresis. Dopamine is widely distributed. It has an onset of action of 5 minutes, a duration of action of 10 minutes, and a plasma half-life of 2 minutes. Metabolized in the liver, kidney, and plasma by monoamine oxidase (MAO) and catechol O-methyltransferase (COMT), with about 25% of the dose being converted to norepinephrine. Primarily excreted in urine.

INDICATIONS AND USES
To correct hemodynamic imbalances, including hypotension resulting from shock syndrome of myocardial infarction, trauma, endotoxic septicemia, open heart surgery, renal failure, and chronic cardiac decompensation. ▪ Drug of choice for hypotension and shock. ▪ AHA guidelines recommend dopamine as the second drug of choice after atropine to treat symptomatic bradycardia.

Unlabeled uses: Chronic obstructive pulmonary disease, congestive heart failure, infant respiratory distress syndrome, symptomatic bradycardia, calcium channel blocker overdose, beta-blocker overdose, and drug-induced hypovolemic shock; consult literature.

CONTRAINDICATIONS
Hypersensitivity to any components (contains sulfites), pheochromocytoma, uncorrected tachyarrhythmias, ventricular fibrillation. Premixed solutions containing dextrose may be contraindicated in patients with known allergies to corn or corn products.

PRECAUTIONS
Avoid bolus administration. ▪ Some preparations contain sulfites; use caution in patients with allergies. ▪ Use with caution in patients with known subclinical or overt diabetes mellitus. ▪ IV administration of fluids may cause fluid overload, resulting in dilution of serum electrolyte concentrations, overhydration, a congested state, or pulmonary edema. ▪ Avoid hypovolemia. ▪ Presence of hypoxia, hypercapnia, or acidosis may reduce the effectiveness of dopamine and/or increase the incidence of dopamine-induced adverse events. ▪ Ventricular arrhythmias have been reported. Reduce dose if possible if an increased number of ectopic beats is observed. ▪ Use caution in patients with a history of occlusive vascular disease (e.g., atherosclerosis, arterial embolism, Raynaud's disease, cold injury, diabetic endarteritis, and Buerger's disease). ▪ Excess administration of potassium-free solutions may result in significant hypokalemia. ▪ See Dose Adjustments and Drug/Lab Interactions.

Monitor: Recognition of signs and symptoms of hemodynamic imbalance and prompt treatment with dopamine will improve prognosis. ▪ Close monitoring of BP, cardiac output, cardiac rhythm, and urine output required. Avoid hypertension. If possible, check central venous pressure or pulmonary wedge pressure before administration and as ordered thereafter. ▪ Use larger veins (antecubital fossa) and avoid extravasation; may cause necrosis and sloughing of tissue. Central vein preferred for continuous infusions; see Antidote. ▪ If possible, correct hypovolemia with IV fluids, whole blood or plasma as indicated; correct acidosis if present. ▪ Monitor for decreased urine output, increased tachycardia, or new arrhythmias. ▪ With high-dose administration, palpate pulses and monitor extremities for signs of peripheral vasoconstriction (e.g., coldness, paresthesias). ▪ Therapy may be continued until the patient can maintain hemodynamic and renal functions. ▪ Monitor changes in fluid balance, electrolyte concentration, and acid-base balance during prolonged parenteral therapy or whenever patient's condition warrants such evaluation. ▪ See Maternal/Child and Drug/Lab Interactions.

Maternal/Child: Safety for use in pregnancy and breast-feeding not established. If used, benefits must outweigh risks. ▪ Safety for use in pediatric patients not established. Has been used, but experience is limited. ▪ Do not administer into an umbilical arterial catheter. Vasospastic events have been reported when dopamine is infused through the umbilical artery.

Elderly: Lower-end initial doses may be appropriate; see Dose Adjustments. ▪ Differences in response compared to younger adults not identified.

DRUG/LAB INTERACTIONS

Alkaline solutions, including sodium bicarbonate, inactivate dopamine. ▪ May cause serious arrhythmias in presence of **cyclopropane or halogen anesthetics.** ▪ May cause severe hypertension with **oxytocic drugs** (e.g., methylergonovine or oxytocin). ▪ **MAO inhibitors** prolong and potentiate the effect of dopamine. Concurrent use may cause hypertensive crisis. ▪ Concurrent administration of low-dose dopamine and diuretic agents may produce an additive or potentiating effect on urine flow. ▪ Antagonizes effects of **guanethidine.** ▪ Cardiac effects may be antagonized by **alpha- or beta-blocking agents.** ▪ **Tricyclic antidepressants** may potentiate the cardiovascular effects of dopamine. ▪ May cause severe bradycardia and hypotension with **phenytoin.** ▪ **Alpha-adrenergic blocking agents** antagonize the peripheral vasoconstriction caused by high-dose dopamine. ▪ **Butyrophenones** (e.g., haloperidol) and **phenothiazines** (e.g., chlorpromazine, prochlorperazine) can suppress the dopaminergic renal and mesenteric vasodilation induced with low-dose dopamine. ▪ See Dose Adjustments.

SIDE EFFECTS

Aberrant conduction/arrhythmias (e.g., atrial fibrillation, ectopic beats, widened QRS complex, ventricular arrhythmias), anginal pain, anxiety, azotemia, bradycardia, dyspnea, headache, hypertension, hypotension, nausea, palpitation, piloerection, tachycardia, vasoconstriction, vomiting. Gangrene of the extremities has occurred with high doses administered for prolonged periods and in patients with occlusive vascular disease receiving a low dose of dopamine.

ANTIDOTE

Notify the physician of all side effects. Decrease infusion rate and notify the physician immediately for decrease in established urine flow rate, disproportionate rise in diastolic BP (i.e., a marked decrease in pulse pressure), increasing tachycardia, or new arrhythmias. For accidental overdosage with hypertension, reduce rate or temporarily discontinue until condition stabilizes. Phentolamine, an alpha-adrenergic blocker, may be useful in an overdose situation that does not respond to discontinuation of dopamine. To prevent sloughing and necrosis in areas where extravasation has occurred, use a fine hypodermic needle to inject 5 to 10 mg of phentolamine (Regitine) diluted in 10 to 15 mL normal saline liberally throughout the tissue in the extravasated area. Begin as soon as extravasation is recognized.

DOXERCALCIFEROL
(**DOX**-err-kal-**sif**-er-ol)

Hectorol Injection

USUAL DOSE
Pretreatment: Baseline studies indicated; see Monitor.

Optimal dose of doxercalciferol must be individualized. The dose is adjusted in an attempt to achieve intact parathyroid hormone (iPTH) levels within a targeted range of 150 to 300 pg/mL. See Precautions and Monitor. Recommended initial dose for a patient with an iPTH level greater than 400 pg/mL is 4 mcg administered as a bolus dose three times weekly at the end of dialysis (approximately every other day). Total weekly dose is 12 mcg/week. Maximum dose was limited to 18 mcg/week in clinical studies.

DOSE ADJUSTMENTS
Adjust dosing based on patient response in order to lower blood iPTH into the range of 150 to 300 pg/mL. The dose may be increased at 8-week intervals by 1 to 2 mcg if iPTH is not lowered by 50% and fails to reach the target range. Doses higher than 18 mcg weekly have not been studied. During titration monitor iPTH, serum calcium, phosphorus, and calcium $\times$ phosphorus product (Ca $\times$ P) weekly. Maximize iPTH suppression while maintaining serum calcium and phosphorus levels in prescribed ranges; see Monitor. ▪ Immediately suspend dosing if hypercalcemia, hyperphosphatemia, or a Ca $\times$ P product of greater than 55 mg^2/dL^2 is noted. Reinitiate therapy at a dose that is 1 mcg lower when parameters have normalized. ▪ Patients with impaired hepatic function may not metabolize doxercalciferol appropriately; see Precautions. ▪ The following chart is a suggested approach to dose titration.

Suggested Dose Adjustment Guidelines for Doxercalciferol	
iPTH Level	**Doxercalciferol Dose Guidelines**
Decreased by <50% and above 300 pg/mL	Increase by 1 to 2 mcg at 8-week intervals as necessary
Decreased by >50% and above 300 pg/mL	Maintain
150 to 300 pg/mL	Maintain
<100 pg/mL	Suspend for 1 week, then resume at a dose that is at least 1 mcg lower

DILUTION
May be given undiluted. Available as a single-use injection containing either 4 mcg/2 mL or 2 mcg/mL and as a multidose injection containing 4 mcg/2 mL.

Storage: Store unopened vials at 25° C (77° F); range: 15° to 30° C (59° to 86° F). Protect from light. Discard unused portion of single-use vial. After initial multidose vial use, the contents remain stable up to 3 days when stored at 2° to 8° C (36° to 46° F). Discard unused portion of multidose vial after 3 days.

COMPATIBILITY
Compatibility information not available from manufacturer; consult a pharmacist.

RATE OF ADMINISTRATION
Administer as a bolus dose at the end of dialysis.

ACTIONS
A synthetic vitamin D analog. Metabolizes to a naturally occurring, biologically active form of vitamin D_2 that regulates blood calcium at levels required for essential body functions (i.e., intestinal absorption of dietary calcium, tubular reabsorption of calcium by the kidney and, in conjunction with the parathyroid hormone [PTH], the mobilization

of calcium from the skeleton). Acts directly on bone cells (osteoblasts) to stimulate skeletal growth and on the parathyroid glands to suppress PTH synthesis and secretion. In uremic patients, deficient production of biologically active vitamin D metabolites leads to secondary hyperparathyroidism, which contributes to the development of metabolic bone disease. Doxercalciferol is activated in the liver. Peak blood levels are reached in 2.1 to 13.9 hours. Mean half-life range is 32 to 96 hours.

INDICATIONS AND USES
Treatment of secondary hyperparathyroidism in patients with chronic kidney disease undergoing dialysis.

CONTRAINDICATIONS
Evidence of vitamin D toxicity, hypercalcemia, hyperphosphatemia, or known hypersensitivity to any ingredient in this product; see Precautions.

PRECAUTIONS
Overdose of any form of vitamin D, including doxercalciferol, is dangerous. Progressive hypercalcemia due to overdose of vitamin D and its metabolites may require emergency attention. Acute hypercalcemia may exacerbate tendencies for cardiac arrhythmias and seizures and may potentiate the action of digoxin drugs. Chronic hypercalcemia can lead to elevated Ca × P product, and generalized vascular and other soft-tissue calcification. If clinically significant hypercalcemia develops, dose should be reduced or held. Do not allow the Ca × P product to exceed 55 mg^2/dL^2. See Side Effects and Antidote. ▪ To avoid possible additive effects and hypercalcemia, vitamin D–related compounds should not be taken concomitantly with doxercalciferol. ▪ Serious hypersensitivity reactions, including fatal outcome, have been reported. ▪ Oversuppression of iPTH levels may lead to a dynamic bone syndrome. ▪ Hyperphosphatemia can exacerbate hyperparathyroidism. ▪ Use caution in patients with impaired hepatic function. More frequent monitoring of iPTH, calcium, and phosphorus levels is recommended. ▪ Patients with higher pretreatment serum levels of calcium (more than 10.5 mg/dL) or phosphorus (more than 6.9 mg/dL) may be more likely to experience hypercalcemia or hyperphosphatemia; see Contraindications.

Monitor: During initiation of therapy, obtain baseline serum iPTH, calcium, and phosphorus levels, and determine levels weekly during the early phase of treatment (i.e., first 12 weeks). For dialysis patients, serum or plasma iPTH and serum calcium, phosphorus, and alkaline phosphatase should be determined periodically. See Dose Adjustments. ▪ Calculate Ca × P (should be less than 55 mg^2/dL^2). ▪ Monitor serum calcium levels weekly after all dose changes and during subsequent dose titration. ▪ Monitor for signs and symptoms of hypercalcemia. See Side Effects. Radiographic evaluation of suspect anatomical regions may be useful in the early detection of generalized vascular or other soft-tissue calcification. ▪ Oral calcium-based or other non–aluminum-containing phosphate binders and a low phosphate diet are indicated to control serum phosphorus levels in dialysis patients. Hyperphosphatemia can lessen the effectiveness of doxercalciferol in reducing blood PTH levels. After initiating doxercalciferol therapy, the dose of calcium-containing phosphate binders should be decreased to correct persistent mild hypercalcemia (10.6 to 11.2 mg/dL for 3 consecutive determinations), or increased to correct persistent mild hyperphosphatemia (7 to 8 mg/dL for 3 consecutive determinations). ▪ Persistent or markedly elevated serum calcium levels may be corrected by dialysis against a reduced calcium or calcium-free dialysate. ▪ Monitor for S/S of hypersensitivity reactions (e.g., anaphylaxis with symptoms of angioedema [involving face, lips, tongue, and airways], cardiopulmonary arrest, chest discomfort, hypotension, shortness of breath, unresponsiveness). ▪ See Precautions and Drug/Lab Interactions.

Patient Education: Report symptoms of hypercalcemia promptly. Dose adjustment or treatment may be required. Strict adherence to dietary supplementation of calcium and restriction of phosphorus is required to ensure optimal effectiveness of therapy. Phosphate-binding compounds (e.g., calcium acetate, sevelamer) may be needed to control serum phosphorus levels in patients with CRF, but excessive use of aluminum-containing products (e.g., aluminum hydroxide gel) should be avoided. ▪ Review all nonprescription drugs with physician.

Maternal/Child: Category B: safety for use in pregnancy not established; use only if clearly needed. ▪ Discontinue breast-feeding. ▪ Safety and effectiveness for use in pediatric patients not established.

Elderly: No overall differences in effectiveness or safety observed.

DRUG/LAB INTERACTIONS

Specific interaction studies have not been performed. ▪ **Digoxin** toxicity is potentiated by hypercalcemia. Use caution when doxercalciferol is prescribed concomitantly with digoxin compounds. ▪ **Phosphate or vitamin D**–related compounds should not be taken concomitantly with doxercalciferol. ▪ May reduce serum total **alkaline phosphatase levels.** ▪ **Magnesium-containing antacids** may cause hypermagnesemia; concomitant use is not recommended. ▪ Concomitant use with **cytochrome P$_{450}$ enzyme inducers** (e.g., phenobarbital, phenytoin, rifampin) may affect hydroxylation of doxercalciferol and require dose adjustments. ▪ Concomitant use with **cytochrome P$_{450}$ enzyme inhibitors** (e.g., erythromycin, ketoconazole) may inhibit metabolism of the active form of vitamin D, decreasing effectiveness.

SIDE EFFECTS

Dose-limiting side effects are hypercalcemia, hyperphosphatemia, and oversuppression of iPTH (less than 150 pg/mL). Overdose or chronic administration may lead to hypercalcemia. Signs and symptoms of vitamin D intoxication associated with hypercalcemia include: *Early:* anorexia, bone pain, constipation, dry mouth, headache, metallic taste, muscle pain, nausea, somnolence, vomiting, and weakness. *Late:* albuminuria, anorexia, apathy, arrested growth, cardiac arrhythmias, conjunctivitis (calcific), death, decreased libido, dehydration, ectopic calcification, elevated AST and ALT, elevated BUN, hypercholesterolemia, hypertension, hyperthermia, nocturia, overt psychosis (rare), pancreatitis, photophobia, polydipsia, polyuria, pruritus, rhinorrhea, sensory disturbances, urinary tract infections, and weight loss.

Post-Marketing: Hypersensitivity reactions, including fatal outcome (e.g., anaphylaxis with symptoms of angioedema [involving face, lips, tongue, and airways], cardiopulmonary arrest, chest discomfort, hypotension, shortness of breath, unresponsiveness).

Overdose: Hypercalcemia, hypercalciuria, hyperphosphatemia, and oversuppression of PTH secretion leading in certain cases to adynamic bone disease. High intake of calcium and phosphate concomitant with doxercalciferol may lead to similar abnormalities. High levels of calcium in the dialysate bath may contribute to hypercalcemia.

ANTIDOTE

Notify physician of any side effects. Treatment of patients with clinically significant hypercalcemia (more than 1 mg/dL above the upper limit of normal range) consists of immediate dose reduction or interruption of the therapy and includes a low-calcium diet, withdrawal of calcium supplements, patient mobilization, attention to fluid and electrolyte imbalances, assessment of electrocardiographic abnormalities (critical in patients receiving digoxin), forced diuresis, and hemodialysis or peritoneal dialysis against a calcium-free dialysate, as warranted. Monitor serum calcium levels frequently until calcium levels return to within normal limits. Not removed from blood during hemodialysis. When serum calcium levels return to within normal limits (usually 2 to 7 days), therapy may be restarted at a dose that is at least 1 mcg lower than prior therapy. Should a hypersensitivity reaction occur, discontinue doxercalciferol and initiate appropriate treatment and monitoring as indicated.

DOXORUBICIN HYDROCHLORIDE BBW ▪ DOXORUBICIN HYDROCHLORIDE LIPOSOMAL INJECTION BBW

Antineoplastic (anthracycline antibiotic)

(dox-oh-**ROO**-bih-sin hy-droh-**KLOR**-eyed)
(dox-oh-**ROO**-bih-sin hy-droh-**KLOR**-eyed **LIP**-oh-sohm-ul)
ADR, Adriamycin ▪ Doxil

pH 3.8 to 6.5 ▪ pH 6.5

USUAL DOSE

Pretreatment: Verify pregnancy status. Assessment required before dosing; see Precautions and Monitor.

CONVENTIONAL DOXORUBICIN

60 to 75 mg/M^2 once every 21 days as a *single agent.* When used in *combination* with other agents, the most common dose of doxorubicin is 40 to 75 mg/M^2 every 21 to 28 days.

Breast cancer with lymph node involvement after resection: Doxorubicin 60 mg/M^2 in combination with cyclophosphamide 600 mg/M^2 given IV sequentially on Day 1 of each 21-day treatment cycle. Four cycles have been administered.

Adjuvant treatment of operable node-positive breast cancer: Treatment protocol includes doxorubicin, cyclophosphamide, and docetaxel. Administer doxorubicin 50 mg/M^2 and cyclophosphamide 500 mg/M^2. One hour later, give docetaxel 75 mg/M^2. Repeat every 3 weeks for 6 cycles. See docetaxel and cyclophosphamide monographs.

DOXIL (LIPOSOMAL DOXORUBICIN)

Do not substitute Doxil for conventional doxorubicin.

AIDS-related Kaposi's sarcoma: 20 mg/M^2 as an IV infusion over 60 minutes every 21 days until disease progression or unacceptable toxicity.

Ovarian cancer: 50 mg/M^2 as an IV infusion over 60 minutes every 28 days until disease progression or unacceptable toxicity.

Multiple myeloma: Given in combination with bortezomib (Velcade).

Bortezomib: Administer 1.3 mg/M^2 as an IV bolus on Days 1, 4, 8, and 11 of each 21-day cycle; see bortezomib monograph.

Doxil: Administer 30 mg/M^2 as an IV infusion over 60 minutes on Day 4 of each 21-day cycle following bortezomib. Continue regimen for 8 cycles or until disease progression or the occurrence of unacceptable toxicity.

Breast cancer (unlabeled): 50 mg/M^2 as an IV infusion over 60 minutes every 4 weeks. Other combination protocols are in use.

PEDIATRIC DOSE

CONVENTIONAL DOXORUBICIN:
In combination with other chemotherapeutic agents as first-line treatment, 30 to 60 mg/M^2 every 21 to 42 days. See Maternal/Child.

DOXIL:
Safety for use in pediatric patients not established.

DOSE ADJUSTMENTS

CONVENTIONAL DOXORUBICINS:
Reduce dose in patients with impaired hepatic function. *Elevated serum bilirubin:* Give 50% of above doses for serum bilirubin from 1.2 to 3 mg/mL and 25% of above doses for serum bilirubin above 3 mg/mL. Discontinue therapy for serum bilirubin greater than 5 mg/dL. ▪ See Precautions. ▪ Consider lower-end doses or longer intervals between cycles for heavily pretreated patients, elderly patients, or obese patients.

Breast cancer with lymph node involvement after resection: Reduce dose to 75% of the starting dose for neutropenic fever/infection. If necessary, delay the next cycle of treatment until the ANC is 1,000 cells/mm^3 or more and the platelet count is 100,000 cells/mm^3 or more and nonhematologic toxicities have resolved.

DOXIL: Reduce dose for serum bilirubin of 1.2 or higher. ▪ Dose adjustments are required in hematologic toxicity (see the following chart) and in patients with stomatitis or

hand-foot syndrome (HFS) (see product literature for guidelines). Adjust or delay a dose as described in the product literature at the first sign of a Grade 1 or higher adverse event.
- Do not increase Doxil dose after a dose reduction for toxicity.

	Doxil Dosing Based on Hematologic Toxicity (Neutropenia or Thrombocytopenia)
Grade	**Modification**
1	No dose reduction.
2	Delay until ANC ≥1,500 and platelets ≥75,000; resume treatment at previous dose.
3	Delay until ANC ≥1,500 and platelets ≥75,000; resume treatment at previous dose.
4	Delay until ANC ≥1,500 and platelets ≥75,000; resume at 25% dose reduction or continue previous dose with prophylactic granulocyte growth factor.

Dose adjustments for Doxil in combination therapy with bortezomib for treatment of multiple myeloma are listed in the following chart. See bortezomib monograph for bortezomib dose adjustments.

Dose Adjustments for Doxil in Combination Therapy With Bortezomib	
Patient Status	**Doxil**
Fever ≥38° C and ANC <1,000/mm³	Withhold dose for this cycle if before Day 4. Decrease dose by 25% if after Day 4 of previous cycle.
On any day of drug administration after Day 1 of each cycle: • Platelet count <25,000/mm³ • Hemoglobin <8 Gm/dL • ANC <500/mm³	Withhold dose for this cycle if before Day 4. Decrease dose by 25% if after Day 4 of previous cycle AND if bortezomib is reduced for hematologic toxicity.
Grade 3 or 4 nonhematologic drug-related toxicity	Do not dose until recovered to Grade <2, then reduce dose by 25%.
Neuropathic pain or peripheral neuropathy	No dose adjustments for Doxil. Refer to bortezomib prescribing information.

DILUTION

Specific techniques required; see Precautions.

Conventional Doxorubicin: Each 10 mg must be diluted with 5 mL of NS to obtain a final concentration of 2 mg/mL. Do not use bacteriostatic diluent. Shake gently to dissolve completely. Also available in preservative-free solutions. May be further diluted in 50 mL or more D5W or NS and given as a continuous infusion through a central venous line.

DOXIL: Doses up to 90 mg must be diluted in 250 mL D5W. Not a clear solution, but a translucent red liposomal dispersion. Do not use filters. Doses over 90 mg should be diluted in 500 mL D5W. See Compatibility.

Filters: *Conventional doxorubicin:* Data not available from manufacturer; however, one source indicates no evidence of drug loss when administered through a 0.2-micron in-line nylon filter, and another source indicates no significant drug loss using various types of 0.2-micron filters.

Doxil: Do not use filters during preparation or administration.

Storage: *Conventional doxorubicin:* Retain vials in carton until time of use. Refrigerate unopened vials containing solution. Refrigeration can result in the formation of a gelled product. If this occurs, place vial at RT for 2 to 4 hours to return the product to a slightly viscous mobile solution. Vials containing lyophilized powder may be stored at CRT. All forms should be protected from light.

Doxil: Refrigerate unopened vials at 2° to 8° C (36° to 46° F). Do not freeze. Refrigerate diluted solution and use within 24 hours.

COMPATIBILITY

CONVENTIONAL DOXORUBICIN

Manufacturer lists fluorouracil and heparin as **incompatible** and states mixing with other drugs is not recommended unless specific **compatibility** data available. Avoid contact with alkaline solutions; can lead to hydrolysis of doxorubicin.

Other sources suggest specific **compatibilities** dependent on concentration and manufacturer; consult a pharmacist.

DOXIL

Manufacturer states, "Do not mix Doxil with other drugs. Do not use any other diluent (use D5W only). Do not use any bacteriostatic agents (e.g., benzyl alcohol)."

Other sources suggest specific **compatibilities** dependent on concentration and manufacturer; consult a pharmacist.

RATE OF ADMINISTRATION

CONVENTIONAL DOXORUBICIN

IV injection: A single dose of properly diluted medication over a minimum of 3 to 10 minutes. Should be given through a central line or a secure and free-flowing peripheral venous line containing NS, $^1/_2$ NS, or D5W. Slow injection rate further for erythematous streaking along the vein or facial flushing.

Continuous infusion: Central venous line required. Equally distributed over time interval outlined in given protocol.

DOXIL

Do not administer as an undiluted suspension or as an IV bolus. For IV infusion only. Rapid infusion may increase risk of acute infusion-related reactions. Primarily occurs during the first infusion; may resolve with a reduced rate or may take up to a day after infusion completed to resolve.

Begin with an initial rate of 1 mg/min to minimize the risk of infusion reactions. If no adverse infusion-related effects, the rate may be increased from the initial rate of 1 mg/min to evenly distribute and complete infusion over 1 hour. Avoid rapid flushing of the infusion line.

ACTIONS

CONVENTIONAL DOXORUBICIN: A highly cytotoxic anthracycline topoisomerase II inhibitor that is cell-cycle specific for the S phase. Widely distributed and rapidly cleared from plasma, it interferes with cell division by binding with DNA to slow production of nucleic acid synthesis. Metabolized in the liver. Elimination half-life is 20 to 48 hours. Does not cross blood-brain barrier. Slowly excreted in bile and urine. Secreted in breast milk.

DOXIL: Doxorubicin encapsulated in long-circulating STEALTH liposomes (phospholipids). The small size of these liposomes and their persistence in the circulation enable them to evade immune system detection and penetrate the often altered and/or compromised vasculature of tumors. Once distributed to tumor tissue, the doxorubicin is released by an unknown mechanism. It differs from conventional doxorubicin because it mostly confines itself to vascular fluid volume. Metabolized and eliminated renally. Plasma clearance is slower. Half-life is extended to 55 hours. Concentration in Kaposi's sarcoma lesions is much higher than in normal skin (range is 3 to 53 times higher).

INDICATIONS AND USES

CONVENTIONAL DOXORUBICIN: Adjuvant therapy in females with evidence of axillary lymph node involvement following resection of primary breast cancer. ▪ Treatment of acute lymphoblastic leukemia, acute myeloblastic leukemia, Hodgkin lymphoma, non-Hodgkin lymphoma, metastatic breast cancer, metastatic Wilms' tumor, metastatic neuroblastoma, metastatic soft tissue sarcoma, metastatic bone sarcoma, metastatic ovarian carcinoma, metastatic transitional cell bladder carcinoma, metastatic thyroid carcinoma, metastatic gastric carcinoma, metastatic bronchogenic carcinoma.

DOXIL: Treatment of AIDS-related Kaposi's sarcoma in patients after failure of prior systemic chemotherapy or in patients who are intolerant to such therapy. ▪ Treatment of patients with ovarian cancer whose disease has progressed or recurred after platinum-based chemotherapy (e.g., cisplatin, carboplatin). ▪ Treatment of multiple myeloma in combination with bortezomib (Velcade) in patients who have received one prior therapy but have not previously received bortezomib.

Unlabeled uses: *Doxil:* Treatment of refractory metastatic breast cancer.

CONTRAINDICATIONS

CONVENTIONAL DOXORUBICIN: Severe myocardial insufficiency, recent myocardial infarction (occurring within the last 4 to 6 weeks), severe persistent drug-induced myelosuppression, severe hepatic impairment (Child-Pugh Class C or serum bilirubin level greater than 5 mg/dL).

ALL DOXORUBICINS: History of hypersensitivity to conventional or liposomal formulations of doxorubicin or to their components.

PRECAUTIONS

ALL DOXORUBICINS: Follow guidelines for handling cytotoxic agents and patient excreta. Precautions recommended for up to 5 days after a dose. See Appendix A, p. 1308. ■ Usually administered by or under the direction of a physician specialist, with facilities for monitoring the patient and responding to any medical emergency. ■ For IV use only. Do not give IM or SQ. ■ *Do Not Substitute* Doxil for conventional doxorubicin. Severe side effects have resulted. Differences in liposomal products as well as conventional products can substantially affect the functional properties of these agents; do not substitute one agent for another. ■ Use extreme caution in pre-existing drug-induced bone marrow suppression, existing heart disease, hepatic impairment, previous treatment with other anthracyclines (e.g., daunorubicin), anthracenediones (e.g., mitoxantrone), other cardiotoxic agents (e.g., bleomycin), concurrent cyclophosphamide therapy, or radiation therapy encompassing the heart; risk of cardiotoxicity increased and may occur at lower doses. ■ All forms of doxorubicin may cause cardiotoxicity. May be manifest by acute (e.g., arrhythmias, including life-threatening arrhythmias, ECG abnormalities) or delayed (e.g., reduction in LVEF, CHF) events. Life-threatening or fatal left ventricular failure may occur during therapy or months after therapy is completed. Cardiotoxicity occurs with increasing frequency as cumulative doses increase above 300 mg/M^2. The risk of developing CHF increases rapidly with increasing total cumulative doses above 400 mg/M^2; see Antidote. Prior use of other anthracyclines or anthracenediones should be included in calculations of total cumulative dose. Patients with active or dormant cardiovascular disease or patients who have received radiotherapy to the mediastinal area or concomitant therapy with other anthracyclines (e.g., daunorubicin, idarubicin), anthracenediones, or other cardiotoxic agents (e.g., bleomycin, cyclophosphamide, mitoxantrone, mitomycin C, trastuzumab) may be at greater risk. Patients receiving doxorubicin after stopping treatment with trastuzumab may also be at an increased risk of developing cardiotoxicity. Trastuzumab may persist in the circulation for up to 7 months. When possible, avoid anthracycline-based therapy for up to 7 months after stopping trastuzumab. If anthracyclines are used before this time, carefully monitor cardiac function. Consider the use of dexrazoxane to reduce the incidence and severity of cardiomyopathy due to doxorubicin in patients who have received a cumulative dose of 300 mg/M^2 and who will continue to receive doxorubicin. ■ May cause severe myelosuppression resulting in serious infection, septic shock, required transfusions, hospitalization, hemorrhage, and death. ■ See Maternal/Child and Side Effects.

CONVENTIONAL DOXORUBICIN: In addition to cardiomyopathy, pericarditis and myocarditis have been reported during or after therapy with doxorubicin. ■ Secondary acute myelogenous leukemia (AML) and myelodysplastic syndrome (MDS) have been reported and generally occur within 1 to 3 years of treatment. ■ Tumor lysis syndrome may occur; see Monitor.

DOXIL: Benefits must outweigh risks if Doxil is used in patients with a history of cardiovascular disease. ■ Serious, life-threatening and fatal infusion-related reactions and serious, sometimes life-threatening or fatal hypersensitivity/anaphylactoid-like reactions have been reported; see Monitor. ■ Has caused hand-foot syndrome (HFS). Incidence may be increased with higher doses or increased frequency. Generally seen after 2 or 3 cycles but may occur earlier. May be severe and require a dose adjustment or discontinuation of Doxil. ■ Secondary oral cancers, primarily squamous cell carcinoma, have been reported in patients who have received Doxil for a year or longer. Malignancies have been diagnosed both during treatment and up to 6 years after completion of therapy. ■ Severe, additive myelosuppression may occur in Kaposi's sarcoma patients and may be dose limiting.

Monitor: ALL DOXORUBICINS: Monitoring of CBC including differential and platelet count, uric acid levels, electrolytes, liver function (AST, ALT, alkaline phosphatase, and bilirubin), kidney function, ECG, chest x-ray, echocardiogram, and left ventricular ejection fraction (LVEF) is necessary before and during therapy. At a minimum, CBC with platelets should be monitored before each dose. Testing for renal and hepatic function may also be indicated; see Dose Adjustments. ▪ Observe for S/S of cardiotoxicity (e.g., fast or irregular HR, shortness of breath, swelling of the feet or lower legs). Endomyocardial biopsy or gated radionuclide scans have been used to monitor potential cardiac toxicity. Increase frequency of assessment as cumulative dose exceeds 300 mg/M^2. Use same method of assessment of LVEF at all time points. ▪ Be alert for signs of bone marrow suppression, bleeding, or infection. ▪ Monitor for thrombocytopenia (platelet count less than 50,000/mm^3). Initiate precautions to prevent excessive bleeding (e.g., inspect IV sites, skin, and mucous membranes; use extreme care during invasive procedures; test urine, emesis, stool, and secretions for occult blood). ▪ Use of prophylactic antibiotics may be indicated pending C/S in a febrile, neutropenic patient. Sepsis in a neutropenic patient has resulted in discontinuation of treatment and, in rare cases, death. ▪ Prophylactic antiemetics are indicated. ▪ See Drug/Lab Interactions.

CONVENTIONAL DOXORUBICIN: Monitor for tumor lysis syndrome. S/S include hyperkalemia, hyperphosphatemia, hyperuricemia, hypocalcemia, metabolic acidosis, urate crystalluria, and renal failure. Prevent or alleviate tumor lysis syndrome with appropriate supportive and pharmacologic measures. ▪ Maintain adequate hydration. ▪ Uric acid–lowering drugs (e.g., allopurinol [Aloprim]) may prevent formation of uric acid crystals. ▪ Use only large veins. Avoid veins over joints or in extremities with compromised venous or lymphatic drainage. Determine absolute patency of vein. A stinging or burning sensation indicates extravasation; severe cellulitis and tissue necrosis will result. *Extravasation may occur with or without stinging or burning and even if blood returns well on aspiration of infusion needle.* Observe and touch site frequently to feel air and/or liquid under the skin. If extravasation occurs, discontinue injection; use another vein; see Antidote.

DOXIL: Monitor for S/S of acute infusion reactions and/or hypersensitivity (e.g., apnea, asthma, back pain, bronchospasm, chills, cyanosis, facial swelling, fever, flushing, headache, hypotension, pruritus, rash, shortness of breath, syncope, tachycardia, tightness in the chest or throat). The majority of infusion-related reactions occur during the first infusion. ▪ Monitor for HFS (skin eruptions characterized by swelling, pain, erythema, and possible desquamation of the skin on the hands and feet). ▪ Monitor for the presence of oral ulceration or oral discomfort that may be indicative of secondary oral cancer. ▪ Extravasation may cause irritation at infusion site. Discontinue and use another vein.

Patient Education: ALL DOXORUBICINS: Urine and other body fluids will be reddish for several days (from dye, not hematuria). ▪ Effective birth control required for females of reproductive potential during treatment and for 6 months after the last dose and for males with female partners of reproductive potential during treatment and for 3 months after the last dose. May cause infertility in both males and females. ▪ Effects may be additive with current medications. Review all medications (prescription and nonprescription) with nurse and/or physician. ▪ Promptly report cough, fast heartbeat, shortness of breath, and/or swelling of the feet or lower legs. ▪ Report S/S of infection (e.g., chills, fever, painful urination), stomatitis, bothersome side effects, or any unusual bleeding (e.g., bruising, tarry stools). ▪ Report IV site burning, stinging, puffiness, or the feeling of liquid under the skin and any other side effects promptly. ▪ Report tingling, burning, redness, flaking, swelling, blisters or small sores on the palms of hands or soles of feet. ▪ See Precautions. ▪ See Appendix D, p. 1311.

Maternal/Child: ALL DOXORUBICINS: Avoid pregnancy. Based on its mechanism of action, can cause fetal harm. ▪ Has been used only when benefits outweigh risks (see Doxil). ▪ Discontinue breast-feeding during treatment and for 10 days after the final dose.

CONVENTIONAL DOXORUBICIN: Treatment during childhood may result in abnormal cardiac function. ▪ Infants and children are at increased risk for developing delayed cardiotoxicity; follow-up cardiac evaluation is recommended; see Precautions. ▪ In infants under 2 years of age, doxorubicin clearance is similar to adults, but clearance may be increased in pediatric patients over 2 years of age. ▪ May contribute to prepubertal growth failure and/or gonadal impairment (which is usually temporary). ▪ See Precautions, extended recommendations for handling patient excreta.

Doxil: If use during pregnancy is considered, avoid use during the first trimester. ▪ Safety for use in pediatric patients not established.

Elderly: All Doxorubicins: Response similar to that seen in younger adults, but greater sensitivity of some older individuals cannot be ruled out. ▪ Cardiotoxicity and myelotoxicity may be more severe in patients over 70 years of age. ▪ Consider age-related organ impairment and concomitant disease and/or drug therapy; see Dose Adjustments.

DRUG/LAB INTERACTIONS

Studies not yet completed for Doxil; interactions may be similar to conventional doxorubicins. ▪ Doxorubicin is a major substrate for cytochrome P_{450} CYP3A4 and CYP2D6 and P-glycoprotein. Clinically significant interactions have been reported with inhibitors of CYP3A4 and CYP2D6 and P-glycoprotein (e.g., **verapamil**), resulting in increased concentrations and clinical effects of doxorubicin. Inducers of CYP3A4 (e.g., **phenobarbital, phenytoin, St. John's wort**) and P-glycoprotein may decrease the concentration of doxorubicin. Avoid concurrent use with **inhibitors or inducers of CYP3A4 and CYP2D6 and P-glycoprotein.** ▪ Avoid concurrent administration of doxorubicin and **trastuzumab**; results in an increased risk of cardiac dysfunction. Patients receiving doxorubicin after stopping treatment with trastuzumab may also be at an increased risk of developing cardiotoxicity. Trastuzumab may persist in the circulation for up to 7 months. When possible, avoid anthracycline-based therapy for up to 7 months after stopping trastuzumab. If anthracyclines are used before this time, carefully monitor cardiac function. ▪ May exacerbate **cyclophosphamide**-induced hemorrhagic cystitis or increase hepatotoxicity of **6-mercaptopurine.** ▪ May increase bone marrow toxicity of **other chemotherapeutic agents and radiation.** ▪ **Barbiturates** increase clearance and decrease effects. ▪ May decrease serum levels of **digoxin.** ▪ May decrease serum levels of **anticonvulsants** (e.g., phenytoin, carbamazepine, valproate). ▪ Risk of cardiotoxicity increased in patients previously treated with **other anthracyclines** (e.g., idarubicin) **and/or radiation encompassing the heart.** ▪ **Cyclosporine and streptozocin** may decrease clearance and increase toxicity of doxorubicin. ▪ **Paclitaxel** appears to decrease the clearance of doxorubicin. Administration of doxorubicin before paclitaxel is recommended to prevent increased toxicity. ▪ Coadministration with high-dose **progesterone** may increase doxorubicin toxicity. ▪ Many drug interactions possible; observe patient closely. ▪ Do not administer **live virus vaccines** to patients receiving antineoplastic drugs. ▪ Increased toxicity to mucosa, myocardium, skin (including redness and exfoliative changes), and liver possible when given concurrently **with or after radiation.** ▪ **Dexrazoxane** is given with doxorubicin to reduce cardiotoxic effects. May also decrease antitumor effectiveness if given before a cumulative dose of doxorubicin 300 mg/M^2 is reached or other chemotherapeutic agents are included in the protocol (e.g., fluorouracil). ▪ See Precautions.

SIDE EFFECTS

All Doxorubicins: Abdominal pain; alopecia (complete); anorexia; asthenia; bone marrow suppression (e.g., anemia, hypochromic anemia, leukopenia, neutropenia [ANC less than 1,000/mm^3], thrombocytopenia may be dose-limiting); cardiac toxicity (e.g., CHF); constipation; decreased serum calcium; depressed QRS voltage; diarrhea; dry skin; esophagitis; fatigue; fever; gonadal suppression; headache; hyperpigmentation of nail beds and dermal creases; hypersensitivity reactions (including life-threatening or fatal anaphylaxis); hyperuricemia; increase in alkaline phosphatase, ALT, AST, bilirubin, BUN, glucose, SCr; infection; mucositis; nausea; oral moniliasis; paresthesia; prolonged PT; rash; recall of skin reactions due to prior radiotherapy; stomatitis; weakness; vomiting.

Doxil: In addition to all of the above, acute infusion reactions, hand-foot syndrome, secondary oral cancer. *Kaposi's sarcoma* patients may be taking numerous other drugs that may confuse the overall side effect picture (e.g., didanosine [ddI], stavudine [D4T], sulfamethoxazole/trimethoprim, zalcitabine [ddC], zidovudine [AZT, Retrovir]).

Post-Marketing: Muscle spasms, myelogenous leukemia, pulmonary embolism, and skin and subcutaneous tissue disorders (e.g., erythema multiforme, Stevens-Johnson syndrome, and toxic epidermal necrolysis).

Overdose: ALL DOXORUBICINS: Increase in bone marrow suppression and mucositis.

ANTIDOTE

ALL DOXORUBICINS: Most side effects will either be tolerated or treated symptomatically. Keep the physician informed. Bone marrow toxicity may require cessation of therapy. Administration of whole blood products (e.g., packed RBCs, platelets, leukocytes) and/or blood modifiers (e.g., darbepoetin alfa, epoetin alfa, filgrastim, pegfilgrastim, sargramostim) may be indicated to treat bone marrow toxicity. Acute cardiac failure occurs suddenly (most common when total cumulative dosage approaches 550 mg/M^2) and frequently does not respond to currently available treatment (digoxin, diuretics [e.g., furosemide], ACE inhibitors [e.g., enalapril]). Close monitoring of accumulated dosage, bone marrow, ECG, chest x-ray, echocardiography, and systolic ejection fraction may prevent most serious and potentially fatal cardiac side effects. There is no specific antidote. Supportive therapy as indicated will help sustain the patient in toxicity. Treat hypersensitivity reactions as required; discontinue therapy if severe.

CONVENTIONAL DOXORUBICIN: Discontinue doxorubicin in patients who develop signs or symptoms of cardiomyopathy. For extravasation, attempt to aspirate extravasated fluid before removing needle. Do not flush line or apply pressure to site. Elevate the extremity and apply ice for 15 minutes four times a day for 3 days. If appropriate, administer dexrazoxane at the site of extravasation as soon as possible and within the first 6 hours after extravasation. Site should be observed promptly by a reconstructive surgeon.

DOXIL: In addition to all of the above, treatment may have to be interrupted or discontinued for severe hand-foot syndrome or acute infusion reactions. Infusion reactions may resolve with slowing of infusion rate. May be able to control hand-foot syndrome by allowing it to resolve and by increasing intervals between subsequent cycles. For extravasation, discontinue infusion and apply ice over site for 30 minutes to alleviate local reaction.

DOXYCYCLINE HYCLATE
(dox-ih-**SYE**-kleen **HI**-klayt)

Antibacterial
(tetracycline)
Antiprotozoal
Antimalarial

Doxy 100, Doxy 200, Vibramycin

pH 1.8 to 3.3

USUAL DOSE

Pretreatment: Verify pregnancy status; see Contraindications.

Parenteral therapy is indicated only when oral therapy is not indicated. Transfer to oral therapy as soon as practical.

ADULTS AND PEDIATRIC PATIENTS WEIGHING 45 KG OR MORE

200 mg the first day in one or two infusions followed by 100 to 200 mg/24 hr on subsequent days with 200 mg administered in one or two infusions. Depends on severity of the infection.

Primary and secondary syphilis: 300 mg daily for at least 10 days.

Acute pelvic inflammatory disease: 100 mg every 12 hours. Used in combination with cefoxitin 2 Gm every 6 hours.

Treatment of inhalational anthrax (postexposure): 100 mg every 12 hours. Continue therapy for 60 days.

PEDIATRIC DOSE
ALL DOSES ARE FOR PEDIATRIC PATIENTS WEIGHING LESS THAN 45 KG
4.4 mg/kg of body weight on the first day of treatment, administered in one or two infusions. Subsequent daily dose is 2.2 mg/kg to 4.4 mg/kg of body weight/day given as one or two infusions depending on the severity of the infection. Transfer to oral therapy as soon as practical. Do not exceed adult dose. See Maternal/Child.

Treatment of inhalational anthrax (postexposure): 2.2 mg/kg of body weight every 12 hours. Do not exceed adult dose. Continue therapy for 60 days.

DOSE ADJUSTMENTS
See Drug/Lab Interactions.

DILUTION
Each 100 mg or fraction thereof is diluted with 10 mL of SWFI or NS (may also be reconstituted with any of the **compatible** solutions listed for further dilution). Further dilute each 100 mg (10 mL) with 100 to 1,000 mL of a **compatible** infusion solution such as NS, D5W, R, LR, D5LR, 10% invert sugar in water, Normosol-M or Normosol-R in 5% dextrose in water, or other **compatible** solutions (see literature). Recommended concentrations 0.1 to 1 mg/mL. 100 mg in 1,000 mL of solution equals 0.1 mg/mL, 100 mg in 100 mL equals 1 mg/mL.

Storage: Store vials at CRT in carton; protect from light. Stable for 48 hours when diluted with NS or D5W to concentrations between 0.1 and 1 mg/mL and stored at 25° C (77° F). Protect from direct sunlight during storage and infusion. These dilutions may be stored for 72 hours if refrigerated and protected from sunlight *and* artificial light. Infusion must be completed within 12 hours. Solutions must be used within these time periods or discarded. See manufacturer's prescribing information for stability data when mixed with other solutions.

COMPATIBILITY
Compatibility information not available from manufacturer.

Other sources suggest specific **compatibilities** dependent on concentration and manufacturer; consult a pharmacist.

RATE OF ADMINISTRATION
Avoid rapid administration. Duration of infusion may vary with dose but is usually 1 to 4 hours. The recommended minimum infusion time for 100 mg of a 0.5 mg/mL solution is 1 hour.

ACTIONS
A broad-spectrum tetracycline antibiotic, bacteriostatic against many microorganisms, including gram-positive, gram-negative, anaerobic, atypical, and parasitic organisms. Thought to interfere with the protein synthesis of microorganisms. Doxycycline is well distributed in most body tissues and is highly bound to plasma protein. Half-life is 18 to 22 hours. Concentrated by the liver in the bile and excreted in urine and feces. Crosses the placental barrier. Secreted in breast milk.

INDICATIONS AND USES
Infections caused by susceptible strains of several microorganisms, including many gram-positive, gram-negative, anaerobic, atypical bacteria (e.g., *Rickettsia, Chlamydia, Chlamydophila, Mycoplasma*) or parasites (e.g., *Balantidium coli, Entamoeba* species). Types of infections treated may include GU infections, including those caused by *Chlamydia trachomatis* and *Neisseria gonorrhoeae;* respiratory tract infections, including *Mycoplasma pneumonia;* skin and soft tissue infections; syphilis; and others. ■ To substitute for contraindicated penicillin or sulfonamide therapy. ■ Adjunct to amebicides in acute intestinal amebiasis. ■ Prevention and/or treatment of anthrax in all its forms, including cutaneous and inhalation anthrax postexposure.

CONTRAINDICATIONS
Known hypersensitivity to tetracyclines. Not recommended in pediatric patients under 8 years or in pregnancy or breast-feeding.

PRECAUTIONS

Sensitivity studies indicated to determine susceptibility of the causative organism to doxycycline. ■ To reduce the development of drug-resistant bacteria and maintain its effectiveness, doxycycline should be used to treat or prevent only those infections proven or strongly suspected to be caused by bacteria. ■ Continue for at least 2 to 3 days after all symptoms of infection subside. ■ Avoid prolonged use of drug; superinfection caused by overgrowth of nonsusceptible organisms may result. ■ *Clostridium difficile*–associated diarrhea (CDAD) has been reported. May range from mild to life threatening. Consider in patients who present with diarrhea during or after treatment with doxycycline. ■ Initiate oral therapy as soon as possible. ■ Cross-resistance with other tetracyclines is common. ■ Intracranial hypertension (IH, pseudotumor cerebri) has been associated with the use of tetracyclines, including doxycycline. Clinical manifestations include headache, blurred vision, diplopia, vision loss, and papilledema. Females of childbearing age who are overweight or have a history of IH are at greater risk for developing tetracycline-associated IH. ■ In venereal diseases in which coexistent syphilis is suspected, perform a dark-field examination before initiating treatment. Repeat blood serology monthly for at least 4 months. ■ The antianabolic action of tetracyclines may cause an increase in BUN. Studies to date indicate that this does not occur with the use of doxycycline in patients with impaired renal function. ■ All infections due to group A beta-hemolytic streptococci should be treated for at least 10 days.

Monitor: Determine absolute patency of vein and avoid extravasation; thrombophlebitis may occur. ■ Monitor for S/S of intracranial hypertension. If visual symptoms develop during treatment with doxycycline, prompt ophthalmologic evaluation is warranted. Intracranial pressure can remain elevated for weeks after drug cessation. Continue ophthalmologic monitoring until patient stabilizes. Permanent vision loss can occur. ■ Monitor hematopoietic, renal, and hepatic studies periodically in long-term therapy. ■ Monitor for S/S of hypersensitivity reactions. ■ See Drug/Lab Interactions.

Patient Education: Report severe diarrhea, S/S of hypersensitivity reactions, or S/S of IH promptly. ■ Alert patient to photosensitive skin reaction. ■ Consider birth control options.

Maternal/Child: Avoid pregnancy; see Contraindications. ■ May cause retardation of skeletal development in the fetus and in infants. ■ Exposure during the last half of pregnancy, infancy, and childhood to the age of 8 years may cause permanent discoloration of the teeth. Avoid exposure in this age-group unless potential benefits are expected to outweigh the risks in severe or life-threatening infections (e.g., anthrax, Rocky Mountain spotted fever), particularly when there are no alternative therapies. ■ Discontinue breast-feeding.

DRUG/LAB INTERACTIONS

May render **oral contraceptives** less effective; may result in pregnancy or breakthrough bleeding. ■ Interferes with bactericidal action of **all penicillins** (e.g., ampicillin, oxacillin). Avoid concomitant use. ■ Serum levels decreased by **barbiturates, carbamazepine, hydantoins** (e.g., phenytoin), and others. ■ May depress **plasma prothrombin activity;** a reduction in **anticoagulant** dose may be indicated. ■ Avoid concomitant use with **isotretinoin**.

SIDE EFFECTS

Relatively nontoxic in average doses. More toxic in large doses or if given too rapidly. Anogenital lesions, anorexia, blood dyscrasias (eosinophilia, hemolytic anemia, neutropenia, thrombocytopenia), diarrhea, dysphagia, elevated BUN, enterocolitis, glossitis, nausea, skin rashes, vomiting.

Major: Hypersensitivity reactions (including anaphylaxis, angioneurotic edema, exacerbation of systemic lupus erythematosus, pericarditis, and urticaria), bulging fontanels in infants, CDAD, drug rash with eosinophilia and systemic symptoms (DRESS), exfoliative dermatitis, hepatotoxicity, intracranial hypertension (blurred vision, diplopia, headache, papilledema, vision loss), photosensitivity, systemic candidiasis, thrombophlebitis.

ANTIDOTE

Notify the physician of all side effects. If minor side effects are progressive or any major side effect occurs, discontinue the drug, treat hypersensitivity reactions as indicated, or resuscitate as necessary. Mild cases of CDAD may respond to discontinuation of doxycycline. Treat antibiotic-related CDAD with fluid, electrolytes, protein supplements, and appropriate antibiotics (e.g., oral vancomycin) as indicated. Not removed by hemodialysis.

DURVALUMAB

(dur-**VAL**-ue-mab)

Imfinzi

Antineoplastic agent
Monoclonal antibody (Anti-PD-L1)

USUAL DOSE

Pretreatment: Baseline studies indicated; see Monitor.

Premedication: May be considered in subsequent infusions in patients who experience a Grade 1 or 2 infusion-related reaction.

Urothelial carcinoma: 10 mg/kg as an IV infusion over 60 minutes every 2 weeks until disease progression or unacceptable toxicity.

Non–small-cell lung cancer: 10 mg/kg as an IV infusion over 60 minutes every 2 weeks until disease progression, unacceptable toxicity, or a maximum of 12 months.

DOSE ADJUSTMENTS

No dose reductions are recommended for durvalumab. Withhold and/or discontinue durvalumab to manage adverse reactions as described in the following chart.

Recommended Treatment Modifications for Durvalumab Adverse Reactions			
Treatment-Related Adverse Reaction	**Severity of Adverse Reaction[a]**	**Durvalumab Treatment Modification**	**Corticosteroid Treatment Unless Otherwise Specified**
Pneumonitis	Grade 2	Withhold dose until Grade 1 or resolved and corticosteroid dose is less than 10 mg/day (or equivalent)[b]	Initial dose of 1 to 2 mg/kg/day prednisone or equivalent followed by a taper
	Grade 3 or 4	Permanently discontinue	Initial dose of 1 to 4 mg/kg/day prednisone or equivalent followed by a taper
Hepatitis	ALT or AST >3 but ≤8 × ULN or total bilirubin >1.5 but ≤5 × ULN	Withhold dose until Grade 1 or resolved and corticosteroid dose is less than 10 mg/day (or equivalent)[b]	Initial dose of 1 to 2 mg/kg/day prednisone or equivalent followed by a taper
	ALT or AST >8 × ULN or total bilirubin >5 × ULN OR Concurrent ALT or AST >3 × ULN and total bilirubin >2 × ULN with no other cause	Permanently discontinue	

Recommended Treatment Modifications for Durvalumab Adverse Reactions —cont'd			
Treatment-Related Adverse Reaction	**Severity of Adverse Reaction[a]**	**Durvalumab Treatment Modification**	**Corticosteroid Treatment Unless Otherwise Specified**
Colitis or diarrhea	Grade 2	Withhold dose until Grade 1 or resolved and corticosteroid dose is less than 10 mg/day (or equivalent)[b]	Initial dose of 1 to 2 mg/kg/day prednisone or equivalent followed by a taper
	Grade 3 or 4	Permanently discontinue	
Hypothyroidism	Grades 2 to 4		Initiate thyroid hormone replacement as clinically indicated
Hyperthyroidism	Grades 2 to 4	Withhold dose until clinically stable	Medical management
Adrenal insufficiency, hypophysitis/ hypopituitarism	Grades 2 to 4	Withhold dose until clinically stable	Initiate 1 to 2 mg/kg/day prednisone or equivalent followed by a taper and hormone replacement as clinically indicated
Type 1 diabetes mellitus	Grades 2 to 4	Withhold dose until clinically stable	Initiate treatment with insulin as clinically indicated
Nephritis	Creatinine >1.5 to 3 × ULN	Withhold dose until Grade 1 or resolved and corticosteroid dose is less than 10 mg/day (or equivalent)[b]	Initial dose of 1 to 2 mg/kg/day prednisone or equivalent followed by a taper
	Creatinine >3 × ULN	Permanently discontinue	
Rash or dermatitis	Grade 2 for >1 week or Grade 3	Withhold dose until Grade 1 or resolved and corticosteroid dose is less than 10 mg/day (or equivalent)[b]	Consider initial dose of 1 to 2 mg/kg/day prednisone or equivalent followed by a taper
	Grade 4	Permanently discontinue	
Infection	Grade 3 or 4	Withhold dose until clinically stable	Treat with anti-infectives for suspected or confirmed infections
Infusion-related reactions	Grade 1 or 2	Interrupt or slow the rate of the infusion	Consider premedications with subsequent doses
	Grade 3 or 4	Permanently discontinue	

Continued

	Recommended Treatment Modifications for Durvalumab Adverse Reactions—cont'd		
Treatment-Related Adverse Reaction	**Severity of Adverse Reaction[a]**	**Durvalumab Treatment Modification**	**Corticosteroid Treatment Unless Otherwise Specified**
Other immune-mediated adverse reactions	Grade 3	Withhold dose until Grade 1 or resolved and corticosteroid dose is less than 10 mg/day (or equivalent)[b]	Initial dose of 1 to 2 mg/kg/day prednisone or equivalent followed by a taper
	Grade 4	Permanently discontinue	Consider initial dose of 1 to 4 mg/kg/day prednisone or equivalent followed by a taper
Persistent Grade 2 or 3 adverse reactions (excluding endocrinopathies)	Grade 2 or 3 adverse reaction that does not recover to Grade 0 or 1 within 12 weeks after last durvalumab dose	Permanently discontinue	
Inability to taper corticosteroids	Inability to reduce to prednisone ≤10 mg/day (or equivalent) within 12 weeks after last durvalumab dose	Permanently discontinue	
Recurrent Grade 3 or 4 adverse reaction	Recurrent Grade 3 or 4 (severe or life-threatening) adverse reaction	Permanently discontinue	

[a]Toxicity was graded per the National Cancer Institute Common Terminology Criteria for Adverse Events (CTCAE), Version 4.03.

[b]Based on the severity of the adverse reactions, durvalumab should be withheld and corticosteroids administered. For adverse reactions that do not result in permanent discontinuation, resume treatment when adverse reaction returns to ≤Grade 1, and the corticosteroid dose has been reduced to ≤10 mg prednisone or equivalent per day.

- No pharmacokinetic differences were observed in patient subgroups defined by age, body weight, gender, albumin levels, LDH levels, creatinine levels, race, soluble PD-L1, tumor type, mild renal impairment (CrCl 60 to 89 mL/min), moderate renal impairment (CrCl 30 to 59 mL/min), mild hepatic impairment (bilirubin less than or equal to the ULN and AST greater than the ULN or bilirubin greater than 1 to 1.5 times the ULN and any AST), or ECOG performance status. ■ The effect of severe renal impairment (CrCl 15 to 29 mL/min), moderate hepatic impairment (bilirubin greater than 1.5 to 3 times the ULN and any AST), or severe hepatic impairment (bilirubin greater than 3 times the ULN and any AST) on the pharmacokinetics of durvalumab is unknown. ■ See Monitor and Precautions.

DILUTION

Available as a 120 mg/2.4 mL (50 mg/mL) and 500 mg/10 mL (50 mg/mL), clear to opalescent, colorless to slightly yellow solution in a single-dose vial. *Do not shake.* Withdraw the required volume from the vial(s) and transfer into an IV bag containing NS or D5W. Mix diluted solution by gentle inversion. *Do not shake.* The final concentration of the diluted solution should be between 1 and 15 mg/mL.

Filters: Use of sterile, nonpyrogenic, low–protein-binding, in-line filter (pore size of 0.2 or 0.22 micron) required.

Storage: Before use, refrigerate vials at 36° to 46° F (2° to 8° C) in original carton to protect from light. *Do not freeze or shake.* Immediate use of prepared solution is preferred. If solution is not administered immediately, the total time from vial puncture to start of administration should not exceed 24 hours if stored in a refrigerator or 4 hours if stored at RT. Discard any partially used or empty vials.

COMPATIBILITY
Manufacturer states, "Do not coadminister other drugs through the same infusion line."

RATE OF ADMINISTRATION
A single dose equally distributed over 60 minutes through an IV line containing a sterile, nonpyrogenic, low–protein-binding, in-line filter (pore size of 0.2 or 0.22 micron). Interrupt or slow the rate of infusion for mild or moderate infusion-related reactions; see Dose Adjustments.

ACTIONS
A human IgG1 kappa monoclonal antibody. Durvalumab is a programmed cell death–ligand 1 (PD-L1) blocking antibody. Durvalumab binds PD-L1 and blocks the interaction between PD-L1 and its receptors PD-1 and B7.1. This interaction releases the inhibitory effects of PD-L1 on the immune response without inducing antibody-dependent cell-mediated cytotoxicity. This results in the restoration of immune responses, including antitumor immune responses. Terminal half-life is 18 days.

INDICATIONS AND USES
Treatment of patients with locally advanced or metastatic urothelial carcinoma who have disease progression during or following platinum-containing chemotherapy or who have disease progression within 12 months of neoadjuvant or adjuvant treatment with platinum-containing therapy. (This indication is approved under accelerated approval based on tumor response and duration of response. Continued approval may be contingent on verification and description of clinical benefit in confirmatory trials.) ■ Treatment of patients with unresectable Stage III non–small-cell lung cancer (NSCLC) whose disease has not progressed following concurrent platinum-based chemotherapy and radiation therapy.

CONTRAINDICATIONS
Manufacturer states, "None."

PRECAUTIONS
Immune-mediated pneumonitis and interstitial lung disease with fatalities have been reported. ■ Immune-mediated hepatitis with fatalities has been reported. ■ Durvalumab can cause immune-mediated colitis. ■ Durvalumab can cause immune-mediated endocrinopathies (e.g., adrenal insufficiency, thyroid disorders [hypothyroidism/hyperthyroidism], type 1 diabetes mellitus, and hypophysitis/hypopituitarism). ■ Durvalumab can cause immune-mediated thyroid disorders. Thyroid disorders can occur at any time during treatment. Manage hypothyroidism with hormone replacement therapy, if indicated. Initiate medical management for control of hyperthyroidism, if indicated. ■ Durvalumab can cause diabetes, including type 1 diabetes mellitus. Withhold durvalumab and administer antihyperglycemics or insulin in patients with severe or life-threatening hyperglycemia. ■ Immune-mediated nephritis with fatalities has been reported. ■ Immune-mediated dermatologic reactions (e.g., bullous dermatitis, Stevens-Johnson syndrome [SJS]/toxic epidermal necrolysis [TEN]) have been reported with other products in this class. ■ Durvalumab has caused other immune-mediated adverse reactions, including aseptic meningitis, hemolytic anemia, immune thrombocytopenic purpura, myocarditis, myositis, and ocular inflammatory toxicity (e.g., uveitis and keratitis). Immune-mediated reactions may involve any organ. They usually occur during treatment with durvalumab but may also manifest after discontinuation of therapy; see Dose Adjustments. ■ Serous infections, including fatal cases, have been reported. ■ Severe or life-threatening infusion-related reactions have been reported. ■ A protein substance; has a potential for immunogenicity.

Monitor: Obtain baseline serum creatinine, serum glucose, liver function tests, and thyroid function tests before initiating treatment and monitor periodically during treatment and as indicated based on clinical evaluation. Repeat serum creatinine and liver function tests before each cycle. ■ Monitor for S/S of pneumonitis. Evaluate patients with suspected pneumonitis with radiographic imaging. ■ Monitor for S/S of colitis. Antidiarrheal agents may be used in addition to corticosteroids and treatment modifications as outlined in Dose Adjustments. ■ Monitor for S/S of adrenal insufficiency during and after treatment. S/S may include fatigue, hyperkalemia, hyponatremia, hypotension, low cortisol concentrations, nausea, and vomiting. Administer corticosteroids and hormone replacement as appropriate for adrenal insufficiency. ▪ Monitor for hyperglycemia or other S/S of diabetes. For patients with severe or life-threatening hyperglycemia, resume treatment with durvalumab when metabolic control is achieved with insulin replacement or antihyperglycemics. ▪ Monitor for S/S of hypophysitis or hypopituitarism (e.g., fatigue, headache, low levels of the hormones produced by the pituitary gland [adrenocorticotropic hormone (ACTH), thyroid-stimulating hormone (TSH), follicle-stimulating hormone (FSH), luteinizing hormone (LH), growth hormone (GH), prolactin]). Administer corticosteroids and hormone replacement as clinically indicated. ▪ Monitor for S/S of rash. ▪ Monitor for other possible immune-mediated adverse reactions. Evaluate to confirm or rule out an immune-mediated adverse reaction and to exclude other causes. Use of high-dose corticosteroids and/or hormone replacement therapy may be indicated. ▪ Monitor for S/S of infection. Initiate treatment with anti-infectives for suspected or confirmed infections. ▪ Monitor for S/S of infusion-related reactions, including back pain, chills, dizziness, dyspnea, fever, flushing, hypotension, pruritus, rash, urticaria, and wheezing. Interrupt or slow the rate of infusion in patients with mild or moderate infusion reactions. ▪ Administer corticosteroids followed by a corticosteroid taper for Grade 2 or greater colitis, hepatitis, nephritis, pneumonitis, dermatitis, or other immune-mediated reactions; see Precautions and Dose Adjustments.

Patient Education: Review manufacturer's medication guide. ▪ Avoid pregnancy; females of childbearing potential should use effective contraception during treatment with durvalumab and for at least 3 months after the last dose. ▪ Promptly report S/S of pneumonitis (e.g., chest pain, new or worsening cough, or shortness of breath). ▪ Promptly report S/S of hepatitis (e.g., easy bruising or bleeding, jaundice, lethargy, pain on the right side of abdomen, or severe nausea or vomiting). ▪ Promptly report S/S of colitis (e.g., blood or mucus in stools, diarrhea, or severe abdominal pain). ▪ Promptly report S/S of endocrinopathies (e.g., adrenal insufficiency, diabetes mellitus, hyperthyroidism, hypophysitis, or hypothyroidism). ▪ Promptly report S/S of nephritis and renal dysfunction (e.g., blood in urine, decreased urine output, loss of appetite, swelling in ankles, and any other symptoms of renal dysfunction). ▪ Promptly report S/S of other possible immune-mediated adverse reactions (e.g., aseptic meningitis, hemolytic anemia, myocarditis, myositis, rash, thrombocytopenic purpura, uveitis, and keratitis). ▪ Promptly report S/S of infection (e.g., chills, fever). ▪ Promptly report S/S of infusion-related reactions (e.g., chills, fever, hives, and shortness of breath or wheezing).

Maternal/Child: Based on its mechanism of action, durvalumab can cause fetal harm. Females of reproductive potential should use effective contraception during treatment with durvalumab and for at least 3 months after the last dose. ▪ Discontinue breast-feeding during therapy with durvalumab and for at least 3 months after final dose. ▪ Safety and effectiveness for use in pediatric patients has not been established.

Elderly: The majority of patients in studies were 65 years of age or older. Differences between elderly patients and younger patients were not identified.

DRUG/LAB INTERACTIONS
Formal drug interaction studies have not been conducted.

SIDE EFFECTS
The most common side effects reported were constipation, cough, decreased appetite, dyspnea, fatigue, musculoskeletal pain, nausea, peripheral edema, pneumonitis/radiation pneumonitis, rash, upper respiratory tract infection, and urinary tract infection. The most common Grade 3 or Grade 4 adverse reactions were abdominal pain, dehydration, fatigue, general physical health deterioration, musculoskeletal pain, and urinary tract infection. Other side effects reported were diarrhea/colitis, fever, hypothyroidism, pneumonia, and pruritus. Laboratory abnormalities included anemia; hypercalcemia; hyperglycemia; hyperkalemia; hypermagnesemia; hypoalbuminemia; hypokalemia; hyponatremia; increased alkaline phosphatase, ALT, AST, bilirubin, creatinine, GGT; lymphopenia; and neutropenia. Serious infections, infusion-related reactions, immune-mediated colitis,

immune-mediated dermatologic reactions, immune-mediated endocrinopathies, immune-mediated hepatitis, immune-mediated nephritis and renal dysfunction, immune-mediated pneumonitis, and other immune-mediated reactions have occurred.

ANTIDOTE

No overdose information is available. Keep physician informed of all side effects. May constitute a medical emergency or will be treated symptomatically as indicated; see Dose Adjustments. For life-threatening infusion reactions, immediately and permanently stop durvalumab and administer appropriate supportive treatment. For less severe infusion reactions, management may involve temporarily stopping the infusion, reducing the infusion rate, and/or administering symptomatic treatment (e.g., IV saline, diphenhydramine, bronchodilators such as albuterol, and acetaminophen). Resuscitate if indicated.

ECULIZUMAB BBW

(eck-you-**LIZ**-you-mab)

Soliris

Monoclonal antibody
Complement inhibitor

pH 7

USUAL DOSE

Pretreatment: *A meningococcal vaccine must be administered at least 2 weeks before initial dosing with eculizumab to all patients who have not been previously vaccinated. A booster dose may be required for patients previously vaccinated. Revaccinate according to current medical guidelines. If eculizumab must be initiated immediately and vaccines are administered less than 2 weeks before starting eculizumab therapy, provide patients with 2 weeks of antibacterial drug prophylaxis.* Baseline laboratory studies indicated; see Monitor.

Administer eculizumab at the recommended dosage regimen time points or within 2 days of these time points.

Paroxysmal nocturnal hemoglobinuria (PNH) in patients 18 years of age or older: Administer 600 mg as an infusion weekly for the first 4 weeks, followed by 900 mg for the fifth dose 1 week later, then 900 mg every 2 weeks thereafter.

Atypical hemolytic uremic syndrome (aHUS) in patients 18 years of age or older: Administer 900 mg as an infusion weekly for the first 4 weeks, followed by 1,200 mg for the fifth dose 1 week later, then 1,200 mg every 2 weeks thereafter.

Generalized myasthenia gravis in adults (gMG): Administer 900 mg as an infusion weekly for the first 4 weeks, followed by 1,200 mg for the fifth dose 1 week later, then 1,200 mg every 2 weeks thereafter.

PEDIATRIC DOSE

See general comments under Usual Dose.

Atypical hemolytic uremic syndrome (aHUS) in patients under 18 years of age: Administer eculizumab based on body weight as outlined in the following chart.

Atypical Hemolytic Uremic Syndrome (aHUS) Dose in Patients Under 18 Years of Age		
Patient Body Weight	Induction	Maintenance
40 kg and over	900 mg weekly × 4 doses	1,200 mg at week 5; then 1,200 mg every 2 weeks
30 kg to less than 40 kg	600 mg weekly × 2 doses	900 mg at week 3; then 900 mg every 2 weeks
20 kg to less than 30 kg	600 mg weekly × 2 doses	600 mg at week 3; then 600 mg every 2 weeks
10 kg to less than 20 kg	600 mg × 1 dose	300 mg at week 2; then 300 mg every 2 weeks
5 kg to less than 10 kg	300 mg × 1 dose	300 mg at week 2; then 300 mg every 3 weeks

DOSE ADJUSTMENTS

A variance of 1 to 2 days in the scheduled administration time points is allowed if indicated. ▪ Age, gender, race, and renal function do not appear to influence the pharmacokinetics of eculizumab. ▪ Supplemental dosing of eculizumab is required in patients with aHUS and adult patients with gMG in the setting of concomitant support with PE/PI (plasmapheresis or plasma exchange, or fresh frozen plasma infusion). See the following chart for supplemental dosing based on the type of intervention.

Supplemental Dose of Eculizumab After PE/PI			
Type of Plasma Intervention	Most Recent Eculizumab Dose	Supplemental Eculizumab Dose with Each PE/PI Intervention	Timing of Supplemental Eculizumab Dose
Plasmapheresis or plasma exchange	300 mg	300 mg per each plasmapheresis or plasma exchange session	Within 60 minutes after each plasmapheresis or plasma exchange
Plasmapheresis or plasma exchange	600 mg or more	600 mg per each plasmapheresis or plasma exchange session	Within 60 minutes after each plasmapheresis or plasma exchange
Fresh frozen plasma (FFP) infusion	300 mg or more	300 mg per each infusion of FFP	60 minutes before each infusion of FFP

DILUTION

Available in 300 mg/30 mL single-use vials (10 mg/mL). A clear, colorless solution. Withdraw the required dose of eculizumab (2 vials are required for the 600-mg dose, 3 vials are required for the 900-mg dose, and 4 vials are required for the 1,200-mg dose) and transfer it to an infusion bag. Must be further diluted to a 5 mg/mL concentration by adding an amount of NS, ½NS, D5W, or Ringer's injection to the infusion bag equal to the total volume of the eculizumab.

Preparation and Reconstitution of Eculizumab		
Eculizumab Dose	Diluent Volume	Final Volume
300 mg	30 mL	60 mL
600 mg	60 mL	120 mL
900 mg	90 mL	180 mL
1,200 mg	120 mL	240 mL

Invert gently to ensure thorough mixing. Allow the diluted solution to reach room temperature before infusion. Do not use an artificial heat source (e.g., microwave). Discard unused portions; contains no preservatives.

Filters: Specific information not available.

Storage: Refrigerate vials in original carton at 2° to 8° C (36° to 46° F) and protect from light. Vials may be held in the original carton at RT (not more than 25° C [77° F]) for only a single period up to 3 days. Do not use beyond the expiration date on the vial. Diluted solution is stable for 24 hours refrigerated or at RT. Do not freeze or shake.

COMPATIBILITY

Compatibility information not available from manufacturer; consult a pharmacist.

RATE OF ADMINISTRATION

Do not administer as an IV push or a bolus injection. For infusion via gravity feed, syringe-type pump, or infusion pump.

Adults: A single dose as an infusion over 35 minutes. If infusion is slowed or stopped for any reason, the total infusion time should not exceed 2 hours.

Pediatric patients: A single dose as an infusion over 1 to 4 hours.

ACTIONS

A recombinant, DNA-derived, humanized IgG monoclonal antibody. A genetic mutation in patients with paroxysmal nocturnal hemoglobinuria (PNH) leads to the generation of abnormal RBCs (known as PNH cells) that are deficient in terminal complement inhibitors; this deficiency makes these RBCs sensitive to persistent terminal complement-mediated destruction. Ongoing destruction of these RBCs is called hemolysis. Eculizumab, a complement inhibitor, specifically binds to the complement protein C5 and prevents complement-mediated intravascular hemolysis. It improves the lives of patients suffering from this disease by directly targeting the underlying disease process and markedly decreasing the ongoing RBC destruction that causes the hemolysis responsible for the S/S of PNH. In aHUS, impairment in the regulation of complement activity leads to uncontrolled terminal complement activation, resulting in platelet activation, endothelial cell damage, and thrombotic microangiopathy. Eculizumab inhibits the complement-mediated thrombotic microangiopathy (TMA) in patients with aHUS. Half-life is 270 to 375 hours. Plasma exchange or infusion increases clearance of eculizumab and reduces the half-life to 1.26 hours.

INDICATIONS AND USES

A complement inhibitor for the treatment of patients with paroxysmal nocturnal hemoglobinuria (PNH) to reduce hemolysis. PNH is a rare, disabling, and life-threatening genetic mutation blood disorder defined by chronic RBC destruction (hemolysis). Symptoms may include anemia; disabling fatigue; dysphagia; dyspnea; erectile dysfunction; hemoglobinuria; jaundice; recurrent pain in the abdomen, back, or head; renal dysfunction; and thromboses. Average age of onset is the early 30s. ▪ Treatment of adult patients with generalized myasthenia gravis (gMG) who are anti–acetylcholine receptor (AchR) antibody-positive. ▪ Treatment of patients with atypical hemolytic uremic syndrome (aHUS) to inhibit complement-mediated thrombotic microangiography; see Limitation of Use.

Limitation of use: Eculizumab is NOT indicated for treatment of patients with Shiga toxin *E. coli*–related hemolytic uremic syndrome (STEC-HUS).

CONTRAINDICATIONS

Do not use in patients with unresolved serious *Neisseria meningitidis* infection or in patients not currently vaccinated against *N. meningitidis* unless the risk of delaying eculizumab therapy outweighs the risk of developing meningococcal infection.

PRECAUTIONS

For IV infusion only; do not administer by IV push or bolus injection.

▪ Life-threatening and fatal meningococcal infections have occurred in patients treated with eculizumab. Susceptibility to serious meningococcal infections (septicemia and/or meningitis) is increased approximately 2,000-fold in comparison to the general U.S. population. Meningococcal infections may become rapidly life threatening or fatal if not recognized and treated early. ▪ Comply with the most current Advisory Committee on Immunization Practices (ACIP) recommendations for meningococcal vaccination in patients with complement deficiencies. Revaccinate according to current medical guidelines, considering the duration of eculizumab therapy. ▪ A meningococcal vaccine must be administered at least 2 weeks before initial dosing with eculizumab to all patients who have not been previously vaccinated unless the risks of delaying eculizumab therapy outweigh the risks of developing meningococcal infection. If urgent eculizumab therapy is indicated in an unvaccinated patient, administer the meningococcal vaccine as soon as possible and provide patients with 2 weeks of antibacterial drug prophylaxis. In clinical studies, such patients received antibiotics for prophylaxis of meningococcal infection until at least 2 weeks after vaccination. Benefits and risks of antibiotic prophylaxis not established. Vaccination reduces, but does not eliminate, the risk of meningococcal infections. ▪ Use caution in patients with any systemic infection. ▪ Serious infections with *Neisseria species* (other than *N. meningitides*), including disseminated gonococcal infections, have been reported. Eculizumab blocks terminal complement activation; therefore patients may have increased susceptibility to infections, especially with encapsulated bacteria. *Aspergillus* infections have occurred in immunocompromised and neutropenic patients. Pediatric patients may be at increased risk of developing serious infections due to *Streptococcus pneumoniae* or *Haemophilus influenzae* type B (Hib). Administer vaccinations for prevention of these infections according to guidelines of the Advisory Committee on Immunization Practices (ACIP). ▪ Serious hemolysis or thrombotic microangiopathy (TMA) may occur in patients who discontinue eculizumab therapy; see Monitor and Antidote. ▪ A protein product; infusion reactions may occur. Hypersensitivity reactions, including anaphylaxis, are possible; however, infusion reactions severe enough to discontinue eculizumab did not occur during clinical trials. ▪ Has a potential for immunogenicity. Low titers of antibodies to eculizumab have been detected but did not appear to correlate to clinical response. ▪ Continue established anticoagulant therapy during eculizumab treatment; the effect of withdrawal of anticoagulant therapy during eculizumab therapy has not been established. ▪ Eculizumab is available through a restricted program under a Risk Evaluation and Mitigation Strategy (REMS). Prescribers must be enrolled in the program. Contact manufacturer for further information.

Monitor: Obtain baseline and periodic CBC with differential and platelets, lactic dehydrogenase (LDH), SCr, bilirubin, and urinalysis. ▪ LDH levels increase during hemolysis and with TMA. Monitoring may assist in determining the effectiveness of eculizumab therapy. ▪ Monitor for early S/S of meningococcal infections (moderate to severe headache with nausea or vomiting, fever, or a stiff neck or stiff back; fever of 103° F [39.4° C] or higher; fever and a rash; confusion; and/or severe muscle aches with flu-like symptoms and light sensitivity). Evaluate immediately and treat with antibiotics if indicated. Discontinue eculizumab during treatment of serious meningococcal infections. ▪ Monitor for other types of infections. ▪ Monitor for S/S of an infusion or hypersensitivity reaction (e.g., chills, dyspnea, pruritus) during infusion and for at least 1 hour postinfusion. Slow or temporarily discontinue the infusion as indicated. ▪ Monitor patients with PNH who discontinue eculizumab for a minimum of 8 weeks to detect serious hemolysis (S/S may include blood clots; chest pain; confusion; decreased hemoglobin, hematocrit, and haptoglobin; difficulty breathing; elevated LDH, bilirubin, or SCr; free serum hemoglobin; and hemoglobinuria with pink/red urine). ▪ Monitor patients with aHUS who discontinue eculizumab for S/S of TMA complications for a minimum of 12 weeks. Clinical S/S of TMA may include angina, dyspnea, mental status changes, seizures, or thrombosis. Changes in laboratory parameters that may indicate TMA include a decrease in platelet count by 25% or more compared with baseline or nadir during eculizumab treatment or an increase in SCr and LDH by 25% or more compared with baseline or nadir during eculizumab treatment.

Patient Education: Read the patient medication guide before initiating eculizumab and before each dose. ▪ Meningococcal vaccination is required before initiating therapy. Previously vaccinated individuals may require a booster dose. Vaccination may not prevent meningococcal infection. Important to receive and stay up-to-date on all recommended immunizations. Discuss immunization status with physician. ▪ Eculizumab affects the immune system and can lower the ability to fight infections. Immediately report S/S of a meningococcal infection (moderate to severe headache with nausea or vomiting, fever, or a stiff neck or stiff back; fever of 103° F [39.4° C] or higher; fever and a rash; confusion; and/or severe muscle aches with flu-like symptoms and light sensitivity). Manufacturer supplies a patient safety card that lists these symptoms. Card should be carried at all times during treatment and for 3 months after the last dose of eculizumab is administered. Share card with all health care providers treating you. ▪ Promptly report other S/S of an infection. ▪ Prevent gonorrheal infections; patients at risk should be tested regularly. ▪ Promptly report chills, dyspnea, and/or itching during or soon after an infusion. ▪ Report a suspected pregnancy and/or tell your doctor if you are breast-feeding. ▪ Stopping the infusions may have serious side effects and requires prolonged monitoring for development of hemolysis or TMA. Increased risk of meningococcal infection continues for several weeks after eculizumab is discontinued.

Maternal/Child: Use during pregnancy only if the benefits justify the potential risk to the fetus. There are risks to the mother and fetus associated with untreated PNH and aHUS. PNH in pregnancy is associated with adverse maternal outcomes, including bleeding, cytopenias (worsening), infections, miscarriages, thrombotic events, and increased maternal mortality, as well as adverse fetal outcomes, including fetal death and premature delivery. aHUS in pregnancy is associated with adverse maternal outcomes, including pre-eclampsia and preterm delivery, and adverse fetal/neonatal outcomes, including intrauterine growth restriction (IUGR), low birth weight, and fetal death. Treatment with eculizumab may increase fetal survival and decrease maternal complications. ▪ Use caution if breast-feeding; IgG is secreted in breast milk. There is insufficient information on the presence of eculizumab in human milk or the effects on breast-fed infants or human milk production. Consider risks to infant versus benefits of breast-feeding. ▪ Safety and effectiveness have been established for use in pediatric patients for treatment of aHUS ▪ Safety and effectiveness for use in pediatric patients have NOT been established for treatment of PNH or gMG. ▪ Follow ACIP guidelines for vaccinations for prevention of infections due to *Neisseria meningitidis, Streptococcus pneumoniae,* and Hib.

Elderly: Limited experience did not identify age-related differences in safety and effectiveness.

DRUG/LAB INTERACTIONS

Formal drug interaction studies have not been completed. ▪ **Intravenous immunoglobulin (IVIG)** treatment may interfere with the endosomal neonatal Fc receptor (FcRn) recycling mechanism of monoclonal antibodies, such as eculizumab, and decrease serum eculizumab concentrations. ▪ Continue established anticoagulant therapy during eculizumab treatment; the effect of withdrawal of anticoagulant therapy during eculizumab therapy has not been established.

SIDE EFFECTS

PNH and aHUS: Meningococcal infections (meningitis and/or septicemia) are the most serious side effects reported; may be life threatening and may occur in patients who have been vaccinated.

PNH: The most commonly reported side effects are back pain, headache, nasopharyngitis, and nausea. The most serious reactions include anemia, fever, headache, infection (including viral infections), and the progression of PNH. Other reported side effects include constipation, cough, fatigue, herpes simplex infections, influenza-like illness, myalgia, pain in extremity, respiratory tract infection, and sinusitis.

aHUS: The most commonly reported side effects are abdominal pain, anemia, cough, diarrhea, fever, headache, hypertension, nasopharyngitis, nausea, peripheral edema, upper respiratory infection, UTI, and vomiting. The most serious reactions include chronic renal failure, hypertension, infections, renal impairment, upper respiratory tract infection, and viral gastroenteritis. Other reported side effects include arthralgia, asthenia, back pain, bronchitis, fatigue, gastroenteritis, hypokalemia, hypotension, insomnia, leukopenia, neoplasms (benign, malignant, and unspecified), proteinuria, pruritus, rash, and renal impairment.

gMG: The most commonly reported side effect is musculoskeletal pain. Other reported side effects include abdominal pain, arthralgia, fever, headache, diarrhea, infections, nasopharyngitis, nausea, peripheral edema, and upper respiratory tract infection.

Post-Marketing: Cases of serious or fatal infections (e.g., *Neisseria gonorrhoeae, Neisseria meningitidis, Neisseria sicca/subflava, Neisseria* spp unspecified) have been reported.

ANTIDOTE

Keep physician informed of all side effects. Some will be treated symptomatically. Potential meningococcal infections must be evaluated immediately and treated with antibiotics promptly; may be life threatening. Treat hypersensitivity or infusion reactions as indicated; may respond to slowing or temporarily discontinuing the infusion or may require the use of epinephrine, corticosteroids, diphenhydramine bronchodilators (e.g., albuterol, aminophylline), IV saline, oxygen, and/or acetaminophen. Interrupt infusion and institute appropriate supportive measures if signs of cardiovascular instability or respiratory compromise occur. Total infusion time should not exceed 2 hours. If TMA complications occur after eculizumab is discontinued, consider reinstitution of treatment, plasma therapy (plasmapheresis, plasma exchange or FFP infusion [PE/PI]), or appropriate organ-specific supportive measures. Resuscitate as necessary.

EDARAVONE
(e-**DAR**-a-vone)

Free radical scavenger

Radicava

pH 4

USUAL DOSE

Initial treatment cycle: 60 mg as an IV infusion over 60 minutes once daily for 14 days, followed by a 14-day drug-free period.

Subsequent treatment cycles: 60 mg as an IV infusion over 60 minutes once daily for 10 days out of 14-day periods, followed by a 14-day drug-free period.

DOSE ADJUSTMENTS

The effect of renal or hepatic impairment on the pharmacokinetics of edaravone has not been studied. No dose adjustment is needed in patients with renal impairment or mild or moderate hepatic impairment. No specific dosing recommendations can be provided for patients with severe hepatic impairment. ■ Age, gender, and race have not been found to affect the pharmacokinetics of edaravone.

DILUTION

Available as a 60 mg/100 mL (0.6 mg/mL) clear, colorless, sterile solution in a single-dose polypropylene bag. Each bag is overwrapped with polyvinyl alcohol secondary packaging containing an oxygen absorber and oxygen indicator, which should be pink to reflect appropriate oxygen levels.

Filters: Data are not available.

Storage: Store at CRT. Protect from light. Store in overwrapped package to protect from oxygen degradation until time of use. The oxygen indicator will turn blue or purple if the oxygen has exceeded acceptable levels. Do not use if the oxygen indicator has turned blue or purple before opening the package. Once the overwrap package is opened, use within 24 hours.

COMPATIBILITY

Manufacturer states, "Other medications should not be injected into the infusion bag or mixed with edaravone."

RATE OF ADMINISTRATION
A single dose equally distributed over 60 minutes.

ACTIONS
The mechanism by which edaravone exerts its therapeutic effect in patients with amyotrophic lateral sclerosis (ALS) is unknown. The maximum plasma concentration is reached by the end of the infusion. Edaravone is highly bound to plasma proteins, primarily albumin. It is metabolized to inactive sulfate and glucuronide conjugates and is excreted mainly in the urine as the glucuronide conjugate. Terminal elimination half-life is 4.5 to 6 hours.

INDICATIONS AND USES
Treatment of amyotrophic lateral sclerosis.

CONTRAINDICATIONS
History of hypersensitivity to edaravone or any of the inactive ingredients of this product.

PRECAUTIONS
For IV infusion only. ▪ Hypersensitivity reactions, including anaphylaxis, have been reported. ▪ Edaravone contains sodium bisulfite, a sulfite that may cause allergic-type reactions, including anaphylactic symptoms and life-threatening or less severe asthmatic episodes in susceptible people; use caution in patients with asthma.
Monitor: Monitor for S/S of hypersensitivity reactions (e.g., dyspnea, erythema multiforme, hypotension, urticaria, wheals).
Patient Education: Read FDA-approved patient information. ▪ Promptly report S/S of a hypersensitivity reaction (e.g., breathing problems; dizziness; hives; itching; swelling of the face, lips, or tongue; wheezing). ▪ Edaravone contains sodium bisulfite. ▪ Notify health care provider if pregnant or breast-feeding or if you intend to become pregnant or breast-feed.
Maternal/Child: There are no adequate data on the developmental risk associated with the use of edaravone in pregnant women. Adverse developmental effects (e.g., increased mortality, decreased growth, delayed sexual development, and altered behavior) have been observed in animal studies. ▪ Use caution in breast-feeding. Data on the presence of edaravone in human milk and safety in breast-feeding are not available. ▪ Safety and effectiveness for use in pediatric patients have not been established.
Elderly: No overall differences in safety or effectiveness were observed between patients over 65 years of age and younger patients, but greater sensitivity of some older individuals cannot be ruled out.

DRUG/LAB INTERACTIONS
The pharmacokinetics of edaravone is not expected to be significantly affected by inhibitors of CYP enzymes, UGTs, or major transporters. ▪ Edaravone and its metabolites are not expected to induce CYP1A2, CYP2B6, or CYP3A4.

SIDE EFFECTS
The most common adverse reactions are contusion, gait disturbance, and headache. Other commonly reported adverse reactions include dermatitis, eczema, glycosuria, hypoxia, respiratory failure, and tinea infection.
Post-Marketing: Hypersensitivity reactions, including anaphylaxis.

ANTIDOTE
Discontinue the infusion at the first S/S consistent with a hypersensitivity reaction. Treat per standard of care (e.g., oxygen, diphenhydramine, epinephrine, corticosteroids, vasopressors, and/or fluids) and monitor until condition resolves. Resuscitate as necessary.

EFGARTIGIMOD ALFA
(**EF**-gar-**TIG**-i-mod **AL**-fa)

Vyvgart

Neonatal Fc receptor
antagonist

USUAL DOSE
10 mg/kg/dose every week for 4 weeks. Further infusions based on clinical response, but no sooner than 50 days from the start of the previous treatment cycle. Maximum dose 1.2 gm.

PEDIATRIC DOSE
No pediatric dosages provided by manufacturer.

DOSE ADJUSTMENTS
Renal: No dosage adjustments provided by manufacturer.
Hepatic: No dosage adjustments provided by manufacturer.

DILUTION
Dilute the required dose from each vial, which contains 400 mg in NS, to make 125 mL total volume. Gently invert bag; *do not shake*.

COMPATIBILITY
Do not administer simultaneously with any other medication or IV solutions other than NS.

RATE OF ADMINISTRATION
Allow infusion to reach room temperature and infuse over 1 hour using a 0.22-micron filter. Flush entire line with NS.

ACTIONS
Efgartigimod afla is a human IgG1 antibody fragment that binds to the neonatal Fc receptor, resulting in a reduction of circulating IgG.

INDICATIONS AND USES
Myasthenia gravis.

CONTRAINDICATIONS
None given by manufacturer.

PRECAUTIONS
Ensure patient is up-to-date on vaccinations before starting therapy; live vaccines must be avoided during therapy. Infections may occur.
Monitor: Monitor for S/S of infusion-related reactions (anaphylaxis, fever, chills, hypotension, rash, pruritus) throughout infusion and for 1 hour after infusion.
Patient Education: Used for myasthenia gravis. May cause cold symptoms, headache, muscle pain. Contact physician with signs of infection (fever, chills), urinary tract infection, or a burning and numbness that is not normal.
Maternal/Child: Other agents for myasthenia gravis are recommended if patient is pregnant or lactating.
Elderly: Refer to Usual Dose and Precautions.

DRUG/LAB INTERACTIONS
Bacille Calmette-Guérin (BCG) vaccine, baricitnib, brincidofovir, cladribine, COVID-19 vaccines (may decrease effectiveness), moderate and strong CYP3A4 inducers (may decrease effectiveness of efgartigimod; avoid), denosumab, Echinacea, fexinidazole, fingolimod, inebilizumab, influenza vaccines (may decrease effectiveness), leflunomide, natalizumab, ocrelizumab, ofatumumab, ozanimod, pidotimod, pimecrolimus (avoid), pneumococcal vaccine, polio vaccine (avoid), rabies vaccine, rubella or varicella live vaccines (avoid), ruxolitinib topical (avoid), sipuleucel-T, tacrolimus topical (avoid), talimogene laherparepvec (avoid), tertomotide (avoid), tofacitinib, typhoid vaccine (avoid), upadacitinib (avoid), live vaccines (avoid), varicella virus vaccine (avoid).

Inactivated vaccines may have reduced response; give prior to therapy start. Please refer to package insert for further information.

SIDE EFFECTS

Angioedema; antibody development; cold symptoms; decreased neutrophils, WBC count; headache; hypersensitivity; lymphocytopenia; muscle pain; myalgia; paresthesia; respiratory tract infection.

ANTIDOTE

Discontinue infusion and treat appropriately for severe hypersensitivity reactions.

EMAPALUMAB-lzsg

Monoclonal Antibody

(**EM**-a-**PAL**-ue-mab)

Gamifant

USUAL DOSE

Pretreatment: Pretesting required and baseline studies indicated; see Monitor.

Premedications: Administer prophylaxis for herpes zoster, *Pneumocystis jirovecii,* and for fungal infections before emapalumab-lzsg administration.

Concomitant medications: For patients who are not already receiving baseline dexamethasone treatment, begin dexamethasone at a daily dose of at least 5 to 10 mg/M^2 the day before emapalumab-lzsg treatment begins. Patients who are already receiving baseline dexamethasone may continue their regular dexamethasone dose provided that the dose is at least 5 mg/M^2. Dexamethasone can be tapered according to the judgment of the treating physician.

Emapalumab-lzsg: The recommended starting dose is 1 mg/kg as an IV infusion over 1 hour twice per week (every 3 to 4 days). Subsequent doses may be increased based on clinical and laboratory criteria; see Dose Adjustments. Administer emapalumab-lzsg until hematopoietic stem cell transplantation (HSCT) is performed or there is unacceptable toxicity. Discontinue emapalumab-lzsg when the patient no longer requires therapy for the treatment of hemophagocytic lymphohistiocytosis (HLH).

DOSE ADJUSTMENTS

Titrate the dose upward as outlined in the following chart if disease response is unsatisfactory. After the patient's clinical condition is stabilized, decrease the dose to the previous level to maintain clinical response.

Emapalumab-lzsg Dose Titration Criteria		
Treatment Day	**Emapalumab-lzsg Dose**	**Criteria for Dose Increase**
Day 1	Starting dose of 1 mg/kg	N/A
On Day 3	Increase to 3 mg/kg	Unsatisfactory improvement in clinical condition as assessed by a health care provider AND at least one of the following:
From Day 6 onward	Increase to 6 mg/kg	• Fever: persistence or recurrence • Platelet count If baseline <50,000/mm^3 and no improvement to >50,000/mm^3 If baseline >50,000/mm^3 and <30% improvement If baseline >100,000/mm^3 and decrease to <100,000/mm^3 • Neutrophil count If baseline <500/mm^3 and no improvement to >500/mm^3 If baseline 500-1,000/mm^3 and decrease to <500/mm^3 If baseline 1,000-1,500/mm^3 and decrease to <1,000/mm^3 • Ferritin (ng/mL) If baseline ≥3,000 ng/mL and <20% decrease If baseline <3,000 ng/mL and any increase to >3,000 ng/mL • Splenomegaly: any worsening • Coagulopathy (both D-dimer and fibrinogen must apply) D-dimer: if abnormal at baseline and no improvement Fibrinogen (mg/mL) If baseline levels ≤100 mg/dL and no improvement If baseline levels >100 mg/dL and any decrease to <100 mg/dL
From Day 9 onward	Increase to 10 mg/kg	Assessment by a health care provider that, based on initial signs of response, a further increase in emapalumab-lzsg dose can be of benefit

No clinically significant differences in the pharmacokinetics of emapalumab-lzsg were observed based on age, sex, race, renal impairment (including dialysis), or hepatic impairment (mild, moderate, and severe).

DILUTION
Available in 10 mg/2 mL and 50 mg/10 mL (5 mg/mL) single-dose vials. Solution is clear to slightly opalescent, colorless to slightly yellow. Calculate the dose (mg/kg) of emapalumab-lzsg, the total volume (mL) required, and the number of vials needed based on patient actual body weight. Withdraw the necessary volume of solution and dilute with NS to a maximum concentration of 2.5 mg/mL. Do not dilute product to less than 0.25 mg/mL. The diluted solution can be placed in either a syringe or an infusion bag depending on the volume needed. Use a gamma-irradiated, latex-free, polyvinyl chloride (PVC)-free syringe or a non-PVC polyolefin infusion bag. Do not use with ethylene oxide–sterilized syringes.

Filters: Administer through an IV line containing a sterile, nonpyrogenic, low–protein-binding, 0.2-micron in-line filter.

Storage: Store emapalumab-lzsg in a refrigerator at 2° to 8° C (36° to 46° F) in original carton to protect from light. Do not freeze or shake. If not administered immediately, store the diluted solution under refrigeration at 2° to 8° C (36° to 46° F) for no more than 4 hours from the time of dilution. Allow refrigerated solution to come to room temperature before administration. Do not freeze. Do not shake. Discard any unused solution contained in the vial or diluted for infusion.

COMPATIBILITY
Manufacturer states, "Do not infuse emapalumab-lzsg concomitantly with other agents and do not add any other product to the infusion bag or syringe." Use a gamma-irradiated, latex-free, polyvinyl chloride (PVC)-free syringe or a non-PVC polyolefin infusion bag. Do not use with ethylene oxide–sterilized syringes.

RATE OF ADMINISTRATION

A single dose administered as an IV infusion over 1 hour. Administer through an IV line containing a sterile, nonpyrogenic, low–protein-binding, 0.2-micron in-line filter. In the event of an infusion-related reaction, the infusion may be interrupted and re-initiated at a slower rate.

ACTIONS

Emapalumab-lzsg is an interferon gamma (IFNγ) blocking antibody produced by recombinant DNA technology that binds to and neutralizes IFNγ. Nonclinical data suggest that IFNγ plays a pivotal role in the pathogenesis of HLH by being hypersecreted. Emapalumab-lzsg exhibits target-mediated clearance dependent on INFγ production, which can vary between and within patients as a function of time and can affect the recommended dosage. Half-life is approximately 22 days in healthy subjects and ranged from 2.5 to 18.9 days in HLH patients. The metabolic pathway of emapalumab-lzsg has not been characterized. As with other proteins, it is expected to be degraded into small peptides and amino acids via catabolic pathways.

INDICATIONS AND USES

Treatment of adult and pediatric (newborn and older) patients with primary hemophagocytic lymphohistiocytosis (HLH) with refractory, recurrent, or progressive disease or intolerance with conventional HLH therapy.

CONTRAINDICATIONS

Manufacturer states, "None."

PRECAUTIONS

May increase the risk of fatal and serious infections to include specific pathogens favored by IFNγ neutralization, including mycobacteria, herpes zoster virus, and *Histoplasma capsulatum*. Do not administer emapalumab-lzsg in patients with infections caused by these pathogens until appropriate treatment has been initiated. ▪ Serious infections, including sepsis, bacteremia, pneumonia, disseminated histoplasmosis, necrotizing fasciitis viral infections, and perforated appendicitis have been reported. Reported pathogens were bacterial, viral, fungal, and of unknown origin. ▪ Infusion-related reactions have been reported and were rated as mild to moderate in severity. ▪ As with all therapeutic proteins, there is the chance for immunogenicity. ▪ See Drug/Lab Interactions.

Monitor: Test for latent tuberculosis infections using the purified protein derivative (PPD) or IFNγ release assay. ▪ Evaluate patients for tuberculosis risk factors before initiating therapy. Administer tuberculosis prophylaxis to patients at risk for tuberculosis or known to have a positive PPD test result or positive IFNγ release assay. ▪ Obtain baseline and periodic neutrophil count, platelet count, ferritin, D-dimer, and fibrinogen to help guide therapy; see Dose Adjustments. ▪ Monitor for persistent or recurrent fever. ▪ Monitor for tuberculosis, adenovirus, EBV, and CMV every 2 weeks and as clinically indicated. ▪ Closely monitor for other S/S of infection. Initiate a complete diagnostic workup appropriate for an immunocompromised patient and initiate antimicrobial therapy as indicated. ▪ Monitor for S/S of an infusion related reaction (e.g., drug eruption, erythema, fever, hyperhidrosis, rash). One-third of reported reactions occurred during the first infusion.

Patient Education: Read the FDA-approved patient medication guide. ▪ Report S/S of infection. ▪ Review vaccination status with provider; see Drug/Lab Interactions. ▪ Report S/S of infusion-related reactions.

Maternal/Child: Information on use in pregnancy and breast-feeding is not available. Use with caution and evaluate risk versus benefit. ▪ Safety and effectiveness have been established in pediatric patients, newborn and older, with primary HLH that is reactivated or refractory to conventional therapies.

Elderly: Clinical studies did not include sufficient numbers of patients 65 years of age and older to determine whether they respond differently from younger patients. Differences have not been identified.

DRUG/LAB INTERACTIONS

Do not administer live or live-attenuated vaccines to patients receiving emapalumab-lzsg and for at least 4 weeks after the last dose of emapalumab-lzsg. Safety of immunization with live vaccines during or after therapy has not been studied. ▪ The formation of CYP450 enzymes may be suppressed by increased levels of cytokines such as IFNγ. By neutralizing IFNg, emapalumab-lzsg may normalize CYP450 activities, which may reduce the efficacy of drugs that are **CYP450 substrates** due to increased metabolism. Monitor for reduced efficacy and adjust dosage of CYP450 substrate drugs as appropriate when emapalumab-lzsg therapy is initiated or discontinued.

SIDE EFFECTS

The most commonly reported adverse reactions were fever, hypertension, infections, and infusion-related reactions. The most commonly reported serious reactions were GI hemorrhage, infections, and multiple organ dysfunction. Other adverse reactions included abdominal pain, constipation, cough, cytomegalovirus infection, diarrhea, hypokalemia, irritability, lymphocytosis, rash, tachycardia, and tachypnea. Other reactions were reported in fewer than 10% of study patients.

ANTIDOTE

Notify physician of all side effects. Most will be treated symptomatically. Interrupt the infusion for an infusion-related reaction and institute appropriate medical management before continuing the infusion at a slower rate.

ENALAPRILAT BBW
(en-**AL**-ah-prill-at)

ACE inhibitor
Antihypertensive
Vasodilator

pH 6.5 to 7.5

USUAL DOSE

Pretreatment: See Maternal/Child.

Enalaprilat: 1.25 mg every 6 hours. Doses up to 5 mg every 6 hours have been tolerated for up to 36 hours, but clinical studies have not shown a need for dosage over 1.25 mg. Dosage is the same (1.25 mg) when converting from oral to IV therapy. Resume oral therapy as soon as tolerated. See Precautions.

PEDIATRIC DOSE (UNLABELED)

Infants and pediatric patients: 5 to 10 mcg/kg/dose every 8 to 24 hours, not to exceed 1.25 mg/dose. Dose and frequency determined by clinical response.

Adolescents: 0.625 to 1.25 mg every 6 hours. See Maternal/Child.

DOSE ADJUSTMENTS

Reduce initial dose to 0.625 mg in patients taking diuretics, patients with CHF, hyponatremia, severe volume or salt depletion, a CrCl less than 30 mL/min, and dialysis patients; see Rate of Administration. If the 0.625 dose is not clinically effective after 1 hour, it may be repeated. Additional doses of 1.25 mg may be administered at 6-hour intervals. ▪ Blood levels may be increased in the elderly; dose selection should be cautious. Consider decreased cardiac, hepatic, and renal function; concomitant disease; or other drug therapy. ▪ See Drug/Lab Interactions and Precautions.

DILUTION

May be given undiluted through the port of a free-flowing infusion of NS, D5W, D5NS, D5LR, or Isolyte E. May also be diluted in up to 50 mL of any of the same solutions and given as an infusion.

Storage: Store at CRT. Stable for up to 24 hours after dilution.

COMPATIBILITY

Compatibility information not available from manufacturer.

Other sources suggest specific **compatibilities** dependent on concentration and manufacturer; consult a pharmacist.

RATE OF ADMINISTRATION

A single dose must be evenly distributed over 5 minutes. Extend rate of infusion up to 1 hour in patients at risk for severe hypotension (e.g., heart failure, hyponatremia, high-dose diuretic therapy, recent intensive diuresis or increase in diuretic dose, renal dialysis, or severe volume and/or salt depletion of any etiology).

ACTIONS

An antihypertensive agent. The active metabolite of the orally administered prodrug enalapril maleate. An angiotensin-converting enzyme (ACE) inhibitor that prevents conversion of angiotensin I to the vasoconstrictor substance angiotensin II. Angiotensin II also stimulates aldosterone secretion by the adrenal cortex. Inhibition of ACE results in decreased plasma angiotensin II, which leads to decreased vasopressor activity and decreased aldosterone secretion. A decrease in aldosterone secretion results in a small increase of serum potassium. Administration of enalaprilat results in a decrease of both supine and standing systolic and diastolic BP, usually with no orthostatic component. Onset of action is usually within 15 minutes. Peak BP reduction occurs in 1 to 4 hours, and effects last up to 6 hours. Peak effects after the first dose may not occur for up to 4 hours after administration. Peak effects of subsequent doses may be greater than the initial dose. Excreted in urine. Crosses placental barrier. Secreted in breast milk.

INDICATIONS AND USES

Treatment of hypertension when oral therapy is not practical.

Unlabeled uses: Treatment of pediatric hypertensive urgency or emergency.

CONTRAINDICATIONS

Hypersensitivity to enalaprilat or its components. ▪ A history of angioedema related to previous treatment with an ACE inhibitor, or hereditary or idiopathic angioedema. ▪ Coadministration of aliskiren with enalaprilat in patients with diabetes. ▪ Administration in combination with a neprilysin inhibitor (e.g., sacubitril/valsartan); see Drug/Lab Interactions.

PRECAUTIONS

Excessive hypotension is rare in uncomplicated hypertensive patients but may occur in patients who are severely salt/volume depleted. Patients at risk for excessive hypotension include those with the following conditions or characteristics: heart failure, hyponatremia, high-dose diuretic therapy, recent intensive diuresis or increase in diuretic dose, renal dialysis, or severe volume and/or salt depletion of any etiology. Excessive hypotension may be associated with oliguria and/or progressive azotemia and, rarely, with acute renal failure and/or death. In patients at risk, consider discontinuing the diuretic, decreasing the diuretic dose, or increasing salt intake cautiously, if possible, before initiating enalaprilat therapy. ▪ Use caution in patients with ischemic heart or cerebrovascular disease; an excessive fall in blood pressure could result in MI or stroke. ▪ Angioedema of the face, extremities, lips, tongue, glottis, and/or larynx has been reported and may occur at any time during treatment. Angioedema associated with laryngeal edema may be fatal. See Drug/Lab Interactions. ▪ Intestinal angioedema has been reported. Patients may present with abdominal pain, with or without nausea and vomiting. ▪ Use caution in patients with aortic stenosis or hypertrophic cardiomyopathy. ▪ Use caution in patients with collagen vascular disease and renal disease; neutropenia and/or agranulocytosis have been reported with captopril, another ACE inhibitor. Monitoring of WBC may be indicated. ▪ Use caution in surgery, with anesthesia, or with agents that produce hypotension. ▪ May rarely cause a syndrome that starts with cholestatic jaundice, progresses to hepatic necrosis, and may progress to death. Discontinue in patients who develop elevated liver enzymes or jaundice. ▪ May cause oliguria or progressive azotemia in patients with severe congestive heart failure whose renal function is dependent on the activity of the renin-angiotensin-aldosterone system. Acute renal failure and death are possible. ▪ Increases in BUN and SCr have been observed and are more likely to occur in patients with pre-existing renal impairment. Dose reduction and/or discontinuation of diuretic therapy may be required. ▪ ACE inhibitors often cause a persistent, nonproductive cough, which should resolve when drug is discontinued. ▪ In clinical trials, ACE inhibitors had less of an effect on blood pressure in Black patients compared with non-Black patients. In addition, Black patients have been reported to have a higher incidence of angioedema compared with non-Black patients. ▪ Has been used intravenously for up to 7 days. ▪ Average dose for conversion to oral therapy is 5 mg/day as a single dose. When a reduced dose of enalaprilat IV has been indicated (e.g., diuretics, impaired renal function [CrCl ≤30 mL/min], dialysis), reduce initial oral dose to 2.5 mg/day as a single daily dose. Adjust dose based on BP response. ▪ See Monitor and Drug/Lab Interactions.

Monitor: Monitor vital signs frequently. May cause excessive drop in BP following the first dose. ▪ Use extreme caution in patients with volume and/or salt depletion. ▪ Monitor BUN and SCr. ▪ Monitor serum potassium levels; may cause hyperkalemia. May cause a significant increase in serum potassium with concurrent use of potassium-sparing diuretics or potassium supplements. Use with caution and only for documented hypokalemia. Use salt substitutes with caution. ▪ Monitor for S/S of angioedema. Intestinal angioedema has been diagnosed by abdominal CT scan or ultrasound or during surgery. ▪ Monitoring of WBC may be indicated in patients with collagen vascular disease or renal disease. ▪ See Drug/Lab Interactions.

Patient Education: Consider birth control options. ▪ May cause dizziness; avoid sudden changes in posture and request assistance for ambulation if necessary. Promptly report S/S of any adverse reaction (e.g., difficulty breathing, rash, swelling of face, tongue, or other body parts).

Maternal/Child: Category D. Drugs that act directly on the renin-angiotensin system can cause injury and death to the developing fetus. These adverse outcomes are usually associated with use in the second and third trimester of pregnancy. When pregnancy is detected, discontinue enalaprilat as soon as possible; see prescribing information for further information. ▪ Observe any infant with in utero exposure for hypotension and oliguria. ▪ Discontinue breastfeeding. ▪ Safety for use in pediatric patients not established but has been used. ▪ May contain benzyl alcohol, which has been associated with a fatal "gasping syndrome" in neonates.

Elderly: Dose selection should be cautious; see Dose Adjustments and Precautions/Monitor.

DRUG/LAB INTERACTIONS

Use caution in surgery, with **anesthesia,** or with any **agents that produce hypotension.** ▪ Dual blockade of the renin-angiotensin system (RAS) with **angiotensin receptor blockers, ACE inhibitors,** or **aliskiren** is associated with increased risks of hypotension, hyperkalemia, and changes in renal function (including acute renal failure) compared with monotherapy. In general, combined use of **RAS inhibitors** should be avoided. ▪ Has been used with other cardiovascular agents, including digitalis, beta-adrenergic–blocking agents, methyldopa, nitrates, calcium-blocking agents, hydralazine, and prazosin, without evidence of clinically significant adverse interactions. ▪ **Diuretics** given concomitantly may cause an excessive drop in BP, especially in at-risk patients. ▪ **Antihypertensive agents that cause renin release** (e.g., diuretics) potentiate the antihypertensive effect of enalaprilat. ▪ May cause hyperkalemia with **potassium-sparing diuretics, potassium supplements,** or **potassium-containing salt substitutes**. ▪ In patients who are elderly, volume depleted (including those receiving diuretic therapy), or have compromised renal function, concurrent use with **NSAIDs** may result in further deterioration of renal function, including acute renal failure. ▪ Concurrent use with **NSAIDs** may also decrease the hypotensive effects of enalaprilat by inhibiting the renal prostaglandin synthesis and/or by causing sodium and fluid retention. ▪ May increase **lithium** concentration, resulting in lithium toxicity. ▪ Nitritoid reactions (symptoms include facial flushing, nausea, vomiting, and hypotension) have been reported rarely in patients receiving therapy with **injectable gold** (sodium aurothiomalate) and concomitant ACE inhibitor therapy. ▪ Coadministration of an ACE inhibitor and an **mTOR inhibitor** (e.g., temsirolimus, sirolimus, everolimus) may increase the risk for angioedema. ▪ Patients taking a concomitant **neprilysin inhibitor** (e.g., sacubitril/valsartan) may be at increased risk for angioedema. Do not administer enalaprilat within 36 hours of switching to or from sacubitril/valsartan. ▪ Concomitant use with **aliskiren** is contraindicated in patients with diabetes and should be avoided in all patients with GFR <60 mL/min. ▪ See Precautions and Monitor.

SIDE EFFECTS

Hypotension was the most frequently reported adverse event, followed by headache and nausea. Other reported adverse reactions include abdominal pain, alopecia, angina, angioedema, anorexia, anosmia (absence of sense of smell), asthenia, asthma, ataxia, atrial fibrillation, blurred vision, bone marrow suppression, bradycardia, bronchitis, bronchospasm, cardiac arrest, cerebrovascular accident, chest pain, confusion, conjunctivitis, constipation, cough (persistent, dry), decreases in hemoglobin and hematocrit, depression, diaphoresis, diarrhea, dizziness, dream abnormality, dry eyes, dry mouth, dyspepsia, dyspnea, elevated LFTs, eosinophilic pneumonitis, erythema multiforme, exfoliative dermatitis, fatigue, fever, flank pain, flushing, glossitis, gynecomastia, hepatotoxicity, herpes zoster, hoarseness, hyperkalemia, hyponatremia, hypotension (severe), ileus, impotence, increased SCr and BUN, insomnia, melena, MI, muscle cramps, nervousness, neutropenia, oliguria, palpitations, pancreatitis, pemphigus, peripheral neuropathy, photosensitivity, pneumonia, pruritus, pulmonary edema, pulmonary embolism and infarction, pulmonary infiltrates, rash, Raynaud's phenomenon, renal dysfunction, renal failure (reversible), rhinorrhea, somnolence, sore throat, Stevens-Johnson syndrome, stomatitis, syncope, taste disturbances, tearing, thrombocytopenia, toxic epidermal necrolysis, upper respiratory infection, urinary tract infection, urticaria, vertigo, vomiting. Anaphylaxis has been reported.

ANTIDOTE

For minor side effects, notify the physician. Most will be tolerated or treated symptomatically. If symptoms progress or any major side effect occurs (angioedema, excessive hypotension), discontinue drug and notify the physician immediately. If hypotension occurs, place the patient in the supine position and, if necessary, administer an IV infusion of NS. Other drugs in the regimen (e.g., diuretics) may need to be discontinued or the dosage reduced. Epinephrine, diphenhydramine, and hydrocortisone may be used to treat angioedema. Maintain the patient as indicated. If cardiac arrhythmias occur, treat appropriately. Hemodialysis may be useful in toxicity.

EPHEDRINE SULFATE
(eh-**FED**-rin **SUL**-fayt)

Alpha- and beta-adrenergic agonist
Vasopressor

Akovaz, Corphedra

pH 4.5 to 7

USUAL DOSE
5 to 10 mg; administer additional boluses as needed, titrating to effect. Do not exceed a total dose of 50 mg.

PEDIATRIC DOSE (UNLABELED)
One source recommends 0.1 to 0.2 mg/kg/dose by slow IV push; administer as needed to maintain blood pressure, not to exceed a total dose of 25 mg.

DOSE ADJUSTMENTS
Lower-end initial doses may be appropriate in the elderly based on the potential for decreased renal function and concomitant disease or drug therapy. See Drug/Lab Interactions.

DILUTION
Available as a 50 mg/mL single-dose vial. Must be diluted to a final concentration of 5 mg/mL with D5W or NS before administration by withdrawing 1 mL (50 mg) of ephedrine and diluting with 9 mL of D5W or NS. Withdraw appropriate volume of diluted solution to provide desired dose (e.g., 1 mL equals a 5-mg dose) and administer as an IV bolus.

Filters: No data available from manufacturer.

Storage: Store at CRT in carton until time of use to protect from light.

COMPATIBILITY
Compatibility information not available from manufacturer. Other sources suggest a few specific **compatibilities** dependent on concentration and manufacturer; consult a pharmacist.

RATE OF ADMINISTRATION
Administer as a slow IV push. Rate not specified by manufacturer.

ACTIONS
A sympathomimetic drug that stimulates both alpha- and beta-adrenergic receptors and stimulates the release of norepinephrine. Pressor effects by direct alpha- and beta-adrenergic receptor activation are mediated by increases in arterial pressures, cardiac output, and peripheral resistance. Indirect adrenergic stimulation is caused by norepinephrine release from sympathetic nerves. It is less potent but longer acting than epinephrine. Stimulates heart rate and cardiac output and variably increases peripheral resistance; as a result, ephedrine usually increases blood pressure. Widely distributed in body fluids. Metabolized in the liver (exact metabolic pathway unknown) and excreted in urine. Urinary excretion is dependent on pH of urine; see Drug/Lab Interactions. Crosses the placental barrier and is secreted in breast milk.

INDICATIONS AND USES
Treatment of clinically important hypotension occurring in the setting of anesthesia.

CONTRAINDICATIONS
Manufacturer states, "None."

PRECAUTIONS
Repeated administration of ephedrine can result in tachyphylaxis. An alternative pressor should be available, if needed, to mitigate unacceptable responsiveness. ▪ When used to *prevent* hypotension (prophylactic use), ephedrine has been associated with an increased incidence of hypertension compared with when it is used to *treat* hypotension.

Monitor: Check BP and HR. ▪ In patients with renal impairment, elimination half-life may be increased, resulting in prolonged pharmacologic effect and potential adverse reactions. Monitor carefully after initial bolus. ▪ See Drug/Lab Interactions.

Maternal/Child: Limited published data; determine risk versus benefit. Cases of potential metabolic acidosis in newborns at delivery with maternal ephedrine exposure have been reported; monitoring of newborn for S/S of metabolic acidosis may be required. ▪ Safety for use in breast-feeding not established. ▪ Safety and effectiveness for use in pediatric patients not established.

Elderly: Differences in response have not been identified between the elderly and younger patients. In general, dose range for the elderly should be cautious, usually starting at the low end of the dosing range.

DRUG/LAB INTERACTIONS

Serious postpartum hypertension has been reported in patients who received both a vasopressor (e.g., ephedrine) and an **oxytocic** (e.g., methylergonovine, ergonovine, oxytocin). Monitor BP in patients who receive both ephedrine and an oxytocic. ▪ Do not use concomitantly with **other sympathomimetic agents** (e.g., dopamine, dobutamine, epinephrine). Additive effects may cause toxicity. ▪ **Atropine, clonidine, MAO inhibitors**, and **propofol** increase pressor response. Monitor BP carefully. ▪ **Digoxin** may sensitize myocardium and increase the risk of arrhythmias. ▪ **Alpha-adrenergic antagonists, beta-adrenergic antagonists, reserpine**, and **quinidine** are examples of drugs that may antagonize the pressor effects of ephedrine, decreasing its effectiveness. Monitor blood pressure. ▪ Antihypertensive effect of **guanethidine** may be decreased; monitor carefully. ▪ May reduce the onset of neuromuscular blockade when used for intubation with **rocuronium** if administered simultaneously with the anesthetic induction. ▪ May decrease the efficacy of **epidural anesthesia blockade** by hastening the regression of sensory analgesia. Monitor and treat the patient according to clinical practice. ▪ Use with **theophylline** may increase cardiac, CNS, and GI side effects. ▪ Interacts with many other drugs.

SIDE EFFECTS

The most common adverse reactions are nausea, vomiting, and tachycardia. Other reported adverse reactions include bradycardia, dizziness, palpitations, reactive hypertension, restlessness, and ventricular ectopics.

ANTIDOTE

If side effects occur, discontinue drug and notify physician. Side effects may be treated symptomatically. Monitor BP carefully. If BP continues to rise to an unacceptable level, parenteral antihypertensive agents can be administered at the discretion of the clinician. Resuscitate as necessary.

EPINEPHRINE HYDROCHLORIDE
(ep-ih-**NEF**-rin hy-droh-**KLOR**-eyed)

Alpha/beta adrenergic agonist
Vasopressor

Adrenalin Chloride

pH 2.5 to 5

USUAL DOSE

Hypotension associated with septic shock: 0.05 to 2 mcg/kg/min. Titrate in increments of 0.05 to 0.2 mcg/kg/min every 10 to 15 minutes to achieve a desired mean arterial pressure (MAP). ACLS guidelines recommend an initial dose of 0.1 to 0.5 mcg/kg/min with titration to desired response. After hemodynamic stabilization, wean the epinephrine infusion incrementally over time, such as by decreasing doses every 30 minutes over a 12- to 24-hour period.

Treatment of anaphylaxis: *IM administration in the thigh is preferred* in the setting of anaphylaxis. IV administration should be reserved for patients who are unresponsive or profoundly hypotensive and who have failed to respond to IV fluid replacement and several epinephrine injections.

Slow IV bolus: 0.1 mg using a **0.1 mg/mL** solution administered over 5 to 10 minutes.

Continuous infusion: Initiate at 2 to 15 mcg/min (with crystalloid administration).

Bradycardia (symptomatic; unresponsive to atropine or pacing): ACLS guidelines recommend an epinephrine infusion at 2 to 10 mcg/min **or** 0.1 to 0.5 mcg/kg/min. Titrate to desired effect.

Cardiac arrest: ACLS guidelines recommend 1 mg (10 mL of a 0.1 mg/mL concentration) IV; may repeat every 3 to 5 minutes. Follow each dose with a 20-mL IV flush to ensure delivery to systemic circulation. See Compatibility. Doses up to 0.2 mg/kg have been used for specific indications (beta-blocker or calcium channel blocker overdose). May also be given as a continuous infusion by adding 1 mg of epinephrine (1 mL of a 1 mg/mL solution) to 500 mL NS or D5W. Begin with an infusion rate of 0.1 to 0.5 mcg/kg/min and titrate to response. The dose for a 70-kg patient would be 7 to 35 mcg/min. Higher doses of epinephrine (greater than 1 mg) are controversial; have not been shown to improve survival or neurologic outcomes compared with standard dose epinephrine and are not recommended.

Endotracheal: A diluted solution may be given through the endotracheal tube before an IV is established. ACLS guidelines recommend 2 to 2.5 mg (of a 1 mg/mL solution) diluted in 10 mL NS.

PEDIATRIC DOSE

Hypersensitivity reactions or bronchospasm in infants and children: See comments under Usual Dose. 0.01 mg/kg (0.1 mL/kg of a 0.1 mg/mL concentration). May repeat at 20-minute to 4-hour intervals. One source suggests a maximum dose of 0.3 mg.

Severe anaphylactic shock in infants and children: One source suggests 0.1 mg IV of a 0.01 mg/mL concentration (0.1 mL of a 1 mg/mL concentration diluted in 10 mL NS) given over 5 to 10 minutes. Another source suggests 0.01 mL/kg of a 1 mg/mL concentration SC. Maximum 0.5 mL/dose.

Bradycardia (symptomatic; unresponsive to atropine or pacing) in infants and children: PALS guidelines recommend 0.01 mg/kg (0.1 mL/kg of a 0.1 mg/mL concentration) (maximum dose: 1 mg) every 3 to 5 minutes as needed. If IV access is not readily available, guidelines recommend 0.1 mg/kg (0.1 mL/kg of a 1 mg/mL concentration) via ET (maximum single dose: 2.5 mg) every 3 to 5 minutes as needed.

Asystolic or pulseless arrest in infants and children: PALS guidelines recommend 0.01 mg/kg (0.1 mL/kg of a 0.1 mg/mL concentration) (maximum single dose: 1 mg). Repeat every 3 to 5 minutes during arrest. May be given via ET (0.1 mg/kg [0.1 mL/kg of a 1 mg/mL concentration]) (maximum single dose: 2.5 mg) every 3 to 5 minutes until IV established, then begin with first IV dose.

Asystolic or pulseless arrest in neonates: PALS guidelines recommend 0.01 to 0.03 mg/kg (0.1 to 0.3 mL/kg of a 0.1 mg/mL concentration) initially. May repeat every 3 to 5 minutes.

DOSE ADJUSTMENTS

Lower-end initial dosing may be appropriate in the elderly based on the potential for decreased organ function and concomitant disease or drug therapy. ▪ See Drug/Lab Interactions.

DILUTION

New changes in labeling eliminate the use of ratios; what was previously a 1:1,000 solution will now be referred to only as a 1 mg/mL solution, a 1:10,000 solution will now be referred to only as a 0.1 mg/mL solution, and a 1:100,000 solution will now be referred to only as a 0.01 mg/mL solution.

Check label. Not all epinephrine solutions can be given IV. The 1 mg/mL strength is for SC or IM use only. It must be further diluted with 9 mL of NS to prepare a 0.1 mg/mL solution before IV or ocular use.

1 mg (1 mL) mixed in 9 mL = 1 mg/10 mL = 0.1 mg/mL solution

1 mg (1 mL) mixed in 99 mL = 1 mg/100 mL = 0.01 mg/mL

IV injection: Available prediluted (0.1 mg/mL) in 10-mL syringes. Available in a 30-mL vial (30 mg [1 mg/mL solution]). Each 1 mg (1 mL) of 1 mg/mL solution must be diluted in 9 mL of NS to prepare a 0.1 mg/mL solution.

Infusion: Manufacturer recommends diluting 1 mg in 1000 mL of D5W or a 5% dextrose and sodium chloride solution to provide an infusion solution with a final concentration of 1 mcg/mL. Other commonly used infusion concentrations are 1 mg in 250 mL (concentration: 4 mcg/mL) or 4 mg in 250 mL (concentration: 16 mcg/mL). In pediatric patients, commonly used infusion concentrations are 16 mcg/mL, 32 mcg/mL, or 64 mcg/mL. See chart on inside back cover for additional **compatible** solutions.

Filters: No data available from manufacturer.

Storage: Store at CRT unless otherwise specified by manufacturer. Do not refrigerate. Do not use if colored or cloudy or contains particulate matter. Deteriorates rapidly. Protect from light and freezing.

COMPATIBILITY

Manufacturer states, "Readily destroyed and precipitate forms with alkalis, alkaline solutions (e.g., sodium bicarbonate and oxidizing agents)." *If coadministration with sodium bicarbonate is indicated, give at separate sites.* Manufacturer also states that dilution in dextrose-containing solutions provides protection against significant loss of potency by oxidation and that *administration in saline solution alone is not recommended.* (However, another source says that epinephrine is stable in NS.) Unstable in any solution with a pH over 5.5 (e.g., aminophylline, ampicillin, lidocaine, warfarin). Administration of whole blood or plasma, if needed, should be given through a separate line.

Other sources suggest specific **compatibilities** dependent on concentration and manufacturer; consult a pharmacist.

RATE OF ADMINISTRATION

IV injection: Some sources recommend giving IV doses for treatment of hypersensitivity reactions over 5 to 10 minutes. May be given more rapidly in cardiac resuscitation; follow with 20-mL IV flush.

Infusion: See Usual Dose. Must be delivered by central venous access (preferred) or through a large vein. Use an infusion pump to control rate.

ACTIONS

A naturally occurring hormone secreted by the adrenal glands. A sympathomimetic drug, it imitates almost all actions of the sympathetic nervous system. Stimulates both alpha- and beta-adrenergic receptors. The mechanism of the rise of blood pressure is threefold: (1) a direct myocardial stimulation that increases the strength of the ventricular contraction (positive inotropic action), (2) an increased heart rate (positive chronotropic action), and (3) peripheral vasoconstriction. Most vascular beds are constricted, including renal, splanchnic, mucosal, and skin. Decreases in systemic vascular resistance and diastolic BP are seen at lower doses. At higher doses, alpha-mediated vasoconstriction leads to an increase in diastolic BP. Onset of action for elevating blood pressure is less than 5 minutes. Time to offset of blood pressure response occurs within 20 minutes. When used for treatment of anaphylaxis, epinephrine lessens the vasodilation and increased vascular permeability that occurs during anaphylaxis and can lead to a loss of intravascular fluid volume and hypotension. Epinephrine causes bronchial smooth muscle relaxation and helps alleviate bronchospasm, wheezing, and dyspnea. It also helps to alleviate pruritus, urticaria, and angioedema and may relieve gastrointestinal and genitourinary symptoms because of its relaxant effects on the smooth muscle of the stomach, intestine, uterus, and urinary bladder. Has a rapid onset of action. Steady state is achieved within 10 to 15 minutes of starting an infusion. Half-life is less than 5 minutes. It is rapidly and extensively metabolized and is excreted in changed form in the urine. Crosses placental barrier.

INDICATIONS AND USES

Treatment of hypotension associated with septic shock in adult patients. (Used to increase mean arterial pressure [MAP].) ▪ Emergency treatment of type I allergic reactions (including anaphylaxis) that may result from allergic reactions to insect stings, insect bites, foods, drugs, sera, diagnostic testing substances, and other allergens, as well as idiopathic anaphylaxis or exercise-induced anaphylaxis. S/S associated with anaphylaxis include flushing, apprehension, syncope, tachycardia, thready or unobtainable pulse associated with hypotension, convulsions, vomiting, diarrhea and abdominal cramps, involuntary voiding, airway swelling, laryngospasm, bronchospasm, pruritus, urticaria or angioedema, and swelling of the eyelids, lips, and tongue. ■ Induction and maintenance of mydriasis during intraocular surgery (given as an intraocular irrigation).

Unlabeled indications: Acute, severe asthma unresponsive to an inhaled beta-agonist; asystole/pulseless arrest, ventricular fibrillation, or pulseless ventricular tachycardia; bradycardia unresponsive to atropine or pacing; hypotension/shock unresponsive to volume resuscitation; inotropic support.

CONTRAINDICATIONS

One manufacturer states, "None." Some manufacturers and sources list the following potential contraindications: anesthesia with halogenated hydrocarbons or cyclopropane, cerebral arteriosclerosis, diabetes, hypersensitivity to sympathomimetic amines, hypertension and other cardiovascular disorders, labor and delivery if maternal BP exceeds 130/80 mm Hg, labor (may delay second stage), narrow-angle glaucoma, nonanaphylactic shock, organic brain damage. There are no absolute contraindications in a life-threatening situation.

PRECAUTIONS

Usual route is SC or IM except in cardiac resuscitation or as a vasopressor infusion. ■ Correct blood volume depletion as fully as possible before administration. In an emergency situation (e.g., intra-aortic pressures must be maintained to prevent cerebral or coronary artery ischemia), epinephrine can be administered before and concurrently with blood volume replacement. ■ Because of varying responses to epinephrine, dangerously high blood pressure can occur; see Monitor and Drug/Lab Interactions. ■ Tissue necrosis can occur with extravasation. Blanching along the course of the vein, sometimes without obvious extravasation, may be attributed to constriction of the vasa vasorum (small blood vessels that supply or drain the walls of the larger arteries and veins and connect with a branch of the same vessel or a neighboring vessel). This constriction may result in increased permeability of the vein wall, permitting some leakage that, rarely, may progress to a superficial slough. If blanching occurs, consider changing infusion site. ■ Pulmonary edema may occur as a result of the peripheral constriction and cardiac stimulation that is produced; see Antidote. Constriction of renal blood vessels may result in decreased urine formation. ■ Epinephrine may induce cardiac arrhythmias and angina pectoris. Risk is increased in patients with coronary artery disease, organic heart disease, cerebrovascular disease, or hypertension or in patients who are receiving drugs that sensitize the myocardium. ■ Use caution in elderly patients, pregnant women, and patients with diabetes (may experience transient increases in blood sugar), hyperthyroidism, pheochromocytoma, and Parkinson's disease (may experience psychomotor agitation or a temporary worsening of symptoms). ■ Higher doses may be required to treat poison-induced shock. ■ Manufacturer lists additional precautions for nonintravenous routes.

Monitor: Monitor vital signs. Invasive arterial blood pressure monitoring and central venous pressure monitoring are recommended. Dangerously high blood pressure can occur with IV administration. ■ Monitoring of ECG and serum potassium and glucose concentrations may be indicated. ■ Epinephrine is a vesicant. Frequent monitoring of IV infusion site is required. Whenever possible, administer infusion into a large vein; central line administration is preferred. Avoid administering in areas of limited blood supply (e.g., fingers, toes) or if peripheral vascular disease is present. Occlusive vascular diseases (e.g., atherosclerosis, arteriosclerosis, diabetic endarteritis, Buerger's disease) are more likely to occur in the lower extremity than in the upper extremity; avoid veins of the legs in elderly patients or in patients suffering from occlusive vascular diseases. ■ Monitor urinary output. ■ See Drug/Lab Interactions.

Patient Education: Review potential side effects with patient or caregiver (e.g., anxiety, apprehension, difficulty breathing, dizziness, forceful heartbeat, headache, increase in HR, nausea, nervousness, pallor, palpitations, shakiness, sweating, vomiting, and weakness). These S/S usually subside rapidly, especially with rest, quiet, and recumbent positioning. ▪ Symptoms of anaphylaxis may recur following successful treatment. Seek medical help if needed. ▪ Increases in blood glucose levels may occur following administration of epinephrine.

Maternal/Child: Category C: assess risk versus benefit; may cause fetal anoxia, spontaneous abortion, or both. ▪ Avoid use in obstetrics when maternal blood pressure exceeds 130/80 mm Hg. ▪ Use caution during labor and delivery. Inhibits spontaneous or oxytocin-induced contractions and may delay the second stage of labor. In doses sufficient to reduce uterine contraction, epinephrine may cause a prolonged period of uterine atony with hemorrhage. Although epinephrine improves maternal hypotension associated with anaphylaxis, it may result in uterine vasoconstriction, decreased uterine blood flow, and fetal anoxia. ▪ Use caution in breast-feeding. ▪ Safety and effectiveness in pediatric patients with septic shock have not been established. Clinical use data support weight-based dosing for treatment of anaphylaxis and suggest that the adverse reactions seen in children are similar in nature and extent to those reported for adults.

Elderly: Data are limited. May be more sensitive to the effects of beta-adrenergic receptor agonists (e.g., hypertension, hypokalemia, tachycardia, tremor). Patients with cardiac disease may be at increased risk for adverse effects. ▪ Dose selection should be cautious in the elderly; see Dose Adjustments and Precautions.

DRUG/LAB INTERACTIONS

May be used alternately with isoproterenol (Isuprel), but they may not be used together. Both are direct cardiac stimulants, and concomitant use may increase the risk of arrhythmia. Adequate interval between doses must be maintained. ▪ **Oxytocics** (e.g., oxytocin), **other sympathomimetic agents** (e.g., ephedrine, dopamine), **MAO inhibitors, nonselective beta-adrenergic blockers** (e.g., propranolol), **tricyclic antidepressants, catechol-O-methyltransferase (COMT) inhibitors** (e.g., entacapone), **and clonidine** potentiate the pressor effects of epinephrine; may result in hypertension or cause hypertensive crisis. ▪ **Alpha-blockers, vasodilators** (e.g., nitrates), **diuretics, antihypertensives, and ergot alkaloids** may antagonize the pressor effects of epinephrine. ▪ Epinephrine may antagonize the neuronal blockade produced by **guanethidine**, resulting in a decreased antihypertensive effect and requiring increased dosage of the latter. ▪ Epinephrine should not be used to counteract circulatory collapse or hypotension caused by **phenothiazines**, because a reversal of the pressor effects of epinephrine may result in further lowering of blood pressure. ■ **Hydrocarbon anesthetics** (e.g., enflurane, halothane), **digoxin, nonselective beta-adrenergic blockers** (e.g., propranolol), **antihistamines, thyroid hormone, diuretics, and quinidine** may increase the risk of arrhythmias; monitor patients who must receive concomitant use. ■ Use with **theophylline, potassium-depleting diuretics, and corticosteroids** may potentiate the hypokalemic effects of epinephrine. ■ Interacts with many other drugs.

SIDE EFFECTS

The most commonly reported adverse reactions associated with the IV administration of epinephrine include anxiety, apprehensiveness, dizziness, headache, nausea, pallor, palpitations, peripheral coldness, restlessness, respiratory difficulties, sweating, tremor, vomiting, and weakness. Arrhythmias (including fatal ventricular fibrillation), rapid rises in blood pressure producing cerebral hemorrhage, and angina have occurred. Other reported reactions include chest pain, diaphoresis, excitability, extravasation, hyperglycemia, hypoglycemia, hypokalemia, insulin resistance, lactic acidosis, limb ischemia, MI, myocardial ischemia, nervousness, paresthesia, piloerection, pulmonary edema, rales, renal insufficiency, skin blanching, skin necrosis with extravasation, stroke, supraventricular tachycardia, tachycardia, ventricular arrhythmias.

Overdose (frequently caused by too-rapid injection): Arrhythmia (atrial and ventricular), bradycardia (transient followed by tachycardia), cardiomyopathy, cerebrovascular hemorrhage, extreme pallor and coldness of the skin, hypertension, metabolic acidosis due to elevated lactic acid levels, myocardial ischemia or infarction, pulmonary edema, pupillary dilation, renal failure, tachycardia, death.

ANTIDOTE

Treatment is primarily supportive. If side effects from the average dose become progressively worse, discontinue the drug and notify the physician. IM or SC route may be preferable. To prevent sloughing and necrosis in areas in which extravasation has occurred, use a fine hypodermic needle to inject 5 to 10 mg of phentolamine diluted in 10 to 15 mL NS liberally throughout the tissue in the affected area. Begin as soon as extravasation is recognized. Treatment of pulmonary edema consists of a rapidly acting alpha-adrenergic blocking agent (such as phentolamine) and respiratory support. Pressor effects may be counteracted by rapidly acting vasodilators (e.g., nitrates) or alpha-adrenergic blocking agents (e.g., phentolamine). If prolonged hypotension follows such measures, it may be necessary to administer another pressor drug. Treat cardiac arrhythmias with a beta-adrenergic blocker. Resuscitate as necessary.

EPIRUBICIN HYDROCHLORIDE BBW

(ep-ee-**ROO**-bih-sin hy-droh-**KLOR**-eyed)

Ellence ▪ **Pharmorubicin PFS** ♣

Antineoplastic
(anthracycline antibiotic)

pH 3 ▪ pH 4 to 5.5

USUAL DOSE

ELLENCE

Pretreatment: Verify pregnancy status. Preassessment and baseline studies required; see Monitor.

Premedication: Consider use of antiemetics before administration of epirubicin or when clinically indicated to reduce nausea and vomiting, particularly when given in conjunction with other emetigenic drugs.

Epirubicin: Recommended starting dose is 100 to 120 mg/M^2. Administer as an IV injection over 15 to 20 minutes through Y-tube of a free-flowing infusion of NS or D5W. Patients receiving the 120-mg/M^2 dose should also receive prophylactic antibiotic therapy with sulfamethoxazole/trimethoprim or a fluoroquinolone (e.g., ciprofloxacin [Cipro]). Ellence is usually given in repeated 3- to 4-week cycles. Total dose may be given on Day 1 of each cycle or equally divided and given on Days 1 and 8 of each cycle.

One regimen used is 60 mg/M^2 of epirubicin intravenously on Days 1 and 8 given in a regimen with oral cyclophosphamide 75 mg/M^2 on Days 1 to 14 and fluorouracil 500 mg/M^2 on Days 1 and 8. Repeat every 28 days for six cycles. Another regimen used is 100 mg/M^2 of epirubicin intravenously together with fluorouracil 500 mg/M^2 and cyclophosphamide 500 mg/M^2. All three agents are given on Day 1 and are repeated every 21 days for 6 cycles. In either regimen the total dose of epirubicin may be given on Day 1 of each cycle or equally divided and given on Days 1 and 8 of each cycle.

♣PHARMORUBICIN PFS

Metastatic breast cancer: *Single agent:* 75 to 90 mg/M^2 once every 21 days. This dose may be divided and given on Day 1 and Day 2. An alternative weekly dose schedule of 12.5 to 25 mg/M^2 has been used and has been reported to produce less clinical toxicity than higher doses given every 3 weeks. *Combination therapy:* 50 mg/M^2. Used in combination with cyclophosphamide and fluorouracil.

Early-stage breast cancer (Stage II-IIIA): 50 to 60 mg/M^2 given on Days 1 and 8 every 4 weeks. Used in combination with cyclophosphamide and fluorouracil.

Small-cell lung cancer: *Single agent:* 90 to 120 mg/M^2 once every 3 weeks. *Combination therapy:* 50 to 90 mg/M^2. Several combinations have been used (e.g., with either cisplatin or ifosfamide; with cyclophosphamide and vincristine; with cyclophosphamide and etoposide; or with cisplatin and etoposide).

Non–small-cell lung cancer: *Single agent:* 120 to 150 mg/M^2 on Day 1 every 3 to 4 weeks. *Combination therapy:* 90 to 120 mg/M^2 on Day 1 every 3 to 4 weeks. Used in combination with cisplatin, etoposide, mitomycin, and vinblastine.

Non-Hodgkin lymphoma: *Single agent:* 75 to 90 mg/M^2 once every 3 weeks. *Combination therapy:* 60 to 75 mg/M^2. Used in combination with cyclophosphamide, prednisone, and vincristine with or without bleomycin for the treatment of newly diagnosed non-Hodgkin lymphoma.

Hodgkin disease: *Combination therapy:* 35 mg/M^2 once every 2 weeks or 70 mg/M^2 once every 3 to 4 weeks. Used in combination with bleomycin, dacarbazine, and vinblastine.

Ovarian cancer: *Single agent:* 50 to 90 mg/M^2 once every 3 or 4 weeks in patients who have had prior therapy. *Combination therapy:* 50 to 90 mg/M^2 once every 3 or 4 weeks can be added to their regimen in patients who have had prior therapy; or the same dose in combination with cisplatin and cyclophosphamide is used for initial therapy of ovarian cancer.

Locally unresectable or metastatic gastric cancer: *Single agent:* 75 to 100 mg/M^2 once every 3 weeks. *Combination therapy:* 80 mg/M^2 once every 3 to 4 weeks. Used in combination with fluorouracil.

DOSE ADJUSTMENTS

ALL FORMULATIONS: Reduced dose required with elevated serum bilirubin. Give 50% of a dose for serum bilirubin from 1.2 to 3 mg/dL or AST 2 to 4 times the ULN. Give 25% of a dose for serum bilirubin greater than 3 mg/mL or AST greater than 4 times the ULN.
ELLENCE: Consider reducing starting dose to 75 to 90 mg/M^2 in heavily pretreated patients, those with pre-existing bone marrow suppression, or in the presence of neoplastic bone marrow infiltration. ▪ Consider reduced dose in patients with severe renal impairment (SCr greater than 5 mg/dL). ▪ Base dose adjustments after the first treatment cycle on hematologic response during treatment cycle nadir and nonhematologic toxicities. In patients who received the full dose on Day 1, reduce dose to 75% of initial first dose in subsequent cycles for platelet count less than 50,000/mm^3, absolute neutrophil count (ANC) less than 250/mm^3, neutropenic fever, or Grade 3 or 4 nonhematologic toxicity. Delay dose in subsequent treatment cycles until platelet count recovers to at least 100,000/mm^3, ANC recovers to at least 1,500/mm^3, and nonhematologic toxicities have recovered to equal to or less than Grade 1. For patients receiving a divided dose, reduce the Day-8 dose to 75% of the Day-1 dose if platelet counts are 75,000 to 100,000/mm^3 and ANC is 1,000 to 1,499/mm^3. Omit the Day-8 dose if platelet counts are less than 75,000/mm^3, ANC less than 1,000/mm^3, or Grade 3 or 4 nonhematologic toxicity has occurred.
❦**PHARMORUBICIN PFS:** Use lower dose in range for patients with inadequate marrow reserves due to old age, prior therapy, or neoplastic marrow infiltration. ▪ Reduced dose, delay, or suspension of epirubicin may be required based on hematologic toxicity; manufacturer provides no specific recommendations. ▪ No dose adjustment required in impaired renal function.

DILUTION

Specific techniques required; see Precautions.
ELLENCE: Available as 2 mg/mL in 25-mL and 100-mL vials. A ready-to-use, preservative-free solution; further dilution not required. Must be given through Y-tube of a free-flowing infusion of NS or D5W.
❦**PHARMORUBICIN PFS:** Available as 2 mg/mL in 5-mL, 25-mL, and 100-mL vials. Use of the 100-mL vial should be restricted to a pharmacy admixture program using a sterile transfer or dispensing device. Enter any vial only once and withdraw desired dose into a syringe. No further dilution is required.
FILTERS: Manufacturer indicates that studies show some initial potency loss in the first few minutes with the use of cellulose ester membrane or nylon filters; however, the total amount of drug loss is negligible. A second source has a similar statement.
Storage: *Ellence:* Refrigerate vials at 2° to 8° C (34° to 46° F); protect from light. Do not freeze. Refrigeration may result in a gel-formed product; will return to a slightly viscous to mobile solution within 2 to 4 hours. Must be used within 24 hours of removal from refrigeration. Discard unused solution.
❦*Pharmorubicin:* Store unopened PFS vials in refrigerator; keep in original cartons to protect from light. Use any filled syringe within 24 hours if stored at room temperature and within 48 hours if refrigerated. Syringes prepared from the pharmacy bulk vial must be used within 24 or 48 hours of the initial puncture of that vial based on method of storage. Once the transfer set has been inserted in the bulk vial, any remaining undispensed drug must be discarded in 8 hours.

COMPATIBILITY

Manufacturers recommend not mixing with other drugs in the same syringe. Avoid prolonged contact with alkaline solutions; will result in hydrolysis of all forms of epirubicin. Do not mix with heparin or fluorouracil (5-FU); may precipitate. **Incompatible** with ifosfamide (Ifex) when combined in syringe or solution with mesna (Mesnex). Can be used with other antitumor agents, but do not mix in the same syringe.

Other sources suggest a few specific **compatibilities** dependent on concentration and manufacturer; consult a pharmacist.

RATE OF ADMINISTRATION

IV injection: *All formulations:* An initial starting dose of 100 to 120 mg/M^2 should be infused over 15 to 20 minutes. Lower starting doses or modified doses may be administered over a minimum of 3 minutes and up to 20 minutes. Must be given through Y-tube of a free-flowing infusion of NS or D5W. Slow injection rate further for erythematous streaking along the vein or facial flushing.

ACTIONS

A semi-synthetic, anthracycline, antineoplastic antibiotic agent. Exact method of action is unknown. Rapidly and widely distributed into tissue. Inhibits DNA, RNA, and protein synthesis and interferes with replication and transcription. Free radicals cause further cytotoxic activity. Metabolized in the liver and by other organs and cells, including RBCs. WBC nadir is reached in 10 to 14 days and should return to normal by Day 21. Elimination half-life is 30 to 40 hours. Does not cross blood-brain barrier. Primarily excreted in bile; some excretion in urine.

INDICATIONS AND USES

ELLENCE: A component of adjuvant therapy in patients with evidence of axillary-node tumor involvement following resection in primary breast cancer.
♣**PHARMORUBICIN:** Treatment of metastatic as well as early-stage breast cancer, small-cell lung cancer (both limited and extensive disease), advanced non–small-cell lung cancer, non-Hodgkin lymphoma, Hodgkin disease, Stage III and IV ovarian cancer, and metastatic and locally unresectable gastric cancers. May be used as a single agent or in combination with other chemotherapeutic agents.
UNLABELED USES: All Formulations: Treatment of soft-tissue sarcomas in combination with other agents. Treatment of esophageal and esophagogastric junction cancers in combination with other agents. Ellence has been used in place of Pharmorubicin for various indications.

CONTRAINDICATIONS

Patients with severe myocardial insufficiency, recent myocardial infarction, or severe arrhythmias. ▪ Severe persistent drug-induced myelosuppression. ▪ Severe hepatic impairment (defined as Child-Pugh Class C or serum bilirubin level greater than 5 mg/dL). Contraindicated in patients who have received previous treatment with maximum recommended cumulative doses of epirubicin, other anthracyclines, or anthracenediones (e.g., daunorubicin [Cerubidine], doxorubicin [Adriamycin], idarubicin [Idamycin], mitoxantrone [Novantrone], or mitomycin C). ▪ Severe hypersensitivity to epirubicin, other anthracyclines, or anthracenediones.

PRECAUTIONS

Follow guidelines for handling cytotoxic agents. See Appendix A, p. 1308. ▪ Administered by or under the direction of the physician specialist, with facilities for monitoring the patient and responding to any medical emergency. ▪ For IV use only. Do not give IM or SC. ▪ May cause severe myelosuppression, resulting in serious infection, septic shock, requirement of transfusions, hospitalizations and death may occur. ▪ Epirubicin and other anthracycline drugs can result in early (acute) or late (delayed) cardiac toxicity. ▪ Prior history of cardiovascular disease, prior or concomitant radiotherapy to the mediastinal/pericardial area, previous therapy with other anthracyclines or anthracenediones, and concomitant use of other cardiotoxic drugs increase the risk of developing late cardiac toxicity. ▪ Cumulative doses of 900 mg/M^2 should generally be avoided. ▪ Myocardial damage, including acute left ventricular failure, can occur. ▪ The risk of cardiomyopathy is further increased with concomitant cardiotoxic therapy. ▪ Cardiotoxicity may occur at lower cumulative doses whether or not cardiac risk factors are present. ▪ Patients are at increased risk of developing cardiotoxicity with epirubicin after stopping treatment with other cardiotoxic drugs, especially those with long half-lives (e.g., trastuzumab). ▪ Epirubicin can increase radiation-induced toxicity to the myocardium, mucosa, skin, and liver. Radiation recall, including but not limited to cutaneous and pulmonary toxicity, can occur in patients after prior radiation therapy. ▪ Secondary acute myelogenous leukemia (AML) and myelodysplastic syndrome (MDS) occur at a higher Incidence in patients treated with anthracyclines. The cumulative probability of developing AML/MDS is particularly increased in patients who have received more than 720 mg/M^2 of epirubicin or more than 6,300 mg/M^2 of cyclophosphamide. ▪ Thrombophlebitis and thromboembolic events, including pulmonary embolism, have been reported.

Monitor: Obtain baseline CBC, including differential and platelet count; serum calcium, phosphate, and potassium; SCr; uric acid level; liver function tests (AST, ALT, alkaline phosphatase, and serum bilirubin). ▪ Obtain baseline cardiac evaluations with an ECG and evaluation of left ventricular ejection fraction (LVEF). ▪ Monitor LVEF during the course of treatment and consider discontinuation if LVEF decreases or S/S of CHF develop. ▪ Monitor lab values during therapy, especially before each dose. ▪ Monitor ECG, chest x-ray, echocardiogram, and/or radionuclide angiography in patients who have had mediastinal radiation, other anthracycline or anthracene therapy, those with pre-existing cardiac disease or S/S of impending heart disease, or those who have received prior epirubicin cumulative doses exceeding 550 mg/M^2. ▪ Monitor for signs of cardiac toxicity (e.g., rapid or irregular HR, shortness of breath, swelling of abdomen, feet, and lower legs); early signs usually include sinus tachycardia and nonspecific ST-T wave changes in the ECG; late signs include reduced LVEF and or S/S of CHF. If late cardiac toxicity occurs, it usually develops late during therapy or within 2 to 3 months after completion of treatment, but occurrences of months to years after treatment have happened. ▪ Closely monitor patients with other risk factors for cardiac toxicity, particularly prior administration of anthracycline or anthracenedione. ▪ Use only large veins. Avoid veins over joints or in extremities with compromised venous or lymphatic drainage. Determine absolute patency of vein. Extravasation may occur with or without stinging or burning along the injection site even if blood returns well on aspiration of the infusion needle. Observe site frequently. Extravasation can result in severe local tissue injury and tissue necrosis; if it occurs, discontinue injection. Use another vein; see Antidote. ▪ Prevention and treatment of hyperuricemia due to tumor lysis syndrome may be accomplished with adequate hydration and, if necessary, uric acid–lowering drugs (e.g., allopurinol [Aloprim]). ▪ Be alert for signs of bone marrow suppression, bleeding, or infection. ▪ Use of prophylactic antibiotics may be indicated pending C/S in a febrile neutropenic patient. ▪ Monitor for thrombocytopenia (platelet count less than 50,000/mm^3). Initiate precautions to prevent excessive bleeding (e.g., inspect IV sites, skin, and mucous membranes; use extreme care during invasive procedures; test urine, emesis, stool, and secretions for occult blood). ▪ Prophylactic antiemetics are indicated. ▪ See Drug/Lab Interactions.

Patient Education: Urine will be reddish for several days (from drug, not hematuria). ▪ Females of reproductive potential must use effective contraception during treatment and for 6 months after the last dose. ▪ Male patients with female partners of reproductive potential must use effective contraception during treatment and for 3 months after the last dose. Male patients with pregnant partners must use condoms during treatment and for at least 7 days after the last dose. May cause amenorrhea and premature menopause in women and oligospermia, azoospermia, and permanent loss of fertility in men. ▪ Report IV site burning, stinging, or puffiness promptly. ▪ Report dizziness, lightheadedness, rapid or irregular HR, shortness of breath, and swelling of the abdomen, feet, or lower legs. ▪ Report vomiting, dehydration, fever, or other evidence of infection. ▪ Review side effects; may be severe (e.g., nausea and vomiting, cardiotoxicity). ▪ See Appendix D, p. 1311.

Maternal/Child: Based on its mechanism of action, can cause fetal harm. Avoid pregnancy. ▪ Discontinue breast-feeding during treatment and for at least 7 days after the last dose. ▪ Information on safety for use in pediatric patients not available. Some studies suggest that pediatric patients may be at greater risk for anthracycline-induced acute cardiotoxicity and/or late cardiovascular dysfunction.

Elderly: No overall difference in safety and effectiveness compared with younger patients. ■ See Dose Adjustments. ■ There is a major decrease in plasma clearance of epirubicin in elderly female patients; monitor closely for signs of toxicity.

DRUG/LAB INTERACTIONS

May increase bone marrow and GI toxicity of other **chemotherapeutic agents.** ■ Increased toxicity including skin redness and exfoliative changes possible when given concurrently with or after **radiation.** ■ Monitoring of cardiac function may be indicated in patients taking **medications that may cause heart failure** (e.g., calcium channel blockers such as verapamil), beta-blockers (e.g., propranolol). ■ Plasma clearance decreased and serum levels increased by **cimetidine**; discontinue cimetidine. ■ Epirubicin is extensively metabolized in the liver; **changes in hepatic function induced by concomitant therapies** may affect epirubicin metabolism, pharmacokinetics, effectiveness, and toxicity. ■ Risk of cardiotoxicity increased in patients previously treated with maximum cumulative doses of **other anthracyclines** (e.g., doxorubicin, idarubicin) **and/or radiation encompassing the heart.** ■ **Trastuzumab** may persist in circulation for up to 7 months. Avoid anthracycline-based therapy for up to 7 months after stopping trastuzumab when possible. Monitor cardiac function closely if anthracyclines are used before this time. ■ Risk of cardiotoxicity is also increased when epirubicin is administered with **other cardiotoxic agents;** if possible, delay epirubicin-based therapy until other cardiotoxic agents have been cleared from the circulation. Careful cardiac monitoring is required if delay is not feasible. ■ Concomitant administration with other cytotoxic drugs may produce additive toxicity, especially hematologic and GI effects. ■ Leukopenic and/or thrombocytopenic effects may be increased with **drugs that cause blood dyscrasias** (e.g., anticonvulsants [e.g., carbamazepine, phenytoin], NSAIDs [e.g., ibuprofen, naproxen]). ■ Administration of epirubicin immediately before or after **paclitaxel** increased the systemic exposure (AUC) of epirubicin. The mean AUC of epirubicin's metabolites increased when paclitaxel was administered immediately after epirubicin. Epirubicin had no effect on the exposure of paclitaxel. ■ Administration of epirubicin immediately before or after **docetaxel** had no effect on the systemic exposure of epirubicin. However, the mean AUC of epirubicin's metabolites increased when docetaxel was administered immediately after epirubicin. Epirubicin had no effect on the AUC of docetaxel. ■ Do not administer **live virus vaccines** to patients receiving antineoplastic agents. Killed or inactivated vaccines may be administered; however, the response to these vaccines may be diminished. ■ See Precautions.

SIDE EFFECTS

Acute adverse events occurring in 10% or more of patients included alopecia, amenorrhea, conjunctivitis/keratitis, diarrhea, hematologic toxicity (anemia, leukopenia, neutropenia, thrombocytopenia), infection, lethargy, local toxicity, mucositis, nausea/

vomiting, and rash/itch. Dose-limiting toxicities are infection, myelosuppression, and cardiotoxicity (usually delayed, manifested by reduced LVEF and/or S/S of CHF [e.g., ascites, dependent edema, dyspnea, gallop rhythm, hepatomegaly, pleural effusion, pulmonary edema, tachycardia]). Other serious cardiovascular adverse reactions that have occurred include AV block, bradycardia, bundle branch block, thromboembolism, and ventricular tachycardia. Severe cellulitis, vesication, local pain, and tissue necrosis can occur with extravasation. Venous sclerosis may result from injection into small veins or repeated injection into the same vein. Other side effects are anorexia, febrile neutropenia, fever, hot flashes, malaise, mucositis (esophagitis, stomatitis), phlebitis, recall of skin reaction associated with prior radiation. Hypersensitivity reactions have been reported.

Overdose: May cause an acute myocardial dysfunction within 24 hours. Bone marrow aplasia, gastrointestinal bleeding, Grade 4 mucositis, hyperthermia, lactic acidosis, multiple organ failure, and death have been reported following significant overdoses.

Post-Marketing: Anaphylaxis; chills; dehydration; erythema; fever; flushing; GI disorders (e.g., bleeding, burning, pain, ulceration); hyperpigmentation of the skin, nails, and oral mucosa; hyperuricemia; photosensitivity; pneumonia; pulmonary embolism; radiation recall; red coloration of urine for 1 to 2 days; sepsis; urticaria; and vascular disorders (arterial embolism, hemorrhage, phlebitis, shock, and thrombophlebitis).

ANTIDOTE

Most side effects will either be tolerated or treated symptomatically. Keep the physician informed. Discontinue in patients who develop S/S of cardiomyopathy. Hematopoietic toxicity (leukopenia, thrombocytopenia) may require dose reduction or cessation of therapy, antibiotics, platelet and granulocyte transfusions, darbepoetin alfa, epoetin alfa, filgrastim, pegfilgrastim, or sargramostim. Acute cardiac failure occurs suddenly (most common when total cumulative doses approach 900 mg/M^2) and frequently does not respond to currently available treatment. Close monitoring of accumulated dose, bone marrow, ECG, chest x-ray, echocardiography, and systolic ejection fraction may prevent most serious and potentially fatal cardiac side effects. There is no specific antidote. Supportive therapy as indicated will help sustain the patient in toxicity. Dexrazoxane is currently available to prevent cardiotoxicity of doxorubicin in specific situations; in the future it may be considered with epirubicin. If extravasation occurs, discontinue immediately, and attempt aspiration of the infiltrated epirubicin. Elevate the extremity and apply local intermittent ice compresses for up to 3 days. If appropriate, administer dexrazoxane (Totect) at the site of extravasation as soon as possible and within the first 6 hours after extravasation. Observe the site frequently. Should be seen by a reconstructive surgeon if local pain persists or skin changes progress after 3 to 4 days. Ulceration may require early wide excision of the involved area and skin grafting. Treat hypersensitivity reactions as indicated.

EPOETIN ALFA BBW ∎
EPOETIN ALFA-epbx[a] BBW
(ee-**POH**-ee-tin **AL**-fah)

Recombinant human erythropoietin
Erythropoiesis-stimulating agent
(ESA) Hematopoietic agent

EPO, Epogen, Erythropoietin, Procrit, Retacrit[a]

pH 5.8 to 7.2

USUAL DOSE

Epoetin alfa-epbx[a] is a biosimilar drug of epoetin alfa (Epogen, Procrit). Unless specifically stated otherwise, information in this monograph applies to all formulations of epoetin-alfa.

Pretreatment: In all situations, rate of hematocrit increase is dose dependent and varies among patients. Availability of iron stores, baseline hematocrit, and concurrent medical problems affect the rate and extent of response. Correct or exclude other causes of anemia (e.g., vitamin deficiency, metabolic or chronic inflammatory conditions, bleeding) before initiating epoetin alfa. Use the lowest dose for each patient that will gradually increase the hemoglobin concentration to avoid the need for RBC transfusion; see Precautions and Monitor.

Anemia associated with chronic kidney disease (CKD) for patients on dialysis: Initiate epoetin when the hemoglobin level is less than 10 Gm/dL. ***Starting dose:*** 50 to 100 units/kg of body weight three times a week. May be given by IV or SC injection or into the venous line at the end of a dialysis session. The IV route is recommended in patients on hemodialysis; see Precautions.

Anemia associated with chronic kidney disease (CKD) for patients NOT on dialysis: Consider initiating epoetin only when the hemoglobin level is less than 10 Gm/dL and the following two considerations apply: (1) the rate of hemoglobin decline indicates the likelihood of requiring a RBC transfusion, and (2) reducing the risk of alloimmunization and/or other RBC transfusion-related risks is a goal. ***Starting dose:*** 50 to 100 units/kg of body weight three times a week.

Anemia in zidovudine-treated, HIV-infected patients: May be given IV or SC. 100 units/kg 3 times a week. Obtain endogenous serum erythropoietin level (before transfusion) before initiating therapy; see Monitor. Serum erythropoietin levels in adults should be equal to or less than 500 mUnits/mL, and the zidovudine dose should be equal to or less than 4,200 mg/week.

Anemia associated with cancer patients on chemotherapy: SC injection recommended. ESAs shortened overall survival and/or increased the risk of tumor progression or recurrence in clinical studies of patients with certain types of cancer; see Precautions. Initiate epoetin in patients on cancer chemotherapy only if the hemoglobin is less than 10 Gm/dL and there is a minimum of 2 additional months of planned chemotherapy. Use the lowest dose necessary to avoid RBC transfusions. ***Starting dose:*** 150 units/kg of body weight 3 times a week until completion of chemotherapy course. An alternative schedule is 40,000 units weekly until completion of chemotherapy course.

Reduction of allogeneic blood transfusions in surgery patients: SC injection recommended. Obtain hemoglobin before initiating therapy. Should be greater than 10 Gm/dL but less than or equal to 13 Gm/dL. 300 units/kg/day for 10 days before surgery, on the day of surgery, and for 4 days after surgery. An alternate regimen is 600 units/kg once each week on Days 21, 14, and 7 before surgery and again on the day of surgery. Deep venous thrombosis prophylaxis is recommended during epoetin therapy (e.g., enoxaparin [Lovenox]); see Precautions.

PEDIATRIC DOSE

May be given by IV or SC injection. The IV route is recommended in patients on hemodialysis; see Precautions. Use the lowest dose for each patient that will gradually increase the hemoglobin concentration to avoid the need for RBC transfusion; see Precautions and Monitor.

---

[a]Please see p. xi for more information about biosimilars.

Anemia of CKD in pediatric patients 1 month to 16 years of age: Initiate epoetin when the hemoglobin level is less than 10 Gm/dL. *Starting dose:* 50 units/kg of body weight 3 times a week. May be given into the venous line at the end of the dialysis session.

Anemia in zidovudine-treated, HIV-infected pediatric patients 8 months to 17 years (unlabeled): Doses of 50 to 400 units/kg 2 to 3 times a week have been reported. See all comments under the similar section in Usual Dose. Adjust dose to achieve and maintain the lowest hemoglobin level sufficient to avoid the need for RBC transfusion; see Dose Adjustments.

Anemia associated with pediatric cancer patients on chemotherapy, ages 5 to 18 years: See comments under Usual Dose. *Starting dose:* 600 units/kg IV weekly until completion of chemotherapy course. Do not exceed 40,000 units.

DOSE ADJUSTMENTS

Dose adjustment is based on hemoglobin. Adjust dose to achieve and maintain the lowest hemoglobin level sufficient to avoid the need for RBC transfusion.

All adult and pediatric patients with CKD: When adjusting therapy, consider hemoglobin rate of rise, hemoglobin rate of decline, ESA responsiveness, and hemoglobin variability. A single hemoglobin excursion may not require a dose adjustment. Dose should be started slowly and adjusted for each patient to achieve and maintain the lowest hemoglobin level sufficient to avoid the need for RBC transfusion. Allow sufficient time before adjusting a dose; increased hemoglobin levels may not be observed for 2 to 6 weeks. ▪ Do not increase the dose more frequently than once every 4 weeks. Decreases in dose can occur more frequently. ▪ If the hemoglobin rises rapidly (e.g., more than 1 Gm/dL in any 2-week period), reduce the dose by 25% or more as needed to reduce rapid responses. ▪ For patients who do not respond adequately after 4 weeks of therapy (e.g., the hemoglobin has not increased by more than 1 Gm/dL), increase the dose by 25%. ▪ For patients who do not respond adequately over a 12-week escalation period, increasing the dose further is unlikely to improve response and may increase risks. Discontinue epoetin if responsiveness does not improve.

Adult patients with CKD on dialysis: If the hemoglobin level approaches or exceeds 11 Gm/dL, reduce or interrupt the dose of epoetin.

Adult patients with CKD NOT on dialysis: If the hemoglobin level exceeds 10 Gm/dL, reduce or interrupt the dose of epoetin.

Pediatric patients with CKD: If the hemoglobin level approaches or exceeds 12 Gm/dL, reduce or interrupt the dose of epoetin.

Zidovudine-treated, HIV-infected patients and cancer patients on chemotherapy: If hemoglobin does not increase after 8 weeks of therapy, increase dose by 50 to 100 units/kg. May increase dose at 4- to 8-week intervals until hemoglobin reaches a level needed to avoid RBC transfusions or dose reaches 300 units/kg. ▪ Withhold dose if the hemoglobin exceeds 12 Gm/dL. Restart dose at 25% below previous dose when hemoglobin falls to less than 11 Gm/dL. ▪ Discontinue epoetin if increase in hemoglobin is not achieved at a dose of 300 units/kg for 8 weeks.

Cancer patients on chemotherapy: *Reduce dose* by 25% when the hemoglobin reaches a level needed to avoid transfusion or increases more than 1 Gm/dL in any 2-week period. *Withhold dose* if the hemoglobin exceeds a level needed to avoid transfusion, and restart at 25% below the previous dose when the hemoglobin approaches a level at which transfusions may be required. ▪ Increase **adult dose** to 300 units/kg three times a week or 60,000 units weekly if hemoglobin increases by less than 1 Gm/dL and remains below 10 Gm/dL after the initial 4 weeks of therapy. Increase **pediatric dose** to 900 units/kg weekly if hemoglobin increases by less than 1 Gm/dL and remains below 10 Gm/dL after the initial 4 weeks of therapy. Do not exceed a dose of 60,000 units. ▪ Discontinue epoetin after 8 weeks if no response as measured by hemoglobin levels or by continued need for RBC transfusions.

DILUTION

Available as a clear, colorless solution in numerous concentrations from 2,000 units /mL to 40,000 units/mL; check dose on vial carefully. May be given undiluted as an IV injection. Do not dilute (see exception below). *Do not shake* during preparation; will render it biologically inactive. Single-dose vial contains no preservatives. Use only 1 dose per vial, then discard. Never re-enter a preservative-free vial. Epogen and Procrit are available in a multidose vial with preservative (benzyl alcohol); sterile technique imperative. Do not use vials that have been shaken or frozen. Epogen and Procrit single-dose preservative-free vials may be admixed in a syringe with bacteriostatic NS in a 1:1 ratio at the time of administration except when administered to pregnant or lactating women, neonates, or infants.

Storage: Store all vials in refrigerator at 2° to 8° C (36° to 46° F) in original carton to protect from light. Refrigerate multiple-dose vial after initial use. Discard multiple-dose vial 21 days after initial entry. Do not freeze or shake any vial of epoetin-alfa.

Filters: Specific information not available for all formulations.

COMPATIBILITY

Manufacturers state, "Do not dilute or administer in conjunction with other drug solutions." One source indicates there may be protein loss from adsorption to PVC containers and tubing. Manufacturer suggests it may be mixed 1-to-1 with bacteriostatic NS in a syringe when prepared from a single-dose vial.

RATE OF ADMINISTRATION

A single dose over at least 1 minute.

ACTIONS

An amino acid glycoprotein manufactured by recombinant DNA technology. Has the same biologic effects as erythropoietin produced naturally by the kidneys. Stimulates bone marrow to produce RBCs, increasing the reticulocyte count within 10 days and the red cell count, hemoglobin, and hematocrit within 2 to 6 weeks. Normal iron stores are necessary because it steps up RBC production to a rate above what the body usually makes. New cells need iron, which is quickly depleted. Half-life is 4 to 13 hours. Continued therapy will maintain improved RBC levels and decrease need for transfusions.

INDICATIONS AND USES

Treatment of anemia associated with chronic kidney disease in adults and pediatric patients, including patients on dialysis and not on dialysis, to decrease the need for red blood cell (RBC) transfusion. ■ Treatment of anemias related to zidovudine (AZT, Retrovir) therapy in HIV-infected patients. ■ To reduce the need for allogeneic blood transfusions among patients with perioperative hemoglobin greater than 10 to less than or equal to 13 Gm/dL who are at high risk for perioperative blood loss from elective, noncardiac, nonvascular surgery. ■ Treatment of chemotherapy-induced anemia in adult cancer patients who have nonmyeloid malignancies in which anemia is due to the effect of concomitant myelosuppressive chemotherapy and who, upon initiation of therapy, have a minimum of 2 additional months of planned chemotherapy.

Limitations of use: Not indicated for use in patients receiving hormonal agents, therapeutic biologic products, or radiotherapy unless receiving concomitant myelosuppressive chemotherapy. ■ Not indicated for patients receiving myelosuppressive therapy when the anticipated outcome is cure; see Precautions. ■ Not indicated for patients with cancer who are receiving myelosuppressive chemotherapy and in whom the anemia can be managed by transfusion. ■ Has not been shown to improve quality of life, fatigue, or patient well-being. ■ Not indicated in patients scheduled for surgery who are willing to donate autologous blood. ■ Not indicated in patients undergoing cardiac or vascular surgery. ■ Not indicated as a substitute for a RBC transfusion in patients who require immediate correction of anemia.

Unlabeled uses: Anemia of prematurity.

CONTRAINDICATIONS

Known hypersensitivity to epoetin alfa, uncontrolled hypertension, pure red cell aplasia (PRCA). Epoetin alfa from multidose vials containing benzyl alcohol is contraindicated in neonates, infants, pregnant women, and nursing mothers.

PRECAUTIONS

May be given IV or SC in patients not receiving dialysis. May be given to dialysis patients into the venous line at the end of the dialysis procedure to eliminate additional venous access. ■ Erythropoiesis-stimulating agents (ESAs) increase the risk of death, MI, stroke, congestive heart failure, and thrombosis of hemodialysis vascular access and other thromboembolic events. ■ In clinical trials of patients with CKD, patients experienced greater risks of these adverse events when ESAs were administered to target a hemoglobin of greater than 11 Gm/dL. No trial has identified a hemoglobin target level, an epoetin alfa dose, or a dosing strategy that does not increase these risks. Use the lowest epoetin alfa dose sufficient to reduce the need for RBC transfusions. Providers and patients should weigh the possible benefits of decreasing transfusions against the increased risks of death and other serious cardiovascular adverse reactions. ■ Use with caution in patients with coexistent cardiovascular disease and stroke. Patients with CKD who have an insufficient hemoglobin response to ESA therapy may be at even greater risk for cardiovascular reactions and mortality than other patients. ■ In clinical trials, ESAs increased the risk of death in patients undergoing CABG surgery and the risk of deep venous thrombosis in patients undergoing orthopedic procedures. ■ Increases in hemoglobin of greater than 1 Gm/dL during any 2-week period have been associated with an increased incidence of cardiac arrest, exacerbations of hypertension, congestive heart failure (CHF), vascular thrombosis/ischemia/infarction, acute MI, deep vein thrombosis (DVT), pulmonary embolus, and fluid overload/edema and may be associated with neurologic events (e.g., seizures, stroke). See Dose Adjustments. ■ For lack or loss of hemoglobin response to epoetin alfa, initiate a search for causative factors (e.g., bleeding, infection, inflammation, iron deficiency). If typical causes of lack or loss of hemoglobin response are excluded, evaluate for pure red cell aplasia (PRCA). In the absence of PRCA, follow dosing recommendations for management of patients with an insufficient hemoglobin response to epoetin alfa therapy. ■ Not intended for use in anemias caused by iron or folate deficiencies, hemolysis, or GI bleeding or for use in treating symptoms of anemia, including dizziness, fatigue, low energy, poor quality of life, or shortness of breath. ■ PRCA and severe anemia, with or without other cytopenias, in association with neutralizing antibodies to native erythropoietin have been observed. Most often reported in patients with CKD who are receiving epoetin alfa by SC injection. Any patient who develops a sudden loss of response to epoetin alfa accompanied by severe anemia and low reticulocyte count should be evaluated. Physicians may contact manufacturer (Amgen) for help with the evaluation of these patients. ■ Administration of erythropoiesis-stimulating agents (ESAs) to cancer patients shortened the overall survival and/or increased the risk of tumor progression or recurrence in clinical studies of some patients with breast, cervical, head and neck, lymphoid, and non–small-cell lung malignancies; see prescribing information for specific studies. To minimize these risks, as well as the risks of serious cardiovascular and thromboembolic events, use the lowest dose needed to avoid a red blood cell transfusion. Use only to treat anemia due to concomitant myelosuppressive chemotherapy, and discontinue after completion of a chemotherapy course. ■ BP may increase during therapy with epoetin. Hypertensive encephalopathy and seizures have been observed. ■ Patients with uncontrolled hypertension should not be treated with epoetin until BP has been adequately controlled. ■ Epoetin increases the risk of seizures in patients with CKD. Use with caution in patients with a seizure disorder. ■ Serious hypersensitivity reactions, including anaphylaxis, have been reported. ■ Blistering and skin exfoliation reactions, including erythema multiforme and Stevens-Johnson syndrome/toxic epidermal necrolysis (SJS/TEN), have been reported. ■ Epogen and Procrit contain albumin and carry a risk for transmission of viral diseases or Creutzfeldt-Jakob disease. However, donor screening and manufacturing processes make this risk extremely remote. ■ Retacrit contains 0.5 mg of phenylalanine in each 1-mL single-dose vial (all concentrations) and may be harmful to patients with phenylketonuria (PKU). Consider combined daily amount of phenylalanine from all sources before prescribing Retacrit.

Monitor: Monitor hemoglobin weekly in patients who are initiating therapy. Continue until stable and the maintenance dose has been established, then monitor at least monthly. ■ Monitor hemoglobin weekly for at least 4 weeks following adjustment of therapy. Once stabilized, continue to monitor at least monthly. ■ A biologic product. Monitor for S/S of hypersensitivity reactions. ■ Monitor BP routinely; initiation or intensification of antihypertensive therapy and dietary restrictions may be necessary. If BP is difficult to control by pharmacologic or dietary measures, the dose of epoetin should be reduced or withheld. ▪ Normal iron stores required to support epoetin-stimulated erythropoiesis. Transferrin saturation should be at least 20% and ferritin at least 100 ng/mL. Monitor before and during therapy. Supplemental iron is usually required to increase and maintain transferrin saturation. Administration of IV parenteral iron may be necessary in some patients. ▪ Monitor for the presence of premonitory neurologic symptoms during initiation of therapy or when dose is adjusted. Seizures have been reported; see Precautions. ▪ Monitor patients with pre-existing vascular disease carefully (especially those with CKD); increase in hematocrit may precipitate a cerebrovascular accident, transient ischemic attack, or myocardial infarction. ▪ Dialysis patients may require additional anticoagulation with heparin to prevent clotting of artificial kidney or clotting of the vascular access (AV shunt) and to maintain efficiency of the dialysis procedure.

Patient Education: Risk of seizures, especially during first 90 days of therapy. Contact provider for new-onset seizures, premonitory symptoms, or a change in seizure frequency. ▪ Additional instruction (e.g., equipment, techniques) will be required in patients who will self-administer (manufacturer supplies brochure). ▪ Stress importance of compliance with diet, iron, and vitamin (e.g., folic acid, B_{12}) supplementation and BP control. Close monitoring of BP and Hgb is imperative. ▪ Promptly report S/S of hypersensitivity or skin reactions, pain or swelling in legs, SOB, increase in BP, dizziness, or loss of consciousness. ▪ Increased risk of mortality, serious cardiovascular events, thromboembolic events, and tumor progression or recurrence. ▪ Read Medication Guide carefully. All patients should discuss the risks of using an ESA with a health care professional.

Maternal/Child: May present risk to fetus; benefits must justify risk. ▪ Some formulations contain benzyl alcohol. Serious and fatal reactions, including "gasping syndrome," can occur in neonates and infants treated with drugs preserved in benzyl alcohol. There is a potential for similar risks to fetuses and infants exposed to benzyl alcohol in utero or in breast-fed milk, respectively; see Contraindications. ▪ Use caution in nursing mothers. ▪ Indicated in pediatric patients ages 1 month to 16 years of age for the treatment of anemia associated with CKD requiring dialysis. Use of epoetin alfa in pediatric patients with CKD not requiring dialysis is supported by efficacy in pediatric patients requiring dialysis. ▪ Safety and effectiveness for use in infants under 1 month of age not established. ▪ Indicated in pediatric cancer patients ages 5 to 18 years for the treatment of anemia due to myelosuppressive chemotherapy. ▪ Has been used in zidovudine-treated and anemic pediatric patients ages 8 months to 17 years. Data limited. ▪ Pharmacokinetics (absorption, distribution, metabolism, and excretion) in children and adolescents similar to adults. ▪ Limited data available for use in neonates. Clearance may be increased compared to adults.

Elderly: *Epogen and Procrit:* Response similar to that found in younger patients; however, elderly patients may have a greater sensitivity to its effects. *Retacrit:* Response unknown due to insufficient numbers in studies.

DRUG/LAB INTERACTIONS
Specific information not available.

SIDE EFFECTS
Generally well tolerated. Occur most frequently in patients with chronic renal failure. Increased hypertension is common, and hypertensive encephalopathy and seizures can occur. Clotted vascular access (AV shunt) and clotting of the artificial kidney may occur during dialysis. Allergic reactions have been reported. Other reported side effects are those common to the underlying disease and not necessarily attributable to epoetin and include arthralgias, asthenia, bone marrow fibrosis, bone pain, cerebrovascular accident or transient ischemic attack (CVA/TIA), chest pain, chills, cough, deep vein thrombosis, depression, diarrhea, dizziness, dysphagia, edema, fatigue, fever, headache, hyperglycemia, hyperkalemia, hypokalemia, injection site irritation or pain, insomnia, muscle spasm, myocardial infarction, nausea, polycythemia, pruritus, rash, respiratory congestion,

shortness of breath, stomatitis, tachycardia, upper respiratory tract infection, vomiting, and weight decrease. PRCA and severe anemia, with or without other cytopenias, in association with neutralizing antibodies have been reported; see Precautions.

ANTIDOTE

Notify physician of all side effects; most will be treated symptomatically. Excessive hypertension may require discontinuation of epoetin until BP is controlled or may respond to reduction in dose of epoetin or to an increase in antihypertensive therapy. Reduce dose of epoetin in patients with an increase in hemoglobin over 1 Gm/dL in any 2-week period. Consider phlebotomy in toxicity. If overdose or polycythemia does occur, monitor closely for cardiovascular events and hematologic abnormalities. When resuming therapy, monitor closely for evidence of rapid increases in hemoglobin concentration (greater than 1 Gm/dL within 14 days) and reduce dose as indicated. Additional heparin may be required during dialysis to prevent clotting. Permanently discontinue therapy in patients with antibody-mediated anemia or severe cutaneous reactions. Patients should not be switched to other erythropoietic proteins because antibodies may cross-react. Treat minor hypersensitivity reactions symptomatically. Discontinue drug and treat anaphylaxis as indicated; resuscitate as necessary.

EPOPROSTENOL SODIUM
(eh-poh-**PROST**-en-ohl **SO**-dee-um)

Flolan, Veletri

Prostaglandin
Vasodilating agent
Antihypertensive (pulmonary)

pH 10.2 to 13

USUAL DOSE

Acute dose initiation and chronic continuous infusion: May be given through a peripheral line on a temporary basis until a central venous line is established. A central venous catheter should be put in place as soon as possible and must be used for continuous long-term 24-hour administration with an ambulatory infusion pump. Begin infusion at 2 ng/kg/min. Increase in increments of 1 to 2 ng/kg/min every 15 minutes or longer until dose-limiting pharmacologic effects occur or until a tolerance limit to the drug is established and further increases in the infusion rate are not clinically warranted; see Dose Adjustments. Most common S/S of dose-limiting effects include abdominal pain, flushing, headache, hypotension, nausea, respiratory disorders, sepsis, and vomiting. If dose-limiting pharmacologic effects occur, decrease infusion rate slowly until pharmacologic effects are tolerated; see Dose Adjustments. If the initial dose of 2 ng/kg/min is not tolerated, use a lower dose. May be given concomitantly with anticoagulant therapy in selected patients; see Monitor.

DOSE ADJUSTMENTS

Changes in the chronic infusion rate are to be expected. If symptoms of primary pulmonary hypertension (PPH) persist, recur, or worsen, increase infusion rate promptly by 1 to 2 ng/kg/min. Wait at least 15 minutes to assess clinical response. Observe patient for several hours to confirm patient tolerance, and take BP and HR in supine and standing positions. ■ Occurrence of dose-related side effects that do not resolve may require a decrease in the chronic infusion rate. Reduce dose gradually in 2-ng/kg/min increments and wait at least 15 minutes to assess clinical response. Use extreme caution if decreasing the dose; abrupt withdrawal or sudden large reductions may cause a rapid return of PPH symptoms and may precipitate death. ■ In patients receiving lung transplants, doses were tapered after the initiation of cardiopulmonary bypass. ■ Dose selection for the elderly should be cautious. ■ Asymptomatic increases in pulmonary artery pressure with increases in cardiac output may occur during acute dose initiation; consider dose adjustment. ■ See Precautions.

DILUTION

Infusion pump required. It must be small and lightweight; able to adjust infusion rates in increments of 2 ng/kg/min; have occlusion, end of infusion, and low battery alarms; be accurate to ±6% of the programmed rate; be positive-pressure driven (continuous or pulsatile) with intervals between pulses not exceeding 3 minutes at rates required to deliver drug; and have a disposable reservoir cassette made of polyvinyl chloride, polypropylene, or glass with a capacity of at least 100 mL. Pumps used during trials were manufactured by Pharmacia Deltec, Medfusion, Inc., and Baxter Health Care. The infusion pump used in the most recent clinical trials was the CADD-1 HFX 5100 (SIMS Deltec). A 60-inch microbore non-DEHP extension set with proximal antisiphon valve, low priming volume (0.9 mL), and in-line 0.22-micron filter was used during clinical trials. Preparation and administration materials containing polyethylene terephthalate (PET) or polyethylene terephthalate glycol (PETG) may become damaged when used with **Flolan prepared with pH 12 sterile diluent for Flolan** and therefore must not be used.

Available in 0.5- and 1.5-mg single-dose vials. The diluents specified for each product are to be used for reconstitution and dilution. *Flolan:* Sterile diluent for Flolan or pH 12 sterile diluent for Flolan is provided by the manufacturer. Do not use any other diluent. *Generic:* Sterile diluent for epoprostenol is provided by the manufacturer. Do not use any other diluent. *Veletri:* Reconstitute and dilute with SWFI or NS (not provided by manufacturer). A concentration should be selected that is **compatible** with the infusion pump being used with respect to minimum and maximum flow rates, reservoir capacity, and the infusion pump criteria. See Rate of Administration. Two vials of the manufacturer-supplied sterile diluent for *Flolan and generic* will be required to prepare each 24-hour dose in each of the concentrations in the following chart.

Guidelines for Dilution of Epoprostenol to Various Concentrations	
To Make 100 mL of Solution With Final Concentration (ng/mL) of:	**Directions**
3,000 ng/mL	Dissolve contents of one 0.5-mg vial with 5 mL of product-specific diluent. Withdraw 3 mL and add to sufficient identical diluent to make a total of 100 mL.
5,000 ng/mL	Dissolve contents of one 0.5-mg vial with 5 mL of product-specific diluent. Withdraw entire vial contents and add sufficient identical diluent to make a total of 100 mL.
10,000 ng/mL	Dissolve contents of two 0.5-mg vials each with 5 mL of product-specific diluent. Withdraw entire vial contents and add sufficient identical diluent to make a total of 100 mL.
15,000 ng/mL[a]	Dissolve contents of one 1.5-mg vial with 5 mL of product-specific diluent. Withdraw entire vial contents and add sufficient identical diluent to make a total of 100 mL.
30,000 ng/mL[a]	Dissolve contents of two 1.5-mg vials each with 5 mL of product-specific diluent. Withdraw entire vial contents and add sufficient volume of the identical diluent to make a total of 100 mL.

[a]Higher concentrations may be prepared for patients who receive epoprostenol long-term.

Prepare in a drug delivery reservoir appropriate for the infusion pump with a total reservoir volume of at least 100 mL. In general, 3,000 ng/mL and 10,000 ng/mL concentrations should be satisfactory to deliver between 2 and 16 ng/kg/min in adults.

Filters: An in-line 0.22-micron filter was used during clinical trials.

Storage: *All products:* Vials are for single use only; discard any unused diluent or unused reconstituted solution. *Flolan and generic:* Unopened vials of epoprostenol may be stored at 15° to 25° C (59° to 77° F [*generic* at CRT]) in the carton to protect from light. Diluent may be stored at 15° to 25° C (59° to 77° F [*generic* at CRT]). Protection from light not required. Do not freeze. See expiration dates on both. *Flolan and generic diluted with sterile diluent:* When used at room temperature, reconstituted solutions are stable for up to 8 hours following reconstitution or removal from refrigeration and may be stored for up to 40 hours before use if refrigerated. When used with a cold pack, reconstituted solutions are stable for up to 24 hours, or may be refrigerated before use as long as the total time of refrigerated storage and infusion does not exceed 48 hours. Change cold packs every 12 hours. Before use, reconstituted solutions *(Flolan and generic)* must be refrigerated and protected from light. Do not freeze. *Flolan diluted with pH 12 sterile diluent:* Freshly prepared reconstituted solutions or reconstituted solutions that have been refrigerated at 2° to 8° C (36° to 46° F) for no longer than 8 days can be administered from 12 to 72 hours at specific temperatures; see prescribing information. Protect from light and do not freeze.

Veletri: Unopened vials may be stored at 20° to 25° C (68° to 77° F) in the carton to protect from direct sunlight. Vials reconstituted with 5 mL of SWFI or NS and further diluted with the identical diluent must be protected from light and can be refrigerated at 2° to 8° C (36° to 46° F) for as long as 8 days. Maximum duration of administration ranges from 24 to 72 hours and is dependent on ambient temperature, final concentration, and duration of refrigerated storage before administration; see Prescribing Information.

COMPATIBILITY

Manufacturer states, "Stable only when reconstituted with the provided or recommended diluent. Must not be reconstituted or mixed with any other parenteral medications or solutions prior to or during administration." Manufacturer states, "Preparation and administration materials containing polyethylene terephthalate (PET) or polyethylene terephthalate glycol (PETG) may become damaged when used with **Flolan prepared with pH 12 sterile diluent for Flolan** and therefore must not be used. Consult the manufacturer of the sets to confirm that they are considered **compatible** with highly alkaline solutions, such as Flolan prepared with pH 12 sterile diluent for Flolan."

One source suggests **compatibility** at the **Y-site** with bivalirudin (Angiomax).

RATE OF ADMINISTRATION

Administered by a continuous IV infusion through a central venous catheter using an ambulatory infusion pump. Peripheral access may be used temporarily until a central line can be placed. Do not administer bolus injections of epoprostenol. Titrate dose as outlined in Usual Dose and Dose Adjustments. If dose-limiting pharmacologic effects occur, decrease infusion rate slowly until pharmacologic effects are tolerated; see Dose Adjustments. The infusion rate may be calculated using the following formula:

$$\text{Infusion rate (mL/hr)} = \frac{\text{Dose (ng/kg/min)} \times \text{Weight in kg} \times 60 \text{ min/hr}}{\text{Final concentration (ng/mL)}}$$

Example calculations for infusion rates are as follows:

Example 1: For a 60-kg person at the recommended initial dose of 2 ng/kg/min using a 3,000 ng/mL concentration, the infusion rate would be as follows:

$$\text{Infusion rate (mL/hr)} = \frac{[2 \text{ (ng/kg/min)} \times 60 \text{ (kg)} \times 60 \text{ min/hr}]}{3,000 \text{ (ng/mL)}} = 2.4 \text{ (mL/hr)}$$

Example 2: For a 70-kg person at a dose of 16 ng/kg/min using a 15,000 ng/mL concentration, the infusion rate would be as follows:

$$\text{Infusion rate (mL/hr)} = \frac{[16 \text{ (ng/kg/min)} \times 70 \text{ (kg)} \times 60 \text{ min/hr}]}{15,000 \text{ (ng/mL)}} = 4.48 \text{ (mL/hr)}$$

ACTIONS

A naturally occurring prostaglandin. It directly vasodilates pulmonary and systemic arterial vascular beds and inhibits platelet aggregation. Produces dose-related increases in cardiac index and stroke volume and dose-related decreases in pulmonary vascular resistance, total pulmonary resistance, and mean systemic arterial pressure. Has been shown to increase exercise capacity, improve hemodynamic status, and extend survival. Onset of action is immediate. Half-life is approximately 6 minutes at body pH of 7.4. Rapidly hydrolyzed and is also subject to enzymatic degradation. Excreted in urine and feces.

INDICATIONS AND USES

Treatment of pulmonary arterial hypertension (PAH [WHO Group 1]) to improve exercise capacity. Effectiveness established predominantly in patients with NYHA Functional Class III-IV symptoms and etiologies of idiopathic or heritable PAH or PAH associated with connective tissue diseases.

CONTRAINDICATIONS

Heart failure due to severe left ventricular systolic dysfunction. ▪ Known hypersensitivity to epoprostenol, related compounds, or any component of the formulation. ▪ Patients who develop pulmonary edema during dose initiation **(Veletri)**.

PRECAUTIONS

Administered by or under the direction of the physician specialist. ▪ During dose initiation, facilities for monitoring the patient and responding to any medical emergency must be available. ▪ Abrupt withdrawal, interruptions in drug delivery, or sudden large reductions in dose may result in rebound pulmonary hypertension. Symptoms may include dyspnea, dizziness, and weakness. Death of one patient was attributed to these causes. Backup medication and equipment must always be available. ▪ Use of a multilumen catheter should be considered if other IV therapy is used. ▪ Not recommended for patients who develop pulmonary edema during acute dose initiation. Consider the possibility of associated pulmonary veno-occlusive disease in these patients; see Contraindications. ▪ Asymptomatic increases in pulmonary artery pressure with increases in cardiac output may occur during acute dose initiation; consider dose adjustment. ▪ Cardiac catheterization may be used for acute dose initiation but is not necessary; consider benefit versus risk. ▪ In patients undergoing lung transplants, it is recommended that the dose of epoprostenol be tapered after initiation of cardiopulmonary bypass. ▪ A potent inhibitor of platelet aggregation; an increased risk for hemorrhagic complications may occur, particularly in patients with other risk factors for bleeding. ▪ See Monitor, Patient Education, Drug/Lab Interactions.

Monitor: Frequent monitoring of vital signs recommended during acute dose initiation. ▪ Monitor standing and supine HR and BP for several hours after any dose adjustment. ▪ Observe for dose-limiting side effects (e.g., abdominal pain, dizziness, flushing, headache, hypotension, nausea, respiratory disorder, sepsis, vomiting). ▪ Monitor for S/S of hemorrhagic complications. ▪ To reduce the risk of pulmonary thromboembolism or systemic embolism through a patent foramen ovale, anticoagulant therapy is recommended concomitantly unless contraindicated. ▪ Therapy may be required for months or years; consideration must be given to the ability of the patient and family to manage this care. ▪ Thorough patient teaching and continued support services are imperative to facilitate a good clinical outcome. ▪ See Precautions, Patient Education, Drug/Lab Interactions.

Patient Education: After initial dose titration and training, this is a self-administered drug. Must assume responsibility for drug reconstitution, drug administration, and care of the permanent central venous catheter. Follow all dilution and storage requirements for the product that is being used. ▪ Aseptic technique during reconstitution and with routine care of permanent indwelling central venous catheter is imperative to prevent infection. ▪ Report fever or any sign of infection at catheter site (e.g., redness, warmth). ▪ Report any unusual bruising or bleeding. ▪ Delivery of medication cannot be interrupted. Interruption will cause a rapid return of PPH symptoms. ▪ Should have access to a backup infusion pump and intravenous infusion sets to avoid potential interruption in drug delivery. ▪ Dose adjustments should be made only under the direction of the physician except in an emergency situation (e.g., unconsciousness, collapse).

Maternal/Child: Category B: *(Veletri). All formulations:* use only if clearly needed. No evidence of fetal harm in animal studies to date. Pregnant women with untreated PAH are at risk for heart failure, stroke, preterm delivery, and maternal and fetal death. Consider risk versus benefit. ▪ Use during labor and delivery has not been adequately studied. ▪ Use caution in nursing mothers; safety not established. ▪ Safety for use in pediatric patients not established.

Elderly: See Dose Adjustments. Decreased organ function (cardiac, hepatic, renal), concomitant disease, and other drug therapy may cause concern. Differences in response of younger patients versus the elderly not documented.

DRUG/LAB INTERACTIONS

Has been used with digoxin, diuretics, anticoagulants, oral vasodilators, and oxygen. ▪ Hypotension may be increased with **diuretics, antihypertensive agents, or other vasodilators.** ▪ Risk of bleeding may be increased with **antiplatelet agents, anticoagulants, or NSAIDs.** ▪ May decrease clearance of **furosemide** and **digoxin;** monitor digoxin levels.

SIDE EFFECTS

Acute dose initiation: The most common S/S of dose-limiting effects include flushing, headache, hypotension, nausea, and vomiting. Abdominal pain, agitation, anorexia, anxiety/nervousness, back pain, bradycardia, chest pain, dizziness, dyspepsia, dyspnea, hyperesthesia, hyperkinesias, musculoskeletal pain, myalgia, paresthesia, respiratory disorders, sepsis, sweating, tachycardia, tremor, urticaria, and many other side effects may occur.

Chronic continuous infusion: Any of the above and arthralgia, bleeding at various sites, chills, diarrhea, fever, flu-like symptoms, infection (may be local at site of catheter insertion), jaw pain, pallor, pulmonary edema, rash, sepsis, thrombocytopenia.

Overdose: Hypotension, hypoxemia, respiratory arrest, and death may occur.

Post-Marketing: Anemia, hepatic failure, high-output cardiac failure, hypersplenism, hyperthyroidism, pancytopenia, pulmonary embolism, splenomegaly, thrombocytopenia.

ANTIDOTE

Continuous maintenance of drug flow imperative. Keep physician informed of all side effects. Most will be treated with dose reduction; some may require symptomatic treatment. Discontinue therapy if pulmonary edema develops.

EPTIFIBATIDE
(**ep**-tih-**FY**-beh-tide)

Antiplatelet agent

Integrilin

pH 5.35

USUAL DOSE
Pretreatment: Baseline studies indicated; see Monitor.

Used in combination with heparin and aspirin. A calculated CrCl greater than or equal to 50 mL/min is required in patients receiving the following doses. Use of the Cockroft-Gault equation is recommended for calculating CrCl. Discontinue eptifibatide infusion before CABG surgery and in patients requiring thrombolytic therapy.

ACUTE CORONARY SYNDROME
Eptifibatide: 180 mcg/kg as an IV bolus as soon as possible following diagnosis. Follow with a continuous infusion of 2 mcg/kg/min until hospital discharge or initiation of coronary artery bypass graft (CABG) surgery for up to 72 hours. Alternately, if a patient is to undergo a percutaneous coronary intervention (PCI) while receiving eptifibatide, the infusion should be continued up to hospital discharge or for 18 to 24 hours after the procedure, whichever comes first. Patient may receive up to 96 hours of therapy. See Dosing Chart by Weight on the following page and Dose Adjustments. Dose in patients with a calculated CrCl greater than or equal to 50 mL/min weighing more than 121 kg should not exceed a bolus of 22.6 mg or an infusion rate of 15 mg/hr.

Aspirin: 160 to 325 mg PO initially and daily thereafter.

Heparin: *Medical management:* Suggested heparin dose to achieve the target aPTT of 50 to 70 seconds during medical management is *Weight 70 kg or more,* 5,000 units as an IV bolus followed by an infusion of 1,000 units/hr. *Weight less than 70 kg,* 60 units/kg as an IV bolus followed by an infusion of 12 units/kg/hr.

Patients undergoing PCI: Target ACT is 200 to 300 seconds during PCI. If heparin is initiated before PCI, give additional boluses during PCI as needed to keep ACT in range. Heparin infusion after PCI is discouraged.

PERCUTANEOUS CORONARY INTERVENTION (PCI)
Eptifibatide: 180 mcg/kg as an IV bolus immediately before initiation of PCI followed by a continuous infusion of 2 mcg/kg/min. Repeat bolus of 180 mcg/kg 10 minutes after the first bolus. Continue infusion until hospital discharge or for up to 18 to 24 hours, whichever comes first. A minimum of 12 hours of infusion is recommended. See the following chart and Dose Adjustments. Dose in patients with a calculated CrCl greater than or equal to 50 mL/min weighing more than 121 kg should not exceed a bolus of 22.6 mg or an infusion rate of 15 mg/hr.

Aspirin: 160 to 325 mg PO 1 to 24 hours before PCI and daily thereafter.

Heparin: Target ACT is 200 to 300 seconds during PCI. In patients not treated with heparin within 6 hours of PCI, give 60 units/kg as a bolus. Give additional boluses as needed during PCI to keep ACT in range. Heparin infusion is discouraged after PCI.

FOR BOTH INDICATIONS
Refer to the following Eptifibatide Dosing Chart by Weight.

Eptifibatide Dosing Chart by Weight					
Patient Weight	180 mcg/kg Bolus Volume	2 mcg/kg/min Infusion Rate		1 mcg/kg/min Infusion Rate	
	From 2 mg/mL Vial	From 2 mg/mL 100-mL Vial	From 0.75 mg/mL 100-mL Vial	From 2 mg/mL 100-mL Vial	From 0.75 mg/mL 100-mL Vial
37–41 kg	3.4 mL	2 mL/hr	6 mL/hr	1 mL/hr	3 mL/hr
42–46 kg	4 mL	2.5 mL/hr	7 mL/hr	1.3 mL/hr	3.5 mL/hr
47–53 kg	4.5 mL	3 mL/hr	8 mL/hr	1.5 mL/hr	4 mL/hr
54–59 kg	5 mL	3.5 mL/hr	9 mL/hr	1.8 mL/hr	4.5 mL/hr
60–65 kg	5.6 mL	3.8 mL/hr	10 mL/hr	1.9 mL/hr	5 mL/hr
66–71 kg	6.2 mL	4 mL/hr	11 mL/hr	2 mL/hr	5.5 mL/hr
72–78 kg	6.8 mL	4.5 mL/hr	12 mL/hr	2.3 mL/hr	6 mL/hr
79–84 kg	7.3 mL	5 mL/hr	13 mL/hr	2.5 mL/hr	6.5 mL/hr
85–90 kg	7.9 mL	5.3 mL/hr	14 mL/hr	2.7 mL/hr	7 mL/hr
91–96 kg	8.5 mL	5.6 mL/hr	15 mL/hr	2.8 mL/hr	7.5 mL/hr
97–103 kg	9 mL	6 mL/hr	16 mL/hr	3 mL/hr	8 mL/hr
104–109 kg	9.5 mL	6.4 mL/hr	17 mL/hr	3.2 mL/hr	8.5 mL/hr
110–115 kg	10.2 mL	6.8 mL/hr	18 mL/hr	3.4 mL/hr	9 mL/hr
116–121 kg	10.7 mL	7 mL/hr	19 mL/hr	3.5 mL/hr	9.5 mL/hr
>121 kg	11.3 mL	7.5 mL/hr	20 mL/hr	3.7 mL/hr	10 mL/hr

DOSE ADJUSTMENTS
ACUTE CORONARY SYNDROME
In patients with a calculated CrCl less than 50 mL/min, give a bolus of 180 mcg/kg. Decrease rate of the continuous infusion to 1 mcg/kg/min. In patients with a calculated CrCl less than 50 mL/min or a SCr greater than 2 mg/dL and weighing more than 121 kg, a maximum bolus of 22.6 mg followed by a maximum infusion rate of 7.5 mg/hr should be administered.

PCI
In patients with a calculated CrCl less than 50 mL/min, give a bolus of 180 mcg/kg. Decrease rate of the continuous infusion to 1 mcg/kg/min. Repeat bolus of 180 mcg/kg 10 minutes after the first bolus. In patients with a calculated CrCl less than 50 mL/min or a SCr greater than 2 mg/dL and weighing more than 121 kg, a maximum bolus of 22.6 mg followed by a maximum infusion rate of 7.5 mg/hr should be administered.

ALL DIAGNOSES
Dose reduction may be indicated in patients over 75 years of age weighing less than 50 kg. ■ See Dosing Chart by Weight in Usual Dose. ■ See Contraindications.

DILUTION
The 10-mL vial contains 20 mg of eptifibatide; the 100-mL vials contain 75 mg or 200 mg of eptifibatide.

IV bolus: Given undiluted. Withdraw total bolus dose (usually from the 10-mL vial) into a syringe.

Infusion: Usually given undiluted directly from the 75 mg/100 mL (0.75 mg/mL) or the 200 mg/100 mL (2 mg/mL) vials using an IV infusion pump. The 100-mL vial should be spiked with a vented infusion set. Center the spike within the circle on the stopper top. May be diluted with NS or D5NS. Use of a metriset or infusion pump appropriate.

Storage: Refrigerate vials at 2° to 8° C (36° to 46° F) or they may be kept at CRT for up to 2 months. Protect from light until administration. Do not use beyond the expiration or discard date. Discard any unused portion left in the vial.

COMPATIBILITY

Manufacturer lists furosemide as **incompatible** and states "is **incompatible** with any solution or drug not specifically listed as **compatible**."

Manufacturer lists as **compatible** at **Y-site** with NS or D5NS with or without up to 60 mEq/L of potassium chloride as well as with alteplase, atropine sulfate, dobutamine, heparin, lidocaine, meperidine, metoprolol, midazolam, morphine, nitroglycerin IV, verapamil.

Other sources suggest a few specific **compatibilities** dependent on concentration and manufacturer; consult a pharmacist.

RATE OF ADMINISTRATION

IV bolus: A single dose IV push over 1 to 2 minutes.

Infusion: See Dosing Charts by Weight under Usual Dose.

ACTIONS

A cyclic heptapeptide (amino acid) that reversibly binds to the platelet receptor glycoprotein GP IIb/IIIa of human platelets and inhibits platelet aggregation by preventing the binding of fibrinogen, von Willebrand factor, and other adhesive ligands to GP IIb/IIIa. Inhibits platelet aggregation in a dose- and concentration-dependent manner. Recovery of platelet function after termination of the eptifibatide infusion is rapid. Administered alone, eptifibatide has no measurable effect on PT or aPTT. Does not exert a pharmacologic effect on other integrins. Recommended regimens of a bolus followed by an infusion produce immediate inhibition of platelet aggregation and an early peak level, followed by a small decline, with steady state achieved within 4 to 6 hours. This decline can be prevented by administering a second bolus. Plasma elimination half-life is approximately 2.5 hours. 50% cleared from plasma by the kidneys. Balance of clearance is by nonrenal mechanisms. Has been shown to reduce clinical events (e.g., acute MI, need for urgent intervention) in patients undergoing PCI during drug administration and in those receiving medical management alone.

INDICATIONS AND USES

Used in combination with heparin, aspirin and, in selected situations, a thienopyridine (e.g., clopidogrel, prasugrel). ▪ Treatment of patients with acute coronary syndrome (unstable angina or non–ST-segment elevation MI), including those who are to be managed medically and those undergoing PCI. In this setting, has been shown to decrease the rate of a combined endpoint of death or new MI. ▪ Treatment of patients undergoing PCI, including those undergoing intracoronary stenting. In this setting has been shown to decrease the rate of a combined endpoint of death, new MI, or need for urgent intervention.

CONTRAINDICATIONS

Known hypersensitivity to any component of the product. ▪ Current or planned administration of another parenteral glycoprotein GPIIb/IIIa inhibitor (e.g., tirofiban). ▪ Dependency on renal dialysis. ▪ History of bleeding diathesis or evidence of active abnormal bleeding within the previous 30 days. ▪ History of stroke within 30 days or any history of hemorrhagic stroke. ▪ Major surgery within the preceding 6 weeks. ▪ Severe hypertension (systolic BP greater than 200 mm Hg or diastolic BP greater than 110 mm Hg) not adequately controlled on antihypertensive therapy.

PRECAUTIONS

Use caution when given with drugs that affect hemostasis (e.g., NSAIDs, clopidogrel, dipyridamole, warfarin). Limited data on the use of eptifibatide in patients receiving thrombolytic agents (e.g., alteplase), reteplase, streptokinase) do not allow an estimate of the bleeding risk associated with concomitant use. Systemic thrombolytic therapy should be used with caution in patients who have received eptifibatide. See Drug/Lab Interactions. ▪ Use with caution in patients with renal insufficiency; clearance is reduced and plasma levels are elevated; see Dose Adjustments. There is no experience in patients dependent on dialysis. ▪ Bleeding is the most common complication encountered during therapy. ▪ Risk of major bleeding increased inversely with patient weight, especially for patients weighing less than 70 kg. ▪ Most major bleeding occurs at the arterial access site for cardiac catheterization or from the GI or GU tracts. ▪ Acute profound thrombocytopenia has been reported; see Monitor. ▪ Because eptifibatide is readily reversible, procedures such as emergency CABG may be performed safely shortly after discontinuation of an infusion without the need for platelet transfusions. ▪ Development of antibodies to eptifibatide and immune-mediated thrombocytopenia have been reported; may be associated with hypotension and/or other signs of hypersensitivity. ▪ No clinical experience in patients with a baseline platelet count less than 100,000/mm³. Monitor closely if use is indicated.

Monitor: Before therapy obtain platelet count, hemoglobin or hematocrit, SCr, and PT/aPTT. Obtain ACT in patients undergoing PCI. ▪ Maintain target aPTT between 50 and 70 seconds unless PCI is to be performed. During PCI, the ACT should be maintained between 200 and 300 seconds. ▪ The aPTT or ACT should be checked before sheath removal. The sheath should not be removed unless the aPTT is less than 45 seconds or the ACT is less than 150 seconds. In patients treated with heparin, bleeding can be minimized by close monitoring of the aPTT. ▪ If acute profound thrombocytopenia occurs or the platelet count drops to less than 100,000/mm³, heparin and eptifibatide should be discontinued. Monitor serial platelet counts, assess the presence of drug-dependent antibodies, and initiate appropriate therapy as indicated. ▪ Monitor the patient for signs of bleeding; take vital signs (avoiding automatic BP cuffs); observe any invaded sites at least every 15 minutes (e.g., sheaths, IV sites, cutdowns, punctures, Foleys, NGs); watch for hematuria, hematemesis, bloody stool, petechiae, hematoma, flank pain, muscle weakness. Perform neuro checks frequently. If during therapy bleeding cannot be controlled with pressure, heparin and eptifibatide should be discontinued. ▪ Use care in handling patient; minimize use of urinary catheters, nasotracheal intubation, and nasogastric tubes. Avoid arterial puncture, venipuncture, and IM injection. Use extreme precautionary methods and only compressible sites if these procedures are absolutely necessary (i.e., avoid subclavian or jugular veins). Apply pressure for 30 minutes to any invaded site and then apply pressure dressings. Saline or heparin locks suggested to facilitate blood draws. ▪ See Precautions.

Additional monitoring for patients receiving PCI: After PCI, eptifibatide should be continued until hospital discharge or for up to 18 to 24 hours, whichever comes first. See suggested time frames under each dose. Heparin use is discouraged after the PCI procedure. The femoral artery sheath may be removed during eptifibatide infusion, but only after heparin has been discontinued and its effects largely reversed. Heparin should be discontinued 3 to 4 hours before pulling the sheath, and an aPTT less than 45 seconds or an ACT of less than 150 seconds should be documented. ▪ Care should be taken to obtain proper hemostasis after removal of the sheath using standard compressive techniques followed by close observation. Sheath hemostasis should be achieved at least 2 to 4 hours before hospital discharge.

Patient Education: Compliance with all measures to minimize bleeding (e.g., strict bed rest, positioning) is imperative. ▪ Avoid use of razors, toothbrushes, and other sharp items. ▪ Use caution while moving to avoid excessive bumping. ▪ Report all episodes of bleeding and apply local pressure if indicated. ▪ Expect oozing from IV sites.

Maternal/Child: Category B: safety for use in pregnancy not established; use only if clearly needed. ▪ It is not known whether eptifibatide is excreted in breast milk; use caution if administered to a nursing mother. ▪ Safety and effectiveness for use in pediatric patients not established.

Elderly: Dose adjusted by weight; see Dosing Charts by Weight in Usual Dose. ▪ Clearance decreased and plasma levels increased in older patients; incidence of bleeding complications was higher and eptifibatide-associated bleeding was greater in the elderly during studies. ▪ No apparent difference in effectiveness between older and younger patients.

DRUG/LAB INTERACTIONS

All studies with eptifibatide included the use of **aspirin and heparin.** In the ESPRIT study, **clopidogrel** was administered routinely starting the day of PCI. Concomitant use, although indicated, increases the risk of bleeding. ▪ Use caution when given with **drugs that affect hemostasis** such as **thrombolytics, oral anticoagulants, NSAIDs, dipyridamole, clopidogrel, selected antibiotics** (e.g., cefotetan). ▪ Avoid concomitant treatment with **other inhibitors of platelet receptor glycoprotein GPIIb/IIIa** (e.g., tirofiban); may have potentially serious additive effects. See Contraindications.

SIDE EFFECTS

Bleeding is the most frequent adverse event; may occur more frequently in patients undergoing CABG or PCI, or in the elderly or those weighing less than 70 kg. Bleeding is usually reported as mild oozing, but major bleeding (e.g., GI bleeding, pulmonary hemorrhage, intracranial hemorrhage, and stroke) may occur. Fatal bleeding events have been reported. Laboratory findings related to bleeding include decrease in hemoglobin, hematocrit, and platelet count and occult blood in urine and feces. Other side effects that have been reported include hypersensitivity reactions, hypotension, and thrombocytopenia (acute and profound). Incidence in studies similar to that seen with placebo.

Acute toxicity: Specific information not available for humans, but decreased muscle tone, dyspnea, loss of righting reflex, petechial hemorrhages in the femoral and abdominal areas, and ptosis occurred in animals.

Post-Marketing: Immune-mediated thrombocytopenia.

ANTIDOTE

Keep physician informed of laboratory values and side effects. Discontinue the infusion of eptifibatide and heparin if any serious bleeding not controllable with pressure occurs, if CABG surgery is initiated, and/or if patient requires thrombolytic therapy. If acute profound thrombocytopenia occurs or the platelet count drops to less than $100,000/mm^3$, heparin and eptifibatide should be discontinued. Monitor serial platelet counts, assess the presence of drug-dependent antibodies, and initiate appropriate therapy as indicated. Monitor closely; platelet transfusion may be required. If a hypersensitivity reaction should occur, discontinue the infusion and treat as indicated by severity (e.g., epinephrine, dopamine, theophylline, antihistamines such as diphenhydramine, and/or corticosteroids as necessary). No specific antidote is available. Platelet inhibition reverses rapidly when infusion is discontinued. Hemodialysis may be useful in an overdose situation.

EPTINEZUMAB-jjmr
(**EP**-ti-**NEZ**-ue-mab)

Vyepti

Antimigraine agent
Calcitonin gene-related peptide
(CGRP) receptor antagonist
Monoclonal antibody
CGRP antagonist

USUAL DOSE
100 mg every 3 months; some patients may require 300 mg every 3 months.

PEDIATRIC DOSE
Not established.

DOSE ADJUSTMENTS
Renal: No dosage adjustment is provided by the manufacturer.
Hepatic: No dosage adjustments are provided by the manufacturer.

DILUTION
IV infusion: Dilute only in 100 mL NS. *Do not shake*; gently invert the diluted solution to mix; discard unused portion remaining in vial. Infusion bags must be made of polyvinyl chloride, polyethylene, or polyolefin.
100-mg dose: Withdraw 1 mL of eptinezumab and dilute in a 100-mL NS bag, which gives a final concentration of 1 mg/mL.
300-mg dose: Withdraw 3 mL eptinezumab and dilute in a 100-mL NS bag to a final concentration of 3 mg/mL.

COMPATIBILITY
Do not administer simultaneously with any other medication or IV solutions other than normal saline.

RATE OF ADMINISTRATION
After dilution, infuse IV over 30 minutes. Do not give as an IV push or bolus injection. Use an infusion set with a 0.2-micron or 0.22-micron in-line or add-on sterile filter. Do not mix or infuse other medications in the same infusion set. Flush line with 20 mL NS after infusion.

ACTIONS
Eptinezumab is a monoclonal antibody that binds to calcitonin gene-related peptide ligand and blocks its binding to the receptor.

INDICATIONS AND USES
Migraine prophylaxis.

CONTRAINDICATIONS
Hypersensitivity to eptinezumab or any component of the formulation.

PRECAUTIONS
Hypersensitivity reactions, including angioedema, facial flushing, itching, and rash, have occurred. Some dosage forms may contain polysorbate 80 (also known as *Tween 80*) which may cause hypersensitivity reactions, usually a delayed reaction.
Monitor: Monitor for signs and symptoms of hypersensitivity reactions.
Patient Education: Promptly report any signs of hypersensitivity (e.g., rash, hives, itching, wheezing, trouble breathing or swallowing, chest tightness, hoarseness, swelling of mouth, face, lips or tongue).
Maternal/Child: There are no adequate data on developmental risks associated with the use of eptinezumab in pregnant or lactating women.
Elderly: Refer to adult dosing and precautions.

DRUG/LAB INTERACTIONS
There are no significant drug interactions.

SIDE EFFECTS
Antibody development, nausea, hypersensitivity reactions, fatigue, nasopharyngitis.

ANTIDOTE
There is no antidote. Stop infusion at the first sign of hypersensitivity and treat appropriately.

ERAVACYCLINE

(er-a-va-**SYE**-kleen)

Antibacterial (tetracycline)

Xerava

pH 5.5 to 7

USUAL DOSE

1 mg/kg as an IV infusion over approximately 60 minutes every 12 hours. The recommended duration of treatment with eravacycline for a complicated intra-abdominal infections (cIAI) is 4 to 14 days. The duration of therapy should be guided by the severity and location of infection and the patient's clinical response.

DOSE ADJUSTMENTS

In patients with severe hepatic impairment (Child-Pugh C), administer eravacycline 1 mg/kg IV every 12 hours on Day 1 followed by 1 mg/kg every 24 hours on Day 2 for a total duration of 4 to 14 days. ▪ No dose adjustment is warranted in patients with mild to moderate hepatic impairment (Child-Pugh A and Child-Pugh B), in patients with any degree of renal impairment, or based on age. ▪ With concomitant use of a strong CYP3A inducer, administer eravacycline 1.5 mg/kg every 12 hours for a total duration of 4 to 14 days. No dosage adjustment is warranted in patients with concomitant use of a weak or moderate CYP3A inducer; see Drug/Lab Interactions.

DILUTION

Available as a yellow to orange, lyophilized powder in single-dose vials containing 50 mg of eravacycline. Calculate the dose of eravacycline based on the patient weight (1 mg/kg). Reconstitute the required number of vials needed to make the dose by injecting 5 mL of SWFI into each vial (final concentration 10 mg/mL). Swirl the vial(s) gently to dissolve. **Do not shake.** The reconstituted product should be a clear, pale-yellow to orange solution. The reconstituted solution must be further diluted with NS to a target final concentration of 0.3 mg/mL (range 0.2 to 0.6 mg/mL). To dilute the reconstituted solution, withdraw the calculated dose and add it to a NS infusion bag to generate an infusion solution with the target concentration (e.g., a 70-kg patient will require a 70-mg dose. Add 70 mg [7 mL] to a 250 mL bag of NS to provide a final concentration of approximately 0.27 mg/mL). **Do not shake the bag.**

Filter: Data not available.

Storage: Store unopened vials in original carton at 2° to 8° C (36° to 46° F). The reconstituted and diluted solutions must be infused within 6 hours if stored at RT or within 24 hours if stored at 2° to 8° C (36° to 46° F). Do not freeze. Discard unused portions of the reconstituted or diluted solution.

COMPATIBILITY

Manufacturer states, "Eravacycline is compatible with NS. **Compatibility** with other drugs and infusion solutions has not been established. Eravacycline should not be mixed with other drugs or added to solutions containing other drugs."

RATE OF ADMINISTRATION

Administer as an IV infusion over approximately 60 minutes. May be administered through a dedicated line or through a Y-site. If the same IV line is used for sequential infusion of several drugs, the line should be flushed with NS before and after the infusion of eravacycline.

ACTIONS

A synthetic fluorocycline antibacterial within the tetracycline class of antibacterial drugs. Eravacycline disrupts bacterial protein synthesis by binding to the 30s ribosomal subunit, thus preventing the incorporation of amino acid residues into elongating peptide chains. In general, eravacycline is bacteriostatic against gram-positive bacteria (e.g., *Staphylococcus aureus* and *Enterococcus faecalis*); however, in vitro bactericidal activity has been demonstrated against certain strains of *Escherichia coli* and *Klebsiella pneumoniae*. Active against selected gram-positive and gram-negative aerobic and anaerobic bacteria;

see prescribing information and Indications. Protein binding to human plasma proteins increases with increasing plasma concentrations. Metabolized primarily by CYP3A4- and FMO-mediated oxidation. Half-life is 20 hours. Excreted in urine and feces.

INDICATIONS AND USES

Treatment of complicated intra-abdominal infections (cIAI) caused by susceptible microorganisms in patients 18 years or older. Organisms that may be susceptible include: *E. coli, K. pneumoniae, Citrobacter freundii, Enterobacter cloacae, Klebsiella oxytoca, E. faecalis, Enterococcus faecium, S. aureus, Streptococcus anginosus* group, *Clostridium perfringens, Bacteroides* species, and *Parabacteroides distasonis*.

Limitation of use: Eravacycline is not indicated for treatment of a complicated urinary tract infection (cUTI).

CONTRAINDICATIONS

Known hypersensitivity to eravacycline, tetracycline-class antibacterial drugs, or to any of the excipients. Not recommended in pediatric patients under 8 years or in breast-feeding.

PRECAUTIONS

For IV use only. ■ To reduce the development of drug-resistant bacteria and maintain its effectiveness, eravacycline should be used to treat or prevent only those infections proven or strongly suspected to be caused by bacteria. ■ Sensitivity studies indicated to determine susceptibility of the causative organism to eravacycline. ■ Life-threatening hypersensitivity (anaphylactic) reactions have been reported. Eravacycline is structurally similar to other tetracycline-class antibacterial drugs and should be not be administered to patients with known hypersensitivity to any drug in this class. ■ Exposure during the last half of pregnancy, infancy, and childhood to the age of 8 years may cause permanent discoloration of the teeth. This adverse reaction is more common during long-term use of the tetracycline-class drugs but has also been observed following repeated short-term courses. Enamel hypoplasia has also been reported with the tetracycline-class drugs. ■ The use of eravacycline during the second and third trimester of pregnancy, infancy, and childhood up to the age of 8 years may cause reversible inhibition of bone growth. All tetracyclines form a stable calcium complex in any bone-forming tissue. ■ Eravacycline is structurally similar to tetracycline-class antibacterial drugs and may have similar adverse reactions. Adverse reactions including photosensitivity, pseudotumor cerebri, and anti-anabolic action leading to increased BUN, azotemia, acidosis, hyperphosphatemia, pancreatitis, and abnormal liver function tests have been reported for other tetracycline-class antibacterial drugs and may occur with eravacycline. ■ Avoid prolonged use of drug; superinfection caused by overgrowth of nonsusceptible organisms may result. ■ *Clostridium difficile*–associated diarrhea (CDAD) has been reported. May range from mild to life threatening. Consider in patients who present with diarrhea during or after treatment with eravacycline. ■ May be active against some organisms that are normally resistant to other tetracyclines.

Monitor: Monitor for S/S of hypersensitivity reactions. ■ Determine absolute patency of vein and avoid extravasation; thrombophlebitis may occur. ■ Monitor hematopoietic, renal, and hepatic studies periodically in long-term therapy. ■ See Drug/Lab Interactions.

Patient Education: Promptly report severe diarrhea, S/S of hypersensitivity reactions, or any other side effect. ■ May cause permanent tooth discoloration of deciduous teeth and reversible inhibition of bone growth when administered during the second and third trimesters of pregnancy. Tell your health care provider right away if you become pregnant during treatment. ■ Alert patient to the possibility of a photosensitive skin reaction. ■ May impair spermiation and sperm maturation. Long-term effects on male fertility have not been studied.

Maternal/Child: Data on use in pregnant women are limited. May cause permanent tooth discoloration of deciduous teeth and reversible inhibition of bone growth when administered during the second and third trimesters of pregnancy. Consider risk versus benefit. ■ Discontinue breast-feeding during treatment and for 4 days after the last dose.

- Safety and effectiveness of eravacycline in pediatric patients have not been established. Due to the adverse effects on tooth development and bone growth, use in pediatric patients less than 8 years of age is not recommended.

Elderly: No overall differences in safety or efficacy were observed between elderly patients and younger patients.

DRUG/LAB INTERACTIONS

Concomitant use of **strong CYP3A inducers** (e.g., rifampin decreases the exposure of eravacycline, which may reduce its efficacy. Increase eravacycline dose if concomitant use of a strong CYP3A inducer is required; see Dose Adjustments. ■ Because tetracyclines have been shown to depress plasma prothrombin activity, patients who are on **anticoagulant therapy** may require downward adjustment of their anticoagulant dosage. ■ In vitro studies have not demonstrated antagonism between eravacycline and other commonly used antibacterial drugs for the indicated pathogens.

SIDE EFFECTS

The most common adverse reactions are infusion site reactions, nausea, and vomiting. Less commonly reported adverse reactions included diarrhea, hypotension, and wound dehiscence. Several other adverse reactions were reported in fewer than 1% of patients. *C. difficile*–associated diarrhea, hypersensitivity reactions, inhibition of bone growth, tetracycline-class adverse reactions and tooth discoloration have been reported; see Precautions.

ANTIDOTE

Notify the physician of all side effects. Discontinue eravacycline at the first sign of a hypersensitivity reaction or if the development of any tetracycline-class adverse drug reaction is suspected. Treat hypersensitivity reactions as indicated (e.g., antihistamines, epinephrine, corticosteroids) and resuscitate as necessary. Treat CDAD with fluids, electrolytes, protein supplements, and appropriate antibiotics (e.g., oral vancomycin) as indicated. In severe cases, surgical evaluation may be indicated. Significant quantities are not expected to be removed by hemodialysis.

ERIBULIN MESYLATE
(ER-ih-BUE-lin MES-ih-late)

Halaven

Antineoplastic
(antimicrotubular)

pH 6.5 to 8.5

USUAL DOSE

Pretreatment: Verify pregnancy status. Baseline studies indicated; see Monitor.

1.4 mg/M^2 IV over 2 to 5 minutes on Days 1 and 8 of a 21-day cycle.

DOSE ADJUSTMENTS

Dose adjustment not required based on age, gender, or race. ■ Reduce dose in patients with mild hepatic impairment (Child-Pugh Class A) to 1.1 mg/M^2 IV. ■ Patients with moderate hepatic impairment (Child-Pugh Class B) should receive 0.7 mg/M^2 IV. ■ Patients with moderate or severe renal impairment (CrCl 15 to 49 mL/min) should receive 1.1 mg/M^2 IV. ■ Do not administer dose on Day 1 or Day 8 in patients with an ANC less than 1,000/mm^3, platelets less than 75,000/mm^3, or Grade 3 or 4 nonhematologic toxicities. ■ The Day 8 dose may be delayed for a maximum of 1 week. If toxicities do not resolve or improve to Grade 2 or less by Day 15, omit the dose. If toxicities resolve or improve to Grade 2 or less by Day 15, administer at a reduced dose as outlined in the following chart and initiate the next cycle no sooner than 2 weeks later. ■ If a dose has been delayed for toxicity and the toxicities have recovered to Grade 2 severity or less, resume eribulin as outlined in the following chart. ■ Do not re-escalate eribulin dose after it has been reduced.

Recommended Dose Reductions for Eribulin Mesylate	
Event Description	Recommended Eribulin Dose
Permanently reduce the 1.4 mg/M² eribulin dose for any of the following: • ANC <500/mm³ for >7 days • ANC <1,000/mm³ with fever or infection • Platelets <25,000/mm³ • Platelets <50,000/mm³ requiring transfusion • Nonhematologic Grade 3 or 4 toxicities[a] • Omission or delay of Day 8 eribulin dose in previous cycle for toxicity	1.1 mg/M²
Occurrence of any event requiring permanent dose reduction while receiving 1.1 mg/M²	0.7 mg/M²
Occurrence of any event requiring permanent dose reduction while receiving 0.7 mg/M²	Discontinue eribulin

[a]Toxicities graded in accordance with National Cancer Institute (NCI) Common Terminology Criteria for Adverse Events (CTCAE), Version 3.0.

DILUTION

Specific techniques required; see Precautions. Available in a single-use vial containing 1 mg/2 mL (0.5 mg/mL). Withdraw calculated dose and administer undiluted or may dilute in 100 mL NS.

Filter: Information not available.

Storage: Store unopened vials in carton at CRT. Do not freeze. Store undiluted solution drawn up into a syringe for up to 4 hours at RT or 24 hours under refrigeration (4° C [40° F]). Store diluted solution for up to 4 hours at RT or 24 hours under refrigeration (4° C [40° F]). Discard unused portion of vial.

COMPATIBILITY

Manufacturer states, "Do not dilute in or administer through an IV line containing solutions with dextrose. Do not administer in the same intravenous line concurrent with other medicinal products."

RATE OF ADMINISTRATION

An IV injection evenly distributed over 2 to 5 minutes.

ACTIONS

A synthetic analog of halichondrin B, a product isolated from a marine sponge. Eribulin is a non-taxane microtubule inhibitor. Inhibits the growth phase of microtubules without affecting the shortening phase and sequesters tubulin into nonproductive aggregates. Exerts its effects via a tubulin-based antimitotic mechanism leading to G_2/M cell-cycle block, disruption of mitotic spindles and, ultimately, apoptotic cell death after prolonged mitotic blockage. Plasma protein binding is 49% to 65%. Mean elimination half-life is approximately 40 hours. There are no major human metabolites. Is eliminated primarily in feces unchanged. Small amount excreted as unchanged drug in urine.

INDICATIONS AND USES

Treatment of patients with metastatic breast cancer who have previously received at least two chemotherapeutic regimens for the treatment of metastatic disease. Prior therapy should have included an anthracycline and a taxane in either the adjuvant or metastatic setting. ▪ Treatment of patients with unresectable or metastatic liposarcoma who have received a prior anthracycline-containing regimen.

CONTRAINDICATIONS

Manufacturer states, "None." ▪ Do not administer in patients with an ANC less than 1,000/mm³, platelets less than 75,000/mm³, or Grade 3 or 4 nonhematologic toxicities. ▪ Should be avoided in patients with congenital long QT syndrome.

PRECAUTIONS

Follow guidelines for handling cytotoxic agents. See Appendix A, p. 1308. ▪ May cause severe neutropenia (ANC less than 500/mm^3) lasting more than 1 week. Higher incidence of Grade 4 neutropenia and febrile neutropenia seen in patients with ALT or AST greater than 3 times the ULN and in patients with a bilirubin greater than 1.5 times the ULN. Deaths from complications of febrile neutropenia and neutropenic sepsis have been reported. In clinical trials, the mean time to nadir was 13 days, and the mean time to recovery from severe neutropenia was 8 days. ▪ Grades 3 and 4 peripheral neuropathy have been reported. Peripheral neuropathy was the most common toxicity leading to discontinuation of therapy. Neuropathy may not be reversible. ▪ QT prolongation, independent of eribulin concentration, was observed on Day 8 in an uncontrolled, open-label ECG study. ▪ Has not been studied in patients with severe hepatic impairment (Child-Pugh Class C). ▪ See Dose Adjustments.

Monitor: Obtain baseline CBC with platelets, bilirubin, liver function tests, SCr, and electrolytes. ▪ Obtain CBC with platelets before each dose. Increase frequency of hematologic monitoring in patients who develop severe cytopenias (Grade 3 or 4); see Dose Adjustments. ▪ Assess for peripheral motor and sensory neuropathy before each dose; see Dose Adjustments. ▪ ECG monitoring is recommended in patients with CHF or bradyarrhythmias; in patients taking drugs that prolong the QT interval, such as Class Ia and III antiarrhythmics (e.g., amiodarone, disopyramide, dofetilide, ibutilide, *N*-acetyl-procainamide, procainamide, quinidine, sotalol); and in patients with electrolyte abnormalities. Correct hypokalemia or hypomagnesemia before initiating therapy, and monitor electrolytes periodically during therapy. ▪ Monitor for nausea and vomiting. Use prophylactic antiemetics to reduce nausea and vomiting and increase patient comfort. ▪ Observe closely for signs of infection. Prophylactic antibiotics may be indicated pending results of C/S in a febrile neutropenic patient. ▪ In patients with thrombocytopenia (platelet count less than 50,000/mm^3), initiate precautions to prevent excessive bleeding (e.g., inspect IV sites, skin, and mucous membranes; use extreme care during invasive procedures; test urine, emesis, stool, and secretions for occult blood).

Patient Education: Read FDA-approved patient information. ▪ Avoid pregnancy. Women should use effective contraception during treatment with eribulin and for 2 weeks following the final dose. Males with female partners of reproductive potential should use effective contraception during treatment and for 3.5 months following the final dose. ▪ May result in damage to male reproductive tissues, leading to impaired fertility of unknown duration. ▪ Promptly report S/S of infection (e.g., fever, chills, cough, burning or pain on urination). ▪ Report symptoms of peripheral neuropathy (e.g., numbness, tingling, or burning in hands or feet).

Maternal/Child: Can cause fetal harm. ▪ Discontinue breast-feeding. ▪ Safety and effectiveness for use in pediatric patients not established.

Elderly: No overall differences in safety were observed between older and younger patients. ▪ Consider age-related cardiac, hepatic, or renal dysfunction.

DRUG/LAB INTERACTIONS

No drug-drug interactions are expected with CYP3A4 inhibitors, CYP3A4 inducers, or P-glycoprotein (P-gp) inhibitors. ▪ A substrate and a weak inhibitor of the drug efflux transporter P-gp in vitro.

SIDE EFFECTS

The most common side effects were abdominal pain, alopecia, anemia, asthenia, constipation, fatigue, fever, nausea, neutropenia, and peripheral neuropathy. The most common serious side effects were febrile neutropenia and neutropenia. The most common side effects resulting in discontinuation of eribulin were fatigue, peripheral neuropathy, and thrombocytopenia. Grade 3 or 4 laboratory abnormalities included hypocalcemia, hypokalemia, and neutropenia. Other reported side effects included anorexia, arthralgia, cough, diarrhea, dyspnea, headache, liver function test abnormalities, mucosal inflammation, myalgia, pain (back, bone, extremity), UTI, vomiting, and weight loss. Less frequently reported side effects included anxiety, depression, dizziness, dry mouth, dysgeusia, dyspepsia, hyperglycemia, hypophosphatemia, hypotension, increased lacrimation, insomnia, muscle spasm or weakness, oropharyngeal pain, peripheral edema, rash, stomatitis, and upper respiratory tract infection.

Post-Marketing: Dehydration, hepatotoxicity, hypersensitivity, hypomagnesemia, interstitial lung disease, lymphopenia, neutropenic sepsis, pancreatitis, pneumonia, pruritus, sepsis, Stevens-Johnson syndrome, and toxic epidermal necrolysis.

ANTIDOTE

Keep physician informed of all side effects. Most will be treated symptomatically as indicated. Neutropenia can be profound. Colony-stimulating factors (G-CSF [filgrastim], GM-CSF [sargramostim]) have been administered to aid in neutrophil recovery. Severe peripheral neuropathies may necessitate discontinuation of eribulin. There is no specific antidote for overdose. Supportive therapy will help sustain the patient in toxicity. Resuscitate if indicated.

ERTAPENEM

(er-tah-**PEN**-em)

Invanz

**Antibacterial
(carbapenem)**

pH 7.5

USUAL DOSE

Pretreatment: Baseline studies indicated; see Monitor.

Duration of therapy is based on diagnosis as listed in the following chart. May be given IV for up to 14 days or IM for up to 7 days.

Ertapenem Dosing Guidelines			
Infection[a]	Daily Dose (IV or IM) in Adults and Pediatric Patients 13 Years of Age and Older	Daily Dose (IV or IM) in Pediatric Patients 3 Months to 12 Years of Age	Duration
Complicated intra-abdominal infections	1 Gm	15 mg/kg q 12 hr[b]	5–14 days
Complicated skin and skin structure infections, including diabetic foot infections[c]	1 Gm	15 mg/kg q 12 hr[b]	7–14 days[d]
Community-acquired pneumonia	1 Gm	15 mg/kg q 12 hr[b]	10–14 days[e]
Complicated urinary tract infections, including pyelonephritis	1 Gm	15 mg/kg q 12 hr[b]	10–14 days[e]
Acute pelvic infections, including postpartum endomyometritis, septic abortion, and postsurgical gynecologic infections.	1 Gm	15 mg/kg q 12 hr[b]	3–10 days
Prophylaxis of surgical site infection in adults for elective colorectal surgery	1 Gm		Single intravenous dose given 1 hour before surgical incision

[a]Due to designated pathogens.

[b]Not to exceed 1 Gm/24 hr.

[c]Has not been studied in diabetic foot infections with concomitant osteomyelitis.

[d]Adult patients with diabetic foot infections received up to 28 days of treatment (parenteral or parenteral plus oral switch therapy).

[e]Duration includes a possible switch to an appropriate oral therapy, after at least 3 days of parenteral therapy, once clinical improvement has been demonstrated.

DOSE ADJUSTMENTS

Reduce dose to 0.5 Gm (500 mg) daily in adults with a CrCl at or less than 30 mL/min/1.73 M^2, including adults with end-stage renal insufficiency (CrCl $\leq$10 mL/min/1.73 M^2). No dose adjustment indicated in adults with a CrCl at or more than 31 mL/min/1.73 M^2. Give a supplementary dose of 150 mg to patients who received the daily dose within 6 hours of a dialysis session. No data are available for pediatric patients with renal insufficiency or pediatric patients on hemodialysis. No data on patients undergoing peritoneal dialysis or hemofiltration. ■ No dose adjustment indicated based on age or gender. The pharmacokinetics of ertapenem in patients with hepatic impairment have not been established. Dose recommendations are not available. ■ Dosing should be cautious in the elderly, and reduced doses may be indicated based on potential for decreased organ function.

DILUTION

Reconstitute each 1-Gm vial of ertapenem with 10 mL SWFI, NS, BWFI using a syringe equipped with a 21-gauge or smaller diameter needle. Use with a needleless IV system is **not** recommended. Shake well to dissolve, and dilute immediately as outlined below.

Adults and pediatric patients 13 years of age and older: Further dilute in 50 mL of NS.

Pediatric patients 3 months to 12 years of age: Withdraw the volume equal to the 15 mg/kg dose and dilute in NS to a final concentration of 20 mg/mL or less.

Storage: Store unopened vials at or below 25° C (77° F). Dilute reconstituted solution immediately. Use diluted solution within 6 hours when stored at RT. May refrigerate for up to 24 hours and use within 4 hours after removal. Do not freeze.

COMPATIBILITY

Manufacturer states, "Do not mix or co-infuse ertapenem with other medications. Do not use diluents containing dextrose."

Other sources suggest a few specific **compatibilities** dependent on concentration and manufacturer; consult a pharmacist.

RATE OF ADMINISTRATION

A single dose as an infusion equally distributed over 30 minutes.

ACTIONS

A unique, synthetic 1-beta-methyl-carbapenem structurally related to beta-lactam antibiotics. Effective against gram-positive and gram-negative aerobic and anaerobic bacteria. May effectively replace some combination therapies. Does not cover *Pseudomonas* and *Acinetobacter* species. Bactericidal activity results from inhibition of bacterial cell wall synthesis. Stable against hydrolysis by a variety of beta-lactamases, including penicillinases, cephalosporinases, and extended-spectrum beta-lactamases. Hydrolyzed by metallo-beta-lactamases. Widely distributed throughout the body into many body tissues and fluids. Highly protein bound. Average half-life is 4 hours. Primarily excreted in urine (some as unchanged drug). Some excretion in feces. Secreted in breast milk.

INDICATIONS AND USES

Treatment of adult and pediatric patients with moderate to severe infections caused by susceptible strains of microorganisms in conditions that include complicated intra-abdominal infections; complicated skin and skin structure infections, including diabetic foot infections **without** osteomyelitis; community-acquired pneumonia; complicated urinary tract infections, including pyelonephritis; and acute pelvic infections, including postpartum endomyometritis, septic abortion, and postsurgical gynecologic infections.

■ Prophylaxis of surgical site infections in adults following elective colorectal surgery.

■ Not recommended for use in the treatment of meningitis in pediatric patients (lack of sufficient CSF penetration).

CONTRAINDICATIONS

Known hypersensitivity to any component of ertapenem or other drugs in the same class (e.g., imipenem-cilastatin), or in patients who have had anaphylactic reactions to beta-lactams (e.g., penicillins and cephalosporins); see Precautions.

PRECAUTIONS

To reduce the development of drug-resistant bacteria and maintain its effectiveness, ertapenem should be used to treat or prevent only those infections proven or strongly suspected to be caused by bacteria. ■ Culture and sensitivity studies indicated to determine susceptibility of the causative organism to ertapenem. ■ Serious and occasionally fatal hypersensitivity reactions have been reported in patients receiving therapy with beta-lactams. More likely in patients with a history of sensitivity to multiple allergens; obtain a careful history and watch for early symptoms of hypersensitivity reactions. Emergency equipment must be readily available; cross-sensitivity is possible. ■ Prolonged use may cause superinfection because of overgrowth of nonsusceptible organisms. ■ CNS stimulation and seizures have been reported. Use with caution in patients with CNS disorders (e.g., brain lesions or history of seizures) and/or compromised renal function. ■ *Clostridium difficile*–associated diarrhea (CDAD) has been reported. May range from mild diarrhea to fatal colitis. Consider in patients who present with diarrhea during or after treatment with ertapenem. ▪ See Monitor and Drug/Lab Interactions.

Monitor: Monitor closely for S/S of hypersensitivity reactions (e.g., difficulty breathing, itching, rash, swelling of eyelids, lips, or face). ▪ Obtain baseline CBC with differential and platelets, and baseline kidney and liver studies (e.g., CrCl, serum creatinine, ALT, AST, serum bilirubin). Monitor periodically during prolonged therapy. ▪ Monitor patients who are at risk for CNS stimulation or are receiving anticonvulsant therapy. If focal tremors, myoclonus, or seizures occur, neurologic evaluation and dose reduction or discontinuation of ertapenem may be indicated. ▪ Monitor IV site carefully and rotate as indicated. ▪ See Precautions.

Patient Education: Promptly report S/S of hypersensitivity reaction (e.g., rash, shortness of breath, hives), fever, sore throat, unusual bleeding or bruising, severe stomach cramps, seizures, and pain or discomfort at the injection site. ▪ Promptly report diarrhea or bloody stools that occur during treatment or up to several months after an antibiotic has been discontinued; may indicate CDAD and require treatment. ▪ Patients with a history of seizures should review medication profile with physician before taking ertapenem; see Drug/Lab Interactions.

Maternal/Child: Available data insufficient to inform any drug-associated risks for major birth defects, miscarriage, or adverse maternal or fetal outcomes. Use during pregnancy only if clearly needed. ▪ There are no data on the effects on the breast-fed infant or the effects on milk production; is found in breast milk. Benefits must outweigh risks to infant (e.g., diarrhea, candidiasis, or allergic response). Undetectable in breast milk 5 days after ertapenem is discontinued. ▪ Following a 1-Gm daily IV dose, plasma concentrations and half-life of ertapenem in pediatric patients 13 to 17 years of age are comparable to those in adults. ▪ Compared to plasma clearance in adults, plasma clearance (mL/min/kg) in pediatric patients 3 months to 12 years of age is approximately twofold higher. 30 mg/kg/24 hr (15 mg/kg every 12 hours) is comparable to a 1-Gm dose daily in adults. Half-life in pediatric patients 3 months to 12 years of age is 2.5 hours compared to 4 hours for adults and pediatric patients 13 years of age or older. ▪ Not recommended for use in infants under 3 months; no data available; see Indications and Uses.

Elderly: Dosing should be cautious in the elderly; see Dose Adjustments. ▪ Response similar to that seen in younger patients, but may be more sensitive to side effects. ▪ Monitoring of renal function may be indicated.

DRUG/LAB INTERACTIONS

Carbapenems may reduce serum **valproic acid** concentrations to subtherapeutic levels, resulting in a loss of seizure control. Monitor valproic acid levels. Consider alternative antibacterial therapy. If administration of ertapenem is necessary, supplemental anticonvulsant therapy should be considered. ▪ **Probenecid** reduces the renal clearance of ertapenem, resulting in increased plasma concentrations. Coadministration is not recommended.

SIDE EFFECTS

Adults: Diarrhea, headache, infusion site reactions, nausea, and vaginitis in females were most common and described as mild to moderate. Other side effects that were reported in greater than 2% of patients included abdominal pain, altered mental status, constipation, dizziness, dyspnea, edema/swelling, fever, hypotension, insomnia, pruritus, rash, and vomiting. The most commonly reported laboratory abnormalities were elevated ALT, AST, and alkaline phosphatase; decreased hemoglobin and hematocrit; and increased platelets and eosinophils. Serious but less frequently reported adverse events included CDAD, CNS stimulation (e.g., aggressive behavior, anxiety, depression, insomnia, nervousness, seizures, tremor), hypersensitivity reactions (e.g., anaphylaxis, cardiovascular collapse, death, dyspnea, edema [facial, laryngeal, or pharyngeal], hypotension, itching, rash, shock, urticaria), and pseudomembranous colitis. Numerous other side effects occurred in fewer than 1% of patients.

Pediatric patients: Side effects similar to adults. Diarrhea, infusion site pain, erythema, and vomiting were most common.

Post-Marketing: Abnormal coordination, acute generalized exanthematous pustulosis (AGEP), altered mental status (including aggression, delirium, and hallucinations), anaphylaxis, depressed level of consciousness, drug rash with eosinophilia and systemic symptoms (DRESS syndrome), dyskinesia, gait disturbance, muscular weakness, myoclonus, teeth staining, tremor.

ANTIDOTE

Keep physician informed of all side effects. Most minor side effects will be treated symptomatically. Discontinue ertapenem at the first sign of hypersensitivity (e.g., skin rash). Treat hypersensitivity reactions as indicated; may require epinephrine, airway management, oxygen, IV fluids, antihistamines, corticosteroids, and pressor amines (e.g., dopamine). Treat CNS symptoms as indicated; may require dose reduction and/or anticonvulsants (e.g., phenytoin, diazepam) for seizures. Mild cases of CDAD may respond to discontinuation of the drug. Treat CDAD with fluids, electrolytes, protein supplements, and appropriate antibiotics (e.g., oral vancomycin), as indicated. In severe cases, surgical evaluation may be indicated. Ertapenem is partially removed by hemodialysis.

ERYTHROMYCIN LACTOBIONATE

(eh-**rih**-throw-**MY**-sin **LAK**-to-**bye**-oh-nayt)

Erythrocin

Antibacterial
(macrolide)

pH 6.5 to 7.7

USUAL DOSE

IV formulation used when oral administration is not possible or when the severity of the infection requires immediate high serum levels of erythromycin. Begin oral therapy as soon as practical.

Antibacterial: 15 to 20 mg/kg of body weight/24 hr in equally divided doses every 6 hours (3.75 to 5 mg/kg every 6 hours). Range is 350 to 500 mg every 6 hours. Continuous infusion over 24 hours is preferred. Up to 4 Gm/24 hr has been given for severe infections. See Elderly.

Legionnaires' disease: 1 to 4 Gm/day in divided doses (250 mg to 1 Gm every 6 hours). Optimum doses not established.

Pelvic inflammatory disease: 500 mg every 6 hours for 3 days. Follow with oral erythromycin 250 mg every 6 hours for 7 days.

Diabetic gastroparesis (unlabeled): 200 mg immediately before each meal. When practical, continue treatment with oral erythromycin 3 times daily, 30 minutes before meals, for 4 weeks.

PEDIATRIC DOSE

15 to 20 mg/kg of body weight/24 hr in equally divided doses every 6 hours is recommended (3.75 to 5 mg/kg every 6 hours). Another source recommends 20 to 50 mg/kg/24 hr in equally divided doses every 6 hours (5 to 12.5 mg/kg every 6 hours). See Maternal/Child.

DOSE ADJUSTMENTS

Reduced dose may be required in impaired liver function.

DILUTION

Each 500 mg must be reconstituted with 10 mL of SWFI without preservatives to avoid precipitation. Forms a 5% solution. Shake well to ensure dilution. May be further diluted with NS, Normosol, or LR. If a dextrose solution is used, add sodium bicarbonate (Neut) 1 mL for each 100 mL of solution.

Continuous infusion (preferred): Further dilute to a 1 mg/mL solution (e.g., each 1 Gm in 1,000 mL of NS, Normosol, or LR).

Intermittent infusion: Dilute to a final concentration of 1 to 5 mg/mL. No less than 100 mL of IV diluent should be used (1 Gm in 1,000 mL equals 1 mg/mL; 1 Gm in 200 mL equals 5 mg/mL).

Storage: Store unopened vials at CRT. Solutions diluted from *lyophilized powder vials* are stable for 8 hours at CRT.

COMPATIBILITY

Compatibility information not available from manufacturer. Other sources suggest specific **compatibilities** dependent on concentration and manufacturer; consult a pharmacist.

RATE OF ADMINISTRATION

Administer with a volume control set. A slow infusion rate is recommended to reduce pain along the injection site.

Continuous infusion (preferred): A 0.1% to 0.2% solution equally distributed over 6 to 24 hours.

Intermittent infusion: 1 Gm or fraction thereof in at least 100 mL over 20 to 60 minutes.

Diabetic gastroparesis (unlabeled): 1 to 3 mg/kg/hr, usually approximately over 15 minutes.

ACTIONS

Macrolide antibiotic, bactericidal and bacteriostatic. Effective against a number of gram-positive and some gram-negative organisms as well as *Mycoplasma pneumoniae*. Inhibits protein synthesis by binding to ribosomal subunits of susceptible organisms. Diffuses readily into most bodily fluids. Metabolized by the liver and excreted in urine and bile. Crosses placental barrier. Secreted in breast milk.

INDICATIONS AND USES

Treatment of mild to moderate infections of the upper and lower respiratory tract, skin and skin structures, and gynecologic infections caused by susceptible organisms. ▪ Alternative treatment in several sexually transmitted diseases in females with a history of penicillin sensitivity. ▪ Legionnaires' disease. ▪ Additional indications listed for oral formulation.

Unlabeled uses: Diabetic gastroparesis.

CONTRAINDICATIONS

Known erythromycin sensitivity. See Drug/Lab Interactions. ▪ Coadministration with ritonavir is contraindicated. Contraindicated when used concomitantly with HMG-CoA reductase inhibitors (statins) that are extensively metabolized by cytochrome P_{450} isoform 3A4 (lovastatin or simvastatin) due to the increased risk of myopathy, including rhabdomyolysis.

PRECAUTIONS

IV formulation used when oral administration is not possible or when the severity of the infection requires immediate high serum levels of erythromycin. Switch to oral therapy when appropriate. ▪ Sensitivity studies indicated to determine susceptibility of the causative organism to erythromycin. ▪ To reduce the development of drug-resistant bacteria and maintain its effectiveness, erythromycin should be used to treat or prevent only those infections proven or strongly suspected to be caused by bacteria. ▪ Superinfection may occur from overgrowth of nonsusceptible organisms. ▪ Use caution in impaired liver function. ▪ Hepatic dysfunction, with or without jaundice, has been reported in patients taking oral erythromycin. ▪ Use caution in patients with a history of cardiac disease. Life-threatening episodes of ventricular tachycardia associated with prolonged QT intervals (torsades de pointes) have been reported. ▪ Use caution in patients with myasthenia gravis; weakness may be aggravated. ▪ *Clostridium difficile*–associated diarrhea (CDAD) has been reported. May range from mild diarrhea to fatal colitis. Consider in patients who present with diarrhea during or after treatment with erythromycin. ▪ Hypersensitivity reactions, including anaphylaxis have occurred; emergency equipment, medications, and supplies must be available.

Monitor: Monitor vital signs. ▪ Monitor for development of torsades de pointes related to electrolyte imbalance, hepatic dysfunction, myocardial ischemia, left ventricular dysfunction, idiopathic QT prolongation, and concurrent antiarrhythmic therapy. ▪ Monitor IV site for redness and inflammation. ▪ Monitor for S/S of hypersensitivity reactions (e.g., hypotension, rash, urticaria, tightness of the chest, wheezing). ▪ See Drug/Lab Interactions.

Patient Education: Promptly report diarrhea or bloody stools that occur during treatment or up to several months after an antibiotic has been discontinued; may indicate CDAD and require treatment.

Maternal/Child: Use during pregnancy only if clearly needed. ▪ Considered safe for use in breast-feeding; use caution. ▪ Some products contain benzyl alcohol; not recommended for use in neonates.

Elderly: When doses of 4 Gm/day or higher are used, the risk of developing erythromycin-induced hearing loss is increased in elderly patients, particularly those with impaired renal or hepatic function. ▪ May be more susceptible to development of torsades de pointes. ▪ May experience increased effects of oral anticoagulation; see Drug/Lab Interactions.

DRUG/LAB INTERACTIONS

Contraindicated with **ritonavir.** ▪ Antibacterial activity is antagonized by coadministration of **clindamycin, lincomycin, and chloramphenicol.** ▪ May inhibit **penicillins.** ▪ Will increase serum levels and potentiate the effects of **alfentanil, anticoagulants, bromocriptine, carbamazepine, cyclosporine, digoxin, disopyramide, ergot alkaloids, methylprednisolone, midazolam, phenytoin, theophyllines, triazolam, and valproate;** serious toxicity may result. ▪ Plasma concentrations of erythromycin may be increased by **antifungal agents** metabolized by CYP3A4 isoenzymes (e.g., fluconazole, itraconazole). May result in an increase in QT prolongation and ventricular arrhythmias. ▪ Severe **vinblastine** toxicity has been reported in conjunction with erythromycin. ▪ May increase serum levels of **sildenafil.** ▪ Contraindicated when used concomitantly with **HMG-CoA reductase inhibitors** (statins) that are extensively metabolized by cytochrome P_{450} isoform 3A4 (e.g., lovastatin or simvastatin). ▪ Coadministration results in increased serum levels of the antihyperlipidemic agent and increases the risk of severe myopathy and rhabdomyolysis. ▪ Concurrent use with **theophylline** (aminophylline) may decrease plasma levels of erythromycin. ▪ Serotonin syndrome has been reported with coadministration of erythromycin and **serotonin-uptake inhibitors.** ▪ May interfere with fluorometric determination of **urinary catecholamines.**

SIDE EFFECTS

Relatively free from side effects when given as directed. Nausea and vomiting, urticaria, and mild local venous discomfort. Increased incidence of usually reversible ototoxicity with larger doses. CDAD; QT prolongation and ventricular arrhythmias, including ventricular tachycardia and torsades de points, and skin reactions ranging from mild eruptions to erythema multiforme, Stevens-Johnson syndrome, and toxic necrolysis have been reported. Hypersensitivity reactions, including anaphylaxis, may occur.

ANTIDOTE

Notify the physician of early or mild symptoms. For severe symptoms, discontinue the drug, treat hypersensitivity reactions, or resuscitate as necessary and notify physician. Treat CDAD with fluids, electrolytes, protein supplements, and appropriate antibiotics (e.g., oral vancomycin) as indicated. In severe cases, surgical evaluation may be indicated. Not removed by peritoneal dialysis or hemodialysis.

ESMOLOL HYDROCHLORIDE
(**EZ**-moh-lohl hy-droh-**KLOR**-eyed)

Brevibloc

Beta-adrenergic blocking agent
Antiarrhythmic

pH 4.5 to 5.5

USUAL DOSE

Supraventricular tachycardia (SVT) or noncompensatory sinus tachycardia: Administer by continuous IV infusion with or without a loading dose. Additional loading doses and/or titration of the maintenance infusion (stepwise dosing) may be necessary based on desired ventricular response.

Esmolol Stepwise Dosing for Supraventricular Tachycardia or Noncompensatory Sinus Tachycardia	
Step	**Action**
1	Optional loading dose (500 mcg/kg over 1 minute), then 50 mcg/kg/min for 4 min
2	Optional loading dose if necessary, then 100 mcg/kg/min for 4 min
3	Optional loading dose if necessary, then 150 mcg/kg/min for 4 min
4	If necessary, increase dose to 200 mcg/kg/min

In the absence of loading doses, continuous infusion of a single concentration of esmolol reaches a pharmacokinetic and pharmacodynamic steady-state in about 30 minutes. Effective maintenance dose for continuous and stepwise dosing is 50 to 200 mcg/kg/min, although doses as low as 25 mcg/kg/min have been adequate. Doses greater than 200 mcg/kg/min provide little additional lowering of heart rate, and the rate of adverse reactions increases. Maintenance infusions may be continued for up to 48 hours. See Precautions/Monitor.

Intraoperative and postoperative tachycardia and/or hypertension: *Immediate control:* 1 mg/kg over 30 seconds. Follow with an infusion of 150 mcg/kg/min (0.15 mg/kg/min) if necessary. Adjust as required to maintain desired HR and/or BP.

Gradual control: Use procedure listed for SVT.

Immediate and gradual control: Higher doses (250 to 300 mcg/kg/min [0.25 to 0.3 mg/kg/min]) may be required to control hypertension. Maintenance infusion doses greater than 200 mcg/kg/min are not recommended for the treatment of tachycardia. They provide little additional lowering of heart rate, and the rate of adverse reactions increases.

Transition to alternative drugs: After control of HR and BP is achieved and clinical status is stable,

1. Administer the first dose of the alternative drug. In 30 minutes, reduce the esmolol infusion rate by one-half (50%).
2. After administration of the second dose of the alternative drug, monitor patient response carefully. If control is satisfactory and is maintained for 1 hour, discontinue the esmolol infusion.

PEDIATRIC DOSE

See Maternal/Child.

Antiarrhythmic (unlabeled): *Pediatric patients 1 to 12 years of age:* A loading dose of 100 to 500 mcg/kg (0.1 to 0.5 mg/kg) administered over 1 minute. Follow with a maintenance infusion of 25 to 100 mcg/kg/min (0.025 to 0.1 mg/kg/min). Titrate doses upward to response by 50 to 100 mcg/kg/min (0.05 to 0.1 mg/kg/min) at 5- to 10-minute intervals as needed. Dose requirements may be higher than in adults. Doses as high as 1,000 mcg/kg/min have been administered to pediatric patients 1 to 12 years of age.

Antihypertensive (postoperative [unlabeled]): *Pediatric patients 1 to 12 years of age:* A loading dose of 500 mcg/kg (0.5 mg/kg) administered over 1 minute. Follow with a maintenance infusion of 50 to 250 mcg/kg/min (0.05 to 0.25 mg/kg/min). Titrate doses upward 50 to 100 mcg/kg/min (0.05 to 0.1 mg/kg/min) as needed. Titrate to individual desired response. Dose requirements may be higher than in adults. Doses as high as 1,000 mcg/kg/min have been administered to pediatric patients 1 to 12 years of age.

DOSE ADJUSTMENTS
Reduced dose may be required in impaired renal function. No dose adjustment required if the maintenance infusion does not exceed 150 mcg/kg/min for more than 4 hours; no data available for higher doses or longer duration. ▪ No dose adjustment indicated in impaired hepatic function. ▪ Reduction required with transfer to alternate agent; see Monitor. ▪ See Drug/Lab Interactions.

DILUTION
Available premixed as 10 mg/mL in 100 mL NS or as 20 mg/mL in 100 mL NS (double strength). Single-dose vials are available as 100 mg/10 mL and may be given by IV injection without further dilution or may be further diluted in D5W, D5R, D5LR, D5NS, D5/½NS, NS, LR, ½NS, or D5W with KCl 40 mEq/L. Premixed solutions have a delivery port and a medication port (for withdrawing the initial bolus only). Ready-to-use vials may be used to administer initial and subsequent boluses.

Storage: Store vials and premix at CRT; protect from freezing and avoid excessive heat. Diluted solution stable at room temperature for 24 hours. If a bolus has been removed from the premixed bag, the bag should be used within 24 hours.

COMPATIBILITY
Manufacturer lists as **incompatible** with sodium bicarbonate and furosemide and states, "Do not add any additional medications to the bag" (premixed injection).

Other sources suggest specific **compatibilities** dependent on concentration and manufacturer; consult a pharmacist.

RATE OF ADMINISTRATION
IV injection: See Usual Dose.

Infusion: Titrate infusion according to procedure outlined in Usual Dose.

ACTIONS
A short-acting, B_1-selective adrenergic blocking agent with antiarrhythmic effects. Decreases HR and BP in a dose-related titratable manner. Hemodynamically similar to propranolol, but vascular resistance is not increased. Onset of action occurs within 1 to 2 minutes. Half-life is approximately 9 minutes, and the effects last about 20 to 30 minutes. Metabolized via esterases in RBCs and excreted in urine.

INDICATIONS AND USES
Management of supraventricular tachycardia (atrial fibrillation or atrial flutter) in situations requiring short-term control of ventricular rate with a short-acting agent (perioperative, postoperative, or other emergent circumstances). ▪ Management of noncompensatory tachycardia when HR requires specific intervention. ▪ Management of intraoperative and postoperative tachycardia and/or hypertension.

Limitation of use: Intended only for short-term use.

CONTRAINDICATIONS
Cardiogenic shock. ▪ Decompensated heart failure. ▪ Heart block greater than first degree. ▪ Hypersensitivity reactions, including anaphylaxis, to esmolol or any of its inactive ingredients (cross-sensitivity between beta-blockers is possible). ▪ IV administration of cardiodepressant calcium-channel antagonists (e.g., verapamil) and esmolol in close proximity (i.e., while the cardiac effects of the other drug are still present). ▪ Pulmonary hypertension. ▪ Severe sinus bradycardia. ▪ Sick sinus syndrome.

PRECAUTIONS
For IV use only. ▪ May cause hypotension at any dose but is dose related; risk is increased in patients with hemodynamic compromise, in patients receiving interacting medications, and with doses above 200 mcg/kg/min. Severe reactions may include loss of consciousness, cardiac arrest, and death. ▪ Use caution in patients with first-degree AV block, sinus node dysfunction, or conduction disorders. May be at increased risk for bradycardia. Sinus pause, heart block, severe bradycardia, and cardiac arrest have

occurred. ■ May further depress cardiac contractility and precipitate heart failure and cardiogenic shock. ■ Use caution in patients whose BP is primarily driven by vasoconstriction associated with hypothermia (e.g., intraoperative and postoperative tachycardia and hypertension). ■ Use with extreme caution in patients with reactive airway disease (e.g., asthma), diabetes mellitus and/or hypoglycemia, Prinzmetal's angina, pheochromocytoma, hypovolemia, peripheral circulatory disorders (Raynaud's disease, peripheral occlusive vascular disease), coronary artery disease, impaired renal function, metabolic acidosis, and hyperthyroidism. ■ In general, patients with reactive airway disease (e.g., asthma) should not receive beta-blockers. Titrate to the lowest possible effective dose. ■ In patients with hypoglycemia or diabetes who are receiving insulin or hypoglycemic agents, beta-blockers may mask tachycardia of hypoglycemia, but other manifestations of hypoglycemia such as dizziness and sweating may still be observed. ■ May exacerbate angina attacks in patients with Prinzmetal's angina; do not use nonselective beta-blockers (e.g., propranolol). ■ A paradoxical increase in BP may occur if beta-blockers are administered to patients with pheochromocytoma. If use is necessary, administer an alpha-blocker (e.g., phentolamine) before the beta-blocker. ■ Can worsen reflex tachycardia and increase the risk of hypotension in hypovolemic patients. ■ May increase serum potassium levels, causing hyperkalemia. Risk is increased in patients with renal impairment and is potentially life threatening in hemodialysis patients. ■ Use caution in patients with metabolic acidosis; hyperkalemic renal tubular acidosis has been reported. ■ Beta-adrenergic blockade may mask the clinical signs of hyperthyroidism (e.g., tachycardia). Abrupt withdrawal may precipitate thyroid storm. ■ Patients at risk for hypersensitivity reactions may be more reactive to allergen exposure when receiving beta-blockers and may be unresponsive to the usual doses of epinephrine used to treat anaphylactic or anaphylactoid reactions; see Drug/Lab Interactions. ■ Infusion site reactions, including irritation, inflammation, and severe reactions (e.g., thrombophlebitis, necrosis, and blistering), have occurred; avoid infusion into small veins or through a butterfly catheter. ■ Although it has not been a problem with esmolol, it is recommended that the dose of beta-adrenergic blockers be reduced gradually to avoid rebound angina, MI, or ventricular arrhythmias. Use caution, especially in patients with coronary artery disease. ■ Intended for short-term use only. Transfer to an alternative antiarrhythmic agent (e.g., digoxin, verapamil) is required after stable clinical status and HR control are obtained; see Usual Dose. ■ See Drug/Lab Interactions, Monitor, and Antidote.

Monitor: Continuous observation of the patient and ECG and BP monitoring are mandatory during administration. Hypotension should reverse within 30 minutes after decreasing the infusion rate or discontinuing the drug. ■ Avoid infusion into small veins or through a butterfly catheter. Well tolerated if administered through a central vein. Monitor for infusion site reaction and prevent extravasation. Restart at an alternate infusion site. ■ Titrate BP slowly in patients whose BP is primarily driven by vasoconstriction associated with hypothermia (e.g., intraoperative and postoperative tachycardia and hypertension). ■ May mask symptoms of hypoglycemia; monitor blood glucose in patients with diabetes. ■ Monitor electrolytes as indicated. Monitor patients with increased risk factors very closely; see Precautions. ■ See Drug/Lab Interactions and Contraindications.

Maternal/Child: Category C: safety for use in pregnancy not established. Use only when clearly indicated. ■ Discontinue breast-feeding. ■ Safety and effectiveness for use in pediatric patients not established.

Elderly: Numbers in clinical studies are insufficient to determine if the elderly respond differently from younger subjects. Consider age-related organ impairment (e.g., bone marrow reserve, renal, hepatic); monitor and reduce dose if indicated.

DRUG/LAB INTERACTIONS

The effects of esmolol on BP, contractility, and impulse propagation can be increased with concomitant use of other drugs that can lower BP, reduce myocardial contractility, or interfere with sinus node function or electrical impulse propagation in the myocardium. May result in severe hypotension, cardiac failure, severe bradycardia, sinus pause, sinoatrial block, atrioventricular block, and/or cardiac arrest. ■ **Sympathomimetic drugs having beta-adrenergic agonist activity** (e.g., epinephrine, norepinephrine) will counteract the effects of esmolol. ■ Use with **calcium channel blockers** may potentiate both drugs and result in severe depression of myocardium and AV conduction, severe hypotension, and fatal cardiac arrest. ■ Increases **digoxin** blood levels, synergistic with digoxin; both drugs slow AV conduction. Concomitant use increases the risk of bradycardia. ■ Esmolol should not be used in patients receiving **vasoconstrictive or inotropic drugs** (e.g., norepinephrine, digoxin) because of the potential for reduced cardiac contractility when the systemic vascular resistance is high. ■ Concomitant use with certain **antihypertensive agents** (e.g., clonidine, guanfacine) may precipitate increased withdrawal effects (withdrawal rebound hypertension). If antihypertensive therapy is to be interrupted or discontinued, discontinue the beta-blocker first and then gradually discontinue the antihypertensive agent. ■ Concomitant use with **catecholamine-depleting drugs** (e.g., reserpine) may produce additive effects. Monitor for hypotension and bradycardia. ■ May prolong neuromuscular blockade produced by **succinylcholine** and moderately prolong neuromuscular blockade produced by **mivacurium**. ■ May mask S/S of developing hypoglycemia in patients on **insulin or oral antidiabetic agents.** ■ Concurrent use with **xanthines** (e.g., aminophylline, theophyllines) may result in mutual inhibition of therapeutic effects. ■ Patients taking **beta-blockers** who are exposed to a potential allergen may be unresponsive to the usual dose of epinephrine used to treat a hypersensitivity reaction.

SIDE EFFECTS

Symptomatic hypotension (dizziness, excessive sweating) and asymptomatic hypotension are most common. Inflammation or induration of the infusion site, nausea, and somnolence are also fairly common. Abdominal discomfort, abnormal thinking, agitation, anxiety, confusional state, constipation, convulsions (with one death), depression, dry mouth, dyspepsia, flushing, headache, light-headedness, pallor, paresthesia, peripheral ischemia, speech disorders, syncope, urinary retention, and vomiting have occurred. **Overdose:** Cardiac effects (e.g., atrioventricular block [first-, second-, third-degree], bradycardia, cardiac failure [including cardiogenic shock], cardiac arrest/asystole, decreased cardiac contractility, hypotension, intraventricular conduction delays, junctional rhythms, and pulseless electrical activity); CNS effects (e.g., fatigue, lethargy, respiratory depression, seizures, sleep and mood disturbances, and coma). In addition, bronchospasm, hyperkalemia, hypoglycemia (especially in children), mesenteric ischemia, and peripheral cyanosis may occur. **Post-Marketing:** Angioedema, cardiac arrest, coronary arteriospasm, psoriasis, urticaria.

ANTIDOTE

Notify the physician of all side effects. Decrease rate or discontinue drug if hypotension occurs. Hypotension should reverse within 30 minutes. Trendelenburg position may be appropriate. May require treatment with IV fluids or vasopressors (e.g., dopamine, norepinephrine [Levophed]), but protracted severe hypotension may result. Unresponsive hypotension and bradycardia may be reversed by glucagon 5 to 10 mg over 30 seconds followed by a continuous infusion of 5 mg/hr. Reduce rate as condition improves. Decrease rate of or discontinue esmolol if severe bradycardia develops. Treat with an anticholinergic drug (e.g., atropine) or cardiac pacing. Discontinue esmolol at the first S/S of cardiac failure and start supportive treatment (e.g., digoxin and diuretics). In shock resulting from inadequate cardiac contractility, consider IV dobutamine or dopamine. Glucagon may be useful. Discontinue the infusion if bronchospasm occurs. Administer a beta$_2$-stimulating agent (e.g., epinephrine, albuterol) and/or a theophylline derivative and monitor ventricular rate. Treat other side effects symptomatically and resuscitate as necessary.

ESOMEPRAZOLE SODIUM
(es-oh-**MEP**-rah-zohl **SO**-dee-um)

Proton pump inhibitor (PPI)
(gastric acid inhibitor)
Substituted benzimidazole

Nexium IV

pH 9 to 11

USUAL DOSE
Gastroesophageal reflux disease (GERD) with erosive esophagitis: Given as an alternative to oral therapy. Resume oral therapy as soon as practical. Safety and efficacy of IV use for more than 10 days not established. Dose and serum levels similar by IV or oral route.
Adults: 20 or 40 mg as an IV injection or infusion once daily for up to 10 days.
Risk reduction of rebleeding gastric or duodenal ulcers following therapeutic endoscopy in adults: 80 mg as an IV infusion over 30 minutes followed by a continuous infusion of 8 mg/hr for 71.5 hours (a total treatment duration of 72 hours). Therapy is for management of the acute initial bleeding of gastric or duodenal ulcers and does not constitute full treatment. Follow with oral acid-suppressive therapy.

PEDIATRIC DOSE
GERD with erosive esophagitis: Administered as an infusion over 10 to 30 minutes. See comments under Usual Dose.
1 to 17 years of age: WEIGHT LESS THAN 55 KG: 10 mg. WEIGHT 55 KG OR MORE: 20 mg.
1 month to less than 1 year of age: 0.5 mg/kg.

DOSE ADJUSTMENTS
GERD with erosive esophagitis: No dose adjustment is required based on age or gender, in the elderly, in patients with renal insufficiency, or in patients with mild to moderate liver impairment (Child-Pugh Classes A and B). ■ Do not exceed a dose of 20 mg in patients with severe liver impairment (Child-Pugh Class C [10 or over]).
Risk reduction of rebleeding gastric or duodenal ulcers following therapeutic endoscopy in adults: No adjustment of the initial 80-mg dose is required. Reduce the continuous infusion rate to a maximum of 6 mg/hr for patients with mild to moderate liver impairment (Child-Pugh Classes A and B) and to a maximum of 4 mg/hr for patients with severe liver impairment (Child-Pugh Class C). Do not exceed these maximum doses.

DILUTION
GERD with erosive esophagitis:
Injection (adults): Each 40-mg vial must be reconstituted with 5 mL of NS. Mix gently until powder is dissolved.
Infusion (adult and pediatric patients 1 month to less than 1 year of age): To determine the dose needed for patients 1 month to less than 1 year of age, first calculate the dose (0.5 mg/kg). Reconstitute a 40-mg vial with 5 mL of NS, D5W, or LR. Further dilute to a final volume of 50 mL with NS. Withdraw desired dose to administer as an infusion.
40-MG VIAL: Concentration is 0.8 mg/mL; withdraw 25 mL for a 20-mg dose and 12.5 mL for a 10-mg dose. Adjust infusion amount as needed to provide the correct dose (0.5 mg/kg) for pediatric patients 1 month to less than 1 year of age.
Risk reduction of rebleeding gastric or duodenal ulcers following therapeutic endoscopy in adults:
30-minute infusion: Two 40-mg vials required for the 80-mg dose. Reconstitute each 40-mg vial with 5 mL of NS and add contents of both vials to 100 mL of NS.
Continuous infusion: Two 40-mg vials required. Reconstitute each 40-mg vial with 5 mL of NS and add contents of both vials to 100 mL of NS. Administer at a rate of 8 mg/hr for 71.5 hours; see Dose Adjustments.
Filters: Not required or recommended; no additional data available from manufacturer.
Storage: Before use, store in carton at CRT and protect from light. Reconstituted and diluted solutions may be stored at CRT. Administer reconstituted solutions within

12 hours of reconstitution. Administer diluted solutions within 6 hours if diluted in D5W and within 12 hours if diluted in NS or LR. Discard any unused solution.

COMPATIBILITY
Manufacturer states, "Should not be administered concomitantly with any other medications through the same IV site and/or tubing." Flush the IV line with a **compatible** IV solution (NS, LR, or D5W) before and after administration of esomeprazole.

RATE OF ADMINISTRATION
Flush the IV line with a **compatible** IV solution (NS, LR, or D5W) before and after administration of esomeprazole.
GERD with erosive esophagitis: *Injection (adults):* A single 20- or 40-mg dose evenly distributed over no less than 3 minutes.
Infusion (adults and pediatric patients): A single dose properly diluted as an infusion and evenly distributed over 10 to 30 minutes.
Risk reduction for rebleeding of gastric or duodenal ulcers following therapeutic endoscopy in adults: *Initial dose:* A single 80-mg dose evenly distributed over 30 minutes.
Continuous infusion: Administer at a rate of 8 mg/hr over 71.5 hours; see Dose Adjustments.

ACTIONS
A proton pump inhibitor. It suppresses gastric acid secretion by specific inhibition of the H^+/K^+-ATPase in the gastric parietal cell. It blocks the final step in acid production, thus reducing gastric acidity. Effect is dose-related. Highly bound to serum protein. Extensively metabolized in the liver by the cytochrome P_{450} isoenzyme system (CYP2C19 and CYP3A4 isoenzymes). Half-life is 1.1 to 1.4 hours and is prolonged with increasing doses. Primarily excreted as metabolites in urine with some excretion in feces. Secreted in breast milk.

INDICATIONS AND USES
Short-term treatment of GERD with erosive esophagitis in adults and pediatric patients 1 month to 17 years of age. Used as an alternative to oral therapy when oral esomeprazole is not possible or appropriate. ▪ Risk reduction for rebleeding in patients following therapeutic endoscopy for acute bleeding gastric or duodenal ulcers in adults.

CONTRAINDICATIONS
Known hypersensitivity to esomeprazole (Nexium) or other substituted benzimidazoles (e.g., omeprazole [Prilosec], pantoprazole [Protonix]) or to any component of the formulation. ▪ Contraindicated in patients receiving rilpivirine-containing products (e.g., systemic rilpivirine, emtricitabine/rilpivirine).

PRECAUTIONS
For IV use only; do not give IM or SC. ▪ Discontinue as soon as the patient is able to resume oral therapy. ▪ Gastric malignancy may be present even though patient's symptoms improve. Consider additional follow-up and diagnostic testing in adult patients who have a suboptimal response or an early symptomatic relapse after completing treatment with a PPI. In older patients, also consider an endoscopy. ▪ Decreased gastric acidity may increase bacterial count in GI tract. Risk of GI infections (e.g., *Salmonella* and *Campylobacter*) may be slightly increased. ▪ May be associated with an increased risk of *Clostridium difficile*–associated diarrhea (CDAD), especially in hospitalized patients. Consider in patients who develop diarrhea that does not improve. ▪ May be associated with an increased risk for osteoporosis-related fractures of the hip, wrist, or spine. Risk increased in patients receiving high-dose (multiple daily doses) and long-term therapy (a year or longer). Use lowest dose and shortest duration of therapy appropriate for the condition being treated. ▪ Cutaneous lupus erythematosus (CLE) and systemic lupus erythematosus (SLE) have been reported in patients taking PPIs. These events have occurred as both new onset and as an exacerbation of existing autoimmune disease. Subacute CLE is more common and occurs weeks to years after continuous PPI therapy in patients ranging from infants to the elderly. In general, histologic findings were observed without organ involvement. PPI-induced systemic lupus erythematosus (SLE) is usually milder than non–drug-induced SLE and occurs days to years after initiating PPI

therapy, primarily in patients ranging from young adults to the elderly. Most patients present with rash, but arthralgia and cytopenia have also been reported. Discontinue esomeprazole if S/S of CLE or SLE develop, and refer patient to the appropriate specialist. Most patients improve within 4 to 12 weeks of PPI discontinuation. ▪ Hypomagnesemia, both symptomatic and asymptomatic, has been reported rarely (usually with the use of PPIs for 3 months to more than a year). Arrhythmias, seizures, and tetany have occurred. Magnesium replacement and discontinuation of esomeprazole may be required. ▪ Patients should use the lowest dose and shortest duration of PPI therapy appropriate for the condition being treated. ▪ Acute interstitial nephritis has been observed. Is generally attributed to an idiopathic hypersensitivity reaction and may occur at any time during therapy. Discontinue esomeprazole if it occurs. ▪ PPI use is associated with an increased risk of fundic gland polyps that increases with long-term use, especially beyond 1 year. Most patients were asymptomatic and polyps were identified incidentally on endoscopy. ▪ To avoid complications, use the shortest duration of PPI therapy appropriate to the condition being treated. ▪ See Drug/Lab Interactions.

Monitor: Observe for S/S of a hypersensitivity reaction (e.g., anaphylaxis, anaphylactic shock, angioedema, bronchospasm, acute interstitial nephritis, urticaria). ▪ Monitor vital signs, pain levels, and injection site. ▪ Consider obtaining baseline and periodic magnesium levels if prolonged therapy is indicated or in patients taking digoxin or medications that may cause hypomagnesemia (e.g., diuretics). ▪ Serologic testing (e.g., antinuclear antibody [ANA] titers) may be indicated in patients who present with S/S of CLE or SLE.

Patient Education: Review prescription and nonprescription drugs with physician. ▪ Oral route preferred. ▪ Promptly report cardiovascular or neurologic symptoms, including dizziness, palpitations, seizures, or tetany; may be signs of hypomagnesemia.

Maternal/Child: Use during pregnancy only if the potential benefit justifies the potential risk to the fetus. ▪ Esomeprazole may be secreted in human milk; use with caution during breast-feeding. ▪ Safety and effectiveness for use of IV formulation for short-term treatment of GERD with erosive esophagitis in pediatric patients established for ages 1 month to 17 years. Safety and effectiveness for use in neonates (0 to 1 month of age) not established.

Elderly: Safety and effectiveness similar to that seen in younger adults. ▪ Consider potential for impaired liver function; see Dose Adjustments.

DRUG/LAB INTERACTIONS

Extensively metabolized by CYP2C19 and CYP3A4. ▪ Because of profound and long-lasting inhibition of gastric acid secretion, esomeprazole may interfere with the absorption of drugs in which gastric pH is an important determinant of their bioavailability. Absorption of **atazanavir, erlotinib, iron salts, ketoconazole,** and **mycophenolate mofetil** can decrease; other drugs (e.g., digoxin) can increase. Monitor digoxin concentrations and adjust the dose, if needed, to maintain therapeutic drug concentrations. ▪ Avoid concurrent use with **clopidogrel**; esomeprazole may interfere with the conversion of clopidogrel into its active form and decrease its effectiveness. ▪ Exposure of **citalopram** is increased, leading to an increased risk of QT prolongation. Limit the dose of citalopram to a maximum of 20 mg/day. Coadministration of **mycophenolate mofetil** and **omeprazole** in transplant patients receiving MMF reduces the exposure to MMF's active metabolite, mycophenolic acid; see Precautions. ▪ Increases in INR and PT have been reported when administered concurrently with **warfarin;** monitoring of INR and PT indicated. ▪ Concurrent use with **selected protease inhibitors** such as atazanavir and nelfinavir is not recommended. Coadministration of proton pump inhibitors results in a significant reduction in plasma concentrations of atazanavir and nelfinavir, thus inhibiting their antiviral therapeutic effect and promoting the development of drug resistance. In contrast, elevated plasma concentrations have been reported with **other protease inhibitors** (e.g., saquinavir); dose reduction of saquinavir should be considered. Unchanged serum levels have been reported with some other antiretroviral drugs. ▪ The metabolism of **diazepam** may be decreased and serum levels increased by esomeprazole; not considered clinically significant. ▪ Administration with a **combined inhibitor of CYP2C19**

and CYP3A4 (e.g., voriconazole) may more than double the exposure (concentration) of esomeprazole. With recommended doses of esomeprazole, a dose adjustment is not normally required; however, it may be indicated in patients who require higher doses. ▪ Concurrent administration of **oral contraceptives, diazepam, phenytoin, or quinidine** did not change the pharmacokinetic profile of esomeprazole. ▪ Drugs that **induce CYP2C19 or CYP3A4** (e.g., rifampin, St. John's wort) can substantially decrease esomeprazole concentrations. Avoid concomitant use. ▪ Concomitant administration of esomeprazole and **tacrolimus** may increase serum levels of tacrolimus. Monitoring of serum levels may be indicated. ▪ Studies suggest no clinically significant interactions with other drugs metabolized by the cytochrome P_{450} system (e.g., amoxicillin, clarithromycin, phenytoin, quinidine). ▪ Coadministration with **cilostazol** may increase concentrations of cilostazol and its metabolite. Consider a dose reduction of cilostazol from 100 mg to 50 mg twice daily. ▪ Concomitant use of proton pump inhibitors with high-dose **methotrexate** may elevate and prolong serum levels of methotrexate and/or its metabolite. May lead to methotrexate toxicity; consider withdrawal of esomeprazole. ▪ Serum chromogranin A (CgA) levels increase secondary to drug-induced decreases in gastric acidity. Increased CgA levels may cause a false-positive result in diagnostic tests for neuroendocrine tumors. Temporarily discontinue esomeprazole at least 14 days before assessing CgA levels, and consider repeating the test (using the same commercial laboratory) if the initial CgA level is high.

SIDE EFFECTS
Generally well tolerated. The most commonly reported side effects include abdominal pain, constipation, diarrhea, dizziness/vertigo, dry mouth, flatulence, headache, injection site pain or reaction (including erythema, phlebitis, superficial phlebitis, swelling, and thrombophlebitis), nausea, and pruritus. Cough, duodenal ulcer hemorrhage, and fever were also reported. Numerous other side effects may occur in fewer than 1% of patients.
Post-Marketing: Aggression, agitation, agranulocytosis, alopecia, anaphylaxis (rare), blurred vision, bone fracture, bronchospasm, CDAD, CLE, depression, GI candidiasis, gynecomastia, hallucinations, hepatic encephalopathy, hepatic failure, hepatitis with or without jaundice (rare), hyperhidrosis, hypomagnesemia with or without hypocalcemia and/or hypokalemia, interstitial nephritis, microscopic colitis, muscular weakness, myalgia, pancreatitis, pancytopenia, serious dermatologic reactions (including erythema multiforme, photosensitivity, Stevens-Johnson syndrome, and toxic epidermal necrolysis [some fatal]), shock, SLE, stomatitis, and taste disturbance.
Overdose: Ataxia, changes in respiratory frequency, decreased motor activity, intermittent clonic convulsions, tremor.

ANTIDOTE
Keep physician informed of all side effects. May be treated symptomatically. If hypomagnesemia develops, magnesium replacement and discontinuation of esomeprazole may be required. Discontinue esomeprazole if acute interstitial nephritis, CLE, or SLE occurs. Discontinue and initiate appropriate treatment if hypersensitivity reactions, S/S associated with post-marketing reports, or overdose occurs; see Side Effects. Not removed by hemodialysis.

ETEPLIRSEN
(e-**TEP**-lir-sen)

Antisense oligonucleotide

Exondys 51

pH 7.5

USUAL DOSE
Pretreatment: Pretesting indicated; see Monitor.

Eteplirsen: 30 mg/kg administered once weekly as a 35- to 60-minute IV infusion. If a dose of eteplirsen is missed, it may be administered as soon as possible after the scheduled time. Consider application of a topical anesthetic cream to the infusion site before administration of eteplirsen.

PEDIATRIC DOSE
See Usual Dose.

DOSE ADJUSTMENTS
Eteplirsen has not been studied in patients with renal or hepatic impairment. Dosing recommendations in these patient populations have not been provided by the manufacturer.

DILUTION
Available as a 100 mg/2 mL and 500 mg/10 mL (50 mg/mL) solution in a single-dose vial. Calculate the total dose of eteplirsen administered based on the patient's weight. Determine the volume of eteplirsen needed and the correct number of vials to supply the calculated dose. Allow vials to warm to RT. Mix the contents of each vial by gently inverting the vial 2 or 3 times. **Do not shake**. Visually inspect each vial. Eteplirsen is a clear, colorless solution that may have some opalescence. Do not use if the solution is discolored or if particulate matter is present. Withdraw the calculated volume of eteplirsen from the appropriate number of vials using a syringe fitted with a 21-gauge or smaller noncoring needle. Dilute the withdrawn eteplirsen in NS to make a total volume of 100 to 150 mL. For example, a 70-kg patient would require 2,100 mg (30 mg/kg $\times$ 70 kg = 2,100 mg). 2,100 mg $\div$ 50 mg/mL = 42 mL. Warm four 500 mg/10 mL vials and one 100 mg/2 mL vial to RT and further dilute in 100 mL of NS.

Storage: Store unopened vials in original carton at 2° to 8° C (36° to 46° F). Protect from light. Do not freeze. Immediate use preferred. Complete infusion of diluted solution within 4 hours of dilution. If immediate use is not possible, the diluted solution may be stored for up to 24 hours at 2° to 8° C (36° to 46° F). Discard unused eteplirsen.

COMPATIBILITY
Manufacturer states, "Do not mix other medications with eteplirsen or infuse other medications concomitantly via the same intravenous access line."

RATE OF ADMINISTRATION
A single dose as an infusion equally distributed over 35 to 60 minutes. Flush the intravenous access line with NS before and after the eteplirsen infusion. If a hypersensitivity reaction occurs, consider slowing the infusion or interrupting the eteplirsen therapy.

ACTIONS
Duchenne's muscular dystrophy (DMD) is a rare progressive disease characterized by the virtual absence of functional dystrophin, a protein essential for maintaining muscle cell membrane integrity. Eteplirsen is an antisense oligonucleotide of the phosphorodiamidate morpholino oligomer (PMO) subclass. PMOs are synthetic molecules in which the five-membered ribofuranosyl rings found in natural DNA and RNA are replaced by a six-membered morpholino ring. Eteplirsen is designed to bind to exon 51 of dystrophin pre-mRNA, resulting in exclusion of this exon during mRNA processing in patients with genetic mutations that are amenable to exon 51 skipping. Exon skipping is intended to allow for production of an internally truncated but functional dystrophin protein. The peak plasma concentration of eteplirsen occurs near the end of infusions following single or multiple IV infusions. Plasma protein binding is low. Eteplirsen does not appear to be metabolized by hepatic microsomes. Renal clearance of eteplirsen accounts for

approximately two-thirds of the administered dose within 24 hours of IV administration. The elimination half-life of eteplirsen is 3 to 4 hours.

INDICATIONS AND USES

Treatment of Duchenne's muscular dystrophy (DMD) in patients who have confirmed mutation of the DMD gene that is amenable to exon 51 skipping. ▪ This indication is approved under accelerated approval based on an increase in dystrophin in skeletal muscle observed in some patients treated with eteplirsen. A clinical benefit of eteplirsen has not been established. Continued approval for this indication may be contingent on verification of a clinical benefit in confirmatory trials.

CONTRAINDICATIONS

Manufacturer states, "None."

PRECAUTIONS

Hypersensitivity reactions have occurred.

Monitor: Confirmation of mutation of the DMD gene that is amenable to exon 51 skipping indicated. ▪ Monitor for S/S of any adverse reactions; treat as indicated. ▪ Monitor for S/S of a hypersensitivity reaction (bronchospasm, cough, dyspnea, flushing, hypotension, rash, and urticaria).

Patient Education: Report any S/S of a hypersensitivity reaction (e.g., itching, rash, wheezing) and/or changes in balance.

Maternal/Child: Eteplirsen has not been studied in females. There are no human or animal data available to assess eteplirsen during pregnancy. ▪ There are no human or animal data available to assess the effect of eteplirsen on milk production, the presence in milk, or the effects of eteplirsen on the breast-fed infant. ▪ DMD is largely a disease of children and young adults. Approved indication includes use in pediatric patients.

Elderly: DMD is largely a disease of children and young adults; therefore there is no geriatric experience with eteplirsen.

DRUG/LAB INTERACTIONS

Based on in vitro data on plasma protein binding, CYP or drug transporter interactions, and microsomal metabolism, eteplirsen is expected to have a low potential for drug-drug interactions in humans.

SIDE EFFECTS

The most common adverse reactions were balance disorder and vomiting. Other adverse reactions (reported in 10% or more of patients) were arthralgia, catheter site pain, contact dermatitis, contusion, excoriation, rash, and upper respiratory tract infection. Hypersensitivity reactions have also occurred.

ANTIDOTE

Notify physician of any side effects; treat as indicated. If a hypersensitivity reaction occurs, based on severity, institute appropriate medical treatment and/or consider slowing the infusion or interrupting the eteplirsen therapy. There is no experience with overdose of eteplirsen.

ETOMIDATE
(eh-**TOM**-ih-dayt)

Amidate

Anesthetic, general
Anesthesia adjunct

pH 4 to 7

USUAL DOSE
Rapid sequence intubation and/or induction of anesthesia: Dose must be individualized. 0.3 mg/kg IV (range: 0.2 to 0.6 mg/kg). Titrate to effect. Smaller, incremental doses may be administered to adult patients during short operative procedures to supplement subpotent anesthetic agents, such as nitrous oxide.

Procedural sedation: 0.1 to 0.2 mg/kg has been used effectively. Subsequent doses of 0.05 mg/kg every 3 to 5 minutes may be administered as needed. If analgesia is required, concurrent administration of fentanyl may be used.

PEDIATRIC DOSE
Rapid sequence intubation and/or induction of anesthesia: *Pediatric patients up to 10 years of age:* Safety and effectiveness have not been established.
Pediatric patients 10 years of age and older: See Usual Dose.
Procedural sedation (unlabeled): 0.1 to 0.3 mg/kg. Repeat doses may be needed based on the length of the procedure. If analgesia is required, concurrent administration of fentanyl may be used.

DOSE ADJUSTMENTS
Dose must be individualized for each patient. ▪ Caution and lower-end dosing suggested in the elderly; consider decreased organ function and concomitant disease or drug therapy. ▪ See Drug/Lab Interactions.

DILUTION
May be given undiluted. Solution must be clear.
Filters: No data available from manufacturer.
Storage: Store at CRT. Discard unused portion.

COMPATIBILITY
Compatibility information not available from manufacturer. Other sources suggest a few specific **compatibilities** dependent on concentration and manufacturer; consult a pharmacist.

RATE OF ADMINISTRATION
A single dose equally distributed over 30 to 60 seconds. More-rapid injections may produce hypotension.

ACTIONS
A short-acting, nonbarbiturate general anesthetic without analgesic activity. Does not cause significant cardiovascular or respiratory depression. Has little or no effect on myocardial metabolism, cardiac output, peripheral circulation, or pulmonary circulation. Produces a slight increase in $Paco_2$. Does not elevate plasma histamine or cause signs of histamine release. Decreases cerebral blood flow and lowers intracranial pressure. Usually lowers intraocular pressure moderately. Onset of action is within 1 minute. Duration of action is dose dependent, usually 3 to 5 minutes at a dose of 0.3 mg/kg. Metabolized in the liver and excreted primarily in the urine. Half-life is approximately 75 minutes.

INDICATIONS AND USES
Induction of general anesthesia. Usefulness of hemodynamic properties should be weighed against the high frequency of transient skeletal muscle movements. ▪ Supplementation of subpotent anesthetic agents (e.g., nitrous oxide in oxygen) during maintenance of anesthesia for short operative procedures such as dilation and curettage or cervical conization.
Unlabeled uses: Procedural sedation, rapid sequence intubation (RSI).

CONTRAINDICATIONS
Hypersensitivity to etomidate. ▪ Not recommended for use during labor and delivery.

PRECAUTIONS

For IV use only. ■ Should be administered by or under the direct supervision of persons trained in the administration of general anesthetics and in the management of complications encountered during general anesthesia (e.g., anesthesiologists, emergency department physicians) in a facility with adequate diagnostic and treatment facilities to monitor the patient and respond to any medical emergency. ■ Induction doses of etomidate have been associated with the reduction of plasma cortisol and aldosterone concentrations that may last for 6 to 8 hours. Because of the hazards of prolonged suppression, etomidate is not intended for administration by prolonged infusion. Exogenous replacement (e.g., methylprednisolone) should be considered if concern exists for patients undergoing severe stress or for patients receiving chronic oral corticosteroid therapy (e.g., prednisone). **Monitor:** Monitor airway and vital signs. ■ Monitor injection site. Use of larger, more proximal arm veins is recommended to lessen incidence and severity of pain on injection. Avoid use of wrist or hand veins if possible. ■ See Precautions and Drug/Lab Interactions. **Patient Education:** Avoid alcohol or other CNS depressants (e.g., antihistamines, benzodiazepines) for 24 hours following administration. ■ Do not perform tasks requiring mental alertness (e.g., driving, operating hazardous machinery) for 24 hours following administration. ■ Discuss with parents or caregivers the risks, benefits, timing, and duration of surgery or procedures requiring anesthetic and sedation drugs; see Maternal/Child.
Maternal/Child: Safety for use in pregnancy not established; benefit must justify potential risks to fetus; see Contraindications. ■ Safety for use during breast-feeding not established; effects unknown. Use caution. ■ Safety and effectiveness for use in pediatric patients under 10 years of age not established. ■ Published studies suggest that repeated or prolonged exposures to anesthetic agents in utero (third trimester) and early in life (up to 3 years of age) may have negative effects on the developing brain, resulting in adverse cognitive or behavioral effects; see prescribing information for further discussion. Balance the benefits of appropriate anesthesia in pregnant women, neonates, and young children who require procedures with the potential risks described.
Elderly: See Dose Adjustments. ■ May be more sensitive to effects. Administration in elderly patients, particularly in those with hypertension, may induce cardiac depression as evidenced by a decrease in heart rate, cardiac index, and mean arterial BP.

DRUG/LAB INTERACTIONS

Administration of **fentanyl** 0.1 mg before induction with etomidate may shorten the immediate recovery period and decrease the incidence of disturbing skeletal muscle movements. ■ May have additive effects with concomitant **anesthetics, sedatives, hypnotics, and/or opiates** (e.g., fentanyl); reduced doses of etomidate may be indicated. ■ Does not significantly alter the usual dosage requirements of **neuromuscular blocking agents** (e.g., vecuronium, rocuronium).

SIDE EFFECTS

The most common adverse reactions are transient venous pain on injection and transient skeletal muscle movements, including myoclonus, averting movements, and eye movements. Less frequently reported side effects include apnea of short duration (5 to 90 seconds with spontaneous recovery), arrhythmia, bradycardia, hiccups and/or snoring (may indicate partial airway obstruction), hypertension, hyperventilation, hypotension, hypoventilation, laryngospasm, postoperative nausea and vomiting, and tachycardia.

ANTIDOTE

Discontinue drug if significant side effects or overdose occur. Support patient. Establish and maintain an airway; administer oxygen with assisted ventilation if needed. Resuscitate as necessary.

ETOPOSIDE BBW
(eh-**TOH**-poh-syd)

Antineoplastic
(topoisomerase inhibitor)

Etopophos PF, Etoposide Phosphate, VP-16-213

pH 2.9 to 4

USUAL DOSE
Pretreatment: Verify pregnancy status. Baseline studies indicated; see Monitor.
Testicular cancer: 50 to 100 mg/M^2 daily for 5 days or 100 mg/M^2/day on Days 1, 3, and 5. Repeat at 3- to 4-week intervals. Used in combination with other chemotherapy agents.
Small-cell lung cancer: 35 mg/M^2/day for 4 days to 50 mg/M^2/day for 5 days. Repeat at 3- to 4-week intervals. Used in combination with other chemotherapy agents.

DOSE ADJUSTMENTS
Modify dose if indicated based on myelosuppressive effects of other drugs administered in combination and any previous radiation therapy or chemotherapy (compromised bone marrow reserve). Frequently given in combination with cisplatin, bleomycin, and doxorubicin. ▪ Withhold dose if platelets less than 50,000/mm^3 or absolute neutrophil count less than 500/mm^3. Do not restart until adequate recovery. ▪ Dose selection should be cautious in the elderly. ▪ Reduce dose by 25% if CrCl is 15 to 50 mL/min. Further reduction may be indicated if the CrCl is less than 15 mL/min. One source recommends decreasing dose by 50% if CrCl is less than 10 mL/min. ▪ Dose reduction may be required in impaired hepatic function. One source recommends a dose reduction of 50% with a bilirubin of 1.5 to 3 or an AST greater than 3 times the ULN. Use in severe hepatic impairment is contraindicated in the Canadian product labeling.

DILUTION
Specific techniques required; see Precautions.
NONPHOSPHATE PRODUCTS (E.G., VEPESID): Each 100 mg (5 mL) must be diluted in at least 250 mL of D5W or NS and given as an infusion (0.4 mg/mL). 500 mL of solution will yield 0.2 mg/mL. Maximum concentration to prevent precipitation is 0.4 mg/mL. Monitor closely for precipitation from dilution to completion of infusion. Undiluted etoposide has caused acrylic or ABS plastic devices to crack and leak; handle carefully during dilution process.
PHOSPHATE PRODUCT (E.G., ETOPOPHOS): Reconstitute each 100-mg vial with 5 or 10 mL of SWFI, D5W, or NS (with or without benzyl alcohol). 5 mL of diluent will yield 20 mg/mL, 10 mL will yield 10 mg/mL. Further dilute to concentrations as low as 0.1 mg/mL with D5W or NS for administration. A 1-mg/mL solution has a pH of 2.9.
Storage: *Nonphosphate Products (e.g., VePesid):* May be stored at CRT before dilution. Stable after dilution at CRT for 96 hours (0.2 mg/mL solution) or 24 hours (0.4 mg/mL) in D5W or NS. *Phosphate Products (e.g., Etopophos):* Refrigerate in carton until use to protect from light. Store reconstituted solutions under refrigeration at 2° to 8° C (36° to 46° F) for 7 days. Solutions reconstituted with nonbacteriostatic diluents may be stored at CRT for up to 24 hours. Solutions reconstituted with bacteriostatic diluents may be stored at CRT for up to 48 hours. Store fully diluted solutions under refrigeration or at CRT for up to 24 hours.

COMPATIBILITY
NONPHOSPHATE PRODUCTS (E.G., VEPESID)
Hydrolysis may occur in alkaline solutions.
    Other sources suggest specific **compatibilities** dependent on concentration and manufacturer; consult a pharmacist.
PHOSPHATE PRODUCTS (E.G., ETOPOPHOS)
Other sources suggest specific **compatibilities** dependent on concentration and manufacturer; consult a pharmacist.

RATE OF ADMINISTRATION

NONPHOSPHATE PRODUCTS (E.G., VEPESID): Total desired dose, properly diluted (0.2 to 0.4 mg/mL) and evenly distributed over at least 30 to 60 minutes. Rapid infusion may cause marked hypotension. May be extended if fluid volume is a concern.

PHOSPHATE PRODUCTS (E.G., ETOPOPHOS): Total desired dose, properly reconstituted and diluted, may be given evenly distributed over as little as 5 minutes or up to 3.5 hours. Do not give as a bolus injection.

ACTIONS

A semi-synthetic derivative of podophyllotoxin. A topoisomerase II inhibitor that is cell cycle–specific for the G_2 phase. Appears to cause DNA strand breaks. Etopophos (phosphate) is a phosphate ester of etoposide that promptly converts to etoposide in plasma. The pharmacokinetics and pharmacodynamics of etoposide are similar after administration of either the phosphate or non-phosphate products. Half-life is from 4 to 11 hours (average is 7 hours). Bound to human plasma proteins, primarily albumin. Metabolized in the liver. Primarily excreted as unchanged drug or metabolites through urine and bile (feces).

INDICATIONS AND USES

Treatment of refractory testicular tumors (used in combination with other chemotherapeutic drugs). ▪ Treatment of small-cell lung cancer (used in combination with cisplatin as first-line treatment).

Unlabeled uses: Conditioning regimen for hematopoietic cell transplantation. Treatment of acute lymphocytic leukemias (ALL), Hodgkin lymphoma, non-Hodgkin lymphomas, carcinoma of the breast, neuroblastoma, Wilms' tumor, and many malignancies. Used alone or in combination with other agents.

CONTRAINDICATIONS

Hypersensitivity to etoposide, etoposide phosphate, or any other component of the formulations.

PRECAUTIONS

Follow guidelines for handling cytotoxic agents. See Appendix A, p. 1308. Always wear impervious gloves when handling vials containing etoposide. If a solution of etoposide contacts the skin, wash the skin immediately and thoroughly with soap and water. If there is contact with mucous membranes, flush thoroughly with water. ▪ For IV infusion only; do not give as a bolus injection. ▪ Usually administered by or under the direction of the physician specialist. ▪ Severe myelosuppression with resulting infection or bleeding may occur. Deaths have been reported. ▪ A low serum albumin may result in an increase of free (active) etoposide, resulting in an increased risk of toxicity. Occurs more frequently in pediatric patients. ▪ Hypersensitivity reactions have been reported. Higher-than-recommended concentration, the presence of polysorbate 80, and a rapid rate of infusion may contribute to the development of these reactions. ▪ Secondary leukemias have occurred with long-term use. ▪ Use with caution in hepatic or renal impairment; see Dose Adjustments. ▪ Oral dose of nonphosphate product (e.g., etoposide) is usually twice the IV dose.

Monitor: Determine absolute patency and quality of vein and adequate circulation of extremity. Avoid extravasation; may result in cellulitis, pain, swelling, and necrosis, including skin necrosis. ▪ Obtain baseline CBC with differential and platelets. Monitor before each dose and between courses. See Dose Adjustments. ▪ Monitor vital signs during infusion. ▪ Examine patient's mouth for ulceration before each dose. ▪ Monitor hepatic and renal function before and during therapy. ▪ Bone marrow recovery from a course is usually complete within 21 days. No cumulative toxicity has been reported as yet. ▪ Be alert for signs of bone marrow suppression or infection. ▪ Monitor for S/S of hypersensitivity reactions (e.g., bronchospasm, chills, dyspnea, fever, hypotension, pruritus, rash, tachycardia, urticaria). ▪ Monitor for thrombocytopenia (platelet count less than 50,000/mm^3). Initiate precautions to prevent excessive bleeding (e.g., inspect IV sites, skin, and mucous membranes; use extreme care during invasive procedures; test urine, emesis, stool, and secretions for occult blood). ▪ Prophylactic antibiotics may be indicated pending results of C/S in a febrile neutropenic patient. ▪ Maintain adequate hydration. ▪ Prophylactic antiemetics may increase patient comfort.

Patient Education: Female patients should use effective contraception during treatment and for at least 6 months after the final dose. Males with female sexual partners of reproductive potential should use condoms during treatment and for 4 months after the final dose. ▪ Notify provider of known or suspected pregnancy. ▪ Periodic monitoring of blood counts is required. ▪ Promptly report new onset of bleeding, fever, or S/S of infection. ▪ Report IV site burning or stinging promptly. ▪ Report chills, difficult breathing, fever, and rapid heartbeat promptly. See Appendix D, p. 1311.

Maternal/Child: Avoid pregnancy. Can cause fetal harm. ▪ May cause infertility. In male patients, may result in oligospermia, azoospermia, and permanent loss of fertility. May damage spermatozoa and testicular tissue, resulting in possible genetic fetal abnormalities. In female patients, may cause infertility and result in amenorrhea and premature menopause; see Patient Education. ▪ Discontinue breast-feeding. ▪ Has been used in pediatric patients, but safety and effectiveness not established. Higher rates of anaphylactic-like reactions have occurred in pediatric patients who have received infusions of etoposide at higher-than-recommended concentrations. See Precautions. ▪ Depending on the preparation, VePesid may contain benzyl alcohol or polysorbate 80.

Elderly: Numbers in clinical studies insufficient to determine if elderly patients respond differently than do younger subjects. ▪ Monitor renal, hepatic, and hematologic function closely. ▪ See Dose Adjustments.

DRUG/LAB INTERACTIONS

All products: Concurrent or consecutive use with other **bone marrow suppressants** (e.g., bleomycin, cisplatin, doxorubicin) **and/or radiation therapy** may produce additive bone marrow suppression. See Dose Adjustments. ▪ Antineoplastic activity of etoposide and **cisplatin** may be synergistic against some tumors. ▪ Do not administer **live virus vaccines** to patients receiving antineoplastic drugs. ▪ Clearance decreased and toxicity increased by **cyclosporine.** ▪ May potentiate **warfarin**; monitor PT/INR. ▪ Concomitant use of **antiepileptic medications**, including phenytoin, phenobarbital, carbamazepine, and valproic acid, may increase clearance and reduce efficacy of etoposide. ▪ Phenylbutazone, sodium salicylate, and aspirin-displaced protein-bound etoposide in vitro. ▪ May be a substrate of the P-glycoprotein (P-gp) transporter system based on in vitro studies.

PHOSPHATE PRODUCT (E.G., ETOPOPHOS): Use caution with drugs that are **known to inhibit phosphatase activities** (e.g., levamisole [Ergamisol]).

SIDE EFFECTS

Bone marrow toxicity (e.g., leukopenia, neutropenia, thrombocytopenia) can be severe, is dose related, and may be dose limiting. Side effects are usually reversible: abdominal pain, aftertaste, alopecia, anaphylactic-like reactions (bronchospasm, chills, diaphoresis, dyspnea, facial flushing, fever, hypertension or hypotension, pruritus, rash, tachycardia), anemia, anorexia, asthenia, back pain, constipation, coughing, cyanosis, diarrhea, dizziness, dysphagia, elevated liver function tests (e.g., AST, ALT), facial/tongue swelling, hepatic toxicity, hypertension, hypotension, interstitial pneumonitis/pulmonary fibrosis, laryngospasm, local soft tissue toxicity following extravasation, malaise, mucositis, nausea, neuritic pain, optic neuritis, paralytic ileus, peripheral neurotoxicity, pigmentation, radiation recall dermatitis, seizures, Stevens-Johnson syndrome, stomatitis, taste alteration, thrombophlebitis, toxic epidermal necrolysis, transient cortical blindness, urticaria, vomiting. Hepatic toxicity and metabolic acidosis have occurred with higher-than-recommended doses.

Post-Marketing: Acute renal failure and extravasation.

Overdose: No antidote has been established for overdose. In animal studies, overdosage may result in neurotoxicity.

ANTIDOTE

Notify the physician of all side effects; symptomatic treatment is often indicated, and dose reduction or discontinuation may be necessary. For extravasation, discontinue the drug immediately and administer into another vein. No specific treatment for extravasation is recommended. Hypotension is usually due to a rapid infusion rate. Discontinue infusion. Trendelenburg position and IV fluids should reverse the hypotension; vasopressors (e.g., dopamine) may be required. After recovery, restart at slower rate. Administration of whole blood products (e.g., packed RBCs, platelets, leukocytes) and/or blood modifiers (e.g., darbepoetin alfa, epoetin alfa, filgrastim, pegfilgrastim, sargramostim) may be indicated to treat bone marrow toxicity. Discontinue infusion at the first sign of a hypersensitivity reaction; antihistamines, corticosteroids, pressor agents, or volume expanders may be indicated. Permanently discontinue in patients who experience a severe hypersensitivity reaction. Resuscitate as necessary.

FACTOR IX (HUMAN) ▪ FACTOR IX COMPLEX (HUMAN)

Antihemorrhagic

(**FAK**-tor **NINE**)

AlphaNine SD ▪ **Bebulin VH, Profilnine SD**

pH 7 to 7.4 ▪

USUAL DOSE

(International units [units])

ALL FORMULATIONS

Completely individualized based on patient's circumstances, condition, degree of deficiency, and desired blood level percentage. Specific products may be indicated or preferred in some situations; see Indications and Uses. Range is 10 to 75 International units (units)/kg of body weight. May be repeated every 12 hours in some situations, required only every 2 or 3 days in others. Actual number of International units contained shown on each bottle or vial. Units required to raise blood level percentages can be calculated as follows:

$$\text{Body weight (kg)} \times \text{Desired increase (\% of normal)} \times 1 \text{ Unit/kg}$$

(70 kg × 40% increase × 1 units/kg = 2,800 units). To maintain levels above 25%, calculate each dose to raise level to 40% to 60% of normal.

Minor hemorrhage: A single injection calculated to increase plasma level to 20% to 30%. May be repeated in 24 hours if indicated.

Major trauma or surgery: Increase plasma level to 25% to 50% and maintain at that level for a minimum of 1 week or as indicated. May require daily injections (every 18 to 30 hours).

Dental extraction: Increase plasma level to 50% before procedure; repeat if indicated.

Prophylaxis: 10 to 20 units/kg once or twice a week or increase plasma level to 20% to 30%.

FACTOR IX COMPLEX

Reversal of coumarin effect: 15 units/kg.

DILUTION

Diluent usually provided. Some preparations also supply double-ended needles for dilution and filter needle for aspiration into a syringe. Sterile technique imperative. Confirm expiration date. Use plastic syringes to prevent binding to glass surfaces. Factor IX and diluent should be at room temperature. Direct diluent from above to side of vial to gently moisten all contents. Swirl gently to dissolve; avoid foaming. Do not shake. May take 1 to 5 minutes. Should be clear and colorless. Must be used within 3 hours to avoid bacterial contamination. The addition of 2 to 3 units of heparin/mL factor IX complex may reduce the incidence of thrombosis. May be given through an IV administration set (often provided) if multiple vials are required. Discard any unused contents. Discard all administration equipment after single use; do not attempt to resterilize.

AlphaNine SD: Follow general directions above. After diluent is drawn through double-ended needle, remove diluent bottle first; then remove double-ended needle. *Do not invert concentrate vial until ready to withdraw contents!* Air from syringe into vial required to withdraw contents. Withdraw through filter.

Mononine: Follow general directions listed previously. After diluent is drawn through double-ended needle, remove diluent bottle first; then remove double-ended needle. *Use only the provided self-venting filter spike to transfer Mononine to a syringe! Do not inject any air into Mononine vial; could cause product loss.* Discard filter and use only provided wing needle and micropore tubing to administer.

Filters: Usually supplied by manufacturer. If more than one vial is required for a dose, multiple vials may be drawn into the same syringe; however, a new filter needle must be used to withdraw the contents of each vial of factor IX and/or factor IX complex (Human). Manufacturers of *AlphaNine SD* and *Mononine* provide a filter needle, which is to be used to withdraw reconstituted solution into a syringe. Discard filter needle after aspiration into the syringe. No further filtering is required for administration.

Storage: Store lyophilized powder at 2° to 8° C (36° to 46° F); do not freeze. Do not refrigerate after dilution. *Mononine* may be stored at room temperature before dilution for up to 30 days.

COMPATIBILITY

Compatibility information not available from manufacturer; consult a pharmacist.

RATE OF ADMINISTRATION

Average rate is 2 to 3 mL or 100 units/min. Completely individualized according to patient's condition. Decrease rate of administration for side effects such as burning or pain at injection site, chills, fever, flushing, headache, tingling, or changes in BP or pulse. Never exceed 10 mL/min.

ACTIONS

A lyophilized concentrate of human coagulation factors: IX (plasma thromboplastin and antihemophilic factor B), II (prothrombin), VII (proconvertin), and X (Stuart-Prower factor). In contrast to other products, AlphaNine SD and Mononine are highly purified factor IX and contain only minimal amounts of the other factors. All products are obtained from fresh human plasma and prepared, irradiated, and dried by specific processes. Additional processes are used to prepare AlphaNine SD and Mononine that markedly reduce the possibility of viral contamination. Concentration of 25 units/mL is 25 times greater than normal plasma. Preparations contain varying amounts of total protein in each vial. Half-life is approximately 24 hours (range 18 to 36 hours).

INDICATIONS AND USES

All factor IX products: Prevention/control of bleeding in patients with factor IX deficiency due to hemophilia B. Indicated to correct or prevent a dangerous bleeding episode or to perform surgery. ▪ Prophylaxis to prevent spontaneous bleeding in patients with proven specific congenital deficiency (hemophilia B).

Factor IX (human): Preferred for surgical coverage; treatment of crush injuries and/or large IM hemorrhages requiring several days of replacement therapy; and treatment in neonates, individuals with severe hepatocellular dysfunction, or those with a history of thrombotic complications associated with factor IX complex.

Factor IX complex: Prevention/control of bleeding in patients with hemophilia A who have inhibitors to factor VIII. ▪ Reversal of coumarin effect (fresh frozen plasma preferred unless risk of hepatitis transfer would be life threatening). ▪ Hemorrhage caused by hepatitis-induced lack of production of liver-dependent coagulation factors. ▪ Proplex T is used for prevention or control of bleeding episodes in patients with factor VII deficiency.

CONTRAINDICATIONS
Factor IX complex: Known liver disease with suspicion of intravascular coagulation or fibrinolysis. ▪ Factor VII deficiency except for Proplex T.
Mononine: Known hypersensitivity to mouse protein. ▪ No other known contraindications for **AlphaNine SD** or **Bebulin VH.** ▪ **AlphaNine SD, Bebulin VH,** and **Mononine** are not indicated for replacement of any other coagulation factors.

PRECAUTIONS
Used when plasma infusions would result in hypervolemia and/or proteinemia or when blood volume or RBC replacement is not indicated. ▪ Use extreme caution in newborns, infants, postoperative patients, and patients with liver disease. Factor IX (human) (e.g., AlphaNine SD, Mononine) would be preferred because studies show no incidence of thrombin generation. ▪ Fresh frozen plasma may be required in addition to factor IX complex when prompt reversal is required. ▪ Danger of thromboembolic episodes (DIC, myocardial infarction, pulmonary embolism, venous thrombosis) increases with plasma levels over 50%. ▪ Large or frequently repeated doses of factor IX complex may cause intravascular hemolysis in patients with type A, B, or AB blood.
Monitor: Monitor the patient's levels of coagulation factors before, after, and between administrations. ***Do not overdose;*** see Side Effects. ▪ AIDS or hepatitis is possible for the recipient. Health care professionals should exercise caution in handling. Possibility markedly reduced with additional preparation process of AlphaNine SD and Mononine. ▪ Observe for signs and symptoms of postoperative thrombosis or disseminated intravascular coagulation (DIC). Risk multiplies with repeated administrations except for AlphaNine, AlphaNine SD, and Mononine.
Patient Education: Alert to possible risk of HIV virus and hepatitis. ▪ Report early signs of hypersensitivity promptly (burning or pain along injection site, hives, rash, tightness of chest, wheezing). ▪ Notify physician if medication seems less effective. May be developing antibodies to factor IX. ▪ Carry identification card. ▪ Proper preparation and administration imperative if given in home.
Maternal/Child: Category C: safety for use during pregnancy not established; use only if clearly indicated; see Precautions. ▪ Use extreme caution in neonates with hepatitis; high rate of morbidity.

DRUG/LAB INTERACTIONS
Concurrent use of **aminocaproic acid** may increase risk of thrombosis.

SIDE EFFECTS
Burning or pain along injection site, changes in BP, chills, fever, flushing, headache, nausea, tingling, urticaria, vomiting.
Major: Anaphylaxis, DIC, hepatitis, myocardial infarction, postoperative thrombosis (rare with pure factor IX [Human] products), pulmonary embolism. Consider risk potential of contracting AIDS and hepatitis; markedly reduced with pure factor IX (Human) products (AlphaNine, AlphaNine SD, and Mononine).

ANTIDOTE
Temporarily discontinue or decrease rate of administration for minor side effects. For major symptoms, discontinue, and notify physician. Treat hypersensitivity reactions as indicated; a different lot may not cause reaction. For thrombosis or DIC, anticoagulation with heparin may be indicated.

FACTOR IX (RECOMBINANT)

Antihemorrhagic

(**FAK**-tor **NINE** [re-**KOM**-be-nant])

Alprolix, BeneFIX, IDELVION, IXINITY, RIXUBIS

USUAL DOSE

(International units [units])

Available recombinant factor IX products include:

Alprolix (recombinant): A coagulation factor IX Fc fusion protein consisting of the human coagulation factor IX sequence covalently linked to the Fc domain of human immunoglobulin G_1 (IgG_1). Does not contain proteins derived from animal or human sources.

BeneFIX (recombinant), IXINITY (recombinant), RIXUBIS (recombinant): Coagulation factor IX proteins produced by a genetically engineered mammalian cell line derived from Chinese hamster ovary (CHO) cells. No human or animal proteins are added during any stage of manufacturing.

IDELVION (recombinant): A coagulation factor IX, albumin fusion protein (rIX-FP) comprising genetically fused recombinant coagulation factor IX and recombinant albumin. Does not contain proteins derived from animal or human sources.

Adults and pediatric patients: Completely individualized based on the degree of deficiency, the location and extent of bleeding, the patient's clinical condition and age, and the pharmacokinetic parameters of factor IX, such as incremental recovery and half-life. Base dose and frequency on individual clinical response. Units required to raise blood level percentages are somewhat increased with recombinant products compared with other factor IX products and can be calculated using the following formulas:

Number of factor IX units required = Body weight (in kg) × Desired factor IX increase (% of normal or units/dL) × Reciprocal of observed recovery (units/kg per units/dL)

The observed recovery for the various products is as follows:

Alprolix: One unit of recombinant product/kg of body weight increases the circulating level of factor IX by 1% (units/dL).

BeneFIX: One unit of recombinant product/kg of body weight increases the circulating level of factor IX by 0.8% (units/dL) for adults and by 0.7% (units/dL) in pediatric patients under 15 years of age.

IDELVION: One unit of recombinant product/kg of body weight is expected to increase the circulating level of factor IX by 1.3% (units/dL) in patients 12 years of age or older and by 1% (units/dL) in pediatric patients under 12 years of age.

IXINITY: One unit of recombinant product/kg of body weight increases the circulating level of factor IX by 0.98% (units/dL).

RIXUBIS: One unit of recombinant product/kg of body weight increases the circulating level of factor IX by 0.9% (units/dL) for patients 12 years of age or older and by 0.7% (units/dL) in pediatric patients under 12 years of age.

In the presence of an inhibitor, higher doses may be required. See examples of dose calculation in prescribing information.

The following chart may be used to guide dosing in the prevention of bleeding episodes.

Factor IX (Recombinant) Dosing Guidelines for Prevention and Control of Bleeding in Adults and Pediatric Patients			
Type of Bleeding Episodes	**Circulating Factor IX Activity Required (% of normal or units/dL)**	**Dosing Interval (hours)**	**Duration of Therapy (days)**
Minor Uncomplicated or early bleeds: hemarthroses, superficial muscle (except iliopsoas) with no neurovascular compromise, other soft tissue, or oral bleeding	**Alprolix** 30 to 60	48 hours	Repeat every 48 hours if there is further evidence of bleeding
	BeneFIX 20 to 30	12 to 24 hours	1 to 2 days
	IDELVION[a] 30 to 60	48 to 72 hours	At least 1 day until bleeding stops and healing is achieved A single dose should be sufficient for the majority of bleeds
	IXINITY 30 to 60	24 hours	1 to 3 days until healing is achieved
	RIXUBIS 20 to 30	12 to 24 hours	At least 1 day until healing is achieved
Moderate Intramuscular or soft tissue with dissection, mucous membranes, dental extractions, hematuria, hemarthrosis of longer duration, recurrent hemarthrosis, deep lacerations	**Alprolix** 30 to 60	48 hours	Repeat every 48 hours if there is further evidence of bleeding
	BeneFIX and RIXUBIS 25 to 50	12 to 24 hours	Treat until bleeding stops and healing begins, about 2 to 7 days
	IDELVION[a] 30 to 60	48 to 72 hours	At least 1 day until bleeding stops and healing is achieved A single dose should be sufficient for the majority of bleeds
	IXINITY 40 to 60	24 hours	2 to 7 days until healing is achieved
Major Life-threatening or limb-threatening hemorrhage, iliopsoas and deep muscle with neurovascular injury or substantial blood loss, pharyngeal, retropharyngeal, retroperitoneal, CNS	**Alprolix** 80 to 100	Consider a repeat dose after 6 to 10 hours and then every 24 hours for the first 3 days	Due to the long half-life of Alprolix, the dose may be reduced and frequency may be extended after Day 3 to every 48 hours or longer until bleeding stops and healing is achieved
	BeneFIX and RIXUBIS 50 to 100	12 to 24 hours	7 to 10 days until bleeding stops and healing is achieved
	IDELVION[a] 60 to 100	48 to 72 hours	7 to 14 days until bleeding stops and healing is achieved Maintenance dose weekly
	IXINITY 60 to 100	12 to 24 hours	2 to 14 days until healing is achieved

Units, International units.
[a]Adapted from the WFH Guidelines for the Management of Hemophilia.
Source: Roberts and Eberst and Srivastava et al. 2013.

Dosing for perioperative management is provided in the following chart.

Factor IX (Recombinant) Dosing for Perioperative Management in Adults and Pediatric Patients			
Type of Surgery	**Circulating Factor IX Level Required (% or units/dL)**	**Dosing Interval (hours)**	**Duration of Therapy (days)**
Minor (e.g., tooth extraction)	**Alprolix** 50 to 80	A single infusion may be sufficient	Repeat as needed after 24 to 48 hours until bleeding stops and healing is achieved
	BeneFIX 20 to 30	12 to 24 hours	1 to 2 days until bleeding stops and healing is achieved
	IDELVION[a] 50 to 80	48 to 72 hours	At least 1 day or until healing is achieved. A single dose should be sufficient for the majority of minor surgeries
	IXINITY **Preoperative:** 50 to 80 **Postoperative:** 30 to 80	24 hours	1 to 5 days depending on type of procedure
	RIXUBIS 30 to 60	24 hours	At least 1 day until healing is achieved
Major (e.g., intracranial, intra-abdominal, intrathoracic, joint replacement, pharyngeal, retropharyngeal, retroperitoneal)	**Alprolix** 60 to 100 (initial level)	Consider a repeat dose after 6 to 10 hours and then every 24 hours for the first 3 days	Due to the long half-life of Alprolix, the dose may be reduced and frequency in the postsurgical setting may be extended after Day 3 to every 48 hours or longer until bleeding stops and healing is achieved
	BeneFIX 50 to 100	12 to 24 hours	7 to 10 days until bleeding stops and healing is achieved
	IDELVION[a] 60 to 100 (initial level)	48 to 72 hours	7 to 14 days or until bleeding stops and healing is achieved. Repeat dose every 48 to 72 hours for the first week or until healing is achieved. Maintenance dose 1 to 2 times per week
	IXINITY **Preoperative:** 60 to 80 **Postoperative:** 40 to 60 **Postoperative:** 30 to 50 **Postoperative:** 20 to 40	8 to 24 hours	1 to 3 days 4 to 6 days 7 to 14 days
	RIXUBIS 80 to 100	8 to 24 hours	7 to 10 days until bleeding stops and healing is achieved

[a]Adapted from the WFH Guidelines for the Management of Hemophilia.

Routine prophylaxis dosing is as follows:

Alprolix dosing for routine prophylaxis in adults and pediatric patients: Routine starting regimens are either 50 units/kg once weekly or 100 units/kg once every 10 days. Adjust dose based on patient response.

IDELVION dosing for routine prophylaxis in patients 12 years of age or older: Recommended dose is 25 to 40 units/kg every 7 days. Patients who are well-controlled on this regimen may be switched to a 14-day interval at 50 to 75 units/kg.

IDELVION dosing for routine prophylaxis in pediatric patients under 12 years of age: Recommended dose is 40 to 55 units/kg every 7 days.

RIXUBIS dosing for routine prophylaxis in adults: Dose for previously treated patients is 40 to 60 units/kg twice weekly for patients 12 years of age and older and 60 to 80 units/

kg twice weekly for patients under 12 years of age. Dose titration may be necessary based on individual patient's age, bleeding pattern, and physical activity.

DOSE ADJUSTMENTS

Adjust dose and frequency of repeated infusions by using factor IX activity and pharmacokinetic parameters such as half-life and incremental recovery, as well as by taking the clinical situation into consideration. ▪ Patients at the lower end of the observed factor IX recovery range may require upward dose adjustment; see Monitor. ▪ Dose adjustment may be necessary in pediatric patients under 12 years of age; see Maternal/Child.

DILUTION   (International units [units])

Actual number of International units (units) contained is shown on each bottle or vial. **Alprolix** is supplied in a kit that includes single-use vials containing 500, 1,000, 2,000, or 3,000 units/vial. **BeneFIX** is supplied in a kit that includes single-use vials containing 250, 500, 1,000, 2,000, or 3,000 units/vial. **IDELVION** is available in a kit that includes single-use vials containing 250, 500, 1,000, or 2,000 units/vial. **IXINITY** is available in single-use vials containing 500, 1,000, or 1,500 units/vial. **RIXUBIS** is available in single-use vials containing 250, 500, 1,000, 2,000, or 3,000 units/vial. Sterile technique imperative. Confirm expiration date. Plastic syringes may be indicated to prevent binding to glass surfaces. Factor IX and diluent should be at room temperature. Provided diluent, dilution, and transfer equipment are specific to each product; consult manufacturer's detailed preparation and reconstitution process in prescribing information. When diluted, solution should be clear and colorless. (**IDELVION** may be yellow to colorless.) Multiple vials may be drawn in the same larger syringe per manufacturer's specific directions. Most products must be used within 3 hours of reconstitution. **IDELVION** must be used within 4 hours of reconstitution.

Filters: Supplied by manufacturer if indicated. If more than one vial is required for a dose, multiple vials may be drawn into the same syringe; see Dilution.

Storage: *Alprolix:* Refrigerate kit at 2° to 8° C (36° to 46° F). Store in original package and protect from light. *Do not refrigerate after reconstitution.*

BeneFIX: If product is labeled for RT storage, it may be stored at CRT or refrigerated at 2° to 8° C (36° to 46° F). If product is labeled for refrigeration, store at 2° to 8° C (36° to 46° F).

IDELVION: Store in original carton to protect from light in the refrigerator or at RT (2° to 25° C [36° to 77° F]). Do not freeze. *Do not refrigerate after reconstitution.*

IXINITY: Store at 2° to 25° C (36° to 77° F) in original carton to protect from light. *Do not refrigerate after reconstitution.*

RIXUBIS: Refrigerate at 2° to 8° C (36° to 46° F) for up to 24 months.

All products: Avoid freezing. Do not use after the expiration date. Discard unused product.

All products except IDELVION: Must be used within 3 hours of reconstitution. **IDELVION** must be used within 4 hours of reconstitution. **Alprolix, BeneFIX,** and **RIXUBIS** may be stored at room temperature not exceeding 30° C (86° F) for up to 6 months (12 months for RIXUBIS) before expiration (mark date removed from refrigerator on carton). Do not return to the refrigerator.

COMPATIBILITY

Alprolix, IXINITY: Manufacturer states, "Do not administer in the same tubing or container with other medications."

BeneFIX: Do not administer in the same tubing or container with other medicinal products. Do not allow blood to enter the syringe; if red blood cell agglutination is observed, discard everything and start over with new product and supplies.

IDELVION: Manufacturer states, "Do not mix or administer in the same tubing or container with other medicinal products."

RIXUBIS: Specific information not available. Consider specific use; consult pharmacist and note **compatibility** under BeneFIX.

RATE OF ADMINISTRATION

Alprolix, IDELVION, IXINITY, RIXUBIS: Administer as an IV bolus infusion. Rate of administration should be determined by patient's comfort level and no faster than 10 mL/min.

BeneFIX: Administer over a period of several minutes. Adapt to the comfort level of each individual patient.

All products: Record the name and batch number of the product in the patient record.

ACTIONS

An antihemorrhagic. A purified protein produced by recombinant DNA technology for use in the treatment of factor IX deficiency. Its primary amino acid sequence is identical to a form of plasma-derived factor IX, and it has structural and functional characteristics similar to those of endogenous factor IX. Inherently free from the risk of transmission of human bloodborne pathogens such as HIV, hepatitis viruses, and parvovirus. Factor IX is the specific clotting factor deficient in patients with hemophilia B and in patients with acquired factor IX deficiencies. Factor IX (recombinant) increases plasma levels of factor IX and can temporarily correct the coagulation defect in these patients, restoring hemostasis. Normalizes aPTT. Average half-life of *Alprolix* is 86 hours. Half-life of *BeneFIX* ranges from 11 to 36 hours. The fusion of the recombinant coagulation factor IX with recombinant albumin extends the half-life of factor IX with *IDELVION*. The half-life of *IDELVION* ranges from 104 to 118 hours in adults and from 87 to 93 hours in pediatric patients under 18 years of age (depending on dose). *IXINITY* half-life ranges from 17 to 31 hours. *RIXUBIS* half-life ranges from 16 to 42 hours.

INDICATIONS AND USES

All Products: Control and prevention of bleeding episodes in adult and pediatric patients with hemophilia B (congenital factor IX deficiency or Christmas disease). ▪ Perioperative management in adult and pediatric patients with hemophilia B. **IXINITY** use is limited to patients 12 years of age or older.

Alprolix, IDELVION, RIXUBIS: Routine prophylaxis to prevent or reduce the frequency of bleeding episodes in adults and pediatric patients with hemophilia B.

Limitations of use: *All Products:* Not indicated for induction of immune tolerance in patients with hemophilia B; see Precautions.

BeneFIX: Not indicated for treatment of other factor deficiencies (e.g., factors II, VII, VIII, and X), hemophilia A patients with inhibitors to factor VIII, reversal of coumarin-induced anticoagulation, or bleeding due to low levels of liver-dependent coagulation factors.

CONTRAINDICATIONS

Alprolix: Known history of hypersensitivity reactions (including anaphylaxis) to the product or its excipients.

BeneFIX, IDELVION, IXINITY, RIXUBIS: Known history of hypersensitivity to the products or their excipients, including hamster protein.

RIXUBIS: Disseminated intravascular coagulation (DIC) and/or signs of fibrinolysis.

PRECAUTIONS

All Products: For IV bolus infusion only; see Rate of Administration. Safety and effectiveness of continuous infusion have not been established. ▪ Usually administered under the supervision of a physician experienced in the treatment of hemophilia B. ▪ Hypersensitivity reactions, including anaphylaxis, have been reported. Risk may be highest during the early phases of initial exposure in previously untreated patients. An association between the occurrence of factor IX inhibitor and allergic reactions has been reported. ▪ Thromboembolic episodes (e.g., disseminated intravascular coagulation [DIC], myocardial infarction, pulmonary embolism, arterial or venous thrombosis) have been reported with factor IX concentrates. Most have been reported in patients receiving factor IX complex concentrates or factor IX via continuous infusions. ▪ Because of potential thromboembolic problems, use caution in patients with liver disease, patients with signs of fibrinolysis, patients in the perioperative or postoperative period, neonates, or patients at risk for thromboembolic phenomena or DIC. Benefit must be weighed against risk. ▪ Factor IX inhibitors may develop; see Monitor. ▪ Nephrotic syndrome has been reported following attempted immune tolerance induction in hemophilia B patients with factor IX inhibitors. Safety for use in immune tolerance induction not established.

Monitor: *All Products:* To ensure desired factor IX activity levels are achieved and maintained, precise monitoring using the one-stage factor IX activity assay is recommended, especially during surgical intervention. Adjust dose and frequency as required. *Do not overdose;* see Side Effects. ▪ Monitor vital signs. ▪ Monitor for S/S of hypersensitivity reaction (e.g., angioedema, chest pain, dizziness, dyspnea, fever, flushing, hypotension, nausea, pruritus, rash, rigors, urticaria, wheezing). ▪ Monitor for early signs of thrombotic events and consumptive coagulopathy; see Precautions. ▪ Monitor for development of factor IX inhibitors. Failure to attain the expected factor IX activity plasma levels or to control bleeding with an appropriate dose may indicate development of factor IX inhibitors. Assays used to determine if factor IX inhibitor is present should be titered in Bethesda units (BUs). ▪ Patients dosed with high-purity factor IX products who develop inhibitors are at increased risk for anaphylaxis with repeat doses. Evaluate patients who experience a hypersensitivity reaction for the presence of an inhibitor.

Patient Education: *All Products:* Read manufacturer-supplied patient product information. ▪ Hypersensitivity reactions can occur. Promptly report difficulty breathing, hives, itching, tightness of the chest, and/or wheezing. If self-administering, discontinue use and contact physician immediately. ▪ Contact provider for lack of clinical response. May indicate development of inhibitors.

Maternal/Child: *All Products:* Use during pregnancy only if clearly indicated and/or the potential benefit justifies the potential risk. ▪ Use caution during breast-feeding. ▪ Pediatric patients may have higher factor IX body weight–adjusted clearance, shorter half-life, and lower recovery. Higher dose per kilogram of body weight or more frequent dosing may be needed. ▪ Safety and effectiveness of IXINITY for use in pediatric patients under 12 years of age not established.

Elderly: *All Products:* Numbers in clinical studies insufficient to determine whether the elderly respond differently than do younger subjects.

DRUG/LAB INTERACTIONS

Specific information not available. Factor IX activity measurements in the clinical lab may be affected by the type of activated partial thromboplastin time (aPTT) reagent or laboratory standard used.

SIDE EFFECTS

Alprolix: Headache and oral paresthesia were most common. Breath odor, dizziness, dysgeusia, fatigue, hypotension, infusion site pain, obstructive uropathy, and palpitations have been reported. No inhibitors were detected and no events of anaphylaxis were reported during clinical studies.

BeneFIX: Dizziness, headache, injection site pain, injection site reaction, nausea, and rash were most common. Blurred vision, cellulitis at IV site, chest tightness, drowsiness, dry cough, factor IX inhibition, fever, flushing, hives, hypoxia, phlebitis at IV site, renal infarct, shaking, taste perversion, and vomiting have been reported. Hypersensitivity reactions (including bronchospastic reactions and/or hypotension and anaphylaxis) and the development of high-titer inhibitors requiring alternate treatments to factor IX therapy are the most serious.

IDELVION: Most commonly reported reaction is headache. Dizziness, eczema, hypersensitivity reactions, and rash have been reported.

IXINITY: Most commonly reported reaction is headache. Apathy, asthenia, depression, dysgeusia, influenza, injection site discomfort, lethargy, and pruritic rash have been reported.

RIXUBIS: Dysgeusia, pain in extremity, and positive furin antibody test were most common during clinical studies.

All Products: Anaphylaxis, angioedema, dyspnea, hypotension, inadequate factor IX recovery, inhibitor development, and thrombosis may occur.

Post-Marketing: *BeneFIX:* Anaphylaxis, angioedema, dyspnea, hypotension, and thrombosis. *RIXUBIS:* Hypersensitivity (including dyspnea, pruritus), rash, and urticaria.

ANTIDOTE

Temporarily discontinue or decrease rate of administration for minor side effects. If any major symptoms appear, discontinue drug, notify physician, and consider alternative hemostatic measures. Treat hypersensitivity reactions as indicated. For thrombosis or DIC, anticoagulation with heparin may be indicated.

FACTOR XIII CONCENTRATE (HUMAN)

Antihemorrhagic

(**FAK**-tor **THIR**-teen **KON**-sen-trayt **HUE**-man)

Corifact

USUAL DOSE

Dose must be individualized based on body weight, laboratory values, and patient's clinical condition.

Initial dose in adult and pediatric patients: 40 units/kg.

Subsequent doses in adult and pediatric patients: Should be guided by the most recent trough factor XIII (coagulation factor XIII) activity level. Dose every 28 days (4 weeks) to maintain a trough factor XIII activity level of approximately 5% to 20%. Recommended dosing adjustments of ±5 units/kg should be based on trough factor XIII activity levels as shown in the chart in Dose Adjustments and on the patient's clinical condition.

DOSE ADJUSTMENTS

Guide dose adjustments based on a specific assay used to determine factor XIII levels (e.g., Berichrom Activity Assay).

Dose Adjustment of Factor XIII Concentrate Using the Berichrom Activity Assay	
Factor XIII Activity Trough Level (%)	**Dosage Change**
One trough level of <5%	Increase by 5 units/kg
Trough level of 5% to 20%	No change
Two trough levels of >20%	Decrease by 5 units/kg
One trough level of >25%	Decrease by 5 units/kg

DILUTION

Available as a single-use vial containing 1,000 to 1,600 units of factor XIII as a lyophilized concentrate. Actual units of potency stated on vial label. Sterile diluent and Mix2Vial filter transfer set provided. Sterile technique imperative. Confirm expiration date. Record the batch number of the product in the patient's medical record with each infusion. Bring factor XIII concentrate and diluent to RT. Place vial, diluent, and Mix2Vial transfer set on a flat surface. Remove flip caps on vial and diluent, and wipe stoppers with provided alcohol swab; allow to dry. Peel away the lid on the Mix2Vial transfer set, but leave it in the clear package. Hold the diluent vial tightly on a flat surface and pick up the Mix2Vial transfer set by its clear package. Push the plastic spike at the blue end of the Mix2Vial transfer set through the center of the diluent vial stopper. Carefully remove only the clear packaging from the transfer set. Invert the diluent vial with the Mix2Vial transfer set attached, and push the plastic spike of the transparent adapter firmly through the center of the factor XIII concentrate. Diluent will automatically transfer into the vial. With all parts still attached, gently swirl to fully dissolve. ***Do not shake.*** Solution should be colorless to slightly yellowish and slightly opalescent. Grasp the factor XIII side with one hand and the diluent side with the other and unscrew the set into 2 pieces. Draw air into an empty 20-mL sterile syringe. With the factor XIII vial upright, screw the syringe to the Mix2Vial transfer set. Inject air into the factor XIII vial. Keep the syringe plunger pressed, and invert the system upside down to draw the concentrate into the syringe by pulling the plunger back slowly. Keep the plunger facing down and remove syringe from transfer set. Attach the syringe to a suitable IV administration set. If the same patient is to receive more than one vial, contents of multiple vials may be pooled. Use a separate, unused Mix2Vial transfer set for each vial. Must be used within 4 hours of reconstitution.

Filters: Mix2Vial filter transfer set provided.

Storage: Protect from light; refrigerate vials and diluent in carton at 2° to 8° C (36° to 46° F). Do not freeze. Stable for 24 months up to the expiration date on the carton under refrigeration. May be stored at RT not to exceed 25° C (77° F) for up to 6 months; however, it cannot be returned to refrigeration. Mark date removed from refrigeration. Do not use beyond expiration date on carton and vial labels or beyond end of RT storage, whichever comes first. Must be used within 4 hours of reconstitution. Do not refrigerate or freeze the reconstituted solution. Contains no preservatives; a single-use vial; discard partially used vials.

COMPATIBILITY

Manufacturer states, "Do not mix with other medicinal products, and administer through a separate infusion line."

RATE OF ADMINISTRATION

Initial dose: Do not exceed 4 mL/min.

ACTIONS

A heat-treated, lyophilized factor XIII (coagulation factor XIII) concentrate made from pooled human plasma. Several manufacturing steps are used to inactivate or remove both enveloped and nonenveloped viruses. Factor XIII circulates in blood and is present in platelets, monocytes, and macrophages. Activated factor XIII (factor XIIIa) promotes cross-linking of fibrin during coagulation and is essential to the physiologic protection of the clot against fibrinolysis. Cross-linked fibrin is the end result of the coagulation cascade and provides tensile strength to a primary hemostatic platelet plug. Half-life is approximately 6.6 ± 2.29 days. The increase in plasma levels of factor XIII after administration lasts approximately 28 days.

INDICATIONS AND USES

Routine prophylactic treatment of congenital factor XIII deficiency in adult and pediatric patients. To be effective, a trough factor XIII activity level of approximately 5% to 20% should be maintained.

Limitation of use: There are no controlled trials demonstrating a direct benefit on treatment of bleeding episodes.

CONTRAINDICATIONS

Known anaphylactic or severe hypersensitivity reactions to human plasma–derived products or to any components of the product.

PRECAUTIONS

For IV use only. ▪ Hypersensitivity reactions have occurred; emergency equipment, medications, and supplies must be available. ▪ Neutralizing inhibitory antibodies against factor XIII have been detected in patients receiving factor XIII. ▪ Thromboembolic complications have been reported. Assess benefit versus risk in pregnant women because of their hypercoagulable state and potential for increased risk of thromboembolic events. ▪ Made from human plasma and may contain infectious agents (e.g., HIV, Creutzfeldt-Jakob disease, hepatitis B, or hepatitis C). Numerous steps in the manufacturing process are used to reduce the potential for infection. ▪ Consider appropriate vaccination against hepatitis A and B.

Monitor: Monitor trough factor XIII activity levels as outlined in Usual Dose and Dose Adjustments. ▪ Monitor for S/S of hypersensitivity reactions (e.g., chest pain, dizziness, dyspnea, fever, flushing, hypotension, nausea, pruritus, rash, rigors, urticaria). ▪ Monitor for possible development of inhibitory antibodies (e.g., response to treatment is inadequate, expected plasma factor XIII activity levels are not attained, or breakthrough bleeding occurs). ▪ Monitor for thromboembolic complications (e.g., chest pain, dyspnea, edema, hemoptysis, leg pain, or positive Homans' sign). ▪ Monitor for S/S of viral infection (e.g., chills, drowsiness, fever, runny nose followed by joint pain and rash or abdominal pain, dark urine, jaundice, nausea, vomiting).

Patient Education: Manufactured from pooled human plasma. Possibility of viral transmission exists. Promptly report S/S of viral infections (e.g., chills, drowsiness, fever, runny nose followed by joint pain and rash or abdominal pain, dark urine, jaundice, nausea, vomiting). ▪ Promptly report difficulty breathing, pruritus, or rash. ▪ Promptly report breakthrough bleeding.

Maternal/Child: Category C: use only if clearly needed; see Precautions. ▪ Use only if clearly needed in breast-feeding women. ▪ No apparent differences in the safety profile in pediatric patients compared with adults. Pediatric patients under 16 years of age had a shorter half-life and faster clearance compared with adults.

Elderly: Numbers in clinical studies insufficient to determine whether elderly patients respond differently than younger subjects.

DRUG/LAB INTERACTIONS
Specific information not available.

SIDE EFFECTS
The most commonly reported side effects included arthralgia, chills, elevated thrombin-antithrombin levels, fever, headache, hypersensitivity reactions (including allergy, erythema, pruritus, and rash), and increased hepatic enzymes. Other reported side effects included abdominal pain, diarrhea, epistaxis, flu-like syndrome, hematoma, URT infection, and vomiting.

Post-Marketing: Hypersensitivity reactions (including anaphylaxis), factor XIII inhibition (neutralizing antibodies), thrombotic events (e.g., embolism, thrombosis), viral infection (possible).

ANTIDOTE
Keep physician informed of side effects; most will be treated symptomatically. Discontinue administration and treat hypersensitivity reactions as indicated. A different lot may not cause a reaction. For thrombosis, anticoagulation may be indicated. Resuscitate as necessary.

FAMOTIDINE
(fah-**MOH**-tih-deen)

Antiulcer agent
(H₂ antagonist)
Gastric acid inhibitor

Famotidine PF, Pepcid   pH 5.7 to 6.4

USUAL DOSE
20 mg every 12 hours. Increase frequency of dose, not amount, if necessary for pain relief. In hypersecretory states (e.g., Zollinger-Ellison syndrome), higher doses may be required. Adjust dose to individual patient needs.

PEDIATRIC DOSE
Age 1 to 16 years: Starting dose is 0.25 mg/kg every 12 hours. Treatment duration and dose must be individualized based on clinical response, pH determination, and/or endoscopy. Doses up to 0.5 mg/kg every 12 hours may be required for gastric acid suppression. Another source suggests 0.6 to 0.8 mg/kg/24 hr (0.3 to 0.4 mg/kg every 12 hours or 0.2 to 0.27 mg/kg every 8 hours). May need to reduce interval to every 8 hours because of increased elimination. Maximum dose is 40 to 80 mg/24 hr based on diagnosis.
Neonate (unlabeled): 0.5 mg/kg/dose/24 hr.

DOSE ADJUSTMENTS
Reduce dose by one-half or increase the dosing interval to 36 to 48 hours in patients with moderate or severe renal dysfunction (CrCl less than 50 mL/min). Adjust based on patient response. Half-life may exceed 20 hours if CrCl less than 10 mL/min.

DILUTION
IV injection: Available in vials containing 10 mg/mL and as premixed solution 20 mg/50 mL. Each 20-mg vial may be diluted with 5 to 10 mL of NS or other **compatible** infusion solutions for injection (e.g., D5W, D10W, LR, SWFI). Many references state famotidine may be administered undiluted.

Intermittent infusion: Each 20 mg may be diluted in 100 mL of D5W or other **compatible** infusion solution and given piggyback.

Storage: Refrigerate vials before dilution. Manufacturer recommends use of diluted solutions within 48 hours. However, studies suggest diluted solutions are physically and chemically stable at RT for 7 days. Store premixed Galaxy containers at CRT; avoid excessive heat. If solution freezes, bring to RT; allow sufficient time to solubilize.

COMPATIBILITY

May form a precipitate with sodium bicarbonate in concentrations greater than 0.2 mg/mL.

Other sources suggest specific **compatibilities** dependent on concentration and manufacturer; consult a pharmacist.

RATE OF ADMINISTRATION

IV injection: Each 20 mg or fraction thereof over at least 2 minutes.

Intermittent infusion: Each 20-mg dose over 15 to 30 minutes.

ACTIONS

A histamine H_2 antagonist, it inhibits both daytime and nocturnal basal gastric acid secretion. It also inhibits gastric acid secretion stimulated by food and pentagastrin. Onset of action occurs within 30 minutes and lasts for 10 to 12 hours. No cumulative effect with repeated doses. 30 to 60 times more potent than cimetidine. Elimination half-life is 2.5 to 3.5 hours. Eliminated by renal and other metabolic routes. Crosses placental barrier. Secreted in breast milk.

INDICATIONS AND USES

Short-term treatment of active duodenal ulcers, benign gastric ulcers, and pathologic hypersecretory conditions in hospitalized patients or in patients unable to take oral medication. ▪ Used orally for short-term treatment of gastroesophageal reflux disease (GERD), including erosive or ulcerative esophagitis.

Unlabeled uses: GI bleeding. ▪ Stress ulcer prophylaxis.

CONTRAINDICATIONS

Known hypersensitivity to H_2 receptor antagonists or their components; cross-sensitivity has occurred.

PRECAUTIONS

Use with caution in patients with moderate or severe renal dysfunction; see Dose Adjustments. ▪ CNS adverse effects have been reported in patients with impaired renal function. ▪ Gastric malignancy may be present even though patient is asymptomatic. ▪ Effects maintained with oral dosage. Total treatment usually discontinued after 4 to 8 weeks.

Monitor: Use antacids concomitantly to relieve pain. ▪ See Precautions.

Patient Education: Stop smoking or at least avoid smoking after last dose of the day. ▪ Gastric pain and ulceration may recur after medication is stopped.

Maternal/Child: Category B: use during pregnancy only when clearly needed. ▪ Advisable to discontinue breast-feeding. ▪ Plasma clearance is reduced and half-life is increased in pediatric patients under 3 months of age compared to older pediatric patients with pharmacokinetic parameters similar to adults.

Elderly: Response similar to that seen in younger patients; however, greater sensitivity in the elderly cannot be ruled out. ▪ Consider risk of renal dysfunction; reduced doses and monitoring of renal function may be indicated; see Dose Adjustments.

DRUG/LAB INTERACTIONS

May inhibit gastric absorption of **ketoconazole.** ▪ May decrease **cyclosporine** serum levels when famotidine is given concurrently with ketoconazole and cyclosporine.

SIDE EFFECTS

Constipation, diarrhea, dizziness, and headache are the most common side effects. Hypersensitivity reactions (bronchospasm, fever, pruritus, rash, eosinophilia) can occur. Abdominal discomfort, agitation, alopecia, anorexia, anxiety, arthralgias, confusion, decreased libido, depression, dry mouth, dry skin, elevated ALT, flushing, grand mal seizure, hallucinations, insomnia, interstitial pneumonia, malaise, muscular pain, nausea and vomiting, orbital edema, palpitations, paresthesias, somnolence, taste disorder, thrombocytopenia, tinnitus, and toxic epidermal necrolysis/Stevens-Johnson syndrome (very rare) have been reported. Convulsions in patients with impaired renal function have been reported rarely.

ANTIDOTE

Notify physician of all side effects. May be treated symptomatically or may respond to decrease in frequency of dosage. Resuscitate as necessary for overdosage.

FAT EMULSION, INTRAVENOUS BBW

Clinolipid 20%, Intralipid 20% & 30%, Liposyn II 10% & 20%, Nutrilipid 20%

Nutritional supplement
(fatty acid)

pH 6 to 8.9

USUAL DOSE

Dose depends on energy expenditure and on patient's clinical status, body weight, tolerance, and ability to metabolize fat emulsion. For partial parenteral nutrition, energy supplied by oral or enteral nutrition must be taken into account. Some solutions may contain aluminum; see Precautions.

Caloric source (as a component of parenteral nutrition): *Initial dose:* 1 to 1.5 Gm/kg/day (not to exceed 500 mL of Intralipid 20% on the first day). *Maximum daily dose:* 2.5 Gm/kg/day. Do not exceed 60% of the patient's total caloric intake. Amino acids and carbohydrates should account for the remaining caloric input.

Essential fatty acid deficiency (Intralipid and Nutrilipid): 8% to 10% of the caloric input should be supplied as a fat emulsion to provide adequate amounts of essential fatty acids; see Dose Adjustments.

PEDIATRIC DOSE

Some solutions may contain aluminum; see Precautions. The American Society of Enteral and Parenteral Nutrition recommends the following doses for pediatric patients.

Caloric source (as a component of parenteral nutrition): *Infants (preterm and term to less than 1 year of age):* 1 to 2 Gm/kg/day as an initial dose. Increase dose by 0.5 to 1 Gm/kg/day each day to a maximum daily dose of 3 Gm/kg/day. Infuse daily dose over 24 hours. *Pediatric patients (1 to 10 years of age):* 1 to 2 Gm/kg/day as an initial dose. Increase dose by 0.5 to 1 Gm/kg/day each day to a maximum daily dose of 2 to 3 Gm/kg/day. Infuse daily dose over 24 hours. *Adolescents:* 1 Gm/kg/day as an initial dose (not to exceed 500 mL of Intralipid 20% on the first day). Increase dose by 1 Gm/kg/day each day to a maximum daily dose of 2.5 Gm/kg/day. Infuse daily dose over 12 to 24 hours.

Do not exceed 60% of total caloric intake. Amino acids and carbohydrates should account for the remaining caloric input.

Premature infants: *Intralipid:* Treatment of premature and low-birth-weight infants must be based on careful benefit-risk assessment. Strict adherence to the recommended total daily dose is mandatory. Hourly infusion rate should be as slow as possible. Never exceed 1 Gm/kg in 4 hours. Begin with 0.5 Gm fat/kg/24 hr (2.5 mL/kg/24 hr of 20% solution). May be increased based on infant's ability to eliminate fat. See comments under Pediatric Dose, Rate of Administration, Precautions, and Maternal/Child. *Nutrilipid:* See infant dose.

Essential fatty acid deficiency: See Usual Dose and Dose Adjustments.

DOSE ADJUSTMENTS

Lower initial starting doses and smaller incremental advances are suggested in patients with elevated triglyceride levels. Checking of triglycerides is recommended before each incremental advance. ▪ If essential fatty acid deficiency occurs together with stress, dose may need to be increased. ▪ Reduce dose in patients who develop serum triglyceride concentrations above 400 mg/dL to prevent consequences associated with hypertriglyceridemia. (Serum triglyceride levels above 1,000 mg/dL have been associated with an increased risk of pancreatitis.)

DILUTION

Follow manufacturer's specific instructions for preparation of each individual brand. Must be given as prepared by manufacturer; check labels for aluminum content; see Precautions. Do not use if there appears to be an oiling out of the emulsion. **Intralipid 30% is not to be given by direct IV infusion.** Packaged for bulk use in a pharmacy admixture program. Must be specifically combined with dextrose solutions and amino acids (TPN) so total fat content does not exceed 20%. When combined with dextrose, check mixture closely for the presence of precipitates. Prepared for an individual patient in the pharmacy.

Filters: Do not use filters of less than 1.2 microns with lipid emulsions. Use of a 1.2-micron in-line filter during administration (alone or as part of an admixture) is recommended.

Storage: Must be stored at temperatures not exceeding 25° C (77° F). Specific storage conditions required (see literature). Do not freeze. Use only freshly opened solutions; discard remainder of partial dose.

COMPATIBILITY

Consider any drug NOT listed as compatible to be INCOMPATIBLE until consulting a pharmacist; specific conditions may apply.

Lipids may extract phthalates from phthalate-plasticized PVC (DEHP). Non-phthalate infusion sets recommended.

Manufacturer recommends not mixing with any electrolyte or other nutrient solution. Infuse separately; do not disturb emulsion; no additives or medications are to be placed in bottle or tubing with the exception of heparin 1 to 2 units/mL (may be added before administration [activates lipoprotein lipase]). In actual practice, carbohydrates, amino acids, and fat emulsion are mixed in specific percentages and in a specific order to meet individual total parenteral nutritional needs but should be prepared in the pharmacy. Any addition of supplemental vitamins, minerals, or electrolytes (e.g., calcium, magnesium, phosphates) may cause a precipitate unless a specific order is followed. Precipitates are difficult to detect in lipids. The prime destabilizers of emulsions are excessive acidity (such as pH below 5) and inappropriate electrolyte content. Divalent cations (calcium and magnesium) have been shown to cause emulsion instability. Amino acid solutions exert buffering effects that protect the emulsion.

RATE OF ADMINISTRATION

May be infused through a peripheral or central line. Lipids may extract phthalates from phthalate-plasticized PVC (DEHP). Non-phthalate infusion sets recommended.

May be administered via a Y-tube near the infusion site. Rates of both solutions (fat emulsion and amino acid products) should be controlled by infusion pumps.

Do not hang flexible plastic containers in series connection, do not pressurize to increase flow rates without first fully evacuating residual air from the container, and do not use vented IV administration sets. All may result in air embolism. In general, administration rate should be adjusted taking into account the dose being administered, the daily volume intake, and the duration of the infusion. Most doses are administered over 12 to 24 hours.

Adult: *20%:* 0.5 mL/min or 0.1 Gm fat/min for the first 15 to 30 minutes. If no untoward effects after 30 minutes, the rate may be increased gradually to the required rate (***Nutrilipid:*** 0.5 mL/kg/hr).

Premature infants: *Intralipid:* 0.5 Gm fat/kg/24 hr (2.5 mL of 20%/kg/24 hr). Hourly infusion rate should be as slow as possible. Adjust rate and/or increase amount based on the infant's ability to eliminate fat. ***Nutrilipid:*** Initial rate of 0.05 mL/min for the first 10 to 15 minutes. If no untoward effects, rate may be increased to 0.75 mL/kg/hr. Never exceed 1 Gm/kg in 4 hours. See comments under Usual Dose and Maternal/Child.

Pediatric: *Intralipid:* Initial rate of 0.05 mL/min for the first 10 to 15 minutes. If no untoward effects, rate may be increased to 0.5 mL/kg/hr. *Nutrilipid:* Initial rate of 0.05 mL/min for the first 10 to 15 minutes. If no untoward effects, rate may be increased to 0.75 mL/kg/hr (1 to 10 years of age) or 0.5 mL/kg/hr (over 10 years of age).

ACTIONS

An isotonic nutrient that serves as an important substrate for energy production. Used as a source of calories and essential fatty acids. Fatty acids are important for membrane structure and function as precursors for bioactive molecules (e.g., prostaglandins) and as regulators of gene expression. Total caloric value (fat, phospholipid, and glycerol) is 1.1 cal/mL for the 10% emulsion and 2 cal/mL for the 20% emulsion. The various formulations contain different components (see manufacturer's prescribing information for actual ingredients). The fatty acids, phospholipids, and glycerol found in lipid emulsions are metabolized by cells to carbon dioxide and water. This metabolism results in the generation of energy. Increases heat production and oxygen consumption. Decreases respiratory quotient. Some lipids are excreted through the biliary system.

INDICATIONS AND USES

To provide additional calories and essential fatty acids for patients requiring parenteral nutrition who will be receiving parenteral nutrition over extended periods (usually over 5 days) or when oral or enteral nutrition is not possible, is insufficient, or is contraindicated. ▪ To prevent essential fatty acid deficiency (Intralipid and Nutrilipid only).

Limitation of use: *Clinolipid* is not indicated for use in pediatric patients because there are insufficient data to demonstrate that it provides sufficient amounts of essential fatty acids in this population.

CONTRAINDICATIONS

Severe hyperlipidemia (serum triglycerides above 1,000 mg/dL) or severe disorders of lipid metabolism, such as pathologic hyperlipemia, lipoid nephrosis, and acute pancreatitis with hyperlipemia. ▪ Known hypersensitivity to any component in the product (e.g., *Clinolipid* and *Nutrilipid*: egg or soybean proteins).

PRECAUTIONS

Isotonic; may be administered by a peripheral vein or central venous infusion; when administered with dextrose and amino acids, choice of peripheral or central vein is based on osmolarity of the final infusate. ▪ Fatty acids displace bilirubin bound to albumin. Use caution in jaundiced or premature infants. ▪ Deaths in preterm infants have been reported; see Maternal/Child. ▪ Use caution in pulmonary disease, liver disease, anemia, or blood coagulation disorders or when there is any danger of fat embolism. ▪ Patients requiring parenteral nutrition may be at higher risk for infection due to malnutrition, underlying disease state, and/or catheter access. ▪ Hypersensitivity reactions are possible. ▪ Fat overload syndrome has been reported (rare); see Monitor. ▪ Parenteral nutrition–associated liver disease has been reported with use for extended periods of time, especially in preterm infants. May present as cholestasis or steatohepatitis. ▪ Administration of parenteral nutrition to severely undernourished patients may result in refeeding syndrome. Initiate parenteral nutrition therapy slowly and monitor closely. ▪ Some solutions may contain aluminum. In impaired kidney function, aluminum may reach toxic levels. Premature neonates are particularly at risk because of their immature kidneys and requirement for calcium and phosphate, which also contain aluminum. Research indicates that patients with impaired renal function who receive more than 4 to 5 mcg/kg/day of parenteral aluminum are at risk for developing CNS or bone toxicity associated with aluminum accumulation. ▪ See Maternal/Child.

Monitor: Monitor lipids routinely; lipemia should clear daily. ▪ Correct severe water and electrolyte disorders, severe fluid overload states, and severe metabolic disorders before administration. ▪ Obtain baseline values and monitor blood glucose, fluid and electrolyte status, blood coagulation, liver and kidney function, triglycerides, CBC and platelet count, and serum osmolarity as indicated, especially in neonates. Discontinue use for significant abnormality. ▪ Monitor for S/S of hypersensitivity (e.g., altered mentation, bronchospasm, chills, cyanosis, dizziness, dyspnea, erythema, fever, flushing, headache, hypotension, hypoxia, nausea, rash, sweating, tachycardia, tachypnea, urticaria, vomiting). ▪ Monitor for S/S of infection. ▪ Monitor for S/S of fat overload syndrome. Reduced or limited ability to metabolize and clear lipids may result in a sudden deterioration of patient condition accompanied by anemia, coagulation disorders, deteriorating liver function, fever, hepatomegaly, hyperlipidemia, leukopenia, thrombocytopenia, and CNS manifestations (e.g., coma). ▪ For severely undernourished patients initiating parenteral nutrition therapy, monitor closely for S/S of refeeding syndrome. May be characterized by the intracellular shift of potassium, phosphorus, and magnesium; thiamine deficiency; and fluid retention. ▪ Monitor for S/S of essential fatty acid deficiency. ▪ Monitor catheter site. ▪ See Maternal/Child.

Patient Education: Inform parents that deaths in premature infants after infusion of IV fat emulsion have been reported. ▪ Laboratory monitoring is required. ▪ Promptly report any S/S of hypersensitivity reactions (e.g., bronchospasm, chills, dyspnea, hypotension, hypoxia, nausea, rash, urticaria). ▪ Promptly report any S/S of infection (e.g., fever, chills, pain at infusion site). ▪ Review other possible side effects.

Maternal/Child: Category C: use in pregnancy only when clearly needed; safety not established. Severe malnutrition in a pregnant woman is associated with preterm delivery, low birth weight, intrauterine growth restriction, congenital malformations, and perinatal mortality. Parenteral nutrition should be considered if a pregnant woman's nutritional requirements cannot be fulfilled by oral or enteral intake. ▪ Use caution if fat emulsion is administered to a woman who is breast-feeding. ▪ Use extreme caution in neonates; death from intravascular fat accumulation in the lungs has occurred. Strict adherence to dose and rate of administration is imperative. Premature and small-for-gestational-age infants have poor clearance. Administration of less than the maximum recommended dose should be considered in these patients to decrease the likelihood of intravenous fat overload. Monitor serum triglycerides and/or plasma free fatty acid levels to assess infant's ability to eliminate infused fat from the circulation; must clear between daily infusions. Frequent, even daily, platelet counts are recommended in neonatal patients receiving TPN with IV fat emulsion. *Clinolipid:* Safety and effectiveness for use in pediatric patients, including preterm infants, have not been established. Use in pediatric patients is not recommended.

Elderly: *Clinolipid and Nutrilipid:* No overall differences in safety and/or effectiveness. Dose selection should be cautious, usually starting at the low end of the dosing range.

DRUG/LAB INTERACTIONS
Intralipid: No specific information available; see Dilution. *Clinolipid:* Drug interaction studies not performed. ▪ Olive and soybean oils contain vitamin K_1. May decrease the anticoagulant activity of **coumarin derivatives** (e.g., warfarin). ▪ May interfere with certain **lab tests** if samples are taken before the lipids are eliminated from the serum (5 to 6 hours).

SIDE EFFECTS
Intralipid: Back pain, chest pain, cyanosis, dizziness, dyspnea, flushing, headache, hypercoagulability, hyperlipemia, hypersensitivity reactions, hyperthermia, irritation at injection site, nausea and vomiting, sepsis (from contamination of IV catheter), sleepiness, slight pressure over eyes, sweating, thrombophlebitis (from concurrent parenteral nutrition fluids), thrombocytopenia in neonates (rare), and transient increase in liver enzymes may occur.

Clinolipid: Abnormal liver function tests, hyperglycemia, hyperlipidemia, hypoproteinemia, nausea, and vomiting were most common. Hypersensitivity, infectious complications (e.g., fever of unknown origin, septicemia, UTI), and refeeding syndrome have been reported.

All formulations with long-term therapy: Abnormal liver function tests, hepatomegaly, jaundice due to central lobular cholestasis, leukopenia, overloading syndrome, splenomegaly, thrombocytopenia, and deposition of brown pigment in the reticuloendothelial tissue of the liver may occur.

Post-Marketing: Diarrhea, pruritus.

ANTIDOTE

Notify physician of all side effects. Many will be treated symptomatically. Treat hypersensitivity reactions promptly and resuscitate as necessary. For accidental overdose, stop the infusion. Obtain blood sample for inspection of plasma, triglyceride concentration, or measurement of plasma light-scattering activity by nephelometry. Repeat blood samples until the lipid has cleared. Stop infusion immediately for any signs of acute respiratory distress. May represent pulmonary embolus or interstitial pneumonitis, which may be caused by an unseen precipitate of electrolytes (e.g., calcium and phosphates) in the solution. Lipids administered and fatty acids produced are not dialyzable.

FENOLDOPAM MESYLATE

(feh-**NOL**-doh-pam **MES**-ih-layt)

Antihypertensive
Vasodilator

Corlopam

USUAL DOSE

Initiate dosing at 0.01 to 0.3 mcg/kg/min as a continuous infusion. Titrate in increments of 0.05 to 0.1 mcg/kg/min every 15 minutes or longer until target blood pressure is reached. The maximum infusion rate reported in clinical studies was 1.6 mcg/kg/min. Doses lower than 0.1 mcg/kg/min and slow up-titration have been associated with less reflex tachycardia. Maintenance infusions may be continued for up to 48 hours. Transition to oral therapy with another agent can begin any time after blood pressure is stable during fenoldopam infusion. Avoid hypotension and rapid decreases in BP.

PEDIATRIC DOSE

Initiate dosing at 0.2 mcg/kg/min as a continuous infusion. Titrate dose by 0.3 to 0.5 mcg/kg/min every 20 to 30 minutes to a maximum dose of 0.8 mcg/kg/min. Higher doses generally produced no further decreases in mean arterial pressure (MAP) but did worsen tachycardia. See Maternal/Child.

DOSE ADJUSTMENTS

Dose adjustment is not required in end-stage renal disease; in patients on continuous ambulatory peritoneal dialysis (CAPD); in severe hepatic failure; or by age, gender, or race. Effects of hemodialysis have not been evaluated. ■ Caution and lower-end dosing suggested in elderly patients. Consider decreased organ function and concomitant disease or drug therapy.

DILUTION

Each 10 mg (1 mL) must be diluted with 250 mL of NS or D5W and given as a continuous infusion. (10 mg in 250 mL, 20 mg in 500 mL, or 40 mg in 1,000 mL all yield 40 mcg/mL.) Use of an infusion pump is recommended.

Pediatric dilution: Mix to yield a final concentration of 60 mcg/mL (6 mg in 100 mL, 15 mg in 250 mL, or 30 mg in 500 mL of D5W or NS). Use of an infusion pump capable of delivering low infusion rates is required.

Storage: Store unopened ampules or vials at 2° to 30° C (35.6° to 86° F). Discard diluted solution if not being administered to a patient after 4 hours at RT or after 24 hours refrigerated.

COMPATIBILITY

Compatibility information not available from manufacturer. Other sources suggest specific **compatibilities** dependent on concentration and manufacturer; consult a pharmacist.

RATE OF ADMINISTRATION

Do not give as a bolus injection; must be given as an infusion. See Usual Dose and Pediatric Dose for recommended initial infusion rate, titration, and maximum recommended infusion rate. Use of an infusion pump is recommended. To calculate the infusion rate in mL/hr, use the following formula:

$$\text{Infusion rate (mL/hr)} = \frac{[\text{Dose (mcg/kg/min)} \times \text{Weight (kg)} \times 60 \text{ min/hr}]}{\text{Concentration (mcg/mL)}}$$

Example: For a 60-kg patient at an initial dose of 0.01 mcg/kg/min using the 40 mcg/mL concentration, the infusion rate would be:

$$\text{Infusion rate (mL/hr)} = \frac{[0.01 \text{ mcg/kg/min} \times 60 \text{ kg} \times 60 \text{ min/hr}]}{40 \text{ mcg/mL}} = 0.9 \text{ mL/hr}$$

Avoid hypotension and rapid decreases in BP. Manufacturer's prescribing information contains charts of infusion rates per hour for a range of doses and a range of weights for both adult and pediatric patients.

ACTIONS

A peripherally acting rapid-acting vasodilator. Is an agonist at the D_1 receptor and binds with moderate affinity to the alpha$_2$ adrenoreceptor. Causes a dose-dependent fall in systolic and diastolic BP. May cause a reflex increase in HR. Decreases peripheral vascular resistance. Increases renal blood flow, diuresis, and natriuresis. Onset of action begins within 5 minutes, and with continuous infusion, steady-state concentrations (peak effects) are reached in 15 to 20 minutes. Elimination half-life is about 5 minutes. Metabolized in the liver primarily by conjugation (without cytochrome P_{450} enzymes). Primarily eliminated in urine; some excretion in feces.

INDICATIONS AND USES

Adult patients: In-hospital, short-term (up to 48 hours) management of severe hypertension when rapid, but quickly reversible, emergency reduction of BP is indicated, including malignant hypertension with deteriorating end-organ function.
Pediatric patients: In-hospital, short-term (up to 4 hours) for reduction in BP.
Unlabeled uses: Renal protection before study with contrast dye.

CONTRAINDICATIONS

Manufacturer states, "None known."

PRECAUTIONS

Use limited to the hospital. Adequate personnel and appropriate equipment must be available for continuous monitoring. ▪ Use extreme caution in patients with open-angle glaucoma or intraocular hypertension. Has caused a dose-dependent increase in intraocular pressure. Upon discontinuation of fenoldopam, intraocular pressure returned to baseline values within 2 hours. ▪ Causes a dose-related tachycardia with infusion rates above 0.1 mcg/kg/min in adults. May diminish over time in adults but is consistent at higher doses. Has not been reported but could lead to ischemic cardiac events or worsened heart failure. ▪ Tachycardia occurred in pediatric patients at doses greater than or equal to 0.8 mcg/kg/min. ▪ Rapidly decreases serum potassium leading to hypokalemia; see Monitor. ▪ Use caution; contains sulfites. Sulfite sensitivity is seen more frequently in asthmatic individuals. ▪ See Drug/Lab Interactions.
Monitor: Determine patency of vein; avoid extravasation. ▪ Monitor BP and HR frequently, especially during titration. Avoid hypotension. ▪ Monitor serum electrolytes frequently; hypokalemia has been observed after less than 6 hours of fenoldopam infusion. Oral or intravenous supplements may be required. ▪ Transfer to oral antihypertensive agents when BP is stable. May be added during fenoldopam infusion or following its discontinuation; monitor effects carefully. ▪ See Precautions and Drug/Lab Interactions.
Patient Education: Report IV site burning or stinging promptly. ▪ Request assistance with ambulation.
Maternal/Child: Category B: use only if clearly needed. ▪ Discontinue breast-feeding; not known if fenoldopam is secreted in breast milk (is secreted in milk of rats). ▪ Antihypertensive effects have been studied in pediatric patients under 1 month of age (at least

2 kg or full term) to 12 years of age. Pharmacokinetics are independent of age when corrected for body weight. Clinical studies did not include adolescents (12 to 16 years of age). Dose selection for this group should consider clinical condition and concomitant drug therapy.

Elderly: Dose selection should be cautious; see Dose Adjustments. ▪ Response similar to other age-groups.

DRUG/LAB INTERACTIONS

No specific drug interaction studies have been conducted. ▪ Concurrent use not recommended with **beta-adrenergic blocking agents**. May cause unexpected hypotension from beta-blocker inhibition of the reflex response to fenoldopam (e.g., tachycardia). Monitor BP frequently if concurrent use is required.

SIDE EFFECTS

Dose-dependent side effects may include hypotension with resulting tachycardia, flushing, headache, and nausea. Additional side effects unrelated to dose include abdominal pain or fullness; angina; anxiety; cardiac failure; chest pain; diaphoresis; diarrhea; dizziness; ECG T-wave inversion; extrasystoles; fever; hypokalemia; increased BUN, SCr, glucose, transaminases, and lactate dehydrogenase; injection site reaction; insomnia; ischemic heart disease; muscle spasm; MI; nasal congestion; nervousness; oliguria; palpitations; postural hypotension; urinary infection; and vomiting.

Post-Marketing: Abdominal distension, cardiogenic shock, decreased oxygen saturation, ECG ST-segment depression, hypotension.

ANTIDOTE

Keep physician informed of all side effects. Most will be treated symptomatically. Use oral and/or intravenous potassium to treat hypokalemia. Reduce dose gradually as desired BP is reached. Discontinue fenoldopam immediately for excessive hypotension. Half-life is short. Recovery should begin within 5 to 15 minutes; support patient as indicated (e.g., Trendelenburg position, IV fluids if appropriate). With short half-life the need for vasopressors is unlikely. Discontinue fenoldopam and treat life-threatening arrhythmias as indicated.

FENTANYL CITRATE BBW

(**FEN**-tah-nil **SIT**-rayt)

Fentanyl, Fentanyl Citrate PF

Opioid analgesic
(agonist)
Anesthesia adjunct

pH 4 to 7.5

USUAL DOSE

Pretreatment: See Maternal/Child.

Dose should be individualized, taking into account factors such as age, body weight, physical status, concomitant drugs or diseases, type of anesthesia to be used, and type of surgery or procedure to be performed. In all situations, use smallest effective dose at maximum intervals.

Premedication in adults: 50 to 100 mcg (0.05 to 0.1 mg) IM or IV 30 to 60 minutes before surgery.

Adjunct to regional anesthesia: 50 to 100 mcg (0.05 to 0.1 mg) IM or IV slowly over 1 to 2 minutes when additional analgesia is required.

Adjunct to general anesthesia: *Low dose:* 2 mcg/kg (0.002 mg/kg) of body weight. Additional doses are usually not necessary for these minor procedures.

Moderate dose: 2 to 20 mcg/kg (0.002 to 0.02 mg/kg) of body weight. Additional doses of 25 to 100 mcg may be administered as needed.

High dose: 20 to 50 mcg/kg (0.02 to 0.05 mg/kg) of body weight. Additional doses from 25 mcg to one-half the initial loading dose may be administered as needed.

General anesthetic: 50 to 100 mcg/kg (0.05 to 0.1 mg/kg) of body weight administered with oxygen and a muscle relaxant. Doses up to 150 mcg/kg (0.15 mg/kg) may be necessary. Used in open heart surgery and/or certain complicated neurologic or orthopedic procedures.

Postoperative pain management (recovery room): 50 to 100 mcg (0.05 to 0.1 mg) IM for control of pain, tachypnea, and emergence delirium. Repeat in 1 to 2 hours as needed.

Pain management as an IV injection (unlabeled): An initial dose of 25 to 100 mcg (0.025 to 0.1 mg). Titrate to effect.

Pain management as an infusion (unlabeled): Used postoperatively with a patient-controlled analgesic (PCA) device. One source suggests a concentration of 10 mcg/mL, with a starting patient-controlled dose of 10 to 20 mcg and a lockout interval of 4 to 10 minutes. See pain literature.

Pain management in critically ill patients (unlabeled): Initiated as a continuous infusion at 25 to 50 mcg/hr. Titrate to desired effect. Doses up to 700 mcg/hr have been used. Several regimens are in use. See pain literature.

PEDIATRIC DOSE

Induction and maintenance in pediatric patients 2 to 12 years of age: A reduced dose as low as 2 to 3 mcg/kg is recommended. See Maternal/Child.

Pain management (unlabeled): 0.5 to 2 mcg/kg/dose every 2 to 4 hours as needed. Titrate to effect.

DOSE ADJUSTMENTS

Reduce dose in patients receiving other CNS depressants, such as general anesthetics, alcohol, anticholinergics, antihistamines, barbiturates, hypnotics, sedatives, psychotropic agents, and narcotic analgesics. When concurrent administration is required, consider reducing the dose of one or both drugs. ▪ Reduce dose or increase intervals for elderly, debilitated, and poor-risk patients or those with impaired pulmonary, hepatic, or renal function. ▪ See Drug/Lab Interactions.

DILUTION

Small volumes may be given undiluted. May be given through Y-tube of infusion set. May be further diluted with NS and administered as an infusion or PCA (unlabeled).

Storage: Store at room temperature and protect from light before dilution. Use promptly.

COMPATIBILITY

Compatibility information not available from manufacturer. Other sources suggest specific **compatibilities** dependent on concentration and manufacturer; consult a pharmacist.

RATE OF ADMINISTRATION

Administer over 1 to 2 minutes. Too-rapid administration may result in apnea or respiratory paralysis. Rate must be titrated by desired dose and patient response.

ACTIONS

A potent opioid agonist whose principal actions of therapeutic value are analgesia and sedation. Binds to receptors in the CNS, increasing the pain threshold and altering the perception of pain. Produces respiratory depression by direct action on brain stem respiratory centers. Produces peripheral vasodilation, which may result in orthostatic hypotension or syncope. Fentanyl is approximately 100 times more potent than morphine milligram for milligram (100 **mcg** of fentanyl is approximately equivalent to 10 **mg** of morphine). It has respiratory-depressant actions that may outlast its analgesic effect. Duration and degree of respiratory depression are dose related. Onset of action is almost immediate; however, the maximal analgesic and respiratory depressant effect may not be noted for several minutes. The usual duration of action of analgesic effect is 30 to 60 minutes after a single IV dose of up to 100 mcg. Effects are cumulative with repeat doses. Half-life is approximately 3.6 hours. Metabolized in the liver and excreted in the urine. Crosses the placental barrier. Secreted in breast milk.

INDICATIONS AND USES
A narcotic analgesic supplement in general and regional anesthesia. ▪ Short-term analgesia during perioperative period. ▪ For administration with a neuroleptic such as droperidol as an anesthetic premedication, for the induction of anesthesia, and as an adjunct in the maintenance of general and regional anesthesia. ▪ For use as an anesthetic agent with oxygen in selected high-risk patients, such as those undergoing open heart surgery or certain complicated neurologic or orthopedic procedures. ▪ Useful in short-duration minor surgery in outpatients and in diagnostic procedures or treatments that require the patient to be awake or very lightly anesthetized (e.g., bronchoscopy, radiologic studies, burn dressings, cystoscopy).

Unlabeled use: Treatment of severe pain. Has been administered as an intermittent injection, as an epidural injection or infusion, and as patient-controlled analgesia (PCA).

CONTRAINDICATIONS
Patients with known intolerance to fentanyl and other opioid agonists.

PRECAUTIONS
Fentanyl exposes patients and other users to the risks of opioid addiction, abuse, and misuse, which can lead to overdose and death. Assess each patient's risk before prescribing fentanyl, and monitor all patients regularly for the development of these behaviors and conditions. Strategies to reduce the risk of diversion or misuse should be used by health care facilities that use this and other controlled substances. ▪ See prescribing information for further discussion regarding abuse, addiction, physical dependence, and tolerance. ▪ Should be administered only by persons specifically trained in the use of IV anesthetics and management of the respiratory effects of potent opioids. ▪ Serious, life-threatening, or fatal respiratory depression may occur with the use of fentanyl. ▪ Adequate facilities should be available for monitoring and ventilation. An opioid antagonist (e.g., naloxone), resuscitative and intubation equipment, and oxygen should be readily available. ▪ The respiratory depressant effect of fentanyl may persist longer than the analgesic effect. The total dose of all opioid agonists administered should be considered before ordering opioid analgesics during recovery from anesthesia. ▪ Use caution in patients with pulmonary disease or cor pulmonale and in those with decreased respiratory reserve, hypoxia, hypercapnia, or pre-existing respiratory depression; these patients are at increased risk for decreased respiratory drive, including apnea. ▪ Sleep-related breathing disorders, including central sleep apnea (CSA) and sleep-related hypoxemia, can occur. Opioid use increases the risk of CSA in a dose-dependent fashion. ▪ Use caution in cachectic or debilitated patients, in elderly patients, and in patients with impaired hepatic or renal function; these patients may be at an increased risk for adverse effects, including respiratory depression. Reduced dose may be indicated. ▪ May cause muscle rigidity, particularly with muscles of respiration. Incidence and severity of muscle rigidity is rate- and dose-related. The incidence of muscle rigidity may be reduced by (1) administration of up to one-fourth of the full paralyzing dose of a nondepolarizing neuromuscular blocking agent just before administration of fentanyl, (2) administration of a full paralyzing dose of a neuromuscular blocking agent following loss of eyelash reflex when fentanyl is used in anesthetic doses titrated by slow IV infusion, or (3) simultaneous administration of fentanyl and a full paralyzing dose of a neuromuscular blocking agent when fentanyl is used in rapidly administered anesthetic doses. ▪ In patients with circulatory shock, fentanyl may cause vasodilation, which can further reduce cardiac output and blood pressure. ▪ Cases of serotonin syndrome have been reported during concomitant use of fentanyl with serotonergic drugs. ▪ Cases of adrenal insufficiency have been reported with opioid use, more often following more than 1 month of use. If adrenal insufficiency is diagnosed, treat with physiologic replacement doses of corticosteroids, and wean the patient off the opioid to allow adrenal function to recover. Another opioid may be tried; some cases reported use of a different opioid without recurrence of adrenal insufficiency. ▪ Use caution in patients with head injury, brain tumors, or increased intracranial pressure. Respiratory depression may cause an increased PCO_2, cerebral vasodilation, and increased intracranial pressure. Clinical course of head injury may be obscured. ▪ Use caution in patients with biliary

tract disease, including acute pancreatitis. May cause spasm of the sphincter of Oddi. Opioids may cause increases in amylase. ▪ Fentanyl may increase the frequency of seizures in patients with seizure disorders. ▪ Use caution when administered with a neuroleptic agent (e.g., droperidol [Inapsine]). Neuroleptics have been associated with QT prolongation, torsades de pointes, and cardiac arrest. Use extreme caution in patients at risk for prolonged QT syndrome, such as patients with clinically significant brady-cardia (less than 50 bpm) or clinically significant cardiac disease (including baseline-prolonged QT interval), patients treated with Class I (e.g., disopyramide, quinidine) and Class III antiarrhythmics (e.g., amiodarone, ibutilide, sotalol), patients treated with MAO inhibitors, patients undergoing concomitant treatment with other agents known to pro-long the QT interval, patients with electrolyte imbalance (particularly hypokalemia and hypomagnesemia), or patients treated with concomitant agents (e.g., diuretics) that may cause electrolyte imbalance. Cardiac dysrhythmias, cardiac arrest, and death have been reported. ▪ May cause severe bradycardia, hypotension, and syncope. Use caution in patients with bradyarrhythmias. ▪ See Drug/Lab Interactions.

Monitor: Monitor for respiratory depression, especially during initiation of therapy or after a dose increase. Oxygen, controlled respiratory equipment, naloxone, and neuromuscular block-ing agents (e.g., succinylcholine) must always be available. May cause rigidity of respi-ratory muscles; may require a muscle relaxant to permit artificial ventilation. ▪ Observe patient frequently; monitor vital signs and oxygenation. Patient may appear to be asleep and may forget to breathe unless commanded to do so. ▪ Monitor patient for breathing disorders (e.g., CSA and sleep-related hypoxemia), and consider decreasing the opioid dosage using best practices for opioid taper. ▪ Keep patient supine; orthostatic hypoten-sion and fainting may occur. ▪ In patients with circulatory shock, monitor for signs of hypotension after initiating or titrating the dosage of fentanyl. ▪ Monitor patients who may be susceptible to the intracranial effects of CO_2 retention for increasing intracranial pressure and signs of sedation and respiratory depression. ▪ Monitor patients with bili-ary tract disease for worsening symptoms. ▪ Monitor patients with a history of seizure disorders for worsening seizure control. ▪ ECG monitoring indicated when a neurolep-tic drug is administered with fentanyl. ▪ Monitor for S/S of serotonin syndrome (e.g., mental status changes [e.g., agitation, coma, hallucinations], autonomic instability [e.g., hyperthermia, labile blood pressure, tachycardia], neuromuscular aberrations [e.g., hy-perreflexia, incoordination, rigidity], and/or GI symptoms [e.g., diarrhea, nausea, vomit-ing]). Onset of symptoms may occur within hours to days of concomitant use of opioids with serotonergic drugs. ▪ See Precautions.

Patient Education: Avoid use of alcohol or other CNS depressants (e.g., antihistamines, benzodiazepines). ▪ Promptly report S/S of serotonin syndrome. ▪ Use caution per-forming any task requiring alertness; may cause dizziness, euphoria, and sedation. ▪ May result in severe constipation. Scheduled bowel regimen recommended. ▪ May result in addiction, abuse, and misuse, even when taken as recommended. ▪ Blurred vision, diz-ziness, drowsiness, or light-headedness may occur; request assistance with ambula-tion. ▪ Review all medications for interactions.

Maternal/Child: Safety for use in pregnancy and labor and delivery not established. Fen-tanyl is not recommended for use in pregnant women during or immediately before labor when other analgesic techniques are more appropriate. ▪ Prolonged use of opioid anal-gesics during pregnancy can result in neonatal opioid withdrawal syndrome, which may be life threatening if not recognized and treated. ▪ Use caution with breast-feeding. Monitor infants exposed to fentanyl through breast milk for excess sedation and respira-tory depression. Withdrawal symptoms can occur in breast-fed infants when maternal administration of an opioid analgesic is stopped or when breast-feeding is stopped. ▪ Safety for use in pediatric patients under 2 years of age not established; rare cases of clinically significant methemoglobinemia have been reported in premature neonates; see Precautions.

Elderly: See Dose Adjustments and Precautions. ▪ May be more sensitive to effects (e.g., respiratory depression, urinary retention, constipation). Respiratory depression is the chief risk in elderly patients. ▪ Lower doses may provide effective analgesia. ▪ Consider age-related organ impairment; may delay postoperative recovery.

DRUG/LAB INTERACTIONS

Concomitant use of fentanyl with **benzodiazepines** (e.g., diazepam, midazolam) and other **CNS depressants** (e.g., sedative/hypnotics, anxiolytics, tranquilizers, muscle relaxants, general anesthetics, antipsychotics, other opioids, alcohol) may result in profound sedation, respiratory depression, coma, and death. Hypotension can also occur. Reserve concomitant use for patients for whom alternative treatment options are inadequate. Limit dose and duration of treatment to the minimum required, and monitor patients carefully for S/S of respiratory depression and sedation. When such combinations are administered, IV fluids and other measures to manage hypotension should be available. ▪ Use caution with concomitant use of fentanyl and **CYP3A4 inhibitors** (e.g., macrolide antibiotics, azole antifungals, and protease inhibitors) or when discontinuing a **CYP3A4 inducer** (e.g., rifampin, carbamazepine, phenytoin) in a fentanyl-treated patient. May increase plasma concentration of fentanyl and increase or prolong opioid adverse effects, and may cause potentially fatal respiratory depression. Dose reduction may be indicated. ▪ Alternatively, concomitant use of fentanyl with CYP34A4 inducers or discontinuation of a CYP34A4 inhibitor could result in lower than expected fentanyl plasma concentration and decreased efficacy. An increase in the dose of fentanyl may be required. ▪ Serotonin syndrome has been reported with the concomitant use of opioids, including fentanyl, and other **drugs that affect the serotonergic neurotransmitter system** (e.g., selective serotonin reuptake inhibitors [SSRIs], serotonin and norepinephrine reuptake inhibitors [SNRIs], tricyclic antidepressants [TCAs], triptans, 5-HT$_3$ receptor antagonists, mirtazapine, trazodone, tramadol, certain muscle relaxants [e.g., cyclobenzaprine, metaxalone], MAO inhibitors, linezolid, and intravenous methylene blue). Careful observation, particularly during treatment initiation and dose adjustment, is required with concomitant use. ▪ Severe and unpredictable potentiation of **MAO inhibitors** (e.g., selegiline, phenelzine, tranylcypromine, linezolid) has been reported. MAO inhibitor interactions may manifest as serotonin syndrome or opioid toxicity (e.g., respiratory depression, coma). Use of fentanyl is not recommended for patients taking MAOIs or within 14 days of stopping such treatment. ▪ **Mixed agonist/antagonist analgesics and partial agonists** (e.g., buprenorphine, butorphanol, nalbuphine) may reduce the analgesic effect of fentanyl and/or precipitate withdrawal symptoms. Avoid concomitant use. ▪ Fentanyl may enhance the neuromuscular blocking action of **skeletal muscle relaxants** (e.g., cyclobenzaprine, orphenadrine), increasing the degree of respiratory depression. Monitor patient and decrease dose if indicated. ▪ Opioids can reduce the efficacy of **diuretics** by inducing the release of antidiuretic hormone. Increase dose of diuretic if needed. ▪ Concomitant use with **anticholinergic drugs** may increase the risk of urinary retention and/or severe constipation, which may lead to paralytic ileus. ▪ Cardiovascular depression may result from concurrent use of **diazepam** or **nitrous oxide** and high-dose fentanyl. ▪ Concurrent use with **neuroleptic agents** may cause elevated BP, with or without pre-existing hypertension.

SIDE EFFECTS

Apnea, bradycardia, respiratory depression, and respiratory muscle rigidity are the most common serious adverse reactions. Untreated, they may lead to respiratory arrest, circulatory depression, and cardiac arrest. Blurred vision, bronchoconstriction, diaphoresis, dizziness, hypersensitivity reactions (e.g., anaphylaxis, laryngospasm, pruritus, urticaria), hypertension, hypotension, nausea, respiratory depression (slight), and vomiting have been reported. Cases of adrenal insufficiency, androgen deficiency, and serotonin syndrome have been reported.

Overdose: Atypical snoring; bradycardia; cold, clammy skin; death; hypotension; partial or complete airway obstruction; pinpoint pupils of eyes; pulmonary edema; respiratory depression; skeletal muscle flaccidity; somnolence progressing to stupor or coma. Marked mydriasis rather than miosis may be seen with hypoxia in overdose situations.

ANTIDOTE

With increasing severity of any side effect or onset of symptoms of overdose, discontinue the drug and notify the physician. Naloxone will reverse serious respiratory depression. Because the duration of opioid reversal is expected to be less than the duration of action of fentanyl, careful monitoring is necessary and repeat doses of naloxone may be required. A patent airway, artificial ventilation, oxygen therapy, and other symptomatic treatment must be instituted promptly. Treat hypotension with a Trendelenburg position and IV fluids or vasopressors (e.g., dopamine, norepinephrine) as needed. Avoid epinephrine if a neuroleptic agent has also been administered. May paradoxically decrease BP when given with neuroleptics that block alpha-adrenergic activity. A fast-acting muscle relaxant (e.g., succinylcholine) may be required to facilitate ventilation. Use atropine to treat bradycardia. Muscle rigidity during anesthesia induction or surgery must be controlled with neuromuscular blocking agents and controlled ventilation with oxygen. Use a neuromuscular blocking agent prophylactically to prevent muscle rigidity or to induce muscle relaxation after rigidity occurs. Resuscitate as necessary.

FERRIC CARBOXYMALTOSE INJECTION

(**FER**-ik kar-box-ee **MAWL**-tose)

Hematinic
Iron supplement
Antianemic

Injectafer

pH 5 to 7

USUAL DOSE

Dose is expressed in terms of mg of elemental iron. Each course consists of 2 doses given at least 7 days apart. Treatment may be repeated if iron deficiency recurs.

Patients weighing 50 kg or more: Give in 2 doses separated by at least 7 days. Give each dose as 750 mg for a total cumulative dose not to exceed 1,500 mg of iron per course.

Patients weighing less than 50 kg: Give in 2 doses separated by at least 7 days. Give each dose as 15 mg/kg body weight for a total cumulative dose not to exceed 1,500 mg of iron per course.

DILUTION

Available in a 750 mg/15 mL (50 mg/mL) single-use vial. May be given undiluted as a slow intravenous push or further diluted in NS and given as an infusion. When administering as an infusion, dilute dose in no more than 250 mL of NS. Do not dilute to concentrations below 2 mg/mL.

Filters: No data available from manufacturer.

Storage: Store unopened vials at CRT. Do not freeze. Solutions diluted with NS to a concentration of 2 to 4 mg/mL are stable for 72 hours at RT. Vials are single use. Discard any unused product.

COMPATIBILITY

Compatibility information not available from manufacturer; consult a pharmacist.

RATE OF ADMINISTRATION

Slow IV push: A single undiluted dose at a rate of 100 mg/min (7.5 minutes for a 750-mg dose).

Infusion: Administer over at least 15 minutes.

ACTIONS

A colloidal iron (III) hydroxide in complex with carboxymaltose, a carbohydrate polymer that releases iron. Used to replenish the total body iron stores in patients with iron deficiency. Iron is critical for normal hemoglobin synthesis to maintain oxygen transport and necessary for metabolism and synthesis of DNA and various other processes. Rapidly cleared from the plasma following administration. Iron distributes into liver, spleen, and bone marrow. Because the disappearance of iron from serum depends on the need for iron in the iron stores and iron-utilizing tissues of the body, serum clearance of iron is expected to be more rapid in patients with iron deficiency as compared with healthy individuals. Terminal half-life is 7 to 12 hours. Renal elimination of iron is negligible. Excreted in breast milk.

INDICATIONS AND USES

Treatment of iron deficiency anemia in adult patients who have intolerance to oral iron or have had an unsatisfactory response to oral iron and in adult patients who have non–dialysis dependent chronic kidney disease.

CONTRAINDICATIONS

Known hypersensitivity to ferric carboxymaltose or any of its components.

PRECAUTIONS

Serious hypersensitivity reactions, including anaphylactic-type reactions, some of which have been life-threatening and fatal, have been reported. Patients may present with shock, clinically significant hypotension, loss of consciousness, and/or collapse. Other serious reactions potentially associated with hypersensitivity have included pruritus, rash, urticaria, and wheezing. ▪ Administer in a facility with adequate diagnostic and treatment facilities to monitor the patient and respond to any medical emergency. ▪ Transient elevations in systolic blood pressure, sometimes occurring with dizziness, facial flushing, or nausea, have been reported. ▪ Avoid extravasation. Brown discoloration of extravasation site may be long lasting.

Monitor: Confirm IV placement. If extravasation occurs, discontinue administration at that site. ▪ Monitor for S/S of hypersensitivity reactions (e.g., acute respiratory distress, angioedema, chest tightness, hypotension, lethargy, nausea, paresthesia, pruritus, restlessness, urticaria, vomiting, wheezing) during and after administration for at least 30 minutes and until clinically stable; see Precautions. ▪ Monitor vital signs and monitor for S/S of hypertension following administration. ▪ Periodic monitoring of hematologic and hematinic parameters (hemoglobin, hematocrit, serum ferritin, and transferrin saturation) is indicated during parenteral iron replacement therapy; see Drug/Lab Interactions.

Patient Education: Review any possible reactions to past parenteral iron therapy. ▪ Report S/S of a hypersensitivity reaction promptly (e.g., hypotension, rash, urticaria, tightness of the chest, wheezing).

Maternal/Child: Use in pregnancy only if clearly needed and if potential benefit justifies the potential risk to the fetus. Untreated iron deficiency anemia (IDA) in pregnancy is associated with adverse maternal outcomes such as postpartum anemia. Adverse pregnancy outcomes associated with IDA include increased risk for preterm delivery and low birth weight. ▪ Iron is present in breast milk. There is no information on the effects of use on milk production. Consider developmental and health benefits of breast-feeding along with the mother's clinical need for ferric carboxymaltose. Monitor breast-fed infants for gastrointestinal toxicity (constipation, diarrhea). ▪ Safety and effectiveness for use in pediatric patients not established.

Elderly: Differences in response between elderly and younger patients have not been identified, but greater sensitivity of some older individuals cannot be ruled out.

DRUG/LAB INTERACTIONS

Specific information not available. ▪ In the 24 hours following administration of ferric carboxymaltose, laboratory assays may overestimate serum iron and transferrin-bound iron by also measuring the iron in ferric carboxymaltose.

SIDE EFFECTS

The most common side effects are dizziness, flushing, hypertension, hypophosphatemia, and nausea. Less frequently reported side effects include abdominal pain, constipation, diarrhea, dysgeusia, elevated ALT and gamma glutamyl transferase, headache, hypersensitivity reactions, hypertension, hypotension, injection site discoloration and pain/irritation, paresthesia, rash, sneezing, and vomiting.

Overdose: Hemosiderosis.

Post-Marketing: Angioedema, arthralgia, back pain, chest discomfort, chills, dyspnea, erythema, fever, pruritus, syncope, tachycardia, urticaria.

ANTIDOTE

Keep physician informed of all side effects. Discontinue drug if severe hypersensitivity reactions occur. Treat hypersensitivity reactions as indicated; may require epinephrine, airway management, oxygen, IV fluids, antihistamines (e.g., diphenhydramine), corticosteroids (e.g., hydrocortisone sodium succinate), and pressor amines (e.g., dopamine). Treat hypertension as indicated. Resuscitate as needed.

FERUMOXYTOL BBW

(**FER**-ue-**MOX**-i-tol)

Feraheme

Antianemic
Iron supplement

pH 6 to 8

USUAL DOSE

An initial IV dose of 510 mg followed by a second IV dose of 510 mg 3 to 8 days later. Administer as an IV infusion over at least 15 minutes. After 1 month and an evaluation of the hematologic response, the recommended dose may be repeated in patients with persistent or recurrent iron deficiency anemia. Administer to hemodialysis patients at least 1 hour into dialysis session, after blood pressure has stabilized. Patient should receive infusion in a reclined or semi-reclined position; see Monitor. See Drug/Lab Interactions.

DOSE ADJUSTMENTS

No dose adjustment is required and no gender differences have been observed.

DILUTION

Available in a single-use vial containing 510 mg of elemental iron in 17 mL (30 mg/mL of elemental iron). Black to reddish brown in color. This single dose must be further diluted in 50 to 200 mL of NS or D5W for administration as an IV infusion.

Filters: Specific information not available.

Storage: Store unopened vials at CRT. When added to D5W or NS at concentrations of 2 to 8 mg of elemental iron/mL, may be stored at RT for up to 4 hours or refrigerated for up to 48 hours. However, immediate use is preferred. Discard unused portion.

COMPATIBILITY

Compatibility information not available from manufacturer; consult a pharmacist. Given as an IV infusion. Consider flushing the IV line with NS before and after infusion.

RATE OF ADMINISTRATION

Administer as an IV infusion over at least 15 minutes.

ACTIONS

An iron-replacement product. A superparamagnetic iron oxide that is coated with a carbohydrate shell. The shell helps to isolate the bioactive iron from plasma components until the iron-carbohydrate complex enters the reticuloendothelial system macrophages of the liver, spleen, and bone marrow. The iron is released from the complex within the macrophages and then either enters the intracellular storage iron pool (e.g., ferritin) or is transferred to plasma transferrin for transport to erythroid precursor cells for incorporation into hemoglobin. Exhibits dose-dependent, capacity-limited elimination from plasma with a half-life of approximately 15 hours.

INDICATIONS AND USES

Treatment of iron deficiency anemia (IDA) in adult patients who have intolerance to oral iron or have had unsatisfactory response to oral iron or who have chronic kidney disease (CKD).

CONTRAINDICATIONS

Known hypersensitivity to ferumoxytol or any of its components. ■ History of allergic reaction to any intravenous iron product. ■ Should not be used in patients with evidence of iron overload or in patients with anemia not caused by iron deficiency.

PRECAUTIONS

Fatal and serious hypersensitivity reactions, including anaphylaxis, have been reported. Reactions have occurred after the first dose or subsequent doses of ferumoxytol in patients in whom a previous dose was tolerated. Patients with a history of multiple drug allergies may have a greater risk of anaphylaxis. Consider risk versus benefit of administration. ■ Facilities for monitoring the patient and responding to any medical emergency must be available. ■ Use only when truly indicated. Excessive therapy with parenteral iron can lead to excess storage of iron with the possibility of iatrogenic hemosiderosis. One source recommends discontinuing oral iron before administering parenteral iron. ■ Clinically significant hypotension has been reported. ■ May transiently affect the diagnostic ability of MRI studies. Anticipated MRI studies should be conducted before administration of ferumoxytol. Alteration of MRI studies may last for up to 3 months after the last ferumoxytol dose. See manufacturer's prescribing information if MRI studies must be obtained after ferumoxytol administration. Ferumoxytol does not interfere with x-ray, computed tomography (CT), positron emission tomography (PET), single photon emission computed tomography (SPECT), ultrasound, or nuclear medicine imaging.

Monitor: Patient should be in a reclined or semi-reclined position during and after administration to prevent postural hypotension. ■ BP should be stable in patients receiving hemodialysis before dose is administered. ■ Monitor BP and HR during and after dose administration. ■ Observe for hypersensitivity reactions (e.g., anaphylaxis, cardiac or cardiopulmonary arrest, clinically significant hypotension, pruritus, rash, syncope, unresponsiveness, urticaria, or wheezing) during and for at least 30 minutes and until clinically stable after administration. ■ Evaluate hematologic response (hemoglobin, hematocrit, ferritin, iron, and transferrin saturation) at least 1 month after the second dose. Regularly monitor response during parenteral iron therapy. Avoid evaluation of therapy immediately after therapy. In the 24 hours following administration, laboratory assays may overestimate serum iron and transferrin-bound iron by also measuring the iron in the ferumoxytol complex.

Patient Education: Review FDA-approved patient package insert. ■ Review any possible reactions to past parenteral iron therapy. ■ Promptly report S/S of a hypersensitivity reaction (e.g., hives, itching, rash, shortness of breath, wheezing).

Maternal/Child: Use during pregnancy only if potential benefit to the mother justifies the potential risk to the fetus. There are risks to the mother and fetus associated with untreated iron deficiency anemia. Adverse outcomes may include maternal postpartum anemia, preterm delivery, and low birth weight. ■ There are no data on the presence of ferumoxytol in human milk, the effects on the breast-fed infant, or the effects on milk production. Consider risk versus benefit. ■ Safety and effectiveness for use in pediatric patients not established.

Elderly: No overall differences in safety and efficacy were observed between older and younger patients. However, greater sensitivity of older patients cannot be ruled out. Elderly patients with multiple or serious comorbidities who experience hypersensitivity reactions and/or hypotension after administration of ferumoxytol may have more severe outcomes. Consider risk versus benefit of administration.

DRUG/LAB INTERACTIONS

Drug-drug interaction studies have not been conducted. ■ May reduce the absorption of concomitantly administered **oral iron** preparations. ■ Allow at least 30 minutes between administration of ferumoxytol and administration of other medications that could potentially cause serious hypersensitivity reactions and/or hypotension (e.g., chemotherapeutic agents or monoclonal antibodies).

SIDE EFFECTS

The most common side effects are constipation, diarrhea, dizziness, headache, hypotension, nausea, and peripheral edema. Serious side effects may include hypersensitivity reactions (e.g., anaphylaxis, pruritus, rash, urticaria, or wheezing) and hypotension. Other reported side effects are abdominal pain, back pain, chest pain, cough, dyspnea, ecchymosis, edema, fatigue, fever, infusion site swelling, muscle spasm, vomiting.

Post-Marketing: Anaphylactic/anaphylactoid reactions (fatal, life-threatening, or serious), angioedema, cardiac/cardiopulmonary arrest, CHF, cyanosis, hypotension (clinically significant), ischemic myocardial events, loss of consciousness, syncope, tachycardia/rhythm abnormalities, and unresponsiveness.

ANTIDOTE

Notify the physician of significant side effects. Treat hypersensitivity reactions, or resuscitate as necessary. Epinephrine and diphenhydramine should always be available. In overdose, monitor CBC, iron studies, vital signs, blood gases, glucose, and electrolytes. Maintain fluid and electrolyte balance. Consultation with a poison control center may be warranted. Deferoxamine is an iron chelating agent and may be useful in iron toxicity or overdose. Dialysis will not remove iron alone but will remove the iron deferoxamine complex and is indicated if oliguria or anuria is present.

FIBRINOGEN CONCENTRATE (HUMAN)

Coagulation factor I

(fi-**BRIN**-oh-gen **KON**-sen-trayt)

RiaSTAP

USUAL DOSE

Individualize dosing, duration of dosing, and frequency of administration based on the extent of bleeding, laboratory values, and clinical condition. A target fibrinogen level of 100 mg/dL should be maintained until hemostasis is obtained.

Dose when baseline fibrinogen level IS known: Calculate individually for each patient based on the target plasma fibrinogen level, which is based on the type of bleeding, actual measured plasma fibrinogen level, and body weight using the following formula:

$$\text{Dose (mg/kg)} = \frac{(\text{Target level [mg/dL]} - \text{Measured level [mg/dL]})}{1.7 \ (\text{mg/dL per mg/kg body weight})}$$

Dose when baseline fibrinogen level IS NOT known: 70 mg/kg.

DILUTION

Available as a single-use vial containing 900 to 1,300 mg lyophilized fibrinogen concentrate powder. Fibrinogen potency for each lot is printed on the vial label and carton. Bring fibrinogen concentrate to room temperature. Reconstitute with 50 mL SWFI. Gently swirl until the powder is completely dissolved. Solution should be colorless and may be clear or slightly opalescent. Do not shake. Administer within 24 hours of reconstitution.

Filters: Specific information not available.

Storage: Store in carton between 2° and 25° C (36° and 77° F). Protect from light. Do not freeze in powder or reconstituted form. Do not use beyond expiration date on vial. Reconstituted solution is stable for 24 hours at CRT. Discard partially used vials.

COMPATIBILITY

Manufacturer states, "Do not mix with other medicinal products or intravenous solutions, and should be administered through a separate injection site."

RATE OF ADMINISTRATION

A single dose is to be given at a rate not to exceed 5 mL/min.

ACTIONS

Fibrinogen (factor I) is a soluble plasma glycoprotein made from cryoprecipitate derived from pooled human plasma. It is a physiologic substrate of three enzymes—thrombin, factor XIIIa, and plasmin—and is an essential part of the coagulation cascade required for forming blood clots and preventing bleeding. In patients with congenital fibrinogen deficiency, it replaces the missing or low coagulation factor (normal levels range from 200 to 400 mg/dL). Less than 100 mg/dL can be associated with spontaneous bleeding; without treatment, these patients are at risk for potentially life-threatening bleeding. Half-life is 78.7 $\pm$ 18.13 hours (range 55.73 to 117.26 hours).

INDICATIONS AND USES
Treatment of acute bleeding episodes in patients with congenital fibrinogen deficiency, including afibrinogenemia and hypofibrinogenemia. ▪ Not indicated for use in dysfibrinogenemia (malfunction of fibrinogen in the blood).

CONTRAINDICATIONS
Known hypersensitivity to fibrinogen concentrate or its components.

PRECAUTIONS
For IV use only. ▪ Administration under the supervision of a physician is recommended. ▪ Severe hypersensitivity reactions, including anaphylaxis, may occur. Administer in a facility capable of monitoring the patient and responding to any medical emergency. Epinephrine should be immediately available. ▪ Thrombotic events (e.g., myocardial infarction, pulmonary embolism, arterial thrombosis, deep vein thrombosis) have occurred in patients with congenital fibrinogen deficiency with or without the use of fibrinogen concentrate therapy. Consider benefit versus risk. ▪ Made from human plasma and may contain infectious agents (e.g., HIV, Creutzfeldt-Jakob disease, hepatitis B, or hepatitis C). Numerous steps in the manufacturing process are used to reduce the potential for infection.

Monitor: Monitor fibrinogen levels during treatment. A target fibrinogen level of 100 mg/dL should be maintained until hemostasis is obtained. ▪ Observe for symptoms of a hypersensitivity reaction (e.g., chest pain, dizziness, dyspnea, fever, flushing, hypotension, nausea, pruritus, rash, rigors, urticaria). ▪ Monitor patients for S/S of thrombotic events.

Patient Education: Inform patient of risks for infectious agent transmission and of safety precautions taken during the manufacturing process. ▪ Promptly report symptoms of a hypersensitivity reaction (e.g., difficulty breathing, feeling faint, hives, itching, tightness in the chest, wheezing). ▪ Promptly report symptoms of a possible thrombosis (e.g., altered consciousness or speech; loss of sensation or motor power; new-onset swelling and pain in abdomen, chest, or limbs; shortness of breath).

Maternal/Child: Category C: safety and effectiveness for use during pregnancy, labor and delivery, and breast-feeding not studied; use only if clearly needed. ▪ Clinical studies included 5 patients between 8 and 16 years of age; a shorter half-life and faster clearance were noted in these patients.

Elderly: Numbers in clinical studies are insufficient to determine whether the elderly respond differently than younger subjects.

DRUG/LAB INTERACTIONS
No drug interaction studies have been conducted.

SIDE EFFECTS
The most common side effects reported include chills, fever, headache, hypersensitivity reactions, nausea, and vomiting. The most serious side effects include hypersensitivity reactions (e.g., anaphylaxis, dyspnea, hives, hypotension, rash, tightness of the chest, urticaria, and wheezing) and thrombotic events (e.g., myocardial infarction, pulmonary embolism, arterial thrombosis, deep vein thrombosis).

ANTIDOTE
Keep the physician informed of all side effects. Interrupt or discontinue injection, if indicated, until symptoms subside; then resume at a tolerated rate. ▪ Discontinue fibrinogen concentrate if anaphylaxis or thrombotic events occur. Treat thrombotic events as indicated. Treat anaphylaxis with oxygen, epinephrine, antihistamines (e.g., diphenhydramine), vasopressors (e.g., dopamine), corticosteroids, albuterol, IV fluids, and ventilation equipment as indicated. Resuscitate as necessary.

FILGRASTIM ▪ FILGRASTIM-aafi[a] ▪ FILGRASTIM-sndz[a]

Colony-stimulating factor
Hematopoietic agent

(fill-**GRASS**-tim)

G-CSF, Human Granulocyte Colony-Stimulating Factor, Neupogen ▪ Nivestym[a] ▪ Releuko[a] ▪ Zarxio[a]

pH 4

USUAL DOSE

Filgrastim-aafi[a] (Nivestym) and Filgrastim-sndz (Zarxio)[a] and filgrastim-ayow (Releuko) are bio-similar drugs of filgrastim (Neupogen). **Unless specifically stated otherwise, monograph information and the use of the name** *filgrastim* or *filgrastim product(s)* **applies to all formulations.**

Filgrastim products: Do not use 24 hours before to 24 hours after the administration of cytotoxic chemotherapy because of the potential sensitivity of rapidly dividing myeloid cells to cytotoxic chemotherapy. Safety and effectiveness for use with concurrent radiation therapy have not been evaluated; simultaneous use should be avoided.

Pretreatment: Baseline studies indicated and diagnosis confirmation may be indicated; see Monitor.

Cancer patients receiving myelosuppressive chemotherapy or induction and/or consolidation chemotherapy for acute myeloid leukemia (AML): The recommended starting dose is 5 mcg/kg/24 hr administered as a single daily injection by subcutaneous injection, short intravenous infusion, or continuous intravenous infusion. Administer daily for up to 2 weeks or until the ANC has reached 10,000/mm³ following the expected chemotherapy-induced neutrophil nadir. Duration of therapy needed may be dependent on the myelosuppressive potential of the chemotherapy regimen employed. Expect a transient increase in neutrophil counts 1 to 2 days after initiation of therapy. In clinical trials, efficacy was observed at doses of 4 to 8 mcg/kg/day. See Monitor.

Bone marrow transplant (BMT): 10 mcg/kg/24 hr as an IV infusion over no longer than 24 hours. Give the first dose at least 24 hours after cytotoxic chemotherapy and 24 hours after bone marrow infusion.

Nivestym and Zarxio: Direct administration of less than 0.3 mL (180 mcg) is not recommended due to the potential for dosing errors. The spring mechanism of the BD UltraSafe Passive™ Needle Guard apparatus interferes with the visibility of the graduated markings corresponding to 0.1 mL and 0.2 mL.

DOSE ADJUSTMENTS

Consider dose escalation in increments of 5 mcg/kg for each chemotherapy cycle, according to the duration and severity of the ANC nadir. Discontinue filgrastim if the ANC surpasses 10,000/mm³ after the chemotherapy-induced ANC nadir has occurred. ▪ During neutrophil recovery after BMT, titrate the daily dose against the neutrophil response as shown in the following chart.

Filgrastim Dose Adjustments During Neutrophil Recovery Following a Bone Marrow Transplant (BMT)	
Absolute Neutrophil Count (ANC)	**Filgrastim Dose**
When ANC >1,000/mm³ for 3 consecutive days	Reduce to 5 mcg/kg/day[a]
Then: If ANC remains >1,000/mm³ for 3 more consecutive days	Discontinue filgrastim[a]
Then: If ANC decreases to <1,000/mm³	Resume at 5 mcg/kg/day

[a]If ANC decreases to less than 1,000/mm³ at any time during the 5 mcg/kg/day administration, increase filgrastim to 10 mcg/kg/day; the above steps should then be followed.

▪ Consider dose reduction and/or interruption of therapy in patients who develop glomerulonephritis or cutaneous vasculitis thought to be related to filgrastim therapy; see Antidote.

[a]Please see p. xi for more information on biosimilars.

DILUTION

Neupogen and Nivestym: Available as a single-dose vial with either 300 mcg/mL or 480 mcg/1.6 mL and as a prefilled syringe with an UltraSafe Needle Guard® as 300 mcg/0.5 mL or 480 mcg/0.8 mL.

Zarxio: Available as a prefilled syringe with an UltraSafe Passive™ Needle Guard as 300 mcg/0.5 mL or 480 mcg/0.8mL.

Filgrastim products: Remove from refrigerator to allow to warm to room temperature for a minimum of 30 minutes and a maximum of 24 hours.

Neupogen and Nivestym (vials): Confirm expiration date to ensure valid product. Avoid shaking. Contains no preservatives; use sterile technique, entering vial only once to withdraw a single dose. May dilute with D5W to concentrations of 5 to 300 mcg/mL. With concentrations from 5 to 15 mcg/mL, filgrastim must be combined with albumin to a final concentration of 2 mg/mL to prevent adsorption to plastic (e.g., add 2 mL of 5% albumin to each 50 mL of D5W). Discard any unused portion. Should be clear and colorless. Do not dilute to less than 5 mcg/mL.

Filgrastim products in prefilled syringes: Primarily used for SC administration; however, **Zarxio** syringes may be diluted for IV use in D5W to concentrations between 5 and 15 mcg/mL. With concentrations from 5 to 15 mcg/mL, Zarxio also must be combined with albumin to a final concentration of 2 mg/mL to prevent adsorption to plastic (e.g., add 2 mL of 5% albumin to each 50 mL of D5W). Do not dilute to less than 5 mcg/mL.

Storage: Before use, store filgrastim in refrigerator in original packaging to protect from light. Avoid freezing; if frozen, thaw in the refrigerator before administration. Discard if frozen more than once. Do not expose to direct sunlight. Avoid shaking. Discard any vial, diluted solution, or prefilled syringe left at RT for more than 24 hours, including administration time.

COMPATIBILITY

Filgrastim products: Manufacturers state, *"Do not dilute with saline at any time; product may precipitate."* **Incompatible** with saline.

Other sources suggest specific **compatibilities** for **Neupogen** dependent on concentration and manufacturer; consult a pharmacist.

RATE OF ADMINISTRATION

Intermittent infusion: A single dose over 15 to 30 minutes.

Continuous infusion: A single dose over no more than 24 hours. In all situations, flush IV line with D5W before and after administration.

ACTIONS

A human granulocyte colony-stimulating factor (G-CSF) manufactured by recombinant DNA technology. Colony-stimulating factors are glycoproteins that bind to specific hematopoietic cell surface receptors and stimulate proliferation, differentiation commitment, and some end-cell functional activation. Endogenous granulocyte colony-stimulating factor is produced by monocytes, fibroblasts, and endothelial cells. G-CSF is lineage-specific with selectivity for the neutrophil lineage. It regulates the production of neutrophils within the bone marrow and affects neutrophil progenitor proliferation, differentiation, and selected end-cell functions. In studies, administration of filgrastim products resulted in a dose-dependent increase in circulating neutrophil counts. Absolute monocyte counts also increased in a dose-dependent manner; however, the percentage of monocytes in the differential count remained within the normal range. With discontinuation of therapy, neutrophil counts returned to baseline in most cases within 4 days. The elimination half-life is approximately 3.5 hours. Filgrastim and filgrastim-sndz have been shown to be safe and effective in accelerating the recovery of neutrophil counts following a variety of chemotherapy regimens. In studies, benefits to therapy were shown to be prevention of infection as manifested by febrile neutropenia, decreased hospitalization, and decreased IV antibiotic usage. The incidence, severity, and duration of severe neutropenia (absolute neutrophil count [ANC] less than 500/mm^3) following chemotherapy were all significantly reduced.

INDICATIONS AND USES

Decrease the incidence of infection (febrile neutropenia) in patients with nonmyeloid malignancies receiving myelosuppressive anticancer drugs associated with a significant incidence of severe neutropenia with fever. ■ Reduce the time to neutrophil recovery and the duration of fever, following induction or consolidation chemotherapy treatment of adults with AML. ■ Decrease duration of neutropenia and related clinical problems (e.g., febrile neutropenia) in patients with nonmyeloid malignancies receiving myeloablative chemotherapy followed by BMT. ■ Used SC to treat severe chronic neutropenia (e.g., congenital, cyclic, or idiopathic) after all diseases associated with neutropenia have been ruled out. Administered chronically to reduce the incidence and duration of sequelae of neutropenia (e.g., fever, infections, oropharyngeal ulcers) in symptomatic patients. ■ Used SC to mobilize autologous hematopoietic progenitor cells into the peripheral blood for collection by leukapheresis with transplantation after myeloablative chemotherapy.

Neupogen: Used SC to increase survival in patients acutely exposed to myelosuppressive doses of radiation. (Efficacy studies could not be conducted in humans with acute radiation syndrome for ethical and feasibility reasons. Approval of this indication was based on efficacy studies conducted in animals and on data supporting the use of filgrastim for other approved indications.)

CONTRAINDICATIONS

Serious hypersensitivity reaction to human granulocyte colony-stimulating factors such as filgrastim or pegfilgrastim.

PRECAUTIONS

Should be administered under the direction of a physician knowledgeable about appropriate use for each indication (e.g., expert in bone marrow transplantation). ■ Frequently given by SC injection. ■ Use extreme caution in any malignancy with myeloid characteristics. The possibility that filgrastim can act as a growth factor for any tumor type, particularly myeloid malignancies, cannot be excluded. Safety in chronic myeloid leukemia (CML) and myelodysplasia has not been established. ■ When filgrastim is used to mobilize peripheral blood progenitor cells (PBPCs), tumor cells may be released from the marrow and subsequently collected in the leukapheresis product. The effect of reinfusion of tumor cells has not been well studied. Data are inconclusive. ■ Acute respiratory distress syndrome (ARDS) has been reported. ■ Hypersensitivity reactions have been reported. Majority have occurred with initial exposure. Allergic reactions, including anaphylaxis, can recur within days after the discontinuation of initial antiallergic treatment; see Monitor. ■ Splenic rupture has been reported; fatalities have occurred. ■ Glomerulonephritis has occurred in patients receiving filgrastim. ■ Severe sickle cell crises have been reported with the use of filgrastim in patients with sickle cell trait or sickle cell disease. Fatalities have occurred. Consider risk versus benefit. ■ Capillary leak syndrome (CLS) has been reported. Episodes vary in frequency and severity and may be life threatening if treatment is delayed. ■ Use caution in patients with congenital severe chronic neutropenia (SCN); risk of developing cytogenetic abnormalities, myelodysplastic syndromes (MDS), and acute myelogenous leukemia (AML) may be increased. If a patient with SCN develops abnormal cytogenetics or myelodysplasia, the risk versus benefit of continuing filgrastim therapy should be considered. ■ Alveolar hemorrhage manifesting as pulmonary infiltrates and hemoptysis and requiring hospitalization has been reported in healthy donors undergoing peripheral blood progenitor cell (PBPC) mobilization. Hemoptysis resolved when filgrastim was discontinued. Use of filgrastim for PBPC mobilization in healthy donors is not an approved indication. ■ Moderate to severe cutaneous vasculitis has been reported in patients treated with filgrastim. Most reports involved patients with SCN receiving long-term filgrastim therapy. ■ As with any therapeutic protein, potential for immunogenicity exists. ■ Thrombocytopenia has been reported; see Monitor. ■ Removable needle cap of Zarxio prefilled syringes contains latex. Safe use in latex-sensitive individuals has not been studied. Nivestym needle caps are not made with natural rubber latex.

Monitor: Obtain a CBC and platelet count before chemotherapy begins and twice weekly thereafter to monitor the neutrophil count and to avoid leukocytosis. ■ Increase frequency of monitoring of CBC and platelet count after bone marrow infusion. ■ Because higher doses of chemotherapy may be tolerated, side effects associated with the chemotherapeutic drug may be more pronounced; observe carefully. ■ Observe for S/S of hypersensitivity reactions (e.g., hypotension, rash, tightness of the chest, urticaria, wheezing). ■ Evaluate patients complaining of left upper abdominal pain and/or shoulder pain for an enlarged spleen or splenic rupture. ■ Monitor respiratory status. Evaluate for ARDS if fever, lung infiltrates, or respiratory distress develop. ■ Monitor for S/S of CLS (e.g., edema, hypoalbuminemia, hypotension, and hemoconcentration). ■ Monitor for glomerulonephritis. Has been diagnosed based on the development of azotemia, hematuria, and proteinuria and with renal biopsy. ■ See Precautions.

Patient Education: Promptly report any symptoms of infection (e.g., fever), abdominal or left shoulder pain, bruising, hypersensitivity reaction (itching, redness, swelling at the injection site) or dyspnea, with or without fever. ■ Promptly report symptoms of glomerulonephritis (e.g., swelling of face or ankles, dark-colored urine or blood in the urine, decrease in urine production) or cutaneous vasculitis (e.g., purpura, erythema). ■ Promptly report symptoms of cutaneous vasculitis (e.g., erythema, purpura) or aortitis (abdominal pain, back pain, fever, malaise). ■ May be self-injected SC by the patient at home; requires instruction. Literature includes a patient handout.

Maternal/Child: An association with filgrastim use during pregnancy and major birth defects, miscarriage, or adverse maternal or fetal outcomes has not been seen in observational studies. ■ Secreted in breast milk but not orally absorbed by the neonate. Consider risks versus benefits. ■ Safety and effectiveness for use in pediatric patients with severe chronic neutropenia (SCN) have been established. Experience in pediatric patients similar to adult population in patients with cancer. May cause bone pain, fever, or rash. ■ The relationship is unclear; however, pediatric patients with congenital neutropenia have developed cytogenetic abnormalities and have undergone transformation to MDS and AML while receiving chronic filgrastim therapy.

Elderly: Age-related differences in safety and efficacy have not been observed.

DRUG/LAB INTERACTIONS

Filgrastim products: Interaction with other drugs has not been evaluated. ■ Increased hematopoietic activity of the bone marrow in response to growth factor therapy has been associated with transient positive bone-imaging changes. Consider when interpreting **bone-imaging results.** ■ Increases in **LDH, serum alkaline phosphatase, and serum uric acid** have been seen.

SIDE EFFECTS

Cancer patients receiving myelosuppressive chemotherapy: Most common adverse reactions were cough, dyspnea, fever, pain, and rash.

Patients with acute myeloid leukemia (AML) receiving induction or consolidation chemotherapy: Most common adverse reactions were epistaxis, pain, and rash. Bone marrow transplant (BMT): Most common adverse reaction was rash.

Other reported reactions included arthralgia, back pain, bone pain, chest pain, dizziness, fatigue, headache, increased alkaline phosphatase and lactate dehydrogenase, nausea, pain in an extremity, and thrombocytopenia. Hypersensitivity reactions (itching, redness, swelling at the injection site) have occurred; anaphylaxis is possible. Complaints of dose-related bone pain are common and may require analgesics. Serious side effects include acute respiratory distress syndrome (ARDS), alveolar hemorrhage and hemoptysis, capillary leak syndrome, cutaneous vasculitis, glomerulonephritis, leukocytosis, sickle cell disorders, splenic rupture, and thrombocytopenia.

Post-Marketing: Acute respiratory distress syndrome (ARDS), alveolar hemorrhage and hemoptysis, anaphylaxis, aortitis, capillary leak syndrome, cutaneous vasculitis, glomerulonephritis, leukocytosis, splenic rupture, splenomegaly, Sweet's syndrome (acute febrile neutrophilic dermatosis), and thrombocytopenia. Decreased bone density and osteoporosis have been reported in pediatric patients with severe chronic neutropenia (SCN) receiving chronic therapy.

ANTIDOTE

Notify physician promptly if any signs of infection (fever) or other potential side effects occur. Monitor potential leukocytosis with twice-weekly CBCs. Discontinue therapy after ANC surpasses 10,000/mm^3 and the chemotherapy nadir has occurred. Discontinue filgrastim and notify physician immediately if a generalized hypersensitivity reaction should occur. Treat hypersensitivity reactions as indicated. Withhold or discontinue for other side effects (e.g., ARDS, hemoptysis). Patients who experience CLS should receive standard symptomatic treatment, which may include the need for intensive care. Hold filgrastim therapy in patients with cutaneous vasculitis. May restart at reduced dose when symptoms resolve and ANC has decreased. Consider dose reduction and/or interruption of therapy in patients who develop glomerulonephritis. Discontinue filgrastim if leukocyte count rises to greater than 100,000/mm^3 during administration of filgrastim for PBPC mobilization or if aortitis is suspected.

FISH OIL TRIGLYCERIDES INJECTABLE EMULSION

Nutritional supplement (fatty acid)

(fish oyl tri-glyc-er-ides in-**JEK**-tuh-buhl e-**MUL**-shun)

Omegaven   pH 6 to 9

PEDIATRIC DOSE

Pretreatment: Baseline studies indicated; see Monitor. Correct severe water and electrolyte disorders before administration.

Dose depends on energy requirements, which may be influenced by patient's clinical status, body weight, tolerance, and ability to metabolize and eliminate lipids. The energy supplied by dextrose and amino acids from parenteral nutrition (PN), oral or enteral nutrition, and lipid-based medications must also be taken into account. May be administered alone or as part of a PN admixture. May be infused through a peripheral or central line; see Precautions.

Fish oil triglycerides: 1 Gm/kg/day is the recommended and maximum daily dose. Initiate as soon as direct bilirubin (DBil) or conjugated bilirubin levels are 2 mg/dL or greater in pediatric patients who are expected to be PN-dependent for at least 2 weeks. Administer until DBil levels are less than 2 mg/dL or until the patient no longer requires PN.

DOSE ADJUSTMENTS

If hypertriglyceridemia (triglycerides greater than 250 mg/dL in neonates and infants or greater than 400 mg/dL in older pediatric patients) develops once fish oil triglycerides has been initiated at the recommended dose, consider stopping the administration for 4 hours and then obtain a repeat serum triglyceride level. Resume fish oil triglycerides based on new result as indicated. ■ In patients with elevated triglyceride levels, consider other reasons for hypertriglyceridemia (e.g., renal disease, other drugs). If triglycerides remain at elevated levels, consider a reduced dose of 0.5 to 0.75 Gm/kg/day with an incremental increase to 1 Gm/kg/day.

DILUTION

Fish oil triglycerides (Omegaven) is a white, homogenous, sterile emulsion supplied in 5 Gm/50 mL and 10 Gm/100 mL single-dose glass bottles.

Fish oil triglycerides as a single agent: Before infusion, visually inspect for particulate matter and discoloration; discard if observed. Gently invert the bottle before use. Emulsion should be homogeneous and the container undamaged. Do not use if there appears to be an oiling out of the emulsion. See Rate of Administration for tubing, filter, and connection requirements and specific procedures. Hang the bottle using the attached hanger and start infusion.

Fish oil triglycerides as a component of parenteral nutrition (PN): Follow manufacturer's specific instructions for preparation when used in combination with dextrose and amino acids. See Rate of Administration.

Filters: Use of a 1.2-micron in-line filter required.

Storage: Store below 25° C (77° F). Avoid excessive heat. Do not freeze. If accidentally frozen, discard product. Once connected to infusion set, use immediately and complete within 12 hours when using a Y-connector and within 24 hours when used as part of an admixture. Admixtures should be used immediately but may be stored for up to 6 hours at RT or up to 24 hours under refrigeration. Complete infusion within 24 hours after removal from storage. For single use only; discard any unused portion.

COMPATIBILITY

Manufacturer states, "Do not use infusion sets and lines that contain di-2-ethylhexyl phthalate (DEHP). Infusion sets that contain polyvinyl chloride (PVC) components have DEHP as a plasticizer." Lipids may extract phthalates from phthalate-plasticized PVC infusion sets and lines. Emulsions are destabilized by excessive acidity (such as a pH less than 5) and by inappropriate electrolyte content. Divalent cations (e.g., calcium and magnesium) have been shown to cause emulsion instability.

RATE OF ADMINISTRATION

May be infused through a peripheral or central line. Solutions with an osmolarity of 900 mOsm/L or greater must be infused through a central vein. Administer through a dedicated peripheral or central line with a 1.2-micron in-line filter via a Y-connector located closest to the infusion site. Flow rates of both solutions (fat emulsion and dextrose–amino acid products) should be controlled by separate infusion pumps. Avoid multiple connections; do not connect multiple medications in series. Turn off pump before the bottle runs dry. A vented infusion set is used when fish oil emulsion is infused from the bottle. Use caution to avoid air embolism.

Fish oil triglycerides: Initial rate of infusion should not exceed 0.05 mL/min for the first 15 to 30 minutes. If tolerated, gradually increase until reaching the required rate after 30 minutes. Maximum infusion rate should not exceed 1.5 mL/kg/hr, corresponding to 0.15 Gm/kg/hr. The recommended duration for infusion is between 8 and 24 hours depending on the clinical situation.

ACTIONS

A sterile, nonpyrogenic, white, homogenous emulsion for IV infusion that provides a biologically utilizable source of calories and essential fatty acids. Fatty acids serve as an important substrate for energy production. Fatty acids are also important for membrane structure and function, as precursors for bioactive molecules (such as prostaglandins), and as regulators of gene expression. Total energy content is 112 kcal/100 mL (1.12 kcal/mL), including lipids, phospholipids, and glycerol. Approximate osmolarity is 342 mOsm/kg water (which represents an osmolarity of 273 mOsm/L).

INDICATIONS AND USES

A source of calories and fatty acids in pediatric patients with parenteral nutrition–associated cholestasis (PNAC).

Limitations of use: Not indicated for the prevention of PNAC. It has not been proven that fish oil triglycerides prevents PNAC in PN-dependent patients. ■ It has not been demonstrated that clinical outcomes observed in patients treated with this product are a result of the omega-6:omega-3 fatty acid ratio of the product.

CONTRAINDICATIONS

Known hypersensitivity to fish or egg protein or to any of the active ingredients or excipients. ■ Severe hemorrhagic disorders due to a potential effect on platelet aggregation. ■ Severe hyperlipidemia or severe disorders of lipid metabolism characterized by hypertriglyceridemia (serum triglyceride concentrations greater than 1,000 mg/dL).

PRECAUTIONS

Can be administered alone or as part of a PN admixture by central or peripheral IV infusion. When administered with dextrose and amino acids, the choice of a central or peripheral venous route should depend on the osmolarity of the final infusate. Solutions with an osmolarity of 900 mOsm/L or greater must be infused through a central vein. ▪ Deaths in preterm infants due to pulmonary lipid accumulation after infusion of soybean oil–based IV lipid emulsions (e.g., Intralipid) have been reported. The risk of pulmonary lipid accumulation with fish oil triglycerides is unknown. ▪ Preterm and small-for-gestational age infants have poor clearance of IV lipid emulsion and increased free fatty acid plasma levels following lipid emulsion infusion. Consider administration of less than the maximum recommended dose in these patients to decrease the likelihood of IV fat overload; see Monitor and Dose Adjustments. ▪ Hypersensitivity reactions may occur. ▪ Patients requiring PN may be at higher risk for infection (e.g., septicemia) due to malnutrition-associated immunosuppression, long-term use and poor maintenance of IV catheters, or immunosuppressive effects of other conditions or concomitant drugs. In addition, lipid emulsions can support microbial growth and are an independent risk factor for the development of bloodstream infections. ▪ Fat overload syndrome has been reported (rare). Most frequently observed when the recommended lipid dose is exceeded but has occurred with correct dosing. Usually reversible when lipid emulsion infusion is stopped; see Monitor. ▪ Administration of PN to severely undernourished patients may result in refeeding syndrome. ▪ Impaired lipid metabolism with hypertriglyceridemia may occur in conditions such as inherited lipid disorders, obesity, diabetes mellitus, and metabolic syndrome. Serum triglyceride levels greater than 1,000 mg/dL have been associated with an increased risk of pancreatitis. ▪ This product contains no more than 25 mcg/L of aluminum. With prolonged PN and impaired kidney function, aluminum may reach toxic levels. Premature neonates are particularly at risk because of their immature kidneys and requirement for calcium and phosphate, which also contain aluminum. Research indicates that patients with impaired renal function who receive more than 4 to 5 mcg/kg/day of parenteral aluminum are at risk for developing CNS or bone toxicity associated with aluminum accumulation. May occur at lower rates of administration. ▪ Contains 0.15 to 0.3 mg/mL of di-alpha-tocopherol. Take this into account when determining the need for additional supplementation of vitamin E.

Monitor: Obtain baseline values of blood glucose, electrolytes, blood coagulation parameters, liver and kidney function, serum triglycerides, CBC, and platelet count and monitor throughout treatment. ▪ Correct severe water and electrolyte disorders. ▪ Monitor for laboratory evidence of essential fatty acid deficiency (EFAD) ▪ Measure serum osmolarity as indicated, especially in neonates. Discontinue use for significant abnormality. ▪ Use of aseptic technique imperative in the preparation and administration of Fish Oil Emulsion and in catheter placement and maintenance. ▪ Monitor for S/S of infection (e.g., chills, fever, laboratory test results that might indicate infection [including leukocytosis and hyperglycemia]) and frequently inspect the IV catheter insertion site for discharge, edema, and redness. ▪ Monitor for S/S of pleural or pericardial effusion. ▪ Monitor for S/S of a hypersensitivity reaction (e.g., altered mentation, bronchospasm, chills, cyanosis, dizziness, dyspnea, erythema, fever, flushing, headache, hypotension, hypoxia, nausea, rash, sweating, tachycardia, tachypnea, vomiting, urticaria). ▪ Monitor for S/S of fat overload syndrome. Reduced or limited ability to metabolize and clear lipids may result in a sudden deterioration of patient condition accompanied by anemia, coagulation disorders, deteriorating liver function, fever, hepatomegaly, hyperlipidemia, leukopenia, thrombocytopenia, and CNS manifestations (e.g., coma). Serum triglycerides and/or plasma free fatty acid levels are monitored to assess infant's ability to eliminate infused fat from the circulation; must clear between daily infusions; see Dose Adjustments. ▪ For severely undernourished patients initiating PN therapy, monitor closely for S/S of refeeding syndrome. May be characterized by the intracellular shift of potassium, phosphorus, and magnesium; thiamine deficiency; and fluid retention. Initiate PN therapy slowly and monitor closely.

Patient Education: Inform parents that deaths in premature infants after infusion of IV fat emulsion have been reported. ■ Review other possible complications. ■ Laboratory monitoring is required. ■ Parents or pediatric patients should promptly report any S/S of hypersensitivity reactions (e.g., bronchospasm, chills, dyspnea, hypotension, hypoxia, nausea, rash, urticaria). ■ Parents or pediatric patients should promptly report any S/S of infection (e.g., fever, chills, pain at infusion site).

Maternal/Child: Not intended for use in pregnancy, labor, or lactation. No data available. ■ Safety and effectiveness established for use in pediatric patients; see Precautions.

DRUG/LAB INTERACTIONS

Prolonged bleeding time has been reported in patients taking **antiplatelet agents** or **anticoagulants** (e.g., heparin) **and oral omega-3 fatty acids.** Prolongation of bleeding times in studies did not exceed normal limits, and there were no clinically significant bleeding episodes. Periodic monitoring of bleeding time in patients receiving concomitant antiplatelet agents or anticoagulants is recommended. ■ May interfere with some **laboratory blood tests** (e.g., bilirubin, hemoglobin, lactate dehydrogenase, and oxygen saturation) if blood is sampled before lipids have cleared from the bloodstream. Lipids are normally cleared after 5 to 6 hours once the lipid infusion is stopped.

SIDE EFFECTS

Agitation, apnea, bradycardia, viral infections, and vomiting are most common. Abscess, erythema, hypertonia, incision site erythema, neutropenia, and rash have been reported. Serious adverse reactions may include death due to pulmonary lipid accumulation, hypersensitivity reactions, infections, fat overload syndrome, refeeding syndrome, hypertriglyceridemia, and aluminum toxicity.

Post-Marketing: Life-threatening hemorrhage following a central venous catheter change was reported in one infant with no prior history of bleeding, coagulopathy, or portal hypertension.

ANTIDOTE

Notify physician of all side effects. Many will be treated symptomatically. See Dose Adjustments. In the event of a hypersensitivity reaction, stop the infusion immediately and initiate appropriate treatment and supportive measures. For accidental overdose, stop the infusion. Obtain blood sample for inspection of serum triglyceride concentration. Repeat blood samples until the lipid has cleared. Lipids are not dialyzable.

FLUCONAZOLE

(flew-**KON**-ah-zohl)

Diflucan

Antifungal

(azole derivative)

pH 3.5 to 8

USUAL DOSE

Daily dose should be based on the infecting organism and the patient's response to therapy. Treatment should be continued until clinical parameters or laboratory tests indicate that active fungal infection has subsided. IV dose has been used for a maximum of 14 days. Plasma levels are similar with IV or oral, so oral dose can replace IV dose at any time. See Monitor.

Pretreatment: Baseline studies indicated; see Monitor. See Maternal/Child.

Oropharyngeal candidiasis: Initial dose of 200 mg followed by 100 mg/day for a minimum of 14 days. PO maintenance therapy usually required in AIDS patients to prevent relapse.

Esophageal candidiasis: Initial dose of 200 mg followed by 100 mg/day for a minimum of 21 days and for at least 2 weeks after symptoms subside. Up to 400 mg/24 hr may be used.

Urinary tract or peritoneal candidiasis: 50 to 200 mg/day has been used.

Systemic candidiasis: Optimum therapeutic dose and duration of therapy not established. Doses up to 400 mg/day have been used.

Treatment of acute cryptococcal meningitis: Initial dose of 400 mg followed by 200 mg/day for a minimum of 10 to 12 weeks after CSF culture becomes negative.

Suppression of cryptococcal meningitis: 200 mg/day. Usually required in patients with AIDS to prevent relapse.

Prevention of candidiasis in bone marrow transplant: 400 mg/day. If severe neutropenia (less than 500/mm³) is expected, begin fluconazole prophylaxis several days ahead of expected neutropenia. Continue for 7 days after neutrophils reach 1,000/mm³.

PEDIATRIC DOSE
Experience with pediatric patients is limited; see Maternal/Child.

In pediatric patients, 3 mg/kg is equivalent to an adult dose of 100 mg, 6 mg/kg to 200 mg, and 12 mg/kg to 400 mg. Some older pediatric patients may have clearance similar to an adult. Do not exceed 600 mg/day.

Oropharyngeal candidiasis: Initial dose of 6 mg/kg of body weight followed by 3 mg/kg/day for a minimum of 14 days.

Esophageal candidiasis: Initial dose of 6 mg/kg of body weight followed by 3 mg/kg/day for a minimum of 21 days and for at least 2 weeks after symptoms subside. Up to 12 mg/kg has been used.

Systemic candidiasis: 6 to 12 mg/kg/day. See Comments in Usual Dose.

Treatment of acute cryptococcal meningitis: Initial dose of 12 mg/kg of body weight followed by 6 mg/kg/day for a minimum of 10 to 12 weeks after CSF culture becomes negative. Up to 12 mg/kg/day has been used.

Suppression of cryptococcal meningitis: 6 mg/kg/day.

NEONATAL DOSE
Experience is limited to pharmacokinetic studies in premature newborns; see Maternal/Child.

Birth to 2 weeks of age in premature neonates: Manufacturer suggests using pediatric doses and extending the intervals to once every 72 hours. Prolonged half-life is seen in premature newborns (gestational age 26 to 29 weeks). After 2 weeks, dose may be given every 24 hours.

DOSE ADJUSTMENTS
In all adult situations, the infecting organism and response to therapy may justify increased doses up to 400 mg daily. ▪ After the initial loading dose, reduce each dose by 50% in patients with a CrCl at or less than 50 mL/min. ▪ Give 100% of the recommended dose after each dialysis in patients receiving regular dialysis. ▪ Dose reduction in pediatric patients with renal insufficiency should parallel that recommended for adults. ▪ See Drug/Lab Interactions.

DILUTION
Packaged prediluted and ready for use as an iso-osmotic solution containing 2 mg/mL in both glass bottles and Viaflex Plus plastic containers. Do not remove moisture barrier overwrap of plastic container until ready for use. Tear overwrap down side at slit to open, and remove sterile inner bag. Plastic may appear somewhat opaque due to sterilization process but will clear. Squeeze inner bag firmly to check for leaks. Discard if leakage noted; sterility is impaired. Do not use if cloudy or precipitated.

Storage: Store glass bottles between 5° C (41° F) and 30° C (86° F); store plastic containers between 5° C (41° F) and 25° C (77° F). Protect both from freezing.

COMPATIBILITY
Manufacturer states, "Do not add supplementary medication."

Other sources suggest specific **compatibilities** dependent on concentration and manufacturer; consult a pharmacist.

RATE OF ADMINISTRATION
A single dose as a continuous infusion at a rate not to exceed 200 mg/hr. Do not use plastic containers in series connections; air embolism could result.

ACTIONS

A synthetic, broad-spectrum, bis-Triazole antifungal agent. Inhibits fungal growth of *Candida* and *Cryptococcus neoformans* by acting on a key enzyme and depriving the fungus of ergosterol; the cell membrane becomes unstable and can no longer function normally. Human sterol synthesis is not affected. Peak plasma concentrations achieved in 1 to 2 hours; half-life extends for 30 hours (range 20 to 50 hours). Administration of a loading dose (on Day 1) of twice the usual daily dose results in a plasma concentration close to steady state by Day 2 when given IV or PO. Penetrates into all body fluids studied (see prescribing information) in similar and effective concentrations and remains constant with daily single-dose administration. 80% excreted as unchanged drug and about 11% excreted as metabolites in the urine. Secreted in breast milk.

INDICATIONS AND USES

Oropharyngeal and esophageal candidiasis. ▪ Serious candidal infections, including GU tract infections, peritonitis, and systemic *Candida* infections including candidemia, disseminate candidiasis, and pneumonia. May be an appropriate and less toxic alternative to amphotericin B. ▪ Cryptococcal meningitis, including suppressive therapy to prevent relapse. ▪ Prevention of candidiasis in bone marrow transplant patients. ▪ Used orally for additional indications (e.g., candidiasis prophylaxis).

Unlabeled uses: Has been used in many other fungal or parasitic infections.

CONTRAINDICATIONS

Hypersensitivity to fluconazole or any of its components. Use caution in patients hypersensitive to other azoles (e.g., ketoconazole). ▪ Coadministration with drugs known to prolong the QT interval that are metabolized via the enzyme CYP3A4, such as erythromycin, pimozide, and quinidine.

PRECAUTIONS

For IV use only; do not give IM. ▪ Specimens for fungal culture and serologic and histopathologic testing should be obtained before therapy to isolate and identify causative organisms. Therapy may begin as soon as all specimens are obtained and before results are known. ▪ Inadequate treatment may lead to a recurrence of active infection; continue treatment until clinical parameters or laboratory tests indicate that active fungal infection has subsided. See specific recommendations in Usual Dose. ▪ Use caution in patients with pre-existing liver disease. ▪ Serious hepatotoxicity may occur. Causal relationship uncertain, but many patients are taking hepatotoxic drugs for treatment of malignancies and AIDS. Note any abnormal liver function tests (e.g., AST). If any clinical signs and symptoms consistent with liver disease develop, discontinue drug. Has caused deaths. ▪ Associated with prolongation of the QT interval. Rare cases of torsades de pointes have been reported. More common in seriously ill patients with multiple confounding factors, such as heart disease, electrolyte abnormalities, and concomitant medications that may have been contributory (e.g., Class IA antiarrhythmic agents [e.g., quinidine, procainamide] and Class III antiarrhythmic agents [e.g., amiodarone, sotalol]). ▪ Exfoliative skin disorders have been reported. Fatalities have occurred in patients with serious underlying diseases. ▪ Use with caution in patients with renal dysfunction; see Dose Adjustment. ▪ Anaphylaxis has been reported rarely. ▪ See Drug/Lab Interactions.

Monitor: Obtain baseline liver function tests and SCr; monitor periodically during treatment. ▪ Observe for S/S of hypersensitivity or skin reactions. Closely monitor patients with deep-seated fungal infections who develop rashes; discontinue fluconazole if lesions progress; see Antidote. ▪ Consider ECG monitoring in patients at risk for QT prolongation. ▪ See Drug/Lab Interactions.

Patient Education: May cause serious problems with selected medications; review prescription and nonprescription drugs with physician or pharmacist. ▪ May cause dizziness or seizures. Do not drive or operate hazardous machinery until effects of fluconazole are known.

Maternal/Child: Category D: safety for use in pregnancy and breast-feeding not established. There have been rare cases of distinct congenital anomalies in infants exposed in utero to high-dose maternal fluconazole during most or all of the first trimester. ▪ Use caution if administered to nursing mothers. ▪ Safety profile has been studied in pediatric patients ages 1 day to 17 years. Efficacy in pediatric patients under 6 months of age has not been established. However, a small number of patients ranging from age 1 day to 6 months have been treated safely (unlabeled).

Elderly: Differences in response compared to younger adults not identified; however, may be at increased risk for side effects (e.g., acute renal failure, anemia, diarrhea, rash, and vomiting). ▪ Use caution; consider decreased cardiac, hepatic, or renal function and effects of concomitant disease or other drug therapy. ▪ See Dose Adjustments and Drug/Lab Interactions.

DRUG/LAB INTERACTIONS

A potent CYP2C9 inhibitor and a moderate CYP3A4 inhibitor. Closely monitor patients who are treated concomitantly with **drugs with a narrow therapeutic index metabolized by CYP2C9 or CYP3A4.** The enzyme-inhibiting effect of fluconazole can last for 4 to 5 days after it is discontinued. ▪ Avoid concurrent use with **erythromycin**; may increase the risk of cardiotoxicity (prolonged QT interval, torsades de pointes) and, consequently, sudden death. ▪ Potentiated by **hydrochlorothiazide**; decreases renal clearance of fluconazole. ▪ Inhibits metabolism and increases serum levels of **phenytoin, sirolimus, oral tacrolimus, and theophyllines;** careful monitoring of their plasma levels is required; nephrotoxicity has been reported with tacrolimus. ▪ Inhibits metabolism and increases serum levels of **cyclosporine.** Monitor levels and SCr. Cyclosporine dose reduction may be indicated with concomitant use. ▪ Potentiates **warfarin**; monitor PT and INR frequently. ▪ Potentiates **sulfonylureas**; monitor blood glucose levels. Adjust the dose of the oral hypoglycemic agent as indicated. ▪ **Rifampin** increases metabolism; fluconazole dose may need to be increased. One source recommends avoiding concurrent use. ▪ Increases serum levels of **zidovudine.** Dose reduction may be necessary. ▪ Increases serum levels of **rifabutin.** Uveitis has been reported in patients receiving rifabutin and fluconazole concomitantly. Monitoring is recommended. ▪ Risk of cardiac arrhythmias increased with **erythromycin, pimozide,** and **quinidine**; concurrent use not recommended; see Contraindications. ▪ Fluconazole may inhibit metabolism and increase plasma concentrations of **carbamazepine**; monitor carbamazepine concentrations. ▪ Avoid concomitant use with **voriconazole.** Potential for voriconazole toxicity remains if voriconazole is initiated within 24 hours of the last dose of fluconazole. ▪ May decrease metabolism and increase serum concentrations of **celecoxib** and other **NSAIDs.** Monitor for toxicity related to NSAIDs and adjust dose as needed. ▪ May decrease metabolism and increase serum concentrations of **selected benzodiazepines** that are metabolized by the cytochrome P_{450} system. ▪ May increase serum concentrations and adverse effects of **alfentanil, buspirone, calcium channel blockers, corticosteroids, fentanyl, haloperidol, methadone, nisoldipine, tolterodine, tricyclic antidepressants, and vinca alkaloids** (e.g., vincristine). Reduce doses of the above drugs as indicated to avoid toxicity. Dose may need to be increased when fluconazole is discontinued. **Tolterodine** dose should be limited to no more than 1 mg twice daily when coadministered with fluconazole. ▪ Inhibits metabolism of **losartan** to its active metabolite. Monitor BP closely. ▪ Coadministration may increase plasma levels of some **protease inhibitors** (e.g., nelfinavir, saquinavir), increasing the risk of toxicity. ▪ Increases serum levels of **HMG-CoA reductase inhibitors**; rhabdomyolysis has been reported. **Pravastatin** levels may be the least affected. ▪ Increases systemic exposure to **tofacitinib.** Dose reduction required with coadministration; see tofacitinib prescribing information. ▪ May increase the plasma concentrations and therapeutic effects of **zolpidem.** ▪ An increase in serum bilirubin and creatinine has been observed with concurrent use of **cyclophosphamide** and fluconazole. Use caution and monitor if combined use is required. ▪ No significant pharmacokinetic interaction between fluconazole and **azithromycin** has been observed. ▪ May **elevate liver function tests** (e.g., ALT, AST, alkaline phosphatase, and bilirubin).

SIDE EFFECTS

Abdominal pain, diarrhea, dizziness, dry mouth, dyspepsia, exfoliative skin disorders, headache, hepatic reactions, hypercholesterolemia, hypersensitivity reactions (including anaphylaxis with angioedema, face edema, and pruritus), hypertriglyceridemia, hypokalemia, increased appetite, increased sweating, leukopenia (including neutropenia and agranulocytosis), nausea, pallor, QT prolongation, rash, seizures, taste perversion, thrombocytopenia, torsades de pointes, tremor, vomiting.

Overdose: Cyanosis, decreased motility, decreased respirations, hallucinations, lacrimation, loss of balance, salivation, urinary incontinence. Clonic convulsions preceded death in experimental animals. Changes in renal and hematologic function test results and hepatic abnormalities have been seen in some patients, particularly those with serious underlying diseases such as AIDS and cancer. Clinical significance and relationship to treatment are unclear.

Post-Marketing: Asthenia, cholestasis, fatigue, fever, hepatocellular damage, insomnia, malaise, myalgia, paresthesia, somnolence.

ANTIDOTE

Notify physician of all side effects; most will be treated symptomatically. Discontinue drug and notify physician of abnormal liver function tests progressing to clinical signs and symptoms of liver disease. Rash may be the first sign of an exfoliative skin disorder in immunocompromised patients; discontinue drug and notify physician. In overdose a 3-hour dialysis session will decrease plasma levels by 50%. Treat anaphylaxis or resuscitate if indicated.

FLUDARABINE PHOSPHATE `BBW`
(floo-**DAIR**-ah-bean **FOS**-fayt)

Fludara

Antineoplastic
(antimetabolite)

pH 7.2 to 8.2 (lyophilized)
pH 7.3 to 7.7 (liquid)

USUAL DOSE

Pretreatment: Verify pregnancy status. Baseline studies indicated; see Monitor.

Fludarabine: 25 mg/M^2/day for 5 consecutive days. Repeat every 4 weeks. Optimum duration of treatment not established. If there is no major toxicity, treat until maximum response achieved, then administer three additional complete cycles.

PEDIATRIC DOSE

Safety and effectiveness for use in pediatric patients not established; see Maternal/Child.

Pediatric acute lymphocytic leukemia (ALL) patients (unlabeled): Give an initial loading bolus of 10.5 mg/M^2 on Day 1 followed by a continuous infusion of 30.5 mg/M^2/day on Days 1 through 5.

Pediatric patients with solid tumors (unlabeled): Dose-limiting myelosuppression was observed with a loading dose of 8 mg/M^2 on Day 1 followed by a continuous infusion of 23.5 mg/M^2/day on Days 1 through 5. Maximum tolerated dose in solid tumor pediatric patients was a loading dose of 7 mg/M^2/day followed by a continuous infusion of 20 mg/M^2/day for 5 days.

DOSE ADJUSTMENTS

Decrease or delay dose based on evidence of hematologic or nonhematologic toxicity. Increased toxicity may occur in the elderly and in patients with renal insufficiency or bone marrow impairment. Monitor closely and adjust dose as indicated. ■ Adjust initial starting doses for patients with renal impairment as indicated in the following chart.

Fludarabine Starting Dose Adjustment for Renal Impairment	
Creatinine Clearance	**Starting Dose**
≥80 mL/min	25 mg/M^2 (full dose)
50–79 mL/min	20 mg/M^2
30–49 mL/min	15 mg/M^2
<30 mL/min	Do not administer

DILUTION
Specific techniques required; see Precautions. Available as a sterile solution 50 mg/2 mL (25 mg/mL) or as a lyophilized solid cake (50 mg) requiring reconstitution with 2 mL of SWFI (25 mg/mL). Should dissolve within 15 seconds. In clinical studies, each single dose was further diluted in 100 to 125 mL of NS or D5W and given as an infusion over 30 minutes. **Filters:** Specific information from studies not available; contact manufacturer for further information.
Storage: Refrigerate between 2° and 8° C (36° to 46° F) before dilution. No preservative; use within 8 hours of dilution.

COMPATIBILITY
Manufacturer states, "Should not be mixed with other drugs."

Other sources suggest specific **compatibilities** dependent on concentration and manufacturer; consult a pharmacist.

RATE OF ADMINISTRATION
Single daily dose properly diluted for infusion over 30 minutes.

ACTIONS
A potent antineoplastic agent. A fluorinated nucleotide analog of the antiviral agent vidarabine. Rapidly converts to the active metabolite 2-fluoro-ara-ATP and interferes with the synthesis of DNA. Actual mechanism of action unknown and may be multifaceted. Median time to response in studies of patients with refractory chronic lymphocytic leukemia (CLL) was 7 to 21 weeks (range 1 to 68 weeks). Elimination half-life is approximately 20 hours. Total body clearance of the active metabolite is correlated with the CrCl, indicating the importance of renal excretion for drug elimination.

INDICATIONS AND USES
Treatment of patients with B-cell CLL who have not responded to or progressed during treatment with at least one standard alkylating agent–containing regimen. ▪ Safety and effectiveness in previously untreated or nonrefractory patients with CLL not established. **Unlabeled uses:** Treatment of non-Hodgkin lymphoma, acute lymphocytic leukemia, acute myeloid leukemia, prolymphocytic leukemia or prolymphocytoid variant of CLL, mycosis fungoides, hairy-cell leukemia, and Waldenström's macroglobulinemia. Dose and/or efficacy not established.

CONTRAINDICATIONS
Hypersensitivity to fludarabine or its components (e.g., mannitol and sodium hydroxide). ▪ Not recommended for use in patients with severely impaired renal function (CrCl less than 30 mL/min). ▪ Not recommended for use in combination with pentostatin (Nipent); see Drug/Lab Interactions.

PRECAUTIONS
Follow guidelines for handling cytotoxic agents. See Appendix A, p. 1308. ▪ Administered by or under the direction of the physician specialist. ▪ Use with caution in advanced age, renal insufficiency, or bone marrow impairment, or in patients with immunodeficiency or a history of opportunistic infection. ▪ Severe myelosuppression (anemia, neutropenia, and thrombocytopenia) is common. Median time to nadir counts was 13 days for granulocytes and 16 days for platelets. ▪ Most patients have hematologic impairment at baseline because of disease or prior myelosuppressive therapy. Myelosuppression may be severe and cumulative. ▪ Several instances of trilineage bone marrow hypoplasia or aplasia resulting in pancytopenia, sometimes resulting in death, have been reported. Clinically

significant cytopenias lasted from 2 months to 1 year and occurred in untreated and previously treated patients. ▪ Use of irradiated blood product is recommended for patients requiring transfusions during fludarabine therapy because transfusion-associated graft-versus-host disease has been reported. ▪ Use caution in patients with large tumor burdens; may cause tumor lysis syndrome. Response can occur within 1 week. ▪ Life-threatening and sometimes fatal cases of autoimmune phenomena, such as hemolytic anemia, autoimmune thrombocytopenia/thrombocytopenic purpura (ITP), Evans syndrome, and acquired hemophilia, have been reported; see Antidote. ▪ Serious, sometimes fatal infections, including opportunistic infections and reactivations of latent viral infections (e.g., varicella zoster virus [VZV], Epstein-Barr virus, and JC virus [progressive multifocal leukoencephalopathy]), as well as disease progression and transformation (e.g., Richter's syndrome) have been reported. ▪ Severe neurotoxicity characterized by delayed blindness, coma, and death has been reported in patients who received doses that were approximately 4 times greater than the recommended dose. Significant neurotoxicity has also been reported in patients receiving doses in the recommended range. Symptoms may appear 7 to 225 days after the last dose. ▪ Do not administer **live virus vaccines** during or after treatment with fludarabine. ▪ See Side Effects.

Monitor: Observe closely for signs of toxicity, both hematologic and nonhematologic. ▪ Obtain baseline CBC, including differential and platelet count. Repeat regularly to monitor hematopoietic suppression (especially neutrophils and platelets) and hemolysis. ▪ Obtain baseline CrCl. ▪ Observe closely for all signs of infection and any fever of unknown origin. ▪ Prophylactic antibiotics may be indicated pending results of C/S in a febrile neutropenic patient. ▪ Consider prophylactic therapy in patients at risk for developing opportunistic infections. ▪ Nausea and vomiting usually less severe than with many other antineoplastics; prophylactic administration of antiemetics may be indicated. ▪ Monitor for early signs of tumor lysis syndrome (e.g., flank pain, hematuria). Prevention and treatment of hyperuricemia due to tumor lysis syndrome may be accomplished with adequate hydration and, if necessary, with uric acid–lowering drugs (e.g., allopurinol [Aloprim]). ▪ Monitor for evidence of hemolysis. ▪ Monitor for S/S of neurotoxicity (e.g., agitation, coma, confusion, seizures). ▪ Monitor for thrombocytopenia (platelet count less than 50,000/mm^3). Initiate precautions to prevent excessive bleeding (e.g., inspect IV sites, skin, and mucous membranes; use extreme care during invasive procedures; test urine, emesis, stool, and secretions for occult blood).

Patient Education: Avoid pregnancy; effective birth control recommended for both males and females during therapy and for at least 6 months after fludarabine regimen has been completed. ▪ Use caution while driving or operating machinery. Agitation, confusion, fatigue, seizures, visual disturbances, and weakness have been reported. ▪ Adherence to periodic blood count monitoring is imperative. ▪ See Appendix D, p. 1311.

Maternal/Child: Category D: both males and females should use effective contraception and avoid pregnancy; may cause fetal harm; see Patient Education. ▪ Discontinue breast-feeding. ▪ Safety and effectiveness for use in pediatric patients not established; however, data have been submitted to the FDA using the doses described under Pediatric Dose. In pediatric patients, platelet counts appeared to be more sensitive than hemoglobin and WBCs to the effects of fludarabine.

Elderly: See Precautions and Dose Adjustments.

DRUG/LAB INTERACTIONS

Do not use with **pentostatin** (Nipent); may increase risk of fatal pulmonary toxicity. ▪ Do not administer **live virus vaccines** during or after treatment with fludarabine.

SIDE EFFECTS

Are frequent, may be dose limiting, and may cause death. The most common side effects include myelosuppression (anemia, neutropenia, thrombocytopenia), chills, cough, diarrhea, fatigue, fever, infection (including opportunistic and pneumonia), mucositis, nausea and vomiting, and weakness. The most serious side effects include CNS toxicity, hemolytic anemia, pulmonary toxicity, and severe bone marrow suppression. Other reported side effects include agitation, anorexia, arrhythmia, bone marrow aplasia or hypoplasia (may result in pancytopenia), cerebral hemorrhage, coma, confusion, dyspnea, dysuria, edema, elevated hepatic enzymes, esophagitis, GI bleeding/hemorrhage, headache, heart failure, hemorrhagic cystitis, infection, malaise, myalgia, pain, paresthesia, peripheral neuropathy, pulmonary toxicity (ARDS, dyspnea, interstitial pulmonary infiltrate, pulmonary fibrosis, pulmonary hemorrhage, respiratory distress and failure), rashes, seizures, sinusitis, stomatitis, visual disturbances. Onset of flank pain and hematuria may indicate tumor lysis syndrome (hyperkalemia, hyperphosphatemia, hyperuricemia, hypocalcemia, metabolic acidosis, urate crystalluria, and renal failure); one reported.

Overdose: Severe bone marrow suppression (neutropenia and thrombocytopenia). Severe neurologic toxicity including delayed blindness, coma, and death occurred from 21 to 60 days after the last dose in 36% of patients treated with doses only 4 times greater than the recommended dose. Has occurred (in no more than 0.2% of patients) with average doses.

Post-Marketing: Erythema multiforme, Stevens-Johnson syndrome, toxic epidermal necrolysis, and pemphigus (some with fatal outcomes); rare cases of myelodysplastic syndrome and acute myeloid leukemia associated with prior, concomitant, or subsequent treatment with alkylating agents, topoisomerase inhibitors (e.g., irinotecan [Camptosar]), or irradiation; progressive multifocal leukoencephalopathy (PML) within a few weeks to a year (most with a fatal outcome; some patients had prior and/or concurrent chemotherapy); trilineage bone marrow hypoplasia or aplasia resulting in pancytopenia and death; and worsening or flare-up of pre-existing skin cancer lesions and/or new onset of skin cancer during or after treatment with fludarabine.

ANTIDOTE

Notify physician of all side effects. Most will be treated symptomatically. Some toxicity is necessary to produce remission. Delay or discontinue the drug for serious hematologic depression. Administration of whole blood products (e.g., packed RBCs, platelets, leukocytes) and/or blood modifiers (e.g., darbepoetin alfa, epoetin alfa, filgrastim, pegfilgrastim, sargramostim) may be indicated to treat bone marrow toxicity. Restart as soon as signs of bone marrow recovery occur. Delay or discontinue if neurotoxicity occurs. There is no specific antidote; supportive therapy as indicated will help sustain the patient in toxicity. Symptoms of pulmonary toxicity may improve with the use of corticosteroids; rule out an infectious origin before use. Steroids may or may not be useful in controlling hemolytic episodes.

FLUOROURACIL BBW

(flew-roh-**YOUR**-ah-sill)

Adrucil, 5-Fluorouracil, 5-FU

Antineoplastic
(antimetabolite)

pH 9.2

USUAL DOSE

Pretreatment: Verify pregnancy status. Baseline studies indicated; see Monitor.

Fluorouracil: Many dosing regimens are in use. May be given as an injection or as a continuous infusion. Manufacturer recommends 12 mg/kg of body weight/24 hr for 4 days. Total dose should not exceed 800 mg/24 hr. If no toxicity is observed, one-half dose (6 mg/kg) is given on Days 6, 8, 10, and 12 unless toxicity occurs. No medication is given on Days 5, 7, 9, or 11. Discontinue therapy on Day 12, even if no toxicity is apparent. See Precautions/Monitor. The most common form of maintenance therapy is to repeat the entire course of therapy beginning 30 days after the previous course is completed and any toxicity has subsided or to give a single dose of 10 to 15 mg/kg/week, not to exceed 1 Gm/week. Dose adjustments of subsequent doses are made depending on side effects and tolerance.

Advanced colorectal cancer (unlabeled dose): Various protocols have been used. Examples are leucovorin calcium 20 mg/M² followed by fluorouracil 425 mg/M², or leucovorin calcium 200 mg/M^2 followed by fluorouracil 370 mg/M^2 daily for 5 days. Repeat at 4-week intervals twice, then repeat every 28 to 35 days based on complete recovery from toxic effects. Do not initiate or continue in any patient with GI toxicity until completely subsided. Reduce fluorouracil dose based on tolerance to previous course; reduce 20% for moderate hematologic or GI toxicity, 30% for severe toxicity. Increase fluorouracil dose 10% if no toxicity. Leucovorin calcium dose is not adjusted. Alternatively, fluorouracil may also be used in combination with levoleucovorin; dose is different; see levoleucovorin monograph. Fluorouracil and leucovorin calcium are also used in combination with irinotecan (Camptosar); see irinotecan monograph.

Breast cancer (unlabeled dose): Various protocols have been used. An example is fluorouracil 600 mg/M^2 on Days 1 and 8 of each cycle combined with cyclophosphamide (Cytoxan) 100 mg/M^2 on Days 1 through 14 of each cycle and methotrexate 40 mg/M^2 on Days 1 and 8 of each cycle. Repeat cycles monthly (allowing a 2-week rest between cycles). Repeat for 6 to 12 cycles (6 to 12 months). Doxorubicin (Adriamycin) has also been included in this regimen. In patients older than 60 years of age, reduce the fluorouracil dose to 400 mg/M^2 and the initial methotrexate dose to 30 mg/M^2.

DOSE ADJUSTMENTS

For poor-risk patients or those in a poor nutritional state, either reduce dose by one-half or more throughout a course of therapy or give 6 mg/kg/day for 3 days. If no toxicity observed, give 3 mg/kg on Days 5, 7, and 9. Give nothing on Days 4, 6, or 8. Do not exceed 400 mg/day. ■ Dose based on ideal body weight in presence of edema, ascites, or obesity. ■ Reduce dose in patients who have received high-dose pelvic irradiation or other cytotoxic drug therapy with alkylating agents (e.g., cisplatin, ifosfamide). ■ One source recommends a dose adjustment in patients with impaired hepatic function. Give the full dose if the bilirubin is 5 or less on the day of administration; omit the dose if the bilirubin is greater than 5. ■ Used with other antineoplastic drugs in reduced doses to achieve tumor remission. ■ See Usual Dose.

DILUTION

Specific techniques required; see Precautions. May be slightly discolored without affecting safety and potency. Dissolve any precipitate by heating to 60° C (140° F) and shaking vigorously. Let cool to body temperature before using.

IV injection: May be given undiluted. May inject through Y-tube of a free-flowing infusion.

Infusion: May be further diluted with D5W or NS and given as an infusion. Doses up to 2 Gm are being given with extreme caution under the specific supervision of experienced specialists. Leucovorin calcium has been mixed into the solution with fluorouracil.

Storage: Store at room temperature; protect from light.

COMPATIBILITY

Compatibility information not available from manufacturer. Other sources suggest a few specific **compatibilities** dependent on concentration and manufacturer; consult a pharmacist.

RATE OF ADMINISTRATION

IV injection: A single dose over 1 to 15 minutes.

Infusion: A single dose is usually administered over 24 hours. Toxicity may be lessened by extended administration.

ACTIONS

An antimetabolite. A fluorinated pyrimidine antagonist, cell cycle specific, that interferes with the synthesis of DNA and RNA. Through various chemical processes this deprivation acts more quickly on rapidly growing cells and causes their death. Distributes into tumors, intestinal mucosa, bone marrow, liver, and readily crosses the blood-brain barrier into cerebrospinal fluid and brain tissue. Metabolized by the liver within 3 hours. Half-life is approximately 16 minutes. Excretion is through the urine and as respiratory CO_2.

INDICATIONS AND USES

To suppress or slow neoplastic growth. Palliative treatment of cancers of the breast, colon, pancreas, rectum, and stomach. May be used alone or in combination with other agents.

Unlabeled uses: Has been used for the treatment of bladder, cervical, endometrial, esophageal, head and neck, ovarian, prostatic, skin (topical), and other cancers. Consult oncology literature for protocols in use.

CONTRAINDICATIONS

Potentially serious infections, depressed bone marrow function, poor nutritional state, hypersensitivity, major surgery within the previous month.

PRECAUTIONS

Follow guidelines for handling cytotoxic agents. See Appendix A, p. 1308. ■ Administered by or under the direction of the physician specialist with facilities for monitoring the patient and responding to any medical emergency. Hospitalization, at least during the initial course of therapy, is recommended. ■ Use caution in patients who have had high-dose pelvic irradiation, previous alkylating agents (e.g., cisplatin), other antimetabolic drugs (e.g., methotrexate), metastatic tumor involvement of the bone marrow, impaired hepatic or renal function, or dihydropyrimidine dehydrogenase deficiency. ■ Pseudomembranous colitis has been reported. May range from mild to life threatening. Consider in patients who present with diarrhea during or after treatment with fluorouracil.

Monitor: Confirm patency of vein. Avoid extravasation. Change peripheral injection site every 48 hours. ■ Obtain a CBC with differential and platelet count before each dose. When given with leucovorin calcium, repeat weekly the first two courses and then at the time of anticipated WBC nadir in following courses. Electrolytes and liver function tests should be done before the first three courses, then every other course. ■ Be alert for signs of bone marrow suppression or infection. Prophylactic antibiotics may be indicated pending results of C/S in a febrile neutropenic patient. ■ Examine mouth and lips daily for sores or other signs of stomatitis. ■ Prophylactic antiemetics may reduce nausea and vomiting and increase patient comfort. ■ Toxicity increased by any form of therapy that adds to stress, poor nutrition, and bone marrow suppression. ■ Monitor for thrombocytopenia (platelet count less than 50,000/mm^3). Initiate precautions to prevent excessive bleeding (e.g., inspect IV sites, skin, and mucous membranes; use extreme care during invasive procedures; test urine, emesis, stool, and secretions for occult blood). ■ See Drug/Lab Interactions.

Patient Education: Effective birth control recommended. ■ See Appendix D, p. 1311. ■ Report IV site burning and stinging promptly. ■ Drink at least 2 liters of fluid each day.

Maternal/Child: Category D: avoid pregnancy; can cause fetal harm. ■ Discontinue breastfeeding. ■ Safety for use in pediatric patients not established.

Elderly: May be more sensitive to toxic effects of the drug. Consider age-related organ impairment. ■ See Dose Adjustments.

DRUG/LAB INTERACTIONS

Potentiates **anticoagulants.** ■ Do not administer **live virus vaccines** to patients receiving antineoplastic drugs. ■ **Cimetidine** (Tagamet), **interferon-alfa, and leucovorin calcium** may increase toxicity. ■ Additive bone marrow suppression may occur with **radiation therapy, other bone marrow–suppressing agents** (e.g., azathioprine, chloramphenicol, irinotecan, melphalan, vinorelbine), **and/or agents that cause blood dyscrasias** (e.g., metronidazole). ■ **Thiazide diuretics** (e.g., chlorothiazide) may prolong antineoplastic-induced leukopenia. ■ May decrease metabolism and increase serum levels of **phenytoin.**

SIDE EFFECTS

Abnormal bromsulphalein (BSP), prothrombin, total protein, sedimentation rate; alopecia (reversible), anaphylaxis, bleeding, bone marrow suppression (agranulocytosis, anemia, leukopenia, pancytopenia, thrombocytopenia), cerebellar syndrome, cramps, dermatitis, diarrhea, disorientation, dry lips, erythema, esophagopharyngitis and stomatitis (may lead to sloughing and ulceration), euphoria, frequent stools, GI ulceration and bleeding, headache, hemorrhage from any site, increased skin pigmentation, infection, lacrimal duct stenosis, mouth soreness and ulceration, myocardial ischemia, nail changes, nausea, palmar-plantar erythrodysesthesia syndrome (tingling of hands and feet followed by pain, redness, and swelling), photophobia, photosensitivity, pneumopathy (cough, shortness of breath), thrombophlebitis, visual changes, vomiting (intractable). Diarrhea and stomatitis are most common and may be more severe with a prolonged duration in patients on combination therapy. Pseudomembranous colitis has been reported.

ANTIDOTE

Keep physician informed of any side effects. Discontinue the drug and notify physician promptly at the first sign of toxicity (e.g., bleeding, diarrhea, esophagopharyngitis, gastritis, intractable vomiting, rapidly falling white count, sores in or around the lips or mouth, stomatitis). Nadir of leukocyte count occurs around Days 9 to 14. Recovery should be by Day 30. Discontinue the drug if the WBC count is less than 3,500/mm^3 or platelets are less than 100,000/mm^3; should reach 4,000/mm^3 and 130,000/mm^3 respectively in 2 weeks; if they do not, discontinue treatment. Administration of whole blood products (e.g., packed RBCs, platelets, leukocytes, and/or blood modifiers [e.g., darbepoetin alfa, epoetin alfa, filgrastim, pegfilgrastim, sargramostim]) may be indicated to treat bone marrow toxicity. Continue to monitor for 4 weeks. Palmar-plantar erythrodysesthesia syndrome has been treated with oral pyridoxine (vitamin B$_6$), 100 to 150 mg daily. Death may occur from the progression of many side effects. There is no specific antidote; supportive therapy as indicated will help sustain the patient in toxicity.

FOLIC ACID
(**FOH**-lik **AS**-id)

Nutritional supplement
(vitamin)
Antianemic

pH 8 to 11

USUAL DOSE

Pretreatment: Baseline studies indicated; see Monitor.

Therapeutic dose: 0.1 to 1 mg daily (never give less than 0.1 mg). Larger doses may be required.

Maintenance dose: 0.4 mg daily. *Pregnant or lactating females:* 0.8 mg daily.

PEDIATRIC DOSE

See Maternal/Child.

Therapeutic dose: 0.1 to 1 mg daily (never give less than 0.1 mg).

Maintenance dose: *Infants:* 0.1 mg daily. *Under 4 years of age:* Up to 0.3 mg daily. *Over 4 years of age:* Same as adult.

DOSE ADJUSTMENTS

Increased initial and maintenance doses may be required in alcoholism, hemolytic anemia, anticonvulsant therapy, or chronic infection.

DILUTION

Each dose (up to 5 mg) should be diluted in at least 50 mL of SWFI, D5W, or NS. May be added to most IV solutions and given as an infusion.

Storage: Protect from light and freezing.

COMPATIBILITY

Consider any drug NOT listed as compatible to be INCOMPATIBLE until consulting a pharmacist; specific conditions may apply.

Manufacturer lists as **incompatible** with calcium gluconate (even though a precipitate cannot be seen), doxapram, heavy metal ions, iron sulfate, oxidizing agents, reducing agents, solutions with a pH less than 5.

RATE OF ADMINISTRATION

Usually given over 30 minutes or more in an infusion.

ACTIONS

Folic acid is part of the vitamin B complex. In humans, exogenous folate is required for nucleoprotein synthesis and the maintenance of normal erythropoiesis. It is the precursor of tetrahydrofolic acid, an important cofactor involved in the synthesis of amino acids and DNA. Stimulates the production of RBCs, WBCs, and platelets. Metabolized in the liver and excreted in the urine. Crosses the placental barrier. Secreted in breast milk.

INDICATIONS AND USES

For prevention and treatment of folic acid deficiency. Megaloblastic anemias resulting from folic acid deficiency may be seen in sprue; anemias of malnutrition, pregnancy, infancy, and childhood; developmental or surgical anomalies of the GI tract; and other conditions.

CONTRAINDICATIONS

Pernicious anemia unless used in combination with diagnostic testing.

PRECAUTIONS

Folic acid is not commonly administered by the IV route. Oral or IM administration provides adequate absorption in most cases. ▪ Obscures the peripheral blood picture and prevents the diagnosis of pernicious anemia. May actually aggravate the neurologic symptoms.

Monitor: Obtain CBC before and during therapy.

Maternal/Child: Category A: an important vitamin before and during pregnancy. Folate-deficient mothers have a higher incidence of fetal anomalies and complications of pregnancy. ▪ Safe for use during breast-feeding; infant may require supplementation if mother is folate deficient. ▪ Some products contain benzyl alcohol as a preservative. Avoid use in neonates.

Elderly: More likely to have folate deficiency.

DRUG/LAB INTERACTIONS

Toxic effects of antineoplastic folic acid antagonists are blocked by **folinic acid** (leucovorin calcium) but not by folic acid IV. ▪ Increases **phenytoin** metabolism; seizures may result. ▪ Inhibited by **dihydrofolate reductase inhibitors** (e.g., methotrexate, trimethoprim), **pyrimethamine, and triamterene** and by depressed **hematopoiesis, alcoholism,** and deficiencies of **vitamins B_6, B_{12}, C, and E.** ▪ **Aminosalicylic acid** or **sulfasalazine** may decrease serum folate levels. ▪ **Oral contraceptives** may inhibit folate metabolism.

SIDE EFFECTS

Almost nonexistent. Confusion, some slight flushing or feeling of warmth, nausea; anaphylaxis can occur.

ANTIDOTE

If anaphylaxis occurs, discontinue drug, treat anaphylaxis, and notify physician. Resuscitate as necessary.

FOMEPIZOLE INJECTION

Antidote

(foh-**MEP**-ih-zoll in-**JEK**-shun)

Antizol

USUAL DOSE

Begin fomepizole treatment immediately upon suspicion of ethylene glycol or methanol ingestion based on patient history and/or anion gap metabolic acidosis, increased osmolar gap, visual disturbances, or oxalate crystals in the urine, or a documented serum ethylene glycol or methanol concentration greater than 20 mg/dL. Ethylene glycol is the main component of antifreeze and coolants. Methanol is the main component of windshield washer fluid and a component of products such as Sternol (for fondue pots), Heet (gasoline antifreeze), and various paint products.

Adults with blood concentrations over 20 mg/dL but less than 50 mg/dL: Administer a loading dose of 15 mg/kg as a slow intravenous infusion. Follow with 10 mg/kg every 12 hours times 4 doses, then 15 mg/kg every 12 hours until ethylene glycol or methanol concentrations are undetectable or have been reduced below 20 mg/dL and the patient is asymptomatic with normal pH.

Adults with blood concentrations of 50 mg/dL or higher, renal failure, or significant or worsening metabolic acidosis: In addition to dosing as above, dialysis should be considered to correct metabolic abnormalities and to lower the ethylene glycol or methanol concentrations below 50 mg/dL.

Dosage with renal dialysis: Amount of loading dose and following doses (mg/kg) remains the same, but fomepizole is dialyzable and the frequency of dosing should be increased to every 4 hours during hemodialysis. Base frequency on the following chart.

Fomepizole Dosing in Patients Requiring Dialysis	
DOSE AT THE BEGINNING OF HEMODIALYSIS	
If <6 hours since last fomepizole dose Do not administer dose	If ≥6 hours since last fomepizole dose Administer next scheduled dose
DOSING DURING HEMODIALYSIS	
Dose every 4 hours	
DOSING AT THE TIME HEMODIALYSIS IS COMPLETED	
Time between last dose and the end of the hemodialysis	
<1 hour	Do not administer dose at the end of hemodialysis
1–3 hours	Administer one-half of next scheduled dose
>3 hours	Administer next scheduled dose
MAINTENANCE DOSING OFF HEMODIALYSIS	
Give next scheduled dose 12 hours from last dose administered	

DOSE ADJUSTMENTS

Fomepizole has not been studied sufficiently to determine whether the pharmacokinetics differ for the elderly (see Elderly), pediatric patients, between genders, in renal insufficiency (excreted renally), or in hepatic insufficiency (metabolized by the liver).

DILUTION

Fomepizole solidifies at temperatures less than 25° C (77° F). If it is solidified, liquefy by running the vial under warm water or by holding in the hand. Solidification does not

affect the efficacy, safety, or stability. Withdraw the appropriate dose. Each single dose *must be diluted* in at least 100 mL of NS or D5W and given as an infusion. Mix well.
Storage: Store vials at CRT 20° to 25° C (68° to 77° F). Diluted solutions are stable refrigerated or at CRT for 48 hours; however, manufacturer states should be used within 24 hours of dilution.

COMPATIBILITY

Compatibility information not available from manufacturer; consult a pharmacist.

RATE OF ADMINISTRATION

Each single dose must be given as a slow intravenous infusion equally distributed over 30 minutes. *Do not give undiluted or by bolus injection;* has caused serious venous irritation and phlebosclerosis.

ACTIONS

A synthetic competitive alcohol dehydrogenase inhibitor. Effectively blocks formation of toxic metabolites (glycolic and oxalic acids [ethylene glycol] and formic acid [methanol]). These toxins can induce metabolic acidosis, nausea and vomiting, seizures, stupor, coma, calcium oxaluria, acute tubular necrosis, blindness, and death. Has shown minimal CNS depressant effects. Plasma half-life varies with dose and has not been calculated. Rapidly distributes into total body water. Metabolized in the liver by the P_{450} mixed-function oxidase system. Significant increases in the elimination rate occur after 30 to 40 hours. Excreted in urine.

INDICATIONS AND USES

An antidote for ethylene glycol (antifreeze) or methanol (windshield wiper fluid) poisoning, or for use in suspected ethylene glycol or methanol ingestion either alone or in combination with hemodialysis.

CONTRAINDICATIONS

Known serious hypersensitivity to fomepizole or other pyrazoles (e.g., sulfinpyrazone).

PRECAUTIONS

Acute ethylene glycol or methanol poisoning is a medical emergency that is characterized by a syndrome that can include CNS depression, severe metabolic acidosis, renal failure, and coma. Can be lethal if left untreated or when treatment is delayed due to delayed diagnosis. The lethal dose of ethylene glycol is approximately 1.4 mL/kg. The lethal dose of methanol is approximately 1.2 mL/kg. ▪ If ethylene glycol or methanol poisoning is left untreated, the natural progression of the poisoning leads to accumulation of toxic metabolites, including glycolic and oxalic acids (ethylene glycol) and formic acid (methanol). These metabolites can induce metabolic acidosis, nausea and vomiting, seizures, stupor, coma, calcium oxaluria, acute tubular necrosis, and death. ▪ The diagnosis of these poisonings may be difficult because ethylene glycol and methanol levels diminish in the blood as they are metabolized. ▪ The ethylene glycol or methanol concentrations and the acid-base balance, as determined by serum electrolyte (anion gap) and/or arterial blood gas analysis, should be frequently monitored and used to guide treatment. ▪ Fomepizole has caused minor hypersensitivity reactions (mild rash, eosinophilia).

Monitor: Maintain a patent airway and support ventilation as indicated; CNS and respiratory distress may occur suddenly. ▪ Gastric lavage may be indicated if performed soon after ingestion or in patients who are comatose or at risk for seizures. ▪ Patients must be managed for metabolic acidosis, acute renal failure (ethylene glycol), adult respiratory distress syndrome, visual disturbances (methanol), and hypocalcemia (may result in tetany). Sodium bicarbonate may be required to treat metabolic acidosis. Correct electrolyte imbalance and maintain adequate urine output with IV fluids. A decrease in the amount of fluids will be required in impending renal failure to prevent fluid overload; monitor closely. ▪ Potassium supplementation and oxygen administration are usually necessary. ▪ Administer IV calcium to patients with seizures or tetany that may be caused by decreased calcium, but do not attempt to correct hypocalcemia itself (may increase precipitation of calcium oxalate crystals in the tissues). ▪ Hemodialysis is necessary in the anuric patient and should be considered in patients with severe metabolic acidosis or azotemia and in any patient with high ethylene glycol or methanol concentrations (equal to or greater than 50 mg/dL). ■ ECG should be continuous to monitor for cardiac irregularities. ■ EEG may be required in the comatose patient. ■ The effective inhibition of alcohol dehydrogenase requires fomepizole plasma concentrations in the range of 100 to 300 micromol/L (8.6 to 24.6 mg/L). ■ To assess treatment success, obtain baseline and frequently monitor measurements of blood gases, pH, electrolytes, BUN, creatinine, and urinalysis in addition to other laboratory tests as indicated by each patient's condition. ■ To assess the status of ethylene glycol or methanol and their respective metabolite clearances, obtain baseline ethylene glycol or methanol plasma and urine concentrations and presence of urinary oxalate crystals (ethylene glycol) and monitor frequently. ■ Obtain baseline and monitor hepatic enzymes and WBC counts during treatment; transient increases in serum transaminase levels and eosinophilia have been noted with repeated fomepizole dosing. ■ Monitor for signs of hypersensitivity reactions; see Precautions.

Patient Education: Monitoring of urine output imperative. ■ Cooperation with adequate hydration and frequent laboratory analysis required. ■ Request assistance with ambulation.

Maternal/Child: Category C: use during pregnancy only if clearly needed. ■ Decreased testicular mass in rats. ■ Use caution during breast-feeding; not known if fomepizole is secreted in breast milk. ■ Safety and effectiveness for use in pediatric patients not established.

Elderly: Risk of toxic reactions may be greater in patients with impaired renal function; consider age-related renal impairment.

DRUG/LAB INTERACTIONS

Has not been studied, but reciprocal interactions (increasing or decreasing clearance, effects, or toxicity) may occur with concomitant use of **drugs that induce or inhibit the cytochrome P$_{450}$ system**. Ethanol decreased the rate of elimination of fomepizole (by 50%).

SIDE EFFECTS

The most common side effects are dizziness, headache, and nausea. Abdominal pain, abnormal smell, anemia, anorexia, arrhythmias (bradycardia, tachycardia), back pain (lower), blurred vision, decreased awareness of surroundings, diarrhea, DIC, feeling of drunkenness, fever, hangover, heartburn, hiccups, hypersensitivity reactions (e.g., mild rash, eosinophilia), hypotension, injection site reaction, light-headedness, lymphangitis, multisystem organ failure, nystagmus, pharyngitis, phlebitis, phlebosclerosis, seizure, shock, slurred speech, somnolence, taste changes (bad or metallic), vertigo, visual problems, vomiting occurred in up to 6% of patients.

Overdose: Dizziness, nausea, and vertigo occurred in healthy volunteers given 3 to 6 times the recommended dose.

ANTIDOTE

Keep physician informed of all side effects, laboratory results, and concurrent medical problems. Dialysis may be indicated for changes in patient condition (e.g., renal failure, significant or worsening metabolic acidosis, or a measured ethylene glycol or methanol concentration of greater than 50 mg/dL) or in the treatment of overdose. Treat side effects symptomatically as indicated. Resuscitate as necessary.

FOSAPREPITANT DIMEGLUMINE
(fos-ap-**RE**-pi-tant dye-**MEG**-loo-meen)

Emend

USUAL DOSE

150 mg as IV infusion over 20 to 30 minutes, completing the infusion approximately 30 minutes before chemotherapy. Given in combination with dexamethasone and a 5-HT$_3$ antagonist.

PEDIATRIC DOSE

Single-Dose Regimen of Fosaprepitant for Injection for Pediatric Patients 6 Months[a] to 17 Years of Age for the Prevention of Nausea and Vomiting Associated With Single-Day Regimens of HEC or MEC		
Drug	**Age-Group**	**Regimen**
Fosaprepitant for injection	12 years to 17 years	150 mg IV over 30 minutes[b]
	2 years to <12 years	4 mg/kg (maximum dose 150 mg) IV over 60 minutes[b]
	6 months to <2 years	5 mg/kg (maximum dose 150 mg) IV over 60 minutes[b]

[a]Dosing in pediatric patients less than 6 kg is not recommended.
[b]Complete fosaprepitant infusion on Day 1 approximately 30 minutes before chemotherapy.

Pediatric Patients 6 Months[a] to 17 Years of Age Recommended 3-Day Fosaprepitant Dosage Regimen for Prevention of Nausea and Vomiting Associated With Single- or Multi-Day Regimens of HEC or MEC				
Age-Group	**Drug**	**Day 1**	**Day 2**	**Day 3**
12 years to 17 years	Fosaprepitant for injection	115 mg IV over 30 minutes[b]	—	—
	Fosaprepitant capsules[c]	—	80 mg PO	80 mg PO
6 months to <12 years	Fosaprepitant for injection	3 mg/kg (maximum dose 115 mg) IV over 60 minutes[b]	—	—
	Fosaprepitant for oral suspension	—	2 mg/kg PO (maximum 80 mg)	2 mg/kg PO (maximum 80 mg)

[a]Dosing in pediatric patients less than 6 kg is not recommended.
[b]Complete fosaprepitant infusion approximately 30 minutes before chemotherapy.
[c]For patients 12 years to 17 years of age who cannot swallow oral capsules, fosaprepitant for oral suspension can be used instead.

DOSE ADJUSTMENTS

No dose adjustment indicated based on race, gender, body mass index (BMI), renal status (including patients with ESRD on dialysis), or mild to moderate hepatic insufficiency. Data in patients with severe hepatic insufficiency (Child-Pugh score >9) not available.

DILUTION

Reconstitute each 150-mg vial with 5 mL of NS. Direct stream of NS to side of vial to avoid foaming. Swirl gently; do not shake. Prepare an infusion bag with 145 mL of NS. Withdraw entire volume of reconstituted vial and transfer it into the infusion bag. Gently invert the bag 2 to 3 times. Final concentration is 1 mg/mL. Determine the volume to be administered from the prepared infusion bag based on the recommended dose.

Adults: The entire volume of the prepared infusion bag (150 mL) should be administered.

Pediatric patients 12 years of age and older: The volume to be administered is calculated as follows:

$$\text{Volume to administer (mL)} = \text{Recommended dose (mg)}$$

Pediatric patients 6 months to less than 12 years of age: The volume to be administered is calculated as follows:

$$\text{Volume to administer (mL)} = \text{Recommended dose (mg/kg)} \times \text{weight (kg)}$$
Note: Do not exceed the maximum dose

In pediatric patients, the entire volume in the infusion bag may not be required. If necessary, for volumes less than 150 mL, the calculated volume can be transferred to an appropriate-size bag or syringe before administration by infusion.
Storage: Store unopened vials at 2° to 8° C (36° to 46° F). Diluted solution is stable for 24 hours at RT.

COMPATIBILITY
Manufacturer states, "Do not mix or reconstitute with solutions for which physical and chemical **compatibility** have not been established. Fosaprepitant (Emend) for injection is **incompatible** with any solutions containing divalent cations (e.g., calcium or magnesium), including lactated Ringer's solution and Hartmann's solution."

Other sources suggest a few specific **compatibilities** dependent on concentration and manufacturer; consult a pharmacist.

RATE OF ADMINISTRATION
Adults: A single dose as an infusion equally distributed over 20 to 30 minutes.
Pediatric patients 12 to 17 years of age: A single dose as an infusion through a central venous catheter over 30 minutes.
Pediatric patients 6 months to less than 12 years of age: A single dose as an infusion through a central venous catheter over 60 minutes.

ACTIONS
A prodrug of aprepitant, a substance P/neurokinin$_1$ (NK$_1$) receptor antagonist. Has little or no affinity for 5-HT$_3$, dopamine, and corticosteroid receptors (the targets of existing therapies for chemotherapy-induced nausea and vomiting). Fosaprepitant is rapidly converted to aprepitant following IV administration. Aprepitant inhibits emesis induced by cytotoxic chemotherapeutic agents, such as cisplatin, via central actions. Crosses the blood-brain barrier and occupies brain NK$_1$ receptors. Augments the antiemetic activity of the 5-HT$_3$-receptor antagonist ondansetron and the corticosteroid dexamethasone and inhibits both the acute and delayed phases of cisplatin-induced emesis. Highly protein bound. Undergoes extensive metabolism, primarily by CYP3A4 and to a lesser extent by CYP1A2 and CYP2C19. Eliminated primarily by metabolism; not renally excreted. Half-life is approximately 9 to 13 hours.

INDICATIONS AND USES
Given in combination with other antiemetics in adult and pediatric patients 6 months of age and older for the prevention of acute and delayed nausea and vomiting associated with initial and repeat courses of highly emetogenic cancer chemotherapy, including high-dose cisplatin and delayed nausea and vomiting associated with initial and repeat courses of moderately emetogenic cancer chemotherapy.
Limitation of use: Has not been studied for treatment of established nausea and vomiting.

CONTRAINDICATIONS
Hypersensitivity to fosaprepitant or any components of the product. ▪ Concurrent use with pimozide; see Drug Interactions.

PRECAUTIONS
Fosaprepitant is rapidly converted to aprepitant, which is a substrate, inhibitor, and inducer of CYP3A4. Use with caution in patients receiving concomitant medications that are primarily metabolized through CYP3A4; see Drug Interactions. ▪ Use with caution in patients with severe hepatic insufficiency (Child-Pugh score >9); see Dose Adjustments.

- Serious hypersensitivity reactions, including anaphylaxis and anaphylactic shock, during or soon after infusion have been observed; see Monitor. ▪ Infusion site reactions (ISR) have been reported. The majority of severe ISRs (e.g., thrombophlebitis, vasculitis) have been reported with concomitant vesicant (anthracycline-based) chemotherapy administration, particularly when associated with extravasation. Necrosis was also reported with concomitant vesicant chemotherapy. Most ISRs occurred with the first, second, or third exposure to single doses of fosaprepitant, and in some cases reactions lasted for up to 2 weeks. Avoid infusion of fosaprepitant for injection into small veins or through a butterfly catheter; see Monitor and Drug/Lab Interactions.

Monitor: Monitor for S/S of hypersensitivity reactions during and after the infusion (e.g., anaphylaxis, anaphylactic shock, dyspnea, erythema, flushing, hypotension, and syncope). ▪ Monitor IV site for reactions. ▪ See Drug/Lab Interactions.

Patient Education: Read manufacturer-supplied patient package insert before starting therapy. ▪ Discontinue use of fosaprepitant and promptly report S/S of a hypersensitivity reaction (e.g., difficulty breathing or swallowing, dizziness, feeling faint, flushing, hives, itching, rapid or weak heartbeat, rash, skin peeling, or sores). ▪ Efficacy of hormonal contraceptives may be reduced during and for 28 days following administration of the last dose of fosaprepitant; includes birth control pills, skin patches, implants, and certain IUDs. Alternative or backup methods of contraception should be used during treatment and for 1 month following the last dose of fosaprepitant. ▪ Numerous drug interactions possible. A complete review of all prescription, nonprescription, and herbal products is required before each dose. ▪ Patients on chronic warfarin therapy should have their INR checked in the 2-week period, particularly at 7 to 10 days, following initiation of fosaprepitant with each chemotherapy cycle. ▪ Report new or worsening infusion site reactions (e.g., edema, erythema, necrosis, pain, thrombophlebitis, or vasculitis).

Maternal/Child: Should be used during pregnancy only if clearly needed. ▪ Information on use during breast-feeding not available. Use caution. ▪ Safety and effectiveness of a single-dose regimen and a 3-day IV/oral regimen of fosaprepitant have been established for use in pediatric patients 6 months to 17 years of age for the prevention of acute and delayed nausea and vomiting associated with initial and repeat courses of HEC and MEC. ▪ Safety and effectiveness of fosaprepitant injection administered on consecutive days has not been established in pediatric patients 6 months to 17 years of age for the prevention of acute and delayed nausea and vomiting associated with initial and repeat courses of HEC and MEC. ▪ Safety and effectiveness for the prevention of nausea and vomiting associated with HEC or MEC have not been established in patients under 6 months of age.

Elderly: Response similar to that seen in younger patients, but greater sensitivity of some older individuals cannot be ruled out.

DRUG/LAB INTERACTIONS

Fosaprepitant is rapidly converted to aprepitant. When given as a single 150-mg dose, it is a **weak inhibitor of CYP3A4,** and the weak inhibition of CYP3A4 continues for 2 days after the single dose. Single-dose fosaprepitant does not induce CYP3A4. **Aprepitant is a substrate, inhibitor, and inducer of CYP3A4. It is also an inducer of CYP2C9.** ▪ Efficacy of **hormonal contraceptives** may be reduced during and for 28 days following administration of the last dose of fosaprepitant or aprepitant; see Patient Education. ▪ Patients on chronic **warfarin** therapy should be closely monitored over a 2-week period, particularly at 7 to 10 days following initiation of fosaprepitant with each chemotherapy cycle. Co-administration may result in a clinically significant decrease in INR. ▪ Concurrent use with **pimozide** is **contraindicated.** Inhibition of CYP3A4 by fosaprepitant or aprepitant could result in elevated plasma concentrations of pimozide, potentially causing serious or life-threatening reactions, including prolongation of the QT interval; see Contraindications. ▪ Fosaprepitant/aprepitant can increase plasma concentrations of **dexamethasone and methylprednisolone.** When given concurrently with fosaprepitant or aprepitant, reduce the dexamethasone and methylprednisolone PO doses by approximately 50% and the methylprednisolone IV dose by approximately 25%. (Dexamethasone doses listed in Usual Dose take drug interaction into account.) ▪ Coadministration of fosaprepitant or aprepitant with **chemotherapy agents metabolized by CYP3A4** (e.g., irinotecan, ifosfamide, imatinib, vinblastine, and vincristine) should be done with caution and careful monitoring. In clinical studies, the oral aprepitant regimen was commonly administered with etoposide, vinorelbine, paclitaxel, and docetaxel. Dose adjustments were not required. ▪ May increase plasma levels of **benzodiazepines** (e.g., alprazolam, midazolam). Monitor for sedation or other benzodiazepine-related adverse reactions. ▪ Aprepitant is a CYP2C9 inducer. Has been shown to induce metabolism of **CYP2C9 substrates** (e.g., phenytoin, tolbutamide, warfarin), thus decreasing plasma concentrations. Monitor patients receiving CYP2C9 substrates as indicated (e.g., plasma drug concentrations, therapeutic effect/efficacy, blood sugar control). ▪ Concurrent use with **CYP3A4 inhibitors** (e.g., clarithromycin, diltiazem, itraconazole, ketoconazole, nefazodone, nelfinavir, ritonavir) may increase aprepitant or fosaprepitant plasma concentrations and increase the risk of adverse reactions. Use caution. ▪ Coadministration with **CYP3A4 inducers** (e.g., carbamazepine, phenytoin, rifampin) may decrease fosaprepitant or aprepitant plasma concentrations and decrease efficacy. ▪ Aprepitant is a moderate **inhibitor of CYP3A4**. Use with caution in patients receiving concomitant medications that are primarily metabolized through CYP3A4.

SIDE EFFECTS

Adults: The most common side effects reported include anemia, asthenia, diarrhea, dyspepsia, fatigue, neutropenia, pain in extremity, peripheral neuropathy, and urinary tract infections. Other reported side effects include infusion site reactions (e.g., erythema, induration, pain, pruritus, infusion site thrombophlebitis).

Pediatric patients: Adverse reactions in pediatric patients are similar to those for adults. In pediatric patients (6 months to 17 years) the most common side effects were anemia, febrile neutropenia, neutropenia, and thrombocytopenia.

Post-Marketing: Hypersensitivity reactions (including anaphylaxis and anaphylactic shock), pruritus, rash, Stevens-Johnson syndrome, toxic epidermal necrolysis, and urticaria have been reported. Ifosfamide-induced neurotoxicity after fosaprepitant and ifosfamide coadministration have also been reported.

ANTIDOTE

Keep physician informed of all side effects. Most minor side effects will be treated symptomatically. Discontinue fosaprepitant at the first sign of hypersensitivity. Treat hypersensitivity reactions as indicated; may require epinephrine, airway management, oxygen, IV fluids, antihistamines (e.g., diphenhydramine), corticosteroids (e.g., hydrocortisone), and pressor amines (e.g., dopamine). Do not reinitiate therapy in patients who have had a previous hypersensitivity reaction. Discontinue fosaprepitant for a severe ISR. Treatment for a severe ISR consists of medical and possibly surgical intervention. In the event of overdose, discontinue treatment and provide general supportive treatment and monitoring. Because of the antiemetic activity of fosaprepitant, drug-induced emesis may not be effective in cases of overdose. Fosaprepitant is not removed by hemodialysis.

FOSCARNET SODIUM BBW

Antiviral

(fos-**KAR**-net **SO**-dee-um)

Foscavir

pH 7.4

USUAL DOSE

Pretreatment: Baseline studies indicated. Adequate hydration and other specific testing required; see Monitor.

An individualized dose should be calculated based on body weight (mg/kg), renal function, indication of use, and dosing frequency. To reduce the risk of nephrotoxicity, creatinine clearance (mL/min/kg) should be calculated even if SCr is within the normal range.

CMV retinitis: 90 mg/kg every 12 hours or 60 mg/kg every 8 hours for 14 to 21 days. Length of induction treatment based on clinical response. Begin a maintenance dose of 90 mg/kg/day the next day (Day 15 to 22). If retinitis progresses during the maintenance regimen, retreat with the induction and maintenance regimens. Maintenance dose may be increased to 120 mg/kg/day in patients who show excellent tolerance to foscarnet or those who require early re-induction because of retinitis progression. Normal renal function required. Patients who experience a progression of retinitis while receiving foscarnet maintenance therapy may be retreated with the induction and maintenance regimens listed previously or with a combination of foscarnet and ganciclovir. See the Clinical Trials section in the foscarnet sodium prescribing information.

Acyclovir-resistant HSV patients: 40 mg/kg every 8 or 12 hours for 2 to 3 weeks or until healed.

DOSE ADJUSTMENTS

Foscarnet is not recommended in patients undergoing hemodialysis because dosage guidelines have not been established.

Dose must be individualized according to patient's renal function. Safety and efficacy data for patients with baseline SCr greater than 2.8 mg/dL or measured 24-hour CrCl less than 50 mL/min are limited. Dose adjustment may be required during treatment even if the patient had normal renal function initially. Recommended doses based on renal function are listed in the following charts. To use these dosing guides, the actual 24-hour CrCl (mL/min) must be divided by body weight (kg), or the estimated CrCl in mL/min/kg can be calculated from the SCr (mg/dL) using the following formula (modified Cockcroft-Gault equation):

$$\text{For males: CrCl (mL/min/kg)} = (140 - \text{Age}) \div (\text{SCr} \times 72)$$
$$\text{For females: CrCl (mL/min/kg)} = [(140 - \text{Age}) \div (\text{SCr} \times 72)] \times 0.85$$

Foscarnet Dose Adjustment Guide for Induction				
	Acyclovir-Resistant HSV		**CMV Retinitis**	
CrCl (mL/min/kg)	**Dose of 40 mg/kg q 12 hr**	**Dose of 40 mg/kg q 8 hr**	**Dose of 60 mg/kg q 8 hr**	**Dose of 90 mg/kg q 12 hr**
>1.4 mL/min/kg	40 mg/kg q 12 hr	40 mg/kg q 8 hr	60 mg/kg q 8 hr	90 mg/kg q 12 hr
>1–1.4 mL/min/kg	30 mg/kg q 12 hr	30 mg/kg q 8 hr	45 mg/kg q 8 hr	70 mg/kg q 12 hr
>0.8–1 mL/min/kg	20 mg/kg q 12 hr	35 mg/kg q 12 hr	50 mg/kg q 12 hr	50 mg/kg q 12 hr
>0.6–0.8 mL/min/kg	35 mg/kg q 24 hr	25 mg/kg q 12 hr	40 mg/kg q 12 hr	80 mg/kg q 24 hr
>0.5–0.6 mL/min/kg	25 mg/kg q 24 hr	40 mg/kg q 24 hr	60 mg/kg q 24 hr	60 mg/kg q 24 hr
≥0.4–0.5 mL/min/kg	20 mg/kg q 24 hr	35 mg/kg q 24 hr	50 mg/kg q 24 hr	50 mg/kg q 24 hr
<0.4 mL/min/kg	Not recommended	Not recommended	Not recommended	Not recommended

Specific calculation for maintenance dose is shown in the following chart.

Foscarnet Dose Adjustment Guide for Maintenance in CMV Retinitis		
CrCl (mL/min/kg)	90 mg/kg/day (once daily)	120 mg/kg/day (once daily)
>1.4 mL/min/kg	90 mg/kg q 24 hr	120 mg/kg q 24 hr
>1–1.4 mL/min/kg	70 mg/kg q 24 hr	90 mg/kg q 24 hr
>0.8–1 mL/min/kg	50 mg/kg q 24 hr	65 mg/kg q 24 hr
>0.6–0.8 mL/min/kg	80 mg/kg q 48 hr	105 mg/kg q 48 hr
>0.5–0.6 mL/min/kg	60 mg/kg q 48 hr	80 mg/kg q 48 hr
≥0.4–0.5 mL/min/kg	50 mg/kg q 48 hr	65 mg/kg q 48 hr
<0.4 mL/min/kg	Not recommended	Not recommended

DILUTION
Available in a single-use, 250-mL glass bottle containing 6,000 mg of foscarnet (24 mg/mL). An individualized dose at the required concentration (24 mg/mL or 12 mg/mL) for the route administration (central line or peripheral line) must be aseptically prepared before dispensing. Remove any excess quantity of medication from the infusion bottle using aseptic technique. To avoid any possibility of overdose, only the calculated dose should be in the infusion bottle. Discard any excess before administration.
Central line: Standard 24-mg/mL solution may be given undiluted.
Peripheral line: Each 1 mL of a calculated dose must be diluted with 1 mL of D5W or NS (yields a 12-mg/mL solution).
Storage: Store at CRT. Avoid excessive heat and freezing. Use only if vacuum is present and solution is clear and colorless. Use solution within 24 hours of entry into bottle.

COMPATIBILITY
Manufacturer states, "Administer only with NS or D5W solutions; no other drug or supplement should be administered concurrently via the same catheter." Because of chelating properties, a precipitate can occur. Manufacturer specifically lists as **incompatible** with 30% dextrose, solutions containing calcium (e.g., LR, TPN), acyclovir, amphotericin B, diazepam, digoxin, ganciclovir, leucovorin calcium, midazolam, pentamidine, phenytoin, prochlorperazine, sulfamethoxazole/trimethoprim, trimetrexate glucuronate, vancomycin.

Other sources suggest specific **compatibilities** dependent on concentration and manufacturer; consult a pharmacist.

RATE OF ADMINISTRATION
Do not administer by rapid or bolus IV injection. Infusion pump required to deliver accurate dose evenly distributed over specific time frame. Excessive plasma levels and toxicity (including a decrease in ionized calcium) will occur with too-rapid rate of infusion. Slowing the infusion rate may decrease or prevent symptoms. Advisable to clear tubing with NS if possible before and after administration through Y-tube. Never exceed 1 mg/kg/min.
CMV retinitis: *Induction doses:* Each 60-mg/kg dose equally distributed over a minimum of 1 hour. Increase to 1½ to 2 hours for 90-mg/kg dose.
Maintenance dose: Each dose equally distributed over a minimum of 2 hours.
Acyclovir-resistant HSV: Each dose equally distributed over a minimum of 1 hour.

ACTIONS
An antiviral agent capable of inhibiting replication of herpes viruses, including cytomegalovirus (CMV), herpes simplex virus types 1 and 2 (HSV-1, HSV-2), and varicella zoster virus (VZV [unlabeled]). Does not destroy existing viruses but stops them from reproducing and invading healthy cells. Also capable of chelating metal ions (e.g., calcium, magnesium). CMV strains resistant to ganciclovir and HSV strains resistant to

acyclovir may be sensitive to foscarnet. Some penetration into bone and cerebrospinal fluid. Plasma half-life ranges from 2 to 6 hours and increases markedly with renal impairment. Terminal half-life determined by urinary excretion was 87.5 +/− 41.8 hours, possibly due to release of foscarnet from bone. Excreted unchanged in urine.

INDICATIONS AND USES

Treatment of CMV retinitis in patients with AIDS. Most frequently used in patients who do not tolerate or are resistant to ganciclovir. Combination therapy with ganciclovir is indicated for patients who have relapsed after monotherapy with either drug. ▪ Treatment of acyclovir-resistant mucocutaneous HSV infections in immunocompromised patients.

CONTRAINDICATIONS

Hypersensitivity to foscarnet.

PRECAUTIONS

For IV use only. ▪ Safety and efficacy of foscarnet have not been established for treatment of other CMV infections (e.g., pneumonitis, gastroenteritis), congenital or neonatal CMV disease, other HSV infections (e.g., retinitis, encephalitis), congenital or neonatal HSV disease, or CMV or HSV in nonimmunocompromised individuals. Use should be limited to treatment of conditions listed in Indications and Uses above. ▪ Renal impairment is the major toxicity of foscarnet. Frequent monitoring of serum creatinine, with dose adjustment for changes in renal function, and adequate hydration are imperative. Changes can occur at any time, most likely during second week of induction therapy. Elevations in SCr are usually reversible following dose adjustment or discontinuation of therapy. ▪ Use caution in patients with a history of impaired renal function, altered calcium or other electrolyte levels, or neurologic or cardiac abnormalities, and in patients receiving other drugs known to influence minerals and electrolytes; see Drug/Lab Interactions. Has caused hyperphosphatemia, hypocalcemia (and decreased ionized calcium, which may not be reflected in the total serum calcium), hypokalemia, hypomagnesemia, and hypophosphatemia, resulting in cardiac disturbances, seizures, and tetany. ▪ Seizures related to alterations in plasma minerals and electrolytes have been reported and have included cases of status epilepticus. Several cases were associated with death. Risk factors for seizures included impaired baseline renal function, low total serum calcium, and underlying CNS conditions. ▪ Serious acute hypersensitivity reactions have been reported. If an acute hypersensitivity reaction occurs, discontinue therapy and treat as indicated; see Antidote. ▪ Foscarnet has been associated with prolongation of the QT interval. Use with caution in patients who have a history of QT prolongation, in patients taking medication known to prolong the QT interval, in patients with electrolyte disturbances, or in patients who have other risk factors for QT prolongation; see Drug Interactions. ▪ Contains 5.5 mg sodium/mL. Avoid use in patients who may not tolerate a large amount of sodium or water (e.g., patients with cardiomyopathy) or in patients on a controlled-sodium diet. ▪ In controlled clinical trials, anemia was reported in 33% of patients receiving foscarnet. Granulocytopenia was reported in 17% of patients. ▪ Resistance has been reported to develop. May be higher in patients treated for a prolonged period. Consider the possibility of resistance in patients who show poor clinical response. ▪ Amino acid substitutions conferring foscarnet resistance with cross-resistance to ganciclovir, cidofovir, and acyclovir have been identified. ▪ Sensitivity testing of the viral isolate is recommended before repeat treatment and/or to evaluate sensitivity versus development of resistance.

Monitor: Obtain baseline ECG, SCr, and CrCl (either 24-hour measurement or estimated using the modified Cockcroft-Gault equation based on serum creatinine). Baseline calcium, magnesium, potassium, phosphorus, and electrolytes required before treatment begins. Correct any deficiencies. ▪ Repeat entire testing process 2 to 3 times a week during induction therapy and weekly during maintenance therapy. Foscarnet dose must be adjusted as indicated by test results. More frequent testing may be indicated in specific patients. Supplementation of minerals and electrolytes may be required during treatment. ▪ Monitor for S/S of a hypersensitivity reaction (e.g., anaphylactic shock, angioedema, urticaria). ▪ To minimize renal toxicity, hydration adequate to establish diuresis is recommended before and during treatment. Clinically dehydrated patients should be adequately hydrated before initiating therapy. Give 750 to 1,000 mL NS or D5W before the first foscarnet infusion to establish diuresis. With subsequent infusions, give 750 to 1,000 mL concurrently with 90 to 120 mg/kg foscarnet and a minimum of 500 mL concurrently with 40 to 60 mg/kg. Oral rehydration may be considered in certain patients. Hydration fluid may need to be decreased if clinically warranted. ▪ Discontinue foscarnet if CrCl drops below 0.4 mL/min/kg. Monitor patient daily until resolution of renal impairment is ensured. Safety for use in these patients has not been studied. ▪ Phlebitis or pain may occur at site of infusion; confirm patency of vein and use large veins to ensure adequate blood flow for rapid dilution and distribution. ▪ See Drug/Lab Interactions.

Patient Education: Not a cure. ▪ Retinitis may progress during or after treatment; regular ophthalmologic exams imperative. ▪ Complete healing of HSV infections may occur, but most relapse. ▪ Perioral tingling, numbness in the extremities, or paresthesias indicate electrolyte abnormalities; report immediately. ▪ Close monitoring of renal function and electrolyte balance during treatment is imperative. Hydration may help minimize the risk of renal toxicity. ▪ Promptly report any cardiac symptoms (e.g., transient chest pain). ▪ Cases of male and female genital irritation/ulceration have been reported. Adequate hydration and increased personal hygiene may minimize some side effects. ▪ May cause CNS side effects (e.g., dizziness, seizures, somnolence) that could result in impairment. Use caution when driving or operating machinery. ▪ Dose modification or discontinuation may be required for major side effects.

Maternal/Child: Use only if clearly needed; has caused skeletal anomalies in animals. ▪ Discontinue breast-feeding. ▪ Safety for use in pediatric patients not established; deposited in teeth and bones, and deposition greater in young animals. Use only if benefits outweigh risks.

Elderly: Safety and effectiveness not established; however, foscarnet has been used in patients over 65 years of age. Side effects seen are similar to other age-groups. Consider age-related renal impairment in dose selection, and monitor renal function; see Dose Adjustments.

DRUG/LAB INTERACTIONS

Because of physical **incompatibilities,** foscarnet sodium and **ganciclovir sodium** must never be mixed. ▪ Has caused hypocalcemia with parenteral **pentamidine;** deaths have been reported. ▪ Capable of causing calcium or electrolyte disorders. Use particular caution when administering **any drug known to influence serum calcium concentrations, other minerals, or electrolytes** (e.g., hypocalcemic agents [gallium nitrate], diuretics [furosemide, mannitol], adrenocortical steroids). ▪ Elimination of foscarnet may be impaired and toxicity increased by **drugs that inhibit renal tubular secretion.** When **diuretics** are indicated, **thiazides** (e.g., hydrochlorothiazide) are recommended over **loop diuretics** (e.g., furosemide) because the latter inhibit renal tubular secretion. ▪ Avoid concomitant use with other **nephrotoxic drugs** (e.g., acyclovir, aminoglycosides [e.g., gentamicin], amphotericin B, cyclosporine, methotrexate, pentamidine, tacrolimus) unless benefits outweigh risks. ▪ Abnormal renal function has been reported in patients receiving foscarnet and **ritonavir** or foscarnet and **ritonavir and saquinavir.** ▪ There is no clinically significant interaction with zidovudine or probenecid. ▪ The combination antiviral activity of foscarnet and **ganciclovir** or **acyclovir** is not antagonistic in cell culture. ▪ Foscarnet sodium should be avoided in combination with **agents known to prolong the QT interval,** including **Class IA antiarrhythmic agents** (e.g., procainamide or quinidine) or **Class III antiarrhythmic agents** (e.g., amiodarone, dofetilide, sotalol), **phenothiazines** (e.g., chlorpromazine), **tricyclic antidepressants** (e.g., amitriptyline), and certain **macrolide** (e.g., erythromycin) **and fluoroquinolone** (e.g., levofloxacin) **antibiotics.**

SIDE EFFECTS

Impaired renal function, alterations in plasma minerals and electrolytes, and seizures are major side effects and are dose limiting. Abnormal renal function, including acute renal failure, decreased CrCl, and increased SCr; anemia; bone marrow suppression; diarrhea; fatigue; fever; headache; hyperphosphatemia; hypocalcemia (perioral tingling, numbness in extremities, paresthesias, tetany); hypokalemia; hypomagnesemia; hypophosphatemia; irritation at injection site; irritation and ulcerations of penile and vaginal epithelium; nausea; rigors; seizure; vomiting; and death have occurred. All deaths could not be directly related to foscarnet. Abdominal pain, anorexia, anxiety, asthenia, confusion, coughing, depression, dizziness, dyspnea, granulocytopenia, hypoesthesia, infection, involuntary muscle contractions, leukopenia, malaise, neuropathy, pain, rash, sweating, and vision abnormalities have occurred in 5% of patients. Numerous other side effects have occurred in fewer than 5% of patients.

Post-Marketing: Administration site extravasation, crystal-induced nephropathy, diabetes insipidus, esophageal ulcerations, Fanconi syndrome (acquired), gastrointestinal hemorrhage, glomerulonephritis, hypersensitivity reactions (serious, acute, including anaphylactic shock, angioedema, and urticaria), increased lipase, localized edema, muscle disorders (e.g., myopathy, myositis, muscle weakness, rhabdomyolysis), nephrotic syndrome, prolongation of the QT interval, proteinuria, renal calculi, renal tubular acidosis, renal tubular necrosis, status epilepticus, torsades de pointes, ventricular arrhythmia, vesiculobullous eruptions (e.g., erythema multiforme, toxic epidermal necrolysis, Stevens-Johnson syndrome).

ANTIDOTE

There is no specific antidote. Keep physician informed. Adequate hydration and careful monitoring will help reduce potential for renal impairment and may minimize other side effects. Elevations in SCr are usually reversible (within 1 week) with dose adjustment or discontinuation but have caused death. Discontinue foscarnet if CrCl falls below 0.4 mL/min/kg. Monitor daily until resolution of renal impairment is ensured. Discontinue foscarnet if perioral tingling, numbness in the extremities, or paresthesias occur during or after infusion; evaluate calcium and electrolyte levels (decrease in ionized serum calcium may not be reflected in total serum calcium); notify physician. Administration of foscarnet can be resumed following seizures or cardiac disturbances after treatment of underlying disease, electrolyte disturbance, or after dose adjustment. Overdose/toxicity can occur with too-rapid rate of infusion. Hemodialysis and hydration may be useful in overdose. Discontinue the infusion if an acute hypersensitivity reaction occurs. Treat immediately with oxygen, epinephrine, antihistamines (e.g., diphenhydramine), vasopressors (e.g., dopamine), corticosteroids, albuterol, IV fluids, and ventilation equipment as indicated. Resuscitate as necessary.

FOSNETUPITANT AND PALONOSETRON

(fos-net-**UE**-pi-tant and pal-oh-**NOE**-se-tron)

Akynzeo

Antiemetic

(Substance P/NK-1 receptor antagonist/
5-HT$_3$ receptor antagonist)

USUAL DOSE

Pretreatment: See Maternal/Child.

Highly emetogenic chemotherapy, including cisplatin-based chemotherapy: Administer 1 vial (235 mg fosnetupitant/0.25 mg palonosetron) as an IV infusion over 30 minutes starting 30 minutes before chemotherapy on Day 1. Administer 12 mg dexamethasone 30 minutes before chemotherapy on Day 1 and dexamethasone 8 mg once daily on Days 2 through 4.

The oral formulation of fosnetupitant/palonosetron may be substituted for the IV formulation and is also indicated for anthracyclines and cyclophosphamide-based chemotherapy and chemotherapy not considered highly emetogenic; see Limitation of Use.

DOSE ADJUSTMENTS

No dose adjustment necessary for patients with mild to moderate hepatic impairment (Child-Pugh score 5 to 8) or mild to moderate renal impairment (CrCl of 30 to 60 mL/min). Avoid use in patients with severe hepatic or renal impairment or end-stage renal disease.

DILUTION

Available as 235 mg fosnetupitant/0.25 mg palonosetron lyophilized powder in a single-dose vial for reconstitution. Inject 20 mL of D5W or NS into the vial, directing the stream along the vial wall to prevent foaming. Swirl vial gently. Prepare an infusion vial or bag filled with 30 mL of D5W or NS. Withdraw the entire contents of the reconstituted solution and transfer it into the infusion vial or bag containing 30 mL of D5W or NS to yield a total volume of 50 mL. Gently invert the vial or bag until completely dissolved. Discard if particulates and/or discoloration are observed.

Filter: Data not available.

Storage: Before use, refrigerate at 2° to 8° C (35.6° to 46.4° F) in carton to protect from light. Store reconstituted solution and the final diluted solution at RT. The total time from reconstitution to the start of infusion should not exceed 3 hours.

COMPATIBILITY

Manufacturer states, "Fosnetupitant/palonosetron is **incompatible** with any solution containing divalent cations (e.g., calcium, magnesium), including LR and Hartmann's solution."

Limited data are available on the **compatibility** of fosnetupitant and palonosetron with other IV substances, additives, or other medications, and they should not be added to the fosnetupitant and palonosetron solution or infused simultaneously. If the same IV line is used for sequential infusion of several different drugs, flush the line before and after infusion of fosnetupitant and palonosetron with NS.

RATE OF ADMINISTRATION

Administer over 30 minutes as an IV infusion. At the end of the infusion, flush the infusion line with the same carrier solution to ensure complete drug administration.

ACTIONS

Akynzeo for injection is a combination product of fosnetupitant, a prodrug of netupitant (a substance P/neurokinin 1 [NK-1] receptor antagonist), and palonosetron hydrochloride, a serotonin-3 (5-HT$_3$) receptor antagonist. Both are antinausea and antiemetic agents. Palonosetron prevents nausea and vomiting during the acute phase, and fosnetupitant prevents nausea and vomiting during both the acute and delayed phase after cancer chemotherapy. Palonosetron has a strong binding affinity for the 5-HT$_3$ receptor and little or no affinity for other receptors. Chemotherapeutic agents such as cisplatin increase the release of serotonin from specific cells in the GI tract, causing emesis. By antagonizing serotonin receptors both on the vagus nerve in the periphery and centrally in the chemoreceptor trigger zone, the incidence and severity of chemotherapy-induced nausea and vomiting is decreased. Delayed emesis has been largely associated with the activation of tachykinin family neurokinin 1 (NK-1) receptors by substance P. Netupitant inhibits substance P–mediated responses. Palonosetron is partially metabolized by multiple CYP enzymes. Fosnetupitant is converted in vivo to netupitant by metabolic hydrolysis. Netupitant is extensively metabolized by CYP3A4 and to a lesser extent by other CYP enzymes. Palonosetron is excreted mostly through urine. Netupitant is excreted mostly through feces. The terminal half-life of palonosetron is 31 to 85 hours. The terminal half-life of fosnetupitant (as the prodrug) is 0.35 to 1.15 hours, and the terminal half-life of netupitant is 71 to 217 hours.

INDICATIONS AND USES

Indicated in combination with dexamethasone in adults for the prevention of acute and delayed nausea and vomiting associated with initial and repeat courses of highly emetogenic cancer chemotherapy.

Limitation of use: The injection has not been studied for the prevention of nausea and vomiting associated with anthracycline plus cyclophosphamide chemotherapy.

CONTRAINDICATIONS

Manufacturer states, "None."

PRECAUTIONS

Hypersensitivity reactions, including anaphylaxis, have occurred with or without known hypersensitivity to other 5-HT$_3$ antagonists. ■ Serotonin syndrome has been reported with 5-HT$_3$ receptor antagonists. Most reports were associated with concomitant use of serotonergic drugs; see Drug/Lab Interactions.

Monitor: Monitor for S/S of hypersensitivity reactions (e.g., chest pain, dizziness, dyspnea, fever, flushing, hypotension, nausea, pruritus, rash, rigors, urticaria). ▪ Monitor for serotonin syndrome, especially when fosnetupitant/palonosetron is used concurrently with other serotonergic drugs. S/S associated with serotonin syndrome may include mental status changes (e.g., agitation, coma, delirium, hallucinations), autonomic instability (e.g., diaphoresis, dizziness, flushing, hyperthermia, labile blood pressure, tachycardia), neuromuscular symptoms (e.g., hyperreflexia, incoordination, myoclonus, rigidity, tremor), and seizures, with or without GI symptoms (e.g., diarrhea, nausea, vomiting). ▪ See Antidote.

Patient Education: Read FDA-approved patient information. ▪ Review prescription and nonprescription medications with health care provider. ▪ Review other medical conditions with health care provider. ▪ Notify provider of known or suspected pregnancy. ▪ Promptly report S/S of hypersensitivity reactions (e.g., hives, swollen face, trouble breathing, chest pain). ▪ Promptly report S/S of serotonin syndrome (e.g., altered mental status, autonomic instability, and neuromuscular symptoms); see Precautions.

Maternal/Child: Based on animal studies, there may be a potential risk to the fetus when administered during pregnancy. ▪ Safety for use during breast-feeding not established; effects unknown. ▪ The safety and effectiveness for use in patients under 18 years of age have not been established.

Elderly: Safety and effectiveness similar to younger adults; however, greater sensitivity in some elderly patients cannot be ruled out.

DRUG/LAB INTERACTIONS

Netupitant is a moderate inhibitor of CYP3A4. Use fosnetupitant and palonosetron with caution in patients receiving concomitant medications that are primarily metabolized through CYP3A4. A single dose of netupitant 300 mg significantly inhibits CYP3A4 for 6 days. Avoid concomitant use of drugs that are **CYP3A4 substrates** for 1 week, if possible. If not avoidable, consider dose reduction of CYP3A4 substrates. ▪ A single dose of fosnetupitant increased the systemic exposure of concomitant **dexamethasone** more than twofold on Days 2 and 4. Administer a reduced dose of dexamethasone with treatment; see Usual Dose. ▪ Systemic exposure of **benzodiazepines** metabolized via CYP3A4 (e.g., alprazolam, midazolam) is increased with coadministration. ▪ The systemic exposure of **chemotherapy agents metabolized by CYP3A4** (e.g., cyclophosphamide, docetaxel, etoposide, ifosfamide, imatinib, irinotecan, paclitaxel, vinblastine, vincristine, and vinorelbine) can increase when administered in combination with fosnetupitant and palonosetron. Monitor for chemotherapy-related adverse reactions with concomitant use. ▪ The effects of fosnetupitant and palonosetron on INR and prothrombin time have not been studied. With concomitant use of **warfarin** and fosnetupitant and palonosetron, monitor INR and adjust the dosage of warfarin to maintain target INR range as needed. ▪ **Strong CYP3A inducers** (e.g., rifampin) can decrease the effectiveness of fosnetupitant and palonosetron; concomitant use should be avoided. ▪ Use with strong **CYP3A4 inhibitors** (e.g., ketoconazole) can increase the systemic exposure to the netupitant component; no dose adjustment indicated for single-dose administration. ▪ Serotonin syndrome (including altered mental status, autonomic instability, and neuromuscular symptoms) has been reported following the concomitant use of 5-HT$_3$ receptor antagonists and **other serotonergic drugs** (e.g., **selective serotonin reuptake inhibitors, serotonin and norepinephrine reuptake inhibitors, monoamine oxidase inhibitors, mirtazapine, fentanyl, lithium, tramadol,** and intravenous **methylene blue**).

SIDE EFFECTS

The most common adverse reactions with IV infusion or oral capsules are asthenia, constipation, dyspepsia, erythema, fatigue, and headache. Safety profiles are similar. Other side effects included concomitant elevations of transaminases and total bilirubin. Serious side effects include hypersensitivity reactions and serotonin syndrome.

ANTIDOTE

Keep physician informed of all side effects. Most minor side effects will be treated symptomatically. In the event of overdose, discontinue treatment and provide general supportive treatment and monitoring. Dialysis studies have not been performed. Discontinue fosnetupitant and palonosetron if a hypersensitivity reaction occurs and treat as indicated (e.g., oxygen, antihistamines, epinephrine, corticosteroids, vasopressor, and/or fluids). If S/S of serotonin syndrome occur, discontinue treatment and initiate supportive care. Resuscitate as indicated.

FOSPHENYTOIN SODIUM BBW
(**FOS**-fen-ih-toyn **SO**-dee-um)

Cerebyx

Anticonvulsant
(hydantoin)

pH 8.6 to 9

USUAL DOSE

Pretreatment: See Maternal/Child.

1.5 mg of fosphenytoin sodium is equivalent to 1 mg phenytoin sodium and is referred to as 1 mg phenytoin sodium equivalents (PE). The amount and concentration of fosphenytoin is always expressed in terms of mg PE. Fosphenytoin 15 to 20 mg PE/kg is equivalent to phenytoin 15 to 20 mg/kg, or a 1,000-mg PE dose of fosphenytoin is equivalent to a 1,000-mg dose of phenytoin. Because of the risk of severe hypotension and cardiac arrhythmias, fosphenytoin should be administered no faster than 150 mg PE/min; see Rate of Administration, Precautions, and Monitor.

Status epilepticus: Adult loading dose: 15 to 20 mg PE/kg administered at 100 to 150 mg PE/min. Full effect is not immediate; concomitant administration of an IV benzodiazepine (e.g., lorazepam) is usually necessary to control status epilepticus. If seizures are not controlled, consider other anticonvulsants and other measures as needed (e.g., barbiturates or anesthesia).

Nonemergent indications: *Loading dose:* 10 to 20 mg PE/kg. ***Maintenance dose (for status epilepticus and nonemergent situations):*** 4 to 6 mg PE/kg/24 hr in divided doses. After administration of a loading dose, maintenance doses should typically be started at the next identified dosing interval. Because of the risk of cardiac and local toxicity associated with IV fosphenytoin, oral phenytoin should be administered whenever possible. See all comments under Usual Dose. See Elderly.

Substitute for oral phenytoin: May be substituted at the same total daily phenytoin sodium equivalents (PE) dose. (Due to a 10% increase in bioavailability [IV/IM to oral], plasma levels with the IV/IM product may be increased slightly.)

PEDIATRIC DOSE

See comments in Usual Dose.

Status epilepticus loading dose: 15 to 20 mg PE/kg at a rate of 2 mg PE/kg/min (or 150 mg PE/min, whichever is lower).

Nonemergent loading dose: 10 to 15 mg PE/kg at a rate of 1 to 2 mg PE/kg/min (or 150 mg PE/min, whichever is lower).

Maintenance dose (for status epilepticus and nonemergent situations): 4 to 8 mg PE/kg/24 hr divided into 2 equal doses (2 to 4 mg PE/kg every 12 hours). Maintenance doses should be started 12 hours after the loading dose and then continued every 12 hours at a rate of 1 to 2 mg PE/kg/min (or 100 mg PE/min, whichever is lower). Because of the risks of cardiac and local toxicity, oral phenytoin should be used whenever possible. IM administration of fosphenytoin is not recommended in pediatric patients unless IV access is not possible.

DOSE ADJUSTMENTS

After the initial maintenance dose, subsequent maintenance doses should be individualized by monitoring serum levels of phenytoin to achieve a target therapeutic concentration. ▪ Lower or less frequent dosing may be required in elderly patients. ▪ Reduced doses may be required in the elderly, in impaired renal or hepatic function, or in patients with hypoalbuminemia. ▪ See Precautions, Monitor, Drug/Lab Interactions, and Antidote.

DILUTION

Use only clear solutions. Available in a 100 mg PE/2 mL or a 500 mg PE/10 mL single-dose vial (50 mg PE/mL). *Do not confuse the concentration of fosphenytoin with the total amount of the drug in the vial; serious errors have occurred. Do not confuse the amount of drug to be given in PE with the concentration of the drug in the vial.* Should be diluted in D5W or NS to a concentration of 1.5 to 25 mg PE/mL. Dilute each milliliter of fosphenytoin with 1 mL of diluent to equal 25 mg PE/mL. Dilute a 1,000-mg PE dose in 100 mL diluent to equal 10 mg PE/mL.

Storage: Keep refrigerated; do not store at room temperature for more than 48 hours. For single use only. Discard any unused product after opening.

COMPATIBILITY

Compatibility information not available from manufacturer. Other sources suggest a few specific **compatibilities** dependent on concentration and manufacturer; consult a pharmacist.

RATE OF ADMINISTRATION

Although the risk of cardiovascular toxicity increases with infusion rates above the recommended infusion rate, these events have also been reported at or below the recommended infusion rates. Slow the rate of infusion or temporarily stop infusion for cardiovascular side effects or for burning, itching, numbness, or pain along injection site.

Adults: Each 100 to 150 mg PE or fraction thereof over a minimum of 1 minute. Do not exceed a rate of 150 mg PE/min.

Pediatric patients: *Loading dose:* Do not exceed a rate of 2 mg PE/kg/min (or 150 mg PE/min, whichever is lower). *Maintenance doses:* Do not exceed a rate of 1 to 2 mg PE/kg/min (or 100 mg PE/min, whichever is lower).

ACTIONS

A water-soluble prodrug of phenytoin. Maximum fosphenytoin concentrations are achieved at the end of the infusion. Converts to phenytoin, phosphate, and formaldehyde after IV/IM administration, with a conversion half-life of approximately 15 minutes. An anticonvulsant, chemically related to barbiturates. Selectively stabilizes seizure threshold and depresses seizure activity in the motor cortex. Modulation of voltage-dependent sodium channels of neurons thought to be the primary cellular mechanism responsible for anticonvulsant activity. Extensively bound to protein, fosphenytoin displaces phenytoin from protein binding sites and increases free phenytoin (dose and rate dependent). Phenytoin's half-life is 12 to 28.9 hours. It is metabolized in the liver by hepatic cytochrome P_{450} enzymes (CYP2C9 and CYP2C19) and excreted in urine. Crosses the placental barrier. Secreted in breast milk.

INDICATIONS AND USES

Treatment of generalized tonic-clonic status epilepticus. ▪ Treatment or prophylaxis of seizures in neurosurgical patients. ▪ Substitute for oral phenytoin when oral administration is not feasible or prompt increases in antiepileptic drug levels are needed.

CONTRAINDICATIONS

History of hypersensitivity to fosphenytoin or its inactive components or to phenytoin or other hydantoins. Reactions have included angioedema. ▪ Sinus bradycardia, sinoatrial block, second- and third-degree AV block, or Adams-Stokes syndrome because of the effect of parenteral phenytoin or fosphenytoin on ventricular automaticity. ▪ A history of acute hepatotoxicity attributable to fosphenytoin or phenytoin. ▪ Coadministration with delavirdine (Rescriptor); see Drug/Lab Interactions.

PRECAUTIONS

Doses of fosphenytoin are expressed in terms of milligrams of phenytoin equivalents (mg PE) to avoid the need to perform molecular weight–based adjustments when substituting fosphenytoin for phenytoin or vice versa; no adjustment required when substituting fosphenytoin or vice versa. Labeling of fosphenytoin has been updated by the manufacturer to reduce the incidence of dosing errors. To ensure accuracy, confirm actual dose and volume to be administered with a pharmacist or another RN. ▪ Advantages of fosphenytoin over present phenytoin products include solubility in IV solutions, improved infusion site tolerance, more rapid rate of administration, and well-tolerated IM option. ▪ IV route indicated in emergency situations (e.g., status epilepticus). May be given IM to adults in nonemergency situations. ▪ Oral phenytoin is preferred in nonemergency situations because of the risks of cardiac and local toxicity associated with IV fosphenytoin. Adverse cardiovascular reactions have occurred during and after infusions and have been reported with infusion rates above the recommended rate as well as with infusion rates at or below the recommended rate. ▪ May cause severe cardiovascular reactions (e.g., severe hypotension, bradycardia, various degrees of AV block, QT interval prolongation, ventricular tachycardia, ventricular fibrillation) that have resulted in asystole, cardiac arrest, and death; use extreme caution in elderly or seriously ill patients and in patients with hypotension or severe myocardial insufficiency. Risk of severe hypotension and cardiac arrhythmias increased by higher IV doses and/or rapid administration. ▪ Intended for short-term parenteral use (up to 5 days). ▪ Transfer to oral phenytoin therapy as soon as feasible. ▪ Abrupt withdrawal of antiepileptic drugs may cause increased seizure activity, including status epilepticus. Gradually reduce dose, discontinue, or substitute alternative antiepileptic agents. ▪ Discontinue immediately for hypersensitivity reactions; with caution rapidly substitute a nonhydantoin anticonvulsant. ▪ Angioedema has been reported. ▪ In patients who have experienced phenytoin hypersensitivity, alternatives to structurally similar drugs such as carbamazepine, barbiturates, succinimides, and oxazolidinediones should be considered. ▪ May exacerbate porphyria. ▪ Drug reaction with eosinophilia and systemic symptoms (DRESS), also known as multiorgan hypersensitivity, has been reported. DRESS usually presents with fever, rash, and/or lymphadenopathy and/or facial swelling in association with other organ system involvement such as hepatitis, nephritis, hematologic abnormalities, myocarditis, or myositis. Eosinophilia is often present. Deaths have been reported. ▪ May cause acute phenytoin hepatotoxicity, which may manifest as elevated liver function tests, jaundice, hepatomegaly, leukocytosis, eosinophilia, and/or acute hepatic failure. These events may be part of the spectrum of DRESS or may occur in isolation. Discontinue immediately, do not readminister, and substitute alternate anticonvulsant therapy. ▪ Has caused hematopoietic complications (e.g., agranulocytosis, granulocytopenia, leukopenia, thrombocytopenia, or pancytopenia with or without bone marrow suppression). ▪ Some reports suggest a relationship between phenytoin and the development of lymphadenopathy (local or generalized), including benign lymph node hyperplasia, pseudolymphoma, lymphoma, and Hodgkin disease. Lymph node involvement may occur with or without S/S resembling DRESS. In all cases of lymphadenopathy, follow-up observation for an extended period is indicated, and alternative anticonvulsant therapy should be strongly considered. ▪ Sensory disturbances, including severe burning, itching, and paresthesia, have been reported; more common with higher doses and/or rates. The occurrence and intensity of discomfort may be lessened by slowing or temporarily stopping the infusion. No permanent sequelae have been reported. ▪ Purple glove syndrome (edema, discoloration, and pain distal to the injection site) has occurred and may or may not be associated with extravasation. The syndrome may not develop for several days. ▪ Severe cutaneous adverse reactions (SCARs) have been reported, including toxic epidermal necrolysis (TEN), Stevens-Johnson syndrome (SJS), acute generalized exanthematous pustulosis (AGEP), and DRESS. Deaths have occurred. Onset of symptoms is usually within 28 days but may occur later. Discontinue fosphenytoin at the first sign of a rash unless the rash is clearly not drug related. If a rash develops, the patient should be evaluated for S/S of SCARs. ▪ Selected patients of Asian ancestry with a specific human leukocyte antigen allele (HLA-B*1502) may have an increased risk of serious skin reactions (e.g., Stevens-Johnson syndrome, toxic epidermal necrolysis) from phenytoin therapy. ▪ Use caution in patients with impaired renal or hepatic function or in patients with hypoalbuminemia. After an IV loading dose, fosphenytoin clearance to phenytoin may be increased without a similar increase in phenytoin clearance. This, together with an increased fraction of unbound phenytoin in these patient populations, may increase the incidence and frequency of adverse reactions. ▪ Use caution with low serum albumin levels, and adjust dose as indicated. Phenytoin is highly bound to serum protein, and a reduced albumin causes an increase in free drug availability and may increase toxicity. ▪ Not effective for absence seizures; combined therapy required if both conditions present. ▪ Not indicated for seizures due to hypoglycemia or other metabolic causes. ▪ Inhibits insulin release and may increase serum glucose; monitoring indicated in diabetics. ▪ May lower serum folate levels. ▪ Antiepileptic drugs (AEDs) increase the risk of suicidal thoughts or behavior in patients taking these drugs for any indication. Patients treated with any AED for any indication should be monitored for the emergence or worsening of depression, suicidal thoughts or behavior, and/or any unusual changes in mood or behavior. Some psychotic symptoms and/or behavioral changes resolved without intervention. Others required dose reduction or discontinuation of the antiepileptic agent. ▪ Confusional states referred to as delirium, psychosis, encephalopathy or, rarely, irreversible cerebellar dysfunction and/or cerebellar atrophy have been reported when plasma phenytoin concentrations are sustained above the optimum range. At the first sign of acute toxicity, determination of plasma phenytoin concentration is recommended. Reduce dose if indicated. If symptoms persist, discontinue fosphenytoin. ▪ A small percentage of patients may be slow metabolizers of phenytoin. This appears to be genetically determined. If early signs of dose-related CNS toxicity develop, obtain serum levels immediately.

Monitor: Monitor ECG, BP, and respirations continuously during loading dose and for at least 10 to 20 minutes after infusion is complete. ▪ Allow fosphenytoin time to convert to phenytoin; accurate serum levels are not available until 2 hours after the end of an IV infusion or 4 hours after IM injection. Narrow margin of error between therapeutic and toxic dose. Plasma levels above 10 mcg/mL usually control seizure activity. The acceptable range is 5 to 20 mcg/mL (unbound phenytoin concentration of 1 to 2 mcg/mL). Toxicity usually begins with nystagmus at levels exceeding 20 mcg/mL. ▪ Because the unbound fraction of phenytoin is increased in patients with renal or hepatic disease or in those with hypoalbuminemia, the monitoring of phenytoin serum levels should be based on the unbound fraction. ▪ Periodic monitoring of CBC, liver function, and blood glucose levels recommended. ▪ Monitor for S/S of hypersensitivity reactions. Observe for rash and discontinue if one appears. If rash is mild, fosphenytoin may be resumed when the rash has completely disappeared. Discontinue fosphenytoin if the mild rash occurs again, if the initial rash is serious in nature (e.g., exfoliative, purpuric, bullous), or if Stevens-Johnson syndrome or toxic epidermal necrolysis is suspected. Do not resume; consider alternative therapy. ▪ Monitor for symptoms of angioedema (e.g., facial, perioral, or upper airway swelling). ▪ Phosphate is produced as a metabolite; monitor in patients who require phosphate restriction (e.g., renal impairment). ▪ Monitor patients who are gravely ill, have impaired liver or renal function or hypoalbuminemia, or are elderly. May show early signs of toxicity. ▪ Determine absolute patency of vein; avoid extravasation. Not as alkaline as phenytoin. ▪ Observe patient closely for signs of CNS side effects; see Precautions.

Patient Education: Effective birth control required for women of childbearing potential who are not planning a pregnancy. Hormonal contraceptive efficacy may be decreased; see Maternal/Child. ▪ Capable of numerable drug interactions. Review list of over-the-counter and prescription medications and alcohol use with provider. ▪ Promptly report burning, itching, numbness, pain, or rash. ▪ Promptly report chills and/or fever and S/S of cardiovascular toxicity, an infusion reaction, a hypersensitivity reaction (e.g., chest pain, dizziness, feeling faint, flushing, hives, nausea, shortness of breath), or S/S of angioedema (e.g., facial, perioral, or upper airway swelling). ▪ May increase the risk of suicidal thoughts and behavior. Promptly report emergence or worsening of the S/S of depression, any unusual changes in mood or behavior, or thoughts about self-harm. ▪ Women who are pregnant or who become pregnant should be encouraged to enroll in the North American Antiepileptic Drug (NAAED) Pregnancy Registry.

Maternal/Child: Avoid pregnancy. Prenatal exposure to phenytoin may increase the risk of congenital malformations and other adverse developmental outcomes. Consider risk versus benefit. ▪ Decreased serum concentrations of phenytoin may occur during pregnancy and may result in increased seizure frequency. Periodic serum phenytoin concentrations should be performed based on the unbound fraction because of potential changes in protein binding during pregnancy; adjust dose as indicated. ▪ Newborns whose mothers received phenytoin during pregnancy may develop a life-threatening bleeding disorder that can be prevented by giving vitamin K to the mother before delivery and to the neonate after birth. ▪ Active metabolite of fosphenytoin (phenytoin) is secreted in breast milk; consider risk versus benefit. ▪ Safety and effectiveness for use in pediatric patients has been established. ▪ See Patient Education.

Elderly: See Dose Adjustments. ▪ Sensitivity and/or toxicity may be increased because serum concentrations may be elevated due to reduced clearance, or low serum albumin may cause a decrease in protein binding and an increase in free phenytoin.

DRUG/LAB INTERACTIONS

No drugs are known to interfere with the conversion of fosphenytoin to phenytoin, although phosphatase activity may have an impact. ▪ *Capable of innumerable catastrophic drug interactions; review of drug profile by pharmacist imperative.* In all situations, monitoring of phenytoin serum levels may be indicated. ▪ Phenytoin is highly protein bound and is prone to competitive displacement. ▪ Phenytoin is metabolized by CYP2C9 and CYP2C19 and is particularly susceptible to inhibitory drug interactions because it is subject to saturable metabolism. Inhibition of metabolism may produce significant increases in circulating phenytoin concentrations, increasing the risk of toxicity. ▪ Coadministration with **delavirdine** is contraindicated. Has the potential for loss of virologic response and possible resistance to delavirdine or to the class of nonnucleoside reverse transcriptase inhibitors. ▪ Serum levels and toxicity of phenytoin may be increased by **alcohol (acute intake), amiodarone, antiepileptic agents** (e.g., felbamate, topiramate, oxcarbazepine), **azoles** (e.g., fluconazole, itraconazole, ketoconazole, miconazole, voriconazole), **capecitabine, chloramphenicol, chlordiazepoxide, disulfiram, estrogens, fluorouracil, fluoxetine, fluvastatin, fluvoxamine, H$_2$ antagonists, halothane, isoniazid, methylphenidate, omeprazole, phenothiazines, salicylates** (aspirin), **sertraline, succinimides** (e.g., ethosuximide), **sulfonamides** (e.g., sulfamethizole, sulfamethoxazole/trimethoprim), **tolbutamide, trazodone, and warfarin**. ▪ Serum levels and effectiveness of phenytoin may be decreased by **anticancer drugs, antivirals** (e.g., fosamprenavir, nelfinavir, ritonavir), **carbamazepine, chronic alcohol abuse, diazepam, diazoxide, folic acid, reserpine, rifampin, St. John's wort, theophylline, and vigabatrin**. ▪ Serum levels of phenytoin may be increased or decreased by **phenobarbital, valproate sodium, valproic acid.** Similarly, phenytoin may unpredictably affect the levels and efficacy of these drugs. ▪ Phenytoin will inhibit the effects of **azole antifungals** (e.g., fluconazole, posaconazole, voriconazole), **corticosteroids, doxycycline, estrogens, furosemide, irinotecan, oral contraceptives, paclitaxel, paroxetine, quinidine, rifampin, sertraline, teniposide, theophylline, and vitamin D.** Dose adjustment of these agents may be indicated. ▪ Decreases plasma concentrations of **active metabolites of albendazole, antiepileptic agents, atorvastatin,** certain **HIV antivirals** (e.g., efavirenz, lopinavir/ritonavir, indinavir, nelfinavir, ritonavir, saquinavir), **chlorpropamide, clozapine, cyclosporine, digoxin, fluvastatin, folic acid, methadone, mexiletine, nifedipine, nimodipine, nisoldipine, praziquantel, quetiapine, simvastatin,** and **verapamil.** Adjust doses of these agents as indicated. ▪ May increase or decrease PT/INR responses when coadministered with **warfarin**. ▪ When given with **fosamprenavir** alone, phenytoin may decrease the concentration of **amprenavir,** the active metabolite. When given in combination with **fosamprenavir and ritonavir**, phenytoin may increase the concentration of **amprenavir**. ■ Resistance to the neuromuscular blocking action of the **nondepolarizing neuromuscular blocking agents** pancuronium, vecuronium, rocuronium, and cisatracurium has occurred in patients receiving long-term administration of phenytoin. Monitor for more rapid than expected recovery from neuromuscular blockade. ■ Alters some **clinical laboratory tests** (e.g., may decrease T_4, increase glucose, alkaline phosphatase, and gamma-glutamyl transferase (GGT); may produce low results in dexamethasone or metyrapone tests).

SIDE EFFECTS
Transient ataxia, dizziness, nystagmus, paresthesia, pruritus, and somnolence are the most common side effects in adults and are dose- and rate-related. Ataxia, nystagmus, and vomiting are the most common side effects in pediatric patients. Risks of side effects increased with upper-end doses given at upper-end rates. The more important adverse clinical events caused by IV use of fosphenytoin are cardiovascular collapse and/or CNS depression. Coma, hyperreflexia, hypotension, lethargy, nausea, slurred speech, tremor, and vomiting are also signs of increased toxicity. Confusional states (e.g., delirium, encephalopathy, psychosis) and, rarely, irreversible cerebellar dysfunction can occur with high plasma concentrations. Fosphenytoin breaks down into formate and phosphate metabolites that may cause formate and phosphate toxicity in overdose situations (hypocalcemia, metabolic acidosis, muscle spasms, paresthesia, and seizures). Psychotic symptoms, including aggression, agitation, anger, anxiety, apathy, depersonalization, depression, emotional lability, hallucinations, hostility, irritability, and suicidal tendencies, have occurred with antiepileptic agents. Several other adverse reactions have been reported.

Overdose: Arrhythmias (e.g., asystole, bradycardia, cardiac arrest, tachycardia), ataxia, coma, dysarthria, hepatotoxicity, hyperreflexia, hypocalcemia, hypotension, lethargy, metabolic acidosis, nausea, nystagmus, slurred speech, syncope, tremor, and vomiting. Deaths from circulatory and respiratory depression have been reported. The lethal dose of phenytoin in adults is estimated to be 2 to 5 Gm. The lethal dose in pediatric patients is not known.

Post-Marketing: Anaphylactoid reactions, including anaphylaxis and angioedema; dyskinesia; laboratory test abnormalities, including decreased serum concentrations of T4, lower than normal values for dexamethasone or metyrapone tests, and increased serum levels of GGT.

ANTIDOTE
Notify physician of any side effects. Obtain serum plasma levels at first signs of toxicity; reduce dose. If serum levels are excessive, symptoms persist or major side effects appear, discontinue fosphenytoin and notify physician. Treat symptomatically, maintain a patent airway, and resuscitate as necessary. Discontinue fosphenytoin at the first sign of a rash unless the rash is clearly not drug related. If TEN or SJS is suspected, do not rechallenge; consider alternate therapy. Discontinue immediately if symptoms of angioedema develop. Evaluate for multiorgan hypersensitivity reactions (DRESS). Cardiovascular toxicity, including hypotension or cardiac arrhythmias, may respond to a decrease in infusion rate. Consider hemodialysis in overdose (phenytoin [the active metabolite of fosphenytoin] is not completely bound to plasma proteins). Total exchange transfusion has been used in the treatment of severe intoxication in pediatric patients. In acute overdose, consider the possibility of other CNS depressants, including alcohol. In overdose, measure ionized free calcium levels to guide treatment in phosphate toxicity.

FUROSEMIDE BBW

(fur-**OH**-seh-myd)

Lasix

Diuretic (loop)

pH 8 to 9.3

USUAL DOSE

Adjust dose and dose schedule to individual patient needs. Reserve parenteral therapy for emergent situations or for patients unable to take oral therapy. Switch to oral therapy as soon as practical.

Pretreatment: Patient assessment may be indicated; see Precautions.

Edema: 20 to 40 mg. May be repeated in 2 hours. If necessary, increase dosage by 20-mg increments (under close medical supervision and no sooner than 2 hours after previous dose) until desired diuresis is obtained. After the initial diuresis the minimum effective dose may be given once or twice every 24 hours as required for maintenance.

Acute pulmonary edema: 40 mg. Dose may be increased to 80 mg after 1 hour if satisfactory response is not obtained. AHA guidelines recommend 0.5 mg/kg to 1 mg/kg over 1 to 2 minutes. If no response, increase to 2 mg/kg. For **new-onset pulmonary edema with hypovolemia**, a dose of less than 0.5 mg/kg is recommended. Additional therapy (e.g., digoxin, oxygen) may be administered concurrently as needed.

Hypertensive crisis (unlabeled): AHA guidelines recommend 0.5 to 1 mg/kg over 1 to 2 minutes. If no response, increase dose to 2 mg/kg.

PEDIATRIC DOSE

See Maternal/Child.

Diuretic: 1 mg/kg of body weight. After 2 hours increase by 1-mg/kg increments to effect desired response. Do not exceed 6 mg/kg/dose. Effective dose may be given every 6 to 12 hours. Another source suggests 1 to 2 mg/kg/dose every 6 to 12 hours.

NEONATAL DOSE

Diuretic: 0.5 to 1 mg/kg/dose every 8 to 24 hours. Maximum dose is 2 mg/kg/dose. Literature reports suggest that the maximum dose for premature infants should not exceed 1 mg/kg/day. See Maternal/Child.

DOSE ADJUSTMENTS

Higher doses may be required in renal insufficiency and acute or chronic renal failure. ▪ Reduced dose or extended intervals may be appropriate in the elderly. ▪ Extend dosing intervals in neonates because half-life is prolonged. ▪ See Drug/Lab Interactions.

DILUTION

May be given undiluted. May be given through Y-tube of infusion set. Not usually added to IV solutions, but large doses may be added to NS, LR, or D5W and given as an infusion. Another source suggests it can be diluted with D5NS. pH of solution must be over 5.5. Some sources recommend protecting diluted solutions from light to prevent photodegradation (minimized at pH 7).

Filters: One source found no significant drug loss when filtered through a 0.22-micron filter.

Storage: Store vials at CRT. Protect from light. If diluted for infusion, discard after 24 hours.

COMPATIBILITY

Furosemide may precipitate at a pH below 7. Manufacturer states, "Acid solutions, including other parenteral medications (e.g., amrinone, ciprofloxacin, labetalol, milrinone), must not be administered concurrently in the same infusion." Additionally, "Furosemide should not be added to an IV line containing any of these acidic products."

Other sources suggest specific **compatibilities** dependent on concentration and manufacturer; consult a pharmacist.

RATE OF ADMINISTRATION
IV injection: Each 40 mg or fraction thereof should be given over 1 to 2 minutes.
Infusion: One source recommends the following: **Adults:** 0.1 mg/kg/hr. **Pediatric patients:** 0.05 mg/kg/hr. Titrate to effect. High-dose therapy in an infusion should not exceed a rate of 4 mg/min.

ACTIONS
A potent loop diuretic, structurally related to sulfonamides. Onset of action is prompt, usually within 5 minutes. Duration of action and half-life are approximately 2 hours. Inhibits the reabsorption of sodium and chloride in the proximal and distal tubules and in the loop of Henle, causing increased excretion of water, sodium, chloride, magnesium, and calcium. Highly protein bound. Metabolized and excreted in the urine. Crosses the placental barrier. Secreted in breast milk.

INDICATIONS AND USES
Parenteral therapy should be reserved for patients unable to take oral medications or for emergency clinical situations. ▪ Edema associated with congestive heart failure, cirrhosis of the liver, and renal disease, including nephrotic syndrome. Particularly useful when an agent with a greater diuretic potential is required. ▪ Adjunctive therapy in acute pulmonary edema. Indicated when rapid onset of diuresis is necessary (e.g., acute pulmonary edema).

CONTRAINDICATIONS
Anuria, hypersensitivity to furosemide.

PRECAUTIONS
A potent diuretic; may precipitate excessive diuresis with water and electrolyte depletion. Careful medical supervision is required. ▪ Use caution and improve basic condition first in hepatic coma, electrolyte depletion, and advanced cirrhosis of the liver. Sudden alterations of fluid and electrolyte balance in patients with cirrhosis may precipitate hepatic coma. Supplemental potassium chloride and, if required, an aldosterone antagonist (e.g., spironolactone) are helpful in preventing hypokalemia and metabolic alkalosis. ▪ Excessive diuresis may cause dehydration and blood volume reduction with circulatory collapse and possibly vascular thrombosis and embolism, particularly in the elderly. ▪ If increasing azotemia and oliguria develop during treatment of severe progressive renal disease, furosemide should be discontinued. ▪ Use caution in known sulfonamide sensitivity. Manufacturer states that patients allergic to sulfonamides may also be allergic to furosemide. However, current literature suggests that the potential for cross-reactivity between antibiotic sulfonamides and nonantibiotic sulfonamides is low. ▪ Ototoxicity (tinnitus, reversible or irreversible hearing impairment and deafness) has been reported. Risk increases with higher doses, rapid injection, severe renal dysfunction, hypoproteinemia, or concurrent use with other ototoxic drugs; see Drug/Lab Interactions. ▪ In patients with hypoproteinemia (e.g., associated with nephrotic syndrome), the effect of furosemide may be weakened and its ototoxicity potentiated. ▪ May activate or exacerbate systemic lupus erythematosus. ▪ Use caution in patients with severe symptoms of urinary retention (because of bladder emptying disorders, prostatic hypertrophy, urethral narrowing). May experience acute urinary retention related to increased production and retention of urine. Careful monitoring required, especially during the initiation of therapy.
Monitor: Monitor BP frequently, especially during initial therapy. ▪ May precipitate excessive diuresis with water and electrolyte imbalance (hyponatremia, hypochloremic alkalosis, hypokalemia, hypomagnesemia, or hypocalcemia). Routine checks on electrolyte panel, CO_2, SCr, and BUN are necessary during therapy. Electrolyte replacement may be required. ▪ May increase blood glucose and has precipitated diabetes mellitus (rare). Monitoring may be indicated, especially in patients with diabetes or suspected latent diabetes. ▪ Periodic monitoring of CBC and liver function tests are indicated to monitor for blood dyscrasias or liver damage. ▪ Monitor for other S/S of fluid or electrolyte imbalance, which may include arrhythmia, drowsiness, dryness of the mouth, hypotension, lethargy, muscle cramps or fatigue, nausea or vomiting, oliguria, restlessness, tachycardia,

thirst, and weakness. ▪ May lower serum calcium level; may cause tetany. ▪ Hyperuricemia can occur. Rarely precipitates acute gout attack. ▪ See Drug/Lab Interactions.

Patient Education: Hypotension may cause dizziness; request assistance with ambulation. ▪ Report cramps, dizziness, muscle weakness, or nausea promptly. ▪ May cause a decrease in potassium levels and require a supplement. ▪ Skin may become photosensitive; avoid unprotected exposure to sun. ▪ Therapy for diabetes may require adjustment; monitoring of serum glucose required.

Maternal/Child: Category C: use during pregnancy only when clearly needed and benefits outweigh potential risks to fetus. Treatment during pregnancy requires monitoring of fetal growth because of the potential for higher fetal birth weights. ▪ Use caution in breast-feeding; may inhibit lactation. ▪ May precipitate nephrocalcinosis and nephrolithiasis in premature infants. Has also been observed in pediatric patients under 4 years of age who have been treated chronically with furosemide. Monitor renal function. Renal ultrasonography may be indicated. ▪ Administration in the first few weeks of life may increase risk of persistent patent ductus arteriosus in preterm infants with respiratory distress syndrome. ▪ Premature infants receiving doses exceeding 1 mg/kg/day may develop plasma levels that could be associated with toxicity, including ototoxicity. Hearing loss in neonates has been associated with the use of furosemide.

Elderly: Protein binding and clearance are decreased in the elderly. ▪ Consider increased sensitivity to hypotensive and electrolyte effects. Dose selection should be cautious, starting at the lower end of the dosing range. ▪ May be more susceptible to dehydration; observe carefully. ▪ Avoid rapid contraction of plasma volume and hemoconcentration. May cause thromboembolic episodes (e.g., CVA, pulmonary emboli). ▪ The initial diuretic effect in older patients is decreased relative to younger patients.

DRUG/LAB INTERACTIONS

Concomitant use with **amphotericin B, corticosteroids, ACTH, licorice** in large amounts, or prolonged use of **laxatives** may increase the risk of hypokalemia. ▪ Potentiates **antihypertensive drugs** (e.g., angiotensin II receptor blockers, nitroglycerin, nitroprusside sodium); reduced dose of the antihypertensive agent or both drugs may be indicated. In addition to hypotension, concomitant use with angiotensin-converting enzyme inhibitors (ACEIs) or angiotensin II receptor blockers (ARBs) may lead to deterioration in renal function, including renal failure. An interruption or reduction in the dose of furosemide, ACEI, or ARB may be necessary. ▪ May cause transient or permanent deafness with doses exceeding the usual or when given in conjunction with **other ototoxic drugs** (e.g., aminoglycosides [e.g., gentamicin], cisplatin), especially in the presence of renal impairment; avoid concomitant use if possible. Do not use concomitantly with **ethacrynic acid** (Edecrin); risk of ototoxicity markedly increased. ▪ Nephrotoxicity increased by **other nephrotoxic agents** (e.g., aminoglycosides, cephalosporins, cisplatin, cyclosporine, radiocontrast agents, vancomycin). Monitor renal function closely. ▪ Diuretics reduce the renal clearance of **lithium**, increasing the risk of toxicity. ▪ May cause cardiac arrhythmias with **amiodarone or digoxin** (potassium depletion). ▪ May enhance or inhibit actions of **nondepolarizing muscle relaxants**. ▪ May potentiate the action of **succinylcholine**. ▪ Effects may be inhibited by **NSAIDs** (e.g., ibuprofen) **or probenecid**. ▪ May cause profound diuresis and serious electrolyte abnormalities with **thiazide diuretics** because of synergistic effects. ▪ **Furosemide** may increase serum levels of salicylates, increasing the risk of toxicity. ▪ May decrease arterial responsiveness to **norepinephrine**. Dose adjustment may be required. ▪ May enhance adverse effects of **chloral hydrate**. Concomitant use not recommended. ▪ **Methotrexate** and other drugs that undergo significant renal tubular secretion may decrease the effectiveness of furosemide. ▪ Furosemide may decrease renal elimination of other drugs that undergo tubular secretion. High-dose treatment of both furosemide and these other drugs may result in elevated serum levels and may potentiate toxicity. ▪ Concomitant use of **cyclosporine** and furosemide has been associated with increased risk of gouty arthritis secondary to furosemide-induced hyperuricemia and cyclosporine impairment of renal urate excretion. ▪ Simultaneous administration of sucralfate and furosemide injection may reduce the natriuretic and antihypertensive effects of furosemide. Separate doses by at least 2 hours and monitor for desired effect. ▪ High doses (greater than 80 mg) of furosemide may inhibit the binding of **thyroid hormones** to carrier proteins and result in a transient increase in free thyroid hormones followed by an overall decrease in total thyroid hormone levels. ▪ See Precautions.

SIDE EFFECTS

Usually occur in prolonged therapy, seriously ill patients, or following large doses.

The most serious side effects include anaphylactic or anaphylactoid reactions (severe or with shock), aplastic anemia, drug rash with eosinophilia and systemic symptoms (DRESS), erythema multiforme, exanthematous pustulosis (acute, generalized), hepatic encephalopathy in patients with hepatocellular insufficiency, orthostatic hypotension (may be aggravated by alcohol, barbiturates, or narcotics), Stevens-Johnson syndrome, tinnitus and hearing loss, and toxic epidermal necrolysis. Anorexia; blurred vision; bullous pemphigoid; constipation; cramping; diarrhea; dizziness; exfoliative dermatitis; headache; hematologic reactions (agranulocytosis, anemia, eosinophilia, hemolytic anemia, GI cramping, leukopenia, thrombocytopenia); increased cholesterol, liver enzymes, and triglyceride serum levels; interstitial nephritis; jaundice (intrahepatic cholestatic jaundice); nausea; necrotizing angiitis; oral and gastric irritation; pancreatitis; paresthesias; photosensitivity; pruritus; purpura; rash; thrombocytopenia; urticaria; vasculitis (systemic); vertigo; vomiting; and xanthopsia have occurred. Fever, glycosuria, hyperglycemia, hyperuricemia, muscle spasms, restlessness, thrombophlebitis, transient injection site pain following IM injection, urinary bladder spasm, and weakness have also been reported.

Overdose: Blood volume reduction, dehydration, electrolyte imbalances, hypochloremic alkalosis, and hypotension.

ANTIDOTE

If minor side effects are noted, notify the physician, who may treat the side effects symptomatically and continue the drug. If side effects are progressive or any major side effect occurs, discontinue the drug immediately and notify the physician. Treatment of major side effects is symptomatic and aggressive. Monitor serum electrolytes, carbon dioxide level, and BP frequently, and replace excessive fluid and electrolyte losses as needed. Hemodialysis does not accelerate furosemide elimination. Resuscitate as necessary.

GANCICLOVIR SODIUM BBW

(gan-**SYE**-kloh-veer **SO**-dee-um)

Antiviral

Cytovene IV, Ganzyk-RTU

pH 9 to 11, pH 7.5

USUAL DOSE

Pretreatment: Verify pregnancy status. Adequate hydration and specific testing required; see Monitor.

CMV retinitis in adults: Induction dose: 5 mg/kg of body weight every 12 hours for 14 to 21 days.

Maintenance dose: Begin a maintenance dose the next day (Day 15 to 22) of 5 mg/kg daily for 7 days each week or 6 mg/kg daily for 5 days each week. See Precautions/Monitor. Do not exceed recommended dose or infusion rate. Larger doses or increased rates of infusion have resulted in increased toxicity. For patients who have relapsed after induction and re-induction monotherapy with either ganciclovir or foscarnet, practitioners may consider an unlabeled combination therapy that adds the alternate drug to the regimen. Information on this combination regimen is available from the manufacturer and in the Clinical Trials section of the foscarnet sodium prescribing information.

Prevention of CMV disease in adult transplant recipients: *Induction dose:* 5 mg/kg every 12 hours for 7 to 14 days.

Maintenance dose: Follow with maintenance regimen of 5 mg/kg once daily for 7 days per week or 6 mg/kg once daily for 5 days per week until 100 to 120 days posttransplantation. CMV disease may occur if treatment is stopped prematurely.

PEDIATRIC DOSE

Safety for use in pediatric patients not established. ■ Use extreme caution; long-term carcinogenicity and reproductive toxicity are probable. Benefit must outweigh risks. See Indications and Maternal/Child.

CMV retinitis in pediatric patients over 3 months of age (unlabeled): *Induction dose:* 5 mg/kg of body weight every 12 hours for 14 to 21 days. May be increased to 7.5 mg/kg/dose every 12 hours.

Maintenance dose: Begin a maintenance dose the next day (Day 15 to 22) of 5 mg/kg daily for 5 to 7 days each week.

Prevention of CMV disease in transplant recipients (unlabeled): See Usual Dose.

DOSE ADJUSTMENTS

Dose selection should be cautious in elderly patients. Reduced doses may be indicated based on the potential for decreased organ function and concomitant disease or drug therapy; see Elderly. ■ Use is not recommended in patients with an absolute neutrophil count (ANC) less than 500 cells/mm^3, hemoglobin less than 8 gm/dL, or platelet count less than 25,000 cells/mm^3. ■ See Drug/Lab Interactions. ■ With impaired renal function, reduce dose according to the following chart.

Ganciclovir Induction and Maintenance Dose Guidelines in Impaired Renal Function					
Creatinine Clearance (mL/min)	Ganciclovir IV Induction Dose (mg/kg)	Dosing Interval (hours)	Ganciclovir Maintenance Dose (mg/kg)	Dosing Interval (hours)
≥70	5 mg/kg	12 hours	5 mg/kg	24 hours
50–69	2.5 mg/kg	12 hours	2.5 mg/kg	24 hours
25–49	2.5 mg/kg	24 hours	1.25 mg/kg	24 hours
10–24	1.25 mg/kg	24 hours	0.625 mg/kg	24 hours
<10	1.25 mg/kg	3 times per week following hemodialysis	0.625 mg/kg	3 times per week following hemodialysis

DILUTION

Specific techniques required; see Precautions.

Cytovene IV: Initially dissolve the 500-mg vial with 10 mL SWFI (50 mg/mL). Do not use bacteriostatic water containing parabens; will cause precipitation. Gently swirl the vial. Continue swirling until a clear reconstituted solution is obtained. Discard if particulate matter or discoloration observed. Withdraw desired dose and further dilute with NS, D5W, Ringer's, or LR to provide a concentration less than 10 mg/mL (70-kg adult at 5 mg/kg equals 350 mg; dissolved in 100 mL of solution equals 3.5 mg/mL).

Ganzyk-RTU: Premixed, ready-to-use, single-dose polymeric bag containing 500 mg ganciclovir in 250 mL of solution (2 mg/mL).

Filters: Use not required by manufacturer; however, use of a filter would not have an adverse effect.

Storage: *Cytovene IV:* Store at CRT before use. Reconstituted solution in vial stable at RT ($25°$ C [$77°$ F]) for 12 hours. Do not refrigerate or freeze. Solution fully diluted for administration must be refrigerated at $2°$ to $8°$ C ($36°$ to $46°$ F) and used within 24 hours to reduce incidence of bacterial contamination. Do not freeze.

Ganzyk-RTU: Store at CRT before use. Discard any unused portion.

COMPATIBILITY

Manufacturer of Ganzyk-RTU states, "Do not add supplemental medication to the intravenous bag."

Because of physical **incompatibilities,** ganciclovir sodium and *foscarnet sodium* must never be mixed.

Other sources suggest a few specific **compatibilities** dependent on concentration and manufacturer; consult a pharmacist.

RATE OF ADMINISTRATION

A single dose must be administered at a constant rate over 1 hour as an infusion, preferably via plastic cannula. *Do not give by rapid or bolus IV injection.* Excessive plasma levels and toxicity will occur with a too-rapid rate of injection. Advisable to clear tubing with NS before and after administration through Y-tube.

ACTIONS

An antiviral agent with virustatic activity against CMV. Inhibits DNA synthesis and stops cytomegalovirus (CMV) from multiplying. Widely distributed in tissues and body fluids. Crosses the placental barrier. Suspected to be secreted in breast milk. Half-life is 2.6 to 4.4 hours. Approximately 90% excreted unchanged in urine in patients with normal renal function.

INDICATIONS AND USES

Treatment of CMV retinitis in immunocompromised adult individuals, including patients with AIDS. ▪ CMV disease prevention in at-risk adult transplant patients.

Unlabeled uses: Treatment of other CMV infections (e.g., gastroenteritis, hepatitis, pneumonitis) in immunocompromised patients. ▪ Combination therapy (ganciclovir and foscarnet) to treat progressive retinitis refractory to single-agent therapy.

CONTRAINDICATIONS

Patients who have experienced a clinically significant hypersensitivity reaction (e.g., anaphylaxis) to ganciclovir, valganciclovir, or any component of the formulation. ▪ Use is not recommended in patients with neutrophil count less than 500 cells/mm^3, hemoglobin less than 8 gm/dL, or platelet count less than 25,000 cells/mm^3.

PRECAUTIONS

A nucleoside analog; follow guidelines for handling and disposal of cytotoxic agents. See Appendix A, p. 1308. ▪ For IV use only; IM or SQ administration will cause severe tissue irritation. ▪ Hematologic toxicity (anemia, granulocytopenia, pancytopenia, thrombocytopenia) has been reported; see Monitor. ▪ Use with caution in patients with pre-existing cytopenias and in patients receiving myelosuppressive drugs or irradiation. ▪ Use with caution in patients with renal impairment. Increased SCr has been reported in elderly patients and in transplant patients receiving concomitant nephrotoxic medications (e.g., cyclosporine and amphotericin B). ▪ Ganciclovir is not a cure for CMV infections. Maintenance therapy is almost always necessary to prevent relapse in patients with AIDS. ▪ Resistance has been reported to develop. May be higher in patients treated for a prolonged period. The possibility of resistance should be considered in patients who show poor clinical response or experience persistent viral excretion during therapy. ▪ May cause temporary or permanent inhibition of spermatogenesis in males and suppression of fertility in females. ▪ Based on animal data, has the potential to cause cancer in humans.

Monitor: Confirm diagnosis of CMV retinitis by indirect ophthalmoscopy. Diagnosis may be supported by cultures of CMV (e.g., urine, blood, throat); negative culture does not rule out CMV retinitis. ▪ Continue ophthalmologic exams during induction and maintenance treatment to monitor CMV status. ▪ CBC with differential and platelet counts are required before treatment is initiated. ▪ Monitor CBC, differential, and platelet counts frequently in all patients, especially in patients who have renal impairment and/or are undergoing hemodialysis, patients who have experienced previous cytopenias from ganciclovir or other nucleoside analogs, or patients who have fewer than 1,000 cells/mm^3 neutrophils at the beginning of treatment. ▪ Obtain baseline SCr and CrCl. Monitor during therapy and adjust dose as needed. Monitoring renal function during therapy is essential for all patients but especially for elderly patients and patients receiving concomitant agents that may cause nephrotoxicity. ▪ Maintain adequate hydration and urine flow before and during infusion. ▪ Phlebitis or pain may occur at site of infusion; confirm patency of vein and use small needles and large veins to ensure adequate blood flow for rapid dilution and distribution. ▪ Neutropenia usually occurs during the first or second week of treatment but may occur at any time; recovery should begin within 3 to 7 days of discontinuing ganciclovir. ▪ See Drug/Lab Interactions.

Patient Education: Pregnancy testing required before initiation of treatment in females of childbearing potential, and effective contraception should be used during treatment and for at least 30 days after treatment. Males should use barrier contraception during treatment and for at least 90 days after treatment. ▪ May cause temporary or permanent infertility. ▪ Not a cure; retinitis may still progress. Frequent ophthalmoscopic examinations are important. ▪ Cooperation for close monitoring of blood cell counts and renal function is imperative to control possible side effects (e.g., anemia, neutropenia, thrombocytopenia, increased SCr). ▪ Promptly report any unexpected side effects (e.g., chills, fever, unusual bleeding or bruising). ▪ Patients with AIDS receiving zidovudine (AZT, Retrovir) may not tolerate ganciclovir. ▪ Review all medications (prescription, over the counter, and herbal) with health care provider. ▪ Ganciclovir may affect cognitive abilities, including the ability to drive and operate machinery. Seizures, dizziness, and/or confusion have been reported.

Maternal/Child: Avoid pregnancy. Has the potential to cause birth defects in humans. Do not use during pregnancy unless risk is justified. ▪ Breast-feeding is not recommended because of the potential for serious adverse reactions in nursing infants. The CDC recommends HIV-infected mothers not breast-feed to avoid potential postnatal transmission of HIV. ▪ Safety and efficacy in pediatric patients have not been established. Long-term carcinogenicity and reproductive toxicity are probable. Benefit must outweigh risks.

Elderly: Dose selection should be cautious; see Dose Adjustments. Monitor renal function during therapy and adjust dose as indicated.

DRUG/LAB INTERACTIONS
Because of physical **incompatibilities,** ganciclovir and **foscarnet** must never be mixed. ▪ Additive toxicity may occur with concurrent or consecutive use with **other bone marrow suppressants** (e.g., dapsone, doxorubicin, flucytosine, hydroxyurea, pentamidine, sulfamethoxazole/trimethoprim, tacrolimus, vinblastine, vincristine, zidovudine). Consider risk versus benefit. ▪ May cause severe anemia and neutropenia with **zidovudine**. Combination used in patients with AIDS may not be tolerated. ▪ Concurrent treatment with **didanosine** may cause increased didanosine levels. Monitor for didanosine toxicity. ▪ May cause seizures with **imipenem-cilastatin**; coadministration not recommended. ▪ Potentiated by **probenecid and other drugs that may reduce renal clearance;** monitor for evidence of ganciclovir toxicity. ▪ Risk of renal toxicity increased with concurrent use of other **nephrotoxic agents** (e.g., cyclosporine, amphotericin B). Monitor renal function.

- Increased risk of hematologic and renal toxicity when given concomitantly with **myco-phenolate mofetil**. Monitoring required.

SIDE EFFECTS

Abdominal pain, anemia, asthenia, cough, decreased appetite, diarrhea, dyspnea, fever, headache, hyperhidrosis, increased blood creatinine, leukopenia, nausea, and sepsis are most common. Anorexia, chills, infection, neuropathy, neutropenia, pain and infection at injection site, phlebitis, pruritus, rash, retinal detachment, sweating, thrombocytopenia, and vomiting occur in some patients. Hypersensitivity reactions have been reported. Numerous additional side effects may occur.

Overdose: Abdominal pain, acute renal failure, bone marrow failure, diarrhea, hepatitis, leukopenia, liver function disorder, myelosuppression, seizures, vomiting, and worsening in pre-existing renal impairment have occurred.

ANTIDOTE

Notify physician of all side effects; most will be treated symptomatically. Filgrastim has been used to increase the neutrophil count. Hydration and hemodialysis (up to 50% removal) are useful in overdose. Treat anaphylaxis and resuscitate as necessary.

GEMCITABINE HYDROCHLORIDE

(jem-**SIGHT**-ah-been hy-droh-**KLOR**-eyed)

Gemzar, Infugem

Antineoplastic
(miscellaneous)

pH 2.7 to 3.3

USUAL DOSE

Pretreatment: Verify pregnancy status. Baseline studies indicated; see Monitor. Review monographs of indicated antineoplastics that are to be used in combination with gemcitabine for additional information.

Pancreatic cancer: 1,000 mg/M^2 as outlined in the following treatment schedule:

Weeks 1-8: Weekly dosing for the first 7 weeks followed by 1 week of rest.

After Week 8: Weekly dosing on Days 1, 8, and 15 of 28-day cycles.

Non–small-cell lung cancer (NSCLC): 1,000 mg/M^2 as an infusion on Days 1, 8, and 15 of each 28-day cycle. Given in combination with cisplatin. Administer cisplatin 100 mg/M^2 IV on Day 1 after the infusion of gemcitabine. An alternate schedule is gemcitabine 1,250 mg/M^2 on Days 1 and 8 of each 21-day cycle. Administer cisplatin 100 mg/M^2 IV on Day 1 after the infusion of gemcitabine.

Breast cancer: 1,250 mg/M^2 as an infusion on Days 1 and 8 of each 21-day cycle. Given in combination with paclitaxel. On Day 1, administer paclitaxel 175 mg/M^2 as a 3-hour infusion before the gemcitabine infusion.

Ovarian cancer: 1,000 mg/M^2 as an infusion on Days 1 and 8 of a 21-day cycle. Given in combination with carboplatin. On Day 1 of the 21-day cycle, administer carboplatin at AUC 4 after gemcitabine administration.

Bladder cancer (unlabeled): 1,000 mg/M^2 on Days 1, 8, and 15. Repeat cycle every 28 days. Given in conjunction with cisplatin. Alternatively, 1,000 mg/M^2 on Days 1 and 8. Repeat cycle every 21 days. Given in combination with carboplatin.

Hodgkin lymphoma (relapsed) or non-Hodgkin lymphoma (refractory) (unlabeled): 1,000 mg/M^2 on Days 1 and 8 of a 21-day cycle. Given in combination with other agents.

Head and neck cancer (unlabeled): 1,000 mg/M^2 on Days 1, 8, and 15 every 28 days or 1,000 mg/M^2 on Days 1 and 8 every 21 days. Given in combination with vinorelbine.

Adenocarcinoma of the pancreas: Given in combination with Abraxane; see paclitaxel protein-bound particles for injectable suspension monograph.

DOSE ADJUSTMENTS

Clearance decreased in females and the elderly. May be less likely to progress to subsequent cycles; see Precautions and Elderly.

Gemcitabine Dose Modifications for Nonhematologic Adverse Reactions
Permanently discontinue gemcitabine for any of the following: • Unexplained dyspnea or other evidence of severe pulmonary toxicity • Severe hepatic toxicity • Hemolytic-uremic syndrome (HUS) or severe renal impairment • Capillary leak syndrome (CLS) • Posterior reversible encephalopathy syndrome (PRES) • Withhold gemcitabine or reduce dose by 50% for other severe (Grade 3 or 4) nonhematologic toxicity until resolved **Gemzar:** No dose modifications are recommended for alopecia, nausea, or vomiting.

Treatment of pancreatic cancer and NSCLC: Reduce dose based on the degree of hematologic toxicity according to the following chart.

Recommended Gemcitabine Dose Modifications for Myelosuppression in Pancreatic Cancer and NSCLC			
Absolute Neutrophil Count (× 10⁶/L)		**Platelet Count (× 10⁶/L)**	**% of Full Dose to Be Administered**
≥1,000	and	≥100,000	100%
500–999	or	50,000–99,999	75%
<500	or	<50,000	Hold

Treatment of breast cancer (combination with paclitaxel): Reduce dose based on degree of hematologic toxicity according to the following chart.

Recommended Dose Modifications for Gemcitabine for Myelosuppression on Day of Treatment in Breast Cancer[a]				
Treatment Day	**Absolute Neutrophil Count (× 10⁶/L)**		**Platelet Count (× 10⁶/L)**	**% of Full Dose**
Day 1	≥1,500	and	≥100,000	100%
	<1,500	or	<100,000	Hold
Day 8	≥1,200	and	>75,000	100%
	1,000–1,199	or	50,000–75,000	75%
	700–999	and	≥50,000	50%
	<700	or	<50,000	Hold

[a]See paclitaxel monograph for additional dose adjustment guidelines.

Treatment of ovarian cancer in combination with carboplatin: Reduce dose based on the degree of hematologic toxicity according to the following charts.

Recommended Dose Modifications for Gemcitabine for Myelosuppression on Day of Treatment in Ovarian Cancer[a]				
Treatment Day	**Absolute Neutrophil Count (× 10⁶/L)**		**Platelet Count (× 10⁶/L)**	**% of Full Dose**
Day 1	≥1,500	and	≥100,000	100%
	<1,500	or	<100,000	Delay treatment cycle
Day 8	≥1,500	and	≥100,000	100%
	1,000–1,499	or	75,000–99,999	50%
	<1,000	or	<75,000	Hold

[a]See carboplatin monograph for additional dosing guidelines.

Gemcitabine dose modification for myelosuppression in previous cycle in ovarian cancer: Reduce dose based on myelosuppression occurrence according to the following chart:

Continued

Recommended Gemcitabine Dose Modifications for Myelosuppression in Previous Cycle in Ovarian Cancer[a]		
Occurrence	Myelosuppression During Treatment Cycle	Dose Modification
Initial occurrence	• Absolute neutrophil count <500 × 10⁶/L for more than 5 days or • Absolute neutrophil count <100 × 10⁶/L for more than 3 days or • Febrile neutropenia or • Platelets <25,000 × 10⁶/L or • Cycle delay of more than 1 week due to toxicity	Permanently reduce dose to 800 mg/M² on Day 1 and Day 8
Subsequent occurrence	Occurrence of any of the above toxicities after the initial dose reduction	Permanently reduce dose to 800 mg/M² on Day 1 only

[a]See carboplatin monograph for additional dosing guidelines.

DILUTION

Specific techniques required; see Precautions. Gemzar: Available in single-use vials containing 200 mg or 1 Gm of gemcitabine. A white to off-white lyophilized powder. Each 200 mg must be reconstituted with 5 mL NS without preservatives (25 mL NS for 1 Gm). Yields 38 mg/mL. Shake to dissolve. Do not use less solution to reconstitute; dissolution will be incomplete. The appropriate dose *must* be further diluted with NS to concentrations as low as 0.1 mg/mL. 1,500 mg diluted in 250 mL yields 6 mg/mL. 750 mg in 100 mL yields 7.5 mg/mL.

Infugem: Provided in premixed bags (10 mg/mL) that are ready for infusion and do not require any further preparation before use. Do not dilute before use. Do not remove or add medication. Infugem is a clear, colorless solution. Check for leaks by squeezing inner bag firmly. If leaks are found, discard the bag. Select the gemcitabine premixed bag(s) that allow for a variance of up to 5% of the BSA-calculated dose for all indications. See manufacturer's prescribing information for charts showing specific size of infusion bags to use based on BSA range.

Filters: Specific information not available.

Storage: *Gemzar:* Store unopened vials at CRT. Reconstituted or diluted solutions are stable at CRT for 24 hours. Do not refrigerate in any form; may crystallize. Discard unused portion.

Infugem: Unopened infusion bags are stable until the expiration date on the package when stored at RT. Do not freeze, as crystallization can occur.

COMPATIBILITY

Gemzar: Manufacturer states, "No **incompatibilities** observed with IV bottles or PVC bags and administration sets."

Infugem: Manufacturer states, "Do not remove or add medication."

Other sources suggest **compatibilities** for Gemzar dependent on concentration and manufacturer; consult a pharmacist.

RATE OF ADMINISTRATION

Gemzar: A single dose as an infusion equally distributed over 30 minutes.

Infugem: Infuse all doses of gemcitabine over 30 minutes. If two premixed infusion bags are required to achieve the prescribed dose, infuse the total volume of both bags over 30 minutes.

Gemzar and Infugem: Do not extend infusion time beyond 60 minutes; will increase toxicity.

ACTIONS

A nucleoside metabolic inhibitor with antineoplastic activity. Metabolized intracellularly to two active nucleosides. Cell phase specific, these nucleosides induce internucleosomal DNA fragmentation, primarily killing cells undergoing DNA synthesis (S-phase) and also blocking the progression of cells through the G_1/S-phase boundary. Very little is bound to plasma protein. Volume of distribution is increased by infusion length. Half-life is shorter (42 to 94 minutes) with a short infusion (less than 70 minutes), and longer (245 to 638 minutes) with a long infusion (more than 70 minutes). Half-life is slightly longer and rate of clearance is lower in females and in the elderly, resulting in higher concentrations for any given dose. Primarily excreted in urine.

INDICATIONS AND USES

First-line treatment for patients with locally advanced (nonresectable Stage II or Stage III) or metastatic (Stage IV) adenocarcinoma of the pancreas in patients previously treated with fluorouracil. ▪ First-line treatment in combination with cisplatin for the treatment of inoperable, locally advanced (Stage IIIA or IIIB) or metastatic (Stage IV) non–small-cell lung cancer. ▪ First-line treatment in combination with paclitaxel for treatment of metastatic breast cancer after failure of previous anthracycline chemotherapy unless anthracyclines (e.g., doxorubicin [Adriamycin], idarubicin [Idamycin]) were clinically contraindicated. ▪ Treatment in combination with carboplatin for patients with advanced ovarian cancer that has relapsed at least 6 months after completion of platinum-based therapy.

Unlabeled uses: Treatment of metastatic bladder cancer. ▪ Treatment of testicular cancer. ▪ Treatment of cancer of the head and neck. ▪ Treatment of Hodgkin lymphoma (relapsed) or non-Hodgkin lymphoma (refractory).

CONTRAINDICATIONS

Hypersensitivity to gemcitabine or any of its components.

PRECAUTIONS

Follow guidelines for handling cytotoxic agents. See Appendix A, p. 1308. ▪ Administered by or under the direction of the physician specialist. ▪ Adequate diagnostic and treatment facilities must be available. ▪ For IV use only. May be administered on an outpatient basis. ▪ Prolongation of the infusion time beyond 60 minutes and more frequent than weekly dosing have been shown to increase toxicity (e.g., clinically significant hypotension, severe flu-like symptoms, myelosuppression, and asthenia). ▪ Myelosuppression (e.g., anemia, neutropenia, and thrombocytopenia) is the dose-limiting toxicity. Occurs with gemcitabine as a single agent, and the risk increases when it is combined with other cytotoxic drugs; see Dose Adjustments. ▪ Clearance in females and the elderly is reduced; females, especially older females, were more likely not to proceed to a subsequent cycle and to experience Grade 3 or 4 neutropenia and thrombocytopenia. No age or gender dose adjustments recommended. ▪ Use with caution in impaired renal or hepatic function. Clear dose recommendations are not available; data from clinical studies insufficient. ▪ Hepatotoxicity, including liver failure and death, has been reported. Use in patients with concurrent liver metastases or a history of alcoholism, hepatitis, or liver cirrhosis may lead to exacerbation of the underlying hepatic insufficiency. ▪ Hemolytic-uremic syndrome (HUS) and/or renal toxicity, including renal failure leading to death or requiring dialysis, has been reported. Serious cases of thrombotic microangiopathy other than HUS have been reported. ▪ Gemcitabine is a potent radiosensitizer. Concurrent use of gemcitabine with radiation therapy (or using 7 or fewer days apart from radiation therapy) may cause severe, life-threatening mucositis, especially esophagitis and pneumonitis. Data suggest that gemcitabine can be administered if given more than 7 days before or after radiation therapy. Radiation recall has been reported in patients who receive gemcitabine after prior radiation. ▪ Pulmonary toxicity (e.g., adult respiratory distress syndrome [ARDS], interstitial pneumonitis, pulmonary edema, pulmonary fibrosis) has been reported. Fatalities have occurred. Onset of pulmonary symptoms may occur up to 2 weeks after the last dose of gemcitabine. Discontinue gemcitabine in patients who develop unexplained dyspnea, with or without bronchospasm, or who have any evidence of pulmonary toxicity. ▪ Capillary leak syndrome (CLS) and posterior reversible encephalopathy syndrome (PRES) have been reported. ▪ Use caution in patients who have had previous cytotoxic chemotherapy or radiation therapy.

Monitor: Monitor for bone marrow suppression. Obtain a CBC, including differential and platelet count, before each dose; see Dose Adjustments. ▪ Obtain baseline renal function (e.g., SCr) and liver function tests (e.g., AST, ALT) and repeat periodically. ▪ Monitor serum calcium, magnesium, potassium, and SCr during combination therapy with cisplatin. ▪ Monitor vital signs. ▪ Monitor respiratory status. ▪ Maintain adequate hydration. ▪ Nausea and vomiting are frequent and were severe in 15% of patients; prophylactic administration of antiemetics will increase patient comfort. ▪ Observe closely for S/S of infection. May cause fever in the absence of infection, or prophylactic antibiotics may be indicated pending results of C/S in a febrile or nonfebrile patient. ▪ Monitor for thrombocytopenia (platelet count less than 50,000/mm³). Initiate precautions to prevent excessive bleeding (e.g., inspect IV sites, skin, and mucous membranes; use extreme care during invasive procedures; test urine, emesis, stool, and secretions for occult blood). ▪ Consider a diagnosis of HUS if anemia with evidence of microangiopathic hemolysis, elevation of bilirubin or LDH, reticulocytosis, severe thrombocytopenia, and/or evidence of renal failure (elevation of SCr or BUN) develops; discontinue gemcitabine. ▪ Monitor for S/S of CLS (sudden edema, rapid drop in blood pressure, shock, hemoconcentration, hypoalbuminemia). ▪ Monitor for S/S of PRES (blindness, confusion, headache, hypertension, lethargy, seizure, or other visual or neurologic disturbances). Confirm diagnosis of PRES with MRI. ▪ Not a vesicant, but monitor injection site for inflammation and/or extravasation.

Patient Education: Effective birth control is recommended for females of reproductive potential and males with female partners of reproductive potential during and for 6 months (females) and for 3 months (males) after the last dose of gemcitabine. ▪ May impair fertility in males of reproductive potential. ▪ Report any unusual or unexpected symptoms or side effects (e.g., shortness of breath, cough, wheezing, blood in stool or urine, change in color or volume of urine, S/S of infection, jaundice, pain/tenderness in the right upper abdominal quadrant, unusual bruising or bleeding) as soon as possible. ▪ See Appendix D, p. 1311.

Maternal/Child: Avoid pregnancy. May cause fetal harm. ▪ Discontinue breast-feeding during treatment and for at least 1 week after the last dose. ▪ Safety and effectiveness for use in pediatric patients not established.

Elderly: Clearance reduced in the elderly; hematologic toxicity requiring reduction, delay, or omission of subsequent doses is higher than in younger adults; however, incidence of nonhematologic toxicity is similar. Elderly males and females are more likely to experience Grade 3 or 4 thrombocytopenia. Elderly females are also more likely to experience Grade 3 or 4 neutropenia. Usual dose adjustments based on toxicity are considered appropriate. Age-related impaired renal function may further reduce clearance and increase toxicity.

DRUG/LAB INTERACTIONS

Interaction of gemcitabine with other drugs has not been adequately studied. ▪ Do not administer **live virus vaccines** to patients receiving antineoplastic agents.

SIDE EFFECTS

The most common side effects are anemia, dyspnea, fever, hematuria, increased alkaline phosphatase, AST and ALT, nausea, neutropenia, peripheral edema, proteinuria, rash, thrombocytopenia, and vomiting. Less frequently reported side effects include alopecia, anorexia, arthralgia, bone marrow toxicity (e.g., anemia, leukopenia, neutropenia, thrombocytopenia), bone pain, bronchospasm, cerebrovascular accident, constipation, diarrhea, edema, elevated lab tests (e.g., BUN, creatinine, hematuria, proteinuria), fatigue, febrile neutropenia, flu syndrome (e.g., anorexia, chills, cough, headache, myalgia, weakness), hemorrhage, hepatotoxicity, hypertension, increased liver function tests (e.g., ALT, AST, GGT, alkaline phosphatase, and bilirubin), infection, injection site reaction, myalgia, neuropathy (motor and sensory), pain, paresthesias, pruritus, pulmonary toxicity (including respiratory failure), radiation recall reactions, somnolence, and stomatitis. Anaphylaxis and hemolytic-uremic syndrome have been reported.

Post-Marketing: Adult respiratory distress syndrome (ARDS), arrhythmias, capillary leak syndrome, cellulitis, congestive heart failure, gangrene, hepatic failure, hepatic venoocclusive disease, interstitial pneumonitis, myocardial infarction, peripheral vasculitis, posterior reversible encephalopathy syndrome (PRES), pseudocellulitis, pulmonary edema, pulmonary eosinophilia, pulmonary fibrosis, severe skin reactions (including desquamation and bullous skin eruptions), supraventricular arrhythmias, and thrombotic microangiopathy (TMA).

ANTIDOTE

Keep physician informed of all side effects. Symptomatic and supportive treatment is indicated. Permanently discontinue gemcitabine if any of the following occur: unexplained dyspnea or other evidence of severe pulmonary toxicity, severe hepatic toxicity, hemolytic uremic syndrome or severe renal impairment, capillary leak syndrome, or posterior reversible encephalopathy syndrome (PRES). Reduce dose or withhold gemcitabine until myelosuppression improves to specific criteria; see Dose Adjustments. Anemia may require RBC transfusions. Other whole blood products (e.g., platelets, leukocytes) and/or blood modifiers (e.g., darbepoetin alfa, epoetin alfa, filgrastim, pegfilgrastim, sargramostim) may be indicated to treat bone marrow toxicity. Most side effects are reversible with dose reduction or temporary withholding of gemcitabine. No known antidote for overdose. If hemolytic-uremic syndrome occurs, discontinue gemcitabine; renal failure may not be reversible even with discontinuation of therapy, and dialysis may be required. Treat hypersensitivity reactions as indicated; may require epinephrine, airway management, oxygen, IV fluids, antihistamines (e.g., diphenhydramine), corticosteroids (e.g., hydrocortisone sodium succinate), and pressor amines (e.g., dopamine).

GENTAMICIN SULFATE BBW

(jen-tah-**MY**-sin **SUL**-fayt)

Antibacterial
(aminoglycoside)

pH 3 to 5.5

USUAL DOSE

Pretreatment: See Monitor and Maternal/Child.

Gentamicin: 3 mg/kg of body weight/24 hr equally divided into 3 doses (1 mg/kg every 8 hours). Reduce to usual dose as soon as feasible. Gentamicin can also be dosed as 5 to 7 mg/kg/day. **Dosage based on adjusted body weight.** Studies suggest a single daily dose of 4 to 7 mg/kg (instead of divided into 2 to 3 doses) may provide higher peak levels and enhance drug effectiveness while actually reducing or having no adverse effects on risk of toxicity. Various procedures for monitoring blood levels are in use. Some health facilities are monitoring with trough levels; others may draw levels at predetermined times and plot the concentration on nomograms. Depending on the protocol in place, doses or intervals may be adjusted. See Dose Adjustments and Precautions/Monitor.

Prevention of bacterial endocarditis in dental, respiratory tract, GI or GU tract surgery or instrumentation: 1.5 mg/kg 30 minutes before procedure. Do not exceed 80 mg. Repeat in 8 hours. Given concurrently with ampicillin, vancomycin, or amoxicillin.

Pelvic inflammatory disease: 2 mg/kg as an initial dose. Follow with 1.5 mg/kg every 8 hours for 4 days or 48 hours after patient improves. Given concurrently with clindamycin.

PEDIATRIC DOSE

See Maternal/Child.

6 to 7.5 mg/kg of body weight/24 hr (2 to 2.5 mg/kg every 8 hours). A single daily dose is also being used in pediatric patients. See comments under Usual Dose. 10 mg/mL product available for pediatric use.

Prevention of bacterial endocarditis in dental, respiratory tract, GI or GU tract surgery or instrumentation: 2 mg/kg. See Usual Dose for instructions.

NEONATAL DOSE

See Maternal/Child.

2.5 mg/kg. Intervals adjusted based on age as follows:

0 to 7 days of age; less than 28 weeks' gestation: Every 24 hours.

28 to 34 weeks' gestation: Every 18 hours.

Over 34 weeks' gestation: Every 12 hours.

Over 7 days of age; less than 28 weeks' gestation: Every 18 hours.

28 to 34 weeks' gestation: Every 12 hours.

Over 34 weeks' gestation: Every 8 hours.

Another source suggests that higher doses (4 to 5 mg/kg/dose) at extended intervals (24 to 48 hours) may be used.

DOSE ADJUSTMENTS

Reduce daily dose commensurate with amount of renal impairment. Other protocols are in use; see literature. ■ Once-daily dosing is not usually used for patients with ascites, burns covering more than 20% of the total body surface area, CrCl less than 40 mL/min (including patients requiring dialysis), CrCl greater than 120 mL/min, cystic fibrosis, endocarditis, mycobacterium infections, or in infants or during pregnancy. ■ Reduced dose or extended intervals may be indicated in elderly adults.

Dosing and dose adjustments are generally done by hospital pharmacists. ▪ See Monitor and Drug/Lab Interactions.

The recommended dose at the end of each dialysis period is 1 to 1.7 mg/kg depending on the severity of the infection. 2 mg/kg may be administered to pediatric patients. The amount of gentamicin removed by dialysis may vary; however, an 8-hour dialysis session may reduce serum concentrations by 50%.

High-dose therapy: Interval may be extended (e.g., every 48 hours) in patients with moderate renal impairment (CrCl 30 to 59 mL/min) and/or adjusted based on serum level determinations.

DILUTION
Available premixed in several concentrations. Vials equal 10 or 40 mg/mL. Further dilute each single dose in 50 to 200 mL of IV NS or D5W. Decrease volume of diluent for pediatric patients. Commercially diluted solutions available.

COMPATIBILITY
Manufacturer states, "Do not physically premix with other drugs; administer separately." Inactivated in solution with beta-lactam antibiotics (e.g., cephalosporins, penicillins) and vancomycin. Do not mix in the same solution. Appropriate spacing required because of physical **incompatibilities.** See Drug/Lab Interactions.

Other sources suggest specific **compatibilities** dependent on concentration and manufacturer; consult a pharmacist.

RATE OF ADMINISTRATION
Each single dose, properly diluted, over 30 to 60 minutes, up to 2 hours in pediatric patients. Studies suggest bolus dosing (versus infusion over 30 minutes) may produce an earlier bactericidal effect, which is sustained. No dose, dilution, or rate recommendations are available at this time.

ACTIONS
Aminoglycoside antibiotic with neuromuscular blocking action. Bactericidal against specific gram-negative bacilli, including *Escherichia coli, Klebsiella, Proteus,* and *Pseudomonas.* Not effective for fungi or viral infections. Well distributed throughout all body fluids; serum and urine levels remain adequate for 6 to 12 hours. Usual half-life is 2 hours. Half-life prolonged in infants, postpartum females, fever, liver disease and ascites, spinal cord injury, cystic fibrosis, and the elderly; shorter in severe burns. Crosses placental barrier. Excreted through kidneys.

INDICATIONS AND USES
Treatment of serious infections of the GI (peritonitis), respiratory, and urinary tracts; CNS (meningitis); skin; bone; soft tissue (burns); septicemia; and bacterial neonatal sepsis. ▪ Primarily used when penicillin and other less toxic antibiotics are ineffective or contraindicated. ▪ Prevention of bacterial endocarditis in dental, respiratory tract, GI, or GU surgery or instrumentation. ▪ Used concurrently with clindamycin to treat pelvic inflammatory disease. ▪ Considered initial therapy after culture and sensitivity is drawn in suspected or confirmed gram-negative infections or other serious infections. ▪ Treat suspected infection in the immunosuppressed patient. ▪ May be used synergistically in gram-positive infections. ▪ Used concurrently with penicillin for endocarditis and neonatal sepsis.

CONTRAINDICATIONS
Known gentamicin or aminoglycoside sensitivity, renal failure. Sulfite sensitivity may be a contraindication.

PRECAUTIONS
Sensitivity studies indicated to determine susceptibility of the causative organism to gentamicin. ▪ Use extreme caution if therapy is required over 7 to 10 days. ▪ Superinfection may occur from overgrowth of nonsusceptible organisms. ▪ Use caution in

infants, children, and the elderly. ▪ Advanced age and dehydration may increase risk of toxicity. ▪ May contain sulfites; use caution in patients with asthma. ▪ Aminoglycosides are nephrotoxic; risk for nephrotoxicity is increased in patients with impaired renal function and in patients who receive high doses or prolonged therapy. ▪ Use extreme caution in patients with end-stage renal disease. ▪ Single daily dosing has been used effectively in abdominal, pelvic inflammatory, and GU infections in patients with normal renal function. Not recommended in bacteremia caused by *Pseudomonas aeruginosa,* endocarditis, meningitis, during pregnancy, or in patients less than 6 weeks postpartum. Limited data available for use in all other situations (e.g., burns, cystic fibrosis, elderly, pediatrics, renal impairment). ▪ Potentially nephrotoxic, ototoxic, and neurotoxic. Risk of neurotoxicity (e.g., auditory and vestibular ototoxicity) is increased in patients with pre-existing renal damage or in normal renal function with prolonged use. Partial or total irreversible deafness may continue to develop after gentamicin is discontinued. ▪ *Clostridium difficile*–associated diarrhea (CDAD) has been reported. May range from mild diarrhea to fatal colitis. Consider in patients who present with diarrhea during or after treatment with gentamicin.

Monitor: Narrow range between toxic and therapeutic levels. Periodically monitor peak and trough concentrations. Therapeutic level is between 4 and 8 mcg/mL. Avoid trough levels above 2 mcg/mL and prolonged peak levels above 12 mcg/mL; adjust dose as indicated. Risk of renal and eighth cranial nerve toxicity increased. Monitor frequently in patients with impaired renal function. ▪ Watch for decrease in urine output and rising BUN and SCr. May require decreased dose. ▪ Routine gentamicin serum levels and evaluation of hearing are recommended. ▪ Closely monitor renal and eighth cranial nerve function, especially in patients with known or suspected reduced renal function at onset of therapy and in patients who develop signs of renal dysfunction during therapy. Monitor urine for decreased specific gravity, increased protein, and the presence of cells or casts. Serial audiograms are recommended, particularly in high-risk patients. ▪ Maintain good hydration. ▪ Monitor serum calcium, magnesium, sodium, and potassium; levels may decline. Depressed levels have caused mental confusion, paresthesia, positive Chvostek and Trousseau signs (provoked spasm of facial muscles and other muscles; occurs in tetany), and tetany in adults; muscle weakness and tetany in infants. ▪ Closely monitor patients with impaired renal function for nephrotoxicity and neurotoxicity (e.g., auditory and vestibular ototoxicity, convulsions, muscle twitching, numbness, tingling); nephrotoxicity may be reversible. ▪ In extended treatment, daily monitoring of serum levels, electrolytes, and renal, auditory, and vestibular functions is recommended. ▪ See Drug/Lab Interactions.

Patient Education: Report promptly: dizziness, hearing loss, weakness, or any changes in balance. ▪ Promptly report diarrhea or bloody stools that occur during treatment or up to several months after an antibiotic has been discontinued; may indicate CDAD and require treatment. ▪ Consider birth control options.

Maternal/Child: Category D: avoid pregnancy. Potential hazard to fetus. ▪ Safety for use during breast-feeding not established; use extreme caution. ▪ Peak concentrations are generally lower in infants and young children.

Elderly: Consider less toxic alternatives. Half-life prolonged. Longer intervals between doses may be more important than reduced doses. ▪ Advanced age and dehydration may increase risk for toxicity. ▪ Monitor renal function and drug levels carefully. Measurement of CrCl more useful than BUN or SCr to assess renal function. ▪ See Precautions.

DRUG/LAB INTERACTIONS

Inactivated in solution with **penicillins** but is synergistic when used in combination with **beta-lactam antibiotics** and **vancomycin.** Do not mix in the same solution. Dose adjustment and appropriate spacing required because of physical **incompatibilities** and interactions. Synergism may be inconsistent; measure aminoglycoside levels. ■ Concurrent and/or sequential use topically or systemically with any other **neurotoxic or nephrotoxic agent** should be avoided (e.g., amikacin, cisplatin, colistin, neomycin, polymyxin B, tobramycin, vancomycin). ■ May have dangerous additive effects with **anesthetics** (e.g., enflurane), **other neuromuscular blocking antibiotics** (e.g., kanamycin, streptomycin), **beta-lactam antibiotics** (e.g., cephalosporins), **diuretics** (e.g., furosemide), **vancomycin,** and many others. ■ **Neuromuscular blocking muscle relaxants** are potentiated by aminoglycosides. *Apnea can occur.* ■ Aminoglycosides are also potentiated by **anticholinesterases** (e.g., edrophonium), **antineoplastics** (e.g., nitrogen mustard, cisplatin). ■ May be antagonized by **bacteriostatic antibiotics** (e.g., chloramphenicol, erythromycin, tetracyclines); bactericidal action may be impacted.

SIDE EFFECTS

Occur more frequently with impaired renal function, higher doses, or prolonged administration, in dehydrated or elderly patients, and in patients receiving other ototoxic or nephrotoxic drugs.

Anorexia, burning, dizziness, fever, headache, hypertension, hypotension, itching, lethargy, muscle twitching, nausea, numbness, rash, roaring in ears, seizures, tingling sensation, tinnitus, urticaria, vomiting, weight loss.

Major: Acute organic brain syndrome; blood dyscrasias; CDAD; convulsions; elevated bilirubin, BUN, SCr, AST, and ALT; hearing loss; laryngeal edema; neuromuscular blockade; oliguria; respiratory depression or arrest.

ANTIDOTE

Notify the physician of all side effects. If minor side effects persist or any major symptom appears, notify the physician; may require dose adjustment or discontinuation of gentamicin. Treatment is symptomatic. In overdose or toxic reactions, hemodialysis may be indicated. Rate of gentamicin removal is lower with peritoneal dialysis. Monitor fluid balance, CrCl, and plasma levels carefully. Complexation with ticarcillin may be as effective as hemodialysis. Consider exchange transfusion in the newborn. Calcium salts or neostigmine may reverse neuromuscular blockade. Treat CDAD with fluids, electrolytes, protein supplements, and appropriate antibiotics (e.g., oral vancomycin) as indicated. In severe cases, surgical evaluation may be indicated. Resuscitate as necessary.

GLUCAGON
(**GLOO**-kah-gon)

GlucaGen, Glucagon for Injection, Baqsimi

pH 2.5 to 3.5

USUAL DOSE

Pretreatment: Pretesting for patients suspected of having glucagonoma indicated; see Monitor. **Hypoglycemia in adults and pediatric patients weighing more than 20 kg (Glucagon [44 lb]) to 25 kg (GlucaGen [55 lb]):** 1 mg. May be given IV, IM, or SQ. May be repeated if needed. For severe hypoglycemia or when patient fails to respond to glucagon, IV glucose must be administered. After patient responds to treatment, give fast-acting and long-acting oral carbohydrates to restore liver glycogen and prevent the recurrence of hypoglycemia.

Diagnostic aid: stomach, duodenal bulb, duodenum, and small bowel: 0.2 to 0.5 mg IV or 1 mg IM before procedure begins. When diagnostic procedure is over, administer oral carbohydrates to patients who have been fasting if this is compatible with the diagnostic procedure.

Diagnostic aid: colon: 0.5 to 0.75 mg IV or 1 to 2 mg IM before procedure begins. When diagnostic procedure is over, administer oral carbohydrates to patients who have been fasting if this is compatible with the diagnostic procedure.

Management of cardiac effects of beta-blocker or calcium channel blocker overdose (unlabeled): 3 to 10 mg (0.05 to 0.15 mg/kg) over 3 to 5 minutes. May be followed by an infusion of 3 to 5 mg/hr (0.05 to 0.1 mg/kg/hr). Titrate to patient response.

PEDIATRIC DOSE

Hypoglycemia in infants and children weighing less than 20 kg (Glucagon [44 lb]) to 25 kg (GlucaGen [55 lb]): 20 to 30 mcg/kg or 0.5 mg. See comments under Usual Dose. If the weight is unknown, use 0.5 mg for pediatric patients younger than 6 years of age and 1 mg for those 6 years of age and older.

DOSE ADJUSTMENTS

For uses other than hypoglycemia, lower-end doses may be indicated in the elderly; consider impaired organ function and concurrent disease or other drug therapy.

DILUTION

Dilute 1 unit (1 mg) with 1 mL sterile water for reconstitution (SWFR [if supplied]) or SWFI to achieve a final concentration of approximately 1 mg/mL. Shake vial gently until completely dissolved. Concentrations greater than 1 mg/mL are not recommended. Do not add to IV solutions. May be given through Y-tube of infusion set if a dextrose solution is infusing.

Reverse effects of beta-blockade: Reconstitute each 1 unit (1 mg) with 1 mL SWFI. For *continuous infusion* this reconstituted solution may be further diluted in D5W to deliver 1 to 5 mg/hr.

Storage: Use immediately after reconstitution. Discard any unused portion. Before reconstitution, may be stored at CRT for up to 24 months in original package to protect from light. Do not freeze. If solution shows any sign of gel formation or particles after reconstitution, it should be discarded. Do not use after the expiration date on vials.

COMPATIBILITY

May form a precipitate with saline solutions and solutions with a pH of 3 to 9.5. Consider specific use; consult pharmacist.

RATE OF ADMINISTRATION

Too-rapid rate of injection or doses over 1 mg may increase incidence of side effects (e.g., nausea and vomiting).

1 unit (1 mg) or fraction thereof over 1 minute. *Gvoke is given subcutaneously only. Do not give IV.*

ACTIONS

An antihypoglycemic agent and a gastrointestinal motility inhibitor for SQ, IM, or IV use. A polypeptide hormone identical to naturally occurring human glucagon produced by recombinant DNA technology. Induces liver glycogen breakdown, releasing glucose from the liver. Glucagon acts only on liver glycogen; hepatic stores of glycogen are necessary for glucagon to produce an antihypoglycemic effect. Blood glucose is raised within 10 minutes. Maximum glucose concentrations are seen about 30 minutes after administration. Duration of antihypoglycemic effect is 60 to 90 minutes. Extrahepatic effect produces relaxation of the smooth muscle of the stomach, duodenum, small bowel, and colon, inhibiting GI motility. Onset of smooth muscle relaxation is less than 1 minute. Duration of smooth muscle relaxation is dose-dependent and ranges from 9 to 25 minutes. Has a half-life of 8 to 18 minutes. Degraded in the liver, kidney, and plasma. Does not cross the placental barrier.

INDICATIONS AND USES

Treatment of severe hypoglycemia (e.g., during insulin therapy in the management of diabetes mellitus). ▪ As a diagnostic aid during radiologic examinations to temporarily inhibit movement of the gastrointestinal tract; see Drug/Lab Interactions.
Unlabeled uses: May be helpful in reversing adverse beta-blockade of beta-adrenergic blocking agents (e.g., propranolol) in overdose situations. ▪ If conventional therapy is ineffective, may be helpful in reversing myocardial depression of calcium channel blockers (e.g., diltiazem).

CONTRAINDICATIONS

Glucagon for injection: Known hypersensitivity to glucagon or its components, patients with known pheochromocytoma, insulinoma, or glucagonoma. **GlucaGen:** Known hypersensitivity to GlucaGen, lactose, or any of its components; patients with pheochromocytoma or insulinoma.

PRECAUTIONS

Easily absorbed IM or SQ. ▪ If glucagon and glucose do not awaken patient, coma is probably caused by a condition other than hypoglycemia. ▪ Use caution in patients with a history suggestive of glucagonoma; secondary hypoglycemia may occur. Treat with adequate carbohydrate intake; see Contraindications and Monitor. ▪ May cause the release of catecholamines in patients with pheochromocytoma. Use is contraindicated; see Antidote. ▪ Should not be administered to patients suspected of having insulinoma; see Contraindications. Administration may produce an initial increase in blood glucose; however, it may directly or indirectly stimulate exaggerated insulin release from the insulinoma, producing hypoglycemia. Administer IV or oral glucose to a patient who develops symptoms of hypoglycemia. ▪ Treatment with glucagon in patients with diabetes mellitus may cause hyperglycemia. ▪ Evaluation by a physician is recommended for all patients who experience severe hypoglycemia. ▪ Use caution in patients with conditions that result in low levels of releasable glucose (e.g., adrenal insufficiency, chronic hypoglycemia, prolonged fasting, starvation). Insufficient glucose stores will result in inadequate reversal of hypoglycemia. Treatment with dextrose is recommended. ▪ Use caution; hypersensitivity reactions have occurred, usually in association with endoscopic examination during which other agents are administered (e.g., contrast media, local anesthetics). ▪ When used to inhibit gastrointestinal motility, use caution in patients with known cardiac disease. Glucagon exerts positive inotropic and chronotropic effects and may cause tachycardia and hypertension. ▪ Necrolytic migratory erythema (NME), a skin rash commonly associated with glucagon-producing tumors, has been reported following continuous glucagon infusion. ▪ Hypotension has been reported for up to 2 hours after use as premedication for upper GI endoscopy procedures. ▪ Not all products are packaged with the syringe and diluent necessary for rapid preparation and administration during an emergency outside a health care facility. Ensure that correct product is prescribed and dispensed for outpatient use. ▪ See Drug/Lab Interactions.
Monitor: Prolonged hypoglycemia may result in damage to the central nervous system. Monitor blood glucose levels and mentation. Repeat dose and supplement with IV dextrose (50%) if needed. ▪ Monitor BP and HR. In patients with cardiac disease, cardiac monitoring may be indicated. ▪ Test patients suspected of having glucagonoma for

glucagon levels before treatment, and monitor for changes in blood glucose levels during treatment. ▪ Monitor for S/S of NME (e.g., scaly, pruritic erythematous plaques, bullae, and erosions). May affect the face, groin, perineum, and legs or be more widespread. Symptoms have resolved with the discontinuation of the continuous glucagon infusion. Use of corticosteroids not effective. Should NME occur, consider benefits of continuous glucagon infusion versus risk. ▪ Emesis on awakening is common. Prevent aspiration by turning patient face down. ▪ Depletes glycogen stores, especially in children and adolescents; supplement with fast-acting and long-acting oral carbohydrates on awakening (if able to swallow) to replenish liver glycogen and to prevent recurrence of hypoglycemia. ▪ Monitor for S/S of hypersensitivity (e.g., dizziness, dyspnea, fever, flushing, hypotension, nausea, pruritus, rash, rigors, urticaria). ▪ In patients with diabetes mellitus, monitor for hyperglycemia. Administration of insulin may be indicated.
Patient Education: Eat some form of sugar if hypoglycemia recurs. ▪ Report episodes of hypoglycemia and glucagon use at home. Dose adjustment of diabetes medications may be indicated. ▪ Hypoglycemia may impair ability to concentrate or react. Do not drive or operate machinery until oral carbohydrates have been consumed and hypoglycemic episode has resolved. ▪ Teach patient and family proper storage and preparation of glucagon from kits. Include signs of hypoglycemia and procedures to be followed after administration to an unconscious patient.
Maternal/Child: Use during pregnancy only if clearly needed. Use caution during breastfeeding. Not absorbed through the GI tract; it would be unlikely to have any effect on the infant. ▪ Does not cross the placental barrier. ▪ Safety and effectiveness for treatment of severe hypoglycemia in pediatric patients have been demonstrated; however, safety and effectiveness for use in pediatric patients as a diagnostic aid have not been established.
Elderly: Cautious dosing may be indicated in the elderly; see Dose Adjustments. ▪ Differences in response compared with younger adults not identified. ▪ If used to inhibit gastrointestinal motility, use caution in elderly patients with known cardiac disease.

DRUG/LAB INTERACTIONS
Beta-blockers may cause a temporary increase in BP and pulse; treatment may be required in patients with coronary artery disease or pheochromocytoma. ▪ Concurrent use with **indomethacin** may cause glucagon to lose its ability to raise blood glucose and may even produce hypoglycemia. ▪ Coadministration with **anticholinergic** agents (e.g., atropine) is not recommended due to increased GI side effects. ▪ May increase the anticoagulant effects of **warfarin**. ▪ **Insulin** reacts antagonistically toward glucagon; use caution when glucagon is used as a diagnostic aid in patients with diabetes.

SIDE EFFECTS
Rare in recommended doses: hyperglycemia (in diabetic patients), hypersensitivity reactions (e.g., anaphylaxis, dyspnea, hypotension, rash), hypoglycemia, hypoglycemic coma, hypotension, increased BP, increased HR, nausea, vomiting. Increases in BP and HR may be greater in patients taking beta-blockers.
Post-Marketing: Necrolytic migratory erythema in patients receiving continuous glucagon infusions.
Overdose: Nausea and vomiting, increase in BP and HR, inhibition of GI tract motility, hypokalemia.

ANTIDOTE
Nausea and vomiting are tolerable and do occur in hypoglycemia. Antiemetics are indicated when larger doses are given. Increased BP and HR may require treatment in patients with coronary heart disease or pheochromocytoma. Treat sudden increases in BP with phentolamine 5 to 10 mg IV. In overdose situations, glucagon may decrease serum potassium levels; supplemental potassium may be indicated. For any other side effects, discontinue the drug and notify the physician. Treat hypersensitivity reaction as appropriate (e.g., oxygen, antihistamines, epinephrine, corticosteroids, vasopressors, and/or fluids). Insulin administration may be indicated in acute overdose. Effects of dialysis unknown; unlikely to provide benefit because of the short half-life of glucagon and the nature of the symptoms of overdose. Resuscitate as indicated.

GLUCARPIDASE
(gloo-**KAR**-pi-dase)

Voraxaze

USUAL DOSE
Pretreatment: Baseline studies indicated; see Monitor.
Glucarpidase: 50 units/kg as a single intravenous injection over 5 minutes.

PEDIATRIC DOSE
See Usual Dose.

DOSE ADJUSTMENTS
No dose adjustment is recommended in patients with renal impairment. ▪ Has not been studied in patients with hepatic impairment.

DILUTION
Available in a vial containing 1,000 units of lyophilized powder. Reconstitute with 1 mL of NS to provide a solution containing 1,000 units/vial. Roll and tilt vial gently to mix. *Do not shake.* Solution should be clear and colorless. Withdraw calculated dose from vial for administration as an IV injection.
Storage: Refrigerate unopened vials at 2° to 8° C (36° to 46° F). Do not freeze. Do not use beyond expiration date on vial. Use reconstituted solution immediately or store under refrigeration for up to 4 hours. Discard any unused product.

COMPATIBILITY
Compatibility information not available from manufacturer; consult a pharmacist.

RATE OF ADMINISTRATION
Administer as an injection evenly distributed over 5 minutes. Flush IV line before and after administration.

ACTIONS
A carboxypeptidase enzyme produced by recombinant DNA technology. Hydrolyzes the carboxyl-terminal glutamate residue from folic acid and classic antifolates such as methotrexate. Converts methotrexate to its inactive metabolite, 4-deoxy-4-amino-N10-methylpteroic acid (DAMPA) and glutamate. Glucarpidase provides an alternate nonrenal pathway for methotrexate elimination in patients with renal dysfunction during high-dose methotrexate treatment. The desired endpoint of therapy is a rapid and sustained clinically important reduction (RSCIR) in methotrexate concentration, which is defined as attaining a plasma methotrexate concentration less than or equal to 1 μmol/L at 15 minutes and sustaining it for up to 8 days after administration of glucarpidase. The likelihood of attaining a RSCIR correlates with the pre-glucarpidase methotrexate concentration. However, even patients with methotrexate concentrations greater than 50 μmol/L were able to achieve greater than 95% reduction in methotrexate concentrations for up to 8 days following glucarpidase administration. Glucarpidase distribution is restricted to the plasma volume. Mean elimination half-life is 5.6 hours.

INDICATIONS AND USES
Reduce toxic plasma methotrexate concentrations (greater than 1 μmol/L) in adult and pediatric patients with delayed methotrexate clearance (plasma methotrexate concentrations greater than 2 standard deviations of the mean methotrexate excretion curve specific for the dose of methotrexate administered) due to impaired renal function.
Limitation of use: Not recommended for use in patients who exhibit the expected clearance and expected plasma methotrexate concentration. Reducing plasma methotrexate concentration in these patients may result in subtherapeutic exposure to methotrexate.

CONTRAINDICATIONS
Manufacturer states, "None."

PRECAUTIONS

Serious hypersensitivity reactions, including anaphylaxis, have been reported. ▪ Efficacy of a second dose of glucarpidase in patients with markedly elevated pre-glucarpidase methotrexate concentrations was not demonstrated in studies. ▪ Continue hydration, alkalinization of the urine, and leucovorin rescue as indicated; see Monitor and methotrexate and leucovorin monographs. ▪ A protein substance, it has the potential to produce immunogenicity. Anti-glucarpidase antibodies have been detected in a small number of patients treated with glucarpidase.

Monitor: Obtain baseline and periodic renal function tests (e.g., SCr and BUN). ▪ Watch for early S/S of hypersensitivity or infusion reactions (e.g., chills, dyspnea, fever, flushing, headache, hives, itching, numbness, rash, throat tightness). ▪ Monitor methotrexate concentrations. During the first 48 hours after glucarpidase administration, methotrexate concentrations can be reliably measured only by a chromatographic method. During this period, DAMPA (the inactive metabolite of methotrexate) interferes with the measurement of methotrexate concentration using immunoassays. ▪ When administering glucarpidase concomitantly with leucovorin, administer leucovorin at least 2 hours before or 2 hours after the glucarpidase dose; see Drug/Lab Interactions. ▪ For 48 hours after glucarpidase administration, determine the leucovorin dose based on the patient's pre-glucarpidase methotrexate concentration (i.e., administer the same leucovorin dose given before the glucarpidase dose). Beyond 48 hours, administer leucovorin based on the measured methotrexate concentration. Do not discontinue leucovorin based on the determination of a single methotrexate concentration below the leucovorin rescue threshold. Continue therapy with leucovorin until the methotrexate concentration has been maintained below the leucovorin treatment threshold for a minimum of 3 days; see leucovorin monograph. Monitor for S/S of potential methotrexate toxicity (e.g., abdominal distress, chills, dizziness, fever, leukopenia, malaise, nausea, stomatitis, undue fatigue). ▪ Continue IV hydration and urinary alkalinization as indicated.

Patient Education: Promptly report any S/S of a hypersensitivity reaction or an infusion reaction (e.g., chills, feeling hot, fever, flushing, headache, hives, itching, numbness, rash, throat tightness or breathing problems, tingling). ▪ Continued monitoring of methotrexate levels and renal status is imperative.

Maternal/Child: Safety for use during pregnancy and breast-feeding not established. Administered in combination with methotrexate, which can cause embryo-fetal harm. See methotrexate monograph. ▪ Effectiveness in pediatric patients has been established in clinical studies. No overall differences in safety were observed between pediatric patients (age 1 month to 17 years of age) and adult patients.

Elderly: No overall differences in safety or effectiveness were observed between elderly patients and younger patients.

DRUG/LAB INTERACTIONS

Leucovorin is a substrate for glucarpidase. Do not administer leucovorin within 2 hours before or after a dose of glucarpidase. Glucarpidase can decrease leucovorin concentration, which may decrease the effect of leucovorin rescue unless leucovorin is dosed as recommended. ▪ Other potential exogenous substrates of glucarpidase include **reduced folates and folate antimetabolites, other folate analogs or folate analog metabolic inhibitors.** ▪ During the first 48 hours after glucarpidase administration, methotrexate concentrations can be reliably measured only by a chromatographic method. During this period, DAMPA (the inactive metabolite of methotrexate) interferes with the measurement of methotrexate concentration using immunoassays.

SIDE EFFECTS
The most commonly reported side effects included flushing, headache, hypotension, nausea, paraesthesia, and vomiting. Other reported adverse reactions included blurred vision, diarrhea, hypersensitivity reactions (including anaphylaxis), hypertension, rash, throat irritation or tightness, and tremor.

ANTIDOTE
Notify the physician of any side effects. Discontinue the drug if indicated. Treat hypersensitivity reactions as indicated (airway, oxygen, IV fluids, antihistamines [e.g., diphenhydramine], corticosteroids [e.g., hydrocortisone sodium succinate], epinephrine, pressor amines [e.g., dopamine]) and resuscitate as necessary.

GLYCOPYRROLATE
(**GLYE**-koh-**pye**-roh-layt)

GLYRX-PF

Anticholinergic
Antidote

pH 2 to 3

USUAL DOSE
Dose equivalents in mL are based on the 0.2 mg/mL concentration. Check vial for correct concentration.
Preanesthetic medication: 0.004 mg/kg (0.02 mL/kg) of body weight IM 30 to 60 minutes before anesthesia induction. Usually given at the same time as the preanesthetic narcotic and/or sedative.
Intraoperative medication: 0.1 mg (0.5 mL) IV. Repeat as needed at 2- to 3-minute intervals to counteract drug-induced or vagal reflexes and associated arrhythmias (e.g., bradycardia). Attempt to determine the etiology of arrhythmia and the procedures required to correct parasympathetic imbalance.
Reversal of neuromuscular blockade: 0.2 mg (1 mL) IV for each 1 mg of neostigmine or 5 mg of pyridostigmine; to minimize the bradycardia and excessive secretions caused by these agents used to reverse the neuromuscular blockade of nondepolarizing muscle relaxants. May be administered simultaneously and may be mixed in the same syringe.
Peptic ulcer: 0.1 mg (0.5 mL) at 4-hour intervals 3 to 4 times/day. May be given IV or IM. Adjust frequency of administration based on patient response. Some may require only a single dose. If a more profound effect is required, dose may be increased to 0.2 mg (1 mL).

PEDIATRIC DOSE
See Maternal/Child.
Preanesthetic medication: Same as Usual Dose. *Infants 1 month to 2 years of age:* May require up to 0.009 mg/kg (0.045 mL/kg) of body weight.
Intraoperative medication: Rarely needed in pediatric patients because of the long duration of action from the preanesthetic dose. If required, administer 0.004 mg/kg (0.02 mL/kg) of body weight IV. Do not exceed 0.1 mg (0.5 mL) in a single dose. Repeat as needed at 2- to 3-minute intervals to counteract drug-induced or vagal traction reflexes and associated arrhythmias (e.g., bradycardia). Attempt to determine the etiology of arrhythmia and the procedures required to correct parasympathetic imbalance.
Reversal of neuromuscular blockade: Same as Usual Dose.
Peptic ulcer: Not recommended for treatment of peptic ulcer in pediatric patients; see Maternal/Child.

DOSE ADJUSTMENTS
Caution and lower-end dosing suggested for elderly patients based on potential for decreased organ function and concomitant disease or drug therapy. ▪ Elimination prolonged in patients with renal failure. Dose adjustment not provided; see Precautions. ▪ See Drug/Lab Interactions.

DILUTION

May be given undiluted. Administer through Y-tube of infusion tubing containing D5 or D10 in water or saline, D5/½NS, NS, or Ringer's. May be further diluted with D5 or D10 in water or saline.

Filters: No data available from manufacturer.

Storage: Store at CRT.

COMPATIBILITY

Manufacturer lists as **incompatible** with lactated Ringer's and states, "Stability is questionable above a pH of 6". Do not combine in the same syringe with chloramphenicol, dexamethasone, diazepam, dimenhydrinate, methohexital, pentobarbital, secobarbital, sodium bicarbonate, thiopental; will result in a pH above 6 and may result in gas production or precipitation.

Other sources suggest a few specific **compatibilities** dependent on concentration and manufacturer; consult a pharmacist.

RATE OF ADMINISTRATION

0.2 mg or fraction thereof over 1 to 2 minutes.

ACTIONS

A synthetic anticholinergic agent. It inhibits the action of acetylcholine. It reduces the volume and free acidity of gastric secretions and controls excessive pharyngeal, tracheal, and bronchial secretions. Antagonizes muscarinic symptoms (e.g., bronchorrhea, bronchospasm, bradycardia, and intestinal hypermotility) induced by cholinergic drugs. Onset of action is within 1 minute. Vagal blocking effects last 2 to 3 hours, and antisialagogic (inhibited saliva flow) effects last up to 7 hours. Metabolism has not been studied. Half-life is 0.7 to 0.96 hours. Excreted primarily in urine and to a small extent in bile. Does not effectively cross the blood-brain barrier. Crosses the placental barrier in very small amounts.

INDICATIONS AND USES

Indicated during anesthesia (for all ages) for (1) reduction of salivary, tracheobronchial, and pharyngeal secretions; reduction of volume and acidity of gastric secretions; and blockade of cardiac inhibitory reflexes during induction of anesthesia and intubation; (2) intraoperatively to counteract surgically or drug-induced or vagal reflex–associated arrhythmias; and (3) for protection against peripheral muscarinic effects of cholinergic agents such as neostigmine and pyridostigmine given to reverse the neuromuscular blockade due to nondepolarizing agents. ▪ Adjunctive therapy for the treatment of peptic ulcer in adults when rapid anticholinergic effect is desired or when oral medication is not tolerated.

CONTRAINDICATIONS

Known hypersensitivity to glycopyrrolate or any of its inactive ingredients. ▪ Peptic ulcer patients with the following concurrent conditions: glaucoma, obstructive uropathy, obstructive disease of the GI tract, paralytic ileus, intestinal atony of the elderly or debilitated, unstable cardiovascular status in acute hemorrhage, severe ulcerative colitis, toxic megacolon complicating ulcerative colitis, and myasthenia gravis. ▪ Glycopyrrolate formulations that contain benzyl alcohol are contraindicated in neonates.

PRECAUTIONS

Use IV only when immediate drug effect is essential. ▪ Use extreme caution in autonomic neuropathy, asthma, glaucoma, pregnancy, breast-feeding, cardiac arrhythmias, congestive heart failure, coronary artery disease, hepatic or renal disease, hiatal hernia, hypertension, hyperthyroidism, incomplete intestinal obstruction (diarrhea may be an early symptom), ulcerative colitis, and prostatic hypertrophy. Anticholinergic drugs may aggravate these conditions. ▪ Obtain cardiac history before administration of glycopyrrolate; may exacerbate pre-existing tachycardia. ▪ Heat prostration can occur with the use of anticholinergic agents in the presence of fever or high environmental temperatures. Pediatric patients and the elderly are at increased risk.

Monitor: Urinary retention can be avoided if the patient voids just before each dose. ▪ Monitor patient for abdominal distension, dyspepsia, early satiety, increased abdominal pain, and vomiting. Discontinue treatment if these symptoms develop or worsen. ▪ See Drug/Lab Interactions.

Patient Education: Inform health care provider of all current medications. ▪ Use caution if a task requires alertness; may cause blurred vision, dizziness, or drowsiness. ▪ Promptly report constipation, difficulty urinating, dry mouth, flushing, increased light sensitivity, pain and reddening of the eyes (accompanied by dilated pupils), or skin rash. ▪ Use caution during exercise or hot weather. Increased heat sensitivity may result in heatstroke. ▪ Protect eyes from light after receiving treatment.

Maternal/Child: Limited data on safety for use in pregnancy. ▪ It is not known whether this drug is secreted in breast milk; may suppress lactation; use caution. ▪ Safety and effectiveness for use in pediatric patients not established for management of peptic ulcer. ▪ Dysrhythmias have been observed in pediatric patients. ▪ Pediatric patients may have an increased response to anticholinergics and be at increased risk for side effects (e.g., paradoxical hyperexcitability). Infants and young children, patients with Down syndrome, and pediatric patients with spastic paralysis or brain damage are especially susceptible to this increased response. ▪ *Do not use glycopyrrolate formulations that contain benzyl alcohol in neonates.* See Contraindications.

Elderly: Differences in response compared to younger adults not observed. ▪ Dosing should be cautious; see Dose Adjustments. ▪ May produce excitement, agitation, confusion, or drowsiness in the elderly. ▪ May precipitate undiagnosed glaucoma. ▪ Risk of urinary retention and constipation increased. ▪ May increase memory impairment.

DRUG/LAB INTERACTIONS

Potentiated by other drugs with **anticholinergic activity, antiparkinson drugs, atropine, phenothiazines,** and **tricyclic antidepressants**. Reduced dose of either or both drugs may be indicated. ▪ Concomitant administration with **KCl** in a wax matrix may increase the risk and severity of KCl-induced GI lesions (due to slower GI transit time). ▪ May decrease antipsychotic effects of **phenothiazines.** Dose adjustment may be required. ▪ Risk of ventricular arrhythmias increased when given in presence of **cyclopropane.** Risk is less than with atropine and when given in doses of 0.1 mg or less. ▪ Potentiates **atenolol** and **digoxin.**

SIDE EFFECTS

Anaphylaxis, bloated feeling, blurred vision, confusion or excitement, constipation, cycloplegia, decreased sweating, dizziness, drowsiness, dry mouth, dry skin, headache, impotence, increased ocular tension, insomnia, loss of taste, nausea and vomiting, nervousness, palpitation, photophobia, pruritus, suppression of lactation, tachycardia, urinary hesitancy and retention, urticaria, weakness.

Post-Marketing: Cardiac arrest, cardiac arrhythmias, hypertension, hypotension, malignant hyperthermia, respiratory arrest, seizures.

Overdose: A curare-like action may occur (i.e., neuromuscular blockade leading to muscular weakness and possible paralysis).

ANTIDOTE

Notify physician of all side effects. May be treated symptomatically or drug may be discontinued. Treat hypotension with IV fluids and/or pressor agents (e.g., dopamine). Initiate artificial respiration if overdose with paralysis of respiratory muscles occurs. Neostigmine, in 0.25-mg increments, may be used to counteract peripheral anticholinergic effects. May repeat every 5 to 10 minutes to a maximum dose of 2.5 mg. Need for repetitive doses of neostigmine should be based on close monitoring of the decrease in HR and the return of bowel sounds. Physostigmine, in increments of 0.5 to 2 mg, may be used to counteract CNS effects. May repeat as needed to a maximum dose of 5 mg. Proportionately smaller doses should be used in pediatric patients. Resuscitate as necessary.

GOLIMUMAB BBW

(goe-**LIM**-ue-mab)

Monoclonal antibody
Antirheumatic agent
TNF-blocker

Simponi Aria

pH 5.5

USUAL DOSE

Pretreatment: Preliminary patient evaluation and testing required; see Monitor.

Golimumab: Begin with an initial dose of 2 mg/kg as an infusion over 30 minutes. Repeat at Week 4 and then every 8 weeks thereafter. Given in combination with methotrexate in patients with rheumatoid arthritis (RA). See methotrexate monograph. Patients with RA may continue taking other nonbiologic disease-modifying antirheumatic drugs (DMARDs), corticosteroids, NSAIDs, and/or analgesics. In patients with psoriatic arthritis (PsA) or ankylosing spondylitis (AS), golimumab may be given with or without methotrexate or other nonbiologic DMARDs. Corticosteroids, NSAIDs, and/or analgesics may be continued.

The efficacy and safety of switching between IV and SQ formulations and routes of administration of golimumab have not been established.

DILUTION

Available as a 50 mg/4 mL concentrated solution for infusion (12.5 mg/mL). Determine the number of vials required using the following calculations:

$$\text{(Weight in kg} \times \text{dose/kg)} \div 50 \text{ mg} = \text{\# of vials required}$$

For a 60-kg patient: $[(60 \text{ kg}) \times (2 \text{ mg/kg})] \div 50 \text{ mg/vial} = 2.4$ vials. After patient is weighed and appropriate dose is calculated, remove sufficient vials from the refrigerator. Aseptic technique imperative. Solution should be colorless to light yellow and may develop a few translucent particles because golimumab is a protein. Do not use if opaque particles, discoloration, or other foreign particles are present. Withdraw the calculated dose (9.6 mL in above example) from the required number of vials. This calculated dose must be further diluted in NS or 0.45% NS to a final total volume of 100 mL. Withdraw and discard a volume of NS or 0.45% NS equal to the calculated volume of golimumab from a 100-mL bottle or bag of solution and slowly add golimumab. Mix gently.

Filters: Must be administered through an infusion set with an in-line, sterile, nonpyrogenic, low–protein binding filter (pore size 0.22 micrometer or less).

Storage: Refrigerate at 2° to 8° C (36° to 46° F) in original carton to protect from light. Do not freeze or shake. The diluted product may be stored at RT for up to 4 hours. Do not use beyond expiration date. Discard any unused product remaining in vials.

COMPATIBILITY

Manufacturer states, "Do not infuse concomitantly in the same IV line with other agents. No **compatibility** studies have been conducted."

RATE OF ADMINISTRATION

Use of an infusion set with an in-line, sterile, nonpyrogenic, low–protein binding filter (pore size 0.22 micrometer or less) is required. Use of an infusion pump is helpful. Administer a single dose as an infusion over 30 minutes. Flush the IV line with NS at the end of the infusion to ensure the total dose is received.

ACTIONS

A human monoclonal antibody that binds to both the soluble and transmembrane bioactive forms of human tumor necrosis factor alpha (TNFα). This interaction prevents the binding of TNFα to its receptors, thereby inhibiting the biologic activity of TNFα (a cytokine protein). There has been no evidence of the golimumab antibody binding to other TNF superfamily ligands. Elevated TNFα levels in the blood, synovium, and joints have been implicated in the pathophysiology of rheumatoid arthritis (RA), psoriatic arthritis, and ankylosing spondylitis. Golimumab is thought to be distributed primarily in the circulatory system with limited extravascular distribution. Elimination pathways have not been characterized. Mean terminal half-life is estimated to be 9 to 15 days in healthy subjects and 10 to 18 days in patients with RA. Crosses the placental barrier.

INDICATIONS AND USES

Treatment of adult patients with moderate to severely active rheumatoid arthritis. Used in combination with methotrexate. ▪ Treatment of adult patients with active psoriatic arthritis. ▪ Treatment of adult patients with active ankylosing spondylitis.

CONTRAINDICATIONS

Manufacturer states, "None."

PRECAUTIONS

TNFα mediates inflammation and modulates cellular immune response. Anti-TNF therapies, including golimumab, may affect normal immune responses. ▪ Administered under the direction of a physician knowledgeable in its use in a facility with adequate diagnostic and treatment facilities to monitor the patient and respond to any medical emergency. ▪ Patients treated with golimumab are at increased risk for developing serious infection that may lead to hospitalization or death. Most patients who developed these infections were taking concomitant immunosuppressant therapy (e.g., methotrexate, corticosteroids) that, in addition to their underlying disease, may predispose them to infection. Treatment with golimumab should not be initiated in patients with an active infection, including clinically important localized infections. ▪ Discontinue golimumab if a patient develops a serious infection. Reported infections with TNF-blockers include active tuberculosis, including reactivation of latent tuberculosis (TB); invasive fungal infections (e.g., histoplasmosis, coccidioidomycosis, candidiasis, aspergillosis, blastomycosis, and pneumocystosis); and bacterial, viral, and other infections due to opportunistic pathogens, including *Legionella* and *Listeria*. ▪ Patients with TB have frequently presented with disseminated or extrapulmonary disease. ▪ Patients with histoplasmosis or other invasive fungal infections may present with disseminated, rather than localized, disease. Antigen and antibody testing for histoplasmosis may be negative. ▪ Consider the risks and benefits of golimumab treatment before initiating therapy in patients with chronic or recurrent infection, patients who have been exposed to TB, patients with a history of an opportunistic infection, patients who have resided or traveled in areas of endemic tuberculosis or endemic mycoses (e.g., histoplasmosis, coccidioidomycosis, or blastomycosis), or patients with underlying conditions that may predispose them to infection. ▪ Has been associated with the reactivation of hepatitis B virus (HBV) in patients who are chronic hepatitis B carriers (i.e., surface antigen–positive). Fatalities have been reported. ▪ Lymphoma and other malignancies, some fatal, have been reported in pediatric, adolescent, and young adult patients treated with TNF-blockers; most of these patients were receiving concomitant immunosuppressants. ▪ Rare post-marketing cases of hepatosplenic T-cell lymphoma (HSTCL) have been reported in patients treated with TNF-blocking agents. This rare type of T-cell lymphoma has a very aggressive disease course and is usually fatal. Nearly all cases have occurred in adolescents and young adult males with Crohn's disease or ulcerative colitis who have been treated with azathioprine or 6-mercaptopurine concomitantly with a TNF-blocker at or before diagnosis. ▪ Consider risk versus benefit in adult patients with a known malignancy other than a successfully treated nonmelanoma skin cancer (NMSC) or when considering continuing a TNF-blocker in patients who develop a malignancy. ▪ In controlled trials, more cases of lymphoma were seen in patients receiving anti-TNF treatment compared with the control group. Patients with RA and other chronic inflammatory diseases, particularly patients with highly active disease and/or chronic exposure to immunosuppressant therapies, may be at higher risk than the general population for developing lymphoma and other malignancies. Melanoma and Merkel cell carcinoma have also been reported in patients treated with TNF-blocking agents. ▪ Concurrent use with abatacept or anakinra is not recommended; see Drug/Lab Interactions. ▪ Cases of worsening CHF and new-onset CHF have been reported with TNF-blockers, including golimumab. Some incidents have resulted in hospitalization and increased mortality. Use with caution in patients with a history of CHF. Discontinue if new or worsening symptoms of CHF appear. ▪ TNF-blockers have been associated with rare cases of new onset or exacerbation of CNS demyelinating disorders, including multiple sclerosis and peripheral demyelinating disorders such as Guillain-Barré syndrome. Use with caution if indicated in these patients. Consider discontinuation of golimumab if these disorders develop. ▪ Treatment with TNF-blockers, including golimumab, may result in the formation of antinuclear antibodies. Rarely, treatment with TNF-blockers may result in a lupus-like syndrome. If symptoms suggestive of a lupus-like syndrome develop, discontinue golimumab. ▪ Use caution if switching from one biologic product to another (e.g., abatacept, adalimumab, infliximab, golimumab, rituximab); overlapping biologic activity may further increase the risk of infection. ▪ Use caution in patients who have or have had significant cytopenias; agranulocytosis, aplastic anemia, leukopenia, neutropenia, thrombocytopenia, and pancytopenia have been reported. ▪ May receive vaccinations, except for live virus vaccines; see Drug/Lab Interactions. ▪ Hypersensitivity reactions have been reported. ▪ Has not been studied in patients with impaired hepatic or renal function.

Monitor: Before initiating TNF-blocker therapy, including golimumab therapy, patients should be tested for HBV infection. If the test is positive, consultation with a physician with expertise in the treatment of hepatitis B is recommended before beginning treatment. Consider risk versus benefit in patients who are carriers of HBV. ▪ In patients who are carriers of HBV and require treatment with TNF-blockers, closely monitor for clinical and laboratory signs of active HBV throughout treatment and for several months after completion of treatment. If HBV reactivation occurs, discontinue golimumab; see Antidote. ▪ Evaluate patients for active and latent TB before and throughout therapy. Initiate treatment for latent TB before therapy with golimumab. ▪ Antituberculosis treatment of patients with a reactive TB skin test may reduce the risk of TB reactivation in patients receiving golimumab. Consider antituberculosis therapy before initiation for patients with a history of latent or active TB (if an adequate course of treatment cannot be confirmed) and for patients with a negative TB test who have risk factors for TB infection. Consultation with a physician with expertise in the treatment of TB is recommended. ▪ Consider a diagnosis of TB in patients who develop a new infection during treatment. ▪ Monitor for S/S of infection during and after treatment with golimumab, including the possible development of TB in patients who tested negative for latent TB before initiating therapy. Discontinue if a serious infection, an opportunistic infection, or sepsis occurs; see Precautions and Antidote. ▪ A prompt and complete diagnostic workup appropriate for an immunocompromised patient is indicated for patients who develop a new infection during treatment. Monitor closely and initiate appropriate antimicrobial therapy. Consider empiric antifungal therapy in patients at risk for invasive fungal infections who develop severe systemic illness. ▪ Monitor patients for S/S of malignancy. Periodic skin examination is recommended for all patients, particularly those with risk factors for skin cancer. ▪ Closely monitor patients with S/S of CHF. ▪ Monitor for S/S of a hypersensitivity reaction (e.g., anaphylaxis, dyspnea, hives, nausea, and pruritus). Most hypersensitivity reactions occurred during or within 1 hour of the infusion. Some reactions occurred after the first administration of golimumab.

Patient Education: Read the manufacturer's medication guide before starting therapy with golimumab and each time the prescription is renewed. ▪ Tell health care professionals about heart conditions, previous or current infections, and recent or past exposure to TB or histoplasmosis. ▪ Review all medicines and disease history with pharmacist or physician before initiating treatment. ▪ Lymphoma and other malignancies may occur while receiving golimumab. ▪ Promptly report S/S of infection (e.g., burning on urination; chills; cough; diarrhea; fever; stomach pain; warm, red, or painful skin; or sores on body). ▪ Promptly report S/S of tuberculosis, invasive fungal infections, and/or hepatitis B reactivation. ▪ Promptly report new or worsening conditions such as heart failure (e.g., shortness of breath, swelling feet), demyelinating disorders, autoimmune diseases, liver disease, cytopenias, or psoriasis. ▪ Report S/S of hypersensitivity reactions (e.g., itching, rash, swelling in the throat). ▪ Report changes of growths on your skin during or after golimumab treatment. ▪ Promptly report possible symptoms of lupus (e.g., excessive tiredness, new joint or muscle pain, rash on cheeks, sun sensitivity). ▪ Report recently receiving or being scheduled to receive a live virus vaccine or treatment with weakened bacteria (such as BCG for bladder cancer) to your physician. ▪ Consider potential benefit and risks of golimumab. ▪ See Appendix D.

Maternal/Child: Use during pregnancy only if clearly needed. ▪ There is no information regarding the presence of golimumab in human milk, the effects on the breast-fed infant, or the effects on milk production. ▪ Safety and effectiveness for use in pediatric patients under 18 years of age not established. ▪ Infants exposed to golimumab in utero and infants born to mothers treated with golimumab during pregnancy may be at increased risk for infection for up to 6 months. Administration of live virus vaccines is not recommended for 6 months after the last dose of golimumab that was administered to the mother during pregnancy.

Elderly: Numbers in clinical studies insufficient to determine whether the elderly respond differently than younger subjects. ▪ Patients over 65 years of age and those with comorbid conditions may be at increased risk for infections.

DRUG/LAB INTERACTIONS

Golimumab should be used with **methotrexate**. Following IV administration, concomitant administration of methotrexate decreased golimumab clearance by reducing the development of anti-golimumab antibodies. ▪ Concurrent administration with **other biologic products,** including **anakinra** or **abatacept**, may be associated with an increased risk of serious infections without any increase in benefit. Anakinra is also associated with an increased risk of neutropenia. Concurrent administration of TNF-blocking agents (e.g., golimumab) with other biologics approved to treat RA, including anakinra or abatacept, is not recommended. ▪ Concomitant use of **NSAIDs** (e.g., ibuprofen, naproxen), **oral corticosteroids** (e.g., prednisone), or **sulfasalazine** did not influence golimumab SQ clearance. ▪ **Live virus vaccines** and **therapeutic infectious agents** (e.g., BCG bladder instillation for treatment of cancer) should not be given concurrently with golimumab. Could result in clinical infection, including disseminated infections. In addition, for infants who had in utero exposure to golimumab, it is recommended that live vaccines not be given for at least 6 months after the last golimumab infusion administered to the mother during pregnancy; see Precautions and Maternal/Child. ▪ Cytochrome P_{450} enzymes may be suppressed by increased levels of cytokines during chronic inflammation. Golimumab antagonizes cytokine activity, and the formation of the CYP_{450} enzyme may be normalized. When initiating or discontinuing golimumab in patients treated with **CYP_{450} substrates with a narrow therapeutic index,** monitoring of the effect (e.g., **warfarin**) or drug concentrations (e.g., **cyclosporine** or **theophylline**) is recommended. Dose adjustment may be necessary.

SIDE EFFECTS

The most common side effects are bronchitis, decreased neutrophil count, hypertension, increased liver function tests (e.g., ALT, AST), rash, upper respiratory tract infections, and viral infections. The most serious were malignancies (e.g., lymphoma, skin cancer) and serious infections (e.g., abscess, cellulitis, invasive fungal infections, opportunistic infections, pneumonia, sepsis, and tuberculosis). Other less common side effects include bullous skin reactions, constipation, dizziness, fever, infusion reactions (e.g., rash), leukopenia, lower respiratory tract infection (pneumonia), paresthesia, pyelonephritis, sinusitis, superficial fungal infections.

Post-Marketing: Bullous skin reactions, infusion-related reactions, interstitial lung disease, lichenoid reactions, melanoma, Merkel cell carcinoma, sarcoidosis, serious systemic hypersensitivity reactions (including anaphylactic reactions), skin exfoliation. Rare cases of hepatosplenic T-cell lymphoma have been reported with TNF-blockers.

ANTIDOTE

Notify physician of any side effects; most will be treated symptomatically. Discontinue golimumab if patient experiences a serious infection, a serious hypersensitivity reaction, new or worsening S/S of heart failure, new or worsening S/S of CNS demyelinating disorders (multiple sclerosis [MS]), peripheral demyelinating disorders (including Guillain-Barré syndrome), or a lupus-like syndrome. Treat a hypersensitivity reaction with oxygen, epinephrine, antihistamines (e.g., diphenhydramine), vasopressors (e.g., dopamine), corticosteroids, albuterol, IV fluids, and ventilation equipment as indicated. Discontinue golimumab in patients who develop HBV reactivation, and initiate antiviral therapy with appropriate supportive treatment. Safety of resuming therapy after HBV is controlled is not known; use caution if resumption of therapy is considered and monitor closely.

GRANISETRON HYDROCHLORIDE

(gran-**ISS**-eh-tron hy-droh-**KLOR**-eyed)

Antiemetic
(5-HT₃ receptor antagonist)

pH 4 to 6

USUAL DOSE

Chemotherapy-induced nausea and vomiting (prophylaxis): A single dose of 10 mcg/kg of body weight as an injection or as an infusion. Begin within 30 minutes before giving emetogenic cancer chemotherapy (e.g., cisplatin, carboplatin) and only on the day(s) chemotherapy is given. Clinical trials used doses up to 40 mcg/kg with effects similar to the recommended 10-mcg/kg dose. Some studies question the effectiveness of a 10-mcg/kg dose. Repeat doses are frequently required to prevent nausea with chemotherapy. Oral granisetron is available.

Prevention and treatment of postoperative nausea and vomiting: 1 mg before induction of anesthesia, immediately before reversal of anesthesia, or postoperatively.

PEDIATRIC DOSE

Chemotherapy-induced nausea and vomiting (prophylaxis) in pediatric patients 2 to 16 years of age: Identical to adult dose. See Maternal/Child.

DOSE ADJUSTMENTS

No dose adjustment required for the elderly or in renal failure or impaired hepatic function.

DILUTION

Read label carefully. Available in two concentrations (0.1 mg/mL and 1 mg/mL). The 0.1-mg/mL vial contains no preservatives. The 1-mg/mL single-dose and multidose vials contain benzyl alcohol. Sterile technique imperative when withdrawing a single dose from the multidose vial; see Storage.

A single dose may be given undiluted by IV injection or further diluted to a total volume of 20 to 50 mL with NS or D5W and given as an infusion.

Storage: Store vials at CRT or below. Do not freeze; protect from light. Should be administered after dilution (preservative free) but is stable up to 24 hours at room temperature. Discard multidose vial within 30 days of initial penetration.

COMPATIBILITY

Manufacturer recommends not mixing in solution with other drugs as a general precaution.

Other sources suggest specific **compatibilities** dependent on concentration and manufacturer; consult a pharmacist.

RATE OF ADMINISTRATION

IV injection: A single dose over 30 seconds.

Intermittent infusion: A single dose equally distributed over 5 minutes.

ACTIONS

An antinauseant and antiemetic agent. A selective antagonist of specific serotonin (5-HT$_3$) receptors. Chemotherapeutic agents such as cisplatin increase the release of serotonin from specific cells in the GI tract, causing emesis. By antagonizing these receptors, chemotherapy-induced nausea and vomiting are prevented. Has little effect on BP, HR, ECG, plasma prolactin, or aldosterone concentrations. Moderately bound to protein (65%). Distributes freely between plasma and RBCs. Metabolized in the liver by hepatic cytochrome P$_{450}$ enzymes. Mean half-life is approximately 9 hours. Excreted in urine and feces.

INDICATIONS AND USES

Prevention of nausea and vomiting associated with initial and repeat courses of emetogenic cancer therapy, including high-dose cisplatin. Has been shown to be effective with most emetogenic antineoplastic agents. ▪ Prevention and treatment of postoperative nausea and vomiting in adults.

Unlabeled uses: Prevention of nausea and vomiting associated with total body radiation or fractional abdominal radiation.

CONTRAINDICATIONS

Known hypersensitivity to granisetron.

PRECAUTIONS

Stool softeners or laxatives may be required to prevent constipation. ▪ See Drug/Lab Interactions. ▪ Hypersensitivity reactions have been reported. Use caution in patients who have exhibited hypersensitivity to other selective 5-HT$_3$ receptor antagonists. Cross-sensitivity has been reported between dolasetron and other agents in this class (e.g., granisetron, ondansetron). ▪ The use in patients following abdominal surgery or in patients with chemotherapy-induced nausea and vomiting may mask a progressive ileus and/or gastric distension. ▪ Does not stimulate GI motility and should not be used instead of NG suction. ▪ QT prolongation has been reported. Use with caution in patients with pre-existing arrhythmias, cardiac conduction disorders, or electrolyte abnormalities or in patients who are taking other medications that can prolong the QT interval; see Drug/Lab Interactions. ▪ Serotonin syndrome has been reported with 5-HT$_3$ receptor antagonists. Most reports were associated with concomitant use of serotonergic drugs (e.g., selective serotonin reuptake inhibitors, serotonin and norepinephrine reuptake inhibitors, monoamine oxidase inhibitors, mirtazapine, fentanyl, lithium, tramadol, and intravenous methylene blue). Some cases were fatal. ▪ Not recommended if nausea and vomiting are not expected postoperatively unless nausea and vomiting must be avoided during the postoperative period.

Monitor: Ambulate slowly to avoid orthostatic hypotension. ▪ Monitor for S/S of hypersensitivity (e.g., anaphylaxis, hypotension, shortness of breath, urticaria). ▪ Monitor ECG in patients at risk for prolongation of the PR and QRS interval; see Precautions. ▪ Monitor for serotonin syndrome, especially when dolasetron is used concurrently with other serotonergic drugs. Symptoms associated with serotonin syndrome may include the following combination of S/S: mental status changes (e.g., agitation, coma, delirium, hallucinations), autonomic instability (e.g., diaphoresis, dizziness, flushing, hyperthermia, labile blood pressure, tachycardia), neuromuscular symptoms (e.g., hyperreflexia, incoordination, myoclonus, rigidity, tremor), seizures, with or without GI symptoms (e.g., diarrhea, nausea, vomiting).

Patient Education: Request assistance for ambulation. ▪ Report promptly if nausea persists for more than 10 minutes. ▪ Maintain adequate hydration. ▪ Stool softeners may be required to avoid constipation. ▪ Promptly report S/S of serotonin syndrome (e.g., altered mental status, autonomic instability, and neuromuscular symptoms); see Precautions.

Maternal/Child: Category B: no evidence of impaired fertility or harm to fetus. Benzyl alcohol may cross the placenta; see Dilution. Use during pregnancy only if benefits justify risks. ▪ Use caution if required during breast-feeding. ▪ Safety and effectiveness for use in the treatment of chemotherapy-induced nausea and vomiting in pediatric patients under 2 years of age have not been established. ▪ Not recommended for prevention and treatment of postoperative nausea and vomiting in pediatric patients due to a lack of efficacy and QT prolongation observed in a clinical trial.

Elderly: Response similar to other age-groups. ▪ Clearance lower and half-life prolonged but has no clinical significance.

DRUG/LAB INTERACTIONS

Metabolism may be inhibited by **ketoconazole**. Clinical significance unknown. ▪ Does not induce or inhibit the cytochrome P_{450} drug metabolizing system, but definitive interaction studies have not been done. Its clearance and half-life may be affected by **inducers of these enzymes** such as anticonvulsants or rifampin or by **inhibitors of these enzymes** (e.g., cimetidine, calcium channel blockers, antiviral agents [e.g., indinavir, ritonavir, saquinavir]). ▪ Has been safely administered with **benzodiazepines, neuroleptics**, and **antiulcer drugs** commonly prescribed with antiemetic treatment. ▪ Does not appear to interact with emetogenic cancer chemotherapies. ▪ Concurrent use with **drugs known to prolong the QT interval** (e.g., amiodarone, antihistamines, azole antifungals, disopyramide, fluoroquinolones, ibutilide, mexiletine, phenothiazines, procainamide, quinidine, and tricyclic antidepressants) may result in clinical consequences. ▪ Serotonin syndrome (including altered mental status, autonomic instability, and neuromuscular symptoms) has been reported following the concomitant use of 5-HT$_3$ receptor antagonists and other serotonergic drugs, including selective serotonin reuptake inhibitors (SSRIs) and serotonin and norepinephrine reuptake inhibitors (SNRIs); see Precautions.

SIDE EFFECTS

Asthenia (5%), constipation (3%), diarrhea (4%), headache (14%), somnolence (4%), and weakness (5%) occur most frequently. Hypersensitivity reactions, including anaphylaxis (rare), have occurred. Transient elevation of AST or ALT may occur. Other side effects include abdominal pain, anemia, anxiety, bradycardia, coughing, dizziness, dyspepsia, fever, hypertension, hypotension, infection, insomnia, leukocytosis, oliguria, pain. Other side effects have occurred in fewer than 2% of patients but could not be clearly associated with granisetron.

Post-Marketing: QT prolongation. Serotonin syndrome has been reported as a 5-HT$_3$ class reaction.

ANTIDOTE

Most side effects will be treated symptomatically. Keep physician informed as indicated. There is no specific antidote. If symptoms of serotonin syndrome occur, discontinue granisetron and initiate supportive care. Treat anaphylaxis and resuscitate as necessary.

HEMIN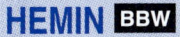

(**HEE**-men)

Panhematin

Porphyrin inhibitor

USUAL DOSE

A single dose of 1 to 4 mg/kg of body weight/24 hr of hematin for 3 to 14 days. This dose could be repeated in 12 hours for severe cases. Never exceed a total dose of 6 mg/kg/24 hr. Length of treatment dependent on severity of symptoms and clinical response. See Precautions.

DILUTION

Each vial containing 313 mg of hemin must be diluted with 43 mL of SWFI (provides 301 mg of hematin). Shake well for 2 to 3 minutes to ensure dissolution. Each 1 mL contains 7 mg hematin. Each 0.14 mL contains 1 mg hematin. May be given directly from vial as an infusion or through Y-tube of infusion set.

Filters: Use of a 0.45-micron or smaller in-line filter recommended.

Storage: Store in refrigerator at 2° to 8° C (36° to 46° F). Contains no preservative, decomposes rapidly; discard unused solution.

COMPATIBILITY

Undergoes rapid chemical decomposition in solution. Manufacturer states, "No drug or chemical agent should be added unless its effect on the chemical and physical stability has been determined." Specific information not available; consult pharmacist.

RATE OF ADMINISTRATION

A single dose evenly distributed over 10 to 15 minutes.

ACTIONS

An iron-containing metalloporphyrin enzyme inhibitor extracted from RBCs. Inhibits rate of porphyria/heme biosynthesis in the liver and bone marrow by an unknown mechanism. Induces remission of symptoms only; not curative. Some excretion occurs in urine and feces.

INDICATIONS AND USES

To control symptoms of recurrent attacks of acute intermittent porphyria in selected patients (often related to the menstrual cycle in susceptible females).

CONTRAINDICATIONS

Hypersensitivity to hemin; porphyria cutanea tarda.

PRECAUTIONS

Confirm diagnosis of acute porphyria before use (positive Watson-Schwartz or Hoechst test). Administered by or under the supervision of a physician experienced in the treatment of porphyrias and in facilities equipped to monitor the patient and respond to any medical emergency. ■ Alternate therapy of 400 Gm glucose/24 hr for 1 to 2 days should be tried before use of hemin is initiated. ■ Give as early as possible with onset of attack to achieve the most benefit. ■ Must be given before irreversible neuronal damage of porphyria has begun. ■ See Drug/Lab Interactions.

Monitor: Use of a large arm vein or central venous catheter recommended to avoid phlebitis. ■ Effectiveness monitored by decrease in urine concentration of S-aminolevulinic acid (ALA), uroporphyrinogen (UPG), or porphobilinogen (PBG).

Maternal/Child: Category C: safety for use during pregnancy, breast-feeding, and in pediatric patients not established.

DRUG/LAB INTERACTIONS

Action inhibited by **estrogens, barbiturates, and steroid metabolites.** Avoid concurrent use. ■ Has mild anticoagulant effects. Avoid concurrent use with **anticoagulants** (e.g., heparin, warfarin).

SIDE EFFECTS

Almost nonexistent with usual dosage and appropriate technique; fever, phlebitis. Reversible renal shutdown has been reported with excessive doses.

ANTIDOTE

Discontinue temporarily if known or questionable side effect appears, and notify physician. Renal shutdown of overdose has responded to ethacrynic acid (Edecrin) and mannitol. Treat anaphylaxis (antihistamines, epinephrine, corticosteroids) and resuscitate as necessary.

HEPARIN SODIUM
(**HEP**-ah-rin **SO**-dee-um)

Anticoagulant

pH 5 to 7.5

USUAL DOSE

Pretreatment: Baseline studies indicated; see Monitor.

Confirm choice of the correct heparin product; see Precautions.

Intermittent injection for therapeutic anticoagulation (based on a 68-kg [150-lb] patient): 10,000 units initially. Dosage is repeated every 4 to 6 hours and adjusted according to coagulation test results. Usually 5,000 to 10,000 units. Initial and repeat doses may be given undiluted or may be diluted in 50 to 100 mL of NS.

IV infusion for therapeutic anticoagulation (based on a 68-kg [150-lb] patient): An initial bolus dose of 5,000 units is required. 20,000 to 40,000 units/24 hr in NS or other **compatible** infusion solution. Adjust dose according to coagulation test results.

Treatment of venous thromboembolism (VTE): American College of Chest Physicians recommends an initial bolus of 80 units/kg (alternately 5,000 units) followed by an initial continuous infusion of 18 units/kg/hr (alternately 1,000 units/hr) for VTE.

Adjuvant therapy in treatment of AMI: AHA guidelines recommend an initial bolus dose of 60 units/kg of body weight (maximum dose 4,000 units). Follow with an infusion of 12 units/kg/hr. The initial maximum recommended infusion rate is 1,000 units/hr. Adjust to maintain aPTT at 1.5 to 2 times control. Other protocols are in use.

Adjuvant therapy during treatment with thrombolytic agents (e.g., alteplase, reteplase, streptokinase) and glycoprotein GPIIb/IIIa receptor antagonists (e.g., abciximab, eptifibatide, tirofiban): See individual monographs for suggested doses.

Open heart surgery: 150 to 400 units/kg of body weight during surgical procedure, depending on duration of procedure. Frequently, a dose of 300 units/kg is administered for procedures estimated to last less than 60 minutes. 400 units/kg may be given for procedures estimated to last longer than 60 minutes.

Disseminated intravascular coagulation: Use and dose of heparin is based on severity of DIC and underlying cause and extent of thrombosis. Several dosing regimens have been used; see literature.

Maintain patency of indwelling venipuncture devices (e.g., heparin-lock, catheter, or implanted port) intended for intermittent use: Consult device manufacturer's instructions for specific requirements regarding its use. 10 unit/mL concentration is commonly used for younger infants (less than 10 kg). Higher concentration of 100 units/1 mL is used in older infants, pediatric patients, and adults. Volume of heparin flush solution should be similar to volume of catheter. May be used after initial placement of the device in the vein, after each medication injection, after withdrawal of blood for laboratory tests, or every 8 to 24 hours to maintain patency of device. Confirm patency by aspirating before each injection. Flush with SWFI or NS before and after any medication **incompatible** with heparin. Re-instill heparin after second flush. If additional medications are not needed, each single dose of heparin will prevent clotting within the lumen of indwelling venipuncture devices for up to 24 hours.

Blood transfusion: 400 to 600 units/100 mL whole blood.

Converting to an oral anticoagulant: When converting from heparin to **warfarin** (Coumadin), begin warfarin on the first or second day of heparin therapy at the usual initial dose and determine PT/INR at the usual intervals. To ensure continuous anticoagulation, continue full heparin therapy for several days until the PT/INR has reached a therapeutic range (INR of 2 or greater) for at least 24 hours. Once target PT/INR has been achieved and maintained, heparin therapy can be discontinued without tapering. When initiating oral therapy with an oral anticoagulant, stop the heparin infusion immediately after the first dose of the oral anticoagulant. For intermittent IV administration of heparin, start the oral anticoagulant 0 to 2 hours before the time that the next dose of intermittent heparin was to have been administered.

PEDIATRIC DOSE
Read label carefully. Comes in many strengths. Confirm use of the correct strength. Fatal hemorrhages have occurred in pediatric patients, including neonates, as a result of medication errors in which heparin sodium injection vials have been confused with heparin-lock flush vials.

Do not use products containing benzyl alcohol in neonates or infants. Preservative-free solution is required for neonates and infants. See Maternal/Child.

Full-dose continuous IV infusion: A *loading dose* of 75 to 100 units/kg administered over 10 minutes and a *maintenance dose* (to maintain an aPTT of approximately 60 to 85 seconds or a range corresponding to an anti-factor Xa level of 0.35 to 0.7) based on age as follows:

Infants under 2 months: (Have the highest requirements) Average 28 units/kg/hr.

Infants 2 months to 1 year of age: 25 to 30 units/kg/hr.

Over 1 year of age: 18 to 20 units/kg/hr.

Older pediatric patients: May require less heparin, similar to the weight-adjusted dose in adults (18 units/kg/hr).

Disseminated intravascular coagulation: Use and dose of heparin are based on severity of DIC and underlying cause and extent of thrombosis. Several dosing regimens have been used; see literature.

Patency of indwelling venipuncture devices: See Maternal/Child. Safety and effectiveness of the 100-USP units/mL heparin-lock flush solution for pediatric patients not established. Patency for peripheral devices (e.g., single- and double-lumen central catheters) is usually accomplished with 10 units/mL heparin solution in younger infants (e.g., less than 10 kg) and with 100 units/mL for older infants, children, and adults. Avoid approaching therapeutic unit/kg dose. Follow catheter manufacturer's guidelines. See all comments under similar section in Usual Dose.

DOSE ADJUSTMENTS
Reduction of initial dose indicated in patients 60 years of age and older (especially females). Adjust dose based on coagulation tests; see Monitor.

DILUTION
May be given undiluted or diluted in any given amount of NS, dextrose, or Ringer's solution for infusion and given by IV injection, as an intermittent IV, or continuous IV infusion. When added to an infusion solution for continuous IV administration, invert container a minimum of 6 times to ensure adequate mixing and to prevent pooling of heparin in the solution. Available in several strengths for administration or dilution as well as in several premixed concentrations and volumes. Unit-dose heparin flush syringes are not for multiple use; discard unused portions.

Intermittent injection or infusion: Usually given undiluted or may be diluted in 50 to 100 mL of NS or D5W.

Continuous infusion: Available in several manufacturer-supplied concentrations. If prepared, may be diluted in 250 to 1,000 mL of **compatible** solution to provide a 24-hour dose. See chart on inside back cover.

Blood transfusion: Add 7,500 units heparin to 100 mL NS. Add 6 to 8 mL of this sterile solution to each 100 mL of whole blood.

Filters: No significant reduction in potency when 10,000 units diluted in D5W or NS was filtered through a 0.22-micron cellulose ester membrane filter.

Storage: Store at CRT. Do not freeze. Do not use if solution is discolored or contains a precipitate. Storage of prepared (diluted) heparin infusion solutions should not exceed 4 hours at RT or 24 hours refrigerated.

COMPATIBILITY

Several sources recommend not mixing or administering through the same IV line with other drugs until **compatibility** confirmed. To avoid precipitation with heparin, they also caution to flush with SWFI or NS before and after any acidic or **incompatible** medication or solution. Manufacturer lists as **incompatible** in solution with alteplase, amikacin, atracurium, ciprofloxacin, cytarabine, daunorubicin, droperidol, erythromycin, gentamicin, idarubicin, kanamycin, mitoxantrone, polymyxin B, promethazine, streptomycin, and tobramycin.

Other sources suggest specific **compatibilities** dependent on concentration and manufacturer; consult a pharmacist.

RATE OF ADMINISTRATION

A single injection (5,000 units or fraction thereof) may be given over 1 minute. A continuous IV infusion may be given over 4 to 24 hours, depending on specific dosage of heparin required, amount of heparin added, and amount of infusion fluid used as a diluent. Continuous IV infusion is the preferred method of administration. Use an infusion pump for accuracy.

ACTIONS

An anticoagulant with immediate and predictable effects on the blood. Inhibits reactions that lead to clotting of blood and the formation of fibrin clots. Heparin combines with other factors in the blood to inhibit the conversion of prothrombin to thrombin and fibrinogen to fibrin. Adhesiveness of platelets is reduced. Well-established clots are not dissolved, but growth is prevented and newer clots may be dissolved. Duration of action is short, about 4 to 6 hours. Average plasma half-life is 30 to 120 minutes. The half-life of the anticoagulant effect of heparin is approximately 1.5 hours and does not increase with dose. Metabolic fate not fully determined. May be partially metabolized in the liver and the reticuloendothelial system. Small amount excreted as unchanged drug in the urine.

INDICATIONS AND USES

Prevention and/or treatment of all types of thromboses and emboli, including deep vein thrombosis (DVT), pulmonary emboli (PE), thromboembolic complications associated with atrial fibrillation (AF), and peripheral arterial embolism. ▪ Treatment of disseminated intravascular coagulation (DIC). ▪ Prevention of clotting in arterial and cardiac surgery and during blood transfusion, extracorporeal circulation, and dialysis procedures. ▪ Maintain patency of an indwelling venipuncture device designed for intermittent injection or infusion therapy or blood sampling (e.g., heparin-lock, catheter, or implanted port).

Unlabeled uses: Adjunct in treatment of coronary occlusion with acute myocardial infarction (MI). ▪ Adjunct to use of glycoprotein GP IIb/IIIa receptor antagonists in percutaneous coronary intervention (PCI). ▪ ST-elevation MI, as an adjunct to thrombolysis.

CONTRAINDICATIONS

History of heparin-induced thrombocytopenia (HIT) and heparin-induced thrombocytopenia and thrombosis (HITT). ▪ Severe thrombocytopenia. ▪ Patients receiving full-dose heparin unless blood coagulation tests can be performed at appropriate intervals. ▪ Hypersensitivity to heparin (or any of its components [may contain sulfites]) or pork products. ▪ Uncontrolled bleeding except in DIC. ▪ Do not administer heparin preparations preserved with benzyl alcohol to neonates, infants, pregnant females, or breast-feeding mothers.

PRECAUTIONS

Read label carefully. Comes in many strengths. Confirm use of the correct strength. Fatal hemorrhages have occurred in pediatric patients, including neonates, as a result of medication errors in which heparin sodium injection vials have been confused with heparin-lock flush vials. ▪ For IV or SQ use only; avoid IM administration (may cause hematomas). ▪ Derived from animal protein (pork). ▪ Avoid using heparin in the presence of major bleeding, except when the benefits of heparin therapy outweigh the potential risks. ▪ Use extreme caution in any disease state or clinical condition in which risk of hemorrhage may be increased, such as subacute bacterial endocarditis; severe hypertension; during or following spinal tap, spinal anesthesia, or major surgery (especially major surgery involving the brain, spinal cord, or eye); hemophilia; thrombocytopenia; gastrointestinal ulcerative lesions; vascular purpuras; patients with hereditary antithrombin III deficiency receiving concurrent antithrombin III therapy (see Drug/Lab Interactions); continuous tube drainage of the stomach or small intestine; menstruation; or severe liver disease with impaired hemostasis. ▪ Resistance to heparin increased in cancer, fever, infections with thrombosing tendencies, MI, patients with antithrombin III deficiency, postsurgical patients, thrombophlebitis, and thrombosis. ▪ May cause thrombocytopenia; monitor closely. ▪ May develop HIT, an antibody-mediated reaction resulting from irreversible aggregation of platelets. HIT may progress to HITT, which involves the development of venous and arterial thromboses. HIT and HITT may occur during heparin treatment or may be delayed for up to several weeks after heparin treatment is discontinued; see Monitor. ▪ See Elderly for additional precautions. ▪ Repeated flushing of an indwelling venipuncture device with heparin may result in a systemic anticoagulant effect. ▪ Heparin-lock flush solution is intended for maintenance of patency of intravenous injection devices only and is not to be used for anticoagulant therapy. ▪ See Maternal/Child.

Monitor: Obtain baseline coagulation studies (e.g., whole blood clotting time [WBCT], activated coagulation time [ACT], activated partial thromboplastin time [aPTT], and INR) and a baseline CBC with platelets. ▪ Dose is considered adequate when the aPTT is 1.5 to 2 times normal or when the WBCT is elevated approximately 2.5 to 3 times the control value. Confirm desired control level with physician. ▪ During the early stages of treatment, coagulation tests are often done before each intermittent injection or every 4 hours with a continuous infusion. Once the patient is adequately anticoagulated and stable, monitoring may be decreased to daily. Reinstitute more frequent monitoring with any dose adjustment, change in patient condition, or change in therapy that might affect anticoagulation status. Notify the physician if aPTT, ACT, or WBCT is above therapeutic level. ▪ Monitor platelet count periodically. Discontinue heparin if it falls below 100,000 or a thrombosis forms. May develop HIT or HITT. Immune-mediated HIT is diagnosed based on clinical findings supplemented by laboratory tests confirming the presence of antibodies to heparin or platelet activation induced by heparin. Thrombotic events may be the initial presentation for HITT and may include DVT, cerebral vein thrombosis, limb ischemia, mesenteric thrombosis, thrombus formation on a prosthetic cardiac valve, or renal artery thrombosis; skin necrosis; gangrene of the extremities that may lead to amputation; MI; pulmonary embolism; stroke; or death. HIT and HITT may occur during heparin therapy or may be delayed. Evaluate patients for HIT and HITT if they present with thrombocytopenia or thrombosis after heparin is discontinued. Can occur up to several weeks after heparin is discontinued. ▪ Also monitor hematocrit and occult blood in stool. ▪ Hemorrhage can occur at any site and is the primary complication. Monitor closely. Consider the possibility of a hemorrhagic event with an unexplained fall in hematocrit, a fall in BP, or any other unexplained symptom. GI or urinary tract bleeding may indicate an underlying lesion. Certain hemorrhagic complications may be difficult to detect and can be very serious (e.g., adrenal [with resultant adrenal insufficiency], ovarian [corpus luteum], and retroperitoneal hemorrhage). ▪ Use extensive precautionary methods to prevent bleeding if patient requires IM injection, arterial puncture, or venipuncture. ▪ Monitor coagulation tests closely in patients who develop resistance to heparin. Adjustment of heparin doses based on anti-Factor Xa levels may be warranted; see Precautions. ▪ Monitor for S/S of a hypersensitivity reaction in patients with allergies; derived from animal tissue, and some products may contain a sulfite preservative.

Patency of indwelling venipuncture devices: Obtain a baseline aPTT prior to insertion of an indwelling venipuncture device. Repeated heparin injections can alter aPTT. ▪ To avoid precipitation, irrigate indwelling venipuncture devices with NS before and after injecting acidic or **incompatible** solutions. ▪ Heparin and/or NS may interfere with blood samples drawn from these devices, especially if drawn on a frequent basis. Clear the heparin flush solution by aspirating and discarding a volume of solution equal to that of the indwelling venipuncture device before the desired blood sample is drawn.

Patient Education: Report all episodes of bleeding and apply local pressure if indicated. ▪ Report tarry stools. ▪ Compliance with all measures to minimize bleeding is very important (e.g., avoid use of razors, toothbrushes, other sharp items). ▪ Use caution while moving to avoid excess bumping. ▪ Promptly report S/S of any other side effects (e.g., hypersensitivity reaction, HIT, HITT).

Maternal/Child: Use with caution. Maternal and fetal outcomes associated with heparin use during pregnancy have been investigated in numerous studies. These studies generally reported normal deliveries with no maternal or fetal bleeding and no other complications. ▪ Not secreted in breast milk. ▪ Some preparations may contain benzyl alcohol; do not use in neonates, infants, pregnant females, or breast-feeding mothers; see Contraindications. ▪ There are no adequate and well-controlled studies on heparin use in pediatric patients. Pediatric dosing recommendations are based on clinical experience. ▪ Use heparin-lock flush with caution in infants with diseases with an increased risk of hemorrhage. The 100 units/mL concentration should not be used in neonates or infants who weigh less than 10 kg because of the risk of systemic anticoagulation. Use minimal doses and preservative-free preparations, and monitor carefully. ▪ See Dose Adjustments and Precautions.

Elderly: Higher plasma levels of heparin and longer aPTTs may occur in patients over 60 years of age. Higher incidence of bleeding in patients 60 years of age and older (especially females). Lower doses of heparin may be indicated; see Dose Adjustments.

DRUG/LAB INTERACTIONS

Increased risk of bleeding with **drugs that can interfere with platelet aggregation and/or increase the risk of bleeding** (e.g., **systemic salicylates** [aspirin], **NSAIDs, platelet aggregation inhibitors, GP IIb/IIIa receptor antagonists, some cephalosporins** [e.g., cefotetan], **dextran, or other thrombolytic agents**); use heparin with caution in patients receiving such agents. ▪ Anticoagulant effect of heparin is enhanced by concurrent treatment with **antithrombin III (human)**. ▪ Inhibited by **antihistamines, digoxin, nicotine, nitrates, tetracyclines, and others;** may counteract anticoagulant action of heparin. ▪ Potentiates **oral anticoagulants** (e.g., apixaban, dabigatran, rivaroxaban, warfarin). ▪ See Precautions/Monitor. ▪ Use caution when administered with or around **other anticoagulants.** Lab data may not provide an accurate baseline. ▪ Numerous **lab values** (e.g., aminotransferase levels [AST, ALT], PT) may be altered. Notify lab of heparin use. Diagnostic results may not be attainable. See Monitor. ▪ When heparin is given concomitantly with warfarin, the PT may be prolonged. Wait at least 5 hours after IV bolus heparin dose before drawing PT. If heparin is being administered as a continuous infusion, may draw PT at any time.

SIDE EFFECTS

The most common side effects are elevations of aminotransferase levels and general hypersensitivity reactions, usually chills, fever, and urticaria (anaphylactoid reactions, including shock, asthma, headache, itching and burning on plantar side of feet, lacrimation, nausea and vomiting, and rhinitis may occur less frequently); hemorrhage (bruising, epistaxis, hematuria, tarry stools [adrenal hemorrhage (with resultant acute adrenal insufficiency), ovarian hemorrhage (corpus luteum hemorrhage that may be fatal), and/or retroperitoneal hemorrhage may be difficult to detect]); HIT and HITTS (including delayed-onset cases); injection site irritation; and thrombocytopenia.

ANTIDOTE

Discontinue drug and notify physician of any side effects. Protamine sulfate is a heparin antagonist and specifically indicated in overdose or desired heparin reversal. Each milligram of protamine neutralizes approximately 100 units heparin. No more than 50 mg should be administered, very slowly, in any 10-minute period. Administration of protamine can cause severe hypotension and anaphylactoid reactions. Use with caution and have emergency equipment and medications readily available. If HIT (with or without thrombosis) is diagnosed or strongly suspected, discontinue all sources of heparin, including heparin flushes. Use an alternative anticoagulant. Any future use of heparin should be avoided, especially within 3 to 6 months after the diagnosis of HIT or HITT and while patients test positive for HIT antibodies. Whole blood transfusion may be indicated. If HIT or white clot syndrome occurs, discontinue heparin and administer a non-heparin anticoagulant (e.g., argatroban, bivalirudin) as an alternate form of anticoagulation. Follow-up with oral anticoagulation (e.g., warfarin) may also be indicated. Avoid use of heparin for at least 3 to 6 months or for as long as the patient tests positive for HIT antibodies.

HEPATITIS B IMMUNE GLOBULIN INTRAVENOUS (HUMAN)

Immunizing agent (passive)

(hep-ah-**TY**-tiss ih-**MUNE GLAW**-byoo-lin IV)

HepaGam B

pH 5.6

USUAL DOSE

(International units [IU])

Pretreatment: Baseline studies indicated; see Monitor.

Prevention of hepatitis B recurrence following liver transplantation: Administered by a set dosing regimen designed to attain serum levels of antibodies to hepatitis B surface antigen (anti-HBs) greater than 500 IU/L. Each dose should contain 20,000 IU calculated from the measured potency as stamped on the vial label. Administer the first dose of 20,000 IU concurrently with grafting of the transplanted liver (the anhepatic phase). Administer each subsequent dose of 20,000 IU as recommended in the following chart.

Hepatitis B IGIV Dosing Regimen			
Anhepatic Phase	**Week 1 Postoperative**	**Weeks 2-12 Postoperative**	**Month 4 Onward**
First dose of 20,000 IU	20,000 IU daily from Day 1 through Day 7; see Dose Adjustments	20,000 IU every 2 weeks from Day 14 (Week 2) through Week 12	20,000 IU monthly

DOSE ADJUSTMENTS

(International units [IU])

Increased doses may be required in patients who fail to reach anti-HBs levels of 500 IU/L within the first week after liver transplantation. Particularly susceptible to an extensive decrease of circulated anti-HBs are patients who have surgical bleeding or abdominal fluid drainage (greater than 500 mL) or those who undergo plasmapheresis. If the desired anti-HBs levels are not reached, increase the dosing regimen to a half-dose (10,000 IU [calculated from the measured potency as stamped on the vial label]) and administer IV every 6 hours until the target anti-HBs level is reached.

DILUTION

A ready-to-use liquid preparation; should be clear to opalescent. Multiple vials will be required. **Do not shake vials; avoid foaming.** Bring to room temperature before administration. Administer through a separate IV line using an IV administration set and an infusion pump.

Filters: No data available from manufacturer.

Storage: Store between 2° and 8° C (36° and 46° F). Do not freeze. Do not use after expiration date. Use within 6 hours of opening the vial, and discard partially used vials.

COMPATIBILITY

Manufacturer states, "Administer through a separate IV line using an IV administration set via infusion pump."

RATE OF ADMINISTRATION

Set infusion pump rate at 2 mL/min. Decrease to 1 mL/min or slower for patient discomfort, infusion-related adverse events, or concern about the speed of infusion.

ACTIONS

A solvent/detergent-treated sterile solution of purified gamma globulin containing anti-HBs. Prepared from plasma donated by healthy, screened donors with high titers of anti-HBs. Purified by an anion-exchange column chromatography manufacturing method. It provides passive immunization for individuals exposed to the hepatitis B virus (HBV) by binding to the surface antigen and reducing the rate of hepatitis B infection. Following liver transplantation, HBV re-infection can occur immediately at the time of liver reperfusion due to a circulating virus or later from a virus retained in extrahepatic sites. Provides an immediate immune response to the HBV. Mechanism of action is not known but may occur through several pathways (e.g., through blockage of a putative HBV receptor, neutralization of circulating virions through immune precipitation and immune complex formation, triggering of an antibody-dependent cell-mediated cytotoxicity response that results in target cell lysis, or binding to hepatocytes and interaction with HBsAg within cells). Clinical effectiveness is dependent on dose, length of administration, and viral replication status of the patient at the time of transplant. Bioavailability is complete and immediate and is distributed quickly between plasma and extravascular fluid. Immune globulins are metabolized by being broken down in the reticuloendothelial system. IM injection results in mean peak concentrations within 4 to 5 days of administration and an elimination half-life of 22 to 25 days. A slightly decreased half-life is expected following IV administration.

INDICATIONS AND USES

Prevention of hepatitis B recurrence following liver transplantation in HBsAg-positive liver transplant patients. Recommended for use in patients who have no or low levels of viral replication at the time of liver transplantation. ▪ Used IM for postexposure prophylaxis in the following settings: acute exposure to blood containing HBsAg, perinatal exposure of infants born to HBsAg-positive mothers, sexual exposure to HBsAg-positive persons, and household exposure to persons with acute HBV infection.

CONTRAINDICATIONS

History of anaphylactic or severe systemic reactions to human globulins. ▪ Weigh benefits versus risk of hypersensitivity reactions in IgA-deficient individuals; see Precautions.

PRECAUTIONS

Administer in a facility with adequate equipment and supplies to monitor the patient and respond to any medical emergency. ▪ Hypersensitivity and/or infusion reactions may occur. ▪ Individuals deficient in IgA may have the potential to develop IgA antibodies and have an anaphylactoid reaction. ▪ Contains maltose, which can interfere with select blood glucose monitoring systems (those based on the glucose dehydrogenase pyrroloquinequinone [GDH-PQQ] method). May cause falsely elevated glucose readings, result in inappropriate insulin administration, and cause life-threatening hypoglycemia. In contrast, cases of true hypoglycemia may go untreated if the hypoglycemic state is masked by falsely elevated results. ▪ Derived from human plasma. Despite screening and purification processes, may have the potential risk of transmitting infectious agents (e.g., viruses [e.g., HIV, hepatitis]) or the Creutzfeldt-Jakob disease agent. ▪ Has not been evaluated in combination with antiviral therapy posttransplantation. ▪ See Patient Education and Drug/Lab Interactions.

Monitor: Hepatitis B IGIV is most effective in patients with no or low levels of HBV replication at the time of transplantation. Monitor serum HBsAg and levels of anti-HBs antibody pre-infusion and regularly to track treatment response and adjust dose when indicated. ▪ Infusion reactions may occur; usually related to rate of infusion. Monitor closely during and following an infusion. ▪ Use caution and observe diabetic patients closely; see Precautions. Only glucose-specific testing systems can be used in patients receiving hepatitis IGIV. Review product information of the blood glucose testing system to confirm that it can be used with maltose-containing parenteral products. ▪ Monitor for S/S of a hypersensitivity reaction.

Patient Education: Regular monitoring of serum HBsAg and anti-HBs antibody levels imperative. ▪ Vaccination with live virus vaccines should be deferred until approximately 3 months after administration of hepatitis B IGIV. Revaccination may be required if the previous vaccination occurred within 2 weeks of the initial hepatitis IGIV dose.

Maternal/Child: Category C: use during pregnancy only if clearly indicated. ▪ Use caution during breast-feeding. ▪ Safety and effectiveness for use in pediatric patients under 18 years of age not established.

Elderly: Safety and effectiveness not established.

DRUG/LAB INTERACTIONS

May reduce the effectiveness of **live virus vaccines** (e.g., measles, mumps, rubella, varicella). Vaccination with live virus vaccines should be deferred until approximately 3 months after administration of hepatitis B IGIV. ▪ Contains **maltose,** which can interfere with select blood glucose monitoring systems (those based on the glucose dehydrogenase pyrroloquinequinone [GDH-PQQ] method). May cause falsely elevated glucose readings. Use only glucose-specific testing systems in patients receiving hepatitis B IGIV. ▪ Passively transferred antibodies may cause a misleading positive result in **serologic testing** (e.g., Coombs' test). ▪ No data available on drug interactions with other medications.

SIDE EFFECTS

Arthralgia, chills, fever, headaches, hypersensitivity reactions, moderate or low back pain, nausea, and vomiting are the most common. Other reported side effects include agitation, amnesia, aphthous stomatitis, diarrhea, dyspepsia, edema, fatigue, gingival hyperplasia, hepatobiliary disease, hyperglycemia, hypertension, hypotension, infectious diarrhea, liver transplant rejection, nocturia, pleural effusion, pneumonia, presbyopia, pruritus, rash, sepsis, splenomegaly, tremors.

ANTIDOTE

Reduce rate of infusion for patient discomfort, infusion-related side effects, or other concerns. Discontinue the drug immediately for any signs of a hypersensitivity reaction. Notify the physician. Antihistamines (e.g., diphenhydramine) or analgesic agents may be indicated for symptoms related to immune complex formation. Resume infusion at a slower rate if symptoms subside. Treat anaphylaxis immediately. Epinephrine, diphenhydramine, corticosteroids, and ventilation equipment must always be available.

HETASTARCH BBW
(**HET**-ah-starch)

Plasma volume expander

Hespan, Hextend

pH 5.5 to 5.9

USUAL DOSE
HESPAN, HEXTEND
Plasma volume expansion: Variable. Total dosage and rate of administration depend on amount of fluid loss and resultant hemoconcentration. Age, weight, and clinical condition of the patient are also considered. Usually 500 to 1,000 mL. Total dose usually does not exceed 1,500 mL/24 hr for the typical 70-kg patient (approximately 20 mL/kg of body weight). Higher doses, usually in conjunction with blood and/or blood products, have been used in postoperative and trauma patients who have had severe blood loss.

HESPAN
Leukapheresis: 250 to 700 mL with citrate anticoagulant in continuous flow centrifugation procedures. Do not use Hextend for leukapheresis.

DOSE ADJUSTMENTS
Avoid use in patients with pre-existing renal impairment. Information on dose adjustment in hepatic impairment is not available.

DILUTION
HESPAN: Available as a 6% solution in 500-mL containers properly diluted in NS and ready for use. Calculated osmolarity is approximately 310 mOsm/L.

HEXTEND: Available as a 6% solution in 500-mL containers properly diluted in lactated electrolyte solution and ready for use. Lactated electrolyte solution contains dextrose, normal physiologic levels of calcium and sodium, and slightly lower than normal physiologic levels of potassium and magnesium.

Storage: Store at CRT. Avoid excessive heat. Do not freeze. Do not use if color is a turbid deep brown or a crystalline precipitate is visible. Discard unused portions.

COMPATIBILITY
HESPAN
Compatibility information not available from manufacturer. Other sources suggest a few specific **compatibilities** dependent on concentration and manufacturer; consult a pharmacist.

HEXTEND
Safety and **compatibility** of other additives not established. Contains calcium; do not administer simultaneously through the same administration set as blood; coagulation likely.

Other sources suggest specific **compatibilities** dependent on concentration and manufacturer; consult a pharmacist.

RATE OF ADMINISTRATION
Variable, depending on indication, present blood volume, and patient response. Initial 500 mL may be given at rates approaching 20 mL/kg of body weight per hour. If additional hydroxyethyl starch is required, reduce flow to lowest rate possible to maintain hemodynamic status. If pressure infusion is used (flexible containers), withdraw all air through medication port before infusing. If a pumping device is used for administration, discontinue pumping action before the container runs dry or air embolism may result.

Leukapheresis: Usually infused at a constant ratio to venous whole blood (i.e., 1:8).

ACTIONS
A synthetic colloid solution. Pharmacologically classified as a plasma volume expander. The amount of plasma volume expansion produced approximates that of 5% albumin and decreases over the succeeding 24 to 36 hours. **Hextend** supports oncotic pressure and provides electrolytes. Its electrolyte content resembles that of normal plasma. **Hespan** supports oncotic pressure and increases erythrocyte sedimentation rate. Improves the

efficiency of granulocyte collection by centrifugal means. Hetastarch molecules are rapidly eliminated by renal excretion.

INDICATIONS AND USES

HESPAN AND HEXTEND: Treatment of hypovolemia when plasma volume expansion is desired.

HESPAN: Adjunct in leukapheresis to improve harvesting and increase yield of granulocytes.

CONTRAINDICATIONS

Do not use in critically ill adult patients, including patients with sepsis. ■ Severe liver disease. ■ Hypersensitivity to hetastarch. ■ Clinical conditions in which volume overload is a potential problem (such as CHF or renal disease with oliguria or anuria not related to hypovolemia). ■ Pre-existing coagulation or bleeding disorders. ■ **Hextend** contains lactate; not for use in leukapheresis or in the treatment of lactic acidosis.

PRECAUTIONS

HESPAN AND HEXTEND: For IV infusion only. ■ Not a substitute for whole blood or plasma proteins. ■ In critically ill adult patients, including patients with sepsis, the use of hydroxyethyl starch (HES) products, including Hespan and Hextend, increases the risk of mortality and renal replacement therapy. ■ Avoid use in patients with pre-existing renal dysfunction. ■ Discontinue use at the first sign of renal injury. ■ Use caution in heart disease, congestive heart failure, pulmonary edema, and liver disease. ■ Anaphylactic reactions have occurred, even after solutions containing hetastarch have been discontinued. Patients allergic to corn may also be allergic to hetastarch. ■ Administration of large volumes may transiently alter the coagulation mechanism due to hemodilution and a mild direct inhibitory action on factor VIII. Hemodilution by isotonic solutions containing 6% hetastarch may also result in a 24-hour decline of total protein, albumin, and fibrinogen levels and in transient prolongation of prothrombin, activated partial thromboplastin, clotting, and bleeding times. Volumes greater than 25% of blood volume within 24 hours may cause significant hemodilution (decreased hematocrit and plasma proteins). Administration of packed RBCs, platelets, or fresh frozen plasma may be indicated. ■ When used over a period of days, hetastarch has been associated with coagulation abnormalities in conjunction with an acquired reversible von Willebrand's–like syndrome and/or factor VIII deficiency. If a severe factor VIII deficiency is identified, replacement therapy may be indicated. If coagulopathy develops, it may take days to resolve. ■ Not recommended for use as a cardiac bypass pump prime, while the patient is undergoing cardiopulmonary bypass, or in the immediate period after the pump has been discontinued. Risk of coagulopathies and bleeding increased.

HEXTEND: Use extreme caution in patients with metabolic or respiratory alkalosis; contains lactate ions. Excessive lactate may result in metabolic alkalosis. ■ Contains electrolytes; use caution in patient populations in which sodium or potassium administration or retention could pose a problem (e.g., renal insufficiency, CHF, hyperkalemia, edema). Use caution in patients receiving corticosteroids and in renal or cardiac disease, particularly in digitalized patients. ■ Contains dextrose; use caution in patients with overt diabetes.

Monitor: *Hespan and Hextend:* Monitor vital signs, hemoglobin, hematocrit, platelet count, prothrombin time, partial thromboplastin time, and renal and liver function tests. ■ Acid-base balance, electrolytes, and serum protein evaluation are also necessary during therapy. ■ Monitor renal function in hospitalized patients for at least 90 days because the use of renal replacement therapy has been reported up to 90 days after administration of hydroxyethyl starch solutions. ■ May reduce coagulability of the circulating blood. Observe patient for increased bleeding and/or circulatory overload. Risk increased with higher doses.

Hespan: Monitor donors undergoing repeated leukapheresis procedures; may have a slight decline in platelet count and hemoglobin levels resulting from hemodilution by hetastarch and saline and the collection of platelets and erythrocytes. Temporary declines in total protein, albumin, calcium, and fibrinogen may also be present. Regular and frequent clinical evaluation and complete blood counts are necessary for proper monitoring of Hespan use during leukapheresis. If frequency of leukapheresis is to exceed the guidelines for whole blood donation, additional testing may be indicated; see manufacturer's prescribing information.

Maternal/Child: Category C: embryocidal to rabbits. Use only if benefit justifies the potential risk to the fetus. ■ Use caution during breast-feeding. ■ Safety and effectiveness for use in pediatric patients not established, but has been used. Increased prothrombin time noted in pediatric patients who received more than 20 mL/kg/24 hr.

Elderly: Differences in response between elderly and younger patients not identified. Risk of toxic reactions may be greater in patients with impaired renal function. Monitoring of renal function suggested in the elderly.

DRUG/LAB INTERACTIONS

Use with caution in patients receiving other drugs that affect coagulation (e.g., **anticoagulants, platelet aggregation inhibitors, glycoprotein GP IIb/IIIa receptor antagonists, plicamycin, valproic acid**). Close monitoring of aPTT and PT indicated. ■ May increase **indirect bilirubin** levels. Total bilirubin remained normal. ■ Elevated serum amylase levels have been observed, although no association with pancreatitis has been demonstrated.

SIDE EFFECTS

The most common adverse reactions are circulatory overload, coagulopathy, hemodilution, hypersensitivity (including anaphylaxis), and metabolic acidosis. Anemia and/or bleeding due to hemodilution and/or factor VIII deficiency, acquired von Willebrand's–like syndrome, and other coagulopathies, including DIC; chills; congestive heart failure; elevated serum amylase; fever; headache; increased urine specific gravity; intracranial bleeding; itching; muscle pains; peripheral edema; pulmonary edema; submaxillary and parotid glandular enlargement; urticaria; and vomiting have been reported.

Post-Marketing: Death, renal failure requiring renal replacement therapy.

ANTIDOTE

Notify the physician of any side effect. Discontinue the drug immediately at the first sign of a hypersensitivity reaction, provided other means of sustaining the circulation are available. Antihistamines such as diphenhydramine are helpful. Epinephrine may also be indicated. Not eliminated by dialysis. Many side effects can result in medical emergencies. Deaths from severe hypersensitivity reactions have occurred. Treat as indicated and resuscitate as necessary.

HYDRALAZINE HYDROCHLORIDE
(hy-**DRAL**-ah-zeen hy-droh-**KLOR**-eyed)

Antihypertensive
Vasodilator

pH 3.4 to 4

USUAL DOSE

10 to 40 mg. Begin with a low dose. Increase gradually as indicated. Repeat every 3 to 6 hours as necessary. Maximum dose is 300 to 400 mg/24 hr.

Eclampsia: 5 to 10 mg every 20 minutes. If no effect after a total dose of 20 mg, use another agent.

PEDIATRIC DOSE

See Maternal/Child (unlabeled).

0.1 to 0.5 mg/kg/dose every 4 to 6 hours. Initial dose should not exceed 20 mg. Maximum IV dose is 0.2 to 0.8 mg/kg/dose up to 40 mg. Another source suggests 0.1 to 0.2 mg/kg/dose (not to exceed 20 mg) every 4 to 6 hours as needed. Up to 1.7 to 3.5 mg/kg/day divided in 4 to 6 doses.

DOSE ADJUSTMENTS

Reduced dose may be required with advanced renal disease and in the elderly. ■ See Drug/Lab Interactions.

DILUTION

May be given undiluted. Do not add to IV solutions. May be given through Y-tube of infusion set. Color changes occur in most 10% dextrose solutions and after drawing through a metal filter. Use immediately after drawing up solution.

Filters: See Dilution.

COMPATIBILITY

Compatibility information not available from manufacturer. Other sources suggest a few specific **compatibilities** dependent on concentration and manufacturer; consult a pharmacist.

RATE OF ADMINISTRATION

Adults: A single dose over 1 minute.

Pediatric patients: A single dose over 3 to 5 minutes.

ACTIONS

A potent antihypertensive drug. It lowers BP by direct relaxation of smooth muscle of arteries and arterioles. Peripheral vasodilation and decreased peripheral vascular resistance result. HR, cardiac output, and stroke volume are all increased. Renal blood flow increased in some cases, while cerebral blood flow maintained. Onset of action is 5 to 20 minutes. Average duration of action is 2 to 6 hours. Metabolized by the liver and excreted in urine. Crosses placental barrier. Secreted in breast milk.

INDICATIONS AND USES

Severe essential hypertension. ▪ Vasodilation in cardiogenic shock. ▪ Drug of choice for pregnancy-induced hypertension (eclampsia).

CONTRAINDICATIONS

Hypersensitivity to hydralazine, coronary artery disease, mitral valvular rheumatic heart disease.

PRECAUTIONS

IV use recommended only when the oral route is not feasible. ▪ Rarely the drug of choice for hypertension unless used in combination (effectiveness increased and side effects decreased) with spironolactone, reserpine, guanethidine, and thiazide diuretics. ▪ Tolerance is easily developed but subsides about 7 days after the drug is discontinued. ▪ Use caution in advanced renal disease, cerebrovascular accidents, congestive heart failure, coronary insufficiency, headache, increased intracranial pressure, and tachycardia. ▪ Use in pregnancy should be limited to treatment of eclampsia.

Monitor: Check BP every 5 minutes until stabilized at the desired level. Check every 15 minutes thereafter throughout crisis. Average maximum decrease occurs in 10 to 80 minutes. ▪ Withdraw drug gradually to avoid rebound hypertension.

Patient Education: Report chest pain, fatigue, fever, joint or muscle pain promptly.

Maternal/Child: Category C: can cause fetal abnormalities; see Indications and Precautions. ▪ Safety for use in pediatric patients not established. ▪ May be used in breast-feeding females.

Elderly: Increased risk of hypotension. ▪ Consider age-related renal impairment.

DRUG/LAB INTERACTIONS

Sometimes used with a **beta-adrenergic blocking drug or diuretics**; use caution; may potentiate effects. ▪ Potentiated by **anesthetics, MAO inhibitors, and other antihypertensive agents**. ▪ Inhibits **epinephrine, levarterenol**. ▪ Use with **diazoxide** can cause profound hypotension. ▪ **NSAIDs** may decrease antihypotensive effect.

SIDE EFFECTS

May often be minimized by initiating therapy with a small dose and increasing the dose gradually.

Anxiety, depression, dry mouth, flushing, headache, nausea, numbness, palpitations, paresthesia, postural hypotension, tachycardia, tingling, unpleasant taste, vomiting.

Major: Angina, blood dyscrasias, chills, coronary insufficiency, delirium, dependent edema, fever, ileus, lupus erythematosus (simulated), myocardial ischemia and infarction, rheumatoid syndrome (simulated), toxic psychosis.

ANTIDOTE

If minor side effects occur, notify the physician, who will probably treat them symptomatically. Beta-adrenergic blocking agents will control tachycardia. Pyridoxine will relieve numbness, tingling, and paresthesia. Antihistamines, barbiturates, and salicylates may be required. Treat hypotension with a vasopressor that is least likely to precipitate cardiac arrhythmias. If side effects are progressive or any major side effects occur, discontinue the drug immediately and notify the physician. Treatment is symptomatic. Resuscitate as necessary. Occasionally methyldopa will be used as a substitute because it is effective for the same indications but has fewer side effects.

HYDROCORTISONE SODIUM SUCCINATE

Hormone (corticosteroid)
Anti-inflammatory

(hy-droh-**KOR**-tih-zohn **SO**-dee-um **SUK**-sih-nayt)

A-Hydrocort, Solu-Cortef

pH 7 to 8

USUAL DOSE

Average dose range is 100 to 500 mg repeated as necessary every 2, 4, or 6 hours depending on patient condition and response. Dosage must be individualized. The IV route is usually used in an emergency situation or when oral dosing is not feasible. Larger doses may be justified by patient condition (doses as high as 8 Gm/day can be found in the literature). High-dose treatment is used until patient condition stabilizes, usually no longer than 48 to 72 hours. When high-dose hydrocortisone therapy must be continued beyond 48 to 72 hours, hypernatremia may occur. Under such circumstances it may be desirable to substitute with a corticoid such as methylprednisolone sodium succinate, which causes little or no sodium retention. Once an adequate clinical response has been achieved, slowly taper dosage downward, using the lowest possible dose required to maintain that response.
Life-threatening shock: 50 mg/kg initially. Repeat in 4 hours and/or every 24 hours as needed *or*

0.5 to 2 Gm initially. Repeat every 2 to 6 hours as needed.
Adrenal insufficiency (acute): 100 mg as an IV bolus. Follow with 200 mg over 24 hours as a continuous IV infusion or in divided doses every 6 hours, then 100 mg over 24 hours the following day. Change to oral dosing when patient is stable. *See literature for additional dosing regimens in use.*

PEDIATRIC DOSE

See Maternal/Child. Dose should be based on the severity of the disease and on patient response rather than on strict adherence to a dose indicated by age, weight, or body surface area.

Average dose range in pediatric patients is 0.56 to 8 mg/kg/day in 3 to 4 divided doses (0.19 to 2.67 mg/kg every 8 hours or 0.14 to 2 mg/kg every 6 hours).

Other sources recommend:
Status asthmaticus: *Loading dose (optional):* 4 to 8 mg/kg up to a maximum dose of 250 mg.
Maintenance dose: 8 mg/kg/24 hr in equally divided doses every 6 hours (2 mg/kg every 6 hours).
Anti-inflammatory: 1 to 5 mg/kg/24 hr, or 0.5 to 2.5 mg/kg every 12 hours, or 30 to 150 mg/M^2/24 hr, or 15 to 75 mg/M^2 every 12 hours.

DOSE ADJUSTMENTS

Use lowest possible dose required to control condition being treated. When dose reduction is possible, decrease dose gradually while monitoring for S/S of disease exacerbation. ▪ Because complications of treatment with glucocorticoids depend on dose and duration of therapy, a risk/benefit decision must be made for each patient regarding dose and duration of treatment and whether daily or intermittent therapy should be used. ▪ Clearance of corticosteroids is decreased in patients with hypothyroidism and increased in patients with hyperthyroidism. Dose adjustment may be required. ▪ See Drug/Lab Interactions.

DILUTION

Available in Act-O-Vials, which are reconstituted by pressing down on the plastic activator to force diluent into the lower compartment. Agitate gently. Remove plastic tab covering center of stopper. Sterilize top of stopper, then insert needle squarely through center of stopper until tip is just visible. Invert vial and withdraw dose. Also available in flip-top vials. For these other preparations, reconstitute each 100 mg with not more than 2 mL bacteriostatic water for injection. Agitate gently to mix solution. May be given by IV injection, or each 100 mg (250 mg, 500 mg, or more) may be further diluted in at least 100 mL (250 mL, 500 mL, or more) but not more than 1,000 mL of D5W, NS, or D5NS to a concentration of 0.1 to 1 mg/mL for IV infusion.

Storage: Store vials and solutions at RT (20° to 25° C [68° to 77° F]). Protect solution from light. Discard unused solutions after 3 days. If fluid restriction is necessary, 100 to 3,000 mg may be added in 50 mL of **compatible** solution. Resultant solution is stable for at least 4 hours.

COMPATIBILITY

Manufacturer states, "Should not be diluted or mixed with other solutions."

Other sources suggest specific **compatibilities** dependent on concentration and manufacturer; consult a pharmacist.

RATE OF ADMINISTRATION

Each 100 mg or fraction thereof over 30 seconds to 1 minute. Extend to 10 minutes for larger doses (500 mg or more). IV injection is usually the route of choice and eliminates the possibility of overloading the patient with IV fluids. At the discretion of the physician, an intermittent or continuous infusion may be given, properly diluted over the specified time desired.

ACTIONS

An anti-inflammatory glucocorticoid secreted by the adrenal cortex. Has both glucocorticoid and mineralocorticoid properties. Glucocorticoids cause profound and varied metabolic effects. In addition, they modify the body's immune response to diverse stimuli. Peak plasma levels achieved promptly. Onset of action is within 1 hour. Metabolized in the liver and excreted as inactive metabolites in the urine. Elimination half-life is 2 hours. Crosses placental barrier. Secreted in breast milk.

INDICATIONS AND USES

Agent of choice for replacement therapy in adrenocortical insufficiency because it has both glucocorticoid and mineralocorticoid activity. ▪ May be used for acute exacerbation of disease for patients on steroid therapy. ▪ Because of their minimal mineralocorticoid activity, synthetic glucocorticoids (e.g., dexamethasone, methylprednisolone) are the preferred agents for anti-inflammatory or immunosuppressive indications. ▪ May be used for the treatment of various diseases or disorders, including allergic states, dermatologic diseases, endocrine disorders, GI diseases, hematologic disorders, neoplastic diseases, nervous system disorders, ophthalmic diseases, renal diseases, respiratory diseases, or rheumatic disorders; see manufacturer's prescribing information.

CONTRAINDICATIONS

Hypersensitivity to hydrocortisone or any of the product components. ▪ Cerebral malaria (no evidence of benefit). ▪ Systemic fungal infections. ▪ Intrathecal administration. ▪ IM administration for idiopathic thrombocytopenic purpura.

PRECAUTIONS

Corticosteroids can produce reversible hypothalamic-pituitary-adrenal (HPA) axis suppression with the potential for glucocorticosteroid insufficiency after withdrawal of treatment. Adrenocortical insufficiency may result from too-rapid withdrawal of corticosteroids and may be minimized by gradual reduction of dosage. This type of relative insufficiency may persist for months after discontinuation of therapy; therefore hormone therapy should be reinstituted in any situation of stress occurring during that period (e.g., surgery, trauma, infection). If the patient is receiving steroids already, dosage may need to be increased. The exception is short-term therapy. ■ Anaphylactoid reactions have occurred (incidence is rare). ■ Should not be used for treatment of traumatic brain injury. May increase mortality. ■ Hypertension, sodium and water retention, and potassium and calcium excretion can occur with average to large doses of corticosteroids. Dietary sodium restriction and potassium supplementation may be necessary. Caution and close monitoring required in patients with existing cardiovascular disease or renal insufficiency. ■ Use with caution in patients who have had a recent MI. May be associated with left ventricular free wall rupture. ■ Prolonged use of corticosteroids may increase susceptibility to infection, reactivate latent infectious diseases, or mask signs of infection. ■ Infections such as chickenpox and measles can have a more serious or even fatal course in pediatric and adult patients on corticosteroids. Patients who have not had these diseases should take care to avoid exposure. If exposed, therapy with varicella zoster immune globulin (VZIG) or IVIG may be indicated. If chickenpox develops, treatment with antiviral agents should be considered. ■ Corticosteroids should be used with great caution in patients with known or suspected *Strongyloides* (threadworm) infestation. Corticosteroid-induced immunosuppression may lead to *Strongyloides* hyperinfection and dissemination with widespread larval migration, often accompanied by severe enterocolitis and potentially fatal gram-negative sepsis. ■ The use of corticosteroids in patients with active tuberculosis should be restricted to cases of fulminating or disseminated tuberculosis in which the corticosteroid is being used for disease management in conjunction with an appropriate antituberculosis regimen. ■ If corticosteroids are indicated in patients with latent tuberculosis or tuberculin reactivity, reactivation of the disease may occur. During prolonged corticosteroid therapy, chemoprophylaxis is indicated. ■ Prolonged use of corticosteroids may produce posterior subcapsular cataracts or glaucoma with possible damage to the optic nerves and may enhance the establishment of secondary ocular infections due to fungi or viruses. ■ Use with caution in patients with ocular herpes simplex; corneal perforation can occur ■ Kaposi's sarcoma has been reported in patients receiving corticosteroid therapy, most often for chronic conditions. Clinical improvement may occur if therapy is discontinued. ■ Use with caution in patients with active or latent peptic ulcer disease, diverticulitis, fresh intestinal anastomoses, and nonspecific ulcerative colitis; may increase risk of perforation. ■ Use with caution in cirrhosis; effect of corticosteroids may be enhanced due to decreased metabolism. ■ May induce psychological side effects (e.g., euphoria, insomnia, mood swings, depression, psychosis) or may aggravate existing emotional instability or psychotic tendencies. ■ An acute myopathy has been reported with the use of high doses of corticosteroids, most often in patients with disorders of neuromuscular transmission (e.g., myasthenia gravis) or in patients receiving concomitant therapy with neuromuscular blocking agents. This myopathy is generalized, may involve ocular and respiratory muscles, and may result in quadriparesis. Improvement or recovery after stopping corticosteroids may take weeks to years. ■ Use with caution in patients at risk for osteoporosis. Corticosteroids decrease bone formation, increase bone resorption, and decrease the protein matrix of the bone. May lead to inhibition of bone growth in pediatric patients and the development of osteoporosis at any age. ■ Pheochromocytoma crisis, which can be fatal, has been reported. Use caution and consider risk in patients with suspected pheochromocytoma.

Monitor: Monitor electrolytes. May cause sodium retention and potassium and calcium excretion. Dietary salt restriction and potassium supplementation may be necessary. BP monitoring may be indicated; may cause hypertension secondary to fluid and electrolyte disturbances. ■ Monitor for S/S of infection; S/S may be masked. ■ Patients with latent tuberculosis should be monitored for reactivation of the disease. ■ Monitor blood glucose. May increase insulin needs in diabetes. ■ Periodic ophthalmic exams may be necessary with prolonged treatment. ■ Monitor for S/S of a hypersensitivity reaction. ▪ Elevation of creatine kinase may occur with acute myopathy. Monitor if indicated. ▪ See Drug/Lab Interactions.

Patient Education: Do not discontinue abruptly. ▪ Advise all medical personnel of current or past corticosteroid use. ▪ Report edema, tarry stools, or weight gain promptly. Anorexia, diarrhea, dizziness, fatigue, low blood sugar, nausea, weakness, weight loss, and vomiting may indicate adrenal insufficiency after dose reduction or discontinuation of therapy; report any of these symptoms. ▪ May mask signs of infection and/or decrease resistance. ▪ Patients with diabetes may have an increased requirement for insulin or oral hypoglycemics. ▪ Avoid immunization with live virus vaccines. ▪ Carry ID stating steroid dependent if receiving prolonged therapy.

Maternal/Child: Category C: use with caution; benefits must outweigh risks. ▪ Discontinue breast-feeding. ▪ Observe newborn for hypoadrenalism if mother has received large doses. ▪ Observe growth and development in long-term use in pediatric patients.

Elderly: Use cautiously in the smallest possible dose. ▪ Monitor BP, blood glucose, and electrolytes carefully. ▪ Higher risk of glucocorticoid-induced osteoporosis.

DRUG/LAB INTERACTIONS

Aminoglutethimide may increase the metabolism of hydrocortisone, thereby decreasing therapeutic effects. ▪ Metabolism increased and effects reduced by **hepatic enzyme–inducing agents** (e.g., alcohol, barbiturates, phenytoin, and rifampin); dose adjustment may be required when adding or deleting from drug profile. ▪ Risk of hypokalemia increased with **amphotericin B or potassium-depleting diuretics** (e.g., thiazides, furosemide). Monitor potassium levels and cardiac function. ▪ Increased risk of **digoxin** toxicity secondary to hypokalemia. ▪ May also decrease effectiveness of **potassium supplements;** monitor serum potassium. ▪ **Diuretics** decrease sodium and fluid retention effects of corticosteroids; corticosteroids decrease sodium excretion and diuretic effects of diuretics. ▪ May enhance the adverse/toxic effects of **anticholinesterases** (e.g., neostigmine); increased weakness may occur. ▪ May decrease effectiveness of **isoniazid, salicylates, and somatrem;** dose adjustments may be required. ▪ Clearance decreased and effects increased with **estrogens, oral contraceptives, macrolide antibiotics** (e.g., azithromycin), **and ketoconazole.** ▪ May interact with **anticoagulants, nondepolarizing muscle relaxants, or theophyllines;** may inhibit or potentiate action. ▪ Carefully monitor patients receiving **insulin;** dose adjustments may be required. ▪ Increased activity of both **hydrocortisone and cyclosporine** may occur with concurrent use; convulsions have been reported. ▪ Concurrent use with **aspirin or NSAIDs** may increase the risk of GI side effects. ▪ Administration of **live or live-attenuated vaccines** is contraindicated in patients receiving immunosuppressive dose of corticosteroids. Inactivated vaccines may be administered; however, the response to these vaccines cannot be predicted. ▪ **Corticosteroids** may suppress reactions to skin tests. ▪ See Dose Adjustments.

SIDE EFFECTS

Do occur but are usually reversible: alteration of glucose metabolism including hyperglycemia and glycosuria; Cushing's syndrome (e.g., moon face, fat pads); electrolyte and calcium imbalance; euphoria or other psychic disturbances; fluid retention; hypersensitivity reactions, including anaphylaxis; impaired wound healing; increased BP; increased intracranial pressure; leukocytosis; masking of infection; menstrual irregularities; ophthalmic disorders (glaucoma, increased intraocular pressure); perforation and hemorrhage from aggravation of peptic ulcer; protein catabolism with negative nitrogen balance; spontaneous fractures; sweating, headache, or weakness; thromboembolism; transitory burning or tingling; and many others.

ANTIDOTE

Notify the physician of any side effect. Will probably treat the side effect if necessary. Resuscitate as necessary for anaphylaxis and notify physician. Keep epinephrine immediately available.

HYDROMORPHONE HYDROCHLORIDE BBW

Opioid analgesic
(agonist)

(hy-droh-**MOR**-fohn hy-droh-**KLOR**-eyed)

Dilaudid, Dilaudid HP

pH 3.5 to 5.5, 4.5 to 6.5

USUAL DOSE

Individualize dose, taking into account the patient's severity of pain, response, prior analgesic treatment experience, and risk factors for addiction, abuse, and misuse. Use lowest effective dose for the shortest duration consistent with the patient's treatment goals. *Hydromorphone is approximately 7 times more potent than morphine.*

Dispense with caution; dosing errors due to confusion between different concentrations and between mg and mL could result in accidental overdose and death. Never administer hydromorphone-HP to an opioid-naïve patient. Oral and IV doses of hydromorphone and IV doses with doses of other opioids are *NOT* equivalent; see prescribing information for a discussion on opioid conversion and equianalgesic potency for conversion to hydromorphone injection.

IV injection: Usual starting dose is 0.2 to 1 mg every 2 to 3 hours as needed for pain. Titrate dose to achieve acceptable pain management and tolerable adverse events.

Infusion (unlabeled): Used postoperatively with a patient-controlled analgesic device (PCA) and in selected terminally ill cancer patients. One source suggests a concentration of 0.2 mg/mL, with a starting patient-controlled dose of 0.2 mg (range 0.05 to 0.4 mg) that can be activated at prescribed intervals. Must be administered through a controlled infusion device that may be patient activated. The initial loading dose, the continuous background infusion (if prescribed), additional patient-activated doses with a specific time interval, additional health care professional–provided boluses with a specific time interval, and the total dose allowed per hour must be determined by the physician and individualized for each patient.

PEDIATRIC DOSE

Individualized on the basis of age and weight (unlabeled). One source suggests 0.015 mg/kg/dose every 4 to 6 hours as needed in pediatric patients; see Contraindications and Maternal/Child.

DOSE ADJUSTMENTS

Dose selection should be cautious in elderly, cachectic, and debilitated patients. Reduced initial doses may be indicated based on the potential for increased sensitivity, decreased organ function, and concomitant disease or drug therapy. ▪ Depending on the degree of impairment, one-fourth to one-half the usual starting dose is recommended in patients with impaired renal or hepatic function. ▪ Use lower initial doses in opiate-naïve patients. ▪ Doses appropriate for the general population may cause serious respiratory depression in vulnerable patients. ▪ Increase doses as required if analgesia is inadequate, tolerance develops, or pain severity increases. The first sign of tolerance is usually a reduced duration of effect. ▪ Decrease dose if excessive side effects are observed early in the dosing interval. If this results in breakthrough pain at the end of the dosing interval, the dosing interval may be shortened. ▪ See Drug/Lab Interactions.

DILUTION

Available in more than one concentration (1 mg/mL, 2 mg/mL, and 4 mg/mL) and hydromorphone-HP (a high-potency [10 mg/mL]) formulation. Do not confuse hydromorphone-HP with standard formulations of hydromorphone or other opioids; overdose and death could result. Hydromorphone-HP is usually reserved for compounding in the pharmacy or for use in opioid-tolerant patients. Verify concentration to avoid overdose and/or death.

IV injection: May be given undiluted. May give through Y-tube of infusion set.

Infusion: Each 0.1 to 1 mg is usually diluted in 1 mL NS to provide 0.1 to 1 mg/mL for use in a narcotic syringe infuser system. Dilaudid is available in 1-, 2-, or 4-mg/mL clear ampules. Dilaudid-HP is available in 10-mg/mL amber ampules and as lyophilized powder that must be reconstituted with 25 mL SWFI for a concentration of 10 mg/mL. Generic hydromorphone is available in similar concentrations; check mg/mL carefully. Use concentrated preparations for larger doses. May be diluted in larger amounts of D5W, D5NS, D5/¹/₂NS, or NS for infusion and given through a standard infusion pump (requires very close titration).

Storage: Store unopened product at CRT and protect from light and freezing. May develop a slight yellowish discoloration. No loss of potency has been demonstrated. Stable for 24 hours at 25° C (77° F), protected from light, in most common large-volume parenteral solutions.

COMPATIBILITY

Compatibility information not available from manufacturer. Other sources suggest specific **compatibilities** dependent on concentration and manufacturer; consult a pharmacist.

RATE OF ADMINISTRATION

Rapid IV administration increases the possibility of hypotension and respiratory depression.

IV injection: Administer a single dose over a minimum of 2 to 3 minutes. Frequently titrated according to symptom relief and respiratory rate.

Infusion: All parameters (outlined in Usual Dose) should be ordered by the physician. Any dose requiring a controlled infusion device requires accurate titration and close monitoring.

ACTIONS

A mu-opioid receptor agonist closely related to morphine. Precise mode of action is unknown, but opioids are believed to combine with specific CNS opiate receptors. The principal therapeutic action of hydromorphone is analgesia. Seven times more potent than morphine milligram for milligram. Produces respiratory depression by direct effect on brainstem respiratory centers and reduces the responsiveness to increases in carbon dioxide. Onset of action is prompt, and half-life is about 2.3 hours. Hydromorphone is metabolized in the liver and excreted in the urine. Crosses placental barrier. Secreted in breast milk.

INDICATIONS AND USES

Hydromorphone (1 mg/mL, 2 mg/mL, or 4 mg/mL): Management of pain severe enough to require an opioid analgesic and for which alternate treatments are inadequate.

High-potency hydromorphone (10 mg/mL): For use in opioid-tolerant patients who require higher doses of opioids for the management of pain severe enough to require an opioid analgesic and for which alternate treatments are inadequate. Patients considered opioid-tolerant are those who are taking at least 60 mg oral morphine/day, 25 mcg transdermal fentanyl/hr, 30 mg oral oxycodone/day, 8 mg hydromorphone/day, 25 mg oral oxymorphone/day, 60 mg hydrocodone/day, or an equianalgesic dose of another opioid around-the-clock for 1 week or longer.

Limitations of use: Because of the risk of addiction, abuse, and misuse, even at recommended doses, reserve hydromorphone for use in patients for whom alternative treatment options (e.g., nonopioid analgesics or opioid combination products):

- Have not been tolerated or are not expected to be tolerated
- Have not provided adequate analgesia or are not expected to provide adequate analgesia

CONTRAINDICATIONS

Hypersensitivity to hydromorphone, any of its components, or sulfite-containing medications. ▪ Significant respiratory depression. ▪ Acute or severe bronchial asthma in the absence of resuscitation equipment or in unmonitored settings. ▪ In patients with known or suspected GI obstruction, including paralytic ileus. ▪ Hydromorphone-HP is contraindicated in patients who are not opioid tolerant.

PRECAUTIONS

Hydromorphone-HP is a more concentrated solution of hydromorphone that is for use in opioid-tolerant patients only. Do not confuse hydromorphone-HP formulations with standard formulations of hydromorphone or with other opioids; overdose and death could result. ▪ Hydromorphone exposes patients and other users to the risks of opioid addiction, abuse, and misuse, which can lead to overdose and death. Assess each patient's risk before prescribing hydromorphone, and monitor all patients regularly for the development of these behaviors and conditions. Strategies to reduce the risk of diversion or misuse should be used by health care facilities that utilize hydromorphone and other controlled substances. ▪ See prescribing information for further discussion regarding abuse, addiction, physical dependence, and tolerance. ▪ Serious, life-threatening, or fatal respiratory depression may occur with the use of hydromorphone. Adequate facilities should be available for monitoring and ventilation. An opioid antagonist (e.g., naloxone), resuscitative and intubation equipment, and oxygen should be readily available. ▪ Use with extreme caution in patients with COPD, cor pulmonale, a substantially decreased respiratory reserve, hypoxia, hypercapnia, or pre-existing respiratory depression; these patients are at increased risk for decreased respiratory drive, including apnea, even at recommended doses. Consider using nonopioid analgesics, or administer under careful medical supervision at the lowest effective dose. ▪ Use with caution and reduce initial doses in elderly, cachectic, or debilitated patients and in patients with severe impairment of hepatic, pulmonary, or renal function. ▪ Use caution in patients with head injury, brain tumors, or increased intracranial pressure. Respiratory depression may cause an increased PCO_2, cerebral vasodilation, and increased intracranial pressure. Clinical course of head injury may be obscured. Avoid use in patients with impaired consciousness or coma ▪ May cause severe hypotension in postoperative patients or in any patient whose ability to maintain blood pressure has been compromised by a depleted blood volume or concomitant administration of drugs that can cause hypotension (e.g., anesthetics, phenothiazines). In patients with circulatory shock, hydromorphone-induced vasodilation may further reduce cardiac output and blood pressure. Use should be avoided; see Drug/Lab Interactions. ▪ May produce orthostatic hypotension in ambulatory patients. ▪ Cases of serotonin syndrome have been reported during concomitant use of fentanyl with serotonergic drugs. ▪ Cases of adrenal insufficiency have been reported with opioid use, more often after more than 1 month of use. If adrenal insufficiency is diagnosed, treat with physiologic replacement doses of corticosteroids and wean the patient off the opioid to allow adrenal function to recover. Another opioid may be tried; some cases reported use of a different opioid without recurrence of adrenal insufficiency. ▪ Symptoms of acute abdominal conditions may be masked. Use with caution in patients with biliary tract disease, including acute pancreatitis; may cause spasm of the sphincter of Oddi and diminish biliary and pancreatic secretions. ▪ May increase the frequency of seizures in patients with a convulsive disorder and may induce or aggravate seizures in some clinical settings. ▪ Do not abruptly discontinue hydromorphone in a patient who is physically dependent; dose must be tapered gradually. ▪ Some products may use a latex stopper and some may contain sulfites; may cause a hypersensitivity reaction in susceptible patients. ▪ See Drug/Lab Interactions and Maternal/Child.

Monitor: Monitor for respiratory depression, especially during initiation of therapy (within the first 24 to 72 hours) or after a dose increase. Oxygen, naloxone, and equipment to establish and maintain an airway must be available. ▪ Assess baseline pain, reassess after administration of hydromorphone, and adjust dose or interval as required. ▪ Monitor vital signs and oxygenation and observe patient frequently. ▪ Keep patient supine; orthostatic hypotension and fainting may occur; less likely with continuous low doses, but observe closely during ambulation. ▪ Monitor patients who may be susceptible to the intracranial effects of CO_2 retention for increasing intracranial pressure and signs of sedation and respiratory depression. ▪ Monitor patients with biliary tract disease for worsening of symptoms. ▪ Monitor patients with a history of seizure disorders for worsening seizure control. ▪ Monitor for S/S of serotonin syndrome (e.g., mental status changes [e.g., agitation, coma, hallucinations], autonomic instability [e.g., hyperthermia, labile blood pressure, tachycardia], neuromuscular aberrations [e.g., hyperreflexia, incoordination, rigidity], and/or GI symptoms [e.g., diarrhea, nausea, vomiting]). Onset of symptoms may occur within hours to days of concomitant use of opioids with serotonergic drugs. ▪ Uncontrolled pain causes sleep deprivation, decreases pain threshold, and increases pain. When pain is finally controlled, expect the patient to sleep more until recovery from sleep deprivation. ▪ Laxatives with or without stool softeners will be required to avoid constipation and fecal impaction, especially with increased doses and extended use. Maintain adequate hydration.

Patient Education: Avoid alcohol or other CNS depressants. Review all medications for interactions. ▪ May cause blurred vision, drowsiness, or dizziness; use caution in tasks that require alertness. ▪ Request assistance with ambulation. ▪ Report unrelieved pain or unacceptable side effects promptly. ▪ Promptly report S/S of serotonin syndrome. ▪ May result in severe constipation. Scheduled bowel regimen recommended. ▪ May result in addiction, abuse, and misuse, even when taken as recommended.

Maternal/Child: Use during pregnancy only if the potential benefit justifies the risk to the fetus. ▪ Use during labor and delivery may produce respiratory depression and a physiologic effect in neonates. May also prolong labor by reducing the strength, duration, and frequency of contractions. Closely monitor neonates exposed to hydromorphone during labor and delivery for signs of excessive sedation and respiratory depression. ▪ Prolonged use of hydromorphone during pregnancy can result in neonatal opioid withdrawal syndrome, which may be life threatening if not recognized and treated. Infants born to mothers receiving hydromorphone during pregnancy should be monitored closely and treated for neonatal opioid withdrawal syndrome, if indicated. See literature for treatment protocols. Infants born to mothers physically dependent on opioids will also be physically dependent and may exhibit respiratory difficulties and withdrawal symptoms (e.g., excessive crying, fever, hyperactive reflexes, increased respiratory rate, increased stools, sneezing, tremors, vomiting, yawning). ▪ Use caution with breast-feeding. Monitor infants exposed to hydromorphone through breast milk for excess sedation and respiratory depression. Withdrawal symptoms can occur in breast-fed infants when maternal administration of an opioid analgesic is stopped or when breast-feeding is stopped. ▪ Safety and effectiveness for use in pediatric patients not established. ▪ Pediatric patients may be more sensitive to effects (e.g., respiratory depression).

Elderly: See Dose Adjustments and Precautions. ▪ May be more susceptible to effects (e.g., respiratory depression, urinary retention, constipation). Respiratory depression is the chief risk for elderly patients treated with opioids. ▪ Lower doses may provide effective analgesia.

DRUG/LAB INTERACTIONS

Concomitant use of hydromorphone with **benzodiazepines** and other **CNS depressants** (e.g., sedative/hypnotics, anxiolytics, tranquilizers, muscle relaxants, general anesthetics, antipsychotics, other opioids, alcohol) may result in profound sedation, respiratory depression, coma, and death. Hypotension can also occur. Reserve concomitant use for patients for whom alternative treatment options are inadequate. Limit dose and duration of treatment to the minimum required, and monitor patients carefully for S/S of respiratory depression and sedation. ▪ Serotonin syndrome has been reported with the concomitant use of opioids, including hydromorphone, and other **drugs that affect the serotonergic neurotransmitter system** (e.g., selective serotonin reuptake inhibitors [SSRIs], serotonin and norepinephrine reuptake inhibitors [SNRIs], tricyclic antidepressants [TCAs], triptans, 5-HT3 receptor antagonists, mirtazapine, trazodone, tramadol, MAO inhibitors (MAOIs), linezolid, and intravenous methylene blue). Careful observation, particularly during treatment initiation and dose adjustment, is required with concomitant use. ▪ Severe and unpredictable potentiation of **MAO Is** has been reported. MAOI interactions may manifest as serotonin syndrome or opioid toxicity (e.g., respiratory depression, coma). Use of hydromorphone is not recommended for patients taking MAOIs or within 14 days of stopping such treatment. If urgent use of an opioid is necessary, use test doses and frequent titration of small doses to treat pain while closely monitoring BP and S/S of CNS and respiratory depression. ▪ **Mixed agonist/**

antagonist analgesics and partial agonists may reduce the analgesic effect of hydromorphone and/or precipitate withdrawal symptoms. Avoid concomitant use. ▪ Hydromorphone may enhance the neuromuscular blocking action of **skeletal muscle relaxants** (e.g., cyclobenzaprine), increasing the degree of respiratory depression. Monitor patient and decrease dose if indicated. ▪ Opioids can reduce the efficacy of **diuretics** by inducing the release of antidiuretic hormone. Increase dose of diuretic if needed. ▪ Concomitant use with **anticholinergic drugs** may increase the risk of urinary retention and/or severe constipation, which may lead to paralytic ileus.

SIDE EFFECTS

The most frequently occurring side effects include dizziness, dry mouth, dysphoria, euphoria, flushing, light-headedness, nausea, pruritus, sedation, sweating, and vomiting. Serious adverse reactions include respiratory depression and apnea and, to a lesser extent, circulatory depression, respiratory arrest, shock, and cardiac arrest. Other side effects may include abnormal dreams; agitation; alteration of moods; anorexia; antidiuretic effects; anxiety; arrhythmias (e.g., bradycardia, palpitations, tachycardia); biliary colic; blurred or impaired vision; bronchospasm; chills; depression; disorientation and hallucination; drug abuse, addiction, and dependence; GI effects (e.g., abdominal pain, constipation, diarrhea, ileus) and effects in sphincter of Oddi; headache; hypotension; increased intracranial pressure; injection site pain and urticaria; insomnia; laryngospasm; miosis; muscle rigidity; nervousness; nystagmus; paresthesia; rash; seizures; shock; taste alteration; tremor; urinary retention or hesitancy; weakness.

Overdose: Apnea, atypical snoring, bradycardia, cardiac arrest, circulatory depression or collapse, cold and clammy skin, constricted pupils, hypotension (severe), partial or complete airway obstruction, respiratory depression or arrest, skeletal muscle flaccidity, somnolence progressing to stupor or coma, and death.

Post-Marketing: Anaphylactic reactions, confused state, convulsions, dyskinesia, dyspnea, erectile dysfunction, increased hepatic enzymes, hyperalgesia, hypersensitivity reactions, injection site reactions, myoclonus, oropharyngeal swelling, peripheral edema, and somnolence.

ANTIDOTE

Notify the physician of any side effect. If minor side effects progress or any major side effect occurs, including the onset of symptoms of overdose, discontinue the drug and notify the physician. Naloxone will reverse serious cardiovascular, CNS, and respiratory reactions. Naloxone use should be reserved for situations in which clinically significant respiratory or circulatory depression is present. Titrate naloxone dose carefully to avoid precipitating an acute abstinence syndrome or uncontrolled pain. The duration of action of hydromorphone may exceed the duration of action of naloxone. Monitor patient carefully. Repeat doses of naloxone may be required. A patent airway, artificial ventilation, oxygen therapy, and other symptomatic treatment must be instituted promptly. Treat anaphylaxis as indicated or resuscitate as necessary.

HYDROXOCOBALAMIN

(hy-**DROX**-oh-koh-**BAL**-ah-min)

Antidote

Cyanokit

pH 3.5 to 6

USUAL DOSE

Pretreatment: Baseline assessment required and baseline studies helpful; see Precautions and Monitor.

Manufacturer provides a quick-use reference guide in carton to facilitate immediate administration. It covers reconstitution, mixing, infusion rate, common S/S of cyanide poisoning with or without smoke inhalation, **incompatibilities,** and alternate diluents.

Initial dose: 5 Gm administered by IV infusion over 15 minutes. Based on severity of poisoning and clinical response, a second 5-Gm dose may be administered for a total dose of 10 Gm.

PEDIATRIC DOSE

Safety and effectiveness for use in pediatric patients not established but has been used outside the United States.

Initial dose (unlabeled): 70 mg/kg.

DOSE ADJUSTMENTS

No dose adjustments required in the elderly. ▪ Potential need for dose adjustment in patients with impaired hepatic or renal function has not been studied.

DILUTION

Each kit contains one 5-Gm, 250-mL glass vial of lyophilized hydroxocobalamin, a sterile transfer spike, a sterile vented infusion tubing, a quick-use reference guide, and a package insert. The glass vial is marked with a fill line for diluent. Using a sterile spike, transfer 200 mL of NS diluent into the glass vial (to the fill line [25 mg/mL]). If NS is not available, LR or D5W may be used. *Do Not Shake!* Invert or rock vial for a least 60 seconds to mix. Solution should be clear and dark red. Attach infusion tubing and begin infusion of the first vial; see Rate of Administration.

Filters: Specific information not available.

Storage: Store kit at CRT. See package insert for allowable storage temperatures for kit transport in extreme weather conditions. Reconstituted product may be held at a temperature not to exceed 40° C (104° F) for up to 6 hours. Do not freeze. Discard any unused portion after 6 hours.

COMPATIBILITY

Manufacturer lists as **incompatible** with ascorbic acid, blood products (whole blood, packed red cells, platelet concentrate, and/or fresh frozen plasma), diazepam (Valium), dobutamine, dopamine, fentanyl, nitroglycerin IV, pentobarbital (Nembutal), propofol (Diprivan), sodium nitrite, sodium thiosulfate. Do not administer simultaneously through the same IV line. Use of a separate line on the opposing extremity is recommended. The safety of administering other cyanide antidotes simultaneously with hydroxocobalamin has not been established; if used *do not administer* through the same IV lines; see preceding comment.

RATE OF ADMINISTRATION

Each 5-Gm dose properly diluted and evenly distributed over 15 minutes. The rate of infusion for the second 5-Gm dose may range from 15 minutes (for a patient in extremis) to 2 hours based on patient condition.

ACTIONS

A high dose of cyanide can result in death within minutes by inhibiting the cells' ability to use oxygen (inhibition of cytochrome oxidase results in arrest of cellular respiration). Specifically, cyanide binds with a component of cytochrome oxidase (cytochrome a3), prevents the cell from using oxygen, and forces anaerobic metabolism; this results in lactate production, cellular hypoxia, and metabolic acidosis. Each molecule of hydroxocobalamin can bind one cyanide ion to form cyanocobalamin (vitamin B_{12}) and reverse the toxic process. Cyanocobalamin is then excreted in urine.

INDICATIONS AND USES

Treatment of known or suspected cyanide poisoning. Administer without delay if clinical suspicion of cyanide poisoning is high. Symptoms of cyanide poisoning include chest tightness, confusion, dyspnea, headache, nausea. Signs of cyanide poisoning include altered mental status (e.g., confusion, disorientation), seizures or coma, mydriasis (excessive dilation of the pupil of the eye), abnormally rapid or deep breathing (early), abnormally slow breathing or apnea (late), hypertension (early), hypotension (late), cardiovascular collapse, vomiting, plasma lactate concentration equal to or greater than 8 mmol/L. Smoke inhalation victims with cyanide poisoning have usually been exposed to fire and smoke in an enclosed area and may present with soot around mouth, nose, and/or oropharynx or an altered mental status. They may have a plasma lactate concentration equal to or greater than 10 mmol/L.

CONTRAINDICATIONS

Manufacturer states, "None"; see Precautions.

PRECAUTIONS

For IV use only. ▪ If clinical suspicion of cyanide poisoning is high, administer hydroxocobalamin without delay. ▪ In addition to treatment with hydroxocobalamin, immediate confirmation of airway patency, adequacy of oxygenation and hydration, cardiovascular support (may be hypotensive or hypertensive), and management of seizure activity is required. Decontamination measures may also be indicated. ▪ Use caution in patients with known hypersensitivity to hydroxocobalamin or cyanocobalamin (vitamin B_{12}). Consider alternative treatments if available (e.g., sodium nitrite and sodium thiosulfate). ▪ Acute renal failure with acute tubular necrosis, renal impairment, and urine calcium oxalate crystals has occurred. In some cases, hemodialysis was required to achieve recovery. ▪ Collection of a pretreatment blood sample would be useful in confirming a diagnosis of cyanide poisoning but should not delay treatment. ▪ May cause photosensitivity. ▪ Use in patients with impaired hepatic or renal function has not been studied. ▪ See Drug/Lab Interactions.

Monitor: Immediately confirm airway patency, adequacy of oxygenation, and adequate hydration. ▪ If feasible, draw a pretreatment blood sample; see Precautions. ▪ Monitor BP (may be hypotensive or hypertensive [BP equal to or greater than 180 mm Hg systolic or equal to or greater than 110 mm Hg diastolic has been reported with this treatment]). Hypertension may occur at the beginning of the infusion, is usually at a maximum by the end of the infusion, and should return to baseline within 4 hours. Note Compatibility if treatment is required. ▪ Monitor for seizures. Note Compatibility if treatment is required. ▪ Monitor for S/S of hypersensitivity reactions (e.g., anaphylaxis, angioneurotic edema, chest tightness, dyspnea, edema, pruritus, rash, urticaria). ▪ Regular monitoring of renal function, including but not limited to BUN and serum creatinine, should be performed for 7 days after treatment.

Patient Education: Skin redness may last up to 2 weeks. Avoid sun exposure while skin is red. ▪ Urine redness may last up to 5 weeks. ▪ An acne-like rash may appear 7 to 28 days after treatment. Has usually resolved without treatment. ▪ Renal function will be monitored for 7 days after treatment or, in the event of renal impairment, until renal function returns to normal. ▪ Discontinue breast-feeding; talk with your physician to see when and if you can resume. ▪ Notify provider if pregnant during therapy. ▪ Report any side effect that is troublesome or doesn't go away.

Maternal/Child: Has caused skeletal and soft tissue abnormalities, including alterations in the CNS in animal studies. Cyanide readily crosses the placenta. Cyanide poisoning can be fatal for the pregnant woman and fetus if left untreated; life-sustaining therapy should not be withheld due to pregnancy. ▪ Breast-feeding is not recommended during treatment. ▪ Safety and effectiveness for use in pediatric patients not established but has been used outside the United States.

Elderly: Safety and effectiveness similar to that seen in younger adults.

DRUG/LAB INTERACTIONS

Formal drug interaction studies have not been conducted. ▪ **Sodium nitrite and sodium thiosulfate** are also used to treat cyanide poisoning. They are **incompatible** with hydroxocobalamin and must be administered in a separate IV line if used concurrently. Safety of coadministration has not been established. ▪ Because of its deep red color, hydroxocobalamin **interferes with numerous clinical laboratory tests.** Effects persist for varying lengths of time depending on test. See package insert for specifics. ▪ Deep red color may cause hemodialysis machines to shut down (an erroneous detection of a "blood leak"). Consider before hemodialysis is initiated in patients treated with hydroxocobalamin.

SIDE EFFECTS

The most common side effects include chromaturia, decreased lymphocytes, erythema, headache, hypertension, injection site reactions, nausea, oxalate crystals in urine, and rash. Hypersensitivity reactions, hypertension, and renal injury are the most serious side effects associated with hydroxocobalamin. Other reactions that may occur include abdominal discomfort, chest discomfort, diarrhea, dizziness, dry throat, dyspepsia, dysphagia, dyspnea, hematochezia (blood in stool), hot flashes, impaired memory, irritation, peripheral edema, pruritus, redness and swelling of the eyes, restlessness, throat tightness, urticaria, and vomiting.

Post-Marketing: Acute renal failure with acute tubular necrosis, renal impairment, and urine calcium oxalate crystals.

ANTIDOTE

Keep physician informed of all side effects; will be treated symptomatically. Note Compatibility before treating hypertension or seizures; use an alternate IV line if indicated. Severe hypersensitivity reactions may require epinephrine, antihistamines (e.g., diphenhydramine), corticosteroids (e.g., hydrocortisone), or bronchodilators (e.g., albuterol, theophylline). Data on overdose not available; manage symptomatically. Hemodialysis may be effective and is indicated for significant hydroxocobalamin toxicity. Cardiac and/or respiratory arrest may occur before treatment has an effect; resuscitate as indicated.

IBALIZUMAB-uiyk
(eye-ba-**LIZ**-ue-mab uiyk)

Trogarzo

Antiretroviral
Monoclonal antibody (Anti-CD4)

pH 6

USUAL DOSE
Loading dose: 2,000 mg as an IV infusion.

Maintenance dose: 800 mg as an IV infusion every 2 weeks following the initial loading dose. If a maintenance dose (800 mg) is missed by 3 days or longer beyond the scheduled dosing day, a loading dose (2,000 mg) should be administered as early as possible. Resume maintenance dosing (800 mg) every 14 days thereafter.

DOSE ADJUSTMENTS
No dose modifications required when administered with any other antiretroviral or any other treatments. ▪ No formal studies conducted to examine the effects of renal or hepatic impairment on the pharmacokinetics of ibalizumab-uiyk. Renal impairment is not anticipated to affect the pharmacokinetics of ibalizumab-uiyk.

DILUTION
Available in a single-dose vial containing 200 mg/1.33 mL (150 mg/mL). Solution is colorless to slightly yellow and clear to slightly opalescent. Ten vials (13.3 mL) are required for the loading dose. Four vials are required for the maintenance dose (5.32 mL). Withdraw 1.33 mL of solution from each vial and transfer into a 250 mL IV bag of NS. Once diluted, the solution should be administered immediately.

Filters: Specific information not available.

Storage: Before use, refrigerate vials at 2° to 8° C (36° to 46° F) in original cartons to protect from light. Do not freeze. Once diluted, the ibalizumab-uiyk solution should be administered immediately. If not administered immediately, store diluted solution at RT (20° to 25° C [68° to 77° F]) for up to 4 hours, or refrigerate (2° to 8° C [36° to 46° F]) for up to 24 hours. If refrigerated, allow the diluted solution to stand at RT for at least 30 minutes but no more than 4 hours before administration. Discard partially used or empty vials and any unused portion of the diluted solution.

COMPATIBILITY
Compatible only with NS. Manufacturer states, "Other IV diluents must not be used to prepare ibalizumab-uiyk solution for infusion."

RATE OF ADMINISTRATION
Do not administer as an IV push or bolus. Manufacturer suggests administration into the cephalic vein of the patient's right or left arm. If cephalic vein is not accessible, an appropriate vein located elsewhere can be used.

Loading dose: The duration of the first infusion (loading dose) should be no less than 30 minutes.

Maintenance dose: If no infusion reactions have occurred with the loading dose, the duration of the subsequent infusions *(maintenance doses)* can be decreased to no less than 15 minutes. After infusion is complete, flush with 30 mL NS.

ACTIONS
Ibalizumab-uiyk is a CD4-directed postattachment HIV-1 inhibitor. It is a recombinant humanized monoclonal antibody that blocks HIV-1 from infecting CD4$^+$ T-cells by binding to domain 2 of CD4 and interfering with the postattachment steps required for the entry of HIV-1 virus particles into host cells and preventing the viral transmission that occurs via cell-cell fusion. The binding specificity of ibalizumab-uiyk to domain 2 of CD4 allows ibalizumab-uiyk to block viral entry into host cells without causing immunosuppression.

INDICATIONS AND USES

Given in combination with other antiretroviral(s) for the treatment of human immunodeficiency virus type 1 (HIV-1) infection in heavily treatment-experienced adults with multidrug-resistant HIV-1 infection who are failing their current antiretroviral regimen.

CONTRAINDICATIONS

Manufacturer states, "None."

PRECAUTIONS

Immune reconstitution inflammatory syndrome has been reported. During the initial phase of combination antiretroviral therapies, patients whose immune systems respond may develop an inflammatory response to indolent or residual opportunistic infections, which may require further evaluation and treatment. ■ Infusion-associated reactions may occur. ■ As with all therapeutic proteins, there is potential for immunogenicity.

Monitor: Monitor during and for 1 hour after completion of ibalizumab-uiyk administration for at least the first infusion. If no infusion-associated adverse reaction is observed, the postinfusion observation time may be reduced to 15 minutes. ■ Monitor patient for any new symptoms after receiving ibalizumab-uiyk.

Patient Education: Read the FDA-approved patient information. ■ Review all medicines being taken, including prescription and nonprescription medications, with health care provider. ■ Immediately report any S/S of infection. ■ It is important to receive ibalizumab-uiyk injections every 2 weeks and not to change the dosing schedule or any antiretroviral medication without consulting with health care provider. Immediately contact health care provider if ibalizumab-uiyk or any other drug in antiretroviral regimen is stopped.

Maternal/Child: No adequate human data are available to establish whether ibalizumab-uiyk poses a risk to pregnancy outcomes. ■ A pregnancy exposure registry has been established; contact manufacturer. ■ Females infected with HIV should be instructed not to breast-feed due to the potential for HIV transmission to the infant. ■ Safety and effectiveness for use in pediatric patients have not been established.

Elderly: No studies have been conducted in elderly patients.

DRUG/LAB INTERACTIONS

No drug interaction studies have been conducted. Based on ibalizumab-uiyk's mechanism of action and target-mediated drug disposition, drug-drug interactions are not expected.

SIDE EFFECTS

The most common side effects were diarrhea, dizziness, nausea, and rash. Severe rash occurred in one patient, and immune reconstitution inflammatory syndrome (manifested as an exacerbation of progressive multifocal leukoencephalopathy) occurred in another. Laboratory abnormalities include elevated bilirubin, direct bilirubin, creatinine, blood glucose, lipase, and uric acid, and decreased hemoglobin, platelets, leukocytes, and neutrophils.

ANTIDOTE

Notify physician of all side effects. Minor side effects may be treated symptomatically. Treat infusion reactions as appropriate based on severity.

IBANDRONATE SODIUM
(i-**BAN**-dro-nate **SO**-dee-um)

Boniva

Bone resorption inhibitor
Bisphosphonate

USUAL DOSE

breast ca, metastatic bone disease: 6 mg infused over 1 to 2 hours every 3 to 4 weeks.

hypercalcemia of malignancy: 2 to 6 mg as a single dose over 1 to 2 hours.

prostate cancer, metastatic, bone pain: 6 mg as a single dose over 15 minutes.

Pretreatment: Baseline studies indicated; see Monitor.

Ibandronate: 3 mg as an IV injection over 15 to 30 seconds every 3 months. Supplemental calcium and vitamin D may be required. See Precautions. Do not administer more frequently than every 3 months; if a dose is missed, administer it as soon as it can be rescheduled, and schedule the next injection for 3 months from that date.

DOSE ADJUSTMENTS

No dose adjustment is indicated based on age, gender, or impaired hepatic function. ▪ No dose adjustment is indicated for impaired kidney function in patients with a CrCl equal to or greater than 30 mL/min; see Contraindications.

DILUTION

May be given undiluted. Available in a prefilled syringe with a 25-gauge needle and a needlestick protection device. Administer only with the provided 25-gauge needle.

Storage: Store at CRT. Syringes are for single use only; discard unused drug.

COMPATIBILITY

Manufacturer states, "Must not be mixed with calcium-containing solutions or other intravenously administered drugs."

RATE OF ADMINISTRATION

A single dose as an IV injection over 15 to 30 seconds.

ACTIONS

A nitrogen-containing bisphosphonate. Action is based on its affinity for hydroxyapatite, which is part of the mineral matrix of bone. Ibandronate inhibits osteoclast activity and reduces bone resorption and turnover. In postmenopausal females with osteoporosis, it increases bone mineral density and reduces the incidence of vertebral fractures. Either rapidly binds to bone (40% to 50% of a dose) or is excreted unchanged in urine (50% to 60%). No evidence that it is metabolized in humans. Eliminated unchanged by the kidneys. Terminal half-life is dose dependent and ranged from 4.6 to 25.5 hours in studies in which 2 and 4 mg of ibandronate were administered. Renal clearance is related to CrCl. Patients with a CrCl less than 30 mL/min have a more than twofold increase in exposure (AUC) than do patients with a CrCl greater than 80 mL/min.

INDICATIONS AND USES

Treatment of osteoporosis in postmenopausal females.

Limitation of use: Safety and effectiveness based on clinical data of 1-year duration; optimal duration of use has not been determined. Re-evaluate on a periodic basis. Consider discontinuing ibandronate after 3 to 5 years of use in patients at low risk for fracture, and re-evaluate risk for fracture periodically in patients who discontinue ibandronate.

CONTRAINDICATIONS

Hypersensitivity to ibandronate or its excipients, uncorrected hypocalcemia, severe impaired renal function (CrCl less than 30 mL/min).

PRECAUTIONS

For IV injection only. Confirm patency of vein. Intra-arterial or paravenous administration could lead to tissue damage. ▪ Anaphylaxis, including fatal events, has been reported. Administer in a facility equipped to monitor the patient and respond to any medical emergency. ▪ Disturbances of bone and mineral metabolism (e.g., hypocalcemia, hypovitaminosis D) must be treated before administration of ibandronate. ▪ Bisphosphonates have been associated with a deterioration in renal function (e.g., increased SCr, acute renal failure [rare]). Use caution in patients who have concomitant diseases or are taking concomitant medications that may have adverse effects on the kidneys. ▪ Osteonecrosis of the jaw (ONJ) has been reported in patients receiving bisphosphonates. The majority of cases have been in cancer patients undergoing dental procedures. However, some cases have been reported in patients with postmenopausal osteoporosis treated with either oral or IV bisphosphonates. Risk factors include cancer, concomitant therapy (e.g., chemotherapy, angiogenesis inhibitors, radiotherapy, corticosteroids), and comorbid conditions (e.g., anemia, coagulopathies, infection, pre-existing oral disease). Risk may increase with duration of exposure to bisphosphonates. Consider dental exam and appropriate preventive dentistry before beginning therapy with bisphosphonates. Avoid invasive dental procedures during bisphosphonate therapy. Dental surgery may exacerbate ONJ in patients who develop ONJ while on bisphosphonate therapy. ▪ Severe and occasionally incapacitating bone, joint, and muscle pain has been reported rarely. Symptoms may occur from 1 day to several months after initiation of treatment. In most cases, pain resolves when ibandronate is discontinued. A subset of patients had recurrence of symptoms when rechallenged with the same drug or another bisphosphonate. ▪ Atypical, low-energy, or low-trauma fractures of the femoral shaft have been reported in bisphosphonate-treated patients. May be bilateral. Many patients report prodromal pain in the affected area, which usually presents as dull, aching thigh pain weeks to months before a complete fracture occurs. Patients presenting with thigh or groin pain should be evaluated to rule out an incomplete femur fracture. Patients presenting with an atypical fracture should also be assessed for S/S of fracture in the contralateral limb.

Monitor: Obtain baseline measurements of serum calcium, magnesium, phosphate, and serum creatinine; see Precautions. ▪ Perform a routine oral examination with appropriate preventive dentistry before administration. ▪ May cause a transient decrease in serum calcium values. ▪ Daily supplements of calcium and vitamin D may be required during therapy with ibandronate if dietary intake is inadequate. ▪ Monitor SCr before each dose. Nephropathy has been reported; see Precautions. Withhold treatment for renal deterioration. ▪ Monitor for S/S of a hypersensitivity reaction (e.g., chest pain, dizziness, dyspnea, fever, flushing, hypotension, nausea, pruritus, rash, rigors, urticaria). ▪ Influenza-like side effects (e.g., bone, muscle, or joint pains; chills; fever; fatigue) consistent with an acute-phase reaction have been reported. Incidence is higher with IV administration. Usually occurs within 3 days of injection and lasts 7 days or fewer. In most cases, symptoms generally subside within 24 to 48 hours, and treatment other than acetaminophen has not been required.

Patient Education: Read manufacturer's patient information sheet before each infusion. ▪ Daily supplements of calcium and vitamin D may be required during therapy with ibandronate. ▪ Discuss your health history (e.g., kidney problems, diabetes, high blood pressure, heart disease, planned tooth extraction) and prescription and nonprescription medications with health care providers, including your dentist. ▪ Promptly report persistent pain and/or nonhealing sores of the mouth or jaw. ▪ Promptly report chills and/or fever and other S/S of a hypersensitivity reaction (e.g., chest pain, dizziness, feeling faint, flushing, hives, itching, nausea, pruritus, rash, shortness of breath). ▪ Report development of bone, joint, or muscle pain promptly. Onset of pain is variable. ▪ Promptly report thigh or groin pain. ▪ Do not administer more frequently than every 3 months; if a dose is missed, administer it as soon as it can be rescheduled, and schedule the next injection for 3 months from that date. ▪ Laboratory monitoring of renal function required before each dose. ▪ Flu-like symptoms may occur within the first 3 days of therapy and usually resolve within 24 to 48 hours. Administration of acetaminophen may reduce incidence of symptoms.

Maternal/Child: Ibandronate is not indicated for use in females of reproductive potential. There are no data regarding use during pregnancy or with breast-feeding. ▪ Safety and effectiveness for use in pediatric patients not established.

Elderly: Response similar to that seen in younger patients; however, greater sensitivity cannot be ruled out. ▪ Monitor renal function. Consider impaired renal function and concomitant disease or drug therapy.

DRUG/LAB INTERACTIONS

Does not inhibit cytochrome P450 isoenzymes. ▪ Bisphosphonates are known to interfere with the use of **bone-imaging agents;** ibandronate has not been studied.

SIDE EFFECTS

Abdominal pain, arthralgia, and back pain are the most common side effects. Other commonly reported side effects include headache, increased SCr, influenza-like illness (bone, muscle, or joint pains; chills; fever; fatigue), and injection site reactions (redness or swelling). Less frequent side effects include bronchitis, constipation, cystitis, depression, diarrhea, dizziness, dyspepsia, extremity pain, gastritis, gastroenteritis, hypertension, hypocalcemia, insomnia, localized osteoarthritis, myalgia, nasopharyngitis, nausea, rash, upper respiratory infection, urinary tract infection.

Overdose: Hypocalcemia, hypomagnesemia, and hypophosphatemia.

Post-Marketing: Acute renal failure; atypical, low-energy, or low-trauma fractures of the femoral shaft; eye inflammation (iritis and uveitis); hypersensitivity reactions, including anaphylaxis (with fatalities), angioedema, asthma exacerbation, bronchospasm, dermatitis bullous, erythema multiforme, rash, and Stevens-Johnson syndrome; osteonecrosis of the jaw and other orofacial sites, including the external auditory canal; severe or incapacitating musculoskeletal pain.

ANTIDOTE

Keep physician informed of side effects. Most will respond to symptomatic treatment. Withhold treatment for renal deterioration. Treat clinically relevant reductions in serum levels of calcium, magnesium, and phosphorus with IV administration of calcium gluconate, magnesium sulfate, and/or potassium or sodium phosphate as indicated. Discontinue ibandronate if severe bone, joint, or muscle pain develops. To be beneficial, dialysis must be administered within 2 hours of overdose. Treat anaphylaxis and/or resuscitate as indicated.

IBUPROFEN BBW

(**EYE**-bue-**PROE**-fen)

NSAID

Caldolor

pH 7.4

USUAL DOSE

Pretreatment: Baseline assessment and studies indicated; see Monitor. See Maternal/Child.

Use the lowest effective dose for the shortest duration of time based on individual needs and response. Re-evaluate after the initial dose. Adjust dose and frequency as indicated. Total daily dose should not exceed 3,200 mg. Adequate hydration and correction of hypovolemia required before administration to reduce the risk of adverse renal reactions.

Analgesia: 400 to 800 mg every 6 hours as necessary.

Antipyretic: 400 mg followed by 400 mg every 4 to 6 hours or 100 to 200 mg every 4 hours as necessary.

PEDIATRIC DOSE

Pediatric Dosing of Ibuprofen for Fever and Pain			
Age-Group	**Dose**	**Dosing Interval**	**Maximum Daily Dose[a]**
6 months to less than 12 years	10 mg/kg up to 400 mg max	Every 4 to 6 hr as needed	40 mg/kg or 2,400 mg
12 to 17 years	400 mg	Every 4 to 6 hr as needed	2,400 mg

[a]Maximum daily dose is 40 mg/kg or 2,400 mg, whichever is less.

See comments under Usual Dose and Maternal/Child.

DOSE ADJUSTMENTS

To minimize the potential risk for an adverse cardiovascular (CV) event, use the lowest effective dose for the shortest duration possible. ▪ Lower-end initial and reduced doses may be indicated in the elderly and/or debilitated. Consider potential for decreased organ function and concomitant disease or drug therapy.

DILUTION

Available as an 800 mg/200 mL (4 mg/mL) single-dose, ready-to-use flexible bag or as an 800 mg/8 mL single-dose vial (100 mg/mL). Vial must be diluted to a final concentration of 4 mg/mL or less for both adult and weight-based pediatric dosing using NS, D5W, or LR. Infusion without dilution can cause hemolysis. The 800 mg/200 mL ready-to-use bag is intended for 800-mg doses only.

Filters: Specific information not available; consult pharmacist.

Storage: Store vials at CRT. Diluted solutions stable for up to 24 hours at 20° to 25° C (68° to 77° F) and with ambient room lighting.

COMPATIBILITY

Compatibility information not available from manufacturer; consult a pharmacist.

RATE OF ADMINISTRATION

Adult: A single dose as an infusion over no less than 30 minutes.

Pediatric: A single dose as an infusion over no less than 10 minutes.

ACTIONS

A nonsteroidal anti-inflammatory drug (NSAID) that has anti-inflammatory, analgesic, and antipyretic activity. Mechanism of action is not completely understood but involves inhibition of cyclooxygenase (COX-1 and COX-2). It inhibits synthesis of prostaglandins, which are potent mediators of inflammation. Highly protein bound; the mean half-life of a

400-mg dose is 2.2 hours, and the mean half-life of an 800-mg dose is 2.44 hours. Metabolized in the liver via oxidation and excreted in the urine.

INDICATIONS AND USES

Management of mild to moderate pain. ▪ Management of moderate to severe pain as an adjunct to opioid analgesics. ▪ Reduction of fever.

CONTRAINDICATIONS

Known hypersensitivity (anaphylactoid reactions, serious skin reactions) to ibuprofen or any component of the product. ▪ Known history of asthma, urticaria, or allergic-type reactions after taking aspirin or other NSAIDs. ▪ In the setting of coronary artery bypass graft (CABG) surgery. ▪ See Maternal/Child.

PRECAUTIONS

For IV infusion only. ▪ NSAIDs increase the risk for serious cardiovascular (CV) thrombotic events, including MI and stroke, which can be fatal. This risk may occur early in treatment and may increase with duration of use. The increase in CV thrombotic risk has been observed most consistently at higher doses. ▪ There is no consistent evidence that concurrent use of aspirin mitigates the increased risk of serious CV thrombotic events associated with NSAID therapy. However, concurrent use does increase the risk of serious GI toxicity. ▪ An increased incidence of MI and stroke was seen in patients who received an NSAID as an analgesic after CABG surgery; see Contraindications. ▪ Avoid the use of ibuprofen in patients with a recent MI or in patients with severe heart failure unless the benefits are expected to outweigh the risks. Studies have shown these patients to be at increased risk for reinfarction, CV-related death, and all-cause mortality. ▪ NSAIDs increase the risk for serious GI adverse events, including ulceration, bleeding, and/or perforation of the stomach or intestines. Can occur at any time, with or without warning symptoms, and can be fatal. Use extreme caution in patients with a prior history of peptic ulcer disease or GI bleeding. Risk is also increased in elderly or debilitated patients, in patients with advanced liver disease, and with concomitant use of aspirin, oral corticosteroids, anticoagulants, alcohol, selective serotonin reuptake inhibitors (SSRIs), or smoking or with longer durations of therapy. ▪ May cause elevations of liver function tests (e.g., ALT, AST). Rare cases of serious, sometimes fatal, hepatic injury (fulminant hepatitis, liver necrosis, hepatic failure) have occurred. ▪ May cause fluid retention and edema; use caution in patients with CHF or edema; see Drug/Lab Interactions. ▪ May precipitate new-onset hypertension or worsen pre-existing hypertension; see Drug/Lab Interactions. ▪ In addition to the usual caution in patients with reduced hepatic or renal function, NSAIDs may cause a dose-dependent reduction in renal prostaglandin formation and, secondarily, in renal blood flow, which can precipitate renal failure. Patients with impaired renal function, heart failure, liver dysfunction, dehydration, or hypovolemia; elderly patients; and patients receiving ACE inhibitors, angiotensin receptor blockers (ARBs), or diuretics are at greatest risk. ▪ Avoid ibuprofen use in patients with advanced renal disease unless the benefits are expected to outweigh the risk. ▪ Increases in serum potassium, including hyperkalemia, have been reported. ▪ Anaphylactic reactions have occurred in patients with and without known hypersensitivity to ibuprofen and in patients with aspirin-sensitive asthma. Cross-reactivity between aspirin and other NSAIDs has been reported in aspirin-sensitive patients; see Contraindications. Use caution in patients with pre-existing asthma (without known aspirin sensitivity), and monitor for changes in S/S of asthma. ▪ May cause serious skin reactions (e.g., exfoliative dermatitis, Stevens-Johnson syndrome, toxic epidermal necrolysis) without warning; some have been fatal. ▪ Anti-inflammatory and antipyretic effects may reduce the utility of these diagnostic signs in detecting infections. ▪ May cause anemia. Anemia may be due to occult or gross GI blood loss, fluid retention, or an incompletely described effect on erythropoiesis. ▪ NSAIDs inhibit platelet aggregation and may increase the risk of bleeding. Risk may be increased with comorbid conditions such as coagulation disorders or with concomitant use of several medications; see Drug/Lab Interactions. ▪ Aseptic meningitis and ophthalmologic effects (e.g., blurred or diminished vision, changes in color vision) have been reported with oral ibuprofen. ▪ See Maternal/Child.

Monitor: Correct hypovolemia before administration and maintain adequate hydration. ▪ Obtain baseline blood pressure and monitor frequently during therapy. ▪ Consider baseline CBC, electrolytes, liver function tests, and SCr or CrCl. Repeat as needed if S/S of toxicity/adverse events develop. ▪ Monitor patients with or without a previous history of CV disease for S/S of CV events (e.g., chest pain, dyspnea, edema, hypertension, limb or facial paralysis). ▪ Monitor for edema or signs of worsening heart failure. ▪ Observe for S/S of GI ulceration or bleeding and/or liver dysfunction. ▪ Monitor renal function, especially in patients with impaired renal function. ▪ Monitor for S/S of hypersensitivity or serious skin reactions (e.g., anaphylaxis, pruritus, rash, urticaria, or wheezing). ▪ Monitor patients who may be adversely affected by alterations in platelet function (e.g., patients with coagulation disorders or patients receiving anticoagulants) for signs of bleeding.

Patient Education: Review FDA-approved medication guide. ▪ Side effects have resulted in extended hospitalization and could be fatal. ▪ Promptly report any S/S of CV thrombotic events (e.g., chest pain, shortness of breath, slurred speech, weakness), GI adverse events (e.g., dyspepsia, epigastric pain, hematemesis, melena), hepatotoxicity (e.g., diarrhea, fatigue, flu-like symptoms, jaundice, lethargy, nausea, pruritus, right upper quadrant tenderness), heart failure (e.g., edema, shortness of breath, weight gain), serious skin reaction, and/or a hypersensitivity reaction (e.g., difficulty breathing, swelling of the face or throat) or any type or rash. ▪ Avoid use of concomitant NSAIDs. Over-the-counter medications for the treatment of fever, cold, and insomnia may contain NSAIDs. Consult pharmacist before use. ▪ Discuss use of low-dose aspirin for cardiac prophylaxis with health care provider before initiating concomitant therapy; may increase risk of GI toxicity. ▪ May be associated with a reversible delay in ovulation. ▪ See Maternal/Child.

Maternal/Child: Avoid use starting at 30 weeks' gestation (third trimester); premature closure of the ductus arteriosus in the fetus may occur. Use before 30 weeks' gestation only if the potential benefit justifies the potential risk to the fetus. ▪ Effects during labor and delivery unknown. ▪ Use with caution during breast-feeding. ▪ Safety and effectiveness for use in pediatric patients under 6 months of age not established.

Elderly: Increased risk for serious NSAID-associated GI, cardiovascular, and/or renal adverse events. ▪ Dosing should be cautious; see Dose Adjustments.

DRUG/LAB INTERACTIONS

Concurrent use with other **NSAIDs, aspirin,** or other **salicylates** is not recommended; may increase the risk of toxicity and serious GI events. ▪ Ibuprofen may interfere with the platelet effect in patients taking low-dose aspirin for cardioprotection, increasing the risk of CV events. In these patients, consider use of an alternate analgesic that does not interfere with the antiplatelet effect of aspirin. ▪ Increased risk of bleeding with concomitant use of **anticoagulants, antiplatelet agents, SSRIs,** and **serotonin-norepinephrine reuptake inhibitors (SNRIs).** Monitor patients closely if concomitant use indicated. ▪ NSAIDs may decrease the effectiveness of **ACE inhibitors, ARBs,** and **beta-blockers**; monitor BP. ▪ Co-administration with an **ACE inhibitor** or **ARB** may result in deterioration of renal function in at-risk patients; monitor renal function. ▪ Ibuprofen can reduce the natriuretic effects of **loop diuretics** (e.g., furosemide) and **thiazide diuretics** (e.g., hydrochlorothiazide); observe for signs of worsening renal function and ensure diuretic/therapeutic effectiveness. ▪ May increase **digoxin** serum concentration and prolong half-life of digoxin; monitor digoxin levels with concomitant use. ▪ Concurrent use of **lithium** with NSAIDs may decrease lithium clearance, increasing plasma levels of lithium; observe for signs of lithium toxicity. ▪ Concurrent use of NSAIDs with **methotrexate** may enhance methotrexate toxicity (e.g., neutropenia, thrombocytopenia, renal dysfunction); monitor for signs of methotrexate toxicity. ▪ Concomitant use with **cyclosporine** may increase cyclosporine's nephrotoxicity; monitor renal function. ▪ Concomitant use with **pemetrexed** may increase the risk of pemetrexed-associated myelosuppression and renal and GI toxicity; avoid concomitant use for 2 to 5 days before pemetrexed administration and for 2 days following administration in patients with mild to moderate renal impairment (CrCl 45 to 79 mL/min). See pemetrexed monograph.

SIDE EFFECTS

Adults: The most common side effects are dizziness, flatulence, headache, hemorrhage, and nausea and vomiting. Other side effects include abdominal discomfort, anemia, bacteremia, bacterial pneumonia, cough, diarrhea, dyspepsia, eosinophilia, hyperkalemia, hypernatremia, hypertension, hypoalbuminemia, hypokalemia, hypoproteinemia, hypotension, increased blood urea, increased lactic dehydrogenase (LDH), neutropenia, peripheral edema, thrombocytosis, urinary retention, and wound hemorrhage. See Precautions for potential major side effects.

Pediatric patients: The most common side effects are anemia, headache, infusion site pain, nausea, and vomiting.

Overdose: Acute renal failure, coma, drowsiness, epigastric pain, GI bleeding, hypertension, lethargy, nausea, respiratory depression, and vomiting.

ANTIDOTE

Keep the physician informed of significant side effects. With increasing severity or onset of symptoms of any major side effect (e.g., CHF; edema; hypersensitivity reactions; GI bleeding, ulceration, or perforation; hepatic or renal effects; hypertension; skin reactions; thrombotic events), discontinue the drug and notify the physician. A patent airway, artificial ventilation, oxygen therapy, and other symptomatic treatment must be instituted promptly if indicated. Treat anaphylaxis with epinephrine, diphenhydramine, and corticosteroids as indicated. No known antidote. Forced diuresis, alkalinization of urine, hemodialysis, or hemoperfusion may not be useful due to high protein binding.

IBUPROFEN LYSINE

(eye-byou-**PROH**-fen **LIE**-seen)

NSAID

(patent ductus arteriosus adjunct)

NeoProfen

pH 7

NEONATAL DOSE

Pretreatment: Baseline studies indicated; see Monitor.

All doses are based on birth weight. A course of therapy is three doses given at 24-hour intervals.

Initial dose: 10 mg/kg. Follow with a dose of 5 mg/kg in 24 hours and repeat at 48 hours; see Dose Adjustments.

After completion of the first course, no further doses are indicated if the ductus arteriosus closes or is significantly reduced in size. If the ductus arteriosus fails to close or reopens, a second course, alternative pharmacologic therapy, or surgery may be necessary.

DOSE ADJUSTMENTS

If urine output is less than 0.6 mL/kg/hr at any time a dose is to be given, withhold dose until lab studies confirm a return to normal renal function.

DILUTION

Each single dose must be diluted to an appropriate volume for administration as an infusion over 15 minutes with dextrose or saline. Prepare for infusion and begin administration within 30 minutes of preparation. A fresh solution should be prepared just before each administration. Contains no preservatives; discard any unused portion.

Filters: Specific information not available.

Storage: Store vials in cartons at CRT and protect from light until use. Use reconstituted solution within 30 minutes of preparation.

COMPATIBILITY

Manufacturer states, "Should not be simultaneously administered in the same IV line with Total Parenteral Nutrition" (TPN). If required, interrupt TPN for 15 minutes before and after ibuprofen administration. Maintain IV line patency with dextrose or saline infusion.

RATE OF ADMINISTRATION

Administer via the IV port nearest the insertion site.

A single dose, properly diluted, and infused continuously over 15 minutes.

ACTIONS

A nonsteroidal anti-inflammatory drug (NSAID). Mechanism of action by which it causes closure of a patent ductus arteriosus (PDA) is unknown; however, in adults it is an inhibitor of prostaglandin synthesis. By closing the PDA, the need for surgical intervention is eliminated. Half-life varies inversely with postnatal age, but in general the half-life in infants is more than 10 times longer than in adults. In low-birth-weight premature infants half-life may range from 20 to 51 hours. Metabolism and excretion have not been studied in premature infants. In adults, it is metabolized in the liver and excreted in the urine and feces.

INDICATIONS AND USES

Closure of a clinically significant PDA in premature infants weighing between 500 and 1,500 Gm who are no more than 32 weeks' gestational age when usual medical management (e.g., fluid restriction, diuretics, respiratory support) is not effective. Consequences beyond 8 weeks after treatment have not been evaluated.

CONTRAINDICATIONS

Preterm infants with proven or suspected infection that is untreated. ■ Preterm infants with congenital heart disease in whom patency of the PDA is necessary for satisfactory pulmonary or systemic blood flow (e.g., pulmonary atresia, severe tetralogy of Fallot, severe coarctation of the aorta). ■ Preterm infants who are bleeding, especially those with active intracranial hemorrhage or gastrointestinal bleeding. ■ Preterm infants with thrombocytopenia. ■ Preterm infants with coagulation defects. ■ Preterm infants with or who are suspected of having necrotizing enterocolitis. ■ Preterm infants with significant impairment of renal function.

PRECAUTIONS

For IV use only; see Monitor. ■ Reserve for infants with clear evidence of a clinically significant PDA. ■ For use only in a highly supervised setting such as an intensive care nursery. ■ No long-term evaluations available. Effects of ibuprofen on neurodevelopmental outcome and growth and on disease processes associated with prematurity (e.g., retinopathy of prematurity, chronic lung disease) have not been assessed. ■ May alter the usual signs of infection. Use with extreme caution in the presence of an existing controlled infection and in infants at risk for infection. ■ Can inhibit platelet aggregation. ■ Can prolong bleeding time in adults; use caution in infants with underlying hemostatic defects; see Contraindications. ■ Can displace bilirubin from albumin-binding sites; use with caution in infants with elevated total bilirubin.

Monitor: Confirm absolute patency of vein. Avoid extravasation; will irritate tissue. Administration via an umbilical arterial line has not been studied. ■ Obtain baseline and monitor vital signs, oxygenation, acid-base status, fluid and electrolyte balance, and kidney function (SCr, BUN, urine output). ■ Can cause a reduction in urine output, increased BUN and SCr, and a decreased CrCl; may progress to oliguria or renal failure. Monitor all infants closely, especially those with some degree of renal impairment. ■ May inhibit platelet aggregation; monitor for signs of bleeding. ■ Monitor for signs of infection. ■ See Drug/Lab Interactions.

Maternal/Child: Safety and effectiveness have been established only for use in premature infants.

DRUG/LAB INTERACTIONS

Ibuprofen may reduce the effects of **diuretics**; diuretics can increase the risk of nephrotoxicity of **NSAIDs** in dehydrated patients. Monitor renal function in patients receiving concomitant diuretics. ▪ Ibuprofen may decrease the clearance of **amikacin**.

SIDE EFFECTS

The most commonly reported side effects include adrenal insufficiency, anemia, apnea, atelectasis, decreased urine output, edema, GI disorders (including non-necrotizing enterocolitis), hematuria, hypernatremia, hypocalcemia, hypoglycemia, increased BUN and SCr, intraventricular hemorrhage and other bleeding, renal failure, renal insufficiency, respiratory failure, respiratory infection, sepsis, skin lesion or irritation, and urinary tract infection. Other side effects of unknown association include abdominal distension, cardiac failure, cholestasis, convulsions, feeding problems, gastritis, gastroesophageal reflux, hypotension, ileus, infections, inguinal hernia, injection site reactions, jaundice, lab abnormalities (e.g., hyperglycemia, neutropenia, thrombocytopenia), and tachycardia.

Post-Marketing: GI perforation, necrotizing enterocolitis, and pulmonary hypertension.

Overdose: Breathing difficulties, coma, drowsiness, hypotension, irregular heartbeat, kidney failure, seizures, and vomiting have occurred in individuals (not necessarily in premature infants) following overdose of oral ibuprofen.

ANTIDOTE

Discontinue the drug and notify the physician of all side effects. Based on severity, side effects may be treated symptomatically or drug will be completely discontinued in favor of surgical intervention. In case of overdose, there is no specific antidote. Treat symptomatically and follow for several days after apparent recovery; GI ulceration and hemorrhage may occur. Resuscitate as necessary.

IBUTILIDE FUMARATE BBW
(ih-**BYOU**-tih-lyd **FU**-mar-ayt)

Antiarrhythmic

Corvert

pH 4.6

USUAL DOSE

Pretreatment: Baseline studies indicated; see Monitor.

Guidelines for Ibutilide Dosing		
Patient Weight	**Initial Infusion (over 10 minutes)**	**Second Infusion**
60 kg (132 lb) or more	1 mg ibutilide fumarate (one vial [10 mL])	If the arrhythmia does not terminate within 10 minutes after the end of the initial infusion, a second 10-minute infusion of equal strength may be administered 10 minutes after completion of the first infusion.
Less than 60 kg (132 lb)	0.01 mg/kg ibutilide fumarate (0.1 mL/kg)	

Discontinue infusion promptly when the presenting arrhythmia is terminated (desired effect). Must also be discontinued immediately if sustained or nonsustained ventricular tachycardia or marked prolongation of QT or QTc occurs (adverse effects). Postconversion treatment with appropriate antiarrhythmics (e.g., digoxin, verapamil, or propranolol) is usually required.

DOSE ADJUSTMENTS

Dose selection should be cautious in the elderly. Reduced doses may be indicated based on the potential for decreased organ function and concomitant disease or drug therapy.

■ No adjustments required in patients with impaired hepatic or renal function; see Monitor. Lower doses may be indicated in post–cardiac surgery patients. In recent studies, one or two infusions of 0.5 mg in patients weighing 60 kg or more or 0.005 mg/kg/dose for patients under 60 kg was effective in terminating atrial fibrillation and/or flutter.

DILUTION

May be given undiluted or may be diluted in 50 mL of NS or D5W and given as an infusion. 1 mg (10 mL of a 0.1-mg/mL solution) of ibutilide in 50 mL diluent yields 0.017 mg/mL.

Storage: Store at CRT in carton until use. Stable after dilution for 24 hours at room temperature, 48 hours if refrigerated.

COMPATIBILITY

Manufacturer lists as **compatible** with NS and D5W packaged in glass, polyvinyl chloride, or polyolefin infusion containers. Additional information not available; consult pharmacist.

RATE OF ADMINISTRATION

A single dose by injection or infusion over 10 minutes.

ACTIONS

A Class III antiarrhythmic agent that produces mild slowing of the sinus rate and atrioventricular conduction. Delays repolarization by activation of a slow inward current (sodium) rather than blocking outward potassium currents. Prolonged atrial and ventricular action potential duration and refractoriness result. Produces dose-related prolongation of the QT interval (may result from dose of ibutilide or rate of injection). Conversion of atrial flutter/fibrillation usually occurs within 30 minutes but may take up to 90 minutes after the start of the infusion. Most patients remain in normal sinus rhythm (NSR) for 24 hours. At recommended doses, ibutilide has no clinically significant effects on cardiac output, mean pulmonary arterial pressure, or pulmonary capillary wedge pressure. Rapidly distributed and metabolized. Elimination half-life is 6 hours (range 2 to 12 hours). Primarily excreted in urine (7% as unchanged drug). Excreted in small amounts in feces.

INDICATIONS AND USES

Rapid conversion of recent-onset atrial fibrillation or atrial flutter to sinus rhythm. Patients with more recent onset of arrhythmia have a higher rate of conversion. Effectiveness was less in those with a longer-duration arrhythmia.

CONTRAINDICATIONS

Known hypersensitivity to ibutilide or any of its components. ■ Not recommended in patients who have had a previous polymorphic ventricular tachycardia (e.g., torsades de pointes). ■ See Drug/Lab Interactions.

PRECAUTIONS

For IV infusion only. ■ Usually administered by or under the direction of the physician specialist. ■ Skilled personnel and proper equipment (e.g., cardiac monitors, intracardiac pacing facilities, cardioverter/defibrillator, emergency drugs) must be immediately available. ■ May cause life-threatening arrhythmias (e.g., torsades de pointes) with or without documented QT prolongation. ■ Correct hypokalemia and hypomagnesemia before use; may exaggerate a prolonged QT and cause arrhythmias. ■ Adequate anticoagulation (usually at least 2 weeks) is required for any patient with atrial fibrillation of more than 2 to 3 days' duration. ■ Select patients carefully; benefits (potential for maintaining sinus rhythm) must outweigh risks. Patients with chronic atrial fibrillation are more likely to revert back to atrial fibrillation after conversion to sinus rhythm. Patients with a QTc interval greater than 440 msec or a serum potassium less than 4.0 mEq/L are at very high risk to develop life-threatening arrhythmias. ■ Patients with a history of CHF may be more susceptible to sustained polymorphic VT. ■ Slightly more effective in atrial flutter than atrial fibrillation. ■ See Drug/Lab Interactions.

Monitor: Obtain weight, baseline vital signs, and ECG before administration. Continuous ECG monitoring during and after infusion indicated to observe for arrhythmias. Watch for QT or QTc prolongation; may cause arrhythmia (torsades de pointes) with or without QT prolongation. ▪ Monitor BP and HR. Bradycardia, a varying HR, and/or hypokalemia may increase risk of arrhythmia. ▪ Arrhythmia occurs most frequently within 40 minutes of completion of infusion but may occur for up to 3 hours after infusion. Monitor ECG for a minimum of 4 hours or until QTc has returned to baseline. Monitor longer if there are any episodes of arrhythmias or if the patient has impaired liver function.

Patient Education: Promptly report any feeling of faintness, difficulty breathing, or pain or stinging along injection site.

Maternal/Child: Category C: benefits must outweigh risks. Caused birth defects and was embryocidal in rats. ▪ Temporarily discontinue breast-feeding. ▪ Safety and effectiveness for use in pediatric patients under 18 years of age not established.

Elderly: No age-related differences observed. Median age in clinical trials was 65 years. ▪ Lower-end initial doses may be indicated; see Dose Adjustments.

DRUG/LAB INTERACTIONS

Should not be given concurrently with **Class Ia antiarrhythmics** (e.g., disopyramide, procainamide, quinidine) **or other Class III antiarrhythmics** (e.g., amiodarone, sotalol). Withhold any of these agents for at least 5 half-lives before ibutilide infusion and for 4 hours after. ▪ Incidence of arrhythmia may be increased with **other drugs that prolong the QT interval** (e.g., phenothiazines [e.g., promethazine], tricyclic antidepressants [e.g., amitriptyline], tetracyclic antidepressants [e.g., maprotiline]). ▪ Monitor **serum digoxin levels** to avoid digoxin toxicity. ▪ Use with **digoxin, beta-blockers, or calcium channel blockers** does not alter safety or effectiveness of ibutilide. However, **sotalol** is a beta-blocker, and its use with ibutilide is restricted because it has Class III antiarrhythmic activity; see first sentence above.

SIDE EFFECTS

Sustained polymorphic VT (1.7%) and nonsustained polymorphic VT (2.7%) can deteriorate into ventricular fibrillation and be fatal. May cause many other arrhythmias (e.g., first-, second-, or third-degree AV block [1.5%], bradycardia [1.2%], bundle branch block [1.9%], nonsustained monomorphic VT [4.9%], prolonged QT segment [1.2%], PVCs [5.1%], tachycardia [2.7%]), CHF (0.5%), headache (3.6%), hypertension (1.2%), hypotension (2%), nausea (1.9%), palpitation (1%).

Overdose: Side effects exaggerated with overdose in humans. Acute overdose in animals resulted in CNS depression; rapid, gasping breathing; and convulsions.

ANTIDOTE

If proarrhythmias occur, discontinue ibutilide; correct electrolyte abnormalities (e.g., potassium and magnesium). Overdrive cardiac pacing, electrical cardioversion, or defibrillation may be required. Infusions of magnesium sulfate may be helpful. Avoid treatment with antiarrhythmic agents. VT that deteriorates to VF will require immediate defibrillation.

IDARUBICIN HYDROCHLORIDE BBW

(eye-dah-**ROOB**-ih-sin hy-droh-**KLOR**-eyed)

Idamycin PFS, Idarubicin PFS, IDR

Antineoplastic
(anthracycline antibiotic)

pH 5 to 7

USUAL DOSE

Pretreatment: Verify pregnancy status. Baseline studies indicated; see Monitor.

Adult acute myeloid leukemia (AML) induction therapy:

Induction: Idarubicin 12 mg/M^2/day for 3 days. Used in combination with cytarabine (Ara-C). Cytarabine 100 mg/M^2/day may be given as a continuous infusion on Days 1 to 7 (daily for 7 days), or alternately the cytarabine may be given as an IV injection of 25 mg/M^2 followed immediately by a continuous infusion of cytarabine 200 mg/M^2/day on Days 1 to 5 (daily for 5 days). See Precautions/Monitor. If unequivocal evidence of leukemia remains after the first course, a second course may be given; see Dose Adjustments. The benefit of an aggressive consolidation and maintenance program in prolonging the duration of remissions and survival has not been proven. See prescribing information for regimens used in clinical trials.

DOSE ADJUSTMENTS

Delay second course until full recovery if severe mucositis has occurred and reduce dose by 25%. ▪ Consider dose reductions in impaired liver and kidney function based on bilirubin and/or creatinine levels above the normal range. Do not administer if bilirubin is above 5 mg/dL. In one Phase III clinical trial, patients with bilirubin levels between 2.6 and 5 mg/dL received a 50% reduction in dose.

DILUTION

Specific techniques required (see Precautions). Idamycin PFS is a liquid formulation; each 5 mg of powdered idamycin must be reconstituted with 5 mL of nonbacteriostatic NS for injection (1 mg/mL). Use extreme caution inserting the needle; vial contents are under negative pressure. Avoid any possibility of inhalation from aerosol or any skin contamination.

Filters: No data available from manufacturer.

Storage: PFS product must be refrigerated. Reconstituted idamycin is stable for 7 days under refrigeration (2° to 8° C [36° to 46° F]) or 3 days (72 hours) at room temperature (15° to 30° C [59° to 86° F]). Discard unused solution appropriately.

COMPATIBILITY

Manufacturer states, "Should not be mixed with other drugs unless specific **compatibility** data are available," and lists as **incompatible** with heparin. Prolonged contact with solutions of an alkaline pH (e.g., sodium lactate, sodium bicarbonate) will result in degradation of idarubicin.

Other sources suggest specific **compatibilities** dependent on concentration and manufacturer; consult a pharmacist.

RATE OF ADMINISTRATION

A single dose of properly diluted medication over 10 to 15 minutes through Y-tube or three-way stopcock of a free-flowing infusion of D5W or NS.

ACTIONS

A highly toxic, synthetic, antibiotic, antineoplastic agent. An analog of daunorubicin. Rapidly distributed; has an increased rate of cellular uptake compared to other anthracyclines. It inhibits synthesis of DNA and interacts with the enzyme topoisomerase II. Results in a greater number of remissions and longer survival than previous protocols (daunorubicin and cytarabine). It is severely immunosuppressive. Extensive extrahepatic metabolism. Half-life averages 20 to 22 hours. Slowly excreted in bile and urine.

INDICATIONS AND USES

Treatment of acute myeloid leukemia (AML) in adults in combination with other approved antileukemic drugs.

Unlabeled uses: Treatment of acute lymphoblastic leukemia in pediatric patients; see Maternal/Child.

CONTRAINDICATIONS

Not absolute; pre-existing bone marrow suppression, impaired cardiac function, pre-existing infection; see Precautions/Monitor. ▪ Do not administer if bilirubin above 5 mg/dL.

PRECAUTIONS

Follow guidelines for handling cytotoxic agents. See Appendix A, p. 1308. ▪ Administered by or under the direction of the physician specialist, with facilities for monitoring the patient and responding to any medical emergency. ▪ For IV use only. Do not give IM or SQ. ▪ Use extreme caution in pre-existing drug-induced bone marrow suppression, existing heart disease, previous treatment with other anthracyclines (e.g., daunorubicin), other cardiotoxic agents (e.g., bleomycin), or radiation therapy encompassing the heart. ▪ Myocardial toxicity may cause potentially fatal acute congestive heart failure, acute life-threatening arrhythmias, or other cardiomyopathies. Cardiac toxicity is more common in patients who have received prior anthracyclines (e.g., doxorubicin) or who have pre-existing cardiac disease. Risk of myocardial toxicity may be higher after concomitant or previous radiation to the mediastinal-pericardial area; or in patients with anemia, bone marrow depression, infections, leukemic pericarditis and/or myocarditis, active or dormant cardiovascular disease, previous therapy with other anthracyclines or anthracenediones; or with concomitant use of drugs with the ability to suppress cardiac contractility or cardiotoxic drugs (e.g., cyclophosphamide, paclitaxel, and trastuzumab). See Drug/Lab Interactions. ▪ May cause severe myelosuppression. ▪ Use with caution in patients with hepatic or renal dysfunction. Metabolism and excretion of idarubicin may be impaired; see Dose Adjustments.

Monitor: Determine absolute patency of vein. A stinging or burning sensation indicates extravasation, but extravasation may occur without stinging or burning; severe cellulitis and tissue necrosis can occur with extravasation. Discontinue injection; use another vein. ▪ Monitoring of WBCs, RBCs, platelet count, liver function, kidney function, ECG, chest x-ray, echocardiography, and systolic ejection fraction indicated before and during therapy. ▪ Severe myelosuppression occurs with effective therapeutic doses. Observe closely for all signs of infection or bleeding. ▪ Monitor for thrombocytopenia (platelet count less than 50,000/mm^3). Initiate precautions to prevent excessive bleeding (e.g., inspect IV sites, skin, and mucous membranes; use extreme care during invasive procedures; test urine, emesis, stool, and secretions for occult blood). ▪ Prophylactic antibiotics may be indicated pending results of C/S in a febrile neutropenic patient. ▪ Prophylactic antiemetics may reduce nausea and vomiting and increase patient comfort. ▪ Monitor uric acid levels; maintain hydration; uric acid-lowering drugs (e.g., allopurinol [Aloprim]) may be indicated. ▪ See Precautions.

Patient Education: Effective birth control recommended. ▪ Report IV site burning or stinging promptly. ▪ See Appendix D, p. 1311.

Maternal/Child: Avoid pregnancy. May produce teratogenic effects on the fetus. Effective contraceptive measures indicated during childbearing years. ▪ Discontinue breast-feeding before taking idarubicin. ▪ Safety and efficacy for use in pediatric patients not established but has been used; consult literature.

Elderly: Cardiotoxicity or myelotoxicity may be more severe. Patients over 60 years of age who were undergoing induction experienced CHF, serious arrhythmias, chest pain, myocardial infarction, and asymptomatic declines in left ventricular ejection fraction more frequently than younger patients. ▪ Monitor renal, hepatic, and hematologic functions closely.

DRUG/LAB INTERACTIONS

Bone marrow toxicity is additive with **other chemotherapeutic agents.** ▪ Risk of cardiotoxicity increased in patients previously treated with maximum cumulative doses of **other anthracyclines** (e.g., doxorubicin, mitoxantrone), **radiation encompassing the heart**, and/or **cardiotoxic drugs** (e.g., cyclophosphamide, paclitaxel, and trastuzumab). Due to the increased risk of cardiotoxicity, avoid concomitant use of idarubicin until the cardiotoxic agent has been discontinued for at least 5 half-lives, and specifically avoid idarubicin for up to 7 months after stopping trastuzumab. ■ Leukopenic and/or thrombocytopenic effects may be increased with **drugs that cause blood dyscrasias** (e.g., anticonvulsants [e.g., carbamazepine, phenytoin], NSAIDs [e.g., ibuprofen, naproxen]). Adjust dose based on differential and platelet count. ■ Do not administer **live virus vaccines** to patients receiving antineoplastic drugs. ■ See Precautions/Monitor.

SIDE EFFECTS

Acute CHF, alopecia (reversible), arrhythmias, bone marrow suppression (marked with average doses), cramping, decrease in systolic ejection fraction, depressed QRS voltage, diarrhea, erythema and tissue necrosis (if extravasation occurs), fever, headache, hemorrhage (severe), hepatic function changes, infection, mucositis, myocarditis, nausea, pericarditis, renal function changes, seizures, skin rash, urticaria (local), vomiting.

ANTIDOTE

Most side effects will be tolerated or treated symptomatically. Keep physician informed. Close monitoring of bone marrow, ECG, chest x-ray, echocardiography, and systolic ejection fraction may prevent most serious and potentially fatal side effects. There is no specific antidote, but adequate supportive care including platelet transfusions, antibiotics, and symptomatic treatment of mucositis is required. For extravasation, elevate the extremity and apply intermittent ice packs over the area immediately and 4 times a day for $\frac{1}{2}$ hour. Continue for 3 days. Consider aspiration of as much infiltrated drug as possible, flooding of the site with NS, and injection of hydrocortisone sodium succinate (Solu-Cortef) throughout extravasated tissue. Use a 27- or 25-gauge needle. Site should be observed promptly by a reconstructive surgeon. If ulceration begins or there is severe persistent pain at the site, early wide excision of the involved area will be considered. Hemodialysis or peritoneal dialysis probably not effective in overdose.

IDARUCIZUMAB

(**EYE**-da-roo-**KIZ**-ue-mab)

Praxbind

Antidote
Monoclonal antibody

pH 5.3 to 5.7

USUAL DOSE

5 Gm provided as two separate vials, each containing 2.5 Gm/50 mL. There are limited data to support administration of an additional 5-Gm dose of idarucizumab; see Precautions.

DOSE ADJUSTMENTS

No dose adjustment is required in renally impaired patients. ■ Formal studies in patients with hepatic impairment have not been conducted.

DILUTION

A colorless to slightly yellow, clear to slightly opalescent solution available as a 2.5 Gm/50 mL injection in a single-use vial. Administer undiluted by withdrawing and injecting the contents of 2 vials with a syringe or by hanging and infusing the contents of 2 vials.

Filter: Specific information not available.

Storage: Store unopened vials in the refrigerator at 2° to 8° C (36° to 46° F). Do not freeze. Do not shake. Before use, the unopened vial may be kept at RT 25° C (77° F) for up to 48 hours if stored in the original package to protect from light or up to 6 hours when exposed to light. Once solution has been removed from the vial, administration should begin promptly or within 1 hour.

COMPATIBILITY

Manufacturer states, "Do not mix with other medicinal products. A pre-existing IV line may be used for administration. The line must be flushed with NS prior to infusion. No other infusion should be administered in parallel via the same IV access."

RATE OF ADMINISTRATION

Administer by bolus injection by injecting both vials consecutively one after another via syringe. Infusion of the vial should take no more than 10 minutes, and the second vial should be given no later than 15 minutes after the first vial completes infusion. Alternatively, may administer as two rapid consecutive infusions by hanging and infusing each vial one after another. Flush IV line with NS before administration of idarucizumab.

ACTIONS

A recombinant humanized monoclonal antibody fragment (Fab); it is derived from an IgG1 isotype molecule whose target is the direct thrombin inhibitor dabigatran. Idarucizumab is a specific reversal agent for dabigatran. It binds to dabigatran and its acylglucuronide metabolites with a higher affinity than the binding affinity of dabigatran to thrombin, thereby neutralizing their anticoagulant effect. In studies, the plasma concentrations of unbound dabigatran were reduced to below the lower limit of quantification immediately after the administration of 5 Gm idarucizumab. Subjects' diluted thrombin time (dTT), ecarin clotting time (ECT), activated partial thromboplastin time (aPTT), thrombin time (TT), and activated clotting time (ACT) parameters returned to baseline levels. Idarucizumab is rapidly eliminated with an initial half-life of 47 minutes and a terminal half-life of 10.3 hours. Some drug is recovered in the urine. The remaining part of the dose is assumed to be eliminated, via protein catabolism, mainly in the kidney. Idarucizumab is thought to be metabolized via pathways that involve the biodegradation of the antibody to smaller peptides or amino acids, which are then reabsorbed and incorporated in the general protein synthesis.

INDICATIONS AND USES

Reversal of the anticoagulant effects of dabigatran (Pradaxa) when reversal is needed for emergency surgery/urgent procedures or in life-threatening or uncontrolled bleeding.

CONTRAINDICATIONS

Manufacturer states, "None."

PRECAUTIONS

For IV use only. ▪ Idarucizumab treatment should be used in conjunction with standard supportive measures. ▪ Reversing dabigatran therapy exposes patients to the thrombotic risk of their underlying disease. To reduce this risk, resumption of anticoagulant therapy should be considered as soon as medically appropriate. Dabigatran treatment can be initiated 24 hours after administration of idarucizumab. No changes in the pharmacokinetics or pharmacodynamics of dabigatran were noted upon reinitiation 24 hours after administration of idarucizumab. ▪ Elevated coagulation parameters (e.g., aPPT, ECT) have been observed between 12 and 24 hours after administration of a 5-Gm dose of idarucizumab in a limited number of patients. Administration of an additional 5-Gm dose of idarucizumab may be considered if the reappearance of clinically relevant bleeding together with elevated coagulation parameters are observed after administration of the initial dose. Similarly, patients who require a second emergency surgery/urgent procedure and have elevated coagulation parameters may receive an additional 5-Gm dose of idarucizumab. The safety and effectiveness of repeat treatment with idarucizumab have not been established. ▪ Adverse events possibly indicative of hypersensitivity reactions have been reported. The risk of using idarucizumab in a patient with known hypersensitivity to idarucizumab (e.g., anaphylactoid reaction) or to any of its excipients needs to be weighed cautiously against the potential benefit of such an emergency treatment. If an anaphylactic reaction or other serious reaction occurs, immediately discontinue administration of idarucizumab. ▪ The recommended dose of idarucizumab contains 4 Gm of sorbitol as an excipient. Patients with the condition of hereditary fructose intolerance (HFI) have experienced serious adverse reactions (e.g., acute liver failure, hypoglycemia, hypophosphatemia, increase in uric acid, metabolic acidosis) after receiving parenteral administration of sorbitol. When prescribing idarucizumab to patients with HFI, consider the combined daily metabolic load of sorbitol/fructose from all sources, including idarucizumab and other drugs containing sorbitol. The minimum amount of sorbitol at which serious adverse reactions may occur in these patients is not known. ■ Idarucizumab is a specific reversal agent for dabigatran, with no impact on the effect of other anticoagulant or antithrombotic therapies. ■ As with all proteins, there is a potential for immunogenicity with idarucizumab. Pre-existing antibodies with cross-reactivity to idarucizumab were detected in some subjects. No impact on the pharmacokinetics or the reversal effect of idarucizumab or on hypersensitivity reactions was observed in these subjects.

Monitor: Monitor coagulation parameters (e.g., aPPT and ECT [if available]). ■ Monitor for S/S of clinically relevant bleeding and thromboembolic events. ■ Monitor for S/S of hypersensitivity reactions (e.g., bronchospasm, fever, pruritus, rash).

Patient Education: Increased thromboembolic risk with reversal of dabigatran. Resume anticoagulant therapy as directed when deemed stable. ■ Seek immediate medical attention for any S/S of bleeding. ■ Seek immediate medical attention for S/S of a hypersensitivity reaction (e.g., rash, wheezing). Reactions may occur during or after administration of idarucizumab. ■ Inform patients with HFI that idarucizumab contains sorbitol. Adverse reactions related to the parenteral administration of sorbitol may occur during or after administration and should be promptly reported.

Maternal/Child: Data unavailable. Administer during pregnancy only if clearly needed. ■ Safety and effectiveness during labor and delivery have not been studied. ■ Use caution during breast-feeding; risk to infant unknown. ■ Safety and effectiveness for use in pediatric patients not established.

Elderly: No overall differences in safety or effectiveness have been observed between elderly patients and younger patients.

DRUG/LAB INTERACTIONS

Formal drug interaction studies have not been conducted. ■ In vitro data suggest that the inhibition of dabigatran by idarucizumab is not affected by coagulation factor concentrates (3-factor or 4-factor prothrombin complex concentrates [PCCs], activated PCC, or recombinant factor VIIa).

SIDE EFFECTS

The most frequently reported adverse reactions were constipation, headache, and nausea. Hypersensitivity reactions (e.g., bronchospasm, fever, hyperventilation, pruritus, and rash) and thromboembolic events have been reported. Most patients experiencing a thrombotic event were not on antithrombotic therapy at the time of the event.

ANTIDOTE

Notify physician of any side effects; most will be treated symptomatically. Discontinue administration at the first sign of a serious hypersensitivity reaction and treat as indicated (e.g., oxygen, diphenhydramine, epinephrine, corticosteroids, vasopressors, and/or fluids). Resuscitate as necessary.

IFOSFAMIDE BBW

(eye-**FOS**-fah-myd)

Antineoplastic
(alkylating agent/
nitrogen mustard)

Ifex

pH 6

USUAL DOSE

Pretreatment: Verify pregnancy status. Pretesting, baseline studies, and adequate hydration required; see Precautions and Monitor.

1.2 Gm/M^2/day for 5 consecutive days. Repeat every 3 weeks as hematologic recovery permits. To prevent hemorrhagic cystitis, ifosfamide should be given with extensive hydration (e.g., at least 2 liters of oral or IV fluid/day), and mesna should be administered with every dose; see Compatibility.

DOSE ADJUSTMENTS

Reduced dose may be required in renal or hepatic impairment. Adequate data not available. ▪ Dosing should be cautious in the elderly. Consider decrease in cardiac, hepatic, and renal function; concomitant disease; or other drug therapy. See Elderly. ▪ Severe myelosuppression is frequent, especially when ifosfamide is given with other chemotherapeutic agents. Dose adjustments of all agents may be required. Adjustment of dose interval may be required. Unless clinically essential, ifosfamide should be held for WBCs less than 2,000/mm^3 and/or platelets less than 50,000/mm^3. See Monitor and Drug/Lab Interactions.

DILUTION

Specific techniques required; see Precautions. Each 1 Gm must be diluted with 20 mL SWFI or bacteriostatic water for injection (parabens or benzyl alcohol-preserved only). 1 Gm in 20 mL or 3 Gm in 60 mL equals 50 mg/mL; shake solution to dissolve. May be further diluted with D5W, NS, LR, or SWFI to a final concentration of 0.6 to 20 mg/mL. Further dilution with D2½W, ½NS, and D5NS is also acceptable for larger volumes. 1 Gm in 50 mL equals 20 mg/mL; 1 Gm in 200 mL equals 5 mg/mL.

Filters: Studies measured potency of ifosfamide in combination with mesna through a 5-micron filter. No significant drug loss for ifosfamide; mesna was not measured.

Storage: Store at CRT 20° to 25° C (68° to 77° F). Protect from temperatures above 30° C (86° F). Reconstituted and further diluted solution should be refrigerated and used within 24 hours. Solutions containing benzyl alcohol can reduce stability.

COMPATIBILITY

Compatibility information not available from manufacturer. Other sources suggest specific **compatibilities** dependent on concentration and manufacturer; consult a pharmacist.

RATE OF ADMINISTRATION

A single dose over a minimum of 30 minutes as an infusion. Extend administration time based on amount of diluent and patient condition.

ACTIONS

An alkylating agent. Chemically related to the nitrogen mustards and a synthetic analog of cyclophosphamide. A prodrug that requires activation by hepatic cytochrome P450 isoenzymes to exert its cytotoxic activity. Exact mechanism of action not determined, but its cytotoxic action is primarily through DNA cross-links caused by alkylation by isophosphoramide mustard at guanine N7 positions. The formation of inter- and intra-strand cross-links in the DNA results in cell death. Distribution takes place with minimal tissue binding. Plasma protein binding is negligible. Extensively bound by red blood cells. Extensively metabolized in the liver (considerable individual variation). Elimination half-life for a usual dose is about 7 hours. Half-life is extended with larger doses. Ifosfamide and its metabolites are excreted in urine. Secreted in breast milk.

INDICATIONS AND USES

Used in combination with other specific antineoplastic agents for third-line chemotherapy of germ cell testicular cancer. Should be used in combination with mesna for prophylaxis of hemorrhagic cystitis.

Unlabeled uses: Bladder, cervical, and ovarian cancers; Ewing sarcoma; Hodgkin and non-Hodgkin lymphoma; osteosarcoma; soft tissue sarcomas.

CONTRAINDICATIONS

Hypersensitivity to ifosfamide; urinary outflow obstruction.

PRECAUTIONS

Follow guidelines for handling cytotoxic agents. See Appendix A, p. 1308. ▪ Usually administered by or under the direction of the physician specialist. ▪ Exclude or correct any urinary tract obstructions; see Contraindications. ▪ Myelosuppression can be severe and lead to fatal infections. Deaths have been reported. Risk of myelosuppression is dose-dependent and is increased in patients with reduced renal function and when ifosfamide is administered as a single high dose compared to fractionated doses. Severe myelosuppression is often observed when ifosfamide is used in combination with other chemotherapeutic/hematotoxic agents and/or radiation therapy. ▪ Administer cautiously, if at all, to patients with an infection (including an active urinary tract infection), severe immunosuppression, or compromised bone marrow reserve as indicated by leukopenia, granulocytopenia, extensive bone marrow metastases, prior radiation therapy, or prior treatment with other cytotoxic agents. ▪ CNS toxicities can be severe and result in encephalopathy and death. ▪ Nephrotoxic and urotoxic. Acute tubular necrosis, acute renal failure, and chronic renal failure have been reported, and deaths have occurred. Benefits must outweigh risks if ifosfamide is used in patients with pre-existing renal impairment or reduced nephron reserve. Glomerular and tubular disorders of renal function are common and may become apparent during therapy or months and years after stopping treatment. They may resolve, remain stable, or progress even after completion of treatment. Hemorrhagic cystitis can be severe and may require blood transfusions. Urotoxic effects can be reduced by the prophylactic use of mesna. Risk of hemorrhagic cystitis is dose-dependent and increases with the administration of single high doses compared to fractionated administration. Past or concomitant radiation of the bladder or busulfan therapy may also increase risk. ▪ Use caution in patients with risk factors for cardiotoxicity or pre-existing cardiac disease. Cardiotoxicity (e.g., supraventricular or ventricular arrhythmias, decreased QRS voltage and ST-segment or T-wave changes, toxic cardiomyopathy leading to heart failure with congestion and hypotension, pericardial effusion, fibrinous pericarditis, epicardial fibrosis), sometimes with fatal outcomes, has been reported. Risk is dose dependent and is increased with prior or concomitant treatment with other cardiotoxic agents or radiation of the cardiac region and, possibly, renal impairment. ▪ Pulmonary toxicity (e.g., interstitial pneumonitis, pulmonary fibrosis, and other forms of pulmonary toxicity) has been reported, sometimes with fatal outcomes. ▪ Hypersensitivity reactions, including anaphylaxis, have been reported. Cross-sensitivity between oxazaphosphorine cytotoxic agents (e.g., cyclophosphamide) has been reported. ▪ May interfere with normal wound healing. ▪ Risk of secondary malignancies is increased. ▪ Veno-occlusive liver disease has been reported. ▪ Studies in patients with hepatic or renal impairment have not been conducted. Use with caution.

Monitor: Monitor CBC with differential and platelet count before each daily dose and at intervals after each treatment cycle. Unless clinically essential, WBC count should be above $2,000/mm^3$ and platelet count above $50,000/mm^3$. ▪ Nadir of the leukocyte count tends to be reached during the second week after administration. ▪ Evaluate glomerular and tubular kidney function before, during, and after treatment. ▪ Monitor urinary sediment regularly for erythrocytes and other signs of urotoxicity/nephrotoxicity. ▪ Urinalysis before each dose is recommended. Withhold drug if RBCs in urine exceed 10 per high-powered field. Reinstitute after complete resolution with vigorous oral or parenteral hydration. Mesna given concurrently should help prevent hemorrhagic cystitis. ▪ Monitor serum and urine chemistries, including phosphorus and potassium, regularly; administer replacement as indicated. ▪ Monitor for S/S of renal dysfunction (e.g., decreased glomerular filtration rate, increased SCr, aminoaciduria, cylindruria, enzymuria, glycosuria, phosphaturia, proteinuria, and tubular acidosis). ▪ Adequate hydration required; encourage fluid intake (minimum of 2 L/day) and frequent voiding to prevent cystitis. ▪ Monitor for S/S of hypersensitivity (e.g., chest pain, dizziness, dyspnea, fever, flushing, hypotension, nausea, pruritus, rash, rigors, urticaria). ▪ Monitor for S/S of pulmonary toxicity and treat as indicated. ▪ Pneumonias as well as other bacterial, fungal, viral, and parasitic infections have been reported, and latent infections can be reactivated. Observe constantly for signs of infection (e.g., fever, sore throat, tiredness) or unusual bleeding or bruising. Antimicrobial prophylaxis may be indicated in certain cases of neutropenia. Antibiotics and/or antimycotics must be given if neutropenic fever occurs. ▪ Monitor for thrombocytopenia (platelet count less than 50,000/mm^3). Initiate precautions to prevent excessive bleeding (e.g., inspect IV sites, skin, and mucous membranes; use extreme care during invasive procedures; test urine, emesis, stool, and secretions for occult blood). ▪ Monitor for CNS toxicity. Blurred vision, coma, confusion, extrapyramidal symptoms, hallucinations, psychotic behavior, seizures, somnolence, and urinary incontinence have been reported. Peripheral neuropathy has also been reported. Neurotoxicity may appear within a few hours to a few days after the first administration and usually resolves within 48 to 72 hours of discontinuing ifosfamide, although symptoms may persist. Recurrence after several uneventful treatment courses has occurred. Discontinue treatment if encephalopathy occurs. ▪ Prophylactic administration of antiemetics recommended. ▪ See Drug/Lab Interactions.

Patient Education: Effective birth control recommended. Females should avoid pregnancy during therapy, and males should not father a child during therapy and for up to 6 months after the end of therapy. ▪ Interferes with oogenesis and spermatogenesis. May cause amenorrhea in females and oligospermia or azoospermia in males. Sterility has been reported. See Maternal/Child. ▪ Review medical history and medications with provider. ▪ Frequent laboratory monitoring required. ▪ CNS toxicity may impair the ability to operate an automobile or other heavy machinery. ▪ Adequate hydration (at least 2 L/day) and frequent voiding are required to help prevent bladder toxicity. ▪ Side effects are numerous and may be fatal; review all potential side effects with your health care professional before treatment. ▪ Promptly report any side effects, including S/S of infection, hypersensitivity reactions, GI toxicity, CNS toxicity, pulmonary toxicity, stomatitis, blood in urine, bleeding, bruising, or visual/auditory disorders. ▪ See Appendix D, p. 1311.

Maternal/Child: Can cause fetal harm. ▪ Discontinue breast-feeding. ▪ Safety and effectiveness for use in pediatric patients not established. Fanconi syndrome, renal rickets, and growth retardation have been reported in pediatric patients. Prepubescent females may become sterile or are at risk for developing premature menopause. Prepubescent males may not develop secondary sexual characteristics normally and may have oligospermia or azoospermia.

Elderly: Consider age-related organ impairment. Dose selection should be cautious; see Dose Adjustments. Monitor renal, hepatic, and hematologic functions closely.

DRUG/LAB INTERACTIONS

See Dose Adjustments. ▪ A substrate for both CYP3A4 and CYP2B6. **CYP3A4 inducers** (e.g., carbamazepine, phenytoin, phenobarbital, rifampin, and St. John's wort) may increase the metabolism of ifosfamide to its active alkylating metabolites and increase the formation of the neurotoxic/nephrotoxic metabolite chloroacetaldehyde. Monitor closely for signs of toxicity; consider dose adjustment. **CYP3A4 inhibitors** (e.g., aprepitant, fluconazole, grapefruit and grapefruit juice, itraconazole, ketoconazole, sorafenib) may decrease the metabolism of ifosfamide to its active alkylating metabolites, perhaps decreasing the effectiveness of treatment. ▪ May have additive effects with **other drugs that act on the CNS** (e.g., antihistamines, antiemetics, narcotics, or sedatives). Use with caution or discontinue if encephalopathy occurs. ▪ Do not administer **live virus vaccines** to patients receiving antineoplastic drugs.

SIDE EFFECTS

Hematuria, hemorrhagic cystitis, and bone marrow suppression are dose-limiting side effects. The most common side effects included alopecia, anemia, CNS toxicity (see Monitor), hematuria, infection, leukopenia, nausea, and vomiting. Other commonly reported side effects were anorexia, constipation, and diarrhea. Cardiotoxicity (e.g., arrhythmias, CHF, pulmonary edema), dermatitis, fever of unknown origin, hypersensitivity reactions, hypertension, hypotension, liver dysfunction, malaise, neutropenia and neutropenic fever, peripheral neuropathy, phlebitis, pulmonary symptoms, rash, renal dysfunction (e.g., acute renal failure; anuria; increased BUN, SCr; oliguria), stomatitis, or thrombocytopenia, may occur.

Overdose: Manifestations of dose-dependent toxicities such as CNS toxicity, mucositis, myelosuppression, nephrotoxicity.

Post-Marketing: Anaphylaxis; angioedema; benign and malignant neoplasms; hematotoxicity (e.g., agranulocytosis, bone marrow failure, DIC, febrile bone marrow aplasia, hemolytic anemia, hemolytic uremic syndrome, methemoglobinemia, neonatal anemia); infections, including reactivation of latent infections (e.g., herpes zoster, *Pneumocystis jiroveci,* progressive multifocal leukoencephalopathy [PML], *Strongyloides,* viral hepatitis, and other viral and fungal infections); pneumonia; sepsis and septic shock (including fatal outcomes); psychiatric disorders; syndrome of inappropriate antidiuretic hormone secretion (SIADH); tumor lysis syndrome; and numerous other serious side effects have been reported.

ANTIDOTE

Minor side effects will be treated symptomatically if necessary. Discontinue ifosfamide and notify physician immediately if hematuria, hemorrhagic cystitis, WBC below 2,000 mm^3, or platelets below 50,000/mm^3 occur. Administration of whole blood products (e.g., packed RBCs, platelets, leukocytes) and/or blood modifiers (e.g., darbepoetin alfa, epoetin alfa, filgrastim, pegfilgrastim, sargramostim) may be indicated to treat bone marrow suppression. Maintain supportive therapy for CNS symptoms until complete resolution; occasionally, recovery has been incomplete. Discontinue treatment if encephalopathy occurs. There is no specific antidote. Supportive therapy as indicated will help sustain the patient in toxicity. Cystitis prophylaxis with mesna may prevent or limit urotoxic effects. Ifosfamide and its metabolites are dialyzable.

IMETELSTAT
(IM e TEL stat)

**Antineoplastic Agent,
Telomerase Inhibitor**

Rytelo

USUAL DOSE
7.1 mg/kg IV once every 4 weeks; discontinue if patient does not experience a decrease in red blood cell (RBC) transfusion burden after 24 weeks (after 6 doses) or for unacceptable toxicity.

PEDIATRIC DOSE
Safety and efficacy have not been established.

DOSE ADJUSTMENTS
Renal: No dosage adjustments provided by manufacturer.

Hepatic: No dosage adjustments are provided in the manufacturer's labeling prior to treatment initiation.

Hepatotoxicity during treatment

Imetelstat Dosage Modifications for Elevated Liver Function Tetst			
Adverse reaction	**Severity**	**Occurrence**	**Imetelstat dosage modification**
Elevated LFTs	Grade 3 or 4	Third	Permanently discontinue imetelstat.
		First and Second	Delay infusion until recovery of adverse reaction to grade 1 or baseline then restart at one dose level lower.

DOSAGE ADJUSTMENTS FOR ADVERSE REACTIONS
Refer to manufacturer prescribing information.

RECONSTITUTION AND DILUTION
Reconstitution: Calculate dose required (based on the patient's body weight) to determine the number of vials needed. Remove vial(s) from the refrigerator and allow to sit for 10 to 15 minutes (not to exceed 30 minutes) to adjust to room temperature. Reconstitute the 47-mg vial with normal saline (NS) 1.8 mL, which gives a reconstituted concentration of 31.4 mg/mL and a deliverable volume of 1.5 mL. Reconstitute the 188-mg vial with NS 6.3 mL, which gives a reconstituted concentration of 31.4 mg/mL and a deliverable volume of 6 mL. Gently swirl each vial to avoid foaming (do not shake); swirl until the powder is fully reconstituted (not to exceed 15 minutes).

Dilution for infusion: Calculate the volume of reconstituted necessary for the appropriate dose. Withdraw a volume equal to the reconstituted solution volume from a 500-mL NS infusion bag and discard it. Add the required imetelstat volume to the bag so that the final volume is ~500 mL. Gently invert bag at least 5 times to ensure that the solution for infusion is well mixed; do not shake.

COMPATIBILITY
None listed in package insert; consult with hospital pharmacist.

RATE OF ADMINISTRATION
Infuse over 2 hours: Premedications with diphenhydramine and hydrocortisone are recommended to reduce or prevent infusion-related reactions. If infusion-related reactions occur, interruption of infusion, decreased infusion rate, and/or discontinuation may be required. Monitor for at least 1 hour after completion of infusion for adverse reactions.

ACTIONS
Imetelstat is a competitive inhibitor of enzymatic telomerase activity. Imetelstat targets cells with increased telomerase activity to selectively induce apoptosis of malignant cells. Imetelstat binds to the RNA component of human telomerase, inhibits telomerase enzymatic activity, and prevents telomere binding, leading to reduction of telomere length, reduction of malignant cell proliferation, and induction of apoptosis.

INDICATIONS AND USES
Myelodysplastic syndromes (MDS), low- to intermediate-1 risk.

CONTRAINDICATIONS
No contraindications listed by manufacturer.

PRECAUTIONS
Infusion-related reactions: The most common infusion-related reaction was headache. Infusion-related reactions usually occur during or shortly after the end of the infusion.

Neutropenia: Imetelstat may cause neutropenia.

Thrombocytopenia: Imetelstat may cause thrombocytopenia (based on laboratory values).

MONITORING PARAMETERS
Monitor complete blood cell counts before treatment initiation, weekly for the first 2 cycles, before each cycle, and as clinically indicated. Monitor RBC transfusion requirement. Monitor liver function tests before treatment initiation, weekly for the first cycle, before each cycle, and as clinically indicated. Verify pregnancy status before treatment initiation. Monitor patients with thrombocytopenia for bleeding. Monitor patients with Grade 3 or 4 neutropenia for infections. Monitor for adverse reactions for at least 1 hour after completion of the infusion.

Patient Education: Imetelstat (Rytelo) is used to treat types of MDS in certain people with anemia.

Call your doctor or get medical help if you are feeling tired or weak or are experiencing back, bone, joint, muscle, neck pain, or headaches that do not go away.

WARNING/CAUTION
Contact your doctor or get medical help immediately if you have any of the following signs or symptoms:
- Bleeding: for example, throwing up or coughing up blood; vomit that looks like coffee grounds; blood in the urine; black, red, or tarry stools; bleeding from the gums; abnormal vaginal bleeding; bruises without a cause or that get bigger; or bleeding you cannot stop.
- Infection: fever, chills, very bad sore throat, ear or sinus pain, cough, more sputum or change in color of sputum, pain with passing urine, mouth sores, or wounds that will not heal.
- Others: fainting or severe dizziness, fast or abnormal heartbeat.
- Infusion reactions, such as stomach pain; diarrhea; back, bone, or joint pain; tiredness or weakness; redness of the skin; headache; chest pain; itching; hives.
- Signs of an allergic reaction, such as rash; hives; itching; red, swollen, blistered, or peeling skin with or without fever; wheezing; tightness in the chest or throat; trouble breathing, swallowing, or talking; unusual hoarseness; or swelling of the mouth, face, lips, tongue, or throat.

Maternal/Child: *Reproductive considerations:* Verify pregnancy status before initiating treatment in patients who could become pregnant. Patients who could become pregnant should use effective contraception during therapy and for 1 week after the last dose of imetelstat.

Pregnancy considerations: Based on data from animal reproduction studies, in utero exposure to imetelstat may cause fetal harm; embryo-fetal mortality was observed in mice following IV doses ~2.5 times the human exposure.

Breast-feeding considerations: It is not known if imetelstat is present in breast milk.

Due to the potential for serious adverse reactions in the breastfed infant, breast-feeding is not recommended by the manufacturer during therapy and for 1 week after the last dose of imetelstat.

Elderly: No specific recommendations; refer to adult dosing.

DRUG/LAB INTERACTIONS
Avoid the following drugs: abrocitinib, baricitinib, BCG products, brivudine, chloramphenicol (systemic), cladribine, deucravacitinib, etrasimod, aexinidazole, filgotinib, live vaccines, nadofaragene firadenovec, natalizumab, pimecrolimus, ritlecitinib, ruxolitinib (topical), tacrolimus (topical), talimogene laherparepvec, tertomotide, tofacitinib, upadacitinib.

SIDE EFFECTS
Most common side effects include decreased neutrophils, platelets, and white blood cells; prolonged prothrombin time. Increased liver function tests, antibody development, fatigue, headache, arthralgia, and myalgias.

ANTIDOTE
There is no antidote; stop infusion for hypersensitivity reactions and treat appropriately.

IMIPENEM-CILASTATIN

(em-ee-**PEN**-em sigh-lah-**STAT**-in)

Primaxin

Antibacterial (carbapenem)

pH 6.5 to 8.5

USUAL DOSE

Range is from 500 mg to 1 Gm every 6 to 8 hours. The maximum total daily dosage should not exceed 4 Gm/day. Dosage is based on susceptibility of pathogens and CrCl. The dosage recommendations in the following chart represent the quantity of imipenem to be administered. An equivalent amount of cilastatin is also present in the solution.

Dosage of Primaxin in Adult Patients With Creatinine Clearance 90 mL/min or Greater	
Suspected or Proven Pathogen Susceptibility	**Dosage of Imipenem-Cilastatin**
Infection is suspected or proven to be due to a susceptible bacterial species	500 mg every 6 hours OR 1,000 mg every 8 hours
Infection is suspected or proven to be due to bacterial species with intermediate susceptibility	1,000 mg every 6 hours

PEDIATRIC DOSE

Not recommended for use in pediatric patients with CNS infections because of the risk of seizures, or in pediatric patients weighing less than 30 kg with impaired renal function (no data available). Do not exceed 4 Gm/24 hr.

Infants 3 months of age or less weighing 1,500 Gm or more: For non-CNS infections:

Less than 1 week of age: 25 mg/kg every 12 hours.

1 to 4 weeks of age: 25 mg/kg every 8 hours.

4 weeks to 3 months of age: 25 mg/kg every 6 hours.

Infants and other pediatric patients over 3 months of age: For non-CNS infections: 15 to 25 mg/kg/dose every 6 hours. See statements in Usual Dose.

Cystic fibrosis and normal renal function: Higher doses up to 100 mg/kg/day have been used. Do not exceed 4 Gm/24 hr.

DOSE ADJUSTMENTS

Dose adjustments are required in adult patients with a CrCl less than 90 mL/min as shown in the following chart.

Dosage of Imipenem-Cilastatin for Adult Patients in Various Renal Function Groups Based on Estimated Creatinine Clearance (CrCl)				
	Creatinine Clearance (mL/min)			
	≥90 mL/min	**≥60 to <90 mL/min**	**≥30 to <60 mL/min**	**≥15 to <30 mL/min**
Infection is suspected or proven to be due to a susceptible bacterial species	500 mg every 6 hours	400 mg every 6 hours	300 mg every 6 hours	200 mg every 6 hours
	OR			
	1,000 mg every 8 hours	500 mg every 6 hours	500 mg every 8 hours	500 mg every 12 hours
Infection is suspected or proven to be due to a bacterial species with intermediate susceptibility	1,000 mg every 6 hours	750 mg every 8 hours	500 mg every 6 hours	500 mg every 12 hours

■ Patients with a CrCl of 15 to less than 30 mL/min may be at increased risk for seizures. ■ Patients with a CrCl less than 15 mL/min should not receive imipenem-cilastatin unless hemodialysis is instituted within 48 hours. ■ For patients with a CrCl less than 15 mL/min who are undergoing dialysis, administer the dose listed for patients with a CrCl of 15 to less than 30 mL/min. Cleared by hemodialysis; administer after hemodialysis. ■ Reduced doses may be required in elderly patients based on decreased renal function. ■ See Precautions/Monitor and Drug/Lab Interactions.

DILUTION

Reconstitute each vial with 10 mL of **compatible** infusion solutions (e.g., D5W, NS, D5NS, D5/½NS, D5 ¼NS). Color of reconstituted solution ranges from colorless to yellow. Shake well and transfer the resulting suspension to 100 mL of the same infusion solution. Rinse vial with an additional 10 mL of infusion solution to ensure complete transfer of vial contents to the infusion solution. Agitate until clear.

Neonatal dilution: Use preservative-free solutions for reconstitution of neonatal doses.

Filters: Manufacturer's data limited; indicates that use of a filter system when withdrawing the suspension from the vial would probably result in filter clogging and decrease the available antibiotic. An in-house study documented **compatibility** of the final diluted solution with a 0.22-micron in-line filter.

Storage: Store dry powder below 25° C (77° F). Diluted solutions are stable at room temperature for 4 hours after preparation or 24 hours if refrigerated. Do not freeze.

COMPATIBILITY

Manufacturer states, "Do not mix with or physically add to other antibiotics." See Drug/Lab Interactions.

Other sources suggest specific **compatibilities** dependent on concentration and manufacturer; consult a pharmacist.

RATE OF ADMINISTRATION

Intermittent IV: Each 500 mg or fraction thereof over 20 to 30 minutes. Doses greater than 500 mg should be infused over 40 to 60 minutes. Slow infusion rate if patient develops nausea. May be given through Y-tube or three-way stopcock of infusion set.

ACTIONS

A potent broad-spectrum antibacterial agent. Imipenem is a carbapenem antibiotic; cilastatin inhibits the kidney enzyme responsible for the metabolism of imipenem. Both components are present in equal amounts. Bactericidal to many gram-negative, gram-positive, and anaerobic organisms. Bactericidal activity results from the inhibition of bacterial wall synthesis. Effective against many otherwise resistant organisms. Has a high degree of stability in the presence of beta-lactamases produced by gram-negative and gram-positive bacteria. Rapidly and widely distributed into many body fluids and tissues. Metabolized in the kidneys. Half-life is approximately 1 hour. Excreted in the urine. May cross the placental barrier.

INDICATIONS AND USES

Treatment of the following serious infections caused by designated susceptible bacteria: lower respiratory tract, urinary tract (complicated and uncomplicated), skin and skin structure, bone and joint, gynecologic, and intra-abdominal infections; bacterial septicemia; and endocarditis.

Limitation of use: Not indicated in patients with meningitis; safety and efficacy have not been established. ■ Not recommended in pediatric patients with CNS infections because of the risk of seizures. ■ Not recommended in pediatric patients under 30 kg with impaired renal function; data not available.

Unlabeled uses: Treatment of cystic fibrosis exacerbations, febrile neutropenia, and melioidosis (a rare infection in humans and animals).

CONTRAINDICATIONS

Known sensitivity to any component of this product. ■ See Maternal/Child and Precautions.

PRECAUTIONS

Specific sensitivity studies are indicated to determine susceptibility of the causative organism to imipenem-cilastatin. ■ To reduce the development of drug-resistant bacteria and maintain its effectiveness, imipenem-cilastatin should be used to treat only those infections proven or strongly suspected to be caused by bacteria. ■ Serious and occasionally fatal hypersensitivity reactions have been reported in patients receiving therapy with beta-lactams (e.g., carbapenems, cephalosporins, penicillins). More likely in patients with a history of sensitivity to multiple allergens; obtain a careful history. Cross-sensitivity is possible. ■ Avoid prolonged use of drug; superinfection caused by overgrowth of nonsusceptible organisms may result. ■ CNS adverse effects, including confusional states, myoclonic activity, and seizures, have been reported. Incidence increases with higher doses, compromised renal function, or pre-existing CNS disorders. ■ For patients on hemodialysis, especially those with underlying CNS disease, benefits of use must outweigh risk of seizures. ■ *Clostridium difficile*–associated diarrhea (CDAD) has been reported. May range from mild diarrhea to fatal colitis. Consider in patients who present with diarrhea during or after treatment with imipenem-cilastatin. ■ See Maternal/Child and Drug/Lab Interactions.

Monitor: May cause thrombophlebitis. Use small needles and large veins, and rotate infusion sites. ■ Electrolyte imbalance and cardiac irregularities resulting from sodium content are possible. Contains 3.2 mEq of sodium/Gm. ■ Monitor renal, hepatic, and hemopoietic systems in prolonged therapy. ■ See Drug/Lab Interactions.

Patient Education: Promptly report diarrhea or bloody stools that occur during treatment or up to several months after an antibiotic has been discontinued; may indicate CDAD and require treatment. ■ Patients with a history of seizures should review medication profile with physician before taking imipenem. ■ Promptly report S/S of hypersensitivity reactions. ■ See Drug/Lab Interactions.

Maternal/Child: Data from a small number of post-marketing cases with use in pregnancy are not sufficient to identify any drug-associated risks for major birth defects, miscarriage, or adverse maternal/fetal outcomes. ■ Insufficient data on the presence of imipenem/cilastatin in human milk, and no data on the effects on the breast-fed child or on the effects on milk production.

Elderly: Response similar to that seen in younger patients; however, greater sensitivity in the elderly cannot be ruled out. ■ Consider age-related renal impairment; see Dose Adjustments.

DRUG/LAB INTERACTIONS

Carbapenems may reduce serum **valproic acid** concentrations to subtherapeutic levels, resulting in loss of seizure control. Increasing the dose of valproic acid may not be sufficient to overcome this interaction. Concomitant use of imipenem and **valproic acid/divalproex sodium** is generally not recommended. Consider alternative antibacterial therapy. If administration of imipenem is necessary, supplemental anticonvulsant therapy should be considered. ▪ May be used concomitantly with **aminoglycosides and other antibiotics**, but these drugs must never be mixed in the same infusion or given concurrently. ▪ Use with **ganciclovir** may cause generalized seizures. Use only if benefit outweighs risk. ▪ Half-life and plasma levels slightly increased by **probenecid.** Avoid concurrent use. ▪ **Cyclosporine** may enhance the neurotoxic effect of imipenem. Imipenem may increase or decrease the serum concentration of cyclosporine.

SIDE EFFECTS

Adults: The most frequently occurring adverse reactions are diarrhea, dizziness, erythema or pain at injection site, fever, hypotension, nausea, phlebitis, pruritus, rash, seizures, somnolence, urticaria, vein induration, and vomiting.

Pediatric patients 3 months of age or older: The most frequently reported adverse reactions include diarrhea, gastroenteritis, IV site irritation, phlebitis, rash, urine discoloration, and vomiting.

Neonates: Convulsions, diarrhea, oliguria/anuria, oral candidiasis, rash, and tachycardia are the most frequently reported adverse reactions.

Reported serious adverse reactions include CDAD, seizures, and a full scope of hypersensitivity reactions, including anaphylaxis, pruritus, rash, and urticaria. Several other reactions have been reported in fewer than 0.2% of patients.

ANTIDOTE

Notify physician of any side effects. Discontinue the drug if indicated. Treat hypersensitivity reactions as indicated; may require epinephrine, airway management, oxygen, IV fluids, antihistamines (e.g., diphenhydramine), corticosteroids (e.g., hydrocortisone sodium succinate), and pressor amines (e.g., dopamine). Resuscitate as necessary. Begin anticonvulsants if focal tremors, myoclonus, or seizures occur. If symptoms continue, decrease dose or discontinue the drug. Infusion rate reactions may respond to a decrease in rate of infusion. Mild cases of CDAD may respond to discontinuation of the drug. Treat CDAD with fluids, electrolytes, protein supplements, and appropriate antibiotics (e.g., oral vancomycin) as indicated. In severe cases, surgical evaluation may be indicated. Both imipenem and cilastatin are removed by hemodialysis. Hemodialysis may be useful in overdose.

IMIPENEM, CILASTATIN, AND RELEBACTAM
(IM-i-**PEN**-em, **SYE**-la-**STAT**-in, and **REL**-e-**BAK**-tam)

Antibacterial (carbapenem, beta-lactamase inhibitor)

Recarbrio

pH 6.5 to 7.6

USUAL DOSE
Pretreatment: Baseline studies indicated; see Monitor.

Imipenem, cilastatin, and relebactam: 1.25 Gm (imipenem 500 mg, cilastatin 500 mg, relebactam 250 mg) every 6 hours as an IV infusion over 30 minutes. Duration of therapy is 4 to 14 days. Duration guided by the severity and location of infection and the patient's clinical response.

DOSE ADJUSTMENTS
Adjust dose in patients with CrCl less than 90 mL/min as outlined in the following chart.

Recommended Dosage of Imipenem, Cilastatin, and Relebactam for Patients With CrCl Less Than 90 mL/min		
Estimated CrCl (mL/min)[a]	**Recommended Dosage of Imipenem, Cilastatin, and Relebactam (mg)[b]**	**Dosing Interval**
60 to 89 mL/min	1 Gm (imipenem 400 mg, cilastatin 400 mg, and relebactam 200 mg)	q 6 hr
30 to 59 mL/min	0.75 Gm (imipenem 300 mg, cilastatin 300 mg, and relebactam 150 mg)	q 6 hr
15 to 29 mL/min	0.5 Gm (imipenem 200 mg, cilastatin 200 mg, and relebactam 100 mg)	q 6 hr
End-stage renal disease (ESRD) on hemodialysis[c]	0.5 Gm (imipenem 200 mg, cilastatin 200 mg, and relebactam 100 mg)	q 6 hr

[a]CrCl calculated using the Cockroft-Gault formula.
[b]Administer by IV over 30 minutes.
[c]Administration should be timed to follow hemodialysis.

■ Patients with a CrCl less than 15 mL/min should not receive imipenem, cilastatin, and relebactam unless hemodialysis is instituted within 48 hours. ■ There is inadequate information to recommend usage of imipenem, cilastatin, and relebactam in patients undergoing peritoneal dialysis. ■ Imipenem, cilastatin, and relebactam is removed from the circulation by hemodialysis. In hemodialysis patients, administer after hemodialysis and at intervals timed from the end of the dialysis session. ■ Reduced dose may be indicated in elderly patients; consider age-related impaired renal function and concomitant disease states. ■ No clinically significant differences in pharmacokinetics of imipenem, cilastatin, and relebactam were observed based on age, gender, or race.

DILUTION
Supplied as a dry white to light yellow sterile powder for reconstitution. Each single-dose vial contains 1.25 Gm (imipenem 500 mg, cilastatin 500 mg, and relebactam 250 mg). May be reconstituted and diluted with NS, D5W, D5NS, D5 ½NS, or D5 ¼NS. Imipenem, cilastatin, and relebactam has low aqueous solubility. To ensure complete dissolution, adhere to the following preparation instructions:

Step 1. For diluents available in 100-mL prefilled infusion bags, proceed to Step 2. For diluents not available in 100-mL prefilled infusion bags, withdraw 100 mL of the desired diluent and transfer it to an empty infusion bag, then proceed to Step 2.

Step 2. Withdraw 20 mL (as two 10-mL aliquots) of diluent from the appropriate infusion bag and reconstitute the vial with one 10-mL aliquot of the diluent. The reconstituted suspension must be further diluted.

Step 3. After reconstitution, shake vial well and transfer resulting suspension into the remaining 80 mL of the infusion bag.

Step 4. Add the second 10-mL aliquot of infusion diluent to the vial and shake well to ensure complete transfer of vial contents; repeat transfer of the resulting suspension to the infusion solution before administering. Agitate the resulting mixture until clear. Diluted solution color ranges from colorless to yellow.

For patients with renal impairment, prepare a reduced dose of imipenem, cilastatin, and relebactam by preparing a 100-mL solution containing 1.25 Gm and then withdrawing and discarding the excess volume as described in the following chart.

Preparation of Reduced Imipenem, Cilastatin, and Relebactam Doses for Intravenous Administration in Patients With Renal Impairment			
Creatinine Clearance (mL/min)	Dosage of Imipenem, Cilastatin, and Relebactam	After Preparation as Instructed Above, Remove From the 100-mL Prepared Bag the Volume Indicated Below and Discard	Resulting Volume That Provides the Indicated Reduced Dose
60 to 89 mL/min	1 Gm (imipenem 400 mg, cilastatin 400 mg, and relebactam 200 mg)	20 mL	80 mL
30 to 59 mL/min	0.75 Gm (imipenem 300 mg, cilastatin 300 mg, and relebactam 150 mg)	40 mL	60 mL
15 to 29 mL/min or ESRD on hemodialysis	0.5 Gm (imipenem 200 mg, cilastatin 200 mg, and relebactam 100 mg)	60 mL	40 mL

Filter: Data not available.

Storage: Store unopened vial in original carton at CRT. Infusion bag maintains satisfactory potency for at least 2 hours at RT (up to 30° C [86° F]) or for at least 24 hours under refrigeration at 2° to 8° C (36° to 46° F). *Do not freeze.* Discard any unused solution from the infusion bag.

COMPATIBILITY

The manufacturer states, "**Incompatible** with propofol in 5% dextrose USP or 0.9% sodium chloride USP." No other **compatibility** information provided; consult a pharmacist.

RATE OF ADMINISTRATION

A single dose as an infusion equally distributed over 30 minutes.

ACTIONS

An antibacterial combination product consisting of imipenem (a carbapenem antibacterial drug), cilastatin (a renal dehydropeptidase inhibitor), and relebactam (a diazabicyclooctane beta lactamase inhibitor). The bactericidal activity of imipenem results from binding to PBP 2 and PBP1 B in Enterobacteriaceae and *Pseudomonas aeruginosa* and the subsequent inhibition of penicillin-binding proteins (PBPs). Inhibition of PBPs leads to the disruption of bacterial cell wall synthesis. Cilastatin and relebactam do not have antibacterial activity. When administered alone, imipenem is metabolized in the kidneys by dehydropeptidase. Cilastatin, an inhibitor of this enzyme, effectively prevents renal metabolism of imipenem. Relebactam protects imipenem from degradation by certain serine beta-lactamases. Protein binding is approximately 20% for imipenem, 40% for cilastatin, and 22% for relebactam. Relebactam is minimally metabolized. All three components are excreted by the kidneys. The half-lives for imipenem and relebactam are 1 hour and 1.2 hours, respectively.

INDICATIONS AND USES

Treatment of complicated urinary tract infections (cUTIs), including pyelonephritis, caused by susceptible gram-negative microorganisms (*Enterobacter cloacae, Escherichia coli, Klebsiella aerogenes, Klebsiella pneumoniae,* and *Pseudomonas aeruginosa*) in patients 18 years of age or older who have limited or no alternative treatment options. ■ Treatment of complicated intra-abdominal infections (cIAIs) caused by susceptible gram-negative microorganisms (*Bacteroides caccae, Bacteroides fragilis, Bacteroides ovatus, Bacteroides stercoris, Bacteroides thetaiotaomicron, Bacteroides uniformis, Bacteroides vulgatus, Citrobacter freundii, Enterobacter cloacae, Escherichia coli, Fusobacterium nucleatum, Klebsiella aerogenes, Klebsiella oxytoca, Klebsiella pneumoniae, Parabacteroides distasonis,* and *Pseudomonas aeruginosa*) in patients 18 years of age or older who have limited or no alternative treatment options.

Approval of these indications is based on limited clinical safety and efficacy data.

CONTRAINDICATIONS
History of known severe hypersensitivity (severe systemic allergic reaction, such as anaphylaxis) to any component of imipenem, cilastatin, and relebactam.

PRECAUTIONS
Serious and occasionally fatal hypersensitivity (anaphylactic) reactions have been reported in patients receiving beta-lactam antibacterial drugs. Check history of previous hypersensitivity reactions to other carbapenems, penicillins, cephalosporins, other beta lactams, and other allergens. Cross-sensitivity among beta-lactam antibacterial drugs has been established. ▪ Specific sensitivity studies indicated to determine susceptibility of causative organism to imipenem, cilastatin, and relebactam. ▪ Cross-resistance with other classes of antibacterial drugs has not been identified; therefore, isolates resistant to other carbapenems, including imipenem, and to cephalosporins may be susceptible to imipenem, cilastatin, and relebactam. ▪ To reduce the development of drug-resistant bacteria and maintain its effectiveness, imipenem, cilastatin, and relebactam should be used to treat or prevent only those infections proven or strongly suspected to be caused by bacteria. ▪ CNS adverse reactions, such as seizures, confusional states, and myoclonic activity, have been reported during treatment with imipenem/cilastatin (a component of imipenem, cilastatin, and relebactam), especially when recommended dosages of imipenem were exceeded. These have been reported most commonly in patients with CNS disorders (e.g., brain lesions or history of seizures) and/or compromised renal function; see Dose Adjustments. Anticonvulsant therapy should be continued in patients with known seizure disorders. ▪ Concomitant use of imipenem, cilastatin, and relebactam with valproic acid or divalproex sodium may increase the risk of breakthrough seizures; see Drug/Lab Interactions. ▪ *Clostridium difficile*–associated diarrhea (CDAD) has been reported. May range from mild diarrhea to fatal colitis. Consider in patients who present with diarrhea during or after treatment with imipenem, cilastatin, and relebactam.

Monitor: Obtain baseline and periodic CBC and SCr. ▪ Monitor CrCl in patients with fluctuating renal function and adjust dosage accordingly; see Dose Adjustments. ▪ Monitor for S/S of a hypersensitivity reaction. ▪ Monitor for S/S of CNS adverse reactions. If CNS adverse reactions (including seizures) occur, patients should undergo a neurologic evaluation to determine whether imipenem, cilastatin, and relebactam should be discontinued.

Patient Education: Review list of allergies, medications, and medical conditions with provider. ▪ Promptly report any symptoms of hypersensitivity (e.g., difficulty breathing, hives, itching, rash) or neurologic symptoms (e.g., confusion, myoclonus, seizures).

- Promptly report diarrhea or bloody stools that occur during treatment or up to several months after an antibiotic has been discontinued; may indicate CDAD and require treatment.

Maternal/Child: Safety for use during pregnancy and breast-feeding have not been established; use caution. ■ Safety and efficacy for use in pediatric patients younger than 18 years of age have not been established.

Elderly: Consider age-related renal impairment; see Dose Adjustments.

DRUG/LAB INTERACTIONS

Generalized seizures have been reported in patients who received **ganciclovir** concomitantly with imipenem/cilastatin (components of imipenem, cilastatin, and relebactam). Avoid concomitant administration unless the potential benefits outweigh the risks. ■ Concomitant use of carbapenems, including imipenem/cilastatin (components of imipenem, cilastatin, and relebactam), with **valproic acid** or **divalproex sodium** may decrease valproic acid concentrations, which may increase the risk of breakthrough seizures. Avoid concomitant use with valproic acid or divalproex sodium. Consider alternative antibacterials other than carbapenems to treat infections in patients whose seizures are well controlled with valproic acid or divalproex sodium. ■ No clinically significant differences in the pharmacokinetics of imipenem or relebactam were observed when imipenem, cilastatin, and relebactam was used concomitantly with **probenecid**. ■ In vitro studies have demonstrated no antagonism between imipenem/relebactam and **amikacin, azithromycin, aztreonam, colistin, gentamicin, levofloxacin, linezolid, tigecycline, tobramycin,** or **vancomycin.**

SIDE EFFECTS

The most common adverse reactions include diarrhea, elevations in AST and ALT, fever, headache, hypertension, nausea, phlebitis/infusion site reactions, and vomiting. Other reported reactions included anemia, CDAD, CNS adverse reactions (agitation, apathy, confusional states, delirium, disorientation, slow speech, and somnolence), and increased lipase and serum creatinine.

ANTIDOTE

Notify physician of any side effects. Discontinue the drug if indicated. Treat hypersensitivity reaction as indicated. If CNS adverse reactions (including seizures) occur, patients should undergo a neurologic evaluation to determine whether imipenem, cilastatin, and relebactam should be discontinued. Mild cases of CDAD may respond to discontinuation of imipenem, cilastatin, and relebactam. Treat CDAD with fluids, electrolytes, protein supplements, and appropriate antibiotics (e.g., oral vancomycin) as indicated. In severe cases, surgical evaluation may be indicated. Imipenem, cilastatin, and relebactam is removed by hemodialysis.

IMMUNE GLOBULIN INTRAVENOUS BBW

Immunizing agent (passive)

(im-**MUNE GLAW**-byoo-lin IV)

Bivigam, Carimune NF, Flebogamma, Gammagard Liquid, Gammagard S/D, Gammaked, Gammaplex, Gamunex-C, IGIV, Octagam, Panzyga (IGIV-ifas), Privigen

pH 4 to 7.2

USUAL DOSE

Pretreatment: Baseline studies indicated; see Monitor.

For all indications, ensure adequate hydration before administration.

PRIMARY IMMUNODEFICIENCY (PID) DISEASES

Bivigam and Gammuplex: 300 to 800 mg/kg as a single-dose IV infusion every 3 to 4 weeks. Monitor clinical response and trough levels to adjust dose as appropriate. Desired trough level of total IgG concentrations is a minimum of 500 mg/dL (target is 600 mg/dL).

Carimune NF: 400 to 800 mg/kg as a single-dose IV infusion. Administer once every 3 to 4 weeks. Use of a 3% solution is recommended for the first infusion in previously untreated agammaglobulinemic or hypogammaglobulinemic patients. Subsequent infusions may be administered at a higher concentration based on patient tolerance.

Flebogamma, Gammagard Liquid, Gammagard S/D, Gammaked, Gamunex-C, Octagam 5%, and Panzyga: 300 to 600 mg/kg as a single-dose IV infusion every 3 to 4 weeks. Individualize dose and interval based on clinical response. If a patient receiving *Gammaked, Gamunex-C,* or *Octagam* is routinely receiving a dose of less than 400 mg/kg and is at risk for measles exposure (i.e., traveling to a measles endemic area), administer a dose of at least 400 mg/kg just before the expected measles exposure. If a patient is exposed to measles, administer a dose of 400 mg/kg as soon as possible after exposure.

Privigen: 200 to 800 mg/kg (2 to 8 mL/kg) as a single-dose IV infusion every 3 to 4 weeks. Adjust dose to achieve desired serum trough levels and clinical response.

IDIOPATHIC THROMBOCYTOPENIC PURPURA (ITP)

All products must be given by IV infusion for ITP patients. Do not administer SQ due to a potential risk of hematoma.

Carimune NF: 400 mg/kg/day for 2 to 5 consecutive days based on platelet count and clinical response. A 6% solution is recommended for use in ITP. May be discontinued in acute ITP of childhood if an initial platelet count response to the first 2 doses is adequate (30,000 to 50,000/mm^3). After induction, if clinically significant bleeding occurs and/or the platelet count falls below 30,000/mm^3, a maintenance dose of 400 mg/kg may be given as a single infusion. If response inadequate, increase to 800 to 1,000 mg/kg. May be given intermittently to maintain platelet count.

Flebogamma 10%: 1 Gm/kg/day for 2 consecutive days.

Gammagard S/D: 1 Gm/kg. Up to 3 doses can be given on alternate days based on clinical response and platelet count.

Gammaked and Gamunex-C: 1 Gm/kg/day (10 mL/kg/day) for 2 consecutive days for a total dose of 2 Gm/kg. May withhold the second 1 Gm/kg dose if an adequate platelet response is seen within 24 hours. Alternately, the 2 Gm/kg total dose can be administered as 400 mg/kg/day (4 mL/kg/day) for 5 consecutive days. The high-dose regimen (1 Gm/kg/day for 1 to 2 days) is not recommended for individuals with expanded fluid volumes or when fluid volume may be a concern.

Gammaplex, Octagam 10%, Privigen, and Panzyga: *Chronic ITP:* 1 Gm/kg/day for 2 consecutive days for a total dose of 2 Gm/kg.

B-CELL CHRONIC LYMPHOCYTIC LEUKEMIA (CLL)

Gammagard S/D: 400 mg/kg every 3 to 4 weeks.

CHRONIC INFLAMMATORY DEMYELINATING POLYNEUROPATHY (CIDP)

Gamunex-C and Gammaked: *Loading dose:* 1 Gm/kg/day (10 mL/kg/day) for 2 consecutive days or 0.5 Gm/kg/day (5 mL/kg/day) for 4 consecutive days. With either regimen, the total dose is 2 Gm/kg. Follow with *maintenance dose* of 1 Gm/kg every 3 weeks. The maintenance dose may be given as a total dose of 1 Gm/kg (10 mL/kg) on Day 1 or divided into 2 doses of 500 mg/kg/day given over 2 consecutive days.

Privigen: *Loading dose:* 2 Gm/kg (20 mL/kg) in divided doses over 2 to 5 consecutive days. Administer a *maintenance dose* of 1 Gm/kg (10 mL/kg) in 1 to 2 infusions on consecutive days every 3 weeks.

MULTIFOCAL MOTOR NEUROPATHY (MMN)

Gammagard Liquid: Dose range is 0.5 to 2.4 Gm/kg/month based on clinical response.

PEDIATRIC DOSE

KAWASAKI SYNDROME

Gammagard S/D: A single dose of 1 Gm/kg as an IV infusion. Alternately, 400 mg/kg/day may be administered for 4 consecutive days. Begin within 7 days of onset of fever. Concomitant administration of aspirin 80 to 100 mg/kg/day in 4 divided doses is indicated.

OTHER INDICATIONS

See specific product manufacturer prescribing information for age restrictions for other indications.

See mg/kg or Gm/kg dose recommendations under Usual Dose. Begin with the lowest recommended dose. With most brands, clinical studies suggested that no difference in dosing is necessary and no special precautions are indicated. According to the manufacturers, infants and neonates were not included in clinical studies for primary immunodeficiency diseases or Kawasaki disease. All age-groups were represented in clinical studies for ITP. See Maternal/Child.

DOSE ADJUSTMENTS

Adjust dose according to IgG levels and clinical response. Frequency and dose will vary from patient to patient. No controlled clinical trials are available to determine optimum trough serum IgG level.

DILUTION

Requirements for dilution of liquid and lyophilized powder preparations are brand specific and vary considerably; see manufacturer's package insert. Some may be further diluted only with D5W or with D5W and/or NS; others cannot be diluted. Some require D5W or NS to flush the infusion line.

All formulations: Do not mix with IGIV products from other manufacturers. Do not mix with other medicinal products. Administer through a separate infusion line or flush line before and after administration. Do not use if solution is cloudy, turbid, or contains particulate matter. Do not freeze. Do not use if previously frozen. Do not use beyond expiration date. For single use only; use promptly or discard unused product. Bring to room temperature before reconstitution (if required) or administration.

Most formulations: *Do not shake.* If large doses are to be administered, several vials may be pooled using aseptic technique (time limits or specific processes may apply); see specific product.

Bivigam, Flebogamma, Gamunex-C, Gammagard Liquid, Gammaked, Gammaplex, Octagam, Panzyga, and *Privigen* are liquid preparations and are ready to use.

Carimune NF is a lyophilized product, *and Gammagard S/D* is a freeze-dried product. Both require reconstitution. Absolute sterile technique is required at all steps of the reconstitution process. Filtration may be required as drawn into a syringe for administration or as administered through IV tubing. Check both brands for specific equipment and specific dilution requirements.

Bivigam: A ready-to-use 10% sterile solution; do not dilute. Available as 5 Gm in 50 mL or 10 Gm in 100 mL. Does not contain sucrose. Warm to room temperature before use and maintain at room temperature during administration. *Do not shake.* Several vials may be pooled using aseptic technique into sterile infusion bags and infused. pH 4 to 4.6.

Carimune NF: Contains sucrose; see Precautions. Available as a lyophilized powder in 3-, 6-, and 12-Gm vials. Reconstitute with NS, D5W, or SWFI. Package insert has a chart with dilution requirements for all concentrations. *Do not shake.* Immediate use is recommended unless reconstituted under a sterile laminar flow hood; then it may be refrigerated and administration must begin within 24 hours. Several reconstituted vials of identical concentration and diluent may be pooled in an empty sterile glass or plastic IV infusion container using aseptic technique. pH 6.4 to 6.8. A 6% solution of *Carimune NF* is recommended for use in ITP.

Flebogamma: Contains sorbitol; does not contain sucrose. A ready-to-use 5% (50 mg/mL) sterile solution; available as 0.5 Gm in 10 mL, 2.5 Gm in 50 mL, 5 Gm in 100 mL, 10 Gm in 200 mL, and 20 Gm in 400 mL. Also available as a ready-to-use 10% (100 mg/mL) sterile solution of 5 Gm in 50 mL, 10 Gm in 100 mL, and 20 Gm in 200 mL concentrations. Further dilution with other solutions not recommended. Using aseptic technique, several vials may be pooled into an empty sterile solution container. See Filters. pH 5 to 6.

Gammagard Liquid: Does not contain sucrose. A ready-to-use 10% solution available as 1 Gm in 10 mL, 2.5 Gm in 25 mL, 5 Gm in 50 mL, 10 Gm in 100 mL, and 20 Gm in 200 mL. Warm to room temperature before use. *Do not shake.* May be further diluted only with D5W. See Filters. pH 4.6 to 5.1.

Gammagard S/D: Does not contain sucrose. A freeze-dried preparation. Must be warmed to room temperature before reconstitution if refrigerated. Diluent (SWFI), transfer device, administration set with integral airway, and filter provided with each single-use vial. Available in 2.5-, 5-, and 10-Gm single-dose vials with diluent. Use full amount of diluent (50, 96, 192 mL) to prepare a 5% solution (50 mg/mL), or remove one-half the amount of diluent (25, 48, 96 mL) to prepare a 10% solution (100 mg/mL). *Do not shake.* Must be used within 2 hours of dilution if prepared outside a laminar flow hood. Administer within 24 hours if prepared aseptically inside a sterile laminar flow hood and stored in the original glass container or pooled into ViaFlex bags under constant refrigeration. Record date and time of reconstitution/pooling. pH 6.4 to 7.2.

Gammaked: Does not contain sucrose. A ready-to-use 10% solution. Available as 1 Gm in 10 mL, 2.5 Gm in 25 mL, 5 Gm in 50 mL, 10 Gm in 100 mL, and 20 Gm in 200 mL. Bring to room temperature before administration if refrigerated. Use an 18-gauge needle or dispensing pin to penetrate the stopper of the 10-mL vial. Use 16-gauge needles or dispensing pins for the 25 mL and larger sizes. May be further diluted with D5W if required. Do not use any other diluent. *Do not shake.* Content of vials may be pooled under aseptic conditions into sterile infusion bags but must be infused within 8 hours of pooling. pH is 4 to 4.5.

Gammaplex: Does not contain sucrose but does contain fructose; see Contraindications. A ready-to-use 5% sterile solution. Available as 2.5 Gm in 50 mL, 5 Gm in 100 mL, and 10 Gm in 200 mL. *Do not shake.* Begin infusion within 2 hours if multiple vials are pooled under aseptic conditions. Bring to room temperature before administration if refrigerated. pH 4.8 to 5.1.

Gamunex-C: Does not contain sucrose. A ready-to-use 10% sterile solution. Available in 1-, 2.5-, 5-, 10-, and 20-Gm single-dose vials. Bring to room temperature before administration if refrigerated. Use an 18-gauge needle to penctrate the stopper of the 1-Gm size. Use a 16-gauge needle to penetrate the stopper of the 2.5- to 20-Gm sizes. Penetration of the stopper in the center of the raised ring and perpendicular to it is recommended. May be further diluted with D5W if required. Do not use any other diluent. Filtration during administration is not required. Use within 8 hours if multiple vials are pooled under aseptic conditions. pH 4 to 4.5.

Octagam: Does not contain sucrose but does contain maltose; see Contraindications. A ready-to-use 5% or 10% sterile solution. The 5% solution is available as 1-, 2.5-, 5-, 10-, and 25-Gm single-dose vials. The 10% solution is available as 2- 5-, 10-, and 20-Gm single-dose vials. *Do not shake.* Use within 8 hours if multiple vials are pooled under aseptic conditions. Bring to room temperature before administration if refrigerated. pH 5.1 to 6 (5%); pH 4.5 to 5 (10%).

Panzyga: Does not contain sucrose. A ready-to-use 10% sterile solution. Available in 1-, 2.5-, 5-, 10-, 20-, and 30-Gm single-dose vials. Use within 8 hours if multiple vials are pooled under aseptic conditions. pH 4.5 to 5.

Privigen: Does not contain sucrose but does contain L-proline; see Contraindications. A ready-to-use 10% sterile solution. Available in 5-, 10-, 20-, and 40-Gm single-dose vials. *Do not shake.* May be further diluted with D5W if required. Do not use any other diluent. Filtration during administration is not required. Content of vials may be pooled under aseptic conditions into sterile infusion bags, but infusion should begin within 8 hours of pooling; contains no preservatives. pH 4.6 to 5.

Filters: Filter or filter needle is provided by most manufacturers. *Carimune NF and Flebogamma* may be filtered with a larger-pore filter size but is not required by manufacturers (filters greater than or equal to 15 microns will be less likely to slow infusion [0.2-micron antibacterial filters may be used with *Carimune NF, Flebogamma, and Octagam*]). *Carimune NF* is nano-filtered. Filtration of *Gamunex-C* during administration is not required; however, use of a non–protein-binding, 0.22-micron filter is permissible. Use of an in-line filter is optional with *Gammagard Liquid and Octagam. Panzyga* does not require filtration; however, it may be filtered with a filter size of 0.2 to 200 microns.

Storage: Storage requirements are brand specific and vary considerably from refrigeration-only to continuous or partial storage at RT not exceeding 30° C (77° F); see manufacturer's package insert. Do not use after expiration date. Discard partially used vials. Do not use if solution is turbid or has been frozen. Some specifically state, "Do not heat or microwave."

COMPATIBILITY

Manufacturers recommend administration through a separate IV line without admixture with other drugs and state, "Do not combine one IGIV product with an IGIV product from another manufacturer." *Gammagard Liquid, Gammaked, Gamunex-C, and Privigen* are **compatible** only with D5W and are **incompatible** with NS. *Flebogamma and Octagam* should not be further diluted with any solution.

Most preparations may be infused sequentially into a primary IV of D5W or NS, or the tubing may be flushed with D5W or NS before and after administration.

Other sources suggest a few specific **compatibilities** dependent on concentration and manufacturer; consult a pharmacist.

RATE OF ADMINISTRATION

All formulations: Too-rapid infusion may cause a precipitous hypotensive reaction. Decrease rate of infusion at onset of patient discomfort or any adverse reactions; see Antidote. Decrease rate in patients at risk for neuromuscular disorders. See Precautions and individual products for suggested decrease in rates for patients at risk for thrombosis or developing renal dysfunction. Administer via separate IV tubing with filter or filter needle (provided by most manufacturers if required). Do not mix with IGIV products from other manufacturers or with other drugs or IV solutions. An infusion pump will facilitate an accurate rate of administration.

Bivigam: Does not contain sucrose. 0.5 mg/kg/min for the first 10 minutes. If no discomfort or adverse effects, may be increased every 20 minutes by 0.8 mg/kg/min up to 6 mg/kg/min. In patients at risk for thrombosis or developing renal dysfunction, administer at the minimum dose and rate of infusion that is practicable.

Carimune NF: Contains sucrose; see Precautions. An initial infusion rate of 0.5 mg/kg/min for 30 minutes. May then be increased to 1 mg/kg/min for the next 30 minutes. May be gradually increased in steps up to a maximum of 3 mg/kg/min as tolerated. The first dose in previously untreated agammaglobulinemic or hypogammaglobulinemic patients must be a 3% solution. After the first dose, subsequent infusions may be administered at a higher concentration as tolerated; see Precautions. In patients at risk for thrombosis or developing renal dysfunction, administer at the minimum dose; the maximum rate of infusion should not exceed 2 mg/kg/min.

Flebogamma: Does not contain sucrose. In patients at risk for thrombosis or developing renal dysfunction, administer at the minimum dose and rate of infusion that is practicable.

Primary immunodeficiency (PI): Initiate 5% solution at 0.01 mL/kg/min (0.5 mg/kg/min) for the first 30 minutes. If no discomfort or adverse effects, may be gradually increased to a maximum rate of 0.1 mL/kg/min (5 mg/kg/min).

Primary immunodeficiency (PI) and idiopathic thrombocytopenic purpura (ITP): Initiate 10% solution at 0.01 mL/kg/min (1 mg/kg/min) for the first 30 minutes. If no discomfort or adverse effects, may be gradually increased to a maximum rate of 0.08 mL/kg/min (8 mg/kg/min).

Gammagard Liquid: Does not contain sucrose. In patients at risk for developing renal dysfunction or thrombotic episodes, the maximum infusion rate should be less than 3.3 mg/kg/min (less than 2 mL/kg/hr).

Primary immunodeficiency (PI): 0.5 mL/kg/hr (0.8 mg/kg/min) for the first 30 minutes. If no discomfort or adverse effects, may be gradually increased every 30 minutes to a maximum rate of 5 mL/kg/hr (8 mg/kg/min).

Multifocal motor neuropathy (MMN): 0.5 mL/kg/hr. (0.8 mg/kg/min) for the first 30 minutes. If no discomfort or adverse effects, may be gradually increased every 30 minutes to a maximum rate of 5.4 mL/kg/hr (9 mg/kg/min).

Gammagard S/D: Does not contain sucrose. 5% solution at 0.5 mL/kg/hr. May be gradually increased to a maximum rate of 4 mL/kg/hr if no discomfort or adverse effects. If 5% solution well tolerated at 4 mL/kg/hr, a 10% solution can be used. Begin with 0.5 mL/kg/hr. If no adverse effects, gradually increase up to a maximum of 8 mL/kg/hr. In patients at risk for developing renal dysfunction, the concentration and infusion rate should be less than 3.3 mg/kg/min (less than 2 mL/kg/hr of 10% or less than 4 mL/kg/hr of 5%).

Gammaked: Does not contain sucrose. In patients at risk for thrombosis or developing renal dysfunction, administer at the minimum dose and rate of infusion that is practicable.

PI and ITP: 1 mg/kg/min (0.01 mL/kg/min). If the infusion is well tolerated, the rate may be gradually increased to a maximum of 8 mg/kg/min (0.08 mL/kg/min).

Chronic inflammatory demyelinating polyneuropathy (CDIP): 2 mg/kg/min (0.02 mL/kg/min). If the infusion is well tolerated, the rate may be gradually increased to a maximum of 8 mg/kg/min (0.08 mL/kg/min).

Gammaplex: Does not contain sucrose. 0.5 mg/kg/min (0.01 mL/kg/min) for the first 15 minutes. If no discomfort or adverse effects, may be gradually increased every 15 minutes to 4 mg/kg/min (0.08 mL/kg/min). In patients at risk for thrombosis or developing renal dysfunction, administer at the minimum dose and rate of infusion that is practicable.

Gamunex-C: Does not contain sucrose. In patients at risk for thrombosis or developing renal dysfunction, administer at the minimum dose and rate of infusion that is practicable.

Primary immunodeficiency (PI) and idiopathic thrombocytopenic purpura (ITP): 1 mg/kg/min (0.01 mL/kg/min) for the first 30 minutes. If no discomfort or adverse effects, may be gradually increased to a maximum rate of 8 mg/kg/min (0.08 mL/kg/min).

Chronic inflammatory demyelinating polyneuropathy (CIDP): 2 mg/kg/min (0.02 mL/kg/min). If no discomfort or adverse effects, may be gradually increased to a maximum rate of 8 mg/kg/min (0.08 mL/kg/min).

Octagam: Does not contain sucrose; does contain maltose. In patients at risk for thrombosis or developing renal dysfunction, administer at the minimum dose and rate of infusion that is practicable.

Primary immunodeficiency (PI): Initiate 5% solution at 0.5 mg/kg/min for the first 30 minutes. If no discomfort or adverse effects, may increase gradually in 30-minute increments to a maximum rate of 3.33 mg/kg/min.

Idiopathic thrombocytopenic purpura (ITP): Initiate 10% solution at 1 mg/kg/min for the first 30 minutes. If no discomfort or adverse effects, may increase gradually in 30-minute increments to a maximum rate of 12 mg/kg/min.

Panzyga: Does not contain sucrose. In patients at risk for thrombosis or for developing renal dysfunction, administer at the minimum dose and rate of infusion that is practicable.

Primary immunodeficiency (PI) and idiopathic thrombocytopenic purpura (ITP): An initial infusion rate of 1 mg/kg/min (0.01 mL/kg/min) is recommended. If no discomfort or adverse effects, may be gradually increased to a maximum rate of 8 mg/kg/min (0.08 mL/kg/min). In patients with ***primary immunodeficiency*** who have received 3 to

6 infusions, the rate may be increased to 12 or 14 mg/kg/min (0.12 or 0.14 mL/kg/min) as tolerated.

Privigen: Does not contain sucrose. IV line may be flushed with D5W or NS. In patients at risk for thrombosis or developing renal dysfunction, administer at the minimum dose and rate of infusion that is practicable.

Primary immunodeficiency: 0.5 mg/kg/min (0.005 mL/kg/min) initially. If no discomfort or adverse effects, may be gradually increased to a maximum rate of 8 mg/kg/min (0.08 mL/kg/min).

Chronic immune thrombocytopenic purpura: 0.5 mg/kg/min (0.005 mL/kg/min) initially. If no discomfort or adverse effects, may be gradually increased to a maximum rate of 4 mg/kg/min (0.04 mL/kg/min).

Chronic inflammatory demyelinating polyneuropathy: 0.5 mg/kg/min (0.005 mL/mg/min) initially. If no discomfort or adverse effects, may be gradually increased to a maximum rate of 8 mg/kg/min (0.08 mL/kg/min).

ACTIONS

A preparation of concentrated human immunoglobulin G (IgG) antibodies. Obtained, purified, and standardized from human plasma. Specific methods during the manufacturing process (e.g., cold ethanol fractionation, detergents, solvents, nanofiltration) inactivate blood-borne viruses (e.g., hepatitis, HIV). Used as replacement therapy in primary and secondary immunodeficiencies. Active against bacterial, viral, parasitic, and mycoplasma antigens. Capable of both opsonization and neutralization of microbes and toxins. Also contains antibodies capable of interacting with and altering the activity of the immune system as well as antibodies capable of reacting with cells such as erythrocytes. (The role of these antibodies and the mechanisms of action of IgG have not been fully clarified.) Provides immediate antibody levels following infusion. The immediate peak in serum IgG is followed by a rapid decay due to equilibration between the plasma and extravascular fluid compartments. Half-life is variable (approximately 3 to 6 weeks) but may be decreased by fever or infection (increased catabolism or consumption). Crosses the placenta.

INDICATIONS AND USES

Selected products are approved for different uses; see Usual Dose. All provide rapid-onset, short-term passive immunization. Labeled uses include: **Primary immunodeficiency diseases:** Replacement therapy in adults, adolescents, and other pediatric patients unable to produce adequate amounts of IgG antibodies, especially in the following situations: need for immediate increase in intravascular immunoglobulin levels, small muscle mass or bleeding tendencies that contraindicate IM injection, and selected disease states (e.g., congenital agammaglobulinemia, common variable immunodeficiency [CVID], combined immunodeficiency, X-linked agammaglobulinemia, Wiskott-Aldrich syndrome). ▪ **Treatment of acute and chronic idiopathic thrombocytopenic purpura (also called immune thrombocytopenic purpura or primary immune thrombocytopenia):** Temporary increase in platelet counts in patients with idiopathic thrombocytopenic purpura and with thrombocytopenia associated with bone marrow transplant. ▪ **Treatment of chronic inflammatory demyelinating polyneuropathy (CIDP):** Improvement of neuromuscular disability and impairment and maintenance therapy to prevent relapse. ▪ **Adjunct in chronic lymphocytic leukemia:** Prevention of bacterial infections in patients with hypogammaglobulinemia or recurrent bacterial infection associated with B-cell CLL. ▪ **Multifocal motor neuropathy (MMN):** To improve muscle strength and disability in adult patients. ▪ **Kawasaki syndrome:** Prevention of coronary artery aneurysms associated with Kawasaki syndrome. ▪ Safety and effectiveness of **Gammagard S/D, Gammaplex, Octagam 10%, and Panzyga** for use in pediatric patients with chronic ITP have **not** been established; see Maternal/Child for additional limitations with other products. ▪ Several formulations are approved for SQ use in specific diagnoses; consult prescribing information.

Unlabeled uses: There are numerous unlabeled uses; consult literature.

CONTRAINDICATIONS

Individuals known to have anaphylactic or severe hypersensitivity responses to the administration of human immune globulin. ■ IgA-deficient patients with pre-existing anti-IgA antibodies and a history of hypersensitivity. ■ *Gammaplex* is contraindicated in patients with hereditary intolerance to fructose; also contraindicated in infants and neonates for whom sucrose or fructose tolerance has *not* been established. ■ *Octagam* is contraindicated in patients with acute hypersensitivity to corn (contains maltose, which is derived from corn). ■ *Privigen* is contraindicated in patients with hyperprolinemia because it contains L-proline as a stabilizer.

PRECAUTIONS

Check label; must state, "For IV use." ■ Some formulations may be given SQ; however, all products must be given by IV infusion for ITP patients. Do not administer SQ due to a potential risk for hematoma. ■ Hypersensitivity reactions have occurred; administer in a facility with adequate equipment and supplies to monitor the patient and respond to any medical emergency. ■ Use extreme caution in individuals with a history of prior systemic hypersensitivity reactions. Incidence of anaphylaxis may be increased, especially with repeated injections. IgA-deficient patients, especially those with antibodies against IgA, are at greater risk for developing severe hypersensitivity reactions. ■ Some packaging of these products may contain latex; use caution in sensitive individuals. ■ IGIV products have been associated with renal dysfunction, acute renal failure, osmotic nephrosis, and death. Use extreme caution in patients with any degree of renal insufficiency; in patients age 65 years and older; in patients with diabetes mellitus, paraproteinemia, sepsis, or volume depletion; and/or in patients receiving known nephrotoxic drugs. If used, should be administered at the minimum dose and rate of infusion practicable. **Products containing sucrose as a stabilizer (e.g., Carimune NF) have demonstrated an increased risk for renal dysfunction.** Consider benefit versus risk before use. ■ Increases in SCr and/or BUN may progress to oliguria and anuria requiring dialysis; however, some patients improve spontaneously with discontinuation of IGIV. ■ May cause aseptic meningitis syndrome (AMS), especially with high doses (greater than 1 Gm/kg) and/or rapid infusion. May begin from 2 hours to 2 days after treatment. Symptoms are drowsiness, fever, headache (severe), nausea and vomiting, nuchal rigidity, painful eye movements, and photophobia. Cerebrospinal fluid (CSF) studies are often positive with pleocytosis, predominantly from the granulocyte series and elevated protein levels. ■ Hyperproteinemia, with resultant changes in serum viscosity, and electrolyte imbalances (e.g., hyponatremia) may occur. Distinguish true hyponatremia from pseudohyponatremia to determine correct treatment. Decreasing serum-free water in patients with pseudohyponatremia may lead to volume depletion with a further increase in serum viscosity, which may predispose to thromboembolic events. ■ IGIV products have been associated with thrombotic events. Risk factors may include advanced age, prolonged immobilization, hypercoagulable conditions, history of venous or arterial thrombosis, use of estrogens, indwelling vascular catheter, hyperviscosity, and cardiovascular risk factors (e.g., cerebrovascular disease, coronary artery disease, diabetes, hypertension). Thrombosis may occur in the absence of known risk factors. If used, should be administered at the minimum dose and rate of infusion practicable. Ensure adequate hydration before administration. ■ Baseline assessment of blood viscosity should be made in patients at risk for hyperviscosity, including those with cryoglobins, fasting chylomicronemia, markedly high triglycerides, or monoclonal gammopathies. ■ May rarely cause hemolysis, which can result in hemolytic anemia due to enhanced RBC sequestration. High doses (greater than 2 Gm/kg) and non-O blood group may be risk factors for hemolysis. Cases of severe hemolysis-related renal dysfunction/failure or DIC have occurred following infusion; see Monitor. ■ Consider risk/benefit before use of high-dose regimens (greater than 1 Gm/kg) in chronic ITP patients at increased risk for acute kidney injury, hemolysis, thrombosis, or volume overload. ■ Hypertension, including hypertensive urgency, has been observed during and/or shortly after infusion. Patients with a history of hypertension may be at greater risk. Elevated BP may resolve within hours of infusion without therapy or may require adjustment in oral antihypertensive medicines. ■ Noncardiogenic pulmonary edema (transfusion-related acute lung injury [TRALI]) has been reported; see Monitor. ▪ Derived from human blood. Despite purification processes, may carry risk of transmitting infectious agents (e.g., viruses [e.g., HIV, hepatitis] or Creutzfeldt-Jakob disease [CJD] agent). ▪ Patients with gammaglobulinemia or extreme hypogammaglobulinemia who have never before received immunoglobulin substitution treatment or patients whose time from the last treatment is greater than 8 weeks may be at risk for developing inflammatory reactions (e.g., chills, fever, nausea, vomiting) on rapid infusion. Initiate slowly and increase rate as tolerated.

Monitor: Use of larger veins recommended to reduce infusion-site discomfort, especially with 10% solutions. ▪ Correct volume depletion before administration in all patients, especially patients with pre-existing renal insufficiency. ▪ Recording of lot number on vials is recommended. ▪ Monitor vital signs and observe patient continuously during infusion. A precipitous drop in BP or anaphylaxis can occur at any time. Emergency equipment and supplies must be at bedside. ▪ Monitor renal function (e.g., BUN, SCr) and urine output in patients at increased risk for renal failure. Obtain baseline studies, monitor at intervals, and discontinue IGIV if renal function deteriorates. See Precautions. ▪ Monitor for hyperproteinemia with resultant changes in serum viscosity and electrolyte imbalances. ▪ Monitor for S/S of thrombosis and assess blood viscosity in patients at risk for hyperviscosity. ▪ Monitor for S/S of hemolysis (e.g., lysis of red blood cells, liberation of hemoglobin), significant drop in hemoglobin or hematocrit, and hemolytic anemia. ▪ Monitor for S/S of TRALI (e.g., fever, hypoxemia, normal left ventricular function, pulmonary edema, severe respiratory distress). Usually occurs within 1 to 6 hours after completion of the infusion. Manage with oxygen and adequate ventilatory support. If TRALI is suspected, both the product and the patient serum should be tested for the presence of antineutrophil antibodies. ▪ Monitor for volume overload.

Patient Education: Report chills, cyanosis, diaphoresis, dyspnea, faintness or light-headedness, fatigue, fever, headache, hives, itching or rash, neck pain or difficulty moving neck, tachycardia, wheezing. ▪ Report chest pain or tightness, pain and/or swelling of an arm or a leg with warmth over the affected area, difficulty passing urine, decreased urine output, fluid retention, edema, shortness of breath, or sudden weight gain. ▪ Remote risk of viral or CJD infection; consider risk versus benefit of therapy. See Drug/Lab Interactions.

Maternal/Child: Category C: use with caution in pregnancy; no adverse effects documented, but adequate studies are not available. ▪ Safety for use in breast-feeding not established. ▪ Response in pediatric patients usually exceeds response in adults. ▪ Safety and effectiveness of *Gammagard S/D* for use in pediatric patients with chronic ITP have not been established. ▪ Safety and effectiveness of *Gammagard S/D* for use in Kawasaki disease have been established. ▪ Use of *Privigen* to treat primary immunodeficiency in pediatric patients under 3 years of age or to treat chronic immune thrombocytopenic purpura in pediatric patients under 15 years of age not established. ▪ Safety and effectiveness of *Privigen* have not been established in pediatric patients with CIPD who are under 18 years of age. ▪ Safety and effectiveness of *Bivigam* for use in pediatric patients under 6 years of age not established. ▪ Safety and effectiveness of *Flebogamma 5% and 10%, Gammaplex, and Panzyga* for use in pediatric patients under 2 years of age have not been established. ▪ Safety and effectiveness of *Octagam 10%* for use in pediatric patients have not been established. ▪ Safety and effectiveness of *Gammagard Liquid* for treatment of PI in pediatric patients under 2 years of age have not been established. ▪ Safety and effectiveness of *Panzyga* for use in pediatric patients with chronic ITP have not been established. ▪ Safety and effectiveness for use in pediatric patients with MMN have not been established. ▪ Safety and effectiveness of *Gammaked* and *Gamunex-C* for use in pediatric patients with CIDP have not been established.

Elderly: Use with extreme caution. Incidence of renal insufficiency, thrombosis, and other side effects increased due to age, potential for decreased organ function, and pre-existing medical conditions. Do not exceed recommended dose, and infuse at the minimum infusion rate practicable; see Precautions.

DRUG/LAB INTERACTIONS

Do not administer **live virus vaccines** from 2 weeks before to at least 3 months after immune globulin IV. Passive transfer of antibodies may transiently interfere with the response to live virus vaccines, such as measles, mumps, rubella, and varicella; see prescribing information if there is a risk of measles exposure or if accidental exposure has occurred. ▪ Provides immediate antibody levels that last for about 3 weeks. In selected patients, may have an immune-modulating effect that may alter their response to **corticosteroids or antineoplastic agents.** ▪ Concurrent use with **nephrotoxic drugs** (e.g., aminoglycosides, amphotericin B, cidofovir, rifampin) may increase risk of renal insufficiency. ▪ Products that contain **maltose** *(Octagam)* may interfere with blood and urine glucose tests. ▪ Various antibody titers may be raised temporarily, resulting in **false-positive serologic testing.** ▪ May cause a positive **direct or indirect antiglobulin (Coombs') test.**

SIDE EFFECTS

Arthralgia, asthenia, back pain, chills, diarrhea, dizziness, fatigue, fever, flushing, headache, hyperhidrosis, hypertension, infusion site pain/reactions, lethargy, nausea and vomiting, pharyngitis, rash, sinusitis, upper abdominal pain, and urticaria were reported most commonly. Full range of hypersensitivity symptoms, including anaphylaxis, is possible. Angioedema, erythema, fever, and urticaria are most frequently observed. Anxiety, chest tightness, cough, decreased diastolic BP, difficulty breathing, elevated ALT and AST (temporary), hemolytic anemia (reversible), increased BUN and SCr (may occur as soon as 1 to 2 days following infusion), leg cramps, light headedness, malaise, migraine, myalgia, pharyngolaryngeal pain, and tachycardia have been reported. Severe reactions (e.g., circulatory collapse, fever, loss of consciousness, nausea and vomiting, sudden onset of dyspnea) have occurred and are more common in patients with antibody deficiencies. Noncardiogenic pulmonary edema (transfusion-related acute lung injury [TRALI]) has been reported. Acute renal failure, acute tubular necrosis, osmotic nephrosis, and proximal tubular nephropathy have been reported; may result in death. Made from human plasma; process attempts to eliminate risk of hepatitis or HIV infection. A precipitous hypotensive reaction can occur and is most frequently associated with too-rapid rate of injection. Aseptic meningitis syndrome and hemolysis occur infrequently. See Precautions.

Post-Marketing: Abdominal pain, apnea, ARDS, back pain, bronchospasm, bullous dermatitis, cardiac arrest, coma, cyanosis, dyspnea, epidermolysis, erythema multiforme, hepatic dysfunction, hypotension, hypoxemia, leukopenia, loss of consciousness, pancytopenia, positive direct antiglobulin (Coombs') test, pulmonary edema, seizures, Stevens-Johnson syndrome, thromboembolism, and tremor have been reported with IGIV products.

ANTIDOTE

Reduce rate for patient discomfort, for any sign of adverse reaction, and in patients at risk for renal insufficiency or thrombosis. If symptoms subside promptly, the infusion may be resumed at a lower rate. Decreasing the volume of subsequent infusions may also prevent or decrease the incidence of adverse reactions. Loop diuretics (e.g., furosemide [Lasix]) may be helpful in the management of fluid overload. Patients who continue to experience adverse reactions after rate and/or volume have been reduced may be premedicated with hydrocortisone 1 to 2 mg/kg 30 minutes before the immune globulin infusion. Pretreatment with acetaminophen and diphenhydramine or trying a different brand of immune globulin may also be useful. Discontinue the drug immediately for any signs of a hypersensitivity reaction, thrombotic event, or renal insufficiency. Notify the physician. May be treated symptomatically and infusion resumed at slower rate if symptoms subside. Treat anaphylaxis immediately. Epinephrine, diphenhydramine, oxygen, vasopressors (e.g., dopamine), corticosteroids, and ventilation equipment must always be available. Manage TRALI with oxygen and ventilatory support. Resuscitate as necessary.

INDOMETHACIN SODIUM
(in-doh-**METH**-ah-sin **SO**-dee-um)

Prostaglandin inhibitor
(patent ductus arteriosus adjunct)

Indocin IV

pH 6 to 7.5

USUAL DOSE
Pretreatment: Confirmation of diagnosis indicated; see Precautions.

Neonates: Three IV doses, specific to age at first dose, given at 12- to 24-hour intervals constitute a course of therapy.

Less than 48 hours of age: First dose (0.2 mg/kg of body weight), second dose (0.1 mg/kg), third dose (0.1 mg/kg).

2 to 7 days of age: 0.2 mg/kg for each of 3 doses.

Over 7 days of age: First dose (0.2 mg/kg), then 0.25 mg/kg for the next 2 doses.

If ductus arteriosus reopens, a second course of 1 to 3 doses as described for each neonate age may be repeated one time given at 12- to 24-hour intervals. If neonate remains unresponsive to indomethacin therapy after 2 courses, surgery may be required for closure of the ductus arteriosus.

DOSE ADJUSTMENTS
If urine output is less than 0.6 mL/kg/hr at any time a dose is to be given, withhold dose until lab studies confirm normal renal function.

DILUTION
Each 1 mg must be diluted with at least 1 mL NS or SWFI without preservatives (0.1 mg/0.1 mL); may be diluted with 2 mL diluent (0.05 mg/0.1 mL). The preservative benzyl alcohol is toxic in neonates. A fresh solution should be prepared just before each administration. Discard any unused portion.

Filters: No data available from manufacturer.

Storage: Store unopened vials in carton at CRT. Protect from light. Use reconstituted solution immediately.

COMPATIBILITY
Manufacturer states, "Prepare only with preservative-free NS or SWFI"; further dilution with IV solutions is not recommended and may precipitate with solutions with a pH below 6.

Other sources suggest a few specific **compatibilities** dependent on concentration and manufacturer; consult a pharmacist.

RATE OF ADMINISTRATION
A single dose, properly diluted, by IV injection over 20 to 30 minutes.

ACTIONS
A potent inhibitor of prostaglandin synthesis. Through an unconfirmed method of action (thought to be inhibition of prostaglandin synthesis), it causes closure of a patent ductus arteriosus (PDA) 75% to 80% of the time, eliminating the need for surgical intervention. Plasma half-life varies inversely with postnatal age and weight and ranges from 12 to 20 hours. Metabolized in the liver and eventually excreted in urine and bile.

INDICATIONS AND USES
Closure of a hemodynamically significant (PDA) in premature infants weighing between 500 and 1,750 Gm if usual medical management (e.g., fluid restriction, diuretics, digoxin, respiratory support) has not been effective after 48 hours.

CONTRAINDICATIONS
Bleeding, especially active intracranial hemorrhage or GI bleeding; coagulation defects; necrotizing enterocolitis; infants with congenital heart disease (e.g., pulmonary atresia, severe coarctation of the aorta, severe tetralogy of Fallot) who require patency of the ductus arteriosus for satisfactory pulmonary or systemic blood flow; proven or suspected untreated infection; significant renal impairment; thrombocytopenia.

PRECAUTIONS

Clinical evidence of a hemodynamically significant (PDA) (respiratory distress, a continuous murmur, a hyperactive precordium, cardiomegaly and pulmonary plethora on chest x-ray) should be present before use is considered. ▪ For use only in a highly supervised setting such as an intensive care nursery. ▪ May increase potential for GI or intraventricular bleeding. ▪ Use caution in presence of existing controlled infection; may mask signs and symptoms of exacerbation. ▪ May suppress water excretion to a greater extent than sodium excretion. Hyponatremia may result. ▪ For IV use only. ▪ Surgery indicated if condition is not responsive to two courses of therapy.

Monitor: Vital signs, oxygenation, acid-base status, fluid and electrolyte balance, and kidney function (SCr, BUN, urine output) must be monitored and maintained. ▪ Can cause marked reduction in urine output (over 50%), increased BUN and SCr, and reduced glomerular filtration rate and CrCl. These symptoms usually disappear when therapy is completed but may cause acute renal failure, especially in infants with impaired renal function from other causes. ▪ May inhibit platelet aggregation; monitor for signs of bleeding. ▪ Discontinue drug if signs of impaired liver function appear. ▪ Confirm absolute patency of vein. Avoid extravasation; will irritate tissue. ▪ See Drug/Lab Interactions.

DRUG/LAB INTERACTIONS

May reduce elimination and increase serum concentrations of **drugs that are renally excreted** (e.g., aminoglycosides, digoxin). Monitor drug levels and adjust doses as needed to avoid toxicity. ▪ Observe neonate closely for signs of **digoxin toxicity;** frequent monitoring of ECG and digoxin serum levels is indicated. ▪ Use with **furosemide** may help to maintain renal function. ▪ Concomitant use with **anticoagulants** may increase risk of bleeding; monitoring of PT suggested. ▪ Coadministration with **ACE inhibitors** (e.g., enalapril) may result in deterioration of renal function, including renal failure.

SIDE EFFECTS

Abdominal distension; acidosis; alkalosis; apnea; bleeding into the GI tract (gross or microscopic); bradycardia; DIC; elevated BUN or creatinine; exacerbation of preexisting pulmonary infection; fluid retention; gastric perforation; hyperkalemia; hypoglycemia; hyponatremia; intracranial bleeding; necrotizing enterocolitis; oliguria; oozing from needle puncture sites; pulmonary hemorrhage; pulmonary hypertension; reduced urine sodium, chloride, potassium, urine osmolality, free water clearance, or glomerular filtration rate; renal failure; retrolental fibroplasia; thrombocytopenia; transient ileus; uremia; vomiting.

ANTIDOTE

Discontinue the drug and notify the physician of all side effects. Based on severity, side effects may be treated symptomatically or drug will be completely discontinued in favor of surgical intervention. Resuscitate as necessary.

INFLIXIMAB BBW ▪ INFLIXIMAB-dyyb[a] BBW ▪ INFLIXIMAB-abda[a] BBW ▪ INFLIXIMAB-axxq[a] BBW ▪ INFLIXIMAB-qbtx[a] BBW

(in-**FLIX**-ih-mab)

Remicade, Inflectra[a], Renflexis[a], Ixifi[a], Avsola[a]

Monoclonal antibody
Inflammatory bowel disease agent
Antirheumatic agent
TNF-blocking agent

pH 7.2 (Avsola, Inflectra, and Remicade) ▪
pH 6.2 (Renflexis) ▪ pH 6 (Ixifi)

USUAL DOSE

Infliximab-dyyb (Inflectra)[a], infliximab-abda (Renflexis)[a], infliximab-qbtx (Ixifi)[a], and infliximab-axxq (Avsola)[a] are biosimilar drugs to infliximab (Remicade). Unless specifically stated otherwise, the use of the name infliximab or infliximab product(s) applies to all formulations.

Pretreatment: Patients should be tested for latent tuberculosis before infliximab use and periodically during therapy. Treatment for latent infection should be initiated before infliximab therapy. Patients should be tested for hepatitis B virus before infliximab use. See Precautions and Monitor.

Premedication: Administer at the physician's discretion. May include antihistamines (e.g., diphenhydramine), H_2 blockers (e.g., famotidine), acetaminophen, and/or corticosteroids (e.g., hydrocortisone).

Crohn's disease and fistulizing Crohn's disease: Begin with an initial dose of 5 mg/kg as an IV infusion. Repeat at 2 and 6 weeks and every 8 weeks thereafter. For patients who respond and then lose their response, consideration may be given to treatment with 10 mg/kg. If there is no response by Week 14, response with continued dosing is unlikely; consider discontinuing infliximab. See Precautions.

Rheumatoid arthritis: 3 mg/kg as an IV infusion. Repeat dose at 2 and 6 weeks, then every 8 weeks thereafter. Given in combination with methotrexate. See methotrexate monograph. If response to infliximab is incomplete, dose may be adjusted up to 10 mg/kg or interval decreased to every 4 weeks. Risk of infection may be increased at higher doses.

Ankylosing spondylitis: 5 mg/kg as an IV infusion. Repeat at 2 and 6 weeks, then every 6 weeks thereafter.

Psoriatic arthritis: 5 mg/kg as an IV infusion. Repeat dose at 2 and 6 weeks, then every 8 weeks thereafter. May be used with or without methotrexate.

Ulcerative colitis: 5 mg/kg as an IV infusion. Repeat dose at 2 and 6 weeks, then every 8 weeks thereafter.

Plaque psoriasis: 5 mg/kg as an IV infusion. Repeat dose at 2 and 6 weeks, then every 8 weeks thereafter.

PEDIATRIC DOSE

Pretreatment: See comments in Usual Dose and Maternal/Child.

Crohn's disease: 5 mg/kg as an IV infusion. Repeat dose at 2 and 6 weeks. Follow with a maintenance regimen of 5 mg/kg every 8 weeks.

Ulcerative colitis: 5 mg/kg as an IV infusion. Repeat dose at 2 and 6 weeks. Follow with a maintenance regimen of 5 mg/kg every 8 weeks.

DOSE ADJUSTMENTS

Do not exceed a dose of 5 mg/kg in patients with moderate to severe congestive heart failure (CHF) (NYHA Class III/IV); see Contraindications.

DILUTION

Each vial contains 100 mg of infliximab. When reconstituted as directed below, each milliliter of solution contains 10 mg of infliximab. Calculate the dose and the number of vials required and the total volume of reconstituted infliximab solution required. Reconstitute each 100-mg vial with 10 mL of SWFI, using a syringe equipped with a 21-gauge

---

[a]Please see p. xi for more information on biosimilars.

or smaller needle. Direct the stream of SWFI to side of vial. Swirl gently; do not shake. Allow reconstituted solution to stand for 5 minutes. Solutions of *Remicade, Avsola, Inflectra,* and *Renflexis* should be colorless to light yellow and opalescent. *Ixifi* should be colorless to light brown and opalescent. All products may develop a few translucent particles, as infliximab is a protein. Do not use if opaque particles, discoloration, or other foreign particles are present. The total dose of reconstituted solution must be further diluted with NS to a final volume of 250 mL. (May withdraw a volume of NS equal to the calculated volume of reconstituted infliximab from a 250-mL bottle or bag of NS and slowly add reconstituted solution.) Do not dilute the reconstituted infliximab solution with any other diluent. Mix gently. Infusion concentration should range between 0.4 mg/mL and 4 mg/mL.

Filters: Must be administered through an infusion set with an in-line, sterile, non-pyrogenic, low-protein binding filter (pore size equal to or less than 1.2 microns). Flush and prime tubing/filter system with NS before administration of infusion.

Storage: Refrigerate unopened vials at 2° to 8° C (36° to 46° F). Protect Avsola from light. Discard any unused portion. Do not use beyond expiration date on vial. The infusion should begin within 3 hours of reconstitution and dilution. *Remicade, Avsola, and Ixifi:* Unopened vials may also be stored at temperatures up to a maximum of 30° C (86° F) for a single period of up to 6 months but not exceeding the original expiration date. The new expiration date must be written on the carton. Upon removal from refrigerated storage, **Remicade, Avsola, and Ixifi** cannot be returned to refrigerated storage.

COMPATIBILITY

Manufacturer recommends not infusing concomitantly in the same IV line with other agents until specific **compatibility** data are available.

RATE OF ADMINISTRATION

Begin the infusion within 3 hours of reconstitution and dilution. Flush and prime tubing/filter system with NS before administration. A single dose should be given over a period of not less than 2 hours. Upon completion of infusion, IV line should be flushed thoroughly with NS to ensure all active drug is delivered to the patient. Patients experiencing a mild to moderate infusion-related reaction may be able to continue therapy at a reduced rate; see Antidote.

ACTIONS

A chimeric IgG1κ monoclonal antibody that binds specifically to human tumor necrosis factor alpha (TNFα). Is composed of human constant and murine variable regions. Produced by a recombinant cell line cultured by continuous perfusion and purified by a series of steps that include measures to inactivate and remove viruses. Neutralizes the biologic activity of TNFα by binding with high affinity to the soluble and transmembrane forms of TNFα and inhibiting binding of TNFα with its receptors. Infliximab does not neutralize TNFβ. Biologic activities attributed to TNFα include induction of pro-inflammatory cytokines such as IL-1 and IL-6, enhancement of leukocyte migration by increasing endothelial layer permeability and expression of adhesion molecules by endothelial cells and leukocytes, activation of neutrophil and eosinophil functional activity, and induction of acute-phase reactants and other liver proteins as well as tissue-degrading enzymes produced by synoviocytes and/or chondrocytes. Elevated concentrations of TNFα have been found in involved tissues and fluids of patients with Crohn disease, rheumatoid arthritis, ankylosing spondylitis, ulcerative colitis, psoriatic arthritis, and plaque psoriasis. These elevated concentrations correlate with elevated disease activity. Treatment with infliximab blocks the biological activities attributed to TNFα. Infliximab is distributed predominantly within the vascular space. Has a prolonged terminal half-life of 7.7 to 9.5 days.

INDICATIONS AND USES

Adult and pediatric patients 6 years of age and older: Reduce the S/S and induce and maintain clinical remission in patients with moderately to severely active Crohn's disease who have had an inadequate response to conventional therapy. ▪ Reduce the S/S and induce and maintain clinical remission and mucosal healing, and eliminate corticosteroid use in patients with moderately to severely active ulcerative colitis who have had an inadequate response to conventional therapy; see Maternal/Child.

Adult patients: Reduce the number of draining enterocutaneous and rectovaginal fistula(s) and maintain fistula closure in fistulizing Crohn's disease. ▪ Given in combination with methotrexate to improve physical function, inhibit progression of structural damage, and reduce S/S in patients with moderately to severely active rheumatoid arthritis. ▪ Reduce S/S in active ankylosing spondylitis. ▪ Reduce the S/S of active arthritis, inhibit progression of structural damage, and improve physical function in patients with psoriatic arthritis. ▪ Used for treatment of patients with chronic severe (i.e., extensive and/or disabling) plaque psoriasis who are candidates for systemic treatment and when other systemic treatments are less appropriate.

CONTRAINDICATIONS

Known hypersensitivity to infliximab, murine proteins, or other components of the product. ▪ Administration of doses exceeding 5 mg/kg in patients with moderate to severe (NYHA Class III/IV) CHF.

PRECAUTIONS

Administer in a facility that is equipped to monitor the patient and respond to any medical emergency. ▪ TNFα mediates inflammation and modulates cellular immune response. Anti-TNF therapies, including infliximab, may affect normal immune responses. ▪ Patients treated with infliximab are at increased risk for developing serious infections that may lead to hospitalization or death. Many of the serious infections have occurred in patients undergoing concomitant immunosuppressive therapy (e.g., methotrexate, corticosteroids) that, in addition to their underlying disease, may predispose them to infections; see Drug/Lab Interactions. Discontinue infliximab if patient experiences a serious infection or sepsis. Reported infections with TNF-blockers include active tuberculosis, including reactivation of latent tuberculosis; invasive fungal infections (e.g., histoplasmosis, coccidioidomycosis, cryptococcus, candidiasis, aspergillosis, blastomycosis, and pneumocystosis); and bacterial, viral, parasitic, and other infections due to opportunistic pathogens, including *Legionella, Listeria,* and *Salmonella.* ▪ Patients with TB have frequently presented with disseminated or extrapulmonary disease. ▪ Cases of tuberculosis reactivation or new tuberculosis infections have been observed in patients receiving infliximab, including patients who have previously received treatment for latent or active tuberculosis. Cases of active tuberculosis have also occurred in patients being treated with infliximab during treatment for latent tuberculosis. ▪ Antituberculosis treatment of patients with a reactive TB skin test reduces the risk of TB reactivation in patients receiving infliximab. ▪ Patients with histoplasmosis or other invasive fungal infections may present with disseminated rather than localized disease. Antigen and antibody testing for histoplasmosis may be negative. ▪ Treatment with infliximab should not be initiated in patients with an active infection, including clinically important localized infections. Consider the risks and benefits of infliximab treatment before initiating therapy in patients with chronic or recurrent infection, patients who have been exposed to TB, patients with a history of an opportunistic infection, patients who have resided in or traveled to areas of endemic tuberculosis or endemic mycoses (e.g., histoplasmosis, coccidioidomycosis, or blastomycosis), or patients with underlying conditions that may predispose them to infection. ▪ Has been associated with the reactivation of hepatitis B virus (HBV) in patients who are chronic hepatitis B carriers (i.e., surface antigen–positive). Fatalities have been reported. ▪ Infliximab therapy has been associated with adverse outcomes in patients with heart failure and should be used in these patients only after consideration of other treatment options. Studies suggest a higher mortality in patients who receive 10 mg/kg and higher rates of cardiovascular adverse events at doses of 5 mg/kg and 10 mg/kg. Do not use doses greater than 5 mg/kg in patients with moderate to severe CHF; see Contraindications. Discontinue for new-onset CHF or for worsening CHF. Use with caution in patients with mild CHF (NYHA Class I/II); monitor closely. ▪ Hypersensitivity reactions characterized by urticaria, dyspnea, and/or hypotension have occurred in association with infliximab infusion. Most occur during or within 2 hours of the infusion. Discontinue infusion if severe reactions occur. Medications for management of hypersensitivity reaction (e.g., acetaminophen, diphenhydramine, corticosteroids [e.g., hydrocortisone] and/or epinephrine) should be readily available. ▪ Serum sickness-like reactions (dysphagia, fever, hand and facial edema, headache, myalgias, polyarthralgias, rash, sore throat) have been reported and have occurred as early as after the second dose and when infliximab was interrupted and then re-initiated after an extended period. These reactions are associated with a marked increase in antibodies to infliximab, a loss of detectable serum concentrations of infliximab, and a possible loss of drug efficacy. ▪ Readministration of infliximab after a period of no treatment resulted in a higher incidence of infusion reactions relative to regular maintenance treatment in clinical trials. Evaluate risk versus benefit of readministration after a period of no treatment, especially if considering a re-induction regimen given at 0, 2, and 6 weeks. For cases in which maintenance therapy for psoriasis has been interrupted, infliximab should be re-initiated with a single dose followed by maintenance therapy. ▪ Serious cerebrovascular accidents, myocardial ischemia/infarction (some fatal), hypotension, hypertension, and arrhythmias have been reported during and within 24 hours of initiation of infliximab infusion. Transient vision loss has been reported during or within 2 hours of initiation of infliximab infusion. ▪ Infliximab therapy may result in formation of autoimmune antibodies and, rarely, in the development of a lupus-like syndrome. Discontinue therapy if this occurs. In clinical studies, symptoms resolved with discontinuation of therapy. ▪ Lymphoma and other malignancies, some fatal, have been reported in children, adolescent, and young adult patients treated with TNF blockers, including infliximab. Most of the affected patients were receiving concomitant immunosuppressants. ▪ Cases of hepatosplenic T-cell lymphoma have been reported. The majority of reported cases have occurred in adolescents and young adult males being treated with infliximab for Crohn's disease or ulcerative colitis. This type of lymphoma has a very aggressive disease course and is usually fatal. Almost all affected patients received concomitant treatment with a TNF-blocker and azathioprine or 6-mercaptopurine (Purinethol) at or before diagnosis. When treating patients with inflammatory bowel disease, particularly adolescents and young adults, the decision whether to use infliximab alone or in combination with other immunosuppressants should consider the possibility that there is a higher risk of developing hepatosplenic T-cell lymphoma (HSTCL) with combination therapy versus an observed increased risk of immunogenicity and hypersensitivity reactions with infliximab monotherapy. ▪ Use caution in patients with moderate to severe COPD; may have an increased risk of malignancy, especially of the lungs and head or neck. ▪ The potential role of TNF-blocking therapy in the development of lymphoma, leukemia, melanoma, Merkel cell carcinoma, and other malignancies is not known. Patients with Crohn's disease, ulcerative colitis, rheumatoid arthritis, or plaque psoriasis, particularly with highly active disease and/or exposure to immunosuppressant therapies, may be at higher risk (up to several-fold) than the general population for the development of lymphoma, leukemia, and other malignancies, even in the absence of TNF-blocking therapy. Use caution when considering infliximab therapy in patients with a history of malignancy or when continuing treatment in patients who develop a malignancy while receiving infliximab. ▪ In clinical trials, nonmelanoma skin cancers were more common in psoriasis patients with previous phototherapy. ▪ Females treated with infliximab for rheumatoid arthritis may have an increased risk of invasive cervical cancer. ▪ Rare cases with CNS manifestations of systemic vasculitis, seizures, and new-onset or exacerbation of clinical symptoms and/or radiographic evidence of CNS demyelinating disorders (e.g., multiple sclerosis, optic neuritis) and peripheral demyelinating disorders (e.g., Guillain-Barré syndrome) have been reported. Use with caution in patients with any of these existing neurologic disorders. Consider discontinuing therapy if any of these disorders develop. ▪ Severe hepatic reactions, including liver failure, jaundice, hepatitis, cholestasis, and autoimmune hepatitis, have been reported. Reactions have occurred anywhere from 2 weeks to more than a year after initiation of treatment and have resulted in death or the need for a liver transplant. ▪ Leukopenia, neutropenia, thrombocytopenia, and pancytopenia, some with fatal outcome, have been reported. ▪ Use caution when switching between biological disease-modifying antirheumatic drugs (e.g., **abatacept, anakinra) or other TNF-blocking agents** (e.g., adalimumab, etanercept, golimumab); overlapping biological activity may further increase the risk of infection; see Drug/Lab Interactions. ▪ Administration of live virus vaccines or therapeutic infectious agents (e.g., BCG bladder instillation for treatment of cancer) concurrently with infliximab is not recommended. Could result in clinical infections, including disseminated infections. ■ See Drug/Lab Interactions and Maternal/Child.

Monitor: Evaluate patients for tuberculosis risk factors and test for latent infection before initiating infliximab and periodically during therapy. Initiate treatment of latent TB before therapy with infliximab. Antituberculosis therapy should also be considered before initiating infliximab in patients with a history of latent or active tuberculosis for whom an adequate course of treatment cannot be confirmed and in patients with a negative test for latent tuberculosis but risk factors for tuberculosis infection. Consultation with a physician with expertise in the treatment of TB is recommended to aid in deciding whether initiating antituberculosis therapy is appropriate for a given patient. ■ During and after treatment, monitor for the development of tuberculosis in patients who tested negative for latent tuberculosis infection before initiating therapy. Tests for latent tuberculosis infection may also be falsely negative while on therapy with infliximab. Tuberculosis should be strongly considered in patients who develop a new infection during infliximab therapy, especially in patients who have previously or recently traveled to countries with a high prevalence of TB or who have had close contact with a person with active TB. ■ Before initiating TNF-blocker therapy, including infliximab, patients should be tested for HBV infection. Consultation with a physician with expertise in the treatment of hepatitis B is recommended if a patient tests positive for hepatitis B surface antigen. ■ In patients who are carriers of HBV and require treatment with TNF-blockers, closely monitor for clinical and laboratory signs of active HBV infection throughout treatment and for several months after completion of treatment. If HBV reactivation occurs, discontinue infliximab; see Antidote. ■ Monitor for S/S of infection during and after treatment; discontinue if a serious infection occurs and initiate appropriate antimicrobial treatment. Empiric antifungal therapy may be appropriate pending results of a diagnostic workup in patients at risk for invasive fungal infections (e.g., patients who reside or travel in regions where mycoses are endemic); see Precautions. ■ Monitor cardiac status closely for new-onset or worsening CHF; see Precautions. ■ Patients may develop antibodies to infliximab. In clinical trials, patients who were antibody-positive were more likely to have higher rates of clearance and reduced efficacy and to experience an infusion reaction than were patients who were antibody-negative. The incidence of antibody development was lower among patients receiving immunosuppressant therapies (e.g., 6-mercaptopurine, azathioprine, corticosteroids). ■ Monitor for S/S of hepatotoxicity (e.g., jaundice and/or marked liver enzyme elevations [equal to or greater than 5 times the upper limit of normal]). ■ Monitor CBC with differential and platelet count periodically. ■ Monitor for S/S of hypersensitivity or infusion reaction (e.g., anaphylaxis, chills, dyspnea, fever, flu-like symptoms, GI symptoms, headache, hypotension, rash). ■ Monitor for S/S of malignancies such as HSTCL (e.g., abdominal pain, hepatomegaly, night sweats, persistent fever, weight loss) and lymphoma. ■ Periodic skin examination is recommended for all patients, particularly those with risk factors for skin cancer. ■ Screen females for cervical cancer periodically.

Patient Education: Read manufacturer's medication guide before each treatment with infliximab. ■ Tell health care professionals of heart conditions, previous or current infections, and recent or past exposure to TB or mycoses (e.g., histoplasmosis, coccidioidomycosis, blastomycosis). ■ Review all medicines and disease history with pharmacist or physician before initiating treatment. ■ Promptly report abdominal pain, fever, S/S of new or worsening heart failure (e.g., shortness of breath, swelling feet, sudden weight gain), infection, numbness, tingling, or visual disturbances. ■ Report S/S of hypersensitivity reactions (e.g., itching, rash, swelling in the throat). Usually occur during or immediately following the infusion but may occur from 3 to 12 days later. ■ Report changes of growths on your skin during or after infliximab treatment. ■ Report symptoms of a cytopenia, such as bruising, bleeding, or persistent fever. ■ Report recently receiving or being scheduled to receive a live virus vaccine or treatment with a weakened bacteria (such as BCG for bladder cancer) to your physician.

Maternal/Child: *Remicade:* Category B: use during pregnancy only if clearly needed. ■ Has potential for harm to the nursing infant; discontinue breast-feeding.

Avsola, Inflectra, Ixifi, and Renflexis: Available data from published literature on the use of infliximab products during pregnancy have not reported a clear association of infliximab products with adverse pregnancy outcomes. ■ Available information is insufficient to inform the amount of infliximab products present in human milk and the effects on the breast-fed infant. There are no data on the effects of infliximab products on milk production. Consider risk versus benefit.

All products: At least a 6-month waiting period following birth is recommended before the administration of any live vaccine to infants exposed in utero to infliximab. Infliximab crosses the placental barrier and has been detected in these infants up to 6 months after the last dose of infliximab to the mother, and these infants may be at increased risk for infection. ■ Safety and effectiveness for use in pediatric patients with ulcerative colitis and/or Crohn's disease who are under 6 years of age not established. ■ Effectiveness of infliximab in inducing and maintaining mucosal healing could not be established in pediatric patients. ■ Safety and effectiveness for use in pediatric patients with juvenile rheumatoid arthritis was evaluated in a multicenter trial. The study failed to establish effectiveness; see prescribing information for details. ■ Before initiating infliximab therapy in pediatric patients with Crohn's disease or ulcerative colitis, all vaccinations should be brought up to date. ■ Long-term (greater than 1 year) safety and effectiveness in pediatric patients with Crohn's disease not established.

Elderly: Specific differences in safety and effectiveness not noted; the incidence of serious side effects may be increased. An increase in the incidence of serious infections has been noted in patients 65 years and older, and because there is a higher incidence of infections in the elderly population in general, caution should be used in treating the elderly. See Precautions.

DRUG/LAB INTERACTIONS

Specific interaction studies have not been performed. ■ Concurrent administration with **anakinra**, an antirheumatic interleukin-1 antagonist, **or abatacept**, an antirheumatic selective T-cell costimulation blocker, may be associated with an increased risk of serious infections. The added benefit of combination therapy has not been documented. Anakinra is also associated with an increased risk of neutropenia. Concurrent administration of TNF α-blocking agents (e.g., infliximab) with anakinra or abatacept is not recommended. ■ May cause increased immunosuppression and increased risk of infection with **tocilizumab**; concurrent use should be avoided. ■ Concurrent use of infliximab with **other biological products** (adalimumab, etanercept, golimumab, rituximab) used to treat the same conditions as infliximab is not recommended; may increase risk of infection. ■ The majority of patients with Crohn's disease, rheumatoid arthritis, or psoriatic arthritis received one or more of the following concomitant medications without evidence of any type of negative drug interaction: aminosalicylates, antibiotics, antivirals, corticosteroids, 6-mercaptopurine (Purinethol), azathioprine, folic acid, methotrexate, narcotics, NSAIDs, and sulfasalazine. ■ Patients receiving **immunosuppressants** (e.g., 6-mercaptopurine, azathioprine, corticosteroids) tended to experience fewer infusion reactions as compared to patients on no immunosuppressants. ■ Concomitant **methotrexate** use may decrease incidence of anti-infliximab antibody production and increase infliximab concentrations. ■ **Live virus vaccines and therapeutic infectious agents** (e.g., BCG for bladder instillation for treatment of cancer) should not be given concurrently with infliximab. Could result in clinical infection, including disseminated infection. In addition, it is also recommended that live vaccines not be given to infants after in utero exposure to infliximab for at least 6 months following birth; see Precautions and Maternal/Child. ■ Cytochrome P_{450} enzymes may be suppressed by increased levels of cytokines during inflammation. Infliximab antagonizes cytokine activity, and the formation of the CYP450 enzymes may be normalized. When initiating or discontinuing infliximab in patients treated with **CYP450 substrates with a narrow therapeutic index,** monitoring of the effect (e.g., warfarin) or drug concentrations (e.g., cyclosporine or theophylline) is recommended. Dose adjustment may be necessary.

SIDE EFFECTS

Adult: The most commonly reported side effects include abdominal pain, headache, infection (e.g., pharyngitis, sinusitis, upper respiratory tract, and urinary tract), and infusion-related reactions. The most common reasons for discontinuation of therapy were infusion-related reactions (e.g., dyspnea, fever, flushing, headache, rash) occurring during or within 2 hours of infusion or infections (bacterial, fungal, parasitic, and viral), including TB and invasive opportunistic infections (e.g., histoplasmosis, listeriosis, and pneumocystosis). See Precautions. Other less common side effects include arthralgia; autoantibodies/lupus-like syndrome; bronchitis; cough; diarrhea; dyspepsia; hepatitis B virus reactivation; hepatotoxicity (autoimmune hepatitis, increased liver function tests, jaundice, liver failure); hypertension; malignancies, including lymphoma; moniliasis; nausea; new-onset or worsening CHF; pain; pruritus; and rash. Hematologic reactions, neurologic reactions, and deaths have been reported. See Precautions.

Pediatric patients with Crohn's disease: Anemia, bacterial infection, bone fracture, flushing, leukopenia, neutropenia, respiratory tract allergic reactions, and viral infections were reported more commonly in pediatric patients than in adult patients receiving similar treatment regimens. Serious side effects were infections (some fatal), including opportunistic infections and tuberculosis; infusion reactions; and hypersensitivity reactions.

Pediatric patients with ulcerative colitis: Adverse reactions were similar to those seen in adult patients.

Post-Marketing: Agranulocytosis (including infants exposed in utero to infliximab); cholestasis; erythema multiforme; hepatitis; idiopathic and/or thrombotic thrombocytopenic purpura; infusion-related reactions (cases of anaphylactic reactions, including anaphylactic shock, laryngeal/pharyngeal edema and severe bronchospasm; seizures; transient vision loss; cerebrovascular accidents; myocardial ischemia/infarction; and arrhythmia); interstitial lung disease (including pulmonary fibrosis/interstitial pneumonitis and rapidly progressive disease); jaundice; liver failure; malignancies (including leukemia, melanoma, Merkel cell carcinoma, and cervical cancer); myocardial ischemia/infarction; neuropathies; neutropenia; pericardial effusion; peripheral demyelinating disorders (e.g., Guillain-Barré syndrome, chronic inflammatory demyelinating polyneuropathy, and multifocal motor neuropathy); psoriasis (including new-onset and pustular, primarily palmar/plantar); Stevens-Johnson syndrome; systemic and cutaneous vasculitis; toxic epidermal necrolysis; transverse myelitis; and vaccine breakthrough infections (including bovine tuberculosis [disseminated BCG infection] following vaccination in an infant exposed in utero to infliximab) have been reported; fatalities have occurred.

Pediatric patients: Hypersensitivity reactions, infections (including opportunistic infections and tuberculosis), infusion reactions, malignancies (including hepatosplenic T-cell lymphomas), lupus-like syndromes and the development of autoantibodies, and transient hepatic enzyme abnormalities.

ANTIDOTE

Notify physician of any side effects; most will be treated symptomatically. Discontinue infliximab if patient experiences a serious infection, significant changes in vital signs, new or worsening S/S of heart failure, hepatotoxicity, a serious hypersensitivity reaction, a lupus-like syndrome (fever, pleuritic pain, pleural effusion), a neurologic disorder, or significant hematologic abnormalities. Treat hypersensitivity and/or infusion reactions with acetaminophen, antihistamines (diphenhydramine), corticosteroids, dopamine, and epinephrine as indicated. Slow or suspend infusion for a mild or moderate infusion-related reaction. Upon resolution of the reaction, re-initiation at a lower infusion rate and/or therapeutic administration of antihistamines, acetaminophen, and/or corticosteroids may be attempted with caution. If patient does not tolerate the infusion after these interventions, infliximab should be discontinued; see Usual Dose. Lupus-like syndrome usually subsides within 10 days of discontinuing infliximab. Discontinue infliximab in patients who develop HBV reactivation; and initiate antiviral therapy with appropriate supportive treatment. Safety of resuming therapy after HBV is controlled is not known; use caution if resumption of therapy is considered, and monitor closely.

INSULIN HUMAN ASPART or LISPRO or GLULISINE
(Rapid-acting insulin)

Aspart: Novolog; Lispro: Humalog, Admelog, Lyumjev; glulisine: Apidra

pH Novolog 7.2-7.6, Humalog/Admelog/ Lyumjev 7.0-7.8, Apidra 7.3

Hormone Antidiabetic agent

USUAL DOSE

Rapid-acting insulin may be given via intravenous, subcutaneous, and insulin pump.

Individualize dose based on route of administration, patient's metabolic needs, blood glucose monitoring results, and glycemic control goal. It is imperative that dosing is individualized and adjusted based on blood glucose determinations; see **Precautions**. Several protocols have been published. Review institution-specific protocol if available.

Glycemic control in hospitalized patient (unlabeled): Rapid-acting insulins have been used for glycemic control via infusion as an alternative to human regular insulin, although subcutaneous use is more common.

Hyperglycemic Crisis: *Diabetic ketoacidosis (DKA) or hyperosmolar hyperglycemic state (HHS) (unlabeled):* A fixed rate of insulin infusion (0.05-0.1 unit/kg/h) is suggested with hourly glucose and every 2 to 4 hours electrolyte monitoring and systematic fluid resuscitation per hospital protocol. Fluid resuscitation (500-1000 mL/h with a crystalloid solution) will also lower blood glucose. An insulin bolus dose is optional 0.1 unit/kg but does not improve time to goal and is generally not advised unless there is a delay to insulin infusion initiation. The goal in DKA is to close the anion gap and raise bicarbonate/normalize pH while reducing glucose (initially decline 50-70 mg/dL/h) and preventing hypoglycemia. Targeting normoglycemia is not necessary in the first 24 to 48 hours, rather target 150 to 200 mg/dL to avoid relative hypoglycemia. The goal in HHS is to replace fluid and normalize electrolytes. Insulin is added when glucose stops declining with those therapies. A fixed rate of insulin 0.1 unit/kg/h is used, and dextrose is initiated when blood glucose is <250 mg/dL.

Potassium should be monitored and replaced as needed to maintain a level of 4 to 5.5 mmol/L. Delay insulin until potassium replacement is initiated if initial potassium is <3.3 mmol/L in DKA/HHS. Long-acting insulin may be continued per home dose.

For DKA a dextrose (5%-10%) infusion is initiated at 100 to 125 mL/h when the blood glucose is <250 mg/dL as a single infusion (one bag) or a two-bag method or when glucose is <300 mg/dL in HHS. The insulin rate may be reduced to 0.05 unit/kg/h if dextrose is unable to prevent glucose from falling.

Insulin is continued in DKA until the anion gap has closed and pH >7.3 and the patient is able to eat or drink. At that point, insulin may be transitioned to a subcutaneous regimen (basal/prandial/correction) with infusion continued for 2 to 4 hours after basal insulin dose (or resumed on insulin pump). If unable to eat/drink, a titrated dose insulin infusion may be used per hospital protocol.

Euglycemic DKA (e.g. with sodium-glucose cotransporter [SGLT] inhibitors) is treated the same as DKA with hyperglycemia, except that 10% glucose infusion is initiated immediately with insulin. If glucose falls despite 10% dextrose infusion, lower insulin infusion rate to 0.05 unit/kg/hr.

Insulin/fluids/dextrose is continued in HHS to maintain glucose 250 to 300 mg/dL until the patient is fluid resuscitated/hyperosmolarity is resolved and can eat or drink.

Mild to moderate DKA may be managed with frequent doses of rapid-acting insulin in some settings.

Hyperkalemia (unlabeled): Insulin may be used in patients with or without diabetes mellitus to treat hyperkalemia in conjunction with 25 to 50 g dextrose. Insulin effect may persist longer than dextrose bolus and hypoglycemia is a risk with this regimen. Frequent blood glucose monitoring (every 1–2 hours for 4–6 hours) should be initiated. Weight <50 kg, renal insufficiency, female gender, age >60 years, or glucose <150 mg/dL before treatment are associated with increased risk of hypoglycemia. An insulin dose of 5 units with 25 to 50 g dextrose is associated with less hypoglycemia than 10 units with comparable effect on potassium.

PEDIATRIC DOSE

Hyperglycemic Crisis: *DKA (unlabeled):* Management of DKA follows the same pattern as adults with weight-based fluid replacement (initial bolus average 70 mL/kg, range 30–100 mL/kg) followed by ongoing replacement over the next 24 to 48 hours. Insulin infusion starts at 0.1 unit/kg/h after 1 hour of fluid resuscitation, although 0.05 unit/kg/h may be preferred in children <6 years or others with greater insulin sensitivity until resolution of ketoacidosis. An insulin bolus is not used at start of therapy. Dextrose is added when glucose is <250 mg/dL like adults using a one- or two-bag method with 10% dextrose. The process for electrolyte monitoring and replacement is comparable to adults. Transition to a basal/prandial/correction subcutaneous insulin regimen is also similar to adults when DKA is resolved, and child is eating/drinking normally.

Hyperosmolar hyperglycemic state (unlabeled): The frequency of HHS related to uncontrolled diabetes in children is increasing. Fluid resuscitation is initiated, and insulin is added once glucose is declining by <50 mg/dL/hr with fluid alone. Insulin is administered at 0.025 to 0.05 unit/kg/hr initially and may be titrated to maintain a decline in glucose of 50 to 75 mg/dL/hr. An insulin bolus is not recommended.

Hyperkalemia (unlabeled): Administer 0.1 unit/kg of insulin with 400 mg/kg of glucose; usual ratio of combination therapy of insulin to glucose is 1 unit of insulin for every 4 g of glucose.

DOSE ADJUSTMENTS

Insulin infusion doses should be adjusted based on local protocol with frequent (every 1–2 hour) glucose checks. Changes in metabolic stress levels, nutrition, and medications such as catecholamines or corticosteroids are important variables.

See comments under *Usual Dose.* Dose requirements may be reduced in patients with renal or hepatic impairment. Dose adjustment may be indicated if it is necessary to change from one insulin product to another. Dose adjustment may be needed when co-administered with certain drugs; see **Drug/Lab Interactions**.

DILUTION

Insulin aspart 0.5 to 1 unit/mL using polypropylene bags, stable in 0.9% NaCl; Lispro 0.1 to 1 unit/mL in 0.9% NaCl; Lispro-aabc 1 unit/mL in normal saline (NS) or dextrose 5% in water (D5W; using 100 unit/mL solution); Glulisine 0.05–1 unit/mL in 0.9% NaCl using polyvinyl chloride bags.

Use only if insulin solution is clear.

Example: 100 units of insulin (1 mL) to 100 mL of NS will yield a solution with a final concentration of 1 unit/mL.

Storage: *Vials:* Store unopened vials in refrigerator. Vials may be stored at room temperature up to 25° C (77° F) for up to 30 days in original carton. Do not place vial back in refrigerator. Discard after 30 days if stored at room temperature. Do not freeze and do not use if it has been frozen. Do not shake. Discard any unused portion. Protect from sunlight and freezing.

Infusions: Insulin is adsorbed to the material of the infusion bag and IV tubing. Prime new tubing and flush an additional 20 mL. The actual amount of insulin delivered is substantially less than apparent. If Y-sited into another solution, chose a site closest to the patient.

Infusion bags Stability: Prepared as indicated in dilution are stable for: Aspart 24 hours at room temperature; Lispro-Humalog 48 hours under refrigeration (36°F-46° F) and then may be used at room temperature for another 48 hours; Lispro-Admelog stable for 24 hours under refrigeration or up to 4 hours at room temperature; Lispro-aabc-Lyumjev 100 unit/mL solution stable for up to 4 days under refrigeration or for up to 12 hours at room temperature; Glulisine stable for 48 hours at room temperature.

Do not shake. Discard any unused portion.

COMPATIBILITY

Do not add supplementary medication or additives.

Other sources suggest specific compatibilities for insulin dependence on concentration and manufacturer; consult a pharmacist.

RATE OF ADMINISTRATION

Administer insulin infusion in conjunction with close monitoring of glucose (every 1–2 hours) and a validated protocol.

ACTIONS

A hormone produced by the pancreas that controls the storage and metabolism of carbohydrates, proteins, and fat. Responsible for regulation of glucose metabolism. Binds to insulin receptors on muscle and fat cells and lowers blood glucose by facilitating cellular uptake of glucose and inhibiting hepatic glucose production. Also inhibits lipolysis, proteolysis, and gluconeogenesis and enhances protein synthesis and conversion of excess glucose into fat. Rapidly and widely distributed. The glucose-lowering activities of regular insulin, insulin aspart, insulin glulisine, and insulin lispro are equipotent when administered by the IV route. The average elimination half-life is dose dependent and ranges from 0.25 to 1 hour, depending on dose and product.

INDICATIONS AND USES

Treatment of patients with diabetes mellitus to improve glycemic control as an alternative to human regular insulin via infusion or for subcutaneous correction/prandial doses or in a continuous subcutaneous pump. Proper medical supervision is required to prevent hypoglycemia and hypokalemia.

CONTRAINDICATIONS

Contraindicated during episodes of hypoglycemia and in patients hypersensitive to regular human insulin, insulin aspart, insulin glulisine, insulin lispro, or one of the excipients of any of these products.

PRECAUTIONS

Rapid-acting insulin: Concomitant oral antidiabetic treatment may need to be adjusted. Hypoglycemia and hypokalemia are potential side effects of insulin therapy. Use caution in patients in whom these side effects may be clinically relevant (e.g., patients who are fasting, have autonomic neuropathy, are using potassium-lowering drugs [e.g., diuretics], or are taking drugs sensitive to serum potassium levels [e.g., digoxin]). Severe hypoglycemia may lead to unconsciousness and/or convulsions and may result in temporary or permanent impairment of brain function or death. Early warning symptoms of hypoglycemia may be different or less pronounced under certain conditions such as long-standing diabetes, diabetic nerve disease, and the use of medications such as beta-blockers. Untreated hypokalemia may cause respiratory paralysis, ventricular arrhythmia, and death. Use with caution in patients with renal or hepatic impairment; may be at a higher risk of hypoglycemia; see **Dose Adjustments**. Frequent monitoring may be required. Insulin requirements may be altered during illness or stress. Anti-insulin antibodies have been reported. Clinical significance of anti-insulin antibodies is unknown. Systemic hypersensitivity reactions have been reported. May include hypotension, pruritus, rash, shortness of breath, sweating, tachycardia, and/or wheezing.

Anaphylaxis has occurred. See **Drug/Lab Interactions**.

Rapid-acting insulin: Insulin potency may be reduced by $\geq$20% and possibly $\geq$80% via the glass or plastic infusion container and plastic IV tubing before reaching the venous system when given by infusion. Use of a syringe pump (instead of infusion containers) reduces surface area for adsorption.

Monitor: Depending on indication for use, response to insulin may be measured by blood glucose, blood pH, ketones, blood urea nitrogen, serum creatinine, fluid status, sodium, potassium, chloride, osmolality, anion gap, and mental status. Monitor patient carefully in all situations. Glucose and potassium levels must be monitored closely during IV administration of insulin to avoid potentially fatal hypoglycemia and hypokalemia. See **Drug/Lab Interactions**.

Patient Education: Monitor blood glucose as directed. Adhere to consistent diet and exercise programs. Avoid alcohol. Review medications or changes in medication regimen with a health care professional. Review signs and symptoms of hypoglycemia and hyperglycemia with a health care professional. Be familiar with the treatment for each. Insulin requirements may change with onset of illness. Monitor glucose carefully and adjust insulin therapy as required.

Maternal/Child: Insulin therapy is the preferred treatment of type 1 and 2 diabetes during pregnancy.

Poorly controlled diabetes in pregnancy increases maternal risk for DKA, preeclampsia, spontaneous abortions, preterm delivery, stillbirth, and delivery complications. Poorly controlled diabetes increases the fetal risk for major birth defects, stillbirth, and macrosomia-related morbidity. Monitor carefully; insulin requirements may change at different stages of pregnancy and may drop immediately postpartum. Use caution in breastfeeding. Breast-feeding may decrease insulin requirements. Inadequately controlled maternal blood glucose late in pregnancy may cause increased insulin production in the fetus. Monitor and treat neonatal hypoglycemia postpartum.

Elderly: No overall differences in safety or effectiveness were observed between elderly and younger patients. Elderly patients may be at increased risk of hypoglycemia due to comorbid conditions and concomitantly administered medications; see **Dose Adjustments** and **Drug/Lab Interactions**. Initial dosing, dose increments, and maintenance dosage should be conservative to avoid hypoglycemia.

DRUG/LAB INTERACTIONS

Hypoglycemic effect may be potentiated by angiotention-converting enzyme inhibitors, anabolic steroids, angiotensin II receptor-blocking agents, disopyramide, fluoxetine, fibrates, guanethidine, monoamine oxidase inhibitors, oral antidiabetic agents, pentoxifylline, salicylates, sulfonamides, and many others. Dose adjustment and increased frequency of glucose monitoring may be required with concomitant use. Drugs that may reduce blood glucose-lowering effects include atypical antipsychotic medications, corticosteroids, danazol, diuretics, estrogen, glucagon, isoniazid (INH), niacin, oral contraceptives, phenothiazine derivatives, protease inhibitors, somatropin, sympathomimetic agents, and thyroid preparations. Dose adjustment and increased frequency of glucose monitoring may be required with concomitant use. Alcohol, beta-adrenergic blockers including via ophthalmic route, clonidine, and lithium may either potentiate or inhibit the blood glucose-lowering effect of insulin. Dose adjustment and increased frequency of glucose monitoring may be required with concomitant use. Will affect serum potassium levels; use caution in patients taking digoxin. Octreotide may alter insulin, glucagon, and growth hormone secretion, resulting in hypoglycemia or hyperglycemia. Monitor serum glucose and adjust insulin dose as indicated. Pentamidine is toxic to the beta cells of the pancreas. Patients may develop hypoglycemia initially as insulin is released. This may be followed by hypoinsulinemia and hyperglycemia with continued pentamidine therapy. Signs and symptoms of hypoglycemia may be masked in the presence of beta-blockers, clonidine, guanethidine, and reserpine. Increased frequency of glucose monitoring may be required with concomitant use. Thiazolidinediones (TZDs) can cause dose-related fluid retention, particularly when used in combination with insulin. Fluid retention may lead to or exacerbate heart failure. Patients receiving concomitant therapy should be monitored for signs and symptoms of heart failure. Dose reduction or discontinuation of the TZD may be indicated if heart failure develops.

SIDE EFFECTS

The most common adverse reactions with IV administration of insulin include hypoglycemia (<70 mg/dL), hypokalemia, and rare hypersensitivity reactions, pruritus, and rash. Other commonly reported reactions are injection site reactions, peripheral edema, and weight gain. Additional side effects reported in studies include abdominal pain, arthralgia, asthenia, back pain, chest pain, diarrhea, dysmenorrhea, fever, headache, hypertension, hyporeflexia, influenza, myalgia, nasopharyngitis, nausea, onychomycosis, pain, sensory disturbances, sinusitis, skin disorders, upper respiratory infections, and urinary tract infections. Severe hypersensitivity reactions may include anaphylaxis, angioedema, bronchospasm, generalized skin reactions, rash, hypotension, and shock.

Overdose: Severe hypoglycemia and hypokalemia. Severe hypoglycemia may result in coma, seizures, or neurologic impairment. Severe, untreated hypokalemia may lead to respiratory paralysis, ventricular arrhythmia, and death.

ANTIDOTE

Discontinue insulin immediately and notify physician of adverse reactions or hypoglycemia. Follow the hospital hypoglycemia management protocol. Glucagon 1 to 2 mg intramuscularly or subcutaneously is the specific antidote for insulin overdose. It may be supplemented by 15 to 20 g dextrose IV and recheck glucose in 5 to 15 minutes. Oral carbohydrates such as glucose tablets or gel or orange juice may be sufficient to combat early symptoms of mild hypoglycemia. A titrated dextrose dose may be calculated to avoid overcorrection during insulin infusion [dextrose g = (100-glucose mg/dL) x 0.2]. Replace potassium as indicated. Resume insulin at a modified dose. Hypersensitivity reactions usually respond to symptomatic treatment.

INSULIN HUMAN INJECTION (REGULAR)
(**IN**-sue-lin)

Hormone
Antidiabetic agent

Humulin R, Novolin ge Toronto ✦ ▪ Myxredlin

pH 7 to 7.8

USUAL DOSE

Only regular human insulin aspart or insulin lispro is given by IV method.

Dose varies greatly. Individualize dose based on route of administration, patient's metabolic needs, blood glucose monitoring results, and glycemic control goal. It is imperative that dosing is individualized and adjusted based on blood glucose determinations because of the marked loss of insulin from adsorption to glass and plastic infusion containers and tubing; see Precautions. Several protocols have been published. Review institution-specific protocol if available.

Diabetic ketoacidosis or hyperosmolar hyperglycemic state (unlabeled): Administer a bolus dose of 0.1 unit/kg (optional) followed by a continuous infusion of 0.1 to 0.14 unit/kg/hr. If serum glucose does not fall by at least 10% in the first hour, administer an IV bolus of 0.14 unit/kg and continue the infusion. In addition, if serum glucose does not fall by 50 to 75 mg/dL in the first hour, increase the insulin infusion rate hourly until a steady glucose decline is achieved. The insulin infusion should be continued at a fixed dose until the anion gap has closed in DKA and glucose is not a factor for conversion to SC. (UK [see citation later in this comment] uses ketone <0.3 mmol/L and venous pH >7.3.) If the glucose has declined to less than ~250 mg/dL, additional dextrose should be given as an infusion, or the insulin infusion rate may be reduced from 0.1 to 0.05 unit/kg/hr.

Hyperkalemia (unlabeled): Insulin may be used in patients with or without diabetes mellitus to treat hyperkalemia. Must be administered with a dextrose solution in nondiabetic patients. 0.1 unit/kg (not to exceed 10 units) as an IV bolus followed by dextrose 25 Gm IV (25 Gm of dextrose is 500 mL of 5% dextrose or 250 mL 10% dextrose or 50 mL of 50% dextrose) over 5 minutes is an example of one regimen in use.

PEDIATRIC DOSE

Diabetic ketoacidosis (unlabeled): Administer 0.05 to 0.1 unit/kg/hr as a continuous infusion until resolution of ketoacidosis. Transition to a subcutaneous insulin regimen.

Hyperosmolar hyperglycemic state (unlabeled): Administer 0.025 to 0.05 unit/kg/hr. Titrate infusion rate to achieve a decrease in serum glucose concentration at a rate of 50 to 75 mg/dL/hr.

Hyperkalemia (unlabeled): Administer 0.1 unit/kg of insulin with 400 mg/kg of glucose; usual ratio of combination therapy of insulin to glucose is 1 unit of insulin for every 4 Gm of glucose.

DOSE ADJUSTMENTS

Dose adjustments may be needed with changes in physical activity, changes in meal patterns, changes in renal or hepatic function, or during acute illness. ▪ A reduced dose of insulin may be indicated when infusions are discontinued and SQ administration is indicated; see comments under Usual Dose. ▪ Dose requirements may be reduced in patients with renal or hepatic impairment. ▪ Dose adjustment may be indicated if it is necessary to change from one insulin product to another. ▪ Dose adjustment may be needed when coadministered with certain drugs; see Drug/Lab Interactions.

DILUTION

Regular insulin: Use only if clear. Dilute with NS to a concentration from 0.1 unit/mL to 1 unit/mL. 100 units of insulin (1 mL) to 100 mL of NS will yield a solution with a final concentration of 1 unit/mL. Also available in a Galaxy premixed single-dose container containing 100 units/100 mL of NS (**Myxredlin**).

Storage: Vials: Store unopened vials in refrigerator. A vial that is in use may be stored at RT for 31 days *(regular insulin).* Protect from sunlight and freezing.

Infusions: Some insulin may be initially adsorbed to the material of the infusion bag. *Regular insulin:* Infusion bags prepared as indicated in dilution are stable for 48 hours refrigerated and then may be used at RT for up to an additional 48 hours.

Premixed: Store in refrigerator in original carton to protect from light until administration. May be stored at RT up to 25° C (77° F) for up to 30 days in original carton. Do not place back in refrigerator. Discard after 30 days if stored at RT. Do not freeze and do not use if it has been frozen. Do not shake. Discard any unused portion.

COMPATIBILITY

Do not add supplementary medication or additives.

Other sources suggest specific **compatibilities** for *regular insulin* dependent on concentration and manufacturer; consult a pharmacist.

RATE OF ADMINISTRATION

When given in an IV infusion, the rate should be ordered by the physician and will depend on insulin and fluid needs. High-dose insulin is an antidote in calcium channel blocker or beta-blocker overdose treatment. After a bolus of 1 unit/kg IV continuous infusion doses may range from 0.5 to 5 unit/kg/hr (or sometimes higher) in conjunction with dextrose infusion to maintain euglycemia. Use in conjunction with a local Poison Control Center protocol and very close monitoring. See Dilution for example. Follow an insulin infusion protocol for infusion titration based on measured blood glucose.

For DKA/HHS, follow physician orders for fixed-rate insulin infusion and concurrent dextrose replacement when blood glucose is less than 250 mg/dL.

ACTIONS

A hormone produced by the pancreas that controls the storage and metabolism of carbohydrates, proteins, and fat. Responsible for regulation of glucose metabolism. Binds to insulin receptors on muscle and fat cells and lowers blood glucose by facilitating cellular uptake of glucose and inhibiting hepatic glucose production. Also inhibits lipolysis, proteolysis, and gluconeogenesis and enhances protein synthesis and conversion of excess glucose into fat. Rapidly and widely distributed. The glucose-lowering activities of regular insulin, insulin aspart, insulin glulisine, and insulin lispro are equipotent when administered by the IV route. The average elimination half-life is dose dependent and ranges from 0.25 to 1 hour depending on dose and product.

INDICATIONS AND USES

Regular insulin: Treatment of patients with diabetes mellitus to improve glycemic control, to treat DKA/HHS, or as an antidote in calcium channel or beta-blocker severe toxicity. Usually used as part of a SQ injection regimen or as a SQ infusion administered via an external insulin pump. May be given IV via push using an insulin-specific luer tip syringe through a needleless injection port or continuous infusion. Consistent glucose monitoring is required to prevent hypoglycemia and hypokalemia.

CONTRAINDICATIONS

Contraindicated during episodes of hypoglycemia and in patients hypersensitive to regular human insulin, insulin aspart, insulin glulisine, insulin lispro, or one of the excipients of any of these products.

PRECAUTIONS

Regular insulin: Concomitant oral antidiabetic treatment may need to be adjusted. ■ Hypoglycemia and hypokalemia are potential side effects of insulin therapy. Use caution in patients in whom these side effects may be clinically relevant (e.g., patients who are fasting, have autonomic neuropathy, are using potassium-lowering drugs [e.g., diuretics], or are taking drugs sensitive to serum potassium levels [e.g., digoxin]). ■ Severe hypoglycemia may lead to unconsciousness and/or convulsions and may result in temporary or permanent impairment of brain function or death. Early warning symptoms of hypoglycemia may be different or less pronounced under certain conditions, such as long-standing diabetes, diabetic nerve disease, and the use of medications such as beta-blockers. ■ Untreated hypokalemia may cause respiratory paralysis, ventricular arrhythmia, and death. ■ Use with caution in patients with renal or hepatic impairment; may be at a higher risk of hypoglycemia; see Dose Adjustments. Frequent monitoring may be required. ▪ Insulin requirements may be altered during illness or stress. ▪ Anti-insulin antibodies have been reported. Clinical significance of anti-insulin antibodies is unknown. ▪ Systemic hypersensitivity reactions have been reported. May include hypotension, pruritus, rash, shortness of breath, sweating, tachycardia, and/or wheezing. Anaphylaxis has occurred. ▪ See Drug/Lab Interactions.

Regular insulin: Insulin potency may be reduced by at least 20% and possibly up to 80% via the glass or plastic infusion container and plastic IV tubing before it actually reaches the venous system when given by infusion. The percentage adsorbed is inversely proportional to the concentration of insulin (the larger the dose, the less adsorption) and takes place within 30 to 60 minutes. Insulin infusion guidelines suggest priming new IV tubing with 20 mL of the insulin infusion solution prior to attaching the tubing to the patient. Do not add other medications or electrolytes to an insulin infusion. Other methods of compensation for insulin loss include the addition of added insulin to saturate binding sites or the use of a syringe pump (instead of infusion containers) to reduce surface area for adsorption.

Monitor: Depending on indication for use, response to insulin may be measured by blood glucose, blood pH, ketones, BUN, SCr, fluid status, sodium, potassium, chloride, osmolality, anion gap, and mental status. Monitor patient carefully in all situations. ▪ Glucose and potassium levels must be monitored closely during IV administration of insulin to avoid potentially fatal hypoglycemia and hypokalemia. ▪ Glycosylated hemoglobin (HgbA1c) may be measured to assess long-term glycemic control. ▪ See Drug/Lab Interactions.

Patient Education: Monitor blood glucose as directed. ▪ Adhere to consistent diet and exercise programs. ▪ Avoid alcohol. ▪ Review medications or changes in medication regimen with a health care professional. ▪ Review S/S of hypoglycemia and hyperglycemia with a health care professional. Be familiar with the treatment for each. ▪ Insulin requirements may change with onset of illness. Monitor glucose carefully and adjust insulin therapy as required.

Maternal/Child: *Regular insulin:* Insulin therapy is the preferred treatment of type 1 and type 2 diabetes during pregnancy. Regular insulin is used IV for glycemic control during labor. Poorly controlled diabetes in pregnancy increases the maternal risk for diabetic ketoacidosis, pre-eclampsia, spontaneous abortions, preterm delivery, stillbirth, and delivery complications. Poorly controlled diabetes increases the fetal risk for major birth defects, stillbirth, and macrosomia-related morbidity. Monitor carefully; insulin requirements may change at different stages of pregnancy and may drop immediately postpartum. ▪ Use caution in breast-feeding. ▪ Breast-feeding may decrease insulin requirements. ▪ Inadequately controlled maternal blood glucose late in pregnancy may cause increased insulin production in the fetus. Monitor and treat neonatal hypoglycemia postpartum.

Elderly: No overall differences in safety or effectiveness were observed between elderly patients and younger patients. Elderly patients may be at increased risk of hypoglycemia due to comorbid conditions and concomitantly administered medications; see Dose Adjustments and Drug/Lab Interactions. Initial dosing, dose increments, and maintenance dosage should be conservative to avoid hypoglycemia.

DRUG/LAB INTERACTIONS

Hypoglycemic effect may be potentiated by **ACE inhibitors, anabolic steroids, angiotensin II receptor–blocking agents, disopyramide, fluoxetine, fibrates, guanethidine, MAO inhibitors, oral antidiabetic agents, pentoxifylline, salicylates, sulfonamides, and many others**. Dose adjustment and increased frequency of glucose monitoring may be required with concomitant use. ▪ Drugs that may reduce blood glucose-lowering effect include **atypical antipsychotic medications, corticosteroids, danazol, diuretics, estrogen, glucagon, isoniazid** (INH), **niacin, oral contraceptives, phenothiazine derivatives, protease inhibitors, somatropin, sympathomimetic agents, thyroid preparations, and others**. Dose adjustment and increased frequency of glucose monitoring may be required with concomitant use. ▪ **Alcohol, beta-adrenergic blockers including ophthalmics, clonidine, and lithium** may either potentiate or inhibit the blood glucose-lowering effect of insulin. Dose adjustment and increased frequency of glucose monitoring may be required with concomitant use. ▪ Will affect serum potassium levels; use caution in patients taking **digoxin**. ▪ **Octreotide** may alter insulin, glucagon, and growth hormone secretion, resulting in hypoglycemia or hyperglycemia. Monitor serum glucose and adjust insulin dose as indicated. ▪ **Pentamidine** is toxic to the beta cells of the pancreas. Patients may develop hypoglycemia initially as insulin is released. This may be followed by hypoinsulinemia and hyperglycemia with continued pentamidine therapy. ▪ S/S of hypoglycemia may be masked in the presence of **beta-blockers, clonidine, guanethidine**. Increased frequency of glucose monitoring may be required with concomitant use. ▪ **Thiazolidinediones** (TZDs) can cause dose-related fluid retention, particularly when used in combination with insulin. Fluid retention may lead to or exacerbate heart failure. Patients receiving concomitant therapy should be monitored for S/S of heart failure. Dose reduction or discontinuation of the TZD may be indicated if heart failure develops.

SIDE EFFECTS

The most common adverse reactions with IV administration of insulin include hypersensitivity reactions, hypoglycemia, pruritus, and rash. Other commonly reported reactions are hypokalemia, injection site reactions, peripheral edema, and weight gain. Additional side effects reported in studies include abdominal pain, arthralgia, asthenia, back pain, chest pain, diarrhea, dysmenorrhea, fever, headache, hypertension, hyporeflexia, influenza, myalgia, nasopharyngitis, nausea, onychomycosis, pain, sensory disturbances, sinusitis, skin disorders, upper respiratory infections, and urinary tract infections. Severe hypersensitivity reactions may include anaphylaxis, angioedema, bronchospasm, generalized skin reactions, rash, hypotension, and shock.

Overdose: Severe hypoglycemia and hypokalemia. Severe hypoglycemia may result in coma, seizures, or neurologic impairment. Severe, untreated hypokalemia may lead to respiratory paralysis, ventricular arrhythmia, and death.

ANTIDOTE

Discontinue the drug immediately and notify physician of adverse reactions or hypoglycemia. *Glucagon* 1 to 2 mg IM or SQ is the specific antidote for insulin overdose. It may be supplemented by dextrose 50% IV. Oral carbohydrates such as glucose tablets or gel or orange juice may be sufficient to combat early symptoms of mild hypoglycemia. Correct hypokalemia as indicated. Hypersensitivity reactions usually respond to symptomatic treatment.

IRINOTECAN HYDROCHLORIDE [BBW] ■
IRINOTECAN LIPOSOME INJECTION [BBW]

Antineoplastic
(topoisomerase 1 inhibitor)

(**eye**-rih-noh-**TEE**-kan hy-droh-**KLOR**-eyed)
(**eye**-rih-noh-**TEE**-kan **LIP**-oh-sohm in-**JEK**-shun)

Camptosar, CPT-11 ■ ONIVYDE

pH 3 to 3.8 (Camptosar)

USUAL DOSE

Pretreatment: *Both formulations (conventional and ONIVYDE):* Verify pregnancy status.

CONVENTIONAL IRINOTECAN

Premedication: *Antiemetics:* Dexamethasone 10 mg and a 5-HT3 blocker (e.g., ondansetron [Zofran] or granisetron [Kytril]) should be given on the day of treatment. Begin at least 30 minutes before giving irinotecan. ***Anticholinergic premedication:*** In addition, prophylactic or therapeutic atropine may be indicated in patients experiencing cholinergic symptoms. See Monitor.

First-line treatment of colorectal cancer: Premedication as described above is recommended. Initiate regimen with the dose of irinotecan over 90 minutes. Follow immediately with the dose of leucovorin calcium (see leucovorin calcium monograph). Follow the leucovorin immediately with the dose of fluorouracil (see fluorouracil monograph). Doses and modified dosing recommendations are outlined in the chart Combination-Agent Dosage Regimens and Dose Modifications. Doses of irinotecan and fluorouracil may require modification based on toxicity.

See the following chart, Combination-Agent Dosage Regimens and Dose Modifications, and see Dose Adjustments, combination therapy, and/or package insert.

Combination-Agent Dosage Regimens and Dose Modifications[a] (Irinotecan/Fluorouracil [5-FU]/Leucovorin Calcium [LV])				
Regimen 1 6-wk cycle with bolus 5-FU/LV (next cycle begins on Day 43)	irinotecan leucovorin 5-FU	125 mg/M^2 IV over 90 min, Day 1, 8, 15, 22 20 mg/M^2 IV bolus, Day 1, 8, 15, 22 500 mg/M^2 IV bolus, Day 1, 8, 15, 22		
	Starting Dose and Modified Dose Levels (mg/M^2)			
		Starting Dose	Dose Level −1	Dose Level −2
	irinotecan	125 mg/M^2	100 mg/M^2	75 mg/M^2
	leucovorin	20 mg/M^2	20 mg/M^2	20 mg/M^2
	5-FU	500 mg/M^2	400 mg/M^2	300 mg/M^2
Regimen 2 6-wk cycle with infusional 5-FU/LV (next cycle begins on Day 43)	irinotecan leucovorin 5-FU bolus 5-FU infusion[b]	180 mg/M^2 IV over 90 min, Day 1, 15, 29 200 mg/M^2 IV over 2 hr, Day 1, 2, 15, 16, 29, 30 400 mg/M^2 IV bolus, Day 1, 2, 15, 16, 29, 30 600 mg/M^2 IV over 22 hr, Day 1, 2, 15, 16, 29, 30		
	Starting Dose and Modified Dose Levels (mg/M^2)			
		Starting Dose	Dose Level −1	Dose Level −2
	irinotecan	180 mg/M^2	150 mg/M^2	120 mg/M^2
	leucovorin	200 mg/M^2	200 mg/M^2	200 mg/M^2
	5-FU bolus	400 mg/M^2	320 mg/M^2	240 mg/M^2
	5-FU infusion[b]	600 mg/M^2	480 mg/M^2	360 mg/M^2

[a]Dose reductions beyond dose level −2 by decrements of ~20% may be warranted for patients continuing to experience toxicity. Provided intolerable toxicity does not develop, treatment with additional cycles may be continued indefinitely as long as patients continue to experience clinical benefit.
[b]Infusion follows bolus administration.

Treatment of colorectal cancer after failure of treatment with fluorouracil: Irinotecan: Administer as an infusion based on the following chart, Irinotecan Single-Agent Regimens and Dose Modifications. See Premedication. After adequate recovery, additional doses may be repeated in a similar cycle and continued indefinitely in patients who attain a response or in those whose disease remains stable.

Irinotecan Single-Agent Regimens and Dose Modifications			
Weekly Regimen[a]	125 mg/M^2 IV over 90 min, Day 1, 8, 15, 22 then 2-wk rest		
	Starting Dose and Modified Dose Levels (mg/M^2)[c]		
	Starting Dose	Dose Level −1	Dose Level −2
	125 mg/M^2	100 mg/M^2	75 mg/M^2
Once-Every-3-Weeks Regimen[b]	350 mg/M^2 IV over 90 min, once every 3 wks[c]		
	Starting Dose and Modified Dose Levels (mg/M^2)		
	Starting Dose	Dose Level −1	Dose Level −2
	350 mg/M^2	300 mg/M^2	250 mg/M^2

[a]Subsequent doses may be adjusted as high as 150 mg/M^2 or to as low as 50 mg/M^2 in 25 to 50 mg/M^2 decrements depending upon individual patient tolerance.

[b]Subsequent doses may be adjusted as low as 200 mg/M^2 in 50 mg/M^2 decrements depending upon individual patient tolerance.

[c]Provided intolerable toxicity does not develop, treatment with additional cycles may be continued indefinitely as long as patients continue to experience clinical benefit.

ONIVYDE (LIPOSOMAL IRINOTECAN)
Do not substitute ONIVYDE for other drugs containing irinotecan HCl.
Administer **ONIVYDE before** administering leucovorin and fluorouracil.
Premedication: Administer a corticosteroid and an antiemetic 30 minutes before the **ONIVYDE** infusion.
Metastatic adenocarcinoma of the pancreas: 70 mg/M^2 as an IV infusion over 90 minutes every 2 weeks. In patients known to be homozygous for the UGT1A1*28 allele, the recommended starting dose is 50 mg/M^2 as an IV infusion over 90 minutes. Increase dose to 70 mg/M^2 as tolerated in subsequent cycles. In clinical trials, a dose of 70 mg/M^2 **ONIVYDE** was followed by leucovorin 400 mg/M^2 IV over 30 minutes, followed by fluorouracil 2,400 mg/M^2 IV over 46 hours every 2 weeks.

DOSE ADJUSTMENTS
CONVENTIONAL IRINOTECAN
A reduction in the starting dose by one dose level may be required in patients with a performance status of 2, in patients who have previously received pelvic/abdominal irradiation, and in patients with increased bilirubin levels; see Elderly. Available information insufficient to recommend a dose for patients with bilirubin greater than 2 mg/dL.
▪ Consider decreasing the **starting dose** by at least one level of irinotecan when administered in combination with other agents or as a single agent to a patient known to be homozygous for the UGT1A1*28 allele (an allele is an alternative form of a gene). The precise dose reduction for this patient population is not known. Subsequent dose modification should be based on individual patient tolerance as outlined in the following charts. Heterozygous patients (patients who carry one variant allele) appear to tolerate normal starting doses. ▪ See Precautions.
Combination therapy: Decrease dose based on toxicity as described in the following chart.

Continued

Guidelines for Dose Adjustments in Combination Schedules (Irinotecan/Fluorouracil [5-FU]/Leucovorin Calcium [LV])		
Patients should return to pretreatment bowel function without requiring antidiarrheal medications for at least 24 hours before the next chemotherapy administration. A new cycle of therapy should also not begin until the granulocyte count has recovered to ≥1,500/mm³ and the platelet count has recovered to ≥100,000/mm³. Treatment should be delayed 1 to 2 weeks to allow for recovery from treatment-related toxicities. If the patient has not recovered after a 2-week delay, consideration should be given to discontinuing therapy.		
Toxicity NCI CTC[a] Grade (Value)	**During a Cycle of Therapy**	**At the Start of Subsequent Cycles of Therapy[b]**
No toxicity	Maintain dose level	Maintain dose level
Neutropenia 1 (1,500 to 1,999/mm³)	Maintain dose level	Maintain dose level
2 (1,000 to 1,499/mm³)	↓1 dose level	Maintain dose level
3 (500 to 999/mm³)	Omit dose until resolved to ≤Grade 2, then ↓1 dose level	↓1 dose level
4 (<500/mm³)	Omit dose until resolved to ≤Grade 2, then ↓2 dose levels	↓2 dose levels
Neutropenic fever	Omit dose, then ↓2 dose levels when resolved	
Other hematologic toxicities	Dose modifications for leukopenia or thrombocytopenia during a cycle of therapy and at the start of subsequent cycles of therapy are also based on NCI toxicity criteria and are the same as previously recommended for neutropenia.	
Diarrhea 1 (2-3 stools/day >pretx[c])	Delay dose until resolved to baseline, then give same dose	Maintain dose level
2 (4-6 stools/day >pretx)	Omit dose until resolved to baseline, then ↓1 dose level	Maintain dose level
3 (7-9 stools/day >pretx)	Omit dose until resolved to baseline, then ↓1 dose level	↓1 dose level
4 (≥10 stools/day >pretx)	Omit dose until resolved to baseline, then ↓2 dose levels	↓2 dose levels
Other nonhematologic toxicities[d] Grade 1	Maintain dose level	Maintain dose level
Grade 2	Omit dose until resolved to ≤Grade 1, then ↓1 dose level	Maintain dose level
Grade 3	Omit dose until resolved to ≤Grade 2, then ↓1 dose level	↓1 dose level
Grade 4	Omit dose until resolved to ≤Grade 2, then ↓2 dose levels	↓2 dose levels
	For mucositis/stomatitis decrease only 5-FU, not irinotecan	*For mucositis/stomatitis decrease only 5-FU, not irinotecan*

[a]National Cancer Institute Common Terminology Criteria (Version 1.0).
[b]Relative to the starting dose of the previous cycle.
[c]Pretreatment.
[d]Excludes alopecia, anorexia, asthenia.

Single-agent therapy: Reduce dose based on toxicity levels in the following chart, Guidelines for Irinotecan Dose Adjustments in Single-Agent Schedules. The most common reasons for dose reduction are late diarrhea, neutropenia, and leukopenia.

Guidelines for Irinotecan Dose Adjustments in Single-Agent Schedules[a]

A new cycle of therapy should not begin until the granulocyte count has recovered to ≥1,500/mm³, the platelet count has recovered to ≥100,000/mm³, and treatment-related diarrhea is fully resolved. Treatment should be delayed 1 to 2 weeks to allow for recovery from treatment-related toxicities. If the patient has not recovered after a 2-week delay, consideration should be given to discontinuing irinotecan.

Worst Toxicity NCI CTC Grade[b] (Value)	During a Cycle of Therapy	At the Start of the Next Cycles of Therapy (After Adequate Recovery). Compared with the Starting Dose in the Previous Cycle[a]	
	Weekly	**Weekly**	**Once Every 3 Weeks**
No toxicity	Maintain dose level	↓25 mg/M² up to a maximum dose of 150 mg/M²	Maintain dose level
Neutropenia			
1 (1,500 to 1,999/mm³)	Maintain dose level	Maintain dose level	Maintain dose level
2 (1,000 to 1,499/mm³)	↓25 mg/M²	Maintain dose level	Maintain dose level
3 (500 to 999/mm³)	Omit dose until resolved to ≤Grade 2, then ↓25 mg/M²	↓25 mg/M²	↓50 mg/M²
4 (<500/mm³)	Omit dose until resolved to ≤Grade 2, then ↓50 mg/M²	↓50 mg/M²	↓50 mg/M²
Neutropenic fever	Omit dose until resolved, then ↓50 mg/M²	↓50 mg/M²	↓50 mg/M²
Other hematologic toxicities	Dose modifications for leukopenia, thrombocytopenia, and anemia during a cycle of therapy and at the start of subsequent cycles of therapy are also based on NCI toxicity criteria and are the same as recommended for neutropenia above.		
Diarrhea			
1 (2-3 stools/day >pretx[c])	Maintain dose level	Maintain dose level	Maintain dose level
2 (4-6 stools/day >pretx)	↓25 mg/M²	Maintain dose level	Maintain dose level
3 (7-9 stools/day >pretx)	Omit dose until resolved to ≤Grade 2, then ↓25 mg/M²	↓25 mg/M²	↓50 mg/M²
4 (≥10 stools/day >pretx)	Omit dose until resolved to ≤Grade 2, then ↓50 mg/M²	↓50 mg/M²	↓50 mg/M²
Other nonhematologic toxicities[d]			
Grade 1	Maintain dose level	Maintain dose level	Maintain dose level
Grade 2	↓25 mg/M²	↓25 mg/M²	↓50 mg/M²
Grade 3	Omit dose until resolved to ≤Grade 2, then ↓25 mg/M²	↓25 mg/M²	↓50 mg/M²
Grade 4	Omit dose until resolved to ≤Grade 2, then ↓50 mg/M²	↓50 mg/M²	↓50 mg/M²

[a]All dose modifications should be based on the worst preceding toxicity.
[b]National Cancer Institute Common Terminology Criteria (Version 1.0).
[c]Pretreatment.
[d]Excludes alopecia, anorexia, asthenia.

ONIVYDE

There is no recommended dose of **ONIVYDE** for patients with serum bilirubin above the upper limit of normal. ▪ Withhold **ONIVYDE** for an absolute neutrophil count below 1,500/mm³ or neutropenic fever. ▪ Withhold **ONIVYDE** for diarrhea of Grade 2 to 4 severity. ▪ See the following chart for dose modifications recommended for adverse reactions.

Continued

Recommended Dose Modifications for Adverse Reactions to ONIVYDE			
Toxicity NCI CTCAE, v 4.0[a]	Occurrence	ONIVYDE Adjustment in Patients Receiving 70 mg/M^2	ONIVYDE Adjustment in Patients Homozygous for UGT1A1*28 Without Previous Increase to 70 mg/M^2
Grade 3 or 4 adverse reactions	1. Withhold ONIVYDE. 2. Initiate loperamide for late-onset diarrhea of **any** severity. 3. Administer IV or SQ atropine 0.25 to 1 mg (unless clinically contraindicated) for early-onset diarrhea of **any** severity. 4. Upon recovery to ≤ Grade 1, resume ONIVYDE at:		
	First	50 mg/M^2	43 mg/M^2
	Second	43 mg/M^2	35 mg/M^2
	Third	Discontinue ONIVYDE	Discontinue ONIVYDE
Interstitial lung disease	First	Discontinue ONIVYDE	Discontinue ONIVYDE
Anaphylactic reaction	First	Discontinue ONIVYDE	Discontinue ONIVYDE

[a]*NCI CTCAE, v 4.0,* National Cancer Institute Common Toxicity Criteria for Adverse Events, Version 4.0.

For recommended dose modifications for fluorouracil (5-FU) and/or leucovorin (LV), refer to their monographs and/or full prescribing information.

DILUTION

Specific techniques required; see Precautions.

Conventional Irinotecan: Available in single-dose vials in 2-mL, 5-mL, and 15-mL sizes with a concentration of 20 mg/mL. Must be diluted for infusion with D5W (preferred) or NS to concentrations between 0.12 and 2.8 mg/mL. Usually diluted in 250 to 500 mL D5W.

ONIVYDE: Available in a single-dose vial containing 43 mg irinotecan free base at a concentration of 4.3 mg/mL. It is a slightly yellow, opaque, liposomal dispersion. Withdraw the calculated volume from the vial and dilute in 500 mL D5W or NS. Mix by gentle inversion. Protect diluted solution from light.

Filters: *Conventional irinotecan:* Specific information not available. *ONIVYDE:* Do not use in-line filters.

Storage: *Conventional irinotecan:* Packaged in a blister pack to protect against accidental breakage and leakage. Store in carton protected from light at CRT. When mixed with D5W, is chemically and physically stable for 48 hours if refrigerated and in ambient fluorescent lighting and for 24 hours at CRT. *Do not refrigerate if mixed with NS;* a precipitate may form. Stable for 24 hours at CRT when mixed in NS. Because of the risk of microbial contamination, the manufacturer recommends that solutions mixed in D5W or NS be used within 4 hours if kept at RT. However, if reconstitution and dilution are performed under strict aseptic conditions (e.g., on a laminar air flow bench), the solution should be used (i.e., infusion completed) within 12 hours at RT or 24 hours (D5W) if refrigerated. Avoid freezing.

ONIVYDE: Refrigerate in carton at 2° to 8° C (36° to 46° F) to protect from light. Do not freeze. Administer diluted solution within 4 hours of preparation when stored at RT or within 24 hours if refrigerated. Allow diluted solution to come to RT before administration. Do not freeze. Discard unused portion.

COMPATIBILITY

CONVENTIONAL IRINOTECAN

Manufacturer states, "Other drugs should not be added to the infusion solution."

Other sources suggest a few **compatibilities** based on concentration and manufacturer; consult a pharmacist.

ONIVYDE

Compatibility information not available from manufacturer; consult a pharmacist.

RATE OF ADMINISTRATION

Both formulations: A single dose as an infusion equally distributed over 90 minutes.
ONIVYDE: Do not use in-line filter.

ACTIONS

CONVENTIONAL IRINOTECAN: A semi-synthetic derivative of camptothecin. An alkaloid extract from plants such as *Camptotheca acuminata*. A class of antineoplastic agent that inhibits the enzyme topoisomerase I required for DNA replication. Together with its active metabolite, SN-38, it causes cell death by damaging DNA produced during the S-phase of the cell cycle. Maximum plasma SN-38 levels are reached within 1 hour of infusion end. Terminal half-life of irinotecan is about 6 to 12 hours; SN-38 is 10 to 20 hours. Irinotecan is moderately bound to plasma proteins (30% to 68%), but SN-38 is highly bound (95%). Metabolic conversion of irinotecan to SN-38 primarily occurs in the liver. SN-38 is conjugated to a glucuronide metabolite by the enzyme UDP-glucuronosyltransferase 1A1 (UGT1A1). Approximately 25% to 50% excreted through bile and urine.

ONIVYDE: A topoisomerase 1 inhibitor encapsulated in a lipid bilayer vesicle or liposome. Topoisomerase 1 relieves torsional strain in DNA by inducing single-strand breaks. Irinotecan and its active metabolite SN-38 bind reversibly to the topoisomerase 1–DNA complex and prevent re-ligation of the single-strand breaks, leading to cell death. 95% of irinotecan remains liposome-encapsulated. Terminal elimination half-life is approximately 25.8 hours. Protein binding is less than 0.44% of the total irinotecan in ONIVYDE. Metabolism and excretion of irinotecan liposome have not been evaluated.

INDICATIONS AND USES

CONVENTIONAL IRINOTECAN: As a component of first-line therapy in combination with 5-fluorouracil (5-FU) and leucovorin (LV) for patients with metastatic carcinoma of the colon or rectum. ■ For patients with metastatic carcinoma of the colon or rectum whose disease has recurred or progressed following initial fluorouracil-based therapy.

ONIVYDE: Treatment of patients with metastatic adenocarcinoma of the pancreas after disease progression following gemcitabine-based therapy. Used in combination with fluorouracil and leucovorin.

Limitation of use of ONIVYDE: Not indicated as a single agent for the treatment of patients with metastatic adenocarcinoma of the pancreas.

CONTRAINDICATIONS

Both formulations: History of hypersensitivity to conventional or liposomal formulations of irinotecan or any of their components.

PRECAUTIONS

Both formulations: Follow guidelines for handling cytotoxic agents. See Appendix A, p. 1308. ■ Administered by or under the direction of the physician specialist. ■ Adequate diagnostic and treatment facilities must be available. ■ Can cause severe or life-threatening neutropenia and fatal neutropenic sepsis. ■ Patients who are homozygous for the UGT1A1*28 allele have decreased UGT1A1 enzyme activity. This leads to a higher exposure to SN-38 and an increased risk for neutropenia; see Dose Adjustments. A laboratory test is available to determine the UGT1A1 status of patients. ■ Can cause severe or life-threatening diarrhea that may be either early or late onset (see discussion under individual agents). ■ Severe hypersensitivity reactions, including anaphylaxis, have been reported. ■ Interstitial pulmonary disease has been reported and can be fatal. Use caution in patients with pleural effusions and/or impaired pulmonary function. Risk factors may include pre-existing lung disease or use of pneumotoxic agents (e.g., amiodarone [Nexterone]), radiation therapy, or colony-stimulating factors; see Antidote.

CONVENTIONAL IRINOTECAN: Can induce both early and late forms of diarrhea that appear to be mediated by different mechanisms. Both forms may be severe. Interrupt therapy and reduce subsequent doses if severe diarrhea occurs; see Dose Adjustments. Late diarrhea may be complicated by colitis, ulceration, bleeding, ileus, obstruction, and infection. Cases of megacolon and intestinal perforation have been reported. Patients must not be treated with irinotecan until resolution of any bowel obstruction. ■ May cause severe myelosuppression. Bacterial, viral, and fungal infections have occurred. Deaths due to sepsis following severe neutropenia have been reported. Patients who have previously received pelvic/abdominal irradiation, patients with a baseline serum total bilirubin level of 1 mg/dL or more, or patients with deficient glucuronidation of bilirubin (e.g., patients with Gilbert syndrome) may be at a greater risk of myelosuppression. ▪ Hepatic dysfunction may impair the metabolism of both irinotecan and SN-38. Patients with a bilirubin of 1 to 2 mg/dL are at increased risk for developing Grade 3 or 4 neutropenia. The manufacturer does not recommend a dose for patients with a bilirubin greater than 2 mg/dL and states that insufficient information is available to recommend dosing. ▪ Use with caution in patients with renal impairment. Has not been studied. Not recommended for use in patients on dialysis. ▪ Renal impairment and acute renal failure have been reported; see Monitor. ▪ Use caution in elderly patients (may have an increased incidence and severity of diarrhea). ▪ Use caution in patients with poor performance status. Patients with a baseline performance status of 2 had higher rates of hospitalization, neutropenic fever, thromboembolism, first-cycle treatment discontinuation, and early deaths than patients with a performance status of 0 or 1. ▪ Contains sorbitol. Do not use in patients with hereditary fructose intolerance. ▪ The regimen of 5-FU/LV (administered for 4 to 5 days every 28 days) should not be used in combination with irinotecan outside a carefully controlled, well-designed clinical study. Regimen has caused increased toxicity and death. ▪ See Monitor.

ONIVYDE: Severe or life-threatening neutropenia, neutropenic fever or sepsis, and fatal neutropenic sepsis have occurred. The incidence of Grade 3 or 4 neutropenia was higher among Asian patients compared with White patients in clinical trials. Withhold ONIVYDE for absolute neutrophil count below 1,500/mm^3 or neutropenic fever; see Monitor. ▪ Severe diarrhea has occurred in patients receiving liposomal irinotecan in combination with fluorouracil and leucovorin. Withhold ONIVYDE for diarrhea of Grade 2 to 4 severity. An individual patient may experience both early- and late-onset diarrhea; see Monitor. ▪ Do not administer ONIVYDE to patients with bowel obstruction. ▪ Not studied in patients with hepatic impairment. ▪ No pharmacokinetic effects noted in patients with mild to moderate renal impairment. Data for severe renal impairment are insufficient.

Monitor: BOTH FORMULATIONS: Prophylactic antiemetics are recommended; see Usual Dose. To reduce nausea and vomiting and increase patient comfort after initial dosing, additional antiemetics should be available (e.g., prochlorperazine, ondansetron, granisetron). ▪ Monitor vital signs. ▪ Obtain an accurate bowel history to evaluate changes in bowel habits after administration of irinotecan. ▪ Monitor for "early" diarrhea. Occurs during or within 24 hours of irinotecan administration and is cholinergic in nature. Usually transient and only infrequently is severe. May be accompanied by other cholinergic symptoms (e.g., abdominal cramping, bradycardia, diaphoresis, flushing, increased salivation, lacrimation, miosis, rhinitis). Patients who have a cholinergic reaction to irinotecan will probably have similar reactions to subsequent doses. Atropine 0.25 to 1 mg IV or SQ may be considered for treatment or for prophylactic use unless clinically contraindicated. ▪ Monitor for "late" diarrhea (more than 24 hours after irinotecan administration), which probably results from cytotoxic effects on GI epithelium. May be prolonged; may cause dehydration, electrolyte imbalances, or sepsis; and can be life-threatening. At first onset, give loperamide 4 mg; give 2 mg every 2 hours (4 mg every 4 hours during the night) until diarrhea-free for a minimum of 12 hours. Monitor carefully; replace fluids and electrolytes as needed; see Patient Education. ▪ Maintain adequate hydration. Orthostatic hypotension or dizziness may indicate dehydration. ▪ Initiate antibiotic therapy in patients who develop ileus, fever, or severe neutropenia. ▪ Be alert for signs of bone marrow suppression or infection. Prophylactic antibiotics may be indicated pending results of C/S in a febrile neutropenic patient. ▪ Monitor for thrombocytopenia (platelet count less than 50,000/mm^3). Initiate precautions to prevent excessive bleeding (e.g., inspect IV sites, skin, and mucous membranes; use extreme care during invasive procedures; test urine, emesis, stool, and secretions for occult blood). ▪ Monitor for S/S of a hypersensitivity reaction (e.g., chest pain, chills, dizziness, dyspnea, fever, flushing, hypotension, nausea, pruritus, rash, urticaria) or an infusion reaction (e.g., asthenia, chills, fatigue, fever, vomiting). ▪ Monitor for S/S of interstitial lung disease. Withhold therapy in patients with new or progressive cough, dyspnea, and fever pending diagnostic evaluation; see Precautions and Antidote. ■ See Dose Adjustments.

CONVENTIONAL IRINOTECAN: Obtain a WBC with differential, hemoglobin, and platelet count before each dose. ■ Obtain baseline electrolytes and liver function tests. Repeat as indicated. ■ Not a vesicant, but monitor injection site for inflammation and/or extravasation. ■ If late-onset diarrhea develops, subsequent weekly chemotherapy treatments should be delayed until pretreatment bowel function has returned for at least 24 hours without the need for antidiarrheal medication. If Grade 2, 3, or 4 late diarrhea recurs, subsequent doses of irinotecan should be decreased; see Dose Adjustments. ■ Avoid use of diuretics and laxatives in patients with diarrhea. ■ Monitor renal function and hydration status. Rare cases of renal impairment or acute renal failure have been reported, usually in patients who became dehydrated from vomiting and/or diarrhea.

ONIVYDE (LIPOSOMAL IRINOTECAN): Prophylactic antiemetics and corticosteroids are recommended 30 minutes before ONIVYDE infusion. ■ Monitor CBC on Days 1 and 8 of every cycle and more frequently if clinically indicated. Withhold ONIVYDE if the absolute neutrophil count (ANC) is below 1,500/mm³ or if neutropenic fever occurs. Resume when the ANC is 1,500 mm³ or above; see Dose Adjustments. ■ Monitor for infusion reactions occurring on the day of administration. S/S have included periorbital edema, pruritus, rash, and urticaria.

Patient Education: *Both formulations:* Review patient counseling information. ■ Report any unusual or unexpected symptoms or side effects as soon as possible. ■ Report black or bloody stools, diarrhea not under control within 24 hours, dry mouth, fever or chills, inability to retain oral fluids due to nausea and vomiting, infections, symptoms of dehydration (e.g., light-headedness, dizziness, fainting), urine changes, or vomiting immediately; each must be treated promptly. Have loperamide available. Dose of loperamide prescribed for late diarrhea is higher than the usual dose recommendation. Limit use at this dose to 48 hours to avoid risk of paralytic ileus. ■ May cause dizziness or visual disturbances (usually within 24 hours of administration); use caution in tasks that require alertness. ■ Compliance with regimen imperative (e.g., taking temperature, obtaining lab work, adequate rest, nourishment, and fluids). ■ *Both formulations:* Effective birth control required. *ONIVYDE:* Advise females of reproductive potential to use effective contraception during treatment and for 1 month after the final dose. Advise males with female partners of reproductive potential to use condoms during treatment and for 4 months after the final dose. ■ Inform health care professionals of any problems with previous treatments. ■ See Appendix D, p. 1311.

Maternal/Child: *Both formulations:* Avoid pregnancy. May cause fetal harm. ■ Discontinue breast-feeding during treatment and for 1 month after the final dose. ■ Safety and effectiveness for use in pediatric patients not established.

Elderly: *Conventional irinotecan:* Half-life slightly extended. ■ Reduce starting dose by one dose level to 300 mg/M² in patients 70 years and older in the single-agent, once-every-3-weeks regimen. No change in the starting dose is recommended for elderly patients receiving the weekly dose schedule of irinotecan. See Usual Dose and Dose Adjustments. ■ Risk of early and late diarrhea increased in the elderly. ■ Monitor carefully; may dehydrate more quickly from diarrhea. Begin loperamide therapy promptly. Avoid laxatives.

ONIVYDE: No overall differences in safety and effectiveness observed between the elderly and younger patients.

DRUG/LAB INTERACTIONS

Interaction of **conventional irinotecan** and/or **ONIVYDE** with other drugs has not been adequately studied.

Both formulations: Concomitant use with **CYP3A4 enzyme-inducing anticonvulsants and strong CYP3A4 inducers** may increase the metabolism of irinotecan, which decreases concentrations and effectiveness. Avoid use of **strong CYP3A4 inducers** (e.g., carbamazepine, oxcarbazepine, phenobarbital, phenytoin, rifampin, rifabutin, St. John's wort) if possible. Substitute non–enzyme inducing therapies at least 2 weeks before initiation of irinotecan therapy. ▪ **CYP3A4 inhibitors** (e.g., clarithromycin, indinavir, itraconazole, ketoconazole, lopinavir/ritonavir, nefazodone, nelfinavir, ritonavir, saquinavir, telaprevir, voriconazole) **and UGT1A1 inhibitors** (e.g., atazanavir, gemfibrozil, indinavir, ketoconazole) may decrease metabolism, which increases serum concentrations and the risk of toxicity. Avoid the use of **strong CYP3A4 or UGT1A1 inhibitors** if possible. Discontinue at least 1 week before starting irinotecan therapy. ▪ Do not administer **live virus vaccines** to patients receiving antineoplastic drugs.

Conventional irinotecan: Additive bone marrow suppression may occur with **radiation therapy and/or other bone marrow–suppressing agents** (e.g., azathioprine, chloramphenicol, melphalan). Dose reduction may be required. ▪ Concurrent administration with **irradiation** is not recommended. ▪ Use caution or withhold **diuretics** (e.g., furosemide) **and laxatives** during treatment; may increase risk of dehydration secondary to vomiting and/or diarrhea.

SIDE EFFECTS

Conventional irinotecan: Myelosuppression (anemia, leukopenia, neutropenia) and diarrhea ("early" [e.g., abdominal cramping or pain, diaphoresis] or "late") occur in patients and are the most common dose-limiting toxicities with irinotecan administration.

Combination therapy: Common adverse reactions (greater than 30%) observed in combination therapy are abdominal pain, abnormal bilirubin, alopecia, anemia, anorexia, asthenia, constipation, diarrhea, fever, infection, leukopenia (including lymphocytopenia), mucositis, nausea, neutropenia, pain, thrombocytopenia, and vomiting.

Single-agent therapy: Common adverse reactions (greater than 30%) observed in single-agent therapy are abdominal pain, alopecia, anemia, anorexia, asthenia, constipation, diarrhea, fever, leukopenia (including lymphocytopenia), nausea, neutropenia, weight loss, and vomiting.

Other reported side effects with irinotecan include abdominal bloating, back pain, chills, confusion, coughing, dehydration, dizziness, dyspepsia, dyspnea, edema, exfoliative dermatitis, flatulence, flushing, headache, hypersensitivity reactions (including anaphylaxis), hyponatremia, hypotension, increased alkaline phosphatase and AST, increased bilirubin, insomnia, interstitial pulmonary disease, muscular contractions or cramps, MI, neutropenic fever, neutropenic infection, paresthesia, pneumonia, pulmonary embolism, rash, rhinitis, somnolence, stomatitis, thrombophlebitis, and weight loss may occur. In addition, ileus without preceding colitis has occurred. Renal impairment or failure has occurred, usually in patients who became volume depleted from severe vomiting and/or diarrhea.

ONIVYDE: Asthenia, decreased appetite, diarrhea, fatigue, fever, lymphopenia, nausea, neutropenia, stomatitis, and vomiting are most common. The most common serious side effects were acute renal failure, dehydration, diarrhea, fever, nausea, neutropenic fever or neutropenic sepsis, pneumonia, sepsis, septic shock, thrombocytopenia, and vomiting. Diarrhea, vomiting, and sepsis were the most common reasons for discontinuing therapy. Anemia, diarrhea, nausea, and neutropenia were the most common reasons for dose reduction.

Post-Marketing: Asymptomatic elevated pancreatic enzymes (e.g., amylase, lipase), dysarthria (transient), ischemic or ulcerative colitis, megacolon, myocardial ischemic events, pancreatitis.

ANTIDOTE

Keep physician informed of all side effects and monitor carefully. Adjust or omit dose as indicated for toxicity; see Dose Adjustments. Treat diarrhea immediately; see Monitor. In the event of an acute onset of new or progressive, unexplained pulmonary symptoms (e.g., cough, dyspnea, fever), interrupt irinotecan and other coprescribed chemotherapeutic agents pending diagnostic evaluation. If interstitial pulmonary disease is diagnosed, discontinue irinotecan and other chemotherapy and initiate appropriate treatment as needed. Administration of whole blood products (e.g., packed RBCs, platelets, leukocytes) and/or blood modifiers (e.g., darbepoetin alfa, epoetin alfa, filgrastim, pegfilgrastim, sargramostim) may be indicated to treat bone marrow toxicity. Death may occur from the progression of many side effects. No known antidote for overdose. Maximum supportive care (e.g., to prevent dehydration due to diarrhea and to treat any infectious complications) will help sustain patient in toxicity. If extravasation occurs, flush site with SWFI, elevate the extremity, and apply ice.

IRON DEXTRAN INJECTION `BBW`

(**EYE**-ern **DEKS**-tran in-**JEK**-shun)

DexFerrum, DexIron♥, InFeD, Infufer♥, Proferdex

Hematinic
Antianemic
Iron supplement

pH 4.5 to 7

USUAL DOSE

Iron deficiency anemia: A test dose is required on the first day. The maximum daily dose is 100 mg/day.

Test dose: 0.5 mL (25 mg) on the first day as a test dose. Wait 1 hour. If no adverse reactions, administer the remainder of the initial therapeutic dose of 1.5 mL (75 mg).

Therapeutic dose: Repeat the total dose of 2 mL (100 mg)/24 hr daily until results achieved or maximum calculated dosage reached (see dosage charts in literature or formula below). A total calculated dose has been given as an infusion. Though not FDA-approved, this method is preferred by some to multiple small-dose infusions or injections. To calculate the total amount of iron dextran (mL) required to restore hemoglobin and to replenish iron stores in adults and pediatric patients weighing over 15 kg (lean body weight [LBW]):

$$\text{Dose (mL)} = 0.0442 \text{ (Desired Hb} - \text{Observed Hb)} \times \text{LBW in kg} + (0.26 \times \text{LBW in kg})$$

If actual weight is less than LBW or in pediatric patients between 5 and 15 kg, use actual weight in kg. Calculated dose is in **mL.**

Iron replacement for blood loss: Dose should represent the equivalent amount of iron represented in blood loss. Begin with a test dose of 0.5 mL (25 mg). Wait 1 hour. If no adverse reactions, calculate the desired dose with the following formula and administer the balance of the replacement dose over 2 to 3 daily doses:

$$\text{Amount of replacement iron } \textbf{(mg)} = \text{Blood loss } \textbf{(mL)} \times \text{Hematocrit}$$

Calculated dose is in **mg;** convert to **mL** before administration.

Formula is based on the approximation that 1 mL of normocytic, normochromic red cells contains 1 mg of elemental iron.

PEDIATRIC DOSE

Injectable iron not normally used in infants under 4 months of age. See Maternal/Child. **Iron deficiency anemia:** *Test dose:* 0.5 mL (25 mg) for pediatric patients or 0.25 mL (12.5 mg) for infants over at least 5 minutes on the first day. Wait 1 hour. If no adverse reactions, may give remainder of daily dose. Direct IV push is not recommended; diluting with NS for infusion may lower the incidence of phlebitis. If actual weight is less than LBW or for pediatric patients between 5 and 15 kg, use actual weight in kg. The following daily doses have been

Continued

recommended for IM injection by one source: *less than 5 kg,* 25 mg; *5 to 10 kg,* 50 mg; *more than 10 kg,* 100 mg. Repeat daily until results achieved or maximum calculated dosage reached (see dosage charts in literature or the formula listed earlier).

Iron replacement for blood loss: Calculate dose by formula used for adult dose. Dose should represent the equivalent amount of iron represented in blood loss. Begin with a test dose of 0.5 mL (25 mg) for pediatric patients or 0.25 mL (12.5 mg) for infants over at least 5 minutes on the first day. Wait 1 hour. If no adverse reactions, administer the balance of the replacement dose over 2 to 3 daily doses.

DILUTION

Given undiluted or up to the total desired dose may be further diluted in 50 to 1,000 mL NS for infusion. D5W may cause additional local pain and phlebitis.

Filters: No data available from manufacturer.

Storage: Store unopened vials at CRT; protect from freezing.

COMPATIBILITY

Manufacturer states, "Do not mix with other medications or add to parenteral nutrition solutions."

RATE OF ADMINISTRATION

Test dose: 25 mg over 5 minutes (DexFerrum) or over 30 seconds (InFeD). Specific rates of test dose infusions not available for other manufacturers.

IV injection: If no adverse reactions to the test dose, administer 1 mL (50 mg) or a fraction thereof over 1 minute or more. Extend injection time in pediatric patients.

Infusion: If no adverse reactions to the test dose, infuse remaining dose over 1 to 8 hours (based on amount of dose, amount of diluent, and patient comfort).

ACTIONS

Iron dextran is removed from the plasma by cells of the reticuloendothelial system, which split the complex into its components of iron and dextran. Iron is immediately bound to protein moieties to form hemosiderin or ferritin, the physiologic forms of iron, or, to a lesser extent, to transferrin. This iron replenishes hemoglobin and depleted iron stores. Serum ferritin peaks approximately 7 to 9 days after iron dextran administration and slowly returns to baseline after about 3 weeks. Dextran is metabolized or excreted. Negligible amounts of iron are lost via the urinary or alimentary pathways after administration of iron dextran. Some placental transfer of iron dextran may occur. Trace amounts of unmetabolized iron dextran are excreted in breast milk.

INDICATIONS AND USES

Iron deficiency anemia in patients for whom oral administration is unsatisfactory or impossible; identify and treat the cause of the anemia.

Unlabeled uses: Iron supplementation for patients taking epoetin alfa (Epogen).

CONTRAINDICATIONS

Manifestation of hypersensitivity reactions; any anemia other than iron deficiency.

PRECAUTIONS

Anaphylactic-type reactions, including fatalities, have been reported. Fatal reactions have occurred both after the test dose and in situations in which the test dose was tolerated. Administer in facilities equipped to monitor the patient and respond to any medical emergency. Patients with a history of drug allergy or multiple drug allergies may be at increased risk for anaphylactic-type reactions. Concomitant use of angiotensin-converting enzyme inhibitors may also increase the risk of reactions. Facilities for monitoring the patient and responding to any medical emergency must be readily available. ■ Iron dextran products are not clinically interchangeable. They differ in chemical characteristics and may differ in clinical and adverse effects. ■ Large IV doses have been associated with an increased incidence of side effects, including arthralgia, backache, chills, dizziness, fever, headache, malaise, myalgia, nausea, and vomiting. The onset of these side effects is often delayed (1 to 2 days) and symptoms generally subside within 3 to 4 days. Maximum daily recommended dose is 100 mg (2 mL) of undiluted iron dextran. ■ Use with caution in patients with severe liver impairment, cardiovascular disease, or a history of significant allergies and/or asthma. ■ Do not administer during the acute phase of infectious kidney disease. ▪ Patients with rheumatoid arthritis may experience increased joint pain and swelling after administration of iron dextran. ▪ Administration of parenteral iron therapy should be limited to patients in whom clinical and laboratory investigations have established an iron-deficient state. Unwarranted therapy may cause excess storage of iron and possible exogenous hemosiderosis.

Monitor: Keep patient lying down after injection to prevent postural hypotension. ▪ Observe continuously for a hypersensitivity reaction during an infusion. Monitor vital signs. ▪ Monitor hemoglobin, hematocrit, reticulocyte count, total iron-binding capacity (TIBC), and percent of saturation of transferrin as indicated to monitor therapy and iron status. May take up to 3 weeks to see response. ▪ Monitor serum ferritin assays in prolonged therapy. Consider possibility of false results for months after injection caused by delayed utilization. ▪ In patients undergoing chronic renal dialysis who are receiving iron dextran complex, the correlation of body iron stores and serum ferritin may not be valid.

Patient Education: Promptly report S/S of hypersensitivity (e.g., rash, itching, SOB). ▪ Promptly report any other side effects, immediate or delayed.

Maternal/Child: Category C: use only if absolutely necessary in pregnancy, breast-feeding, or childbearing years. ▪ Injectable iron not normally used in infants under 4 months of age.

DRUG/LAB INTERACTIONS

Inhibited by **chloramphenicol.** ▪ Concurrent administration of medicinal iron with **dimercaprol** will result in the formation of a toxic complex. Either postpone iron therapy or treat severe iron deficiency with transfusions. ▪ Effectiveness negated by **deferoxamine**, an iron chelating agent. May be affected by **other chelating agents** (e.g., edetate disodium). Give iron dextran at least 2 hours after a chelating agent. ▪ May cause **false serum iron values** within 1 to 2 weeks of large doses of iron dextran. ▪ May cause a **false elevated bilirubin, false decreased calcium, or affect numerous other tests or scans.** ▪ See Monitor.

SIDE EFFECTS

Backache, dizziness, headache, itching, local phlebitis at injection site, malaise, nausea, rash, shivering, transitory paresthesias.

Major: Anaphylaxis (fatalities have occurred); arthritic reactivation; dyspnea; febrile episodes; hypotension; leukocytosis; local phlebitis; lymphadenopathy; peripheral vascular flushing, especially with too-rapid injection; tachycardia; urticaria; shock (severe iron toxicity increases vasodilation and venous pooling and decreases circulating blood volume; results in decreased cardiac output, hypotension, increased peripheral vascular resistance, and shock).

Overdose: Serum iron levels greater than 300 mcg/dL may indicate iron poisoning. Overdose with iron dextran is unlikely. May result in hemosiderosis, and excess iron may increase susceptibility to infection. If acute toxicity is seen, it may present as:

Early: Abdominal pain, diarrhea, vomiting.

Late: Bluish-colored lips, fingernails, and palms of hands; acidosis, drowsiness, shallow and rapid breathing, clammy skin, weak and fast heartbeat, hypotension, hypoglycemia, cardiovascular collapse.

ANTIDOTE

Discontinue the drug and notify the physician of early symptoms. For severe symptoms, discontinue drug, treat hypersensitivity reactions, or resuscitate as necessary, and notify physician. Epinephrine and diphenhydramine should always be available. In overdose, monitor CBC, iron studies, vital signs, blood gases, and glucose and electrolytes. Maintain fluid and electrolyte balance. Correct acidosis with sodium bicarbonate. Deferoxamine is an iron chelating agent and may be useful in iron toxicity or overdose. Dialysis will not remove iron alone but will remove the iron deferoxamine complex and is indicated if oliguria or anuria is present.

IRON SUCROSE
(**EYE**-ern **SOO**-kros)

Venofer

Hematinic
Iron supplement
Antianemic

pH 10.5 to 11.1

USUAL DOSE

Dose is expressed in terms of mg of elemental iron. The usual total treatment course of iron sucrose is 1,000 mg. For all indications, treatment may be repeated if iron deficiency recurs.

Adult patients with hemodialysis-dependent chronic kidney disease (HDD-CKD): 100 mg undiluted as a slow IV injection or diluted as a 15-minute infusion during consecutive hemodialysis sessions. Administered early during the dialysis session. Frequency of dosing should be no more than three times weekly.

Adult patients with non–dialysis-dependent chronic kidney disease (NDD-CKD): 200 mg undiluted as a slow IV injection over 2 to 5 minutes or as an infusion of 200 mg in a maximum of 100 mL of NS over 15 minutes. Administer on 5 different days over a 14-day period to a total cumulative dose of 1,000 mg. Alternately, there is limited experience with administering a 500-mg dose on Day 1 and Day 14 as a 3.5- to 4-hour infusion diluted in a maximum of 250 mL of NS.

Adult patients with peritoneal dialysis-dependent chronic kidney disease (PDD-CKD): 300 mg as an infusion on Day 1 and Day 14. Follow with 400 mg as an infusion on Day 28. A total cumulative dose of 1,000 mg given in 3 doses over 28 days. Each infusion is diluted in a maximum of 250 mL NS and administered over 1.5 to 2.5 hours; see Rate of Administration.

PEDIATRIC DOSE

Pediatric patients (2 years of age and older) with hemodialysis-dependent chronic kidney disease (HDD-CKD) for iron maintenance treatment: The dosing for iron replacement treatment in pediatric patients with HDD-CKD has not been established.

Iron maintenance treatment: 0.5 mg/kg. Do not exceed 100 mg/dose. Administer every 2 weeks for 12 weeks; given undiluted by slow IV injection over 5 minutes or diluted in NS at a concentration of 1 to 2 mg/mL and administered over 5 to 60 minutes. Do not dilute to concentrations below 1 mg/mL. Regimen may be repeated if necessary.

Pediatric patients (2 years of age and older) with non–dialysis-dependent chronic kidney disease (NDD-CKD) or peritoneal dialysis-dependent chronic kidney disease (PDD-CKD) who are undergoing erythropoietin therapy for iron maintenance treatment: The dosing for iron replacement treatment in pediatric patients with NDD-CKD or PDD-CKD has not been established.

Iron maintenance treatment: 0.5 mg/kg. Do not exceed 100 mg/dose. Administer every 4 weeks for 12 weeks; given undiluted by slow IV injection over 5 minutes or diluted in NS at a concentration of 1 to 2 mg/mL and administered over 5 to 60 minutes. Do not dilute to concentrations below 1 mg/mL. Regimen may be repeated if necessary.

DOSE ADJUSTMENTS

Begin at the low end of the dosing range in elderly patients. Consider the potential for decreased organ function and concomitant disease or drug therapy. ▪ Withhold in patients with evidence of tissue iron overload; see Monitor.

DILUTION

Available in several sizes of single-dose vials. Check vial carefully and select the size that is closest to the desired dose. All contain 20 mg/mL of elemental iron. May be given undiluted or further diluted in NS. Do not dilute to concentrations below 1 mg/mL.

Adult patients with hemodialysis-dependent chronic kidney disease (HDD-CKD): 100-mg dose may be given undiluted or may be further diluted in a maximum of 100 mL of NS and given as an infusion.

Adult patients with non–dialysis dependent chronic kidney disease (NDD-CKD): 200-mg dose may be given undiluted or may be further diluted in a maximum of 100 mL of NS. The 500-mg dose may be further diluted in a maximum of 250 mL of NS and given as an infusion.

Adult patients with peritoneal dialysis–dependent chronic kidney disease (PDD-CKD): Each 300- or 400-mg dose must be diluted in a maximum of 250 mL NS and given as an infusion.

Pediatric patients receiving iron maintenance treatment: A single dose may be given undiluted or diluted in NS at a concentration of 1 to 2 mg/mL and given as an infusion. Do not dilute to concentrations below 1 mg/mL; see Usual Dose.

Filters: No data available from manufacturer.

Storage: Store unopened vials in original carton at CRT. Do not freeze. Diluted iron infusions should be used immediately after preparation. Discard any unused portion. When diluted with NS to a concentration of 1 to 2 mg/mL in PVC or non-PVC infusion bags, iron sucrose is stable for 7 days at CRT. When undiluted (20 mg/mL) or diluted with NS to a concentration of 2 to 10 mg/mL and stored in a plastic syringe, iron sucrose is stable for 7 days at CRT or refrigerated.

COMPATIBILITY

Manufacturer states, "Do not mix with other medications or add to parenteral nutrition solutions."

RATE OF ADMINISTRATION

Too-rapid administration may cause hypotension or symptoms of overdose; see Side Effects.

Slow IV injection in adults: A single undiluted dose over 2 to 5 minutes. In dialysis patients, administer into the dialysis line during the dialysis session.

Infusion in adults: This method of administration may reduce the risk of hypotensive episodes.

Adult hemodialysis-dependent chronic kidney disease patients (HDD-CKD): A single 100-mg undiluted dose given as a slow IV injection over 2 to 5 minutes. Alternately may be diluted and given as an infusion equally distributed over at least 15 minutes.

Adult non–dialysis dependent chronic kidney disease patients (NDD-CKD): A single 200-mg undiluted dose as a slow IV injection over 2 to 5 minutes or as an infusion equally distributed over 15 minutes. Has also been administered as an infusion in a 500-mg dose equally distributed over 3.5 to 4 hours.

Adult peritoneal dialysis–dependent chronic kidney disease patients (PDD-CKD): A single 300-mg dose as an IV infusion equally distributed over 1.5 hours or a single 400-mg dose equally distributed over 2.5 hours.

Pediatric patients receiving iron maintenance treatment: A single dose as a slow IV injection over 5 minutes or diluted in NS at a concentration of 1 to 2 mg/mL and administered as an infusion over 5 to 60 minutes. Do not dilute to concentrations below 1 mg/mL; see Usual Dose.

ACTIONS

An aqueous complex of polynuclear iron (III)-hydroxide in sucrose. Used to replenish the total body iron stores in patients with iron deficiency. Iron is critical for normal hemoglobin synthesis to maintain oxygen transport and is necessary for various other processes. Following intravenous administration, iron sucrose is dissociated by the reticuloendothelial system into iron and sucrose. Iron distributes into liver, spleen, and bone marrow. Half-life of the iron component is 6 hours. The sucrose component is eliminated mainly by urinary excretion. Most iron is stored in the body. Small amounts are eliminated in the urine. Significant increases in serum iron and ferritin and significant decreases in total iron-binding capacity occur within 4 weeks of beginning iron sucrose treatment.

INDICATIONS AND USES

Treatment of iron deficiency anemia (IDA) in patients with chronic kidney disease (CKD).

CONTRAINDICATIONS
Known hypersensitivity to iron sucrose or any of its inactive components.

PRECAUTIONS
Use only when truly indicated to avoid excess storage of iron. Not recommended for use in patients with iron overload. ▪ Potentially fatal hypersensitivity reactions characterized by anaphylactic shock, loss of consciousness, collapse, and/or hypotension (clinically significant) have been reported. Medications and equipment for resuscitation must be readily available. ▪ Hypotension has been reported frequently and may be related to rate of administration and/or total dose administered. Follow guidelines for dosing and administration. See Usual Dose and Rate of Administration.

Monitor: Confirm IV placement and avoid extravasation; injection site discoloration has been reported following extravasation. ▪ Monitor vital signs during and immediately following administration. Recumbent position during and after administration may help to prevent postural hypotension. Hypotensive effects may be additive to transient hypotension during dialysis and/or from too-rapid rate of administration. ▪ Monitor for S/S of hypersensitivity reactions during and after administration for at least 30 minutes and until clinically stable; see Precautions. Reactions may occur after the first dose or subsequent doses of iron sucrose. ▪ Periodic monitoring of hematologic and iron parameters (hemoglobin, hematocrit, serum ferritin and transferrin saturation) is indicated during parenteral iron replacement therapy. Takes about 4 weeks of treatment to see increased serum iron and ferritin and decreased TIBC (total iron-binding capacity) and about 2 to 4 weeks to see an increase in hemoglobin. Transferrin saturation values increase rapidly after IV administration of iron sucrose; wait at least 48 hours after an IV dose to obtain serum iron measurements.

Patient Education: Review any possible reactions to past parenteral iron therapy. ▪ Report S/S of a hypersensitivity reaction promptly.

Maternal/Child: Use in pregnancy only if clearly needed. Iron deficiency anemia (IDA) during pregnancy should be treated. Untreated IDA has been associated with adverse maternal outcomes such as postpartum anemia and an increased risk for preterm delivery and low birth weight. ▪ Safety for use during breast-feeding not established. Use caution and monitor breast-fed infant for GI toxicity (constipation, diarrhea). ▪ Safety and effectiveness for iron replacement treatment in pediatric patients with dialysis-dependent or non–dialysis-dependent CKD have not been established. Safety and effectiveness for iron maintenance treatment have been established for pediatric patients with dialysis-dependent or non–dialysis-dependent CKD 2 years of age and older. Has not been studied in patients younger than 2 years of age. ▪ Necrotizing enterocolitis in 5 premature infants (weight less than 1,250 Gm) with 2 deaths has been reported in one country in which iron sucrose is approved for use in pediatric patients. No causal relationship to drugs could be established; it may be a complication of prematurity in very-low-birth-weight infants.

Elderly: Differences in response between elderly and younger patients have not been identified. Lower-end initial doses may be appropriate in the elderly; see Dose Adjustments.

DRUG/LAB INTERACTIONS
Drug interactions involving iron sucrose have not been studied. May reduce the absorption of concomitantly administered **oral iron preparations;** concurrent use not recommended.

SIDE EFFECTS
Adult patients: Arthralgia, back pain, chest pain, diarrhea, dizziness, headache, hypotension, injection site burning or pain, muscle cramps, nausea, pain in extremity, peripheral edema, pruritus, and vomiting are most common. Other side effects varied according to the type of chronic kidney disease patient who was receiving iron sucrose (e.g., hemodialysis dependent, peritoneal dialysis-dependent, non–dialysis dependent) and included abdominal pain, asthenia, conjunctivitis, cough, dysgeusia, dyspnea, ear pain, feeling abnormal, fluid overload, gout, graft complications, hyperglycemia, hypersensitivity

reactions, hypertension, hypoglycemia, injection site extravasation, myalgia, nasal congestion, nasopharyngitis, pharyngitis, sinusitis, upper respiratory tract infection.

Pediatric patients: Arteriovenous fistula thrombosis, cough, dizziness, fever, headache, hypertension, hypotension, nausea, peritonitis, respiratory tract viral infection, and vomiting occurred.

Overdose: May result in hemosiderosis. Excess iron may increase susceptibility to infection. If acute toxicity is seen, it may present as abdominal and muscle pain, cardiovascular collapse, dizziness, dyspnea, edema, headache, hemosiderosis, hypotension, joint aches, nausea, pale eyes, paresthesia, sedation, vomiting.

Post-Marketing: Life-threatening hypersensitivity reactions (e.g., anaphylactic-type reactions, angioedema, bronchospasm, collapse, convulsions, dyspnea, loss of consciousness, shock), back pain, bradycardia, cardiac failure, chromaturia, confusion, dysgeusia, lightheadedness, sepsis, sweating, swelling of joints.

ANTIDOTE

Reduce rate of infusion for hypotension or other symptoms. Most symptoms are successfully treated with IV fluids, hydrocortisone sodium succinate, and/or antihistamines. Keep physician informed of all side effects. Discontinue drug if severe hypersensitivity reactions occur. Treat hypersensitivity reactions as indicated; may require epinephrine, airway management, oxygen, IV fluids, antihistamines (e.g., diphenhydramine), corticosteroids (e.g., hydrocortisone), and pressor amines (e.g., dopamine). Resuscitate as needed. Not removed by dialysis.

ISATUXIMAB
(**EYE**-sa-**TUX**-i-mab)

Sarclisa

Antineoplastic agent
Monoclonal antibody (Anti-CD38)

USUAL DOSE

Premedicate with dexamethasone, famotidine, diphenhydramine, and acetaminophen prior to each dose.

Cycle 1: 10 mg/kg on Days 1, 8, 15, and 22 of a 28-day cycle in combination with pomalidomide and dexamethasone or carfilzomib and dexamethasone.

Cycle 2: 10 mg/kg on Days 1 and 15 of a 28-day cycle in combination with combination with pomalidomide and dexamethasone or carfilzomib and dexamethasone. Continue until disease progression or unacceptable toxicity. Available through authorized specialty distributors and specialty pharmacies.

PEDIATRIC DOSE

Safety and efficacy have not been established.

DOSE ADJUSTMENTS

Renal: No dosage adjustments provided by manufacturer.

Hepatic: No dosage adjustments are necessary.

DILUTION

Calculate required isatuximab dose and dose volume. Remove an amount from a 250-mL NS or D5W infusion bag that is equal to the required volume of isatuximab. Withdraw the necessary isatuximab volume and add to the NS or D5W infusion bag (for a total infusion bag volume of 250 mL). Invert bag gently to mix; *do not shake*. Infusion bag must be made of polyolefins, polyethylene, polypropylene, polyvinyl chloride (PVC) with di-(2-ethylhexyl)-phthalate (DEHP), or ethyl vinyl acetate (EVA).

Use IV tubing infusion set made of polyethylene, polyvinyl chloride (PVC) with or without di-2-ethylhexyl phthalate (DEHP), polybutadiene, or polyurethane with a 0.22-micron in-line polyethersulfone, polysulfone, or nylon filter.

COMPATIBILITY

Do not administer simultaneously with any other medication or IV solutions.

RATE OF ADMINISTRATION

Administer as an IV infusion. Infusion duration depends on the rate of infusion.

First infusion: Initiate at 25 mL/hr for 60 minutes; if tolerated, increase rate by 25 mL/hr every 30 minutes to a maximum rate of 150 mL/hr.

Second infusion: Initiate at 50 mL/hr for 30 minutes; if tolerated, increase rate by 50 mL/hr for 30 minutes, then increase rate by 100 mL/hr to a maximum rate of 200 mL/hr.

Subsequent infusions: Initiate at 200 mL/hr; maximum rate: 200 mL/hr.

ACTIONS

Isatuximab is an IgG-1–derived monoclonal antibody directed against CD38. It has antitumor activity, cell-mediated cytotoxicity, complement-dependent cytotoxicity, and antibody-dependent cellular phagocytosis and directly inhibits activity of CD38 ectoenzymes.

INDICATIONS AND USES

Multiple myeloma.

CONTRAINDICATIONS

Severe hypersensitivity to isatuximab or any component of the formulation.

PRECAUTIONS

Bone marrow suppression, infusion reactions (including anaphylaxis), secondary malignancy, false-positive indirect Coombs test.

Monitor: Blood type and screening prior to first dose; consider phenotyping. Screen for hepatitis B.

Patient Education: Advise patients to call physician if they feel very tired or weak or experience infection, fever, chills, sore throat, sinus pain, increased or a change in sputum production, bleeding, shortness of breath, or signs of allergic reaction.

Maternal/Child: May cause fetal harm, thus contraindicated. Breast-feeding is not recommended.

Elderly: Refer to Usual Dose and Precautions.

DRUG/LAB INTERACTIONS

5-ASA, abrocitinib, bacille Calmette-Guérin (BCG) vaccine, baricitinib, brincidofovir, chloramphenicol ophthalmic, cladribine, clozapine, COVID-19 vaccines (may decrease effectiveness), moderate and strong CYP3A4 inducers (may decrease effectiveness of isatuximab; avoid), strong CYP3A4 inhibitors (may increase serum concentration of isatuximab; avoid), deferiprone, denosumab, dipyrone, echinacea, fexinidazole, fingolimod, inebilzumab, leflunomide, natalizumab, ocrelizumab, ofatumumab, ozanimod, pidotimod, pimecrolimus (avoid), pneumococcal vaccine, polio vaccine (avoid), promazine, rabies vaccine, ropeginterferon alfa 2b, rubella or varicella live vaccines (avoid), sipuleucel-T, tacrolimus topical (avoid), talimogene laherparepvec (avoid), tertomotide, tofacitinib, typhoid vaccine (avoid), upadacitinib (avoid), live vaccines (avoid), varicella virus vaccine (avoid). Inactivated vaccines may have reduced response; give prior to therapy start. Please refer to package insert for further information.

SIDE EFFECTS

Anemia, antibody development, bronchitis, cardiac failure, cough, diarrhea, dyspnea, fatigue, febrile neutropenia, hypertension, infection, infusion-related reactions, lymphocytopenia, malignant neoplasm of skin, nausea, neutropenia, solid tumor, thrombocytopenia, upper respiratory tract infection, vomiting.

ANTIDOTE

Discontinue infusion and treat appropriately for severe hypersensitivity reactions.

ISAVUCONAZONIUM SULFATE
(eye-sah-vew-koh-nah-**ZOH**-nee-um **SUL**-fayt)

Cresemba

USUAL DOSE

Pretreatment: Obtain specimens for fungal culture and other relevant lab studies (including histopathology) to isolate and identify causative organism(s) before initiating therapy. Institute antifungal therapy and adjust based on results of culture and lab studies. See Maternal/Child.

Loading dose: 372 mg (1 vial) as an infusion every 8 hours for 6 doses.

Maintenance dose: 372 mg (1 vial) as an infusion once daily. Initiate 12 to 24 hours after the last loading dose. Oral formulation (2 capsules = 372 mg) may be substituted when appropriate.

DOSE ADJUSTMENTS

No dose adjustment is required based on age, gender, or race or in patients with mild, moderate, or severe renal impairment, including ESRD. ▪ No dose adjustment is required with mild to moderate hepatic impairment.

DILUTION

Available as a lyophilized powder containing 372 mg isavuconazonium sulfate (equivalent to 200 mg isavuconazole). Reconstitute 1 vial with 5 mL of SWFI. Gently shake to dissolve the powder completely. Solution should be clear and free of particulates. Withdraw 5 mL from the reconstituted vial and inject into a 250-mL bag of NS or D5W. Final concentration is approximately 1.5 mg/mL. Diluted solution may have visible translucent to white particulates, which will be removed by in-line filtration. Use gentle mixing or roll bag to minimize the formation of particulates. Avoid unnecessary vibration or vigorous shaking of the solution. Do not use a pneumatic transport system.

Filters: Must be administered using an infusion set that contains a sterile, nonpyrogenic, in-line filter (pore size of 0.2 to 1.2 micrometers).

Storage: Before use, refrigerate at 2° to 8° C (36° to 46° F). Reconstituted solution should be further diluted and used immediately but may be stored below 25° C for a maximum of 1 hour before further dilution. Diluted solution must be used within 6 hours if kept at RT or may be immediately refrigerated. Complete the infusion within 24 hours. Do not freeze.

COMPATIBILITY

Manufacturer states, "Do not infuse isavuconazonium with other intravenous medications." **Compatible** only with NS or D5W.

RATE OF ADMINISTRATION

Do not administer as an IV bolus; for use as a diluted IV infusion only. Administer a single dose as an infusion equally distributed over a minimum of 60 minutes. Flush the IV line before and after each isavuconazonium infusion with NS or D5W. Administer through an infusion set that contains a sterile, nonpyrogenic, in-line filter (pore size of 0.2 to 1.2 micrometers).

ACTIONS

Isavuconazonium is a prodrug of isavuconazole, an azole antifungal drug. Acts by inhibiting the synthesis of ergosterol, a key component of fungal cell membranes. Rapidly hydrolyzed in blood to isavuconazole by esterases, predominantly by butylcholinesterase. Extensively distributed and highly protein bound, predominantly to albumin. Following IV administration, maximum plasma concentrations of the prodrug and inactive products were detectable during infusion and declined rapidly following the end of administration. Mean plasma half-life is 130 hours. CYP3A4, CYP3A5 and, subsequently, uridine diphosphate-glucuronosyltransferase (UGT) are involved in the metabolism of isavuconazole. Primarily excreted as metabolites in urine and feces.

INDICATIONS AND USES

Treatment of invasive aspergillosis and invasive mucormycosis in patients 18 years of age and older.

CONTRAINDICATIONS

Known hypersensitivity to isavuconazole. ▪ Coadministration of strong CYP3A4 inhibitors such as ketoconazole or high-dose ritonavir (Norvir [400 mg every 12 hours]). ▪ Coadministration of strong CYP3A4 inducers such as rifampin, carbamazepine, St. John's wort, or long-acting barbiturates (e.g., phenobarbital). ▪ Patients with familial short QT syndrome. ▪ See Drug/Lab Interactions.

PRECAUTIONS

Do not administer as an IV bolus; for use as a diluted IV infusion only. ▪ Elevations in liver function tests (e.g., ALT, AST, alkaline phosphatase, total bilirubin) have been reported, were generally reversible, and did not require discontinuation of isavuconazonium. ▪ Severe hepatic reactions (e.g., cholestasis, hepatitis, or hepatic failure, including death) have been reported in patients with serious underlying medical conditions (e.g., hematologic malignancy) during treatment with azole antifungal agents, including isavuconazonium. ▪ Has not been studied in patients with severe hepatic impairment (Child-Pugh Class C); use in these patients only when benefits outweigh risks. ▪ Infusion-related reactions have been reported. ▪ Serious hypersensitivity and severe skin reactions, such as anaphylaxis or Stevens-Johnson syndrome, have been reported with other azole antifungal agents. There is no information regarding cross-sensitivity between isavuconazole and other azole antifungal agents. Use caution in patients with hypersensitivity to other azoles. ▪ In vitro and animal studies suggest cross-resistance between isavuconazole and other azoles. Relevance of cross-resistance to clinical outcome has not been fully characterized. Patients failing prior azole therapy may require alternative antifungal therapy. ▪ See Drug/Lab Interactions.

Monitor: Obtain specimens for fungal culture and other relevant lab studies (including histopathology) to isolate and identify causative organism(s) before initiating therapy. Institute antifungal therapy and adjust based on results of culture and lab studies. ▪ Obtain baseline liver function tests and repeat as necessary. Monitor more frequently in patients who develop abnormal liver function tests and when treating patients with severe hepatic impairment. ▪ Monitor for infusion-related reactions (e.g., chills, dizziness, dyspnea, hypoesthesia, hypotension, and paresthesia). ▪ Monitor for S/S of hypersensitivity reactions (e.g., hypotension, rash, tightness of the chest, urticaria, wheezing). ▪ Monitor for S/S of skin reactions (e.g., rash, blisters).

Patient Education: Review manufacturer's medication guide. ▪ Review of health history and medication profile is imperative. ▪ Avoid pregnancy; effective birth control recommended; see Drug/Lab Interactions. Should pregnancy occur, notify physician and discuss potential hazards. ▪ Promptly report S/S of a hypersensitivity/infusion reaction (e.g., itching, hives, shortness of breath, or a serious skin reaction [e.g., rash]).

Maternal/Child: Category C: may cause fetal harm. Use during pregnancy only if the potential benefit to the patient outweighs the risk to the fetus. Report a suspected pregnancy. ▪ Discontinue breast-feeding. ▪ Safety and effectiveness for use in patients under 18 years of age have not been established.

Elderly: Response similar to that seen in younger adults.

DRUG/LAB INTERACTIONS

Isavuconazole is a sensitive substrate of CYP3A4. CYP3A4 inhibitors or inducers may alter the plasma concentrations of isavuconazole. Isavuconazole is a moderate inhibitor of CYP3A4, a mild inhibitor of P-glycoprotein (P-gp), and an organic cation transporter 2 (OCT2). ▪ Coadministration of isavuconazonium with **strong CYP3A4 inhibitors** such as ketoconazole or high-dose ritonavir is ***contraindicated***. Strong CYP3A4 inhibitors can significantly increase the plasma concentration of isavuconazole. ▪ Coadministration of isavuconazonium with **strong CYP3A4 inducers** such as rifampin, carbamazepine, St. John's wort, or long-acting barbiturates is ***contraindicated***. Strong CYP3A4 inducers can significantly decrease the plasma concentration of isavuconazole. ▪ Coadministration with **lopinavir/ritonavir** can significantly increase the plasma concentration of isavuconazole, and **isavuconazole** may decrease the antiviral effectiveness of lopinavir/ritonavir. ▪ Coadministration with **atorvastatin** may increase atorvastatin exposure and toxicity. ▪ Coadministration with **cyclosporine, mycophenolate, sirolimus,** and **tacrolimus** may increase exposure of these drugs. Monitor drug concentrations of these drugs and/or drug-related toxicities and adjust doses as needed. ▪ May increase exposure of **midazolam**. Consider dose reduction of midazolam with concomitant administration. ▪ May decrease exposure of **bupropion**. Dose increase of bupropion may be necessary with co-administration; do not exceed the maximum recommended dose. ▪ Concomitant administration with **digoxin** increases digoxin exposure. Monitor serum digoxin concentrations and adjust dose as necessary.

SIDE EFFECTS

The most commonly reported side effects include back pain; constipation; cough; diarrhea; dyspnea; elevated ALT, AST, alkaline phosphatase, total bilirubin, and GGT; headache; hypokalemia; nausea and vomiting; and peripheral edema. Hepatic adverse drug reactions, infusion-related or hypersensitivity reactions, and embryo-fetal toxicity are considered the most serious. Abdominal pain, acute respiratory failure, anxiety, chest pain, decreased appetite, delirium, dyspepsia, fatigue, hypomagnesemia, hypotension, injection site reaction, insomnia, pruritus, rash, and renal failure have also been reported.

ANTIDOTE

Notify physician of all side effects; most will be treated symptomatically. If a hypersensitivity reaction, infusion reaction, or severe cutaneous reaction occurs, discontinue the infusion and treat as indicated. Discontinue isavuconazonium if clinical S/S consistent with liver disease develop that may be attributable to isavuconazonium. No known specific antidote. Not removed by hemodialysis.

ISOPROTERENOL HYDROCHLORIDE

(**eye**-so-**PROH**-ter-ih-nohl hy-droh-**KLOR**-eyed)

Cardiac stimulant
(inotropic/chronotropic)
Bronchodilator
Antiarrhythmic

Isuprel

pH 3.5 to 4.5

USUAL DOSE

In all situations, adjust the rate of infusion based on HR, CVP, BP, respiratory rate, and urine output.

Recommended Isoproterenol Dose for Adults With Atropine-Resistant Hemodynamically Significant Bradycardia, Heart Block, Adams-Stokes Attacks, and Cardiac Arrest			
Route of Administration	**Preparation of Dilution**	**Initial Dose**	**Subsequent Dose Range[a]**
Bolus intravenous injection	Dilute 1 mL (0.2 mg) to 10 mL with NS or D5W	0.02 to 0.06 mg (1 to 3 mL of diluted solution)	0.01 to 0.2 mg (0.5 to 10 mL of diluted solution)
Intravenous infusion	Dilute 10 mL (2 mg) in 500 mL D5W (4 mcg/mL)	5 mcg/min (1.25 mL of diluted solution per minute)	
Intracardiac	Use solution 0.2 mg/mL undiluted	0.02 mg (0.1 mL)	

[a]Subsequent dose depends on the ventricular rate and the rapidity with which the cardiac pacemaker can take over when the drug is gradually withdrawn.
AHA recommendation is 2 to 10 mcg/min if an external pacemaker is not available.

Recommended Isoproterenol Dose for Adults With Shock (Cardiogenic, CHF, Hypoperfusion [Low Cardiac Output], Hypovolemic, Septic)		
Route of Administration	**Preparation of Dilution[a]**	**Infusion Rate[b]**
Intravenous infusion	Dilute 5 mL (1 mg) in 500 mL of D5W (2 mcg/mL)	0.5 to 5 mcg/min (0.25 to 2.5 mL of diluted solution)

[a]Concentrations up to 10 times greater have been used when limitation of volume is essential.
[b]Rates over 30 mcg/min have been used in advanced stages of shock. Adjust infusion rate based on HR, CVP, BP, and urine flow. If HR exceeds 110 beats/min, consider decreasing rate or temporarily discontinue the infusion.

Recommended Isoproterenol Dose for Adults With Bronchospasm Occurring During Anesthesia			
Route of Administration	**Preparation of Dilution**	**Initial Dose**	**Subsequent Dose**
Bolus intravenous injection	Dilute 1 mL (0.2 mg) to 10 mL with NS or D5W	0.01 to 0.02 mg (0.5 to 1 mL of diluted solution)	Repeat initial dose as necessary

Complete heart block following closure of ventricular septal defects: 0.04 to 0.06 mg (2 to 3 mL of a 0.02 mg/mL dilution) as a bolus injection. May maintain a sinus rhythm with a HR above 90 to 100 beats/min or may relapse into complete heart block again.
Diagnosis of mitral regurgitation (unlabeled): 4 mcg/min as an infusion (1 mL/min of a 4 mcg/mL dilution).
Diagnosis of coronary artery disease or lesions (unlabeled): 1 to 3 mcg/min as an infusion (0.25 to 0.75 mL/min of a 4 mcg/mL dilution).
Refractory torsades de pointes, bradycardia in heart transplant patients, beta-adrenergic blocker poisoning: AHA recommends 2 to 10 mcg/min (0.5 to 2.5 mL/min of a 4 mcg/mL dilution).

Titrate to adequate heart rate. In torsades de pointes, titrate to increase heart rate until VT is suppressed.

PEDIATRIC DOSE

See Dilution and Maternal/Child.

0.05 to 2 mcg/kg/min. Begin with 0.1 mcg/kg/min as an infusion. Increase by 0.1 mcg/kg/min until desired effect. Titrate to patient response and monitor cardiac status carefully. Maximum dose is 2 mcg/kg/min. Another source suggests a maximum dose of 1 mcg/kg/min.

Complete heart block after closure of ventricular septal defects in infants: 0.01 to 0.03 mg (0.5 to 1.5 mL of a 0.02 mg/mL solution) as a bolus injection. See comments in Usual Dose.

DOSE ADJUSTMENTS

Lower-end initial doses may be appropriate in the elderly; consider the potential for decreased organ function and concomitant disease or drug therapy.

DILUTION

IV injection: Available in a 0.2 mg/mL solution. Dilute 1 mL of a 0.2 mg/mL solution with 10 mL NS or D5W to provide a concentration of 0.02 mg/mL.

Infusion: *Atropine-resistant, hemodynamically significant bradycardia, heart block, Adams-Stokes attacks, and cardiac arrest:* Dilute 10 mL (2 mg of a 0.2 mg/mL solution) in 500 mL D5W (4 mcg/mL). **Shock:** Dilute 5 mL (1 mg of a 0.2 mg/mL solution) in 500 mL D5W (2 mcg/mL). Use an infusion pump or microdrip (60 gtts equals 1 mL) to administer. Less diluent may be used to reduce fluid intake.

Filters: No data available from manufacturer. Another source cites no significant loss in drug potency in several studies using various types and sizes of filters from 0.22 to 5 microns in size.

Storage: Store between 8° and 15° C (46° to 59° F) unless otherwise specified by manufacturer. Do not use if pink or brown in color or contains a precipitate.

COMPATIBILITY

Compatibility information not available from manufacturer. Other sources suggest specific **compatibilities** dependent on concentration and manufacturer; consult a pharmacist.

RATE OF ADMINISTRATION

IV injection: Each 1 mL of a 0.02 mg/mL solution or fraction thereof over 1 minute. Follow with a 20-mL flush of NS if indicated to ensure distribution to circulation.

Infusion: Titrate to desired dose, HR, and rhythm; see the following infusion rate chart. Decrease rate of infusion as necessary. Ventricular rate generally should not exceed 110 beats/min.

Isoproterenol (Isuprel) Infusion Rates						
Desired Dose	1 mg in 500 mL D5W (2 mcg/mL)			1 mg in 250 mL D5W 2 mg in 500 mL D5W (4 mcg/mL)		
mcg/min	mcg/hr	mL/min	mL/hr	mcg/hr	mL/min	mL/hr
2	120	1	60	120	0.5	30
5	300	2.5	150	300	1.25	75
10	600	5	300	600	2.5	150
15	900	7.5	450	900	3.75	225
20	1,200	10	600	1,200	5	300
25	1,500	12.5	750	1,500	6.25	375
30	1,800	15	900	1,800	7.5	450

ACTIONS

A nonselective synthetic cardiac beta receptor stimulant (sympathomimetic amine) similar to epinephrine and norepinephrine. Has positive inotropic and chronotropic actions more potent than those of epinephrine. It increases cardiac output, cardiac work, coronary flow, and venous return. Improves atrioventricular conduction. Stimulates only the higher ventricular foci, allowing a more normal cardiac pacemaker to take over, thus suppressing ectopic pacemaker activity. Decreases peripheral vascular resistance by relaxing arterial smooth muscle and is a most effective bronchial smooth muscle relaxant. Onset of action is immediate and lasts 1 to 2 hours. Metabolized by the liver and inactivated by various enzyme systems. Excreted in the urine.

INDICATIONS AND USES

Treatment of mild or transient episodes of heart block that do not require cardioversion or pacemaker therapy. ▪ Treatment of serious episodes of heart block and Adams-Stokes attacks (except when caused by VT or VF). ▪ May be used in cardiac arrest until defibrillation or pacemaker (the treatments of choice) is available. ▪ Bronchospasm during anesthesia. ▪ Management of shock (cardiogenic, CHF, hypoperfusion [low cardiac output], hypovolemic, septic). Adequate fluid and electrolyte replacement required. ▪ AHA recommends cautious use in symptomatic bradycardia if a pacemaker is not available, treatment of refractory torsades de pointes unresponsive to magnesium sulfate, temporary control of bradycardia in heart transplant patients (denervated heart unresponsive to atropine), and treatment of poisoning from beta-adrenergic blockers (e.g., metoprolol).

Unlabeled uses: Aid in diagnosis of the etiology of mitral regurgitation. ▪ Aid in diagnosis of coronary artery disease or lesions. ▪ Pulmonary embolism to increase pulmonary blood volume and decrease pulmonary arterial pressure and vascular resistance.

CONTRAINDICATIONS

Tachyarrhythmias, patients with tachycardia or heart block caused by digoxin intoxication, angina pectoris, ventricular arrhythmias that require inotropic therapy.

PRECAUTIONS

IV injection in cardiac standstill must be accompanied by cardiac massage to perfuse drug into the myocardium. Current JAMA recommendations do not include isoproterenol in the treatment of cardiac arrest or hypotension. ▪ Fourth-line agent for bradycardia; considered possibly helpful but may be harmful. ▪ Can cause a severe drop in BP and can be very harmful in bradycardia. ▪ Use extreme caution when inhalant anesthetics (e.g., cyclopropane) are being administered and supplementary to digoxin administration. ▪ Use caution in coronary insufficiency, diabetes, hyperthyroidism, known sensitivity to sympathomimetic amines, history of seizures, hypertension, and pre-existing cardiac arrhythmias with tachycardia. ▪ Increased cardiac output and work can increase ischemia and worsen arrhythmias. ▪ Contains sulfites; use caution in allergic patients.

Monitor: Decrease rate of infusion as necessary. Ventricular rate generally should not exceed 110 beats/min. Maintain adequate blood volume and correct acidosis. ▪ Continuous cardiac monitoring, central venous pressure readings, BP, respiratory rate, and urine flow measurements are advisable during therapy with isoproterenol. ▪ Monitoring of serum glucose, magnesium, and potassium may be indicated. ▪ See Drug/Lab Interactions and Maternal/Child.

Maternal/Child: Category C: safety for use in pregnancy or breast-feeding not established. Benefits must outweigh risks. ▪ Safety and effectiveness in pediatric patients not established. ▪ In asthmatic pediatric patients, IV infusion of isoproterenol has caused clinical deterioration, myocardial necrosis, CHF, and death. Risks of cardiac toxicity may be increased by other factors such as acidosis, hypoxemia, coadministration of corticosteroids or methylxanthines (e.g., aminophylline). Continuous assessment of VS, frequent ECGs, and daily measurement of cardiac enzymes (e.g., CPK, MB) is suggested if isoproterenol infusion is required.

Elderly: Difference in response from younger adults not known. May be more sensitive to the effects of beta-adrenergic agents (e.g., hypertension, hypokalemia, tachycardia,

tremor). Patients with cardiac disease may be at increased risk for cardiac effects.
■ Lower-end initial doses may be appropriate; see Dose Adjustments.

DRUG/LAB INTERACTIONS
May be used alternately with epinephrine, but they may not be used together. Both are direct cardiac stimulants; serious arrhythmias and death may result. An adequate interval between doses must be maintained. ■ Do not use concomitantly with other **sympathomimetic agents** (e.g., ephedrine, dopamine). Additive effects may cause toxicity. May be used after effects of previous drug have subsided. ■ Simultaneous use with **oxytoxics** may cause hypertensive crisis. ■ May cause hypertension with **guanethidine** (Ismelin). ■ **Digoxin, quinidine, and halogenated hydrocarbon anesthetics** (e.g., halothane) may sensitize myocardium and cause serious arrhythmias. ■ Antagonized by **propranolol.** May be used to treat tachycardia caused by isoproterenol, but tachycardia and hypotension secondary to peripheral vasodilation may occur. ■ Potentiated by **tricyclic antidepressants**. ■ Concomitant use with **theophylline** increases the risk of cardiotoxicity. ■ See Contraindications.

SIDE EFFECTS
Anginal pain, cardiac arrhythmias, flushing, headache, hyperglycemia, hypokalemia, nausea, nervousness, palpitations, sweating, tachycardia, vomiting. Cardiac dilation, marked hypotension, pulmonary edema, and death may occur with prolonged use or overdose. Adams-Stokes attacks have been reported.

ANTIDOTE
Notify the physician of any side effect. Treatment will probably be symptomatic. For ventricular rate over 110 beats/min, PVCs, or ECG changes, decrease rate of infusion or discontinue drug. Vasodilators (e.g., nitrates) may be useful for treatment of hypertension. For accidental overdose, discontinue drug immediately, resuscitate and sustain patient, and notify physician.

IXABEPILONE BBW
(ix-ab-**EP**-i-lone)

**Antineoplastic
(microtubule inhibitor)**

Ixempra Kit

USUAL DOSE
Pretreatment: Verify pregnancy status. Baseline studies indicated; see Monitor.
Premedication: An H_1 antagonist (e.g., diphenhydramine) and an H_2 antagonist (e.g., famotidine) should be administered orally 60 minutes prior to ixabepilone to minimize the chance of a hypersensitivity reaction. Patients who experience a hypersensitivity reaction require premedication with a corticosteroid (e.g., dexamethasone 20 mg IV 30 minutes before infusion or orally 60 minutes before infusion) in addition to pretreatment with the H_1 and H_2 antagonists.
Ixabepilone: 40 mg/M^2 as an infusion over 3 hours every 3 weeks. Doses for patients with a body surface area (BSA) greater than 2.2 M^2 should be calculated based on 2.2 M^2. Administered alone or in combination with capecitabine (Xeloda) 1,000 mg/M^2 twice daily for 2 weeks followed by 1 week of rest.

DOSE ADJUSTMENTS
If toxicities are present, therapy should be delayed to allow recovery. ▪ Dosing adjustment guidelines for monotherapy and combination therapy are listed in the following chart. *If toxicities recur, an additional 20% dose reduction should be made.*

Dose Adjustments Guidelines	
Ixabepilone (Monotherapy or Combination Therapy)	**Ixabepilone Dose Modification**
NONHEMATOLOGIC	
Grade 2 neuropathy (moderate) lasting ≥7 days	Decrease the dose by 20%
Grade 3 neuropathy (severe) lasting <7 days	Decrease the dose by 20%
Grade 3 neuropathy (severe) lasting ≥7 days or disabling neuropathy	Discontinue treatment
Any Grade 3 toxicity (severe) other than neuropathy	Decrease the dose by 20%
Transient Grade 3 arthralgia/myalgia or fatigue	No change in dose required
Grade 3 hand-foot syndrome (palmar-plantar erythrodysesthesia)	No change in dose required
Any Grade 4 toxicity (disabling)	Discontinue treatment
HEMATOLOGIC	
Neutrophils <500 cells/mm^3 for ≥7 days	Decrease the dose by 20%
Febrile neutropenia	Decrease the dose by 20%
Platelets <25,000/mm^3 or platelets <50,000/mm^3 with bleeding	Decrease the dose by 20%
Capecitabine (When Used in Combination With Ixabepilone)	**Capecitabine Dose Modification**
NONHEMATOLOGIC	Follow capecitabine prescribing information
HEMATOLOGIC	
Platelets <25,000/mm^3 or platelets <50,000/mm^3 with bleeding	Hold for concurrent diarrhea or stomatitis until platelet count >50,000/mm^3, then continue at same dose
Neutrophils <500 cells/mm^3 for ≥7 days or febrile neutropenia	Hold for concurrent diarrhea or stomatitis until neutrophil count >1,000/mm^3, then continue at same dose

Dose adjustments at the start of a cycle should be based on nonhematologic toxicity or blood counts from the preceding cycle following the previous guidelines. Patients should not begin a new cycle unless the neutrophil count is at least 1,500 cells/mm³, the platelet count is at least 100,000 cells/mm³, and nonhematologic toxicities have improved to Grade 1 (mild) or have resolved. ▪ Combined use with capecitabine is contraindicated in patients who have AST or ALT greater than 2.5 times the ULN or bilirubin greater than 1 times the ULN; see Contraindications and Precautions. ▪ Patients with hepatic impairment who are receiving monotherapy should be dosed according to the guidelines listed in the following chart.

Dose Adjustments for Ixabepilone as Monotherapy in Patients With Hepatic Impairment					
	Transaminase Levels			**Bilirubin Levels[a]**	**Ixabepilone Dose[b] (mg/M²)**
Mild	AST and ALT ≤2.5 × ULN	and		≤1 × ULN	40
	AST or ALT ≤10 × ULN	and		≤1.5 × ULN	32
Moderate	AST and ALT ≤10 × ULN	and		>1.5 × ULN to ≤3 × ULN	20–30
Severe	AST or ALT >10 × ULN	or		>3 × ULN	Not recommended

[a]Excluding patients whose total bilirubin is elevated due to Gilbert disease.
[b]Dosage recommendations are for the first course of therapy; further decreases in subsequent courses should be based on individual tolerance.

Patients with moderate hepatic impairment should start with 20 mg/M². The dose in subsequent cycles may be increased up to, but should not exceed, 30 mg/M² if tolerated. ▪ Reduce dose to 20 mg/M² when coadministered with a strong CYP3A4 inhibitor; see Drug/Lab Interactions. If the strong inhibitor is discontinued, wait for at least 1 week before adjusting the ixabepilone dose upward to the indicated dose. ▪ If coadministration of a strong CYP3A4 inducer is required and alternatives are not feasible (e.g., the patient has been maintained on a strong CYP3A4 inducer), the dose may be gradually increased from 40 mg/M² to 60 mg/M² if tolerated; see Drug/Lab Interactions. Increase infusion duration of 60 mg/M² dose to 4 hours and monitor patient closely for toxicity. If CYP3A4 inducer is discontinued, return to original dose. ▪ No dose adjustment indicated based on age, race, and gender. ▪ Minimally excreted by the kidney; no studies conducted in patients with renal impairment.

DILUTION
Specific techniques required; see Precautions. Available as a 15-mg or 45-mg Ixempra Kit that contains two vials; one vial contains the indicated amount of ixabepilone, and the other contains a manufacturer-supplied diluent. Only the manufacturer-supplied diluent may be used for reconstitution. Calculate dose and remove required number of kits from refrigerator. Let stand at RT for approximately 30 minutes. A white precipitate may appear in the diluent vial. This will dissolve as the vial warms to RT. Withdraw diluent and slowly inject it into the ixabepilone vial. (The 15-mg vial is reconstituted with 8 mL of diluent, and the 45-mg vial is reconstituted with 23.5 mL.) Gently swirl and invert until completely dissolved. Concentration of reconstituted solution is 2 mg/mL. Must be further diluted to a final concentration of 0.2 to 0.6 mg/mL with LR, Plasma-Lyte A Injection pH 7.4, or NS 250 to 500 mL (the pH of the NS must be adjusted to between 6 and 9 by adding 2 mEq [i.e., 2 mL of an 8.4% w/v solution or 4 mL of a 4.2% w/v solution] of sodium bicarbonate injection before adding the ixabepilone). A 250-mL bag will be sufficient for most doses. Withdraw the calculated dose from the ixabepilone vials and transfer to a DEHP-free IV bag containing an appropriate volume of infusion solution to achieve the final desired concentration. Thoroughly mix by manual rotation. Should be administered through a DEHP-free, polyethylene-lined administration set.
Filter: Must be administered through an in-line filter with a microporous membrane of 0.2 to 1.2 microns.

Storage: Store unopened vials at 2° to 8° C (36° to 46° F) in original carton. Protect from light. Reconstituted solution may be stored in vial for 1 hour at RT and room light. Once diluted, solution is stable for a maximum of 6 hours at RT. Administration must be completed within this 6-hour period.

COMPATIBILITY

Manufacturer states, "DEHP-free infusion containers and administration sets must be used." Must be reconstituted with manufacturer-supplied diluent only and further diluted with the infusion solutions noted in Dilution. Indicated solutions have a pH between 6 to 9, which is required for ixabepilone stability.

RATE OF ADMINISTRATION

A single dose as an infusion equally distributed over 3 hours. In patients who experience a hypersensitivity reaction, increase duration of infusion and premedicate with corticosteroids and H_1 and H_2 antagonists; see Usual Dose. Increase duration of infusion to 4 hours in patients receiving 60 mg/M^2 dose; see Dose Adjustments.

ACTIONS

A microtubule inhibitor belonging to a class of antineoplastic agents, the epothilones. A semi-synthetic analog of epothilone B. Binds directly to β-tubulin subunits on microtubules, leading to suppression of microtubule dynamics. Blocks cells in the mitotic phase of the cell division cycle, leading to cell death. Has antitumor activity against multiple human tumor xenografts and is active in xenografts that are resistant to multiple agents, including taxanes, anthracyclines, and vinca alkaloids. Has demonstrated synergistic antitumor activity in combination with capecitabine. In addition to direct antitumor activity, ixabepilone has antiangiogenic activity. 67% to 77% bound to plasma proteins. Extensively metabolized in the liver, primarily by CYP3A4. Eliminated primarily as metabolized drug in feces and urine. Half-life is approximately 52 hours.

INDICATIONS AND USES

In combination with capecitabine for the treatment of patients with metastatic or locally advanced breast cancer resistant to treatment with an anthracycline and a taxane or for patients whose cancer is taxane resistant and for whom further anthracycline therapy is contraindicated. Anthracycline resistance is defined as progression while on therapy or within 6 months in the adjuvant setting or 3 months in the metastatic setting. Taxane resistance is defined as progression while on therapy or within 12 months in the adjuvant setting or 4 months in the metastatic setting. ▪ As monotherapy for the treatment of metastatic or locally advanced breast cancer in patients whose tumors are resistant or refractory to anthracyclines, taxanes, and capecitabine.

CONTRAINDICATIONS

History of severe (CTCAE Grade 3 or 4) hypersensitivity reaction to agents containing Cremophor EL or its derivatives. ▪ Neutrophil count less than 1,500 cells/mm^3 or platelet count less than 100,000 cells/mm^3. ▪ In combination with capecitabine in patients with AST or ALT greater than 2.5 times the ULN or bilirubin greater than 1 times the ULN.

PRECAUTIONS

Follow guidelines for handling cytotoxic agents. See Appendix A, p. 1308. ▪ Should be administered by or under the direction of the physician specialist in facilities equipped to monitor the patient and respond to any medical emergency. ▪ Ixabepilone in combination with capecitabine is contraindicated in patients with significant hepatic insufficiency due to increased risk of toxicity and neutropenia-related death; see Contraindications. ▪ Use caution in patients with hepatic insufficiency receiving monotherapy. Risk of toxicity is increased and data are limited; see Dose Adjustments. ▪ Premedication is required to minimize the chance of a hypersensitivity reaction; see Usual Dose. ▪ Peripheral neuropathy is a common side effect and was the most common cause of treatment discontinuation in clinical studies. It is cumulative and generally reversible. May require dose reduction or delay in therapy; see Dose Adjustments. Use caution in patients with diabetes mellitus or pre-existing peripheral neuropathy. Risk of severe neuropathy may be increased. ▪ Myelosuppression is dose dependent and primarily manifested as neutropenia. Hold therapy in patients with a neutrophil count less than 1,500 cells/mm^3; see Dose Adjustments and Contraindications. ▪ Use caution in patients with a history of cardiac disease. Adverse cardiac events (e.g., myocardial ischemia, ventricular dysfunction, and supraventricular arrhythmias) have been reported. ▪ Not studied in patients with renal impairment.

Monitor: Obtain baseline and periodic CBC with differential and platelet count. ▪ Obtain baseline and periodic bilirubin, AST, and ALT. ▪ Monitor for S/S of a hypersensitivity reaction (e.g., bronchospasm, dyspnea, flushing, rash). ▪ Monitor for S/S of peripheral neuropathy (primarily sensory [e.g., burning sensation, discomfort, hyperesthesia, hypo-esthesia, neuropathic pain or paresthesia]). Most cases of new-onset or worsening neuropathy occurred during the first 3 cycles. ▪ Monitor for thrombocytopenia (platelet count less than 50,000/mm^3); see Dose Adjustments and Contraindications. Initiate precautions to prevent excessive bleeding (e.g., inspect IV sites, skin, and mucous membranes; use extreme care during invasive procedures; test urine, emesis, stool, and secretions for occult blood).

Patient Education: Promptly report any numbness or tingling of feet, S/S of infection (fever, chills cough), or S/S of a hypersensitivity reaction (chest tightness, dyspnea, flushing, pruritus, rash, urticaria). ▪ Avoid pregnancy. Use of effective birth control is required. ▪ Promptly report chest pain, difficulty breathing, palpitations, or unusual weight gain; these may be signs of adverse cardiac events.

Maternal/Child: Category D: avoid pregnancy; may cause fetal harm. ▪ Discontinue breast-feeding. ▪ Effectiveness for use in pediatric patients not established. Evaluation in two clinical studies suggests that pediatric patients have a safety profile consistent with that seen in adults.

Elderly: The incidence of Grade 3 and 4 adverse reactions was higher when used in combination with capecitabine in clinical studies. As monotherapy, no overall difference in safety was seen in the elderly compared with younger adults.

DRUG/LAB INTERACTIONS

Use of concomitant strong **CYP3A4 inhibitors** (e.g., amprenavir, atazanavir, clarithromycin, delavirdine, indinavir, itraconazole, ketoconazole, nefazodone, nelfinavir, ritonavir, saquinavir, telithromycin, or voriconazole [VFEND]) may increase plasma concentrations of ixabepilone. Avoid concomitant use if possible. If required, decrease dose of ixabepilone to 20 mg/M^2 and monitor closely for acute toxicity. If strong inhibitor is discontinued, wait for at least 1 week before adjusting ixabepilone dose upward to indicated dose. ▪ **Grapefruit juice** may increase plasma concentrations of ixabepilone and should be avoided. ▪ **Rifampin**, a potent CYP3A4 inducer, decreases ixabepilone plasma concentrations. Other strong **CYP3A4 inducers** (e.g., carbamazepine, dexamethasone, phenobarbital, phenytoin, rifabutin) may also decrease ixabepilone plasma concentrations, decreasing effectiveness. Avoid use if possible; see Dose Adjustments. ▪ **St. John's wort** may decrease ixabepilone plasma concentrations, decreasing effectiveness. Avoid use. ▪ Ixabepilone does not inhibit CYP enzymes and is not expected to alter plasma concentrations of other drugs.

SIDE EFFECTS

The most common side effects in patients receiving monotherapy included alopecia, anemia, arthralgia, asthenia, diarrhea, fatigue, leukopenia, mucositis, musculoskeletal pain, myalgia, nausea, neutropenia, peripheral sensory neuropathy, stomatitis, thrombocytopenia, and vomiting. In combination therapy, the following additional side effects were commonly reported: abdominal pain, anorexia, constipation, nail disorder, and hand-foot syndrome (palmar-plantar erythrodysesthesia). Other less commonly reported side effects included chest pain, cough, dehydration, dizziness, dyspnea, edema, febrile neutropenia, fever, gastroesophageal reflux disease, headache, hot flush, hypersensitivity reactions (including anaphylaxis), increased lacrimation, infection, insomnia, pain, pruritus, rash, skin exfoliation, skin hyperpigmentation, taste disorder.

Overdose: Fatigue, GI symptoms (e.g., abdominal pain, anorexia, diarrhea, nausea, stomatitis), musculoskeletal pain/myalgia, and peripheral neuropathy.

Post-Marketing: Radiation recall has been reported.

ANTIDOTE

Keep physician informed of all side effects. Most minor side effects will be treated symptomatically. Monitor patient closely. Discontinuation should be considered in patients who develop cardiac ischemia or impaired cardiac function. Discontinue ixabepilone at the first sign of a severe hypersensitivity reaction. Treat hypersensitivity reactions as indicated; may require epinephrine, airway management, oxygen, IV fluids, antihistamines (e.g., diphenhydramine), corticosteroids (e.g., hydrocortisone sodium succinate), and pressor amines (e.g., dopamine). Patients who experience a hypersensitivity reaction may be able to continue therapy. Rate reduction and additional pretreatment with corticosteroids may be attempted in subsequent cycles (see Usual Dose).

KETOROLAC TROMETHAMINE BBW

NSAID

(kee-toh-**ROH**-lack tro-**METH**-ah-meen)

Toradol

pH 6.9 to 7.9

USUAL DOSE

Pretreatment: See Monitor.

Adults under 65 years: 30 mg. May repeat every 6 hours. Maximum dose is 120 mg/24 hr. Do not increase the dose or frequency for breakthrough pain. Ketorolac oral may be used only as continuation therapy to parenteral dosing. Maximum oral dose is 40 mg/24 hr. Do not administer for longer than 5 days (IV/intramuscular (IM) alone or combined use with oral).

Adults over 65 years, patients with impaired renal function, and/or patients under 50 kg (110 lb): 15 mg. May repeat every 6 hours. Maximum dose is 60 mg in 24 hours. Note all restrictions for adults under 65 years outlined above.

PEDIATRIC DOSE

See Maternal/Child.

Pediatric patients 2 to 16 years of age: One dose of 0.5 mg/kg up to a maximum dose of 15 mg. 0.5 mg/kg IV every 6 hours has been administered in a limited number of patients (unlabeled).

Short-term postoperative pain management (unlabeled): 1 mg/kg alone or as an adjunct.

DOSE ADJUSTMENTS

Required for patients under 50 kg (110 lb), patients over 65 years of age, and patients with reduced renal function (moderately elevated serum creatinine [SCr] (see Usual Dose). Further dose reductions may be required with high-dose salicylates (see Drug/Lab Interactions).

DILUTION

Confirm IV use. Some 2-mL tubex syringes are for IM use only. May be given undiluted through Y-tube of infusion set. Administration through a free-flowing IV is preferred.

Storage: Store at controlled room temperature (CRT); protect from light.

COMPATIBILITY

May form a precipitate if admixed with drugs with a low pH (e.g., meperidine, morphine, promethazine).

Other sources suggest a few specific **compatibilities** dependent on concentration and manufacturer; consult a pharmacist.

RATE OF ADMINISTRATION

A single dose over a minimum of 15 seconds.

ACTIONS

A nonsteroidal anti-inflammatory drug (NSAID) with peripheral analgesic, anti-inflammatory, and antipyretic actions. Inhibits prostaglandin synthesis. Studies reflect less drowsiness, nausea, and vomiting. Not a narcotic agonist or antagonist. Cardiac and hemodynamic parameters are not altered. Onset of action is 30 to 60 minutes. Half-life varies from 3.8 to 8.6 hours based on age and clinical status. Relief in some patients may last 6 to 8 hours. Excreted primarily in urine. Secreted in breast milk.

INDICATIONS AND USES
Short-term management of moderately severe, acute pain (no longer than 5 days). ■ NOT indicated for minor or chronic painful conditions.

Unlabeled uses: Postoperative short-term pain management in pediatric patients.

CONTRAINDICATIONS
Hypersensitivity to ketorolac, its components, or to acetylsalicylic acid (ASA) or other NSAIDs; labor and delivery; breastfeeding; preoperative or intraoperative medication when hemostasis is critical due to increased risk of bleeding; patients currently receiving ASA or NSAIDs (e.g., ibuprofen [Advil, Motrin], naproxen [Aleve, Naprosyn]); active peptic ulcer disease; recent gastrointestinal (GI) bleeding or perforation; patients with a history of peptic ulcer disease or GI bleeding; suspected or confirmed cerebrovascular bleeding; hemorrhagic diathesis; incomplete hemostasis; high risk of bleeding; advanced renal impairment; or patients at risk for renal failure because of volume depletion. Do not use for epidural or intrathecal administration; contains alcohol (see Drug/Lab Interactions).

PRECAUTIONS
Use only recommended doses; increased doses will not be more effective and will increase the risk of serious adverse events. ■ Hypersensitivity reactions, including anaphylaxis, have been reported. Administer in a facility with adequate diagnostic and treatment facilities to monitor the patient and respond to any medical emergency. ■ NSAIDs may increase the risk of serious cardiovascular (CV) thrombotic events, myocardial infarction, and stroke, which can be fatal. This risk may occur early in treatment and may increase with duration of use. Patients with cardiovascular disease or risk factors for cardiovascular disease may be at greater risk. ■ Inhibits platelet aggregation and may prolong bleeding time. ■ May cause serious GI ulceration and bleeding without warning. ■ In addition to the usual caution in patients with reduced hepatic or renal function, ketorolac may also cause a dose-dependent reduction in renal prostaglandin formation. Can precipitate renal failure in patients with impaired renal function, heart failure, or liver dysfunction; in the elderly; or in patients receiving diuretics. ■ Use caution in patients with cardiac decompensation, hypertension, or similar conditions; may cause fluid retention and edema. ■ Use caution in patients with pre-existing asthma, especially aspirin-sensitive asthma. Severe bronchospasm has been reported.

Monitor: Correct hypovolemia before giving ketorolac and maintain adequate hydration. ■ Observe patient frequently, especially for heartburn or signs and symptoms of GI upset or bleeding, and monitor vital signs. ■ Monitor blood urea nitrogen (BUN), SCr, liver enzymes, occult blood loss, urinalysis, urine output, and signs of pain relief (e.g., increased appetite and activity). ■ Observe closely during ambulation. ■ Low doses of narcotics may be required to treat breakthrough pain.

Patient Education: Side effects have resulted in extended hospitalization and could be fatal. ■ Discard any remaining oral ketorolac at end of 5-day total cumulative maximum time for use.

Maternal/Child: See Contraindications. ■ Category C: safety for use not established. Use only if other alternatives are not available. ■ Discontinue breastfeeding. ■ Multiple-dose treatment in pediatric patients has not been studied; limited data available.

Elderly: See Dose Adjustments and Precautions. ■ More sensitive to side effects. ■ Incidence of GI bleeding and acute renal failure increases with age.

DRUG/LAB INTERACTIONS
Probenecid inhibits clearance and may triple plasma levels of ketorolac. Concomitant use is contraindicated. ■ Potentiated by **salicylates** (especially high-dose regimens). May double plasma levels of ketorolac. Reduce dose of ketorolac by half. ■ May decrease clearance and increase toxicity of **methotrexate**. ■ Additive if used with other **NSAIDs** (see Contraindications); side effects may increase markedly. ■ May potentiate **lithium** levels. ■ May increase risk of bleeding, especially from the GI tract, when given concomitantly with **anticoagulants** or **thrombolytic agents**. ■ May increase risk of bleeding when given with **agents that may cause thrombocytopenia or inhibit or interfere with platelet aggregation** (e.g., clopidogrel, valproic acid) and **serotonin reuptake inhibitors (SSRIs)**. ■ Can precipitate

failure concomitantly with **diuretics**; see Precautions. ▪ Can reduce response to **furosemide or other diuretics** in normovolemic healthy individuals. ▪ May increase risk of renal impairment with **ACE inhibitors** (e.g., enalapril). ▪ Nephrotoxicity of both agents may be increased with **other nephrotoxic agents** (e.g., aminoglycosides, cyclosporine). ▪ May potentiate **nondepolarizing muscle relaxants**. ▪ Has caused seizures in a few patients taking **antiepileptics**. ▪ May cause hallucinations with **antipsychotics or antidepressants**. ▪ May cause **elevations of liver function tests** AST and ALT.

SIDE EFFECTS

Average dose: Diarrhea, dizziness, dyspepsia, drowsiness, edema, GI bleeding, GI pain, headache, injection site pain, nausea, renal failure, and sweating are most common. Capable of all side effects of other NSAIDs, especially with extended use: abnormal taste, abnormal vision, asthenia, asthma, confusion, constipation, depression, dry mouth, dyspnea, euphoria, excessive thirst, flatulence, inability to concentrate, insomnia, liver function abnormalities, melena, myalgia, nervousness, oliguria, pallor, paresthesia, peptic ulcer, rectal bleeding, stimulation, stomatitis, pruritus, purpura, urinary frequency, urticaria, vasodilation, vertigo, vomiting.

Overdose: Abdominal pain, diarrhea, labored breathing, metabolic acidosis, pallor, peptic ulcer, rales, vomiting.

ANTIDOTE

With increasing severity of any side effect or onset of symptoms of overdose, discontinue the drug and notify the physician. A patent airway, artificial ventilation, oxygen therapy, and other symptomatic treatment must be instituted promptly if indicated. Treat anaphylaxis with epinephrine, diphenhydramine, and corticosteroids as indicated. Not significantly cleared by dialysis.

LABETALOL HYDROCHLORIDE
(lah-**BET**-ah-lohl hy-droh-**KLOR**-eyed)

Alpha/beta-adrenergic blocking agent
Antihypertensive

pH 3 to 4.5

USUAL DOSE

Dose must be individualized based on degree of hypertension and patient response.

20 mg as an initial dose by IV injection. May repeat with injections of 40 to 80 mg at 10-minute intervals until desired BP is achieved, or may be diluted and given as a continuous infusion. Usually effective with 50 to 200 mg. Do not exceed a total dose of 300 mg. Initiate oral labetalol after desired BP has been achieved and the supine diastolic pressure starts to rise. See literature for dose regimen. AHA recommends 10 mg IV over 1 to 2 minutes. May repeat or double dose every 10 minutes to a maximum dose of 150 mg. Or initial dose may be given by IV injection followed by an infusion of 2 to 8 mg/min. Titrate slowly to achieve desired results without exceeding maximum dose.

DOSE ADJUSTMENTS

See Precautions and Drug/Lab Interactions.

DILUTION
IV injection: May be given undiluted in a 5 mg/mL concentration.

Continuous infusion: May be diluted in most commonly used IV solutions (see chart on inside back cover). Addition of 200 mg (40 mL) to 160-mL solution yields 1 mg/mL, 300 mg (60 mL) to 240 mL yields 1 mg/mL, or 200 mg (40 mL) to 250 mL yields 2 mg/3 mL. Amount of solution may be decreased if required by fluid restrictions of the patient.

Storage: Store unopened vial between 2° and 30° C (36° and 86° F). Do not freeze. Protect from light. Stable after dilution for 24 hours at room temperature or refrigerated.

COMPATIBILITY
Manufacturer lists 5% sodium bicarbonate as **incompatible** and indicates to use care when administering alkaline drugs, including furosemide.

Other sources suggest specific **compatibilities** dependent on concentration and manufacturer; consult a pharmacist.

RATE OF ADMINISTRATION
IV injection: Each 20 mg or fraction thereof over at least 2 minutes.

Continuous infusion: Begin at 2 mg/min. Adjust according to orders of physician and BP response. Another source suggests 0.5 to 2 mg/min. Use of a microdrip (60 drops/mL) or an infusion pump may be helpful.

ACTIONS
An adrenergic receptor blocking agent with both selective alpha-1-adrenergic and nonselective beta-adrenergic receptor blocking activity. Causes dose-related falls in BP without reflex tachycardia or significant reduction in HR. Maximum effect of each dose is reached in 5 minutes. Half-life is 5.5 hours, but some effects last up to 16 hours. Metabolized and excreted as metabolites in urine and through bile to feces. Crosses the placental barrier. Present in small amounts in breast milk.

INDICATIONS AND USES
Control of BP in severe hypertension.

Unlabeled uses: Treatment of clonidine withdrawal hypertension. ▪ Decrease BP and relieve symptoms in patients with pheochromocytoma.

CONTRAINDICATIONS
Obstructive airway disease including asthma, cardiogenic shock, greater than first-degree heart block, overt cardiac failure, severe bradycardia, other conditions associated with severe and prolonged hypotension, and hypersensitivity to labetalol or its components.

PRECAUTIONS
Use caution in impaired liver function. ▪ Hepatic injury has been reported. Has occurred after both short-term and long-term treatment. Usually reversible, but hepatic necrosis and death have been reported. ▪ Use extreme caution in patients with any degree of cardiac failure; may further depress myocardial contractility. Does not alter effectiveness of digoxin on heart muscle. ▪ Effective in lowering BP in pheochromocytoma but has caused a paradoxical hypertensive response in some patients. ▪ Use with extreme caution in diabetics or patients with a history of hypoglycemia. May mask the symptoms of hypoglycemia and reduce the release of insulin in response to hyperglycemia. ▪ Routine withdrawal of chronic beta-blocker therapy before surgery is not recommended. However, the effect of the alpha-adrenergic activity of labetalol has not been evaluated in the surgical setting. Deaths have occurred when labetalol has been used during surgery. ▪ Intraoperative floppy iris syndrome has been observed during cataract surgery in some patients treated with alpha-1 blockers. Characterized by a combination of a flaccid iris, progressive miosis despite preoperative dilation with standard mydriatic drugs, and potential prolapse of the iris. Modification of the surgical technique may be required. ▪ See Drug/Lab Interactions.

Monitor: Keep patient supine. Postural hypotension can occur for up to 3 hours after administration. Ambulate with care and assistance. ▪ Monitor BP before and 5 and 10 minutes after each direct IV injection. Monitor at least every 5 minutes during infusion. Avoid rapid or excessive falls in either systolic or diastolic BP. When severely elevated BP drops too rapidly, catastrophic reactions can occur (e.g., cerebral infarction, optic nerve infarction, angina, ischemic ECG changes). ▪ Monitor for S/S of CHF. ▪ Although rebound angina, myocardial infarction, or ventricular arrhythmias have not been a problem with labetalol, it is recommended that the dose of beta-adrenergic blockers be reduced gradually to avoid these conditions. ▪ See Drug/Lab Interactions.

Patient Education: Report cough, dizziness, irregular pulse, or shortness of breath promptly. ▪ May cause dizziness or fainting; request assistance with ambulation.

Maternal/Child: Category C: use in pregnancy only when clearly indicated and benefit outweighs risk. Hypotension, bradycardia, hypoglycemia, and respiratory depression have been reported in infants of mothers who were treated with labetalol for hypertension during pregnancy. Has been used during labor and delivery. ▪ Use caution during breast-feeding. ▪ Safety and effectiveness for use in pediatric patients not established.

Elderly: Use with caution in age-related peripheral vascular disease; risk of hypothermia increased. ▪ May exacerbate mental impairment.

DRUG/LAB INTERACTIONS

Amiodarone may enhance the bradycardic effect of beta-blockers. ▪ Inhibits **beta-agonist bronchodilators** (e.g., albuterol); increased doses may be required, especially in patients with asthma. ▪ Synergistic with **halothane anesthesia**. ▪ Potentiated by **cimetidine**. ▪ May blunt the reflex tachycardia produced by **nitroglycerin.** May cause further hypotension with **nitroglycerin.** ▪ The use of labetalol with **calcium channel blockers** may potentiate both drugs and result in severe depression of myocardium, AV conduction, and severe hypotension. ▪ May mask the hypoglycemic effects of **insulin and other antidiabetic agents.** May inhibit the mobilization of glucose from hepatic stores. Monitor glucose carefully in diabetic patients. ▪ Patients receiving beta-blockers who have a history of severe anaphylactic reaction to a variety of allergens may be unresponsive to the usual doses of **epinephrine** used to treat an allergic reaction. ▪ May interfere with lab tests in the **diagnosis of pheochromocytoma.** ▪ May cause a **false-positive urine test** for amphetamine use.

SIDE EFFECTS

Diaphoresis, dizziness, flushing, moderate hypotension, numbness, severe postural hypotension, nausea, somnolence, tingling of scalp, and ventricular dysrhythmias (e.g., intensified atrioventricular block) occur most frequently.

ANTIDOTE

Notify the physician of all side effects. Decrease rate or discontinue drug if hypotension occurs. Notify physician immediately. Trendelenburg position may be appropriate. May require treatment with IV fluids or vasopressors (e.g., norepinephrine, dopamine). Use atropine or epinephrine for severe bradycardia; digoxin, diuretics, dopamine, or dobutamine for cardiac failure; norepinephrine for hypotension; epinephrine and/or albuterol for bronchospasm; and diazepam for seizures. Unresponsive hypotension and bradycardia may be reversed by glucagon 5 to 10 mg over 30 seconds followed by a continuous infusion of 5 mg/hr. Reduce rate as condition improves. Treat other side effects symptomatically and resuscitate as necessary. Hemodialysis is not effective.

LACOSAMIDE

(la-**KOE**-sa-mide)

Anticonvulsant

Vimpat

pH 3.5 to 5

USUAL DOSE

Pretreatment: Baseline studies indicated; see Monitor.

Serum levels similar by oral or IV route; no dose or frequency adjustment is necessary. Transfer to oral therapy as soon as practical. Twice-daily IV infusions have been used for up to 5 days.

Monotherapy: Begin with an initial dose of 100 mg twice daily (200 mg/day); dose should be increased by 50 mg twice daily (100 mg/day) every week up to a recommended maintenance dose of 150 to 200 mg twice daily (300 to 400 mg/day). Alternatively, lacosamide may be initiated with a single loading dose of 200 mg* followed approximately 12 hours later by 100 mg twice daily (200 mg/day); this dose regimen should be continued for 1 week. Based on individual response and tolerability, the dose can be increased at weekly intervals by 50 mg twice daily (100 mg/day) until the recommended maintenance dose of 150 to 200 mg twice daily (300 to 400 mg/day) is achieved. For patients who are already on a single antiepileptic and are converting to lacosamide monotherapy, the therapeutic dose of 150 to 200 mg twice daily should be maintained for at least 3 days before initiating withdrawal of the concomitant antiepileptic drug. A gradual withdrawal of the concomitant antiepileptic drug over at least 6 weeks is recommended.

Adjuvant therapy: Begin with an initial dose of 50 mg twice daily (100 mg/day). Based on individual patient response and tolerability, the dose may be increased at weekly intervals by 50 mg twice daily (100 mg/day). The recommended maintenance dose is 100 to 200 mg twice daily (200 to 400 mg/day). Alternatively, lacosamide may be initiated with a single loading dose of 200 mg* followed approximately 12 hours later by 100 mg twice daily (200 mg/day); this dose regimen should be continued for 1 week. Based on individual response and tolerability, the dose can be increased at weekly intervals by 50 mg twice daily (100 mg/day) as needed until the maximum recommended maintenance dose of 200 mg twice daily (400 mg/day) is achieved.

***Monotherapy and adjuvant therapy:** The loading dose should be administered with medical supervision because of the increased incidence of CNS adverse reactions. There is no evidence that doses greater than 400 mg/day offer additional benefit, and they have been associated with a higher incidence of side effects.

Transfer from an IV dose to an oral dose: Transfer at the equivalent daily dose and frequency of the IV dose.

DOSE ADJUSTMENTS

Titrate dose with caution in patients with renal or hepatic impairment and in the elderly.
- No dose adjustment is indicated for patients with mild to moderate renal impairment.
- 300 mg is the maximum recommended dose for patients with severe renal impairment (a CrCl equal to or less than 30 mL/min) and for patients with end-stage renal disease. A supplemental dose of up to 50% should be considered after a 4-hour hemodialysis treatment. ■ A maximum dose of 300 mg/day is recommended for patients with mild or moderate hepatic impairment. ■ Not recommended for patients with severe hepatic impairment. ■ Patients with renal or hepatic impairment who are taking strong inhibitors of CYP3A4 and CYP2C9 may have a significant increase in exposure of lacosamide. Consult with pharmacist. Dose reduction may be required. ■ Dose adjustment not required based on gender or race or in the elderly; see Elderly.

DILUTION

Available as a 200 mg/20 mL (10 mg/mL) solution for injection.

May be given undiluted or may be further diluted with NS, D5W, or LR. See Rate of Administration.

Filters: Specific information not available.

Storage: Store unopened vials at CRT. Do not freeze. Diluted solutions should not be stored for more than 4 hours at RT. Discard unused portions of vial.

COMPATIBILITY

Solutions: Compatible with NS, D5W, and LR. Additional information not available; consult a pharmacist.

RATE OF ADMINISTRATION

A single dose as an infusion over 30 to 60 minutes is preferred. When medically necessary, may be infused over 15 minutes. Incidence of CNS side effects (e.g., dizziness, paresthesia, and somnolence) may be higher with the 15-minute infusion.

ACTIONS

An antiepileptic (anticonvulsant) drug. The precise mechanism of action is unknown. In vitro studies have shown that it selectively enhances the slow inactivation of voltage-gated sodium channels, resulting in stabilization of hyperexcitable neuronal membranes and inhibition of repetitive neuronal firing. Some effects are reached at the end of infusion. Steady-state plasma concentrations are achieved after 3 days of administration. Doses above 400 mg/day do not appear to have additional benefit. Less than 15% bound to plasma proteins. Partially metabolized. Half-life is approximately 13 hours. Excreted as metabolites and as unchanged drug in urine.

INDICATIONS AND USES

Monotherapy or adjunctive therapy in the treatment of partial-onset seizures in adult patients (17 years of age and older) with epilepsy. IV injection is used as a temporary alternative to oral therapy. May be used alone or in combination with other antiepileptic drugs (AEDs).

CONTRAINDICATIONS

Manufacturer indicates none; see Precautions.

PRECAUTIONS

For IV use only. ▪ AEDs increase the risk of suicidal thoughts or behavior in patients taking these drugs for any indication. Patients treated with any AED for any indication should be monitored for the emergence or worsening of depression, suicidal thoughts or behavior, and/or any unusual changes in mood or behavior. In an analysis of AED clinical trials, symptoms occurred as early as 1 week after starting AEDs and persisted for the duration of treatment. May require a dose reduction or discontinuation of lacosamide. Many illnesses for which AEDs are prescribed, including epilepsy, are associated with morbidity and mortality and an increased risk of suicidal thoughts and behavior. Consider that these symptoms may also be related to the illness being treated. ▪ May cause dizziness and ataxia. Dizziness was the adverse event most frequently leading to discontinuation of therapy. Onset of symptoms commonly observed during titration. ▪ Dose-dependent prolongations in PR intervals have been observed. AV heart block, bradycardia, and ventricular tachyarrhythmias have been reported. Use caution in patients with underlying proarrhythmic conduction problems such as known conduction problems (e.g., marked first-degree AV block, second-degree or higher AV block, and sick sinus syndrome without a pacemaker), sodium channelopathies (e.g., Brugada syndrome), or severe cardiac disease such as myocardial ischemia, heart failure, or structural heart disease. ▪ May cause atrial arrhythmias (atrial fibrillation or atrial flutter), especially in patients with diabetic neuropathy or cardiovascular disease. ▪ Syncope or loss of consciousness was reported. Often associated with changes in orthostatic hypotension, atrial flutter/fibrillation (and associated tachycardia), or bradycardia. Most commonly seen in patients with a history of risk factors for cardiac disease, in patients receiving medications that slow AV conduction, and in patients with diabetic neuropathy. Most cases were associated with doses above the recommended 400 mg/day. ▪ Drug reaction with eosinophilia and systemic symptoms (DRESS), also known as multiorgan hypersensitivity, has been reported. Usually presents with fever, rash, lymphadenopathy, and/or facial swelling in association with other organ system involvement such as hematologic abnormalities, hepatitis, nephritis, myocarditis, or myositis. Eosinophilia is often present.

Deaths have been reported. S/S of early hypersensitivity (e.g., fever, lymphadenopathy) may be present even though a rash is not evident. If S/S appear, evaluate patient and discontinue lacosamide if an alternative etiology for the S/S cannot be established. ▪ Not recommended for patients with severe hepatic impairment. ▪ To minimize the potential for increased seizure frequency, withdraw AEDs (including lacosamide) gradually (over a minimum of 1 week). ▪ Physical dependence has not been demonstrated; however, psychological dependence cannot be excluded because of the ability of lacosamide to produce a euphoria-type response.

Monitor: Baseline CBC, CrCl, bilirubin, and liver function tests indicated; monitor as needed. ▪ Monitor vital signs. ▪ Monitor for seizure activity. ▪ Monitor for the emergence or worsening of depression, suicidal thoughts or behavior, and/or any unusual changes in mood or behavior. ▪ Observe patient closely for signs of CNS side effects, prolonged PR interval, and/or symptoms of DRESS; see Precautions. ▪ Obtain a baseline ECG in patients with known underlying proarrhythmic conditions or concomitant medications that affect cardiac conduction. Repeat ECG after lacosamide is titrated to steady-state concentrations.

Patient Education: Read patient information guide provided by manufacturer. ▪ May cause dizziness, fainting, and somnolence; use caution performing tasks that require alertness (e.g., operating machinery, driving). ▪ Inform your healthcare professional if you are pregnant or breast-feeding. ▪ May increase the risk of suicidal thoughts and behavior. Promptly report emergence or worsening of S/S of depression, any unusual changes in mood or behavior, or thoughts about self-harm. ▪ Has caused atrial arrhythmias. Promptly report palpitations, rapid pulse, and/or shortness of breath. ▪ May cause various degrees of heart block. Report slow or irregular pulse, light-headedness, chest pain, or fainting. ▪ Promptly report S/S of hypersensitivity (e.g., fever, rash) or liver toxicity (e.g., fatigue, jaundice, dark urine). ▪ Females who are pregnant or who become pregnant should be encouraged to enroll in the North American Antiepileptic Drug (NAAED) Pregnancy Registry. ▪ Review prescription and nonprescription drugs with your physician.

Maternal/Child: Animal studies demonstrated developmental toxicity (increased embryofetal and perinatal mortality, growth deficit). Use during pregnancy only if the potential benefit justifies the potential risk to the fetus. Manufacturer has established a pregnancy registry to evaluate safety and outcomes; see manufacturer's literature and Patient Education. ▪ Effects during labor and delivery unknown. ▪ No data on the presence of lacosamide in human milk, the effects on the breast-fed infant, or the effects on milk production. ▪ Safety and effectiveness for use in pediatric patients under 17 years of age not established.

Elderly: Higher plasma concentrations seen in the elderly may be due to differences in total body water and age-associated impaired renal function. Although dose adjustment based on age is not necessary, dose titration should be performed with caution; see Usual Dose.

DRUG/LAB INTERACTIONS

Use with caution in patients taking concomitant **medications that affect cardiac conduction** (e.g., beta-blockers, calcium channel blockers), potassium channel blockers, sodium channel blockers, and medications that prolong the PR interval. Increased risk of AV block, bradycardia, and ventricular tachyarrhythmia. Baseline ECG and repeat ECG following titration to steady state recommended. ▪ No evidence of any relevant drug/drug interaction with **other antiepileptic drugs**. ▪ Patients with renal or hepatic impairment who are taking **strong inhibitors of CYP3A4** (e.g., ritonavir, clarithromycin, ketoconazole) **and CYP2C9** (e.g., fluconazole) may have a significant increase in exposure of lacosamide. Dose reduction may be necessary.

SIDE EFFECTS

The most common side effects are diplopia, dizziness, headache, and nausea. Ataxia, blurred vision, diplopia, dizziness, nausea, vertigo, and vomiting led to discontinuation of lacosamide. Incidence of side effects increased with doses above 400 mg/day. Most side effects at recommended doses were considered mild or moderate and included abnormal coordination; anemia; asthenia; balance disorder; cerebellar syndrome; chest pain; confusion; constipation; depression; diarrhea; dry mouth; dyspepsia; elevated liver function tests (e.g., ALT, AST); falls; fatigue; feeling drunk; fever; gait disturbance; hyperhidrosis; hypoanesthesia; injection site pain, discomfort, irritation, or erythema; muscle spasms; nystagmus; oral hypoanesthesia; palpitations; paresthesia; pruritus; skin laceration; somnolence; tinnitus; and tremor. Psychiatric disorders, including aggression, agitation, anger, anxiety, apathy, depersonalization, depression, emotional lability, hallucinations, hostility, irritability, and suicidal tendencies, have been reported. May produce euphoria-type reactions. Other serious adverse reactions include ataxia and dizziness, cardiac rhythm and conduction abnormalities, multiorgan hypersensitivity reactions, and syncope.

Post-Marketing: Aggression, agitation, agranulocytosis, angioedema, hallucinations, insomnia, new or worsening seizures, psychotic disorder, rash, Stevens-Johnson syndrome, toxic epidermal necrolysis, urticaria.

ANTIDOTE

Keep physician informed of all side effects. Some may not require intervention, and others may improve with a reduced dose or discontinuation of lacosamide; see Precautions and Side Effects. Discontinue lacosamide for symptoms of DRESS; use of an alternate treatment is recommended. Support patient as required in treatment of overdose. No specific antidote in overdose; however, hemodialysis will remove approximately 50% of a dose in 4 hours.

LEFAMULIN

(le-**FAM**-ue-lin)

Xenleta

Antibacterial
(pleuromutilin)

pH 4.5 to 5.5

USUAL DOSE

Pretreatment: Verify pregnancy status.

Lefamulin: 150 mg every 12 hours as an IV infusion over 60 minutes for 5 to 7 days **OR** 600 mg PO every 12 hours for 5 days; see Precautions. May switch to oral therapy at a dose of 600 mg PO every 12 hours to complete a treatment course.

DOSE ADJUSTMENTS

Reduce dose to 150 mg IV every 24 hours in patients with severe hepatic impairment (Child-Pugh Class C). No adjustment is needed for patients with mild (Child-Pugh Class A) or moderate (Child-Pugh Class B) hepatic impairment. ■ No clinically significant differences in pharmacokinetics of lefamulin were observed based on age, gender, race, weight, or renal impairment, including patients receiving hemodialysis.

DILUTION

Lefamulin injection is available as a clear, colorless solution in a single-dose vial containing 150 mg/15 mL (10 mg/mL). It is supplied with a diluent bag containing 250 mL of 10 mM citrate-buffered 0.9% sodium chloride. Dilute the entire 15-mL vial of lefamulin into the supplied diluent bag. Mix thoroughly. Do not use the diluent bag in series connections.

Filter: Data not available.

Storage: Store unopened vials under refrigeration at 2° to 8° C (36° to 46° F). *Do not freeze.* The diluent bag may be stored at CRT. After dilution, may be stored for up to 24 hours at RT and up to 48 hours when refrigerated at 2° to 8° C (36° to 46° F).

COMPATIBILITY

The manufacturer states, "Do not add other additives to the diluent bag because their **compatibilities** with lefamulin have not been established."

RATE OF ADMINISTRATION

A single dose as an infusion equally distributed over 60 minutes. Do not exceed the recommended rate of administration; may increase the magnitude of QT prolongation; see Precautions. Do not use the diluent bag in series connections.

ACTIONS

A semi-synthetic systemic pleuromutilin antibacterial that inhibits bacterial protein synthesis through various interactions with the 50S ribosomal subunit. Lefamulin is bactericidal in vitro against *Streptococcus pneumoniae, Haemophilus influenzae,* and *Mycoplasma pneumoniae* (including macrolide-resistant strains) and is bacteriostatic against *Staphylococcus aureus* and *Streptococcus pyogenes* at clinically relevant concentrations.

Lefamulin is not active against Enterobacteriaceae and *Pseudomonas aeruginosa.* Plasma protein binding is 94.8% to 97.1%. Lefamulin is primarily metabolized by CYP3A4. The mean elimination half-life is approximately 8 hours (range 3 to 20 hours). Excreted primarily in feces and to a lesser extent in urine.

INDICATIONS AND USES

Treatment of adults with community-acquired bacterial pneumonia (CABP) caused by the following susceptible microorganisms: *S. pneumoniae, S. aureus* (methicillin-susceptible isolates), *H. influenzae, Legionella pneumophila, M. pneumoniae,* and *Chlamydophila pneumoniae.*

CONTRAINDICATIONS

History of known severe hypersensitivity to lefamulin, pleuromutilin class drugs, or to any component of lefamulin.

PRECAUTIONS

May prolong the QT interval of the electrocardiogram (ECG) in some patients. Avoid use in patients with known prolongation of the QT interval, patients with ventricular arrhythmias (including torsades de pointes), patients receiving Class IA (e.g., quinidine, procainamide) or Class III (e.g., amiodarone) antiarrhythmic agents, or patients receiving other drugs that prolong the QT interval such as antipsychotics, erythromycin, pimozide, moxifloxacin, and tricyclic antidepressants. ▪ Use with caution in patients with renal failure who require dialysis and in patients with any degree of hepatic impairment. Metabolic disturbances may lead to QT prolongation; see Monitor. ▪ The magnitude of QT prolongation may increase with increasing concentrations of lefamulin or increasing rate of infusion. Do not exceed recommended dose or rate of administration. ▪ Specific sensitivity studies indicated to determine susceptibility of causative organism to lefamulin. ▪ Some isolates resistant to beta-lactams, glycopeptides, macrolides, mupirocin, quinolones, tetracyclines, and trimethoprim-sulfamethoxazole may be susceptible to lefamulin. ▪ To reduce the development of drug-resistant bacteria and maintain its effectiveness, lefamulin should be used to treat or prevent only those infections proven or strongly suspected to be caused by bacteria. ▪ *Clostridium difficile*–associated diarrhea (CDAD) has been reported. May range from mild diarrhea to fatal colitis. Consider in patients who present with diarrhea during or after treatment with lefamulin.

Monitor: Monitor patients with hepatic impairment for adverse reactions associated with lefamulin. ▪ Monitor ECG in patients at risk for QT prolongation; see Precautions. ▪ Monitoring of electrolytes may be indicated in patients at risk for QT prolongation due to metabolic disturbances related to impaired renal or hepatic impairment.

Patient Education: Verify pregnancy status. Females of reproductive potential should use effective contraception during treatment and for 2 days after the final dose. The manufacturer has a surveillance program for pregnant females who have inadvertently taken lefamulin during pregnancy; see prescribing information. ▪ Review list of medications with provider. ▪ Nausea and vomiting are common adverse reactions seen with lefamulin. ▪ Promptly report any symptoms of hypersensitivity (e.g., difficulty breathing, hives, itching, rash). ▪ Promptly report diarrhea or bloody stools that occur during treatment or up to several months after an antibiotic has been discontinued; may indicate CDAD and require treatment.

Maternal/Child: Based on animal studies, lefamulin may cause fetal harm when administered to pregnant females. ▪ Because of the potential for serious adverse reactions, including QT prolongation, a woman should pump and discard breast milk for the duration of treatment with lefamulin and for 2 days after the final dose. ▪ Safety and efficacy for use in pediatric patients younger than 18 years of age have not been established.

Elderly: Safety and efficacy are similar to that seen in younger patients.

DRUG/LAB INTERACTIONS

Concomitant use of lefamulin with **strong CYP3A4 inducers or P-GP inducers** (e.g., rifampin) decreases lefamulin AUC and C_{max}, which may reduce the efficacy of lefamulin. Avoid concomitant use unless the benefit outweighs the risks. ▪ The pharmacodynamic interaction potential to prolong the QT interval between lefamulin and other drugs that affect cardiac conduction is unknown. Avoid concomitant use of lefamulin with **drugs that can prolong the QT interval** (e.g., Class IA and III antiarrhythmics, antipsychotics, erythromycin, moxifloxacin, tricyclic antidepressants); see Precautions and Monitor. ▪ In vitro studies have demonstrated no antagonism between lefamulin and amikacin, azithromycin, aztreonam, ceftriaxone, levofloxacin, linezolid, meropenem, penicillin, tigecycline, trimethoprim/sulfamethoxazole, and vancomycin. ▪ Lefamulin has demonstrated synergy in vitro with **doxycycline** against *S. aureus.*

SIDE EFFECTS

The most common adverse reactions include headache, hepatic enzyme elevation, hypokalemia, injection site reactions, insomnia, and nausea. Other reported reactions include abdominal pain, anemia, anxiety, atrial fibrillation, CDAD, constipation, diarrhea, dyspepsia, epigastric discomfort, erosive gastritis, increased creatine phosphokinase, oropharyngeal candidiasis, QT prolongation, palpitations, somnolence, thrombocytopenia, urinary retention, vomiting, and vulvovaginal candidiasis.

ANTIDOTE

Notify physician of any side effects. Discontinue the drug if indicated. Treat hypersensitivity reactions as indicated. Mild cases of CDAD may respond to discontinuation of lefamulin. Treat CDAD with fluids, electrolytes, protein supplements, and appropriate antibiotics (e.g., oral vancomycin) as indicated. In severe cases, surgical evaluation may be indicated. Lefamulin and its primary metabolite are not dialyzable.

LETERMOVIR

Antiviral

(le-**TERM**-oh-vir)

Prevymis

pH 7.5

USUAL DOSE

480 mg PO or IV once daily. Initiate between Day 0 and Day 28 posttransplantation (before or after engraftment) and continue through Day 100 posttransplantation. Reserve IV formulation for patients unable to take oral preparation. Transfer to oral dosing as soon as practical. IV and oral dose may be used interchangeably at the discretion of the physician. No dose adjustment necessary when switching formulations.

DOSE ADJUSTMENTS

If cyclosporine is initiated after starting letermovir, decrease letermovir to 240 mg once daily beginning with the next scheduled dose. ▪ If cyclosporine is discontinued after starting letermovir, increase letermovir to 480 mg once daily beginning with the next scheduled dose. ▪ If cyclosporine dosing is interrupted due to high cyclosporine levels, no dose adjustment of letermovir is required. ▪ No dose adjustment required based on renal impairment for patients with a creatinine clearance (CrCl) greater than 10 mL/min. ▪ Data insufficient to make dosing recommendations in patients with CrCl 10 mL/min or less or in patients on dialysis. ▪ No dose adjustment required for patients with mild or moderate hepatic impairment. Not recommended for patients with severe hepatic impairment. ▪ No dose adjustment indicated based on age, body weight (up to 100 kg), gender, or race.

DILUTION

Available in single-dose vials containing 240 mg/12 mL or 480 mg/24 mL (both are 20 mg/mL). Do not shake the vial. Withdraw the desired dose and add to an IV bag containing 250 mL of NS or D5W; see Compatibility. Mix gently. Do not shake. May be colorless to slightly yellow.

Filters: Specific information not available.

Storage: Store single-dose vials at CRT in carton to protect from light. Diluted solutions are stable for up to 24 hours at RT or up to 48 hours under refrigeration (time includes time in storage through completion of the infusion).

COMPATIBILITY

Consider any item NOT listed as compatible to be INCOMPATIBLE.

Manufacturer states, "Should not be coadministered through the same IV line or cannula with other drug products and diluent combinations except those specifically listed."

Compatible With:

IV Bags: Polyvinyl chloride (PVC), ethylene vinyl acetate (EVA), polyolefin (polypropylene and polyethylene).

Infusion Sets: PVC, polyethylene (PE), polybutadiene (PBD), silicone rubber (SR), styrene-butadiene copolymer (SBC), styrene-butadiene-styrene copolymer (SBS), polystyrene (PS).

Plasticizers: Diethylhexyl phthalate (DEHP), tris (2-ethylhexyl) trimellitate (TOTM), benzyl butyl phthalate (BBP).

Catheters: Radiopaque polyurethane.

Y-site:

Diluted with NS: Ampicillin, ampicillin/sulbactam, caspofungin, daptomycin, fentanyl citrate, fluconazole, furosemide, human insulin, magnesium sulfate, methotrexate, micafungin.

Diluted with D5W: Amphotericin B, anidulafungin, cefazolin, ceftaroline, ceftriaxone, doripenem, famotidine, folic acid, ganciclovir, hydrocortisone sodium succinate, morphine, norepinephrine, pantoprazole, potassium chloride, potassium phosphate, tacrolimus, telavancin, tigecycline.

RATE OF ADMINISTRATION

A single dose as an infusion at a constant rate over 1 hour. May be infused via a peripheral catheter or a central venous line.

ACTIONS

Letermovir is an antiviral drug against cytomegalovirus (CMV). It inhibits the CMV DNA terminase complex, which is required for viral DNA processing and packaging. 99% bound to human plasma proteins in vitro. Metabolized in the liver via UGT1A1/1A3. Mean terminal half-life is 12 hours. Primarily eliminated in feces (93%) as unchanged drug (70%) with minimal excretion in urine.

INDICATIONS AND USES

Prophylaxis of CMV infection and disease in adult CMV-seropositive recipients [R+] of an allogeneic hematopoietic stem cell transplantation (HSCT).

CONTRAINDICATIONS

Patients receiving pimozide or ergot alkaloids. ▪ Concomitant use with pitavastatin and simvastatin when coadministered with cyclosporine; see Drug/Lab Interactions.

PRECAUTIONS

Do not administer an IV bolus injection. ▪ Concomitant use of letermovir and certain drugs may result in potentially significant drug interactions, which may lead to adverse reactions (letermovir or concomitant drug) or decreased therapeutic effect of letermovir or the concomitant drug; see Contraindications and Drug/Lab Interactions.

Monitor: See Drug/Lab Interactions for specific monitoring requirements when letermovir is administered with other drugs. ▪ See Contraindications. ▪ After the completion of letermovir prophylaxis, monitoring for CMV reactivation is recommended. ▪ Monitor SCr in patients with a CrCl less than 50 mL/min. Accumulation of the IV vehicle (hydroxypropyl betadex) can occur.

Patient Education: Interacts with many drugs. Report the use of all prescription and nonprescription medications and herbal products to a healthcare provider.

Maternal/Child: Data on safety for use in pregnancy not available; benefit must justify potential risks to fetus. ▪ There are no data on the presence of letermovir in human milk, the effects on breast-fed infants, or the effects on milk production. Consider risk versus benefit. ▪ Safety and effectiveness for use in pediatric patients not established.

Elderly: Safety and effectiveness similar across older and younger subjects.

DRUG/LAB INTERACTIONS

The following drug interactions apply only to coadministration of letermovir alone (without cyclosporine) unless otherwise noted. The magnitude of letermovir drug interactions on coadministered drugs may be different when letermovir is coadministered with cyclosporine; see cyclosporine monograph.

Potentially Significant Drug Interactions of Letermovir When Administered Without Cyclosporine[a]		
Concomitant Drug Class and/or Clearance Pathway and Drug Name	**Effect on Concentration**	**Clinical Comments Suggested When Letermovir Administered With Each Drug**
Antiarrhythmic Agents		
Amiodarone	Concentration of amiodarone increased	Monitor closely for amiodarone side effects. Monitor amiodarone concentrations frequently.
Antibiotics		
Nafcillin	Concentration of letermovir decreased	Coadministration not recommended.
Anticoagulants		
Warfarin	Concentration of warfarin decreased	Monitor INR frequently.
Anticonvulsants		
Carbamazepine	Concentration of letermovir decreased	Coadministration not recommended.
Phenobarbital	Concentration of letermovir decreased	Coadministration not recommended.
Phenytoin	Concentration of letermovir decreased Concentration of phenytoin decreased	Coadministration not recommended.
Antidiabetic Agents		
Glyburide, repaglinide, rosiglitazone, others	Concentration of all three agents increased	Monitor glucose concentrations frequently. If letermovir is coadministered with cyclosporine, use of repaglinide is not recommended.
Antifungals		
Voriconazole	Concentration of voriconazole decreased	Monitor closely for reduced effectiveness of voriconazole.
Antimycobacterials		
Rifabutin	Concentration of letermovir decreased	Coadministration not recommended.
Rifampin	Concentration of letermovir decreased	Coadministration not recommended.
Antipsychotics		
Pimozide	Concentration of pimozide increased	Contraindicated due to risk of QT prolongation and torsades de pointes.
Thioridazine	Concentration of letermovir decreased	Coadministration not recommended.
Endothelin Antagonists		
Bosentan	Concentration of letermovir decreased	Coadministration not recommended.

Continued

Potentially Significant Drug Interactions of Letermovir When Administered Without Cyclosporine[a]—cont'd		
Concomitant Drug Class and/or Clearance Pathway and Drug Name	**Effect on Concentration**	**Clinical Comments Suggested When Letermovir Administered With Each Drug**
Ergot Alkaloids		
Ergotamine, dihydroergotamine	Concentration of ergot alkaloids increased	Contraindicated due to risk of ergotism.
Herbal Products		
St. John's wort (*Hypericum perforatum*)	Concentration of letermovir decreased	Coadministration not recommended.
HIV Medications		
Efavirenz	Concentration of letermovir decreased	Coadministration not recommended.
Etravirine	Concentration of letermovir decreased	Coadministration not recommended.
Nevirapine	Concentration of letermovir decreased	Coadministration not recommended.
HMG-CoA Reductase Inhibitors		
Atorvastatin	Concentration of atorvastatin increased	Do not exceed an atorvastatin dose of 20 mg daily. Monitor closely for myopathy and rhabdomyolysis. If letermovir is coadministered with cyclosporine, use of atorvastatin is not recommended.
Pitavastatin, simvastatin	Concentration of HMG-CoA reductase inhibitors increased	Coadministration not recommended. Contraindicated if letermovir is coadministered with cyclosporine because of significant increases of concentrations of pitavastatin and simvastatin and risk of myopathy or rhabdomyolysis.
Fluvastatin, lovastatin, pravastatin, rosuvastatin	Concentration of HMG-CoA reductase inhibitors increased	A statin dose reduction may be necessary. Monitor closely for myopathy and rhabdomyolysis. If letermovir is coadministered with cyclosporine, use of lovastatin is not recommended. Refer to the prescribing information for other statins for specific statin dosing recommendations.
Immunosuppressants		
Cyclosporine	Concentration of cyclosporine and letermovir increased	Decrease dose of letermovir to 240 mg once daily. Monitor cyclosporine whole blood concentrations frequently during treatment and after discontinuation of letermovir, and adjust dose of cyclosporine accordingly.
Sirolimus	Concentration of sirolimus increased	Monitor sirolimus whole blood concentrations frequently during treatment and after discontinuation of letermovir, and adjust dose of sirolimus accordingly. If letermovir is coadministered with cyclosporine and sirolimus, refer to the sirolimus prescribing information for specific sirolimus dosing recommendations.

Potentially Significant Drug Interactions of Letermovir When Administered Without Cyclosporine[a] —cont'd		
Concomitant Drug Class and/or Clearance Pathway and Drug Name	Effect on Concentration	Clinical Comments Suggested When Letermovir Administered With Each Drug
Tacrolimus	Concentration of tacrolimus increased	Monitor tacrolimus whole blood concentrations frequently during treatment and after discontinuation of letermovir, and adjust dose of tacrolimus accordingly.
Proton Pump Inhibitors		
Omeprazole Pantoprazole	Concentration of omeprazole and pantoprazole decreased	Clinical monitoring and dose adjustment may be needed.
Wakefulness-Promoting Agents		
Modafinil	Concentration of letermovir decreased	Coadministration not recommended.
CYP3A Substrates		
Alfentanil, fentanyl, midazolam, quinidine, others	Concentration of CYP3A substrate increased	When letermovir is coadministered with a CYP3A substrate, refer to the prescribing information for dosing of the CYP3A substrate with a moderate CYP3A inhibitor. When letermovir is coadministered with cyclosporine, the combined effect on CYP3A substrates may be similar to a strong CYP3A inhibitor. Refer to the prescribing information for dosing of the CYP3A substrate with a strong CYP3A inhibitor. CYP3A substrates pimozide and ergot alkaloids are contraindicated.

[a]Table is not all-inclusive.

- Letermovir is an inhibitor of OATP1B1/3 transporters; coadministration with drugs that are substrates of OATP1B1/3 transporters may result in clinically relevant increases in the plasma concentrations of the substrates. ▪ If dose adjustments of concomitant medications are made due to treatment with letermovir, doses should be readjusted after treatment with letermovir is completed. Clinically significant interactions were **not** observed with acyclovir, digoxin, mycophenolate mofetil, fluconazole, posaconazole, ethinyl estradiol, and levonorgestrel.

SIDE EFFECTS
Abdominal pain, cough, diarrhea, fatigue, headache, nausea, peripheral edema, and vomiting are most common. Cardiac events (atrial fibrillation, tachycardia) have been reported. Laboratory abnormalities include decreased ANC), hemoglobin, and platelets and increased serum creatinine. A hypersensitivity reaction with associated moderate dyspnea occurred in one subject after the first infusion of letermovir, leading to discontinuation. Nausea was the most common reason for drug discontinuation.

ANTIDOTE
Notify physician of all side effects; most will be treated symptomatically. There is no specific antidote for overdose, and the effects of dialysis on removal of letermovir from the systemic circulation are unknown. Monitor drug/drug interactions closely for risk of increased side effects or reduced therapeutic effect. Should a hypersensitivity reaction occur, treat as necessary (e.g., antihistamines, epinephrine, corticosteroids). Resuscitate if indicated.

LEUCOVORIN CALCIUM
(loo-koh-**VOR**-in **KAL**-see-um)

Antidote
Antineoplastic adjunct

**Citrovorum Factor, Folinic Acid,
Leucovorin Calcium PF**

pH 6 to 8.1

USUAL DOSE
May be given IV/IM or PO. If GI toxicity is present, should be administered parenterally. **Delayed excretion or overdose of methotrexate (MTX):** 10 mg/M^2 every 6 hours until the serum MTX level is less than 0.05 micromolar. Milligram for milligram or greater than the dose of MTX is common. Administer within the first hour (or as soon as possible) in overdose or within 24 hours of MTX dose if there is delayed excretion. At least every 24 hours, obtain a SCr and MTX level. If SCr is more than 50% above pretreatment level, increase the leucovorin dose to 100 mg/M^2 every 3 hours until the serum MTX level is less than 0.05 micromolar.

Leucovorin rescue after high-dose MTX therapy: With high-dose MTX (12 to 15 Gm/M^2 as an infusion over 4 hours), begin leucovorin 15 mg (approximately 10 mg/M^2) 24 hours after MTX infusion started. Repeat every–6 hours for 10 doses. If MTX elimination is delayed, extend every-6-hour dosing until MTX level is less than 0.05 micromolar. If there is evidence of acute renal injury, increase leucovorin to 150 mg every 3 hours until MTX level is less than 1 micromolar, then 15 mg every 3 hours until MTX level is less than 0.05 micromolar. In both situations obtain SCr and MTX level at least every 24 hours. Other protocols are in use. Amount of leucovorin is dependent on MTX dose, MTX serum levels, and SCr.

Megaloblastic anemia: Up to 1 mg daily.

Advanced colorectal cancer: 200 mg/M^2 followed by fluorouracil (5-FU) 370 mg/M^2 or leucovorin 20 mg/M^2 followed by 5-FU 425 mg/M^2 daily for 5 days. Repeat at 4-week intervals twice, then repeat every 28 to 35 days based on complete recovery from toxic effects. Reduce 5-FU dose based on tolerance to previous course, 20% for moderate hematologic or GI toxicity, 30% for severe. Leucovorin doses remain the same. Increase 5-FU dose 10% if no toxicity. Other protocols are in use. Also approved for use with irinotecan and 5-FU.

Pemetrexed toxicity (unlabeled): A single dose of 100 mg/M^2. Follow with 50 mg/M^2 every 6 hours for 8 days.

DOSE ADJUSTMENTS
See adjustments in Usual Dose; larger reductions may be required in the elderly based on the potential for decreased renal function, especially in combination with fluorouracil. ■ See Precautions/Monitor.

DILUTION
Each 50-mg, 100-mg, or 350-mg vial should be diluted to a 10 mg/mL to 20 mg/mL solution. For total doses less than 10 mg/M^2, dilute with bacteriostatic water for injection (contains benzyl alcohol as a preservative). Use SWFI without a preservative for any dose 10 mg/M^2 or greater. May be further diluted in 100 to 500 mL of D5W, D10W, NS, R, or LR. 1-mL (3-mg) ampules may be given undiluted (contain benzyl alcohol).

Storage: If prepared without a preservative, use immediately; stable up to 7 days with a preservative.

COMPATIBILITY
Several sources, including the manufacturer, cite **incompatibility** with 5-FU as an additive; may form a precipitate.

Other sources suggest specific **compatibilities** dependent on concentration and manufacturer; consult a pharmacist.

RATE OF ADMINISTRATION

Because of calcium content, do not exceed a rate of 160 mg/min (16 mL of a 10-mg/mL or 8 mL of a 20-mg/mL solution). May be given more slowly. Large doses may be infused equally distributed over 1 to 6 hours. Never exceed above limits.

ACTIONS

Potent agent for neutralizing immediate toxic effects of MTX (and other folic acid antagonists) on the hematopoietic system. Preferentially rescues normal cells without reversing the oncolytic effect of methotrexate. Also enhances the therapeutic and toxic effects of fluoropyrimidines (e.g., 5-FU).

INDICATIONS AND USES

Treatment of accidental folic acid antagonist (e.g., MTX) overdose or delayed excretion of MTX. ▪ Folinic acid rescue to prevent or decrease the toxicity of massive MTX doses used to treat resistant neoplasms. ▪ Treatment of megaloblastic anemia due to folic acid deficiency when oral therapy not appropriate. ▪ In combination with fluorouracil or fluorouracil and irinotecan to treat colorectal cancer.

Unlabeled uses: Adjunct in the treatment of Ewing sarcoma, head and neck cancer, non-Hodgkin lymphomas, and trophoblastic tumors. ▪ Treatment of pemetrexed toxicity.

CONTRAINDICATIONS

Pernicious anemia and other megaloblastic anemias secondary to lack of vitamin B_{12}. None when used as indicated for other specific uses.

PRECAUTIONS

Usually administered in the hospital by or under the direction of the physician specialist. ▪ Permits use of massive doses of MTX. ▪ Do not discontinue leucovorin calcium until methotrexate serum levels fall below toxic levels. ▪ Much less effective in accidental overdose after a 1-hour delay. ▪ Delayed MTX excretion may occur from third-space fluid accumulation (ascites, pleural effusion), renal insufficiency, or inadequate hydration. ▪ All doses over 25 mg should be given IM or IV (no more than 25 mg can be absorbed orally). ▪ IM or IV dosing required in presence of GI toxicity, nausea, or vomiting. ▪ Benzyl alcohol associated with gasping syndrome in premature infants.

Monitor: Monitor serum blood levels of MTX and SCr levels at least daily until level is less than 0.05 micromolar. Death can occur in 5 to 10 days if MTX remains at toxic levels longer than 48 hours. ▪ Minimum fluid intake of 3 L/24 hr and alkalinization of urine to a pH of 7 or more with oral sodium bicarbonate recommended. Begin 12 hours before MTX dose and continue for 48 hours after final dose in each sequence. Does not reduce nephrotoxicity of MTX from drug or metabolite precipitation in the kidney. ▪ See MTX or 5-FU monograph.

Maternal/Child: Category C: safety for use in pregnancy and breast-feeding not established. Benefits must outweigh risks. ▪ Contains benzyl alcohol; do not use in neonates or dilute with SWFI if indicated; see Dilution.

Elderly: Response similar to that seen in younger patients; however, use caution; may have greater sensitivity to its toxic effects (e.g., greater risk for GI toxicity and severe diarrhea in combination with 5-FU). Monitoring of renal function suggested. ▪ See Dose Adjustments.

DRUG/LAB INTERACTIONS

May inhibit **phenytoin, phenobarbital, and primidone;** may cause increased frequency of seizures. ▪ Is used in combination with **fluorouracil;** use caution; leucovorin calcium may increase toxic as well as therapeutic effects of 5-FU. ▪ When given with **MTX,** avoid any drug that may interfere with MTX elimination or binding to serum albumin (e.g., **NSAIDs, probenecid, procarbazine, salicylates, sulfonamides**). Consider as a possible cause of toxicity. ▪ High doses of leucovorin may reduce the effectiveness of intrathecally administered **MTX.** ▪ Leucovorin may enhance the toxic effects of **capecitabine**; monitor closely. ▪ Concurrent use with **sulfamethoxazole and trimethoprim** may cause treatment failure and increased morbidity in HIV patients being treated for *Pneumocystis jiroveci* pneumonia.

SIDE EFFECTS
Allergic reactions including anaphylaxis have occurred rarely. MTX or 5-FU may cause many serious and dose-limiting side effects; see individual monographs.

ANTIDOTE
Keep physician informed of patient's condition. Symptomatic treatment indicated.

LEVETIRACETAM INJECTION

Anticonvulsant

(lee-ve-tye-**RA**-se-tam in-**JEK**-shun)

Keppra

pH 5.5

USUAL DOSE
Pretreatment: Baseline studies indicated; see Monitor.

Serum levels similar by oral or IV route; no dose or frequency adjustment is necessary. Transfer to oral therapy as soon as practical. Administer levetiracetam at the same dose and frequency whether given by the IV or oral route. There is no clinical study experience with administration of IV levetiracetam for longer than 4 days.

All indications: *Monotherapy or adjunctive therapy:* Initiate treatment with a daily dose of 1,000 mg/day, given as twice-daily dosing (500 mg twice daily). Monitor for 2 weeks. Dose may be increased by 1,000 mg/day (500 mg twice daily) every 2 weeks to a maximum recommended daily dose of 3,000 mg (1,500 mg twice daily).

Partial-onset seizures in adults 16 years of age and older: There is no evidence that doses *greater* than 3,000 mg/day offer additional benefit.

Myoclonic seizures in adults and adolescents 12 years of age and older with juvenile myoclonic epilepsy and primary generalized tonic-clonic seizures in adults 16 years of age and older: The effectiveness of doses *lower* than 3,000 mg/day has not been adequately studied.

PEDIATRIC DOSE
Partial-onset seizures: *1 month to less than 6 months of age:* Initiate treatment with a daily dose of 14 mg/kg in 2 divided doses (7 mg/kg twice daily). Increase the daily dose every 2 weeks in increments of 14 mg/kg to the recommended daily dose of 42 mg/kg (21 mg/kg twice daily). In the clinical trial, the mean daily dose was 35 mg/kg in this age-group.

6 months to less than 4 years of age: Initiate treatment with a daily dose of 20 mg/kg in 2 divided doses (10 mg/kg twice daily). Increase the daily dose every 2 weeks in increments of 20 mg/kg to the recommended daily dose of 50 mg/kg (25 mg/kg twice daily). If the patient cannot tolerate a daily dose of 50 mg/kg, the daily dose may be reduced. In the clinical trial, the mean daily dose was 47 mg/kg in this age-group.

4 years to less than 16 years of age: Initiate treatment with a daily dose of 20 mg/kg in 2 divided doses (10 mg/kg twice daily). Increase the daily dose every 2 weeks in increments of 20 mg/kg to the recommended daily dose of 60 mg/kg (30 mg/kg twice daily). If the patient cannot tolerate a daily dose of 60 mg/kg, the daily dose may be reduced. In the clinical trial, the mean daily dose was 44 mg/kg in this age-group. The maximum daily dose was 3,000 mg.

Myoclonic seizures in adolescents 12 years of age and older with juvenile myoclonic epilepsy (JME): See Usual Dose.

Primary generalized tonic-clonic seizures: *6 years to less than 16 years of age:* Initiate treatment with a daily dose of 20 mg/kg in 2 divided doses (10 mg/kg twice daily). Increase the daily dose every 2 weeks in increments of 20 mg/kg (10 mg/kg twice daily) to the recommended daily dose of 60 mg/kg (30 mg/kg twice daily). The effectiveness of doses lower than 60 mg/kg/day has not been adequately studied.

DOSE ADJUSTMENTS

No dose adjustment is required for gender, race, or impaired hepatic function. ▪ Dose adjustment may be required in the elderly based on impaired renal function. ▪ Information is unavailable for dosage adjustments in pediatric patients with renal impairment. ▪ Dose adjustment for adults with impaired renal function is calculated based on CrCl adjusted for body surface area using the following formula:

$$\text{CrCl (mL/min/1.73 M}^2) = [\text{CrCl (mL/min)} \div \text{BSA (M}^2)] \times 1.73$$

Adjust dose according to the following chart.

Levetiracetam Dose Adjustment in Adults With Impaired Renal Function		
Creatinine Clearance (mL/min/1.73 M²)	**Dose in mg**	**Frequency**
>80 mL/min/1.73 M²	500 to 1,500 mg	Every 12 hours
50 to 80 mL/min/1.73 M²	500 to 1,000 mg	Every 12 hours
30 to 50 mL/min/1.73 M²	250 to 750 mg	Every 12 hours
<30 mL/min/1.73 M²	250 to 500 mg	Every 12 hours
ESRD patients on dialysis	500 to 1,000 mg[a]	Every 24 hours[a]

[a]Administration of a 250- to 500-mg supplemental dose following dialysis is recommended.

DILUTION

Adults: Each vial contains 500 mg/5 mL (100 mg/mL). A single dose (500, 1,000, or 1,500 mg [1, 2, or 3 vials]) must be diluted in 100 mL of NS, LR, or D5W for infusion. Doses of 500, 1,000, or 1,500 mg are available prediluted in 100 mL of NS.

Pediatric patients: A smaller volume of infusion solution may be required due to limitations around the total daily fluid intake of the patient. The amount of diluent should be calculated such that the final concentration of the levetiracetam solution does not exceed 15 mg/mL. For example, a 1-year-old, 10-kg child beginning therapy for treatment of partial-onset seizures would initiate therapy at 20 mg/kg/day = 200 mg/day = 100 mg twice daily. 100 mg (1 mL) mixed in 24 mL of **compatible** solution will provide a final concentration of 4 mg/mL. In a fluid-restricted patient, the solution volume could be decreased to as low as 5.7 mL [100 mg ÷ (1 mL from drug + 5.7 mL of solution) = 14.9 mg/mL].

Filters: Specific information not available.

Storage: Store at CRT. Diluted solution should not be stored for more than 4 hours at CRT in polyvinyl chloride (PVC) bags. Discard any unused portion of vial.

COMPATIBILITY

Manufacturer lists solutions NS, LR, D5W, and other antiepileptic drugs lorazepam (Ativan), diazepam (Valium), and valproate sodium (Depacon) as **compatible** for 4 hours stored in PVC bags at CRT.

RATE OF ADMINISTRATION

A single dose properly diluted as an infusion over 15 minutes.

ACTIONS

An antiepileptic (anticonvulsant) drug. The precise mechanism of action is unknown. In animal studies it inhibited burst firing without affecting normal neuronal excitability, which suggests that it may selectively prevent hypersynchronization of epileptiform burst firing and propagation of seizure activity in human complex partial seizures. Less than 10% bound to plasma proteins. Not extensively metabolized in humans and not liver (cytochrome P450) dependent. Undergoes enzymatic hydrolysis. Half-life is 6 to 8 hours. Primarily excreted in urine as unchanged drug and metabolites. Crossed the placental barrier in animal studies. Secreted in breast milk.

INDICATIONS AND USES

Treatment of partial-onset seizures in adults and pediatric patients 1 month of age and older. ▪ Adjunctive therapy in the treatment of myoclonic seizures in adults and adolescents 12 years of age and older with JME. ▪ Adjunctive therapy in the treatment of primary generalized tonic-clonic seizures in adults and pediatric patients 6 years of age and older with idiopathic generalized epilepsy.

Limitations of Use: For IV use only as an alternative for patients when oral administration is temporarily not feasible.

CONTRAINDICATIONS
Known hypersensitivity to levetiracetam.

PRECAUTIONS
For IV use only. ▪ Associated with CNS side effects (e.g., somnolence and fatigue, coordination difficulties [abnormal gait, ataxia, incoordination], behavioral abnormalities [e.g., aggression, agitation, anger, anxiety, apathy, depersonalization, depression, emotional lability, hostility, hyperkinesias, irritability, nervousness, neurosis, personality disorders], and psychotic symptoms [paranoia, psychosis, suicidal tendencies]). Somnolence and fatigue and coordination difficulties occurred most frequently within the first 4 weeks of treatment and resolved or improved with dose reduction or discontinuation of levetiracetam. ▪ Antiepileptic drugs (AEDs) increase the risk of suicidal thoughts or behavior in patients taking these drugs for any indication. Patients treated with any AED for any indication should be monitored for the emergence or worsening of depression, suicidal thoughts or behavior, and/or any unusual changes in mood or behavior. Some behavioral changes resolved without intervention. Others required dose reduction or discontinuation of levetiracetam. ▪ Serious dermatologic reactions, including Stevens-Johnson syndrome (SJS) and toxic epidermal necrolysis, have been reported. Median time to onset is 14 to 17 days, but development up to 4 months after initiation of therapy has been reported. ▪ Hypersensitivity reactions, including angioedema and anaphylaxis, have been reported. ▪ To minimize the potential of increased seizure frequency, withdraw antiepileptic drugs (including levetiracetam) gradually. If withdrawal is needed because of a serious adverse reaction, rapid discontinuation can be considered. ▪ Hematologic abnormalities have been reported. ▪ Increase in diastolic BP has been reported in patients 1 month to under 4 years of age who are receiving the oral formulation of levetiracetam. This side effect was not observed in older pediatric patients or adults.

Monitor: Baseline CBC and CrCl indicated; monitor as needed. Decreases in WBC, neutrophils, RBC, hemoglobin (Hgb), and hematocrit (Hct) have been reported, but a change or discontinuation of therapy was not required. Increases in eosinophil counts and cases of agranulocytosis, pancytopenia, and thrombocytopenia have also been reported. A CBC is recommended in patients experiencing significant coagulation disorders, fever, recurrent infections, or significant weakness. ▪ Monitor for psychiatric S/S. ▪ Monitor for somnolence and fatigue. ▪ Monitor for seizure activity. ▪ Observe patient closely for signs of CNS side effects; see Precautions. ▪ Monitor vital signs. Pediatric patients 1 month to under 4 years of age should be monitored for a possible increase in diastolic BP. ▪ Monitor for serious dermatologic reactions. ▪ Monitor for S/S of a hypersensitivity reaction, which can occur with the first dose or any time throughout treatment.

Patient Education: May cause dizziness, coordination difficulties, and somnolence; use caution when performing tasks that require alertness or coordination (e.g., operating machinery, driving). ▪ Inform your healthcare professional if you are pregnant or breastfeeding. ▪ May increase the risk of suicidal thoughts and behavior. Promptly report emergence or worsening of S/S of depression, any unusual changes in mood or behavior, or thoughts about self-harm. ▪ Females who are pregnant or who become pregnant should be encouraged to enroll in the North American Antiepileptic Drug (NAAED) Pregnancy Registry. ▪ May cause serious dermatologic reactions; promptly report development of a rash. ▪ Discontinue levetiracetam and seek medical care if S/S of a hypersensitivity reaction (e.g., facial edema, hives, hypotension, respiratory distress) develop.

Maternal/Child: Although available studies cannot definitively establish the absence of risk, data from the published literature and pregnancy registries have not established an association between levetiracetam use during pregnancy and major birth defects or miscarriage. Animal studies demonstrated evidence of developmental toxicity, including teratogenic effects. ▪ Physiologic changes during pregnancy may decrease levetiracetam concentration. Monitor carefully during pregnancy. Extend monitoring to postpartum period if dose adjustments were required during the pregnancy. ▪ Effects during labor and delivery unknown. ▪ There are no data on the effects of levetiracetam on the breast-fed infant or the effects on milk production. ▪ Safety and effectiveness for use in certain pediatric populations have been established; see Indications. ▪ Pharmacokinetic analysis showed that body weight was significantly correlated to the clearance of levetiracetam in pediatric patients; clearance increased with an increase in body weight.

Elderly: Safety similar to that seen in younger adults; however, total body clearance is decreased and half-life is increased. ▪ Reduced doses may be indicated; see Dose Adjustments. Monitoring of renal function suggested.

DRUG/LAB INTERACTIONS

Manufacturer states that levetiracetam "is unlikely to produce, or be subject to, pharmacokinetic interactions." ▪ An increase in the clearance of levetiracetam was seen in pediatric patients when it was coadministered with **enzyme-inducing AEDs** (e.g., carbamazepine, phenytoin). Dose adjustment was not recommended. ▪ **Probenecid** decreases renal clearance and increases serum concentrations of one of the metabolites of levetiracetam. ▪ Levetiracetam may increase serum concentration of **methotrexate**, resulting in serious adverse events, including acute kidney failure. Careful monitoring of serum levels of methotrexate is recommended.

SIDE EFFECTS

Adults: Asthenia, dizziness, infection, and somnolence occurred most frequently during the first 4 weeks of treatment.

Pediatric patients: Aggression, decreased appetite, fatigue, irritability, and nasal congestion were most commonly reported.

Patients of all ages: Other side effects reported and presenting anywhere from 1 to 4 weeks included amnesia; anorexia; anxiety; ataxia; cough; decreased RBC, WBC, Hct, and Hgb; depersonalization; depression; diarrhea; diplopia; emotional lability; headache; hostility; influenza; insomnia; irritability; mood swings; neck pain; nervousness; pain; paresthesia; pharyngitis; rhinitis; seizures; sinusitis; and vertigo.

Post-Marketing: Abnormal liver function tests, acute kidney injury, agranulocytosis, anaphylaxis, angioedema, choreoathetosis, drug rash with eosinophilia and systemic symptoms (DRESS), dyskinesia, erythema multiforme, hepatic failure, hepatitis, hyponatremia, leukopenia, muscle weakness, neutropenia, pancreatitis, pancytopenia (with bone marrow suppression), panic attack, SJS, suicidal behavior, thrombocytopenia, toxic epidermal necrolysis (TEN), and weight loss. Alopecia has been reported; recovery occurred in the majority of cases if levetiracetam was discontinued.

Overdose: Aggression, agitation, coma, depressed level of consciousness, drowsiness, respiratory depression, and somnolence.

ANTIDOTE

Keep physician informed of all side effects. Some may not require intervention, and others may improve with a reduced dose or discontinuation of levetiracetam; see Precautions and Side Effects. Discontinue at first sign of rash, unless the rash is clearly not drug related. If S/S suggest SJS/TEN, use of this drug should not be resumed and alternative therapy should be considered. Discontinue if a hypersensitivity reaction occurs and treat as indicated. If a clear alternative etiology for the reaction cannot be established, levetiracetam should be discontinued permanently. Support patient as required in treatment of overdose. No specific antidote in overdose; however, hemodialysis will remove approximately 50% of a dose in 4 hours.

LEVOFLOXACIN BBW
(**lee**-voh-**FLOX**-ah-sin)

Levaquin

**Antibacterial
(fluoroquinolone)**

pH 3.8 to 5.8

USUAL DOSE
Pretreatment: Baseline studies indicated; see Monitor.

250 to 750 mg once every 24 hours. Dose and duration of treatment are based on degree of infection and specific diagnosis. CrCl equal to or greater than 50 mL/min is required. Dose and serum levels similar by oral or IV route. Transfer to oral dose as soon as practical.

Levofloxacin Dosing Guidelines		
Type of Infection[a]	**Dose Every 24 Hours[b]**	**Duration (Days)**
Nosocomial pneumonia	750 mg	7-14 days
Community-acquired pneumonia	500 mg or 750 mg	7-14 days / 5 days
Complicated SSSI[c]	750 mg	7-14 days
Uncomplicated SSSI[c]	500 mg	7-10 days
Chronic bacterial prostatitis	500 mg	28 days
Inhalation anthrax (postexposure) in adults and pediatric patients >50 kg[d]	500 mg	60 days[f]
Inhalation anthrax (postexposure) in pediatric patients <50 kg and ≥6 months of age[d]	8 mg/kg q 12 hr[b] (not to exceed 250 mg/dose)	60 days[f]
Plague in adults and pediatric patients >50 kg[d]	500 mg	10-14 days[f]
Plague in pediatric patients <50 kg and ≥6 months of age[d]	8 mg/kg q 12 hr[b] (not to exceed 250 mg/dose	10-14 days[f]
Complicated UTI[e] or acute pyelonephritis	750 mg	5 days
Complicated UTI[e] or acute pyelonephritis	250 mg	10 days
Uncomplicated UTI[e]	250 mg	3 days
Acute bacterial exacerbation of chronic bronchitis (ABEC:B)	500 mg	7 days
Acute bacterial sinusitis (ABS)	750 mg	5 days
Acute bacterial sinusitis (ABS)	500 mg	10-14 days

[a]Due to the designated pathogens (see Indications and Usage in manufacturer's prescribing information).
[b]Frequency is every 12 hours (not 24 hours) for treatment of inhalation anthrax and plague in pediatric patients less than 50 kg and age 6 months or more.
[c]Skin and skin structure infections.
[d]Begin drug administration as soon as possible after suspected or confirmed exposure to aerosolized *Bacillus anthracis* or to *Yersinia pestis*.
[e]Urinary tract infections.
[f]See Precautions and Maternal/Child.

DOSE ADJUSTMENTS
No dose adjustment is required specifically for age, gender, race, or in impaired hepatic function. ▪ Clearance is reduced and half-life is prolonged in patients with a CrCl less than 50 mL/min. See the following chart for dosing guidelines. See Important IV Therapy Facts on p. xix for formula to convert SCr to CrCl. ▪ Supplemental doses are not required after hemodialysis or peritoneal dialysis.

Levofloxacin Dosing Guidelines in Impaired Renal Function			
Dosage in Normal Renal Function Every 24 hours	Creatinine Clearance 20 to 49 mL/min	Creatinine Clearance 10 to 19 mL/min	Hemodialysis or Chronic Ambulatory Peritoneal Dialysis (CAPD)
750 mg	750 mg q 48 hr	750 mg initial dose, then 500 mg q 48 hr	750 mg initial dose, then 500 mg q 48 hr
500 mg	500 mg initial dose, then 250 mg q 24 hr	500 mg initial dose, then 250 mg q 48 hr	500 mg initial dose, then 250 mg q 48 hr
250 mg	No dose adjustment required	250 mg q 48 hr; no dose adjustment required if treating uncomplicated UTI	No information on dose adjustment available

DILUTION

Available in single-use vials and as prediluted, ready-to-use infusions.

Single-use vials: Withdraw desired dose from single-use vial (10 mL for 250 mg, 20 mL for 500 mg, 30 mL for 750 mg). Each 10 mL (250 mg) must be further diluted with a minimum of 40 mL NS, D5W, D5NS, D5LR, or D5/½NS. Desired concentration is 5 mg/mL. No preservatives; enter vial only once. When 500-mg (20-mL) vial is used to prepare two 250-mg doses, withdraw entire contents of vial at once using a single-entry procedure. Prepare and store second dose for subsequent use.

Premix flexible containers: No further dilution necessary. Available as 250 mg in 50 mL, 500 mg in 100 mL, or 750 mg in 150 mL D5W. Instructions for access to and use of premix flexible containers are on its storage carton. Do not use flexible containers in series connections.

Filters: Not required; however, contents of both vials and premixed solutions were filtered during manufacturing with polyvinyl mixed ester cellulose filters. Size not specified by manufacturer. No significant loss of potency expected.

Storage: Store vials at CRT; protect from light. Store premix at or below 25° C (77° F); protect from freezing, light, and excessive heat. Premixed product may also be stored in the refrigerator. Brief exposure up to 40° C (104° F) does not adversely affect the product. Both are stable to expiration date. Solutions diluted from vials are stable at or below 25° C (77° F) for 3 days and for up to 14 days if refrigerated. May be frozen for up to 6 months. Do not force thaw (e.g., microwave or water bath) and do not refreeze. Discard any unused portion of premixed solutions and/or opened vials.

COMPATIBILITY

Manufacturer states, "Limited **compatibility** information available; other intravenous substances, additives, or other medications should not be added to levofloxacin or infused simultaneously through the same intravenous line." Never administer in the same IV or through the same tubing with any solution containing multivalent cations (e.g., calcium, magnesium). Flush line with a **compatible** solution before and after administration of levofloxacin and/or any other drug through the same IV line.

Other sources suggest specific **compatibilities** dependent on concentration and manufacturer; consult a pharmacist.

RATE OF ADMINISTRATION

Each 250- or 500-mg dose must be given over 60 minutes as an infusion. A 750-mg dose must be given over 90 minutes as an infusion. Too-rapid administration may cause hypotension. May be given through a Y-tube of infusion set. Temporarily discontinue other solutions infusing at the same site and flush tubing with **compatible** solutions before and after levofloxacin.

ACTIONS

A synthetic, broad-spectrum, fluoroquinolone antibacterial agent. Bactericidal to aerobic gram-negative and gram-positive organisms through interference with enzymes (type II topoisomerases) needed for bacterial DNA replication, transcription, repair, and recombination. May be active against bacteria resistant to aminoglycosides, beta-lactam antibiotics, and macrolides. Onset of action is prompt, and serum levels are dose related. Mean terminal half-life is 6 to 8 hours. Steady state is achieved within 48 hours. Widely distributed into body tissues, including blister fluid and lung tissues. Moderately bound to serum protein (24% to 38%). Metabolism is minimal; primarily excreted as unchanged drug in urine. Very small amounts found in bile and feces. May cross placental barrier. May be secreted in breast milk.

INDICATIONS AND USES

Treatment of adults with mild, moderate, and severe infections caused by susceptible strains of designated microorganisms in conditions listed in this section. ■ Treatment of nosocomial pneumonia. For cases in which *Pseudomonas aeruginosa* is a documented or presumptive organism, combination therapy with an anti-pseudomonal beta-lactam is recommended. ■ Treatment of community-acquired pneumonia due to many organisms, including *Streptococcus pneumoniae* (including multidrug-resistant strains [MDRSPs]). MDRSP strains are resistant to two or more of the following antibiotics: penicillin, second-generation cephalosporins (e.g., cefuroxime), macrolides, tetracyclines, and sulfamethoxazole/trimethoprim. ■ Treatment of complicated skin and skin structure infections and mild to moderate uncomplicated skin and skin structure infections. ■ Treatment of complicated urinary tract infections and acute pyelonephritis (including cases with concurrent bacteremia). ■ Treatment of uncomplicated urinary tract infections. Because fluoroquinolones, including levofloxacin, have been associated with serious adverse reactions and because for some patients uncomplicated urinary tract infection is self-limiting, reserve levofloxacin for treatment of uncomplicated urinary tract infections in patients who have no alternative treatment options. ■ Treatment of acute bacterial exacerbation of chronic bronchitis (ABECB) and acute bacterial sinusitis (ABS). Because fluoroquinolones, including levofloxacin, have been associated with serious adverse reactions and because for some patients ABECB and ABS are self-limiting, reserve levofloxacin for treatment in patients who have no alternative treatment options. ■ To reduce the incidence or progression of inhalational anthrax following exposure to *Bacillus anthracis* in adults and pediatric patients. Begin administration as soon as possible after suspected or confirmed exposure. Transfer to oral therapy when practical. ■ Treatment of plague, including pneumonic and septicemic plague, due to *Yersinia pestis,* as well as prophylaxis for plague in adults and pediatric patients 6 months of age and older. ■ Treatment of chronic bacterial prostatitis (usually oral therapy).

CONTRAINDICATIONS

History of hypersensitivity to levofloxacin, its components, or any other quinolone antimicrobial agents (e.g., ciprofloxacin, norfloxacin).

PRECAUTIONS

For IV use only. ■ To reduce the development of drug-resistant bacteria and maintain its effectiveness, levofloxacin should be used to treat or prevent only those infections proven or strongly suspected to be caused by bacteria. ■ Culture and sensitivity studies indicated to determine susceptibility of the causative organism to levofloxacin. ■ *P. aeruginosa* may develop resistance during treatment. Ongoing culture and sensitivity studies indicated. ■ The emergence of bacterial resistance to fluoroquinolones and the occurrence of crossresistance with other fluoroquinolones have been observed and are of concern. Proper use of fluoroquinolones and other classes of antibiotics is encouraged to avoid the emergence of resistant bacteria from overuse. ■ Cross-resistance may occur with other fluoroquinolones, but some microorganisms resistant to other fluoroquinolones may be susceptible to levofloxacin. ■ Prolonged use may cause superinfection because of overgrowth of nonsusceptible organisms. ■ Fluoroquinolones, including levofloxacin, have been associated with disabling and potentially irreversible serious adverse reactions that have occurred together in the same patient. Commonly seen adverse reactions include tendinitis and tendon rupture, arthralgia, myalgia, peripheral neuropathy, CNS effects (e.g., anxiety, confusion, depression, hallucinations, insomnia, severe headaches), and hypoglycemia or hyperglycemia.

Due to the potential for side effects, the FDA suggests not using levofloxacin unless there are no other alternatives. These reactions can occur within hours to weeks after starting levofloxacin and have been seen in patients of any age and in patients without any pre-existing risk factors. Discontinue levofloxacin immediately and avoid the use of fluoroquinolones, including levofloxacin, in patients who experience any of these serious adverse reactions. ▪ Fluoroquinolones, including levofloxacin, have been associated with an increased risk of seizures (convulsions), increased intracranial pressure (pseudotumor cerebri), tremors, and light-headedness. May trigger seizures or lower the seizure threshold. Use caution in patients with epilepsy or known or suspected CNS disorders that may predispose patients to seizures or lower the seizure threshold (e.g., severe cerebral arteriosclerosis, previous history of convulsions, reduced cerebral blood flow, altered brain structure, or stroke) or in the presence of other risk factors that may predispose patients to seizures (e.g., drugs that may lower the seizure threshold, renal dysfunction). ▪ Fluoroquinolones, including levofloxacin, have been associated with an increased risk of psychiatric adverse reactions, including toxic psychosis; psychotic reactions progressing to suicidal ideations/thoughts, hallucinations, or paranoia; depression or self-injurious behavior such as attempted or completed suicide; anxiety, agitation, restlessness, or nervousness; confusion, delirium, disorientation, or disturbances in attention; insomnia or nightmares; and memory impairment. These reactions may occur after the first dose. ▪ Use caution in patients with impaired renal function; see Dose Adjustments. ▪ Severe, sometimes fatal hepatotoxicity has been reported. Symptoms appeared within 6 to 14 days of initiating therapy, and most cases were not associated with hypersensitivity. The majority of fatal hepatotoxicity reports occurred in patients 65 years of age or older; see Patient Education and Antidote. ▪ Tendinitis and tendon rupture that required surgical repair or resulted in prolonged disability have been reported in patients of all ages receiving quinolones. Most frequently involves the Achilles tendon but has also been reported with the shoulder, hand, biceps, thumb, and other tendon sites. ▪ Tendon rupture or tendinitis may occur during or up to months after fluoroquinolone therapy and may occur bilaterally. Risk may be increased in patients over 60 years of age; in patients taking corticosteroids; in patients with heart, kidney, or lung transplants; with strenuous physical activity; and in patients with renal failure or previous tendon disorders such as rheumatoid arthritis. Avoid levofloxacin in patients who have a history of tendon disorders or have experienced tendinitis or tendon rupture. Discontinue levofloxacin immediately if patient experiences pain, swelling, inflammation, or rupture of a tendon. ▪ Prolongation of the QT interval on ECG and infrequent cases of arrhythmia (including torsades de pointes) have been reported. The risk of arrhythmia may be reduced by avoiding the use of levofloxacin in patients with known prolongation of the QT interval, uncorrected electrolyte imbalances (e.g., hypokalemia, hypomagnesemia), significant bradycardia, cardiomyopathy, or concurrent treatment with Class Ia antiarrhythmic agents (e.g., quinidine, procainamide) or Class III antiarrhythmic agents (e.g., amiodarone, sotalol) and any other drug that can prolong the QT interval; avoid coadministration; see Drug/Lab Interactions. ▪ Fluoroquinolones have neuromuscular blocking activity and may exacerbate muscle weakness in persons with myasthenia gravis. Serious adverse events, including a requirement for ventilatory support and deaths, have been reported in these patients. Avoid use in patients with a known history of myasthenia gravis. ▪ Fluoroquinolones, including levofloxacin, have been associated with an increased risk of peripheral neuropathy. Cases of sensory or sensorimotor axonal polyneuropathy resulting in paresthesias, hypoesthesias, dysesthesias (impairment of sensitivity or touch), or weakness have been reported. Symptoms may occur soon after initiation of therapy and may be irreversible. Avoid levofloxacin in patients who have previously experienced peripheral neuropathy. ▪ Serious and occasionally fatal hypersensitivity and/or anaphylactic reactions have been reported. Often occur after the first dose. ▪ Other serious events (sometimes fatal) due to hypersensitivity or uncertain etiology have been reported with fluoroquinolones, including levofloxacin; usually occur after multiple doses. Manifestations may include allergic pneumonitis, arthralgia, myalgia, renal or hepatic impairment/

failure, hematologic toxicity, dermatologic toxicity, serum sickness, and vasculitis; see Side Effects, Post-Marketing. Immediately discontinue levofloxacin at the first appearance of a skin rash, jaundice, or other signs of hepatotoxicity or hypersensitivity. ■ *Clostridium difficile*–associated diarrhea (CDAD) has been reported. May range from mild diarrhea to fatal colitis. Consider in patients who present with diarrhea during or after treatment with levofloxacin. ■ Epidemiologic studies report an increased rate of aortic aneurysm and dissection within 2 months after use of fluoroquinolones, particularly in elderly patients. In patients with a known aortic aneurysm or in patients who are at greater risk for aortic aneurysms, levofloxacin use should be limited to cases in which no alternative antibacterial treatments are available. ■ Moderate to severe photosensitivity/phototoxicity reactions have been reported in patients receiving quinolones; see Patient Education. ■ Fluoroquinolones, including levofloxacin, have been associated with disturbances of blood glucose, including symptomatic hyperglycemia and hypoglycemia, usually in patients with diabetes who are receiving concomitant treatment with an oral hypoglycemic agent (e.g., glyburide) or with insulin. In these patients careful monitoring of blood glucose is recommended. Severe cases of hypoglycemia resulting in coma or death have been reported. ■ Not tested in humans for postexposure prevention of inhalation anthrax; however, plasma concentrations are considered to be in a range to produce effective results. ■ Safety for use in adults beyond 28 days or in pediatric patients beyond 14 days not studied; use only for prescribed indication; benefits must outweigh risks. An increased incidence of musculoskeletal adverse events has been observed in pediatric patients.

Monitor: Obtain baseline CBC with differential, CrCl, and blood glucose. Periodic monitoring of organ systems, including hematopoietic, hepatic, and renal, is recommended. ■ Monitor for S/S of a hypersensitivity reaction (e.g., airway obstruction, angioedema, cardiovascular collapse, dyspnea, hypotension/shock, itching, loss of consciousness, seizure, tingling, urticaria, and other serious skin reactions). May cause anaphylaxis with the first or succeeding doses, even in patients without known hypersensitivity. Emergency equipment must always be available; see Precautions. ■ Monitor for S/S of peripheral neuropathy. Discontinue levofloxacin at the first symptoms of neuropathy (e.g., pain, burning, tingling, numbness and/or weakness) or if patient is found to have deficits in light touch, pain, temperature, position sense, vibratory sensation, and/or motor strength. ■ ECG monitoring for QT prolongation may be indicated in select patients. ■ Monitor for CNS adverse effects, including altered mental status, seizures, and changes in mood or behavior. ■ Monitor for S/S of tendinitis or tendon rupture. ■ Maintain adequate hydration to prevent concentrated urine throughout treatment. Crystalluria and cylindruria have been reported with quinolones. ■ Monitor infusion site for inflammation and/or extravasation. ■ Monitor blood glucose, especially in patients with diabetes. ■ See Precautions, Drug/Lab Interactions, and Antidote.

Patient Education: A patient medication guide is available from the manufacturer. ■ Discontinue levofloxacin and promptly report the development of any severe adverse reaction. ■ Review all medicines and disease history with pharmacist or physician before initiating treatment. ■ Inform physician of any history of myasthenia gravis. ■ Patients with a history of myasthenia gravis should avoid the use of levofloxacin. ■ Drink fluids liberally. ■ Promptly report skin rash or any other hypersensitivity reaction. ■ Promptly report pain, burning, tingling, numbness and/or weakness in extremities. Nerve damage can be permanent. ■ Photosensitivity has been reported. Avoid excessive sunlight or artificial ultraviolet light. May cause severe sunburn; wear protective clothing, use sunscreen, and wear dark glasses outdoors. Report a sunburn-like reaction or skin eruption promptly. ■ Promptly report development of any CNS side effects (e.g., convulsions, dizziness, light-headedness, change in mood or behavior). ■ Inform physician of any history of seizures. ■ Request assistance with ambulation; may cause dizziness and light-headedness. Use caution in tasks that require alertness. ■ Effects of caffeine, theophylline preparations, and/or warfarin (Coumadin) may be increased; notify your physician if you take any of these agents. If diabetic and on medication, monitor your blood glucose carefully. If a hypoglycemia reaction occurs, discontinue levofloxacin and consult physician. ▪ Promptly report S/S of liver injury (e.g., dark-colored urine, fever, itching, jaundice [yellowing of skin or whites of eyes], light-colored bowel movements, loss of appetite, nausea, right upper quadrant tenderness, tiredness, vomiting, weakness). ▪ Promptly report tendon pain or inflammation, weakness, or the inability to use a joint; rest and refrain from exercise. ▪ Before initiating therapy, parents should inform their child's physician if their child has a history of joint-related problems, and they should notify their child's physician of any tendon or joint-related problems that occur during or after therapy. ▪ Promptly report diarrhea or bloody stools that occur during treatment or up to several months after an antibiotic has been discontinued; may indicate CDAD and require treatment. ▪ Seek emergency medical care if sudden chest, stomach, or back pain is experienced. ▪ See Precautions, Monitor, Drug/Lab Interactions, and Antidote.

Maternal/Child: Safety for use in pregnancy not established; benefits must outweigh risks. ▪ Discontinue breast-feeding. ▪ Safety for use in pediatric patients under 18 years of age not established. Indicated in pediatric patients 6 months of age or older only for prevention of inhalation anthrax (postexposure) and prevention and treatment of plague. The risk-benefit assessment indicates that administration of levofloxacin to pediatric patients for these indications is appropriate. Safety for use in pediatric patients under 6 months of age not established. ▪ An increased incidence of musculoskeletal disorders (arthralgia, arthritis, tendinopathy, and gait abnormality) compared with controls has been observed in pediatric patients receiving levofloxacin. May erode cartilage of weight-bearing joints or cause other signs of arthropathy in infants and children.

Elderly: Half-life may be slightly extended due to age-related renal impairment. Dose reduction required only in the elderly with a CrCl of less than 50 mL/min. ▪ Safety and effectiveness similar to that in younger adults; however, they may experience an increased risk of side effects (e.g., aortic aneurysm and dissection, CNS effects, hepatotoxicity, tendinitis, tendon rupture, risk of QT prolongation). Monitoring of renal function may be useful. ▪ See Dose Adjustments and Precautions.

DRUG/LAB INTERACTIONS

May cause ventricular arrhythmias or torsades de pointes with **drugs that prolong the QT interval,** such as **Class Ia antiarrhythmic agents** (e.g., quinidine, procainamide), **Class III antiarrhythmic agents** (e.g., amiodarone, sotalol), **phenothiazines** (e.g., chlorpromazine), **tricyclic antidepressants** (e.g., imipramine, amitriptyline). Avoid coadministration. ▪ Risk of CNS stimulation and convulsive seizures may be increased with **NSAIDs.** ▪ May cause hyperglycemia and hypoglycemia with concurrent administration of **antidiabetic agents**; monitoring of blood glucose recommended. ▪ Interactions with **theophylline** that occur with other quinolones have not been noted, but monitoring of theophylline levels is recommended with concomitant use. ▪ May enhance effects of **warfarin**; monitoring of PT or INR is recommended with concomitant use. ▪ May cause **false-positive when testing urine for opiates;** more specific testing methods may be indicated.

SIDE EFFECTS

The most common side effects are constipation, diarrhea, dizziness, headache, insomnia, and nausea. Abdominal pain, chest pain, crystalluria, cylindruria, dyspepsia, dyspnea, edema, injection site reaction, moniliasis, photosensitivity/phototoxicity (sun sensitivity), pruritus, rash, vaginitis, and vomiting have occurred. Abnormal dreaming, abnormal gait, abnormal hepatic function, abnormal renal function, acute renal failure, agitation, anemia, anorexia, anxiety, arthralgia, cardiac arrest, CDAD, confusion, convulsions, depression, epistaxis, esophagitis, gastritis, gastroenteritis, genital moniliasis, glossitis, granulocytopenia, hallucinations, hyperglycemia, hyperkalemia, hyperkinesia, hypersensitivity reactions, hypertonia, hypoglycemia, increased alkaline phosphatase, increased hepatic enzymes, myalgia, nightmares, palpitation, pancreatitis, paresthesia, phlebitis, pseudomembranous colitis, skeletal pain, sleep disorders, somnolence, stomatitis, syncope, tendinitis, thrombocytopenia, tremor, urticaria, ventricular arrhythmia, ventricular tachycardia, and vertigo have also been reported in fewer than 1% of patients.

Post-Marketing: Abnormal EEG; hematologic abnormalities (agranulocytosis, anemia [hemolytic and aplastic], eosinophilia, leukopenia, pancytopenia, thrombocytopenia [including thrombotic thrombocytopenic purpura]); exacerbation of myasthenia gravis; eye disorders (e.g., blurred vision, diplopia, reduced visual acuity, scotoma, uveitis); hepatic failure, including fatal cases; fever; hepatitis; hypersensitivity reactions (sometimes fatal, including angioneurotic edema, anaphylaxis); interstitial nephritis; jaundice; leukocytoclastic vasculitis; multiorgan failure; muscle injury and increased muscle enzymes; paranoia; peripheral neuropathy; photosensitivity/phototoxicity reactions; prolonged INR; prolonged PT; prolonged QT interval; pseudotumor cerebri; psychosis; rhabdomyolysis; serum sickness; severe dermatologic reactions (e.g., acute generalized exanthematous pustulosis [AGEP], fixed drug eruptions, erythema multiforme, toxic epidermal necrolysis [Lyell's syndrome], Stevens-Johnson syndrome); tachycardia; tendon rupture; tinnitus; vasodilation; and isolated reports of allergic pneumonitis, encephalopathy, suicidal ideation, suicide attempts, completed suicide, and torsades de pointes.

ANTIDOTE

Keep physician informed of all side effects. Most minor side effects will be treated symptomatically; monitor closely. Discontinue levofloxacin at the first sign of any major side effect (CDAD, CNS symptoms, dermatologic reactions, hepatotoxicity, hypersensitivity, hypoglycemic reactions, phototoxicity, symptoms of peripheral neuropathy, or tendon rupture). Treat hypersensitivity reactions as indicated with epinephrine, airway management, oxygen, IV fluids, antihistamines (e.g., diphenhydramine), corticosteroids, and pressor amines (e.g., dopamine). Treat CNS symptoms as indicated. Mild cases of CDAD may respond to discontinuation of levofloxacin. Treat CDAD with fluids, electrolytes, protein supplements, and appropriate antibiotics (e.g., oral vancomycin) as indicated. In severe cases, surgical evaluation may be indicated. Complete rest is indicated for an affected tendon until treatment is available. Maintain hydration in overdose. No specific antidote; not removed by hemodialysis or peritoneal dialysis. Maintain patient until drug is excreted and symptoms subside.

LEVOTHYROXINE SODIUM BBW

(lee-voh-thigh-**ROX**-een **SO**-dee-um)

Hormone
(thyroid)

T_4, L-Thyroxine

USUAL DOSE

When oral ingestion is not practical, IV dose should be one-half of any previously established oral dose; see Indications and Uses, Limitation of Use. Adjust in small increments as indicated. Initiate oral treatment as soon as possible.

Hypothyroidism (when oral therapy is not possible): Usual IV starting dose would be 6.25 to 12.5 mcg/day. Increase in increments of 12.5 mcg every 2 to 4 weeks. Base dosing on clinical response and serum thyroid and TSH levels. Average maintenance dose is 50 to 100 mcg/day PO.

Myxedema coma: 300 to 500 mcg as an initial dose. Follow with once-daily IV maintenance doses between 50 and 100 mcg.

PEDIATRIC DOSE

Given orally (may be crushed in food or liquid). See Precautions. Any IV dose should be 50% to 75% of the established oral dose. See pediatric literature for dosing guidelines.

DOSE ADJUSTMENTS

Age, general condition, cardiac risk factors, and clinical severity of myxedema symptoms should be considered when determining the starting and maintenance dosages.
- Reduce dose in elderly, functional, or ECG evidence of cardiovascular disease (including angina), long-standing thyroid disease, other endocrinopathies, and severe hypothyroidism. ■ See Drug/Lab Interactions.

DILUTION

Available in different strengths; read label carefully. Each vial of lyophilized powder is diluted with 5 mL of NS for injection (without preservatives). Shake well to dissolve completely. **Reconstituted concentrations will be 20 mcg/mL for the 100-mcg vial and 100 mcg/mL for the 500-mcg vial.** Do not add to IV solutions. May be given through Y-tube of infusion set.

Storage: Store dry product at CRT and protect from light. Reconstituted solution is preservative-free and stable for 4 hours; any remaining solution is discarded.

COMPATIBILITY

Manufacturer states, "Do not add to other IV fluids."

RATE OF ADMINISTRATION

100 mcg or fraction thereof over 1 minute.

ACTIONS

A synthetic thyroid hormone. Effective replacement for decreased or absent thyroid hormone. Thyroid hormone synthesis and secretion is regulated by the hypothalamic-pituitary-thyroid axis. Thyroid hormones regulate multiple metabolic processes and play an essential role in normal growth and development. Actions are produced predominantly by T_3 (triiodothyronine). Approximately 80% of T_3 is derived from T_4 (levothyroxine) by deiodination in peripheral tissues. The metabolic actions of thyroid hormones include augmentation of cellular respiration and thermogenesis, as well as metabolism of proteins, carbohydrates, and lipids. Circulating thyroid hormones are greater than 99% bound to plasma proteins (thyroxine-binding globulin [TBG], thyroxine-binding prealbumin [TBPA], and albumin [TBA]). The higher affinity of both TBG and TBPA for T_4 partially explains the higher serum levels, slower metabolic clearance, and longer half-life of T_4 (6 to 8 days) compared with T_3 (less than 2 days). The major pathway of thyroid hormone metabolism is through sequential deiodination. The liver is the major site of degradation for both T_4 and T_3. Primary route of elimination is through the kidneys. Small amounts are eliminated into the bile and feces.

INDICATIONS AND USES

Treatment of myxedema coma. ■ Specific replacement therapy for reduced or absent thyroid function due to any cause (usually given orally).

Limitation of use: The relative bioavailability between oral and IV levothyroxine sodium for injection has not been established but has been estimated to be between 48% and 74%. Caution should be used when switching patients from oral products to the parenteral product because adequate dosing conversions have not been studied.

CONTRAINDICATIONS

None. ■ Not indicated for use in treatment of obesity. Risk can outweigh benefit.

PRECAUTIONS

Excessive bolus doses (greater than 500 mcg) are associated with cardiac complications, particularly in the elderly and in patients with underlying cardiac disease; see Dose Adjustments. ■ Patients with undiagnosed endocrine disorders (e.g., adrenal insufficiency, hypopituitarism, diabetes insipidus) may experience new or worsening symptoms of these endocrinopathies. Patients should be treated with replacement glucocorticoids before initiation of treatment with levothyroxine until adrenal function has been adequately assessed. Failure to do so may precipitate an acute adrenal crisis when thyroid hormone therapy is initiated as a result of increased metabolic clearance of glucocorticoids by thyroid hormone. Patients with myxedema coma should be monitored for previously undiagnosed diabetes insipidus. ■ Not indicated for treatment of obesity or for weight loss. Doses within the range of daily hormonal requirements are ineffective for weight reduction.

Larger doses may produce serious or even life-threatening manifestations of toxicity, particularly when given in conjunction with sympathomimetic amines, such as those used for the anorectic effects.

Monitor: Observe patient closely and monitor vital signs. ▪ Monitor thyroid function tests (e.g., free T_4 index, TSH). ▪ TSH and thyroid hormone levels should be measured a few weeks after switching from IV to oral therapy. Adjust dose according to results and clinical status. ▪ Monitor TSH every 6 to 8 weeks until normalized, every 8 to 12 weeks after dose changes, and every 6 to 12 months throughout therapy.

Maternal/Child: Category A: may be used during pregnancy. ▪ Presumed safe in breast-feeding; use caution and observe infant. ▪ Myxedema coma is a disease of the elderly. An approved oral dosage form should be used in pediatric patients for maintaining a euthyroid state in noncomplicated hypothyroidism; see Pediatric Dose.

Elderly: See Dose Adjustments; more sensitive to effects. Atrial fibrillation is a common side effect associated with levothyroxine treatment in the elderly.

DRUG/LAB INTERACTIONS

Addition of levothyroxine to **antidiabetic or insulin** therapy may result in increased antidiabetic or insulin requirements. Monitor glucose values closely, especially when thyroid therapy is initiated, changed, or discontinued. ▪ Levothyroxine increases response to **oral anticoagulant** therapy (e.g., warfarin). Reduction in dose of oral anticoagulant may be required. Monitor PT/INR. ▪ May decrease therapeutic effects of **digoxin**, necessitating an increase in the digoxin dose. Monitor serum digoxin levels. ▪ Concurrent use of **tricyclic** (e.g., amitriptyline) or **tetracyclic** (e.g., maprotiline) **antidepressants** and levothyroxine may increase the therapeutic and toxic effects of both drugs, possibly due to increased receptor sensitivity to catecholamines. ▪ Administration of **sertraline** in patients stabilized on levothyroxine may result in increased levothyroxine requirements. ▪ Concurrent use with **ketamine** may produce marked hypertension and tachycardia. Use caution. ▪ Concurrent use with **sympathomimetics** (e.g., epinephrine, norepinephrine) may increase the effects of sympathomimetics or thyroid hormone. May increase risk of coronary insufficiency. ▪ **Carbamazepine, fosphenytoin, phenytoin, and rifampin** may decrease the serum concentration of thyroid hormones. Monitor levels closely. ▪ Levothyroxine can increase the metabolism of **theophylline**, necessitating an increase in theophylline dose. Monitor theophylline levels. ▪ Changes in TBG concentration must be considered when interpreting T_3 and T_4 values, which necessitates measurement and evaluation of unbound (free) hormone and/or determination of the free levothyroxine index. Several medications and disease states can alter TBG concentrations. See manufacturer's prescribing information.

SIDE EFFECTS

Abdominal cramps, angina, arrhythmias, chest pain, diarrhea, heart palpitations, heat intolerance, increased pulse and BP, insomnia, menstrual irregularities, muscle cramps, nervousness, sweating, tachycardia, tremors, vomiting, and weight loss.

ANTIDOTE

Notify the physician of any side effect. A reduction in dose will usually decrease symptoms. Supportive treatment should be initiated as dictated by the patient's medical status.

LIDOCAINE HYDROCHLORIDE

(**LYE**-doh-kayn hy-droh-**KLOR**-eyed)

Lidocaine PF, Xylocaine PF, Xylocard ✤

Antiarrhythmic

pH 5 to 7 (Injection)
3 to 7 (IV infusion)

USUAL DOSE

1 to 1.5 mg/kg of body weight as a **bolus dose.** ACLS guidelines recommend repeat doses of 0.5 to 0.75 mg/kg every 5 to 10 minutes to desired effect, up to a maximum cumulative dose of 3 mg/kg. Follow with a continuous infusion of 1 to 4 mg/min (0.02 to 0.05 mg/kg/min in an average 70-kg adult). Transition to maintenance oral anti-arrhythmic therapy as soon as possible. Infusions beyond 24 hours should rarely be needed; see Dose Adjustments. Exact dosage regimen is determined by patient characteristics and response.

Perfusing arrhythmia (stable VT, wide-complex tachycardia of uncertain type, significant ectopy): AHA guidelines recommend doses ranging from 0.5 to 0.75 mg/kg and up to 1 to 1.5 mg/kg. Repeat 0.5 to 0.75 mg/kg every 5 to 10 minutes to a maximum total dose of 3 mg/kg. Follow with a continuous infusion of 1 to 4 mg/min (20 to 50 mcg/kg/min).

PEDIATRIC DOSE

See Maternal/Child (unlabeled).

Antiarrhythmic: AHA recommends 1 mg/kg as an IV bolus followed immediately by an infusion of 20 to 50 mcg/kg/min (average of 30 mcg/kg/min). If 15 minutes have elapsed since the initial bolus dose before the infusion is started, administration of an additional bolus (1 mg/kg) is recommended when the infusion is initiated.

DOSE ADJUSTMENTS

Lower-end initial doses may be indicated in elderly patients based on potential for decreased organ function and concomitant disease or drug therapy. ▪ Reduce maintenance dose in patients with impaired liver function or severe renal impairment and in patients receiving drugs that may decrease clearance of lidocaine or decrease liver blood flow (e.g., beta-blockers [propranolol, cimetidine]). ▪ Reduce infusion rate by approximately one-half after prolonged infusion (24 hours) to compensate for decreased rate of clearance (accumulation of the drug) and potential toxicity.

DILUTION

Available premixed in 0.4% or 0.8% solutions (4 or 8 mg/mL) and as prefilled syringes. Label must state "for IV use" and be preservative free. Bolus dose may be given undiluted.

Filters: One PI states "Use of a final filter is recommended, where possible." Another source suggests use of a 0.45 micron cellulose membrane filter.

Storage: Store at CRT. Protect from freezing.

COMPATIBILITY

Manufacturer states, "Because doses of lidocaine are titrated to response, additives should not be introduced into solutions of lidocaine." Should not be added to blood transfusion assemblies because of the possibilities of pseudoagglutination or hemolysis.

Other sources suggest specific **compatibilities** dependent on concentration and manufacturer; consult a pharmacist.

RATE OF ADMINISTRATION

Bolus dose: 25 to 50 mg or fraction thereof over 1 minute.

Infusion: 1 to 4 mg/min (0.02 to 0.05 mg/kg/min in an average 70-kg adult). Use of a calibrated infusion device recommended. Adjust as indicated by progress in patient's condition; see Dose Adjustments.

IV infusions in flexible plastic containers: *With or without a pump:* Do not hang in series connection, do not pressurize to increase flow rates without first fully evacuating residual air from the container, and do not use vented IV administration sets. All may result in air embolism.

ACTIONS

IV lidocaine exerts an antiarrhythmic effect by increasing the electric stimulation threshold of the ventricle during diastole. In usual therapeutic doses, produces no change in myocardial contractility, systemic arterial pressure, or absolute refractory period. Decreases neuronal membrane permeability to sodium ions, resulting in inhibition of depolarization. Plasma protein binding is concentration dependent; fraction bound decreases with increasing concentration. Onset of action should occur within 1 to 2 minutes and last approximately 10 to 20 minutes. Terminal half-life is 1.5 to 2 hours. Primarily metabolized in the liver. Excreted in the urine with about 10% excreted unchanged and 90% excreted as various metabolites. Crosses the blood-brain and placental barriers and is secreted in breast milk.

INDICATIONS AND USES

Acute management of life-threatening ventricular arrhythmias (e.g., ventricular tachycardia [VT], ventricular fibrillation [VF]), such as occur during acute myocardial infarction, or ventricular arrhythmias occurring during cardiac manipulations such as cardiac surgery.

Unlabeled uses: Pediatric ventricular arrhythmias, seizures unresponsive to other therapy.

CONTRAINDICATIONS

Known sensitivity to lidocaine or any other local anesthetic of the amide type. ▪ Patients with Stokes-Adams syndrome, Wolff-Parkinson-White syndrome, or severe degrees of sinoatrial, atrioventricular, or intraventricular block. ▪ Solutions containing dextrose may be contraindicated in patients with known allergies to corn or corn products.

PRECAUTIONS

Administered by healthcare professionals knowledgeable in its use with access to adequate equipment and appropriate emergency drugs to monitor the patient and respond to any medical emergency. ▪ In patients with bradycardia or incomplete heart block, administration of lidocaine for the elimination of ventricular ectopic beats without prior acceleration in heart rate (e.g., by isoproterenol or electric pacing) may promote more frequent and serious ventricular arrhythmias or complete heart block. ▪ Acceleration of ventricular rate may occur in patients with atrial fibrillation or flutter treated with lidocaine. ▪ Use caution in patients with any degree of liver impairment or severe renal impairment; accumulation may occur and lead to toxicity. ▪ Systemic toxicity (usually with plasma levels above 6 mcg/mL) may result in CNS depression (sedation) or irritability (twitching). May progress to frank convulsions with respiratory depression and/or arrest. ▪ Has been associated with malignant hyperthermia. ▪ Hypersensitivity reactions, including anaphylaxis, have been reported.

Monitor: Monitor ECG continuously. ▪ Discontinue lidocaine when patient's cardiac condition is stable or any signs of toxicity become apparent (signs of excessive depression of cardiac conductivity, such as prolongation of the PR interval, widening of the QRS interval, or appearance or aggravation of arrhythmias). ▪ Therapeutic serum levels range from 1.5 to 5 mcg/mL; above 6 mcg/mL is usually toxic. ▪ Monitor electrolytes, fluid balance, and acid-base balance. ▪ Half-life increases over time. Reduce rate of continuous infusion after 24 hours and monitor blood levels. ▪ Keep patient lying down to reduce hypotensive effects. ▪ Monitor for S/S of hypersensitivity (e.g., large hives, rash, shortness of breath or troubled breathing, swelling of eyelids, lips, or face). ▪ Discontinue infusion if malignant hyperthermia develops and treat as appropriate. ▪ See Drug Interactions.

Patient Education: May cause dizziness; remain at bed rest; request assistance if ambulation permitted.

Maternal/Child: Use during pregnancy only if clearly needed. ▪ Present in human milk. Safety for use in breast-feeding, the effects on the breast-fed infant, or the effects on milk production are unknown. Consider risk versus benefit. ▪ Safety for use in pediatric patients not established.

Elderly: Data are limited. Difference in responses between elderly patients and younger patients has not been identified. Lower-end initial dosing may be appropriate. See Dose Adjustments. ▪ Consider age-related renal and hepatic impairment.

DRUG/LAB INTERACTIONS

Administration with other **antiarrhythmic agents** (e.g., amiodarone, procainamide, propranolol, quinidine) may result in additive or antagonistic cardiac effects, and toxic effects may be additive. ▪ Concomitant use with **inhibitors of CYP1A2** (such as fluvoxamine) **and/or CYP3A4** (such as propofol) may decrease lidocaine clearance, increase lidocaine plasma levels, and prolong the elimination half-life. Monitor for toxicity with concurrent use. ▪ Concomitant use with **inducers of CYP1A2 and/or CYP3A4** (e.g., phenytoin) may decrease lidocaine plasma levels, and higher doses of lidocaine may be required. ▪ Concomitant use with a **weak CYP1A2 and CYP3A4 inhibitor** (e.g., cimetidine) may decrease clearance and increase lidocaine plasma levels, by 24% to 75%, resulting in toxic accumulation of lidocaine. Monitor lidocaine serum concentrations and monitor closely for signs of toxicity. ▪ Concomitant use with **beta-adrenergic blockers** may increase lidocaine plasma levels by decreasing hepatic blood flow resulting in decreased lidocaine clearance. Monitor for toxicity when co-administering lidocaine with **drugs that decrease hepatic blood flow**. ▪ May potentiate neuromuscular blockade of succinylcholine. ▪ Monitor toxicity when lidocaine is used in patients with digitalis toxicity accompanied by supraventricular arrhythmia and/or atrioventricular block; see Contraindications.

SIDE EFFECTS

Side effects include agitation; apprehension; asystole; blurred or double vision; bradycardia; cardiac arrest; confusion; convulsions; disorientation; dizziness; drowsiness; dysarthria; euphoria; hypoesthesia (oral); hypotension; light-headedness; malignant hyperthermia (tachycardia, tachypnea, metabolic acidosis, fever); methemoglobinemia; nausea; paresthesia; prolonged PR interval; QRS complex widening; respiratory depression and arrest; sensations of heat, cold, and numbness; tinnitus; tremors; twitching; unconsciousness; ventricular arrhythmia; VF; VT; and vomiting. Hypersensitivity reactions, including anaphylaxis, have been reported (infrequent). Cross-sensitivity between lidocaine and procainamide or between lidocaine and quinidine has not been reported.

Overdose: In addition to many of the previously listed side effects, arrhythmias (including asystole, bradycardia, heart block, tachycardia, and ventricular arrhythmias), cardiorespiratory arrest (sometimes fatal), cardiovascular collapse, CNS depression, coma, myocardial depression, nystagmus, and tingling of the tongue and lips have been reported.

ANTIDOTE

Notify the physician of any side effects. For major side effects, discontinue the drug immediately and institute appropriate measures. Ensure patency of airway and adequacy of ventilation. Treat anaphylaxis immediately with oxygen, epinephrine, antihistamines (e.g., diphenhydramine), vasopressors (e.g., dopamine), corticosteroids, albuterol, IV fluids, and ventilation equipment as indicated. There is no specific antidote for overdose of lidocaine. Maintain and support patient using appropriate corrective, resuscitative, and other supportive measures.

LINEZOLID
(lih-**NAY**-zoh-lid)

Zyvox

Antibacterial
(oxazolidinone)

pH 4.8

USUAL DOSE

Dose and duration of therapy are based on diagnosis and designated pathogens. May be transferred to oral dosing when appropriate; no dose adjustment is necessary. See Precautions.

	Recommended Linezolid Doses in Pediatric and Adult Patients		
	Dosage and Route of Administration		
Infection[a]	**Pediatric Patients[b] (Birth Through 11 Years of Age)**	**Adults and Adolescents (12 Years of Age and Older)**	**Recommended Duration of Treatment (Consecutive Days)**
Complicated skin and skin structure infections	10 mg/kg IV or PO[c] q 8 hr	600 mg IV or PO[c] q 12 hr	10 to 14
Community-acquired pneumonia, including concurrent bacteremia			
Nosocomial pneumonia			
Vancomycin-resistant *Enterococcus faecium* infections, including concurrent bacteremia	10 mg/kg IV or PO[c] q 8 hr	600 mg IV or PO[c] q 12 hr	14 to 28
Uncomplicated skin and skin structure infections	Under 5 years: 10 mg/kg PO[c] q 8 hr 5 to 11 years: 10 mg/kg PO[c] q 12 hr	Adults: 400 mg PO[c] q 12 hr Adolescents: 600 mg PO[c] q 12 hr	10 to 14

[a]Due to the designated pathogens (see Indications and Uses and package insert).

[b]Neonates under 7 days of age: Most preterm neonates under 7 days of age (gestational age under 34 weeks) have lower systemic linezolid clearance values and larger AUC values than many full-term neonates and older infants. These neonates should be initiated with a dosing regimen of 10 mg/kg q 12 hr. Consideration may be given to the use of 10 mg/kg q 8 hr regimen in neonates with a suboptimal clinical response. All neonatal patients should receive 10 mg/kg q 8 hr by 7 days of life.

[c]Oral dosing using either linezolid tablets or linezolid for oral suspension.

PEDIATRIC DOSE

See Usual Dose and Maternal/Child.

DOSE ADJUSTMENTS

Dose adjustment based on age, gender, renal insufficiency, or hepatic insufficiency is not required. ■ 30% of a dose is removed during a 3-hour dialysis session. Administer linezolid after hemodialysis.

DILUTION

Available in ready-to-use flexible plastic infusion bags in a foil laminate overwrap. Available as a 2 mg/mL solution in 200- and 600-mg infusion bags. Before use, remove overwrap and check for leaks by squeezing the bag. Each overwrap contains a peel-off label that should be applied to the infusion bag for barcode scanning before use. Do not use flexible containers in series connections.

Storage: Store at CRT. Protect from light and freezing. Keep in overwrap until ready to use. Solution may exhibit a yellow color that can intensify with time. Will not adversely affect potency.

COMPATIBILITY

Additives should not be introduced into this solution. If administered through the same tubing as other medications, flush line before and after infusion of linezolid with a solution that is **compatible** with linezolid (e.g., D5W, NS, LR) and with any medications administered through the common line. **Incompatible** at the **Y-site** with amphotericin B, ceftriaxone, chlorpromazine, diazepam, erythromycin, pentamidine, phenytoin, and sulfamethoxazole/trimethoprim.

Other sources suggest specific **compatibilities** dependent on concentration and manufacturer; consult a pharmacist.

RATE OF ADMINISTRATION

Administer as an infusion over 30 to 120 minutes. Flush line before and after administration if indicated; see Compatibility.

ACTIONS

A synthetic antibacterial agent. The first agent of a new class of antibiotics, the oxazolidinones. Clinically useful in the treatment of infections caused by aerobic gram-positive bacteria. See Indications and Uses and manufacturer's literature. Inhibits bacterial protein synthesis through a mechanism of action different from that of other antibacterial agents; therefore cross-resistance between linezolid and other classes of antibiotics is unlikely. Bacteriostatic against enterococci and staphylococci. Bactericidal against most strains of streptococci. Readily distributes into well-perfused tissues. Metabolized to two inactive metabolites. Metabolic pathway is not fully understood. Half-life is 4.8 hours. Approximately 30% of a dose is excreted in the urine as linezolid and 50% is excreted as metabolites.

INDICATIONS AND USES

Treatment of adults, adolescents, and other pediatric patients with the following infections caused by susceptible strains of the designated microorganisms: vancomycin-resistant *Enterococcus faecium* infections, including cases with concurrent bacteremia; nosocomial pneumonia caused by *Staphylococcus aureus* (methicillin-susceptible and methicillin-resistant strains) or *Streptococcus pneumoniae* (including multidrug-resistant strains [MDRSP]); complicated skin and skin-structure infections (including diabetic foot infections without concomitant osteomyelitis) caused by *S. aureus* (methicillin-susceptible and methicillin-resistant strains), *Streptococcus pyogenes,* or *Streptococcus agalactiae;* uncomplicated skin and skin-structure infections caused by *S. aureus* (methicillin-susceptible strains only) or *Streptococcus pyogenes;* and community-acquired pneumonia caused by *S. pneumoniae* (including multidrug-resistant strains [MDRSPs] and cases with concurrent bacteremia) or *S. aureus* (methicillin-susceptible strains only). ▪ Treatment of decubitus ulcers has not been studied. ▪ Given orally to treat uncomplicated skin and skin-structure infections. ▪ Not indicated for treatment of gram-negative infections. Critical that specific gram-negative therapy be initiated immediately if a concomitant gram-negative pathogen is documented or suspected. ▪ Not approved for and should not be used for treatment of patients with catheter-related bloodstream infections or catheter-site infections.

CONTRAINDICATIONS

History of hypersensitivity to linezolid or any of its components. ▪ Avoid use in patients taking any medicinal products that inhibit monoamine oxidase A or B (e.g., isocarboxazid, phenelzine) or within 2 weeks of taking any such product. ▪ Unless closely monitored for potential increases in BP, avoid use in patients with uncontrolled hypertension, pheochromocytoma, or thyrotoxicosis and/or in patients taking any of the following types of medications: directly and indirectly acting sympathomimetic agents (e.g., pseudoephedrine), vasopressive agents (e.g., epinephrine, norepinephrine), dopaminergic agents (e.g., dobutamine, dopamine); see Precautions and Drug/Lab Interactions. ▪ Unless closely monitored for S/S of serotonin syndrome or neuroleptic malignant syndrome–like (NMS-like) reactions, avoid use in patients with carcinoid syndrome and/or in patients taking any of the following medications: serotonin reuptake inhibitors, tricyclic antidepressants, serotonin 5-HT$_1$ receptor agonists, meperidine, or buspirone; see Precautions and Drug/Lab Interactions.

PRECAUTIONS

Culture and sensitivity studies are indicated to determine susceptibility of the causative organism to linezolid. ▪ To reduce the development of drug-resistant bacteria and maintain its effectiveness, linezolid should be used to treat only those infections proven or strongly suspected to be caused by bacteria. ▪ Reports of vancomycin-resistant *Enterococcus faecium* (VRE) becoming resistant to linezolid during its clinical use have been published. ▪ There has been a report of methicillin-resistant *S. aureus* (MRSA) developing resistance to linezolid during its clinical use. ▪ Combination therapy may be clinically indicated in treatment of nosocomial pneumonia or complicated skin and skin-structure infections if the documented or presumptive pathogens include gram-negative organisms. ▪ Should not be used for treatment of patients with catheter-related blood-stream infections or catheter site infections. ▪ Myelosuppression (including anemia, leukopenia, pancytopenia, and thrombocytopenia) has been reported; see Monitor. ▪ Hypoglycemia, including symptomatic episodes, has been reported in patients with diabetes who have been treated with insulin or oral hypoglycemic agents and linezolid; see Monitor and Drug/Lab Interactions. ▪ Use with caution in patients with renal failure. Although dose adjustments are not recommended in this patient population, the metabolites may accumulate. The clinical significance of this accumulation is unknown. Dose should be given after hemodialysis. ▪ Use with caution in patients with uncontrolled hypertension, severe hepatic insufficiency, pheochromocytoma, carcinoid syndrome, or untreated hyperthyroidism; see Contraindications. Use has not been studied in these patient populations. ▪ Safety and efficacy of linezolid given for longer than 28 days have not been evaluated. ▪ Neuropathy (peripheral and optic) has been reported, primarily in patients treated for longer than the maximum recommended duration of 28 days. May occur in patients treated with linezolid for shorter periods, as well as in patients treated for more than 28 days. ▪ Superinfection, caused by the overgrowth of nonsusceptible organisms, may occur with antibiotic use. Treat as indicated. ▪ *Clostridium difficile*–associated diarrhea (CDAD) has been reported. May range from mild diarrhea to fatal colitis. Consider in patients who present with diarrhea during or after treatment with linezolid. ▪ Lactic acidosis has been reported. In most cases, patients experienced repeated episodes of N/V. ▪ Serotonin syndrome (including fatal cases) and neuroleptic malignant syndrome–like (NMS-like) reactions have been reported in patients receiving linezolid and concomitant serotonergic agents; see Contraindications, Monitor, and Drug/Lab Interactions. ▪ Convulsions have been reported; however, a history of seizures was reported in some of the cases. ▪ See Monitor, Patient Education, and Drug/Lab Interactions.

Monitor: CBC with differential and platelet count should be monitored weekly, especially in patients who receive linezolid for longer than 2 weeks; those with pre-existing myelosuppression; those receiving concomitant drugs that produce bone marrow suppression (e.g., antineoplastics, chloramphenicol, immunosuppressants) or affect platelet function (e.g., aspirin, NSAIDs, platelet aggregation inhibitors, selected antibiotics, valproic acid); or those with a chronic infection who have received previous or concomitant antibiotics. Consider discontinuing therapy in patients who develop or have worsening myelosuppression. Myelosuppression appears to be reversible following discontinuation of linezolid. ▪ Monitor patients with diabetes who are receiving insulin or hypoglycemic agents for hypoglycemia; see Drug/Lab Interactions. ▪ Monitoring of visual function is recommended in patients taking linezolid for extended periods (3 months or more). Prompt ophthalmic evaluation is recommended if symptoms of visual impairment appear (e.g., blurred vision, changes in visual acuity or color vision, or visual field defect). ▪ Monitor for S/S of lactic acidosis (e.g., recurrent N/V, unexplained acidosis, or a low bicarbonate level); immediate medical evaluation is indicated. ▪ Monitor for S/S of serotonin syndrome or NMS-like reactions (autonomic instability, hyperthermia, myoclonus, rigidity, and mental status changes that include extreme agitation progressing to delirium and coma) when administered concurrently with serotonergic agents; see Drug/Lab Interactions. ▪ Monitor dietary intake of tyramine; see Patient Education. Hypertension may result from excessive tyramine intake (less than 100 mg/day). ▪ See Precautions and Drug/Lab Interactions.

Patient Education: Avoid foods or beverages high in tyramine (e.g., aged cheeses, fermented or air-dried meats, sauerkraut, soy sauce, tap beers, red wines). ▪ Inform physician of any history of hypertension or seizures. See Precautions. ▪ Inform physician if taking any medications containing pseudoephedrine or phenylpropanolamine (found in many cold or allergy preparations or diet aids), if taking serotonin reuptake inhibitors (e.g., fluoxetine, sertraline, paroxetine) or other antidepressants, or if taking an antidiabetic agent (e.g., insulin or an oral hypoglycemic agent). ▪ Promptly report diarrhea or bloody stools that occur during treatment or up to several months after an antibiotic has been discontinued; may indicate CDAD and require treatment. ▪ Promptly report any hypoglycemic reactions (e.g., diaphoresis and tremulousness) along with low blood glucose measurements. ▪ Report any vision changes promptly. See Drug Interactions.

Maternal/Child: Category C: safety for use in pregnancy and breast-feeding not established; benefits must outweigh risks. ▪ Volume of distribution is similar regardless of age in pediatric patients; however, clearance varies as a function of age. With the exception of preterm neonates under 1 week of age, clearance is most rapid in the youngest age-groups (ranging from under 1 week to 11 years of age), resulting in lower single-dose systemic exposure (AUC) and a shorter half-life. ▪ Most preterm neonates under 7 days of age (gestational age under 34 weeks) have lower systemic linezolid clearance values and larger AUC values than many full-term neonates and older infants; see Usual Dose. ▪ AUC values in patients from birth to 11 years of age dosed every 8 hours are similar to adolescents and adults dosed every 12 hours. ▪ Therapeutic concentrations are not consistent in CSF; not indicated for empiric treatment of CNS infections in pediatric patients.

Elderly: No overall difference in safety or effectiveness has been observed between these patients and younger patients. Pharmacokinetics is not significantly altered in the elderly. See Dose Adjustments.

DRUG/LAB INTERACTIONS

Linezolid is a reversible, nonselective inhibitor of monoamine oxidase and therefore has the potential to interact with **adrenergic and serotonergic agents and with tyramine-containing foods.** ▪ A reversible enhancement of the pressor response to **indirect-acting sympathomimetic agents or vasopressor or dopaminergic agents** (e.g., pseudoephedrine, epinephrine, dopamine) may be seen with concomitant use. Initial doses of adrenergic agents, such as epinephrine or dopamine, should be reduced and titrated to achieve the desired response; see Contraindications. ▪ Serotonin syndrome has been reported in patients receiving concurrent therapy with linezolid and **selective serotonin reuptake inhibitors (SSRIs)** or **serotonin norepinephrine reuptake inhibitors** (SNRIs). Linezolid use in patients taking serotonergic drugs should be limited to life-threatening or urgent situations in which linezolid is considered to be the drug of choice (e.g., treatment of vancomycin-resistant enterococcus [VRE] infections, serious infections such as nosocomial pneumonia, or complicated skin and skin structure infections, including cases caused by MRSA). The serotonergic agent should be stopped promptly when linezolid therapy is initiated. Patients should be monitored for the development of serotonin syndrome for 2 weeks (5 weeks if fluoxetine was taken) or until 24 hours after the last dose of linezolid, whichever comes first. If S/S of serotonin syndrome develop, consider discontinuing linezolid. Patients should also be monitored for specific symptoms due to discontinuation of the serotonergic agent; see prescribing information for the specific agent and; Contraindications and Monitor. ▪ May cause hypoglycemia with **insulin or hypoglycemic agents.** Dose reduction or discontinuation of the antidiabetic agent and/or discontinuation of linezolid may be indicated. ▪ **Other strong inducers of hepatic enzymes** (e.g., carbamazepine, phenytoin, phenobarbital) may cause a decrease in linezolid concentration. ▪ Severe myelosuppression may occur with **bone marrow suppressants and other drugs that affect platelet function;** see Monitor.

SIDE EFFECTS

The most common side effects are anemia, diarrhea, headache, nausea, and vomiting. Other reported side effects include abdominal pain; CDAD; constipation; dizziness; dysgeusia (change in sense of taste); dyspepsia; eosinophilia; fever; fungal infection; hypertension; increased AST, BUN, SCr, total bilirubin; insomnia; lactic acidosis; myelosuppression (anemia, leukopenia, neutropenia, pancytopenia, thrombocytopenia); neuropathy (peripheral and optic [optic neuropathy may progress to vision loss]); oral moniliasis; pruritus; rash; seizures; serotonin syndrome (cognitive dysfunction, hyperpyrexia, hyperreflexia, lack of coordination); tongue discoloration; vaginal moniliasis; vertigo; and vomiting.

Post-Marketing: Anaphylaxis; angioedema; bullous skin disorders, including severe cutaneous adverse reactions (SCAR) such as toxic epidermal necrolysis and Stevens-Johnson syndrome; convulsions; hypoglycemia (including symptomatic episodes); sideroblastic anemia; and superficial tooth and tongue discoloration.

ANTIDOTE

Keep physician informed of all side effects. Discontinue drug if indicated. If S/S of serotonin syndrome develop, consider discontinuing linezolid or the serotonergic agent. Consider discontinuing linezolid in patients who develop or have worsening myelosuppression. Mild cases of CDAD may respond to discontinuation of linezolid. Treat CDAD with fluids, electrolytes, protein supplements, and appropriate antibiotics (e.g., oral vancomycin) as indicated. In severe cases, surgical evaluation may be indicated. In the event of an overdose, initiate supportive care and maintain glomerular filtration. Both linezolid and its metabolites are partially removed by hemodialysis.

LORAZEPAM BBW

(lor-**AYZ**-eh-pam)

Ativan, Lorazepam PF

Benzodiazepine
Sedative-hypnotic
Antianxiety agent
Anticonvulsant

USUAL DOSE

Pretreatment: Verify pregnancy status; see Maternal/Child.

Dose must be individualized, especially when used in conjunction with other medications that may cause CNS depression. See Dose Adjustments, Precautions, and Drug/Lab Interactions.

Preoperative sedation/antianxiety/amnestic: 2 mg or 0.044 mg/kg of body weight, whichever is smaller, 15 to 20 minutes before procedure. For greater lack of recall 0.05 mg/kg up to 4 mg may be given. 2 mg is usually the maximum dose for patients over 50 years of age.

Sedation in intubated and mechanically ventilated ICU patients (unlabeled): 0.02 to 0.04 mg/kg (maximum single dose: 2 mg). Follow with a maintenance dose of 0.02 to 0.06 mg/kg every 2 to 6 hours as needed or with an infusion of 0.01 to 0.1 mg/kg/hr. Titrate to achieve adequate sedation. Up to 5 to 10 mg/hr has been used. When sedation is adequate, reduce to lowest amount needed.

Status epilepticus: 4 mg as the initial dose. May repeat once in 10 to 15 minutes if seizures continue or recur. Experience with further doses is very limited. Additional intervention (e.g., concomitant administration of phenytoin) may be required. Another source suggests 0.1 mg/kg of body weight to a total dose of 4 mg. May repeat once in 5 to 10 minutes. If still not effective, use another anticonvulsant agent (e.g., phenytoin).

Management of emetic-inducing chemotherapy (unlabeled): One source recommends 0.5 to 2 mg every 6 hours as needed. Another source suggests 1.5 mg/M² (up to a maximum of

3 mg) over 5 minutes. Administer 30 to 45 minutes before administration of antineoplastic agent. May be given in combination with other antiemetics (e.g., ondansetron [Zofran], dexamethasone).

PEDIATRIC DOSE

Safety for use in pediatric patients under 12 years of age has not been fully studied, but it has been used for status epilepticus in neonates, infants, and children; see Maternal/Child.

Sedation in intubated and mechanically ventilated pediatric ICU patients (unlabeled): 0.025 to 0.05 mg/kg/dose up to a maximum of 2 mg/dose every 2 to 4 hours or as an infusion at a rate of 0.025 mg/kg/hr (up to 2 mg/hr). Titrate to effect.

Status epilepticus (unlabeled; see Maternal/Child): *neonates, infants, and children:* 0.05 to 0.1 mg/kg up to a maximum of 4 mg/dose. Another source suggests a maximum dose of 2 mg/dose. May repeat 0.05 mg/kg once in 10 to 15 minutes if needed.

Antiemetic, adjunct therapy (unlabeled): 0.02 to 0.05 mg/kg/dose up to a maximum of 2 mg/dose. May repeat every 6 hours as needed.

DOSE ADJUSTMENTS

Start with a small dose in the elderly and increase gradually based on response. Consider the potential for decreased organ function and concomitant disease or drug therapy. ▪ Dose adjustments are not required with impaired liver function. ▪ Dose adjustments are not required with impaired renal function unless frequent doses are given over a short period of time. ▪ Reduced dose may be indicated in the presence of other CNS depressants. ▪ Reduce dose by 50% when given concurrently with probenecid or valproate. ▪ See Drug/Lab Interactions.

DILUTION

IV injection: Dilute immediately before use with an equal volume of SWFI, D5W, or NS. Do not shake vigorously; will result in air entrapment. Gently invert repeatedly until completely in solution. May be given by IV injection or through Y-tube of infusion tubing.

Infusion (unlabeled): One source recommends further diluting the 2-mg/mL concentration in a non-PVC (glass or polyolefin) container to a concentration of 1 mg/mL or less using D5W or NS. Alternatively, the 2-mg/mL concentration has been administered undiluted as an infusion using a patient-controlled analgesia infusion pump.

Very viscous; mix well and observe for crystallization. Crystallization does occur and is thought to be due to propylene glycol preservative. May occur more frequently with 4-mg/mL vials of lorazepam base than with 2-mg/mL vials.

Filter: Use of an in-line filter is required with administration of an infusion (unlabeled).

Storage: Refrigerate before dilution; protect from light. Use only freshly prepared solutions; discard if discolored or precipitate forms. Infusions stable at room temperature for 24 hours in glass.

COMPATIBILITY

Compatibility information not available from manufacturer. Other sources suggest specific **compatibilities** dependent on concentration and manufacturer; consult a pharmacist.

RATE OF ADMINISTRATION

IV injection: Each 2 mg or fraction thereof over 1 to 5 minutes.

Infusion: Use a microdrip or infusion pump for accuracy to deliver desired dose and/or titrate to desired level of sedation.

Pediatric rate: 2 mg/min is the maximum rate of administration.

ACTIONS

A benzodiazepine with antianxiety, sedative, and anticonvulsant effects. Inhibits ability to recall events. Interacts with the GABA-benzodiazepine receptor complex in the brain. Effective in 15 to 20 minutes. Effects last an average of 6 to 8 hours but may last as long as 12 to 24 hours. Half-life is 9 to 19 hours. Metabolized by the liver to inactive metabolites; excreted in urine and to a lesser extent in the feces. Crosses the placental barrier. Excreted in breast milk.

INDICATIONS AND USES

Preanesthetic medication for adult patients. Produces sedation, relieves anxiety, and provides anterograde amnesia. ▪ Management of status epilepticus.

Unlabeled uses: Chemotherapy-associated nausea and vomiting (adjunct, breakthrough, or anticipatory). ▪ Treatment of alcohol withdrawal. ▪ Amnestic during endoscopic procedures.

CONTRAINDICATIONS

Hypersensitivity to benzodiazepines or the components (e.g., polyethylene glycol, propylene glycol, or benzyl alcohol). ▪ Patients with acute narrow-angle glaucoma, sleep apnea syndrome, or severe respiratory insufficiency (except patients requiring relief of anxiety and/or diminished recall of events while being mechanically ventilated). ▪ Intra-arterial injection. ▪ Use in premature infants because the formulation contains benzyl alcohol.

PRECAUTIONS

Rapidly and completely absorbed IM. ▪ When given as a sedative, patient is able to respond to simple instructions. ▪ Increased risk of airway obstruction and respiratory depression; airway support, emergency drugs, and equipment must be immediately available. ▪ Dependence is possible with prolonged use or high dose. ▪ Use with extreme caution in the elderly, the very ill, or patients with limited pulmonary reserve; risk of hypoventilation and/or hypoxic cardiac arrest is increased. ▪ Use as a premedicant before local or regional anesthesia may cause excessive drowsiness and interfere with assessment of levels of anesthesia. More likely to occur with doses greater than 0.05 mg/kg or when narcotic agents are used concomitantly. ▪ Use with caution in patients with mild to moderate renal or hepatic disease. Not recommended for use in patients with hepatic and/or renal failure. ▪ There have been reports of possible propylene and polyethylene glycol toxicity (e.g., lactic acidosis, hyperosmolality, hypotension, acute tubular necrosis) when lorazepam has been administered at higher than recommended doses. Patients with renal impairment may be at increased risk of developing toxicity. ▪ Paradoxical reactions may occur. ▪ There are insufficient data to support the use of lorazepam injection for outpatient endoscopic procedures. Inpatient endoscopic procedures require adequate recovery room observation time. ▪ When lorazepam is used for peroral endoscopic procedures, adequate topical or regional anesthesia is recommended to minimize the reflex activity associated with such procedures. ▪ See Antidote (e.g., risk of seizure with flumazenil).

Monitor: To reduce incidence of thrombophlebitis, avoid smaller veins. Extravasation is hazardous; arterial administration may cause arteriospasms and gangrene and/or require amputation. ▪ Monitor patients for respiratory depression and sedation, especially when used concomitantly with opioids and other CNS depressants; see Drug/Lab Interactions. ▪ Monitor and maintain patent airway. Respiratory assistance and flumazenil must be available. ▪ Monitor vital signs. ▪ Monitor depth of sedation in critically ill patients (e.g., Richmond Agitation-Sedation Scale [RASS]). ▪ Contains propylene glycol. Monitor for toxicity if administered as a continuous infusion (e.g., acute renal failure, lactic acidosis, and/or osmol gap). ▪ **Status epilepticus:** Establish an IV and monitor vital signs. In addition to the above, observe for and correct any other possible cause of seizure (e.g., hypoglycemia, hyponatremia, other metabolic disorders). ▪ Sedative effects may add to the impairment of consciousness seen in the post-ictal state (e.g., after a seizure). ▪ Neurologic consult is suggested for any patient who fails to regain consciousness.

Patient Education: May produce drowsiness or dizziness; request assistance with ambulation and use caution when performing tasks that require alertness for 24 to 48 hours or until the effects of the drug have subsided. ▪ Avoid use of alcohol or other CNS depressants (e.g., antihistamines, barbiturates) for 24 to 48 hours or until the effects of the drug have subsided. ▪ Has amnestic potential; may impair memory. ▪ Discuss with parents or caregivers the risks, benefits, timing, and duration of surgery or procedures requiring anesthetic and sedation drugs; see Maternal/Child.

Maternal/Child: Category D: avoid pregnancy. May cause fetal harm. Not recommended during pregnancy except in serious or life-threatening conditions in which safer drugs cannot be used or are ineffective. Status epilepticus may represent a serious and life-threatening condition. Not recommended for use in labor and delivery, breast-feeding, or in pediatric patients under 12 years of age. ▪ Has FDA approval for treatment of status epilepticus in adults over 18 years of age. Safety and effectiveness for use in status epilepticus have not been established in pediatric patients. A randomized, double-blind, superiority-designed clinical trial of lorazepam versus diazepam failed to establish the efficacy of lorazepam for this indication. ▪ There are insufficient data to support the efficacy of injectable lorazepam as a preanesthetic agent in patients under 18 years of age. ▪ May cause paradoxical excitement in pediatric patients. ▪ Seizure activity and myoclonus have been reported in low-birth-weight neonates. ▪ Published studies suggest that repeated or prolonged exposures to certain anesthetic and sedation agents in utero (third trimester) and early in life (up to 3 years of age) may have negative effects on the developing brain, resulting in adverse cognitive or behavioral effects; see prescribing information for further discussion. Balance the benefits of appropriate anesthesia/sedation in pregnant females, neonates, and young children who require procedures with the potential risks described. ▪ Contains benzyl alcohol. Exposure to excessive amounts of benzyl alcohol has been associated with toxicity (hypotension, metabolic acidosis), particularly in neonates, and an increased incidence of kernicterus, particularly in preterm infants. There have been rare reports of death; see Contraindications. ▪ Half-life prolonged in pediatric patients.

Elderly: Dosing should be cautious in the elderly; see Dose Adjustments. ▪ More sensitive to therapeutic and adverse effects (e.g., ataxia, central nervous system depression, dizziness, oversedation, respiratory depression). ▪ See Precautions and Drug/Lab Interactions.

DRUG/LAB INTERACTIONS

Concomitant use of **benzodiazepines and opioids** (e.g., morphine, meperidine, fentanyl) may result in profound sedation, respiratory depression, coma, and death. If used concomitantly with opioids, monitor patients closely for respiratory depression and sedation. ▪ Concurrent use with **other CNS depressants** such as alcohol, antihistamines, barbiturates, MAO inhibitors, phenothiazines, and tricyclic antidepressants may result in additive effects for up to 48 hours. Reduced dose may be indicated. Monitor for S/S of respiratory depression and sedation. ▪ Concurrent administration with **valproate or probenecid** will decrease clearance of lorazepam. Reduce dose of lorazepam by one-half in patients receiving concurrent valproate or probenecid. ▪ Apnea, arrhythmia, bradycardia, cardiac arrest, coma, and death have been reported when used concurrently with **haloperidol.** ▪ May increase serum concentrations of **digoxin and phenytoin**; monitor digoxin and phenytoin serum levels. ▪ **Theophyllines** (aminophylline) antagonize the sedative effects of benzodiazepines. ▪ Marked sedation, excessive salivation, ataxia and, rarely, death have been reported with concomitant use of **clozapine** and lorazepam. ▪ Estrogen-containing **oral contraceptives** increase clearance and decrease the effects of lorazepam. ▪ Inhibits antiparkinson effectiveness of **levodopa.** ▪ Incidence of hallucinations and irrational behavior and an increased incidence of sedation have been observed with concurrent use of scopolamine.

SIDE EFFECTS

Airway obstruction, apnea, blurred vision, central nervous system depression (e.g., drowsiness, excessive sleepiness), confusion, crying, delirium, depression, hallucinations, headache, hypotension, hypoventilation, injection site reaction, paradoxical reactions, respiratory depression/failure, restlessness, somnolence, stupor.

Overdose: Ataxia, coma, hypnosis, hypotension, hypotonia and, very rarely, death.

ANTIDOTE

Notify physician of all symptoms. Reduction of dose may be required. Treat hypotension with dopamine or norepinephrine. In overdose, flumazenil will reverse all sedative effects of benzodiazepines. See flumazenil monograph (risk of seizures). A patent airway, artificial ventilation, oxygen therapy, and other symptomatic and supportive treatment must be instituted promptly. Monitor vital signs and fluid status carefully. Forced diuresis and osmotic diuretics (e.g., mannitol) may increase rate of lorazepam elimination. The value of dialysis has not been adequately determined.

MAGNESIUM SULFATE
(mag-**NEE**-see-um **SUL**-fayt)

Electrolyte replenisher
Anticonvulsant
Antiarrhythmic
Uterine relaxant

pH 3.5 to 7

USUAL DOSE

Individualize dose based on patient requirement and response. Discontinue as soon as desired response is obtained. Doses are expressed as magnesium sulfate unless stated otherwise. 1 Gm of magnesium sulfate = 98.6 mg elemental magnesium = 8.12 mEq of elemental magnesium.

Pre-eclampsia and eclampsia: Several regimens in literature. The recommended loading dose is 4 to 6 Gm over 15 minutes followed by a recommended maintenance dose of 1 to 2 Gm/hr. For patients with eclampsia, therapy should continue until seizures cease. Consider giving an additional 2-Gm dose for patients with recurrent eclampsia.

Another regimen suggests a total initial dose of 10 to 14 Gm. This may be achieved by administering 4 to 5 Gm in 250 mL of D5W or NS IV. Simultaneously, IM doses of up to 10 Gm (5 Gm or 10 mL of the undiluted 50% solution in each buttock) are given. Alternatively, the initial IV dose of 4 Gm may be given by diluting the 50% solution to a 10% or 20% concentration that is injected over 3 to 4 minutes. Subsequent 4- to 5-Gm doses may be given IM every 4 hours as needed, or a continuous infusion of 1 to 2 Gm/hr may be initiated.

Do not exceed 30 to 40 Gm/24 hr. Frequent monitoring required; see Dose Adjustments, Precautions, and Monitor.

Seizures associated with epilepsy, glomerulonephritis, or hypothyroidism: 1 Gm IV.

Hypomagnesemia (mild): 1 Gm IM every 6 hours for 4 doses. Another source recommends 1 to 4 Gm administered IV at a rate of 1 Gm/hr or less.

Hypomagnesemia (severe): 5 Gm (40 mEq) in 1,000 mL D5W or NS as an infusion evenly distributed over 3 hours. Another source recommends 4 to 8 Gm IV administered at a rate of 1 Gm/hr or less for asymptomatic patients. If symptomatic, may administer a dose of 4 Gm or less over 4 to 5 minutes.

Parenteral nutrition in adults: 8 to 24 mEq/24 hr IV (1 to 3 Gm).

Paroxysmal atrial tachycardia (unlabeled): 3 to 4 Gm IV (30 to 40 mL of a 10% solution) over 30 seconds with extreme caution. Reserve for patients in whom simpler measures have failed and in whom there is no evidence of myocardial damage.

Reduction of cerebral edema (unlabeled): 2.5 Gm IV (25 mL of a 10% solution).

Cardiac arrest (hypomagnesemia or torsades de pointes): AHA recommends 1 to 2 Gm (2 to 4 mL of a 50% solution) diluted in 10 mL D5W as a bolus.

Torsades de pointes: AHA recommends a loading dose of 1 to 2 Gm in 50 to 100 mL D5W as an infusion over 5 to 60 minutes. May follow with an infusion of 0.5 to 1 Gm/hr and titrate to control the torsades.

Barium poisoning: 1 to 2 Gm IV.

Alleviate bronchospasm in acute asthma (unlabeled): 2 Gm given IV over 20 minutes. Usually given concurrently with inhaled albuterol (Proventil) and IV corticosteroids.

PEDIATRIC DOSE

All pediatric doses are unlabeled; see Maternal/Child.

Hypomagnesemia: 25 to 50 mg/kg of body weight/dose. May repeat at 6-hour intervals for 2 to 3 doses, then recheck serum magnesium. Maximum recommended single dose is 2 Gm.

Pulseless VT with torsades de pointes: AHA recommends 25 to 50 mg/kg/dose IV push. A 50% solution equals 500 mg/mL. Maximum recommended dose is 2 Gm.

Status asthmaticus: 25 to 75 mg/kg as an infusion over 20 minutes. Maximum recommended dose is 2 Gm.

Parenteral nutrition: 0.3 to 0.5 mEq/kg/day (dose expressed as elemental magnesium).

DOSE ADJUSTMENTS

Reduce dose of other CNS depressants (e.g., narcotics, barbiturates) when given in conjunction with magnesium sulfate. ▪ Reduce dose in impaired renal function and in the elderly. ▪ In patients with severe renal impairment and/or a urine output less than 0.5 mL/kg/hr, initiate prevention or treatment of eclampsia with a loading dose of 4 Gm in D5W followed by a maintenance infusion of 1 Gm/hr. Titrate to maintain the concentration in the target range and monitor closely for S/S of magnesium toxicity. A lower maintenance dose requirement is likely in these patients. Do not exceed the maximum recommended dose of 20 Gm of magnesium sulfate over 48 hours. ▪ Reduce dose by 50% in patients with renal dysfunction being treated for hypomagnesemia; close monitoring is required.

DILUTION

Concentrated solutions must be diluted to a concentration of 20% (200 mg/mL) or less for IV administration. D5W and NS are the most common diluents. Available in various containers in multiple concentrations and also in multiple concentrations as a premixed solution in sterile water for injection or in 5% dextrose. See Usual Dose for specific dilutions. May be given through Y-tube of infusion set.

Storage: Store at CRT. Protect from freezing. Contains no preservative. Discard any unused solution.

COMPATIBILITY

Will form various precipitates with alcohol (in high concentrations), alkali carbonates and bicarbonates, alkali hydroxides, arsenates, barium, calcium, clindamycin, heavy metals, hydrocortisone sodium succinate, phosphates, salicylates, strontium, and tartrates. Use caution; consult pharmacist.

Other sources suggest specific **compatibilities** dependent on concentration and manufacturer; consult a pharmacist.

RATE OF ADMINISTRATION

IV injection: 150 mg (1.5 mL of a 10% solution or its equivalent) over at least 1 minute, must be diluted first, or as directed in Usual Dose.

IV infusion: As directed in Usual Dose.

ACTIONS

An important cofactor for enzymatic reactions and plays an important role in neurochemical transmission and muscular excitability. It prevents or controls seizures by blocking neuromuscular transmission and decreasing the amount of acetylcholine release. Acts peripherally to produce vasodilation and may cause a lowering of BP at higher doses. Has a depressant effect on the CNS but does not adversely affect the woman, fetus, or neonate when used as directed in eclampsia or pre-eclampsia. Onset of anticonvulsant action is immediate and lasts for about 30 minutes. Average half-life in females with pre-eclampsia is approximately 4 to 5 hours. Excreted in the urine. Secreted in breast milk. Crosses the placental barrier.

INDICATIONS AND USES

Replacement therapy in magnesium deficiency (e.g., acute hypomagnesemia accompanied by signs of tetany similar to those seen in hypocalcemia). ▪ Correction or prevention of hypomagnesemia in patients receiving TPN. ▪ Prevention and control of seizures in pre-eclampsia and eclampsia, respectively.

Unlabeled uses: Control of seizures associated with epilepsy, glomerulonephritis, hypothyroidism. ▪ Reduction of cerebral edema. ▪ Acute nephritis in pediatric patients to control hypertension, encephalopathy, and convulsions. ▪ Treatment of torsades de pointes, ventricular tachycardia, and ventricular fibrillation (VT/VF) caused by hypomagnesemia. ▪ Counteract muscle-stimulating effects of barium poisoning. ▪ Treatment of paroxysmal atrial tachycardia. ▪ Treatment of acute asthma in patients who do not respond to conventional therapy.

CONTRAINDICATIONS

Presence of heart block or myocardial damage. ▪ Diabetic coma. ▪ Myasthenia gravis.

PRECAUTIONS

Continuous administration of magnesium sulfate beyond 5 to 7 days to pregnant females can lead to hypocalcemia and bone abnormalities in the developing fetus, including skeletal demineralization, osteopenia, and neonatal fracture. ▪ Patients receiving magnesium sulfate are at risk for magnesium toxicity, including respiratory depression, acute renal failure and, rarely, pulmonary edema. ▪ Use caution in impaired renal function; may result in magnesium toxicity. ▪ Some solutions may contain aluminum. In impaired kidney function, aluminum may reach toxic levels. Premature neonates are particularly at risk because of their immature kidneys and requirement for calcium and phosphate, which also contain aluminum. Research indicates that patients with impaired renal function who receive greater than 4 to 5 mcg/kg/day of parenteral aluminum are at risk for developing CNS or bone toxicity associated with aluminum accumulation. Tissue loading may occur at even lower rates of administration. ▪ Administer with caution if flushing and sweating occur (first signs of vasodilation). ▪ Solutions containing dextrose should be used with caution in patients with known prediabetes or diabetes mellitus given the risk of elevated blood glucose. ▪ Use of magnesium sulfate in patients with underlying myasthenia gravis can precipitate a myasthenic crisis; see Contraindications. ▪ See Drug/Lab Interactions.

Monitor: Discontinue IV administration when the desired therapeutic effect is obtained. ▪ Monitor for clinical signs of magnesium toxicity (e.g., facial edema, diminished strength of deep tendon reflexes, respiratory depression). ▪ Monitor magnesium levels. Normal plasma magnesium levels range from 1.5 to 2.5 mEq/L. Consider targeting maintenance dose to achieve serum magnesium concentrations of 2.5 to 5 mEq/L (3 to 6 mg/100 mL) in patients with eclampsia. Deep tendon reflexes decrease at plasma magnesium levels above 4 mEq/L and disappear as levels approach 10 mEq/L. Respiratory paralysis will occur at this level. ▪ With each repeated dose, test patellar reflex (knee jerks) and observe respirations. If the knee jerk is absent or if respirations are less than 16/min, **do not** give additional magnesium sulfate. ▪ Equipment to maintain artificial ventilation must be available at all times. Patient must be continuously observed. ▪ Maintain minimum of 100 mL of urine or more during the 4 hours preceding each dose.

Patient Education: If magnesium is given for the treatment of preterm labor, inform the woman that the efficacy and safety of such use have not been established and that use beyond 5 to 7 days may cause fetal abnormalities. ▪ Promptly report symptoms of magnesium toxicity (e.g., difficulty breathing, flushing, sweating, weakness).

Maternal/Child: Continuous administration beyond 5 to 7 days to pregnant females can lead to hypocalcemia and bone abnormalities in the developing fetus; see Precautions. Use during pregnancy only if clearly needed. ▪ Administration of magnesium is not approved for treatment for preterm labor. Safety and efficacy have not been established. Administration of magnesium outside its approved indication in pregnant females should be by trained obstetric personnel in a hospital setting with appropriate obstetric care facilities. ■ A continuous infusion given to control convulsions in toxemic mothers before delivery (especially in the 24 hours preceding) may cause signs of magnesium toxicity in the newborn (e.g., neuromuscular or respiratory depression). ■ Use caution during breast-feeding. ■ Safety for use in pediatric patients not established. Safety and effectiveness have been established for the prevention of eclampsia in adolescents with preeclampsia and the treatment of seizures and prevention of recurrent seizures in adolescents with eclampsia.

Elderly: See Dose Adjustments.

DRUG/LAB INTERACTIONS

Additive CNS depressant effects when used concomitantly with **barbiturates, hypnotics, narcotics, or systemic anesthetics.** See Dose Adjustments and Monitor. ■ Potentiation and prolongation of neuromuscular blockade is possible when used with **neuromuscular blocking agents** (e.g., vecuronium, succinylcholine). Monitor patient closely. Dose adjustment of the neuromuscular blocking agent and reversal agent may be necessary. ■ An exaggerated hypotensive response is possible with concomitant use of magnesium and **dihydropyridine calcium channel blockers** (e.g., amlodipine, nicardipine, nifedipine); monitor vital signs frequently. ■ If **calcium** is used to treat magnesium toxicity, use in digitalized patients may cause serious changes in cardiac conduction, resulting in heart block. Use with extreme caution. ■ **Drugs that may induce magnesium loss** (e.g., alcohol, aminoglycosides, amphotericin B, cisplatin, cyclosporine, digitalis, diuretics) may reduce magnesium concentrations, affecting efficacy; monitor magnesium concentrations closely and adjust dose as needed. ■ Avoid use with **unapproved tocolytics** (e.g., beta-adrenergic agents such as terbutaline or calcium channel blockers such as nifedipine); serious adverse events, including pulmonary edema and hypotension, have occurred.

SIDE EFFECTS

Usually the result of magnesium intoxication. Cardiac and CNS depression proceeding to respiratory paralysis, circulatory collapse, depressed or absent knee jerk reflex, flaccid paralysis, flushing, hypocalcemia with signs of tetany, hypotension, hypothermia, and sweating are most common. Other reported side effects include bradycardia, decreased respiratory rate, hypermagnesemia, lethargy, myasthenic crisis, pulmonary edema, sedation, somnolence, and visual disturbances.

ANTIDOTE

Discontinue the drug and notify the physician of the occurrence of any side effect. An intravenous calcium salt (10 to 20 mL of a 5% solution [diluted if desirable with NS]) may be used to counteract the effects of hypermagnesemia. Physostigmine 0.5 to 1 mg SQ may be helpful. Treat hypotension with dopamine. Employ artificial ventilation as necessary and resuscitate as necessary. Hemodialysis is effective in overdose. **Hypermagnesemia in the newborn** may require resuscitation, endotracheal intubation, assisted ventilation, and IV calcium.

MANNITOL
(**MAN**-nih-tol)

Osmitrol

Diuretic
(osmotic)

pH 4.5 to 7

USUAL DOSE
Pretreatment: See Monitor.

Mannitol: Total dose, concentration, and rate of administration should be based on age, weight, and the nature and severity of the condition being treated, including fluid requirements, electrolyte balance, serum osmolality, urine output, and concomitant therapy.

Reduction of intracranial pressure: One manufacturer recommends 0.25 Gm/kg as an IV infusion over 30 minutes. May be repeated every 6 to 8 hours. Another manufacturer recommends 0.25 to 2 Gm/kg as a 15% to 25% solution administered as an IV infusion over 30 to 60 minutes.

Reduction of intraocular pressure: One manufacturer recommends a single dose of 1.5 to 2 Gm/kg of body weight as a 15% or 20% solution administered as an IV infusion over at least 30 minutes. Another manufacturer recommends 0.25 to 2 Gm/kg as a 15% to 25% solution administered as an IV infusion over 30 to 60 minutes. When used preoperatively, administer 60 to 90 minutes before surgery to achieve maximal reduction of intraocular pressure before the operation.

Measurement of glomerular filtration rate (GFR): Dilute 100 mL of a 20% solution (20 Gm) with 180 mL of NS or 200 mL of a 10% solution (20 Gm) with 80 mL of NS. Infuse the 280 mL of diluted solution at a rate of 20 mL /min. See manufacturer's prescribing information for diagnostic procedure/monitoring.

PEDIATRIC DOSE
See Maternal/Child.

Cerebral or ocular edema: 1 to 2 Gm/kg of body weight or 30 to 60 Gm/M^2 of body surface as an IV infusion over 30 to 60 minutes.

DOSE ADJUSTMENTS
Reduce dose in small or debilitated patients. One manufacturer states that a dose of 500 mg/kg may be sufficient. ■ Dose selection in the elderly should be cautious (usually starting at the low end of the dosing range), reflecting the greater frequency of decreased organ function and of concomitant disease or drug therapy.

DILUTION
Available in concentrations of 5%, 10%, 15%, 20%, or 25%. May be in flexible IV bags or in flip-top vials. No further dilution is necessary; however, if there are any crystals present in the solution, they must be completely dissolved before administration. One manufacturer recommends: To dissolve crystals in the flexible container, warm the unit to 70° C (158° F) with agitation. Heat solution using a dry-heat cabinet with overwrap intact. Use of a water bath is not recommended. To dissolve the crystals in the flip-top vial, warm the bottle in hot water at 80° C (176° F). Shake vigorously periodically. 25% mannitol injection may be autoclaved at 121° C (250° F) for 20 minutes at 15 psi. Consult prescribing information; process may differ with specific brands. Let cool to at least body temperature before administration.

Glomerular filtration rate: See Usual Dose.

Filters: Use an in-line filter for 15%, 20%, and 25% solutions.

Storage: One manufacturer recommends storing at CRT. Protect from freezing. Do not remove container from overwrap until intended for use. Consult prescribing information; may be brand specific. Discard unused portions.

COMPATIBILITY
Admixing with other medications is not recommended. Do not administer simultaneously with blood products through the same administration set because of the possibility of pseudoagglutination or hemolysis. Concomitant administration of electrolyte-free

mannitol solutions with whole blood may cause pseudoagglutination. If blood must be given simultaneously, at least 20 mEq of NaCl should be added to each liter of mannitol solution; consult pharmacist. Do not use PVC infusion bags with 25% mannitol; may form a precipitate.

Other sources suggest specific **compatibilities** dependent on concentration and manufacturer; consult a pharmacist.

RATE OF ADMINISTRATION
Variable based on indication and patient condition; see Usual Dose.

ACTIONS
A sugar alcohol effective as an osmotic diuretic. Mannitol hinders the tubular reabsorption of water and enhances excretion of sodium and chloride by elevating the osmolarity of the glomerular filtrate. The increase in extracellular osmolarity induces the movement of intracellular water into the extracellular and vascular spaces. This action is responsible for the ability of mannitol to decrease intracranial pressure and edema and to reduce elevated intraocular pressure. Mannitol is confined to the extracellular space, is only slightly metabolized, and is rapidly excreted by the kidney. It is not reabsorbed or secreted by the tubules of the kidneys. It is excreted almost completely in the urine along with water, sodium, and chloride. Onset of diuresis is 1 to 3 hours. Reduction in intracranial pressure occurs within 15 to 30 minutes. Duration of effect is 1.5 to 6 hours. Half-life is 0.5 to 2.5 hours.

INDICATIONS AND USES
Reduction of intracranial pressure (associated with cerebral edema and/or brain mass) and treatment of cerebral edema. ▪ Reduction of elevated intraocular pressure. ▪ As a diagnostic for measurement of glomerular filtration rate.

CONTRAINDICATIONS
Anuria, hypersensitivity to mannitol, intracranial bleeding except during craniotomy, pre-existing severe pulmonary vascular congestion or pulmonary edema, severe dehydration (hypovolemia).

PRECAUTIONS
For IV use only, preferably into a large central vein. ▪ Serious hypersensitivity reactions, including anaphylaxis, hypotension, and dyspnea resulting in cardiac arrest and death, have been reported. ▪ Renal complications, including irreversible renal failure and osmotic nephrosis, have been reported. Although osmotic nephrosis is in principle reversible, it may potentially proceed to chronic or even end-stage renal failure. Patients with pre-existing renal disease, patients with conditions that put them at risk for renal failure, or patients receiving potentially nephrotoxic drugs or other diuretics may be at increased risk for renal failure. ▪ Patients with oliguric acute kidney injury who subsequently develop anuria while receiving mannitol are at risk of congestive heart failure, pulmonary edema, hypertensive crisis, coma, and death. ▪ CNS toxicity manifested by symptoms such as coma, confusion, and lethargy has been reported. In the presence of impaired renal function, CNS toxicity may result from high serum mannitol concentrations, serum hyperosmolarity resulting in intracellular dehydration within CNS, hyponatremia, or other electrolyte or acid/base disturbances. Deaths have occurred. ▪ At high concentrations, mannitol may cross the blood-brain barrier and interfere with the ability of the brain to maintain the pH of the cerebrospinal fluid, especially in the presence of acidosis. In patients with pre-existing compromise of the blood-brain barrier, the risk of increasing cerebral edema (general and focal) associated with repeated or continued use of mannitol must be weighed against expected benefits. ▪ A rebound increase of intracranial pressure may occur several hours after a mannitol infusion. Patients with a compromised blood-brain barrier are at increased risk. ▪ Depending on dose and duration, mannitol administration may cause hypervolemia, leading to or exacerbating existing congestive heart failure. Accumulation of mannitol due to insufficient renal excretion increases the risk of hypervolemia. Mannitol-induced osmotic diuresis may cause or worsen dehydration/hypovolemia and hemoconcentration. Administration may also cause hyperosmolarity. ▪ Depending on dose and duration, mannitol administration may

cause electrolyte and acid/base imbalances, which may be fatal. Imbalances may include hypernatremia, dehydration, and hemoconcentration; hyponatremia, which can lead to headache, nausea, seizures, lethargy, coma, cerebral edema, and death (acute symptomatic hyponatremic encephalopathy is a medical emergency); hypokalemia or hyperkalemia, which may result in cardiac adverse reactions, especially in patients receiving drugs that are sensitive to such imbalances; other electrolyte disturbances; and metabolic acidosis/alkalosis. ▪ Infusion of mannitol through a peripheral vein at a concentration of 10% or greater may result in peripheral venous irritation, including phlebitis. ▪ Use with caution in neurosurgical patients. May increase cerebral blood flow and increase risk of postoperative bleeding. ▪ Increased cerebral blood flow may worsen intracranial hypertension in pediatric patients who develop a generalized cerebral hyperemia during the first 24 to 48 hours after injury. ▪ See Drug/Lab Interactions.

Monitor: Evaluate renal, cardiac, and pulmonary status and correct fluid and electrolyte imbalances before administration. ▪ During and after infusion for reduction of intracranial pressure, monitor clinical condition; fluid and electrolytes (sodium, potassium, calcium, phosphorus); serum osmolarity; the osmol gap; renal (SCr, urine output); cardiac and pulmonary function; and intracranial pressure. Discontinue if renal, cardiac, or pulmonary status worsen or if CNS toxicity develops. ▪ Monitor for S/S of a hypersensitivity reaction. ▪ Observe infusion site to prevent infiltration.

Patient Education: Promptly report S/S of a hypersensitivity reaction (e.g., dyspnea, itching, rash). ▪ Report any adverse reaction, such as change in mental status, decreasing urine output, difficulty breathing, edema, or new or worsening heart failure. ▪ Report pain at injection site.

Maternal/Child: Safety for use in pregnancy, labor, or delivery not established. Mannitol crosses the placenta and may cause fluid shifts that could potentially result in adverse effects in the fetus. Benefits must outweigh risks. ▪ Use caution in breast-feeding. ▪ Mannitol is approved for use in pediatric patients for the reduction of intracranial and intraocular pressure. Studies have not identified the optimal dose in this patient population. The safety profile for use in pediatric patients is similar to that seen with adults. ▪ Pediatric patients under 2 years of age, particularly preterm and term neonates, may be at higher risk for fluid and electrolyte abnormalities after mannitol administration because of decreased glomerular filtration rate and limited ability to concentrate urine. ▪ See Precautions.

Elderly: Response similar to that seen in younger patients. Lower-end initial doses may be appropriate; see Dose Adjustments.

DRUG/LAB INTERACTIONS

May increase **lithium** excretion, thereby decreasing its effectiveness. May also increase risk of lithium toxicity in patients who develop mannitol-induced hypovolemia or renal impairment. Consider holding lithium during treatment with mannitol. If concomitant administration of lithium and mannitol is required, monitor lithium levels carefully. ▪ Mannitol-induced electrolyte imbalances (e.g., hyperkalemia, hypokalemia) may result in cardiac adverse reactions in patients receiving drugs that are sensitive to such imbalances (e.g., **digoxin, drugs that prolong the QT interval, neuromuscular blocking agents**). ▪ Use with **potentially nephrotoxic drugs** (e.g., aminoglycosides) or other **diuretics** may increase the risk of renal toxicity. Avoid concomitant use, if possible. ▪ Concomitant administration of **systemic neurotoxic drugs** (e.g., aminoglycosides) may potentiate neurotoxicity. Avoid concomitant use, if possible. ▪ High concentrations of mannitol can cause false low results for inorganic phosphorus blood concentrations with certain assays. ▪ Mannitol may produce a false-positive result in tests for blood ethylene glycol concentrations.

SIDE EFFECTS

The most common adverse reactions are CNS toxicity, hypersensitivity reactions, hypokalemia, hyperkalemia, hyponatremia, hypernatremia, hypovolemia, hypervolemia, infusion site reactions, and renal failure; see Precautions. Other reactions may include acidosis, backache, blurred vision, chest pain, chills, convulsions, decreased chloride levels, dehydration, diuresis, dizziness, dryness of mouth, edema, fever, fulminating congestive heart failure, headache, hyperosmolality, hypertension, hypotension, nausea, polyuria then oliguria, pulmonary edema, rhinitis, tachycardia, thirst, thrombophlebitis, and urinary retention.

ANTIDOTE

If minor side effects persist, notify the physician. Discontinue at the first sign of a hypersensitivity reaction and initiate therapeutic measures as clinically indicated. Discontinue for worsening renal function; CNS toxicity; or for fluid, electrolyte, or acid/base abnormalities and notify the physician. Treatment will be supportive to correct fluid and electrolyte imbalances. Hemodialysis may be used to clear mannitol and reduce serum osmolality.

MELOXICAM INJECTION BBW

(mel-**OKS**-i-kam in-**JEK**-shun)

Analgesic
NSAID

USUAL DOSE

Pretreatment: See Monitor and Maternal/Child. To reduce the risk of renal toxicity, patients must be well hydrated before administration.

Use the lowest effective dose for the shortest duration consistent with individual patient treatment goals.

Meloxicam: Recommended dose is 30 mg once daily as an IV bolus injection over 15 seconds. Meaningful pain relief may not occur for 2 to 3 hours after meloxicam injection. A non-NSAID analgesic with a rapid onset of effect may be needed; see Monitor.

DOSE ADJUSTMENTS

No specific dose adjustments recommended. ▪ Has not been studied in patients with hepatic impairment or in patients with moderate or severe renal impairment. ▪ Consider dose reduction in patients who are known or suspected to be poor CYP2C9 metabolizers based on genotype or previous history/experience with other CYP2C9 substrates (e.g., warfarin or phenytoin). May have abnormally high concentrations due to reduced metabolic clearance.

DILUTION

Available as an opaque, pale yellow, aqueous dispersion for IV use supplied as a 1-mL fill (30 mg/mL) in a clear, 2-mL, single-dose vial.

Filters: Specific information not available.

Storage: Store at CRT. Protect from light. *Do not freeze.*

COMPATIBILITY

Compatibility information not available from manufacturer; consult a pharmacist.

RATE OF ADMINISTRATION

A single dose as an IV bolus over 15 seconds.

ACTIONS

A nonsteroidal anti-inflammatory drug (NSAID) that has anti-inflammatory, analgesic, and antipyretic activity. Mechanism of action is not completely understood but may involve inhibition of the cyclooxygenase (COX-1 and COX-2) pathways. Meloxicam is a potent inhibitor of prostaglandin synthesis. Prostaglandins sensitize afferent nerves and potentiate the action of bradykinin in inducing pain in animal models. Prostaglandins are mediators of inflammation. Because meloxicam is an inhibitor of prostaglandin synthesis, its mode of action may result from a decrease of prostaglandins in peripheral tissues. More than 99% bound to serum proteins, primarily albumin. Metabolized extensively in the liver, primarily by CYP2C9. Mean elimination half-life is approximately 24 hours. Excreted as metabolites in urine and feces.

INDICATIONS AND USES

An NSAID indicated in adults for the management of moderate to severe pain alone or in combination with other non-NSAID analgesics.

Limitation of Use: Because of delayed onset of analgesia, meloxicam is not recommended for use when rapid onset of analgesia is required.

CONTRAINDICATIONS

Known hypersensitivity to meloxicam or any components of the drug product. ■ History of asthma, urticaria, or other allergic-type reactions after taking aspirin or other NSAIDs. ■ Contraindicated in the setting of coronary artery bypass graft (CABG) surgery. ■ Moderate to severe renal insufficiency patients who are at risk for renal failure due to volume depletion.

PRECAUTIONS

For IV administration only. ■ Nonsteroidal anti-inflammatory drugs (NSAIDs) cause an increased risk of serious cardiovascular (CV) thrombotic events, including myocardial infarction and stroke, which can be fatal. This risk may occur early in treatment and may increase with duration of use. Patients with CV disease or risk factors for CV disease may be at greater risk. Some observational studies found that this increased risk of serious CV thrombotic events began as early as the first weeks of treatment. The increase in CV thrombotic risk has been observed most consistently at higher doses. To minimize the potential risk, use the lowest effective dose for the shortest duration possible. ■ In observational studies, patients treated with NSAIDs in the post-MI period were at increased risk for re-infarction, CV-related death, and all-cause mortality beginning in the first week of treatment. Avoid use in patients with recent MI unless benefits are expected to outweigh the risk of recurrent CV thrombotic events. ■ There is no consistent evidence that concurrent use of aspirin mitigates the increased risk of serious CV thrombotic events associated with NSAID use. Concurrent use of aspirin and an NSAID does increase the risk of serious GI events. ■ NSAIDs increase the risk of serious GI adverse events, including inflammation, bleeding, ulceration, and perforation of the esophagus, stomach, or intestines, which can be fatal. These events can occur at any time during use and without warning symptoms. Elderly patients and patients with a prior history of peptic ulcer disease and/or GI bleeding are at greater risk for serious gastrointestinal events. ■ Risk of GI events increases with longer duration of use; however, even short-term GI is not without risk. Use with extreme caution in patients with a history of ulcer disease or GI bleeding. ■ Other factors that increase the risk for GI bleeding include concomitant use of oral corticosteroids, aspirin, anticoagulants, or selective serotonin reuptake inhibitors (SSRIs [e.g., fluoxetine]); smoking; use of alcohol; older age; and poor general health. ■ In addition, patients with advanced liver disease and/or coagulopathy are at increased risk for GI bleeding. Most reports of spontaneous fatal GI events are in patients who are elderly or debilitated. Avoid use in patients at higher risk unless benefits are expected to outweigh the increased risk of bleeding. Alternative therapies should be considered. ■ Elevations of ALT or AST 3 or more times the ULN have been reported. In addition, rare, sometimes fatal, cases of severe hepatic injury, including fulminant hepatitis, liver necrosis, and hepatic failure, have been reported. ■ NSAIDs, including meloxicam, can lead to new onset of hypertension or worsening of pre-existing hypertension, either of which may contribute to the increased incidence of CV events. ■ In patients with heart failure, NSAID use increased the risk of MI, hospitalization for heart failure, and death. Avoid use in patients with severe heart failure unless benefits outweigh the risk of worsening heart failure. ■ Fluid retention and edema have been observed. ■ Long-term administration of NSAIDs has resulted in renal papillary necrosis, renal insufficiency, acute renal failure, and other renal injury. Renal toxicity has also been seen in patients in whom renal prostaglandins have a compensatory role in the maintenance of renal perfusion. NSAIDs may cause a dose-dependent reduction in prostaglandin formation and, secondarily, in renal blood flow, which may precipitate overt renal decompensation. Patients at greatest risk are those with impaired renal function, dehydration, hypovolemia, heart failure, or liver dysfunction; those taking diuretics and ACE (angiotensin-converting enzyme) inhibitors or ARBs (angiotensin receptor blockers); and elderly patients. ■ Increases in serum potassium concentration, including hyperkalemia, have been reported. ■ Meloxicam has been associated with hypersensitivity reactions (including anaphylactic reactions) with and without known hypersensitivity to meloxicam and in patients with aspirin-sensitive asthma. ■ Use with caution in patients with asthma. Use is contraindicated in patients with aspirin-sensitive asthma (a subpopulation of patients with asthma that may include chronic rhinosinusitis complicated by nasal polyps; severe, potentially fatal bronchospasm; and/or intolerance to aspirin and other NSAIDs).

Cross-reactivity between aspirin and other NSAIDs has been reported in such aspirin-sensitive patients. ▪ NSAIDs can cause serious skin adverse events such as exfoliative dermatitis, Stevens-Johnson syndrome (SJS), and toxic epidermal necrolysis (TEN), which may occur without warning and can be fatal. ▪ Anemia has occurred in NSAID-treated patients. May be due to occult or gross blood loss, fluid retention, or an incompletely described effect on erythropoiesis. ▪ By reducing inflammation, and possibly fever, meloxicam may diminish the S/S of infection.

Monitor: Correct hypovolemia before administration and maintain adequate hydration. ▪ Obtain baseline blood pressure and monitor frequently during therapy. ▪ Baseline CBC, chemistry profile, liver function tests, and SCr may be useful. Repeat as indicated in patients at risk for toxicity or if symptoms of toxicity develop. ▪ When initiating meloxicam, monitor patient analgesic response. Because the median time to meaningful pain relief was 2 and 3 hours after meloxicam administration in two clinical studies, a non-NSAID analgesic with a rapid onset of effect may be needed, for example, upon anesthetic emergence or resolution of local or regional anesthetic blocks. ▪ Some patients may not experience adequate analgesia for the entire 24-hour dosing interval and may require administration of a short-acting, non-NSAID, immediate-release analgesic. ▪ Monitor renal function in patients with renal or hepatic impairment, heart failure, dehydration, or hypovolemia. ▪ CV events (e.g., MI, stroke, other thrombotic events) may occur even in the absence of previous CV symptoms. Monitor patients with or without a previous history of CV disease for S/S of thromboembolic complications (e.g., altered consciousness, vision, or speech; chest pain; limb or abdominal swelling and/or pain; loss of sensation or motor power; shortness of breath). If used in patients with a recent MI, monitor for signs of cardiac ischemia. ▪ Monitor for edema, weight gain, or signs of worsening heart failure. ▪ To minimize the GI risks in NSAID-treated patients: (1) use the lowest effective dosage for the shortest possible duration; (2) avoid administration of more than one NSAID at a time; (3) avoid use in patients at higher risk unless benefits are expected to outweigh increased risk of bleeding (for such patients, as well as those with active GI bleeding, consider alternative therapies); (4) observe for S/S of GI ulceration or bleeding; (5) promptly initiate evaluation and treatment if a serious GI adverse event is suspected, and discontinue meloxicam until a serious GI event is ruled out; (6) during concomitant use of low-dose aspirin for cardiac prophylaxis, monitor patients more closely for evidence of GI bleeding. ▪ Observe for S/S of liver dysfunction (e.g., abdominal pain, dark urine, diarrhea, elevated LFTs, eosinophilia, fatigue, jaundice, pruritus, rash). ▪ Monitor for S/S of hypersensitivity reactions (e.g., anaphylaxis, pruritus, rash, urticaria, or wheezing). If used in patients with pre-existing asthma (without known aspirin sensitivity), monitor patients for changes in the S/S of asthma. ▪ Monitor for S/S of serious skin reactions (e.g., rash). ▪ Monitor patients who may be at increased risk for bleeding; see Precautions.

Patient Education: Side effects have resulted in extended hospitalization and could be fatal. ▪ Promptly report any unusual S/S suggestive of thromboembolic events, GI toxicity, hepatotoxicity, hypersensitivity reactions, or fluid and electrolyte imbalance (e.g., abdominal pain, bloody emesis, changes in vision, chest pain, dark stools, diarrhea, dizziness, fatigue, flu-like symptoms, jaundice, lethargy, nausea, numbness of face or limbs, pruritus, rash, shortness of breath, unexplained weight gain or edema). ▪ Review medication profile with physician or pharmacist. ▪ May delay or prevent rupture of ovarian follicles, which has been associated with reversible infertility in some females. ▪ May compromise fertility in males of reproductive potential.

Maternal/Child: May cause premature closure of the fetal ductus arteriosus. Avoid use in pregnant females starting at 30 weeks' gestation (third trimester). There are no adequate and well-controlled studies of meloxicam in pregnant females. Use during pregnancy only if the potential benefit justifies the potential risk to the fetus. ▪ There are no studies on the use of meloxicam during labor or delivery. Inhibition of prostaglandin synthesis, delayed parturition, and increased incidence of stillbirth were seen in animal studies. ▪ Use caution during breast-feeding; data unavailable. ▪ Safety and efficacy have not been established for use in pediatric patients.

Elderly: Safety and effectiveness similar to younger patients. However, elderly patients are at greater risk for serious, NSAID-associated cardiovascular, gastrointestinal, and/or renal adverse reactions. If used, monitor closely.

DRUG/LAB INTERACTIONS

Concurrent use with **drugs that interfere with hemostasis** (e.g., aspirin, SSRIs, SNRIs, warfarin, and other NSAIDs) is not recommended; may increase the risk of serious GI events. ■ Concomitant use with analgesic doses of **aspirin** is not generally recommended. In the setting of concomitant use of **low-dose aspirin** for cardiac prophylaxis, monitor patients more closely for evidence of GI bleeding. Meloxicam is not a substitute for low-dose aspirin for cardiovascular protection. ■ The effects of **anticoagulants** (e.g., heparin, warfarin) and NSAIDs on bleeding are synergistic; risk of bleeding increases with concomitant use. ■ NSAIDs may decrease the antihypertensive effect of **ACE inhibitors, angiotensin receptor blockers** (ARBs), and **beta-blockers**. Monitor blood pressure to ensure desired BP is maintained. Monitor renal function to identify possible renal deterioration in elderly patients, volume-depleted patients (including those on diuretic therapy), and/or patients with renal impairment. ■ Use caution if administered concomitantly with **cyclosporine**; cyclosporine nephrotoxicity may be increased. ■ Meloxicam can reduce the natriuretic effects of **loop diuretics** and **thiazide diuretics**. This response is thought to be due to inhibition of renal prostaglandin synthesis; observe for signs of worsening renal function and ensure diuretic effectiveness. ■ Concurrent use of **lithium** with NSAIDs may decrease lithium clearance, increasing plasma levels of lithium; observe for signs of lithium toxicity. ■ Concurrent use of NSAIDs with **methotrexate** may enhance methotrexate toxicity. Observe for signs of methotrexate toxicity (neutropenia, thrombocytopenia, renal dysfunction). ■ Concomitant use of meloxicam and **pemetrexed** may increase the risk of pemetrexed-associated myelosuppression and renal and GI toxicity. ■ Concomitant use with other **NSAIDs or salicylates** (e.g., diflunisal, salsalate) increases the risk of GI toxicity with little or no increase in efficacy. ■ Metabolized by cytochrome P450 enzymes, predominantly by CYP2C9. Coadministration with **CYP2C9 inhibitors** (e.g., amiodarone, fluconazole, voriconazole) may increase the toxicity of meloxicam. Consider dose reduction in patients undergoing treatment with CYP2C9 inhibitors, and monitor for adverse effects.

SIDE EFFECTS

Most common side effects include anemia, constipation, and increased gamma-glutamyl transferase (GGT). Serious side effects include cardiovascular thrombotic events; GI bleeding, ulceration, and perforation; hepatotoxicity; hypertension; heart failure and edema; renal toxicity and hyperkalemia; anaphylactic reactions; serious skin reactions; and hematologic toxicity. Many other side effects have been reported in fewer than 2% of patients during clinical trials.

Overdose: Drowsiness, epigastric pain, lethargy, nausea, and vomiting are common and have been generally reversible with supportive care. Acute renal failure, coma, GI bleeding, hypertension, and respiratory depression have occurred but were rare.

Post-Marketing: Acute urinary retention, agranulocytosis, alterations in mood (such as mood elevation), anaphylactoid reactions (including shock), erythema multiforme, exfoliative dermatitis, interstitial nephritis, jaundice, liver failure, Stevens-Johnson syndrome, toxic epidermal necrolysis, and female infertility.

ANTIDOTE

Keep the physician informed of side effects. With increasing severity or onset of symptoms of any major side effect (e.g., cardiovascular thrombotic events; CHF; edema; GI bleeding, ulceration, or perforation; hepatic or renal toxicity; hypersensitivity reactions; hypertension; skin reactions), discontinue the drug and notify the physician. A patent airway, artificial ventilation, oxygen therapy, and other symptomatic treatment must be instituted promptly if indicated. Treat anaphylaxis with epinephrine, diphenhydramine, and corticosteroids as indicated. Manage overdose with symptomatic and supportive care. No specific antidote. Forced diuresis, alkalinization of urine, hemodialysis, or hemoperfusion may be used in an overdose situation but are unlikely to be useful due to high protein binding. Accelerated removal of meloxicam with cholestyramine 4 Gm three times daily was demonstrated in a clinical trial and may be useful in overdose.

MEROPENEM
(**mer**-oh-**PEN**-em)

Merrem I.V.

USUAL DOSE

Dose ranges from 500 mg to 2 Gm and depends on type and severity of infection.

Complicated skin and skin structure infections in adults and pediatric patients weighing 50 kg or more: 500 mg every 8 hours. Increase to 1 Gm every 8 hours in complicated skin and skin structure infections caused by *Pseudomonas aeruginosa*.

Complicated intra-abdominal infections in adults and pediatric patients weighing 50 kg or more: 1 Gm every 8 hours.

Febrile neutropenia in adults and pediatric patients weighing 50 kg or more (unlabeled): 1 Gm every 8 hours.

Meningitis (unlabeled in adult patients): 2 Gm every 8 hours.

Bloodstream infections (gram-negative bacteremia) (unlabeled): 1 Gm every 8 hours.

Melioidosis *(Burkholderia pseudomallei)* (unlabeled): 1 Gm every 8 hours.

Mild to moderate infection, other severe infections (unlabeled): 500 mg to 1 Gm every 8 hours.

Complicated urinary tract infections (unlabeled): 500 mg to 1 Gm every 8 hours.

PEDIATRIC DOSE

30 to 120 mg/kg/day divided (10 to 40 mg/kg) every 8 hours depending on type and severity of infection. Maximum dose is 6 Gm/day. See Maternal/Child.

Complicated skin and skin structure infections in pediatric patients 3 months of age and older: 10 mg/kg every 8 hours. Maximum single dose every 8 hours is 500 mg. Increase dose to 20 mg/kg every 8 hours in complicated skin and skin structure infections caused by *P. aeruginosa*. Maximum single dose every 8 hours is 1 Gm.

Complicated intra-abdominal infections in pediatric patients 3 months of age and older: 20 mg/kg every 8 hours. Maximum single dose every 8 hours is 1 Gm.

Complicated intra-abdominal infections in pediatric patients under 3 months of age: Dose is based on gestational age (GA) and postnatal age (PNA).

Infants under 32 weeks GA and PNA under 2 weeks: 20 mg/kg every 12 hours.

Infants under 32 weeks GA and PNA 2 weeks and older: 20 mg/kg every 8 hours.

Infants 32 weeks and older GA and PNA under 2 weeks: 20 mg/kg every 8 hours.

Infants 32 weeks and older GA and PNA 2 weeks and older: 30 mg/kg every 8 hours.

Meningitis in pediatric patients over 3 months of age: 40 mg/kg every 8 hours. Maximum single dose every 8 hours is 2 Gm.

Febrile neutropenia in pediatric patients 3 months of age and older and less than 50 kg (unlabeled): 20 mg/kg every 8 hours. Maximum single dose is 1 Gm.

DOSE ADJUSTMENTS

Reduced dose required if CrCl is less than 51 mL/min based on the following chart.

Meropenem Recommended IV Dosage Schedule for Adults With Impaired Renal Function		
Creatinine Clearance (mL/min)	Dose (dependent on type of infection)	Dosing Interval
26–50 mL/min	Recommended dose	Every 12 hours
10–25 mL/min	One-half recommended dose	Every 12 hours
<10 mL/min	One-half recommended dose	Every 24 hours

Consult package insert or front matter of this text for formula to convert SCr to CrCl. ■ No dose adjustment necessary in impaired hepatic function. ■ Reduced dose may be required in the elderly based on decreased renal function. ■ Information is inadequate for use in patients on hemodialysis or peritoneal dialysis. ■ No experience in pediatric patients with renal impairment.

DILUTION

Injection: Reconstitute each 500 mg with 10 mL SWFI (1 Gm with 20 mL). Yields 50 mg/mL. Shake to dissolve and let stand until clear. May be given as an IV injection or further diluted with **compatible** infusion solutions (see Infusion and Compatibility).

Infusion: Available as a premixed solution ready for infusion and as infusion vials that may be directly reconstituted with a **compatible** solution and then infused. Concentration may range from 1 to 20 mg/mL. Do not use flexible container in series connections.

Storage: Store unopened vials (dry powder) at RT (20° to 25° C [68° to 77° F]). Use of freshly prepared solutions preferred. Injection vials reconstituted with SWFI for bolus administration (up to 50 mg/mL) may be stored for up to 3 hours at up to 25° C (77° F) or for 13 hours at up to 5° C (41° F). Solutions prepared for infusion with NS (concentrations ranging from 1 to 20 mg/mL) may be stored for 1 hour at up to 25° C (77° F) or for 15 hours at up to 5° C (41° F). Solutions prepared for infusion with D5W (concentrations ranging from 1 to 20 mg/mL) should be used immediately. Do not freeze.

COMPATIBILITY

Manufacturer states, "Meropenem should not be mixed or physically added to solutions containing other drugs; **compatibility** not established."

Other sources suggest specific **compatibilities** dependent on concentration and manufacturer; consult a pharmacist.

RATE OF ADMINISTRATION

IV injection in adults and pediatric patients over 3 months of age: A single dose (up to 1 Gm [20 mL] after dilution) over 3 to 5 minutes. (Limited safety data are available to support the administration of 40 mg/kg [up to a maximum of 2 Gm] bolus dose.)

Intermittent infusion in adults and pediatric patients over 3 months of age: A single dose over 15 to 30 minutes.

Intermittent infusion in pediatric patients under 3 months of age: A single dose over 30 minutes.

Extended infusion (unlabeled): 0.5 to 2 Gm over 3 hours every 8 hours.

ACTIONS

A synthetic, broad-spectrum, carbapenem antibiotic. Bactericidal to selected gram-negative, gram-positive, and anaerobic organisms. Bactericidal activity results from the inhibition of cell wall synthesis. Readily penetrates the cell wall of susceptible organisms to reach penicillin-binding protein targets. Has significant stability to hydrolysis by penicillinases and cephalosporinases produced by gram-positive and gram-negative bacteria. Peak plasma concentrations reached by the end of an infusion. Penetrates well into most body fluids and tissues, including cerebrospinal fluid. Peak fluid and tissue concentrations reached in 0.5 to 1.5 hours. Minimal protein binding. Elimination half-life averages 1 hour in adults, 1.5 hours in pediatric patients age 3 months to 2 years, and 2.7 hours in infants under 3 months of age. 70% recovered as unchanged drug in urine within 12 hours. Not yet known if it crosses the placental barrier. Secreted in breast milk.

INDICATIONS AND USES

Indicated as single-agent therapy for treatment of the specific infections caused by susceptible organisms. Is useful as presumptive therapy in the indicated infections before identification of the causative organism because of its broad spectrum of activity. ▪ Treatment of complicated intra-abdominal infections (e.g., complicated appendicitis, peritonitis) in adults and pediatric patients. ▪ Treatment of complicated skin and skin structure infections in adults and pediatric patients 3 months of age and older. ▪ Treatment of bacterial meningitis in pediatric patients 3 months of age and older. Meropenem has been found to be effective in eliminating concurrent bacteremia in association with bacterial meningitis.

Unlabeled uses: Empiric anti-infective therapy in febrile neutropenic patients. ▪ Meningitis in adults. ▪ Septicemia. ▪ Complicated urinary tract infections caused by susceptible bacteria. ▪ Bloodstream infections (gram-negative bacteremia). ▪ Respiratory tract infections. ▪ Alternative or concomitant therapy in melioidosis caused by *B. pseudomallei*.

CONTRAINDICATIONS

History of hypersensitivity to meropenem, its components, any other carbapenem antibiotic (e.g., imipenem-cilastatin [Primaxin]), or patients with demonstrated anaphylaxis to beta-lactams; see Precautions.

PRECAUTIONS

Specific sensitivity studies are indicated to determine susceptibility of the causative organism to meropenem. ▪ To reduce the development of drug-resistant bacteria and maintain its effectiveness, meropenem should be used to treat or prevent only those infections proven or strongly suspected to be caused by bacteria. ▪ May have cross-resistance with strains resistant to other carbapenems (e.g., imipenem-cilastatin [Primaxin]). ▪ Localized clusters of infections resulting from carbapenem-resistant bacteria have been reported in some regions. ▪ Serious and occasionally fatal hypersensitivity reactions have been reported in patients receiving therapy with beta-lactams (e.g., penicillins, cephalosporins, carbapenems). More likely in patients with a history of sensitivity to multiple allergens; obtain a careful history. Cross-sensitivity is possible. ▪ Severe cutaneous adverse reactions (SCAR) such as acute generalized exanthematous pustulosis (AGEP), drug reaction with eosinophilia and systemic symptoms (DRESS), erythema multiforme (EM), Stevens-Johnson syndrome (SJS), and toxic epidermal necrolysis (TEN) have been reported. ▪ Seizures and other adverse CNS reactions have been reported. Occurred most commonly in patients with a history of CNS disorders (e.g., brain lesions, history of seizures) or with bacterial meningitis and/or compromised renal function. Use extreme caution; continue administration of anticonvulsants in patients with known seizure disorders. ▪ Use with caution in patients with impaired renal function; thrombocytopenia may occur; see Dose Adjustments. ▪ Has the potential for neuromotor impairment (e.g., delirium, headaches, paresthesias, seizures) that can interfere with mental alertness and/or cause motor impairment; see Patient Education. ▪ Avoid prolonged use of drug; superinfection caused by overgrowth of nonsusceptible organisms may result. ▪ *Clostridium difficile*–associated diarrhea (CDAD) has been reported. May range from mild diarrhea to fatal colitis. Consider in patients who present with diarrhea during or after treatment with meropenem. ▪ See Drug/Lab Interactions.

Monitor: Anaphylaxis has been reported. Emergency equipment must always be available. ▪ Monitor infusion site for inflammation and/or extravasation. May cause thrombophlebitis. ▪ Monitor for S/S of CDAD. ▪ Monitor for S/S of severe SCAR. ▪ Monitor for S/S of CNS reactions (e.g., focal tremors, myoclonus, seizures); see Antidote. ▪ Monitor renal, hepatic, and hemopoietic systems in prolonged therapy. ▪ Each 1 Gm contains 3.92 mEq of sodium; monitoring of electrolytes may be indicated. ▪ See Drug/Lab Interactions and Side Effects.

Patient Education: Review all medications with physician. ▪ Report any itching, rash, shortness of breath, or twitching sensation immediately. ▪ Report any burning, pain, or stinging at injection site. ▪ Promptly report diarrhea or bloody stools that occur during treatment or up to several months after an antibiotic has been discontinued; may indicate CDAD and require treatment. ▪ Patients with a history of seizures should review medication profile with physician before taking meropenem; see Drug/Lab Interactions. ▪ May interfere with mental alertness and/or cause motor impairment. Do not operate machinery or drive until tolerance is established.

Maternal/Child: Safety for use in pregnancy not established; use only if clearly needed. ▪ Use caution during breast-feeding; no information is available on the effects of meropenem on the breast-fed infant or on milk production. ▪ Safety and effectiveness established for pediatric patients 3 months of age and older with complicated skin and skin structure infections and bacterial meningitis and for pediatric patients of all ages with complicated intra-abdominal infections.

Elderly: Consider age-related renal impairment; plasma clearance is decreased with decreased renal function; see Dose Adjustments. Monitoring of renal function is suggested. Response is similar to that seen in younger patients; however, greater sensitivity in the elderly cannot be ruled out. See Precautions.

DRUG/LAB INTERACTIONS

Carbapenems may reduce serum **valproic acid** or **divalproex sodium** concentrations to sub-therapeutic levels, resulting in a loss of seizure control. Monitor valproic acid levels. Consider alternative antibacterial therapy. If administration of meropenem is necessary, supplemental anticonvulsant therapy should be considered. ▪ **Probenecid** inhibits renal excretion and increases serum levels of meropenem, extending its half-life and increasing systemic exposure; coadministration is not recommended. ▪ May be synergistic with **aminoglycosides** against some isolates of *P. aeruginosa*.

SIDE EFFECTS

Toxicity rate is usually low. *Pediatric patients:* The types of clinical adverse effects seen in pediatric patients are similar to those seen in adults. The most commonly reported adverse effects included diarrhea, glossitis, nausea and vomiting, oral moniliasis, and rash (mostly diaper area moniliasis). In neonates and infants under 3 months of age, additional side effects that were reported irrespective of causality were convulsions, hyperbilirubinemia, and vomiting. *Adults:* Anemia, constipation, diarrhea, headache, nausea and vomiting, and rash are most common. Apnea, injection site reactions (e.g., edema, inflammation, pain, phlebitis), pruritus, sepsis, and shock also occurred in more than 1% of patients. Many other side effects—including CDAD; hypersensitivity reactions (including anaphylaxis); increases or decreases in hematologic, hepatic, and renal lab tests; neuromotor impairment; seizures; and thrombocytopenia—may occur in fewer than 1% of patients.

Post-Marketing: Acute generalized exanthematous pustulosis, agranulocytosis, angioedema, drug reaction with eosinophilia and systemic symptoms (DRESS), erythema multiforme, hemolytic anemia, leukopenia, neutropenia, positive direct or indirect Coombs' test, Stevens-Johnson syndrome, and toxic epidermal necrolysis have been reported.

ANTIDOTE

Notify physician of all side effects. Most treated symptomatically. Discontinue immediately if a hypersensitivity reaction occurs. Treat hypersensitivity reactions as indicated; may require epinephrine, airway management, oxygen, IV fluids, antihistamines, corticosteroids, and pressor amines. Discontinue meropenem immediately if S/S of severe cutaneous adverse reactions (SCAR) appear, and consider an alternative treatment. If focal tremors, myoclonus, or seizures occur, evaluate neurologically, initiate anticonvulsant therapy, and decide whether to decrease or discontinue meropenem. Mild cases of CDAD may respond to discontinuation of meropenem. Treat CDAD with fluids, electrolytes, protein supplements, and appropriate antibiotics (e.g., oral vancomycin) as indicated. In severe cases, surgical evaluation may be indicated. Readily removed by hemodialysis.

MEROPENEM AND VABORBACTAM FOR INJECTION

**Antibacterial
(Carbapenem/beta-lactamase inhibitor)**

(mer-oh-**PEN**-em va-bor-**BAK**-tam)

Vabomere

USUAL DOSE

4 Gm (2 Gm meropenem and 2 Gm vaborbactam) every 8 hours as an infusion over 3 hours. An estimated glomerular filtration rate (eGFR) of 50 mL/min/1.73 M^2 or greater is required. Duration of treatment is up to 14 days.

DOSE ADJUSTMENTS

Reduced dose may be indicated in the elderly based on age-related renal impairment.
- In patients with renal impairment who have an eGFR less than 50 mL/min/1.73 M^2, adjust dose as outlined in the following chart.

Dose Adjustments of Meropenem and Vaborbactam in Patients With Renal Impairment		
eGFR (mL/min/1.73 M^2)	**Recommended Dosage Regimen for Meropenem/Vaborbactam[a]**	**Dosing Interval**
30 to 49 mL/min/1.73 M^2	Meropenem and vaborbactam 2 Gm (1 Gm meropenem and 1 Gm vaborbactam)	Every 8 hours
15 to 29 mL/min/1.73 M^2	Meropenem and vaborbactam 2 Gm (1 Gm meropenem and 1 Gm vaborbactam)	Every 12 hours
Less than 15 mL/min/1.73 M^2	Meropenem and vaborbactam 1 Gm (0.5 Gm meropenem and 0.5 Gm vaborbactam)	Every 12 hours

[a]In patients maintained on hemodialysis, administer doses adjusted for renal impairment after the hemodialysis session.

DILUTION

Available as a dried powder in single-dose vials containing 2 Gm Vabomere (1 Gm meropenem and 1 Gm vaborbactam). Select the appropriate number of vials as determined from the following chart. To prepare the required dose for IV infusion, reconstitute each vial with 20 mL of NS by withdrawing the 20 mL from an infusion bag of NS. Reconstituted solution is **NOT** for direct injection and has a final volume of approximately 21.3 mL. Concentration of meropenem is approximately 0.05 Gm/mL, and concentration of vaborbactam is approximately 0.05 Gm/mL. Mix gently to dissolve. Immediately withdraw the full or partial reconstituted vial contents from each vial and add it back into the infusion bag of NS previously used as diluent. Solution will be colorless to light yellow.

Preparation of Meropenem and Vaborbactam Doses				
Meropenem and Vaborbactam Dose	**Number of Vials Required**	**Volume to Withdraw From Each Reconstituted Vial**	**Volume of Infusion Bag**	**Final Infusion Concentration of Meropenem and Vaborbactam**
4 Gm (2 Gm and 2 Gm)	2 vials	Entire contents (approximately 21 mL)	250 mL	16 mg/mL
			500 mL	8 mg/mL
			1,000 mL	4 mg/mL
2 Gm (1 Gm and 1 Gm)	1 vial	Entire contents (approximately 21 mL)	125 mL	16 mg/mL
			250 mL	8 mg/mL
			500 mL	4 mg/mL
1 Gm (0.5 Gm and 0.5 Gm)	1 vial	10.5 mL (discard unused portion)	70 mL	14.3 mg/mL
			125 mL	8 mg/mL
			250 mL	4 mg/mL

Filters: Specific information not available.

Storage: Store vials at CRT (20° to 25° C [68° to 77° F]). Excursions permitted to 15° to 30° C (59° to 86° F). Reconstituted solution must be further diluted immediately. Infusion of the fully diluted solution must be completed within 4 hours if stored at RT or 22 hours if refrigerated at 2° to 8° C (36° to 46° F). Discard unused portions.

COMPATIBILITY

Manufacturer states, "Only **compatible** with NS."

RATE OF ADMINISTRATION

A single dose as an infusion equally distributed over 3 hours.

ACTIONS

Meropenem and vaborbactam is a combination product that contains meropenem (a synthetic carbapenem antibacterial drug) and vaborbactam (a cyclic boronic acid beta-lactamase inhibitor). Bactericidal activity of meropenem results from the inhibition of cell wall synthesis. Meropenem is stable to hydrolysis by most beta-lactamases (including penicillinases and cephalosporinases produced by gram-negative and gram-positive bacteria), with the exception of carbapenem-hydrolyzing beta-lactamases. The vaborbactam component of meropenem and vaborbactam is a beta-lactamase inhibitor that protects meropenem from degradation by certain serine beta-lactamases such as *Klebsiella pneumoniae* carbapenemase (KPC). Vaborbactam does not have any antibacterial activity and does not decrease the activity of meropenem. Protein binding of the combination product is minimal. A minor pathway of meropenem elimination is hydrolysis of the beta-lactam ring. Vaborbactam does not undergo metabolism. The elimination half-life is 1.22 hours and 1.68 hours for meropenem and vaborbactam, respectively. Both are primarily excreted in urine. Meropenem is secreted in breast milk.

INDICATIONS AND USES

Treatment of patients 18 years of age and older with complicated urinary tract infections (cUTIs), including pyelonephritis caused by the following susceptible microorganisms: *Escherichia coli, K. pneumoniae,* and *Enterobacter cloacae* species complex.

CONTRAINDICATIONS

Known hypersensitivity to any components of the product (meropenem and vaborbactam) or to other drugs in the same class, or in patients who have demonstrated anaphylactic reactions to beta-lactam antibacterial drugs.

PRECAUTIONS

For IV infusion only; do not administer as an IV bolus. ▪ To reduce the development of drug-resistant bacteria and maintain its effectiveness, meropenem/vaborbactam should be used to treat only those infections proven or strongly suspected to be caused by bacteria. ▪ Specific sensitivity studies are indicated to determine susceptibility of the causative organism to meropenem and vaborbactam. ▪ No cross-resistance with other classes of antimicrobials has been identified. Some isolates resistant to carbapenems (including meropenem) and to cephalosporins may be susceptible to meropenem and vaborbactam. ▪ Serious and occasionally fatal hypersensitivity (anaphylactic) reactions and serious skin reactions have been reported in patients receiving beta-lactam antibacterial drugs. Before initiating therapy, check the history of previous hypersensitivity reactions to penicillins, cephalosporins, other beta-lactam antibacterial drugs, and other allergens. ▪ Seizures and other adverse CNS reactions have been reported with meropenem. Occurred most commonly in patients with a history of CNS disorders (e.g., brain lesions, history of seizures) or with bacterial meningitis and/or compromised renal function. Close monitoring, adherence to recommended dosing, and continuation of any prescribed anticonvulsant therapy are recommended in patients at risk for adverse CNS reactions. ▪ *Clostridium difficile*–associated diarrhea (CDAD) has been reported. May range from mild diarrhea to fatal colitis. Consider in patients who present with diarrhea during or after treatment with meropenem and vaborbactam. ▪ Thrombocytopenia has been observed in patients with renal impairment who have received meropenem; no clinical bleeding has been reported. ▪ Has the potential for neuromotor impairment (e.g., delirium, headaches, paresthesias, seizures) that can interfere with mental alertness and/or cause motor impairment; see Patient Education. ▪ Avoid prolonged use of drug; superinfection caused by overgrowth of nonsusceptible organisms may result. ▪ See Drug/Lab Interactions.

Monitor: Obtain baseline SCr and CBC with differential and platelets; repeat as indicated. ▪ Monitor serum creatinine and eGFR at least daily in patients with changing renal function, and adjust dosage accordingly. ▪ Monitor for S/S of hypersensitivity reactions (e.g., hypotension, rash, urticaria, tightness of the chest, wheezing). Anaphylaxis has occurred; emergency equipment, medications, and supplies must be available. ▪ If S/S of CNS reactions occur (e.g., focal tremors, myoclonus, seizures), evaluate neurologically, place on anticonvulsant therapy if not already instituted, and reexamine dose of meropenem and vaborbactam to determine if it should be decreased or discontinued.

Patient Education: Promptly report any itching, rash, shortness of breath, or twitching sensation. ▪ Report any burning, pain, or stinging at injection site. ▪ Promptly report diarrhea or bloody stools that occur during treatment or up to several months after meropenem and vaborbactam has been discontinued; may indicate CDAD and require treatment. ▪ Patients with a history of seizures should review medication profile with physician before taking meropenem and vaborbactam; see Drug/Lab Interactions. ▪ May interfere with mental alertness and/or cause motor impairment. Do not operate machinery or drive until tolerance is established.

Maternal/Child: Safety for use in pregnancy not established; benefit must justify potential risks to fetus. There is a drug-associated risk of major birth defects or miscarriages with meropenem and vaborbactam in pregnant females. Fetal malformations have been observed in vaborbactam-treated rabbits. ▪ Meropenem has been reported to be excreted in human milk. No information available on potential effects of meropenem and vaborbactam on breast-fed infants or on milk production. Consider risk versus benefit. ▪ Safety and effectiveness for use in pediatric patients not established.

Elderly: No overall differences in safety or effectiveness observed between the elderly and younger patients. Consider age-related renal impairment; plasma clearance is decreased with decreased renal function; see Dose Adjustments.

DRUG/LAB INTERACTIONS

Coadministration of carbapenems, including meropenem, to patients receiving **valproic acid** or **divalproex sodium** results in a reduction in valproic acid concentrations. Valproic acid concentrations may drop below the therapeutic range, increasing the risk of breakthrough seizures. Increasing the dose of valproic acid or divalproex sodium may not be sufficient to overcome the interaction. If coadministration is necessary, supplemental anticonvulsant therapy should be considered. ▪ **Probenecid** competes with meropenem for active tubular secretion, resulting in increased plasma concentrations of meropenem. Coadministration of probenecid with meropenem and vaborbactam is not recommended.

SIDE EFFECTS

The most common side effects reported are diarrhea, headache, and phlebitis/infusion site reactions. Fever, hypokalemia, increased ALT and AST, and nausea have also been reported, More serious side effects include breakthrough seizures due to drug interaction with valproic acid, CDAD, hypersensitivity reactions, and seizures and other adverse CNS experiences.

ANTIDOTE

Notify physician of any side effects. Most will be treated symptomatically. Discontinue immediately if a hypersensitivity reaction occurs and treat as appropriate (e.g., oxygen, antihistamines, epinephrine, corticosteroids, vasopressors, and/or fluids). If focal tremors, myoclonus, or seizures occur, evaluate neurologically, initiate anticonvulsant therapy, and decide whether to decrease or discontinue meropenem and vaborbactam. Mild cases of CDAD may respond to discontinuation of meropenem and vaborbactam. Treat CDAD with fluids, electrolytes, protein supplements, and appropriate antibiotics (e.g., oral vancomycin) as indicated. In severe cases, surgical evaluation may be indicated. Removed by hemodialysis.

MESNA
(**MEZ**-nah)

Mesnex, Uromitexan ✤

Antidote
Chemoprotective agent

pH 7.5 to 8.5

USUAL DOSE

Pretreatment: Verify pregnancy status. Specific testing recommended before each dose of ifosfamide; see Monitor.

Mesna: Total daily dose is 60% of the ifosfamide dose equally divided into 3 doses. A single dose of mesna equal to 20% of the ifosfamide dose is given at the time of the ifosfamide injection and repeated 4 hours and 8 hours later (e.g., ifosfamide 1.2 Gm/M^2 would require mesna 240 mg/M^2 with the ifosfamide, followed by additional doses of 240 mg/M^2 in 4 hours, and again at 8 hours). The initial mesna dose each day may be mixed with the ifosfamide. Appears to be **compatible**.

Combination of intravenous and oral doses: At the time of the ifosfamide injection, give a single IV dose of mesna equal to 20% of the ifosfamide dose. At 2 hours and at 6 hours after each dose of ifosfamide, administer mesna tablets PO in a dose equal to 40% of the ifosfamide dose (e.g., ifosfamide 1.2 Gm/M^2 would require mesna 240 mg/M^2 IV with the ifosfamide, followed by an oral mesna dose of 480 mg/M^2 in 2 hours and again at 6 hours). The total daily dose of mesna (IV [20%] and PO [80%] combined) is 100% of the ifosfamide dose; see Monitor. The efficacy and safety of this ratio of IV and oral mesna have not been established as being effective for daily doses of ifosfamide higher than 2 Gm/M^2.

DOSE ADJUSTMENTS

Dose of mesna must be repeated each day ifosfamide is administered and adjusted with each increase or decrease of the ifosfamide dose so that the ratio of mesna to ifosfamide remains the same.

DILUTION

Each 100 mg (1 mL) must be diluted in a minimum of 4 mL D5W, D5NS, D5/^{1}/$_4$NS, D5/^{1}/$_3$NS, D5/^{1}/$_2$NS, NS, or LR. Desired concentration is 20 mg/mL.

Filters: Manufacturer's studies measured the potency of ifosfamide in combination with mesna through a 5-micron filter. No significant drug loss for ifosfamide; mesna was not measured.

Storage: Store at CRT before use. Opened multidose vials may be stored at CRT and used for up to 8 days. Diluted solutions are stable for 24 hours at 25° C (77° F).

COMPATIBILITY

Manufacturer states, "Do not mix mesna injection with cyclophosphamide carboplatin, cisplatin, epirubicin, and nitrogen mustard. The benzyl alcohol contained in mesna injection can reduce the stability of ifosfamide. Ifosfamide and mesna may be mixed in the same bag provided the final concentration of ifosfamide does not exceed 50 mg/mL. Higher concentrations of ifosfamide may not be compatible with mesna and may reduce the stability of ifosfamide."

Other sources suggest specific **compatibilities** dependent on concentration and manufacturer; consult a pharmacist.

RATE OF ADMINISTRATION

A single dose over a minimum of 1 minute given as a single agent. Administer at rate for ifosfamide if given together. Another source recommends administering as an infusion over 15 to 30 minutes or as a continuous infusion maintained for 12 to 24 hours after completion of the ifosfamide infusion.

ACTIONS

A detoxifying agent. Reacts chemically with urotoxic ifosfamide metabolites to detoxify them and inhibit hemorrhagic cystitis. Is distributed to total body water (plasma, extracellular fluid, and intracellular water). Rapidly metabolized in the plasma to its major metabolite mesna disulfide (dimesna). Half-life is 0.36 hours. Excreted in the urine as mesna and dimesna.

INDICATIONS AND USES

A prophylactic agent used to reduce the incidence of hemorrhagic cystitis caused by ifosfamide.

Unlabeled uses: May reduce the incidence of hemorrhagic cystitis caused by cyclophosphamide.

CONTRAINDICATIONS

Hypersensitivity to mesna or any of the excipients.

PRECAUTIONS

Hypersensitivity reactions ranging from mild to anaphylaxis have been reported. May occur after the first dose or after several months of exposure. ▪ Dermatologic toxicity, including drug rash with eosinophilia and systemic symptoms (DRESS), Stevens-Johnson syndrome (SJS), or toxic epidermal necrolysis (TEN), has been reported. Other skin and mucosal reactions characterized by angioedema, erythema, periorbital edema, pruritus, rash, stomatitis, and urticaria have also been reported. May occur after the first dose or after several months of exposure. ▪ Mesna is a thiol compound. Hypersensitivity reactions to mesna and to amifostine, another thiol compound, have been reported. It is unclear whether patients who experience an adverse reaction to a thiol compound are at increased risk for a hypersensitivity reaction to mesna. Repeated doses are required to maintain adequate levels of mesna in the kidneys and bladder to detoxify urotoxic ifosfamide metabolites. ▪ Hemorrhagic cystitis caused by ifosfamide is dose dependent. Mesna is most effective when ifosfamide dose is less than 1.2 Gm/M²/24 hr and is somewhat less effective when ifosfamide dose is 2 to 4 Gm/M²/24 hr. If hematuria develops with appropriate doses of mesna, ifosfamide dose may need to be reduced or discontinued. ▪ Does not inhibit any other side effects or toxicities caused by ifosfamide therapy. ▪ Not effective in preventing hematuria caused by other conditions (e.g., thrombocytopenia).

Monitor: Maintain adequate hydration and sufficient urinary output as required for ifosfamide treatment. ▪ Before administering each dose of ifosfamide, obtain a morning specimen of urine and test for hematuria. Depending on the severity of the hematuria, dose reduction or discontinuation of ifosfamide may be required. ▪ If emesis occurs within 2 hours of taking PO mesna, either repeat the PO dose or administer an IV dose. ▪ Monitor for S/S of a hypersensitivity reaction (e.g., acute renal impairment, angioedema, arthralgia, cardiovascular symptoms [hypotension, tachycardia], disseminated intravascular coagulation [DIC], fever, hematologic abnormalities, hypoxia, increased liver enzymes, myalgia, nausea, respiratory distress, urticaria, vomiting). ▪ Monitor for S/S of dermatologic toxicity.

Patient Education: Read FDA-approved patient information. ▪ Verify pregnancy status of females of reproductive potential before initiating therapy. Effective contraception required during treatment with mesna in combination with ifosfamide and for at least 6 months after the last dose. ▪ Advise males with female partners of reproductive potential to use effective contraception during treatment with mesna in combination with ifosfamide and for at least 3 months after the last dose. ▪ Drink at least one to two liters of liquid daily. ▪ Report pink or red urine immediately. Mesna does not prevent hemorrhagic cystitis in all patients and does not prevent or alleviate any of the other adverse reactions associated with ifosfamide. ▪ Take mesna at prescribed times. Report emesis within 2 hours of taking PO mesna. ▪ Promptly report any S/S of a hypersensitivity or dermatologic reaction.

Maternal/Child: Mesna is used in combination with ifosfamide or other cytotoxic agents. Ifosfamide can cause fetal harm when administered to a pregnant woman; see ifosfamide prescribing information for use during pregnancy and lactation. Use during pregnancy only if benefits clearly outweigh risks. ▪ Avoid breast-feeding during treatment and for 1 week after the last dose of mesna or ifosfamide. ▪ Multidose vial contains benzyl alcohol. Serious adverse reactions, including fatal reactions and the "gasping syndrome," have occurred in premature neonates and low-birth-weight infants who have received benzyl alcohol. Do not use in neonates or infants.

Elderly: Dosing should be cautious; however, the ratio of ifosfamide to mesna should remain the same.

DRUG/LAB INTERACTIONS

No clinical drug interactions studies have been conducted. May interfere with several laboratory studies. May cause a false-positive reaction for **urinary ketones.** If a red-violet color develops, glacial acetic acid returns the coloring to violet. ■ May cause a false-negative test for **enzymatic CPK activity.** ■ May cause a false-positive test for **urinary ascorbic acid.**

SIDE EFFECTS

The most common adverse reactions (greater than 10%) when mesna is given with ifosfamide are abdominal pain, alopecia, anemia, anorexia, asthenia, constipation, diarrhea, fatigue, fever, granulocytopenia, headache, leukopenia, nausea, somnolence thrombocytopenia, and vomiting. Less frequently reported reactions include anxiety, back pain, chest pain, confusion, coughing, dehydration, dizziness, dyspepsia, dyspnea, edema, flushing, hematuria, hypersensitivity reactions, hypokalemia, hypotension, injection site reactions, insomnia, pain, pallor, pneumonia, sweating, tachycardia.

Post-Marketing: Convulsions, dysgeusia, hemoptysis, hepatitis, hypertension.

Overdose: Diarrhea, fever, hypersensitivity reactions (including asthma exacerbation), flushing, mild hypotension, rash, shortness of breath, and vomiting.

ANTIDOTE

No specific antidote. Keep physician informed of all side effects. Discontinue mesna and provide supportive care at the first S/S of a significant hypersensitivity or dermatologic reaction. Resuscitate as necessary.

METHOCARBAMOL
(meth-oh-**KAR**-bah-mohl)

Skeletal muscle relaxant (central acting)

Robaxin

pH 3.5 to 6

USUAL DOSE

Dose and frequency should be based on severity of condition and on therapeutic response.

1 Gm (10 mL) every 8 hours for no more than 3 days.

If condition persists, may be repeated after a drug-free interval of 48 hours if indicated.

PEDIATRIC DOSE

Not recommended for pediatric patients under 12 years of age except in tetanus.

DILUTION

May be given undiluted, or a single dose may be given as an IV infusion diluted in no more than 250 mL NS or D5W.

Storage: Store at CRT. Do not refrigerate after dilution.

COMPATIBILITY

Compatibility information not available from manufacturer; consult a pharmacist.

RATE OF ADMINISTRATION

300 mg (3 mL) or fraction thereof over 1 minute or longer. Administer IV infusion while in recumbent position and maintain position for 10 to 15 minutes after infusion.

ACTIONS

A CNS depressant with sedative and musculoskeletal relaxant properties. Exact mode of action is unknown. Diminishes skeletal muscle hyperactivity without altering normal muscle tone. Widely distributed throughout the body. Metabolized in the liver and excreted in the urine.

INDICATIONS AND USES
Relief of discomfort from acute, painful musculoskeletal conditions. Adjunctive to other measures (e.g., rest, physical therapy). ▪ Treatment of neuromuscular manifestations of tetanus. Adjunctive to other measures (e.g., tetanus antitoxin, fluid and electrolyte replacement).

CONTRAINDICATIONS
Hypersensitivity to methocarbamol, known or suspected renal pathology.

PRECAUTIONS
Blood aspirated into syringe will not mix with medication; an expected phenomenon. ▪ Use caution in known or suspected epileptic patients. ▪ In patients with impaired renal function, polyethylene glycol 300 (a component of methocarbamol) may increase pre-existing acidosis and urea retention. Usually occurs with amounts greater than the amount contained in this product. ▪ Vial stopper contains latex. May cause hypersensitivity reactions when handled by or administered to persons with known or suspected latex sensitivity.

Monitor: Observe site of injection continuously. A hypertonic solution; extravasation may cause thrombophlebitis or sloughing. ▪ Keep patient in recumbent position for at least 15 minutes to avoid postural hypotension. ▪ Monitor renal function if duration of treatment is 3 or more days. ▪ See Drug/Lab Interactions.

Patient Education: Avoid alcohol or other CNS depressants. ▪ May cause dizziness, drowsiness, and visual disturbances. Request assistance for ambulation. ▪ Use caution in any task that requires alertness. ▪ Report fever, itching, nasal congestion, or rash promptly. ▪ Urine may discolor to very dark green.

Maternal/Child: Category C: use caution in pregnancy and breast-feeding. Safety for use not established. American Academy of Pediatrics considers it **compatible** with breast-feeding. ▪ There have been rare reports of fetal and congenital abnormalities following in utero exposure to methocarbamol.

Elderly: Males may have sensitivity to anticholinergic effects (e.g., dry mouth, urinary retention). ▪ Consider age-related renal impairment; may preclude use.

DRUG/LAB INTERACTIONS
Potentiated by alcohol, **CNS depressants, MAO inhibitors, and phenothiazines.** ▪ May inhibit the effect of **pyridostigmine.** Use with caution in patients with myasthenia gravis who are receiving anticholinesterase agents. ▪ May interfere with some laboratory tests **(5-HIAA, VMA).**

SIDE EFFECTS
Infrequent but more often associated with too-rapid injection. Blurred vision, conjunctivitis, diplopia, dizziness, drowsiness, fainting, fever, flushing, headache, hypotension, GI upset, light-headedness, metallic taste, muscular incoordination, nasal congestion, nystagmus, pruritus, rash, urticaria, vertigo.

Major: Anaphylactic reaction, bradycardia, convulsions, pain at injection site, sloughing at injection site, syncope, thrombophlebitis.

ANTIDOTE
Notify the physician of minor side effects. If these side effects progress or major side effects occur, discontinue the drug, notify the physician, and treat symptomatically. Supportive measures may include maintenance of an adequate airway, monitoring of urinary output and VS, and administration of IV fluids. Epinephrine, steroids, and antihistamines should be readily available. Resuscitate as necessary.

METHOTREXATE SODIUM BBW
(meth-oh-**TREKS**-ayt **SO**-dee-um)

Antineoplastic (antimetabolite)
Antipsoriatic
Antirheumatic

Methotrexate PF, MTX   pH 8.5

USUAL DOSE
Pretreatment: Baseline studies indicated; see Monitor. Verify pregnancy status; see Contraindications.

Many dose limitations based on patient condition, renal and hepatic function, and concomitant drugs or therapies; see Precautions/Monitor. Doses between 100 and 500 mg/M^2 *may require* leucovorin calcium rescue. Doses over 500 mg/M^2 *require* leucovorin calcium rescue; see leucovorin calcium or levoleucovorin (Fusilev) monograph. Part of numerous protocols that change as new advances in antileukemic therapy and other cancers are developed. Selections from those protocols are included in the following text.

Acute lymphoblastic leukemia: Induction: 3.3 mg/M^2 in combination with prednisone 60 mg/M^2. Give daily if tolerated, and continue for up to 8 weeks or until satisfactory response (usually 4 to 6 weeks). Usually given PO.

Maintenance: Dose individualized; 15 mg/M^2/dose administered 2 times weekly IM or PO (a total weekly dose of 30 mg/M^2) or 2.5 mg/kg IV every 14 days has been used.

Mycosis fungoides: 5 to 50 mg once weekly in the early stages of disease. Adjust dose or discontinue as indicated by patient response and hematologic monitoring. 15 to 37.5 mg twice weekly may be used in patients who respond poorly to weekly therapy. Usually given PO or IM, but combination chemotherapy regimens, including higher doses of IV methotrexate with leucovorin calcium rescue, have been used in advanced stages of the disease.

Breast cancer (unlabeled): One regimen administers methotrexate 40 mg/M^2 on Days 1 and 8 of each cycle. Given in combination with PO cyclophosphamide 100 mg/M^2 on Days 1 through 14 of each cycle and fluorouracil 600 mg/M^2 on Days 1 and 8 of each cycle. In patients over 60 years of age, reduce the initial methotrexate dose to 30 mg/M^2 and the initial fluorouracil dose to 400 mg/M^2. Repeat monthly (allows a 2-week rest period between cycles) for 6 to 12 cycles.

Psoriasis: 10 to 25 mg once a week until adequate response. Some references suggest an initial test dose of 5 to 10 mg/week before initiating therapy to detect sensitivity to adverse reactions. Sources suggest 30 mg/week as a maximum dose. Use smallest effective dose. Usually given PO or IM. May be used in combination with infliximab; see infliximab monograph.

Osteosarcoma: One regimen recommends 12 Gm/M^2 as a single dose given as an infusion over 4 hours. Begin the fourth week after surgery and repeat weekly at Weeks 5, 6, 7, 11, 12, 15, 16, 29, 30, 44, and 45. A peak serum concentration of 1,000 micromolars/L at the end of the infusion is desired. Dose may be increased to 15 Gm/M^2 if required. Must be accompanied by leucovorin calcium rescue; see leucovorin calcium or levoleucovorin (Fusilev) monograph. Leucovorin calcium may be given IV or PO; levoleucovorin is IV only. When methotrexate is given in combination with leucovorin rescue, the serum creatinine must be normal, and creatinine clearance must be greater than 60 mL/min before beginning therapy. *Osteosarcoma also requires combination chemotherapy.* Protocols vary but may include methotrexate in combination with doxorubicin, with cisplatin, and with the combination of bleomycin, cyclophosphamide, and dactinomycin (BCD regimen). These massive doses are highly individualized and require exacting calculations and constant patient monitoring; see Precautions/Monitor.

PEDIATRIC DOSE

Safety for use in pediatric patients is limited to chemotherapy and in polyarticular-course juvenile rheumatoid arthritis. May contain benzyl alcohol; not recommended for use in neonates. See Maternal/Child.

DOSE ADJUSTMENTS

Manufacturer does not provide information on dose adjustment in patients with impaired renal or hepatic function. However, various recommendations are available in the literature. In patients with impaired hepatic function, one source recommends administering 75% of dose if bilirubin is between 3.1 and 5 or if transaminases are greater than 3 times the ULN; if bilirubin above 5, omit dose. ■ Reduced doses may be required in patients with impaired renal function. Suggested guidelines are to administer 50% of a dose with a CrCl of 10 to 50 mL/min, and avoid use with a CrCl of less than 10 mL/min in adult patients. In pediatric patients, administer 50% of a dose with a CrCl of 10 to 50 mL/min and 30% of a dose with a CrCl of less than 10 mL/min/1.73 M^2. ■ Reduced dose may be required in patients with ascites or pleural effusions, in the very young or very elderly, in the debilitated, and in other diseases; see Precautions. ■ Often used with other antineoplastic drugs to achieve tumor remission. ■ See Drug/Lab Interactions.

DILUTION

Specific techniques required; see Precautions. Available in solution or as a lyophilized powder. Reconstitute powder with D5W or NS. The 1-Gm vial should be reconstituted with 19.4 mL to a concentration of 50 mg/mL. When high-dose methotrexate is administered by IV infusion, the total dose is diluted in D5W. 25 mg/mL is the maximum suggested concentration that can be given IV. Reconstitution of each 5 mg with 2 mL of preservative-free D5W or NS is suggested. Each milliliter equals 2.5 mg of methotrexate. Available in preservative-free solution. Do not use formulations or diluents with preservatives (e.g., bacteriostatic) for high-dose therapy or intrathecal injection. 1-Gm vial available for high-dose use with appropriate dilution. Not usually added to IV solutions when given in smaller doses (less than 100 mg). Discard solution if a precipitate forms. May be given through Y-tube of a free-flowing IV.

A single dose may be further diluted with D5W or NS immediately before use as an infusion with higher (100 mg or more) methotrexate doses.

Filters: No data available from manufacturer. Another source indicates no significant drug loss filtered through a nylon 0.2-micron filter.

Storage: Store in unopened container at CRT; protect from light. If prepared without a preservative, use immediately. May be stable up to 24 hours with a preservative.

COMPATIBILITY

Compatibility information not available from manufacturer. Other sources suggest specific **compatibilities** dependent on concentration and manufacturer; consult a pharmacist.

RATE OF ADMINISTRATION

IV injection: Slow IV push no more than 10 mg/minute.

Infusion: A single dose equally distributed over 30 minutes to 4 hours or as prescribed by protocol.

ACTIONS

An antimetabolite and folic acid antagonist. Inhibits dihydrofolic acid reductase. Cell cycle–specific for the S phase. It interferes with DNA synthesis, repair, and cellular replication. Rapidly proliferating tissues are more sensitive to this effect. Widely distributed and is approximately 50% protein bound. Undergoes some hepatic and intracellular metabolism. Half-life is dose dependent and is 3 to 10 hours in patients receiving low-dose antineoplastic therapy and 8 to 15 hours in patients receiving high-dose methotrexate therapy. 80% to 90% of the administered dose is excreted unchanged in the urine within 24 hours. Clearance rates decrease with higher doses. Does not cross blood-brain barrier. Secreted in breast milk.

INDICATIONS AND USES

Used for life-threatening neoplastic disease alone or in combination with other anticancer agents in the treatment of acute lymphocytic leukemia, breast cancer, epidermal tumors of the head and neck, small-cell and squamous cell lung cancer, non-Hodgkin lymphoma, advanced mycosis fungoides (cutaneous T-cell lymphoma). ▪ Severe, recalcitrant disabling psoriasis or rheumatoid arthritis unresponsive to other treatment. Diagnosis of psoriasis should be established by biopsy and/or dermatology consultation before use. ▪ To prolong relapse-free survival in patients with nonmetastatic osteosarcoma who have undergone surgical resection or amputation of the primary tumor. Given as a high-dose regimen with leucovorin rescue in combination with other chemotherapeutic agents. ▪ Given PO or IM for early-stage mycosis fungoides, trophoblastic diseases (gestational choriocarcinoma, chorioadenoma destruens, and hydatidiform mole), polyarticular-course juvenile rheumatoid arthritis, rheumatoid arthritis, and other diagnoses, and given intrathecally for treatment and prophylaxis of meningeal leukemia.

Unlabeled uses: Treatment of bladder and testicular cancer. Treatment of soft tissue sarcomas and CNS tumors. Management of Crohn's disease and ectopic pregnancy and prevention of acute graft-versus-host disease. High-dose regimens for neoplastic diseases other than osteosarcoma are investigational, and therapeutic efficacy is not established.

CONTRAINDICATIONS

Hypersensitivity to methotrexate; breast-feeding mothers. Contraindicated in pregnant females with psoriasis or rheumatoid arthritis and should be used during pregnancy for treatment of neoplastic diseases only when the potential benefit outweighs the risk to the fetus. Contraindicated in psoriasis or rheumatoid arthritis patients with immunodeficiency syndromes, pre-existing blood dyscrasias (e.g., bone marrow hypoplasia, leukopenia, thrombocytopenia, significant anemia), alcoholism, alcoholic liver disease, or other chronic liver disease.

PRECAUTIONS

Follow guidelines for handling cytotoxic agents. See Appendix A, p. 1308. ▪ Administered by or under the direction of the physician specialist. ▪ Methotrexate should be used only in life-threatening neoplastic diseases or in patients with psoriasis or rheumatoid arthritis with severe, recalcitrant, disabling disease that is not responsive to other forms of therapy. ▪ Deaths have been reported with methotrexate use in the treatment of malignancy, psoriasis, and rheumatoid arthritis. ▪ Methotrexate elimination is reduced in patients with impaired renal function, ascites, or pleural effusions. Careful monitoring, dose reduction and, in some cases, discontinuation of therapy are required; consider evacuating excess fluid from ascites and pleural effusions before treatment if possible. ▪ Methotrexate can suppress hematopoiesis, causing anemia, aplastic anemia, pancytopenia, leukopenia, neutropenia, and/or thrombocytopenia. ▪ Serious and sometimes fatal bone marrow suppression, aplastic anemia, and GI toxicity have been reported with concomitant use of methotrexate (usually high doses) and some NSAIDs; see Drug/Lab Interactions. ▪ Leukoencephalopathy has been reported in patients who have received both IV methotrexate and craniospinal irradiation. ▪ A transient stroke-like encephalopathy has been reported with high-dose methotrexate therapy. Symptoms may include confusion, hemiparesis, transient blindness, seizures, and coma. ▪ Methotrexate-induced lung disease, including acute or chronic interstitial pneumonitis, may occur at any time, may occur even with low doses, and has been fatal. Patients may present with fever, dry cough, dyspnea, hypoxemia, and an infiltrate on chest x-ray. May require interruption of therapy and is not always fully reversible. ▪ Severe skin reactions can occur at any time and have been fatal. ▪ Transient elevations in liver enzymes may occur early during treatment. Chronic hepatotoxicity (fibrosis and cirrhosis) occurs more frequently with prolonged use and a total dose of at least 1.5 Gm. Persistent abnormalities in liver function tests and/or depression of serum albumin may be indicators of serious liver toxicity. Has resulted in deaths; see Monitor. ▪ Use with extreme caution in patients with ascites, bone marrow suppression, folate deficiency, GI obstruction, impaired renal or liver function, infection, peptic ulcer, pleural effusion, or ulcerative colitis; in debilitated patients; and in the very young or very elderly. ■ Diarrhea and ulcerative stomatitis will require interrupting therapy; otherwise hemorrhagic enteritis and death from intestinal perforation may occur. ■ Tumor lysis syndrome may occur, and S/S include hyperkalemia, hyperphosphatemia, hyperuricemia, hypocalcemia, metabolic acidosis, urate crystalluria, and renal failure. Prevent or alleviate tumor lysis syndrome with appropriate supportive and pharmacologic measures; see Monitor. ■ Potentially fatal opportunistic infections, especially *Pneumocystis jiroveci* pneumonia, may occur. ■ Risk of soft tissue necrosis and osteonecrosis may be increased with concomitant use of methotrexate and radiotherapy. ■ May cause renal damage that may lead to acute renal failure. Nonreversible oliguric renal failure is likely to develop in patients who experience delayed early methotrexate elimination. ■ Malignant lymphomas have been reported. May occur in patients receiving low-dose methotrexate and may not require cytotoxic treatment; discontinue methotrexate first and initiate appropriate treatment if the lymphoma does not regress. ■ Use caution when administering high-dose methotrexate to patients receiving proton pump inhibitors. ■ Use caution when administering methotrexate after a recent history of nitrous oxide administration. ■ Lesions of psoriasis may be aggravated by concomitant exposure to UV radiation. ■ Radiation dermatitis and sunburn may be "recalled" by methotrexate use. ■ See Drug Interactions.

Monitor: CBC with differential and platelet counts, chest x-ray, and renal and liver function tests before, during, and after therapy are essential to comprehensive treatment. ■ Close patient observation is mandatory. Course of therapy is not repeated until all signs of toxicity from the previous course subside. ■ Monitor closely for bone marrow, liver, lung, kidney, and skin toxicities. ■ Nadir of leukocyte and platelet count usually occurs after 7 to 10 days, with recovery 7 days later. ■ Liver biopsy, pulmonary studies, and bone marrow studies may be indicated in high-dose or long-term therapy. ■ Monitor renal function closely; verify by measurement of serum methotrexate and CrCl levels; see Precautions. Maintain continuing adequate hydration and urine alkalinization. ■ Prevention and treatment of hyperuricemia due to tumor lysis syndrome may be accomplished with adequate hydration and, if necessary, uric acid–lowering drugs (e.g., allopurinol). ■ Monitor serum methotrexate levels. ■ Use prophylactic antiemetics to reduce nausea and vomiting and increase patient comfort. ■ Observe closely for signs of infection. Prophylactic antibiotics may be indicated pending results of C/S in a febrile neutropenic patient. ■ Profound granulocytopenia and fever should be evaluated immediately and usually requires parenteral broad-spectrum antibiotic therapy. ■ Monitor for thrombocytopenia (platelet count less than 50,000/mm^3). Initiate precautions to prevent excessive bleeding (e.g., inspect IV sites, skin, and mucous membranes; use extreme care during invasive procedures; test urine, emesis, stool, and secretions for occult blood). ■ *Administration of high-dose methotrexate* requires the following: a WBC count greater than 1,500/mm^3, neutrophil count greater than 200/mm^3, platelet count greater than 75,000/mm^3, serum bilirubin less than 1.2 mg/dL, alanine aminotransferase (ALT) level less than 450 units, healing of any mucositis, ascites or pleural effusion must be drained dry, normal SCr, CrCl greater than 60 mL/min, 1 L/M^2 of IV fluid over 6 hours before dosing and 3 L/M^2/day on day of infusion and for 2 days after, alkalinization of urine with sodium bicarbonate to maintain pH above 7, and repeat serum methotrexate and SCr levels at least daily until methotrexate level is below 0.05 micromolar. ■ See Drug/Lab Interactions.

Patient Education: Avoid pregnancy. Effective contraception recommended for both females and males. Continue for at least 3 months after treatment is complete in male patients and for at least one ovulatory cycle after therapy is complete for female patients. ■ Avoid alcohol and take only prescribed medications. Reactions can be lethal. ■ Side effects such as dizziness and fatigue may interfere with ability to drive or operate machinery. ■ Review early signs and symptoms of toxicity with health care provider. ■ Close follow-up with physician is imperative. ■ See Appendix D, p. 1311.

Maternal/Child: Category X: avoid pregnancy. Has caused fetal death and congenital anomalies; effective contraception recommended. ■ Discontinue breast-feeding. ■ Safety for use in pediatric patients established for cancer chemotherapy and polyarticular-course juvenile rheumatoid arthritis. ▪ Serious neurotoxicity (e.g., general or focal seizures) has been reported in patients with acute lymphoblastic leukemia who have been treated with intermediate-dose methotrexate. ▪ Administration of formulations containing the preservative benzyl alcohol has been associated with fatal gasping syndrome in neonates. Use preservative-free formulation of methotrexate in neonates.

Elderly: See Dose Adjustments. Dose selection should be cautious and based on the potential for decreased organ function, decreased folate stores, and concomitant disease or drug therapy. ▪ Consider monitoring CrCl and methotrexate levels. ▪ Monitor for early signs of hepatic, renal, or bone marrow toxicity. ▪ In chronic administration, certain toxicities may be decreased by folate supplementation. ▪ Post-marketing experience suggests that the occurrence of bone marrow suppression, thrombocytopenia, and pneumonitis may increase with age.

DRUG/LAB INTERACTIONS

The following drugs may enhance methotrexate toxicity when administered concomitantly: **cyclosporine**, **any hepatotoxic drug** (e.g., azathioprine, retinoids, sulfasalazine), **NSAIDs** (e.g., ibuprofen, ketoprofen, naproxen), **penicillins** (e.g., amoxicillin, nafcillin), **probenecid, salicylates, sulfonamides, phenylbutazone, phenytoin, pyrimethamine, trimethoprim** (component of sulfamethoxazole/trimethoprim), **and vancomycin** (given up to 10 days prior to methotrexate); interactions may be life threatening. Monitoring serum levels and/or reduced doses of methotrexate may be indicated or a longer duration of leucovorin calcium rescue may be required. One source suggests delaying administration of aspirin, NSAIDs, and probenecid for 48 hours after larger doses of methotrexate; see Precautions. ▪ **NSAIDs** are used in the treatment of rheumatoid arthritis in combination with low doses of methotrexate (e.g., 7.5 to 15 mg/week). Do not administer NSAIDs before or concomitantly with high doses of methotrexate (e.g., treatment of osteosarcoma); deaths from severe hematologic and GI toxicity have been reported. ▪ Use caution if high-dose methotrexate is administered in combination with **nephrotoxic chemotherapy agents** (e.g., cisplatin). ▪ Concurrent use of methotrexate (primarily at high dose) with **some proton pump inhibitors** such as esomeprazole, omeprazole, and pantoprazole may cause prolonged elevation of serum levels of methotrexate and its metabolite, hydroxymethotrexate, leading to toxicity. Discontinue several days before methotrexate administration. Consider an H_2 antagonist. ▪ **Doxycycline** may increase toxicity of methotrexate in high-dose regimens. ▪ **Vitamins with folic acid** or its derivatives may inhibit the antifolate effects of methotrexate, decreasing effectiveness. ▪ Use of **nitrous oxide anesthesia** results in the potential for increased toxicity such as myelosuppression, neurotoxicity, and stomatitis. Avoid concomitant administration with methotrexate. ▪ May increase serum levels of **mercaptopurine**; dose adjustment may be required. ▪ Do not administer **live virus vaccines** to patients receiving antineoplastic drugs. ▪ **Procarbazine** may increase nephrotoxicity of methotrexate. Allow 72 hours between last dose of procarbazine and first dose of methotrexate. ▪ Monitor for signs of increased bone marrow suppression with **sulfonamides** (e.g., sulfisoxazole, SMZ-TMP), **bone marrow–suppressing agents** (e.g., antineoplastics), **and radiation therapy.** May also cause SMZ-TMP-induced megaloblastic anemia. ▪ May decrease **theophylline** clearance and increase serum levels; monitor theophylline serum levels with concurrent use. ▪ **Urinary alkalinizers** increase renal excretion and may reduce effectiveness.

SIDE EFFECTS

Toxicity usually dose related. Death can occur from average doses, high doses, drug interactions (e.g., NSAIDs), bone marrow toxicity, GI toxicity, hepatic toxicity, pulmonary toxicity, and/or severe skin reactions. Abdominal distress, chills, decreased resistance to infection, dizziness, fatigue, fever, leukopenia, malaise, nausea, and ulcerative stomatitis occur most frequently. Other side effects reported include abortion (spontaneous), acne, acute hepatitis, agranulocytosis, alopecia, alveolitis, anaphylaxis, anemia, anorexia, aplastic anemia, azotemia, blurred vision, chronic fibrosis and cirrhosis, convulsions, COPD, cystitis, decreased serum albumin, defective oogenesis or spermatogenesis, diabetes, diarrhea, drowsiness, ecchymosis, enteritis, eosinophilia, erythema multiforme, erythematous rashes, exfoliative dermatitis, fetal defects or death, furunculosis, GI ulceration and bleeding, gingivitis, gynecomastia, headache, hematemesis, hematuria, hemiparesis, hepatic failure, hepatotoxicity, hypotension, infertility, interstitial pneumonitis, liver enzyme elevations, lymphadenopathy and lymphoproliferative disorders, melena (passage of dark, tarry stools), menstrual dysfunction, nephropathy (severe), neutropenia, oligospermia (transient), opportunistic infections (e.g., cryptococcosis, cytomegalovirus infection, disseminated *H. simplex*, herpes zoster, histoplasmosis, *H. simplex* hepatitis, nocardiosis, *P. jiroveci* pneumonia, pneumonia, sepsis [including fatal]), pancreatitis, pancytopenia, paresis, pericardial effusion, pericarditis, pharyngitis, photosensitivity, pigmentary changes, proteinuria, pruritus, pseudomembranous colitis, renal failure, respiratory failure, respiratory fibrosis, serious visual changes of unknown etiology, skin necrosis, skin ulceration, speech impairment (aphasia, dysarthria), Stevens-Johnson syndrome, stomatitis, stress fracture, suppressed hematopoiesis (blood cell formation), telangiectasia, thrombocytopenia, thromboembolic events (e.g., arterial thrombosis, cerebral thrombosis, deep vein thrombosis, pulmonary embolus, retinal vein thrombosis, thrombophlebitis), sudden death, toxic epidermal necrolysis, transient blindness, tumor lysis syndrome, urticaria, vaginal discharge, vomiting. Many other rarer side effects, including anaphylactoid reactions, have been reported.

ANTIDOTE

Discontinue methotrexate and notify the physician of any side effects. **Leucovorin calcium (citrovorum factor, folinic acid)** may be given PO, IM, or IV promptly to counteract inadvertent overdose. Leucovorin calcium is also indicated as a planned rescue mechanism for large doses of methotrexate required to treat some malignancies. Doses equal to dose of methotrexate are frequently required. Should be given within 1 hour in overdose, 24 hours in rescue. See specific process for overdose and for rescue for high-dose MTX in leucovorin calcium monograph. Doses up to 150 mg or 100 mg/M^2 every 3 hours may be required if SCr is 50% or greater than baseline measurement before methotrexate administration. Serum methotrexate must come down to below 0.05 micromolar. Continuing hydration and urinary alkalinization are mandatory to prevent precipitation in renal tubules. Monitor fluid and electrolyte status until serum methotrexate has fallen to less than 0.05 micromolar and renal failure has resolved. Glucarpidase (Voraxaze), an antidote indicated for the treatment of toxic methotrexate concentration in patients with delayed methotrexate clearance due to impaired renal function, may also be used. If glucarpidase is used, do not administer leucovorin within 2 hours before or after a dose of glucarpidase because leucovorin is a substrate for glucarpidase; see glucarpidase monograph. Administration of whole blood products (e.g., packed RBCs, platelets, leukocytes) and/or blood modifiers (e.g., darbepoetin alfa, epoetin alfa, filgrastim, pegfilgrastim, sargramostim) may be indicated to treat bone marrow toxicity. Death may occur from the progression of most of these side effects. Symptomatic and supportive therapy is indicated. Charcoal hemoperfusion may be helpful, and/or acute intermittent hemodialysis with a high-flux dialyzer may be used to counteract toxicity or inadvertent overdose.

METHYLERGONOVINE MALEATE
(meth-ill-er-**GON**-oh-veen **MAL**-ee-ayt)

Methergine

Uterine stimulant
(oxytocic)

pH 2.7 to 3.5

USUAL DOSE
1 mL (0.2 mg); repeat doses should be IM or PO.

DILUTION
Check expiration date on vial; methylergonovine deteriorates with age. May be given undiluted. Some clinicians recommend dilution with 5 mL of NS. Do not add to IV solutions. May be given through Y-tube of infusion set.

Filters: No data available from manufacturer; suggests following hospital protocol for filtering from ampules.

Storage: Store in refrigerator (2° to 8° C [36° to 46° F]); protect from light.

COMPATIBILITY
Compatibility information not available from manufacturer. Other sources suggest a few specific **compatibilities** dependent on concentration and manufacturer; consult a pharmacist.

RATE OF ADMINISTRATION
0.2 mg or fraction thereof over 1 minute. Too-rapid injection may cause severe nausea and vomiting. See Precautions.

ACTIONS
A semi-synthetic ergot alkaloid used for prevention and control of postpartum hemorrhage. An oxytocic. It exerts a direct stimulation on the smooth muscle of the uterus. Increases tone, rate, and amplitude of rhythmic contractions. Shortens third-stage labor and reduces blood loss. In therapeutic doses the prolonged initial contraction of the uterus is followed by periods of relaxation and contraction. May also produce vasoconstriction, increase CVP and BP, and may rarely produce peripheral ischemia. Effective within minutes. Half-life approximately 3.4 hours. It is probably metabolized in the liver and excreted in feces. Secreted in breast milk.

INDICATIONS AND USES
Routine management of uterine atony, hemorrhage, and subinvolution of the uterus following delivery of the placenta. ▪ Control of uterine hemorrhage in the second stage of labor following delivery of the anterior shoulder.

CONTRAINDICATIONS
Hypersensitivity, hypertension, pregnancy before third stage of labor (delivery of the placenta) except as stated in Indications, toxemia. ▪ Contraindicated for concomitant use with potent CYP3A4 inhibitors and azole antifungals; see Drug/Lab Interactions.

PRECAUTIONS
IV administration is for emergency use only. IM or oral routes are preferred and should be used after the initial IV dose. ▪ IV use may induce hypertension and/or CVA. Give slowly and monitor BP. ▪ Use caution in presence of sepsis, obliterative vascular disease, and hepatic or renal disease. ▪ Patients with coronary artery disease or risk factors for coronary artery disease (e.g., diabetes, high cholesterol, obesity, smoking) may be more susceptible to developing myocardial ischemia and infarction associated with methylergonovine-induced vasospasm. ▪ Use with caution during the second stage of labor. The necessity for manual removal of a retained placenta should occur rarely with proper technique and adequate allowance of time for a spontaneous separation. ▪ Avoid intra-arterial or periarterial injection. ▪ See Contraindications.

Monitor: Monitor BP. ▪ Observe for signs of excessive bleeding. ▪ See Drug/Lab Interactions.

Maternal/Child: Category C: see Contraindications and Precautions. ▪ Avoid breastfeeding during treatment with methylergonovine. Wait at least 12 hours after administration of the last dose before initiating or resuming breast-feeding. Milk secreted during this period should be discarded. May be given orally with caution during breast-feeding for up to 1 week after delivery. ■ Inadvertent administration of methylergonovine to newborn infants resulting in convulsions, cyanosis, oliguria, and respiratory depression has been reported. Methylergonovine should be stored separately from medications intended for neonatal administration (e.g., vitamin K, hepatitis B vaccine). ■ Safety and effectiveness for use in pediatric patients not established.

Elderly: Difference in safety and effectiveness compared to younger adults not observed. ■ If used in the elderly, dose selection should be cautious.

DRUG/LAB INTERACTIONS

Severe hypertension and cerebrovascular accidents can result with **ephedrine and other vasopressors.** Hydralazine IV will reduce this hypertension. ■ *Do not administer with potent CYP3A4 inhibitors,* such as **macrolide antibiotics** (e.g., erythromycin, clarithromycin), **HIV protease inhibitors** (e.g., indinavir, nelfinavir, ritonavir), **reverse transcriptase inhibitors** (e.g., delavirdine), **or azole antifungals** (e.g., fluconazole). Serum levels increased. Elevated levels of ergot alkaloids can cause ergotism (i.e., risk for vasospasm potentially leading to cerebral ischemia and/or ischemia of the extremities). ■ May be used cautiously with **less potent CYP3A4 inhibitors** (e.g., saquinavir, fluconazole, grapefruit juice, fluoxetine, fluvoxamine, zileuton, and clotrimazole). ■ **Strong CYP3A4 inducers** (e.g., rifampin, nevirapine) may decrease effectiveness of methylergonovine. ■ **Anesthetics** may reduce oxytocic effect of methylergonovine. ■ Produces vasoconstriction and can be expected to reduce the effect of **antianginal drugs** (e.g., nitroglycerin). ■ Concomitant use with **other ergot alkaloids or prostaglandins** will produce additive effects. Use caution.

SIDE EFFECTS

Rare in therapeutic doses but may include the following:

Abdominal pain (caused by uterine contractions), bradycardia, chest pain (temporary), coronary artery spasm, diaphoresis, diarrhea, dilated pupils, dizziness, dyspnea, hallucinations, headache, hematuria, hypersensitivity reactions, hypertension (transient), hypotension, leg cramps, MI, nasal congestion, nausea, palpitations, rash, seizures, tachycardia, thrombophlebitis, tinnitus, vasoconstriction, vasospasm, vomiting, water intoxication, weakness.

Overdose: Cerebrovascular accident, coma, convulsions, hypertension (followed by hypotension in severe cases), hypothermia, numbness, oliguria, palpitations, respiratory depression, severe nausea and vomiting, tachycardia, tingling of the extremities.

Post-Marketing: Angina, atrioventricular block, cerebrovascular accident, paresthesia, ventricular fibrillation, ventricular tachycardia.

ANTIDOTE

Discontinue the drug immediately at the onset of any side effect and notify the physician. Most side effects are transient unless there is severe toxicity and will be treated symptomatically. Use antiemetics for nausea and vomiting. Treat seizures with anticonvulsants. Maintain adequate pulmonary ventilation, especially if convulsions or coma develop. Correct hypotension with pressor drugs. Apply warmth to extremities to control peripheral vasospasm.

METHYLPREDNISOLONE SODIUM SUCCINATE

(meth-ill-pred-**NISS**-oh-lohn **SO**-dee-um **SUK**-sih-nayt)

A-Methapred, Solu-Medrol

Hormone
(corticosteroid)
Anti-inflammatory

pH 7 to 8

USUAL DOSE

Pretreatment: Patient selection and baseline studies indicated; see Precautions and Monitor.

Use the lowest possible dose to control the condition being treated. When reduction in dose is possible, the reduction should be gradual.

Methylprednisolone: Average initial dose range is 10 to 40 mg. May be repeated every 4 to 6 hours as necessary. IV methylprednisolone is usually given in an emergency situation or when oral dosing is not feasible. Larger doses may be justified by patient condition. Repeat until adequate response, then decrease dose as indicated. Total dose usually does not exceed 1.5 Gm/24 hr, but higher doses have been used in acute, life-threatening situations. High-dose treatment is used until patient condition stabilizes, usually no longer than 48 to 72 hours.

High-dose therapy: 30 mg/kg IV over at least 30 minutes. May repeat every 4 to 6 hours for 48 hours.

Anti-inflammatory: 10 to 40 mg. May be repeated every 4 to 6 hours as necessary.

Acute spinal cord injury high-dose therapy (unlabeled): Spinal cord injury must be less than 8 hours old. The earlier methylprednisolone therapy begins, the better the results. *Loading dose:* 30 mg/kg of a specifically diluted solution (see Dilution) evenly distributed over 15 minutes. Maintain IV line with standard IV fluids for 45 minutes, then begin a *maintenance dose* of 5.4 mg/kg/hr for 23 hours. Discontinue 24 hours after loading dose initiated.

Status asthmaticus or asthma exacerbations: Newer asthma guidelines recommend 40 to 80 mg/day in 1 to 2 divided doses until peak expiratory flow is 70% of predicted or personal best.

Acute exacerbation of multiple sclerosis: 160 mg as a single dose each day for 7 days. Follow with 64 mg every other day for 1 month. Another source recommends an unlabeled dose of 1,000 mg IV daily for 3 to 7 days.

***Pneumocystis jiroveci* pneumonia (unlabeled):** Initiate within 24 to 72 hours of initial antibiotic PCP therapy. 30 mg twice daily for 5 days. Follow with 30 mg once daily for 5 days (Days 6 to 10). Then reduce to 15 mg once daily for 11 days (Days 11 to 21) or until antibiotic regimen is complete.

Severe lupus nephritis (unlabeled): 0.5 to 1 Gm as an infusion over 1 hour for 3 days. Follow with long-term prednisolone oral therapy.

PEDIATRIC DOSE

See Maternal/Child. Dose should be based on the severity of the disease and the patient response rather than on strict adherence to a dose indicated by age, weight, or body surface area.

Anti-inflammatory/immunosuppressive: The range of initial doses is 0.11 to 1.6 mg/kg/day (3.2 to 48 mg/M^2/day) in 3 to 4 divided doses (0.0275 to 0.4 mg/kg every 6 hours or 0.036 to 0.53 mg/kg every 8 hours, or 0.8 to 12 mg/M^2 every 6 hours or 1.06 to 16 mg/M^2 every 8 hours). Another source recommends 0.5 to 1.7 mg/kg/day in divided doses every 6 to 12 hours (0.125 to 0.425 mg/kg every 6 hours, or 0.25 to 0.85 mg/kg every 12 hours).

Status asthmaticus or asthma exacerbation: Newer asthma guidelines recommend 1 to 2 mg/kg/day in single or divided doses (maximum 60 mg/day) until peak expiratory flow is 80% of predicted or personal best. Dose should not be less than 0.5 mg/kg every

24 hours. Usually requires 3 to 10 days of treatment. Another source recommends 2 mg/kg as a *loading* dose. *Maintain* with 0.5 to 1 mg/kg every 6 hours for up to 5 days. **Severe lupus nephritis (unlabeled):** 30 mg/kg every other day for 6 doses. Follow with long-term prednisolone oral therapy.

DOSE ADJUSTMENTS

Use lowest possible dose required to control condition being treated. When dose reduction is possible, decrease dose gradually while monitoring for S/S of disease exacerbation. ▪ Because complications of treatment with glucocorticoids are dependent on dose and duration of therapy, a risk/benefit decision must be made for each patient regarding dose and duration of treatment and whether daily or intermittent therapy should be used. ▪ Clearance of corticosteroids is decreased in patients with hypothyroidism and increased in patients with hyperthyroidism. Dose adjustment may be required. ▪ See Precautions and Drug/Lab Interactions.

DILUTION

Available in Act-O-Vials containing 40 mg, 125 mg, 500 mg, and 1,000 mg. Each vial has an appropriate amount of diluent. Reconstitute by pressing down on the plastic activator, allowing the diluent into the lower chamber. Agitate gently. Remove the plastic tab covering the center of the stopper and sterilize the stopper with a suitable germicide. Using sterile technique, insert a needle through the center of the rubber stopper to withdraw diluted solution. To be diluted only with diluent supplied in Act-O-Vial. Also available in vials, including a 2,000-mg dose. Should be diluted with accompanying diluent or BWFI with benzyl alcohol. May be given as direct IV, as an infusion, or further diluted in desired amounts of D5W, D5NS, or NS.

Acute spinal cord injury loading and maintenance doses: Each 1-Gm vial must be diluted to 16 mL with bacteriostatic water to maintain potency and avoid precipitation (62.5 mg/mL). Further dilute in D5W, D5NS, or NS with an amount to facilitate dose of 5.4 mg/kg/hr. (Example for a patient weighing 50 kg: [50 kg × 5.4 mg/hr = 270 mg/hr. 270 mg/hr × 23 hours = 6,210 mg total dose]. With a total dose of 6,210 mg at 62.5 mg/mL, you will have 99.36 [100] mL of reconstituted methylprednisolone. Add an additional 100 mL diluent to achieve 31.25 mg/mL. 270 mg/hr is the desired dose for this patient. 270 mg/hr divided by 31.25 mg/mL [strength of solution] equals 8.6. Administer at 8.6 mL/hr to achieve desired dose over 23 hours.)

Storage: Protect from light. Store both unreconstituted product and solution at RT (20° to 25° C [68° to 77° F]). Use solution within 48 hours of mixing. Heat sensitive; do not autoclave.

COMPATIBILITY

Manufacturer states, "Because of possible physical **incompatibilities,** should not be diluted or mixed with other solutions."

Other sources suggest specific **compatibilities** dependent on concentration and manufacturer; consult a pharmacist.

RATE OF ADMINISTRATION

IV injection: May give as a slow IV injection; rates range from over several minutes to at least 5 minutes for doses less than or equal to 250 mg. Also refer to institution-specific polices. When higher doses are needed, administer up to 30 mg/kg over 30 minutes or more. Too-rapid administration of high doses (greater than 500 mg administered over a period of less than 10 minutes) may precipitate cardiac arrhythmia and sudden death. Direct IV administration of lower doses (10 to 40 mg) is usually the route of choice in emergency situations and eliminates the possibility of overloading the patient with IV fluids. May be given as an *infusion* in its own diluent. At the discretion of the physician, a continuous infusion may be given, properly diluted in D5W, NS, D5NS, or other **compatible** IV solution over a specified time.

Acute spinal cord injury: See Usual Dose and Dilution.

ACTIONS

A glucocorticoid steroid with potent anti-inflammatory actions. A synthetic adrenocortical steroid. Glucocorticoids cause profound and varied metabolic effects. They are primarily used for their potent anti-inflammatory effects on different organ systems and their ability to modify the body's immune response. Methylprednisolone has a greater anti-inflammatory potency than prednisolone and less tendency to cause excessive potassium and calcium excretion and sodium and water retention. Has five times the potency of hydrocortisone sodium succinate. Has minimal mineralocorticoid activity. Demonstrable effects are seen within 1 hour of administration. Primarily metabolized in the liver and excreted in the urine. Dose is almost completely excreted after 12 hours. Therefore it must be dosed every 4 to 6 hours if sustained high blood levels are required. Crosses the placental barrier. Secreted in breast milk.

INDICATIONS AND USES

Includes treatment of allergic states, dermatologic diseases, endocrine disorders, gastrointestinal diseases, hematologic disorders, neoplastic diseases, nervous system disorders, ophthalmic diseases, renal diseases, respiratory diseases, and rheumatic disorders. See prescribing information for a complete list. Used primarily as an anti-inflammatory or immunosuppressant agent. May be used in conjunction with other forms of therapy, such as epinephrine for acute hypersensitivity reactions. Oral therapy should be used when appropriate.

Unlabeled uses: High-dose therapy as an adjunct to traditional spinal cord injury management; to improve neurologic recovery in an acute (less than 8 hours old) spinal cord injury. ▪ Treatment of *Pneumocystis jiroveci* pneumonia as an adjunct to antibiotics.

CONTRAINDICATIONS

Hypersensitivity to any product component, including sulfites; systemic fungal infections. ▪ Solu-Medrol 40 mg contains lactose monohydrate and is contraindicated in patients with a known or suspected hypersensitivity to cow's milk or its components or other dairy products. ▪ Formulations containing benzyl alcohol are contraindicated in premature infants and for intrathecal administration. ▪ Intrathecal administration. ▪ IM administration for idiopathic thrombocytopenic purpura.

PRECAUTIONS

Ruling out latent amebiasis or active amebiasis is recommended before initiating corticosteroid therapy in any patient who has spent time in the tropics or has unexplained diarrhea. ▪ Not the drug of choice to treat acute adrenocortical insufficiency. ▪ Corticosteroids may produce hypothalamic-pituitary-adrenal (HPA) axis suppression, Cushing's syndrome, and hyperglycemia, with resulting glucocorticosteroid insufficiency in patients undergoing chronic or prolonged therapy. To avoid relative adrenocortical insufficiency, do not stop therapy abruptly; taper off. This type of relative insufficiency may persist for months after discontinuation of therapy; therefore hormone therapy should be reinstituted in any situation of stress occurring during that period (e.g., surgery, trauma, infection). If the patient is already receiving steroids, dosage may need to be increased. ▪ Formulation may contain benzyl alcohol; see Contraindications and Maternal/Child. ▪ Rare instances of anaphylactoid reactions have been reported in patients receiving corticosteroid therapy. ▪ Hypersensitivity reactions to cow's milk have been reported; see Contraindications. ▪ In one study, an increase in mortality was seen in patients with cranial trauma who had no other clear indication for corticosteroid treatment. High doses of systemic corticosteroids should not be used for treatment of traumatic brain injury. ▪ Should not be used in cerebral malaria; no evidence of benefit reported. ▪ Use with caution in patients who have had a recent MI. Ventricular free wall rupture has been reported. ▪ Prolonged use of corticosteroids may increase susceptibility to infection, reactivate latent infectious diseases, or mask signs of infection; see Contraindications. ▪ Corticosteroids should be used with great caution in patients with known or suspected Strongyloides (threadworm) infestation. Corticosteroid-induced immunosuppression may lead to Strongyloides hyperinfection and dissemination with widespread larval migration, often accompanied by severe enterocolitis and potentially fatal gram-negative sepsis. ▪ The use of methylprednisolone in patients with active tuberculosis should be restricted to cases of fulminating or disseminated tuberculosis in which the corticosteroid is being used for management of disease in conjunction with an appropriate antituberculosis regimen. ▪ If corticosteroids are indicated in patients with latent tuberculosis or tuberculin reactivity, reactivation of the disease may occur. Chemoprophylaxis is indicated during prolonged corticosteroid therapy. ▪ Infections such as chickenpox and measles can have a more serious or even fatal course in pediatric and adult patients taking corticosteroids. Patients who have not had these diseases should take care to avoid exposure. If exposed, therapy with varicella zoster immune globulin (VZIG) or IVIG may be indicated. If chickenpox develops, treatment with antiviral agents should be considered. ▪ Use with caution in patients with systemic sclerosis. An increased incidence of scleroderma renal crisis has been observed with corticosteroids, including methylprednisolone. ▪ Use with caution in patients with CHF, hypertension, or renal insufficiency. May affect fluid and electrolyte balance. ▪ Steroid-induced liver injury (acute toxic hepatitis) has been reported with high doses of cyclically pulsed IV methylprednisolone (usually for treatment of exacerbations of multiple sclerosis at doses of 1 Gm/day). Recurrence has occurred after rechallenge. ▪ Use with caution in patients with thyroid dysfunction; see Dose Adjustments. ▪ Use with caution in patients with active or latent peptic ulcers, diverticulitis, fresh intestinal anastomoses, and nonspecific ulcerative colitis. May be at increased risk for perforation. ▪ Metabolism of corticosteroids is decreased in patients with cirrhosis; effects may be enhanced. ▪ Use with caution in patients at risk for osteoporosis. Corticosteroids decrease bone formation, increase bone resorption, and decrease protein matrix of the bone. May lead to inhibition of bone growth in pediatric patients and the development of osteoporosis at any age. ▪ An acute myopathy has been reported with the use of high doses of corticosteroids. Most often seen in patients with disorders of neuromuscular transmission (e.g., myasthenia gravis) or in patients receiving concomitant therapy with neuromuscular blocking drugs (e.g., pancuronium). Myopathy is generalized, may involve ocular and respiratory muscles, and may result in quadriparesis. Clinical improvement following discontinuation of corticosteroids may take weeks to years. ▪ May induce psychological changes (e.g., depression, euphoria, insomnia, mood swings, personality changes, psychosis). May aggravate existing emotional instability or psychotic tendencies. ▪ Kaposi's sarcoma has been reported in patients receiving corticosteroid therapy, most often for chronic conditions. Clinical improvement has been seen with discontinuation of the corticosteroid. ▪ Prolonged use of corticosteroids may produce posterior subcapsular cataracts or glaucoma with possible damage to the optic nerves, and it may enhance the establishment of secondary ocular infections due to bacteria, fungi, or viruses. Use with caution in patients with ocular herpes simplex because of corneal perforation. Should not be used in active ocular herpes simplex.

Monitor: Monitor electrolytes. May cause sodium retention and potassium and calcium excretion. Dietary salt restriction and potassium supplementation may be necessary. ▪ May cause hypertension secondary to fluid and electrolyte disturbances. Monitor BP. ▪ Monitor for S/S of infection. May be masked. ▪ Patients with latent tuberculosis should be monitored for reactivation of the disease. ▪ May increase insulin needs in patients with diabetes. Monitor serum glucose. ▪ During prolonged therapy, routine laboratory studies such as urinalysis, 2-hour postprandial blood sugar, BP, body weight assessment, and chest x-ray should be obtained at regular intervals. Upper GI x-rays are suggested for patients with a history of ulcers or significant dyspepsia. ▪ May increase intraocular pressure. Periodic ophthalmic exams may be necessary with prolonged treatment. ▪ Elevation of creatine kinase may occur with acute myopathy. Monitor if indicated. ▪ Monitor for S/S of a hypersensitivity reaction. ▪ See Drug/Lab Interactions.

Patient Education: Report edema, tarry stools, or weight gain promptly. Report anorexia, diarrhea, dizziness, fatigue, low blood sugar, nausea, weakness, weight loss, or vomiting; may indicate adrenal insufficiency after dose reduction or discontinuing therapy. ▪ May mask signs of infection and/or decrease resistance. ▪ Diabetics may have increased requirement for insulin or oral hypoglycemics. ▪ Avoid immunizations with live virus vaccines. ▪ Avoid exposure to measles or chickenpox. Seek immediate medical advice if exposure occurs. ▪ Carry ID stating steroid dependent if receiving prolonged therapy.

Maternal/Child: Use with caution during pregnancy; benefits must outweigh risks. ▪ Discontinue breast-feeding. ▪ Infants born to mothers who received corticosteroids during pregnancy should be carefully monitored for signs of hypoadrenalism. ▪ May contain benzyl alcohol, which has been associated with a fatal "gasping syndrome" in neonates. ▪ Monitor growth and development of pediatric patients receiving prolonged treatment. **Elderly:** Differences in response between the elderly and younger patients have not been identified. Dose selection should be cautious based on the possibility of age-related organ impairment (e.g., bone marrow reserve, renal, hepatic). May be more sensitive to effects.

DRUG/LAB INTERACTIONS

Aminoglutethimide may lead to a loss of corticosteroid-induced adrenal suppression. ▪ Metabolism increased and effects reduced by **hepatic enzyme–inducing agents** (e.g., barbiturates, carbamazepine, phenytoin, rifampin); dose adjustments may be required when adding or deleting from drug profile. ▪ Risk of hypokalemia increased with **amphotericin B or potassium-depleting diuretics** (e.g., thiazides, furosemide, ethacrynic acid). Monitor potassium levels and cardiac function. ▪ Increased risk of **digoxin** toxicity secondary to hypokalemia. ▪ May decrease effectiveness of **potassium supplements;** monitor serum potassium. ▪ **Diuretics** decrease sodium and fluid retention effects of corticosteroids; corticosteroids decrease sodium excretion and diuretic effects of diuretics. ▪ Increased activity of both **cyclosporine** and **corticosteroids** may occur when used concurrently. Convulsions have been reported with concurrent use. ▪ Clearance decreased and effects increased with **estrogens, oral contraceptives, triazole antifungals** (e.g., itraconazole), **and macrolide antibiotics** (e.g., azithromycin, clarithromycin, erythromycin). ▪ Ketoconazole can significantly decrease the metabolism of certain corticosteroids and lead to an increased risk of corticosteroid side effects. ▪ **Cholestyramine** may increase the clearance of corticosteroids. ▪ Coadministration of **aprepitant** may increase methylprednisolone levels. Dose reduction of methylprednisolone may be indicated. ▪ May interact with **anticoagulants, nondepolarizing muscle relaxants, or theophyllines;** may inhibit or potentiate action; monitor carefully. ▪ Monitor patients receiving **antidiabetic agents** carefully; dose adjustments may be required. ▪ May antagonize effects of **isoniazid and salicylates;** dose adjustments may be required. ▪ Administration of **live virus or live-attenuated vaccines** is contraindicated in patients receiving immunosuppressive doses of corticosteroids. Inactivated vaccines may be administered, but the response to such vaccines cannot be predicted. ▪ Concomitant use with **NSAIDs** may increase the risk of adverse GI effects. ▪ Concomitant use with **anticholinesterase agents** (e.g., neostigmine) may produce severe weakness in patients with myasthenia gravis. If possible, anticholinesterase agents should be withdrawn at least 24 hours before initiating corticosteroid therapy. ▪ Corticosteroids may **suppress reactions to skin tests.** ▪ See Dose Adjustments.

SIDE EFFECTS

Do occur but are usually reversible: Cushing's syndrome; electrolyte and calcium imbalance; euphoria; fluid retention; glycosuria; hepatitis; hyperglycemia; hypersensitivity reactions, including anaphylaxis; hypertension; impaired wound healing; increased appetite; increased intracranial pressure; leukocytosis; menstrual irregularities; ophthalmic disorders (glaucoma, increased intraocular pressure); peptic ulcer perforation and hemorrhage; protein catabolism; spontaneous fractures; transitory burning or tingling, sweating, headache, or weakness; thromboembolism; and many others.

ANTIDOTE

Notify the physician of any side effect. Will probably treat the side effect if necessary. Treat acute overdose with supportive and symptomatic therapy. For chronic overdosage in the face of severe disease requiring continuous steroid therapy, the dosage of the corticosteroid may be reduced only temporarily, or alternate day treatment may be introduced. Discontinue methylprednisolone if toxic hepatitis occurs. Do not rechallenge patient. Resuscitate as necessary for anaphylaxis and notify physician. Keep epinephrine immediately available.

METOCLOPRAMIDE HYDROCHLORIDE BBW

(**meh**-toe-kloh-**PRAH**-myd hy-droh-**KLOR**-eyed)

Reglan

GI stimulant
Antiemetic

pH 4.5 to 6.5

USUAL DOSE

Small bowel intubation and/or radiologic examination of the small bowel: 10 mg (2 mL) as a single dose.

Antiemetic: High-dose regimen for highly emetogenic chemotherapy is rarely used; 5-HT$_3$ receptor antagonists (e.g., ondansetron) preferred. 2 mg/kg of body weight 30 minutes before giving emetogenic cancer chemotherapy (e.g., cisplatin, dacarbazine). Repeat every 2 hours for 2 doses, then every 3 hours for 3 doses; see Dose Adjustments. For less emetogenic regimens, 1 mg/kg/dose may be adequate.

Diabetic gastroparesis: 10 mg immediately before each meal and at bedtime. Use IV for up to 10 days if symptoms are severe. Continue treatment PO for 2 to 8 weeks.

Prevention of postoperative nausea and vomiting: 10 mg, usually given IM toward the end of surgery. Up to 20 mg may be used.

PEDIATRIC DOSE

Small bowel intubation and/or radiologic examination of the small bowel: *6 to 14 years:* 2.5 to 5 mg. ***Under 6 years:*** 0.1 mg/kg of body weight.

Gastroesophageal reflux or GI dysmotility (unlabeled): 0.1 to 0.2 mg/kg/dose. May be given every 6 hours if required. Maximum dose 0.8 mg/kg/24 hr (0.2 mg/kg/dose every 6 hours).

Antiemetic (unlabeled): Rarely used. 5-HT$_3$ receptor antagonists preferred. A high-dose regimen for highly emetogenic chemotherapy of 1 to 2 mg/kg/dose every 2 to 6 hours has been administered but is rarely used. Premedicate with diphenhydramine to reduce extrapyramidal symptoms.

DOSE ADJUSTMENTS

Antiemetic dose may be reduced to 1 mg/kg if initial doses suppress vomiting. Initial doses may be reduced to 1 mg/kg for less emetogenic regimens. ■ Reduce initial dose by half in any patient with a CrCl less than 40 mL/min. Adjust subsequent doses as indicated. ■ Caution and lower-end dosing suggested in elderly patients. Consider potential for decreased organ function and concomitant disease or drug therapy. ■ See Drug/Lab Interactions.

DILUTION

May be given undiluted if dose does not exceed 10 mg. For doses exceeding 10 mg dilute in at least 50 mL of D5W, NS, D5/^{1}/$_2$NS, R, or LR, and give as an infusion.

Storage: Light sensitive; store in carton before use. Diluted solutions stable for 24 hours in normal light, 48 hours if protected from light. Do not freeze unless diluted in NS. Discard if color or particulate matter is observed.

COMPATIBILITY

Manufacturer lists as **incompatible** with chloramphenicol and sodium bicarbonate.

Other sources suggest specific **compatibilities** dependent on concentration and manufacturer; consult a pharmacist.

RATE OF ADMINISTRATION

Too-rapid IV injection will cause intense anxiety, restlessness, and then drowsiness.

IV injection: 10 mg or fraction thereof over 2 minutes. Reduce rate of injection in pediatric patients.

Infusion: Administer over a minimum of 15 minutes.

ACTIONS

A dopamine antagonist. Antiemetic properties appear to be the result of antagonism of central and peripheral dopamine receptors. Blocks the stimulation of medullary chemoreceptor trigger zones by dopamine. Inhibits nausea and vomiting. Increases tone and amplitude of gastric contractions, relaxes the lower pyloric sphincter and duodenal bulb, and increases peristalsis of the duodenum and jejunum, resulting in accelerated gastric emptying. Does not stimulate gastric, biliary, or pancreatic secretions. Acts even if vagal innervation not present. Action negated by anticholinergic drugs. Distributes extensively into tissues. Onset of action occurs in 1 to 3 minutes and lasts 1 to 2 hours. Average half-life is 5 to 6 hours. Excreted in urine. Secreted in breast milk.

INDICATIONS AND USES

Facilitate small bowel intubation. ▪ Stimulate gastric and intestinal emptying of barium to permit radiologic examination of the stomach and small intestine. ▪ Prevention of nausea and vomiting associated with emetogenic cancer chemotherapy. ▪ Prophylaxis of postoperative nausea and vomiting when nasogastric suction is not indicated. ▪ Diabetic gastroparesis.

CONTRAINDICATIONS

Situations in which gastric motility is contraindicated (i.e., gastric hemorrhage, obstruction, or perforation); known hypersensitivity to metoclopramide; patients with epilepsy or patients taking drugs that may also cause extrapyramidal reactions; pheochromocytoma.

PRECAUTIONS

May produce sedation, extrapyramidal symptoms, or Parkinson-like symptoms, similar to those seen with phenothiazines. Use caution in patients with pre-existing disease. ▪ Acute dystonic reactions (a type of extrapyramidal symptom [EPS]) are usually seen during the first 24 to 48 hours of treatment and are more common in pediatric patients, in adults under 30 years of age, and at higher doses used for prophylaxis of N/V due to chemotherapy. ▪ Tardive dyskinesia may develop and is usually related to duration of treatment and total cumulative dose. Avoid use for longer than 12 weeks unless benefit outweighs risk of tardive dyskinesia. ▪ Neuroleptic malignant syndrome (NMS) has been reported rarely. Potentially fatal. Discontinue metoclopramide immediately; see Monitor. ▪ Produces a transient increase in plasma aldosterone; patients with cirrhosis or CHF may develop fluid retention and volume overload. If S/S occur, discontinue metoclopramide. ▪ Use with caution in patients with hypertension. May cause release of catecholamines, exacerbating the condition. ▪ A prolactin-elevating compound; may be carcinogenic. Risk with a single dose almost nonexistent. ▪ May cause serious depression and suicidal tendencies; use extreme caution in any patient with a history of depression. ▪ Patients with NADH-cytochrome b_5 reductase deficiency are at increased risk for developing methemoglobinemia and/or sulfhemoglobinemia. In patients with G6PD deficiency who develop methemoglobinemia, methylene blue treatment is not recommended. Can cause hemolytic anemia. ▪ See Maternal/Child.

Monitor: Monitor vital signs. ▪ Pretreatment with diphenhydramine may reduce incidence of extrapyramidal symptoms with larger doses (e.g., antiemetic). ▪ Monitor for S/S of NMS (e.g., hyperthermia, muscle rigidity, altered consciousness, and evidence of autonomic instability [irregular pulse or BP, tachycardia, diaphoresis, and arrhythmias]). ▪ Discontinue therapy in patients who develop S/S of tardive dyskinesia (syndrome of potentially irreversible involuntary movements of the tongue, face, mouth, jaw, trunk, or extremities). ▪ See Precautions and Drug/Lab Interactions.

Patient Education: Use caution performing any task that requires alertness, coordination, or physical dexterity; may produce dizziness and drowsiness. ▪ If any involuntary movement of eyes, face, or limbs occurs, notify physician promptly. ▪ Avoid alcohol or other CNS depressants (e.g., barbiturates, benzodiazepines [e.g., diazepam]).

Maternal/Child: Category B: use caution in pregnancy and breast-feeding. ▪ May increase milk production (elevates prolactin). ▪ Pharmacokinetics highly variable in children and neonates. ▪ Safety and effectiveness for use in pediatric patients not established except when administered to facilitate small bowel intubation. ▪ Dystonic reactions are more common in pediatric patients. ▪ Prolonged clearance in neonates may produce excessive serum concentrations. ▪ May cause methemoglobinemia in premature and full-term neonates at doses exceeding 0.5 mg/kg/24 hr. ▪ See Precautions and Side Effects.

Elderly: May be more sensitive to therapeutic or adverse effects. ■ Long-term use increases risk of extrapyramidal effects (e.g., parkinsonism, tardive dyskinesia). ■ See Dose Adjustments and Precautions.

DRUG/LAB INTERACTIONS

Antagonized by **anticholinergic drugs** (e.g., atropine) **and narcotic analgesics** (e.g., morphine). ■ May potentiate **alcohol and cyclosporine.** ■ Drugs ingested orally may be absorbed more slowly or more rapidly depending on the absorption site (e.g., inhibits **cimetidine, digoxin**). ■ Potentiates **MAO inhibitors**; use extreme caution or do not use. ■ **Insulin** reactions may result from gastric stasis, making diabetic control difficult. Dose or timing of insulin may need adjustment. ■ Extrapyramidal effects may be potentiated with concomitant use of **phenothiazines, butyrophenones, and thioxanthenes** (antipsychotic drugs). ■ Used concurrently, metoclopramide and **levodopa** have opposite effects on dopamine receptors; metoclopramide is inhibited, and levodopa is potentiated.

SIDE EFFECTS

Usually mild, transient, and reversible after metoclopramide is discontinued. Hypersensitivity reactions can occur. Acute CHF, anxiety, arrhythmias, bowel disturbances, confusion, convulsions, depression (severe, may have suicidal tendencies), dizziness, drowsiness, extrapyramidal reactions, fatigue, fluid retention, hallucinations, headache, hypertension, hypotension, insomnia, methemoglobinemia in neonates, nausea, NMS (hyperthermia, muscle rigidity, altered consciousness, and evidence of autonomic instability [irregular pulse or BP, tachycardia, diaphoresis, and arrhythmias]), restlessness, sulfhemoglobinemia in adults, tardive dyskinesia. Numerous other side effects may occur.

Overdose: Disorientation, drowsiness, and extrapyramidal reactions.

ANTIDOTE

Notify physician of all side effects. Most will respond to a reduced dose or discontinuation of metoclopramide. Treat overdose or extrapyramidal reactions with diphenhydramine or benztropine. Symptoms should disappear within 24 hours. To manage NMS, immediately discontinue metoclopramide. Intensive symptomatic treatment and monitoring are required. Discontinue therapy in patients who develop S/S of tardive dyskinesia; symptoms may resolve. Treat methemoglobinemia with IV methylene blue. Hemodialysis is not likely to be useful in an overdose. Resuscitate as necessary.

METOPROLOL TARTRATE BBW
(me-toe-**PROH**-lohl **TAHR**-trayt)

Beta-adrenergic blocking agent
Antiarrhythmic (post MI)

Lopressor

pH 7.5

USUAL DOSE
Pretreatment: See Monitor.

Treatment of myocardial infarction (MI): 5 mg as an IV bolus dose. Initiate as soon as the patient's hemodynamic condition has stabilized. Repeat at 2-minute intervals for 2 more doses; a total dose of 15 mg (AHA recommends 5 mg at 5-minute intervals to a total dose of 15 mg). If IV doses are well tolerated, give 50 mg PO every 6 hours for 48 hours beginning 15 minutes after the last bolus. Follow with an oral maintenance dose of 100 mg twice daily. In patients who do not tolerate the full IV dose start 25 to 50 mg PO within 15 minutes of the last IV dose. Dosage based on degree of intolerance. May have to discontinue metoprolol.

Treatment of atrial fibrillation (unlabeled): 2.5 to 5 mg as an IV injection over 2 to 5 minutes as necessary to control rate up to a total dose of 15 mg in a 10- to 15-minute period if indicated.

Treatment of ventricular rate control/hypertension (unlabeled): 1.25 to 5 mg every 6 to 12 hours. Begin with a lower initial dose and titrate to response. Up to 15 mg every 3 to 6 hours has been used.

DOSE ADJUSTMENTS
See Drug/Lab Interactions. ▪ Not required in impaired renal function. ▪ In patients with impaired hepatic function, start at a low dose and titrate upward slowly.

DILUTION
May be given undiluted.

Storage: Store at CRT. Protect from light.

COMPATIBILITY
Compatibility information not available from manufacturer. Other sources suggest a few specific **compatibilities** dependent on concentration and manufacturer; consult a pharmacist.

RATE OF ADMINISTRATION
A single dose over 1 minute. Monitor ECG, HR, and BP and discontinue metoprolol if adverse symptoms occur (bradycardia less than 45 beats/min, heart block greater than first degree, systolic BP less than 100 mm Hg, or moderate to severe cardiac failure). May also be given by slow infusion (5-10 mg in 50 mL of fluid) over 30 to 60 minutes in non-emergent situations.

ACTIONS
Metoprolol is a cardioselective (B_1) adrenergic receptor blocker. Its mechanism of action in patients with suspected or definite MI is not known, but its use has been shown to reduce the 3-month mortality rate in this patient population. It reduces the incidence of recurrent MI and reduces the size of the infarct and the incidence of fatal arrhythmias. Reduces HR, systolic BP, and cardiac output. Well distributed throughout the body, it acts within 1 to 2 minutes and lasts about 3 to 4 hours. Maximum beta blockade is achieved in approximately 20 minutes. Metabolized in the liver by the cytochrome P_{450} enzyme system, primarily CYP2D6. Excreted as metabolites in the urine. Crosses placental barrier. Secreted in breast milk.

INDICATIONS AND USES
To reduce cardiac mortality in hemodynamically stable individuals with suspected or definite MI (used in conjunction with oral metoprolol maintenance therapy). ▪ Treatment of hypertension, angina pectoris, and CHF in oral dosage form.

Unlabeled uses: Treatment of atrial fibrillation and unstable angina. ▪ Has been used in the perioperative period to reduce cardiac morbidity and mortality in patients at risk. ▪ Treatment of ventricular rate control and hypertension in patients who cannot take PO medications.

CONTRAINDICATIONS

HR below 45 beats/min, second- or third-degree heart block, significant first-degree heart block (PR interval equal to or greater than 0.24 second), systolic BP below 100 mm Hg, or moderate to severe cardiac failure. ■ Hypersensitivity to metoprolol or to any of the excipients. Use caution in patients with hypersensitivity to other beta-blockers. Cross-sensitivity between beta-blockers can occur. ■ Severe peripheral arterial circulatory disorders or sick sinus syndrome in patients with angina or hypertension.

PRECAUTIONS

Use caution in CHF. Beta blockade may depress myocardial contractility and precipitate or exacerbate heart failure and cardiogenic shock. ■ Use caution in presence of heart failure controlled by digoxin. Both drugs slow AV conduction. Bradycardia, sinus pause, heart block, and cardiac arrest have occurred. Patients with first-degree AV block, sinus node dysfunction, or conduction disorders may be at increased risk; see Antidote. ■ May produce significant first- (PR interval equal to or greater than 0.26 second), second-, or third-degree heart block. Acute MI can also cause heart block. ■ Metoprolol decreases sinus heart rate. MI may also produce significant lowering of HR; see Antidote. ■ Routine withdrawal of chronically administered beta-blockers before major surgery is not necessary; however, the risks of general anesthesia and surgical procedures may be increased by the impaired ability of the heart to respond to reflex adrenergic stimuli. ■ Use caution in patients with a history of severe anaphylactic reactions to a variety of allergens; they may be more reactive to repeated challenge (either accidental, diagnostic, or therapeutic) and may be unresponsive to the usual doses of epinephrine used to treat hypersensitivity reactions; see Drug/Lab Interactions. ■ May mask tachycardia occurring with hypoglycemia in diabetes and tachycardia of hyperthyroidism. ■ In general, patients with bronchospastic disease should not receive beta-blockers, including metoprolol. Because of its relative beta selectivity, metoprolol may be used with extreme caution in these patients. Monitor pulmonary function closely; see Antidote. ■ Use with caution in patients with impaired hepatic function; see Dose Adjustments. ■ May cause arrhythmia, angina, MI, or death if stopped abruptly (more of an issue with chronic oral therapy); see prescribing information. ■ May cause severe bradycardia in patients with Wolff-Parkinson-White syndrome. ■ Contraindicated in patients known to have or suspected of having a pheochromocytoma. If metoprolol is required, it should be given in combination with an alpha-blocker (e.g., phenoxybenzamine [Dibenzyline]) and only after the alpha-blocker has been initiated. ■ See Drug/Lab Interactions.

Monitor: Continuous ECG, HR, BP monitoring mandatory with use of IV metoprolol. ■ Hemodynamic status must be closely monitored. If heart failure or hypotension occurs or persists despite appropriate treatment, metoprolol should be discontinued. Assess extent of myocardial damage. Invasive monitoring of central venous, pulmonary capillary wedge, and arterial pressure may be required. ■ See Drug/Lab Interactions and Antidote.

Patient Education: Report any breathing difficulty promptly.

Maternal/Child: Category C: safety for use in pregnancy and breast-feeding and in pediatric patients not established. ■ If a pregnancy occurs, females should inform physician.

Elderly: Age-related differences in safety and effectiveness not identified; however, greater sensitivity of some elderly cannot be ruled out. Dose with caution. ■ May exacerbate mental impairment.

DRUG/LAB INTERACTIONS

Concurrent use with **calcium channel blockers** (e.g., diltiazem, verapamil) may potentiate both drugs and result in severe depression of myocardium and AV conduction and severe hypotension. ■ Concurrent use with **antihypertensive agents,** including **alpha-adrenergic blockers** (e.g., clonidine, methyldopa), may result in excessive hypotension. Dose adjustment may be required. ■ Concurrent administration with **hydralazine** may decrease metabolism and increase concentrations of metoprolol. ■ **Potent inhibitors of the CYP2D6 enzyme** may increase plasma concentrations of metoprolol and decrease its cardioselectivity. These inhibitors include **antidepressants** (e.g., clomipramine, desipramine, fluoxetine, fluvoxamine, paroxetine, sertraline, bupropion), **antipsychotics** (e.g., chlorpromazine, fluphenazine, haloperidol, thioridazine), **antiarrhythmics** (e.g., quinidine, propafenone), **antiretrovirals** (e.g., ritonavir), **antihistamines** (e.g., diphenhydramine), **antimalarials** (e.g., hydroxychloroquine, quinidine), **allylamine antifungals** (e.g., terbinafine). ▪ Concurrent use within 14 days of **MAO inhibitors** may cause severe hypertension. ▪ Use with **sympathomimetic agents** (e.g., epinephrine, norepinephrine, phenylephrine) **or xanthines** (e.g., aminophylline) may negate therapeutic effects of both drugs. ▪ Effects of beta-adrenergic blocking agents may be decreased by **anti-inflammatory drugs** (e.g., NSAIDs), **barbiturates, rifampin, salicylates, and others.** ▪ **Inhalation anesthetics, phenytoin, and quinolone antibiotics** may increase myocardial depressant effects and hypotension. ▪ Beta-adrenergic blocking agents may be continued during the perioperative period in most patients; however, use caution with **selected anesthetic agents** that may depress the myocardium. ▪ Potentiates effects of **oral antidiabetics, catecholamine-depleting drugs** (e.g., reserpine), insulin, lidocaine, and skeletal muscle relaxants; monitor carefully. Dose adjustment may be required. ▪ Concurrent use with **clonidine** may precipitate acute hypertension if one or both agents are stopped abruptly. Withdraw metoprolol first. ▪ Effects decreased when hypothyroid patient is **converted to a euthyroid state;** adjust dose as indicated. ▪ Use caution; both **digoxin** and beta-blockers slow AV conduction. May increase risk of bradycardia. ▪ Patients taking beta-blockers who are exposed to a potential allergen may be unresponsive to the usual dose of **epinephrine** used to treat a hypersensitivity reaction. ▪ May enhance the vasoconstrictive action of **ergot alkaloids.** ▪ In general, withhold administration of a beta-blocker before **dipyridamole** testing; monitor HR carefully following dipyridamole injection.

SIDE EFFECTS

Abdominal pain, bradyarrhythmias, bronchospasm, cardiac failure, claudication, confusion, dizziness, dyspnea, elevated liver function tests, first-degree heart block, hallucinations, headache, hepatitis, hypotension, jaundice, nausea, nightmares, pruritus, rash, reduced libido, respiratory distress, second- or third-degree heart block, sleep disturbances, syncopal attacks, tiredness, unstable diabetes, vertigo, visual disturbances.

ANTIDOTE

For any side effect, discontinue drug and notify physician immediately. Patients with MI may be more hemodynamically unstable; treat with caution. Use atropine (0.25 to 0.5 mg) for bradycardia or heart block; use isoproterenol with caution if atropine is not effective. Glucagon 5 to 10 mg IV may be effective if atropine and isoproterenol are not (investigational use). Transvenous cardiac pacing may be needed. Treat hypotension with IV fluids if indicated or vasopressors (dopamine or norepinephrine [Levarterenol]); treat cause of hypotension (e.g., bradycardia). Use all vasopressors with extreme caution; severe hypotension can result. Use digoxin and diuretics at first sign of cardiac failure; dobutamine, isoproterenol, or glucagon may be required. Use aminophylline or isoproterenol (with extreme care) for bronchospasm, and glucagon or IV glucose for hypoglycemia. Treat other side effects symptomatically; resuscitate as necessary.

METRONIDAZOLE HYDROCHLORIDE BBW
(meh-troh-**NYE**-dah-zohl hy-droh-**KLOR**-eyed)

Antibacterial
Antiprotozoal
Amebicide

Metro IV

pH 4.5 to 7

USUAL DOSE

Pretreatment: Baseline studies indicated; see Monitor.

May transfer to oral therapy when condition warrants (usual PO dose is 7.5 mg/kg every 6 hours). Dosage, rate of administration, and duration of treatment are to be individualized and depend on the indication for use; the patient's age, weight, clinical condition, and concomitant treatment; and on the patient's clinical and laboratory response to the treatment.

Anaerobic infections: 500 mg every 6 to 8 hours for 7 to 10 days or longer if indicated. Infections involving bone and joint, lower respiratory tract, and endocardium may require longer treatment. Do not exceed 4 Gm in 24 hours.

Surgical prophylaxis to prevent postoperative infection in contaminated or potentially contaminated colorectal surgery: 500 mg IV within 60 minutes before surgical incision in combination with other antibiotics.

PEDIATRIC DOSE

Safety for use in infants and other pediatric patients not established, but is used for anaerobic infections; see Maternal/Child.

Anaerobic infections: *Pediatric patients more than 7 days of age:* 7.5 mg/kg every 6 hours with a maximum dose of 4 Gm/24 hr.

Another source recommends age- and weight-specific doses as follows:

Less than 7 days of age weighing less than 1.2 kg: 7.5 mg/kg every 48 hours.
Less than 7 days of age weighing 1.2 to 2 kg: 7.5 mg/kg every 24 hours.
Less than 7 days of age weighing 2 or more kg: 7.5 mg/kg every 12 hours.
7 days of age or older weighing less than 1.2 kg: 7.5 mg/kg every 24 hours.
7 days of age or older weighing 1.2 to 2 kg: 7.5 mg/kg every 12 hours.
7 days of age or older weighing 2 or more kg: 15 mg/kg every 12 hours.

DOSE ADJUSTMENTS

Reduce dose by 50% in patients with severe (Child-Pugh Class C) hepatic impairment. ■ Reduce the dose as necessary in patients with severe hepatic encephalopathy who experience an exacerbation of CNS adverse effects. ■ Increase intervals in neonates; see Pediatric Dose. ■ No dose adjustment is indicated in mild to moderate impaired renal function. ■ Dose adjustment not indicated in anuric patients; accumulated metabolites readily removed by dialysis. 40% to 65% of a metronidazole dose can be removed by dialysis depending on length of dialysis session and type of dialyzer membrane used. If metronidazole administration cannot be separated from dialysis session, consider supplemental dose following dialysis. ■ Continuous NG suction may remove sufficient metronidazole in gastric aspirate to reduce serum levels. No dose adjustment is recommended.

DILUTION

All solutions are prediluted and ready to use (5 mg/mL). Do not use plastic containers in series connections. Risk of air embolism is present.

Storage: Store at room temperature (25° C [77° F]). Do not refrigerate. Protect from light. Do not remove premixed product from overwrap until ready for use. After removing overwrap, check for minute leaks by squeezing bag firmly. Discard solution if leaks are found.

COMPATIBILITY

Manufacturer recommends, "Administer separately, discontinue the primary IV during administration, and do not introduce additives into the solution." Do not use equipment containing aluminum (e.g., needles, cannulae) that would come in contact with the drug solution as precipitates may form. Manufacturer lists as **incompatible** (includes but is not limited to) aztreonam, cefoxitin, and penicillin G.

Other sources suggest specific **compatibilities** dependent on concentration and manufacturer; consult a pharmacist.

RATE OF ADMINISTRATION

Must be given as a slow intermittent or continuous IV infusion, each single dose evenly distributed over 1 hour. Discontinue primary IV during administration.

Surgical prophylaxis: Administer each single dose over 30 to 60 minutes.

ACTIONS

A bactericidal agent with cytotoxic effects, active against specific obligate anaerobic bacteria and protozoa. Does not possess any clinically relevant activity against facultative anaerobes or obligate aerobes. Metronidazole enters the organism by passive diffusion and is reduced. The reduced form and free radicals that are produced during the reduction reaction interact with DNA, leading to inhibition of DNA synthesis and to DNA degradation and death of bacteria. The precise mechanism of action is unclear. Metronidazole is widely distributed. Plasma concentrations are directly proportional to dose given. Metabolized in the liver. Half-life is 8 hours. Crosses placental and blood-brain barriers. Excreted primarily in urine, some in feces. Secreted in breast milk.

INDICATIONS AND USES

Treatment of serious infections caused by susceptible strains of anaerobic bacteria, including serious intra-abdominal, skin and skin structure, gynecologic, bone and joint, CNS, and lower respiratory tract infections, bacterial septicemia, and endocarditis. Is effective in *Bacteroides fragilis* infections resistant to clindamycin, chloramphenicol, and penicillin. ▪ Perioperative prophylaxis to reduce infection rates in contaminated or potentially contaminated colorectal surgery. ▪ Given orally for amebiasis, giardiasis, *Helicobacter pylori* eradication, and other indications.

Unlabeled uses: *Clostridium difficile*–associated diarrhea (CDAD), Crohn's disease.

CONTRAINDICATIONS

Hypersensitivity to metronidazole or other nitroimidazole derivatives; use of disulfiram within the last 2 weeks; use of alcohol or products containing propylene glycol during and for at least 3 days after therapy with metronidazole.

PRECAUTIONS

A mixed (anaerobic/aerobic) infection will require use of additional antibiotics targeted for treatment of the aerobic infection. ▪ Sensitivity studies indicated to determine susceptibility of the causative organism to metronidazole. ▪ To reduce the development of drug-resistant bacteria and maintain its effectiveness, metronidazole should be used to treat or prevent only those infections proven or strongly suspected to be caused by bacteria. ▪ Avoid prolonged use of the drug; superinfection caused by overgrowth of nonsusceptible organisms may result. ▪ Symptoms of candidiasis may be exacerbated and require treatment. ▪ Severe neurologic disturbances, including encephalopathy, cerebellar symptoms, convulsive seizures, peripheral neuropathy, optic neuropathy, and aseptic meningitis, have been reported in patients treated with metronidazole. CNS symptoms and lesions are generally reversible within days to weeks after metronidazole is discontinued. ▪ Encephalopathy may manifest as confusion or a decreased level of consciousness and is associated with widespread lesions seen on MRI of the brain. Cerebellar toxicity may manifest as ataxia, dizziness, dysarthria, nystagmus, and saccadic pursuit. Accompanied by T2 flair lesions within the dentate nuclei seen on MRI. ▪ Cerebellar toxicity may occur concurrently with encephalopathy, peripheral neuropathy, or seizures. ▪ Peripheral neuropathy (usually symmetric and mainly sensory with S/S of numbness or paresthesia of extremities) has been reported. Symptoms may be prolonged after metronidazole is discontinued. ▪ Aseptic meningitis may occur within hours of dose administration, and symptoms generally resolve after metronidazole is discontinued. ▪ Use caution in patients predisposed to edema and/or taking corticosteroids or receiving a controlled sodium diet, or in patients with impaired cardiac function (contains 27 to 28 mEq sodium/Gm). ▪ Use caution in patients with CNS disease or hepatic or renal impairment. ▪ *Clostridium difficile*–associated diarrhea (CDAD) has been reported. May range from mild diarrhea to fatal colitis. Consider in patients who present with diarrhea during or after treatment with metronidazole. ▪ Carcinogenic in rodents; avoid unnecessary use and restrict use to approved indications. ▪ Use with caution in patients with evidence of or a history of blood dyscrasias. Agranulocytosis, leukopenia, and neutropenia have occurred. ▪ Severe hepatoxicity/acute hepatic failure (including fatal outcome) with very rapid onset after treatment initiation in patients with Cockayne syndrome have been reported with products containing metronidazole for systemic use. Use in this population only if no alternative treatment is available. ▪ Exacerbation of CNS adverse effects may occur in patients with severe hepatic encephalopathy; see Dose Adjustments.

Monitor: Monitor CBC before, during, and after prolonged or repeated courses of therapy and in patients with symptoms of blood dyscrasias (e.g., agranulocytosis, leukopenia, and neutropenia). ▪ Obtain liver function tests before the start of therapy, within the first 2 to 3 days after the initiation of therapy, frequently during therapy, and after the end of treatment in patients with Cockayne syndrome. ▪ Monitor for S/S of toxicity in patients with hepatic or renal impairment and in the elderly. ▪ Monitor for adverse events when metronidazole is administered to those with severe renal impairment or end-stage renal disease who are not undergoing hemodialysis. ▪ Monitor for S/S of toxicity due to the potential accumulation of metronidazole metabolites in those receiving peritoneal dialysis. ▪ Monitor for neurologic S/S (e.g., ataxia, confusion, dizziness, dysarthrias, numbness, paresthesia, and seizures); see Antidote. ▪ Monitor for S/S of bleeding. ▪ Transfer to oral dosing as soon as practical. ▪ See Drug/Lab Interactions.

Patient Education: Avoid alcohol and alcohol-containing preparations during and for at least 3 days after completion of therapy; toxic reactions will occur. ▪ Review medications with health care provider; see Drug/Lab Interactions. ▪ Promptly report any neurologic side effects (e.g., seizures, numbness, or paresthesia of an extremity). ▪ Promptly report diarrhea or bloody stools that occur during treatment or up to several months after an antibiotic has been discontinued; may indicate CDAD and require treatment. ▪ Patients with Cockayne syndrome should stop taking metronidazole immediately and promptly report any S/S of potential liver injury (e.g., abdominal pain, change in stool color, jaundice, or nausea).

Maternal/Child: Use during pregnancy only if clearly needed. ▪ Discontinue breast-feeding during metronidazole therapy and for 24 hours after therapy ends. ▪ Safety for use in pediatric patients and neonates not established. The elimination half-life, measured during the first 3 days of life, was inversely related to gestational age. Half-life markedly extended in newborns; adjust intervals; see Pediatric Dose.

Elderly: Pharmacokinetics altered in the elderly; monitor for metronidazole-associated adverse events and adjust dose accordingly. Dose selection should be cautious, reflecting the greater frequency of decreased hepatic, renal, or cardiac function and of concomitant disease or other drug therapy.

DRUG/LAB INTERACTIONS

Avoid **alcohol and alcohol-containing preparations** for at least 3 days after taking any dose of metronidazole; a disulfiram-like reaction (abdominal cramps, flushing, headaches, nausea, tachycardia, and vomiting) may occur. ▪ Avoid administration of metronidazole to patients who have taken **disulfiram** within the last 2 weeks. Psychotic reactions and confusion have been reported. ▪ Concurrent use with **drugs that induce microsomal enzyme activity** (e.g., phenobarbital, phenytoin) may increase metabolism of metronidazole and decrease plasma levels, thereby decreasing efficacy. ▪ Administration with **drugs that inhibit microsomal liver enzyme activity** may decrease metronidazole metabolism, increasing metronidazole plasma levels and the risk of toxicity. ▪ Concurrent use with **CYP3A4 substrates** (e.g., amiodarone, carbamazepine, cyclosporine, phenytoin, quinidine, tacrolimus) may increase substrate plasma levels. Monitoring of plasma concentrations of CYP3A4 substrates may be necessary. ▪ Metronidazole decreases the clearance of **5-fluorouracil** and may therefore cause 5-fluorouracil toxicity. ▪ Metronidazole may potentiate the effects of **vecuronium**. ▪ Potentiates the anticoagulant effects of **warfarin**. Monitor PT/INR periodically and adjust anticoagulant dose accordingly. ▪ May increase **lithium** levels and cause toxicity. Frequent monitoring of serum lithium and serum creatinine levels is necessary. ▪ May increase plasma concentrations of **busulfan**, increasing the risk of serious busulfan toxicity such as sinusoidal obstruction syndrome, gastrointestinal mucositis, and hepatic veno-occlusive disease. Avoid concomitant use if possible. If concomitant administration is medically necessary, monitor busulfan plasma concentration and adjust busulfan dose accordingly. ▪ May interfere with **selected chemistry studies** (e.g., AST, ALT, LDH, triglycerides, glucose hexokinase).

SIDE EFFECTS
The most serious side effects include aseptic meningitis, seizures, encephalopathy, and optic and peripheral neuropathy. Abdominal cramping, agranulocytosis, arthralgia, asthenia, ataxia, chest pain, chills, chromaturia, CDAD, confusion, darkened deep red urine, decreased appetite, decreased libido, depression, diarrhea, dizziness, drug reaction with eosinophilia and systemic symptoms (DRESS), dysarthria, dysgeusia, dyspnea, dysuria, eosinophilia, erythema, facial edema, headache, increased hepatic enzyme, hepatoxicity/liver failure in patients with Cockayne syndrome, hyperhidrosis, hypersensitivity reactions (including anaphylaxis), hypoesthesia, injection site reaction, insomnia, jaundice, leukopenia, malaise, myalgia, muscle spasms, nausea, neutropenia (reversible), numbness, nystagmus, painful coitus, palpitation, pancreatitis, paresthesia, peripheral edema, proctitis, pruritus, psychosis, rash, saccadic eye movement, somnolence, Stevens-Johnson syndrome, syncope, tachycardia, thrombocytopenia (reversible), toxic epidermal necrolysis, urticaria, vaginal candidiasis, vertigo, and vomiting have occurred.

Overdose: Nausea, neurotoxic effects (including ataxia, confusion, disorientation, seizures, and peripheral neuropathy), and vomiting.

ANTIDOTE
Notify physician of all side effects. Treatment will be symptomatic and supportive. Evaluate risk versus benefit of continuing therapy in patients who develop abnormal neurologic S/S (e.g., encephalopathy, seizures, or signs of peripheral neuropathy). Discontinue metronidazole in patients with Cockayne syndrome who develop elevated liver function tests. Monitor liver function tests until the baseline values are reached. Removed by hemodialysis. Treat anaphylaxis and resuscitate as necessary.

MICAFUNGIN SODIUM
(my-kah-**FUN**-gin **SO**-dee-um)

Mycamine

USUAL DOSE

Pretreatment: Baseline studies indicated; see Monitor.

Treatment of candidemia, acute disseminated candidiasis, *Candida* peritonitis and abscesses: 100 mg/day as an infusion. Mean duration of treatment during clinical studies was 15 days (range 10 to 47 days).

Treatment of esophageal candidiasis: 150 mg/day as an infusion. Mean duration of treatment during clinical studies was 15 days (range 10 to 30 days).

Prophylaxis of *Candida* infections in hematopoietic stem cell transplant (HSCT) recipients: 50 mg/day as an infusion. Mean duration of treatment in patients who responded successfully during clinical studies was 19 days (range 6 to 51 days).

PEDIATRIC DOSE

Recommended doses for pediatric patients based on indication and weight are outlined in the following chart.

Micafungin Dosage in Pediatric Patients 4 Months of Age or Older		
	Pediatric Dose Given Once Daily	
Indication	**30 kg or less**	**Greater than 30 kg**
Treatment of candidemia, acute disseminated candidiasis, *C.* peritonitis and abscesses	2 mg/kg (maximum daily dose 100 mg)	
Treatment of esophageal candidiasis	3 mg/kg	2.5 mg/kg (maximum daily dose 150 mg)
Prophylaxis of *Candida* infections in HSCT recipients	1 mg/kg (maximum daily dose 50 mg)	

Dosage for pediatric patients under 4 months of age: *Treatment of candidemia, acute disseminated candidiasis, C. peritonitis, and abscesses* without *meningoencephalitis and/or ocular dissemination:* The recommended dose is 4 mg/kg once daily; see Limitations of Use.

DOSE ADJUSTMENTS

No dose adjustment indicated based on gender or race, in the elderly, or in patients with severe renal dysfunction or mild to moderate or severe hepatic insufficiency. ▪ Not dialyzable; a supplementary dose following hemodialysis should not be required. ▪ See Drug/Lab Interactions.

DILUTION

Each 50- or 100-mg vial must be reconstituted with 5 mL of NS (without a bacteriostatic agent) or with D5W. Following reconstitution, the 50-mg vial has a final concentration of 10 mg/mL. The 100-mg vial has a final concentration of 20 mg/mL. The use of strict aseptic technique is required. Swirl vial(s) gently to dissolve. ***Do not shake.*** Do not use if precipitation or foreign matter is observed. Each single adult dose (50, 100, or 150 mg) must be further diluted in 100 mL NS or D5W for infusion. For pediatric patients, calculate the dose in milligrams and withdraw the required volume from the selected concentration (10 mg/mL or 20 mg/mL). Add the withdrawn volume to an infusion bag or syringe containing NS or D5W. Final concentration of diluted solution should be between 0.5 and 4 mg/mL. Concentrations greater than 1.5 mg/mL should be infused through a central line.

Filters: No study data available; if filtering is necessary, contact manufacturer.

Storage: Store unopened vials at CRT. Reconstituted solution in original vial or diluted solution is stable up to 24 hours at 25° C (77° F). Protect diluted solution from light. Discard partially used vials.

COMPATIBILITY

Manufacturer states, "Do not mix or co-infuse micafungin with other medications. Has been shown to precipitate when mixed directly with a number of other commonly used medications." Flush IV line with NS before and after infusion.

Other sources suggest a few specific **compatibilities** dependent on concentration and manufacturer; consult a pharmacist.

RATE OF ADMINISTRATION

Flush IV line with NS before and after infusion.

A single dose as an infusion equally distributed over 1 hour. Rapid infusion may result in more frequent histamine-mediated reactions (e.g., facial swelling, pruritus, rash, vasodilation). To minimize the risk of infusion reactions in pediatric patients, concentrations of greater than 1.5 mg/mL should be administered via a central catheter. Injection site reactions have been reported and occur more often in patients receiving micafungin via peripheral intravenous administration.

ACTIONS

A semi-synthetic lipopeptide. An echinocandin antifungal agent. Acts by inhibiting the synthesis of 1,3-beta-D-glucan, an integral component of the fungal cell wall not present in mammalian cells. The AUC increases as doses are increased (e.g., from 50 to 150 mg or from 3 to 8 mg/kg). Highly protein bound primarily to albumin but does not competitively displace bilirubin binding to albumin. 85% of steady-state concentration achieved after three daily doses. Metabolized in the liver. A substrate and weak inhibitor of CYP3A, but CYP3A is not a major pathway for metabolism. Half-life ranges from approximately 11 to 21 hours in adults and from 5 to 22 hours in pediatric patients. Primarily excreted in feces, with some excretion in urine.

INDICATIONS AND USES

Indicated in adult and pediatric patients 4 months of age and older for treatment of candidemia, acute disseminated candidiasis, *Candida* peritonitis, and abscesses. ▪ Treatment of candidemia, acute disseminated candidiasis, *C.* peritonitis, and abscesses **without** meningoencephalitis and/or ocular dissemination in pediatric patients under 4 months of age; see Limitations of Use. ▪ Treatment of esophageal candidiasis in adult and pediatric patients 4 months of age and older. ▪ Prophylaxis of *Candida* infections in patients undergoing hematopoietic stem cell transplantation.

Limitations of Use: Safety and effectiveness of micafungin have **not** been established for the treatment of candidemia **with** meningoencephalitis and/or ocular dissemination in pediatric patients under 4 months of age as a higher dose may be needed. ▪ Has not been adequately studied in patients with endocarditis, osteomyelitis, and meningitis due to *Candida* infections. ▪ Efficacy against infections caused by fungi other than *Candida* not established.

CONTRAINDICATIONS

Hypersensitivity to micafungin, any of its components, or other echinocandins (e.g., anidulafungin), caspofungin.

PRECAUTIONS

Do not give as an IV bolus; for IV infusion only. ▪ Isolated anaphylactoid reactions (including shock) and anaphylaxis have been reported. ▪ Abnormal liver function tests have been reported. Isolated cases of significant hepatic dysfunction, hepatitis, or worsening hepatic failure have occurred. Incidence may be increased in patients with serious underlying conditions who are receiving additional concomitant medications. Evaluate risk versus benefit of continued micafungin therapy. ▪ Elevations in BUN and creatinine have been reported. Isolated cases of significant renal dysfunction or acute renal failure have occurred. ▪ Intravascular hemolysis and hemoglobinuria have been reported. Isolated cases of significant hemolysis and hemolytic anemia have occurred. Evaluate risk versus benefit of continued micafungin therapy. ▪ Reports of clinical failures resulting from development of drug resistance have been reported. ▪ See Monitor and Antidote.

Monitor: Specimens for fungal culture, serologic testing, and histopathologic testing should be obtained before therapy to isolate and identify causative organisms. Therapy may begin as soon as all specimens are obtained and before results are known. Reassess after test results are known. ▪ Baseline CBC with differential and platelet count, BUN, SCr, and liver function tests (e.g., ALT, AST) may be indicated. ▪ Monitor for S/S of a hypersensitivity reaction (e.g., bronchospasm, dyspnea, hives, hypotension, rash, pruritus, swelling of eyelids, lips, or face); discontinue infusion if a hypersensitivity reaction occurs. ▪ Monitor for evidence of worsening hepatic function (e.g., increased ALT, AST, serum alkaline phosphatase). ▪ Monitor for evidence of worsening renal function (e.g., increased BUN, SCr). ▪ Monitor for S/S of hemolytic anemia, hemolysis, and hemoglobinuria as indicated (lysis of RBCs, liberation of hemoglobin, blood in the urine). ▪ Hematologic, hepatic, and renal effects may require discontinuation of micafungin.

Patient Education: Promptly report shortness of breath, dizziness or fainting, itching, rash, or swelling of extremities. ▪ Report S/S of liver dysfunction (anorexia, fatigue, jaundice, nausea and vomiting, dark urine, or pale stools). ▪ Report any S/S of hemoglobinuria (blood in the urine). ▪ Report S/S of renal dysfunction (decrease in urine output). ▪ Review list of current medications with physician. Drug interactions are possible; see Drug/Lab Interactions.

Maternal/Child: Pregnancy category C: use during pregnancy only if benefits justify risk to fetus. Some abnormalities, including abortion, occurred in animal studies. ▪ Use caution if required during breast-feeding. Secreted in milk of drug-treated rats; not known if micafungin is secreted in human milk. ▪ Safety and effectiveness for use in pediatric patients under 4 months of age not established. ▪ Safety and effectiveness *have* been established for use in pediatric patients under 4 months of age for the treatment of candidemia *without* meningoencephalitis and/or ocular dissemination. Safety and effectiveness have *not* been established for use in the treatment of candidemia *with* meningoencephalitis and/or ocular dissemination in pediatric patients under 4 months of age as a higher dose may be needed.

Elderly: Differences in response compared to younger adults not identified; however, greater sensitivity in the elderly cannot be ruled out.

DRUG/LAB INTERACTIONS

The effects of **itraconazole, nifedipine, and sirolimus** are increased with concurrent administration of micafungin. Monitor for itraconazole, nifedipine, or sirolimus toxicity and reduce their dose as indicated. ▪ Not expected to alter effects of drugs metabolized by the CYP3A system.

SIDE EFFECTS

Side effect profile similar in both adult and pediatric patients. The most common side effects include diarrhea, fever, headache, nausea, thrombocytopenia, and vomiting. The most serious side effects that may occur regardless of indication include acute intravascular hemolysis, decreased WBC, hemoglobinuria, hemolytic anemia, histamine-mediated reactions (e.g., facial swelling, pruritus, rash, vasodilation), hypersensitivity reactions (e.g., anaphylaxis and anaphylactoid reactions [including shock]), significant hepatic dysfunction (e.g., hepatitis, hepatocellular damage, hyperbilirubinemia, or worsening hepatic failure), significant renal dysfunction, and/or acute renal failure. Abdominal pain, anemia, chills, delirium, dizziness, increased liver function tests (e.g., alkaline phosphatase, ALT, AST, BUN, transaminases), injection site reactions (including inflammation, phlebitis, and thrombophlebitis), leukopenia, lymphopenia, neutropenia, and somnolence occurred in patients treated for esophageal candidiasis. In addition, constipation, decreased appetite, dysgeusia (altered sense of taste), dyspepsia, fatigue, febrile neutropenia, flushing, hiccups, hyperbilirubinemia, hypertension, hypocalcemia, hypokalemia, hypomagnesemia, hypophosphatemia, hypotension, increased drug levels, increased SCr, and mucosal inflammation occurred in patients undergoing prophylactic use during HSCT.

Patients with esophageal candidiasis: Also reported rash and phlebitis.

Patients with candidemia and other *Candida* infections and prophylaxis of *Candida* infection in HSCT: Both reported bacteremia, hypertension, hypokalemia, hypomagnesemia, hypotension, peripheral edema, tachycardia, and thrombocytopenia.

Patients with candidemia and other *Candida* infections: Also reported aggravated anemia, atrial fibrillation, bradycardia, decubitus ulcer, hyperkalemia, hypernatremia, hypoglycemia, increased blood alkaline phosphatase, pneumonia, sepsis, septic shock, vascular disorders.

Prophylaxis of *Candida* infection in HSCT: Also reported anorexia, anxiety, constipation, cough, dizziness, dyspepsia, dyspnea, epistaxis, erythema, fatigue, febrile neutropenia, fluid overload, fluid retention, flushing, hypocalcemia, mucosal inflammation, neutropenia, pruritus, rash, and rigors.

Post-Marketing: Disseminated intravascular coagulation (DIC), Stevens-Johnson syndrome, and toxic epidermal necrolysis.

ANTIDOTE

Notify physician of all side effects; most will be treated symptomatically. Hematologic, hepatic, and renal effects may require evaluation for the risk/benefit of continuing micafungin. If a hypersensitivity reaction occurs, discontinue micafungin and treat as indicated. Appropriate treatment may include oxygen, epinephrine, antihistamines, vasopressors, corticosteroids, IV fluids, and ventilation equipment. S/S indicative of hepatic, renal, or hematologic side effects may require evaluation of benefits versus risk of continuing micafungin therapy. Not removed by hemodialysis. Resuscitate as indicated.

MILRINONE LACTATE

(**MILL**-rih-nohn **LAK**-tayt)

Primacor

Antiarrhythmic
Inotropic agent

pH 3.2 to 4

USUAL DOSE

Pretreatment: See Monitor.

50 mcg/kg (0.05 mg/kg) of body weight as the initial loading dose.
Follow with a maintenance infusion according to the following chart.

Milrinone Maintenance Dose Guidelines			
	Infusion Rate (mcg/kg/min)	**Total Daily Dose (24 Hours)**	
Minimum	0.375 mcg/kg/min	0.59 mg/kg	Administer as a continuous IV infusion.
Standard	0.50 mcg/kg/min	0.77 mg/kg	
Maximum	0.75 mcg/kg/min	1.13 mg/kg	

Titrate the infusion dose between 0.375 mcg/kg/min and 0.75 mcg/kg/min (26 mcg/min and 52 mcg/min for a 70-kg person) based on hemodynamic and clinical response. Do not exceed a total dose of 1.13 mg/kg/24 hr. Duration of infusion usually does not exceed 48 hours.

DOSE ADJUSTMENTS

Reduced dose required in impaired renal function based on CrCl according to the following chart.

Milrinone Dose Guidelines in Impaired Renal Function	
Creatinine Clearance (mL/min/1.73 M^2)	**Infusion Rate (mcg/kg/min)**
5 mL/min/1.73 M^2	0.2 mcg/kg/min
10 mL/min/1.73 M^2	0.23 mcg/kg/min
20 mL/min/1.73 M^2	0.28 mcg/kg/min
30 mL/min/1.73 M^2	0.33 mcg/kg/min
40 mL/min/1.73 M^2	0.38 mcg/kg/min
50 mL/min/1.73 M^2	0.43 mcg/kg/min

DILUTION

Loading dose: May be given undiluted, or each 1 mg (1 mL) may be diluted in 1 mL NS or ½NS for injection. Alternately, the loading dose may be diluted with NS, ½NS, or D5W to a total volume of 10 or 20 mL for injection.

Infusion: Dilute with NS, ½NS, or D5W. Available prediluted as 200 mcg/mL in D5W. Amount of diluent may be increased or decreased based on patient fluid requirements. Another source suggests dilution with LR.

Guidelines for Dilution of Milrinone for Infusion			
Desired Infusion Concentration (mcg/mL)	**Milrinone 1 mg/mL (mL)**	**Diluent (mL)**	**Total Volume (mL)**
200 mcg/mL	10 mL	40 mL	50 mL
200 mcg/mL	20 mL	80 mL	100 mL

May be given through Y-tube of IV infusion set but should never come in contact with furosemide. Use only freshly prepared solutions.

Filters: No data available from manufacturer.

Storage: Store at room temperature before dilution; avoid freezing.

COMPATIBILITY

Manufacturer states, "Do not add supplementary medications." Forms an immediate precipitate with furosemide (Lasix).

Other sources suggest specific **compatibilities** dependent on concentration and manufacturer; consult a pharmacist.

RATE OF ADMINISTRATION

Loading dose: A single dose evenly distributed over 10 minutes.

Infusion: Use an infusion pump to deliver milrinone in recommended doses. The following manufacturer's dose chart defines selected dose in mcg/kg/min in infusion rate of mL/hr. Adjust as indicated by physician's orders and progress in patient's condition. Reduce rate or stop infusion for excessive drop in BP.

Milrinone Infusion Rate (mL/hr) Using 200 mcg/mL Concentration										
Maintenance Dose	Patient Body Weight (kg)									
(mcg/kg/min)	30	40	50	60	70	80	90	100	110	120
0.375	3.4	4.5	5.6	6.8	7.9	9	10.1	11.3	12.4	13.5
0.4	3.6	4.8	6	7.2	8.4	9.6	10.8	12	13.2	14.4
0.5	4.5	6	7.5	9	10.5	12	13.5	15	16.5	18
0.6	5.4	7.2	9	10.8	12.6	14.4	16.2	18	19.8	21.6
0.7	6.3	8.4	10.5	12.6	14.7	16.8	18.9	21	23.1	25.2
0.75	6.8	9	11.3	13.5	15.8	18	20.3	22.5	24.8	27

ACTIONS

A class of cardiac inotropic agent different in chemical structure and mode of action from digitalis glycosides and catecholamines. Similar to inamrinone, with fewer side effects. With a loading dose, peak effect occurs within 10 minutes. Continuous administration is required to maintain serum levels. It has positive inotropic action with vasodilator activity. Reduces afterload and preload by direct relaxant effect on vascular smooth muscle. Produces slight enhancement of AV node conduction. Cardiac output is improved without significant increases in HR or myocardial oxygen consumption or changes in arteriovenous oxygen difference. Pulmonary capillary wedge pressure, total peripheral resistance, diastolic BP, and mean arterial pressure are decreased. HR generally remains the same. Mean half-life is 2.4 hours. Primary route of excretion is in urine.

INDICATIONS AND USES

Short-term management of patients with acute decompensated heart failure.

CONTRAINDICATIONS

Hypersensitivity to milrinone or inamrinone.

PRECAUTIONS

Not shown to be safe or effective for use longer than 48 hours. No improvement in symptoms and an increased risk of death have been reported. ▪ Use caution in impaired renal function; serum levels may increase considerably. ▪ May be given to digitalized patients without causing signs of digoxin toxicity; correct hypokalemia with potassium supplements. ▪ May increase ventricular response in atrial flutter/fibrillation. Consider pretreatment with digoxin. ▪ Additional fluids and electrolytes may be required to facilitate appropriate response in patients who have been vigorously diuresed and may have insufficient cardiac filling pressure. Use caution. ▪ Safety for use in the acute phase of myocardial infarction not established. ▪ Should not be used in patients with severe obstructive aortic or pulmonary valvular disease in lieu of surgical relief of the obstruction. May aggravate outflow tract obstruction in hypertrophic subaortic stenosis.

Monitor: Observe closely. Continuous ECG monitoring required to allow for prompt detection and management of cardiac events, including life-threatening ventricular arrhythmias. Emergency equipment must be readily available. ▪ Monitoring of BP, urine output, renal function, fluid and electrolyte changes (especially potassium), liver function tests, and body weight is recommended. ▪ Monitoring of cardiac index, pulmonary capillary wedge pressure, central venous pressure, and plasma concentration is very useful. ▪ Observe for orthopnea, dyspnea, and fatigue. ▪ Reduce rate or stop infusion for excessive drop in BP. ▪ As cardiac output and diuresis improve, a reduction in diuretic dose may be indicated. ▪ Possible risk of arrhythmias. Risk further increased with excessive diuresis and/or hypokalemia. Replace potassium as indicated. ▪ Infusion site reactions may occur. Monitor site carefully.

Maternal/Child: Category C: safety for use during pregnancy, breast-feeding, and in pediatric patients not established. Use during pregnancy only if potential benefit justifies potential risk.

Elderly: Consider impaired renal function; may require a reduced dose.

DRUG/LAB INTERACTIONS

May cause additive hypotensive effects with **any drug that produces hypotension** (e.g., alcohol, benzodiazepines, lidocaine). ▪ See Monitor.

SIDE EFFECTS

Supraventricular and ventricular arrhythmias including nonsustained ventricular tachycardia do occur; rare cases of torsades de pointes have been reported. Abnormal liver function tests, anaphylactic shock (rare), angina, bronchospasm, chest pain, headaches, hypokalemia, hypotension, infusion site reactions, rash, and tremor have been reported.

ANTIDOTE

Notify the physician of any side effect. Based on degree of severity and condition of the patient, may be treated symptomatically, and dose may remain the same, be decreased, or the milrinone may be discontinued. Reduce rate or discontinue the drug at the first sign of marked hypotension and notify the physician. May be resolved by these measures alone or vasopressors (e.g., dopamine) may be required. Treat dysrhythmias with the appropriate drug. Resuscitate as necessary.

MITOMYCIN BBW

(my-toe-**MY**-sin)

MTC, Mutamycin

Antineoplastic

pH 6 to 8

USUAL DOSE

Pretreatment: Baseline studies indicated; see Monitor. See Maternal/Child.

10 to 20 mg/M^2 as a single dose. May be repeated in 6 to 8 weeks after adequate bone marrow recovery; see Dose Adjustments. Discontinue drug if no response after two courses of treatment.

DOSE ADJUSTMENTS

Subsequent doses based on posttreatment leukocyte and platelet counts. Withhold dose for leukocytes below 4,000/mm³ or platelet count below 100,000/mm³. Adjust subsequent doses based on nadir after the prior dose according to the following chart. ▪ Lower usual dose range is indicated when used with other antineoplastic drugs and radiation.

Guide to Mitomycin Dose Adjustment		
Nadir After Prior Dose		
Leukocytes/mm³	Platelets/mm³	Percentage of Prior Dose to Be Given
≥4,000	≥100,000	100%
3,000 to 3,999	75,000 to 99,999	100%
2,000 to 2,999	25,000 to 74,999	70%
<2,000	<25,000	50%

DILUTION

Specific techniques required; see Precautions. Each 5 mg must be diluted with 10 mL SWFI. Allow to stand at room temperature until completely in solution. May be given through Y-tube of a free-flowing infusion of NS or D5W or further diluted in either of the same solutions or sodium lactate ⅙ M and given as an infusion.

Storage: Store unopened vial at CRT. Stable after initial reconstitution at room temperature for 7 days, up to 14 days if refrigerated. When further diluted to a concentration of 20 to 40 mcg/mL, it is stable at room temperature for 3 hours in D5W, 12 hours in NS, and 24 hours in sodium lactate ⅙ M.

COMPATIBILITY

Compatibility information not available from manufacturer. Other sources suggest specific **compatibilities** dependent on concentration and manufacturer; consult a pharmacist.

RATE OF ADMINISTRATION

IV injection: A single dose over 5 to 10 minutes.

Infusion: Rate determined by amount and type of solution, typically 15 to 30 minutes.

ACTIONS

A highly toxic antibiotic, antineoplastic agent. Cell cycle phase–nonspecific, it is most useful in G and S phases. Interferes with cell division by binding with DNA to slow production of RNA. Rapidly distributed to body tissues and ascitic fluid. Does not cross blood-brain barrier. Metabolized primarily in the liver, but some metabolism occurs in other tissues as well. Some excreted in urine.

INDICATIONS AND USES

Treatment of disseminated adenocarcinoma of the stomach or pancreas. Used in combination with other drugs. Used intravesically in bladder cancer.

Unlabeled uses: Combination chemotherapy in anal, cervical, head and neck, metastatic breast, and non–small-cell lung cancers and in malignant mesothelioma.

CONTRAINDICATIONS
Not recommended as single-agent primary therapy. Known hypersensitivity to mitomycin, thrombocytopenia, coagulation disorders, increased bleeding from other causes, potentially serious infections, SCr greater than 1.7 mg/100 mL.

PRECAUTIONS
Follow guidelines for handling cytotoxic agents. See Appendix A, p. 1308. ■ Administered by or under the direction of the physician specialist in a facility with adequate diagnostic and treatment facilities for monitoring the patient and responding to any medical emergency. ■ Use extreme caution in impaired renal function; see Contraindications. ■ Acute shortness of breath and bronchospasm have occurred within minutes to hours following administration of vinca alkaloids (e.g., vincristine) in patients who have received mitomycin previously or are receiving mitomycin simultaneously. Bronchodilators, steroids and/or oxygen may be used to treat respiratory distress. ■ Bone marrow suppression (leukopenia and thrombocytopenia) may be severe and contribute to overwhelming infections in an already compromised patient. ■ Hemolytic uremic syndrome (hemolytic anemia, thrombocytopenia, and irreversible renal failure) has occurred in patients receiving mitomycin as a single agent or in combination with other agents. It can occur at any time during treatment, but most cases have occurred with a cumulative dose greater than 60 mg. Administration of blood products may exacerbate the symptoms.

Monitor: Monitor WBC, RBC, platelet count, PT, bleeding time, differential, and hemoglobin before, during, and 7 to 10 weeks after therapy. ■ Monitor all patients, especially those nearing a cumulative dose of 60 mg, for unexplained anemia with fragmented cells on peripheral blood smear, thrombocytopenia, and decreased renal function; see Precautions. ■ Determine absolute patency of vein; use of an IV catheter is preferred because severe cellulitis and tissue necrosis will result from extravasation. If extravasation occurs, discontinue injection and use another vein. Elevate extremity and apply cold compresses to extravasated area. Delayed erythema with or without ulceration has occurred at or distant to the injection site. May occur weeks to months after mitomycin administration, even when no obvious evidence of extravasation was observed during administration. ■ May precipitate acute respiratory distress syndrome. Oxygen can be toxic to the lungs; monitor intake carefully and use only enough to provide adequate arterial saturation. ■ Monitor fluid balance; avoid overhydration. ■ Be alert for signs of bone marrow suppression or infection. ■ Monitor for thrombocytopenia (platelet count less than 50,000/mm^3). Initiate precautions to prevent excessive bleeding (e.g., inspect IV sites, skin, and mucous membranes; use extreme care during invasive procedures; test urine, emesis, stool, and secretions for occult blood). ■ Prophylactic antibiotics may be indicated pending results of C/S in a febrile neutropenic patient. ■ Prophylactic antiemetics may reduce nausea and vomiting and increase patient comfort. ■ See Precautions and Drug/Lab Interactions.

Patient Education: Effective birth control recommended. ■ Report shortness of breath and IV site burning and stinging promptly. ■ See Appendix D, p. 1311.

Maternal/Child: Avoid pregnancy; may produce teratogenic effects on the fetus. ■ Information on safety in breast-feeding or in pediatric patients not available; discontinue breast-feeding.

Elderly: Consider diminished hepatic function; monitor for early signs of toxicity.

DRUG/LAB INTERACTIONS
Do not administer **live virus vaccines** to patients receiving antineoplastic drugs. ■ May cause shortness of breath, severe bronchospasm, and acute pneumonitis with **vinca alkaloids** (e.g., vinblastine).

SIDE EFFECTS
Alopecia, anaphylaxis, anorexia, bleeding, blurring of vision, cellulitis at injection site, confusion, CHF (patient has usually received doxorubicin [Adriamycin, Doxil]), coughing, diarrhea, drowsiness, dyspnea with nonproductive cough, edema, elevated BUN or SCr, fatigue, fever, headache, hematemesis, hemolytic uremic syndrome (microangiopathic

hemolytic anemia [hematocrit less than 25%], irreversible renal failure [SCr greater than 1.6 mg/dL], and thrombocytopenia [less than 100,000/mm³]), hemoptysis, hypertension, leukopenia, mouth ulcers, nausea, paresthesias, pneumonia, pruritus, pulmonary edema, purple discoloration of vein, radiographic evidence of pulmonary infiltrates, rash, renal failure, respiratory distress syndrome (acute), skin toxicity, stomatitis, syncope, thrombocytopenia, thrombophlebitis, vomiting.

ANTIDOTE

Most side effects will be treated symptomatically. Keep the physician informed. All are potentially serious and many can be life threatening. Hematopoietic depression requires cessation of therapy until recovery occurs. Discontinue drug if dyspnea, nonproductive cough, or radiographic evidence of pulmonary infiltrates is present. Discontinue drug for any symptoms of hemolytic uremic syndrome. There is no specific antidote. Supportive therapy as indicated will help sustain the patient in toxicity. Administration of whole blood products (e.g., packed RBCs, platelets, leukocytes) and/or blood modifiers (e.g., darbepoetin alfa, epoetin alfa, filgrastim, pegfilgrastim, sargramostim) may be indicated to treat bone marrow toxicity; see Precautions. If extravasation has occurred, L.A. dexamethasone injected into the indurated area with a fine hypodermic needle may be helpful; elevate extremity.

MITOXANTRONE HYDROCHLORIDE BBW

(my-toe-**ZAN**-trohn hy-droh-**KLOR**-eyed)

Antineoplastic

Novantrone

pH 3 to 4.5

USUAL DOSE

Pretreatment: Preliminary evaluations and testing required; see Monitor. Verify pregnancy status; see Maternal/Child.

Combination initial therapy for acute nonlymphocytic leukemia (ANLL) in adults: Induction: 12 mg/M²/day of mitoxantrone on Days 1 through 3 and cytarabine 100 mg/M²/day as a continuous 24-hour infusion on Days 1 through 7. Should a complete remission not be achieved, repeat mitoxantrone, 12 mg/M²/day for only 2 days, and cytarabine 100 mg/M²/day for 5 days after all signs or symptoms of severe or life-threatening nonhematologic toxicity have cleared.

Consolidation: After full hematologic recovery (usually 6 weeks after induction therapy), administer mitoxantrone 12 mg/M²/day by IV infusion on Days 1 and 2 and cytarabine 100 mg/M²/day as a continuous 24-hour infusion on Days 1 to 5. May repeat in 4 weeks. Severe myelosuppression occurred in these subsequent courses. See Monitor.

Prostate cancer: 12 to 14 mg/M² as a short IV infusion once every 21 days. Used concurrently with steroids.

Multiple sclerosis (MS): 12 mg/M² as an infusion over 5 to 15 minutes. Repeat every 3 months. May be given for up to 2 years or until a cumulative dose of 140 mg/M² has been administered.

DOSE ADJUSTMENTS

Adjust dose based on clinical response and development and severity of toxicity. ■ Clearance is reduced by impaired hepatic function. Treat patients with impaired hepatic function with caution; dose adjustment may be indicated. Specific recommendations not available; see Precautions.

DILUTION

Specific techniques required; see Precautions. A single dose must be diluted with at least 50 mL of NS or D5W. May be further diluted in NS, D5W, or D5NS. Must be given through Y-tube of a free-flowing infusion of D5W or NS, or may be diluted in larger amounts of the same solutions and given as a continuous infusion.

Filters: No data available from manufacturer.

Storage: Store unopened vial at RT (15° to 25° C [59° to 77° F]). Do not freeze. Diluted solution should be used immediately. After penetration of the stopper on a multidose vial, the undiluted mitoxantrone may be stored at RT for 7 days or refrigerated for up to 14 days. Do not freeze.

COMPATIBILITY

Manufacturer recommends not mixing in the same infusion with other drugs until **compatibility** data are available and states that it may form a precipitate if mixed in the same infusion with heparin.

Other sources suggest specific **compatibilities** dependent on concentration and manufacturer; consult a pharmacist.

RATE OF ADMINISTRATION

IV injection: A single dose of properly diluted medication over at least 3 to 5 minutes. Must be given through Y-tube of a free-flowing infusion of D5W or NS.

Intermittent infusion: A single dose over 15 to 30 minutes.

Infusion: Sometimes a single dose is given as a continuous infusion over 24 hours. Is combined with cytarabine.

ACTIONS

An anthracenedione, a synthetic antibiotic antineoplastic agent. Has achieved complete remissions with a single course of combination therapy. Has a cytocidal effect on proliferating and nonproliferating cells. Probably not cell-cycle specific. Inhibits DNA and RNA synthesis. Thought to reduce the number of relapses and slow down progression of MS through its ability to suppress the activity of T-cells, B-cells, and macrophages. These cells attack the myelin sheath around nerve cells, causing the symptoms of MS. Improves the presentation of brain lesions on MRI studies. Extensive distribution to tissue occurs rapidly. Partially metabolized. Exact pathways unknown. Half-life varies from 23 to 213 hours (median 75 hours). Slowly excreted in bile, urine, and feces as either unchanged drug or as inactive metabolites.

INDICATIONS AND USES

Treatment of acute nonlymphocytic leukemia in adults; includes erythroid, monocytic, myelogenous, and promyelocytic acute leukemias. Given in combination with other approved drugs. ■ Treatment of bone pain in patients with advanced prostate cancer resistant to hormones. Used concurrently with steroids. ■ To reduce neurologic disability and/or the frequency of clinical relapses in patients with secondary (chronic) progressive, progressive relapsing, or worsening relapsing-remitting multiple sclerosis (i.e., patients whose neurologic status is significantly abnormal between relapses). Not indicated in the treatment of patients with primary progressive MS.

Unlabeled uses: Treatment of acute lymphocytic leukemia (ALL), breast cancer, Hodgkin lymphoma, non-Hodgkin lymphomas, myelodysplastic syndrome, pediatric acute leukemias, pediatric sarcoma, and part of a conditioning regimen for autologous hematopoietic stem cell transplantation (HSCT).

CONTRAINDICATIONS

Hypersensitivity to mitoxantrone or other anthracyclines. ■ Not for intrathecal use; severe injury with permanent sequelae can result.

PRECAUTIONS

For IV use only. Do not administer SQ, IM, intra-arterially, or intrathecally. ■ Follow guidelines for handling cytotoxic agents. See Appendix A, p. 1308. ■ Use of goggles, gloves, and protective gown recommended. Flush skin copiously with warm water should any contact occur. Irrigate eyes immediately in case of contact. Clean spills with 5.5 parts calcium hypochlorite to 13 parts by weight of water for each 1 part of mitoxantrone. ■ Usually administered by or under the direction of the physician specialist with facilities for monitoring the patient and responding to any medical emergency. ■ Will cause severe myelosuppression; use extreme caution in pre-existing drug-induced bone marrow suppression. ■ Should not be given to patients with baseline neutrophil counts of less than 1,500 cells/mm^3 (except for the treatment of acute nonlymphocytic leukemia). ■ MS patients with a baseline left ventricular ejection fraction

(LVEF) below the lower limit of normal or patients who have received a cumulative dose equal to or greater than 140 mg/M^2 should not be treated with mitoxantrone. ▪ May cause severe cardiac toxicity (e.g., acute congestive heart failure) in all patients, even if cardiac risk factors are not present. May occur early during therapy or months to years after completion. Risk increased with cumulative doses (equal to or greater than 140 mg/M^2), in patients with pre-existing heart disease, and in patients previously treated with anthracyclines (see Drug/Lab Interactions), other cardiotoxic drugs, or radiation therapy encompassing the heart. ▪ Use caution in impaired liver function. Clearance is decreased; see Dose Adjustments. Patients with MS who have hepatic impairment should ordinarily not be treated with mitoxantrone. ▪ Use caution if renal function is impaired; has not been studied. ▪ Urine and sclera may turn bluish in color. ▪ Therapy with mitoxantrone increases the risk of developing secondary leukemia in patients with MS and in patients with cancer. Most commonly reported types are acute promyelocytic leukemia and acute myelocytic leukemia. The occurrence is more common when mitoxantrone is given in combination with other cytotoxic agents and/or radiotherapy or when doses of anthracyclines (e.g., doxorubicin, idarubicin) have been escalated. ▪ Rapid lysis of cancer cells may cause tumor lysis syndrome. ▪ See Monitor.

Monitor: Obtain baseline CBC with differential and platelet count; repeat before each dose and if S/S of infection occur. ▪ Complete a physical exam and ECG and obtain a complete history to assess for S/S of pre-existing cardiac disease. ▪ In all patients, obtain an evaluation of left ventricular ejection fraction (LVEF) by echocardiogram or MUGA (multiple-gated acquisition) before therapy begins. ▪ Evaluation of LVEF and assessment of cardiotoxicity by history, physical exam, and ECG should be repeated before each dose in MS patients. ▪ Obtain repeat LVEF as indicated in all patients. ▪ Mitoxantrone should not ordinarily be administered to MS patients who have received a cumulative dose equal to or greater than 140 mg/M^2 or to patients who experience a drop in LVEF to below the lower limit of normal or a clinically significant reduction in LVEF. MS patients should have an annual quantitative evaluation of LVEF after discontinuing mitoxantrone therapy to monitor for late-occurring cardiotoxicity. ▪ Monitoring of liver function is indicated before and during therapy. ▪ Because of rapid lysis of cancer cells, initiate hypouricemic therapy with allopurinol or similar agents before beginning treatment. Monitor uric acid levels, maintain hydration, and uric acid–lowering drugs (e.g., allopurinol) may be indicated. ▪ Observe closely and frequently for all signs of bleeding or infection. ▪ Prophylactic antibiotics may be indicated pending results of C/S in a febrile neutropenic patient. ▪ Determine absolute patency of vein. Severe local tissue damage may occur with extravasation. Phlebitis at the infusion site has also been reported. Should extravasation or phlebitis occur, discontinue injection and use another vein. ▪ Prophylactic antiemetics may reduce nausea and vomiting and increase patient comfort. ▪ Monitor for thrombocytopenia (platelet count less than 50,000/mm^3). Initiate precautions to prevent excessive bleeding (e.g., inspect IV sites, skin, and mucous membranes; use extreme care during invasive procedures; test urine, emesis, stool, and secretions for occult blood). ▪ Monitor for S/S of acute leukemia (secondary leukemia); may include excessive bruising, bleeding, and recurrent infections. ▪ See Precautions and Drug/Lab Interactions.

Patient Education: Effective birth control recommended; see Maternal/Child. ▪ Blood and cardiac tests are imperative; keep all appointments. ▪ Report IV site burning or stinging promptly. ▪ Urine may turn blue-green for 24 hours following administration. Bluish discoloration of sclera may also occur. ▪ Medication guide available; read before beginning treatment with mitoxantrone. ▪ See Appendix D, p. 1311.

Maternal/Child: Category D: avoid pregnancy. May produce teratogenic effects on the fetus. Females with MS who are biologically capable of becoming pregnant should have a pregnancy test before each dose of mitoxantrone regardless of other methods of birth control used, including birth control pills. ▪ Secreted in breast milk. Discontinue breast-feeding. ▪ Safety for use in pediatric patients not established.

Elderly: Specific age-related differences have not been identified; consider age-related organ impairment (e.g., bone marrow reserve, renal, hepatic) and possibility of increased sensitivity.

DRUG/LAB INTERACTIONS

Additive bone marrow suppression may occur with **radiation therapy and/or other bone marrow–suppressing agents** (e.g., azathioprine, chloramphenicol, melphalan). Dose reduction may be required. ▪ Risk of cardiotoxicity increased in patients previously treated with maximum cumulative doses of **other anthracyclines** (e.g., doxorubicin, epirubicin, idarubicin) **and/or radiation encompassing the heart.** ▪ Do not administer **live virus vaccines** to patients receiving antineoplastic drugs.

SIDE EFFECTS

Alopecia (reversible), bladder infections, menstrual disorders, mucositis, and nausea occur frequently. Other side effects include abdominal pain, acute congestive heart failure, altered electrolytes, altered liver function tests (e.g., increased ALT, AST, BUN), arrhythmias, arthralgias, bleeding, bone marrow suppression (severe with standard doses), cardiotoxicity, conjunctivitis, cough, decrease in LVEF, diarrhea, dyspnea, erythema, fever, GI bleeding, headache, hematuria, hypersensitivity reactions (e.g., dyspnea, hypotension, rash, urticaria), infections, injection site burning, jaundice, leukemia (including secondary acute myelogenous leukemia [AML]), mucositis, myalgias, nail bed changes, phlebitis, renal failure, seizures, skin discoloration, stomatitis, swelling, vomiting. Interstitial pneumonitis has been reported. Anaphylaxis has been reported rarely.

Post-Marketing: Secondary acute myelogenous leukemia (AML).

ANTIDOTE

There is no specific antidote. Notify physician of all side effects. Most will be treated symptomatically. Blood and blood products, antibiotics, and other adjunctive therapies must be available. Blood modifiers (e.g., darbepoetin alfa, epoetin alfa, filgrastim, pegfilgrastim, sargramostim) may be indicated to treat bone marrow toxicity. Nadir of leukocyte count occurs within 10 days. Recovery is within 21 days. For extravasation, elevate extremity and apply ice. Monitor closely and obtain surgical consult if necessary. Overdose has resulted in death. Peritoneal dialysis or hemodialysis not effective. Supportive therapy as indicated will help sustain the patient in toxicity.

MORPHINE SULFATE BBW
(**MOR**-feen **SUL**-fayt)

Opioid analgesic
(agonist)
Adjunct, pulmonary edema
Anesthesia adjunct

Astramorph PF, Duramorph PF

pH 2.5 to 6.5

USUAL DOSE

Individualize dose, taking into account the patient's severity of pain, patient response, prior analgesic treatment experience, and risk factors for addiction, abuse, and misuse. Use lowest effective dose for the shortest duration consistent with the patient's treatment goals.

IV injection: One manufacturer recommends an initial dose of 2 to 10 mg/70 kg of body weight. Repeat every 3 to 4 hours as necessary. Another manufacturer recommends a starting dose of 0.1 to 0.2 mg/kg every 4 hours as needed. Titrate to the lowest possible dose that provides adequate analgesia and minimizes adverse reactions. Administration of smaller, more frequent doses (e.g., 2 to 3 mg every 5 minutes) may be an appropriate way to achieve pain control and/or manage the development of adverse events (e.g., sedation, decreased oxygen saturation) when treating acute moderate to severe pain in a closely monitored setting such as the emergency department or the postanesthesia care unit. When this is done, orders should contain a maximum cumulative dose to trigger reassessment of pain and continued therapy.

Acute MI (unlabeled): 4 to 8 mg initially. May give additional doses of 2 to 8 mg at 5- to 15-minute intervals as needed (AHA guidelines).

Infusion (unlabeled): Used postoperatively with a patient-controlled analgesic device (PCA) and/or as a continuous infusion in select terminally ill cancer patients. **Continuous infusion (opioid tolerant):** 0.8 to 10 mg/hr. Higher doses have been used. A continuous infusion is not recommended in opioid-naïve patients. **PCA infusion:** One source suggests a concentration of 1 mg/mL, with a starting patient-controlled dose of 1 mg (range: 0.5 to 2.5 mg) that can be activated at prescribed intervals (e.g., every 5 to 10 minutes). Must be administered through a controlled infusion device that may be patient activated. The initial loading dose, the continuous background infusion (if prescribed), additional patient-activated doses with a specific time interval, additional health care professional–provided boluses with a specific time interval, and the total dose allowed per hour must be determined by the physician and individualized for each patient. In select cancer or chronic pain patients, these doses may be considerably higher.

Dyspnea during end-of-life care (unlabeled): 2 to 5 mg IV every 2 to 4 hours as needed.

PEDIATRIC DOSE

Analgesic: Usual range is 0.05 to 0.1 mg/kg. Administer very slowly.

Postoperative analgesia: 0.01 to 0.04 mg/kg/hr (10 to 40 mcg/kg/hr).

Select pediatric patients with severe chronic cancer pain or during sickle cell crisis: 0.025 to 2.6 mg/kg/hr (average 0.04 to 0.07 mg/kg/hr).

NEONATAL DOSE

Elimination is reduced in neonates, and they have an increased susceptibility to CNS side effects.

Analgesia/tetralogy (cyanotic) spells (unlabeled): 0.05 to 0.2 mg/kg/dose every 4 hours. Titrate to individual response. Another source suggests an **IV injection** of 0.05 to 0.1 mg/kg/dose every 4 to 8 hours or an **IV infusion** of 0.01 to 0.02 mg/kg/hr. Titrate to individual response.

DOSE ADJUSTMENTS

Reduced dose and/or extended intervals may be required in impaired renal or hepatic function and in elderly, cachectic, or debilitated patients. ▪ Doses appropriate for the general population may cause serious respiratory depression in vulnerable patients. ▪ Increase doses as required if analgesia is inadequate, tolerance develops, or pain severity increases. The first sign of tolerance is usually a reduced duration of effect. ▪ Higher doses may be required in patients with chronic pain. ▪ See Drug/Lab Interactions.

DILUTION

Morphine is available in several concentrations for direct injection, infusion, and PCA use. Dosing errors can result in accidental overdose and death. Avoid dosing errors that may result from confusion between mg and mL and confusion with morphine products of different concentrations when prescribing, dispensing, and administering morphine.

IV injection: May be given undiluted. May be given through Y-tube of infusion set.

Infusion: Each 0.1 to 1 mg is usually diluted in 1 mL NS or D5W and administered via a controlled infusion device. Infusion may be administered at a set rate or may be administered using a PCA system. Higher concentrations may be used in opioid-tolerant patients or for end-of-life infusions. Products for infusion are available in multiple sizes and concentrations. Some products are manufactured for specific infusion devices (i.e., are **compatible** with one brand of infusion device). (***Astramorph PF and Duramorph*** are preservative-free and expensive; can be used IV, but are the only choice for epidural or intrathecal injection; see drug literature. ***Duramorph*** is **NOT** for use in continuous microinfusion devices. ***Infumorph*** is **NOT** for IV use.) Fluid restriction or high doses may require more concentrated solutions.

Storage: Store at CRT. Protect from light and freezing.

COMPATIBILITY

Compatibility information not available from manufacturer. Other sources suggest specific **compatibilities** dependent on concentration and manufacturer; consult a pharmacist.

RATE OF ADMINISTRATION

Frequently titrated according to symptom relief and respiratory rate. Side effects markedly increased if rate of injection is too rapid. Because of a delay in maximum CNS effect with an intravenously administered drug (30 minutes), rapid IV administration may result in overdosing. Rapid IV administration may result in chest wall rigidity.

IV injection: A single dose over 4 to 5 minutes.

Infusion: All parameters (outlined in Usual Dose) should be ordered by the physician. Any dose requiring a controlled infusion device requires accurate titration and close monitoring.

ACTIONS

A mu-opioid receptor agonist. Precise mode of action is unknown, but opioids are believed to combine with specific CNS opiate receptors. Produces a wide spectrum of pharmacologic effects, including analgesia, diminished GI mobility, dysphoria, euphoria, peripheral vasodilation, respiratory depression, and somnolence. Relieves pulmonary congestion, lowers myocardial oxygen requirements, and reduces anxiety. The principal therapeutic action of morphine is analgesia. Pain relief is effected almost immediately. Metabolized in the liver. Excreted in the urine and to a lesser extent in feces. Elimination half-life is 1.5 to 2 hours (range: 1.5 to 4 hours). Crosses the blood-brain barrier, but plasma concentration is higher than CSF concentration. Crosses the placental barrier. Secreted in breast milk.

INDICATIONS AND USES

Management of pain severe enough to require an opioid analgesic and for which alternative treatments are inadequate.

Unlabeled uses: Pain associated with MI, acute pulmonary edema, and analgesia in critically ill patients. Treatment of dyspnea in end-of-life care. ▪ Control of postoperative pain in neonates.

Limitations of use: Because of the risk of addiction, abuse, and misuse, even at recommended doses, reserve morphine for use in patients for whom alternative treatment options (e.g., nonopioid analgesics or opioid combination products):
- Have not been tolerated or are not expected to be tolerated
- Have not provided adequate analgesia or are not expected to provide adequate analgesia

CONTRAINDICATIONS

Hypersensitivity to morphine sulfate or any component of the formulation. ▪ Significant respiratory depression. ▪ Acute or severe bronchial asthma in the absence of resuscitation equipment or in unmonitored settings. ▪ In patients with known, or suspected to have, GI obstruction, including paralytic ileus. ▪ Concurrent use of monoamine oxidase inhibitors (MAOIs) within the last 14 days. ▪ Specific formulations may have additional contraindications; see prescribing information. ▪ **Duramorph** is **NOT** for use in continuous microinfusion devices.

PRECAUTIONS

Morphine exposes patients and other users to the risks of opioid addiction, abuse, and misuse, which can lead to overdose and death. Assess each patient's risk before prescribing morphine, and monitor all patients regularly for the development of these behaviors and conditions. Strategies to reduce the risk of diversion or misuse should be used by health care facilities that use this and other controlled substances. ▪ See prescribing information for further discussion regarding abuse, addiction, physical dependence, and tolerance. ▪ Serious, life-threatening, or fatal respiratory depression may occur with the use of morphine. Because of a delay in maximum CNS effect with an intravenously administered drug (30 minutes), rapid IV administration may result in overdosing. Adequate facilities should be available for monitoring and ventilation. An opioid antagonist (e.g., naloxone), resuscitative and intubation equipment, and oxygen should be readily available. ▪ Although low doses of IV morphine have little effect on cardiovascular stability, high doses are excitatory and result from sympathetic hyperactivity and an increase in circulatory catecholamines. Use caution in patients with atrial flutter and other supraventricular tachycardias because of a possible vagolytic action that may produce a significant increase in ventricular response rate. ▪ Use with extreme caution in patients with COPD, cor pulmonale, a substantially decreased respiratory reserve, hypoxia, hypercapnia, or pre-existing respiratory depression; these patients are at increased risk for decreased respiratory drive, including apnea, even at recommended doses. Consider using nonopioid analgesics, or administer under careful medical supervision at the lowest effective dose. ▪ Use with caution and reduce initial doses in elderly, cachectic, or debilitated patients and in patients with severe impairment of hepatic, pulmonary, or renal function. Consider using nonopioid analgesics. ▪ Cases of serotonin syndrome have been reported during concomitant use of morphine with serotonergic drugs. ▪ Cases of adrenal insufficiency have been reported with opioid use, more often after more than 1 month of use. If adrenal insufficiency is diagnosed, treat with physiologic replacement doses of corticosteroids and wean the patient off the opioid to allow adrenal function to recover. Another opioid may be tried, because some cases reported use of a different opioid without recurrence of adrenal insufficiency. ▪ May cause severe hypotension, including orthostatic hypotension and syncope, in ambulatory patients or in any patient whose ability to maintain blood pressure has been compromised by depleted blood volume or concomitant administration of drugs that can cause hypotension (e.g., anesthetics, phenothiazines); see Drug/Lab Interactions. In patients with circulatory shock, morphine-induced vasodilation may further reduce cardiac output and blood pressure. Use should be avoided. ▪ Use caution in patients with head injury, brain tumors, or increased intracranial pressure. Respiratory depression may cause an increased P_{CO_2}, cerebral vasodilation, and increased intracranial pressure. Clinical course of head injury may be obscured. Avoid use in patients with impaired consciousness or coma. ▪ Use with caution in patients with biliary tract disease, including acute pancreatitis; may cause spasm of the sphincter of Oddi and diminish biliary and pancreatic secretions. ▪ May increase the frequency of seizures in patients with a convulsive disorder and may induce or aggravate seizures in some clinical settings. ▪ Do not abruptly discontinue morphine in a patient who is physically dependent; dose must be tapered gradually.

Monitor: Monitor for respiratory depression, especially during initiation of therapy (within the first 24 to 72 hours) or after a dose increase. Oxygen, naloxone, and equipment to establish and maintain an airway must be available. ▪ Assess baseline pain, reassess after administration of morphine, and adjust dose or interval as required. ▪ Monitor vital signs and oxygenation and observe patient frequently. ▪ Keep patient supine; orthostatic hypotension and fainting may occur; less likely with continuous low doses, but observe closely during ambulation. ▪ Monitor patients who may be susceptible to the intracranial effects of CO_2 retention for increasing intracranial pressure and signs of sedation and respiratory depression. ▪ Monitor patients with biliary tract disease for worsening of symptoms. ▪ Monitor patients with a history of seizure disorders for worsening seizure control. ▪ Monitor for S/S of serotonin syndrome (e.g., mental status changes [e.g., agitation, coma, hallucinations], autonomic instability [e.g., hyperthermia, labile blood pressure, tachycardia], neuromuscular aberrations [e.g., hyperreflexia, incoordination, rigidity], and/or GI symptoms [e.g., diarrhea, nausea, vomiting]). Onset of symptoms may occur within hours to days of concomitant use of opioids with serotonergic drugs. ▪ Uncontrolled pain causes sleep deprivation, decreases pain threshold, and increases pain. When pain is finally controlled, expect the patient to sleep more until recovery from sleep deprivation. ▪ Adhere to prescribed bowel care regimen to avoid constipation and/or impaction. Maintain adequate hydration. ▪ See Drug/Lab Interactions.

Patient Education: Avoid alcohol or other CNS depressants (e.g., barbiturates, benzodiazepines [e.g., diazepam]). Review all medications for interactions. ▪ May cause blurred vision, dizziness, or drowsiness; use caution in tasks that require alertness. ▪ Request assistance with ambulation. ▪ Promptly report unrelieved pain or unacceptable side effects. ▪ Promptly report S/S of serotonin syndrome. ▪ May result in severe constipation. Scheduled bowel regimen recommended. ▪ May result in addiction, abuse, and misuse, even when taken as recommended.

Maternal/Child: Use during pregnancy only if the potential benefit justifies the risk to the fetus. ▪ Use during labor and delivery may produce respiratory depression and a physiologic effect in neonates. Closely monitor neonates exposed to morphine during labor and delivery for signs of excessive sedation and respiratory depression. May also prolong labor by reducing the strength, duration, and frequency of contractions. ▪ Prolonged use of morphine during pregnancy can result in neonatal opioid withdrawal syndrome, which may be life threatening if not recognized and treated. Infants born to mothers receiving morphine during pregnancy should be monitored closely and treated for neonatal opioid withdrawal syndrome, if indicated. See literature for treatment protocols. Infants born to mothers physically dependent on opioids will also be physically dependent and may exhibit respiratory difficulties and withdrawal symptoms (e.g., excessive crying, fever, hyperactive reflexes, increased respiratory rate, increased stools, sneezing, tremors, vomiting, yawning). ▪ Use caution with breastfeeding. Monitor infants exposed to morphine through breast milk for excess sedation and respiratory depression. Withdrawal symptoms can occur in breast-fed infants when maternal administration of an opioid analgesic is stopped or when breast-feeding is stopped. ▪ Safety and effectiveness for use in pediatric patients not established. ▪ Pediatric patients may be more sensitive to effects, especially respiratory depressant effects.

Elderly: See Dose Adjustments and Precautions. ▪ May be more sensitive to effects (e.g., respiratory depression, constipation, urinary retention). Respiratory depression is the chief risk for elderly patients treated with opioids. ▪ Lower doses may provide effective analgesia. ▪ Consider age-related organ impairment.

DRUG/LAB INTERACTIONS

Concomitant use of morphine with **benzodiazepines** and other **CNS depressants** may result in profound sedation, respiratory depression, coma, and death. Hypotension can also occur. Reserve concomitant use for patients for whom alternative treatment options are inadequate. Limit dose and duration of treatment to the minimum required, and monitor patients carefully for S/S of respiratory depression and sedation. ▪ Serotonin syndrome has been reported with the concomitant use of opioids, including morphine, and other **drugs that affect the serotonergic neurotransmitter system** (e.g., selective serotonin reuptake inhibitors [SSRIs], serotonin and norepinephrine reuptake inhibitors [SNRIs], tricyclic antidepressants [TCAs], triptans, 5-HT3 receptor antagonists, mirtazapine, trazodone, tramadol, MAO inhibitors, and linezolid). Careful observation, particularly during treatment initiation and dose adjustment, is required with concomitant use. ■ Severe and unpredictable potentiation of **MAO inhibitors** (e.g., linezolid) has been reported. MAO inhibitor interactions may manifest as serotonin syndrome or opioid toxicity (e.g., respiratory depression, coma). Use of morphine is not recommended for patients taking MAOIs or within 14 days of stopping such treatment. If urgent use of an opioid is necessary, use test doses and frequent titration of small doses to treat pain while closely monitoring BP and S/S of CNS and respiratory depression. ■ **Mixed agonist/antagonist analgesics and partial agonists** may reduce the analgesic effect of morphine and/or precipitate withdrawal symptoms. Avoid concomitant use. ■ Morphine may enhance the neuromuscular blocking action of **skeletal muscle relaxants**, increasing the degree of respiratory depression. Monitor patient and decrease dose if indicated. ■ Opioids can reduce the efficacy of **diuretics** by inducing the release of antidiuretic hormone. Increase dose of diuretic if needed. ■ Concomitant use with **anticholinergic drugs** may increase the risk of urinary retention and/or severe constipation, which may lead to paralytic ileus. ■ Concomitant administration with **cimetidine** may precipitate apnea, confusion, and muscle twitching.

SIDE EFFECTS

The most frequently reported adverse reactions are constipation, diaphoresis, dizziness, light-headedness, nausea, sedation, and vomiting. Serious adverse reactions include respiratory depression and apnea and, to a lesser degree, circulatory depression, respiratory arrest, shock, and cardiac arrest. Anaphylactoid reactions have been reported rarely. Other reported adverse reactions include agitation, biliary tract spasm, bradycardia, depression of cough reflex, dysphoria, euphoria, faintness, headache, histamine-related reactions (e.g., local tissue irritation, pruritus, urticaria, wheals), hypersensitivity reactions, increased intracranial pressure, interference with thermal regulation, oliguria, orthostatic hypotension, palpitations, serotonin syndrome, syncope, tachycardia, transient hallucinations and disorientation, tremors, uncoordinated muscle movement, urinary retention, visual disturbances, and weakness.

Overdose: Apnea, atypical snoring, bradycardia, cardiac arrest, circulatory depression or collapse, cold and clammy skin, constricted pupils, hypotension (severe), partial or complete airway obstruction, pulmonary edema, respiratory depression or arrest, skeletal muscle flaccidity, somnolence progressing to stupor or coma, and death.

ANTIDOTE

With increasing severity of any side effect or onset of symptoms of overdose, discontinue the drug and notify the physician. Naloxone will reverse cardiovascular, CNS, and respiratory reactions. Naloxone use should be reserved for situations in which clinically significant respiratory or circulatory depression is present. Titrate naloxone dose carefully to avoid precipitating an acute abstinence syndrome or uncontrolled pain. The duration of action of morphine may exceed the duration of action of naloxone. Monitor patient carefully. Repeat doses of naloxone may be required. A patent airway, artificial ventilation, oxygen therapy, and other symptomatic treatment must be instituted promptly. Resuscitate as necessary.

MOSUNETUZUMAB
(moe SUN e TOOZ ue mab)

Lunsumio

USUAL DOSE

Premedicate before each dose in cycles 1 and 2. Give premedications in cycle 3 and beyond if patient experiences cytokine release syndrome (CRS) with the previous dose.

Premedication should include a corticosteroid (methylprednisolone 80 mg IV or dexamethasone 20 mg IV), which should be completed at least 1 hour before infusion, an antihistamine (diphenhydramine 50 to 100 mg oral or IV) at least 30 minutes before infusion, and acetaminophen 500 to 1000 mg orally at least 30 minutes before infusion.

Ensure patients are well hydrated before initiation. Do not administer to patients with active infection. Administer prophylactic antimicrobials according to local practice guidelines. Consider prophylactic granulocyte colony-stimulating factor administration, as appropriate.

Follicular lymphoma, relapsed or refractory

Mosunetuzumab IV Dosing Schedule (21-Day Treatment Cycles)			
Cycle number	Day of Treatment	Mosunetuzumab Dose	Infusion Duration
Cycle 1	Day 1	1 mg IV	At least 4 hours
	Day 8	2 mg IV	At least 4 hours
	Day 15	60 mg IV	At least 4 hours
Cycle 2	Day 1	60 mg IV	Infuse over 2 hours if cycle 1 infusions were well-tolerated
Cycle 3 and beyond	Day 1	30 mg IV	Infuse over 2 hours if cycle 1 infusions were well-tolerated

[a]Administer for 8 cycles (in the absence of disease progression or unacceptable toxicity); no further treatment is required after 8 cycles if complete response is achieved. For patients achieving a partial response or with stable disease in response to treatment after 8 cycles, an additional 9 cycles (for a total of 17 cycles) should be administered if no progression of disease or unacceptable toxicity.

Recommendations for Restarting Mosunetuzumab IV After a Dosing Delay		
Last Dose Administered	Time Since Last Dose	Action for Next Mosunetuzumab Dose
Cycle 1, day 1 (1 mg)	1 to 2 weeks	Administer 2 mg (cycle 1, day 8), then resume the planned treatment schedule.
	>2 weeks	Repeat 1 mg (cycle 1, day 1), then administer 2 mg (cycle 1, day 8) and resume the planned treatment schedule.
Cycle 1, day 8 (2 mg)	1 to 2 weeks	Administer 60 mg (cycle 1, day 15), then resume the planned treatment schedule.
	>2 to <6 weeks	Repeat 2 mg (cycle 1, day 8), then administer 60 mg (cycle 1, day 15) and resume the planned treatment schedule.
	≥6 weeks	Repeat 1 mg (cycle 1, day 1) and 2 mg (cycle 1, day 8), then administer 60 mg (cycle 1, day 15) and resume the planned treatment schedule.

Continued

Recommendations for Restarting Mosunetuzumab IV After a Dosing Delay		
Last Dose Administered	**Time Since Last Dose**	**Action for Next Mosunetuzumab Dose**
Cycle 1, day 15 (60 mg)	1 to <6 weeks	Administer 60 mg (cycle 2, day 1), then resume the planned treatment schedule.
	≥6 weeks	Repeat 1 mg (cycle 2, day 1) and 2 mg (cycle 2, day 8), then administer 60 mg (cycle 2, day 15), followed by 30 mg (cycle 3, day 1), and then resume the planned treatment schedule.
Cycle 2, day 1 (60 mg)	3 to <6 weeks	Administer 30 mg (cycle 3, day 1), then resume the planned treatment schedule.
	≥6 weeks	Repeat 1 mg (cycle 3, day 1) and 2 mg (cycle 3, day 8), then administer 30 mg (cycle 3, day 15),[a] followed by 30 mg (cycle 4, day 1) and then resume the planned treatment schedule.
Cycle 3 and beyond (30 mg)	3 to <6 weeks	Administer 30 mg, then resume the planned treatment schedule.
	≥6 weeks	Repeat 1 mg on day 1 and 2 mg on day 8 during the next cycle, then administer 30 mg on day 15,[a] followed by 30 mg on day 1 of subsequent cycles.

PEDIATRIC DOSE
Efficacy and safety have not been established.

DOSE ADJUSTMENTS
Renal: No dosage adjustments provided by manufacturer.

Hepatic: No dosage adjustments provided by manufacturer.

Dosage adjustments for adverse effects: *Cytokine release syndrome:* If CRS is suspected, stop mosunetuzumab until resolved; manage according to the table below and per clinical practice guidelines. Supportive therapy for CRS may include intensive care for severe or life-threatening CRS.

Mosunetuzumab-Related CRS Management		
CRS Grade	**Symptoms**	**Actions**
Grade 1	Temperature ≥38°C (≥100.4°F), attributed to CRS	Stop mosunetuzumab infusion and manage per practice guidelines. If symptoms resolve, restart infusion at the same rate. Ensure CRS symptoms are resolved for at least 72 hours before the next mosunetuzumab dose. Administer premedication before the next mosunetuzumab dose and monitor more frequently.
Grade 2	Temperature ≥38°C (≥100.4°F) with: hypotension not requiring vasopressors and/or hypoxia requiring low-flow oxygen (<6 L/min) via nasal cannula or blow-by	Stop mosunetuzumab infusion and manage per practice guidelines. If symptoms resolve, restart infusion at the 50% rate. Ensure CRS symptoms are resolved for at least 72 hours before the next dose. Administer premedication before the next dose and consider infusing the next dose at 50% rate. For the next dose, monitor more frequently and consider hospitalization.
Grade 2, recurrent		Manage per Grade 3 CRS.

Mosunetuzumab-Related CRS Management		
CRS Grade	**Symptoms**	**Actions**
Grade 3	Temperature ≥38°C (≥100.4°F) with: hypotension requiring a vasopressor (with or without vasopressin) and/or hypoxia requiring high-flow oxygen (≥6 L/min) via nasal cannula, face mask, non-rebreather mask, or Venturi mask	Withhold mosunetuzumab and manage per practice guidelines and provide supportive therapy, which may include intensive care. Ensure CRS symptoms are resolved for at least 72 hours before the next dose. Administer premedication before the next dose and infuse the next dose at 50% rate. Hospitalize for the next mosunetuzumab dose.
Grade 3, recurrent		Permanently discontinue mosunetuzumab. Manage CRS per practice guidelines and provide supportive therapy, which may include intensive care.
Grade 4	Temperature ≥38°C (≥100.4°F) with: Hypotension requiring multiple vasopressors (excluding vasopressin) and/or Hypoxia requiring oxygen via positive pressure, intubation, and mechanical ventilation	Permanently discontinue mosunetuzumab. Manage CRS per practice guidelines and provide supportive therapy, which may include intensive care.

CRS, cytokine release syndrome.

Neurologic toxicity

Stop mosunetuzumab infusion at the first sign of neurologic toxicity, including immune effector cell-associated neurotoxicity syndrome (ICANS), and consider neurology evaluation. Provide supportive therapy, which may include intensive care.

Mosunetuzumab-Related Neurologic Toxicity Management (Including ICANS)		
Adverse Reaction	**Severity**	**Actions**
Neurologic toxicity (including ICANS)	Grade 2	Hold mosunetuzumab until neurologic toxicities/symptoms improve to Grade 1 or baseline for at least 72 hours. Provide supportive therapy. If ICANS, manage per practice guidelines.
	Grade 3	Hold mosunetuzumab until neurologic toxicities/symptoms improve to Grade 1 or baseline for at least 72 hours. Provide supportive therapy, which may include intensive care; consider neurology evaluation. If grade 3 neurologic toxicity recurs, permanently discontinue.
	Grade 4	Permanently discontinue. Provide supportive therapy, which may include intensive care; consider neurology evaluation.

Recommended Mosunetuzumab Dosage Modifications for Other Adverse Reactions		
Adverse Reaction	**Severity**	**Actions**
Hematologic toxicity	ANC <500/mm³	Hold until ANC is ≥500/mm³. Consider prophylactic granulocyte colony-stimulating factor administration as appropriate.
	Other cytopenias	Hold or permanently discontinue based on the severity.

Continued

Recommended Mosunetuzumab Dosage Modifications for Other Adverse Reactions		
Adverse Reaction	**Severity**	**Actions**
Infections	Grades 1 to 4	Hold or consider permanently discontinuing based on severity. Manage infection appropriately and as clinically indicated. Hold in patients with active infection until infection resolves. For grade 4 infection, consider permanently discontinuing.
Compression or obstruction due to tumor flare	Any	Institute standard treatment as clinically indicated.
Other adverse reactions	Grade 3 or higher	Hold until adverse reaction resolves to grade 1 or baseline.

ANC, absolute neutrophil count; **ICANS,** immune effector cell-associated neurotoxicity syndrome.

DILUTION

Withdraw a volume equal to the volume of the dose from an infusion bag containing sodium chloride 0.9% or sodium chloride 0.45%. Use infusion bags made only of polyvinyl chloride (PVC) or polyolefin. Do not use if solution is discolored, cloudy, or contains visible foreign particles. Withdraw the dose from vial and add to infusion bag. Mix gently by slowly inverting the bag; do not shake. Do not mix with other medications.

Infusion Bag Volume Based on Mosunetuzumab Dose	
Mosunetuzumab Dose (and volume)	**Size of Infusion Bag**
1 mg (1 mL)	50 or 100 mL
2 mg (2 mL)	50 or 100 mL
30 mg (30 mL)	50, 100, or 250 mL
60 mg (60 mL)	100 or 250 mL

ADMINISTRATION

Infuse IV over at least 4 hours in cycle 1; if cycle 1 infusions are tolerated, infuse over 2 hours in cycle 2 and beyond. Do not infuse through an inline filter, although drip chamber filters may be used. Do not infuse other medications through the same IV line. Give only in a facility with appropriate support to manage severe reactions.

ACTIONS

Mosunetuzumab is a T-cell engaging bispecific humanized monoclonal antibody that binds to the CD3 receptor expressed on the surface of T cells and CD20 expressed on the surface of lymphoma cells and some healthy B-lineage cells. It also activates T cells, releasing proinflammatory cytokines, and inducing B-cell lysis.

INDICATIONS AND USES

Treatment of relapsed or refractory follicular lymphoma after at least 2 lines of systemic therapy.

CONTRAINDICATIONS

No contraindications are listed by manufacturer.

PRECAUTIONS

Mosunetuzumab has a black box warning regarding CRS, including serious or life-threatening reactions. Dose mosunetuzumab using step-up dosing schedule to reduce the risk for CRS. Withhold until CRS resolves or permanently discontinue based on severity.

Other precautions include:
- Serious or severe cytopenias (including neutropenia, anemia, and thrombocytopenia).
- Serious or fatal infections, including opportunistic infections. Do not give in the presence of active infection.
- Neurologic toxicity (including ICANS). The most frequent neurologic toxicities were headache, peripheral neuropathy, dizziness, and mental status changes (including confusion, attention disturbance, cognitive disorder, delirium, encephalopathy, and somnolence).

Mosunetuzumab may cause serious or severe tumor flare in a small percentage of patients.

Monitoring Parameters: Complete blood count with differential (monitor throughout treatment). Monitor for S/S of CRS and neurologic toxicity, including ICANS. Monitor hydration status. Monitor for S/S of infection (including opportunistic infections) before and during treatment and for S/S of tumor flare, including compression or obstruction due to mass effect secondary to tumor flare; patients with bulky tumors or disease located in close proximity to airways or a vital organ should be monitored closely during initial therapy.

Patient Education: *Contact physician with any of the following adverse effects:* Feeling tired or weak, itching, muscle or joint pain, stomach pain or diarrhea or signs of a common cold.

The following adverse effects are more serious, and a physician should be contacted **immediately**:
- CRS: fever, chills, dizziness or fainting, fast or abnormal heartbeat, trouble breathing, headache, upset stomach or vomiting, or wheezing.
- Infections: fever, chills, very bad sore throat, ear or sinus pain, cough, more sputum or change in color of sputum, pain upon passing urine, mouth sores, or wound that will not heal.
- Bleeding: vomiting or coughing up blood; vomit that looks like coffee grounds; blood in the urine; black, red, or tarry stools; bleeding from the gums; abnormal vaginal bleeding; bruises without a cause or that get bigger; or bleeding you cannot stop.
- Urinary tract infection: blood in the urine, burning or pain when passing urine, feeling the need to pass urine often or right away, fever, lower stomach pain, or pelvic pain.
- Electrolyte problems: mood changes; confusion; muscle pain, cramps, or spasms; weakness; shakiness; changes in balance; an abnormal heartbeat; seizures; loss of appetite; or severe upset stomach or vomiting.
- High blood sugar: confusion, feeling sleepy, unusual thirst or hunger, frequent passing of urine, flushing, fast breathing, or breath that smells like fruit.
- Swelling
- Shortness of breath
- Nervous system problems: headache; feeling sleepy; trouble sleeping; a burning, numbness, or tingling feeling; shakiness; dizziness or fainting; feeling confused; seizures; not able to focus or understand things; muscle problems or weakness; forgetting things; changes in balance; or trouble walking, speaking, reading, or writing.
- Signs of an allergic reaction: rash; hives; itching; red, swollen, blistered, or peeling skin with or without fever; wheezing; tightness in the chest or throat; trouble breathing, swallowing, or talking; unusual hoarseness; or swelling of the mouth, face, lips, tongue, or throat.

Do not drive if any of these neurologic issues occur, such as dizziness or drowsiness.

Maternal/Child: Verify pregnancy status before starting treatment. Patients who could become pregnant should use effective contraception during therapy and for 3 months after the last dose.

Pregnancy considerations

Animal reproduction studies have not been conducted. Based on the mechanism of action, in utero exposure to mosunetuzumab may cause B-cell lymphocytopenia in exposed infants and compromise pregnancy maintenance.

Breastfeeding considerations

It is not known if mosunetuzumab is present in breast milk.

Elderly: No specific recommendations; refer to adult dosing.

DRUG/LAB INTERACTIONS

Avoid the following drugs: abrocitinib, baricitinib, Bacillus Calmette-Guérin (BCG) vaccine, brivudine, chloramphenicol, cladribine, live vaccines, deucravacitinib, etrasimod, fexinidazole, filgotinib, nadofaragene firadenovec, natalizumab, pimecrolimus, ritlecitinib, ruxolitinib (topical), tacrolimus (topical), talimogene laherparepvec, tertomotide, tofacitinib, typhoid vaccine, upadacitinib

SIDE EFFECTS

Most common side effects include edema, pruritus, skin rash, xeroderma; decreased serum magnesium, phosphshate, and potassium; increased glucose and uric acid; abdominal pain, diarrhea, and nausea; decreased hemoglobin, white blood cells, neutrophils, lymphocytopenia, and thrombocytopenia; elevated liver function tests; CSR; chills, dizziness, fatigue, headache, insomnia, peripheral neuropathy, arthralgia, musculoskeletal pain, cough, dyspnea, upper respiratory tract infection, and fever.

ANTIDOTE

There is no antidote; stop infusion for hypersensitivity reactions and treat appropriately.

MOXIFLOXACIN HYDROCHLORIDE BBW

(mox-ee-**FLOX**-ah-sin hy-droh-**KLOR**-eyed)

**Antibacterial
(fluoroquinolone)**

Avelox

pH 4.1 to 4.6

USUAL DOSE

Pretreatment: Baseline studies indicated; see Monitor. See Maternal/Child.

400 mg once every 24 hours. Duration of therapy is based on diagnosis as listed in the following chart. Serum levels similar by oral or IV route. Transfer to oral therapy as soon as practical; no dose adjustment necessary. The magnitude of QT prolongation may increase with increasing serum concentrations. Do not exceed recommended dose.

Moxifloxacin Dosing Guidelines		
Infection[a]	Daily Dose (mg)	Duration (days)
Community-acquired pneumonia	400 mg	7–14 days
Uncomplicated skin and skin structure infections	400 mg	7 days
Complicated skin and skin structure infections	400 mg	7–21 days
Complicated intra-abdominal infections	400 mg	5–14 days
Plague	400 mg	10–14 days
Acute bacterial sinusitis (ABS)	400 mg	10 days
Acute bacterial exacerbation of chronic bronchitis (ABECB)	400 mg	5 days

[a]Due to the designated pathogens.

DOSE ADJUSTMENTS

Dose adjustment is not indicated based on age, gender, or race; in impaired renal function (including patients on hemodialysis or continuous ambulatory peritoneal dialysis (CAPD)); or in mild, moderate, or severe impaired hepatic function (Child-Pugh Classes A, B, and C). See Precautions.

DILUTION

Available in ready-to-use, latex-free flexibags containing 400 mg moxifloxacin in 0.8% saline. No further dilution is necessary. Refer to directions provided with administration set.

Filters: No data available from manufacturer.

Storage: Store at CRT. Do not refrigerate; a precipitate will form. Discard unused portions.

COMPATIBILITY

Limited **compatibility** data available. Manufacturer states, "Other IV substances, additives, or other medications should not be added to moxifloxacin or infused simultaneously through the same IV line." Flush line with a solution **compatible** to both drugs before and after administration of moxifloxacin and/or any other drug through the same IV line. May be administered through a Y-tube. Temporarily discontinue other solutions infusing at the same site.

Y-site: Manufacturer lists as **compatible** with NS, D5W, D10W, SWFI, LR at ratios from 1:10 to 10:1.

Other sources suggest a few specific **compatibilities** dependent on concentration and manufacturer; consult a pharmacist.

RATE OF ADMINISTRATION

Single dose equally distributed over 60 minutes as an infusion. Avoid rapid or bolus IV infusion. Incidence and magnitude of QT prolongation may increase with increasing concentrations or increasing rates of infusion. Do not exceed the recommended rate of infusion. Flush tubing before and after moxifloxacin with a **compatible** solution.

ACTIONS

A synthetic broad-spectrum fluoroquinolone antibacterial agent. Effective against a wide range of gram-negative and gram-positive organisms, including common respiratory pathogens such as *Streptococcus pneumoniae, Haemophilus influenzae,* and *Moraxella catarrhalis,* and atypicals such as *Chlamydophila pneumoniae* and *Mycoplasma pneumoniae*. Bactericidal action results from inhibition of topoisomerase II and IV, which are required for bacterial DNA replication, transcription, repair, and recombination. Mechanism of action of fluoroquinolones differs from that of aminoglycosides, cephalosporins, macrolides, beta-lactams, and tetracyclines, and fluoroquinolones may be active against pathogens resistant to these antibiotics. There is no cross-resistance between fluoroquinolones and these other antibiotics. Widely distributed throughout the body. Concentrations in most target tissues are higher than those found in plasma. Mean half-life is approximately 8.5 to 17 hours. Partially metabolized in the liver by glucuronide and sulfate conjugation. Excreted as unchanged drug and metabolites in feces and urine. May be secreted in breast milk.

INDICATIONS AND USES

Treatment of adults with infections caused by susceptible strains of designated microorganisms in conditions listed in this section. ▪ Treatment of community-acquired pneumonia caused by many organisms, including *S. pneumoniae* (including multidrug-resistant strains [MDRSP]). MDRSP strains are resistant to two or more of the following antibiotics: penicillin, second-generation cephalosporins (e.g., cefuroxime), macrolides, tetracyclines, and sulfamethoxazole/trimethoprim. ▪ Treatment of complicated and uncomplicated skin and skin structure infections. ▪ Treatment of complicated intra-abdominal infections, including polymicrobial infections such as abscess. ▪ Treatment of the plague, including pneumonic and septicemic plague, and prophylaxis of plague in adult patients. ▪ Treatment of acute bacterial exacerbation of chronic bronchitis (ABECB) and acute bacterial sinusitis (ABS). Because fluoroquinolones, including moxifloxacin, have been associated with serious adverse reactions and because for some patients ABECB and ABS are self-limiting, reserve moxifloxacin for treatment in patients who have no alternative treatment options.

CONTRAINDICATIONS

History of hypersensitivity to moxifloxacin or other quinolone antibiotics (e.g., ciprofloxacin, levofloxacin, norfloxacin).

PRECAUTIONS

For IV use only. ▪ To reduce the development of drug-resistant bacteria and maintain its effectiveness, moxifloxacin should be used to treat or prevent only those infections proven or strongly suspected to be caused by bacteria. ▪ C/S studies indicated to determine susceptibility of the causative organism to moxifloxacin. ▪ Cross-resistance has been observed between moxifloxacin and other fluoroquinolones against gram-negative bacteria. However, gram-positive bacteria resistant to other fluoroquinolones may still be susceptible to moxifloxacin. ▪ Observed emergence of bacterial resistance to fluoroquinolones and the occurrence of cross-resistance with other fluoroquinolones are of concern. Proper use of fluoroquinolones and other classes of antibiotics is encouraged to avoid the emergence of resistant bacteria from overuse. ▪ Prolonged use may cause superinfection because of overgrowth of nonsusceptible organisms. ▪ Fluoroquinolones, including moxifloxacin, have been associated with disabling and potentially irreversible serious adverse reactions that have occurred together in the same patient. Commonly seen adverse reactions include tendinitis and tendon rupture, arthralgia, myalgia, peripheral neuropathy, and CNS effects (e.g., anxiety, confusion, depression, hallucinations, insomnia, severe headaches). These reactions can occur within hours to weeks after starting moxifloxacin and have been seen in patients of any age and in patients without any pre-existing risk factors. Discontinue moxifloxacin immediately and avoid the use of fluoroquinolones, including moxifloxacin, in patients who experience any of these serious adverse reactions. ▪ Prolongation of the QT interval on ECG and infrequent cases of arrhythmia (including torsades de pointes) have been reported. The risk of arrhythmia may be reduced by avoiding the use of moxifloxacin in patients with known prolongation of the QT interval, uncorrected electrolyte imbalances (e.g., hypokalemia, hypomagnesemia), significant bradycardia, cardiomyopathy, ventricular arrhythmias (including torsade de pointes), myocardial ischemia, or in patients being treated with Class Ia antiarrhythmic agents (e.g., quinidine, procainamide) or Class III antiarrhythmic agents (e.g., amiodarone, sotalol) or any other drug that can prolong the QT interval; see Drug/Lab Interactions. ▪ Use caution in patients with mild, moderate, or severe hepatic insufficiency; associated metabolic disturbances may lead to QT prolongation. ▪ Fluoroquinolones, including moxifloxacin, have been associated with an increased risk of seizures (convulsions), increased intracranial pressure (pseudo-tumor cerebri), tremors, and light-headedness. May trigger seizures or lower the seizure threshold. Use caution in patients with epilepsy or known or suspected CNS disorders that may predispose patients to seizures or lower the seizure threshold (e.g., severe cerebral arteriosclerosis, previous history of convulsions, reduced cerebral blood flow, altered brain structure, or stroke) or in the presence of other risk factors that may predispose patients to seizures (e.g., drugs that may lower the seizure threshold, renal dysfunction). ▪ Fluoroquinolones, including moxifloxacin, have been associated with an increased risk of psychiatric adverse reactions, including toxic psychosis; psychotic reactions progressing to suicidal ideations/thoughts, hallucinations, or paranoia; depression, or self-injurious behavior such as attempted or completed suicide; anxiety, agitation, restlessness, or nervousness; confusion, delirium, disorientation, or disturbances in attention; insomnia or nightmares; and memory impairment. These reactions may occur after the first dose. ▪ Tendinitis and tendon rupture that required surgical repair or resulted in prolonged disability have been reported in patients of all ages receiving quinolones. Most frequently involves the Achilles tendon but has also been reported with the shoulder, hand, biceps, thumb, and other tendon sites. ▪ Tendinitis or tendon rupture may occur during or for up to months after fluoroquinolone therapy and may occur bilaterally. Risk may be increased in patients over 60 years of age; in patients taking corticosteroids; in patients with heart, kidney, or lung transplants; with strenuous physical activity; and in patients with renal failure or previous tendon disorders such as rheumatoid arthritis. Avoid moxifloxacin in patients who have a history of tendon disorders or have experienced tendinitis or tendon rupture. Discontinue moxifloxacin immediately if patient experiences pain, swelling, inflammation, or rupture of a tendon. ▪ Fluoroquinolones have neuromuscular blocking activity and may exacerbate muscle weakness in persons with myasthenia gravis. Serious adverse events, including requirement for ventilatory support and deaths, have been reported in these patients. Avoid use in patients with a known history of myasthenia gravis. ▪ Fluoroquinolones, including moxifloxacin, have been associated with an increased risk of peripheral neuropathy. Cases of sensory or sensorimotor axonal polyneuropathy resulting in paresthesias, hypoesthesias, dysesthesias (impairment of sensitivity or touch), or weakness have been reported. Symptoms may occur soon after initiation of therapy and may be irreversible. Avoid moxifloxacin in patients who have previously experienced peripheral neuropathy. ▪ Serious and occasionally fatal hypersensitivity and/or anaphylactic reactions have been reported. Often occur after the first dose. ▪ Other serious events (sometimes fatal) due to hypersensitivity or uncertain etiology have been reported with fluoroquinolones, including moxifloxacin. Usually occur following multiple doses. Manifestations may include things such as allergic pneumonitis, renal impairment/failure, hematologic toxicity, hepatic necrosis/failure, vasculitis, and dermatologic toxicity; see Side Effects, Post-Marketing. Discontinue moxifloxacin at the first appearance of a skin rash, jaundice, or other signs of hepatotoxicity or hypersensitivity. ▪ Epidemiologic studies report an increased rate of aortic aneurysm and dissection within 2 months after use of fluoroquinolones, particularly in elderly patients. In patients with a known aortic aneurysm or in patients who are at greater risk for aortic aneurysms, moxifloxacin use should be limited to those cases in which no alternative antibacterial treatments are available. ▪ Fluoroquinolones, including moxifloxacin, have been associated with disturbances of blood glucose, including symptomatic hyperglycemia and hypoglycemia, usually in patients with diabetes who are receiving concomitant treatment with an oral hypoglycemic agent (e.g., glyburide [DiaBeta]) or with insulin. In these patients, careful monitoring of blood glucose is recommended. Severe cases of hypoglycemia resulting in coma or death have been reported. ▪ Moderate to severe photosensitivity/phototoxicity reactions have been reported in patients receiving quinolones; see Patient Education. ▪ *Clostridium difficile*–associated diarrhea (CDAD) has been reported. May range from mild diarrhea to fatal colitis. Due to the potential serious side effects, the FDA recommends not to use fluoroquinolones if other options are available. ▪ See Monitor.

Monitor: Obtain baseline and periodic CBC with differential and blood glucose. ▪ Monitor for S/S of a hypersensitivity reaction (e.g., cardiovascular collapse, dyspnea, itching, loss of consciousness, pharyngeal or facial edema, tingling, urticaria). May be seen with first or subsequent doses. Emergency equipment must be readily available; see Side Effects. ▪ Monitor for S/S of peripheral neuropathy. Discontinue moxifloxacin at first symptoms of neuropathy (e.g., pain, burning, tingling, numbness and/or weakness) or if patient has deficits in light touch, pain, temperature, position sense, vibratory sensation, and/or motor strength. ▪ ECG monitoring for QT prolongation may be indicated in select patients. ▪ Monitor for CNS adverse effects, including altered mental status, seizures, and changes in mood or behavior. ▪ Monitor for S/S of tendinitis or tendon rupture. ▪ Maintain adequate hydration to prevent concentrated urine throughout treatment. Other quinolones have formed crystals. ▪ Monitor blood glucose closely, especially in patients with diabetes. ▪ See Precautions, Drug/Lab Interactions, and Antidote.

Patient Education: A patient medication guide is available from the manufacturer. ▪ Discontinue moxifloxacin and promptly report the development of any severe adverse reaction. ▪ Review medicines and disease states with physician or pharmacist before initiating therapy. ▪ Drink fluids liberally. ▪ Inform physician of any history of myasthenia gravis. ▪ Patients with a history of myasthenia gravis should avoid use of moxifloxacin. ▪ Report skin rash or any other hypersensitivity reaction promptly. ▪ Promptly report development of any CNS side effects (e.g., convulsions, dizziness, light-headedness, change in mood or behavior). ▪ Inform physician of any history of seizures. ▪ Request assistance with ambulation; may cause dizziness and light-headedness. Use caution in tasks that require alertness. ▪ Promptly report tendon pain or inflammation, weakness, or inability to use a joint; rest and refrain from exercise. ▪ Promptly report burning, numbness, pain, tingling, or weakness in extremities. Nerve damage can be permanent. ▪ Promptly report S/S of liver injury (e.g., dark-colored urine, fever, itching, jaundice [yellowing of skin or whites of eyes], light-colored bowel movements, loss of appetite, nausea, right upper quadrant tenderness, tiredness, vomiting, weakness). ▪ May produce changes in ECG. Report fainting spells or palpitations promptly. ▪ May alter glucose control in diabetic patients on insulin or oral therapy. Monitor glucose carefully. Discontinue moxifloxacin and contact physician if hypoglycemic reaction occurs. ▪ Photosensitivity has occurred in patients receiving other quinolones and, infrequently, moxifloxacin. It is best to avoid excessive sunlight or artificial ultraviolet light. May cause severe sunburn; wear protective clothing, use sunscreen, and wear dark glasses outdoors. Report a sunburn-like reaction or skin eruption promptly. ▪ Promptly report diarrhea or bloody stools that occur during treatment or up to several months after an antibiotic has been discontinued; may indicate CDAD and require treatment. ▪ Seek emergency medical care if sudden chest, stomach, or back pain is experienced. ▪ See Precautions, Monitor, Drug/Lab Interactions, and Antidote.

Maternal/Child: Safety for use in pregnancy not established. Based on animal studies, moxifloxacin may cause fetal harm. Benefit must outweigh risk to fetus. ▪ Use caution if breast-feeding infants; consider risk versus benefit. ▪ Safety and effectiveness for use in pediatric patients under 18 years of age not established. ▪ Quinolones have caused erosion of cartilage in weight-bearing joints and other signs of arthropathy in juvenile animals; however, they have been used in infants and children to treat serious infections unresponsive to other antibiotic regimens.

Elderly: Safety and effectiveness similar to that of younger adults; however, elderly may experience an increased risk of side effects (e.g., aortic aneurysm and dissection, CNS effects, tendinitis, tendon rupture, risk of QT prolongation). ■ See Precautions.

DRUG/LAB INTERACTIONS

May cause ventricular arrhythmias or torsades de pointes with **drugs that prolong the QT interval,** such as **Class Ia antiarrhythmic agents** (e.g., quinidine, procainamide), **Class III antiarrhythmic agents** (e.g., amiodarone, sotalol), **phenothiazines, tricyclic antidepressants**. Use with caution; see Precautions. ■ Risk of CNS stimulation and seizures may be increased with concurrent use of **NSAIDs.** ■ May cause hyperglycemia and hypoglycemia with concurrent administration of **antidiabetic agents**; monitoring of blood glucose recommended. ■ May enhance the effects of **warfarin**; monitoring of PT or INR is recommended with concomitant use. ■ See literature for additional drug/drug interactions on transfer to oral moxifloxacin. ■ May cause a false-positive when **testing urine for opiates;** more specific testing methods may be indicated.

SIDE EFFECTS

Diarrhea, dizziness, headache, and nausea were most common and described as mild to moderate in severity. Other side effects reported in 1% or more of patients included abdominal pain, anemia, constipation, dyspepsia, elevated alanine aminotransferase, fever, hypokalemia, insomnia, and vomiting. Capable of numerous other reactions in fewer than 1% of patients. Some of these reactions include cardiovascular effects (e.g., cardiac arrest, palpitations, QT interval prolongation, tachycardia, torsades de pointes, vasodilation, ventricular tachyarrhythmias); CDAD; CNS stimulation (e.g., anxiety, confusion, depression, hallucinations, insomnia, nightmares, paranoia, restlessness, seizures, suicidal thoughts, tremor); hepatic failure; hepatitis and jaundice (predominantly cholestatic); hyperglycemia or hypoglycemia; hypersensitivity reactions (e.g., anaphylaxis, cardiovascular collapse, death, dyspnea, edema [facial, laryngeal, or pharyngeal], hypotension, itching, rash, shock, urticaria); hypotension; increased bilirubin; increased intracranial pressure; pain, inflammation, and ruptures of the shoulder, hand, and Achilles tendon; peripheral neuropathy (e.g., pain, burning, tingling, numbness and/or weakness [see Precautions, Monitor]); photosensitivity/phototoxicity; prolonged PT and INR; Stevens-Johnson syndrome; syncope; and toxic psychoses; see Precautions.

Post-Marketing: Acute renal insufficiency or failure, allergic pneumonitis; arthralgia; exacerbation of myasthenia gravis; hearing impairment, including deafness (reversible in most); hematologic abnormalities (agranulocytosis, anemia [hemolytic and aplastic], leukopenia, pancytopenia, thrombocytopenia, thrombotic thrombocytopenic purpura); interstitial nephritis; liver abnormalities (e.g., acute hepatic necrosis or failure, hepatitis, jaundice); muscle weakness; myalgia; peripheral neuropathy; polyneuropathy; rash; serum sickness; severe dermatologic reactions (e.g., toxic epidermal necrolysis [Lyell's syndrome], Stevens-Johnson syndrome); suicidal ideation/thoughts; vasculitis; vision loss (transient in most cases).

ANTIDOTE

Keep physician informed of all side effects. Most minor side effects will be treated symptomatically or will resolve with continued dosing (e.g., dizziness, light-headedness); monitor closely. Discontinue at first sign of hypersensitivity (e.g., skin rash), CDAD, CNS symptoms, dermatologic reactions, hypoglycemic reactions, phototoxicity, symptoms of peripheral neuropathy, or tendon rupture. Treat hypersensitivity reactions as indicated with epinephrine, airway management, oxygen, IV fluids, antihistamines, corticosteroids, and pressor amines. Treat CNS symptoms as indicated. Mild cases of CDAD may respond to discontinuation of drug. Treat CDAD with fluids, electrolytes, protein supplements, and appropriate antibiotics (e.g., oral vancomycin) as indicated. In severe cases, surgical evaluation may be indicated. Complete rest is indicated for an affected tendon until treatment is available. Discontinue if photosensitivity occurs. Monitoring of the ECG and adequate hydration are indicated in overdose. No specific antidote. Less than 10% of moxifloxacin and its glucuronide metabolite are removed by CAPD or hemodialysis.

MULTIVITAMIN INFUSION
(mul-ti-**VI**-tah-min in-**FU**-zhun)

Nutritional supplement
(vitamin)

Infuvite Adult, Infuvite Pediatric, M.V.I.-12, M.V.I. Adult, M.V.I. Pediatric

USUAL DOSE

Multiples of the daily dose may be given or additional doses of individual vitamins in patients (adult and pediatric patients) with multiple vitamin deficiencies or markedly increased requirements. Individual components may be indicated in specific or long-standing deficiencies. Monitor blood vitamin concentrations to ensure maintenance of adequate levels. Formulations differ in the amount of each vitamin supplied and in their content (some contain vitamin K [e.g., *M.V.I. Adult and Pediatric, Infuvite (Adult and Pediatric)*], and others do not [e.g., *M.V.I.-12*]); see Drug/Lab Interactions.

All adult formulations: One 5- to 10-mL dose every 24 hours.

PEDIATRIC DOSE

See Maternal/Child.

INFUVITE PEDIATRIC

Supplemental vitamin A may be required for low-birth-weight infants.

Less than 1 kg: 30% of the contents of vial 1 and vial 2 (1.2 mL of vial 1 and 0.3 mL of vial 2).

1 to 3 kg: 65% of the contents of vial 1 and vial 2 (2.6 mL of vial 1 and 0.65 mL of vial 2).

Over 3 kg to 11 years of age: Entire contents of vial 1 (4 mL) and entire contents of vial 2 (1 mL).

M.V.I. PEDIATRIC

Less than 1 kg: 1.5 mL/24 hr.

1 to 3 kg: 3.25 mL/24 hr.

Over 3 kg to 11 years of age: 5 mL/24 hr.

DILUTION

Various preparations, including pharmacy bulk packages. Most may be reconstituted with 5 mL of SWFI or supplied diluent. All preparations must be further diluted in at least 500 mL but preferably 1,000 mL of IV fluids. Soluble in commonly used infusion fluids, including dextrose, saline, electrolyte replacement fluids, plasma, and selected protein amino acid products. Do not use if any crystals have formed. When reconstituted as directed, *Infuvite Adult* contains no more than 70 mcg/L of aluminum. M.V.I.-12 also contains aluminum.

Pediatric dilution: *Infuvite Pediatric and M.V.I. Pediatric:* Each dose should be added to at least 100 mL of dextrose, saline, or other **compatible** infusion solution. When reconstituted as directed, *M.V.I. Pediatric* contains no more than 42 mcg/L of aluminum, and *Infuvite Pediatric* contains no more than 30 mcg/L of aluminum; see Precautions. See Maternal/Child.

Storage: Before use, refrigerate at 2° to 8° C (36° to 46° F) protected from light. Manufacturers recommend immediate use of fully diluted Infuvite Pediatric and M.V.I. Adult and Pediatric. Fully diluted M.V.I.-12 and Infuvite Adult should be refrigerated and used within 24 hours. Once a pharmacy bulk vial has been penetrated, complete dispensing within 4 hours. Mixed solution may be stored for up to 4 hours refrigerated.

COMPATIBILITY

Compatibility may vary with preparation; consult prescribing information for specifics of a preparation. Direct addition to IV fat emulsions is not recommended. Some manufacturers suggest that admixture or **Y-site** administration with vitamin solutions should be avoided. Alkaline or other alkaline solutions (e.g., acetazolamide, aminophylline, chlorothiazide, sodium bicarbonate), as well as ampicillin and tetracycline, are listed as

incompatible by one manufacturer. Folic acid may be unstable with calcium salts. *All formulations must be diluted in infusion solutions.*

Other sources suggest a few specific **compatibilities** dependent on concentration and manufacturer; consult a pharmacist.

RATE OF ADMINISTRATION

A single dose given as an infusion at prescribed rate of infusion fluids. **Do not administer** as a direct, undiluted IV injection; may cause dizziness, faintness, and tissue irritation.

ACTIONS

A multiple vitamin solution containing fat-soluble and water-soluble vitamins in an aqueous solution. Provides B complex and vitamins A, D, and E. Some multivitamin preparations presently available do not contain vitamin K. *Infuvite Adult, M.V.I. Adult, Infuvite Pediatric, and M.V.I. Pediatric* do contain vitamin K. Provides daily requirements or corrects an existing deficiency.

INDICATIONS AND USES

A daily multivitamin maintenance supplement for patients receiving parenteral nutrition. Provides the necessary vitamins required to maintain the body's normal resistance and repair processes. Also used in situations such as surgery, trauma, burns, severe infectious disease, and comatose states, which may provoke a stress response and alteration in the body's metabolic demands. Used when oral administration is contraindicated, not possible, or insufficient. Solutions without vitamin K are indicated for patients on warfarin anticoagulant therapy who are receiving parenteral nutrition.

CONTRAINDICATIONS

Known hypersensitivity to thiamine hydrochloride or other product components; pre-existing hypervitaminosis. ■ Contraindicated prior to blood sampling for detection of megaloblastic anemia. Folic acid and cyanocobalamin in formulation may mask serum deficits.

PRECAUTIONS

Solutions containing multivitamins may contain aluminum. In patients with renal impairment, aluminum may reach toxic levels. Premature neonates are particularly at risk because of their immature kidneys and requirement for calcium and phosphate, which also contain aluminum. Patients with impaired renal function who receive more than 4 to 5 mcg/kg/day of parenteral aluminum are at risk for developing CNS or bone toxicity associated with aluminum accumulation. ■ Blood draws for the detection of folic acid and cyanocobalamin deficiencies are indicated before administration to patients with megaloblastic anemia. ■ See Drug/Lab Interactions.

Monitor: Monitor VS. ■ Monitor for any symptoms of a hypersensitivity reaction. ■ Moderate increase in ALT may occur in patients with active inflammatory enterocolitis. Usually reversible following discontinuation of vitamin infusion. Monitoring of ALT levels suggested. ■ Monitor vitamin A levels in patients with liver disease and/or high alcohol consumption. ■ Monitor renal function, aluminum, calcium, phosphorous, and vitamin A levels in patients with impaired renal function. ■ Measure blood vitamin concentrations periodically in patients receiving parenteral nutrition to determine if vitamin deficiencies or excesses are developing. Blood levels of A, C, D, and folic acid may decline in patients receiving parenteral multivitamins as their sole source of vitamins for 4 to 6 months. ■ See Precautions, Maternal/Child, and Drug/Lab Interactions.

Patient Education: Report any S/S of hypersensitivity reactions (e.g., digital edema, periorbital edema, urticaria). ■ Patients with renal impairment should promptly report any nausea, vomiting, headache, dizziness, or blurred vision. ■ Promptly report agitation, anxiety, dizziness, double vision, erythema, headache, itching, and rash. ■ Periodic monitoring of blood vitamin concentrations is indicated.

Maternal/Child: Recommendations for use during pregnancy vary by product. ■ Recommendations for use during breast-feeding vary by product use caution if required during breast-feeding. ■ Safety and effectiveness of adult formulations and M.V.I.-12 for use in pediatric patients under 11 years of age have not been established. ■ See Precautions.

Elderly: Consider age-related decreased organ function and/or medical problems. No identified differences in response between the elderly and younger patients.

DRUG/LAB INTERACTIONS
See specific vitamins for detailed information.

SIDE EFFECTS
Rare when administered as recommended: Agitation; allergic reactions including anaphylaxis, angioedema, periorbital and digital edema, shortness of breath, urticaria, and wheezing; anxiety; diplopia; dizziness; erythema; fainting; headache; pruritus; rash. Vitamin A and vitamin D hypervitaminosis (symptomatology related to hypercalcemia) may occur with prolonged use of significant doses.

ANTIDOTE
With onset of any side effect, discontinue administration immediately and notify physician. Treat anaphylaxis or resuscitate as necessary.

MYCOPHENOLATE MOFETIL HYDROCHLORIDE BBW

Immunosuppressant

(**my**-koh-**FEN**-oh-layt **MAH**-fuh-teel hy-droh-**KLOR**-eyed)

CellCept Intravenous

pH 2.4 to 4.1

USUAL DOSE
Pretreatment: Baseline studies indicated; see Monitor. Verify pregnancy status; see Maternal/Child.

Used in combination with cyclosporine (Sandimmune) and corticosteroids. Oral form should be used as soon as tolerated by the patient. Initial dose should be given within 24 hours of transplantation. The IV preparation may be used for up to 14 days.

Kidney or liver transplant: 1 Gm as an infusion twice daily (total daily dose of 2 Gm).

Heart transplant: 1.5 Gm as an infusion twice daily (total daily dose of 3 Gm).

PEDIATRIC DOSE
Limited data available; see Indications and Uses and product insert. Safety and efficacy of IV formulation not established. Usually given orally.

DOSE ADJUSTMENTS
No dose adjustments are indicated in renal transplant patients who experience delayed graft function postoperatively. ■ Avoid doses greater than 1 Gm twice daily in renal transplant patients with severe chronic renal impairments (GFR less than 25 mL/min/1.73 M^2) outside the immediate posttransplant period. ■ Data not available for cardiac or hepatic transplant patients with severe chronic renal impairment; potential benefits must outweigh risks. ■ Reduce dose or interrupt the dosing cycle if neutropenia (ANC less than 1.3×10^3 [1,300 cells/mm^3]) occurs. ■ Dose adjustment not indicated in impaired liver function. ■ See Precautions/Monitor.

DILUTION
Specific techniques required; see Precautions. Use caution in handling and preparation. Avoid skin contact with the solution. If skin contact occurs, wash thoroughly with soap and water; rinse eyes with plain water.

Reconstitute each 500-mg vial with 14 mL of D5W (500 mg/15 mL). Shake gently to dissolve. Discard if particulate matter or discoloration is observed or if a lack of vacuum in vial is noted when diluent is added. To achieve a final concentration of 6 mg/mL, each 500 mg must be further diluted with 70 mL of D5W (1 Gm with 140 mL; 1.5 Gm with 210 mL).

Filters: Not required by manufacturer; however, no significant loss of potency is expected with the use of a filter.

Storage: Store powder and reconstituted or diluted solutions at 15° to 30° C (59° to 86° F). Most desired storage temperature is 25° C (77° F). Reconstituted or diluted solutions are best used immediately after preparation. Keep reconstituted or diluted solutions at CRT; the infusion must begin within 4 hours of reconstitution/dilution.

COMPATIBILITY

Manufacturer states, "Mycophenolate is **incompatible** with other IV solutions and should not be mixed or administered concurrently via the same infusion catheter with other intravenous drugs or infusion admixtures."

Other sources suggest a few specific **compatibilities** dependent on concentration and manufacturer; consult a pharmacist.

RATE OF ADMINISTRATION

A single dose must be given as an infusion over a minimum of 2 hours. **Must not be** administered by rapid or bolus IV injection. Rapid infusion increases the risk of local adverse reactions such as phlebitis and thrombosis.

ACTIONS

A hydrochloride salt of mycophenolate mofetil. An antimetabolite immunosuppressive agent. Has a potent cytostatic effect on lymphocytes, inhibiting proliferation of both B- and T-lymphocytes. It also suppresses antibody formation by B-lymphocytes. Rapidly and completely metabolized to mycophenolic acid (MPA), its active metabolite. MPA is then metabolized predominantly to its inactive metabolite, mycophenolic acid glucuronide (MPAG). Secondary peak in plasma MPA concentration is usually noted 6 to 12 hours postdose. Enterohepatic recirculation is thought to contribute to MPA concentrations. Both MPA and MPAG are highly bound to albumin. In patients with renal impairment or delayed graft function, levels of MPAG may be elevated. Binding of MPA may then be reduced as a result of competition between MPAG and MPA. Plasma concentrations of metabolites are increased in patients with renal impairment. Half-life is 11.4 to 24.4 hours. Excreted primarily as MPAG in urine. Small amount excreted in feces.

INDICATIONS AND USES

Used as part of an immunosuppressive regimen that includes cyclosporine and corticosteroids. ▪ Prophylaxis of acute organ rejection in patients receiving allogeneic kidney, heart or liver transplants. ▪ Capsules, tablets, and oral solution approved for prevention of rejection in pediatric renal transplant patients.

CONTRAINDICATIONS

Hypersensitivity to mycophenolate mofetil, mycophenolic acid, any component of the drug product, or polysorbate 80 (TWEEN).

PRECAUTIONS

For IV use only. ▪ Use caution in handling and preparation. Avoid skin contact with the solution. If contact occurs, wash thoroughly with soap and water; rinse eyes with plain water. Follow guidelines for handling cytotoxic agents. See Appendix A, p. 1308. ▪ Usually administered by or under the direction of a physician experienced in immunosuppressive therapy and the management of organ transplant patients. Adequate laboratory and supportive medical resources must be available. ▪ Risk of developing lymphoproliferative diseases, lymphomas, and other malignancies, particularly of the skin, is increased. Appears to be related to the intensity and duration of immunosuppression rather than to any specific agent. ▪ Posttransplant lymphoproliferative disorder has been reported in organ transplant patients receiving mycophenolate with other immunosuppressants. Most cases appear to be related to Epstein-Barr virus (EBV) infection. Risk is greatest in patients who are EBV seronegative. ▪ Patients receiving immunosuppressants have increased susceptibility to bacterial, viral, fungal, and protozoal infections, including opportunistic infections and viral reactivation of hepatitis B and C, which may lead to hospitalizations and fatal outcomes. Serious viral infections that have been reported include polyomavirus-associated nephropathy (PVAN), JC virus–associated progressive multifocal leukoencephalopathy (PML), cytomegalovirus (CMV) infections, and reactivation of hepatitis B (HBV) or hepatitis C (HCV). Reduction in immunosuppression should be considered for patients who develop evidence of new or reactivated viral infections. Physicians should also consider the risk that reduced immunosuppression presents to the functioning allograft. ▪ PML has been reported. PML is a serious progressive neurologic disorder caused by infection of the CNS by JC virus, a member of the polyomavirus family. It typically occurs in immunocompromised patients. PML is rare but may result in irreversible neurologic deterioration and death, and there is no known effective treatment. Hemiparesis, apathy, confusion, cognitive deficiencies, and ataxia are the most commonly observed clinical signs. ▪ PVAN, is associated with serious outcomes, including deterioration in renal function and renal graft loss. Reduction in immunosuppression may be indicated. ▪ Risk of CMV viremia and CMV disease is highest among transplant recipients who are seronegative for CMV at time of transplant and receive a graft from a CMV-seropositive donor. ▪ Severe neutropenia has been reported; see Monitor. ▪ Pure red cell aplasia (PRCA) has been reported in patients receiving mycophenolate in combination with other immunosuppressive agents. May be reversible with dose reduction or discontinuation of mycophenolate. In transplant patients, reduced immunosuppression may place the graft at risk. ▪ Has been associated with an increased incidence of GI adverse effects (e.g., GI tract ulceration, hemorrhage, and/or perforation). Use caution in patients with active serious GI disease. ▪ Use with caution in patients with hepatic insufficiency. Metabolism of MPA may be affected by certain types of hepatic disease. ▪ Use caution in patients with severe chronic renal impairment; see Dose Adjustments. ▪ Avoid use in patients with selected rare hereditary deficiencies of hypoxanthine-guanine phosphoribosyl-transferase, such as Lesch-Nyhan and Kelley-Seegmiller syndromes; may exacerbate disease symptoms. ▪ See Monitor, Patient Education, and Maternal/Child.

Monitor: Obtain baseline CBC with differential before treatment. Repeat weekly during the first month, twice monthly for the second and third months, then monthly thereafter for the first year. ▪ Monitor for neutropenia. Has been observed most frequently in the period from 31 to 180 days posttransplant. May be due to mycophenolate, concomitant medications, viral infections, or some combination of these causes. If neutropenia develops (ANC less than 1,300 cells/mm^3), mycophenolate should be interrupted or the dose reduced. Appropriate diagnostic tests and treatment should be instituted. ▪ Monitor for S/S of infection. ▪ Assess neurologic status frequently. ▪ Monitor patients infected with HBV or HCV for clinical and laboratory signs suggestive of reactivation of infection. ▪ Monitor for S/S of organ rejection. ▪ Monitor for S/S of lymphoma or other malignancies. ▪ Monitor patients with severe chronic renal impairment and patients with delayed graft function closely. See Dose Adjustments and Actions.

Patient Education: Read the manufacturer's medication guide before beginning treatment with mycophenolate. ▪ In females of childbearing age, a pregnancy test is required immediately before starting mycophenolate. Test should be repeated in 8 to 10 days. Repeat pregnancy tests should be performed during routine follow-up visits. Effective contraception must be used during therapy and for 6 weeks following cessation of therapy. Females with reproductive potential must be counseled regarding pregnancy prevention and planning. Females with reproductive potential include girls who have entered puberty and all females who have a uterus and have not passed through menopause (menopause must be confirmed). See manufacturer's prescribing information for acceptable contraceptive methods. Birth control pills alone may be ineffective. If a pregnancy occurs, do not stop mycophenolate; call your health care provider. See Maternal/Child. ▪ Alternative immunosuppressants with less potential for embryo-fetal toxicity should be considered in patients who are considering pregnancy. ▪ Promptly report any S/S of infection or bone marrow suppression (e.g., unexpected bruising, bleeding). May cause serious infections. ▪ May increase risk of lymphoproliferative disease and some other malignancies. ▪ Risk of skin cancer may be increased. Reduce exposure to sunlight and UV light. Wear protective clothing and use a sunscreen with a high protection factor. ▪ Promptly report any S/S of GI toxicity (e.g., abdominal pain, bleeding). ▪ Cooperation with repeated laboratory tests imperative. ■ Review medications with the physician responsible for mycophenolate therapy. ■ Do not donate blood during therapy or for at least 6 weeks after discontinuation of mycophenolate because the blood or blood product could be administered to a woman of reproductive potential or to a pregnant woman. ■ Sexually active male patients and/or their female partners should use effective contraception during treatment of the male patient and for at least 90 days after cessation of treatment. ■ Do not donate semen during therapy and for 90 days after discontinuation of mycophenolate. ■ May affect ability to drive or operate machinery. Avoid tasks that require alertness if somnolence, confusion, dizziness, tremor, or hypotension is experienced during treatment with mycophenolate. ■ See Appendix D, p. 1311.

Maternal/Child: Increased risk of first-trimester pregnancy loss and increased risk of congenital malformations, especially external ear and other facial abnormalities (including cleft lip and palate) and anomalies of the distal limbs, heart, esophagus, kidney, and nervous system. See manufacturer's literature for details. Avoid use of mycophenolate during pregnancy if safer treatment options are available. Use during pregnancy only if benefit justifies risk; should pregnancy occur during treatment, discuss the desirability of continuing the pregnancy. Females using mycophenolate at any time during pregnancy are encouraged to enroll in the National Transplantation Pregnancy Registry. Patients considering pregnancy should discuss with their physician appropriate alternative immunosuppressants with less potential for embryo-fetal toxicity. A negative serum or urine pregnancy test with a sensitivity of at least 25 mIU/mL immediately before beginning therapy is indicated in all females of childbearing age. Repeat testing required. Effective contraception required before, during, and after use. See Patient Education. ■ There are no data on the presence of mycophenolate in human milk or the effects on milk production; use caution. ■ Safety and effectiveness of IV formulation for use in pediatric patients not established but has been used; see Indications.

Elderly: No specific recommendations. Consider age-related decreased organ function and/or additional medical problems and medications. May be at increased risk for certain adverse reactions (e.g., certain infections [including CMV tissue invasive disease] and possibly GI hemorrhage and pulmonary edema). Observe carefully.

DRUG/LAB INTERACTIONS

Several drugs have the potential to alter systemic mycophenolic acid (MPA) exposure when coadministered with mycophenolate. Determination of MPA plasma concentrations before and after making changes to immunosuppressive therapy, or when adding or discontinuing concomitant medications, may be appropriate to ensure MPA concentrations remain stable. ■ **Cyclosporine** may decrease serum levels of MPA (mycophenolate). Monitor levels closely when cyclosporine is added or removed from a drug regimen containing mycophenolate. ■ Use caution with **drugs that interfere with enterohepatic recirculation or alter the intestinal flora** (e.g., cholestyramine, rifampin, sulfamethoxazole/trimethoprim, selected antimicrobial classes [e.g., aminoglycosides, cephalosporins, fluoroquinolones, and penicillins]); may decrease MPA systemic exposure, reducing mycophenolate efficacy. ■ When given concomitantly with **drugs that undergo renal tubular secretion** (e.g., acyclovir, ganciclovir, probenecid, valacyclovir, valganciclovir), mycophenolate's metabolite (MPAG) may compete with secretion of these drugs, increasing plasma concentrations and/or adverse reactions associated with these drugs; monitoring of drug-related adverse reactions is recommended. ■ **Oral contraceptives and other hormonal contraceptives** (e.g., transdermal patch, vaginal ring, injection, and implant) may be less effective; use additional barrier contraceptive measures; see manufacturer's prescribing information. ■ Concomitant administration of **drugs that induce glucuronidation** (e.g., telmisartan) decreases MPA systemic exposure, potentially reducing mycophenolate efficacy. ■ Concomitant administration of **drugs that inhibit glucuronidation** (e.g., isavuconazole) increases MPA systemic exposure, potentially increasing the risk of mycophenolate-related adverse reactions. ■ Do not use **live virus vaccines** in patients receiving mycophenolate; vaccinations may be less effective. See Patient Education.

SIDE EFFECTS

Diarrhea, infection, leukopenia, and vomiting occur most frequently. Other reactions that occurred in at least 20% of patients during clinical trials included abdominal pain, asthenia, bone marrow suppression (e.g., anemia, ecchymosis, leukocytosis, leukopenia, neutropenia, thrombocytopenia), constipation, cough, creatinine and BUN increase, decreased appetite, depression, dizziness, dyspepsia, dyspnea, edema, fever, headache, hypercholesterolemia, hyperglycemia, hyperkalemia, hypertension, hypocalcemia, hypokalemia, hypomagnesemia, hypotension, infection, insomnia, lactic dehydrogenase increase, liver function test abnormalities, and nausea. 2 Gm/day demonstrated an overall better safety profile than 3 Gm/day. Serious adverse reactions included blood dyscrasias, embryo-fetal toxicity, GI complications, lymphomas and other malignancies, PML, renal impairment, and serious infections; see Precautions.

Post-Marketing: Bone marrow failure, bronchiectasis, colitis, embryo-fetal toxicity (including congenital malformations and spontaneous abortions [mainly in the first trimester]; see manufacturer's prescribing information), hypogammaglobulinemia, infections (e.g., atypical mycobacterial infections; endocarditis; meningitis; polyomavirus-associated neuropathy [PVAN], especially due to BK virus; progressive multifocal leukoencephalopathy [PML]; protozoal infections; TB; viral reactivation in patients infected with HBV or HCV), interstitial lung disorders (including fatal pulmonary fibrosis), lymphocele, pancreatitis, pure red cell aplasia, venous thrombosis.

ANTIDOTE

Notify the physician of all side effects. Most can be treated symptomatically. Drug may be decreased or discontinued or other immunosuppressive agents utilized. Some side effects (e.g., neutropenia) may require temporary reduction of dosage or withholding of treatment. Consider reducing the amount of immunosuppression in patients who develop PML, taking into account the risk this may represent to the graft. At clinically encountered concentrations, MPA and MPAG are not usually removed by hemodialysis. However, at high concentrations (greater than 100 mcg/mL) small amounts of MPAG are removed. MPA may be removed by bile acid sequestrants such as cholestyramine.

NAFCILLIN SODIUM

(naf-**SILL**-in **SO**-dee-um)

Nallpen ✤

Antibacterial
(penicillinase-resistant penicillin)

pH 6 to 8.5

USUAL DOSE

Pretreatment: Baseline studies indicated; see Monitor.

Nafcillin: 500 mg to 1 Gm every 4 hours. Up to 12 Gm in 24 hours has been used in severe infections. Duration of therapy varies with the type and severity of infection and with the overall condition of the patient; determine by the clinical and bacteriologic response. Usual duration of therapy is at least 14 days for severe staphylococcal infections and longer (4 to 6 weeks) for endocarditis and osteomyelitis.

Endocarditis, meningitis, osteomyelitis, or pericarditis: 1.5 to 2 Gm every 4 to 6 hours.

PEDIATRIC DOSE

Safety and effectiveness for use in pediatric patients not established. All pediatric IV doses are unlabeled; see Maternal/Child. Limited clinical experience with IV route in neonates and infants. Maximum dose is 12 Gm/24 hr.

Pediatric patients over 1 month of age: *Moderate infections:* 100 to 150 mg/kg/day in equally divided doses every 6 hours (25 to 37.5 mg/kg every 6 hours). Maximum daily dose is 4 Gm/day.

Severe infections: 150 to 200 mg/kg/24 hr in equally divided doses every 4 to 6 hours (25 to 33.3 mg/kg every 4 hours or 37.5 to 50 mg/kg every 6 hours). Use the higher dose (e.g., 200 mg/kg/day in equally divided doses every 4 to 6 hours [33.3 mg/kg every 4 hours or 50 mg/kg every 6 hours]) in infections such as meningitis and endocarditis. Maximum dose is 12 Gm/day.

NEONATAL DOSE

Safety and effectiveness for use in neonates not established. All pediatric doses are unlabeled; see Maternal/Child. Limited clinical experience with IV route in neonates and infants.

25 mg/kg with the interval adjusted based on age and weight as follows:

0 to 7 days of age and under 2,000 Gm: Every 12 hours.

Over 7 days of age and under 1,200 Gm: Every 12 hours.

Over 7 days of age and 1,200 to 2,000 Gm: Every 8 hours.

0 to 7 days of age and over 2,000 Gm: Every 8 hours.

Over 7 days of age and over 2,000 Gm: Every 6 hours.

Increase dose to 50 mg/kg every 6, 8, or 12 hours in meningitis.

DOSE ADJUSTMENTS

Dose adjustment not required for patients with renal dysfunction, including those receiving hemodialysis.

DILUTION

Each 500-mg vial is reconstituted with 1.7 mL of SWFI, NS, or BWFI (1-Gm vial with 3.4 mL, 2-Gm vial with 6.6 mL). Each 1 mL equals 250 mg. Further dilute each dose with a minimum of 15 to 30 mL of SWFI, NS, $^1/_2$NS, or other **compatible** IV solutions (see chart on inside back cover or literature). Further dilution and final concentration determined by method of administration (direct IV injection, IVPB, or infusion). Concentration may range from 2 to 250 mg/mL. Available prediluted and in ADD-Vantage vials for use with ADD-Vantage infusion containers. May be given through Y-site or with additive tubing or may be added to larger volume of **compatible** solutions.

Filters: Not required by manufacturer. Premixed and frozen solutions are filtered during manufacturing.

Storage: Store unopened vials at CRT. Stability after reconstitution or further dilution is dependent on concentration, solution, and storage conditions; see individual manufacturer's prescribing information. Frozen, premixed solutions should be stored at $-20°$ C ($-4°$ F). Thaw at room temperature or under refrigeration. Thawed solutions are stable for 72 hours at RT or 21 days refrigerated. Do not refreeze.

COMPATIBILITY

Inactivated in solution with aminoglycosides (e.g., amikacin, gentamicin). Do not mix in the same solution. Appropriate spacing and/or separate sites required. See Drug/Lab Interactions.

Other sources suggest specific **compatibilities** dependent on concentration and manufacturer; consult a pharmacist.

RATE OF ADMINISTRATION

IV injection: May be infused over 5 to 10 minutes.

Intermittent IV: Administration over 30 to 60 minutes may decrease incidence of thrombophlebitis.

Infusion: When diluted in large volumes of infusion fluids, give at rate prescribed.

ACTIONS

A semi-synthetic penicillinase-resistant penicillin, used for its bactericidal activity against gram-positive organisms, primarily penicillinase-producing staphylococci (methicillin-susceptible isolates only). Mode of action involves inhibition of bacterial cell wall biosynthesis. Highly resistant to inactivation by staphylococcal penicillinase. Readily distributes into most body fluids and tissues except the aqueous humor of the eye and spinal fluid. Binds to serum proteins, primarily albumin. Mainly eliminated by hepatic inactivation and excretion in bile; a small amount is excreted in urine. Half-life is 33 to 61 minutes. Crosses the placental barrier. Secreted in breast milk.

INDICATIONS AND USES
Treatment of infections caused by penicillinase-producing staphylococci.

CONTRAINDICATIONS
Known hypersensitivity to any penicillin or cephalosporin (not absolute); see Precautions. Prediluted solutions containing dextrose may be contraindicated with known allergies to corn products.

PRECAUTIONS
Sensitivity studies necessary to determine susceptibility of the causative organism to penicillinase-resistant penicillins. Nafcillin should not be used in infections caused by an organism susceptible to penicillin G. If susceptibility tests indicate that infection is due to methicillin-resistant *Staphylococcus* species, therapy should be discontinued and alternative therapy provided. Modify antimicrobial treatment as indicated by C/S. ▪ To reduce the development of drug-resistant bacteria and maintain its effectiveness, nafcillin should be used to treat or prevent only those infections proven or strongly suspected to be caused by bacteria. ▪ Use with caution in patients with both impaired hepatic and renal function; elevated serum concentrations may cause neurotoxic reactions. See Dose Adjustments. ▪ Hypersensitivity reactions, including fatalities, have been reported in patients receiving beta-lactam antibacterial drugs; most likely to occur in patients with a history of penicillin hypersensitivity or sensitivity to multiple allergens. There have been reports of individuals with a history of penicillin hypersensitivity experiencing severe reactions when treated with cephalosporins. Check history of previous hypersensitivity reactions to penicillins, cephalosporins, or other allergens. Actual incidence of cross-allergenicity not established but may be more common with first-generation cephalosporins. ▪ Avoid prolonged use of the drug; superinfection caused by overgrowth of non-susceptible organisms may result. ▪ *Clostridium difficile*–associated diarrhea (CDAD) has been reported. May range from mild diarrhea to fatal colitis. Consider in patients who present with diarrhea during or after treatment with nafcillin. ▪ Manufacturer's premixed solutions contain dextrose; may be contraindicated in patients with an allergy to corn or corn products.

Monitor: Obtain baseline CBC with differential, SCr, BUN, and urinalysis, and monitor during treatment. ▪ Obtain baseline serum bilirubin, AST, ALT, alkaline phosphate, and gamma glutamyl transferase, and monitor periodically during therapy, especially with high nafcillin doses. In worsening hepatic function, risk versus benefit of continued use should be re-evaluated. ▪ Watch for early symptoms of a hypersensitivity reaction, especially in individuals with a history of allergic problems. ▪ May cause thrombophlebitis, especially in the elderly or with too-rapid injection. Limit peripheral IV treatment to 24 to 48 hours when possible. Change to oral therapy as soon as practical. ▪ Electrolyte imbalance and cardiac irregularities from sodium content are possible. Contains up to 3.3 mEq sodium/Gm. May aggravate CHF. Observe for hypokalemia. ▪ See Drug/Lab Interactions.

Patient Education: May require alternate birth control. ▪ Promptly report diarrhea or bloody stools that occur during treatment or up to several months after an antibiotic has been discontinued; may indicate CDAD and require treatment.

Maternal/Child: Use only if clearly needed. ▪ May cause diarrhea, candidiasis, or allergic response in nursing infants. ▪ Safety and effectiveness for the use of IV nafcillin in pediatric patients not established, but it is used; see Pediatric Dose. ▪ Elimination rate markedly reduced in neonates and infants due to immature hepatic and renal function.

Elderly: Response similar to that seen in younger adults. Consider age-related organ impairment and concomitant disease or drug therapy. Elderly patients may respond with a blunted natriuresis to salt loading, which can be clinically important with regard to diseases such as CHF. ▪ May be at increased risk for thrombophlebitis. ▪ See Precautions/Monitor and Dose Adjustments.

DRUG/LAB INTERACTIONS
May be antagonized by **bacteriostatic antibiotics** (e.g., chloramphenicol, erythromycin, tetracyclines); may interfere with bactericidal action. ▪ Potentiated by **probenecid;** toxicity

may result. ■ Synergistic when used in combination with **aminoglycosides** (e.g., amikacin, gentamicin). Synergism may be inconsistent; see Compatibility. ■ May decrease serum levels and effectiveness of **cyclosporine**. Monitor cyclosporine levels during concomitant use. ■ Inhibits effectiveness of **oral contraceptives;** breakthrough bleeding or pregnancy could result. ■ High doses (9 to 12 Gm daily) may decrease effects of **warfarin;** monitor PT up to 30 days after nafcillin completed. ■ May reduce effectiveness of **nifedipine** by reducing its serum plasma levels. ■ May cause **false values in common lab tests;** see literature.

SIDE EFFECTS

Bleeding abnormalities, bone marrow suppression (e.g., agranulocytosis, neutropenia), CDAD, diarrhea, hypersensitivity reactions (e.g., anaphylaxis, angioedema, bronchospasm, hypotension, laryngospasm, pruritus, rash, serum sickness–like symptoms, urticaria [may be immediate or delayed]), interstitial nephritis, local reactions (e.g., pain, phlebitis, thrombophlebitis, and occasionally skin sloughing with extravasation), nausea and vomiting, and renal tubular damage have been reported. Larger doses may cause neurologic adverse reactions, including convulsions, especially with concomitant impaired hepatic insufficiency and renal dysfunction. Elevation of liver transaminases and/or cholestasis may occur, specifically with higher doses.

ANTIDOTE

Notify physician immediately of any adverse symptoms. For severe symptoms discontinue the drug, treat hypersensitivity reaction (antihistamines, epinephrine, corticosteroids), and resuscitate as necessary. Hemodialysis or peritoneal dialysis is minimally effective in overdose. Treat CDAD with fluids, electrolytes, protein supplements, and appropriate antibiotics (e.g., oral vancomycin) as indicated. In severe cases, surgical evaluation may be indicated. Mild cases may respond to drug discontinuation alone.

NALBUPHINE HYDROCHLORIDE BBW

(**NAL**-byoo-feen hy-droh-**KLOR**-eyed)

Narcotic analgesic
(agonist-antagonist)
Anesthesia adjunct

Nubain ♣

pH 3.5 to 3.7

USUAL DOSE

Individualize dose, taking into account the patient's severity of pain, patient response, prior analgesic treatment experience, and risk factors for addiction, abuse, and misuse. Use lowest effective dose for the shortest duration consistent with the patient's treatment goals.

Pain control: 10 mg/70 kg. May repeat every 3 to 6 hours. In nontolerant patients, the recommended single maximum dose is 20 mg. Maximum total daily dose is 160 mg. Titrate to a dose and interval that provides adequate analgesia and minimizes adverse reactions; see Dose Adjustments.

Supplement to balanced anesthesia: A loading dose of 0.3 to 3 mg/kg over 10 to 15 minutes. Maintain desired level of balanced anesthesia with 0.25 to 0.5 mg/kg as required. Administered only under the direction of the anesthesiologist.

DOSE ADJUSTMENTS

Reduced dose may be required in elderly, cachectic, or debilitated patients; in impaired liver or renal function; in patients with limited pulmonary reserve; and in the presence of other CNS depressants. ■ See Drug/Lab Interactions.

DILUTION
May be given undiluted.

Filters: No data available from manufacturer.

Storage: Store at CRT. Avoid freezing and/or prolonged exposure to light.

COMPATIBILITY
Manufacturer lists as **incompatible** with nafcillin and ketorolac.

Other sources suggest specific **compatibilities** dependent on concentration and manufacturer; consult a pharmacist.

RATE OF ADMINISTRATION
Pain control: Each 10 mg or fraction thereof over at least 2 to 3 minutes. Frequently titrated according to symptom relief and respiratory rate.

Supplement to balanced anesthesia: See Usual Dose.

ACTIONS
A synthetic narcotic agonist-antagonist analgesic. Binds to kappa and mu receptors. Acts as an agonist at kappa receptors and as an antagonist at mu receptors. It equals morphine in analgesic effect. May produce the same degree of respiratory depression as an equianalgesic dose of morphine. However, it exhibits a ceiling effect such that dose increases greater than 30 mg do not produce further respiratory depression in the absence of other CNS-active medications that affect respiration. Has potent opioid antagonist activity at doses equal to or lower than its analgesic dose. When administered after or concurrently with a mu agonist opioid analgesic (e.g., morphine, oxymorphone, fentanyl), nalbuphine may partially reverse or block opioid-induced respiratory depression from the mu agonist analgesic. May precipitate withdrawal in patients dependent on opioid drugs. Onset of pain relief occurs within 2 to 3 minutes and lasts about 3 to 6 hours. Metabolized in the liver. Some excretion in feces and urine. Crosses the placental barrier. Secreted in breast milk.

INDICATIONS AND USES
Management of pain severe enough to require an opioid analgesic and for which alternative treatments are inadequate. ▪ Preoperative and postoperative analgesia. ▪ Supplement to balanced anesthesia. ▪ Obstetric analgesia during labor and delivery.

Unlabeled uses: Opioid-induced pruritus.

Limitations of use: Because of the risk for addiction, abuse, and misuse, even at recommended doses, reserve nalbuphine for use in patients for whom alternative treatment options (e.g., nonopioid analgesics or opioid combination products):
* Have not been tolerated or are not expected to be tolerated
* Have not provided adequate analgesia or are not expected to provide adequate analgesia

CONTRAINDICATIONS
Significant respiratory depression. ▪ Acute or severe bronchial asthma in an unmonitored setting or in the absence of resuscitative equipment. ▪ Known or suspected GI obstruction, including paralytic ileus. ▪ Hypersensitivity to nalbuphine or its components.

PRECAUTIONS
Serious, life-threatening, or fatal respiratory depression may occur, particularly when used concomitantly with other opioids or CNS depressants. Respiratory depression may occur at any time, but risk is greatest during initiation of therapy or after a dose increase. To reduce the risk of respiratory depression, proper dosing and titration are essential. Overestimating the nalbuphine dose when converting patients from another opioid product can result in a fatal overdose with the first dose. ▪ Adequate facilities should be available for monitoring and ventilation. An opioid antagonist (e.g., naloxone), resuscitative and intubation equipment and oxygen should be readily available. ▪ Use with extreme caution in patients with COPD, cor pulmonale, a substantially decreased respiratory reserve, hypoxia, hypercapnia, or pre-existing respiratory depression; these patients are at increased risk for decreased respiratory drive, including apnea, even at recommended doses. Consider using nonopioid analgesics, or administer under careful medical supervision at the lowest effective dose. ▪ Use with caution and reduce initial doses in elderly, cachectic, or

debilitated patients and in patients with severe impairment of hepatic, pulmonary, or renal function. Consider using nonopioid analgesics. ▪ Cases of serotonin syndrome have been reported during concomitant use of nalbuphine with serotonergic drugs ▪ Cases of adrenal insufficiency have been reported with opioid use, more often after more than 1 month of use. If adrenal insufficiency is diagnosed, treat with physiologic replacement doses of corticosteroids and wean the patient off the opioid to allow adrenal function to recover. Another opioid may be tried; some cases reported use of a different opioid without recurrence of adrenal insufficiency. ▪ May cause severe hypotension, including orthostatic hypotension and syncope, in ambulatory patients or in any patient whose ability to maintain blood pressure has been compromised by depleted blood volume or concomitant administration of drugs that can cause hypotension (e.g., anesthetics, phenothiazines); see Drug/Lab Interactions. In patients with circulatory shock, nalbuphine-induced vasodilation may further reduce cardiac output and blood pressure. Use should be avoided. ▪ Use caution in patients with head injury, brain tumors, or increased intracranial pressure. Respiratory depression may cause an increased P_{CO_2}, cerebral vasodilation, and increased intracranial pressure. Clinical course of head injury may be obscured. Avoid use in patients with impaired consciousness or coma. ▪ Use with caution in patients with biliary tract disease, including acute pancreatitis; may cause spasm of the sphincter of Oddi and diminish biliary and pancreatic secretions. ▪ May increase the frequency of seizures in patients with a convulsive disorder, and may induce or aggravate seizures in some clinical settings. ▪ Use caution in patients with myocardial infarction who have nausea and vomiting or compromised cardiac function; effect on heart not fully evaluated. ▪ When used with anesthesia, a high incidence of bradycardia has been reported in patients who did not receive atropine preoperatively. ▪ Should be administered as a supplement to general anesthesia only by persons specifically trained in the use of IV anesthetics and in the management of the respiratory effects of potent opioids. ▪ Do not abruptly discontinue nalbuphine in patients who are physically dependent; dose must be tapered gradually. ▪ Nalbuphine exposes patients and other users to the risks of opioid addiction, abuse, and misuse, which can lead to overdose and death. Assess each patient's risk before prescribing nalbuphine, and monitor all patients regularly for the development of these behaviors and conditions. Strategies to reduce the risk of diversion or misuse should be used by health care facilities that use this and other controlled substances. ▪ See prescribing information for further discussion regarding abuse, addiction, physical dependence, and tolerance. ▪ Do not abruptly discontinue nalbuphine in patients who are physically dependent; dose must be tapered gradually.

Monitor: Naloxone, oxygen, and equipment to establish and maintain an airway must be available. ▪ Monitor for respiratory depression, especially during initiation of therapy (within the first 24 to 72 hours) or after a dose increase. ▪ Assess baseline pain, reassess after administration of nalbuphine, and adjust dose or interval as required. ▪ Monitor vital signs and oxygenation and observe patient frequently. ▪ Keep patient supine to minimize side effects; orthostatic hypotension and fainting may occur. Observe closely during ambulation. ▪ Monitor patients who may be susceptible to the intracranial effects of CO_2 retention for increasing intracranial pressure and signs of sedation and respiratory depression. ▪ Monitor patients with biliary tract disease for worsening of symptoms. ▪ Monitor patients with a history of seizure disorders for worsening seizure control. ▪ Monitor for S/S of serotonin syndrome (e.g., mental status changes [e.g., agitation, coma, hallucinations], autonomic instability [e.g., hyperthermia, labile blood pressure, tachycardia], neuromuscular aberrations [e.g., hyperreflexia, incoordination, rigidity], and/or GI symptoms [e.g., diarrhea, nausea, vomiting]). Onset of symptoms may occur within hours to days of concomitant use of opioids with serotonergic drugs. ▪ Adhere to prescribed bowel care regimen to avoid constipation and/or impaction. Maintain adequate hydration. ▪ See Drug/Lab Interactions.

Patient Education: Avoid use of alcohol, MAO inhibitors, or other CNS depressants. Review all medications for interactions. ▪ Request assistance for ambulation. ▪ Use caution performing any task that requires alertness; may cause dizziness, euphoria, and sedation. ▪ Report unrelieved pain or side effects or S/S of serotonin syndrome. ▪ May result in severe constipation. Scheduled bowel regimen recommended. ▪ May result in addiction, abuse, and misuse.

Maternal/Child: Use during pregnancy (other than labor and delivery) only if benefits justify risks. ▪ Prolonged use of opioids during pregnancy can result in neonatal opioid withdrawal syndrome, which may be life-threatening if not recognized and treated. Infants born to mothers receiving nalbuphine during pregnancy should be monitored closely and treated for neonatal opioid withdrawal syndrome if indicated. See literature for treatment protocols. ▪ Severe fetal bradycardia has been reported when nalbuphine is administered during labor. Take appropriate measures (e.g., fetal monitoring) to detect and manage potential adverse effects to the fetus. ▪ Fetal and neonatal bradycardia, respiratory depression at birth, apnea, cyanosis, hypotonia, and a sinusoidal fetal heart rate pattern have been reported. Some of these events have been life-threatening. Maternal or neonatal administration of naloxone may reverse these effects. Permanent neurologic damage attributed to fetal bradycardia has occurred. Fetal death has been reported when mothers received nalbuphine during labor and delivery. Use during labor and delivery only if clearly indicated and if benefit outweighs risk. Use during or immediately before labor is not recommended when other analgesic techniques are more appropriate. Newborns should be monitored for respiratory depression, apnea, bradycardia, and arrhythmias if nalbuphine has been used. ▪ Use caution with breastfeeding. Monitor infants exposed to nalbuphine through breast milk for excess sedation and respiratory depression. Withdrawal symptoms can occur in breastfed infants when maternal administration of an opioid analgesic is stopped or when breastfeeding is stopped. ▪ Safety and effectiveness in pediatric patients under 18 years of age have not been established.

Elderly: May be more sensitive to effects (e.g., respiratory depression, constipation, dizziness, urinary retention). Respiratory depression is the chief risk for elderly patients treated with opioids. ▪ Analgesia should be effective with lower doses. ▪ Consider age-related organ impairment.

DRUG/LAB INTERACTIONS
Although nalbuphine possesses opioid antagonist activity, there is evidence that it will not antagonize an opioid analgesic administered just before, concurrently, or just after an injection of nalbuphine in nondependent patients. Therefore due to additive pharmacologic effects, the concomitant use of other opioid analgesics, benzodiazepines, or other CNS depressants may result in profound sedation, respiratory depression, coma, and death. Reserve concomitant use for patients for whom alternative treatment options are inadequate. Use minimum effective dose for the shortest duration possible, and monitor for S/S of respiratory depression and sedation. ▪ Serotonin syndrome has been reported with the concomitant use of opioids, including nalbuphine, and other **drugs that affect the serotonergic neurotransmitter system** (e.g., selective serotonin reuptake inhibitors [SSRIs], serotonin and norepinephrine reuptake inhibitors [SNRIs], tricyclic antidepressants [TCAs], triptans, 5-HT$_3$ receptor antagonists, mirtazapine, trazodone, tramadol, MAO inhibitors, linezolid, and IV methylene blue). Careful observation, particularly during treatment initiation and dose adjustment, is required with concomitant use. ▪ Severe and unpredictable potentiation of **MAO inhibitors** has been reported. MAO inhibitor interactions may manifest as serotonin syndrome or opioid toxicity (e.g., respiratory depression, coma). Use of nalbuphine is not recommended for patients taking MAOIs or within 14 days of stopping such treatment. If urgent use of an opioid is necessary, use test doses and frequent titration of small doses to treat pain while closely monitoring BP and S/S of CNS and respiratory depression. ▪ Nalbuphine may enhance the neuromuscular blocking action of **skeletal muscle relaxants**, increasing the degree of respiratory depression. Monitor patient and decrease dose if indicated. ▪ Opioids can reduce the efficacy of **diuretics** by inducing the release of antidiuretic hormone. Increase dose of diuretic if needed. ▪ Concomitant use with

anticholinergic drugs may increase the risk of urinary retention and/or severe constipation, which may lead to paralytic ileus. ■ Use in patients who are receiving a full **opioid agonist** analgesic may reduce the analgesic effect and/or precipitate withdrawal symptoms. Avoid concomitant use. ■ Depending on the test used, nalbuphine may interfere with enzymatic methods for the detection of **opiates**.

SIDE EFFECTS

Sedation is the most commonly reported adverse reaction. Less frequent adverse reactions are dizziness/vertigo, dry mouth, headache, nausea and vomiting, and sweaty/clammy skin. Adverse reactions that occur in 1% or fewer of patients are abdominal cramps, asthma, bitter taste, blurred vision, bradycardia, burning, CNS effects (e.g., confusion, crying, depression, dysphoria, euphoria, faintness, feeling of heaviness, floating, hallucinations, hostility, nervousness, restlessness, tingling, unreality, and unusual dreams), dyspepsia, dyspnea, flushing and warmth, hypersensitivity reactions (e.g., anaphylaxic/anaphylactoid reactions, bronchospasm, diaphoresis, edema, nausea and vomiting, pruritus, rash, shakiness, stridor, weakness, and wheezing), hypertension, hypotension, itching, respiratory depression, speech difficulties, tachycardia, urinary urgency, and urticaria.

Post-Marketing: Abdominal pain, adrenal insufficiency, agitation, anxiety, depressed level of consciousness, fever, injection site reaction, pulmonary edema, seizures, serotonin syndrome, somnolence, and tremor. Death from severe allergic reactions has been reported. Fetal death has been reported when mothers received nalbuphine during labor and delivery.

Overdose: Acute overdose with nalbuphine alone can be manifested by dysphoria and respiratory depression. Acute overdose with nalbuphine and other opioids or CNS depressants can be manifested by apnea, atypical snoring, bradycardia, cardiac arrest, circulatory depression or collapse, cold and clammy skin, constricted pupils, hypotension (severe), partial or complete airway obstruction, pulmonary edema, respiratory depression or arrest, skeletal muscle flaccidity, somnolence progressing to stupor or coma, and death.

ANTIDOTE

With increasing severity of any side effect or onset of symptoms of overdose, discontinue the drug and notify the physician. Naloxone hydrochloride will reverse severe cardiovascular, CNS, and respiratory reactions. Naloxone use should be reserved for situations in which clinically significant respiratory or circulatory depression is present. Titrate naloxone dose carefully to avoid precipitating an acute abstinence syndrome or uncontrolled pain. The duration of action of nalbuphine may exceed the duration of action of naloxone. Monitor patient carefully. Repeat doses of naloxone may be required. A patent airway, artificial ventilation, oxygen therapy, and other symptomatic treatment (e.g., fluids, vasopressors) must be instituted promptly. Resuscitate as necessary.

NALOXONE HYDROCHLORIDE
(nal-**OX**-ohn hy-droh-**KLOR**-eyed)

Antidote
Narcotic antagonist

pH 3 to 4

USUAL DOSE
Narcotic overdose: 0.4 to 2 mg. Repeat in 2 to 3 minutes if indicated. The diagnosis of narcotic overdose should be questioned if no response is observed after 10 mg of naloxone. If effective, dosage may be repeated as necessary for recurrence of symptoms.
Postoperative narcotic depression: 0.1 to 0.2 mg at 2- to 3-minute intervals to desired response. Titrate to avoid excessive reduction of narcotic analgesic action.
Challenge test for suspected opioid dependence: 0.2 mg. Observe for 30 seconds for S/S of withdrawal (e.g., abdominal cramps, diaphoresis, dysphoria, nausea and vomiting, rhinorrhea). If no evidence of withdrawal, inject 0.6 mg of naloxone and observe for an additional 20 minutes. Monitor VS and observe patient again for S/S of opiate withdrawal.

PEDIATRIC DOSE
Ampules containing 0.02 mg/mL are available, but larger doses are frequently required. Adult strength is often used to reduce amount of injection and to effect desired response, which may require increased or repeat doses. One source states, "Up to 10 times a dose has been required."
Narcotic overdose: *Weight less than 20 kg:* 0.01 to 0.1 mg/kg of body weight initially. Based on estimated degree of overdose and respiratory depression. May repeat every 2 to 3 minutes. May dilute with SWFI. American Academy of Pediatrics recommends 0.1 mg/kg. Manufacturer recommends 0.01 mg/kg.
Weight over 20 kg or over 5 years of age: 2 mg. Repeat every 2 to 3 minutes as needed. A continuous infusion may be used after initial effective dose. Add 75% to 100% of effective dose to a specific amount of IV fluid and infuse evenly distributed over 1 hour. For some overdoses (e.g., methadone), weaning in 50% increments may take up to 48 hours. For others, 6 to 12 hours is adequate. If symptoms recur, rebolus and go back to 100%.
Postoperative narcotic depression: 0.005 to 0.01 mg IV at 2- to 3-minute intervals to desired response.

NEONATAL DOSE
Neonatal opiate depression: Administration into umbilical vein is preferred. 0.01 to 0.1 mg/kg of body weight initially. Based on estimated degree of overdose and respiratory depression. May repeat every 2 to 3 minutes to achieve a satisfactory response. May dilute with SWFI. American Academy of Pediatrics recommends 0.1 mg/kg repeated every 2 to 3 minutes. Manufacturer recommends 0.01 mg/kg repeated every 2 to 3 minutes. Another source suggests an initial dose of 0.01 mg/kg. If response is not satisfactory, increase subsequent doses to 0.1 mg/kg.

DILUTION
May be given undiluted, diluted with SWFI, or further diluted in NS or D5W and given as an infusion (2 mg in 500 mL equals a concentration of 0.004 mg/mL). Discard infusions after 24 hours.
Storage: Store below 40° C. Protect from light.

COMPATIBILITY
Manufacturer lists as **incompatible** with bisulfites, sulfites, long-chain or high-molecular-weight anions, solutions with an alkaline pH.

Other sources suggest a few specific **compatibilities** dependent on concentration and manufacturer; consult a pharmacist.

RATE OF ADMINISTRATION
Each 0.4 mg or fraction thereof over 30 seconds. Titrate infusion to patient response.

ACTIONS

A potent narcotic antagonist. Overcomes effects of narcotic overdose including respiratory depression, sedation, and hypotension. Unlike other narcotic antagonists, it does not have any narcotic effect itself. Onset of action is within 2 minutes. Duration of action is dependent on dose and route of naloxone administration. Requirement for repeat doses is dependent on amount, type, and route of narcotic administration. Metabolized in the liver and excreted in urine.

INDICATIONS AND USES

Reversal of narcotic depression. ▪ Antidote for natural (e.g., morphine) and synthetic narcotics (e.g., butorphanol, methadone, nalbuphine, and pentazocine). ▪ Diagnosis of suspected opioid tolerance or acute opiate overdose.

Unlabeled uses: Reversal of alcoholic coma and improvement of circulation in refractory shock.

CONTRAINDICATIONS

Known hypersensitivity to naloxone. ▪ The naloxone challenge test should not be performed in patients showing S/S of withdrawal or whose urine contains opioids.

PRECAUTIONS

Does not produce respiratory depression with nonnarcotic drug overdose, a beneficial action. ▪ It is ineffective against respiratory depression caused by barbiturates, anesthetics, other nonnarcotic agents, or pathologic conditions. ▪ Will precipitate acute withdrawal symptoms in narcotic addicts; use caution, especially in newborns of narcotic-dependent mothers. ▪ Use caution in cardiac disease patients or those receiving cardiotoxic drugs.

Monitor: Symptomatic treatment with oxygen and artificial ventilation as necessary should be continued until naloxone is effective. Observe patient continuously. Duration of narcotic action may exceed that of naloxone.

Maternal/Child: Category B: use in pregnancy and breastfeeding only when clearly needed. Safety for use not established. ▪ See Precautions.

DRUG/LAB INTERACTIONS

Specific information not available.

SIDE EFFECTS

Hypertension, irritability and increased crying in the newborn, nausea and vomiting, sweating, tachycardia, tremulousness. Overdose postoperatively may result in excitement, hypertension, hypotension, pulmonary edema, reversal of analgesia, ventricular tachycardia, and fibrillation.

ANTIDOTE

Notify the physician of any side effect. Treatment will probably be symptomatic. Resuscitate as necessary.

NATALIZUMAB BBW

(nah-tah-**LIZZ**-u-mab)

Tysabri

Monoclonal antibody
Immunomodulator

pH 6.1

USUAL DOSE

Pretreatment: Baseline studies indicated; see Precautions and Monitor.

Multiple sclerosis (MS): 300 mg as an infusion every 4 weeks.

Crohn disease (CD): 300 mg as an infusion every 4 weeks. Discontinue if no benefit is seen after 12 weeks of therapy. For patients with CD who initiate natalizumab therapy while on chronic corticosteroids, begin steroid tapering as soon as therapeutic benefit of natalizumab has occurred. Discontinue natalizumab if the patient cannot be tapered off steroids within 6 months. Consider discontinuing therapy in patients who require more than 3 months of steroid use (excluding the original 6-month taper) in a calendar year to control their CD. Aminosalicylates may be continued during therapy with natalizumab.

DOSE ADJUSTMENTS

None indicated. Pharmacokinetics has not been studied in patients with renal or hepatic insufficiency.

DILUTION

Available in 300 mg/15 mL single-use vials. Solution is a colorless, clear to slightly opalescent concentrate. Do not use if particulates are present or if solution is discolored. Withdraw 15 mL of concentrate (300 mg) from the vial and inject into 100 mL of NS to prepare a solution with a final concentration of 2.6 mg/mL. Gently invert to mix completely. Do not shake. No other IV diluents may be used to prepare the solution.

Filters: Use of filtration devices during administration not evaluated.

Storage: Refrigerate vials at 2° to 8° C (36° to 46° F). Do not use beyond the expiration date on the vial. Do not shake or freeze. Protect from light. Following dilution, solution should be infused immediately. However, it may be refrigerated and used within 8 hours of preparation. If refrigerated, allow to warm to room temperature before infusion.

COMPATIBILITY

Manufacturer states, "Other medications should not be injected into infusion set side ports or mixed with natalizumab." Flush line with NS before and after infusion.

RATE OF ADMINISTRATION

Do not administer as an IV push or bolus injection. Infuse over approximately 1 hour. Flush line with NS before and after infusion.

ACTIONS

A recombinant humanized IgG4κ monoclonal antibody produced in murine myeloma cells. An integrin receptor antagonist. Natalizumab is thought to bind to a subunit on the surface of all leukocytes except neutrophils and inhibit the adhesion of leukocytes to their counter-receptors. The receptors for the α4 family of integrin include vascular cell adhesion molecule-1 (VCAM-1), which is expressed on activated vascular endothelium, and mucosal addressin cell adhesion molecule-1 (MAdCAM-1), which is present on vascular endothelial cells of the GI tract. Disruption of these molecular interactions prevents transmigration of leukocytes across the endothelium into inflamed parenchymal tissue. Specific mechanisms of how natalizumab exerts its effects in multiple sclerosis (MS) and CD have not been fully defined. In MS, lesions are believed to occur when activated inflammatory cells, including T-lymphocytes, cross the blood-brain barrier (BBB). Leukocyte migration across the BBB involves the interaction between adhesion molecules on inflammatory cells and their counter-receptors on the endothelial cells of the vessel wall. The clinical effect of natalizumab in MS may be secondary to blockade of the molecular interaction of α4β1 integrins expressed by inflammatory cells with VCAM-1 on vascular endothelial cells and with CS-1 and/or osteopontin expressed by parenchymal cells in the brain. In clinical trials, natalizumab reduced the rate of clinical relapse and the appearance of new or newly enlarging T2 hyperintense lesions on MRI studies. The number of gadolinium-enhancing lesions on the 1-year MRI scan follow-up was also reduced. In CD, the interaction of the α4β7 integrin with the endothelial receptor MAdCAM-1 has been implicated as an important contributor to the chronic inflammation seen in CD. MAdCAM-1 expression has been found to be increased at active sites of inflammation in the mucosa and to contribute to the inflammatory response characteristic of CD. It is mainly expressed on gut endothelial cells. The action of natalizumab may be secondary to blockade of molecular interaction of the α4β7-integrin receptor with MAdCAM-1 expressed on the venular endothelium at inflammatory foci. Distribution is limited primarily to vascular space (plasma volume). Half-life is 3 to 17 days.

INDICATIONS AND USES

Monotherapy for the treatment of relapsing forms of MS, including clinically isolated syndrome, relapsing-remitting disease, and active secondary progressive disease, in adults. ▪ Induction and maintenance of clinical response and remission in adults with moderately to severely active CD with evidence of inflammation who have had an inadequate response to or are unable to tolerate conventional therapy and inhibitors of TNFα (e.g., infliximab). Should not be used in combination with immunosuppressants (e.g., 6-mercaptopurine, azathioprine, cyclosporine, or methotrexate) or inhibitors of TNFα; see Precautions.

CONTRAINDICATIONS

Hypersensitivity to natalizumab or any of its components. ▪ Patients who have or have had progressive multifocal leukoencephalopathy (PML).

PRECAUTIONS

Natalizumab increases the risk of PML, a rare opportunistic viral infection of the brain caused by the JC virus (JCV) that usually leads to death or severe disability. PML typically occurs only in patients who are immunocompromised. Risk factors for the development of PML include duration of therapy (especially beyond 2 years), prior use of immunosuppressants (e.g., azathioprine, cyclophosphamide, methotrexate, mitoxantrone, or mycophenolate), and the presence of anti-JCV antibodies. Patients who are anti–JCV antibody positive have a higher risk of developing PML. These factors should be considered in the context of expected benefits when initiating and continuing treatment with natalizumab. ▪ There are no known interventions that can reliably prevent PML or adequately treat PML if it occurs. Because of the risk of PML, natalizumab is available only through a special restricted distribution program called the TOUCH™ Prescribing Program. See prescribing information, or contact the manufacturer for specific details and requirements. Retrospective analyses of post-marketing data suggest that the risk of developing PML may be associated with relative levels of serum anti-JCV antibody compared to a calibrator as measured by ELISA (often described as an anti-JCV antibody index value). ▪ Infection by the JCV is required for the development of PML. ▪ Anti-JCV antibody testing should not be used to diagnose PML. Testing positive for anti-JCV antibodies means that a person has been exposed to JCV in the past. Consider testing patients before treatment or during treatment if antibody status is unknown. Patients who test negative for anti-JCV antibodies have a lower risk of PML but are still at risk for the development of PML because of the potential for a new JCV infection or a false-negative test result. Periodic retesting of antibody status should be considered in patients previously determined to be anti–JCV antibody negative. Anti–JCV testing should not be performed for at least 2 weeks after plasma exchange due to the removal of antibodies from the serum. After an IVIG infusion, wait at least 6 months for the IVIG to clear to avoid a false-positive anti-JCV antibody test result. ▪ PML has been reported after discontinuation of natalizumab in patients who did not have findings suggestive of PML at the time of discontinuation. Patients should continue to be monitored for any new S/S suggestive of PML for at least 6 months after discontinuing natalizumab. ▪ JC virus infection of granule cell neurons in the cerebellum (i.e., JCV granule cell neuronopathy [JCV GCN]) has been reported and can cause cerebellar dysfunction (e.g., apraxia, ataxia, incoordination, visual disorders). ▪ Patients who develop PML and have discontinued natalizumab have developed immune reconstitution inflammatory syndrome

(IRIS). In most cases IRIS occurred after plasma exchange was used to eliminate circulating natalizumab. This syndrome has not been seen in patients discontinuing treatment for reasons unrelated to PML. ▪ Has been associated with hypersensitivity reactions, including anaphylaxis. Reactions usually occur within 2 hours of the start of the infusion. Generally associated with antibodies to natalizumab. ▪ In studies, persistent antibody positivity resulted in a substantial decrease in the effectiveness of natalizumab and an increased incidence of hypersensitivity/infusion-related reactions. Patients who receive natalizumab for a short exposure (1 to 2 infusions) followed by an extended period without treatment are at higher risk for developing anti-natalizumab antibodies and/or hypersensitivity reactions on re-exposure compared with patients who received regularly scheduled treatments. Given that patients with persistent antibodies to natalizumab experience reduced efficacy and that hypersensitivity reactions are more common in such patients, consideration should be given to testing for the presence of antibodies in patients who want to resume therapy after a dose interruption. ▪ Effects on immune system may increase the risk of infection, including opportunistic infection. ▪ Risk for developing encephalitis and meningitis caused by herpes simplex and varicella zoster viruses is increased. Serious, life-threatening, and sometimes fatal cases have been reported. ▪ Acute retinal necrosis (ARN), a fulminant viral infection of the retina caused by the family of herpes viruses (e.g., varicella zoster, herpes simplex virus), has been reported. May lead to blindness. ▪ Liver injury has been reported; it has occurred as early as 6 days after the first dose and after multiple doses. The combination of ALT, AST, and bilirubin elevations without evidence of obstruction is generally recognized as an important predictor of severe liver injury that may lead to death or the need for liver transplantation. ▪ No data available on secondary transmission of infections by live virus vaccines.

Monitor: Obtain baseline CBC and differential. Monitor periodically during treatment. Increases in circulating lymphocytes, monocytes, eosinophils, basophils, and nucleated red blood cells and mild decreases in hemoglobin levels have been observed. ▪ Obtain a baseline MRI before initiating treatment and periodically throughout treatment. In MS patients it may be helpful in differentiating subsequent MS symptoms from PML and assessing disease progression. In CD patients it may be helpful in distinguishing pre-existing lesions from newly developed lesions. Cases of PML have been reported that were diagnosed based on MRI findings and on the detection of JCV DNA in the CSF in the absence of clinical S/S specific to PML (i.e., MRI findings may be apparent before clinical S/S of PML). Periodic monitoring for radiographic signs consistent with PML should be considered to allow for an early diagnosis of PML. Lower PML-related mortality and morbidity have been reported following natalizumab discontinuation in patients with PML who were initially asymptomatic compared with patients with PML who had characteristic clinical S/S at diagnosis. It is not known whether these differences are due to early detection and discontinuation of natalizumab or due to differences in disease in these patients. ▪ Consider determining anti-JCV antibody status before initiating natalizumab. Reassess status periodically; see Precautions. ▪ Observe patients during the infusion and for 1 hour after the infusion is complete. Discontinue infusion at the first sign of any hypersensitivity reaction (e.g., chest pain, dizziness, dyspnea, fever, flushing, hypotension, nausea, pruritus, rash, rigors, urticaria). ▪ Anti-natalizumab antibodies detected within the first 6 months of therapy may be transient and disappear. Repeat testing in 3 months. If antibodies are persistent, consider risk versus benefit of continued therapy; see Precautions. ▪ Assess neurologic status frequently for S/S of PML and JCV GCN. S/S associated with PML are diverse and occur over days to weeks. May include progressive weakness on one side of the body, clumsiness of limbs, disturbances of vision, or changes in thinking, memory, and orientation leading to confusion and personality changes. Progression of deficits usually leads to severe disability or death over weeks to months. Withhold natalizumab if PML is suspected. ▪ Use of a gadolinium-enhanced MRI scan of the brain is recommended for diagnosis of PML and JCV GCN. When indicated, CSF analysis for JC viral DNA may also be used to aid in diagnosis. If clinical suspicion of PML remains after initial evaluations are negative, continue to withhold natalizumab, and repeat evaluations. Continue to monitor for S/S suggestive of PML for approximately 6 months after discontinuation of natalizumab. ▪ Monitor for S/S of IRIS; may occur within days to weeks after plasma exchange. IRIS presents as a clinical decline in condition (may occur after clinical improvement); decline may be rapid, can lead to serious neurologic complications or death, and is often associated with characteristic changes in the MRI. ▪ Monitor for S/S of infection. ▪ Monitor for S/S of meningitis and encephalitis (e.g., confusion, fever, headache). ▪ Monitor for S/S of ARN (e.g., decreased visual acuity, eye pain, redness). Patients presenting with eye symptoms should be referred for retinal screening. ▪ Monitor for S/S of liver injury (e.g., elevated bilirubin or liver function tests, jaundice). ▪ Monitor for signs of clinical relapse.

Patient Education: Read medication guide carefully. ▪ Review medical conditions and medications with health care provider. ▪ Promptly report any new medical problems (e.g., new or sudden change in thinking, eyesight, balance, or strength). ▪ Report infections. ▪ Promptly report S/S of encephalitis and meningitis (e.g., confusion, fever, headache) or acute retinal necrosis (e.g., decreased visual acuity, eye pain, or redness). ▪ Promptly report S/S of hepatotoxicity (e.g., anorexia, dark urine, fatigue, jaundice, right upper abdominal discomfort), meningitis, or encephalitis (e.g., confusion, fever, headache). ▪ Immediately report any symptoms of infusion or hypersensitivity reactions (e.g., difficulty breathing, dizziness, feeling faint, itching, nausea). ▪ Discuss potential risks and benefits of treatment (e.g., risk of PML). ▪ Your physician may order a blood test to see if you have ever been exposed to JCV. Risk of PML is greatest if you have all three known risk factors; see Precautions. ▪ Scheduled follow-up visits are required as part of the TOUCH™ Program. ▪ PML has been reported following discontinuation of natalizumab. Monitor for S/S suggestive of PML for approximately 6 months after discontinuation of therapy.

Maternal/Child: Use during pregnancy only if the potential benefit justifies the potential risk to the fetus. ▪ Has been detected in breast milk. Risk of this exposure to infant is unknown. ▪ Safety and effectiveness for use in pediatric patients with MS or CD under 18 years of age not established.

Elderly: Studies did not include sufficient numbers of patients 65 years of age and older to determine whether they respond differently than younger patients. Differences have not been identified in clinical practice.

DRUG/LAB INTERACTIONS

Formal studies not completed. Concurrent use with **antineoplastic, immunosuppressant, or immunomodulating agents** may further increase the risk of infection, including PML and other opportunistic infections, over the risk observed with the use of natalizumab alone. Safety and efficacy of natalizumab in combination with any of these agents not established. ▪ Concurrent use of short courses of **corticosteroids** was associated with an increase in infections in clinical trials. Corticosteroids should be tapered in patients with CD who are initiating natalizumab therapy; see Usual Dose. ▪ No data are available on the effects of **vaccination** in patients receiving natalizumab. ▪ Increases circulating **lymphocytes, monocytes, eosinophils, basophils, and nucleated red blood cells.** A return to baseline usually occurs within 16 weeks after the last dose. Elevations of **neutrophils** are not observed. ▪ May induce mild decreases in **hemoglobin,** frequently transient.

SIDE EFFECTS

The most commonly reported adverse reactions were abdominal discomfort, arthralgia, depression, diarrhea, fatigue, gastroenteritis, headache, infections (UTI, upper and lower respiratory tract), nausea, pain in extremities, rash, and vaginitis. The most commonly reported serious adverse reactions were infections, hypersensitivity reactions (including anaphylaxis), depression (including suicidal ideation), and cholelithiasis. The most commonly reported adverse reactions resulting in clinical intervention (i.e., discontinuation of natalizumab) were urticaria and other hypersensitivity reactions. Infusion-related reactions (defined as any adverse event occurring within 2 hours of the start of an infusion) included headache, dizziness, fatigue, hypersensitivity reactions, nausea, pruritus, rigors, urticaria, and vomiting. Other reported adverse reactions included abnormal liver function tests, amenorrhea, antibody formation, aphthous stomatitis, back pain, chest discomfort, constipation, cough, dermatitis, dry skin, dyspepsia, flatulence, infections (including bacterial, viral, and opportunistic), influenza-like illness, irregular menstruation/dysmenorrhea, joint swelling, local bleeding, muscle cramps, night sweats, peripheral edema, pharyngolaryngeal pain, pruritus, somnolence, syncope, tonsillitis, tremor, urinary urgency, frequency and incontinence, and vertigo. Adverse reactions reported in persistently antibody-positive patients included anxiety, dyspnea, hypertension, infusion-related/hypersensitivity reactions, myalgia, and tachycardia.

Post-Marketing: Acute retinal necrosis (ARN), eosinophilia (resolved with discontinuation of therapy), hemolytic anemia, herpes simplex virus encephalitis and meningitis, herpes zoster virus meningitis, JCV GCN, PML in patients treated with natalizumab monotherapy.

ANTIDOTE

Keep physician informed of all side effects. Most will be treated symptomatically. Consider discontinuation of natalizumab in patients who are diagnosed with ARN. Treatment for ARN may include antiviral therapy and surgery. Discontinue natalizumab at the first sign of liver injury, with S/S of meningitis or encephalitis, with S/S suggestive of PML, or with any change in neurologic status. Discontinue infusion if any S/S of a hypersensitivity or infusion reaction occur. Treat with epinephrine, corticosteroids, diphenhydramine, bronchodilators, and oxygen as indicated. Patients who experience a hypersensitivity reaction should not be retreated with natalizumab.

NECITUMUMAB BBW

(neh-**CIT**-ue-mew-mab)

Antineoplastic
(Monoclonal antibody,
epidermal growth factor
receptor [EGFR] inhibitor)

Portrazza

pH 6

USUAL DOSE

Pretreatment: Verify pregnancy status. Baseline studies required; see Monitor.

Premedication: For patients who have experienced a previous Grade 1 or 2 infusion-related reaction (IRR), premedicate with diphenhydramine or equivalent before all subsequent necitumumab infusions. For patients who have experienced a second occurrence of Grade 1 or 2 IRR, premedicate before all subsequent necitumumab infusions with diphenhydramine (or equivalent), acetaminophen (or equivalent), and dexamethasone (or equivalent).

Necitumumab: 800 mg as an IV infusion over 60 minutes on Days 1 and 8 of each 3-week cycle. Administer before gemcitabine (Gemzar) and cisplatin infusions. Continue until disease progression or unacceptable toxicity. Refer to gemcitabine and cisplatin monographs for premedication, hydration, dose recommendations, precautions, monitoring, and other requirements before administration.

DOSE ADJUSTMENTS

Reduce the infusion rate of necitumumab by 50% for a Grade 1 IRR. ▪ Stop the infusion for a Grade 2 IRR. When signs and symptoms have resolved to Grade 0 or 1, resume necitumumab at a 50% reduced rate for all subsequent infusions. ▪ Permanently discontinue necitumumab for a Grade 3 or 4 IRR. ▪ Withhold necitumumab for Grade 3 dermatologic toxicity (e.g., rash or acneiform rash) until symptoms resolve to Grade 2 or less, then resume necitumumab at a reduced dose of 400 mg for at least 1 treatment cycle. If symptoms do not worsen, dose may be increased to 600 mg and 800 mg in subsequent cycles. ▪ Permanently discontinue necitumumab for dermatologic toxicity if (1) the Grade 3 rash or acneiform rash does not resolve to Grade 2 or less within 6 weeks, (2) reactions worsen or become intolerable at a dose of 400 mg, (3) patient experiences a Grade 3 skin induration/fibrosis, or (4) patient experiences Grade 4 dermatologic toxicity. ▪ Withhold necitumumab for Grade 3 or 4 electrolyte abnormalities. Administer subsequent cycles once electrolyte abnormalities have improved to Grade 2 or less. ▪ No dose adjustment necessary based on body weight.

DILUTION

Available as a preservative-free solution in a single-dose vial containing 800 mg/50 mL (16 mg/mL). Solution should be clear. Discard if discolored or particulate matter is present. Withdraw the desired dose and further dilute to a final volume of 250 mL with NS. Do not use solutions containing dextrose. Gently invert the container to ensure adequate mixing. *Do not freeze or shake.*

Filters: Specific information not available.

Storage: Before use, refrigerate at 2° to 8° C (36° to 46° F) in original carton to protect from light. *Do not freeze or shake the vial.* Diluted solution may be stored for no more than 24 hours if refrigerated or no more than 4 hours at RT. Discard any unused portion left in the vial.

COMPATIBILITY

Manufacturer states, "Do not dilute with solutions other than NS or co-infuse with other electrolytes or medication." Use of a separate line required.

RATE OF ADMINISTRATION

Administer as an infusion over 60 minutes using an infusion pump through a separate infusion line. Flush the line with NS at the end of the infusion. Reduce rate or discontinue infusion for IRR; see Dose Adjustments.

ACTIONS

A recombinant human IgG1 monoclonal antibody that specifically binds to the human epidermal growth factor receptor (EGFR) and blocks the binding of EGFR to its ligands. Expression and activation of EGFR have been correlated with malignant progression, induction of angiogenesis, and inhibition of apoptosis. Binding of necitumumab induces EGFR internalization and degradation in vitro and also leads to antibody-dependent cellular cytotoxicity in EGFR-expressing cells. Elimination half-life is approximately 14 days. The predicted time to reach steady state is approximately 100 days.

INDICATIONS AND USES

First-line treatment of patients with metastatic squamous non–small-cell lung cancer in combination with gemcitabine and cisplatin. **Limitation of use:** Not indicated for treatment of nonsquamous non–small-cell lung cancer. These patients experienced more serious and fatal toxicities, including cardiopulmonary arrest/sudden death, within 30 days when administered necitumumab in combination with pemetrexed and cisplatin.

CONTRAINDICATIONS

Manufacturer states, "None."

PRECAUTIONS

Administered by or under the direction of a physician specialist in a facility with adequate diagnostic and treatment facilities to monitor the patient and respond to any medical emergency. ▪ Cardiopulmonary arrest and/or sudden death has been reported with necitumumab used in combination with gemcitabine and cisplatin. Some of these deaths occurred within 30 days of the last dose of necitumumab in patients with comorbid conditions, including a history of coronary artery disease, hypomagnesemia, COPD, and/or hypertension. ▪ Hypomagnesemia occurred in most patients receiving necitumumab in combination with gemcitabine and cisplatin and was severe in 20% of patients. The median time to development of hypomagnesemia and accompanying electrolyte abnormalities was 6 weeks after initiation of necitumumab. ▪ Venous and arterial thromboembolic events (VTEs and ATEs), some fatal, have been observed. The most common VTEs were pulmonary embolism and deep vein thrombosis. The most common ATEs were cerebral stroke and ischemia and myocardial infarction. Risk is higher in patients with a reported history of VTEs or ATEs. ■ Dermatologic toxicities, some severe, have been reported. ■ Infusion-related reactions have been reported. Most IRRs occurred after the first or second administration of necitumumab; see Premedication and Monitor. ■ As with all therapeutic proteins, there is a potential for immunogenicity. ■ Renal function and mild to moderate hepatic impairment have no influence on the exposure to necitumumab based on population pharmacokinetic analysis; however, no formal studies have been conducted. No patients with severe hepatic impairment were enrolled in clinical trials.

Monitor: Obtain serum electrolytes (including serum magnesium, potassium, and calcium) before each dose of necitumumab. Closely monitor for hypomagnesemia, hypocalcemia, and hypokalemia during treatment and for at least 8 weeks after the last dose is administered, with aggressive replacement when warranted during and after administration of necitumumab. ■ Withhold necitumumab for Grade 3 or 4 electrolyte abnormalities. ■ Monitor for S/S of venous and arterial thromboembolic events (e.g., chest pain, limb or abdominal swelling and/or pain, shortness of breath, loss of sensation or motor power, or altered consciousness, vision, or speech). ■ Monitor for dermatologic toxicities (e.g., acne, dermatitis acneiform, dry skin, erythema, generalized rash, maculopapular rash, rash, skin fissures). Usually develop within the first 2 weeks of therapy and resolve within 17 weeks after onset; see Dose Adjustments and Antidote. ■ Monitor for S/S of IRRs (e.g., chills, dyspnea, fever, hypotension, rash, tightness of the chest, urticaria, wheezing) during and after infusion; see Dose Adjustments and Antidote.

Patient Education: Blood levels of magnesium, potassium, and calcium may be decreased. Take medicines to replace these electrolytes exactly as advised by the physician. ■ Risk of venous and arterial thromboembolic events is increased. Promptly report chest pain, limb or abdominal swelling and/or pain, shortness of breath, loss of sensation or motor power, or altered consciousness, vision, or speech. ■ To reduce the risk of dermatologic reactions, minimize sun exposure with the use of protective clothing and sunscreen during treatment. ■ Immediately report S/S of an infusion-related reaction (e.g., breathing problems, chills, fever, rash, tightness of the chest, urticaria, wheezing). ■ There is a potential risk to a fetus and to postnatal development. Effective contraception is required in females of reproductive potential during treatment and for 3 months after the final dose. ■ See Maternal/Child.

Maternal/Child: Based on its mechanism of action, necitumumab can cause fetal harm or developmental anomalies. Effective contraception required; see Patient Education. ▪ Discontinue breastfeeding during treatment and for 3 months after the final dose. ▪ Safety and effectiveness for use in pediatric patients not established.

Elderly: There was a higher incidence of venous thromboembolic events, including pulmonary embolism, in patients age 70 years and over compared with younger patients.

DRUG/LAB INTERACTIONS

When used in combination with gemcitabine, the dose-normalized area under the curve (AUC) of gemcitabine was increased. Exposure to cisplatin was unchanged. Gemcitabine and cisplatin had no effect on the exposure of necitumumab.

SIDE EFFECTS

The most common adverse reactions (all grades) observed more frequently in patients treated with necitumumab than with gemcitabine and cisplatin alone were dermatitis acneiform, diarrhea, hypomagnesemia, rash, and vomiting. The most common severe (Grade 3 or higher) adverse events were thromboembolic events (including pulmonary embolism), rash, and vomiting. Acne, conjunctivitis, dry skin, electrolyte abnormalities (including hypocalcemia, hypokalemia, and hypophosphatemia), headache, hemoptysis, paronychia, pruritus, skin fissures, stomatitis, VTE, and weight decrease have been reported.

ANTIDOTE

Keep physician informed of all side effects. May constitute a medical emergency or will be treated symptomatically as indicated. Reduce the infusion rate of necitumumab by 50% for Grade 1 IRRs. Stop the infusion for Grade 2 IRRs. Treat infusion-related reactions as indicated and provide premedication (e.g., diphenhydramine, acetaminophen, corticosteroids) for subsequent infusions; see Usual Dose. When signs and symptoms have resolved to Grade 0 or 1, resume necitumumab at a 50% reduced rate for all subsequent infusions. Withhold necitumumab for Grade 3 or 4 electrolyte abnormalities. Permanently discontinue necitumumab for any of the following: (1) Grade 3 or 4 IRR, (2) Grade 3 rash or acneiform rash that does not resolve to Grade 2 or less within 6 weeks, (3) dermatologic reactions that worsen or become intolerable at a dose of 400 mg, (4) Grade 3 skin induration/fibrosis, or (5) Grade 4 dermatologic toxicity. See Dose Adjustments, Precautions, and Monitor.

NEOSTIGMINE METHYLSULFATE
(nee-oh-**STIG**-meen **METH**-ill-**SUL**-fayt)

Acetylcholinesterase inhibitor

Bloxiverz

pH 5.5

USUAL DOSE
Pretreatment: Doses should be individualized. A peripheral nerve stimulator should be used to determine when neostigmine should be initiated and if additional doses are needed. Before neostigmine administration and up until complete recovery of normal ventilation, the patient should be well ventilated and a patent airway maintained. An anticholinergic agent (e.g., atropine or glycopyrrolate) should be administered before or concomitantly with neostigmine using a separate syringe.

Atropine: 0.6 to 1.2 mg IV for each 0.5 to 2 mg of neostigmine **OR**

Glycopyrrolate: 0.2 mg IV for each 1 mg of neostigmine; see Precautions.

Neostigmine: 0.03 to 0.07 mg/kg. This dose will generally achieve a train-of-four (TOF) twitch ratio of 90% within 10 to 20 minutes of administration. The recommended maximum total dose is 0.07 mg/kg or up to a total of 5 mg, whichever is less. Dose selection should be based on the extent of spontaneous recovery that has occurred at the time of administration, the half-life of the neuromuscular blocking agent (NMBA) being reversed, and whether there is a need to rapidly reverse the NMBA.

The 0.03 mg/kg dose is recommended for:
- Reversal of NMBAs with shorter half-lives (e.g., rocuronium) **OR**
- When the first twitch response to the TOF stimulus is substantially greater than 10% of baseline or when a second twitch is present.

The 0.07 mg/kg dose is recommended for:
- Reversal of NMBAs with longer half-lives (e.g., pancuronium or vecuronium) **OR**
- When the first twitch response is relatively weak (i.e., not substantially greater than 10% of baseline) **OR**
- There is need for more rapid recovery.

PEDIATRIC DOSE
See Usual Dose and Maternal/Child.

DOSE ADJUSTMENTS
Individualize dose based on extent of spontaneous recovery at time of administration, the half-life of the NMBA being reversed, and whether or not there is a need to rapidly reverse the NMBA. ▪ Use with caution and with minimum effective dose in pediatric patients and in patients with coronary artery disease, cardiac arrhythmias, recent acute coronary syndrome, or myasthenia gravis; see Maternal/Child. ▪ Reduce dose if recovery from neuromuscular blockade is nearly complete. See Precautions and Monitor.

DILUTION
Available in 0.5 mg/mL and 1 mg/mL in 10-mL multiple-dose vials. May be given undiluted through Y-tube of infusion set.

Storage: Store at CRT in carton. Protect from light.

COMPATIBILITY
Compatibility information not available from manufacturer. Other sources suggest a few specific **compatibilities** dependent on concentration and manufacturer; consult a pharmacist.

RATE OF ADMINISTRATION
Inject slowly over a period of at least 1 minute.

ACTIONS
A competitive cholinesterase inhibitor and antagonist of nondepolarizing neuromuscular blocking agents. Inhibits the enzyme cholinesterase. By reducing the breakdown of acetylcholine, neostigmine induces an increase in acetylcholine in the synaptic cleft. Acetylcholine competes for the same binding sites as nondepolarizing NMBAs and reverses the

neuromuscular blockade. The increase in acetylcholine levels results in the potentiation of both muscarinic and nicotine cholinergic activity. Does not cross the blood-brain barrier so does not significantly affect cholinergic function in the CNS. Metabolized by microsomal enzymes in the liver. Half-life ranges from 24 to 113 minutes. Excreted primarily in urine.

INDICATIONS AND USES
Reversal of the effects of nondepolarizing neuromuscular blocking agents after surgery. **Unlabeled use:** Treatment of myasthenia gravis.

CONTRAINDICATIONS
Known hypersensitivity to neostigmine (known hypersensitivity reactions have included urticaria, angioedema, erythema multiforme, generalized rash, facial swelling, peripheral edema, fever, flushing, hypotension, bronchospasm, bradycardia, and anaphylaxis). ■ Peritonitis or mechanical obstruction of the intestinal or urinary tract.

PRECAUTIONS
For IV administration only. ■ Should be administered by a trained health care provider familiar with the use, actions, characteristics, and complications of neuromuscular blocking agents and neuromuscular block reversal agents. ■ Neostigmine has been associated with bradycardia. In the presence of bradycardia, it is recommended that the anticholinergic agent (atropine or glycopyrrolate) be administered before neostigmine. ■ Cardiovascular effects such as bradycardia, hypotension, or dysrhythmia are anticipated with acetylcholinesterase inhibitors such as neostigmine. Use with caution in patients with coronary artery disease, cardiac arrhythmias, recent acute coronary syndrome, or myasthenia gravis. Risk of blood pressure and heart rate complications may be increased in these patients. ■ Because of the possibility of hypersensitivity, atropine and medications to treat anaphylaxis should be readily available. ■ Large doses of neostigmine administered when neuromuscular blockade is minimal can produce neuromuscular dysfunction. The dose of neostigmine should be reduced if recovery from neuromuscular blockade is nearly complete. ■ It is important to distinguish between myasthenic crisis and cholinergic crisis caused by overdose of neostigmine. Both result in extreme muscle weakness but require radically different treatment; see Antidote. ■ Use with caution in patients with renal and hepatic impairment. Dose adjustment is not required, but duration of action of NMBAs that are renally or hepatically eliminated may be prolonged. Patients must be carefully monitored to ensure that the effects of the NMBA do not persist beyond those of neostigmine.

Monitor: A peripheral nerve stimulation device capable of delivering a TOF stimulus is required. There must be a twitch response to the first stimulus in the TOF of at least 10% of its baseline level (i.e., the response prior to the NMBA) before administering neostigmine. ■ TOF monitoring alone should not be relied on to determine the adequacy of reversal of neuromuscular blockade as related to a patient's ability to adequately ventilate and maintain a patent airway following tracheal extubation. Satisfactory recovery should be judged by adequacy of skeletal muscle tone and respiratory measurements in addition to the response to the peripheral nerve stimulator. ■ Continue monitoring for adequacy of reversal for a period that will ensure full recovery based on the patient's medical condition and the pharmacokinetics of neostigmine and the NMBA used.

Maternal/Child: It is not known whether neostigmine can cause fetal harm when administered to a pregnant female use during pregnancy, labor, or delivery only if clearly needed. Acetylcholinesterase drugs, including neostigmine, may cause uterine irritability and induce premature labor when given to pregnant females who are near term. ■ The effect of neostigmine on the mother and fetus with regard to labor, delivery, the need for forceps delivery or other intervention, or resuscitation of the newborn is not known. ■ Use caution during breastfeeding. ■ Recovery of neuromuscular activity occurs more rapidly with smaller doses of acetylcholinesterase inhibitors in pediatric patients than in adults. However, infants and small children may be at greater risk for complications from incomplete reversal of neuromuscular blockade due to decreased respiratory reserve. The risks associated with incomplete reversal outweigh any risk from giving higher doses of neostigmine. ▪ Because blood pressure in pediatric patients, particularly infants and neonates, is sensitive to changes in heart rate, the effects of an anticholinergic agent (e.g., atropine) should be observed before administration of neostigmine to lessen the probability of bradycardia and hypotension.

Elderly: Duration of action is prolonged in the elderly. However, the elderly also experience a slower spontaneous recovery from NMBAs. Dose adjustment is not generally needed, but an extended monitoring period to ensure complete reversal may be warranted.

DRUG/LAB INTERACTIONS

Pharmacokinetic interactions between neostigmine and other drugs have not been studied. ▪ Metabolized by microsomal enzymes in the liver. Use with caution when using with other drugs that may alter the activity of metabolizing enzymes or transporters.

SIDE EFFECTS

Usually attributable to exaggerated pharmacologic effects at the muscarinic receptor. The most common side effects are bradycardia, nausea, and vomiting. Other side effects include dizziness, dry mouth, dyspnea, headache, hypotension, incision site complications, insomnia, oxygen desaturation, pharyngolaryngeal pain, postoperative shivering, procedural complications, procedural pain, prolonged neuromuscular blockade, pruritus, and tachycardia.

Overdose: Bradycardia, nausea, vomiting, diarrhea, increased bronchial and salivary secretions, muscle weakness (including muscles of respiration), sweating, death (symptoms of cholinergic crisis).

Post-Marketing: Hypersensitivity reactions, anaphylaxis, arthralgia, bowel cramps, bronchospasm, cardiac arrest, cardiac arrhythmias, convulsions, diaphoresis, diarrhea, drowsiness, dysarthria, fasciculation, flatulence, flushing, hypotension, increased peristalsis, increased secretions, loss of consciousness, miosis, muscle cramps, nonspecific ECG changes, rash, respiratory depression or arrest, spasms, syncope, urinary frequency, urticaria, visual changes, weakness.

ANTIDOTE

If side effects occur, discontinue drug and notify the physician. The use of an anticholinergic agent (atropine or glycopyrrolate) may prevent or mitigate most side effects, including cardiovascular complications (bradycardia, hypotension, or dysrhythmia). In the event of an overdose, ventilation should be supported by artificial means until adequacy of spontaneous respiration is assured, and cardiac function should be monitored. Treat anaphylaxis immediately with oxygen, epinephrine, antihistamines (e.g., diphenhydramine), vasopressors (e.g., dopamine), corticosteroids, albuterol, IV fluids, and ventilation equipment as indicated. Resuscitate as necessary.

NICARDIPINE HYDROCHLORIDE

(nye-**KAR**-dih-peen hy-droh-**KLOR**-eyed)

Cardene IV

Calcium channel blocker
Antihypertensive

pH 3.5 to 4.7

USUAL DOSE

Must be individualized based on the severity of hypertension and the response of each patient. Blood pressure decrease is dependent on the rate of infusion and frequency of dose adjustments. Gradual reduction based on clinical situation is best. Avoid too-rapid or excessive drop in BP. See Precautions and Monitor. Transfer to oral medication as soon as clinical condition permits.

To substitute for oral nicardipine therapy: 0.5 mg/hr will achieve similar plasma concentration to an oral dose of 20 mg every 8 hours; 1.2 mg/hr to an oral dose of 30 mg every 8 hours; 2.2 mg/hr to an oral dose of 40 mg every 8 hours.

Gradual reduction of BP in a drug-free patient: Initiate therapy at 5 mg/hr. May be increased by 2.5 mg/hr every 15 minutes until desired BP reduction is achieved. Do not exceed 15 mg/hr.

Rapid reduction of BP in a drug-free patient: Initiate a 5-mg/hr dose as above, but increases of 2.5 mg/hr may be given every 5 minutes until desired BP reduction is achieved (AHA guidelines recommend 5 to 15 minutes). Do not exceed 15 mg/hr.

Maintenance: Adjust as needed to maintain desired response.

Transfer to an oral antihypertensive agent: The first dose of oral nicardipine should be given 1 hour before discontinuing infusion. Initiate any other oral antihypertensive agent on discontinuation of infusion.

DOSE ADJUSTMENTS

Lower doses and slower titration suggested in heart failure and impaired hepatic or renal function; see Precautions. ▪ Lower-end initial doses may be indicated in the elderly. Consider potential for decreased organ function and concomitant disease or drug therapy. ▪ Discontinue infusion if hypotension or tachycardia develop. When blood pressure and heart rate stabilize, restart infusion at a lower dose and titrate to desired response.

DILUTION

Available as a premixed solution containing a final concentration of 0.1 mg/mL or 0.2 mg/mL in D5W or NS. Also available in a vial that requires further dilution. Each vial (25 mg in 10 mL) must be diluted with 240 mL of **compatible** infusion solution to equal a concentration of 0.1 mg/mL; in this 0.1 mg/mL concentration, 2.5 mg/hr equals 25 mL/hr, 3 mg/hr equals 30 mL/hr, 5 mg/hr equals 50 mL/hr, and 15 mL/hr equals 150 mL/hr. **Compatible** in ½NS, NS, D5W, D5/½NS, D5NS. Also **compatible** in D5W with 40 mEq of potassium added.

Fluid-restricted or pediatric patients: One source recommends mixing up to 50 mg in 100 mL (0.5 mg/mL). To avoid superficial phlebitis, administration via a central line is recommended for this concentration.

Filters: No data available from manufacturer.

Storage: Store vials in carton, protected from light at CRT. Has a light yellow color. Diluted solution is stable at room temperature for 24 hours. Store prediluted solutions at CRT; protect from light and excessive heat.

COMPATIBILITY

Manufacturer states, "Do not combine with any product in the same IV line or premixed container. Do not add supplementary medication to the bag." Manufacturer lists as **incompatible** with sodium bicarbonate 5% and LR.

Other sources suggest specific **compatibilities** dependent on concentration and manufacturer; consult a pharmacist.

RATE OF ADMINISTRATION

Must be administered as a slow, continuous infusion. Adjust as indicated in Usual Dose and Dose Adjustments.

ACTIONS

The first dihydropyridine calcium channel blocker for IV use. Inhibits influx of calcium ions into cardiac muscle and smooth muscle without altering serum calcium. Contractile processes are dependent on calcium movement through specific channels. Effects seen are more selective to vascular smooth muscle than cardiac muscle. Causes coronary and peripheral blood vessels to dilate and relax, reducing systemic vascular resistance. Increases cardiac output, coronary blood flow, and myocardial oxygen supply without increasing cardiac oxygen demand. Reduces BP without significantly affecting cardiac conduction and usually does not depress cardiac function. Produces dose-dependent decreases in BP. Begins to reduce BP in minutes; achieves 50% of ultimate decrease in 45 minutes. When discontinued, can lose 50% of effect within 30 minutes, but gradually decreasing effects persist for many hours. Effects more prominent in hypertensive than in normotensive volunteers. Highly protein bound. Extensively metabolized in the liver by the hepatic cytochrome P450 enzymes CYP2C8, 2D6, and 3A4. Half-life is 14 hours. Excreted in urine and feces. Crosses placental barrier. Minimally secreted in breast milk.

INDICATIONS AND USES
Short-term treatment of hypertension when oral therapy is not feasible or not desirable.

CONTRAINDICATIONS
Advanced aortic stenosis (reduced diastolic pressure may worsen rather than improve myocardial oxygen balance). ■ Known hypersensitivity to nicardipine.

PRECAUTIONS
Use caution in patients with coronary artery disease. May cause increase in frequency, duration, or severity of angina. ■ Has improved left ventricle function after beta-blockade. ■ Use caution and titrate slowly in patients with heart failure or significant left ventricular dysfunction, particularly when used in combination with a beta-blocker; possible negative inotropic effects may occur. ■ Use caution with impaired hepatic or renal function; lower doses, slower titration, and close monitoring indicated. ■ May produce symptomatic hypotension or tachycardia. Avoid systemic hypotension (systolic BP less than 90 mm Hg), and use with caution in patients with acute cerebral infarction or hemorrhage. ■ Experience with use in patients with hypertension from pheochromocytoma is limited.

Monitor: To reduce the possibility of venous thrombosis, phlebitis, local irritation, swelling, extravasation, and/or vascular impairment, administer through a central vein or large peripheral vein rather than a small peripheral vein. Avoid intra-arterial administration. If administered via a peripheral vein, change the infusion site every 12 hours. ■ Avoid tachycardia or too-rapid or excessive reduction in either systolic or diastolic BP. Monitor BP and HR continually during infusion and frequently after infusion. Additional monitoring of BP and HR is indicated when used in combination with a beta-blocker in patients with HF or significant left ventricular dysfunction ■ Transfer to oral therapy as soon as clinical condition permits. ■ See Precautions and Drug/Lab Interactions.

Patient Education: Request assistance to change position or ambulate.

Maternal/Child: Category C: use during pregnancy only if benefit justifies potential risk to the fetus. Has been used for the treatment of severe hypertension in pregnancy and preterm labor. Changes in fetal heart rate and neonatal hypotension and acidosis have been reported. If treatment for hypertension during pregnancy is needed, other agents may be preferred. ■ Use caution during breastfeeding; infant exposure may occur. Some manufacturers do not recommend breastfeeding. ■ Safety and effectiveness for use in pediatric patients under 18 years of age not established.

Elderly: Response similar to that seen in younger adults; however, greater sensitivity in the elderly cannot be ruled out. ■ See Dose Adjustments.

DRUG/LAB INTERACTIONS
May cause possible negative inotropic effects with concurrent administration of a **beta-blocker**; see Precautions. ■ **Cimetidine** increases oral nicardipine plasma concentrations; monitor patients receiving IV nicardipine. ■ May increase plasma levels of **cyclosporine** and **tacrolimus** through inhibition of hepatic microsomal enzymes, including CYP3A4; monitor levels and adjust dose if indicated. ■ May potentiate the effects of **other antihypertensives.** Monitor BP closely and adjust doses as indicated. ■ Metabolism may be increased and serum concentrations decreased by **rifampin.** Adjust dose as needed.

SIDE EFFECTS
Average dose: The most common side effects include headache, hypotension, nausea and vomiting, and tachycardia. Many other side effects, including ECG abnormality (e.g., angina pectoris, atrioventricular block, ST-segment depression, inverted T wave), confusion, conjunctivitis, deep vein thrombophlebitis, dyspepsia, ear disorder, fever, hypertonia, hypophosphatemia, neck pain, peripheral edema, respiratory difficulties, thrombocytopenia, tinnitus, and urinary frequency, occurred in fewer than 3% of patients. Hypersensitivity reactions (e.g., angioedema, rash, wheezing) have been reported.

Overdose: Bradycardia (following initial tachycardia), confusion, drowsiness, flushing, hypotension (marked), palpitations, slurred speech.

Post-Marketing: Decreased oxygen saturation (possible pulmonary shunting).

ANTIDOTE

Keep physician informed of all side effects. Headache, hypotension, and tachycardia have required a reduction in dose or discontinuation of nicardipine. When symptoms subside, nicardipine may be restarted at low doses (e.g., 3 to 5 mg/hr [30 to 50 mL/hr of a 0.1 mg/mL solution or 15 to 25 mL/hr of a 0.2 mg/mL solution]) and adjusted to maintain desired BP. In overdose, monitor BP and cardiac and respiratory functions; put patients in Trendelenburg position; use vasopressors (e.g., dopamine) for excessive hypotension. IV calcium gluconate may reverse effects of calcium entry blockade. Not removed by hemodialysis.

NITROGLYCERIN IV

(NYE-troe-GLIS-er-in)

Antianginal
Antihypertensive
Vasodilator

pH 3 to 6.5

USUAL DOSE

See Compatibility; these doses are recommended for use with non-PVC administration sets. Increased doses are required if using PVC administration sets. Dose must be individualized based on patient condition and response to therapy. Initiate infusion at 5 mcg/min. Subsequent titration must be guided by clinical results, with dose increments becoming more cautious as partial response is seen. Initial titration should be in 5-mcg/min increments at intervals of 3 to 5 minutes. If no response is seen at 20 mcg/min, increments of 10 mcg/min and even 20 mcg/min can be used. Once some hemodynamic response is observed, dosage increments should be smaller and less frequent.

Note: If the concentration of nitroglycerin is changed, the tubing must be disconnected from the patient and flushed with the new solution before therapy is continued. If this precaution is not taken, then it might take several hours before nitroglycerin is delivered at the desired rate depending on the tubing, pump, and flow rate used.

PEDIATRIC DOSE

0.25 to 0.5 mcg/kg/min initially. May increase by 0.5 to 1 mcg/kg/min increments every 3 to 5 minutes until desired response. Maximum dose suggested is 20 mcg/kg/min. See Maternal/Child. AHA guidelines recommend titrating by 1 mcg/kg/min every 15 to 20 minutes and state that the typical dose range is 1 to 5 mcg/kg/min. Maximum dose suggested is 10 mcg/kg/min.

DOSE ADJUSTMENTS

Lower-end initial doses may be appropriate in the elderly based on potential for decreased organ function, concomitant disease, or other drug therapy.

DILUTION

Available premixed in D5W with various concentrations of nitroglycerin. Do not use premixed solution if vacuum is not present. All other preparations must be diluted before administration as an infusion. Use only non-PVC plastic (EXCEL or PAB) or glass infusion bottles and specific (nonpolyvinyl chloride) infusion tubing. Do not use filters. Dilute in a given amount of D5W or NS for infusion. Concentration is dependent on initial preparation and patient fluid tolerances. Lower concentrations of nitroglycerin in D5W increase the potential for precision of dosing but increase the total fluid volume that must be administered. Total fluid load may be an important consideration in patients with compromised heart, hepatic, or renal function.

Filters: Some in-line IV filters absorb nitroglycerin; these filters should be avoided.

Storage: Store at CRT. Protect from light and freezing. Discard any unused portion of vial or premixed solution. Solution stable for up to 24 hours.

COMPATIBILITY

Manufacturer states, "Do not admix with any other drug." See Dilution. Non-PVC plastic or glass infusion bottles and nonpolyvinyl chloride infusion tubing are required to deliver accurate dosing with minimal absorption. Calculated dose will not be correct if other infusion containers or tubing are used because of excess absorption.

Other sources suggest specific **compatibilities** dependent on concentration and manufacturer; consult a pharmacist.

RATE OF ADMINISTRATION

Use of an infusion pump is required. Rate is dependent on patient response and effective dose. Specific adjustments required; see Usual Dose. Use extreme caution in patients responsive to initial 5 mcg/min dose. Decrease dose increments and increase time between dose adjustments as patient begins to respond.

Adult infusion rate may be calculated using the following equation:

Infusion rate (mL/hr) = [Dose (mcg/min) × 60 min/hr] ÷ Final concentration (mcg/mL)

Pediatric infusion rate may be calculated using the following equation:

Infusion rate (mL/hr) =
[Dose (mcg/kg/min) × Weight (kg) × 60 min/hr] ÷ Final concentration (mcg/mL)

(Use of the 100 mcg/mL [25 mg/250 mL] concentration is recommended.)

ACTIONS

The principal action of nitroglycerin is relaxation of vascular smooth muscle and consequent dilation of peripheral arteries and veins, especially the latter. Dilation of the veins promotes peripheral pooling of blood and decreases venous return to the heart, thereby reducing left ventricular end-diastolic pressure and pulmonary capillary wedge pressure (preload). Arteriolar relaxation reduces systemic vascular resistance, systolic arterial pressure, and mean arterial pressure (afterload). Dilation of the coronary arteries also occurs. The relative importance of preload reduction, afterload reduction, and coronary dilation remains undefined. Widely distributed throughout the body. Onset of action is immediate. Duration of effect is 3 to 5 minutes. Undergoes both hepatic and nonhepatic metabolism and is excreted in urine.

INDICATIONS AND USES

Treatment of perioperative hypertension. ■ Control of heart failure in the setting of acute myocardial infarction. ■ Treatment of angina pectoris if patient is unresponsive to sublingual nitroglycerin and beta-blockers. ■ Induction of intraoperative hypotension.

CONTRAINDICATIONS

Hypersensitivity to nitrates or any component of the product (dextrose is derived from corn). ■ Patients with pericardial tamponade, restrictive cardiomyopathy, constrictive pericarditis, or cardiac output that is dependent on venous return. ■ Patients with increased intracranial pressure or uncorrected hypovolemia. ■ Concurrent use with phosphodiesterase-5 (PDE-5) inhibitors (e.g., avanafil, sildenafil, tadalafil, or vardenafil) or with soluble guanylate cyclase stimulators (e.g., riociguat).

PRECAUTIONS

Use of polyvinyl chloride (PVC) tubing in infusion sets may lead to loss of active ingredient due to absorption of nitroglycerin by PVC tubing; therefore dosage is affected. Nitroglycerin absorption by PVC tubing is increased when the tubing is long, flow rates are low, and nitroglycerin concentration is high. PVC tubing was used in most published studies of IV nitroglycerin. The delivered fraction of the solution's original nitroglycerin content has been 20% to 60% in published studies. Relatively nonabsorptive IV administration sets are available. **If IV nitroglycerin is administered through nonabsorptive tubing, doses based on published reports will generally be too high.** ■ Severe hypotension and shock may occur with even small doses of nitroglycerin. Hypotension induced by nitroglycerin may be accompanied by paradoxical bradycardia and increased angina pectoris. ■ Nitrate therapy may aggravate angina caused by hypertrophic cardiomyopathy.

- Tolerance development and occurrence of cross-tolerance to other nitro compounds have been reported. ■ Lower concentrations of nitroglycerin in D5W increase the potential for precision of dosing but increase the total fluid volume that must be administered. Total fluid load may be an important consideration in patients with compromised heart, hepatic, or renal function. ■ Methemoglobinemia has been reported (rare); see Antidote.

Monitor: Continuous monitoring of BP and HR required. ■ Monitoring of pulmonary capillary wedge pressure may be indicated. ■ Closely monitor patients who may be volume depleted or who, for whatever reason, are already hypotensive. ■ Monitor blood glucose in patients with known subclinical or overt diabetes mellitus when using solutions containing dextrose. ■ Headache may improve with analgesics or slightly lower dose; usually improves with time. ■ See Drug/Lab Interactions.

Maternal/Child: Safety for use in pregnancy and breastfeeding and in pediatric patients not established. Consider risk versus benefit for each indication.

Elderly: Differences in response compared with younger patients not identified. ■ Lower-end initial doses may be indicated; see Dose Adjustments.

DRUG/LAB INTERACTIONS

Concurrent use with **PDE-5 inhibitors** (e.g., avanafil, sildenafil, tadalafil, or vardenafil) is contraindicated. Concomitant use can cause severe hypotension, syncope, or myocardial ischemia. ■ Concurrent use with **soluble guanylate cyclase stimulators** (e.g., riociguat) is contraindicated. Concomitant use can cause hypotension. ■ Potentiated by **alcohol, antihypertensives** (including **beta-adrenergic blockers** and **calcium channel blockers**), **other vasodilators, phenothiazines, and tricyclic antidepressants**. ■ **Dihydroergotamine** may diminish the vasodilatory effect of nitroglycerin. ■ May cause marked orthostatic hypotension with **calcium channel blockers**. ■ At higher doses, nitroglycerin may antagonize anticoagulant effects of **heparin;** monitor. ■ Concurrent use with **alteplase** (tPA) reduces the thrombolytic effects of alteplase. ■ **Serum triglyceride assays** that rely on glycerol oxidase may give falsely elevated results in patients receiving nitroglycerin in D5W.

SIDE EFFECTS

In general, side effects are dose-related, and almost all are the result of nitroglycerin's activity as a vasodilator. Headache is the most commonly reported adverse reaction. Other reactions include abdominal pain, angina, dizziness, dyspnea, hypersensitivity reactions (e.g., itching, tracheobronchitis, wheezing), hypotension, light-headedness, methemoglobinemia, nausea, postural hypotension, rebound hypotension, syncope, tachycardia, vomiting.

Overdose: Bloody diarrhea, colic, coma, confusion, diaphoresis, dyspnea, fever, flushing, heart block, increased intracranial pressure, nausea and vomiting, palpitations, paradoxical bradycardia, paralysis, seizure, shock, syncope, tachycardia, visual disturbances, and death.

ANTIDOTE

Notify physician of all side effects. There is no specific antidote for overdose of nitroglycerin. The risk of overdose can be minimized by close monitoring during treatment. For significant adverse reactions, reduce rate or temporarily discontinue until condition stabilizes. Lower head of bed (Trendelenburg position). Administration of IV fluids may be useful but must be done with caution in patients with renal disease or heart failure. Invasive monitoring of hemodynamic status may be indicated to help guide therapy. Use O_2 and assisted ventilation if indicated. Epinephrine and related compounds (dopamine) are contraindicated. Monitor levels and treat methemoglobinemia if indicated with methylene blue 1 to 2 mg/kg IV and high-flow oxygen. Treat anaphylaxis and resuscitate as necessary.

NITROPRUSSIDE SODIUM BBW

(nye-troh-**PRUS**-eyed **SO**-dee-um)

Antihypertensive
Vasodilator

Nipride RTU, Nitropress

pH 3.5 to 6

USUAL DOSE

Continuous BP monitoring required.

Begin with 0.3 mcg/kg of body weight/min. Titrate in increments of 0.5 mcg/kg/min to a higher or lower dose to achieve the desired BP. Evaluate BP for at least 5 minutes before titrating to the next dose. (3 mcg/kg/min is the average effective dose; range is 0.1 to 10 mcg/kg/min.) AHA guidelines recommend beginning with 0.1 mcg/kg/min. Titrate upward every 3 to 5 minutes to desired effect (up to 5 mcg/kg/min). Small adjustments can lead to major fluctuations in BP. Dose may be titrated upward until the desired dose effect is achieved, the systemic BP cannot be further reduced without compromising the perfusion of vital organs, or the maximum recommended infusion rate of 10 mcg/kg/min has been reached, whichever occurs first. If 10 mcg/kg/min does not promote adequate BP reduction in 10 minutes, discontinue administration and use another antihypertensive agent. Cyanide toxicity can occur with as little as 2 mcg/kg/min and could begin to occur after 10 minutes at the maximum dose.

PEDIATRIC DOSE

Begin with 0.3 mcg/kg/min. Adjust slowly to individual response as in Usual Dose. AHA guidelines recommend 0.3 to 1 mcg/kg/min initially; titrate up to 8 mcg/kg/min as needed.

DOSE ADJUSTMENTS

Limit the mean infusion rate to less than 3 mcg/kg/min in patients with an eGFR less than 30 mL/min/1.73 M^2 and to 1 mcg/kg/min in anuric patients. ▪ Reduced dose may be required in elderly patients.

DILUTION

Available as a ready-to-use (RTU) single-use vial containing 50 mg/100 mL of NS (0.5 mg/mL) and 10 mg/50 mL of NS (0.2 mg/mL). Also available in a concentrated liquid formulation (50 mg/2 mL). Must be further diluted in a minimum of 250 mL of D5W and administered as an infusion. Larger amounts of solution may be used. 50 mg in 250 mL equals 200 mcg/mL. 50 mg in 500 mL equals 100 mcg/mL. Immediately after mixing, wrap infusion bottle in opaque material (e.g., aluminum foil) to protect from light. Discard solution 24 hours after dilution. ▪ Solution should be a clear, colorless to red/brown color; discard immediately if highly colored, blue, green, or bright red.

COMPATIBILITY

Manufacturer states, "Do not administer other drugs in the same solution with sodium nitroprusside."

Other sources suggest specific **compatibilities** dependent on concentration and manufacturer; consult a pharmacist.

RATE OF ADMINISTRATION

Use of an infusion pump (volumetric preferred) required to regulate dose accurately. Increase mcg/kg/min rate as outlined in Usual Dose to reduce BP gradually to preset or desired levels. Do not exceed maximum dose. Response should be noted almost immediately.

ACTIONS

A potent, rapid-acting antihypertensive agent. Produces peripheral vasodilation through direct action on smooth muscle of the blood vessels. Reduces left ventricular end diastolic pressure and pulmonary capillary wedge pressure (preload) and systemic vascular resistance, systolic arterial pressure, and mean arterial pressure (afterload). Effective almost immediately. May increase HR and/or cardiac output slightly. Effectiveness ends when IV infusion is stopped. BP will return to pretreatment levels in 1 to 10 minutes. Rapidly converted to thiocyanate and eventually excreted in the urine.

INDICATIONS AND USES

For the immediate reduction of blood pressure in adults and pediatric patients in hypertensive crises. ▪ For induction and maintenance of controlled hypotension in adult and pediatric patients to reduce bleeding during surgery. ▪ Treatment of acute heart failure to reduce left ventricular end-diastolic pressure, pulmonary capillary wedge pressure, peripheral vascular resistance, and mean arterial BP.

Unlabeled uses: Hypertension during acute ischemic stroke.

CONTRAINDICATIONS

Diseases with compensatory hypertension (e.g., arteriovenous shunt or coarctation of the aorta). ▪ Should not be used to produce hypotension during surgery in patients with known inadequate cerebral circulation or in moribund patients (ASA Class 5E) coming to emergency surgery. ▪ Patients with congenital (Leber's) optic atrophy or tobacco amblyopia. ▪ Acute heart failure associated with reduced peripheral vascular resistance. ▪ Concomitant use with sildenafil, tadalafil, vardenafil, or riociguat.

PRECAUTIONS

Precipitous decreases in BP can occur quickly. Can lead to irreversible ischemic injuries or death. Hypotension should resolve within 1 to 10 minutes after discontinuation of the nitroprusside infusion. If hypotension persists, consider other causes. Use only when adequate personnel and appropriate equipment are available for continuous monitoring. ▪ Nitroprusside metabolism produces dose-related cyanide, which can be lethal. ▪ At infusions above 2 mcg/kg/min, cyanide ion is generated faster than the body can normally eliminate it. ▪ A patient's ability to buffer cyanide will be exceeded in less than 1 hour at the maximum dose rate (10 mcg/kg/min); limit infusions at the maximum rate to as short a duration as possible. Patients with hepatic dysfunction are more susceptible to cyanide toxicity. ▪ Most of the cyanide produced during metabolism of nitroprusside is eliminated in the form of thiocyanate. Thiocyanate is mildly neurotoxic at serum levels of 1 mmol/L (60 mg/L) and is life-threatening when levels reach approximately 200 mg/L. ▪ Nitroprusside infusions cause conversion of hemoglobin to methemoglobin in a dose-dependent manner. Clinically significant methemoglobinemia is infrequent. Suspect methemoglobinemia in patients who have received greater than 10 mg/kg of nitroprusside and who exhibit signs of impaired oxygen delivery despite adequate cardiac output and adequate arterial Po_2. ▪ As with other vasodilators, nitroprusside can cause increases in intracranial pressure. ▪ Use caution in hypothyroidism, increased intracranial pressure, liver or renal impairment, and elderly patients. ▪ When nitroprusside (or any other vasodilator) is used for controlled hypotension during anesthesia, the patient's capacity to compensate for anemia and hypovolemia may be diminished. If possible, correct pre-existing anemia and hypovolemia before administration.

Monitor: Determine patency of vein; avoid extravasation. ▪ Continuous automatic BP monitoring is mandatory (intra-arterial pressure sensor preferred). ▪ An early manifestation of cyanide toxicity is increasing dosage requirements to maintain blood pressure control. Metabolic acidosis may not be evident for more than an hour after toxic cyanide levels accumulate. ▪ Monitor for S/S of thiocyanate toxicity (hyperreflexia, miosis, tinnitus). ▪ Routine monitoring of thiocyanate plasma levels is recommended in patients with normal renal function when cumulative nitroprusside doses exceed 7 mg/kg/day; see Dose Adjustments. ▪ Measure methemoglobin levels if indicated. Levels greater than 10% are considered clinically significant.

Patient Education: Promptly report IV site burning or stinging.

Maternal/Child: Safety for use in pregnancy not established. Information is limited. Prolonged use and large doses of nitroprusside during pregnancy may result in cyanide toxicity that may be fatal to the fetus. Consider risk versus benefit. Use should generally be avoided unless there is no appropriate alternative therapy. ▪ Has been used in pediatric patients. Efficacy established, and safety concerns have not been identified. ▪ Information on safety with breastfeeding not available. One source recommends that breastfeeding be discontinued.

Elderly: See Dose Adjustments and Precautions. ▪ May be more sensitive to the hypotensive effects. ▪ Consider age-related renal impairment.

DRUG/LAB INTERACTIONS

Potentiated by most **other hypotensive agents**, including **ganglionic blocking agents**, **inhaled anesthesics**, and **negative inotropic agents**.

SIDE EFFECTS

Usually occur with too-rapid rate of infusion and are reversible. The most common adverse reactions are hypotension and cyanide toxicity. Less common adverse reactions include abdominal pain, apprehension, bradycardia, decreased platelet aggregation, diaphoresis, dizziness, ECG changes, flushing, headache, hypotension (profound), hypothyroidism, ileus, increased intracranial pressure, irritation at the infusion site, muscle twitching, nausea, palpitations, rash, restlessness, retching, retrosternal discomfort, tachycardia, venous streaking. Excessive hypotension, cyanide intoxication (air hunger, bright red venous blood, confusion, elevated cyanide levels, marked clinical deterioration, lactic acidosis, and death), or thiocyanate toxicity can occur with prolonged therapy or overdose. Methemoglobinemia (chocolate-brown blood, impaired oxygen delivery even though cardiac output and arterial Po_2 are adequate) can also occur.

ANTIDOTE

At first sign of side effects, decrease rate of administration. If BP begins to rise or side effects persist, notify the physician. For hypotension, slow or discontinue administration and put the patient in Trendelenburg position. Should improve in 1 to 10 minutes. If cyanide toxicity develops, discontinue nitroprusside and consider specific treatment for cyanide toxicity. For overdose with signs of cyanide toxicity or tachyphylaxis, discontinue nitroprusside sodium. Administer 3% sodium nitrite intravenously at a dose of 4 to 6 mg/kg over 2 to 4 minutes. Sodium nitrite provides a buffer for cyanide by converting hemoglobin into methemoglobin. Monitor BP carefully; may cause hypotension that will also require treatment. Next, inject sodium thiosulfate 150 to 200 mg/kg (usually about 12.5 Gm or 50 mL of the 25% solution) in 50 mL of D5W intravenously over 10 minutes. Sodium thiosulfate converts cyanide into thiocyanate, which is then excreted in urine. Observe patient. If signs of overdose reappear, may repeat the previously described process after 2 hours using one-half the original dosage. Treat methemoglobinemia with methylene blue 1 to 2 mg/kg. Hemodialysis is ineffective in the removal of cyanide but will eliminate thiocyanate in cases of severe toxicity.

NIVOLUMAB

(nye-**VOL**-ue-mab)

Opdivo

Antineoplastic
(Monoclonal antibody, anti-PD-1 monoclonal antibody)

pH 6

USUAL DOSE

Pretreatment: Verify pregnancy status. Baseline studies indicated; see Monitor. Pretesting may be indicated based on diagnosis; see Indications and Uses.

Melanoma (single agent): 240 mg every 2 weeks or 480 mg every 4 weeks. Administered as an IV infusion over 30 minutes until disease progression or unacceptable toxicity.

Gastric cancer: 240 mg IV every 2 weeks or 360 mg IV every 3 weeks (in combination with other chemotherapy).

Esphageal cancer: 240 mg IV every 2 weeks or 360 mg IV every 3 weeks or 480 mg IV every 4 weeks, depending on stage.

Head and neck, squamous cell cancer: 240 mg IV every 2 weeks or 480 mg IV every 4 weeks.

Hodgkin lymphoma: 240 mg IV every 2 weeks or 480 mg IV every 4 weeks.

Urothelial carcinoma: 240 mg IV every 2 weeks or 480 mg IV every 4 weeks.

Melanoma in combination with ipilimumab: *Nivolumab:* 1 mg/kg as an IV infusion over 30 minutes, followed by *ipilimumab* 3 mg/kg as an IV infusion over 90 minutes on the same day every 3 weeks for a maximum of 4 doses or until unacceptable toxicity, which-ever occurs earlier. The recommended subsequent dose of nivolumab as a single agent is 240 mg every 2 weeks or 480 mg every 4 weeks. Administered as an IV infusion over 30 minutes until disease progression or unacceptable toxicity. Review impilimumab monograph before initiating therapy.

Adjuvant treatment of melanoma: 240 mg every 2 weeks or 480 mg every 4 weeks. Admin-istered as an IV infusion over 30 minutes until disease recurrence or unacceptable toxic-ity for up to 1 year.

Non–small-cell lung cancer (NSCLC), classical Hodgkin lymphoma (cHL), squamous cell carci-noma of the head and neck (SCCHN), urothelial carcinoma, and hepatocellular carcinoma (HCC): 240 mg every 2 weeks or 480 mg every 4 weeks. Administered as an IV infusion over 30 minutes until disease progression or unacceptable toxicity.

Small-cell lung cancer (SCLC): 240 mg administered as an IV infusion over 30 minutes every 2 weeks until disease progression or unacceptable toxicity.

Renal cell carcinoma (RCC) (single agent): 240 mg every 2 weeks or 480 mg every 4 weeks. Administered as an IV infusion over 30 minutes until disease progression or unaccept-able toxicity.

Renal cell carcinoma (RCC) in combination with ipilimumab: *Nivolumab:* 3 mg/kg as an IV infusion over 30 minutes, followed by *ipilimumab* 1 mg/kg as an IV infusion over 30 min-utes on the same day every 3 weeks for 4 doses. The recommended subsequent dose of nivolumab as a single agent is 240 mg every 2 weeks or 480 mg every 4 weeks. Admin-istered as an IV infusion over 30 minutes until disease progression or unacceptable toxic-ity. Review impilimumab monograph before initiating therapy.

Microsatellite instability–high (MSI-H) or mismatch repair deficient (dMMR) metastatic colorectal cancer (CRC) (single agent): *Adult and pediatric patients 12 years of age and older and weighing 40 kg or more:* 240 mg administered as an IV infusion over 30 minutes every 2 weeks or 480 mg administered as an IV infusion over 30 minutes every 4 weeks, until disease progression or unacceptable toxicity. *Pediatric patients 12 years of age and older and weigh-ing less than 40 kg:* 3 mg/kg administered as an IV infusion over 30 minutes every 2 weeks until disease progression or unacceptable toxicity.

Microsatellite instability–high (MSI-H) or mismatch repair deficient (dMMR) metastatic colorectal cancer (CRC) in combination with ipilimumab: *Nivolumab:* 3 mg/kg as an IV infusion over 30 minutes, followed by *ipilimumab* 1 mg/kg as an IV infusion over 30 minutes on the same day every 3 weeks for 4 doses.

After completing 4 doses of combination therapy, administer nivolumab as single agent until disease progression or unacceptable toxicity. *Adult and pediatric patients 12 years of age and older weighing 40 kg or more:* 240 mg as an IV infusion over 30 minutes every 2 weeks or 480 mg as an IV infusion over 30 minutes every 4 weeks. *Pediatric patients 12 years of age and older weighing less than 40 kg:* 3 mg/kg administered as an IV infusion over 30 minutes every 2 weeks. Review impilimumab monograph before initiating therapy.

PEDIATRIC DOSE

Microsatellite instability–high (MSI-H) or mismatch repair deficient (dMMR) metastatic colorectal cancer (mCRC) in pediatric patients 12 years of age and older (single agent or in combination with ipilimumab): see Usual Dose.

DOSE ADJUSTMENTS

Recommendations for nivolumab dose modifications are provided in the following chart. When nivolumab is administered in combination with ipilimumab, ipilimumab should be withheld if nivolumab is withheld. Review ipilimumab monograph for recommended dose modifications. ■ Initiate corticosteroid therapy for immune-mediated reactions and/or hormone replacement as outlined in Monitor.

Recommended Dose Modifications for Nivolumab		
Adverse Reaction	**Severity[a]**	**Dose Modification**
Colitis	Grade 2 diarrhea or colitis	Withhold dose[b]
	Grade 3 diarrhea or colitis	Withhold dose[b] when administered as a single agent
		Permanently discontinue when administered with ipilimumab
	Grade 4 diarrhea or colitis	Permanently discontinue
Pneumonitis	Grade 2 pneumonitis	Withhold dose[b]
	Grade 3 or 4 pneumonitis	Permanently discontinue
Hepatitis/non-HCC	AST or ALT more than 3 and up to 5 × ULN or total bilirubin more than 1.5 and up to 3 × ULN	Withhold dose[b]
	AST or ALT more than 5 × ULN or total bilirubin more than 3 × ULN	Permanently discontinue
Hepatitis/HCC	AST/ALT within normal limits at baseline and increases to more than 3 and up to 5 × ULN AST/ALT more than 1 and up to 3 × ULN at baseline and increases to more than 5 and up to 10 × ULN AST/ALT more than 3 and up to 5 × ULN at baseline and increases to more than 8 and up to 10 × ULN	Withhold dose[c]
	AST or ALT increases to more than 10 × ULN or total bilirubin increases to more than 3 × ULN	Permanently discontinue
Hypophysitis	Grade 2 or 3 hypophysitis	Withhold dose[b]
	Grade 4 hypophysitis	Permanently discontinue
Adrenal insufficiency	Grade 2 adrenal insufficiency	Withhold dose[b]
	Grade 3 or 4 adrenal insufficiency	Permanently discontinue
Type 1 diabetes mellitus	Grade 3 hyperglycemia	Withhold dose[b]
	Grade 4 hyperglycemia	Permanently discontinue
Nephritis and renal dysfunction	SCr more than 1.5 and up to 6 × ULN	Withhold dose[b]
	SCr more than 6 × ULN	Permanently discontinue
Skin	Grade 3 rash or suspected Stevens-Johnson syndrome (SJS) or toxic epidermal necrolysis (TEN)	Withhold dose[b]
	Grade 4 rash or confirmed SJS or TEN	Permanently discontinue
Encephalitis	New-onset moderate or severe neurologic S/S	Withhold dose[b]
	Immune-mediated encephalitis	Permanently discontinue

Continued

Recommended Dose Modifications for Nivolumab—cont'd		
Adverse Reaction	Severity[a]	Dose Modification

Other	Other Grade 3 adverse reaction
	  First occurrence
	  Recurrence of the same Grade 3 adverse
	    reaction
		Withhold dose[b]
		Permanently discontinue

	Life-threatening or Grade 4 adverse reaction	Permanently discontinue
	Grade 3 myocarditis	Permanently discontinue
	Requirement of 10 mg/day or greater prednisone or equivalent for more than 12 weeks	Permanently discontinue
	Persistent Grade 2 or 3 adverse reactions lasting 12 weeks or longer	Permanently discontinue

[a]Toxicity graded per National Cancer Institute Common Terminology Criteria for Adverse Events, v4.0 (NCI CTCAE v4).
[b]Resume treatment when adverse reactions return to Grade 0 or 1.
[c]Resume treatment when AST/ALT returns to baseline.
[d]*HCC*, Hepatocellular carcinoma.

■ No recommended dose modifications for hypothyroidism or hyperthyroidism. ■ The pharmacokinetics of nivolumab do not appear to be affected by age, weight, sex, race, baseline LDH, PD-L1 expression, solid tumor type, tumor size, renal impairment (eGFR greater than or equal to 15 mL/min/1.73 M^2), mild hepatic impairment (total bilirubin [TB] less than or equal to the ULN and AST greater than ULN or TB greater than 1 to 1.5 times ULN and any AST), or moderate hepatic impairment (TB greater than 1.5 to 3 times ULN and any AST). Nivolumab has not been studied in patients with severe hepatic impairment (total bilirubin greater than 3 times the ULN and any AST). ■ See Monitor and Antidote.

DILUTION
Available as a solution in single-use vials containing 40 mg/4 mL, 100 mg/10 mL, or 240 mg/24 mL (10 mg/mL). Discard the vial if the solution is cloudy or discolored or contains extraneous particulate matter other than a few translucent-to-white, protein-aceous particles. Calculate the number of vials required for the recommended dose, and withdraw the required volume of nivolumab and transfer into an IV bag or container of NS or D5W to prepare an infusion with a final concentration ranging from 1 to 10 mg/mL. For adult and pediatric patients with body weight equal to or greater than 40 kg, do not exceed a total volume of infusion of 160 mL. For adult and pediatric patients with body weight less than 40 kg, the total volume of infusion must not exceed 4 mL/kg of body weight. Mix diluted solution by gentle inversion. ***Do not shake.***
Filters: Must be administered using IV tubing that contains a sterile, nonpyrogenic, low–protein-binding, in-line filter (pore size of 0.2 to 1.2 micrometers).
Storage: Before use, refrigerate at 2° to 8° C (36° to 46° F) in original package to protect from light. Do not freeze or shake. Nivolumab does not contain a preservative. After preparation, store the prepared infusion at room temperature for no more than 8 hours or refrigerate for no more than 24 hours from the time of preparation. Administration time is included in storage time. Do not freeze. Discard partially used vials.

COMPATIBILITY
Manufacturer states, "Do not coadminister other drugs through the same intravenous line."

RATE OF ADMINISTRATION
A single dose as an infusion equally distributed over 30 minutes. Interrupt or slow rate of administration in patients with mild or moderate infusion reactions. If a common IV line is used to administer other drugs in addition to nivolumab, flush the IV line before and after each nivolumab infusion with NS or D5W. Administer through an IV tubing that contains a

sterile, nonpyrogenic, low–protein-binding, in-line filter (pore size of 0.2 to 1.2 micrometers). When administered in combination with ipilimumab, infuse nivolumab first, followed by ipilimumab on the same day. Use separate infusion bags and filters for each infusion.

ACTIONS

An antineoplastic agent. Nivolumab is a programmed death receptor-1 (PD-1) blocking antibody; a human immunoglobulin G4 (IgG4) monoclonal antibody that binds to the PD-1 receptor and blocks its interaction with PD-L1 and PD-L2, thereby releasing PD-1 pathway–mediated inhibition of the immune response, including the antitumor immune response. In syngeneic mouse tumor models, blocking PD-1 activity resulted in decreased tumor growth. Combining nivolumab with ipilimumab results in enhanced T-cell function that is greater than the effects of either antibody alone and results in improved antitumor responses in metastatic melanoma and advanced RCC. Mean elimination half-life is 25 days. Steady-state concentrations were reached by 12 weeks when administered at 3 mg/kg every 2 weeks.

INDICATIONS AND USES

As a single agent or in combination with ipilimumab (Yervoy) for the treatment of patients with unresectable or metastatic melanoma. ▪ Adjuvant treatment of patients with melanoma with involvement of lymph nodes or metastatic disease who have undergone complete resection. ▪ Treatment of patients with metastatic NSCLC with progression on or after platinum-based chemotherapy. Before receiving nivolumab, patients with EGFR or ALK genomic tumor aberrations should have experienced disease progression while undergoing FDA-approved therapy for these aberrations. ▪ Treatment of patients with metastatic SCLC with progression after platinum-based chemotherapy and at least one other line of therapy; see Limitation of Use. ▪ As a single agent for the treatment of patients with advanced RCC who have received prior antiangiogenic therapy. ▪ In combination with ipilimumab (Yervoy) for the treatment of patients with intermediate or poor risk, previously untreated advanced RCC. ▪ Treatment of patients with classical Hodgkin lymphoma (cHL) that has relapsed or progressed after autologous hematopoietic stem cell transplantation (HSCT) and brentuximab vedotin (Adcetris) or 3 or more lines of systemic therapy that includes autologous HSCT; see Limitation of Use. ▪ Treatment of patients with recurrent or metastatic SCCHN with disease progression on or after platinum-based therapy. ▪ Treatment of patients with locally advanced or metastatic urothelial carcinoma who have disease progression during or after platinum-containing chemotherapy or who have disease progression within 12 months of neoadjuvant or adjuvant treatment with platinum-containing chemotherapy; see Limitation of Use. ▪ As a single agent or in combination with ipilimumab (Yervoy) for the treatment of adult and pediatric patients 12 years of age and older with microsatellite instability–high (MSI-H) or mismatch repair deficient (dMMR) metastatic CRC that has progressed after treatment with fluoropyrimidine, oxaliplatin, and irinotecan; see Limitation of Use. ▪ Treatment of patients with hepatocellular carcinoma (HCC) who have been previously treated with sorafenib; see Limitation of Use.

Limitation of use: Specified indications have received accelerated approval. This accelerated approval is based on progression-free survival, tumor response rate, duration of response, or overall response rate. Continued approval may be contingent on verification and description of clinical benefit in the confirmatory trials.

CONTRAINDICATIONS

Manufacturer states, "None."

PRECAUTIONS

Severe immune-mediated pneumonitis, including fatal cases, has occurred with nivolumab treatment. ▪ Severe immune-mediated colitis (including cytomegalovirus [CMV] infection/reactivation) has been reported. ▪ Immune-mediated hepatitis and liver test abnormalities (elevated ALT, AST, alkaline phosphatase, total bilirubin) have occurred with nivolumab treatment. ▪ Immune-mediated nephritis has occurred with nivolumab treatment. ▪ Pneumonitis, colitis, hepatitis, and nephritis (renal dysfunction or Grade 2 or higher increased SCr) were defined as immune-mediated when corticosteroids were required for treatment and there was no clear alternate etiology. ▪ Immune-mediated endocrinopathies, including hypophysitis, adrenal insufficiency, type 1 diabetes mellitus (with possible diabetic ketoacidosis), hypothyroidism, and hyperthyroidism, have been reported. ▪ Immune-mediated skin adverse reactions can occur. Rare cases of Stevens-Johnson syndrome (SJS) and toxic epidermal necrolysis (TEN) have been reported. ▪ Immune-mediated encephalitis with no clear alternate etiology can occur with nivolumab treatment. ▪ Numerous other immune-mediated adverse reactions, some with fatal outcome, were reported in fewer than 1% of patients. ▪ Severe infusion reactions have been reported. ▪ Complications (e.g., acute, chronic or hyperacute graft-versus-host disease [GVHD], steroid-requiring febrile syndrome, hepatic veno-occlusive disease [VOD]), including fatal events, occurred in patients who received allogeneic HSCT despite intervening therapy with a PD-1 receptor–blocking antibody. ▪ Increased mortality occurred in patients with multiple myeloma when nivolumab is added to a thalidomide analog and dexamethasone. ▪ See Dose Adjustments, Monitor, and Antidote for required Dose Adjustments, indicated criteria and medications for treatment, and criteria for withholding or discontinuation of nivolumab. ▪ Nivolumab has not been studied in patients with severe hepatic impairment. ▪ A protein substance; has a potential for immunogenicity.

Monitor: Obtain serum electrolytes and glucose, baseline liver function tests (e.g., ALT, AST, alkaline phosphatase, total bilirubin), serum creatinine, and thyroid function tests before initiating treatment, and monitor periodically during treatment and as indicated based on clinical evaluation. ▪ Monitor for infusion reactions; see Dose Adjustments and Rate of Administration. Infusion reactions have occurred up to 48 hours after the infusion and may lead to dose delay, withholding of nivolumab, or permanent discontinuation. ▪ Monitor patients for S/S of pneumonitis (e.g., abnormal chest x-ray, chest pain, new or worsening cough, or shortness of breath). Administer corticosteroids at a dose of 1 to 2 mg/kg/day prednisone equivalents for moderate (Grade 2) or more severe (Grade 3 or 4) pneumonitis, followed by corticosteroid taper. Withhold nivolumab until resolution for moderate (Grade 2) pneumonitis; see Dose Adjustments. ▪ Monitor patients for colitis. Administer corticosteroids at a dose of 0.5 to 1 mg/kg/day prednisone equivalents followed by corticosteroid taper for moderate (Grade 2) colitis of more than 5 days' duration; if worsening or no improvement occurs despite initiation of corticosteroids, increase dose to 1 to 2 mg/kg/day prednisone equivalents. Administer corticosteroids at a dose of 1 to 2 mg/kg/day prednisone equivalents followed by corticosteroid taper for severe (Grade 3) or life-threatening (Grade 4) colitis. Withhold nivolumab for moderate (Grade 2) or severe (Grade 3) colitis when used as a single agent or for moderate (Grade 2) colitis when used in combination with ipilimumab; see Dose Adjustments. ▪ In cases of corticosteroid-refractory colitis, consider repeating infectious workup to exclude alternative etiologies. Addition of an alternative immunosuppressive agent to the corticosteroid therapy, or replacement of the corticosteroid therapy, should be considered if other causes are excluded. ▪ Monitor for S/S of hepatitis (e.g., easy bruising or bleeding, jaundice, lethargy, pain on the right side of the abdomen, severe nausea or vomiting, abnormal LFTs). Administer corticosteroids at a dose of 0.5 to 1 mg/kg/day prednisone equivalents for moderate (Grade 2) transaminase elevations. Administer corticosteroids at a dose of 1 to 2 mg/kg/day prednisone equivalents followed by corticosteroid taper for severe (Grade 3) or life-threatening (Grade 4) transaminase elevations, with or without concomitant elevations in total bilirubin. For patients without HCC, withhold nivolumab for moderate (Grade 2) immune-mediated hepatitis and permanently discontinue for severe (Grade 3) or life-threatening (Grade 4) immune-mediated hepatitis. For patients with HCC, permanently discontinue, withhold, or continue nivolumab based on severity of immune-mediated hepatitis and baseline AST and ALT levels as outlined in Dose Adjustments. In addition, administer corticosteroids at a dose of 1 to 2 mg/kg/day prednisone equivalents followed by corticosteroid taper when nivolumab is withheld or discontinued due to immune-mediated hepatitis; see Dose Adjustments. ▪ Monitor renal function periodically. For moderate (Grade 2) or severe (Grade 3) SCr elevation, withhold nivolumab and administer corticosteroids at a dose of 0.5 to 1 mg/kg/day prednisone equivalents followed by corticosteroid taper; if worsening or no improvement occurs, increase dose of corticosteroids to 1 to 2 mg/kg/day prednisone equivalents. Administer corticosteroids at a dose of 1 to 2 mg/kg/day prednisone equivalents followed by corticosteroid taper for life-threatening (Grade 4) SCr elevation, and permanently discontinue nivolumab; see Dose Adjustments. ▪ Monitor for S/S of hypophysitis (e.g., fatigue, headache, low levels of the hormones produced by the pituitary [adrenocorticotropic hormone (ACTH), thyroid-stimulating hormone (TSH), follicle-stimulating hormone (FSH), luteinizing hormone (LH), growth hormone (GH), prolactin]). Administer hormone replacement as clinically indicated and corticosteroids at a dose of 1 mg/kg/day prednisone equivalents for moderate (Grade 2) or higher hypophysitis. Withhold nivolumab for moderate (Grade 2) or severe (Grade 3) hypophysitis; see Dose Adjustments. ▪ Monitor for S/S of adrenal insufficiency (e.g., fatigue, nausea, vomiting, hypotension, hyponatremia, hyperkalemia, low cortisol concentrations). Administer corticosteroids at a dose of 1 to 2 mg/kg/day prednisone equivalents followed by corticosteroid taper for severe (Grade 3) or life-threatening (Grade 4) adrenal insufficiency. Hormone replacement therapy was required in more than half of patients who developed adrenal insufficiency. Withhold nivolumab for moderate (Grade 2) adrenal insufficiency; see Dose Adjustments. ▪ Monitor for changes in thyroid function. Administer hormone replacement therapy for hypothyroidism. Initiate medical management for control of hyperthyroidism (e.g., methimazole, propylthiouracil). Administration of corticosteroids was required in some patients; see Dose Adjustments. ▪ Monitor for hyperglycemia. Administer insulin when clinically indicated. Withhold nivolumab for severe (Grade 3) hyperglycemia until metabolic control is achieved; see Dose Adjustments. ▪ Monitor for development of a rash. Administer corticosteroids at a dose of 1 to 2 mg/kg/day prednisone equivalents followed by corticosteroid taper for severe (Grade 3) or life-threatening (Grade 4) rash. Withhold nivolumab for suspected SJS or TEN or severe (Grade 3) rash; see Dose Adjustments. ▪ Monitor for changes in neurologic status. Withhold nivolumab in patients with new-onset moderate to severe neurologic signs or symptoms. Evaluate patient to rule out infectious or other causes of moderate to severe neurologic deterioration. Evaluation may include, but is not limited to, consultation with a neurologist, brain MRI, and lumbar puncture. If other etiologies are ruled out, administer corticosteroids at a dose of 1 to 2 mg/kg/day prednisone equivalents, followed by a prednisone taper; see Dose Adjustments. ▪ Monitor patient for any other clinically significant immune-mediated adverse reactions. Immune-mediated adverse reactions may occur after nivolumab is discontinued. Examples of other immune-mediated adverse reactions that have occurred include aplastic anemia, autoimmune neuropathy, demyelination, duodenitis, facial and abducens nerve paresis, gastritis, Guillain-Barré syndrome, histiocytic necrotizing lymphadenitis, hypopituitarism, iritis, motor dysfunction, myasthenic syndrome, myocarditis, myositis, pancreatitis, pericarditis, polymyalgia rheumatica, rhabdomyolysis, sarcoidosis, systemic inflammatory response syndrome, uveitis, and vasculitis. If uveitis occurs in combination with other immune-mediated adverse reactions, consider a Vogt-Koyanagi-Harada–like syndrome, which may require treatment with systemic steroids to reduce the risk of permanent vison loss. For any suspected immune-mediated adverse reactions, exclude other causes. Based on the severity of the adverse reaction, withhold or discontinue nivolumab, administer high-dose corticosteroids and, if appropriate, initiate hormone-replacement therapy. Upon improvement to Grade 1 or less, initiate corticosteroid taper and continue to taper over at least 1 month. Consider restarting nivolumab after completion of corticosteroid taper based on the severity of the event. ▪ Monitor for early evidence of HSCT-related complications such as hyperacute GVHD, severe acute GVHD, steroid-requiring febrile syndrome, hepatic VOD, and other immune-mediated adverse reactions, and intervene promptly.

Patient Education: Review manufacturer's medication guide. ▪ Effective contraception required during treatment with nivolumab and for at least 5 months following the last dose of nivolumab. ▪ Promptly report a known or suspected pregnancy. ▪ Some side effects may require corticosteroid treatment and interruption or discontinuation of nivolumab. ▪ Promptly report any S/S of an infusion-related reaction. ▪ Promptly report S/S of pneumonitis (e.g., chest pain, new or worsening cough, or shortness of breath). ▪ Promptly report S/S of colitis (e.g., diarrhea or severe abdominal pain). ▪ Promptly report S/S of hepatitis (e.g., easy bruising or bleeding, jaundice, lethargy, pain on the right side of the abdomen, severe nausea or vomiting). ▪ Promptly report S/S of kidney dysfunction (e.g., blood in urine, decreased urine output, loss of appetite, swelling in ankles). ▪ Promptly report S/S of hypophysitis, adrenal insufficiency, hypothyroidism, hyperthyroidism, or diabetes mellitus; see Monitor. ▪ Promptly report S/S of encephalitis; see Monitor. ▪ Promptly report development of a rash. ▪ Keeping scheduled appointments for blood work or other laboratory tests is imperative.

Maternal/Child: Avoid pregnancy. Based on mechanism of action and data from animal studies, nivolumab can cause fetal harm when administered to a pregnant female. Human IgG4 is known to cross the placental barrier, and nivolumab is an IgG4. Effects of nivolumab are likely to be greater during the second and third trimesters of pregnancy. ▪ Do not breast-feed during treatment and for 5 months after the last dose. ▪ Safety and effectiveness as a single agent and in combination with ipilimumab have been established in pediatric patients 12 years of age and older with MSI-H or dMMR mCRC that has progressed after treatment with fluoropyrimidine, oxaliplatin, and irinotecan. Safety and effectiveness have not been established in pediatric patients under 12 years of age with MSI-H or dMMR mCRC or in pediatric patients of any age for other approved indications.

Elderly: No overall differences in safety or efficacy were reported between elderly patients and younger patients.

DRUG/LAB INTERACTIONS
No formal pharmacokinetic drug-drug interaction studies conducted with nivolumab.

SIDE EFFECTS
Several immune-mediated reactions have been reported, including colitis, encephalitis, endocrinopathies, hepatitis, nephritis and renal dysfunction, pneumonitis, and adverse skin reactions/rash; see Precautions, Monitor, and Antidote.

Single agent: The most common adverse reactions were abdominal pain, arthralgia, asthenia, back pain, constipation, cough, decreased appetite, diarrhea, dyspnea, fatigue, fever, headache, musculoskeletal pain, nausea, pruritus, rash, upper respiratory infection, and vomiting. Other reported side effects included arrhythmia (ventricular), dizziness, dry skin, edema, erythema multiforme, exfoliative dermatitis, general physical health deterioration, infusion-related reactions, insomnia, iridocyclitis, myositis (including polymyositis), peripheral and sensory neuropathy, peripheral edema, pneumonia, psoriasis, sepsis, small intestine obstruction, urinary tract infection, vitiligo, and weight loss. Laboratory abnormalities included anemia; hypercalcemia, hyperglycemia; hyperkalemia; hypocalcemia; hypomagnesemia; hyponatremia; increased alkaline phosphate, ALT, amylase, AST, bilirubin, cholesterol, creatinine, lipase, and triglycerides; leukopenia; lymphopenia; neutropenia; thrombocytopenia. Other side effects may occur based on diagnosis.

Combination therapy: The most common adverse reactions were abdominal pain, arthralgia, cough, decreased appetite, diarrhea, dyspnea, fatigue, fever, musculoskeletal pain, nausea, pruritis, rash, upper respiratory tract infection, and vomiting. Other reported side effects included constipation, dizziness, dry skin, edema, headache, insomnia, myositis (including polymyositis), and weight loss. Laboratory abnormalities included anemia; hyperglycemia; hyperkalemia; hypocalcemia; hypomagnesemia; hyponatremia; increased alkaline phosphate, ALT, amylase, AST, creatinine, and lipase; and lymphopenia.

Post-Marketing: Treatment refractory, severe acute and chronic GVHD, Vogt-Koyanagi-Harada (VKH) syndrome.

ANTIDOTE
Keep physician informed of all side effects. May constitute a medical emergency or will be treated symptomatically as indicated. Treat side effects aggressively; see Monitor. Follow guidelines for withholding or discontinuing therapy as outlined in Dose Adjustments. Interrupt or slow the rate of administration in patients with mild or moderate infusion reactions. Discontinue in patients with a severe or life-threatening infusion reaction and treat as

indicated. Initiate corticosteroid therapy as outlined in Monitor for immune-mediated reactions (e.g., pneumonitis, colitis, hepatitis/HCC, renal dysfunction, hypophysitis, adrenal insufficiency, hyperthyroidism or hypothyroidism, rash, neurologic status, and other clinically significant immune-mediated adverse reactions). Hormone replacement may also be indicated; see Monitor. In clinical studies, infliximab was added to high-dose corticosteroid therapy for treatment of colitis, encephalitis, and pneumonitis in select patients. Mycophenolic acid was added for select patients with hepatitis. Resuscitate if indicated.

NIVOLUMAB AND RELATLIMAB

(nye-**VOL**-ue-mab and rel-**AT**-li-mab)

Opdualag

Antineoplastic agent; anti-LAG-3 monoclonal antibody: anti-PD-1 monoclonal antibody; immune checkpoint inhibitor

Check label to ensure that the appropriate product is being administered; "nivolumab and relatlimab" and "nivolumab" are different products and not interchangeable.

USUAL DOSE

Nivolumab 480 mg and relatlimab 160 mg IV once every 4 weeks until disease progression or unacceptable toxicity

PEDIATRIC DOSE

Children greater than or equal to 12 years and adolescents weighing at least 40 kg: nivolumab 480 mg and relatlimab 160 mg IV once every 4 weeks until disease progression or unacceptable toxicity

DOSE ADJUSTMENTS

Renal: No dosage adjustments are provided by the manufacturer, unless the patient develops nephritis with kidney dysfunction during treatment; refer to package insert for details.

Hepatic: No dosage adjustments are provided by the manufacturer, unless the patient develops hepatotoxicity during treatment; refer to package insert for details.

Adverse reactions during treatment: Refer to package insert for details.

DILUTION

Nivolumab and relatlimab may be administered diluted or undiluted. Withdraw the required volume of nivolumab and relatlimab and transfer to an empty IV container made of DEHP-plasticized PVC, ethyl vinyl acetate, or polyolefin. If diluting prior to administration, dilute with NS or D5W and gently invert to mix (do not shake). The concentration for administration should range from 3 to 12 mg/mL (nivolumab component) and from 1 to 4 mg/mL (relatlimab component); the maximum infusion volume should be 160 mL (if weight $\geq$ 40 kg) or 4 mL/kg (if weight $<$ 40 kg). Solution should be clear to opalescent, colorless to slightly yellow; discard vial if cloudy or discolored or contains extraneous particulate matter (other than a few translucent-to-white particles).

COMPATIBILITY

Do not administer simultaneously with any other medication or IV solutions.

RATE OF ADMINISTRATION

Infuse over 30 minutes via an IV containing a sterile, nonpyrogenic, low-protein-binding polyethersulfone nylon or polyvinylidene fluoride 0.2- to 1.2-micrometer in-line filter. Flush IV line at the end of the infusion. Do not administer other medications through the same IV line. Monitor for S/S of infusion-related reactions.

ACTIONS

Relatlimab is a human IgG4 monoclonal antibody that binds to the LAG-3 receptor and blocks interaction between LAG-3 and its ligands to reduce LAG-3 pathway-mediated immune response inhibition; antagonism of this pathway promotes T-cell proliferation and cytokine secretion. Nivolumab is a human IgG monoclonal antibody that binds to the PD-1 receptor and blocks interaction with its ligands PD-L1 and PD-L2 and reduces PD-1 pathway-mediated inhibition of the immune response, including the anti-tumor immune response. Binding of the PD-1 ligands PD-L1 and PD-L2 to the PD-1 receptor found on T-cells inhibits T-cell proliferation and cytokine production. Upregulation of PD-1 ligands occurs in some tumors: therefore signaling through this pathway can contribute to inhibition of active T-cell immune surveillance of tumors. Combining nivolumab (anti-PD1) and relatlimab (anti-LAG-3) results in increased T-cell activation compared to the activity of either antibody alone.

INDICATIONS AND USES
Treatment of unresectable or metastatic melanoma in adult and pediatric patients $\geq$ 12 years of age.

CONTRAINDICATIONS
No contraindications listed in the manufacturer's labeling.

PRECAUTIONS
Hypersensitivity: Immediately discontinue infusion with any signs of allergic reaction and institute appropriate care.

Hypernatremia and hypokalemia: Monitor serum sodium and potassium at baseline and as clinically indicated. Withhold infusion if serum sodium is greater than 145 mmol/L.

Nausea and vomiting: Administer antiemetics prior to each infusion.

Monitor: Monitor hepatic ALT, AST, and total bilirubin at baseline and periodically during treatment and renal function and thyroid function at baseline and periodically during treatment. Monitor for hyperglycemia. Verify pregnancy status prior to treatment. Monitor closely for S/S of immune-mediated adverse reactions, including adrenal insufficiency, hypophysitis, thyroid disorders, diabetes, diarrhea/colitis (consider initiating or repeating infectious workup in patients with corticosteroid-refractory immune-mediated colitis to exclude alternative causes), myocarditis, pneumonitis, rash/dermatologic toxicity, neurotoxicity, and ocular disorders. If suspected immune-mediated reactions occur, initiate appropriate workup to exclude alternative causes (including infection). If patient has received or is receiving a hematopoietic stem cell transplant, monitor closely for early S/S of transplant-related complications. Monitor for S/S of infusion-related reactions. Screen for hepatitis B.

Patient Education: Notify provider immediately if the patient shows signs of: ■ *High blood sugar*, such as confusion, feeling sleepy, greater thirst, hungrier, passing urine more often, flushing, fast breathing, or breath that smells like fruit. ■ *Infection*, such as fever, chills, or sore throat. ■ *Liver problems*, such as dark urine, feeling tired, not hungry, upset stomach, light-colored stools, throwing up, or yellow skin or eyes. ■ *Kidney problems*, such as not being able to pass urine, change in how much urine is passed, bloody brown or foamy urine, shortness of breath or cough, or puffy or swollen face, feet, or hands. ■ *Eye problems*, such as changes in eyesight, eye pain or irritation. ■ *Thyroid, pituitary, or adrenal gland problems*, such as change in mood or behavior, change in weight or taste, constipation, deeper voice, dizziness, fainting, feeling cold, feeling tired, hair loss, sever headache, change in desire for sex, eye problems, fast heartbeat, more sweating, fast or deep breathing, sweet-smelling breath, change in smell of urine or sweat, or passing urine more often. ■ *Severe skin reactions*, such as red, swollen, blistered, or peeling skin (with or without fever); red or irritated eyes; or sores in mouth throat, nose, or eyes. ■ *Pancreas problems*, such as stomach pain, very bad back pain, or throwing up. ■ *Lung or breathing problems*, such as shortness of breath or other trouble breathing, cough, or fever. ■ *Heart problems*, such as chest pain; fast, slow, abnormal heartbeat; or shortness of breath. ■ *Nervous system problems*, such as change in balance, change in mood or behavior, feeling confused or sleepy, fever, memory problems, severe muscle weakness, numbness or tingling in arms or legs, seizures, stiff neck, or being bothered by bright lights. ■ *Bowel problems*, such as black, tarry, or bloody stools; fever; mucus in stools; throwing up blood or vomit that looks like coffee grounds; severe stomach pain; or constipation or diarrhea. ■ *Low sodium levels*, as indicated by headache; trouble focusing; memory problems; feeling confused; weakness; seizures or change in balance; any unexplained bruising or bleeding; swelling in arms or legs; muscle cramps. ■ *Signs of an allergic reaction*, such as hives; itching; red, swollen, blistered or peeling skin with or without fever; wheezing; tightness of chest; trouble with breathing, swallowing, or talking; unusual hoarseness; or swelling of mouth, face, lips, tongue, or throat.

Maternal/child: Verify pregnancy status prior to treatment initiation. Patients who could become pregnant should use effective contraceptive measures during treatment and for at least 5 months after last dose. Based on animal data, in utero exposure may cause fetal harm. It is not known whether the drug is present in breast milk. Due to the potential for serious adverse reaction, breastfeeding is not recommended during treatment and for at least 5 months after the last dose.

Elderly: No specific recommendations; refer to adult dosing.

DRUG/LAB INTERACTIONS

Acetaminophen, systemic steroids, proton pump inhibitors, and efgartigimod alfa may diminish the effects of nivolumab and relatlimab. Desmopressin may have enhanced hyponatremic effects. Ketoconazole may have enhanced hepatotoxicity.

SIDE EFFECTS

High blood sugar, indicated by confusion, feeling sleepy, greater thirst, hungrier, passing urine more often, flushing, or fast breathing or breath that smells like fruit. ■ *Infection*, indicated by fever, chills, or sore throat. ■ *Liver problems*, indicated by dark urine, feeling tired, not hungry, upset stomach, light-colored stools, throwing up, or yellow skin or eyes. ■ *Kidney problems*, indicated by not being able to pass urine; change in how much urine is passed, bloody brown or foamy urine, shortness of breath or cough, or puffy or swollen face, feet, or hands. ■ *Eye problems*, indicated by changes in eyesight, eye pain, or eye irritation. ■ *Thyroid, pituitary, or adrenal gland problems*, indicated by change in mood or behavior, change in weight or taste, constipation, deeper voice, dizziness, fainting, feeling cold, feeling tired, hair loss, severe headache, change in desire for sex, eye problems, fast heartbeat, more sweating, fast or deep breathing, sweet-smelling breath, change in smell of urine or sweat, or passing urine more often. ■ *Severe skin reactions*, indicated by red, swollen, blistered, or peeling skin (with or without fever); red or irritated eyes; or sores in mouth throat, nose, or eyes. ■ *Pancreas problems*, indicated by stomach pain, very bad back pain, or throwing up. ■ *Lung or breathing problems*, indicated by shortness of breath or other trouble breathing, cough, or fever. ■ *Heart problems*, indicated by chest pain; fast, slow, abnormal heartbeat; or shortness of breath. ■ *Nervous system problems*, indicated by change in balance, change in mood or behavior, feeling confused or sleepy, fever, memory problems, severe muscle weakness, numbness or tingling in arms or legs, seizures, stiff neck, or being bothered by bright lights. ■ *Bowel problems*, indicated by black, tarry, or bloody stools; fever; mucus in stools; throwing up blood or vomit looking like coffee grounds; severe stomach pain; or constipation or diarrhea. ■ *Low sodium levels*, indicated by headache, trouble focusing, memory problems, feeling confused, weakness, seizures, or change in balance; any unexplained bruising or bleeding; swelling in arms or legs; muscle cramps. ■ *Signs of an allergic reaction*, indicated by hives; itching, red, swollen, blistered, or peeling skin with or without fever; wheezing; tightness of chest; trouble breathing, swallowing, or talking; unusual hoarseness; or swelling of mouth, face, lips, tongue, or throat.

ANTIDOTE

There is no antidote; stop infusion for hypersensitivity reactions and treat appropriately.

NOREPINEPHRINE BITARTRATE `BBW`

(**nor**-ep-ih-**NEF**-rin by-**TAR**-trayt)

Levarterenol Bitartrate, Levophed

Vasopressor

pH 3 to 4.5

USUAL DOSE

Weight based: 0.05 to 0.15 mcg/kg/min titrated to desired BP range.

Non–weight based: 5 to 15 mcg/min (based on 80-kg patient) and titrated to BP range.

Larger doses may be given safely as long as the patient remains hypotensive and blood volume depletion is corrected. Up to 30 mcg/min may be required in patients with refractory shock.

PEDIATRIC DOSE
Safety and effectiveness for use in pediatric patients not established.
Begin with an initial dose of 0.05 to 0.1 mcg/kg/min as a continuous IV infusion. Titrate to desired effect up to a maximum dose of 2 mcg/kg/min.

DOSE ADJUSTMENTS
Lower-end initial doses may be indicated in the elderly based on potential for decreased organ function and concomitant disease or drug therapy.

DILUTION
Must be diluted in 250 to 1,000 mL of D5W or D5NS and given as infusion. Final concentration based on fluid volume requirements of the patient. Administration in a dextrose solution reduces loss of potency resulting from oxidation. NS without dextrose is not recommended.

Storage: Before dilution, store at CRT; protect from light.

COMPATIBILITY
Consult pharmacist; may be inactivated by solutions with a pH above 6. **Incompatible** with whole blood; administer through **Y-site** or a separate IV line. Avoid contact with iron salts, alkalis, or oxidizing agents.

Other sources suggest specific **compatibilities** dependent on concentration and manu-facturer; consult a pharmacist.

RATE OF ADMINISTRATION
See Usual Dose. Use the slowest possible flow rate to correct hypotension gradually and maintain adequate or preset BP. Some response should be noted within 1 to 2 minutes of IV administration. Use of an infusion pump or microdrip is an aid to correct evaluation of dose. Reduce infusion rate gradually. Avoid sudden discontinuation.

Norepinephrine (Levophed) Infusion Rate						
Desired Dose	4 mg in 1,000 mL D5W or D5NS 2 mg in 500 mL D5W or D5NS 4 mcg/mL			8 mg in 1,000 mL D5W or D5NS 4 mg in 500 mL D5W or D5NS 8 mcg/mL		
mcg/min	mcg/hr	mL/min	mL/hr	mcg/hr	mL/min	mL/hr
2 mcg/min	120	0.5	30	120	0.25	15
3 mcg/min	180	0.75	45	180	0.375	22.5
4 mcg/min	240	1	60	240	0.5	30
6 mcg/min	360	1.5	90	360	0.75	45
8 mcg/min	480	2	120	480	1	60
9 mcg/min	540	2.25	135	540	1.125	67.5
10 mcg/min	600	2.5	150	600	1.25	75
11 mcg/min	660	2.75	165	660	1.375	82.5
12 mcg/min	720	3	180	720	1.5	90

ACTIONS
Levarterenol is the levo-isomer of norepinephrine. It is a sympathomimetic drug that functions as a peripheral vasoconstrictor (alpha-adrenergic action) and inotropic stimula-tor of the heart and dilator of coronary arteries (beta-adrenergic action). Dilates the coro-nary arteries more than twice as much as epinephrine can. It is rapidly inactivated in the body by various enzymes and excreted in changed form in the urine.

INDICATIONS AND USES
All hypotensive states, including those associated with spinal anesthesia, blood reactions, drug reactions, hemorrhage, myocardial infarction, pheochromocytomectomy, septice-mia, surgery, sympathectomy, and trauma. ▪ Adjunct in treatment of cardiac arrest and profound hypotension.

CONTRAINDICATIONS

Do not use in hypotension from blood loss unless an emergency, in mesenteric or peripheral vascular thrombosis, or with cyclopropane or halothane (inhalant) anesthesia.

PRECAUTIONS

Whole blood or plasma should be given in a separate IV site. May be given through Y-tube connection. ▪ Use caution in the elderly and in those with peripheral vascular disease or ischemic heart disease. ▪ Use caution in previously hypertensive patients; see Monitor. ▪ Use caution in patients with allergies; some formulations contain sulfites. ▪ Therapy may be continued until the patient can maintain own BP. Decrease dosage gradually.

Monitor: Check BP every 2 minutes until stabilized at the desired level. Check every 5 minutes thereafter during therapy. Avoid hypertension. One source suggests limiting rise in BP in previously hypertensive patients to no more than 40 mm Hg below previous systolic normal. ▪ Observe for hypovolemia and replace fluids immediately. In an emergency, norepinephrine can be effective in a hypovolemic state before fluid replacement has been accomplished. ▪ Check flow rate and injection site constantly. ▪ Infusion should be through a large vein, preferably the antecubital vein, to prevent complications of prolonged peripheral vasoconstriction. Avoid veins in the hands, ankles, and legs. Use of the femoral vein may be considered. ▪ Causes severe tissue necrosis, sloughing, and gangrene. Insert a plastic IV catheter or similar intravascular device at least 6 inches long well into the large vein chosen to prevent extravasation into any surrounding tissue; see Dilution. ▪ Blanching along the vein pathway is a preliminary sign of extravasation. Change the injection site. ▪ See Drug/Lab Interactions.

Patient Education: Report IV site burning or stinging promptly. ▪ Request assistance to ambulate.

Maternal/Child: Category C: use only if clearly needed; benefits must outweigh risks. ▪ Use caution in breastfeeding.

Elderly: See Precautions. ▪ Lower-end initial doses may be indicated; see Dose Adjustments. ▪ Differences in response versus younger patients not documented.

DRUG/LAB INTERACTIONS

Pressor effects may be potentiated by **amphetamines, anesthetics, antihistamines, tricyclic antidepressants, thyroid preparations, and methylphenidate.** ▪ May cause severe hypertension with **ergot alkaloids and guanethidine** and severe prolonged hypertension with **MAO inhibitors.** ▪ May cause hypotension and bradycardia with **phenytoin.** ▪ **Halogenated hydrocarbon anesthetics** (e.g., halothane) may cause serious arrhythmias. ▪ Interacts in numerous and sometimes contradictory ways with many drugs.

SIDE EFFECTS

Rare when used as directed; anxiety, arrhythmias (e.g., bradycardia and VT), chest pain, decreased cardiac output, dyspnea, headache, ischemia, necrosis caused by extravasation, pallor, photophobia, seizures, vomiting. Persistent headache may indicate overdose and severe hypertension. Gangrene has been reported.

ANTIDOTE

To prevent sloughing and necrosis in areas where extravasation has occurred, use a fine hypodermic needle to inject 5 to 10 mg of phentolamine (Regitine) diluted in 10 to 15 mL of NS liberally throughout the tissue in the extravasated area. Phentolamine causes immediate and conspicuous local hyperemic changes if the area is infiltrated within 12 hours. Treatment should be started as soon as extravasation is recognized. Atropine may be used to counteract the bradycardia. Notify physician of any side effect. Should a sudden or uncontrolled hypertensive state occur, discontinue levarterenol, notify the physician and, if necessary, treat with an adrenergic blocking agent (e.g., phentolamine or phenoxybenzamine).

OCRELIZUMAB

Monoclonal antibody
(Anti-CD20 monoclonal antibody)

Ocrevus

pH 5.3

USUAL DOSE

Pretreatment: Verify pregnancy status. Preassessment required; see Monitor.

Premedication: To reduce the incidence and severity of infusion-related reactions, premedicate with *methylprednisolone* 100 mg IV (or equivalent steroid) 30 minutes before each ocrelizumab infusion. Premedicate with an *antihistamine* (e.g., diphenhydramine) approximately 30 to 60 minutes before the infusion to further reduce the frequency and severity of infusion reactions. Administration of an *antipyretic* (e.g., acetaminophen) may also be considered.

Ocrelizumab: *Initial dose:* 300 mg as an IV infusion followed 2 weeks later by a second 300-mg IV infusion. *Subsequent doses:* 600 mg as an IV infusion every 6 months. The recommended dose, infusion rate, and infusion duration for ocrelizumab are outlined in the following chart.

Recommended Dose, Infusion Rate, and Infusion Duration of Ocrelizumab for Relapsing or Primary Progressive Multiple Sclerosis		Amount and Volume	Infusion Rate and Duration[a]
Initial Dose (two infusions)	Infusion 1	300 mg in 250 mL	Start at 30 mL/hr
	Infusion 2 (2 weeks later)	300 mg in 250 mL	Increase by 30 mL/hr every 30 minutes Maximum: 180 mL/hr Duration: 2.5 hr or longer
Subsequent Doses (one infusion)	One infusion every 6 months[b]	600 mg in 500 mL	Start at 40 mL/hr Increase by 40 mL/hr every 30 minutes Maximum: 200 mL/hr Duration: 3.5 hr or longer

[a]Infusion time may take longer if the infusion is interrupted or slowed.
[b]Administer the first subsequent dose 6 months after Infusion 1 of the initial dose.

DOSE ADJUSTMENTS

If a planned dose is missed, administer as soon as possible; do not wait until the next scheduled dose. Reset the dose schedule to administer the next sequential dose 6 months after the missed dose. Doses of ocrelizumab must be separated by at least 5 months. ▪ For mild to moderate infusion reactions, reduce the infusion rate to half the rate at the onset of the infusion reaction, and maintain the reduced rate for at least 30 minutes. If this rate is tolerated, increase the rate as described in the previous chart. ▪ For severe infusion reactions, immediately interrupt the infusion and administer appropriate supportive treatment as necessary; see Antidote. Restart the infusion only after all symptoms have resolved. When restarting, begin at half of the infusion rate at the time of onset of the infusion reaction. If this rate is tolerated, increase the rate as described in the previous chart. ▪ For life-threatening infusion reactions, immediately stop and permanently discontinue ocrelizumab. Provide appropriate supportive treatment; see Antidote.

DILUTION

Available in a 300-mg/10 mL (30-mg/mL) single-dose vial. Solution is clear or slightly opalescent and colorless to pale brown. For initial doses, withdraw 300 mg (10 mL) and inject into 250 mL of NS. For subsequent doses, withdraw 600 mg (20 mL) and inject into 500 mL of NS. Mix gently. ***Do not shake.*** Contents of the infusion bag should be at RT before the start of the IV infusion.

Filter: Administration through a 0.2- or 0.22-micron in-line filter is required.

Storage: Store vials at 2° to 8° C (36° to 46° F) in the outer carton to protect from light. Do not freeze or shake. Immediate use of prepared solution is preferred. If not used immediately, may store up to 24 hours in the refrigerator and 8 hours at RT, which includes infusion time. If an IV infusion cannot be completed on the same day, discard the remaining solution.

COMPATIBILITY

Manufacturer states, "Do not use other diluents to dilute ocrelizumab since their use has not been tested. No **incompatibilities** between ocrelizumab and polyvinyl chloride or polyolefin bags and IV administration sets have been observed."

RATE OF ADMINISTRATION

Use of a 0.2- or 0.22-micron in-line filter required. See chart in Usual Dose for recommended rate of administration.

ACTIONS

A recombinant humanized monoclonal antibody directed against CD20-expressing B-cells. The precise mechanism by which ocrelizumab exerts its therapeutic effects in multiple sclerosis is unknown but is presumed to involve binding to CD20, a cell surface antigen present on pre-B and mature B-lymphocytes. Following cell surface binding to B-lymphocytes, ocrelizumab results in antibody-dependent cellular cytolysis and complement-mediated lysis. $CD19^+$ B-cell counts are reduced in the blood within 14 days of ocrelizumab administration. In one clinical study, the median time for B-cell counts to return to either baseline or the lower limit of normal was 72 weeks. The pharmacokinetics of ocrelizumab is essentially linear and dose proportional between 400 and 2000 mg. Terminal elimination half-life is 26 days.

INDICATIONS AND USES

Treatment of adult patients with relapsing forms of multiple sclerosis, including clinically isolated syndrome, relapsing-remitting disease, and active secondary progressive disease. ▪ Treatment of adult patients with primary progressive multiple sclerosis.

CONTRAINDICATIONS

Active hepatitis B virus (HBV) infection. ▪ A history of life-threatening infusion reaction to ocrelizumab.

PRECAUTIONS

Ocrelizumab should be administered by or under the direction of the physician specialist in facilities equipped to monitor the patient and respond to any medical emergency. ▪ Ocrelizumab can cause infusion reactions that include bronchospasm, dizziness, dyspnea, erythema, fatigue, fever, flushing, headache, hypotension, nausea, oropharyngeal pain, pharyngeal or laryngeal edema, pruritus, rash, tachycardia, throat irritation, and urticaria. Incidence of reactions was highest with the first infusion and may occur despite premedication; see Monitor and Antidote. ▪ In clinical trials, a higher proportion of ocrelizumab-treated patients experienced infections compared with patients taking Rebif (interferon beta-1a) or placebo. Infections included upper respiratory tract infections, lower respiratory tract infections, skin infections, and herpes-related infections. However, ocrelizumab was not associated with an increased risk of serious infections in MS patients. Delay ocrelizumab administration in patients with an active infection until the infection has resolved; see Monitor. ▪ Progressive multifocal leukoencephalopathy (PML) is an opportunistic viral infection of the brain caused by the JC virus. It is a rare, progressive, demyelinating disease of the CNS that usually leads to death or severe disability, and there is no effective treatment. Although no cases of PML were identified in ocrelizumab trials, JC virus infection resulting in PML has been observed in patients treated with other anti-CD20 antibodies and other MS therapies and has been associated with some risk factors (e.g., immunocompromised patients, polytherapy with immunosuppressants). ▪ There have been no reports of hepatitis B reactivation in MS patients treated with ocrelizumab, but fulminant hepatitis B, hepatic failure, and death caused by

HBV reactivation have occurred in patients treated with other anti-CD20 antibodies; see Contraindications and Monitor. ▪ Vaccination with live-attenuated or live vaccines is not recommended during treatment with ocrelizumab or after discontinuation of ocrelizumab until B-cell repletion; see Monitor. ▪ An increased risk of malignancy, including breast cancer, may exist with ocrelizumab therapy. In controlled trials, breast cancer occurred more frequently in ocrelizumab-treated patients. ▪ A protein substance; potential for immunogenicity exists. ▪ See Drug/Lab Interactions.

Monitor: Review vaccination status. Complete any required live or live-attenuated vaccinations at least 4 weeks and, whenever possible, non-live vaccinations at least 2 weeks before beginning therapy with ocrelizumab. ▪ Screen all patients for HBV infection before treatment initiation; see Contraindications. Consult a liver disease specialist for patients who are negative for surface antigen [HBsAg] and positive for HB core antibody [HBcAb+] or who are carriers of HBV [HBsAg+]. ▪ Assess patient for any S/S of an active infection before every infusion. Delay therapy in the presence of an active infection until the infection resolves. ▪ Monitor patient during and for at least 1 hour after completion of the infusion for any S/S of an infusion reaction. ▪ Assess neurologic status frequently. Consider PML in patients with new-onset neurologic manifestations. At the first S/S suggestive of PML, withhold ocrelizumab and perform an appropriate diagnostic evaluation; consultation with a neurologist, brain MRI, and lumbar puncture may be required for diagnosis. ▪ Follow standard breast cancer screening guidelines.

Patient Education: Read FDA-approved medication guide. ▪ Avoid pregnancy; females of childbearing age should use effective birth control during treatment and for 6 months after completion of treatment. ▪ Promptly report any S/S of an infusion reaction. Reactions can occur up to 24 hours after the infusion. ▪ Promptly report any S/S of infection (e.g., fever, chills, constant cough, or signs of herpes such as cold sores, shingles, or genital sores). ▪ New neurologic S/S (e.g., changes in vision, loss of balance or coordination, disorientation, or confusion) could be warning signs of PML. Report them promptly. ▪ May cause reactivation of HBV infection. Monitoring may be required in patients at risk. ▪ Discuss vaccination status with physician. Complete any required live or live-attenuated vaccinations at least 4 weeks and, whenever possible, non-live vaccinations at least 2 weeks before beginning therapy with ocrelizumab. ▪ An increased risk of malignancy, including breast cancer, may exist. Follow standard breast cancer screening guidelines.

Maternal/Child: Information on the developmental risk associated with the use of ocrelizumab in pregnant females is not available. However, transient peripheral B-cell depletion and lymphocytopenia have been reported in infants born to mothers exposed to other anti-CD-20 antibodies during pregnancy. Ocrelizumab is a humanized monoclonal antibody of an IGG1 subtype, and immunoglobulins are known to cross the placental barrier. ▪ Use caution if breastfeeding; weigh risk versus benefit. ▪ Safety and effectiveness for use in pediatric patients not established. ▪ In infants of mothers exposed to ocrelizumab during pregnancy, do not administer live or live-attenuated vaccinations before confirming recovery of B-cell counts as measured by $CD19^+$ B-cells. Administration of non-live vaccines may be completed before B-cell recovery, but consultation with a qualified specialist to assess whether a protective immune response was mounted should be considered.

Elderly: Clinical trials did not include sufficient numbers of subjects 65 years of age or older to determine whether they respond differently than do younger subjects.

DRUG/LAB INTERACTIONS

When initiating ocrelizumab after an immunosuppressive therapy or when initiating an immunosuppressive therapy after ocrelizumab, consider the potential for increased immunosuppressive effects. The concomitant use of ocrelizumab and other **immune-modulating or immunosuppressive therapies**, including immunosuppressant doses of **corticosteroids,** is expected to increase the risk of immunosuppression; consider the risk of additive immune system effects. ▪ The safety of immunization with **live or live-attenuated vaccines** following ocrelizumab therapy has not been studied and is not recommended during treatment and until B-cell repletion; see Monitor. ■ An attenuated antibody response was seen with concomitant use of ocrelizumab and several **non-live vaccines**. The impact of the observed attenuation on vaccine effectiveness is unknown; see Monitor.

SIDE EFFECTS

The most common adverse reactions were infusion reactions, respiratory tract infections (lower and upper), and skin infections. Other frequently reported reactions included back pain, cough, decreased total immunoglobulin (with the greatest decline seen in IgM levels), decreased neutrophil counts, depression, diarrhea, herpes-associated infections, pain in extremities, and peripheral edema.

ANTIDOTE

Keep physician informed of all side effects. May constitute a medical emergency or will be treated symptomatically as indicated. For life-threatening infusion reactions, immediately and permanently stop ocrelizumab and administer appropriate supportive treatment. For less severe infusion reactions, management may involve temporarily stopping the infusion, reducing the infusion rate, and/or administering symptomatic treatment (e.g., IV saline, diphenhydramine, bronchodilators such as albuterol, and acetaminophen). Resuscitate if indicated.

OCTREOTIDE ACETATE

(ok-**TREE**-oh-tide **AS**-ah-tayt)

Octreotide Acetate PF, Sandostatin

Antidiarrheal
Growth hormone suppressant

pH 3.9 to 4.5

USUAL DOSE

Pretreatment: Baseline studies indicated; see Monitor.

Usually given SC. Check label and confirm for IV use; Sandostatin LAR Depot is for IM use only; see Precautions. In most situations begin with a lower dose to allow gradual tolerance to GI side effects. Increase gradually based on patient response and tolerance. Begin SC or IM (LAR Depot) dosing as soon as practical.

Growth hormone suppression (acromegaly): 50 mcg every 8 hours is the initial dose. Increase dose gradually as indicated by IGF-1 levels; see Monitor. The dose most commonly found to be effective is 100 mcg 3 times daily, but some patients require up to 500 mcg 3 times daily for maximum effectiveness.

Carcinoid tumors: 100 to 600 mcg/24 hr in equally divided doses 2 to 4 times daily during first 2 weeks of therapy (50 to 300 mcg every 12 hours or 25 to 150 mcg every 6 hours). Average total daily dose is 300 mcg. In clinical studies, the median daily maintenance dose was approximately 450 mcg, but therapeutic response was obtained with ranges from 50 to 750 mcg. Up to 1,500 mcg/day has been used in selected patients. Experience with doses above 750 mcg/day is limited.

Vasoactive intestinal peptide tumors: 200 to 300 mcg/24 hr in equally divided doses 2 to 4 times daily during the first 2 weeks of therapy (100 to 150 mcg every 12 hours or 50 to 75 mcg every 6 hours). Therapeutic response is usually achieved with doses at or under 450 mcg/24 hr.

Carcinoid crisis (unlabeled): 500 to 1,000 mcg as an IV bolus. May be given to treat carcinoid crisis during surgery or given before induction of anesthesia as a prophylactic measure. If required intraoperatively, may repeat bolus every 5 minutes as needed to control symptoms. Alternatively, a bolus of 500 to 1,000 mcg may be followed by 50 to 200 mcg/hr as a continuous infusion.

Treatment of esophageal varices bleeding (unlabeled): Begin with a loading dose of 50 to 100 mcg. Follow with a continuous infusion of 25 to 50 mcg/hr for 2 to 5 days.

PEDIATRIC DOSE

Experience is limited, and doses are **unlabeled.** See Maternal/Child.

Intractable diarrhea: 1 to 10 mcg/kg of body weight every 12 hours. Dose may be increased within the recommended range by 0.3 mcg/kg/dose every 3 days as needed. Maximum dose is 1,500 mcg/24 hr.

DOSE ADJUSTMENTS

In all situations dose adjustment may be required on a daily basis to maintain symptomatic control. After initial 2 weeks of therapy, gradually decrease dose to achieve therapeutically effective maintenance dose. ▪ Dose reduction may be required in the elderly; half-life extended and clearance decreased. Start at the lower end of the dosing range. Consider the greater frequency of decreased organ function and of concomitant disease or drug therapy. ▪ Half-life markedly extended in severe renal failure requiring dialysis. Reduction of maintenance dose may be indicated. ▪ See Drug/Lab Interactions.

DILUTION

Available in several different concentrations and formulations; read label carefully. May be given undiluted or may be diluted with 50 to 200 mL of NS or D5W and given as an intermittent infusion or further diluted and given as a continuous infusion.

Storage: Before use store in refrigerator (2° to 8° C [36° to 46° F]) or at CRT for 14 days; protect from light. May store at room temperature on day of use. Diluted solution stable for 24 hours. Multidose vial must be dated on opening and discarded after 14 days.

COMPATIBILITY

Manufacturer lists TPN as **incompatible** (forms a conjugate that decreases effectiveness). If used as an additive with insulin, octreotide markedly increases adsorption of insulin and reduces insulin availability.

Other sources suggest a few specific **compatibilities** dependent on concentration and manufacturer; consult a pharmacist.

RATE OF ADMINISTRATION

IV injection: A single dose over 3 minutes.

Intermittent infusion: A single dose over 15 to 30 minutes.

Continuous infusion: Give at a rate consistent with the required hourly dose in an amount of fluid appropriate for the specific patient.

ACTIONS

A long-acting octapeptide. Mimics the actions of the natural hormone somatostatin, suppressing secretion of serotonin, gastroenteropancreatic peptides (e.g., gastrin, vasoactive intestinal peptide, insulin, glucagon, secretin, motilin, pancreatic polypeptide), and growth hormone. Decreases splanchnic blood flow. Stimulates fluid and electrolyte absorption from GI tract and prolongs GI transit time. These pharmacologic actions provide a means of treating the symptoms associated with metastatic carcinoid tumors (flushing and diarrhea) and vasoactive intestinal peptide (VIP)–secreting tumors (watery diarrhea). Other actions include inhibition of gallbladder contractility and bile secretion and suppression of thyroid-stimulating hormone (TSH) secretion. Distribution from plasma is rapid. About 65% bound to plasma protein. Half-life longer than the natural hormone (1.7 to 1.9 hours compared with 1 to 3 minutes). Action may extend to 12 hours. Some excreted unchanged in urine.

INDICATIONS AND USES

To suppress or inhibit the severe diarrhea and flushing episodes associated with carcinoid tumor. ▪ Treatment of profuse watery diarrhea associated with vasoactive intestinal peptide tumors (VIPomas). ▪ Treatment of acromegaly to suppress growth hormone and achieve normalization of growth hormone and somatomedin C (IGF-1) levels.

Unlabeled uses: Treatment of severe diarrhea in patients with AIDS. ▪ Treatment of refractory or severe chemotherapy-induced diarrhea. ▪ Carcinoid crisis during anesthesia. ▪ Adjunct to treatment of sulfonylurea-induced hypoglycemia. ▪ Treatment of gastroesophageal variceal bleeding. ▪ Diarrhea associated with graft versus host disease.

CONTRAINDICATIONS

Sensitivity to octreotide acetate or any of its components.

PRECAUTIONS

IV use is limited to emergency situations. SC injection with rotation of injection sites is preferred route of administration. ▪ Sandostatin LAR Depot must be administered intragluteally but has the advantage of extending the interval between injections to every 4 weeks. ▪ May decrease size of tumors and slow rate of growth and metastases. Data not definitive. ▪ May inhibit gallbladder contractility and decrease bile secretion. Incidence of gallstone or biliary sludge formation was markedly increased in clinical trials. Cholelithiasis resulting in complications requiring cholecystectomy have been reported. ▪ Use caution in patients with diabetes. In patients with Type 1 diabetes, octreotide is likely to affect glucose regulation, and insulin requirements may be decreased. Severe, symptomatic hypoglycemia has been reported. In nondiabetics and Type 2 diabetics with partially intact insulin reserves, octreotide may result in decreased insulin levels and hyperglycemia. Glucose tolerance and antidiabetic treatment should be closely monitored. ▪ Cardiac abnormalities (e.g., arrhythmias, bradycardia, conduction abnormalities, QT prolongation) have been reported. More common in patients with acromegaly; see Side Effects. ▪ Suppresses thyroid-stimulating hormone. May cause hypothyroidism. ▪ Pancreatitis has been reported. Octreotide may alter the absorption of dietary fats in some patients. ▪ Depressed B_{12} levels and abnormal Schilling's tests have been observed.

Monitor: Monitor baseline and periodic thyroid function tests (TSH, total, and/or free T_4), especially in long-term SC therapy. ▪ Monitor fluids and electrolytes carefully. ▪ Observe for transient hyperglycemia or hypoglycemia during induction and dose changes because of changes in balance of hormones (e.g., insulin, glucagon, and growth hormone). ▪ 5-HIAA, plasma serotonin, and plasma substance P may be useful lab studies to evaluate patient response with carcinoid tumor. ▪ Measurement of plasma vasoactive intestinal peptide will be helpful in VIPoma. ▪ In acromegaly, response may be monitored with growth hormone levels at 1- to 4-hour intervals for 8 to 12 hours after a dose. IGF-1 levels every 2 weeks and/or multiple growth hormone levels taken 0 to 8 hours after administration may be used to make dose adjustments. Goal is to achieve growth hormone levels less than 5 ng/mL or IGF-1 levels less than 1.9 units/mL in males and less than 2.2 units/mL in females. After stabilization, IGF-1 or growth hormone levels should be re-evaluated at 6-month intervals. ▪ In patients with acromegaly who have received irradiation, octreotide should be withdrawn yearly for 4 weeks to assess disease activity. If growth hormone or IGF-1 levels increase and S/S recur, octreotide therapy should be resumed. ▪ Can alter fat absorption and decrease gallbladder motility. Monitor for gallbladder disease. GI symptoms are usually present but may not be specific for gallbladder disease. Ultrasound of gallbladder and bile ducts may be indicated in patients with S/S of gallbladder disease. ▪ Monitor for S/S of pancreatitis. ▪ Monitor B_{12} levels in prolonged therapy. ▪ See Dose Adjustments and Drug/Lab Interactions.

Patient Education: Instruct patient and/or family in appropriate skills if self-administration indicated. ▪ In females with acromegaly being treated with octreotide, normalization of GH and IGF-1 may restore fertility. Effective contraception is recommended. ▪ Contact health care provider for experience of S/S of gallstones (e.g., upper right abdominal pain, jaundice, dark urine, clay-colored stools, severe nausea or vomiting).

Maternal/Child: Although studies do not indicate harm to the fetus or infants, use in pregnancy and breastfeeding only if clearly needed. ▪ Safety and effectiveness for use in pediatric patients not established; see Literature. In post-marketing reports, hypoxia, necrotizing enterocolitis, and death have been reported, most notably in pediatric patients under 2 years of age, many of whom had serious underlying comorbid conditions. Relationship to octreotide not established.

Elderly: See Dose Adjustments. ▪ Response similar to that seen in younger patients; however, may be more sensitive to side effects; observe carefully.

DRUG/LAB INTERACTIONS

Use caution in patients receiving concomitant **beta-blockers, calcium channel blockers, insulin, oral hypoglycemic agents, or any agents used for fluid and electrolyte balance**. Dose adjustments may be necessary. ▪ May affect absorption of **orally administered medications**. ▪ May inhibit effectiveness of **cyclosporine** and may result in transplant rejection. ▪ May increase availability of **bromocriptine**. ▪ Suppression of growth hormones may cause a decreased clearance of drugs metabolized by selected cytochrome P450 enzymes. Use caution with concurrent use of **drugs metabolized by CYP3A4** (e.g., HMG-CoA reductase inhibitors, itraconazole, oral midazolam, quinidine).

SIDE EFFECTS

Most side effects are of mild to moderate severity and of short duration. Abdominal pain/discomfort, abnormal stools, backache, blurred vision, bruising, cold and flu symptoms, constipation, depression, diarrhea, dizziness, edema, fat malabsorption, fatigue, flatulence, flushing, gallbladder abnormalities (stones and/or biliary sludge, cholelithiasis), hair loss, headache, hyperglycemia, hypoglycemia, joint pain, nausea, pancreatitis, pollakiuria, pruritus, urinary tract infection, visual disturbances, vomiting, and weakness. In rare cases, GI side effects may resemble intestinal obstruction with progressive abdominal distension, severe epigastric pain, abdominal tenderness, and guarding. Many other side effects occur in fewer than 1% of patients. Side effects that occur more often in patients with acromegaly include cardiac abnormalities (e.g., sinus bradycardia, ECG changes [including QT prolongation], conduction abnormalities, and arrhythmias) and hypothyroidism.

Overdose: Arrhythmia, brain hypoxia, cardiac arrest, diarrhea, flushing, hepatic steatosis, hepatomegaly, hypotension, lactic acidosis, lethargy, pancreatitis, weakness, and weight loss.

Post-Marketing: Cholelithiasis, cholecystitis, cholangitis, and pancreatitis (sometimes requiring cholecystectomy), intestinal obstruction, thrombocytopenia.

ANTIDOTE

Keep physician informed of all side effects. If complications of cholelithiasis are suspected, discontinue and treat appropriately. A dose adjustment of either octreotide or other concomitant therapies may be required. Symptomatic and supportive treatment may be indicated. Overdose will cause hyperglycemia or hypoglycemia depending on tumor involved and endocrine status of patient. Discontinue octreotide temporarily, notify the physician, and monitor the patient carefully. Symptomatic treatment should be sufficient.

OFATUMUMAB BBW

(oh-**FAT**-oo-moo-mab)

Arzerra

Monoclonal antibody
Antineoplastic

pH 5.5

USUAL DOSE

Pretreatment: Baseline studies required; see Monitor.

Premedication: Patients should receive all of the following premedication agents 30 minutes to 2 hours before each infusion of ofatumumab. The premedication schedule is listed in the following chart.

Premedication Schedule for Ofatumumab					
	Previously Untreated CLL, Relapsed CLL, or Extended Treatment in CLL		Refractory CLL		
Infusion number	1 and 2	3 and beyond[a]	1, 2, and 9	3 to 8	10 to 12
IV corticosteroid (prednisolone or equivalent)	50 mg	0 to 50 mg[b]	100 mg	0 to 100 mg[b]	50 to 100 mg[c]
Oral acetaminophen	1,000 mg				
Oral or IV antihistamine	Diphenhydramine 50 mg or cetirizine 10 mg (or equivalent)				

[a]Up to 13 infusions for previously untreated CLL; up to 7 infusions in relapsed CLL; up to 14 infusions for extended treatment in CLL.

[b]Corticosteroid may be reduced or omitted for subsequent infusions if a Grade 3 or greater infusion-related adverse event did not occur with the preceding infusion(s).

[c]Prednisolone may be given at a reduced dose of 50 to 100 mg (or equivalent) if a Grade 3 or greater infusion-related adverse event did not occur with Infusion 9.

Previously untreated chronic lymphocytic leukemia (CLL): 300 mg as the initial dose (Day 1). Follow 1 week later (on Day 8) with 1,000 mg (Cycle 1). Follow with 1,000 mg on Day 1 of subsequent 28-day cycles for a minimum of 3 cycles until best response or a maximum of 12 cycles. Given in combination with chlorambucil.

Relapsed CLL: 300 mg as the initial dose (Day 1). Follow 1 week later (on Day 8) with 1,000 mg (Cycle 1). Follow with 1,000 mg on Day 1 of subsequent 28-day cycles for a maximum of 6 cycles. Given in combination with fludarabine and cyclophosphamide.

Extended treatment in CLL: 300 mg on Day 1. Follow with 1,000 mg 1 week later on Day 8. Follow with 1,000 mg 7 weeks later and every 8 weeks thereafter for up to a maximum of 2 years. Given as a *single-agent* extended treatment.

Refractory CLL: 300 mg as the initial dose (Dose 1). Follow 1 week later with 2,000 mg weekly for 7 doses (Doses 2 through 8), followed 4 weeks later with 2,000 mg every 4 weeks for 4 doses (Doses 9 through 12).

DOSE ADJUSTMENTS

Ofatumumab: Interrupt infusion for an infusion reaction of any severity. Treatment may be resumed at the discretion of the treating physician using the following guidelines. ▪ If an infusion reaction resolves with interruption or remains less than or equal to Grade 2, resume infusion with the following modifications based on the initial grade of the infusion reaction: *Grade 1 or 2:* infuse at one-half of the previous infusion rate. *Grade 3 or 4:* infuse at 12 mL/hr. After resuming the infusion, the rate may be increased according to the chart in Rate of Administration. ▪ Consider permanent discontinuation if the severity of the infusion reaction does not resolve to equal to or less than Grade 2 despite adequate clinical intervention. Permanently discontinue therapy in patients who develop an anaphylactic reaction. ▪ No dose adjustment is indicated for age, body weight, or gender.

DILUTION

Do not shake ofatumumab in vial or solution. Should be a clear to opalescent colorless solution. Prepare all doses in 1000 mL of NS.

300-mg dose: Withdraw and discard 15 mL from a 1,000-mL bag of NS. Withdraw 5 mL from each of 3 (100-mg) vials of ofatumumab and add to the bag of NS.

1,000-mg dose: Withdraw and discard 50 mL from a 1,000-mL bag of NS. Withdraw 50 mL from 1 single-use 1000-mg vial of ofatumumab and add to the bag of NS.

2,000-mg dose: Withdraw and discard 100 mL from a 1,000-mL bag of NS. Withdraw 50 mL from each of 2 (1000-mg) vials of ofatumumab and add to the bag of NS.

Mix all diluted solution by gentle inversion. Administer using an infusion pump and PVC administration sets.

Filters: An in-line filter is no longer provided or required; see latest prescribing information.

Storage: Refrigerate vials and prepared solutions between 2° to 8° C (36° to 46° F). Protect vials from light and do not freeze. Start infusion within 12 hours of preparation and discard the prepared solution after 24 hours.

COMPATIBILITY

Manufacturer states, "Do not mix ofatumumab with, or administer as an infusion with, other medicinal products." Flush the IV line with NS before and after each dose. "No **incompatibilities** observed with polyvinylchloride or polyolefin bags and administration sets."

RATE OF ADMINISTRATION

For IV infusion only. Use of an infusion pump and PVC administration set is required. Flush the IV line with NS before and after each dose. Interrupt infusion for infusion reactions of any severity; see Dose Adjustments.

Previously untreated CLL, relapsed CLL, and extended treatment in CLL: *300-mg dose:* Initiate infusion at a rate of 3.6 mg/hr (12 mL/hr).

1,000-mg dose: Initiate infusion at a rate of 25 mg/hr (25 mL/hr). Reduce to 12 mg/hr if a Grade 3 or greater infusion-related reaction (IRR) occurred during the previous infusion.

If there is no IRR, the rate may be increased every 30 minutes as described in the following chart. Do not exceed these infusion rates.

Ofatumumab Infusion Rates for Previously Untreated CLL, Relapsed CLL, and Extended Treatment in CLL		
Interval After Start of Infusion	**Initial 300-mg Dose[a] (mL/hr)**	**Subsequent Infusions[b] (mL/hr)**
0 to 30 minutes	12 mL/hr	25 mL/hr
31 to 60 minutes	25 mL/hr	50 mL/hr
61 to 90 minutes	50 mL/hr	100 mL/hr
91 to 120 minutes	100 mL/hr	200 mL/hr
121 to 150 minutes	200 mL/hr	400 mL/hr
151 to 180 minutes	300 mL/hr	400 mL/hr
>180 minutes	400 mL/hr	400 mL/hr

[a]**Initial 300 mg:** Median duration of infusion = 4.8 to 5.2 hours.
[b]**Subsequent infusions of 1,000 mg:** Median duration of infusion = 4.2 to 4.4 hours.

Refractory CLL: Dose 1 (300-mg dose): Initiate infusion at a rate of 3.6 mg/hr (12 mL/hr).
Dose 2 (2,000-mg dose): Initiate infusion at a rate of 24 mg/hr (12 mL/hr).
Doses 3 through 12 (2,000-mg doses): Initiate infusion at a rate of 50 mg/hr (25 mL/hr).

If there is no infusion reaction, the rate may be increased every 30 minutes as described in the following chart. Do not exceed these infusion rates.

Ofatumumab Infusion Rates in Refractory CLL		
Interval After Start of Infusion	Infusions 1 and 2[a] (mL/hr)	Subsequent Infusions[b] (mL/hr)
0 to 30 minutes	12 mL/hr	25 mL/hr
31 to 60 minutes	25 mL/hr	50 mL/hr
61 to 90 minutes	50 mL/hr	100 mL/hr
91 to 120 minutes	100 mL/hr	200 mL/hr
>120 minutes	200 mL/hr	400 mL/hr

[a]**Infusions 1 and 2 (300 mg and 2,000 mg):** Median duration of infusion = 6.8 hours.
[b]**Subsequent infusions (2,000 mg):** Median duration of infusion = 4.2 to 4.4 hours.

ACTIONS

A CD20-directed cytolytic monoclonal antibody (also known as an IgGlk human monoclonal antibody). The CD20 molecule is expressed on normal B lymphocytes and on B-cell CLL. Ofatumumab binds specifically to both the small and large extracellular loops of the CD20 molecule, resulting in B-cell lysis. Possible mechanisms of cell lysis include complement-dependent cytotoxicity and antibody-dependent, cell-mediated cytotoxicity. Decreases circulating CD19-positive B-cells. Ofatumumab is eliminated through both a target-independent route and a B-cell–mediated route. With depletion of B-cells, the clearance of ofatumumab decreases substantially after subsequent infusions compared with the first infusion. The mean half-life after repeated infusions was approximately 17.6 days.

INDICATIONS AND USES

Used in combination with chlorambucil for the treatment of previously untreated patients with CLL when fludarabine-based therapy is considered inappropriate. ▪ Used in combination with fludarabine and cyclophosphamide for treatment of patients with relapsed CLL. ▪ Extended treatment of patients who are in complete or partial response after at least two lines of therapy for recurrent or progressive CLL. ▪ Treatment of patients with CLL refractory to fludarabine and alemtuzumab.

CONTRAINDICATIONS

Manufacturer states, "None."

PRECAUTIONS

Do not administer as an IV push or bolus or SC injection. For IV infusion only. ▪ Administered under the supervision of a physician experienced in the use of antineoplastic therapy in a facility equipped to monitor the patient and respond to any medical emergency. ▪ Serious, including fatal, infusion reactions have occurred. Seem to occur more frequently with the first 2 infusions and may occur despite premedication; see Monitor. ▪ Severe cytopenias, including anemia, neutropenia, and thrombocytopenia, have occurred with ofatumumab. Pancytopenia, agranulocytosis, and fatal neutropenic sepsis have occurred in patients receiving ofatumumab in combination with chlorambucil. Grade 3 or 4 late-onset neutropenia (onset at least 42 days after the last treatment dose) and/or prolonged neutropenia (not resolved between 24 and 42 days after the last treatment dose) have been reported. ▪ Progressive multifocal leukoencephalopathy (PML) resulting in death has been reported. ▪ Hepatitis B virus (HBV) reactivation can occur in patients receiving ofatumumab and, in some cases, has resulted in fulminant and fatal hepatitis, hepatic failure, and death. For patients who show evidence of hepatitis B infection, consult physician with expertise in managing hepatitis regarding monitoring and consideration for HBV antiviral therapy. Insufficient data exist regarding the safety of ofatumumab administration in patients who develop HBV reactivation. ▪ Fatal infection due to hepatitis B in patients who have not been previously infected has also been observed. ▪ Tumor lysis syndrome (TLS) has been reported and has required hospitalization. Patients with a high tumor burden and/or high circulating lymphocyte counts (greater than 25,000/mm³) are at greater risk for developing TLS. ▪ A protein substance, it has the potential for producing immunogenicity.

▪ No studies of ofatumumab use in patients with impaired hepatic function or in patients with a CrCl less than 30 mL/min have been conducted; use with caution. ▪ See Monitor. **Monitor:** Obtain baseline CBC and platelet counts and monitor at regular intervals during and after conclusion of therapy. Increase the frequency of monitoring in patients who develop Grade 3 or 4 cytopenias. ▪ Monitor for S/S of infusion reactions. S/S have included abdominal pain, anaphylactoid/anaphylactic reactions, angioedema, back pain, bronchospasm, cardiac events (e.g., acute coronary syndrome, arrhythmia, bradycardia, myocardial ischemia/infarction), cytokine release syndrome, dyspnea, fever, flushing, hypertension, hypotension, laryngeal edema, pulmonary edema, rash, syncope, and urticaria. ▪ Monitor for new onset of or changes in pre-existing neurologic signs or symptoms. Evaluation for PML includes consultation with a neurologist, brain MRI, and lumbar puncture. ▪ Screen patients for HBV before initiating therapy. Monitor patients with evidence of current or prior HBV closely for clinical and laboratory signs of hepatitis or HBV reactivation during treatment and for up to 12 months after the last infusion. Patients without a history of HBV should also be monitored for S/S of hepatitis. ▪ Prevention and treatment of hyperuricemia due to tumor lysis syndrome may be accomplished with adequate hydration and, if necessary, with uric acid–lowering drugs (e.g., allopurinol). Consider initiating prophylaxis 12 to 24 hours before infusion of ofatumumab. Monitor renal function and correct any electrolyte abnormalities that may develop. ▪ Monitor for thrombocytopenia (platelet count less than 50,000/mm^3). Initiate precautions to prevent excessive bleeding (e.g., inspect IV sites, skin, and mucous membranes; use extreme care during invasive procedures; test urine, emesis, stool, and secretions for occult blood). ▪ Use of prophylactic antiemetics may be indicated to reduce nausea and/or vomiting and to increase patient comfort. ▪ Observe closely for signs of infection. Prophylactic antibiotics may be indicated.

Patient Education: Potential for fetal B-cell depletion when given to a pregnant female. ▪ Blood counts will be required at regular intervals. ▪ Avoid vaccination with live virus vaccines. ▪ Additional monitoring and possible need for treatment may be required with a history of hepatitis B infection. ▪ Promptly report symptoms of the following potential side effects: bleeding, easy bruising or petechiae, fatigue, infection (e.g., cough, fever), infusion reactions (e.g., breathing problems, chills, fever, rash that occur within 24 hours of infusion), pallor or worsening weakness, new or worsening abdominal pain or nausea, new or worsening neurologic S/S, worsening fatigue or yellow discoloration of skin or eyes. ▪ See Appendix D, p. 1311.

Maternal/Child: Use during pregnancy only if the potential benefit justifies the potential risk to the fetus. ▪ Use caution if breastfeeding. The effects of local gastrointestinal and limited systemic exposure to ofatumumab are unknown. ▪ May cause fetal B-cell depletion. Avoid administering live vaccines to neonates and infants exposed to ofatumumab in utero until B-cell recovery occurs. ▪ Safety and effectiveness for use in pediatric patients not established.

Elderly: No clinically meaningful differences in efficacy were seen between elderly and younger patients. **_Previously untreated CLL:_** A higher incidence of Grade 3 or greater neutropenia and pneumonia were reported in elderly patients. **_Refractory CLL:_** Numbers of patients over 65 years of age in studies were not sufficient to determine a response that might differ from younger patients.

DRUG/LAB INTERACTIONS

Formal drug-drug interaction studies have not been conducted. ▪ Do not administer **live virus vaccines** to patients who have recently received ofatumumab. ▪ The ability to generate an immune response to any vaccine following administration of ofatumumab has not been studied. ▪ Coadministration with ofatumumab did not result in clinically relevant effects on the pharmacokinetics of fludarabine, cyclophosphamide, or chlorambucil or its active metabolite, phenylacetic acid mustard.

SIDE EFFECTS

Previously untreated CLL: Infusion reactions and neutropenia are most common. Severe cytopenias, including anemia, neutropenia, pancytopenia, thrombocytopenia, agranulocytosis, and fatal neutropenic sepsis, are the most serious side effects in combination with chlorambucil. Other side effects reported included arthralgia, asthenia, headache, herpes simplex, leukopenia, lower respiratory tract infection, and upper abdominal pain.

Relapsed CLL: Febrile neutropenia, infusion reactions, leukopenia, and neutropenia are the most common side effects reported.

Extended treatment in CLL: Infusion reactions, neutropenia, and upper respiratory infections are the most common side effects reported.

Refractory CLL: The most common side effects are anemia, bronchitis, cough, diarrhea, dyspnea, fatigue, fever, nausea, neutropenia, pneumonia, rash, and upper respiratory infections. Fever, infections (some fatal) including pneumonia and sepsis, infusion reactions, and neutropenia were the most common serious side effects.

All diagnoses: Other side effects reported include abdominal pain, arthralgia, asthenia, back pain, chills, edema, headache, hepatitis B infection or reactivation, herpes simplex, herpes zoster, hypertension, hypogammaglobulinemia, hypotension, influenza, insomnia, intestinal obstruction, leukopenia, lower respiratory tract infection, lymphopenia, muscle spasms, nasopharyngitis, peripheral edema, PML, sinusitis, tachycardia, thrombocytopenia, tumor lysis syndrome, and urticaria.

Post-Marketing: Cardiac arrest, porphyria cutanea tarda, Stevens-Johnson syndrome.

ANTIDOTE

Notify physician of significant side effects. Temporarily discontinue the infusion for an infusion reaction. Institute medical management for severe infusion reactions, including angina or other S/S of myocardial ischemia as indicated. Delay therapy for serious infection or serious hematologic toxicity until the infection or adverse event resolves. Treatment of most reactions will be supportive. Discontinue medication permanently for severe reactions, including Grade 4 infusion reactions or S/S of PML or in patients who develop reactivation of HBV. Infusion reactions may be treated with acetaminophen, antiemetics (e.g., ondansetron), antihistamines (e.g., diphenhydramine), or corticosteroids (e.g., hydrocortisone) as indicated. Discontinue ofatumumab and provide supportive therapy in overdose. Treat hypersensitivity reactions with epinephrine, antihistamines, and corticosteroids as needed. Resuscitate as indicated.

OLARATUMAB
(**OH**-lar-**AT**-ue-mab)

Antineoplastic
Monoclonal antibody

Lartruvo pH 5.2 to 6.8

USUAL DOSE
Pretreatment: Verify pregnancy status. Baseline studies required; see Monitor.
Premedication: Administer diphenhydramine 25 to 50 mg IV and dexamethasone 10 to 20 mg IV before administration of olaratumab on Day 1 of Cycle 1.
Olaratumab: 15 mg/kg administered as an IV infusion over 60 minutes on Days 1 and 8 of each 21-day cycle until disease progression or unacceptable toxicity. For the first 8 cycles, olaratumab is administered with doxorubicin. In clinical studies, patients received doxorubicin 75 mg/M² as an IV infusion on Day 1 of each 21-day cycle for a maximum of 8 cycles and were permitted to receive dexrazoxane before doxorubicin in Cycles 5 to 8. See doxorubicin monograph for dosing and dose adjustments.

DOSE ADJUSTMENTS
Interrupt infusion for Grade 1 or 2 infusion-related reactions (IRRs). After resolution, infusion may be resumed at 50% of the initial infusion rate. ▪ Permanently discontinue for Grade 3 or 4 IRR. ▪ For neutropenic fever/infection or Grade 4 neutropenia lasting longer than 1 week, discontinue administration of olaratumab until ANC is 1,000/mm³ or greater and then permanently reduce the dose to 12 mg/kg. ▪ Age, gender, race, and mild to moderate renal or hepatic impairment did not have any clinically important effect on the pharmacokinetics of olaratumab. ▪ Body weight correlates with clearance and volume of distribution.

DILUTION
Available as a 500-mg/50 mL (10-mg/mL) clear to slightly opalescent, colorless to slightly yellow solution in a single-dose vial. Withdraw the calculated dose based on patient weight and further dilute with NS to a final volume of 250 mL. Gently invert. Do not shake.
Filter: No information available.
Storage: Store vials in refrigerator at 2° to 8° C (36° to 46° F). Keep in original carton to protect from light. *Do not freeze or shake vials or diluted solution.* Diluted solution may be stored for up to 24 hours under refrigeration and for up to an additional 4 hours at RT. Storage times include the duration of infusion. If refrigerated, allow the diluted solution to come to RT before administration. Discard any unused portion left in vial.

COMPATIBILITY
Manufacturer states, "Do not use dextrose-containing solutions. Do not co-infuse with electrolytes or other medications through the same IV line."

RATE OF ADMINISTRATION
A single dose as an infusion equally distributed over 60 minutes. Flush IV line with NS at the end of the infusion. If diluted solution has been refrigerated, bring to RT before administration. Decrease rate of infusion by 50% in patients who experience a Grade 1 or 2 IRR.

ACTIONS
Olaratumab is a recombinant human IgG1 antibody that binds platelet-derived growth factor receptor alpha (PDGFR-α). Signaling through this receptor plays a role in cell growth, chemotaxis, and mesenchymal stem cell differentiation. The receptor has also been detected on some tumor and stromal cells, including sarcomas, where signaling can contribute to cancer cell proliferation, metastasis, and maintenance of the tumor microenvironment. The interaction between olaratumab and PDGFR-α prevents binding of the receptor by the PDGF-AA and PDGF-BB ligands as well as PDGF-AA–, PDGF-BB–, and PDGF-CC–induced receptor activation and downstream PDGFR-α pathway signaling. Olaratumab exhibits in vitro and in vivo antitumor activity against selected sarcoma cell

lines and disrupted the PDGFR-α signaling pathway in in vivo tumor implant models. Half-life is approximately 11 days (range 6 to 24 days).

INDICATIONS AND USES

Treatment of adult patients with soft tissue sarcoma (STS) with a histologic subtype for which an anthracycline-containing regimen is appropriate and that is not amenable to curative treatment with radiotherapy or surgery. Given in combination with doxorubicin. This indication was approved under accelerated approval. Continued approval may be contingent on verification and description of clinical benefit in the confirmatory trial.

CONTRAINDICATIONS

Manufacturer states, "None."

PRECAUTIONS

For IV infusion only. Do not administer as an IV push or bolus. ▪ Should be administered by or under the direction of a physician specialist in a facility equipped to monitor the patient and respond to any medical emergency. ▪ IRRs have been reported. Most occurred during the first or second cycle. Premedication required; see Usual Dose, Dose Adjustments, and Antidote. ▪ May cause fetal harm; see Maternal/Child. ▪ The pharmacokinetics of olaratumab in patients with severe renal or hepatic impairment is unknown. ▪ A therapeutic protein; has the potential for immunogenicity.

Monitor: Premedication required; see Usual Dose. ▪ Obtain baseline CBC with differential and platelets and monitor as indicated during therapy. ▪ Monitor patients during and following olaratumab infusion for S/S of IRR (e.g., anaphylactic shock, bronchospasms, cardiac arrest, chills, fever, flushing, hypotension [may be severe], shortness of breath).

Patient Education: Effective contraception required for females of reproductive potential during treatment with and for 3 months after the last dose of olaratumab. ▪ Promptly report S/S of an infusion reaction (e.g., chills, dizziness, fever, flushing, shortness of breath).

Maternal/Child: Based on animal data and its mechanism of action, olaratumab can cause fetal harm when administered to a pregnant female. ▪ May impair male fertility. ▪ Discontinue breastfeeding. ▪ Safety and effectiveness for use in pediatric patients have not been established.

Elderly: Clinical studies did not include sufficient numbers of patients 65 years of age and older to determine whether they respond differently than do younger patients.

DRUG/LAB INTERACTIONS

Formal drug interaction studies have not been conducted. ▪ No clinically relevant changes in the exposure of either olaratumab or doxorubicin were observed when coadministered in recommended doses to patients with solid tumors.

SIDE EFFECTS

The most common adverse reactions seen with olaratumab plus doxorubicin are abdominal pain, alopecia, decreased appetite, diarrhea, fatigue, headache, mucositis, musculoskeletal pain, nausea, neuropathy, and vomiting. The most common laboratory abnormalities were elevated aPTT, hyperglycemia, hypokalemia, hypophosphatemia, lymphopenia, neutropenia, and thrombocytopenia. The most common adverse reaction leading to dose reduction was Grade 3 or 4 neutropenia. Anemia, neutropenia, and thrombocytopenia were the adverse reactions most commonly responsible for a dose delay. The most common adverse reaction leading to discontinuation of olaratumab was IRR. Other commonly reported adverse reactions included anxiety, dry eyes, hypomagnesemia, and increased alkaline phosphatase.

ANTIDOTE

Notify physician of any side effects; most will be treated symptomatically. Permanently discontinue for Grade 3 or 4 IRR. Treat infusion and hypersensitivity reactions as indicated (e.g., oxygen, diphenhydramine, epinephrine, corticosteroids, vasopressors, and/or fluids); see Dose Adjustments. Resuscitate as necessary.

OMADACYCLINE
(ooh-mad-a-**SYE**-kleen)

Antibacterial (tetracycline)

Nuzyra

USUAL DOSE
Administer as outlined in the following chart.

Omadacycline Dosing in Adult Patients With Community-Acquired Bacterial Pneumonia (CABP) and Acute Bacterial Skin and Skin Structure Infection (ABSSSI)			
Diagnosis	**Loading Dose**	**Maintenance Dose**	**Treatment Duration**
Community-acquired bacterial pneumonia (CABP)[a]	200 mg IV over 60 minutes on Day 1 Or 100 mg IV over 30 minutes twice on Day 1	100 mg IV over 30 minutes once daily Or 300 mg PO once daily	7 to 14 days
Acute bacterial skin and skin structure infections (ABSSSI)[a]	200 mg IV over 60 minutes on Day 1 Or 100 mg IV over 30 minutes twice on Day 1 Or 450 mg PO once daily on Day 1 and Day 2	100 mg IV over 30 minutes once daily Or 300 mg PO once daily	7 to 14 days

[a]Administer loading dose for patients with CABP as an IV infusion. The loading dose for patients with ABSSSI may be administered orally or as an IV infusion.

The exposure of omadacycline is similar between a 300-mg oral dose and a 100-mg IV dose.

DOSE ADJUSTMENTS
No dose adjustments are required for patients with renal or hepatic impairment. ▪ No clinically significant differences in the pharmacokinetics of omadacycline were observed based on age, gender, race, or weight.

DILUTION
Available as a yellow to orange, lyophilized powder in single-dose vials containing 100 mg of omadacycline. Reconstitute the required number of vials needed to make the dose by injecting 5 mL of SWFI, NS, or D5W into each vial. Gently swirl the contents and let the vial stand until the cake has completely dissolved and any foam has dispersed. **Do not shake.** The reconstituted product should be a clear, yellow to dark orange solution. Immediately (within 1 hour) withdraw 5 mL (100-mg dose) or 10 mL (200-mg dose) of the reconstituted solution and further dilute in 100 mL of NS or D5W. The concentration of the final diluted infusion solution will be either 1 mg/mL (100-mg dose) or 2 mg/mL (200-mg dose).
Filter: Specific information not available.
Storage: Store unopened vials at CRT. Do not freeze. The reconstituted solution should be diluted within 1 hour of reconstitution. The diluted solution must be infused within 24 hours if stored at RT or within 48 hours if refrigerated at 2° to 8° C (36° to 46° F). Do not freeze. If stored in the refrigerator, the infusion bag should be removed from the refrigerator and incubated in a vertical position at RT for 60 minutes before use. Discard unused portions of the reconstituted or diluted solution.

COMPATIBILITY
Manufacturer states, "Do NOT administer omadacycline with any solution containing multivalent cations (e.g., calcium and magnesium) through the same intravenous line. The compatibility of omadacycline with other drugs and infusion solutions other than D5W or NS has not been established."

RATE OF ADMINISTRATION

Administer through a dedicated line or through a Y-site. If the same IV line is used for sequential infusion of several drugs, the line should be flushed with NS or D5W before and after the infusion of omadacycline.

Loading dose: Administer 200 mg as an IV infusion over 60 minutes.

Maintenance dose: Administer 100 mg as an IV infusion over 30 minutes.

ACTIONS

A semisynthetic aminomethylcycline antibacterial within the tetracycline class of antibacterial drugs. Omadacycline binds to the 30s ribosomal subunit and blocks protein synthesis. In general, omadacycline is considered bacteriostatic; however, in vitro bactericidal activity has been demonstrated against certain strains of *Streptococcus pneumoniae* and *Haemophilus influenzae*. Active against selected gram-positive and gram-negative bacteria; see prescribing information and Indications. Omadacycline distributes into the lungs. Steady-state exposures in alveolar cells and epithelial lining fluid are higher than plasma exposures. Plasma protein binding is approximately 20% and is not concentration dependent. Omadacycline does not appear to be metabolized. Half-life is 16 hours. Excreted in feces and urine.

INDICATIONS AND USES

Treatment of adult patients with community-acquired bacterial pneumonia (CABP) caused by the following susceptible microorganisms: *S. pneumoniae, Staphylococcus aureus* (methicillin-susceptible isolates), *H. influenzae, Haemophilus parainfluenzae, Klebsiella pneumoniae, Legionella pneumophila, Mycoplasma pneumoniae,* and *Chlamydophila pneumoniae.* ▪ Treatment of adult patients with acute bacterial skin and skin structure infections (ABSSSI) caused by the following susceptible microorganisms: *S. aureus* (methicillin-susceptible and methicillin-resistant isolates), *Staphylococcus lugdunensis, Streptococcus pyogenes, Streptococcus anginosus* group (includes *S. anginosus, S. intermedius,* and *S. constellatus*), *Enterococcus faecalis, Enterobacter cloacae,* and *K. pneumoniae.*

CONTRAINDICATIONS

Known hypersensitivity to omadacycline, tetracycline-class antibacterial drugs, or any of the excipients. Not recommended in pediatric patients under 8 years of age or in breastfeeding.

PRECAUTIONS

To reduce the development of drug-resistant bacteria and maintain its effectiveness, omadacycline should be used to treat or prevent only those infections proven or strongly suspected to be caused by bacteria. ▪ Sensitivity studies indicated to determine susceptibility of the causative organism to omadacycline. ▪ Mortality imbalance was observed in the CABP clinical trial, with eight deaths (2%) occurring in patients treated with omadacycline compared with four deaths (1%) in patients treated with moxifloxacin. The cause of the mortality imbalance has not been established. All deaths in both treatment arms occurred in patients greater than 65 years of age; most patients had multiple comorbidities. The causes of death varied and included worsening and/or complications of infection and underlying conditions. ▪ Exposure during the last half of pregnancy, infancy, and childhood to 8 years of age may cause permanent discoloration of the teeth. This adverse reaction is more common during long-term use of the tetracycline-class drugs but has also been observed after repeated short-term courses. Enamel hypoplasia has also been reported with the tetracycline-class drugs. ▪ The use of omadacycline during the second and third trimesters of pregnancy, infancy, and childhood up to 8 years of age may cause reversible inhibition of bone growth. All tetracyclines form a stable calcium complex in any bone-forming tissue. ▪ Life-threatening hypersensitivity (anaphylactic) reactions have been reported with other tetracycline-class antibacterial drugs. Omadacycline is structurally similar to other tetracycline-class antibacterial drugs and should not be administered to patients with known hypersensitivity to any drug in this class; see Contraindications. ▪ *Clostridium difficile*–associated diarrhea (CDAD) has been reported. May range from mild to life-threatening. Consider in patients who present with diarrhea during or after treatment with omadacycline. ▪ Omadacycline is structurally similar to tetracycline-class antibacterial drugs and may have similar adverse reactions. Adverse reactions, including photosensitivity, pseudotumor cerebri, and anti-anabolic action leading to increased BUN, azotemia, acidosis, hyperphosphatemia, pancreatitis, and abnormal liver function tests, have been reported for other tetracycline-class antibacterial drugs and may occur with omadacycline. ▪ Avoid prolonged use of drug; superinfection caused by overgrowth of nonsusceptible organisms may result. ▪ May be active against some organisms that are normally resistant to other tetracyclines.

Monitor: Closely monitor clinical response to therapy in CABP patients, particularly in those at higher risk for mortality. ▪ Monitor for S/S of hypersensitivity reactions. ▪ Determine absolute patency of vein and avoid extravasation; thrombophlebitis may occur. ▪ Monitor hematopoietic, renal, and hepatic studies periodically in long-term therapy.

Patient Education: May cause embryonic or fetal harm. Use of effective contraception advised. ▪ Promptly report severe diarrhea, S/S of hypersensitivity reactions, or any other side effect. ▪ May cause permanent tooth discoloration of deciduous teeth and reversible inhibition of bone growth when administered during the second and third trimesters of pregnancy. Tell your health care provider right away if you become pregnant during treatment. ▪ Alert patient to the possibility of a photosensitive skin reaction.

Maternal/Child: Data on use in pregnant females are limited. May cause permanent tooth discoloration of deciduous teeth and reversible inhibition of bone growth when administered during the second and third trimesters of pregnancy. Consider risk versus benefit. ▪ Discontinue breastfeeding during treatment and for 4 days after the last dose. ▪ Safety and effectiveness of omadacycline in pediatric patients have not been established. Due to the adverse effects on tooth development and bone growth, use in pediatric patients under 8 years of age is not recommended.

Elderly: In clinical trials, numerically lower clinical success rates at an early clinical response time point were observed in CABP patients 65 years of age or older compared with patients under 65 years of age. In addition, all deaths that occurred in the CABP trial occurred in patients 65 years of age or older. ▪ No clinically relevant differences in the pharmacokinetics of omadacycline were observed with respect to age in a population pharmacokinetic analysis of omadacycline.

DRUG/LAB INTERACTIONS

Because tetracyclines have been shown to depress plasma prothrombin activity, patients who are on **anticoagulant therapy** may require downward adjustment of their anticoagulant dosage.

SIDE EFFECTS

The most common adverse reactions are constipation; diarrhea; headache; hypertension; increased ALT, AST, and gamma-glutamyl transferase; infusion site reactions; insomnia; nausea; and vomiting. Several other adverse reactions were reported in fewer than 2% of patients. An imbalance in mortality, *C. difficile*–associated diarrhea, inhibition of bone growth, and tooth discoloration have been reported. The possibility of tetracycline-class adverse reactions exists; see Precautions.

ANTIDOTE

Notify the physician of all side effects. Discontinue omadacycline at the first sign of a hypersensitivity reaction or if the development of any tetracycline class adverse drug reaction is suspected. Treat hypersensitivity reactions as indicated (e.g., antihistamines, epinephrine, corticosteroids) and resuscitate as necessary. Treat CDAD with fluids, electrolytes, protein supplements, and appropriate antibiotics (e.g., oral vancomycin), as indicated. In severe cases, surgical evaluation may be indicated. Significant quantities are not expected to be removed by hemodialysis.

ONDANSETRON HYDROCHLORIDE

(on-**DAN**-sih-tron hy-droh-**KLOR**-eyed)

Ondansetron HCl PF, Zofran, Zofran PF

Antiemetic
5HT$_3$ receptor antagonist

pH 3 to 4

USUAL DOSE

Prevention of nausea and vomiting associated with emetogenic cancer chemotherapy in adult and pediatric patients 6 months of age and older: Three 0.15 mg/kg of body weight doses up to a maximum of 16 mg/dose. Administer the first dose 30 minutes before giving emetogenic cancer chemotherapy (e.g., cisplatin, methotrexate). Given as an intermittent infusion over 15 minutes. Repeat 0.15 mg/kg dose up to a maximum of 16 mg/dose at 4 and 8 hours after the first dose. Concurrent use with dexamethasone may improve the effectiveness of ondansetron in controlling cisplatin-induced nausea and vomiting.

Prevention of postoperative nausea and/or vomiting in adults and pediatric patients 1 month to 12 years of age weighing more than 40 kg: 4 mg *undiluted* before anesthesia induction or postoperatively if the patient did not receive prophylactic antiemetics and experiences nausea or vomiting within 2 hours after surgery. Although repeat doses are not recommended by the manufacturer, they have been given. Benefit of repeat dosing has not been demonstrated in studies.

PEDIATRIC DOSE

See Maternal/Child.

Nausea associated with emetogenic cancer chemotherapy agents in pediatric patients 6 months of age and older: See Usual Dose.

Postoperative nausea in pediatric patients 1 month to 12 years of age: Given immediately before or following anesthesia induction or postoperatively if the patient did not receive prophylactic antiemetics and experiences nausea or vomiting shortly after surgery. See comments under Usual Dose.

Weight 40 kg or less: 0.1 mg/kg.

Weight more than 40 kg: See Usual Dose.

DOSE ADJUSTMENTS

No dose adjustment required for the elderly or in renal disease. ▪ Before emetogenic chemotherapy, a single maximum daily dose of 8 mg is suggested for patients with severe hepatic disease (Child-Pugh score of 10 or greater).

DILUTION

Available in a 20-mL multidose vial (2 mg/mL) and in premixed solutions.

IV injection: Dilution is not required in adult and pediatric patients when given as an IV injection for the prevention of postoperative nausea and vomiting.

Intermittent infusion: Dilution of each single dose in 50 mL of NS or D5W is required in adult and pediatric patients when ondansetron is given for the prevention of nausea and vomiting associated with emetogenic chemotherapy. In pediatric patients 6 months to 1 year of age and/or 10 kg or less, dilute in 10 to 50 mL of D5W or NS depending on patient's fluid needs. See Compatibility for additional diluents.

Storage: Store unopened vials between 2° and 30° C (36° and 86° F). Protect from light. Stable at RT under normal lighting conditions for 48 hours after dilution. However, manufacturer recommends that the dilution not be used beyond 24 hours. Shake vigorously to resolubilize if a precipitate forms at the stopper/vial interface.

COMPATIBILITY

Manufacturer states, "Do not mix with alkaline solutions as a precipitate may form" and lists as **compatible** and stable for up to 48 hours with D5W, NS, D5/½NS, D5NS, or 3% NaCl injection; see Dilution.

Other sources suggest specific **compatibilities** dependent on concentration and manufacturer; consult a pharmacist.

RATE OF ADMINISTRATION

IV injection (postoperative nausea and vomiting in adults and pediatric patients 12 years of age and older): A single 4-mg dose over at least 30 seconds; 2 to 5 minutes preferred.

IV injection (postoperative nausea and vomiting in pediatric patients 1 month to 12 years of age and weighing more than 40 kg): A single 4-mg dose over at least 30 seconds; 2 to 5 minutes preferred.

IV injection (postoperative nausea and vomiting in pediatric patients 1 month to 12 years of age and weighing 40 kg or less): A single 0.1-mg/kg dose over at least 30 seconds; 2 to 5 minutes preferred.

Intermittent infusion adults and pediatric patients: A single dose equally distributed over 15 minutes.

ACTIONS

A selective antagonist of serotonin (5-HT$_3$) receptors. 5-HT$_3$ receptors are found both peripherally on vagal nerve terminals and centrally in the chemoreceptor trigger zone. It is unclear whether antiemetic action in chemotherapy-induced nausea and vomiting is mediated centrally, peripherally, or at both sites. Chemotherapeutic agents such as cisplatin increase the release of serotonin from specific cells in the GI tract, causing emesis. By antagonizing these receptors, chemotherapy-induced nausea and vomiting are prevented. Lacks the activity at dopamine receptors of metoclopramide, so it does not cause the same level of sedation. No correlation between plasma levels and antiemetic activity. Metabolized by specific hepatic enzymes of the cytochrome P$_{450}$ isoenzyme system; onset of action is prompt. Half-life is 3.5 to 5.5 hours. Excreted in feces and urine.

INDICATIONS AND USES

Prevention of nausea and vomiting associated with initial and repeat courses of emetogenic cancer chemotherapy, including high-dose cisplatin in patients 6 months of age and older. ▪ Prevention of postoperative nausea and/or vomiting in patients 1 month of age and older. ▪ Used orally (available as liquid, tablets, and orally disintegrating tablets) for prevention of nausea and vomiting, including postoperative nausea and vomiting, and nausea and vomiting associated with chemotherapy and radiotherapy (including total body irradiation). Approved for IM injection as an alternative to IV in the prevention of postoperative nausea and vomiting.

CONTRAINDICATIONS

Hypersensitivity to ondansetron or any of its components. ▪ Concomitant use of apomorphine.

PRECAUTIONS

Sterile technique imperative in withdrawing a single dose from the multidose vial. Available in single-dose and multidose vials and in 4- and 8-mg tablets. ▪ Hypersensitivity reactions, including anaphylaxis and bronchospasm, have been reported. Cross-sensitivity has been reported between ondansetron and other 5HT$_3$ receptor agonists (e.g., dolasetron or granisetron). ▪ Use with caution in patients with hepatic impairment. Clearance is decreased; see Dose Adjustments. ▪ Not indicated instead of gastric suction. Use in abdominal surgery or in patients with chemotherapy-induced nausea and vomiting may mask a progressive ileus or gastric distension. ▪ May cause ECG changes, including QT-interval prolongation (prolongs the QT interval in a dose-dependent manner). Postmarketing cases of torsades de pointes have been reported. Avoid use in patients with congenital long QT syndrome. Use with caution in patients with electrolyte abnormalities (e.g., hypokalemia, hypomagnesemia), CHF, or bradyarrhythmias or in patients taking other medicines that may lead to QT prolongation; see Monitor and Drug/Lab Interactions. ▪ Serotonin syndrome has been reported with 5-HT$_3$ receptor antagonists. Most reports were associated with concomitant use of serotonergic drugs (e.g., selective serotonin reuptake inhibitors [e.g., paroxetine, escitalopram], serotonin and norepinephrine reuptake inhibitors [e.g., duloxetine, venlafaxine], monoamine oxidase inhibitors, mirtazapine, fentanyl, lithium, tramadol). Some cases were fatal. ▪ Routine prophylaxis is not recommended for patients in whom there is little expectation of postoperative nausea and vomiting. However, for patients in whom nausea and vomiting must be avoided during the postoperative period, prophylaxis is recommended even when the incidence of postoperative nausea and vomiting is low.

Monitor: Observe closely. Ambulate slowly to avoid orthostatic hypotension. ▪ ECG monitoring is recommended in patients with electrolyte abnormalities (e.g., hypokalemia, hypomagnesemia), CHF, or bradyarrhythmias or in patients taking other medicines that may lead to QT prolongation. ▪ Monitor for S/S of a hypersensitivity reaction (e.g., chest pain, dizziness, dyspnea, fever, flushing, hypotension, nausea, pruritus, rash, rigors, urticaria). ▪ Monitor for serotonin syndrome, especially when ondansetron is used concurrently with other serotonergic drugs. Symptoms associated with serotonin syndrome may include the following combination of S/S: mental status changes (e.g., agitation, coma, delirium, hallucinations), autonomic instability (e.g., diaphoresis, dizziness, flushing, hyperthermia, labile blood pressure, tachycardia), neuromuscular symptoms (e.g., hyperreflexia, incoordination, myoclonus, rigidity, tremor), and seizures, with or without GI symptoms (e.g., diarrhea, nausea, vomiting). ▪ Stool softeners or laxatives may be required to prevent constipation. ▪ Monitor for S/S of bowel obstruction in patients after abdominal surgery and in patients with chemotherapy-induced nausea and vomiting.

Patient Education: May cause dizziness or fainting; request assistance to ambulate. ▪ Promptly report difficulty breathing, tightness in the chest, or wheezing. ▪ May cause cardiac arrhythmias; discuss personal and family history and all prescription and nonprescription medications with a health care professional. ▪ Promptly report any S/S consistent with a potential bowel obstruction. ▪ Promptly report S/S of serotonin syndrome (e.g., altered mental status, autonomic instability, and neuromuscular symptoms); see Precautions.

Maternal/Child: No evidence of impaired fertility or harm to fetus. Use in pregnancy only if potential benefit justifies potential risk. ▪ Use caution if required during breastfeeding. ▪ Information limited in pediatric cancer patients under 6 months of age and in pediatric surgical patients under 1 month of age. ▪ In general, pediatric surgical and cancer patients younger than 18 years tend to have a higher clearance compared with adults, leading to a shorter half-life (2.9 hours). Infants 1 to 4 months of age have a lower clearance, resulting in a longer half-life (6.7 hours). Close monitoring of patients younger than 4 months of age is recommended.

Elderly: A reduction in clearance and an increase in elimination half-life are seen in patients over 75 years of age. See Dose Adjustments.

DRUG/LAB INTERACTIONS

Does not appear to induce or inhibit the **cytochrome P450 isoenzyme system**. ▪ **Phenytoin, carbamazepine**, and **rifampin** increase clearance and decrease levels of ondansetron. Dose adjustment not recommended. ▪ Concomitant use of **apomorphine** may result in profound hypotension and loss of consciousness; see Contraindications. ▪ Concomitant use with **tramadol** may result in reduced analgesic activity of tramadol. See Precautions and use extreme caution with **diuretics or antiarrhythmic drugs or other drugs that lead to prolonged QT intervals** (e.g., amiodarone, procainamide, quinidine). ▪ Serotonin syndrome (including altered mental status, autonomic instability, and neuromuscular symptoms) has been reported following the concomitant use of 5-HT$_3$ receptor antagonists and other serotonergic drugs, including selective serotonin reuptake inhibitors (SSRIs) and serotonin and norepinephrine reuptake inhibitors (SNRIs); see Precautions.

SIDE EFFECTS

The most common side effects reported were diarrhea, fever, and headache.

Adults: Agitation, arrhythmias (including ventricular and supraventricular tachycardia, PVCs, atrial fibrillation, and bradycardia), chest pain, cold sensation, constipation, cramps, diarrhea, dizziness, drowsiness, ECG alterations (including second-degree heart block, QT-interval prolongation, and ST segment depression), faintness, fatigue, fever, flushing, headache, hypersensitivity reactions (e.g., anaphylaxis, angioedema, bronchospasm, cardiopulmonary arrest, hypotension, laryngospasm, shock, shortness of breath, stridor, urticaria), hiccups, hypokalemia, injection site reactions, oculogyric crisis, pain (abdominal, joint, musculoskeletal, rib cage, shoulder), palpitations, paresthesia, pruritus, shivering, transient blurred vision or blindness, transient elevation of AST or ALT, urinary retention. Other side effects have occurred (e.g., extrapyramidal reaction, rash) in fewer than 1% of patients. Overdose caused sudden blindness in one patient.

Infants 1 to 24 months: Bronchospasm, diarrhea, fever, postprocedural pain.

Pediatric patients 2 to 12 years of age: Anxiety/agitation, drowsiness/sedation, fever, headache, wound problems.

Post-Marketing: Arthralgia; dyspnea; ECG changes, including QT/QTc interval prolongation; erythema; hepatitis, hepatic necrosis, hepatic failure, and death (in patients receiving potentially hepatotoxic cytotoxic chemotherapy and antibiotics; etiology unclear); hyperhidrosis; increased alkaline phosphatase (ALP), gamma-glutamyl transferase (GGT), and bilirubin; jaundice; laryngeal edema; lethargy; Stevens-Johnson syndrome; torsades de pointes; toxic epidermal necrolysis; ventricular fibrillation. Serotonin syndrome has been reported as a 5-HT$_3$ class reaction.

ANTIDOTE

Most side effects will be treated symptomatically. Keep physician informed as indicated. Overdose of 10 times the usual dose has not caused significant problems. If symptoms of serotonin syndrome occur, discontinue ondansetron and initiate supportive care. Treat anaphylaxis and resuscitate as necessary.

ORITAVANCIN
(**OR**-it-**A**-van-**SIN**)

Orbactiv, Kimyrsa

Antibacterial
(lipoglycopeptide)

pH 3.1 to 4.3

USUAL DOSE

A single 1200-mg dose administered as an infusion over 3 hours for Orbactiv; over 1 hour for Kimyrsa.

DOSE ADJUSTMENTS

No dose adjustment is recommended in patients with mild or moderate renal or hepatic impairment. ■ No dose adjustment recommended based on age, gender, weight, or race.

DILUTION

Available in single-use vials containing 400 mg of oritavancin as a lyophilized powder. Three vials are required to prepare a single dose. Reconstitute each 400-mg vial with 40 mL of SWFI. Gently swirl to avoid foaming, and ensure that all oritavancin powder is completely dissolved. Concentration is 10 mg/mL in each vial. Solution should be clear and colorless to pale yellow. Withdraw and discard 120 mL from a 1,000-mL IV bag of D5W. Withdraw 40 mL from each of the three reconstituted vials and add to the D5W IV bag to bring the volume back to 1,000 mL. Final concentration is 1.2 mg/mL.

Filters: Specific information not available.

Storage: Vials may be stored at CRT. Reconstituted vials and/or fully diluted solutions may be stored at RT for up to 6 hours or refrigerated at 2° to 8° C (36° to 46° F) for up to 12 hours. Total time from reconstitution to dilution to completion of administration should not exceed 6 hours at RT or 12 hours if refrigerated.

COMPATIBILITY

Manufacturer states, "Use only D5W for dilution. Do **NOT** use NS. NS is **incompatible** with oritavancin and may cause precipitation of the drug. Other IV substances, additives, or other medications mixed in NS should not be added to oritavancin single-use vials or infused simultaneously through the same IV line or through a common IV port. In addition, drugs formulated at a basic or neutral pH may be **incompatible** with oritavancin. If the same IV line is used for sequential infusion of additional medications, the line should be flushed before and after infusion of oritavancin with D5W."

Other sources suggest a few specific **compatibilities** dependent on concentration and manufacturer; consult a pharmacist.

RATE OF ADMINISTRATION

A single dose as an infusion equally distributed over 3 hours for Orbactiv and 1 hour for Kimyrsa. If a common IV line is used to administer other drugs in addition to oritavancin, flush the IV line before and after each oritavancin infusion with D5W. If an infusion reaction occurs, temporarily stop or slow the infusion as indicated.

ACTIONS

Oritavancin is a semi-synthetic lipoglycopeptide antibacterial drug. It exerts a concentration-dependent bactericidal activity in vitro against *Staphylococcus aureus, Streptococcus pyogenes,* and *Enterococcus faecalis*. It has three mechanisms of action (1) inhibition of the transglycosylation (polymerization) step of cell wall biosynthesis by binding to the stem peptide of peptidoglycan precursors, (2) inhibition of the transpeptidation (cross-linking) step of cell wall biosynthesis by binding to the peptide bridging segments of the cell wall, and (3) disruption of bacterial membrane integrity, leading to depolarization, permeabilization, and cell death. Approximately 85% bound to plasma proteins. Extensively distributed into tissue. Not metabolized. Terminal half-life is approximately 245 hours. Minimally excreted as unchanged drug in feces and urine.

INDICATIONS AND USES

Treatment of adult patients with acute bacterial skin and skin structure infections (ABSSSI) caused by susceptible isolates of designated Gram-positive microorganisms, including *S. aureus* (both methicillin-susceptible [MSSA] and methicillin-resistant [MRSA] strains).

CONTRAINDICATIONS

Known hypersensitivity to oritavancin. ▪ Use of IV unfractionated heparin sodium is contraindicated for 120 hours (5 days) after oritavancin administration because aPTT test results are expected to remain falsely elevated for up to 120 hours (5 days).

PRECAUTIONS

Oritavancin artificially prolongs the PT and INR for up to 12 hours, making the monitoring of the anticoagulation effect of warfarin unreliable up to 12 hours after an oritavancin dose. Patients receiving both warfarin and oritavancin should be monitored for S/S of bleeding; see Drug/Lab Interactions. ▪ The aPTT has been shown to be artificially prolonged for up to 120 hours, the PT and INR for up to 12 hours, and the activated clotting time (ACT) for up to 24 hours after administration of oritavancin. D-Dimer concentrations have been shown to be elevated for up to 72 hours after administration; see Drug/Lab Interactions. ▪ Serious hypersensitivity reactions have been reported. Check history of previous hypersensitivity reactions to glycopeptides (e.g., dalbavancin, telavancin, vancomycin). Exercise caution in patients with a history of glycopeptide allergy; cross-sensitivity is possible. ▪ Infusion-related reactions have been reported; see Rate of Administration. ▪ To reduce the development of drug-resistant bacteria and maintain its effectiveness, oritavancin should be used to treat only those infections proven or strongly suspected to be caused by bacteria. ▪ Specific sensitivity studies are indicated to determine susceptibility of the causative organism to oritavancin. ▪ *Clostridium difficile*–associated diarrhea (CDAD) has been reported for nearly all systemic antibacterial agents and may range in severity from mild diarrhea to fatal colitis. Consider in patients who present with diarrhea after treatment with oritavancin. ▪ In clinical trials, more cases of osteomyelitis were reported in the oritavancin-treated arm than in the vancomycin-treated arm. If osteomyelitis is suspected or diagnosed, institute appropriate alternate antibacterial therapy. ▪ The pharmacokinetics of oritavancin has not been studied in patients with severe renal or hepatic impairment.

Monitor: Frequently monitor patients on chronic warfarin therapy for signs of bleeding. ▪ Monitoring of the anticoagulation effect of warfarin (e.g., PT, INR) is unreliable for up to 12 hours after oritavancin administration; see Precautions and Drug/Lab Interactions. ▪ If aPTT monitoring is required within 120 hours of oritavancin dosing, use a non–phospholipid-dependent coagulation test such as a factor Xa (chromogenic) assay, or consider an alternative anticoagulant not requiring aPTT monitoring. ▪ Monitor for S/S of hypersensitivity (e.g., hypotension, rash, urticaria, tightness of the chest, wheezing). In clinical trials, the median onset of hypersensitivity reactions was 1.2 days and the median duration of these reactions was 2.4 days. ▪ Monitor for S/S of an infusion reaction. Reactions may include flushing of the upper body, pruritus, rash, and/or urticaria ("redman syndrome"); see Rate of Administration. ▪ Monitor for S/S of osteomyelitis; see Antidote.

Patient Education: Promptly report S/S of a hypersensitivity reaction (e.g., hives, rash, shortness of breath, wheezing) or an infusion reaction (e.g., flushing of the upper body, pruritus, rash, and/or urticaria). ▪ Promptly report diarrhea or bloody stools that occur up to several months after antibiotic therapy; may indicate CDAD and require treatment.

Maternal/Child: Category C: use during pregnancy only if the potential benefit outweighs the potential risk to the fetus. ▪ Use caution during breastfeeding. ▪ Safety and effectiveness for use in pediatric patients not established.

Elderly: Numbers in clinical studies insufficient to determine if the elderly respond differently from younger subjects. Differences have not been identified. However, greater sensitivity of some older individuals cannot be ruled out.

DRUG/LAB INTERACTIONS

Clinical drug-drug interaction studies have not been conducted. ▪ A screening drug-drug interaction study indicated that oritavancin is a nonspecific weak inducer of CYP3A4 and CYP2D6 and a weak inhibitor of CYP2C9 and CYP2C19. Caution should be used when administering oritavancin with drugs that have a narrow therapeutic window and are predominantly metabolized by one of the affected CYP_{450} enzymes (e.g., **warfarin**). Coadministration may increase or decrease concentrations of drugs with a narrow therapeutic range. ▪ Oritavancin has been shown to artificially prolong aPTT for up to 120 hours, PT and INR for up to 12 hours, and ACT for up to 24 hours after administration of a single 1,200-mg dose by binding to and preventing the action of the phospholipid reagents that activate coagulation in commonly used laboratory coagulation tests. Oritavancin has also been shown to elevate D-dimer concentration up to 72 hours after oritavancin administration. ▪ Oritavancin does not affect chromogenic factor Xa assay, thrombin time (TT), or tests that are used for the diagnosis of heparin-induced thrombocytopenia (HIT). ▪ Oritavancin has no effect on the coagulation system in vivo. ▪ In vitro, oritavancin demonstrated synergistic bactericidal activity in combination with gentamicin, linezolid, moxifloxacin, and rifampin against designated organisms.

SIDE EFFECTS

The most common side effects reported are diarrhea, headache, limb and subcutaneous abscesses, and nausea and vomiting. Hypersensitivity and/or infusion reactions and CDAD may be severe. Cellulitis, dizziness, increased ALT and AST levels, infusion site reactions or phlebitis, osteomyelitis, and tachycardia were also reported. Many other side effects occurred in fewer than 1.5% of patients.

ANTIDOTE

Notify physician of any side effects. Discontinue the drug if indicated. Treat hypersensitivity reactions as indicated (e.g., diphenhydramine, epinephrine, albuterol) and resuscitate as necessary. Temporarily discontinue or slow infusion for infusion-related reactions. Mild cases of CDAD may respond to discontinuation of oritavancin. Treat CDAD with fluids, electrolytes, protein supplements, and appropriate antibiotics (e.g., oral vancomycin) as indicated. In severe cases, surgical evaluation may be indicated. If osteomyelitis is suspected or diagnosed, institute appropriate alternate antibacterial therapy. Oritavancin is not removed by hemodialysis.

OXALIPLATIN BBW

(**OX**-al-ee-**plah**-tin)

Antineoplastic

Eloxatin

USUAL DOSE

Pretreatment: Verify pregnancy status. Baseline studies required; see Monitor.

Both indications: Given in combination with 5-FU and leucovorin calcium in a dose schedule that repeats every 2 weeks. When used as adjuvant therapy in patients with stage III colon cancer, a treatment period repeated every 2 weeks for 6 months is recommended (a total of 12 cycles). For advanced disease, treatment is recommended until disease progression or unacceptable toxicity. For information on 5-FU and leucovorin calcium, see respective monographs. Prehydration is not required. Premedication with antiemetics recommended; see Monitor. Some clinicians are administering magnesium and calcium before and after oxaliplatin to decrease neurotoxicity.

Day 1: Oxaliplatin 85 mg/M^2 and leucovorin calcium 200 mg/M^2, both given as an IV infusion over 120 minutes at the same time in separate bags using a Y-line. Follow with 5-FU 400 mg/M^2 IV bolus given over 2 to 4 minutes, followed by 5-FU 600 mg/M^2 in 500 mL D5W (recommended) as a 22-hour continuous infusion.

Day 2: Leucovorin calcium 200 mg/M^2 IV infusion over 120 minutes. Follow with 5-FU 400 mg/M^2 IV bolus given over 2 to 4 minutes, followed by 5-FU 600 mg/M^2 in 500 mL D5W (recommended) as a 22-hour continuous infusion.

DOSE ADJUSTMENTS

Decrease starting dose to 65 mg/M^2 in patients with severe renal impairment (CrCl less than 30 mL/min). ■ Withhold oxaliplatin for sepsis or septic shock, and reduce dose if indicated as outlined in the following sections.

Advanced colorectal cancer: Dose adjustments are based on clinical toxicities. Reduce dose of oxaliplatin to 65 mg/M^2 in patients who experience persistent Grade 2 neurosensory events that do not resolve. (See Monitor for study-specific neurotoxicity scale.) The infusional 5-FU/leucovorin calcium regimen need not be altered. ■ Reduce dose of oxaliplatin to 65 mg/M^2 and 5-FU to a 300 mg/M^2 bolus and 500 mg/M^2 as a 22-hour infusion in patients who develop Grade 3 or 4 gastrointestinal toxicity (despite prophylactic treatment), Grade 4 neutropenia, febrile neutropenia, or Grade 3 or 4 thrombocytopenia. Delay next dose until neutrophils are greater than or equal to 1.5×10^9/L (1500 cells/mm^3) and platelets are greater than or equal to 75×10^9/L (75,000 cells/mm^3).

Adjuvant therapy in stage III colon cancer (postoperative): Reduce dose of oxaliplatin to 75 mg/M^2 in patients who experience persistent Grade 2 neurosensory events that do not resolve (NCICTC scale version 1 used). The infusional 5-FU/leucovorin calcium regimen need not be altered. ■ Reduce dose of oxaliplatin to 75 mg/M^2 and 5-FU to a 300 mg/M^2 bolus and 500 mg/M^2 as a 22-hour infusion in patients who develop Grade 3 or 4 gastrointestinal toxicity (despite prophylactic treatment), Grade 4 neutropenia, febrile neutropenia, or Grade 3 or 4 thrombocytopenia. Delay next dose until neutrophils are greater than or equal to 1.5×10^9/L (1,500 cells/mm^3) and platelets are greater than or equal to 75×10^9/L (75,000 cells/mm^3).

Both indications: Consider discontinuing therapy in patients with persistent Grade 3 neurosensory events.

DILUTION

Specific techniques required; see Precautions.

Do not reconstitute or dilute with a sodium chloride solution (e.g., NS, ½NS, ¼NS) or other chloride-containing solutions. Available as a concentrate for solution. The concentrate for solution must be further diluted with 250 to 500 mL of D5W. ***Do not use NS or any chloride-containing solutions; see Compatibility.*** Do not use needles or administration sets with aluminum parts; a precipitate may form, and potency may decrease.

Storage: Store vials with concentrate in the original carton at CRT. Protect vials with concentrate from light and do not freeze. After final dilution with 250 to 500 mL of D5W, the solution may be stored for up to 6 hours at RT (20° to 25° C [68° to 77° F]) or up to 24 hours under refrigeration.

COMPATIBILITY

Manufacturer states oxaliplatin "is **incompatible** in solution with alkaline medications or media (such as basic solutions of 5-FU) and must not be mixed with these or administered simultaneously through the same infusion line. *The infusion line should be flushed with D5W prior to administration of any concomitant medication.*" Reconstitution or final dilution must not be performed with a sodium chloride solution or other chloride-containing solutions. Do not use needles or administration sets with aluminum parts; a precipitate may form, and potency may decrease.

Other sources suggest a few specific **compatibilities** dependent on concentration and manufacturer; consult a pharmacist.

RATE OF ADMINISTRATION

The infusion line should be flushed with D5W prior to administration of any concomitant medication.

Day 1: Oxaliplatin and leucovorin calcium are given as infusions and equally distributed over 120 minutes. Given at the same time in separate bags using a Y-line. When complete, flush the IV line with D5W. Follow with a **5-FU bolus** administered over 2 to 4 minutes, followed by a **5-FU continuous infusion** equally distributed over 22 hours. ▪ Increasing the infusion time of oxaliplatin from 2 to 6 hours may mitigate acute toxicities. The infusion times for 5-FU and leucovorin calcium need not be altered.

Day 2: Leucovorin calcium is given as an infusion equally distributed over 120 minutes. Follow with a **5-FU bolus** administered over 2 to 4 minutes, followed by a **5-FU continuous infusion** equally distributed over 22 hours.

ACTIONS

A platinum-based antineoplastic agent. Undergoes nonenzymatic conversion to active derivatives that inhibit DNA replication and transcription. Cytotoxicity is cell cycle nonspecific. Rapidly distributed into tissues or eliminated in the urine. Highly protein bound. Undergoes rapid and extensive nonenzymatic biotransformation. No evidence of cytochrome P_{450}-mediated metabolism. Major route of elimination is renal excretion.

INDICATIONS AND USES

Used in combination with infusional 5-FU and leucovorin calcium for the treatment of patients with advanced colorectal cancer and for adjuvant therapy of stage III colon cancer patients who have undergone complete resection of the primary tumor.

CONTRAINDICATIONS

Hypersensitivity to oxaliplatin or other platinum-containing compounds (e.g., carboplatin, cisplatin).

PRECAUTIONS

Follow guidelines for handling cytotoxic agents. See Appendix A, p. 1308. ▪ Administered by or under the direction of the physician specialist. ▪ Adequate diagnostic and treatment facilities and emergency resuscitation equipment and supplies must always be available. ▪ Hypersensitivity and anaphylactic-like reactions, some fatal, have been reported and may occur within minutes of administration and during any cycle. Rechallenge is contraindicated. See Side Effects and Antidote. ▪ Use with caution in patients with renal impairment; see Dose Adjustments. ▪ Associated with two types of neuropathy. *The first type is an acute, reversible, primarily peripheral sensory neuropathy that is of early onset, occurs within hours or 1 to 2 days of dosing, resolves within 14 days, and frequently recurs with further dosing.* Symptoms may be precipitated or exacerbated by exposure to cold temperature or cold objects. Usually presents as transient paresthesia (abnormal sensation [e.g., burning, prickling]), dysesthesia (decreased sensitivity to stimulation), and hypoesthesia (impairment of any sense, especially touch) in the hands, feet, perioral area, or throat. *The second type is a persistent (lasting more than 14 days), primarily peripheral, sensory neuropathy that is usually characterized by paresthesias, dysesthesias, and hypoesthesias but may also include deficits in proprioception (stimulus of the sensory end organs [e.g., muscles, tendons]), which can interfere with daily activities (e.g., writing, buttoning, swallowing, and walking).* May occur without any prior acute neuropathy event. Symptoms may or may not improve with discontinuation of oxaliplatin. ▪ Reversible posterior leukoencephalopathy syndrome (RPLS, also known as PRES [posterior reversible encephalopathy syndrome]) has been reported; see Monitor. ▪ Grade 3 or 4 neutropenia has occurred in patients treated with oxaliplatin. Sepsis, neutropenic sepsis, and septic shock have been reported. Deaths have occurred; see Dose Adjustments. ▪ Has been associated with pulmonary fibrosis, which may be fatal; see Monitor. ▪ Hepatotoxicity has been reported; see Monitor. ▪ QT prolongation and ventricular arrhythmias, including fatal torsades de pointes, have been reported. Avoid oxaliplatin in patients with congenital long QT syndrome; see Monitor and Drug/Lab Interactions. ▪ Rhabdomyolysis, including fatal cases, has been reported. ▪ See Drug/Lab Interactions.

Monitor: CBC with differential, platelet count, and blood chemistries (including ALT, AST, bilirubin, and creatinine) are recommended before each cycle. See Dose Adjustments and Precautions. ▪ Monitor for S/S of a hypersensitivity reaction (e.g., bronchospasm, chest pain, diaphoresis, diarrhea associated with oxaliplatin infusion, disorientation, erythema, flushing, hypotension, pruritus, rash, shortness of breath, syncope, urticaria). ▪ Monitor for S/S of RPLS; may include abnormal vision from blurriness to blindness, altered mental functioning, headache, or seizures with or without associated hypertension. Diagnosis of RPLS is based on confirmation by brain imaging. ▪ Monitor for unexplained respiratory symptoms such as nonproductive cough, dyspnea, crackles, or radiologic pulmonary infiltrates. Discontinue oxaliplatin until pulmonary investigation rules out interstitial lung disease or pulmonary fibrosis. ▪ Monitor for S/S of neuropathy (e.g., transient paresthesia [abnormal sensation (e.g., burning, prickling)], dysesthesia [decreased sensitivity to stimulation], and hypoesthesia [impairment of any sense, especially touch] in the hands, feet, perioral area, or throat). Neurotoxicity scale used during advanced colorectal cancer studies differed from National Cancer Institute toxicity grading. Grading scale for paresthesias/dysesthesias was as follows: Grade 1, resolved and did not interfere with functioning; Grade 2, interfered with function but not daily activities; Grade 3, pain or functional impairment that interfered with daily activities; Grade 4, persistent impairment that is disabling or life-threatening. ▪ Nausea and vomiting may be significant. Prophylactic administration of antiemetics, including 5HT$_3$ blockers (e.g., ondansetron), with or without dexamethasone, is recommended. ▪ Observe closely for signs of infection, sepsis, or septic shock. Prophylactic antibiotics may be indicated pending results of C/S in a febrile neutropenic patient. ▪ Monitor for S/S of hepatotoxicity. Hepatic vascular disorders should be considered in the case of abnormal liver function test results or portal hypertension that cannot be explained by liver metastases. ▪ ECG monitoring is recommended for patients with CHF, bradyarrhythmias, drugs known to prolong the QT interval, and electrolyte abnormalities. Correct hypokalemia and hypomagnesemia before initiating oxaliplatin therapy, and monitor these electrolytes periodically during therapy; see Drug/Lab Interactions. ▪ Monitor for S/S of rhabdomyolysis (muscle pain, weakness, dark urine, elevation in creatinine kinase [CK] and other serum muscle enzymes).

Patient Education: Avoid pregnancy. Effective birth control recommended. ▪ Report any neurologic symptoms (e.g., confusion or a change in the way you think; headache; numbness, pain, or tingling in extremities; seizures; sensitivity to cold; troubled breathing or swallowing; vision problems). Acute neurosensory toxicity may be precipitated or exacerbated by exposure to cold. Avoid cold drinks and use of ice. Cover exposed skin before exposure to cold temperature. ▪ Promptly report persistent vomiting, diarrhea, breathing difficulty, cough, or any sign of infection, allergic reaction, or dehydration. ▪ Use caution while driving or using machines; neurologic symptoms (e.g., dizziness), nausea and vomiting, and vision abnormalities (e.g., transient vision loss) may interfere with abilities. ▪ Manufacturer supplies a patient information leaflet; read before taking oxaliplatin. ▪ See Appendix D, p. 1311.

Maternal/Child: Category D: avoid pregnancy; may cause fetal harm. ▪ Discontinue breastfeeding. ▪ Safety and effectiveness for use in pediatric patients not established. Has been studied in a small number of solid tumors in pediatric patients. No significant response was observed. See manufacturer's literature.

Elderly: The overall rates of adverse events, including Grade 3 and 4 events, were similar for all age-groups. However, the incidence of dehydration, diarrhea, fatigue, Grade 3 to 4 granulocytopenia, hypokalemia, leukopenia, and syncope were higher in patients 65 years of age or older. Adjustment of starting dose is not required.

DRUG/LAB INTERACTIONS

Formal studies have not been performed. ▪ Do not administer **live virus vaccines** to patients receiving antineoplastic agents. ▪ Platinum-containing species are eliminated primarily through the kidney; clearance of these products may be decreased by coadministration of potentially **nephrotoxic compounds** (e.g., aminoglycosides [e.g., gentamicin], amphotericin B [all formulations], NSAIDs [e.g., ibuprofen, naproxen], pamidronate, tacrolimus). ▪ Oxaliplatin is not metabolized by, nor does it inhibit, cytochrome P_{450} isoenzymes. P450-mediated interactions are not anticipated. ▪ A prolonged PT and INR (occasionally associated with hemorrhage) has been reported when oxaliplatin is used concomitantly with **anticoagulants** (e.g., warfarin); close monitoring of PT and INR recommended. ▪ Use caution when administered with **drugs known to prolong the QT interval** (e.g., Class Ia and III antiarrhythmics [e.g., disopyramide, procainamide, quinidine, amiodarone], macrolide antibiotics [e.g., azithromycin, clarithromycin], fluoroquinolones [e.g., ciprofloxacin, levofloxacin], antiemetics [e.g., dolasetron, ondansetron]). ECG monitoring recommended.

SIDE EFFECTS

Are frequent and numerous. The most common adverse reactions are anemia, diarrhea, fatigue, increased liver function tests (e.g., alkaline phosphatase, total bilirubin, and transaminases), nausea, neutropenia, peripheral sensory neuropathies, stomatitis, thrombocytopenia, and vomiting; see Precautions. Other reported reactions include abdominal pain, alopecia, angioedema, anorexia, arthralgia, back pain, chest pain, conjunctivitis, constipation, coughing, deafness, dehydration, dizziness, dyspepsia, dyspnea, dysuria, edema, elevated serum creatinine, epistaxis, fever, flushing, gastroesophageal reflux, hand-foot syndrome, headache, hematuria, hemolytic uremic syndrome, hypersensitivity reactions (e.g., anaphylaxis, angioedema, bronchospasm, erythema, hypotension, laryngospasm, pruritus, rash, urticaria), hypertension, hypokalemia, immunoallergic hemolytic anemia, infection, injection site reaction, insomnia, intestinal obstruction, lacrimation abnormalities, metabolic acidosis, mucositis, pain, pancreatitis, persistent vomiting, pharyngitis, pulmonary fibrosis, rhinitis, rigors, secondary malignancies, taste perversion, thromboembolism, veno-occlusive disease of the liver, visual disorders (e.g., decrease of visual acuity, visual field disturbance, optic neuritis), weight gain. Many other side effects have been reported and may occur.

Overdose: Chest pain, dehydration, diarrhea, dyspnea, enlarged abdomen and Grade 4 intestinal obstruction, hypersensitivity reactions, myelosuppression, nausea and vomiting, neurotoxicity, paresthesia, respiratory failure, severe bradycardia, stomatitis, wheezing, and death.

Post-Marketing: Acute interstitial nephritis, acute renal failure, acute tubular necrosis, colitis (including *Clostridium difficile* diarrhea), convulsions, cranial nerve palsies, dysarthria, fasciculations, hemolytic uremic syndrome, ileus, immunoallergic hemolytic anemia, Lhermitte's sign, loss of deep tendon reflexes, metabolic acidosis, perisinusoidal fibrosis, pulmonary fibrosis and other interstitial lung diseases (sometimes fatal), QT prolongation leading to ventricular arrhythmias (including fatal torsades de pointes), rhabdomyolysis (including fatal outcomes), reversible posterior leukoencephalopathy syndrome (RPLS), septic shock (including fatal cases), severe diarrhea/vomiting resulting in hypokalemia, transient vision loss (reversible after oxaliplatin is discontinued).

ANTIDOTE

Notify physician of all side effects. Oxaliplatin may need to be discontinued permanently or until recovery. Slowing of infusion rate may help mitigate acute toxicities. Symptomatic and supportive treatment is indicated. Administration of whole blood products (e.g., packed RBCs, platelets, leukocytes) and/or blood modifiers (e.g., darbepoetin alfa [Aranesp], epoetin alfa [Epogen], filgrastim [Neupogen, Zarxio], pegfilgrastim [Neulasta], sargramostim [Leukine]) may be indicated to treat bone marrow toxicity. Treat anaphylaxis with epinephrine, corticosteroids, oxygen, and antihistamines (diphenhydramine). There is no specific antidote. Resuscitate as indicated.

OXYTOCIN INJECTION BBW

(ox-eh-**TOE**-sin in-**JEK**-shun)

Pitocin

Oxytocic
Antihemorrhagic

pH 2.5 to 4.5

USUAL DOSE

Determined by uterine response and intended use, dilution, and rate of administration. Dose must be individualized and initiated at a very low level. Piggyback oxytocin into a physiologic electrolyte IV solution (e.g., NS) without oxytocin; see Precautions.

Induction of labor: 0.5 to 1 milliunits/min (equal to 3 to 6 mL/hr of properly diluted solution). See Dilution and Rate of Administration.

Control of postpartum bleeding: See Dilution and Rate of Administration.

Incomplete, inevitable, or elective abortion: A total of 10 milliunits delivered at 10 to 20 milliunits/min. A total dose should not exceed 30 milliunits in a 12-hour period due to the risk of water intoxication. See Dilution and Rate of Administration.

DILUTION

In all situations, rotate gently to distribute medication through solution.

Induction of labor: Dilute 1 mL (10 milliunits) in 1 liter of NS or LR for infusion (10 milliunits/mL).

Control of postpartum bleeding: Dilute 1 to 4 mL (10 to 40 milliunits) in 1 liter of above infusion fluids (10 to 40 milliunits/mL).

Incomplete, inevitable, or elective abortion: Dilute 1 mL (10 milliunits) in 500 mL of NS or D5W.

Storage: Store at CRT.

COMPATIBILITY

Rapidly decomposes in the presence of sodium bisulfate.

Other sources suggest a few specific **compatibilities** dependent on concentration and manufacturer; consult a pharmacist.

RATE OF ADMINISTRATION

Given only as an IV infusion. Use of an infusion pump or other accurate control device is required. In all situations, use the minimum effective rate and monitor strength, frequency, and duration of contractions; resting uterine tone; fetal HR (in induction of labor); and maternal BP; see Monitor.

Induction of labor: Begin with 0.5 to 1 milliunits/min (3 to 6 mL/hr), and increase in increments of 1 to 2 milliunits/min at 30- to 60-minute intervals until contractions simulate normal labor. Maximum dose rarely exceeds 9 to 10 milliunits/min at term; average is 2 to 5 milliunits/min. Reduce by similar increments when desired frequency of contractions is reached and labor has progressed to 5 to 6 cm. 6 milliunits/min provides oxytocin levels similar to spontaneous labor. Preterm induction may require somewhat higher doses due to a lower concentration of oxytocin receptors; use caution.

Control of postpartum bleeding: Adjust rate of infusion to sustain contractions and control uterine atony.

Incomplete, inevitable, or elective abortion: 10 to 20 milliunits/min. Total dose should not exceed 30 milliunits in a 12-hour period due to the risk of water intoxication.

ACTIONS

A synthetic posterior pituitary hormone that will produce rhythmic contraction of uterine smooth muscle. Has specific receptors in the myometrium, and the receptor concentration increases greatly during pregnancy. Promotes contractions by increasing the intracellular calcium. Distributed throughout the extracellular fluid. Onset of action is almost immediate. Half-life is 1 to 6 minutes. Duration of action is approximately 1 hour. Is the drug of choice for induction of delivery. Rapidly removed from plasma via liver and kidney. Only small amounts are excreted in urine unchanged. May exhibit antidiuretic and pressor effects at higher doses. Probably crosses the placental barrier in small amounts.

INDICATIONS AND USES

Antepartum: Indicated for the initiation or improvement of uterine contractions (when these are desirable and considered suitable for reasons of fetal or maternal concern) in order to achieve vaginal delivery. Indicated for (1) induction of labor in patients with a medical indication (e.g., Rh problems, maternal diabetes, pre-eclampsia at or near term) or when membranes are prematurely ruptured and delivery is indicated; (2) stimulation or reinforcement of labor, as in selected cases of uterine inertia; and (3) as adjunctive therapy in the management of incomplete or inevitable abortion. In the first trimester, curettage is generally considered primary therapy. In second-trimester abortion, oxytocin infusion will often be successful in emptying the uterus. However, other means of therapy may be required.

Postpartum: Indicated to produce uterine contractions during the third stage of labor and to control postpartum bleeding or hemorrhage. ▪ Not indicated for elective induction of labor (i.e., the initiation of labor in a pregnant individual who has no medical indication for induction).

CONTRAINDICATIONS

Cephalopelvic disproportion, fetal malpresentation, hypersensitivity, hypertonic uterine contractions, lack of satisfactory progress with adequate uterine activity, obstetrical emergencies in which the benefit-to-risk ratio for either the fetus or the mother favors surgical intervention (e.g., abruptio placentae), or when vaginal delivery is contraindicated (e.g., active herpes genitalis, cord presentation or prolapse, invasive cervical carcinoma, total placenta previa and vasa previa). See Precautions.

PRECAUTIONS

An NS IV without oxytocin should be hung, connected by Y-tube, and ready for use in adverse reactions. ▪ Should be administered only in the hospital under continuous observation by trained personnel; the physician must be immediately available. ▪ The use of oxytocin for fetal distress, hydramnios, partial placenta previa, prematurity, borderline cephalopelvic disproportion, or any condition that may cause uterine rupture (e.g., previous major surgery on the cervix or uterus, including cesarean section, uterine overdistension, grand multiparity, or past history of uterine sepsis or traumatic delivery) is not recommended except in unusual circumstances. ▪ Maternal deaths due to hypertensive episodes, subarachnoid hemorrhage, and uterine rupture, as well as fetal deaths due to various causes, have been reported. ▪ When used for induction or reinforcement of already existing labor, patients should be carefully selected. Evaluate pelvic adequacy and maternal and fetal conditions before use.

Monitor: When properly administered, oxytocin should stimulate uterine contractions comparable to normal labor. Monitor BP, fetal heart tones, strength and timing of contractions, and resting uterine tone. Continuous observation of patient required. ▪ Electronic fetal monitoring provides the best means of early detection of overdose. A fetal scalp electrode provides a more accurate recording of fetal HR than external monitoring. ▪ Has an intrinsic antidiuretic effect, increasing water reabsorption from the glomerular filtrate. Monitor oral fluid intake and observe for signs of water intoxication. ■ See Precautions and Drug/Lab Interactions.

Maternal/Child: There is no indication for use in the first trimester of pregnancy other than in relation to spontaneous or induced abortion. Not expected to present a risk if used as indicated; see Indications and Contraindications.

DRUG/LAB INTERACTIONS

Severe hypertension can result in the presence of a **vasoconstrictor** given in conjunction with a **local or regional anesthetic** (caudal or spinal) **and with dopamine, ephedrine, epinephrine, and other vasopressors.** ■ Concurrent use with **cyclopropane anesthesia** may cause hypotension and/or sinus bradycardia with abnormal atrioventricular rhythms. ■ **Prostaglandins** (e.g., dinoprostone) may potentiate the uterine response to oxytocin, increasing the risk of uterine hyperstimulation and rupture.

SIDE EFFECTS

Maternal: Anaphylaxis; cardiac arrhythmias; fatal afibrinogenemia; fluid retention leading to water intoxication and coma, convulsion, and death; hypertension; increased blood loss; nausea; pelvic hematoma; postpartum hemorrhage; PVCs; severe uterine hypertonicity, spasm, or tetanic contraction; subarachnoid hemorrhage; uterine rupture; vomiting.

Fetal: Bradycardia, brain damage, CNS damage, death, low Apgar scores, neonatal jaundice, PVCs and other arrhythmias, retinal hemorrhage, seizures.

ANTIDOTE

Nausea and vomiting are tolerable and can be treated symptomatically. Immediately call the physician's attention to any side effect noted or suspected; many can be fatal. Discontinue the drug immediately for any signs of fetal distress, uterine hyperactivity, tetanic contractions, uterine resting tone exceeding 15 to 20 mm Hg, or water intoxication. Use of a Y-connection, allowing the oxytocin drip to be discontinued while the vein is kept open, is recommended. Turn mother on side (to prevent fetal anoxia) and administer oxygen. Restriction of fluids, diuresis, hypertonic saline solutions IV, correction of electrolyte imbalance, control of convulsions with cautious use of barbiturates, or the use of magnesium sulfate may be required. These side effects can occur during labor and delivery and into the postpartum period. Careful evaluation and selection of patients eliminate many hazards, but be prepared for an emergency.

PACLITAXEL · PACLITAXEL PROTEIN-BOUND PARTICLES FOR INJECTABLE SUSPENSION (ALBUMIN-BOUND) BBW

Antineoplastic
(taxane)

(**PACK**-lih-**tax**-el)

Onxol, Taxol ■ **Abraxane**

pH 4.4 to 5.6 ■ not available

USUAL DOSE

Pretreatment: Verify pregnancy status. Baseline studies required; see Monitor and Dose Adjustments.

CONVENTIONAL PACLITAXEL

Several regimens of paclitaxel, alone or in combination with other antineoplastics, are in use. Doses vary, depending on the regimen used. Consult literature. ■ For all uses, pre-medication, specific parameters, and specific equipment are required before or during administration; see Premedication, Dose Adjustments, and Precautions/Monitor.

Premedication: Must be premedicated before each dose to prevent severe hypersensitivity reactions. Usual regimen includes oral dexamethasone 20 mg 12 and 6 hours before; IV diphenhydramine 50 mg 30 to 60 minutes before; and an H_2 antagonist (e.g., famotidine 20 mg) 30 to 60 minutes before dosing with paclitaxel. When premedicating patients with AIDS-related Kaposi's sarcoma, reduce the dose of dexamethasone to 10 mg at 12 and 6 hours before paclitaxel. The doses of IV diphenhydramine and IV H_2 antagonists remain as above.

Ovarian cancer in previously untreated patients: 135 mg/M^2 as an infusion over 24 hours. Follow with cisplatin 75 mg/M^2 as an infusion over 6 to 8 hours. Repeat every 3 weeks. An alternative regimen is paclitaxel 175 mg/M^2 as an infusion over 3 hours. Follow with cisplatin 75 mg/M^2 (one source suggests an infusion over 24 hours; another suggests 6 to 8 hours, which would allow for outpatient therapy). Repeat every 3 weeks. See comments under Usual Dose.

Ovarian cancer in patients previously treated with chemotherapy: 135 or 175 mg/M^2 as an infusion over 3 hours. An alternate regimen suggests the same dose given as a 24-hour infusion. Repeat every 3 weeks. Larger doses, with or without filgrastim (G-CSF, Neupogen), have produced similar responses. See comments under Usual Dose.

Adjuvant treatment of node-positive breast cancer: 175 mg/M^2 as an infusion over 3 hours. Repeat every 3 weeks for four courses. Administered sequentially to doxorubicin-containing combination therapy. Clinical trials used four courses of doxorubicin and cyclophosphamide. Administer filgrastim (G-CSF) 5 mcg/kg/dose on Days 3 through 10. See comments under Usual Dose.

Breast cancer in patients previously treated with chemotherapy: 175 mg/M^2 as an infusion over 3 hours. Repeat every 3 weeks. An alternate regimen suggests 175 to 250 mg/M^2 over 3 hours every 3 weeks. See comments under Usual Dose.

First-line treatment of non–small-cell lung cancer: 135 mg/M^2 as an infusion over 24 hours. Follow with cisplatin 75 mg/M^2 over 6 to 8 hours. Repeat every 3 weeks. See comments under Usual Dose. A Canadian source recommends 175 mg/M^2 as an infusion over 3 hours followed with cisplatin 75 mg/M^2 over 6 to 8 hours and repeated every 3 weeks.

AIDS-related Kaposi's sarcoma: 135 mg/M^2 as an infusion over 3 hours. An alternate regimen suggests the same dose given as a 24-hour infusion. Repeat every 3 weeks. Another regimen is 100 mg/M^2 as an infusion over 3 hours repeated every 2 weeks. Toxicity somewhat increased with 135 mg/M^2 dose in clinical studies. See comments under Usual Dose.

ABRAXANE

Premedication: Generally not required; see Precautions.

Metastatic breast cancer (MBC): 260 mg/M^2 as an infusion over 30 minutes every 3 weeks.

Non–small-cell lung cancer (NSCLC): 100 mg/M^2 as an infusion over 30 minutes on Days 1, 8, and 15 of each 21-day cycle. Given in combination with carboplatin on Day 1 only of each 21-day cycle, beginning immediately after the completion of Abraxane administration.

Adenocarcinoma of the pancreas: 125 mg/M^2 as an infusion over 30 to 40 minutes followed by gemcitabine 1,000 mg/M^2 as an infusion over 30 to 40 minutes on Days 1, 8, and 15 of each 28-day cycle.

DOSE ADJUSTMENTS

CONVENTIONAL PACLITAXEL

Reduce dose by 20% for subsequent courses in patients who experience severe peripheral neuropathy or severe neutropenia (neutrophils less than 500 cells/mm^3) for 1 week or longer. ▪ Withhold therapy if neutrophils below 1,500/mm^3 or platelets below 100,000/mm^3. ▪ Dose reduction not required in impaired renal function. ▪ In AIDS-related Kaposi's sarcoma the parameters are slightly different. Initiate or repeat paclitaxel only if neutrophil count is equal to or greater than 1,000/mm^3; reduce dose of dexamethasone to 10 mg/dose; reduce dose of paclitaxel by 20% in patients who experience severe neutropenia (neutrophils less than 500/mm^3 for a week or longer); use concomitant filgrastim (G-CSF) as clinically indicated. ▪ Recommendations for dose adjustment of the initial course of therapy in patients with impaired hepatic function are listed in the following chart.

Guidelines for Dose Adjustment of Paclitaxel in Impaired Hepatic Function[a]			
Degree of Hepatic Impairment			
Transaminase Levels		**Bilirubin Levels[b]**	**Recommended TAXOL Dose[c]**
24-Hour Infusion			
<2 × ULN	and	≤1.5 mg/dL	135 mg/M^2
2 to <10 × ULN	and	≤1.5 mg/dL	100 mg/M^2
<10 × ULN	and	1.6-7.5 mg/dL	50 mg/M^2
≥10 × ULN	or	>7.5 mg/dL	Not recommended
3-Hour Infusion			
<10 × ULN	and	≤1.25 × ULN	175 mg/M^2
<10 × ULN	and	1.26-2 × ULN	135 mg/M^2
<10 × ULN	and	2.01-5 × ULN	90 mg/M^2
≥10 × ULN	or	>5 × ULN	Not recommended

[a]These recommendations are based on clinical trials of dosages for patients without hepatic impairment of 135 mg/M^2 over 24 hours or 175 mg/M^2 over 3 hours; data are not available to make dose adjustment recommendations for other regimens (e.g., for AIDS-related Kaposi's sarcoma).

[b]Differences in criteria for bilirubin levels between the 3- and 24-hour infusion are due to differences in clinical trial design.

[c]Dosage recommendations are for the first course of therapy; further dose reduction in subsequent courses should be based on individual tolerance.

ABRAXANE

Adjustment of starting dose is not necessary in patients with mild to moderate renal impairment (CrCl equal to or greater than 30 to less than 90 mL/min). ▪ Withhold therapy in all patients if neutrophils below 1,500/mm^3. ▪ In patients with MBC, withhold therapy if platelets below 100,000/mm^3. ▪ For MBC, reduce dose to 220 mg/M^2 in patients who experience severe neutropenia (neutrophils less than 500 cells/mm^3 for 7 days or more) or severe sensory neuropathy. Further reduce dose to 180 mg/M^2 for subsequent courses if severe neutropenia (less than 500 cells/mm^3 for 7 days or more) or severe sensory neuropathy recurs. ▪ If Grade 3 sensory neuropathy occurs, withhold treatment until resolution to Grade 1 or

Continued

2 for **MBC** or until resolution to less than or equal to Grade 1 for **NSCLC,** followed by a dose reduction for all subsequent courses. ▪ No dose adjustment is necessary for patients with mild hepatic impairment (total bilirubin greater than the ULN and less than or equal to 1.5 times the ULN and AST less than or equal to 10 times the ULN), regardless of indication. ▪ Do not administer Abraxane to patients with total bilirubin greater than 5 times the ULN or AST greater than 10 times the ULN regardless of indication because these patients have not been studied. ▪ Do not administer Abraxane to patients with metastatic adenocarcinoma of the pancreas who have moderate to severe hepatic impairment. ▪ Recommendations for a starting dose in patients with hepatic impairment are shown in the following chart. Doses for subsequent cycles should be based on patient tolerance.

Abraxane Starting Dose Recommendations for Patients With Hepatic Impairment					
Degree of Hepatic Impairment	SGOT (AST) Levels	Bilirubin Levels	Abraxane Dose[a]		
			MBC	NSCLC[b]	Pancreatic[b] Adenocarcinoma
Mild	<10 × ULN and	>ULN to ≤1.5 × ULN	260 mg/M²	100 mg/M²	125 mg/M²
Moderate	<10 × ULN and	>1.5 to ≤3 × ULN	200 mg/M²c	80 mg/M²c	N/R
Severe	<10 × ULN and	>3 to ≤5 × ULN	200 mg/M²c	80 mg/M²c	N/R
	>10 × ULN or	>5 × ULN	N/R	N/R	N/R

MBC, Metastatic breast cancer; *N/R,* not recommended; *NSCLC,* non–small-cell lung cancer.
[a]Dose recommendations are for the first course of therapy. The need for further dose adjustments in subsequent courses should be based on individual tolerance.
[b]Patients with bilirubin levels above the ULN were excluded from clinical trials for pancreatic or lung cancer.
[c]A dose increase to 260 mg/M² for patients with MBC or to 100 mg/M² for patients with NSCLC in subsequent courses should be considered if the patient tolerates the reduced dose for two cycles.

▪ In patients with NSCLC who develop severe neutropenia or thrombocytopenia, withhold therapy until counts recover to an ANC of at least 1,500 cells/mm³ and platelets of at least 100,000 cells/mm³ on Day 1 or to an ANC of at least 500 cells/mm³ and platelets of at least 50,000 cells/mm³ on Day 8 or 15 of the cycle. Upon resumption of dosing, follow dose reduction outlined in the following chart.

Permanent Abraxane Dose Reductions for Hematologic and Neurologic Adverse Drug Reactions in NSCLC		
Adverse Drug Reaction	Occurrence	Weekly Abraxane Dose (mg/M²)
Neutropenic fever (ANC less than 500/mm³ with fever >38° C) **OR** Delay of next cycle by more than 7 days for ANC less than 1,500/mm³ **OR** ANC less than 500/mm³ for more than 7 days	First	75 mg/M²
	Second	50 mg/M²
	Third	Discontinue treatment
Platelet count less than 50,000/mm³	First	75 mg/M²
	Second	Discontinue treatment
Severe sensory neuropathy (Grade 3 or 4)	First	75 mg/M²
	Second	50 mg/M²
	Third	Discontinue treatment

- Dose-level reductions for patients with adenocarcinoma of the pancreas are outlined in the following chart.

Abraxane Dose-Level Reductions for Patients With Adenocarcinoma of the Pancreas		
Dose Level	**Abraxane (mg/M²)**	**Gemcitabine (mg/M²)**
Full dose	125 mg/M²	1,000 mg/M²
1st dose reduction	100 mg/M²	800 mg/M²
2nd dose reduction	75 mg/M²	600 mg/M²
If additional dose reduction required	Discontinue	Discontinue

- Dose modifications for neutropenia and/or thrombocytopenia for patients with adenocarcinoma of the pancreas are provided in the following chart.

Dose Recommendations and Modifications for Neutropenia and/or Thrombocytopenia for Patients With Adenocarcinoma of the Pancreas				
Cycle Day	**ANC (cells/mm³)**		**Platelet Count (cells/mm³)**	**Abraxane/Gemcitabine**
Day 1	<1,500	or	<100,000	Delay doses until recovery
Day 8	500 to <1,000	or	50,000 to <75,000	Reduce 1 dose level
	<500	or	<50,000	Withhold doses
Day 15: If Day 8 doses were reduced or given without modification:				
	500 to <1,000	or	50,000 to <75,000	Reduce 1 dose level from Day 8
	<500	or	<50,000	Withhold doses
Day 15: If Day 8 doses were withheld:				
	≥1,000	or	≥75,000	Reduce 1 dose level from Day 1
	500 to <1,000	or	50,000 to <75,000	Reduce 2 dose levels from Day 1
	<500	or	<50,000	Withhold doses

ANC, Absolute neutrophil count.

- Dose modifications for other adverse reactions for patients with adenocarcinoma of the pancreas are provided in the following chart.

Dose Modifications for Other Adverse Reactions for Patients With Adenocarcinoma of the Pancreas		
Adverse Drug Reaction	**Abraxane**	**Gemcitabine**
Febrile Neutropenia: Grade 3 or 4	Withhold until fever resolves and ANC ≥1,500; resume at next lower dose level	
Peripheral Neuropathy: Grade 3 or 4	Withhold until improves to ≤Grade 1; resume at next lower dose level	No dose reduction
Cutaneous Toxicity: Grade 2 or 3	Reduce to next lower dose level; discontinue treatment if toxicity persists	
Gastrointestinal Toxicity: Grade 3 mucositis or diarrhea	Withhold until improves to ≤Grade 1; resume at next lower dose level	

DILUTION
Specific techniques required; see Precautions.
CONVENTIONAL PACLITAXEL
Must be diluted and given as an infusion. May leach the toxic plasticizer DEHP from PVC infusion bags or sets; prepare and store in bottles (glass, polypropylene) or plastic

Continued

bags (polypropylene, polyolefin) and administer through polyethylene-lined administration sets. **Compatible** with NS, D5W, D5NS, or D5R. Final concentration of 0.3 to 1.2 mg/mL required. For a 135 mg/M^2 dose, a large adult (body surface about 2 M^2) will receive 270 mg (45 mL of paclitaxel at 6 mg/mL). Will require dilution in an additional 180 mL to make a 1.2 mg/mL concentration or in an additional 855 mL to make a 0.3 mg/mL concentration. Solution may appear hazy. Do not use a chemo-dispensing pin; can cause the stopper to collapse and result in loss of sterility.

ABRAXANE

Available in single-use vials, each containing 100 mg (5 mg/mL after reconstitution with 20 mL of NS). Calculate the exact number of vials needed to achieve the total dosing volume of suspension required.

$$\text{Total \# of vials required} = \text{Total dose (mg)} \div 100 \text{ mg}$$
$$\text{Dosing volume (mL)} = \text{Total dose (mg)} \div 5 \text{ (mg/mL)}$$

For example, an MBC patient with a body surface area (BSA) of 1.73 M^2 would need a dose of 449.8 mg of Abraxane. 449.8 mg divided by 100 mg equals 4.498 vials, so 5 vials of Abraxane would be needed. 449.8 mg divided by 5 (mg/mL) equals a dosing volume of 90 mL of reconstituted solution.

Reconstitute each 100-mg vial with 20 mL of NS. A specific process is required to avoid foaming or clumping. Over a minimum of 1 minute, slowly inject the NS, directing it to the inside wall of the vial. Do not allow the NS to flow directly onto the lyophilized cake (will cause foaming). Allow each vial to sit for a minimum of 5 minutes while the NS wets the cake. Gently swirl and/or invert each vial slowly for at least 2 minutes until complete dissolution. Avoid generation of foam. If foaming or clumping occurs, allow solution to stand for at least 15 minutes until foam subsides. Solution should be milky and homogenous without visible particulates. If particulates are visible, gently invert to ensure complete resuspension before use.

Withdraw the calculated volume and inject into an empty sterile polyvinyl chloride (PVC) container or a PVC or non–PVC-type infusion bag (a total dosing volume of 90 mL in the previous example). The use of medical devices containing silicone oil as a lubricant (i.e., syringes and IV bags) to reconstitute and administer Abraxane may result in the formation of proteinaceous strands. Discard suspension if proteinaceous strands, particulate matter, or discoloration are observed.

Filters: *Conventional paclitaxel:* Use of an in-line filter not greater than 0.22 microns required for administration.

Storage: *Conventional paclitaxel:* May be stored at CRT or refrigerated before dilution (may appear precipitated under refrigeration; will redissolve at room temperature). Diluted for infusion, it is stable at room temperature for up to 27 hours. *Abraxane:* Store vials in original package at 20° to 25° C (68° to 77° F). Protect from light. Refrigeration or freezing does not affect stability of the product. Immediate use of reconstituted solution is preferred, but reconstituted vial may be refrigerated at 2° to 8° C (36° to 46° F) for a maximum of 24 hours if necessary. If refrigeration required, return to original carton to protect from light. Ensure complete resuspension after removing from refrigerator by gently inverting. Discard unused portions of the vial. Reconstituted solution in an infusion bag should be used immediately; however, it may be refrigerated and protected from bright light for a maximum of 24 hours. The total combined refrigerated storage time of reconstituted Abraxane in the vial and in the infusion bag is 24 hours. This may be followed by storage in the infusion bag at ambient temperature and lighting conditions for a maximum of 4 hours.

COMPATIBILITY

CONVENTIONAL PACLITAXEL

Leaches out plasticizers; see Dilution.

Other sources suggest specific **compatibilities** dependent on concentration and manufacturer; consult a pharmacist.

ABRAXANE

Manufacturer states, "Use of specialized DEHP-free solution containers or administration sets is not necessary." The use of medical devices containing silicone oil as a lubricant (i.e., syringes and IV bags) to reconstitute and administer Abraxane may result in the formation of proteinaceous strands. Additional specific information not available.

RATE OF ADMINISTRATION

CONVENTIONAL PACLITAXEL

A single dose properly diluted must be equally distributed over 3 hours or as indicated in Usual Dose. Use of an in-line filter not greater than 0.22 microns required. Use a metriset (60 gtt/mL) or an infusion pump appropriate to control flow. Rate extended to 24 hours in some regimens.

ABRAXANE

A single dose properly reconstituted and equally distributed over 30 minutes.

ACTIONS

ALL FORMULATIONS

An antineoplastic. A novel antimicrotubule inhibitor. Paclitaxel derived from the bark of Pacific yew has now been replaced by paclitaxel produced semi-synthetically from a renewable source (needles and twigs of the Himalayan yew). Both are chemically identical. Through specific processes it stabilizes microtubules by preventing depolymerization. This action inhibits the normal dynamic reorganization of the microtubule network essential for vital interphase and mitotic cellular functions. Also induces abnormal bundles of microtubules throughout the cell cycle and multiple asters of microtubules during mitosis. Distribution and/or tissue binding is extensive. Evidence suggests metabolism in the liver via the cytochrome P_{450} isoenzyme system (CYP2C8 and CYP3A4). Terminal half-life ranges from 13.1 to 27 hours. Excreted primarily as metabolites in feces and, to a lesser extent, in urine.

CONVENTIONAL PACLITAXEL

More active in patients who have not received previous chemotherapy.

ABRAXANE

Consists of albumin-bound paclitaxel nanoparticles. Highly bound to serum proteins; metabolized in the liver, primarily by CYP2C8 and, to a lesser extent, by CYP3A4. Terminal half-life ranges from 13 to 27 hours. Minimal excretion in urine and feces.

INDICATIONS AND USES

CONVENTIONAL PACLITAXEL

First-line and subsequent therapy for the treatment of advanced carcinoma of the ovary. ▪ First-line treatment for ovarian cancer in combination with cisplatin. ▪ Adjuvant treatment of node-positive breast cancer administered sequentially to standard doxorubicin-containing combination chemotherapy. Most effective in estrogen- and progesterone-receptor–negative tumors. ▪ Metastatic breast cancer refractory to initial chemotherapy or for a relapse within 6 months. ▪ First-line treatment, in combination with cisplatin, for non–small-cell lung cancer in patients who are not candidates for potentially curative surgery or radiation therapy. ▪ Second-line treatment of AIDS-related Kaposi's sarcoma.

ABRAXANE

Treatment of breast cancer after failure of combination chemotherapy for metastatic disease or relapse within 6 months of adjuvant chemotherapy. Prior therapy should have included an anthracycline unless clinically contraindicated. ▪ First-line treatment of locally advanced or metastatic non–small-cell lung cancer (NSCLC) (in combination with carboplatin) in patients who are not candidates for curative surgery or radiation therapy. ▪ First-line treatment of patients with metastatic adenocarcinoma of the pancreas, in combination with gemcitabine.

Unlabeled uses: *Conventional paclitaxel:* Advanced head and neck cancer. ▪ Cancers of the bladder and cervix. ▪ Small-cell lung cancer. ▪ In combination with other agents for treatment of metastatic breast cancer. ■ Relapsed or refractory testicular cancer and testicular germ cell tumors. ■ Treatment of (unknown primary) adenocarcinoma. ***Abraxane:*** Recurrent ovarian, fallopian, and primary peritoneal cancers.

CONTRAINDICATIONS

CONVENTIONAL PACLITAXEL

Baseline neutropenia less than 1,500 cells/mm³ in patients with solid tumors or baseline neutropenia less than 1,000 cells/mm³ in patients with AIDS-related Kaposi's sarcoma. History of prior severe hypersensitivity reactions to paclitaxel or other drugs formulated in polyoxyethylated castor oil (Cremophor EL [e.g., cyclosporine, teniposide]).

ABRAXANE

Baseline neutrophil count less than 1,500 cells/mm³. ■ Patients who experience a severe hypersensitivity reaction to Abraxane should not be rechallenged with the drug.

PRECAUTIONS

ALL FORMULATIONS

Follow guidelines for handling cytotoxic agents. See Appendix A. ■ Usually administered by or under the direction of the physician specialist in a facility with adequate diagnostic and treatment facilities to monitor the patient and respond to any medical emergency.

CONVENTIONAL PACLITAXEL

Use caution in patients with cardiac conduction abnormalities, CHF, and MI within previous 6 months. ■ Bradycardia, hypertension, and hypotension have been observed but rarely required treatment. Occasionally the infusion must be interrupted or discontinued because of initial or recurrent hypertension; see Monitor. ■ Pre-existing neuropathies resulting from prior therapies are not a contraindication for paclitaxel therapy. ■ Various studies show that incidence and severity of neurotoxicity and hematologic toxicity increase with dose, especially above 190 mg/M². ■ Use with caution in patients with a total bilirubin greater than 2 times the ULN. May be at increased risk of toxicity, especially profound myelosuppression; see Dose Adjustments. ■ See Drug/Lab Interactions.

ABRAXANE

Do not substitute for or with other paclitaxel formulations. ■ Use of gloves recommended. Wash skin immediately if contact occurs. Flush mucous membranes thoroughly with water if contact occurs. Topical exposure may result in tingling, burning, and redness. ■ Premedication to prevent hypersensitivity reactions is not required but may be needed in patients who have had a prior hypersensitivity reaction to Abraxane. Reports of severe and sometimes fatal hypersensitivity reactions have occurred; see Contraindications; do not rechallenge patients who have had a severe reaction. ■ Neutropenia is dose dependent and is a dose-limiting toxicity. Do not administer Abraxane to patients with a baseline absolute neutrophil count (ANC) of less than 1,500 cells/mm³; see Dose Adjustments. ■ Sensory neuropathy is dose dependent and schedule dependent and occurs frequently; see Dose Adjustments. ■ Sepsis occurred in 5% of patients, with or without neutropenia, who received Abraxane in combination with gemcitabine. Biliary obstruction or the presence of a biliary stent were risk factors for severe or fatal sepsis. ■ Pneumonitis, including some cases that were fatal, has been reported in patients receiving Abraxane in combination with gemcitabine; see Antidote. ■ Has not been studied in patients with severe renal dysfunction or end-stage renal disease. ■ Use with caution in patients with hepatic impairment. May be at increased risk for toxicity, particularly myelosuppression; see Dose Adjustments. ■ Derived from human albumin; may carry a risk of transmission of viral disease or Creutzfeldt-Jakob disease; risk considered extremely remote. ■ Has not been studied in patients who have had a hypersensitivity reaction to conventional paclitaxel.

Monitor: ALL FORMULATIONS: Neutropenia is dose dependent and is the dose-limiting toxicity. Obtain baseline CBC with differential and platelet count. Monitor frequently during therapy and before each dose. ■ Monitor injection site carefully; avoid extravasation. ■ Observe closely for signs of infection. Prophylactic antibiotics may be indicated pending results of C/S in a febrile neutropenic patient. ■ Use prophylactic antiemetics to reduce nausea and vomiting and increase patient comfort. ■ Monitor for thrombocytopenia (platelet count less than 50,000/mm³). Initiate precautions to prevent excessive bleeding (e.g., inspect IV sites, skin, and mucous membranes; use extreme care during invasive procedures; test urine, emesis, stool, and secretions for occult blood).

CONVENTIONAL PACLITAXEL: Neutrophil nadir occurs around Day 11; see Dose Adjustments. ▪ Monitor VS frequently, particularly during the first hour of the infusion. ▪ Consider obtaining a baseline ECG; arrhythmias have occurred. Continuous cardiac monitoring required for all patients with an abnormal baseline ECG or for those who experienced conduction arrhythmias during administration of a previous dose. ▪ Monitoring of cardiac function is recommended when paclitaxel is used in combination with doxorubicin; see doxorubicin monograph. ▪ Anaphylaxis and severe hypersensitivity reactions characterized by dyspnea, hypotension requiring treatment, angioedema, and generalized urticaria have been reported. Fatal reactions have occurred despite premedication. ▪ Most severe hypersensitivity reactions occur in the first hour; chest pain, dyspnea, flushing, and tachycardia were the most frequent initial symptoms; abdominal pain, diaphoresis, extremity pain, and hypertension also occurred. Monitor all vital signs, including BP, continuously for the first 30 minutes of the infusion and at frequent intervals after that. Incidence seems to decrease with subsequent doses. ▪ Treatment can often be continued in patients with mild hypersensitivity reactions if proper premedication is given. ▪ Monitor injection site carefully; avoid extravasation. Incidence of inflammation increased with 24-hour infusions. Injection site reactions may occur during administration or be delayed by 7 to 10 days. Recurrence of skin reactions at a site of previous extravasation following administration of paclitaxel ("recall") has been reported.

ABRAXANE: Limited infusion time (30 minutes) reduces the likelihood of infusion-related reactions; however, they have been reported; monitor for S/S. ▪ Monitor for S/S of hypersensitivity reactions. ▪ Monitor for S/S of sensory neuropathy. ▪ Monitor for S/S of pneumonitis. ▪ Based on patient history, a baseline ECG may be indicated. ▪ See Precautions and Dose Adjustments.

Patient Education: ALL FORMULATIONS: Effective birth control recommended for males and females; see Maternal/Child. ▪ Review of monitoring requirements and adverse events before therapy imperative. ▪ Report any unusual or unexpected symptoms, side effects, pain or burning at injection site, S/S of a hypersensitivity reaction (e.g., bronchospasm, difficulty breathing, rash, urticaria), signs of infection (e.g., chills, fever, night sweats), signs of sensory neuropathy (e.g., numbness, tingling, or burning in hands and/or feet), signs of pneumonitis (e.g., dry, persistent cough or shortness of breath), or signs of bleeding (e.g., bruising, tarry stools, blood in urine, pinpoint red spots on skin) as soon as possible. ▪ Avoid tasks that require mental alertness (e.g., driving, operating machinery) until the effect of the medication is known. Side effects such as fatigue, lethargy, and malaise may affect the ability to perform these tasks. ▪ See Appendix D, p. 1311. ▪ Obtain name and telephone number of a contact person for emergencies, questions, or problems. ▪ Seek resources for counseling or supportive therapy. ▪ Manufacturer provides a patient information booklet.

Maternal/Child: ALL FORMULATIONS: Category D: females should avoid pregnancy, and males should avoid fathering a child. May cause fetal harm. ▪ Discontinue breast-feeding. ▪ Safety and effectiveness for use in pediatric patients not established.

CONVENTIONAL PACLITAXEL: CNS toxicity (rarely associated with death) was reported in one pediatric trial using high-dose paclitaxel. Use of antihistamines and the ethanol contained in the paclitaxel may have contributed to toxicity noted.

Elderly: ALL FORMULATIONS: Studies suggest response is similar to that seen in younger patients.

CONVENTIONAL PACLITAXEL: Incidence of side effects, including myelosuppression, neuropathy, and cardiovascular events, may be increased in the elderly.

ABRAXANE: Increased incidence of dehydration, diarrhea, epistaxis, fatigue, and peripheral edema was seen in elderly patients receiving Abraxane as monotherapy for MBC. Incidence of myelosuppression, neuropathy, and arthralgia was more common in patients receiving Abraxane and carboplatin for treatment of NSCLC. Incidence of decreased appetite, dehydration, diarrhea, and epistaxis was more common in patients receiving Abraxane and gemcitabine for treatment of adenocarcinoma of the pancreas.

DRUG/LAB INTERACTIONS

ALL FORMULATIONS

Do not administer **chloroquine or live virus vaccines** to patients receiving antineoplastic agents.

CONVENTIONAL PACLITAXEL

Formal drug interaction studies have not been conducted. To reduce potential for profound myelosuppression when using paclitaxel and **cisplatin** concurrently, give paclitaxel first, then cisplatin. ■ Neurotoxicity and symptomatic motor dysfunction occurring with higher doses (greater than 250 mg/M^2) may be potentiated by **cisplatin and filgrastim** (G-CSF). ■ May cause additive effects with **bone marrow–suppressing agents, radiation therapy, or agents that cause blood dyscrasias** (e.g., amphotericin B, antithyroid agents [methimazole], azathioprine, chloramphenicol, ganciclovir, interferon, plicamycin, zidovudine). Reduced doses may be required. ■ May increase levels of **doxorubicin** and its active metabolite when drugs are used in combination. ■ Metabolized by **cytochrome P$_{450}$ isoenzymes CYP3A4 and CYP2C8.** Use caution when administered concomitantly with known **substrates** (e.g., buspirone, eletriptan, felodipine, lovastatin, midazolam, sildenafil, simvastatin, and triazolam), **inhibitors** (e.g., atazanavir, clarithromycin, indinavir, itraconazole, ketoconazole, nefazodone, nelfinavir, ritonavir, saquinavir), **and inducers** (e.g., rifampin and carbamazepine) **of CYP3A4.** ■ **Other medications that are substrates and/ or inducers of CYP3A4** may alter the metabolism of paclitaxel but have not been evaluated in clinical trials. ■ Use caution when administered concomitantly with known **substrates** (e.g., repaglinide), **inhibitors** (e.g., gemfibrozil), **and inducers** (e.g., rifampin) **of CYP2C8.**

ABRAXANE

Drug interaction studies have not been conducted. See All Formulations above. ■ Use caution when administering with medicines **known to inhibit or induce CYP2C8 or CYP3A4.** Drugs that may inhibit these enzymes include ketoconazole and other imidazole antifungals, erythromycin, fluoxetine, gemfibrozil, cimetidine, ritonavir, saquinavir, indinavir, and nelfinavir. Drugs that may induce these enzymes include rifampin, carbamazepine, phenobarbital, phenytoin, efavirenz, and nevirapine.

SIDE EFFECTS

CONVENTIONAL PACLITAXEL

Dose dependent and generally reversible, but may be fatal. All patients were premedicated to prevent hypersensitivity reactions. Abnormal ECG, alopecia, arthralgia/myalgia, asthenia, autonomic neuropathy resulting in paralytic ileus, bleeding, bone marrow suppression (anemia, leukopenia, neutropenia, thrombocytopenia), bradycardia, CHF (including cardiac dysfunction and reduction in left ventricular ejection fraction or ventricular failure [more common in patients receiving combination therapy with anthracyclines]), diarrhea, elevated alkaline phosphatase, elevated AST, elevated bilirubin, febrile neutropenia, fever, fluid retention and edema, hypersensitivity reactions (moderate [e.g., dyspnea, flushing, hypotension, rash, tachycardia]; severe [e.g., chest pain, dyspnea requiring bronchodilators, hypotension requiring treatment, generalized urticaria]), hypertension, hypotension, infections including opportunistic infections (chills, fever, night sweats), injection site reactions (cellulitis, fibrosis, induration, necrosis, phlebitis, skin exfoliation), mucositis, nausea and vomiting, numbness, optic nerve and/or visual disturbances, peripheral neuropathy, respiratory reactions (interstitial pneumonia, lung fibrosis, pleural effusions, pulmonary embolism, respiratory failure), Stevens-Johnson syndrome, toxic epidermal necrolysis, and visual disturbances. A grand mal seizure occurred in one patient. Other side effects (e.g., cardiac arrest, cardiac ischemia/infarction, CVA, hepatic necrosis, and hepatic encephalopathy leading to death; intestinal obstruction; intestinal perforation; ischemic colitis; pancreatitis; thrombosis/ embolism) have been reported rarely. A higher incidence of elevated liver function tests and renal toxicity is seen in Kaposi's sarcoma patients.

Post-Marketing: Diffuse edema, thickening, and sclerosing of the skin; exacerbation of S/S of scleroderma; ototoxicity.

ABRAXANE

Single-agent use in patients with MBC: Abnormal ECG, alopecia, anemia, diarrhea, elevation of alkaline phosphate and AST, fatigue/asthenia, infections (oral candidiasis, pneumonia, and respiratory tract), myalgia/arthralgia, nausea, neutropenia, and sensory neuropathy are most common.

Combination use in patients with NSCLC: Alopecia, anemia, fatigue, nausea, neutropenia, peripheral neuropathy, and thrombocytopenia are most common. The most serious side effects reported are anemia and pneumonia. The most common side effects that result in dose reduction, the withholding of a dose, or a delay in dosing are anemia, neutropenia, and thrombocytopenia. Neutropenia, peripheral neuropathy, and thrombocytopenia sometimes resulted in permanent discontinuation of Abraxane.

Combination use in patients with adenocarcinoma of the pancreas: Alopecia, decreased appetite, dehydration, diarrhea, fatigue, fever, nausea, neutropenia, peripheral edema, peripheral neuropathy, rash, and vomiting. The most common serious side effects are dehydration, fever, pneumonia, and vomiting. The most common side effects that result in dose reduction or delay in dosing are anemia, diarrhea, fatigue, neutropenia, peripheral neuropathy, and thrombocytopenia. The most common side effects resulting in permanent discontinuation are fatigue, peripheral neuropathy, and thrombocytopenia.

All diagnoses with Abraxane: Hypersensitivity reactions have occurred but are not usually severe; premedication is not indicated. Other side effects have been reported and include bradycardia, cardiovascular events (e.g., cardiac ischemia/infarction, SVT), dehydration, extravasation, fever, hypotension, pancytopenia, pneumonitis, pneumothorax, Stevens-Johnson syndrome, toxic epidermal necrolysis, and many others. Frequency of sensory neuropathy may increase with cumulative dose.

Post-Marketing: Many of these side effects occur with paclitaxel and Abraxane and include CHF, left ventricular dysfunction, and atrioventricular block; cranial nerve palsies; hepatic necrosis and hepatic encephalopathy; injection site reactions; interstitial pneumonia; intestinal obstruction or perforation; ischemic colitis; pancreatitis; paralytic ileus; pneumonitis; pulmonary embolism; visual disorders (reduced visual acuity); vocal cord paresis. Rare reports of severe hypersensitivity reactions have occurred with Abraxane.

ANTIDOTE

Keep physician informed of all side effects. Most will be treated symptomatically as indicated. Most hypersensitivity reactions will subside with temporary discontinuation of paclitaxel, and incidence seems to decrease with subsequent doses. Moderate reactions such as dyspnea, flushing, hypotension, skin reactions, or tachycardia do not usually require interruption of treatment. Severe reactions may require epinephrine, antihistamines (e.g., diphenhydramine), corticosteroids (e.g., dexamethasone), or bronchodilators (e.g., albuterol, theophylline). Most severe reactions should not be rechallenged, but some patients tolerated subsequent doses of **conventional paclitaxel;** see Contraindications. Neutropenia can be profound, and the nadir usually occurs about Day 11 with **conventional paclitaxel.** Recovery is generally rapid and spontaneous but may be treated with filgrastim or pegfilgrastim. Severe thrombocytopenia (nadir Day 8 or 9 with **conventional paclitaxel**) may require platelet transfusions. Severe anemia (less than 8 Gm/dL) may require packed cell transfusions. Hypotension and bradycardia do not usually occur at the same time except in hypersensitivity. Treat only if symptomatic. Some arrhythmias (e.g., nonspecific repolarization abnormalities, sinus tachycardia, and PVCs) are common and may not require intervention. Promptly treat any serious or symptomatic arrhythmia (e.g., conduction abnormalities, ventricular tachycardia), and monitor continuously during subsequent doses. Neurologic symptoms tend to worsen with each course; see Dose Adjustments. Usually improve within several months. Severe peripheral neuropathies or seizure may necessitate discontinuation of paclitaxel. Permanently discontinue treatment with **Abraxane** and gemcitabine if pneumonitis develops. There is no specific antidote for overdose. Supportive therapy will help sustain the patient in toxicity. Resuscitate if indicated.

PALIFERMIN
(**PAL**-lih-fur-min)

Keratinocyte growth factor

Kepivance

pH 6.5

USUAL DOSE

Administered as an IV bolus injection for 3 consecutive days before and 3 consecutive days after myelotoxic therapy (a total of 6 doses). Do not administer within 24 hours before, during infusion of, or within 24 hours after administration of myelotoxic chemotherapy. Has resulted in increased severity and duration of oral mucositis. Myelotoxic therapy is high-dose chemotherapy, with or without radiation, that is destructive to bone marrow or any of its components. Followed by bone marrow transplant/hematopoietic stem cell support.

Pre-myelotoxic therapy (first 3 doses): Administer 60 mcg/kg/day for 3 consecutive days before beginning myelotoxic therapy, with the third dose 24 to 48 hours before myelotoxic therapy.

Post-myelotoxic therapy (last 3 doses): Administer 60 mcg/kg/day for 3 consecutive days after myelotoxic therapy is complete; the first of these doses should be administered after, but on the same day of, hematopoietic stem cell infusion and at least 7 days after the most recent administration of palifermin. See Precautions.

DOSE ADJUSTMENTS

None indicated. Gender-related differences were not observed. ■ No dose adjustment is recommended in impaired renal function. ■ Pharmacokinetic studies have not been performed for pediatric patients or for patients with hepatic insufficiency.

DILUTION

Available as a lyophilized powder in a 6.25-mg single-dose vial. Reconstitute by slowly injecting 1.2 mL SWFI into vial. Final concentration is 5 mg/mL. Swirl contents gently. **Do not shake.** Dissolution should take less than 3 minutes. Solution is clear and colorless. Do not use if particulates are present or if solution is discolored.

Filters: Manufacturer states, "Do not filter the reconstituted solution during preparation or administration."

Storage: Keep vials in carton until use. Store at 2° to 8° C (36° to 46° F). Protect from light. Do not use beyond expiration date on vial. Reconstituted product should be used immediately but can be stored up to 24 hours if refrigerated and stored in its carton. Do not freeze. Before administration, allow palifermin to reach room temperature for a maximum of 1 hour protected from light. Discard any unused product.

COMPATIBILITY

Manufacturer states, "If heparin is used to maintain an IV line, saline should be used to flush the line before and after administration since palifermin has been shown to bind to heparin in vitro." Additional **compatibility** information not available from manufacturer; consult a pharmacist.

RATE OF ADMINISTRATION

A single dose administered as an IV bolus injection. If heparin is used to maintain an IV line, flush the line with NS before and after administration.

ACTIONS

Human keratinocyte growth factor (KGF) produced by recombinant DNA technology. Binding of KGF to its receptor results in proliferation, differentiation, and migration of epithelial cells. KGF receptors are present on the epithelial cells in many tissues, including the tongue, buccal mucosa, esophagus, stomach, intestine, salivary gland, lung, liver, pancreas, kidney, bladder, mammary gland, skin (hair follicles and sebaceous gland), and the lens of the eye. The KGF receptor is not present on the cells of the hematopoietic lineage. KGF stimulates the growth of cells in tissues such as the skin and the epithelial layer of the mouth, stomach, and colon. Protects the epithelial cells that line the mouth and GI tract from the damage caused by chemotherapy and radiation and stimulates the growth and development of new epithelial cells. Average half-life is 4.5 hours (range: 3.3 to 5.7 hours).

INDICATIONS AND USES

To decrease the incidence and duration of severe oral mucositis in patients with hematologic malignancies who are receiving myelotoxic therapy in the setting of autologous hematopoietic stem cell support. Indicated as supportive care for preparative regimens predicted to result in equal to or greater than WHO Grade 3 mucositis in the majority of patients.

Limitations of use: Safety and efficacy for use in patients with nonhematologic malignancies not established; see Precautions. Palifermin was not effective in decreasing the incidence of severe mucositis in patients with hematologic malignancies receiving myelotoxic therapy in the setting of allogeneic hematopoietic stem cell support. ▪ Not recommended for use with melphalan 200 mg/M^2 as a conditioning regimen.

CONTRAINDICATIONS

Manufacturer states, "None."

PRECAUTIONS

Safety and efficacy have not been established in patients with nonhematologic malignancies. Effect of palifermin on stimulation of KGF receptor–expressing, nonhematopoietic tumors in patients is not known. Has been shown to enhance the growth of human epithelial tumor cell lines in vitro.

Monitor: Monitor improvement in symptoms of oral mucositis. ▪ Monitor for the appearance of mucocutaneous adverse effects (e.g., edema, erythema, oral/perioral dysesthesia [impairment of sensitivity to touch], rash, taste alteration, tongue discoloration, tongue thickening).

Patient Education: Review possible side effects. ▪ Promptly report side effects (e.g., edema, impairment of sensitivity to touch [especially around the mouth], rash, taste alteration, tongue discoloration, tongue thickening). ▪ Inform patient of the evidence of tumor growth and stimulation in cell cultures and animal models of nonhematopoietic human tumors and that safety and efficacy have not been established in patients with nonhematologic malignancies.

Maternal/Child: Category C: potential benefit to mother must justify potential risk to fetus. ▪ Discontinue breast-feeding. ▪ Information on dosing and safety in pediatric patients is limited. However, use in pediatric patients ages 1 to 16 years is supported by evidence from well-controlled studies in adults and from a Phase 1 study that included 27 pediatric patients with acute leukemia undergoing hematopoietic stem cell transplant. Adverse events were similar to those reported for adults, and age did not affect the pharmacokinetics of palifermin.

Elderly: Clinical studies did not include sufficient numbers of subjects 65 years of age and older to determine whether they respond differently than do younger subjects. No dose adjustment is recommended.

DRUG/LAB INTERACTIONS

Formal studies have not been conducted. ▪ Interacts with **unfractionated as well as low-molecular-weight heparins** (e.g., enoxaparin). When coadministered, there was no significant effect of palifermin on heparin activity with respect to aPPT. However, coadministration resulted in an increased palifermin AUC and a decreased palifermin clearance, volume of distribution, and half-life. Despite the changes in palifermin pharmacokinetics, coadministration did not have any noticeable effect on the pharmacodynamics of either drug. If heparin is used to maintain an IV line, NS should be used to flush the line before and after palifermin administration. ▪ Do not administer within 24 hours before, during infusion of, or within 24 hours after administration of **myelotoxic chemotherapy.** Has resulted in increased severity and duration of oral mucositis.

SIDE EFFECTS

The most common side effects are elevated serum amylase, fever, and skin toxicities (edema, erythema, pruritus, skin rash). Other commonly reported reactions include arthralgia, dysesthesia, elevated serum lipase, oral toxicities (alteration in taste, dysesthesia, tongue discoloration and thickening), pain, and paresthesia. The most common serious adverse reaction was skin rash. Has the potential for immunogenicity, but the clinical significance is unknown.

Post-Marketing: Cataracts, palmar-plantar erythrodysesthesia syndrome (dysesthesia, edema on the palms and soles, erythema), and vaginal edema and erythema.

ANTIDOTE
Notify physician of all side effects. Most will be treated symptomatically.

PALONOSETRON
(**pal**-oh-**NOH**-seh-tron)

Aloxi

Antiemetic
(5-HT$_3$ receptor antagonist)

pH 4.5 to 5.5

USUAL DOSE
Adults: 0.25 mg as a single dose; infuse over 30 seconds starting 30 minutes before start of chemotherapy.

Pediatric patients (1 month to less than 17 years of age): 20 mcg/kg/dose, with a maximum of 1.5 mg as a single dose; infuse over 15 minutes starting 30 minutes before start of chemotherapy.

Postoperative nausea and vomiting in adults: A single dose of 0.075 mg immediately before induction of anesthesia.

DOSE ADJUSTMENTS
No dose adjustment required based on age or race or in patients with any degree of renal or hepatic impairment.

DILUTION
Available in 0.25 mg/5 mL and 0.075 mg/1.5 mL single-use vials. Do not dilute.

Filters: No data available from manufacturer.

Storage: Before use, store at CRT. Protect from freezing and light.

COMPATIBILITY
Manufacturer states, "Should not be mixed with other drugs. Flush the infusion line with NS before and after administration."

Other sources suggest specific **compatibilities** dependent on concentration and manufacturer; consult a pharmacist.

RATE OF ADMINISTRATION
Flush the infusion line with NS before and after administration.

Chemotherapy-induced nausea and vomiting in adults and pediatric patients: See Usual Dose.

Postoperative nausea and vomiting in adults: A single dose as an IV injection equally distributed over 10 seconds.

ACTIONS
A long-acting (up to 120 hours [5 days]) antinauseant and antiemetic agent. A selective antagonist of specific serotonin (5-HT$_3$) receptors. Has a strong binding affinity for this receptor and little or no affinity for other receptors. Chemotherapeutic agents such as cisplatin increase the release of serotonin from specific cells in the GI tract, causing emesis. Postoperative nausea and vomiting are also triggered by the release of serotonin. By antagonizing serotonin receptors both on the vagus nerve in the periphery and centrally in the chemoreceptor trigger zone, the incidence and severity of chemotherapy-induced nausea and vomiting and postoperative nausea and vomiting are decreased. 62% bound to plasma protein. Partially metabolized by multiple CYP enzymes; however, palonosetron is not an inhibitor or an inducer of CYP enzyme activity. Eliminated slowly from the body

through both metabolic pathways and renal excretion. Has a prolonged half-life of approximately 40 hours. 80% of a single dose was recovered in urine within 144 hours.

INDICATIONS AND USES

In pediatric patients 1 month to less than 17 years of age, prevention of acute nausea and vomiting associated with initial and repeat courses of *emetogenic* cancer chemotherapy, including *highly emetogenic* cancer chemotherapy. ▪ In adults, prevention of acute and delayed nausea and vomiting associated with initial and repeat courses of *moderately emetogenic* cancer chemotherapy and prevention of acute nausea and vomiting associated with initial and repeat courses of *highly emetogenic* cancer chemotherapy. Studies identified cisplatin in doses equal to or greater than 70 mg/M^2 and cyclophosphamide (Cytoxan) in doses equal to or greater than 1,100 mg/M^2 as *highly emetogenic.* Studies identified cisplatin in doses equal to or less than 50 mg/M^2, cyclophosphamide in doses less than 1,100 mg/M^2, doxorubicin (Adriamycin) in doses greater than 25 mg/M^2, methotrexate in doses greater than 250 mg/M^2, and carboplatin, epirubicin (Ellence), and irinotecan (Camptosar) in standard doses as *moderately emetogenic.* ▪ Prevention of postoperative nausea and vomiting (PONV) in adults for up to 24 hours following surgery. Efficacy beyond 24 hours has not been demonstrated.

CONTRAINDICATIONS

Known hypersensitivity to palonosetron or any of its components. ▪ See Precautions.

PRECAUTIONS

Hypersensitivity reactions, including anaphylaxis, have been reported with or without known hypersensitivity to other 5-HT_3 receptor antagonists. Cross-sensitivity may occur with other selective 5-HT_3 receptor antagonists. ▪ Serotonin syndrome has been reported with 5-HT_3 receptor antagonists. Most reports were associated with concomitant use of serotonergic drugs (e.g., selective serotonin reuptake inhibitors, serotonin and norepinephrine reuptake inhibitors, monoamine oxidase inhibitors, mirtazapine, fentanyl, lithium, and tramadol). Some cases were fatal. ▪ Routine prophylaxis is not recommended for patients in whom there is little expectation of PONV. However, for patients in whom nausea and vomiting must be avoided during the postoperative period, prophylaxis is recommended even when the incidence of PONV is low. ▪ Palonosetron does not appear to have any effect on ECG intervals, including QTc duration.

Monitor: Observe closely. Monitor VS. ▪ Monitor for serotonin syndrome, especially when palonosetron is used concurrently with other serotonergic drugs. Symptoms associated with serotonin syndrome may include the following combination of S/S: mental status changes (e.g., agitation, coma, delirium, hallucinations), autonomic instability (e.g., diaphoresis, dizziness, flushing, hyperthermia, labile blood pressure, tachycardia), neuromuscular symptoms (e.g., hyperreflexia, incoordination, myoclonus, rigidity, tremor), and seizures, with or without GI symptoms (e.g., diarrhea, nausea, vomiting). ▪ Ambulate slowly to avoid orthostatic hypotension. ▪ Stool softeners or laxatives may be required to prevent constipation.

Patient Education: Request assistance with ambulation. ▪ Used to prevent and/or treat both early and late N/V caused by chemotherapy. Report persistent N/V promptly. ▪ Maintain adequate hydration. ▪ Review prescription and nonprescription medications with healthcare provider. Drug interactions are possible, especially with diuretics or antiarrhythmics. ▪ Review other medical conditions with healthcare provider. ▪ Promptly report S/S of serotonin syndrome (e.g., altered mental status, autonomic instability, and neuromuscular symptoms); see Precautions.

Maternal/Child: Category B: use during pregnancy only if clearly needed. ▪ Safety for use during breast-feeding not established; effects unknown, but potential for tumorigenicity is a concern. Discontinue breast-feeding. ▪ Safety and effectiveness have been established for use in pediatric patients 1 month to less than 17 years of age for the prevention of acute nausea and vomiting associated with initial and repeat courses of emetogenic cancer chemotherapy, including highly emetogenic chemotherapy. Pediatric patients require a higher palonosetron dose than adults to prevent chemotherapy-induced nausea and vomiting. However, the safety profile seen in pediatric patients is consistent with the established profile in adults. ▪ Safety and effectiveness have not been established in pediatric patients for prevention of postoperative nausea and vomiting.

Elderly: Safety and effectiveness similar to younger adults; however, greater sensitivity in some elderly cannot be ruled out. No dose adjustment or special monitoring required.

DRUG/LAB INTERACTIONS

Eliminated through both renal excretion and metabolic pathways. Does not induce or inhibit the cytochrome P_{450} drug metabolizing system; potential for clinically significant drug interactions is considered to be low. ▪ Serotonin syndrome (including altered mental status, autonomic instability, and neuromuscular symptoms) has been reported following the concomitant use of 5-HT$_3$ receptor antagonists and other serotonergic drugs, including selective serotonin reuptake inhibitors (SSRIs) and serotonin and norepinephrine reuptake inhibitors (SNRIs). ▪ See Precautions.

SIDE EFFECTS

Chemotherapy-induced nausea and vomiting in adults: The most common side effects are headache and constipation. Other reported side effects include abdominal pain, diarrhea, dizziness, fatigue, and insomnia.

Chemotherapy-induced nausea and vomiting in pediatric patients: Allergic dermatitis, dizziness, dyskinesia, headache, and infusion site pain.

Postoperative nausea and vomiting: The most common side effects, occurring in at least 2% of patients, are bradycardia, constipation, headache, and QT prolongation. Several other side effects are reported in 1% or fewer of patients.

Overdose: Doses more than 20 times the recommended dose did not cause significant problems. Collapse, convulsions, cyanosis, gasping, and pallor occurred in animal studies with rats and mice.

Post-Marketing: Rare cases of hypersensitivity reactions, including anaphylaxis, anaphylactic shock, and injection site reactions (burning, induration, pain). Serotonin syndrome has been reported as a 5-HT$_3$ class reaction.

ANTIDOTE

Most side effects will be treated symptomatically. Keep physician informed. There is no specific antidote. If symptoms of serotonin syndrome occur, discontinue palonosetron and initiate supportive care. Has a large volume of distribution; dialysis not likely to be effective in overdose. Treat hypersensitivity reactions and resuscitate as indicated.

PAMIDRONATE DISODIUM
(pah-**MIH**-droh-nayt **DYE**-so-dee-um)

Bone resorption inhibitor
Antihypercalcemic
(bisphosphonate)

APD, Aredia

pH 6 to 7.4

USUAL DOSE
Pretreatment: Verify pregnancy status. Baseline studies and prehydration required. See Precautions and Monitor.

Do not exceed a 90-mg dose.

Moderate hypercalcemia (corrected serum calcium of 12 to 13.5 mg/dL): One dose of 60 to 90 mg as an infusion.

Severe hypercalcemia (corrected serum calcium greater than 13.5 mg/dL): One dose of 90 mg as an infusion. Serum calcium levels should fall into the normal range (8.5 to 10.5 mg/100 mL, corrected for serum albumin).

Experience is limited, but retreatment with the same dose may be considered if hypercalcemia is not fully corrected or recurs; wait at least 7 days from completion of first infusion to allow full response. Always used in conjunction with adequate hydration and appropriate testing. See Precautions/Monitor.

Paget's disease: 30 mg/day as an infusion for 3 consecutive days (total dose is 90 mg over 3 days). Selected patients have been retreated with the same dose when indicated. Experience limited. Prehydration required; see Precautions and Monitor.

Osteolytic bone lesions of multiple myeloma: 90 mg as an infusion once every 30 days. Optimal duration of therapy not known. Withhold dose if renal function has deteriorated; see Dose Adjustments, Precautions, and Monitor.

Osteolytic bone metastases of breast cancer: 90 mg as an infusion every 3 to 4 weeks. Optimum duration of therapy not known. Withhold dose if renal function has deteriorated; see Dose Adjustments, Precautions, and Monitor.

DOSE ADJUSTMENTS
Accumulation of pamidronate in renally impaired patients is not anticipated if dosed on a monthly schedule. No experience with creatinine above 5 mg/100 mL (1 dL) or in severe hepatic disease. ▪ See Precautions and Elderly.

Osteolytic bone lesions of multiple myeloma and osteolytic bone metastases of breast cancer: Withhold dose if renal function has deteriorated. Renal deterioration is defined as an increase of 0.5 mg/dL in patients with a *normal* baseline creatinine or an increase of 1 mg/dL in patients with *abnormal* baseline creatinine. One study suggests that treatment should not be resumed until SCr has returned to within 10% of baseline value.

DILUTION
Reconstitute each 30- or 90-mg vial with 10 mL SWFI. Dissolve completely (3 or 9 mg/mL).

Hypercalcemia of malignancy: Further dilute a single dose in 1,000 mL NS, $^1/_2$NS, or D5W. A minimum of 500 mL diluent may be used if absolutely necessary in patients with compromised cardiovascular status.

Paget's disease: Further dilute a single daily dose in 500 mL NS, $^1/_2$NS, or D5W.

Osteolytic bone lesions of multiple myeloma: Further dilute each 90-mg dose in 500 mL NS, $^1/_2$ NS, or D5W.

Osteolytic bone metastases of breast cancer: Further dilute each 90-mg dose in 250 mL NS, $^1/_2$ NS, or D5W.

Storage: Before reconstitution, store at CRT. After reconstitution, may be refrigerated for up to 24 hours. Stable after dilution for 24 hours at room temperature.

COMPATIBILITY
Should be given in a single intravenous solution and line separate from all other drugs, and do not mix with calcium-containing solutions (e.g., Ringer's solutions).

RATE OF ADMINISTRATION

Use of a microdrip (60 gtt/mL) or an infusion pump recommended for even distribution. Do not exceed recommended rate of infusion. Duration should be no less than 2 hours. Too-rapid infusion rate may lead to overdose, elevated BUN and creatinine levels, and renal tubular necrosis. Rate recommendations vary considerably. They are based on specific clinical trials for each diagnosis. In some trials a rate of up to 1 mg/min has been used with caution.

Hypercalcemia of malignancy: A 60-mg dose or 90-mg dose equally distributed over 2 to 24 hours. Longer infusion times (i.e., greater than 2 hours) may reduce the risk of renal toxicity, particularly in patients with pre-existing renal insufficiency.

Paget's disease: A single dose over 4 hours.

Osteolytic bone lesions of multiple myeloma: A single dose over 4 hours.

Osteolytic bone metastases of breast cancer: A single dose over 2 hours.

ACTIONS

A bisphosphonate hypocalcemic agent. Reduces serum calcium concentrations by inhibiting bone resorption. Binds to preformed bone surfaces and may block bone mineral dissolution. May also inhibit osteoclast activity. Effectively inhibits accelerated bone resorption resulting from osteoclast hyperactivity induced by various tumors. Does not inhibit bone formation and mineralization. Some reduction in calcium levels seen in 24 to 48 hours, and maximum response in 4 to 7 days. Rapidly adsorbed by bone. Is not metabolized. Half-life is approximately 21 to 35 hours. Slowly excreted in urine.

INDICATIONS AND USES

Treatment of moderate to severe hypercalcemia of malignancy in patients with or without bone metastasis, in conjunction with adequate hydration. Symptoms of hypercalcemia may include anorexia, bone pain, confusion, constipation, dehydration, depression, fatigue, lethargy, muscle weakness, nausea and vomiting, and polyuria. Severe dehydration may lead to renal insufficiency. With high levels of serum calcium, cardiac manifestations (e.g., bradycardia, cardiac arrest, ventricular arrhythmias) and neurologic symptoms (e.g., coma, seizures, and death) may occur. ▪ Treatment of Paget's disease. ▪ Adjunct in treatment of osteolytic lesions of multiple myeloma and osteolytic bone metastases of breast cancer.

Unlabeled uses: Prevention of bone loss associated with androgen deprivation therapy in prostate cancer.

CONTRAINDICATIONS

Hypersensitivity to pamidronate or other bisphosphonates (e.g., alendronate, risedronate, zoledronic acid).

PRECAUTIONS

Calcium is bound to albumin. Total serum calcium levels in patients who have hypercalcemia of malignancy may not reflect the severity of the hypocalcemia because concomitant hypoalbuminemia is commonly present. Measurement with ionized calcium levels is preferred. If unavailable, all calcium measurement should be corrected for albumin to establish a basis for treatment and evaluation of treatment. ▪ Mild or asymptomatic hypercalcemia will be treated with conservative measures (e.g., saline hydration, with or without diuretics [after correcting hypovolemia]). Consider patient's cardiovascular status. Corticosteroids may be indicated if the underlying cancer is sensitive (e.g., hematologic cancers). ▪ May be used adjunctively with chemotherapy, radiation, or surgery. ▪ May cause renal toxicity. Deterioration in renal function progressing to renal failure has been reported and has occurred after the initial or a single dose of pamidronate. Patients with pre-existing renal impairment may be at increased risk for developing toxicity. Do not exceed dose of 90 mg. ▪ Osteonecrosis of the jaw (ONJ) has been reported in patients receiving bisphosphonates. The majority of cases have been in cancer patients. Risk factors include cancer, concomitant therapy (e.g., chemotherapy, radiotherapy, corticosteroids), and comorbid conditions (e.g., anemia, coagulopathies, infection, pre-existing oral disease). Literature and case reports suggest a higher frequency of ONJ based on tumor type (breast cancer, multiple myeloma) and dental status (dental extraction, periodontal disease, local trauma, including poorly fitting dentures). Cancer patients should maintain good oral hygiene. Consider dental exam and appropriate preventive dentistry before beginning therapy with bisphosphonates. Avoid invasive dental procedures during bisphosphonate therapy. Dental surgery may exacerbate ONJ in patients who develop ONJ while on bisphosphonate therapy. ■ Severe and occasionally incapacitating bone, joint, and/or muscle pain has been reported rarely. Onset of symptoms varied from one day to several months after beginning treatment with pamidronate. In most cases, pain resolves when pamidronate is discontinued; however, in some patients symptoms resolved slowly or persisted. ■ Atypical subtrochanteric and diaphyseal femoral fractures have been reported. May occur after minimal or no trauma. Risk may be increased in patients receiving concurrent glucocorticoids (e.g., dexamethasone, prednisone). ■ May be at risk for anemia, leukopenia, or thrombocytopenia; see Monitor. ■ Patients with a history of thyroid surgery may have relative hypoparathyroidism that may predispose them to hypocalcemia with pamidronate. ***Osteolytic bone lesions of multiple myeloma and osteolytic bone metastases of breast cancer:*** Patients being treated for multiple myeloma and bone metastases should have the dose withheld if renal function has deteriorated; see Dose Adjustments. Use is not recommended in patients with severe renal impairment being treated for bone metastases. See Monitor and Dose Adjustments. Limited information available on use in multiple myeloma patients with a CrCl less than 30 mL/min. In clinical trials, patients with a SCr above 3 mg/dL were excluded. ■ In the absence of hypercalcemia, patients with ***multiple myeloma*** or ***Paget's disease of the bone*** or patients with ***predominantly lytic bone metastases*** who are at risk for calcium and vitamin D deficiency should be given oral calcium and vitamin D to reduce the risk of hypocalcemia.

Monitor: Obtain baseline measurements of serum calcium (corrected for serum albumin), electrolytes, phosphate, magnesium, and creatinine and CBC with differential and hematocrit/hemoglobin. Monitor all closely as indicated by baseline results (may be daily). Serum phosphate levels will decrease and may require treatment. ■ Monitor renal function before each treatment; deterioration in renal function has been reported; see Precautions. ■ Monitor serum alkaline phosphatase during therapy for Paget's disease. ■ Patients with cancer-related hypercalcemia are frequently dehydrated. Must be adequately hydrated orally and/or IV before treatment is initiated. Hydration with saline is preferred to facilitate renal excretion of calcium and to correct dehydration. A pretreatment urine output of 2 L/day is recommended. Maintain adequate hydration and urine output throughout treatment. ■ Avoid overhydration in patients with compromised cardiovascular status. Observe frequently for signs of fluid overload. Correct hypovolemia before using diuretics. ■ Monitor patients with pre-existing anemia, leukopenia, or thrombocytopenia very carefully during treatment and for the first 2 weeks following treatment. ■ Monitor for S/S of atypical femoral fractures that may occur with minimal or no trauma. Thigh or groin pain may be experienced weeks to months before a fracture appears. Fractures are often bilateral; examine both femurs. ***Osteolytic bone lesions of multiple myeloma:*** Adequately hydrate patients who have marked Bence-Jones proteinuria and dehydration before pamidronate infusion.

Patient Education: Regular visits and assessment of lab tests imperative. ■ Dietary restriction of calcium and vitamin D may be required. ■ Take only prescribed medications. ■ Report abdominal cramps, chills, confusion, fever, muscle spasms, sore throat, and/or any new medical problems promptly. ■ Report development of bone, joint, or muscle pain promptly. Onset of pain is variable. ■ Avoid pregnancy; use of effective birth control necessary during treatment and for an undetermined time after treatment; see prescribing information.

Maternal/Child: Category D: should not be used during pregnancy. May cause fetal harm. ■ Discontinue breast-feeding. ■ Safety for use in pediatric patients not established.

Elderly: Response similar to that seen in younger patients. ■ Use with caution based on age-related impaired organ function and concomitant disease or drug therapy; monitor renal function closely. See Dose Adjustments. ■ Monitor fluid and electrolyte status carefully to avoid overhydration or electrolyte imbalance. Use of lower fluid volume may be required; see Dilution.

DRUG/LAB INTERACTIONS
Use caution when administered with other **potentially nephrotoxic drugs** (e.g., aminoglycosides, cisplatin). ▪ Effects may be antagonized by **calcium-containing preparations or vitamin D;** avoid use. ▪ Concurrent use with **thalidomide** may increase risk of renal toxicity in patients with multiple myeloma.

SIDE EFFECTS
Average dose: Abdominal pain, anemia, anorexia, bone pain, confusion and visual hallucinations (sometimes in conjunction with electrolyte imbalance), constipation, fever (mild and transient), generalized pain, hypertension, hypocalcemia (abdominal cramps, confusion, muscle spasms), infusion site reaction (e.g., induration and pain on palpation, redness, swelling), musculoskeletal pain (bone, joint, and/or muscle pain), pruritus, rash, renal toxicity, seizures, urinary tract infections, vomiting. Fluid overload, hypokalemia, hypomagnesemia, and hypophosphatemia occur frequently with use of concurrent fluid and diuretics. Rare instances of hypersensitivity reactions, including anaphylaxis, angioedema, dyspnea, and hypotension, have occurred. Osteonecrosis (primarily of the jaw) has been reported (see Precautions). Anemia, leukopenia, and thrombocytopenia may occur.

Overdose: Occurs less frequently with lower dose range (30 to 60 mg). Fever (high), hypocalcemia, hypotension, leukopenia or lymphopenia (fever, chills, sore throat), transient taste perversion. Elevated BUN and CrCl levels and renal tubular necrosis may occur with excessive dose or rate of administration.

Post-Marketing: Adult respiratory distress syndrome (ARDS); atypical subtrochanteric and diaphyseal femoral fractures; bone, joint, and muscle pain (may be severe and incapacitating); conjunctivitis; focal segmental glomerulosclerosis (including the collapsing variant); glomerulonephropathies; hematuria; hypernatremia; influenza-like symptoms; interstitial lung disease; nephrotic syndrome; orbital inflammation; reactivation of herpes simplex and herpes zoster; renal tubular disorders; tubulointerstitial nephritis.

ANTIDOTE
Keep physician informed of side effects. Some may respond to symptomatic treatment. Magnesium, phosphorus, and potassium may require replacement if depletion too severe. If mild, all will probably return toward normal in 7 to 10 days. For asymptomatic or mild to moderate hypocalcemia (6.5 to 8 mg/100 mL corrected for serum albumin), short-term calcium therapy (e.g., calcium gluconate) may be indicated. Consider discontinuing pamidronate in patients who develop atypical fractures of the femur. Unknown if risk continues after stopping treatment. Discontinue drug for any symptoms of overdose. Monitor serum calcium and use vigorous IV hydration, with or without diuretics, for 2 to 3 days. Monitor intake and output to ensure adequacy and balance. Use short-term IV calcium therapy if indicated. High fever may respond to steroids. RBC transfusions may be required in anemia. Treat anaphylaxis and resuscitate as indicated.

PANITUMUMAB BBW
(pan-i-**TUE**-moo-mab)

Antineoplastic
Immunosuppressant
Monoclonal antibody
(EGFR receptor antagonist)

Vectibix

pH 5.6 to 6

USUAL DOSE

Pretreatment: Verify pregnancy status. Pretesting required. Before initiating treatment, assess *RAS* mutational status in colorectal tumors and confirm the absence of a *RAS* mutation in exon 2 (codons 12 and 13), exon 3 (codons 59 and 61), and exon 4 (codons 117 and 146) of both *KRAS* and *NRAS*; see Precautions. See prescribing information for access to FDA-approved tests. Baseline studies required; see Monitor.

Panitumumab: 6 mg/kg as an infusion once every 14 days.

DOSE ADJUSTMENTS

Upon the first occurrence of a Grade 3 (NCI-CTC/CTCAE) dermatologic reaction, withhold 1 to 2 doses of panitumumab. If the reaction improves to less than Grade 3, re-initiate panitumumab at the original dose. ▪ Upon the second occurrence of a Grade 3 (NCI-CTC/CTCAE) dermatologic reaction, withhold 1 to 2 doses of panitumumab. If the reaction improves to less than Grade 3, reinitiate panitumumab at 80% of the original dose. ▪ Upon the third occurrence of a Grade 3 (NCI-CTC/CTCAE) dermatologic reaction, withhold 1 to 2 doses of panitumumab. If the reaction improves to less than Grade 3, re-initiate panitumumab at 60% of the original dose. ▪ Upon the fourth occurrence of a Grade 3 (NCI-CTC/CTCAE) dermatologic reaction, permanently discontinue panitumumab. ▪ Permanently discontinue panitumumab following the occurrence of a Grade 4 dermatologic reaction or for a Grade 3 dermatologic reaction that does not recover after withholding 1 to 2 doses.

DILUTION

Solution may contain a small amount of visible, translucent-to-white, amorphous, and proteinaceous particulates. Do not use if solution is discolored or cloudy or if foreign matter is present. **Do not shake.** Using a 21-gauge or larger gauge (smaller bore) hypodermic needle, withdraw the calculated dose from the vial. Dilute to a total volume of 100 mL with NS. Doses higher than 1,000 mg should be diluted to a volume of 150 mL. (Withdraw a volume of NS equal to the volume of the calculated dose from the infusion bag.) Final concentration should not exceed 10 mg/mL. Mix diluted solution by gentle inversion.

Filters: Must be administered through a low–protein-binding, 0.2- or 0.22-micron, in-line filter.

Storage: Store unopened vials in refrigerator (2° to 8° C [36° to 46° F]) until time of use. Protect from direct sunlight. Do not freeze. Diluted solutions should be used within 6 hours of preparation if stored at RT and within 24 hours if stored in refrigerator. Do not freeze. Single-dose vial; discard any unused product after entry into vial.

COMPATIBILITY

Manufacturer states, "Should not be mixed with, or administered as an infusion with, other medicinal products. No other medications should be added to solutions containing panitumumab."

RATE OF ADMINISTRATION

For IV infusion only. **Do not administer as an IV push or bolus.** Flush line before and after panitumumab administration with NS. Administer with an IV infusion pump using a low–protein-binding, 0.2- or 0.22-micron, in-line filter.

A single dose equally distributed over 60 minutes. If the first infusion is tolerated, administer subsequent infusions over 30 to 60 minutes. Doses over 1,000 mg should be administered over 90 minutes. Reduce rate of infusion by 50% in patients experiencing a Grade 1 or 2 infusion reaction.

ACTIONS

An epidermal growth factor receptor (EGFR) antagonist for IV use and a human IgG2 kappa monoclonal antibody. EGFR is a transmembrane glycoprotein that is expressed in many normal epithelial tissues, including skin and hair follicles. Overexpression of EGFR is detected in many human cancers, including those of the colon and rectum. Interaction of EGFR with its normal ligands leads to a series of reactions that regulate the transcription of molecules involved with cellular growth and survival, motility, proliferation, and transformation. Panitumumab binds to EGFR on both normal and tumor cells, inhibiting the binding of normal ligands to EGFR. This competitive binding results in inhibition of cell growth, induction of apoptosis, decreased proinflammatory cytokine and vascular growth factor production, and internalization of EGFR. The end result is inhibition of growth and survival of selected human tumor cells that express EGFR. Half-life is approximately 7.5 days (range 3.6 to 10.9 days).

INDICATIONS AND USES

Treatment of patients with wild-type *RAS* (defined as wild-type in both *KRAS* and *NRAS* as determined by an FDA-approved test for this use) metastatic colorectal cancer (mCRC). May be used as first-line therapy in combination with FOLFOX (5-fluorouracil, leucovorin, and oxaliplatin) or as monotherapy following disease progression after prior chemotherapy containing fluoropyrimidine (fluorouracil), oxaliplatin, and irinotecan.

Limitation of use: Not indicated for the treatment of patients with *RAS* mutant mCRC or for patients whose *RAS* mutation status is unknown.

CONTRAINDICATIONS

None known. See Precautions.

PRECAUTIONS

Panitumumab should be used only for treatment of patients with *KRAS* wild-type mCRC as determined by an FDA-approved test. In studies, patients with *KRAS*-mutant mCRC tumors receiving panitumumab in combination with FOLFOX experienced some overall survival compared with patients receiving FOLFOX alone. Perform the assessment for *KRAS* mutational status in colorectal cancer laboratories with demonstrated proficiency in the technology required for testing. ■ Dermatologic toxicities were reported in 90% of patients and were severe (NCI-CTC/CTCAE Grade 3 or higher) in 15% of patients. Manifestations included dermatitis acneiform, dry skin, erythema, paronychia, pruritus, rash, skin exfoliation, and skin fissures. Severe dermatologic toxicities were complicated by infection. Life-threatening and fatal infectious complications, including necrotizing fasciitis, abscesses requiring incision and drainage, and sepsis, have been observed. Life-threatening and fatal bullous mucocutaneous disease with blisters, erosions, and skin sloughing has also been reported. It is unclear whether these reactions were directly related to EGFR inhibition or to idiosyncratic immune-related effects (e.g., Stevens-Johnson syndrome or toxic epidermal necrolysis). See Dose Adjustments and Antidote. ■ Sunlight may exacerbate dermatologic toxicity. Protection from sun is advised; see Patient Education. ■ Infusion reactions, some severe, have been reported. Fatal reactions have been reported. Administer in a facility with adequate emergency medical equipment and medications for treating these reactions and for responding to any medical emergency; see Rate of Administration and Antidote. ■ Increased mortality and toxicity were seen in studies in which panitumumab was administered in combination with bevacizumab and chemotherapy; see manufacturer's prescribing information. ■ Electrolyte abnormalities have been reported; see Monitor. ■ Fatal and nonfatal cases of interstitial lung disease (ILD) and pulmonary fibrosis have been reported; see Monitor. In patients with a history of interstitial pneumonitis or pulmonary fibrosis or with evidence of interstitial pneumonitis or pulmonary fibrosis, the benefit of therapy versus the risk of pulmonary complications must be considered. ■ Severe diarrhea and dehydration leading to acute renal failure and other complications have been observed in patients treated with panitumumab in combination with chemotherapy. ■ Keratitis and ulcerative keratitis, known risk factors for corneal perforation, have been reported. ■ A protein substance. Potential for immunogenicity exists. Anti-panitumumab antibodies have been detected in a small number of patients. No evidence of altered safety profiles has been confirmed.

Monitor: Obtain baseline electrolytes and monitor periodically during and for 8 weeks after completion of therapy. Hypomagnesemia, hypocalcemia, and hypokalemia have been reported. Oral or IV electrolyte replacement may be required. ▪ Monitor hydration status. ▪ Monitor vital signs before, during (as needed), and at the completion of the infusion. ▪ Monitor for S/S of hypersensitivity or infusion-related reactions. Severe reactions may include anaphylaxis, bronchospasm, chills, dyspnea, fever, and hypotension; see Side Effects. Mild to moderate infusion reactions may respond to a reduction in the rate of infusion; see Rate of Administration. Utility of premedication to minimize or prevent infusion-related reactions has not been determined. ▪ Monitor skin integrity. Monitor patients who develop dermatologic or soft tissue toxicities for the development of inflammatory or infectious sequelae. ▪ Monitor lung function. Interrupt therapy in the event of acute onset or worsening of pulmonary symptoms. Discontinue therapy if ILD is confirmed. ▪ Monitor for evidence of keratitis or ulcerative keratitis.

Patient Education: Highly effective contraception required during treatment with panitumumab and for at least 2 months after the last dose of panitumumab. ▪ Notify provider of known or suspected pregnancy. ▪ May reduce fertility in females of reproductive potential. ▪ Review side effects, including dermatologic toxicity, infusion reactions, pulmonary fibrosis, and potential for fetal harm. ▪ Promptly report skin or ocular changes, cough, dehydration, diarrhea, dyspnea, infusion-related reactions, or new-onset facial swelling. ▪ Diarrhea and dehydration may lead to acute renal failure and electrolyte depletion when panitumumab is administered in combination with chemotherapy. ▪ Limit sun exposure during and for 2 months after the last dose of panitumumab. Use of sunscreen and hats recommended. ▪ Compliance with periodic lab work required.

Maternal/Child: Avoid pregnancy; based on its mechanism of action and animal studies, panitumumab administration can result in fetal harm. Human IgG monoclonal antibody and may be transferred across the placenta. Therefore it is possible that panitumumab may be transmitted from the mother to the developing fetus. Appropriate contraceptive measures must be used during treatment with panitumumab and for at least 2 months after the last dose; see Patient Education. ▪ Discontinue breast-feeding during and for 2 months after the completion of therapy. ▪ Safety and effectiveness for use in pediatric patients not established.

Elderly: When used as monotherapy, specific differences in safety and effectiveness compared with younger adults not noted. An increased incidence of serious adverse events and an increased incidence of serious diarrhea were seen in patients over the age of 65 when given panitumumab in combination with FOLFOX.

DRUG/LAB INTERACTIONS
Formal drug interaction studies have not been conducted.

SIDE EFFECTS
The most commonly reported side effects of panitumumab as **monotherapy** are diarrhea, fatigue, nausea, paronychia, and skin rash with variable presentations. The most common serious reactions, as well as the reactions that lead most often to discontinuation of therapy, were general physical health deterioration and intestinal obstruction. Side effects occurring in 5% or more of patients receiving panitumumab as monotherapy included acne, acneiform dermatitis, cough, dry skin, dyspnea, erythema, exfoliative rash, mucosal inflammation, nail disorders, rash, skin exfoliation, skin fissures, skin ulcer, stomatitis, and vomiting. The most commonly reported side effects when panitumumab was used **in combination with chemotherapy** were acneiform dermatitis, anorexia, asthenia, diarrhea, dry skin, hypokalemia, hypomagnesemia, mucosal inflammation, paronychia, pruritus, rash, and stomatitis. The most common serious reactions were diarrhea and dehydration. The most commonly reported side effects leading to discontinuation were acneiform dermatitis, diarrhea, fatigue, hypersensitivity, paresthesia, and rash. Side effects occurring in 5% or more of patients receiving panitumumab in combination with chemotherapy included acne, alopecia, conjunctivitis, dehydration, epistaxis, erythema,

nail disorders, palmar-plantar erythrodysesthesia syndrome, skin fissures, and weight decrease. Other serious but less frequently reported side effects as outlined in Precautions included acute renal failure, infusion reactions, interstitial lung disease/pulmonary fibrosis, and ocular toxicity.

Post-Marketing: Angioedema, infusion reactions (fatal), keratitis/ulcerative keratitis, life-threatening and fatal bullous mucocutaneous disease, and skin necrosis.

ANTIDOTE

Notify physician of any side effects; most will be treated symptomatically. Replace electrolytes parenterally or orally as indicated. Reduce infusion rate by 50% if a mild or moderate (Grade 1 or 2) infusion reaction occurs. Discontinue panitumumab for a serious infusion reaction (Grade 3 or 4). Depending on the severity and/or persistence of the reaction, discontinue permanently. Hold or discontinue panitumumab if dermatologic or soft tissue toxicities Grade 3 or higher occur, if they are considered intolerable, or if severe or life-threatening inflammatory or infectious complications occur. See Dose Adjustments for criteria to resume or permanently discontinue treatment. Discontinue if ILD is confirmed. Interrupt or discontinue panitumumab infusion for acute or worsening keratitis. Treat hypersensitivity or infusion reaction as indicated (e.g., oxygen, antihistamines [e.g., diphenhydramine], epinephrine, corticosteroids, vasopressors [e.g., dopamine], ventilation equipment, and/or fluids). Resuscitate as necessary.

PANTOPRAZOLE SODIUM

(pan-**TOH**-prah-zohl **SO**-dee-um)

Protonix IV

Proton pump inhibitor (PPI)
Substituted benzimidazole

pH 9 to 10.5

USUAL DOSE

Given as an alternative to continued oral therapy. Resume oral therapy as soon as practical.

Treatment of gastroesophageal reflux disease (GERD): 40 mg as an infusion once daily for 7 to 10 days.

Treatment of Zollinger-Ellison syndrome (ZES): 80 mg as an infusion every 12 hours. Adjust to patient needs based on acid output measurements. If an increased dose is required, 80 mg every 8 hours is expected to maintain gastric acid output at less than 10 mEq/hr. Daily doses in excess of 240 mg or for more than 6 days have not been studied.

Upper GI bleed (unlabeled): 80 mg as an IV injection followed by a continuous infusion of 8 mg/hr for 72 hours.

DOSE ADJUSTMENTS

No dose adjustments are necessary based on race or gender; in the elderly; in patients with mild, moderate, or severe renal insufficiency; in patients on hemodialysis; or in patients with mild to severe impaired hepatic function. Oral doses higher than 40 mg/day have not been studied in patients with hepatic impairment.

DILUTION

40-mg dose: Reconstitute each single dose with 10 mL NS. May be given as an injection or further diluted with 100 mL D5W, NS, or LR to achieve a final concentration of approximately 0.4 mg/mL for infusion.

80-mg dose: Combining of two 40-mg vials is required; reconstitute each 40-mg vial with 10 mL NS. May be given as an injection, or this total 80-mg dose may be further diluted with 80 mL D5W, NS, or LR (a total volume of 100 mL) to achieve a final concentration of approximately 0.8 mg/mL for infusion.

Filters: No longer required.

Storage: Store unopened vials at CRT. Protect from light. Do not freeze reconstituted product. Vials reconstituted for the 2-minute infusion may be stored for up to 24 hours at RT. Vials reconstituted for the 15-minute infusion may be stored for up to 6 hours at RT prior to further dilution. Fully diluted solution may then be stored at RT but must be used within 24 hours of initial reconstitution. Protection from light is not required for reconstituted or fully diluted solutions.

COMPATIBILITY

Administer through a dedicated line or through a **Y-site**. Should not be simultaneously administered through the same line with other intravenous solutions. See Rate of Administration. *Discontinue if discoloration or precipitation occurs with any drug at the Y-site.*

Other sources suggest specific **compatibilities** dependent on concentration and manufacturer; consult a pharmacist.

RATE OF ADMINISTRATION

Flush IV line before and after administration of pantoprazole with **compatible** infusion solutions (D5W, NS, or LR).

Concentration determines the rate of administration.

40 mg/10 mL or 80 mg/20 mL: As an injection evenly distributed over at least 2 minutes.

40 mg/100 mL or 80 mg/100 mL: As an infusion evenly distributed over at least 15 minutes (approximately 7 mL/min).

ACTIONS

A proton pump inhibitor (PPI) that suppresses the final step in gastric acid production. Acts at the secretory surface of the gastric parietal cell. Inhibits both basal and stimulated gastric acid secretion irrespective of the stimulus. Does not accumulate and pharmacokinetics are not altered with multiple daily dosing. Onset of antisecretory activity is within 15 to 30 minutes. Half-life is approximately 1 hour. However, duration of antisecretory effect persists longer than 24 hours. Distributed mainly in extracellular fluid. Highly bound by serum protein (primarily albumin). Extensively metabolized in the liver through the cytochrome P_{450} system (primarily through CYP2C19 and, to a lesser extent, through CYP3A4, 2D6, and 2C9). Metabolism is independent of the route of administration (intravenous or oral). Primarily excreted in urine with some excretion in feces. Secreted in breast milk.

INDICATIONS AND USES

Short-term treatment (7 to 10 days) of adult patients with gastroesophageal reflux disease (GERD) and a history of erosive esophagitis, as an alternative to oral therapy. ■ Treatment of pathologic hypersecretory conditions, including Zollinger-Ellison syndrome in adults.

Unlabeled uses: Peptic ulcer disease treatment and secondary prevention (upper GI bleed).

CONTRAINDICATIONS

Known hypersensitivity to pantoprazole, esomeprazole, omeprazole, or any component of the formulation. Patients receiving rilpivirine-containing products.

PRECAUTIONS

For IV use only; do not give IM or SC. ■ Hypersensitivity reactions, including anaphylaxis and severe skin reactions (e.g., erythema multiforme, Stevens-Johnson syndrome, and toxic epidermal necrolysis), have been reported. ■ Gastric malignancy may be present even though patient's symptoms improve with pantoprazole therapy. Consider additional follow-up and diagnostic testing in adult patients who have a suboptimal response or an early symptomatic relapse after completing treatment with a PPI. In older patients, also consider an endoscopy. ■ Formulation contains edetate disodium, which can chelate zinc; see Monitor. ■ Discontinue as soon as the patient is able to resume treatment with pantoprazole delayed-release tablets or oral suspension. Safety for treatment of patients with GERD and a history of erosive esophagitis for more than 10 days has not been demonstrated. ■ Data on safe and effective dosing for other conditions (including life-threatening upper GI bleeds) not available. 40 mg IV of pantoprazole daily does not raise gastric pH levels sufficiently to treat such life-threatening conditions. ■ May be associated with an increased risk for osteoporosis-related fractures of the hip, wrist, or spine. Risk increased in patients receiving high-dose (multiple daily doses) and long-term therapy (a year or longer). Use lowest dose and shortest duration of therapy appropriate for the condition being treated. ▪ Hypomagnesemia (symptomatic and asymptomatic) has been reported in patients treated with proton pump inhibitors (PPIs) for at least 3 months and, in most cases, after a year of treatment. Serious adverse events, including arrhythmias, seizures, and tetany, have occurred. Discontinuation of the PPI and magnesium replacement have been required. ▪ Associated with increased risk of fundic gland polyps, which increases with long-term use, especially beyond 1 year. Most patients who developed fundic gland polyps were asymptomatic, and fundic gland polyps were identified on endoscopy. Use the shortest duration of therapy appropriate for the condition being treated. ▪ Serum chromogranin A (CgA) levels increase secondary to drug-induced decreases in gastric acidity; see Drug/Lab Interactions. ▪ May be associated with an increased risk of *Clostridium difficile*–associated diarrhea (CDAD), especially in hospitalized patients. Consider in patients who develop diarrhea that does not improve. Use lowest dose and shortest duration of therapy appropriate for the condition being treated. ▪ Acute interstitial nephritis has been observed and is generally attributed to an idiopathic hypersensitivity reaction. May occur at any time during therapy. Discontinue pantoprazole if it occurs. ▪ Cutaneous lupus erythematosus (CLE) and systemic lupus erythematosus (SLE) have been reported in patients taking PPIs. These events have occurred both as new onset and as an exacerbation of existing autoimmune disease. CLE is more common and occurs weeks to years after continuous PPI therapy in patients ranging from infants to the elderly. PPI-induced SLE is usually milder than non–drug-induced SLE and occurs days to years after initiating PPI therapy, primarily in patients ranging from young adults to the elderly. Most patients present with rash; however, arthralgia and cytopenia have also been reported. Discontinue pantoprazole if S/S of CLE or SLE develop, and refer patient to the appropriate specialist. Most patients improve within 4 to 12 weeks of PPI discontinuation. ▪ See Drug/Lab Interactions.

Monitor: Observe for S/S of a hypersensitivity reaction and/or severe skin reaction (e.g., acute interstitial nephritis, anaphylactic shock, anaphylaxis, angioedema, bronchospasm, urticaria). ▪ Monitor vital signs and pain levels. ▪ Concomitant use of antacids may be indicated. ▪ In hypersecretory states, acid output measurements may be indicated to guide dose adjustment. ▪ Monitor injection site. Thrombophlebitis has been reported. ▪ Zinc supplementation may be indicated in patients who are prone to zinc deficiency; see Precautions. ▪ Monitoring of magnesium levels may be indicated with prolonged PPI therapy; see Precautions and Drug/Lab Interactions. ▪ Serologic testing (e.g., ANA titers) may be indicated in patients who present with S/S of CLE or SLE. ▪ Change to oral dosing when appropriate. ▪ See Drug/Lab Interactions.

Patient Education: Review prescription and nonprescription drugs with your physician. ▪ Oral route preferred. ▪ Promptly report cardiovascular or neurologic symptoms, including dizziness, palpitations, seizures, or tetany; may be signs of hypomagnesemia. ▪ Promptly report any adverse effects, including S/S of hypersensitivity reactions or diarrhea.

Maternal/Child: Available data from observational studies failed to demonstrate an association of adverse pregnancy-related outcomes and pantoprazole use. Use during pregnancy only when clearly needed. ▪ Use caution during breast-feeding. Has been detected in breast milk. Effects on milk production are unknown. ▪ Safety and effectiveness for use in pediatric patients under 18 years of age not established.

Elderly: Safety and effectiveness similar to that of younger patients.

DRUG/LAB INTERACTIONS

Concurrent use with **rilpivirine-containing products** (e.g., rilpivirine, Complera [emtricitabine, rilpivirine, tenofovir disoproxil fumarate], Juluca [dolutegravir, rilpivirine], Odefsey [emtricitabine, rilpivirine, tenofovir alafenamide]) is contraindicated. ▪ Because of profound and long-lasting inhibition of gastric acid secretion, pantoprazole may interfere with the **absorption of drugs in which gastric pH is an important determinant of their bioavailability.** Absorption of **atazanavir, dasatinib, erlotinib, iron salts, ketoconazole, itraconazole, mycophenolate mofetil,** and **nilotinib** can decrease. ▪ Increases in INR and PT have been reported when administered concurrently with **warfarin**; monitoring of INR and PT indicated. Increases in INR and PT may lead to abnormal bleeding and death. Dose adjustment of warfarin may be needed to maintain target INR range. ▪ The effect of proton pump inhibitors on antiretroviral drugs is variable. Coadministration of proton pump inhibitors results in a significant reduction in **atazanavir** or **nelfinavir** plasma concentrations, which may result in a loss of their therapeutic effect and the development of drug resistance. Avoid concomitant use with **nelfinavir.** See prescribing information for atazanavir for dosing information. Increased exposure of **other antiretroviral drugs** (e.g., saquinavir) when used together with pantoprazole sodium may increase toxicity of the antiretroviral drugs. ▪ Long-term use may increase the risk of **digoxin** toxicity secondary to hypomagnesemia. ▪ Patients on long-term therapy receiving concomitant **diuretic therapy** may be at increased risk for hypomagnesemia. ▪ Concomitant use of proton pump inhibitors with high-dose **methotrexate** may elevate and prolong serum concentrations of methotrexate and/or its metabolite. May lead to methotrexate toxicity; consider withdrawal of pantoprazole. ▪ Concomitant administration of pantoprazole and clopidogrel had no clinically significant effect on clopidogrel-induced platelet aggregation. ▪ Studies suggest that with concurrent use, the metabolism and serum concentrations of pantoprazole are not significantly altered by other drugs metabolized by the cytochrome P_{450} system. ▪ CgA levels increase secondary to PPI-induced decreases in gastric acidity. Increased CgA levels may cause false-positive results in diagnostic investigations for neuroendocrine tumors. Stop pantoprazole treatment at least 14 days before assessing CgA levels and consider repeating the test if initial CgA levels are high (same commercial laboratory should be used). ▪ May cause false-positive **urine screening test for tetrahydrocannabinol** (THC).

SIDE EFFECTS
The most frequently occurring side effects are abdominal pain, arthralgias, diarrhea, dizziness, flatulence, headache, nausea, and vomiting. Abscess, blurred vision, chest pain, confusion, dyspnea, gastroenteritis, hemorrhage, hyperglycemia, hypokinesia, increased salivation, injection site reactions including thrombophlebitis, pruritus, rash, speech disorder, tinnitus, transient elevations of serum transaminase, urinary tract infection, and vertigo are reported. Numerous other side effects have been associated with oral pantoprazole.

Post-Marketing: Agranulocytosis, asthenia, bone fracture, CDAD, CLE, confusion, fatigue, fundic gland polyps, hallucinations, hepatocellular damage leading to jaundice and hepatic failure, hypersensitivity reactions (e.g., anaphylaxis, angioedema), hypomagnesemia, hyponatremia, insomnia, interstitial nephritis, malaise, pancytopenia, rhabdomyolysis, severe dermatologic reactions (e.g., erythema multiforme, Stevens-Johnson syndrome, toxic epidermal necrolysis [some fatal]), SLE, somnolence, taste disorders, weight changes.

ANTIDOTE
Keep physician informed of all side effects. May be treated symptomatically. Discontinue and initiate appropriate treatment if S/S associated with serious reactions listed in post-marketing reports occur; see Side Effects. Adverse effects from overdose (up to 240 mg/day in healthy subjects) did not occur during clinical trials. Not removed by hemodialysis.

PAPAVERINE HYDROCHLORIDE
(pah-**PAV**-er-een hy-droh-**KLOR**-eyed)

Vasodilator
(peripheral)

pH 3 to 4.5

USUAL DOSE
1 to 4 mL (30 to 120 mg) every 3 hours as indicated. Second dose may be given in 10 minutes only when treating extrasystoles.

PEDIATRIC DOSE
1.5 mg/kg of body weight every 6 hours; see Maternal/Child.

DOSE ADJUSTMENTS
See Drug/Lab Interactions.

DILUTION
May be given undiluted.

COMPATIBILITY
Will form a precipitate with LR.

Other sources suggest a few specific **compatibilities** dependent on concentration and manufacturer; consult a pharmacist.

RATE OF ADMINISTRATION
1 mL (30 mg) or fraction thereof over 2 minutes. Rapid IV injection may cause arrhythmias and fatal apnea.

ACTIONS
A nonnarcotic opium alkaloid, it is a direct smooth muscle relaxant and antispasmodic. Relaxation is noted in vascular system and bronchial musculature and in GI, biliary, and urinary tracts. More effective on muscle in spasm, it has an affinity for the smooth muscle of blood vessels. Affects cardiac muscle to depress conduction and increase refractory period. Improved circulation and muscle relaxation decrease pain. Metabolized in the liver and excreted in the urine.

INDICATIONS AND USES
Vascular spasm associated with an acute myocardial infarction. ▪ Peripheral or pulmonary embolism. ▪ Peripheral vascular disease and cerebral angiospastic states. ▪ Visceral spasm of ureteral, biliary, or GI colic. ▪ Angina pectoris.

CONTRAINDICATIONS
Complete AV heart block.

PRECAUTIONS
Rarely used; active therapeutic value is questioned. ▪ Rapid IV injection may cause death. ▪ IM injection is preferred. ▪ Use with caution in glaucoma and impaired liver function. ▪ Large doses can depress AV and intraventricular conduction, resulting in arrhythmias.
Monitor: Observe patient continuously; monitor vital signs. ▪ See Drug/Lab Interactions.
Patient Education: Avoid alcohol and other CNS depressants. ▪ May cause dizziness and drowsiness; request assistance for ambulation. ▪ Use caution in any task requiring alertness.
Maternal/Child: Category C: safety for use in pregnancy and breast-feeding and in pediatric patients not established.
Elderly: Risk of hypothermia may be increased.

DRUG/LAB INTERACTIONS
May be used with **narcotics** if the relaxant effect is not adequate to relieve discomfort. Narcotic dosage should be reduced. ▪ Antagonizes effects of **levodopa.**

SIDE EFFECTS

Blurred or double vision, diaphoresis, discomfort (generalized), flushing, hypertension (slight), hypotension, respiratory depth increase, scleral jaundice, sedation, tachycardia.

Major: Respiratory depression, seizures, ventricular ectopic rhythms, sudden death.

ANTIDOTE

Notify the physician of any minor side effects. If minor symptoms progress or any major side effect appears, discontinue the drug immediately and notify the physician. Treatment of toxicity will be symptomatic and supportive. Consider diazepam or phenytoin for convulsions. Anesthesia with thiopental and a neuromuscular blocking agent may be required. Use dopamine for hypotension. Calcium gluconate may reduce toxic cardiovascular effects. Monitor ECG. Resuscitate as necessary.

PARICALCITOL

(pair-ee-**KAL**-sih-tohl)

Vitamin D analog

Zemplar

USUAL DOSE

Pretreatment: Baseline studies indicated; see Monitor.

Before treatment, ensure calcium is not above the upper limit of normal.

Paricalcitol: Recommended initial dose is 0.04 to 0.1 mcg/kg (2.8 to 7 mcg) administered no more frequently than every other day at any time during dialysis. The maximum daily adult dose is 0.24 mcg/kg. Target the maintenance dose to intact parathyroid hormone (PTH) levels within the desired therapeutic range and serum calcium within normal limits.

Information supplied by the manufacturer suggests that the relative dosing of paricalcitol to calcitriol is 4:1. When converting a patient from calcitriol to paricalcitol, the initial dose of paricalcitol should be four times greater than the patient's dose of calcitriol.

PEDIATRIC DOSE

Dose recommendations are based on severity of disease in addition to body weight. A dose is administered at any time during dialysis.

Pediatric patients 5 years of age and older: Administer three times per week, no more frequently than every other day, at any time during dialysis. Target the maintenance dose to intact PTH levels within the desired therapeutic range and serum calcium within normal limits.

Baseline iPTH level less than 500 pg/mL: 0.04 mcg/kg 3 times a week.

Baseline iPTH level equal to or greater than 500 pg/mL: 0.08 mcg/kg 3 times a week.

See Dose Adjustments.

DOSE ADJUSTMENTS

Adults: Monitor serum calcium, phosphorus, and calcium × phosphorus product (Ca × P) frequently during any dose adjustment period. See Monitor.

Pediatric patients: Adjust dose in 0.04-mcg/kg increments based on the levels of serum iPTH, calcium, and Ca × P.

Adults and pediatric patients: Incremental dosing must be individualized and commensurate with PTH, serum calcium, and phosphorus levels. ▪ Titrate the dose based on intact PTH. Before raising the dose, ensure serum calcium is within normal limits. ▪ Suspend or decrease the dose if intact PTH is persistently and abnormally low to reduce the risk of adynamic bone disease or if serum calcium is consistently above the normal range to

Continued

reduce the risk of hypercalcemia. If dose suspension is necessary, restart at a reduced dose after laboratory values have normalized. ▪ Dose adjustment and increased monitoring may be necessary when given concomitantly with drugs that may increase the risk of hypercalcemia. Dose adjustment as well as increased monitoring of serum calcium and intact PTH may be necessary when given concomitantly with strong CYP3A inhibitors; see Drug/Lab Interactions. ▪ No dose adjustment required in patients with mild or moderate hepatic function. Has not been studied in patients with severe hepatic impairment. ▪ The following chart is a suggested approach to dose titration.

Recommended Paricalcitol Adult Dose Titration Based Upon Intact PTH	
Intact PTH Level at Follow-up Visit	Dose Adjustment
Above target and intact PTH increased	Increase[a] by 2 mcg to 4 mcg every 2 to 4 weeks
Above target and intact PTH decreased by <30%	Increase[a] by 2 mcg to 4 mcg every 2 to 4 weeks
Above target and intact PTH decreased by 30% to 60%	No change
Above target and intact PTH decreased by >60%	Decrease per clinical judgment
At target and intact PTH stable	No change

[a]The maximum daily adult dose is 0.24 mcg/kg.

Recommended Paricalcitol Pediatric Dose Titration Based on Intact PTH Patients 5 Years of Age and Older	
Intact PTH Level at Follow-up Visit	Dose Adjustment
Above target and intact PTH decreased by <30%	Increase by 0.04 mcg/kg every 2 to 4 weeks
Intact PTH ≥150 pg/mL and decreased by 30% to 60%	No change
Intact PTH less than 150 pg/mL or decreased by >60%	Decrease by 0.04 mcg/kg weekly, or by 50% if decreased dose equals zero

DILUTION
May be given undiluted. Available as a solution in a 2 mcg/mL and 5 mcg/mL single-dose vial and a 10 mcg/2 mL multiple-dose vial.
Filters: Not required by manufacturer; no further data available.
Storage: Store single-dose and multidose vials at CRT before use. Discard unused portions of single-dose vials. Multidose vial is stable for up to 7 days at CRT after entry into vial.

COMPATIBILITY
Compatibility information not available from manufacturer; consult a pharmacist.

RATE OF ADMINISTRATION
Administer as an IV injection over 30 seconds through a hemodialysis vascular access port at any time during dialysis. May be administered IV if an access port is unavailable.

ACTIONS
A synthetically manufactured active vitamin D analog. Studies have demonstrated that paricalcitol's biologic actions are mediated through binding of the vitamin D receptor (VDR), which results in the selective activation of vitamin D responsive pathways. Vitamin D and paricalcitol reduce PTH levels by inhibiting PTH synthesis and secretions. Studies suggest that paricalcitol may cause less hypercalcemia and hyperphosphatemia than calcitriol. Serum paricalcitol levels decrease rapidly after a bolus injection. Extensively bound to plasma proteins. Extensively metabolized by multiple hepatic and non-hepatic enzymes. Mean half-life is approximately 15 hours. Eliminated primarily by hepatobiliary excretion in feces and, to a much smaller extent, by the kidneys.

INDICATIONS AND USES

Prevention and treatment of secondary hyperparathyroidism in patients 5 years of age and older with chronic kidney disease (CKD) and on dialysis.

CONTRAINDICATIONS

Patients with evidence of vitamin D toxicity, hypercalcemia, or known hypersensitivity to paricalcitol or any of the active ingredients in this product; see Precautions.

PRECAUTIONS

Hypercalcemia may occur during treatment. Severe hypercalcemia may require emergency attention. If clinically significant hypercalcemia develops, dose should be reduced or held. Acute hypercalcemia may increase the risk of cardiac arrhythmias and seizures and may potentiate the effects of digitalis on the heart. ■ Hypercalcemia can increase the risk of digitalis toxicity. Chronic hypercalcemia can lead to generalized vascular calcification and other soft tissue calcification. See Side Effects and Antidote. ■ Hypercalcemia may be exacerbated by concomitant administration of high doses of calcium-containing preparations, thiazide diuretics, or other vitamin D compounds. High intake of calcium and phosphate concomitantly with vitamin D compounds may lead to hypercalciuria and hyperphosphatemia. ■ Adynamic bone disease with subsequent increased risk of fractures may develop if PTH levels are suppressed to abnormally low levels.

Monitor: During initiation of therapy or when adjusting a dose, obtain baseline serum calcium and phosphorus levels and determine levels at least twice a week. Once dosage has been established, serum calcium and phosphorus should be monitored at least monthly. See Dose Adjustments. ■ Calculate Ca $\times$ P (should be less than 75). ■ Measurements of serum or plasma PTH are recommended every 2 to 4 weeks after initiation of therapy or dose adjustment. ■ Monitor for signs and symptoms of hypercalcemia and digitalis toxicity. See Side Effects.

Patient Education: Inform physician of all medications, including prescription and nonprescription drugs, and supplements being taken. ■ Routine monitoring of laboratory parameters (e.g., calcium and intact PTH) will need to be done during treatment. ■ Report symptoms of hypercalcemia promptly (e.g., constipation, difficulty thinking clearly, fatigue, increased thirst, increased urination, loss of appetite, nausea or vomiting, weight loss). Dose adjustment or treatment may be required. Strict adherence to dietary supplementation of calcium and restriction of phosphorus is required to ensure optimal effectiveness of therapy. Phosphate-binding compounds (e.g., calcium acetate, sevelamer) may be needed to control serum phosphorus levels in patients with CKD, but excessive use of aluminum-containing products (e.g., aluminum hydroxide gel) should be avoided.

Maternal/Child: Data are limited for use in pregnant females. There are risks to the mother and fetus associated with CKD in pregnancy. ■ No information available on the presence of paricalcitol in human milk, the effects of the drug on the breast-fed infant, or the effects of the drug on milk production. ■ Has not been studied in pediatric patients under 5 years of age.

Elderly: Studies did not include sufficient numbers of subjects age 65 years and older to determine whether they respond differently from younger subjects. In general, dose selection should be cautious, usually starting at the low end of the dosing range, reflecting the greater frequency of decreased hepatic or cardiac function and of concomitant disease or other drug therapy.

DRUG/LAB INTERACTIONS

Paricalcitol is partially metabolized by the **cytochrome P$_{450}$ enzyme CYP3A.** Use with caution when administered concomitantly **with known inhibitors of this enzyme** (e.g., atazanavir, boceprevir, clarithromycin, conivaptan, grapefruit juice, indinavir, itraconazole, ketoconazole, lopinavir/ritonavir, nefazodone, nelfinavir, posaconazole, ritonavir, saquinavir, voriconazole). ■ Digitalis toxicity is potentiated by hypercalcemia. Monitor for digitalis toxicity and increase frequency of serum calcium monitoring when initiating or adjusting the dose of paricalcitol. ■ **Phosphate or vitamin D–related compounds** should not be taken concomitantly with paricalcitol; see Precautions. ■ Hypercalcemia may be exacerbated by concomitant administration of high doses of calcium-containing preparations, thiazide diuretics, or other vitamin D compounds; requires more frequent monitoring of calcium and may require dose adjustments. ■ May reduce **serum total alkaline phosphatase** levels.

SIDE EFFECTS

The most commonly reported side effects include arthralgia, chills, dry mouth, edema, fever, gastrointestinal hemorrhage, influenza, malaise, nausea, palpitations, pneumonia, sepsis, and vomiting. Many other side effects occurred in fewer than 2% of patients. Overdose or chronic administration may lead to hypercalcemia. Signs and symptoms of vitamin D intoxication associated with hypercalcemia include: **Early:** bone pain, constipation, dry mouth, headache, metallic taste, muscle pain, nausea, somnolence, vomiting, and weakness. **Late:** Anorexia, cardiac arrhythmias, conjunctivitis (calcific), death, decreased libido, ectopic calcification, elevated AST and ALT, elevated BUN, hypercholesterolemia, hypertension, hyperthermia, overt psychosis (rare), pancreatitis, photophobia, pruritus, rhinorrhea, somnolence, and weight loss.

Post-Marketing: Hypersensitivity reactions (e.g., angioedema [including laryngeal edema]), rash, urticaria.

Overdose: Overdose may lead to hypercalcemia, hypercalciuria, and hyperphosphatemia.

ANTIDOTE

Notify physician of any side effects. Treatment should consist of general supportive measures and serial serum electrolyte determinations (especially calcium). Monitor rate of urinary calcium excretion. Treatment of patients with clinically significant hypercalcemia consists of immediate dose reduction or interruption of the therapy and includes a low-calcium diet, withdrawal of calcium supplements, patient mobilization, attention to fluid and electrolyte imbalances, assessment of electrocardiographic abnormalities (critical in patients receiving digoxin), and hemodialysis or peritoneal dialysis against a calcium-free dialysate, as warranted. Monitor serum calcium levels frequently until calcium levels return to within normal limits. Paricalcitol may be restarted at a lower dose when serum calcium levels return to within normal limits. Not significantly removed by dialysis.

PEGLOTICASE BBW

(peg-**LOE**-ti-kase)

Antigout agent

Krystexxa

USUAL DOSE

Pretreatment: Discontinue oral urate-lowering medications before beginning therapy; see Precautions and Drug/Lab Interactions. Screening for G6PD deficiency may be indicated and baseline studies indicated; see Monitor.

Gout flare prophylaxis: Use of an NSAID or oral colchicine is recommended beginning at least 1 week before the start of pegloticase therapy and lasting at least 6 months unless medically contraindicated or not tolerated.

Premedication: Patients should be premedicated before each dose with antihistamines and corticosteroids to reduce the risk of infusion reactions, including anaphylaxis or other hypersensitivity reactions.

Pegloticase: 8 mg as an IV infusion every 2 weeks. Optimum treatment duration not established.

DOSE ADJUSTMENTS

No dose adjustment is required based on age, gender, race, or renal impairment.

DILUTION

Withdraw 1 mL (8 mg) from the 2-mL vial. A clear, colorless solution that must be further diluted by injecting it into a 250-mL bag of NS or $\frac{1}{2}$NS for infusion. Ensure thorough mixing by inverting the infusion bag a number of times. Do not shake. If diluted solution has been refrigerated, bring to RT before administration (do not subject to artificial heating [e.g., hot water, microwave]).

Filters: No study data available; if filtering is necessary, contact manufacturer.

Storage: Before use, refrigerate in carton at 2° to 8° C (36° to 46° F). Protect from light. Do not shake or freeze. Do not use beyond the expiration date stamped. Diluted infusion bags are stable for 4 hours refrigerated or at RT (20° to 25° C [68° to 77° F]). Manufacturer recommends storing under refrigeration (not frozen), protected from light, and used within 4 hours of dilution. Discard unused product remaining in the 2-mL vial.

COMPATIBILITY

Manufacturer states, "Do not mix or dilute with other drugs."

RATE OF ADMINISTRATION

A single dose properly diluted as an infusion over no less than 2 hours. Do not administer by IV push or as a bolus. Administer by gravity feed, with a syringe-type pump or infusion pump. If an infusion reaction occurs, the infusion may be slowed, or stopped and restarted at a slower rate, at the discretion of the physician.

ACTIONS

A uric acid–specific enzyme; a PEGylated product that consists of recombinant modified mammalian urate oxidase (uricase) produced by a genetically modified strain of *Escherichia coli*. Achieves its therapeutic effect by catalyzing the oxidation of uric acid to allantoin, thereby lowering serum uric acid. Duration of suppression of plasma uric acid appears to be dose related. Allantoin is an inert and water-soluble purine metabolite that is readily eliminated, primarily by renal excretion.

INDICATIONS AND USES

Treatment of chronic gout in adult patients refractory to conventional therapy. Gout refractory to conventional therapy occurs in patients who have failed to normalize serum uric acid and in patients whose S/S are inadequately controlled with xanthine oxidase inhibitors (e.g., allopurinol) at the maximum medically appropriate dose or for whom these drugs are contraindicated.

Limitation of use: Not recommended for the treatment of asymptomatic hyperuricemia.

CONTRAINDICATIONS

Patients with glucose-6-phosphate dehydrogenase (G6PD) deficiency.

PRECAUTIONS

Administer under the direction of a physician knowledgeable in its use in a facility with adequate diagnostic and treatment facilities to monitor the patient and respond to any medical emergency. ▪ Anaphylaxis and infusion reactions have been reported to occur during and after administration of pegloticase. ▪ Anaphylaxis may occur with any infusion, including a first infusion, and generally manifests within 2 hours of the infusion. However, delayed-type hypersensitivity reactions have also been reported. ▪ Infusion reactions and anaphylaxis occurred in patients premedicated with one or more doses of an oral antihistamine and an IV corticosteroid and/or acetaminophen. ▪ Risk of infusion reaction and anaphylaxis is higher in patients who have lost therapeutic response (e.g., uric acid levels increase to above 6 mg/dL); see Monitor. ▪ Concomitant use of oral urate-lowering agents (e.g., allopurinol, febuxostat) and pegloticase may blunt the rise of serum uric acid levels. Discontinue oral urate-lowering medications and do not institute oral urate-lowering agents while taking pegloticase. ▪ Life-threatening hemolysis and methemoglobinemia have been reported with pegloticase in patients with G6PD deficiency. ▪ An increase in gout flares is often observed with the initiation of anti-hyperuricemic therapy because changing serum uric acid levels result in the mobilization of urate from tissue deposits. Gout flare prophylaxis with an NSAID or colchicine is recommended. Pegloticase does not need to be discontinued because of a gout flare. ▪ Exacerbation of CHF has occurred; use with caution in patients with CHF. ▪ Data not available for safety and efficacy of retreatment with pegloticase after stopping treatment for longer than 4 weeks. Due to immunogenicity, may increase risk of infusion reactions, including anaphylaxis. ▪ Anti-pegloticase antibodies developed in most patients treated. High titers were associated with a failure to maintain pegloticase-induced normalization of uric acid. These patients also had a higher incidence of infusion reactions. Anti-PEG antibodies were also detected; the impact on patients' responses to other PEG-containing therapeutics is unknown. ▪ Effects of either renal or hepatic impairment on pegloticase pharmacokinetics were not studied.

Monitor: Before initiating treatment, screening for G6PD deficiency is recommended in patients at higher risk (e.g., African or Mediterranean [including Southern European and Middle Eastern] and Southern Asian ancestry); see Contraindications. ▪ Monitor serum uric acid levels before each infusion. Consider discontinuing treatment if levels increase to above 6 mg/dL, particularly when two consecutive levels above 6 mg/dL are observed. ▪ Closely monitor for S/S of potential anaphylaxis for an appropriate period (e.g., during and for at least 1 hour after administration). Manifestations of anaphylaxis have included hemodynamic instability, perioral or lingual edema, and wheezing with or without rash or urticaria. S/S of infusion reactions have included chest discomfort or pain, dyspnea, erythema, flushing, pruritus, and urticaria. S/S of infusion reactions may overlap with those of anaphylaxis. Infusion reactions can occur at any time during therapy, with approximately 3% occurring with the first infusion and approximately 91% occurring during the time of infusion. Slow or stop the infusion (depending on the severity) if an infusion reaction occurs. ▪ Closely monitor patients with a history of CHF during and after infusion. ▪ Patients being restarted on therapy after a drug-free interval longer than 4 weeks should be monitored carefully.

Patient Education: Immediately report S/S of an infusion or hypersensitivity reaction (e.g., chest pain, dizziness, dyspnea, fever, flushing, hypotension, nausea, perioral or lingual edema, pruritus, rash, rigors, urticaria, wheezing). ▪ Review prescription and nonprescription drugs with physician. Discontinue use of any oral urate-lowering agents. ▪ Report side effects of pegloticase that are bothersome or do not go away (e.g., nausea, vomiting). ▪ Patients of African or Mediterranean (including Southern European and Middle Eastern) and Southern Asian descent may require testing for G6PD deficiency. ▪ Gout flares may increase with initiation of pegloticase; prophylactic medications recommended.

Maternal/Child: Use during pregnancy only if clearly needed. ▪ Not recommended for use during breast-feeding. ▪ Safety and effectiveness for use in pediatric patients under 18 years of age not established.

Elderly: Response similar to other age-groups; however, greater sensitivity in the elderly cannot be ruled out.

DRUG/LAB INTERACTIONS

Formal drug interaction studies have not been conducted. ▪ Concomitant use of oral **urate-lowering agents** (allopurinol, febuxostat) and pegloticase may blunt the rise of serum uric acid levels; discontinue oral urate-lowering medications and do not institute oral urate-lowering agents while taking pegloticase.

SIDE EFFECTS

The most common side effects include anaphylaxis, chest pain, constipation, contusion or ecchymosis, gout flares, infusion reactions, nasopharyngitis, nausea, pain, and vomiting. The most serious reactions are anaphylaxis, infusion reactions, and gout flares.

Post-Marketing: Asthenia, malaise, peripheral swelling.

ANTIDOTE

Keep physician informed of all side effects. Some will be tolerated or treated symptomatically. Discontinue immediately for any acute serious infusion or hypersensitivity reaction and treat as appropriate; may require epinephrine, airway management, oxygen, antihistamines, vasopressors, corticosteroids, albuterol, IV fluids, and ventilation equipment as indicated. Resuscitate as necessary. Slow or stop the infusion (depending on the severity) if an infusion reaction occurs. May be restarted at a slower rate if symptoms subside. Pegloticase does not need to be discontinued because of a gout flare. No specific antidote; monitor and support as indicated in overdose. Resuscitate as necessary.

PEMBROLIZUMAB
(**PEM**-broe-**LIZ**-ue-mab)

Antineoplastic
Monoclonal antibody

Keytruda

pH 5.5

USUAL DOSE

Pretreatment: Verify pregnancy status. Pretesting required and baseline studies indicated; see Monitor.

Patient selection for treatment: Select patients for treatment with pembrolizumab as a single agent based on the presence of positive PD-L1 expression in:

- Stage III NSCLC who are not candidates for surgical resection or definitive chemoradiation
- Metastatic NSCLC
- First-line treatment of metastatic or unresectable, recurrent head and neck squamous cell carcinoma (HNSCC)
- Metastatic urothelial carcinoma
- Metastatic gastric cancer. If PD-L1 expression is not detected in an archival gastric cancer specimen, evaluate the feasibility of obtaining a tumor biopsy for PD-L1 testing
- Metastatic esophageal cancer
- Recurrent or metastatic cervical cancer

Information about FDA-approved tests for the detection of PD-L1 expression for these indications is available at http://www.fda.gov/CompanionDiagnostics.

Unresectable or metastatic melanoma: 200 mg administered as an IV infusion over 30 minutes every 3 weeks until disease progression or unacceptable toxicity.

Adjuvant treatment of adult patients with melanoma: 200 mg administered as an IV infusion over 30 minutes every 3 weeks until disease recurrence, unacceptable toxicity, or for up to 12 months in patients without disease recurrence.

Cervical cancer: 200 mg IV every 3 weeks or 400 mg every 6 weeks; continue until disease progression, unacceptable toxicity, or for up to 24 months in patients without disease progression.

Breast cancer, triple negative, high-risk, early stage: In combination with other chemotherapy for 24 weeks: 200 mg IV once every 3 weeks for 8 doses or 400 mg IV once every 6 weeks for 4 doses, or until disease progression or unacceptable toxicity. Can be given as single agent for up to 27 weeks as 200 mg IV every 3 weeks for 9 doses or 400 mg IV every 6 weeks for 5 doses, until disease progression or unacceptable toxicity. Colorectal cancer, esophageal cancer, gastric cancer, head and neck cancer, hepatocellular carcinoma, Hodgkin lymphoma, Merkel cell carcinoma, urothelial carcinoma: 200 mg IV every 3 weeks or 400 mg every 6 weeks; continue until disease progression, unacceptable toxicity, or for up to 24 months in patients without disease progression.

Metastatic non–small-cell lung cancer (NSCLC), small-cell lung cancer (SCLC), head and neck squamous cell carcinoma (HNSCC), classical Hodgkin lymphoma (cHL), primary mediastinal large B-cell lymphoma (PMBCL), urothelial carcinoma, microsatellite instability–high (MSI-H) cancer, gastric cancer, esophageal cancer, cervical cancer, colorecdtal cancer (unresectable or metastatic); cutaneous squamous cell carcinoma, esophageal cancer, melanoma, hepatocellular carcinoma (HCC), and Merkel cell carcinoma (MCC): 200 mg administered as an IV infusion over 30 minutes every 3 weeks or 400 mg IV once every 6 weeks until disease progression or unacceptable toxicity or up to 24 months in patients without disease progression. When administering in combination with chemotherapy to patients with NSCLC and HNSCC, pembrolizumab should be administered before chemotherapy when given on the same day. Also see prescribing information for pemetrexed and carboplatin or cisplatin, as appropriate.

High-risk BCG-unresponsive, non–muscle invasive bladder cancer (NMIBC): 200 mg administered as an IV infusion over 30 minutes every 3 weeks until persistent or recurrent high-risk NMIBC, disease progression, or unacceptable toxicity, or up to 24 months in patients without disease progression.

Renal cell carcinoma (RCC): 200 mg administered as an IV infusion over 30 minutes every 3 weeks or 400 mg IV every 6 weeks in combination with 5 mg axitinib orally twice daily until disease progression, unacceptable toxicity or, for pembrolizumab, up to 24 months in patients without disease progression. When axitinib is used in combination with pembrolizumab, dose escalation of axitinib above the initial 5-mg dose may be considered at intervals of 6 weeks or longer. See Prescribing Information for recommended axitinib dosing information.

Endometrial carcinoma: 200 mg administered as an IV infusion over 30 minutes every 3 weeks in combination with lenvatinib 20 mg orally once daily until disease progression, unacceptable toxicity or, for pembrolizumab, up to 24 months in patients without disease progression. See prescribing information for recommended lenvatinib dosing information.

PEDIATRIC DOSE

Classical Hodgkin lymphoma (cHL), primary mediastinal large B-cell lymphoma (PMBCL), microsatellite instability–high (MSI-H) cancer, and Merkel cell carcinoma (MCC): 2 mg/kg (up to a maximum of 200 mg) administered as an IV infusion over 30 minutes every 3 weeks until disease progression or unacceptable toxicity or up to 24 months in patients without disease progression.

DOSE ADJUSTMENTS

No dose reductions are recommended. Withhold or discontinue pembrolizumab to manage adverse reactions as described in the following chart.

Recommended Dose Modifications of Pembrolizumab for Adverse Reactions		
Adverse Reaction	**Severity[a]**	**Dose Modification for Pembrolizumab**
Immune-mediated pneumonitis	Grade 2	Withhold[b]
	Grades 3 or 4 or recurrent Grade 2	Permanently discontinue
Immune-mediated colitis	Grades 2 or 3	Withhold[b]
	Grade 4	Permanently discontinue
Immune-mediated hepatitis in patients with HCC	Aspartate aminotransferase (AST) or alanine aminotransferase (ALT) $\geq5 \times$ ULN if baseline less than $2 \times$ ULN; AST or ALT >3 times baseline if baseline $\geq2 \times$ ULN Total bilirubin >2 mg/dL if baseline <1.5 mg/dL; or Total bilirubin >3 mg/dL, regardless of baseline levels	Withhold[c]
	ALT or AST $>10 \times$ ULN; or Child-Pugh score ≥9 points; Gastrointestinal bleeding suggestive of portal hypertension; or New onset of clinically detectable ascites; or encephalopathy	Permanently discontinue
Immune-mediated hepatitis in patients without HCC	AST or ALT >3 but no more than $5 \times$ ULN or total bilirubin >1.5 but no more than $3 \times$ ULN	Withhold[b]
For liver enzyme elevations in RCC patients treated with combination therapy, see dosing guidelines that follow this chart	In patients without liver metastases, AST or ALT $>5 \times$ ULN or total bilirubin $>3 \times$ ULN In patients with liver metastasis and Grade 2 AST or ALT at baseline, with an increase in AST or ALT of 50% or more relative to baseline that persists for at least 1 week	Permanently discontinue

Continued

Recommended Dose Modifications of Pembrolizumab for Adverse Reactions—cont'd		
Adverse Reaction	**Severity[a]**	**Dose Modification for Pembrolizumab**
Immune-mediated endocrinopathies	Grades 3 or 4	Withhold until clinically stable
Immune-mediated nephritis	Grade 2	Withhold[b]
	Grades 3 or 4	Permanently discontinue
Immune-mediated skin adverse reactions	Grade 3 or suspected Stevens-Johnson Syndrome (SJS) or toxic epidermal necrolysis (TEN)	Withhold
	Grade 4 or confirmed SJS or TEN	Permanently discontinue
Hematologic toxicity in patients with cHL or PMBCL	Grade 4	Withhold until resolution to Grades 0 or 1
Other immune-mediated adverse reactions	Grades 2 or 3 based on the severity and type of reaction	Withhold[b]
	Grade 3 based on the severity and type of reaction or Grade 4	Permanently discontinue
Recurrent immune-mediated adverse reactions	Recurrent Grade 2 pneumonitis Recurrent Grades 3 or 4	Permanently discontinue
Inability to taper corticosteroid	Requirement for 10 mg/day or greater prednisone or equivalent for more than 12 weeks after last dose of pembrolizumab	Permanently discontinue
Persistent Grade 2 or 3 adverse reaction (excluding endocrinopathy)	Grades 2 or 3 adverse reactions lasting 12 weeks or longer after last dose of pembrolizumab	Permanently discontinue
Infusion-related reactions	Grades 1 or 2	Interrupt or slow the rate of infusion
	Grades 3 or 4	Permanently discontinue

[a]Toxicity was graded per National Cancer Institute Common Terminology Criteria for Adverse Events. Version 4.0 (NCI CTCAE v4).
[b]Resume in patients with complete or partial resolution (Grades 0 to 1) after corticosteroid taper.
[c]Resume in HCC patients when AST or ALT and total bilirubin recover to Grades 0 to 1 or to baseline.

- In patients with RCC being treated with pembrolizumab in combination with axitinib: (1) if ALT or AST 3 or more times the ULN but less than 10 times the ULN without concurrent total bilirubin 2 or more times the ULN, withhold both pembrolizumab and axitinib until these adverse reactions recover to Grades 0 to 1. Consider corticosteroid therapy. Consider rechallenge with a single drug or sequential rechallenge with both drugs after recovery. If rechallenging with axitinib, consider dose reduction as per the axitinib prescribing information. Or (2) if ALT or AST 10 or more times the ULN or more than 3 times the ULN with concurrent total bilirubin 2 or more times the ULN, permanently discontinue both pembrolizumab and axitinib and consider corticosteroid therapy. ■ When administering pembrolizumab in combination with lenvatinib for the treatment of endometrial carcinoma, interrupt one or both as appropriate. No dose reductions are recommended for pembrolizumab. Withhold dose, reduce dose, or discontinue lenvatinib in accordance with the instructions in the lenvatinib prescribing information. ■ No dose adjustment is recommended for patients with renal impairment or mild hepatic impairment. In addition, age, gender, race, and tumor burden do not affect the clearance of pembrolizumab. ■ See Precautions, Monitor, and Antidote.

DILUTION

Available in single-use vials containing 100 mg/4 mL (25 mg/mL) of pembrolizumab as a clear to slightly opalescent, colorless to slight yellow solution. Calculate the number of vials required for the recommended dose. Withdraw the required volume from the vial(s) of pembrolizumab and transfer into an IV bag or container of NS or D5W. Mix diluted solution by gentle inversion. ***Do not shake.*** The final concentration of the diluted solution should be between 1 and 10 mg/mL.

Filters: Must be administered using IV tubing that contains a sterile, nonpyrogenic, low–protein-binding, 0.2- to 5-micron in-line or add-on filter.

Storage: Before use, refrigerate vials at 2° to 8° C (36° to 46° F) in the carton to protect from light. ***Do not freeze or shake.*** Does not contain a preservative. Store the diluted solutions at RT for no more than 6 hours or refrigerate for no more than 96 hours. Storage times reflect time from initial dilution of solution through administration of dose. If diluted solution is refrigerated, allow it to come to RT before administration. Discard any unused portion left in a vial.

COMPATIBILITY

Manufacturer states, "Do not co-administer other drugs through the same infusion line."

RATE OF ADMINISTRATION

A single dose as an infusion equally distributed over 30 minutes. If diluted solution for administration has been refrigerated, allow it to come to RT before administration. If a common IV line is used to administer other drugs in addition to pembrolizumab, flush the IV line before and after each infusion of pembrolizumab with NS. Administer through an IV tubing that contains a sterile, nonpyrogenic, low–protein-binding, 0.2- to 5-micron in-line or add-on filter.

ACTIONS

An antineoplastic agent. Pembrolizumab is a humanized monoclonal antibody and an IgG4 kappa immunoglobulin that binds to the programmed death receptor-1 (PD-1 receptor) found on the T-cells. The PD-1 ligands PD-L1 and PD-L2 normally bind to the PD receptor and inhibit T-cell proliferation and cytokine release. Up-regulation of PD-1 ligands occurs in some tumors, and signaling through this pathway can contribute to the inhibition of active T-cell immune surveillance of tumors. Pembrolizumab binds to the PD-1 receptor and blocks its interaction with PD-L1 and PD-L2, releasing PD-1 pathway–mediated inhibition of the immune response, including the antitumor immune response. In syngeneic mouse tumor models, blocking PD-1 activity resulted in decreased tumor growth. Mean elimination half-life is 22 days. Steady-state concentrations were reached by 16 weeks of repeated dosing.

INDICATIONS AND USES

Treatment of patients with **unresectable or metastatic melanoma.** ▪ Adjuvant treatment of **melanoma with involvement of lymph node(s)** following complete resection. ▪ In combination with pemetrexed and platinum chemotherapy as first-line treatment of patients with **metastatic nonsquamous non–small-cell lung cancer** (NSCLC) with no epidermal growth factor receptor (EGFR) or anaplastic lymphoma kinase (ALK) genomic tumor aberrations. ▪ In combination with carboplatin and either paclitaxel or paclitaxel protein-bound for the **first-line treatment of patients with metastatic squamous NSCLC.** ▪ As a single agent for first-line treatment of patients with **NSCLC expressing PD-L1** (Tumor Proportion Score [TPS] ≥1%) as determined by an FDA-approved test, with no EGFR or ALK genomic tumor aberrations and either (1) stage III in which patients are not candidates for surgical resection or definitive chemoradiation, or (2) metastatic. ▪ As a single agent for the treatment of patients with **metastatic NSCLC** whose tumors express PD-L1 (TPS ≥1%) as determined by an FDA-approved test with disease progression on or after platinum-containing chemotherapy. Patients with EGFR or ALK genomic tumor aberrations should have disease progression on FDA-approved therapy for these aberrations before receiving pembrolizumab. ▪ Treatment of patients with **metastatic small-cell lung cancer** (SCLC) with disease progression on or after platinum-based chemotherapy and at least one other prior line of therapy.[a] ▪ In combination with platinum and fluorouracil (FU), indicated for the first-line treatment of patients with **metastatic or unresectable, recurrent head and neck squamous cell carcinoma** (HNSCC). ▪ As a single agent for the first-line treatment of patients with **metastatic or unresectable, recurrent HNSCC whose tumors express PD-L1** (Combined Positive Score [CPS] ≥1) as determined by an FDA-approved test. ▪ As a single agent for the treatment of patients with **recurrent or metastatic HNSCC** with disease progression on or after platinum-containing chemotherapy. ▪ Treatment of adult and pediatric patients with **refractory classical Hodgkin lymphoma** (cHL) or patients who have relapsed after 3 or more prior lines of therapy.[a] ▪ Treatment of adult and pediatric patients who have **refractory primary mediastinal large B-cell lymphoma** (PMBCL) or who have relapsed after 2 or more prior lines of therapy[a]; see Limitation of Use. ▪ Treatment of patients with **locally advanced or metastatic urothelial carcinoma** who are not eligible for cisplatin-containing chemotherapy and whose tumors express PD-L1 [Combined Positive Score (CPS) ≥10], or in patients who are not eligible for any platinum-containing chemotherapy regardless of PD-L1 status.[a] ▪ Treatment of patients with **locally advanced or metastatic urothelial carcinoma** who have disease progression during or after platinum-containing chemotherapy or within 12 months of neoadjuvant or adjuvant treatment with platinum-containing chemotherapy. ▪ Treatment of patients with *Bacillus* **Calmette-Guérin (BCG)-unresponsive, high-risk, non–muscle invasive bladder cancer** (NMIBC) with carcinoma in situ (CIS) with or without papillary tumors who are ineligible for or have elected not to undergo cystectomy. ▪ Treatment of adult and pediatric patients with **unresectable or metastatic, microsatellite instability–high (MSI-H) or mismatch repair–deficient** (1) solid tumors that have progressed after prior treatment and who have no satisfactory alternative treatment options, or (2) colorectal cancer that has progressed after treatment with fluoropyrimidine, oxaliplatin, and irinotecan[a]; see Limitation of Use. ▪ Treatment of patients with **recurrent locally advanced or metastatic gastric or gastroesophageal junction adenocarcinoma whose tumors express PD-L1** (CPS ≥1) as determined by an FDA-approved test, with disease progression on or after two or more prior lines of therapy, including fluoropyrimidine- and platinum-containing chemotherapy and, if appropriate, HER2/neu-targeted therapy.[a] ▪ Treatment of patients with **recurrent locally advanced or metastatic squamous cell carcinoma of the esophagus whose tumors express PD-L1** (CPS ≥10) as determined by an FDA-approved test, with disease progression after one or more prior lines of systemic therapy. ▪ Treatment of patients with **recurrent or metastatic cervical cancer** with disease progression on or after chemotherapy whose tumors express PD-L1 (CPS ≥1) as determined by an FDA-approved test.[a] ▪ Treatment of patients with **hepatocellular carcinoma** (HCC) who have been previously treated with sorafenib.[a] ▪ Treatment of adult and pediatric patients with **recurrent locally advanced or metastatic Merkel cell carcinoma** (MCC).[a] ▪ In combination with axitinib for the first-line treatment of patients with **advanced renal cell carcinoma** (RCC). ▪ In combination with lenvatinib for the treatment of patients with **advanced endometrial carcinoma that is not MSI-H or dMMR** who have disease progression after prior systemic therapy and are not candidates for curative surgery or radiation.[a]

Limitations of use: Pembrolizumab is not recommended for treatment of patients with PMBCL who require urgent cytoreductive therapy. ▪ Other indications come out often, refer to primary literature of on-line drug references for up to date list of indications. ▪ The safety and effectiveness in pediatric patients with MSI-H central nervous system cancers have not been established.

CONTRAINDICATIONS
Manufacturer states, "None."

PRECAUTIONS
Immune-mediated pneumonitis, including fatal cases, has occurred with pembrolizumab. Pneumonitis occurred more frequently in patients with a prior history of thoracic

---

[a] These indications are approved under accelerated approval based on tumor response rate and durability of response. Continued approval for these indications may be contingent on verification and description of clinical benefit in the confirmatory trials.

irradiation. ▪ Immune-mediated colitis has occurred with pembrolizumab. ▪ Immune-mediated hepatitis has occurred with pembrolizumab. ▪ Hepatic toxicity has occurred with pembrolizumab in combination with axitinib. ▪ Immune-mediated endocrinopathies, including hypophysitis (inflammation of the pituitary gland), thyroid disorders, and type 1 diabetes mellitus (including diabetic ketoacidosis), have occurred with pembrolizumab. ▪ Immune-mediated nephritis has occurred with pembrolizumab. ▪ Immune-mediated skin adverse reactions, including SJS, TEN (some fatal), exfoliative dermatitis, and bullous pemphigoid have occurred. ▪ Numerous other immune-mediated adverse reactions were reported in fewer than 1% of patients. These immune-mediated reactions may involve any organ system and may occur during or after discontinuation of treatment. ▪ Solid organ transplant rejection has been reported in patients treated with pembrolizumab. Consider benefit of treatment with pembrolizumab versus the risk of possible organ rejection in these patients. ▪ Severe and life-threatening infusion-related reactions, including hypersensitivity and anaphylaxis, have been reported. ▪ Immune-mediated complications, including fatal events, have occurred in patients who underwent allogeneic hematopoietic stem cell transplantation (HSCT) after treatment with pembrolizumab. Graft-versus-host disease (GVHD), hyperacute GVHD, and severe hepatic veno-occlusive disease (VOD) have been reported. ▪ See Dose Adjustments and Monitor for required dose adjustments, indicated criteria and medications for treatment of adverse reactions, and criteria for discontinuation of pembrolizumab. ▪ Pembrolizumab has not been studied in patients with moderate or severe hepatic impairment. ▪ A protein substance; has a potential for immunogenicity. ▪ See Drug/Lab Interactions.

Monitor: Obtain serum electrolytes and glucose, baseline liver function tests (e.g., ALT, AST, alkaline phosphatase, total bilirubin), serum creatinine, and thyroid function tests before initiating treatment, and monitor periodically during treatment and as indicated based on clinical evaluation. ▪ Consider more frequent monitoring of liver enzymes in patients taking pembrolizumab in combination with axitinib. ▪ Monitor for S/S of infusion-related reactions (e.g., chills, fever, flushing, hypotension, hypoxemia, pruritus, rash, rigors, and wheezing); see Dose Adjustments. ▪ Monitor patients for S/S of pneumonitis (e.g., chest pain, new or worsening cough, or shortness of breath). Evaluate patients with suspected pneumonitis with radiographic imaging, and administer corticosteroids (initial dose of 1 to 2 mg/kg/day prednisone or equivalent, followed by a taper) for Grade 2 or greater pneumonitis. Withhold pembrolizumab for moderate (Grade 2) pneumonitis; see Dose Adjustments. ▪ Monitor patients for S/S of colitis. Administer corticosteroids (initial dose of 1 to 2 mg/kg/day prednisone or equivalent, followed by a taper) for Grade 2 or greater colitis. Withhold pembrolizumab for moderate (Grade 2) or severe (Grade 3) colitis; see Dose Adjustments. ▪ Monitor patients for changes in liver function and S/S of hepatitis (e.g., easy bruising or bleeding, jaundice, lethargy, pain on right side of the abdomen, severe nausea or vomiting). Administer corticosteroids (initial dose of 0.5 to 1 mg/kg/day [for Grade 2 hepatitis] or 1 to 2 mg/kg/day [for Grade 3 or greater hepatitis] prednisone or equivalent, followed by a taper) and, based on severity of liver enzyme elevations, withhold or discontinue pembrolizumab and axitinib if used in combination; see Dose Adjustments. ▪ Monitor for S/S of hypophysitis, including hypopituitarism and adrenal insufficiency (e.g., fatigue, headache, dizziness or fainting, changes in vision, low levels of the hormones produced by the pituitary [adrenocorticotropic hormone (ACTH), thyroid-stimulating hormone (TSH), follicle-stimulating hormone (FSH), luteinizing hormone (LH), growth hormone (GH), prolactin]). Administer corticosteroids and hormone replacement as clinically indicated. Withhold pembrolizumab for moderate (Grade 2) hypophysitis, and withhold or discontinue pembrolizumab for severe (Grade 3) or life-threatening (Grade 4) hypophysitis; see Dose Adjustments. ▪ Thyroid disorders (hypothyroidism, hyperthyroidism, thyroiditis) can occur at any time during treatment. Monitor patients for changes in thyroid function. Administer replacement hormones for hypothyroidism, and manage hyperthyroidism with thionamides and beta-blockers as appropriate. Withhold or discontinue pembrolizumab for severe (Grade 3) or life-threatening (Grade 4) hyperthyroidism; see Dose

Adjustments. ▪ Monitor for hyperglycemia or other S/S of diabetes (e.g., increased thirst, urination). Administer insulin for type 1 diabetes, and withhold pembrolizumab and administer antihyperglycemics in patients with severe hyperglycemia; see Dose Adjustments. ▪ Monitor patients for changes in renal function. Administer corticosteroids (initial dose of 1 to 2 mg/kg/day prednisone or equivalent, followed by a taper) for Grade 2 or greater nephritis. Withhold pembrolizumab for moderate (Grade 2) nephritis; see Dose Adjustments. ▪ Monitor patients for suspected severe skin reactions and exclude other causes. Based on the severity of the adverse reaction, withhold or permanently discontinue and administer corticosteroids. Withhold pembrolizumab for Grade 3 skin reactions or suspected Stevens-Johnson syndrome (SJS) or toxic epidermal necrolysis (TEN). If SJS or TEN is suspected, refer the patient for specialized care for assessment and treatment. Permanently discontinue pembrolizumab for Grade 4 skin reactions or confirmed SJS or TEN. ▪ Monitor patient for other clinically significant immune-mediated adverse reactions. Examples of immune-mediated adverse reactions that have occurred include arthritis, encephalitis, Guillain-Barré syndrome, hemolytic anemia, myasthenia gravis, myelitis, myocarditis, myositis, pancreatitis, sarcoidosis, uveitis, and vasculitis. ▪ For any suspected immune-mediated adverse reactions, ensure adequate evaluation to confirm etiology or to exclude other causes. Based on the severity of the adverse reaction, withhold pembrolizumab and administer corticosteroids. With improvement to Grade 1 or less, begin corticosteroid taper and continue to taper over at least 1 month. Based on limited data from clinical trials in patients whose immune-related adverse reactions could not be controlled with corticosteroids, administration of other systemic immunosuppressants can be considered. Restart pembrolizumab if the adverse reaction remains at Grade 1 or less following taper; see Dose Adjustments. ▪ Monitor patients who have undergone allogeneic HSCT after pembrolizumab for transplant-related complications such as hyperacute GVHD, severe acute GVHD, hepatic VOD, steroid-requiring febrile syndrome, and other immune-mediated adverse reactions. Prompt intervention required.

Patient Education: Review manufacturer's medication guide. ▪ Highly effective contraception required during treatment with pembrolizumab and for at least 4 months following the last dose of pembrolizumab. ▪ Promptly report a known or suspected pregnancy. ▪ Immediately report any S/S of infusion-related reactions (e.g., chills, fever, flushing, hypotension, hypoxemia, pruritus, rigors, and wheezing). ▪ Some side effects may require corticosteroid treatment and interruption or discontinuation of pembrolizumab. ▪ Promptly report S/S of pneumonitis (e.g., chest pain, new or worsening cough, or shortness of breath). ▪ Promptly report S/S of colitis (e.g., diarrhea or severe abdominal pain). ▪ Promptly report S/S of hepatitis (e.g., easy bruising or bleeding, jaundice, lethargy, pain on right side of the abdomen, severe nausea or vomiting). ▪ Promptly report S/S of hypophysitis (e.g., dizziness or fainting, extreme weakness, persistent or unusual headache, vision changes) or of hypothyroidism, hyperthyroidism, or type 1 diabetes mellitus (e.g., constipation, dizziness or fainting, extreme tiredness, feeling cold, hair loss, headaches that will not go away, increased thirst or urination, weight gain or loss). ▪ Promptly report any S/S of severe skin reactions, SJS, or TEN. ▪ Contact healthcare provider immediately for S/S of organ transplant rejection. ▪ Inform patient about the risk for postallogeneic hematopoietic stem cell transplantation complications. ▪ Promptly report S/S of kidney dysfunction (e.g., blood in urine, decreased urine output, loss of appetite, swelling in ankles). ▪ Keeping scheduled appointments for blood work or other laboratory tests is imperative.

Maternal/Child: Has the potential to be transmitted from the mother to the developing fetus. Based on its mechanism of action and data from animal studies, pembrolizumab can cause fetal harm when administered to a pregnant woman; see Patient Education. ▪ Discontinue breast-feeding during treatment and for 4 months after the final dose. ▪ There is limited experience in pediatric patients. The concentrations of pembrolizumab in pediatric patients were comparable to those observed in adult patients at the same dose regimen of 2 mg/kg every 3 weeks. Abdominal pain, fatigue, hypertransaminasemia, hyponatremia, and vomiting occurred at a higher rate in pediatric patients when compared with adults under 65 years of age. Safety and effectiveness for use in pediatric patients with cHL, PMBCL, and MSI-H cancer have been established. Safety and effectiveness have not been established in other approved indications.

Elderly: No overall differences in safety or efficacy were reported between elderly patients and younger adults.

DRUG/LAB INTERACTIONS

No formal pharmacokinetic drug interaction studies have been conducted with pembrolizumab. ▪ In patients with multiple myeloma, the addition of pembrolizumab to a thalidomide analog plus dexamethasone resulted in increased mortality. This specific therapy is not indicated and is not recommended for use outside of controlled clinical trials.

SIDE EFFECTS

Pembrolizumab as a single agent: The most common adverse reactions (reported in at least 20% of patients) were abdominal pain, constipation, cough, decreased appetite, diarrhea, dyspnea, fatigue, fever, musculoskeletal pain, nausea, pain, pruritus, and rash.

Pembrolizumab in combination with pemetrexed and platinum chemotherapy: The most common adverse reactions (reported in at least 20% of patients) were alopecia, asthenia, constipation, cough, decreased appetite, diarrhea, dyspnea, fatigue, fever, mucosal inflammation, nausea, peripheral neuropathy, rash, stomatitis, and vomiting.

Pembrolizumab in combination with axitinib: The most common adverse reactions (reported in at least 20% of patients) were asthenia, constipation, cough, decreased appetite, diarrhea, dysphonia, fatigue, hepatoxicity, hypertension, hypothyroidism, mucosal inflammation, nausea, palmar-plantar erythrodysesthesia, rash, and stomatitis.

Pembrolizumab in combination with lenvatinib: The most common adverse reactions (reported in at least 20% of patients) were abdominal pain, constipation, cough, decreased appetite, decreased weight, diarrhea, dyspnea, dysphonia, fatigue, headache, hemorrhagic events, hypertension, hypomagnesemia, hypothyroidism, musculoskeletal pain, nausea, palmar-plantar erythrodysesthesia, rash, stomatitis, urinary tract infection, and vomiting. Other reported side effects included anemia; arrhythmia; arthralgia; asthenia; back pain; chills; decreased bicarbonate; dizziness; headache; hematuria; hemorrhage; herpes zoster; hypercholesterolemia; hyperglycemia; hyperkalemia; hypertriglyceridemia; hypoalbuminemia; hypocalcemia; hypoglycemia; hypokalemia; hyponatremia; hypophosphatemia; increased alkaline phosphatase, influenza-like illness, ALT, AST, creatinine; insomnia; leukopenia; lymphopenia; myalgia; neck pain; neutropenia; pain in extremity; peripheral edema; peripheral neuropathy; pneumonia; sepsis; thrombocytopenia; upper respiratory tract infection; urinary tract infection; and vitiligo; see Precautions.

Post-Marketing: Solid organ transplant rejection.

ANTIDOTE

Keep physician informed of all side effects. May constitute a medical emergency or will be treated symptomatically as indicated. Withhold or discontinue pembrolizumab as outlined in Dose Adjustments. Treat side effects aggressively; see Precautions and Monitor. Treat severe infusion reactions as indicated (e.g., epinephrine, diphenhydramine, IV fluids, oxygen).

PEMETREXED
(peh-meh-**TREX**-ed)

Alimta

Antineoplastic
(Antimetabolite)

pH 6.6 to 7.8

USUAL DOSE

Pretreatment: Verify pregnancy status. Baseline studies indicated; see Monitor. See Premedication.

PREMEDICATION REQUIRED

Regimen to mitigate toxicity begins 1 week before the first infusion of pemetrexed.

Folic acid supplementation: Prophylaxis to reduce treatment-related hematologic and GI toxicity (pemetrexed is an antifolate; severe myelosuppression can occur); 400 to 1,000 mcg of folic acid *must* be taken daily for 7 days *before* the first dose of pemetrexed. Must be continued daily throughout treatment regimen and for 21 days after last dose.

Vitamin B$_{12}$ supplementation: Prophylaxis to reduce treatment-related hematologic and GI toxicity; 1,000 mcg of vitamin B$_{12}$ *must* be given as an IM injection 1 week *before* the first dose of pemetrexed. Repeat this dose every 3 cycles (about every 9 weeks) during treatment; subsequent doses may be given on the same day as the pemetrexed infusion. *Do not substitute oral vitamin B$_{12}$ for intramuscular vitamin B$_{12}$.*

Corticosteroid: To reduce incidence and severity of dermatologic toxicity, administer dexamethasone 4 mg PO (or equivalent) twice daily the day before, the day of, and the day after the pemetrexed infusion. Repeat with each planned dose of pemetrexed.

Prehydration: Required with cisplatin; see cisplatin monograph.

PEMETREXED

Malignant pleural mesothelioma: 500 mg/M^2 as an IV infusion over 10 minutes administered before cisplatin on Day 1 of each 21-day cycle until disease progression or unacceptable toxicity.

Nonsquamous non–small-cell lung cancer (NSCLC): *Initial treatment of locally advanced or metastatic NSCLC:* 500 mg/M^2 as an IV infusion over 10 minutes administered before cisplatin on Day 1 of each 21-day cycle for up to 6 cycles in the absence of disease progression or unacceptable toxicity.

Maintenance treatment of locally advanced or metastatic NSCLC: 500 mg/M^2 as an IV infusion over 10 minutes on Day 1 of each 21-day cycle until disease progression or unacceptable toxicity. Given after 4 cycles of platinum-based first-line chemotherapy.

Treatment of recurrent/metastatic disease: 500 mg/M^2 as an IV infusion over 10 minutes on Day 1 of each 21-day cycle until disease progression or unacceptable toxicity.

Initial treatment of metastatic NSCLC: 500 mg/M^2 administered as an IV infusion over 10 minutes; administered after pembrolizumab and before carboplatin or cisplatin on Day 1 of each 21-day cycle for 4 cycles. Following completion of platinum-based therapy, pemetrexed may be administered as maintenance therapy, alone or with pembrolizumab, until disease progression or unacceptable toxicity. Pembrolizumab should be administered before pemetrexed when given on the same day.

Refer to the full prescribing information for cisplatin, pembrolizumab, and carboplatin.

DOSE ADJUSTMENTS

Pemetrexed dosing recommendations are provided for patients with a CrCl of 45 mL/min or greater. There is no recommended dose for patients whose CrCl is less than 45 mL/min. ▪ Other than those recommended for all patients, no dose adjustments are required based on age, gender, or race or in patients with a CrCl equal to or greater than 45 mL/min. ▪ Delay initiation of the next cycle of treatment until the ANC (absolute neutrophil count) is 1,500 cells/mm^3 or higher, the platelet count is 100,000 cells/mm^3 or higher, the CrCl is 45 mL/min or higher, and there is recovery of nonhematologic toxicity to Grade 0 to 2. Upon recovery, modify the dosage of pemetrexed in the next cycle as outlined in the following chart.

Pemetrexed Dose Modifications for Adverse Reactions[a]	
Toxicity in Most Recent Treatment Cycle	**Pemetrexed Dose Modification for Next Cycle**
Myelosuppressive Toxicity	
ANC <500/mm^3 **and** platelets ≥50,000/mm^3 OR Platelet count <50,000/mm^3 without bleeding	75% of previous dose
Platelet count <50,000/mm^3 with bleeding	50% of previous dose
Recurrent Grade 3 or 4 myelosuppression after 2 dose reductions	Discontinue
Nonhematologic Toxicity	
Any Grade 3 or 4 toxicities EXCEPT mucositis or neurologic toxicity OR Diarrhea requiring hospitalization	75% of previous dose
Grade 3 or 4 mucositis	50% of previous dose
Renal toxicity	Withhold until creatinine clearance is 45 mL/min or greater
Grade 3 or 4 neurologic toxicity	Permanently discontinue
Recurrent Grade 3 or 4 nonhematologic toxicity after 2 dose reductions	Permanently discontinue
Severe and life-threatening skin toxicity	Permanently discontinue
Interstitial pneumonitis	Permanently discontinue

[a]National Cancer Institute Common Toxicity Criteria for Adverse Events version 2 (NCI CTCAE v2).

- Refer to prescribing information of agents in combination therapies for indicated dosing modifications.

DILUTION
Specific techniques required; see Precautions. Calculate the dose and number of vials needed. Reconstitute each 100-mg vial with 4.2 mL of preservative-free NS and each 500-mg vial with 20 mL of preservative-free NS. Concentration equals 25 mg/mL. Gently swirl to completely dissolve the powder. Solution ranges in color from colorless to yellow or green-yellow. Withdraw the required volume to provide the calculated dose of pemetrexed. *Must* be further diluted to a total volume of 100 mL with preservative-free NS.
Filters: No data available from manufacturer.
Storage: Store unopened vials at CRT. Reconstituted and diluted solutions are chemically and physically stable for 24 hours refrigerated. Contains no preservatives; discard unused portions.

COMPATIBILITY
Manufacturer states, "Is physically **incompatible** with diluents containing calcium, including lactated Ringer's and Ringer's injection. Co-administration with other diluents has not been studied." **Compatible** with standard PVC administration sets and bags.
     Other sources suggest specific **compatibilities** dependent on concentration and manufacturer; consult a pharmacist.

RATE OF ADMINISTRATION
A single dose as an infusion equally distributed over 10 minutes.

ACTIONS
An antifolate antineoplastic agent. It disrupts folate-dependent metabolic processes essential for cell replication. Transported into cells by both the reduced folate carrier and the

membrane folate-binding protein transport systems. Converts to polyglutamate forms, which are inhibitors of folate-dependent enzymes involved in the de novo biosynthesis of thymidine and purine nucleotides. 81% bound to plasma protein. Not appreciably metabolized. Half-life is 3.5 hours. Primarily eliminated in urine as an unchanged drug.

INDICATIONS AND USES
Used in combination with cisplatin for the initial treatment of malignant pleural mesothelioma in patients whose disease is unresectable or who are not candidates for curative surgery. ▪ Used in combination with cisplatin for the initial treatment of patients with locally advanced or metastatic nonsquamous NSCLC. ▪ In combination with platinum chemotherapy and pembrolizumab for the initial treatment of patients with metastatic nonsquamous NSCLC with no EGFR or ALK genomic tumor aberration. ▪ As a single agent for maintenance treatment of patients with locally advanced or metastatic nonsquamous NSCLC whose disease has not progressed after 4 cycles of platinum-based first-line chemotherapy. ▪ As a single agent for treatment of patients with recurrent, metastatic nonsquamous NSCLC after prior chemotherapy.

Limitation of use: Not indicated for treatment of squamous cell NSCLC.

CONTRAINDICATIONS
History of severe hypersensitivity reaction to pemetrexed or any of its components. ▪ Should not be administered to patients with a CrCl less than 45 mL/min.

PRECAUTIONS
Follow guidelines for handling cytotoxic agents. See Appendix A, p. 1308. ▪ Should be administered by or under the direction of a physician specialist in a facility equipped to monitor the patient and respond to any medical emergency. ▪ Myelosuppression (e.g., anemia, neutropenia, thrombocytopenia) is a dose-limiting toxicity. May result in requirement for transfusions and development of neutropenic infection; see Dose Adjustments. ▪ The risk of myelosuppression is increased in patients who do not receive vitamin supplementation. Folic acid and vitamin B_{12} supplementation are required as a prophylactic measure to reduce treatment-related hematologic and GI toxicity. ▪ Pemetrexed can cause severe and sometimes fatal renal toxicity. ▪ Serious and sometimes fatal, bullous, blistering, and exfoliative skin toxicity, including cases suggestive of Stevens-Johnson syndrome/toxic epidermal necrolysis, have been reported. ▪ Serious interstitial pneumonitis, including fatal cases, can occur. ▪ Radiation recall can occur with pemetrexed in patients who have received radiation weeks to years previously. ▪ Use caution in patients with a CrCl less than 80 mL/min if ibuprofen (Advil, Motrin) is administered concurrently; see Drug/Lab Interactions. ▪ See Dose Adjustments and Contraindications.

Monitor: Pretreatment with folic acid, vitamin B_{12}, dexamethasone, and adequate hydration required; see Usual Dose. ▪ Obtain baseline CrCl and CBC, including platelet count. Repeat CrCl before each dose. Repeat CBC and platelet count on Day 1 before each dose and on Days 8 and 15 of each cycle. Do not begin a new cycle of treatment unless the ANC is equal to or greater than 1,500 cells/mm^3, the platelet count is equal to or greater than 100,000 cells/mm^3, and the CrCl is equal to or greater than 45 mL/min. ▪ Monitor for skin toxicity. ▪ Monitor for S/S of pneumonitis (e.g., cough, dyspnea, fever). Withhold pemetrexed pending diagnostic evaluation; see Dose Adjustments. ▪ Monitor for radiation recall reaction, if indicated. ▪ Monitor patients who have been or are taking ibuprofen carefully for signs of toxicity, especially myelosuppression and renal or GI toxicity; see Drug/Lab Interactions. ▪ Monitor for thrombocytopenia (platelet count less than 50,000/mm^3). Initiate precautions to prevent excessive bleeding (e.g., inspect IV sites, skin, and mucous membranes; use extreme care during invasive procedures; test urine, emesis, stool, and secretions for occult blood). ▪ See Precautions, Drug/Lab Interactions, and Antidote.

Patient Education: Review manufacturer's patient information guide. ▪ Avoid pregnancy; use of effective contraception is recommended for females of reproductive potential during treatment with pemetrexed and for 6 months after the final dose, and for males with partners of reproductive potential during treatment and for 3 months after the final dose. Females should report a suspected pregnancy immediately. ▪ May impair male fertility.

■ Adherence to medication regimen (folic acid, vitamin B_{12}, dexamethasone), avoidance or limiting of ibuprofen, and keeping appointments for required lab work and healthcare provider visits are imperative. ■ Promptly report S/S of anemia, bleeding, cough, decreased urine output, dehydration from diarrhea or vomiting, dyspnea, fatigue, infection (e.g., fever), radiation recall (in patients who have received prior radiation), rash, redness or sores in the mouth, trouble swallowing, or other symptoms. ■ See Appendix D, p. 1311.

Maternal/Child: Based on animal studies and its mechanism of action, pemetrexed can cause fetal harm; avoid pregnancy. ■ Do not breast-feed during treatment and for 1 week after the last dose of pemetrexed. ■ Safety and effectiveness for use in pediatric patients not established.

Elderly: See Dose Adjustments; required only based on general patient criteria. No overall differences in effectiveness were observed between older and younger patients. ■ Incidence of CTCAE Grade 3 and 4 anemia, fatigue, hypertension, neutropenia, and thrombocytopenia was greater in patients 65 years of age or older even though they were fully supplemented with vitamins.

DRUG/LAB INTERACTIONS

Ibuprofen decreases clearance and increases AUC. In patients with a CrCl between 45 and 79 mL/min avoid administration of ibuprofen for 2 days before, the day of, and at least 2 days after a dose of pemetrexed. Monitor for hematologic, renal, and GI toxicity if concomitant use cannot be avoided. ■ Pharmacokinetics of pemetrexed and cisplatin are not affected by each other. ■ Coadministration of oral folic acid or IM vitamin B_{12} does not adversely affect pemetrexed. ■ Is not a clinically significant inhibitor of drugs metabolized by cytochrome P_{450} enzymes. ■ May be used concurrently with aspirin in low to moderate doses (325 mg every 6 hours). Effect of higher doses not known.

SIDE EFFECTS

The most common adverse reactions with single-agent use are anorexia, fatigue, and nausea. When used in combination with cisplatin, the most common adverse reactions include constipation, hematologic toxicity (anemia, leukopenia, lymphopenia, neutropenia, thrombocytopenia), pharyngitis, stomatitis, and vomiting. When used in combination with platinum chemotherapy and pembrolizumab, the most common adverse reactions included asthenia, constipation, cough, decreased appetite, diarrhea, dyspnea, fatigue, fever, nausea, rash, and vomiting. Other side effects, depending on regimen, may include alopecia; arthralgia; chest pain; conjunctivitis; cough; decreased CrCl; dehydration; dizziness; dysgeusia; dyspepsia; dyspnea; edema; elevated alkaline phosphatase, ALT, AST, and creatinine; embolism or thrombosis; fatigue; febrile neutropenia; fever; headache; hyperglycemia; hyperkalemia; hypertension; hypersensitivity reactions; hypertriglyceridemia; hypoalbuminemia; hypocalcemia; hypokalemia; hyponatremia; hypophosphatemia; infection; insomnia; neuropathy (sensory); pruritus; rash/desquamation; renal failure; taste disturbance; and upper respiratory tract infections. Numerous other adverse reactions were reported in less than 5% of patients.

Overdose: Bone marrow suppression (e.g., anemia, neutropenia, thrombocytopenia), diarrhea, infection with or without fever, mucositis, rash.

Post-Marketing: Colitis, edema, esophagitis, immune-mediated hemolytic anemia, interstitial pneumonitis, pancreatitis, radiation recall, serious and fatal bullous skin conditions, Stevens-Johnson syndrome, and toxic epidermal necrolysis.

ANTIDOTE

Keep physician informed of all side effects. Pemetrexed may be delayed or discontinued based on the degree of side effects; see Dose Adjustments. Symptomatic and supportive therapy is indicated. Death may occur from the progression of some side effects. Based on animal studies, administration of leucovorin may mitigate the toxicities of a pemetrexed overdose. Administration of whole blood products (e.g., packed RBCs, platelets, leukocytes) and/or blood modifiers (e.g., darbepoetin alfa [Aranesp], epoetin alfa [Epogen], filgrastim [Neupogen, Zarxio], pegfilgrastim [Neulasta], sargramostim [Leukine]) may be indicated to treat bone marrow toxicity. Effect of hemodialysis on pemetrexed is unknown.

PENICILLIN G AQUEOUS
(pen-ih-**SILL**-in **A**-kwe-us)

Antibacterial
(penicillin)

Penicillin G Potassium, Penicillin G Sodium, Pfizerpen

pH 5.5 to 8

USUAL DOSE

Dose dependent on type and severity of infection. See package insert for dosing for specific indications.

Adults and pediatric patients 12 years of age and older: 1 million to 24 million units/24 hr equally distributed over 24 hours as a continuous infusion or equally divided in 4 to 6 intermittent infusions (250,000 to 6 million units every 6 hours or 166,000 to 4,000,000 units every 4 hours). (400,000 units equals approximately 250 mg.)

Meningococcal meningitis and/or septicemia: Manufacturer recommends a dose of 24 million units/24 hr as 2 million units every 2 hours.

PEDIATRIC DOSE

Administration by intermittent infusion over 15 to 30 minutes is preferred. Dose is based on age or weight and the severity of the infection.

Serious infections (e.g., pneumonia, endocarditis): 25,000 to 50,000 units/kg every 4 hours or 37,500 to 75,000 units/kg every 6 hours (150,000 to 300,000 units/kg/24 hr).

Meningitis: 41,666 units/kg every 4 hours (250,000 units/kg/24 hr). Continue treatment for 7 to 14 days. Maximum dose is 12 to 20 million units/24 hr.

Disseminated gonococcal infections (arthritis), weight less than 45 kg: 25,000 units/kg every 6 hours (100,000 units/kg/24 hr) for 7 to 10 days.

Disseminated gonococcal infections (meningitis), weight less than 45 kg: 41,666 units/kg every 4 hours (250,000 units/kg/24 hr) for 10 to 14 days.

Disseminated gonococcal infections (endocarditis), weight less than 45 kg: 41,666 units/kg every 4 hours (250,000 units/kg/24 hr) for 4 weeks.

Disseminated gonococcal infections (arthritis, meningitis, endocarditis), weight 45 kg or greater: 2,500,000 units every 6 hours (10,000,000 units/24 hr). Duration of therapy is dependent on diagnosis.

Syphilis (congenital or neurosyphilis) after the newborn period: 50,000 units/kg every 4 to 6 hours (200,000 to 300,000 units/kg/24 hr). Continue treatment for 10 to 14 days.

Diphtheria (adjunctive to antitoxin and prevention of carrier state): 37,500 to 62,500 units/kg every 6 hours (150,000 to 250,000 units/kg/24 hr) for 7 to 10 days.

Rat-bite fever, Haverhill fever (caused by a specific organism): 25,000 to 41,666 units/kg every 4 hours (150,000 to 250,000 units/kg/24 hr) for 4 weeks.

The American Association of Pediatrics (AAP) recommends:

Pediatric patients from 1 month to under 12 years of age: *Mild to moderate bacterial infections:* 25,000 to 37,500 units/kg every 6 hours (100,000 to 150,000 units/kg/24 hr).

Severe infections: 33,333 to 50,000 units/kg every 4 hours (200,000 to 300,000 units/kg/24 hr).

NEONATAL DOSE

Administration by intermittent infusion over 15 to 30 minutes is preferred. Dose is based on weight and age and the severity of the infection.

The American Academy of Pediatrics (AAP) has recommended 25,000 to 50,000 units/dose. Adjust the dosing intervals based on the neonate's weight and age as follows:

Moderate to severe bacterial infections:

7 days of age or younger: Every 12 hours.

8 to 28 days of age: Every 8 hours.

Higher doses may be required for the treatment of meningitis.

DOSE ADJUSTMENTS

Reduce dose in severe impaired renal function; additional reductions may be indicated if liver function is also impaired. ■ If CrCl is greater than 10 mL/min/1.73 M^2 in uremic patients, give a full loading dose followed by one-half loading dose every 4 to 5 hours. ■ If CrCl is less than 10 mL/min/1.73 M^2, administer a full loading dose followed by one-half of the loading dose every 8 to 10 hours. Another source recommends giving 75% of a normal dose every 4 to 6 hours to patients with a CrCl of 10 to 50 mL/min and 20% to 50% of a normal dose every 4 to 6 hours to patients with a CrCl less than 10 mL/min. ■ Additional dose modifications may be indicated in patients with impaired hepatic and/or renal function. ■ See Drug/Lab Interactions.

DILUTION

Available as a premixed frozen solution, or reconstitute each vial with SWFI or NS. Direct flow of diluent against sides of the vial while gently rotating vial. Shake vigorously. Directions on vial should be followed to provide desired number of units per milliliter. Available with 1, 5, 10, and 20 million units per vial. May be added to NS or dextrose solutions for infusion. See chart on inside back cover.

Storage: Dry powder stored at CRT. Reconstituted solutions of penicillin G potassium are stable for 1 week if refrigerated. Reconstituted solutions of penicillin G sodium are stable for 3 days if refrigerated. Infusion solutions are stable at CRT for 24 hours. Store premixed frozen solution at or below $-20°$ C $(-4°$ F). The thawed solution is stable for 14 days refrigerated or for 24 hours at RT. Do not refreeze.

COMPATIBILITY

Penicillins are rapidly inactivated in alkaline carbohydrate solutions, reducing agents, alcohols, and glycols; optimum pH range is 6 to 7. To preserve bactericidal action, consult pharmacist before mixing other agents with penicillin in the infusion solution. May form a precipitate with vancomycin. Inactivated in solution with aminoglycosides. Do not mix in the same solution. Appropriate spacing and/or separate sites required. See Drug/Lab Interactions.

Other sources suggest specific **compatibilities** dependent on concentration and manufacturer; consult a pharmacist.

RATE OF ADMINISTRATION

Penicillin is not given by IV injection. Administer as ordered as continuous IV drip; for example, 5 million units in 1,000 mL of D5W over 12 hours. Is sometimes given by intermittent infusion ($^1/_6$ or $^1/_4$ of a daily dose in 100 mL over 15 to 30 minutes every 4 to 6 hours). Because of its short half-life, frequent dosing is required to maintain serum concentration above the MIC (minimum inhibitory concentration) for most of the dosing interval. Too-rapid administration or excessive doses may cause electrolyte imbalance and/or seizures. Stable at room temperature for at least 24 hours.

Pediatric rate: Administration by intermittent infusion over 15 to 30 minutes is preferred for infants and children.

ACTIONS

A natural penicillin, bactericidal against penicillin-sensitive microorganisms during the stage of active multiplication. Inhibits bacterial cell wall synthesis. Distributed into most areas of the body. Distribution into spinal fluid is minimal unless inflammation is present. Half-life is approximately 40 minutes. Crosses the placental barrier. Excreted in the urine via glomerular filtration and tubular secretion. Secreted in breast milk. Available in a potassium salt containing 1.7 mEq of potassium and 1.02 mEq sodium in 1 million units or a sodium salt containing 1.68 mEq sodium in 1 million units.

INDICATIONS AND USES

Serious infections caused by penicillin G–sensitive gram-positive, gram-negative, and anaerobic microorganisms (e.g., empyema, endocarditis, meningitis, pericarditis, pneumonia, septicemia). See manufacturer's prescribing information for a complete list of clinical indications/infecting organisms. Penicillin G is not the drug of choice in the treatment of gram-negative bacillary infections.

Unlabeled uses: Group B streptococcus, maternal dose (neonatal prophylaxis).

CONTRAINDICATIONS

Known sensitivity to any penicillin. ▪ Premixed solutions containing dextrose may be contraindicated in patients with a known allergy to corn or corn products.

PRECAUTIONS

Hypersensitivity reactions, including fatalities, have been reported in patients undergoing penicillin therapy; most likely to occur in patients with a history of penicillin hypersensitivity or sensitivity to multiple allergens. There have been reports of individuals with a history of penicillin hypersensitivity experiencing severe reactions when treated with cephalosporins. Check history of previous hypersensitivity reactions to penicillins, cephalosporins, or other allergens. Actual incidence of cross-allergenicity not established but may be more common with first-generation cephalosporins. ▪ Sensitivity studies necessary to determine susceptibility of the causative organism to penicillin. ▪ To reduce the development of drug-resistant bacteria and maintain its effectiveness, penicillin should be used to treat or prevent only those infections proven or strongly suspected to be caused by bacteria. ▪ Continue treatment for 48 to 72 hours after symptoms subside. To reduce the risk of rheumatic fever, patients being treated for Group A beta-hemolytic streptococcal infections should be treated for at least 10 days. ▪ Avoid prolonged use of drug; superinfection caused by overgrowth of nonsusceptible organisms may result. ▪ *Clostridium difficile*–associated diarrhea (CDAD) has been reported. May range from mild diarrhea to fatal colitis. Consider in patients who present with diarrhea during or after treatment with penicillin. ▪ Potassium penicillin most frequently used. Doses over 10,000,000 units may cause fatal hyperkalemia, especially in patients with renal insufficiency.

Monitor: Periodic evaluation of renal, hepatic, and hematopoietic systems is recommended in prolonged therapy. ▪ Monitor for S/S of hypersensitivity reaction. ▪ Test patients with gonococcal infections and syphilis for HIV. Test patients with gonococcal infections for syphilis. ▪ Electrolyte imbalance from potassium or sodium content is very possible. Monitor closely. Penicillin G potassium contains 1.02 mEq sodium/million units. May aggravate CHF, especially in the elderly. ▪ May cause thrombophlebitis; observe carefully and rotate infusion sites. ▪ See Drug/Lab Interactions.

Patient Education: May require alternate birth control. ▪ Promptly report diarrhea or bloody stools that occur during treatment or up to several months after an antibiotic has been discontinued; may indicate CDAD and require treatment. ▪ Promptly report S/S of a hypersensitivity reaction (e.g., light-headedness, rash, tightness of the chest, urticaria, wheezing).

Maternal/Child: Category B: use only if clearly needed. ▪ Use caution during breast-feeding. May cause diarrhea, candidiasis, or allergic response in nursing infants. ▪ Elimination rate markedly reduced in neonates.

Elderly: Response similar to that seen in younger adults. ▪ Consider age-related organ impairment and concomitant disease or drug therapy. Monitor renal function. ▪ See Dose Adjustments.

DRUG/LAB INTERACTIONS

Synergistic when used in combination with **aminoglycosides**. Synergism may be inconsistent; see Compatibility. ▪ May be antagonized by **bacteriostatic antibiotics** (e.g., chloramphenicol, erythromycin, sulfonamides, tetracyclines); may interfere with bactericidal action. ▪ **ASA, ethacrynic acid, furosemide, indomethacin, sulfonamides, and thiazide diuretics** may interfere with tubular secretion of penicillin, increasing serum concentration and risk of toxicity. ▪ Risk of bleeding with **anticoagulants** (e.g., warfarin) may be increased. ▪ **Probenecid** decreases elimination of penicillin, resulting in prolonged half-life and increased serum levels. May be desirable or may cause toxicity. ▪ May decrease effectiveness of **oral contraceptives;** breakthrough bleeding or pregnancy could result. ▪ Concomitant use with **potassium supplements, potassium-sparing diuretics, or ACE inhibitors** may increase risk of hyperkalemia. ▪ May decrease clearance and increase toxicity of **methotrexate.** ▪ May cause false values in common **lab tests;** see literature.

SIDE EFFECTS

Acute interstitial nephritis, arthralgia, chills, CDAD, convulsions, edema, fever, hemolytic anemia, hyperkalemia, hyperreflexia, hypersensitivity reactions (immediate [e.g., anaphylaxis, angioneurotic edema, bronchospasm, cardiovascular collapse, hypotension, laryngospasm, death] and delayed [e.g., serum sickness–like symptoms and various skin rashes]), Jarisch-Herxheimer reaction (in patients with syphilis or other spirochetal infections), nausea, neurotoxicity, neutropenia, pain at the injection site, skin rash, sodium-induced congestive heart failure, stomatitis, thrombophlebitis, urticaria, vomiting. Higher-than-normal doses may cause neurologic adverse effects including convulsions, especially with impaired renal function.

ANTIDOTE

For all side effects, discontinue the drug, treat hypersensitivity reactions or resuscitate as necessary, and notify the physician. Treat minor side effects symptomatically according to physician's order. Mild cases of CDAD may respond to discontinuation of the drug. Removed by hemodialysis.

PENTAMIDINE ISETHIONATE
(pen-**TAM**-ih-deen is-ah-**THIGH**-oh-nayt)

Antiprotozoal

pH 4.09 to 5.4

USUAL DOSE

Pretreatment: Baseline studies required; see Monitor.

Treatment of *Pneumocystis jiroveci:* 4 mg/kg of body weight once daily for 14 days. See Precautions/Monitor. Has been used up to 21 days; benefits not defined.

Pneumocystis prophylaxis: 4 mg/kg once each month. May be given every 2 weeks if indicated.

Leishmania, visceral (unlabeled): 2 to 4 mg/kg once daily for up to 15 days.

Leishmania, cutaneous (unlabeled): 2 to 4 mg/kg once or twice a week until lesions heal.

Trypanosoma gambiense (unlabeled): 4 mg/kg once daily for 10 days.

PEDIATRIC DOSE

Pneumocystis jiroveci: 4 mg/kg once daily for 12 to 14 days.

Pneumocystis prophylaxis: See Usual Dose.

Leishmania donovani: 2 to 4 mg/kg once daily for 15 days. Up to 21 days have been suggested, but risks with therapy over 14 days may be increased.

Trypanosoma gambiense: See Usual Dose.

DOSE ADJUSTMENTS

Reduced dose in renal failure may be indicated. One source recommends 4 mg/kg every 24 hours with a CrCl of 10 to 50 mL/min or 4 mg/kg every 24 to 36 hours with a CrCl less than 10 mL/min.

DILUTION

Initially dilute each 300 mg or fraction thereof in 3 to 5 mL SWFI or D5W. A single dose must be further diluted in 50 to 250 mL of D5W and given as an infusion.

Storage: Stable at room temperature for 24 hours. Discard unused portion. Protect dry product and reconstituted solution from light.

COMPATIBILITY

Will form a precipitate with NS; do not use for dilution or infusion. Manufacturer states, "Do not mix pentamidine solutions with any other drugs."

Other sources suggest a few specific **compatibilities** dependent on concentration and manufacturer; consult a pharmacist.

RATE OF ADMINISTRATION

A single dose should be evenly distributed over 60 minutes.

Leishmania, visceral and cutaneous: A single dose evenly distributed over 1 to 2 hours.

ACTIONS

An antiprotozoal agent. Specifically active against *Pneumocystis jiroveci*. It is thought to interfere with nuclear metabolism and inhibit the synthesis of DNA, RNA, phospholipids, and proteins. Route of metabolism is unknown. Excreted partially in urine. May accumulate in renal failure.

INDICATIONS AND USES

Treatment and prophylaxis of *Pneumocystis jiroveci* pneumonia (PCP).

Unlabeled uses: Treatment of trypanosomiasis and visceral and cutaneous leishmaniasis. Aerosol used prophylactically to prevent PCP in high-risk patients.

CONTRAINDICATIONS

None if the diagnosis of *Pneumocystis jiroveci* pneumonia is confirmed.

PRECAUTIONS

Specific use only; establish correct diagnosis. ▪ Sulfamethoxazole/trimethoprim is the drug of choice for treatment of *Pneumocystis* pneumonia. Pentamidine causes numerous and serious side effects and is indicated only if the patient does not respond to or tolerate SMZ-TMP. ▪ Use extreme caution in patients with hypertension, hypotension, hypoglycemia, hyperglycemia, hypocalcemia, leukopenia, thrombocytopenia, anemia, hepatic or renal dysfunction, ventricular tachycardia, pancreatitis, and Stevens-Johnson syndrome.

Monitor: Before, during, and after therapy obtain a BUN and SCr (daily), CBC, platelet count, alkaline phosphatase, bilirubin, AST, ALT, serum calcium, and ECG. ▪ Has caused fatalities resulting from severe hypotension, hypoglycemia, and cardiac arrhythmias even with the administration of the first dose. Keep patient supine, observe continuously for any sign of adverse reaction, and monitor BP continuously during infusion and afterward until stable. ▪ Emergency equipment for resuscitation must be immediately available. ▪ Monitor blood glucose levels daily during therapy and several times after therapy is complete. Pancreatic necrosis and very high plasma insulin levels have occurred. May also cause hyperglycemia and diabetes mellitus.

Patient Education: May cause severe hypotension; remain lying down until BP is stable. ▪ Report any unusual bleeding or bruising.

Maternal/Child: Category C: use only when clearly needed during pregnancy and breast-feeding. Hazards to fetus or infant are unknown. ▪ Discontinue breast-feeding.

DRUG/LAB INTERACTIONS

Nephrotoxic effects may be additive with concomitant use with **other nephrotoxic drugs** (e.g., aminoglycosides, amphotericin B, cisplatin, foscarnet, vancomycin). Monitoring of renal function, dose reductions, and/or dose interval adjustments may be required.

SIDE EFFECTS

Occur in over 50% of patients and may be life threatening. Some occur after course of treatment is completed. Acute renal failure, anemia, anorexia, bad taste in mouth, cardiac arrhythmias including ventricular tachycardia, confusion, dizziness, elevated SCr and liver function tests, fever, hallucinations, hyperglycemia, hyperkalemia, hypocalcemia, hypoglycemia, hypotension, leukopenia, nausea, neuralgia, phlebitis, rash, thrombocytopenia.

ANTIDOTE

Discontinue drug for any life-threatening side effects. Notify physician of all side effects. Symptomatic treatment indicated. Resuscitate as necessary.

PENTOBARBITAL SODIUM
(**PEN**-toh-**bar**-bih-tal **SO**-dee-um)

Barbiturate
Sedative-hypnotic
Anticonvulsant

Nembutal Sodium

pH 9 to 10.5

USUAL DOSE

Pretreatment: See Maternal/Child.

Pentobarbital: 100 mg initially. Wait 1 full minute between each dose to determine drug effect. Additional doses in increments of 25 to 50 mg may be given as indicated. Maximum dosage ranges from 200 to 500 mg.

Barbiturate coma: *Loading dose:* 3 to 10 mg/kg over 30 minutes to 3 hours.

Maintenance dose: 1.5 to 2 mg/kg every 1 to 2 hours or an infusion of 0.5 to 3 mg/kg/hr. Adjust to maintain pentobarbital blood level between 110 and 177 mm/L (25 to 40 mg/dL) or ICP below 25 Torr.

PEDIATRIC DOSE

See Maternal/Child.

1 to 3 mg/kg slowly until asleep. Maximum dose 100 mg/24 hr.

Barbiturate coma: See Usual Dose. An alternate source suggests ***Loading dose:*** 10 to 15 mg/kg over 1 to 2 hours. ***Maintenance dose:*** Begin with 1 mg/kg/hr; increase to 2 to 3 mg/kg/hr to maintain EEG burst suppression.

DOSE ADJUSTMENTS

Reduce dose in impaired renal or hepatic function; usually required in the debilitated or elderly. ▪ See Drug/Lab Interactions.

DILUTION

May be given undiluted or, preferably, may be further diluted in SWFI, NS, or Ringer's injection. Any desired amount of diluent may be used. 9 mL of diluent with 1 mL of pentobarbital (50 mg) equals 5 mg/mL. Use only absolutely clear solutions. Central line is preferred for administration.

COMPATIBILITY

Manufacturer states, "Should not be admixed with any other medication or solution." May precipitate in acidic solutions.

Other sources suggest a few specific **compatibilities** dependent on concentration and manufacturer; consult a pharmacist.

RATE OF ADMINISTRATION

No faster than 50 mg/min. More rapid administration can increase risk of adverse events. Titrate slowly to desired effect. Rapid injection rate may cause symptoms of overdose (e.g., serious respiratory depression).

Barbiturate coma: See specific dose recommendations.

ACTIONS

A sedative, hypnotic barbiturate of short duration with anticonvulsant effects. Pentobarbital is a CNS depressant. Onset of action is prompt by the IV route and lasts about 3 to 4 hours. Will effectively depress the motor cortex if adequate doses are administered. Pain perception is unimpaired. Reportedly reduces cerebral blood flow and thus reduces cerebral edema and intracranial pressure. Detoxified in the liver and excreted fairly quickly in the urine in changed form. Crosses the placental barrier. Secreted in breast milk.

INDICATIONS AND USES

Preanesthetic sedation. ▪ Dental and minor surgical sedation. ▪ Control of convulsions caused by disease/drug poisoning. ▪ Short-term hypnotic. ▪ Sedation in psychotic states.

Unlabeled uses: High doses have been used to induce coma in the management of cerebral ischemia and increased intracranial pressure. Has been most effective in patients under 35 years of age or in closed head injuries.

CONTRAINDICATIONS

Acute or chronic pain, delivery (when maximum drug effect would be at the time of delivery), history of porphyria, known hypersensitivity to barbiturates, severely impaired liver function especially with any signs of hepatic coma, severe respiratory disease or respiratory depression.

PRECAUTIONS

IV route usually reserved for critical situations. ▪ Use caution in status asthmaticus, shock, severe renal or liver disease, depressive states after convulsions, shock, and in the elderly. ▪ Use caution in acute or chronic pain. ▪ Status epilepticus can occur from too-rapid withdrawal. ▪ May be habit forming. Use caution in the presence of fever, diabetes, hyperthyroidism, or severe anemia; may increase side effects. ▪ Benzodiazepines are generally preferred for sedation.

Monitor: Record BP, pulse, and respirations every 3 to 5 minutes. Keep patient under constant observation. ▪ Maintain a patent airway. ▪ Monitor for vein irritation at site of injection. ▪ Treat the cause of a convulsion. ▪ Highly alkaline; determine absolute patency of vein; use of large veins preferred to prevent thrombosis. Avoid extravasation. Intra-arterial injection will cause gangrene. ▪ Monitor phenytoin and barbiturate levels when both drugs are used concurrently. ▪ Monitor hematopoietic, renal, and hepatic systems in extended therapy. ▪ See Drug/Lab Interactions.

Patient Education: Avoid alcohol and other CNS depressants (e.g., antihistamines, diazepam). ▪ May be habit forming. ▪ May require alternate birth control.

Maternal/Child: Category D: avoid pregnancy; will cause birth defects. ▪ May cause drowsiness in the nursing infant. ▪ See Contraindications. ▪ May cause paradoxical excitement in pediatric patients.

Elderly: Often have increased sensitivity to barbiturates; may cause marked excitement, depression, confusion, and increased risk of barbiturate-induced hypothermia. ▪ See Dose Adjustments and Precautions. ▪ Consider age-related hepatic or renal impairment and concomitant disease or drug therapy.

DRUG/LAB INTERACTIONS

Use extreme caution if any **other CNS depressants** have been given, such as alcohol, narcotic analgesics, anesthetics, antidepressants, antihistamines, hypnotics, MAO inhibitors, phenothiazines, sedatives, aminoglycoside antibiotics, or tranquilizers; potentiation with respiratory depression may occur. ▪ Inhibits effectiveness of **propranolol, corticosteroids, doxycycline, oral anticoagulants, oral contraceptives, quinidine, and theophylline.** Capable of innumerable interactions with many drugs. ▪ May increase orthostatic hypotension with **furosemide.** ▪ Monitor **phenytoin** and barbiturate levels when both drugs are used concurrently. ▪ May inhibit **vitamin D** metabolism with extended use.

SIDE EFFECTS

Average dose: Depression, dermatitis, facial edema, fever, hypotension, neonatal apnea, pain at or below injection site, respiratory depression (hypoventilation), thrombocytopenic purpura.

Overdose: Apnea, coma, cough reflex depression, flat EEG (reversible unless hypoxic damage has occurred), hypotension, laryngospasm, lowered body temperature, pulmonary edema, renal shutdown, respiratory depression, sluggish or absent reflexes.

ANTIDOTE

Discontinue drug immediately for pain at or below injection site. Notify the physician of any side effects. Symptomatic and supportive treatment is most important in overdose. Maintain an adequate airway with artificial ventilation if indicated. Keep the patient warm. IV volume expanders and IV fluids will help maintain adequate circulation. Diuretics or hemodialysis will promote the elimination of the drug. Vasopressors will maintain BP.

PENTOSTATIN BBW
(**PEN**-toh-**stah**-tin)

Antineoplastic
(antibiotic)

2-Deoxycoformycin, Nipent

pH 7 to 8.5

USUAL DOSE
Pretreatment: Baseline studies and prehydration are required before administration; see Monitor.

Pentostatin: 4 mg/M^2 every other week. Do not exceed recommended dose; see Precautions. If there is no major toxicity and improvement is continuous, treat until a complete response is achieved, then administer two additional doses. Do not treat beyond 12 months.

DOSE ADJUSTMENTS
Reduced dose and benefit-versus-risk assessment may be required with impaired renal function (CrCl below 60 mL/min); insufficient data available. Two patients with impaired renal function (CrCl 50 to 60 mL/min) achieved complete response without unusual adverse events when treated with 2 mg/M^2. ▪ Withhold dose if SCr elevated; obtain CrCl. ▪ Withhold dose if the absolute neutrophil count falls from a baseline of greater than 500 cells/mm^3 before therapy to less than 200 cells/mm^3 during treatment. Resume treatment when count returns to predose levels.

DILUTION
Specific techniques required; see Precautions. Diluent (5 mL SWFI) provided; dissolve completely; will yield 2 mg/mL. May be given by IV injection or further diluted in 25 to 50 mL NS or D5W; 25 mL yields 0.33 mg/mL, 50 mL yields 0.18 mg/mL. Treat spills or waste with a 5% sodium hypochlorite solution before disposal.

Storage: Refrigerate before initial reconstitution. Store at room temperature and use within 8 hours after initial reconstitution or dilution for infusion.

COMPATIBILITY
Does not interact with PVC infusion containers or administration sets at concentrations specified for dilution.

Other sources suggest a few specific **compatibilities** dependent on concentration and manufacturer; consult a pharmacist.

RATE OF ADMINISTRATION
Follow each dose with an additional 500 mL of prehydration infusion fluids.

IV injection: A single dose over 1 minute.

Infusion: A single dose over 20 to 30 minutes.

ACTIONS
Mechanism of action is not known, but it is cytotoxic as a result of its potent inhibition of the enzyme adenosine deaminase (ADA). Blocks DNA and RNA synthesis and causes DNA damage. Average terminal half-life of 6 hours is extended to 18 hours in patients with impaired renal function (CrCl less than 50 mL/min). Inhibits ADA for up to 1 week; actual response may not occur for months. Primarily excreted in urine.

INDICATIONS AND USES
Single-agent treatment of both untreated patients and alpha-interferon–refractory hairy cell leukemia (HCL) patients with active disease as defined by clinically significant anemia, neutropenia, thrombocytopenia, or disease-related symptoms.

Unlabeled uses: Treatment of chronic lymphocytic leukemia, prolymphocytic leukemia, non-Hodgkin lymphoma, cutaneous T-cell lymphoma, and peripheral T-cell lymphomas.

CONTRAINDICATIONS
Hypersensitivity to pentostatin; see Drug/Lab Interactions.

PRECAUTIONS

Follow guidelines for handling cytotoxic agents. See Appendix A, p. 1308. ■ Assess drug profile before administration. ■ Severe renal, liver, pulmonary, and CNS toxicities have occurred at higher doses; do not exceed recommended dose. ■ Usually administered by or under the supervision of a physician specialist. ■ Myelosuppression, especially neutropenia, is most severe during the first few courses of treatment. ■ Must consider risk/benefit in patients with some bone marrow suppression, the possibility of chickenpox or herpes zoster, a history of gout or urate renal stones, renal function impairment, or previous cytotoxic drug or radiation therapy. Use extreme caution. ■ After 6 months of treatment, assess for response; if partial or complete response is not evident, discontinue treatment. If partial response is evident, re-evaluate as indicated but do not treat beyond 12 months.

Monitor: Monitor CBC (including differential and platelet count) and SCr before each dose and as indicated. Blood chemistries, including serum uric acid, and a CrCl assay are required before and during treatment. ■ Prehydration with 500 to 1,000 mL D5/^{1}/$_2$NS or an equivalent is required. An additional 500 mL is required postadministration. ■ Treatment of patients with infection may exacerbate symptoms and cause death. Control infection before treatment is initiated. Withhold treatment if an active infection occurs; resume when infection is controlled. ■ Prophylactic antiemetics recommended (e.g., prochlorperazine, ondansetron); continue for 48 to 72 hours. ■ Observe closely for severe rashes, nervous system toxicity, and myelosuppression (especially after initial cycles); pentostatin may have to be withheld or discontinued. ■ For severe neutropenia beyond the initial cycles, evaluate for disease status, including a bone marrow examination. ■ Assess response to treatment with periodic monitoring of peripheral blood for hairy cells. Bone marrow aspirates and biopsies may be required at 2- to 3-month intervals. ■ Monitor for thrombocytopenia (platelet count less than 50,000/mm^3). Initiate precautions to prevent excessive bleeding (e.g., inspect IV sites, skin, and mucous membranes; use extreme care during invasive procedures; test urine, emesis, stool, and secretions for occult blood).

Patient Education: Consider birth control options; effective birth control recommended. ■ Report rashes, symptoms of infection, or bruising and bleeding immediately. ■ See Appendix D, p. 1311.

Maternal/Child: Category D: avoid pregnancy; can cause fetal harm. ■ Discontinue breastfeeding. ■ Safety for use in pediatric patients under 18 years of age not established.

Elderly: Consider decreased renal function.

DRUG/LAB INTERACTIONS

Assess drug profile before administration. ■ Do not use with **fludarabine**; may increase risk of fatal pulmonary toxicity. ■ Combination therapy with **carmustine, etoposide, and high-dose cyclophosphamide** as part of the ablative regimen for bone marrow transplant has caused acute pulmonary edema and hypotension. Deaths have occurred. ■ Pentostatin enhances the effects of **vidarabine**. Combined use of these agents may result in an increase in adverse reactions associated with each drug. The therapeutic benefit of this drug combination has not been established. ■ May cause skin rash with **allopurinol**. ■ Elevates **liver function tests;** usually reversible. ■ Do not administer **live virus vaccines** to patients receiving antineoplastic drugs. ■ Uric acid levels may increase; increased dose of **gout agents** (e.g., colchicine, probenecid, sulfinpyrazone) may be indicated. ■ Leukopenia and thrombocytopenia increased by **agents causing blood dyscrasias** (e.g., anticonvulsants [phenytoin], penicillins, phenothiazines, and many others).

SIDE EFFECTS

Anemia, anorexia, chills, cough, diarrhea, fatigue, fever, GU disorders, headache, hepatic disorders/elevated liver function tests, hypersensitivity reactions, infection, leukopenia, lung disorders, myalgia, nausea, neurologic disorders/CNS, pain, rashes, skin disorders, thrombocytopenia, upper respiratory infections, and vomiting occur in 10% of patients and may require discontinuation of treatment. Abdominal pain; abnormal ECG; abnormal thinking; abnormal vision; anxiety; arthralgia; asthenia; back pain; bronchitis; cardiac arrhythmias; chest pain; confusion; conjunctivitis; constipation; depression;

dizziness; dry skin; dyspnea; dysuria; ear pain; ecchymosis; eczema; elevated BUN, creatinine, and LDH; epistaxis; eye pain; flatulence; flu syndrome; hematuria; hemorrhage; herpes simplex; herpes zoster; insomnia; lung edema; lymphadenopathy; maculopapular rash; malaise; neoplasm; nervousness; paresthesia; peripheral edema; petechiae; pharyngitis; pneumonia; pruritus; rhinitis; seborrhea; sinusitis; skin discoloration; somnolence; stomatitis; sweating; thrombophlebitis; vesiculobullous rash; weight loss; and death have occurred in 3% to 10% or more of patients.

ANTIDOTE

Keep physician informed of all side effects; most will be treated symptomatically if indicated. Withhold dose and notify physician for elevated SCr, absolute neutrophil count below 200 cells/mm^3, myelosuppression, infection, CNS toxicity, or severe rash. Administration of whole blood products (e.g., packed RBCs, platelets, leukocytes) and/or blood modifiers (e.g., darbepoetin alfa, epoetin alfa, filgrastim, pegfilgrastim, sargramostim) may be indicated to treat bone marrow toxicity. Overdose may cause death due to severe renal, hepatic, pulmonary, or CNS toxicity. There is no specific antidote. Supportive therapy as indicated will help sustain the patient.

PERAMIVIR
(per-**AM**-i-vir)

Rapivab

Antiviral
(Influenza virus
neuraminidase inhibitor)

pH 5.5 to 8.5

USUAL DOSE

Administer peramivir within 2 days of onset of symptoms of influenza.

Adults and adolescents (13 years of age and older): A single dose of 600 mg administered as an IV infusion over 15 to 30 minutes.

PEDIATRIC DOSE

Pediatric patients (2 to 12 years of age): A single 12 mg/kg dose (up to a maximum of 600 mg) administered as an IV infusion over 15 to 30 minutes.

DOSE ADJUSTMENTS

No dose adjustment is required in patients with a creatinine clearance of 50 mL/min or higher. ▪ Reduce dose in patients with a baseline creatinine clearance below 50 mL/min using the recommendations in the following chart.

Dose Adjustment of Peramivir in Patients With Altered Creatinine Clearance			
Recommended Dose Adjustments in Patients With Altered Creatinine Clearance	Creatinine Clearance (mL/min)		
	≥50 mL/min	30 to 49 mL/min	10 to 29 mL/min[a]
Adults and adolescents (13 years of age and older)	600 mg	200 mg	100 mg
Pediatric patients (2 to 12 years of age)[b]	12 mg/kg	4 mg/kg	2 mg/kg

[a]In patients with chronic renal impairment maintained on hemodialysis, administer after dialysis at a dose adjusted based on renal function.
[b]Up to a maximum of 600 mg.

▪ No dose adjustment is required based on gender, impaired hepatic function, weight, or race (was evaluated primarily in Asians and Whites).

DILUTION

Available in single-use vials containing 200 mg/20 mL (10 mg/mL) as a clear, colorless solution. Contains no preservatives. Do not use if seal over bottle opening is broken or missing. Calculate the number of vial(s) required for the recommended dose. Withdraw the required volume of peramivir and dilute with NS, 1/2NS, D5W, or LR to a maximum volume of 100 mL.

Filters: No data available from manufacturer.

Storage: Before use, store in original cartons at CRT. Administer fully diluted solutions immediately or refrigerate at 2° to 8° C (36° to 46° F) for up to 24 hours. If refrigerated, allow the diluted solution to reach room temperature, then administer immediately. Discard any unused diluted solution of peramivir after 24 hours.

COMPATIBILITY

Compatible with NS, 1/2NS, D5W, or LR. Also **compatible** with materials commonly used for administration such as polyvinylchloride (PVC) bags and PVC-free bags, polypropylene syringes, and polyethylene tubing. Manufacturer states, "Do not mix or co-infuse with other intravenous medications."

RATE OF ADMINISTRATION

A single dose as an infusion equally distributed over 15 to 30 minutes.

ACTIONS

Peramivir is an antiviral drug with activity against the influenza virus. It is an inhibitor of the influenza virus neuraminidase, an enzyme that releases viral particles from the plasma membrane of infected cells. Maximum serum concentration is reached by the end of the infusion. In vitro binding to human plasma proteins is less than 30%. Not significantly metabolized in humans. Elimination half-life is approximately 20 hours. Primarily excreted as unchanged drug in urine.

INDICATIONS AND USES

Treatment of acute uncomplicated influenza in patients 2 years of age and older who have been symptomatic for no more than 2 days.

Limitations of use: Efficacy of peramivir is based on clinical trials of naturally occurring influenza in which the predominant influenza infections were influenza A virus; a limited number of subjects infected with influenza B virus were enrolled. ▪ Influenza viruses change over time. Emergence of resistance substitutions could decrease drug effectiveness. Other factors (e.g., changes in viral virulence) might also diminish the clinical benefit of antiviral drugs. Prescribers should consider available information on influenza drug susceptibility patterns and treatment effects when deciding whether to use peramivir. ▪ The efficacy of peramivir could not be established in patients with serious influenza requiring hospitalization.

CONTRAINDICATIONS

Known serious hypersensitivity or anaphylactic reaction to peramivir or any component of the product.

PRECAUTIONS

Rare cases of serious skin reactions, including erythema multiforme, have been reported. Cases of anaphylaxis and Stevens-Johnson syndrome have been reported in post-marketing surveillance. ▪ Influenza can be associated with a variety of neurologic and behavioral symptoms that can include events such as abnormal behavior, delirium, and hallucinations, which in some cases result in fatal outcomes. These events may occur in the setting of encephalitis or encephalopathy but also can occur in uncomplicated influenza. Neuropsychiatric events (e.g., delirium and abnormal behavior) have been reported in patients (primarily pediatric patients) with influenza who are receiving neuraminidase inhibitors, including peramivir. The contribution of peramivir to these events has not been established. ▪ There is no evidence for the efficacy of peramivir in any illness caused by agents other than influenza viruses. Serious bacterial infections may begin with influenza-like symptoms or may coexist with or occur as complications during the course of influenza. Peramivir has not been shown to prevent such complications. ▪ Circulating seasonal influenza strains expressing neuraminidase resistance–associated substitutions have been observed in individuals who have not received peramivir. Prescribers should consider available information from the CDC on influenza virus drug susceptibility patterns and treatment effects when deciding whether to use peramivir. ■ Cross-resistance between peramivir, oseltamivir, and zanamivir was observed in neuraminidase biochemical assays and cell culture assays. The clinical impact of this reduced susceptibility is unknown. ■ Has not been studied in patients with impaired hepatic function; however, because peramivir is cleared in urine by glomerular filtration, no clinically relevant problems are expected.

Monitor: Monitor for serious skin reactions. Appropriate treatment should be instituted if a serious skin reaction occurs or is suspected. ■ Monitor for potential secondary bacterial infections and treat with antibiotics as appropriate. ■ Monitor for S/S of a hypersensitivity reaction (e.g., anaphylaxis, hypotension, rash, tightness of the chest, urticaria, wheezing). ■ Patients with influenza should be closely monitored for signs of abnormal behavior.

Patient Education: There is a risk of serious skin reactions. Seek immediate medical attention if a skin reaction occurs. ■ There is a risk of neuropsychiatric events in patients with influenza. Patients should contact their physician if they experience signs of abnormal behavior after receiving peramivir. ■ Promptly report S/S of a hypersensitivity reaction (e.g., hives, rash, shortness of breath, wheezing).

Maternal/Child: Use during pregnancy only if clearly needed. Pregnant females are at higher risk for severe complications from influenza, which may lead to adverse pregnancy and/or fetal outcomes. ■ There are no data on the presence of peramivir in human milk, the effects on the breast-fed infant, or the effects on milk production. Consider risk versus benefit. ■ Safety and effectiveness in pediatric patients 2 to 17 years of age have been established. ■ Safety and effectiveness in pediatric patients under 2 years of age have not been established.

Elderly: Numbers in clinical studies were insufficient to determine if elderly patients respond differently than do younger subjects.

DRUG/LAB INTERACTIONS

The concurrent use of peramivir with **live attenuated influenza vaccine** (LAIV) intranasal has not been evaluated. Because of the potential for interference between these two products, avoid the use of LAIV within 2 weeks before or 48 hours after administration of peramivir unless medically indicated. For LAIV, antiviral drugs may inhibit viral replication and may reduce vaccine efficacy. ■ Inactivated influenza vaccine can be administered at any time.

SIDE EFFECTS

Adult and pediatric patients: The most common adverse reaction is diarrhea. Serious skin and hypersensitivity reactions (including anaphylaxis) and neuropsychiatric events have occurred. Constipation; decreased neutrophils; hypertension; increased ALT, AST, creatine phosphokinase, and serum glucose; and insomnia were also reported.

Pediatric patients: Fever, proteinuria, tympanic membrane erythema, and vomiting.

Post-Marketing: Abnormal behavior, anaphylaxis/anaphylactoid reactions, exfoliative dermatitis, hallucination, rash, and Stevens-Johnson syndrome.

ANTIDOTE

Notify physician of any side effects. Discontinue the drug if indicated. Treat overdose with general supportive measures, including monitoring of vital signs and observation of the clinical status of the patient. There is no specific antidote. Treat hypersensitivity reactions as indicated (e.g., diphenhydramine, epinephrine, albuterol) and resuscitate as necessary. Removed by hemodialysis.

PERTUZUMAB `BBW`
(per-**TOOZ**-ue-mab)

Recombinant monoclonal antibody
Antineoplastic

Perjeta

pH 6

USUAL DOSE

Pretreatment: Verify pregnancy status. Preassessment is required; see Monitor and Precautions.

Pertuzumab is given in combination with trastuzumab (Herceptin) or trastuzumab hyaluronidase-oysk (Herceptin Hylecta) and docetaxel (Taxotere) or anthracycline-based chemotherapy regimens. See monographs of any concomitantly administered medications; preassessment and premedication indicated. Pertuzumab, the trastuzumab product, and docetaxel should be administered sequentially. Pertuzumab and the trastuzumab product can be given in any order. Docetaxel should be administered after pertuzumab and the trastuzumab product administrations are complete. An observation period of 30 to 60 minutes is recommended after each pertuzumab infusion and before beginning any subsequent administration of the trastuzumab product or docetaxel. In patients receiving anthracycline-based regimen, pertuzumab and the trastuzumab product should be administered after completion of the anthracycline.

METASTATIC BREAST CANCER (MBC)

Initial doses: *Pertuzumab:* 840 mg as an infusion over 60 minutes.

Trastuzumab: 8 mg/kg as an infusion over 90 minutes. **OR**

Trastuzumab hyaluronidase-oysk: When pertuzumab is administered with trastuzumab hyaluronidase-oysk instead of trastuzumab (Herceptin), the recommended initial dose of trastuzumab hyaluronidase-oysk is 600 mg/10,000 units (600 units of trastuzumab and 10,000 units hyaluronidase) administered SC over approximately 2 to 5 minutes once every 3 weeks irrespective of the patient's body weight.

Docetaxel: 75 mg/M^2 as an infusion over 60 minutes.

Subsequent doses: Begin 3 weeks after initial doses.

Pertuzumab: 420 mg administered as an infusion over 30 to 60 minutes and repeated every 3 weeks.

Trastuzumab: 6 mg/kg as an infusion over 30 to 90 minutes and repeated every 3 weeks.

Docetaxel: If the initial dose is well tolerated, the dose may be escalated to 100 mg/M^2 and repeated every 3 weeks.

NEOADJUVANT TREATMENT OF BREAST CANCER

Administer pertuzumab every 3 weeks for 3 to 6 cycles as part of one of the following treatment regimens for early breast cancer. *Actual initial and subsequent doses of pertuzumab, the trastuzumab product, and docetaxel are the same as above in MBC.* Note all comments under Usual Dose.

- Four preoperative cycles of pertuzumab in combination with trastuzumab or trastuzumab hyaluronidase-oysk and docetaxel followed by 3 postoperative cycles of fluorouracil, epirubicin, and cyclophosphamide (FEC).
- Three or four preoperative cycles of FEC alone followed by 3 or 4 preoperative cycles of pertuzumab in combination with docetaxel and trastuzumab or trastuzumab hyaluronidase-oysk.
- Six preoperative cycles of pertuzumab in combination with docetaxel, carboplatin, and trastuzumab (TCH) or trastuzumab hyaluronidase-oysk (escalation of docetaxel above 75 mg/M^2 is not recommended).
- Four preoperative cycles of dose-dense doxorubicin and cyclophosphamide (ddAC) alone followed by 4 preoperative cycles of pertuzumab in combination with paclitaxel and trastuzumab or trastuzumab hyaluronidase-oysk.

Following surgery, patients should continue to receive pertuzumab and the trastuzumab product to complete 1 year of treatment (up to 18 cycles).

ADJUVANT TREATMENT OF BREAST CANCER

Pertuzumab should be administered in combination with trastuzumab or trastuzumab hyaluronidase-oysk every 3 weeks for a total of 1 year (up to 18 cycles) or until disease recurrence or unmanageable toxicity, whichever occurs first, as part of a complete regimen for early breast cancer, including standard anthracycline and/or taxane-based chemotherapy. Pertuzumab and the trastuzumab product should start on Day 1 of the first taxane-containing cycle.

DOSE ADJUSTMENTS

Recommendations Regarding Delayed or Missed Doses			
Time Between Two Sequential Doses	Pertuzumab	Trastuzumab (Intravenous)	Trastuzumab Hyaluronidase-oysk
Less than 6 weeks	Administer pertuzumab 420 mg IV as soon as possible. Do not wait until the next planned dose.	Administer trastuzumab 6 mg/kg IV as soon as possible. Do not wait until the next planned dose.	Administer trastuzumab hyaluronidase-oysk 600 mg/10,000 units SC as soon as possible. Do not wait until the next planned dose.
6 weeks or more	Readminister pertuzumab loading dose of 840 mg IV as a 60-minute infusion, followed by a maintenance dose of 420 mg IV over a period of 30 to 60 minutes every 3 weeks thereafter.	Readminister trastuzumab loading dose of 8 mg/kg IV over approximately 90 minutes, followed by a maintenance dose of 6 mg/kg IV over a period of 30 or 90 minutes every 3 weeks thereafter.	

- Dose reductions are not recommended for pertuzumab. ■ Pertuzumab should be discontinued if trastuzumab or trastuzumab hyaluronidase-oysk treatment is discontinued. ■ Discontinue immediately for a serious hypersensitivity reaction. ■ For chemotherapy dose modifications, see relevant prescribing information. ■ The recommendations on dose modifications in the event of LVEF dysfunction are indicated in the following chart.

Dose Modifications for LVEF Ventricular Dysfunction					
	Pretreatment LVEF	Monitor LVEF	Withhold Pertuzumab and Trastuzumab Product for at Least 3 Weeks for an LVEF Decrease to		Resume Pertuzumab and Trastuzumab Product After 3 Weeks if LVEF Has Recovered to	
Metastatic breast cancer	≥50%	Every 12 weeks	Either		Either	
			<40%	40% to 45% with a fall of ≥10% points below pretreatment value	>45%	40% to 45% with a fall of <10% points below pretreatment value
Early breast cancer	≥55%[a]	Every 12 weeks (once during neoadjuvant therapy)	<50% with a fall of ≥10% points below pretreatment value		Either	
					≥50%	<10% points below pretreatment value

[a]For patients receiving anthracycline-based chemotherapy, an LVEF of ≥50% is required after completion of anthracyclines and before starting pertuzumab and trastuzumab or trastuzumab hyaluronidase-oysk.

- No dose adjustment is indicated in patients with mild or moderate renal impairment. In patients with severe renal impairment (CrCl less than 30 mL/min), no dose adjustments can be recommended because of the limited pharmacokinetic data available. ■ See Rate of Administration, Precautions, Monitor, and Antidote.

DILUTION

Withdraw the calculated dose of pertuzumab from the vial(s) and inject into a 250-mL PVC or non-PVC polyolefin infusion bag of NS. Invert diluted solution gently to mix. *Do not shake.* Dilute only with NS. Do not use D5W. Immediate use is preferred.

Filters: Not required by manufacturer; additional data not available.

Storage: Store vials in carton in refrigerator at 2° to 8° C (36° to 46° F). Do not freeze. Do not shake. Protect from light. Immediate use preferred; if the diluted solution is not used immediately, however, it can be refrigerated for 24 hours.

COMPATIBILITY

Manufacturer states, "Do not mix pertuzumab with other drugs" and lists as **incompatible** with D5W.

RATE OF ADMINISTRATION

For IV infusion only; do not administer as an IV push or IV bolus. The rate of infusion may be slowed or interrupted if the patient develops an infusion-associated reaction. Discontinue immediately for a serious hypersensitivity reaction.

Pertuzumab: Administer the *initial dose* over 60 minutes. Administer *subsequent doses* over 30 to 60 minutes. An observation period of 30 to 60 minutes is recommended after each pertuzumab infusion and before beginning any subsequent administration of trastuzumab or trastuzumab hyaluronidase-oysk, or docetaxel.

Trastuzumab: Administer the *initial dose* over 90 minutes. Administer *subsequent doses* over 30 to 90 minutes. May be administered before or after pertuzumab.

Trastuzumab hyaluronidase-oysk: See Usual Dose.

Docetaxel: Each dose equally distributed over 60 minutes. Administer after pertuzumab and trastuzumab product administrations have been completed.

ACTIONS

A recombinant humanized monoclonal antibody. It targets the human epidermal growth factor receptor 2 protein (HER2) and blocks ligand-dependent heterodimerization of HER2 with other HER family members, including EGFR, HER3, and HER4. By inhibiting specific pathways, cell growth arrest and apoptosis can occur. Pertuzumab also mediates antibody-dependent, cell-mediated cytotoxicity. While using pertuzumab alone inhibits the proliferation of human tumor cells, the combination of pertuzumab and the trastuzumab product greatly augments antitumor activity in HER2-overexpressing xenograft models. Steady-state concentration can be reached after the first maintenance dose. Median half-life was 18 days.

INDICATIONS AND USES

Pertuzumab in combination with trastuzumab or trastuzumab hyaluronidase-oysk and docetaxel is indicated for the treatment of patients with HER2-positive metastatic breast cancer who have not received prior anti-HER2 therapy or chemotherapy for metastatic disease. ▪ Pertuzumab in combination with trastuzumab or trastuzumab hyaluronidase-oysk and chemotherapy is indicated for the neoadjuvant treatment of patients with HER2-positive, locally advanced, inflammatory, or early-stage breast cancer (either greater than 2 cm in diameter or node positive) as part of a complete treatment regimen for early breast cancer; and the adjuvant treatment of patients with HER2-positive early breast cancer at high risk of recurrence.

CONTRAINDICATIONS

Known hypersensitivity to pertuzumab or to any of its excipients.

PRECAUTIONS

For IV infusion only; do not administer as an IV push or IV bolus. ▪ Assess HER2 status before beginning pertuzumab therapy. Testing should be done by a laboratory with demonstrated proficiency in the testing process using FDA-approved tests. In clinical studies, the only patients who have received benefit from pertuzumab therapy are those with HER2 protein. ▪ Can cause fetal harm when administered to pregnant females; see Patient Education and Maternal/Child. ▪ Administered by or under the direction of a physician specialist. ▪ Adequate laboratory and supportive medical resources must be available. ▪ Emergency equipment and drugs for treatment of left ventricular dysfunction and/or hypersensitivity or infusion reactions must be immediately available; see Antidote.

■ Can result in subclinical and clinical cardiac failure. Evaluate left ventricular function in all patients before and during treatment with pertuzumab. Decreases in LVEF with drugs that block HER2 activity, including pertuzumab, have been reported. Patients who have received prior anthracyclines or radiotherapy to the chest wall may be at higher risk for decreased LVEF. ■ Pertuzumab has not been studied in patients with a pretreatment LVEF value of 50% or less, a prior history of CHF, decreases in LVEF to less than 50% during prior trastuzumab therapy, or conditions that could impair left ventricular function such as uncontrolled hypertension, recent MI, serious cardiac arrhythmia requiring treatment, or a cumulative prior anthracycline exposure to greater than 360 mg/M^2 of doxorubicin or its equivalent. ■ Hypersensitivity reactions, including anaphylaxis (and fatal events), and infusion reactions (including fatal events) have occurred. ■ Trastuzumab products and other concomitantly administered antineoplastics also have extensive precautions and monitoring requirements; a review of their monographs is imperative. ■ Effects on patients with severe renal impairment and/or hepatic impairment have not been studied. ■ A protein substance; has the potential for immunogenicity.

Monitor: Assess LVEF before beginning therapy and at regular intervals during treatment to verify that it remains within expected parameters; see Dose Adjustments. ■ Monitor for S/S of a hypersensitivity reaction (e.g., chest pain, chills, dizziness, dyspnea, fever, flushing, hypotension, nausea, pruritus, rash, urticaria) or infusion reaction (e.g., asthenia, chills, dysgeusia, fatigue, fever, headache, myalgia, vomiting). Observe closely for 60 minutes after the first infusion and for at least 30 minutes after subsequent infusions. ■ Trastuzumab products and other concomitantly administered antineoplastics have additional monitoring requirements.

Patient Education: Avoid pregnancy; effective contraception required while receiving therapy and for 7 months following the last dose of pertuzumab in combination with trastuzumab products. ■ During infusion, promptly report chills and/or fever and other S/S of an infusion or hypersensitivity reaction (e.g., chest pain, dizziness, feeling faint, flushing, hives, itching, nausea, pruritus, rash, shortness of breath). ■ Promptly report new onset or worsening of shortness of breath, cough, swelling of ankles/legs, swelling of the face, palpitations, weight gain of more than 5 pounds in 24 hours, dizziness, or loss of consciousness. ■ Report a suspected pregnancy immediately. If a pregnancy occurs during therapy, if pertuzumab is administered during a pregnancy, or if pregnancy occurs within 7 months of the last dose of pertuzumab, report pregnancy immediately to the Genentech Adverse Event Line. ■ See Appendix D, p. 1311.

Maternal/Child: Avoid pregnancy; may cause fetal harm. Exposure can result in embryo-fetal death and birth defects. Studies in animals have resulted in oligohydramnios, delayed renal development, and embryo-fetal deaths. In post-marketing reports for trastuzumab (another HER2 receptor antagonist), use during pregnancy resulted in cases of oligohydramnios and oligohydramnios sequence manifesting as pulmonary hypoplasia, skeletal abnormalities, and neonatal death. Females who receive pertuzumab in combination with trastuzumab products during pregnancy or within 7 months before conception should be monitored for oligohydramnios. If oligohydramnios occurs, perform fetal testing that is appropriate for gestational age and consistent with community standards of care. ■ Consider risk versus benefit with breast-feeding. Consideration should also take into account the elimination half-life of pertuzumab and the trastuzumab wash-out period of 7 months. ■ Safety and effectiveness for use in pediatric patients not established.

Elderly: No overall differences in safety were observed between patients 65 years of age and older and patients under 65 years of age. There are too few patients 75 years of age and older to draw conclusions on the efficacy in this age-group.

DRUG/LAB INTERACTIONS
No formal drug interaction studies have been done.

SIDE EFFECTS
Pertuzumab administered in combination with the trastuzumab product and docetaxel: The most common side effects were alopecia, diarrhea, fatigue, nausea, neutropenia, peripheral neuropathy, and rash. Anemia, thrombocytopenia, and vomiting were reported when carboplatin was added to the regimen. The most common Grade 3 and 4 adverse reactions were anemia, asthenia, diarrhea, fatigue, febrile neutropenia, leukopenia, neutropenia, and peripheral neuropathy.

Pertuzumab in combination with the trastuzumab product and chemotherapy for the adjuvant treatment of breast cancer: The most common side effects included alopecia, diarrhea, fatigue, nausea, peripheral neuropathy, and vomiting. Adverse events occurring in 10% or more of patients treated with pertuzumab include arthralgia, constipation, decreased appetite, dizziness, dry skin, dysgeusia, dyspnea, headache, increased lacrimation, insomnia, itching, mucosal inflammation, myalgia, nail disorders, nasopharyngitis, peripheral edema, paronychia, stomatitis, upper respiratory tract infections, and vomiting. Adverse reactions were reported less frequently after discontinuation of docetaxel treatment. See prescribing information for additional side effects.

Post-Marketing: Tumor lysis syndrome (TLS).

ANTIDOTE

Notify physician of all side effects. Most will be treated symptomatically. If signs of an infusion reaction occur, slow or interrupt the infusion and treat appropriately. Monitor patients carefully until symptoms resolve. Discontinue immediately for a serious hypersensitivity reaction. Discontinue pertuzumab for a confirmed clinically significant decrease in left ventricular function. Administration of whole blood products (e.g., packed RBCs, platelets, leukocytes) and/or blood modifiers (e.g., darbepoetin alfa, epoetin alfa, filgrastim, pegfilgrastim, sargramostim) may be indicated to treat bone marrow toxicity from concurrent antineoplastics. Treat hypersensitivity reactions with epinephrine, antihistamines, corticosteroids, bronchodilators, and oxygen. Resuscitate as indicated.

PHENOBARBITAL SODIUM
(fee-no-**BAR**-bih-tal **SO**-dee-um)

Barbiturate
Sedative-hypnotic
Anticonvulsant

Luminal Sodium

pH 8.5 to 10.5

USUAL DOSE

Pretreatment: See Maternal/Child.

Use only enough medication to achieve the desired effect. May take up to 15 minutes to reach peak levels in the brain; guard against overdose and excessive respiratory depression.

Hypnotic: 100 to 325 mg.

Sedative: 30 to 120 mg/day in 2 or 3 divided doses (15 to 60 mg every 12 hours or 10 to 40 mg every 8 hours).

Anticonvulsant: 200 to 320 mg. May be repeated if necessary. Maximum dose usually does not exceed 600 mg.

Status epilepticus: *Loading dose:* 10 to 20 mg/kg in single or divided doses. May give an additional 5 mg/kg every 15 to 30 minutes up to a maximum dose of 30 mg/kg.

Maintenance dose: 1 to 3 mg/kg/24 hr or 0.5 to 1.5 mg/kg every 12 hours. **Alcohol withdrawal treatment. Refer to specific protocols found on line as its use is off-label.**

PEDIATRIC DOSE

See comments under Usual Dose.

Preoperative sedation: 1 to 3 mg/kg of body weight 60 to 90 minutes before procedure.

Status epilepticus: *Loading dose:* 15 to 18 mg/kg as a single dose or in divided doses. May give an additional 5 mg/kg every 15 to 30 minutes up to a maximum total dose of 30 mg/kg.

Maintenance dose: Infants: 2.5 to 3 mg/kg every 12 hours.

Ages 1 to 5: 3 to 4 mg/kg every 12 hours.

Ages 6 to 12: 2 to 3 mg/kg every 12 hours.

Over 12 years of age: 0.5 to 1.5 mg/kg every 12 hours. Up to 12 mg/kg/24 hours has been used in maintenance doses.

NEONATAL DOSE

See comments under Usual Dose.

Status epilepticus: *Loading dose:* 15 to 20 mg/kg as a single dose or in divided doses.

Maintenance dose: 1.5 to 2 mg/kg every 12 hours; may be increased to 2.5 mg/kg every 12 hours if needed. Therapeutic range is 15 to 40 mg/L. Because of its long half-life, it may take 2 to 3 weeks to reach steady-state levels.

DOSE ADJUSTMENTS

Reduce dose in impaired renal or hepatic function; usually required in the debilitated or elderly. ▪ See Drug/Lab Interactions.

DILUTION

Sterile powder must be slowly diluted with SWFI. Use a minimum of 3 mL of diluent. Also available in sterile vials and tubexes. Solutions from powder form must be freshly prepared. Use only absolutely clear solutions. Discard powder or solution exposed to air for 30 minutes.

COMPATIBILITY

Compatibility information not available from manufacturer. Other sources suggest specific **compatibilities** dependent on concentration and manufacturer; consult a pharmacist.

RATE OF ADMINISTRATION

60 mg or fraction thereof over 1 minute. Titrate slowly to desired effect. Rapid injection rate may cause symptoms of overdose (e.g., serious respiratory depression).
Status epilepticus: A single loading dose over 10 to 15 minutes.

ACTIONS

A sedative, hypnotic barbiturate of long duration with potent anticonvulsant effects. Phenobarbital is a CNS depressant. Onset of action is prompt by the IV route and becomes rapidly more intense. Effects last from 6 to 10 hours. Will effectively depress the motor cortex with small doses. Pain perception is unimpaired. Rapidly absorbed by all body tissues and excreted in changed form in the urine. Excreted more readily in alkaline urine. Crosses the placental barrier. Secreted in breast milk.

INDICATIONS AND USES

Prolonged sedation (medical and psychiatric). ▪ Anticonvulsant.

CONTRAINDICATIONS

History of porphyria, impaired renal function, impaired hepatic function especially with any signs of hepatic coma, known hypersensitivity to barbiturates, previous addiction, severe respiratory depression including dyspnea, obstruction, or cor pulmonale.

PRECAUTIONS

IV route usually reserved for critical situations. ▪ Use caution in elderly and debilitated patients and those with asthma, pulmonary disease, shock, and impaired renal or hepatic function. ▪ Status epilepticus can occur from too-rapid withdrawal. ▪ May be habit forming. Use caution in acute or chronic pain.
Monitor: Keep patient under constant observation. Record vital signs every hour, or more often if indicated. ▪ Maintain a patent airway. ▪ Monitor for vein irritation at injection site. ▪ Monitor hematopoietic, renal and hepatic systems in any extended therapy. ▪ Treat the cause of a convulsion. ▪ Keep equipment for artificial ventilation available. ▪ Highly alkaline. Determine absolute patency of vein; use of large veins preferred to prevent thrombosis. Avoid extravasation. Intra-arterial injection will cause gangrene. ▪ Monitor serum levels as indicated; the therapeutic range in adults is 20 to 40 mcg/mL (15 to 40 mcg/mL in pediatric patients). Because of its long half-life, it may take 2 to 3 weeks to reach steady-state levels. ▪ See Drug/Lab Interactions.
Patient Education: Avoid alcohol or other CNS depressants. May be habit forming. ▪ May require alternate birth control.
Maternal/Child: Category D: avoid pregnancy; will cause birth defects. ▪ May cause drowsiness in the nursing infant. ▪ See Precautions.
Elderly: See Dose Adjustments and Precautions. ▪ Often have increased sensitivity to barbiturates; may cause marked excitement, depression, confusion, and increased risk of barbiturate-induced hypothermia. ▪ Consider age-related hepatic or renal impairment and concomitant disease or drug therapy.

DRUG/LAB INTERACTIONS

Use extreme caution if any other **CNS depressants** have been given, such as alcohol, amino-glycoside antibiotics, narcotic analgesics, anesthetics, antidepressants, antihistamines, hypnotics, MAO inhibitors, phenothiazines, sedatives, tranquilizers. Potentiation with respiratory depression may occur. ■ Inhibits effectiveness of **corticosteroids, doxycycline, oral anticoagulants, oral contraceptives, propranolol, quinidine, and theophylline.** Capable of innumerable interactions with many drugs. ■ May increase orthostatic hypotension with **furosemide.** ■ Monitor **phenytoin, carbamazepine, valproic acid, and phenobarbital** levels when any combination of these drugs is used concurrently. ■ May decrease the pharmacologic effect of **vitamin D.** ■ May decrease plasma concentrations and effectiveness of **triazole antifungals.**

SIDE EFFECTS

Rarely occur with slow injection of average doses.

Average dose: Depression, dermatitis, facial edema, fever, headache, hypotension, nausea, neonatal apnea, respiratory depression (hypoventilation), thrombocytopenic purpura, vertigo.

Overdose: Apnea, coma, cough reflex depression, delirium, flat EEG (reversible unless hypoxic damage has occurred), hypotension, laryngospasm, lowered body temperature, pulmonary edema, renal shutdown, respiratory depression, sluggish or absent reflexes, stupor.

ANTIDOTE

Notify the physician of any side effects. Symptomatic and supportive treatment is most important in overdose. Maintain an adequate airway with artificial ventilation if indicated. Keep the patient warm. IV volume expanders and other IV fluids will help maintain adequate circulation. Diuretics may promote the elimination of the drug. Vasopressors will maintain BP.

PHENYLEPHRINE HYDROCHLORIDE

Vasopressor

(fen-ill-**EF**-rin hy-droh-**KLOR**-eyed)

Neo-Synephrine, Vazculep

pH 3 to 6.5

USUAL DOSE

Perioperative setting: *Bolus:* 40 to 100 mcg by IV bolus administration. May repeat every 1 to 2 minutes as needed, not to exceed a total dose of 200 mcg.

A second manufacturer lists an initial bolus of 50 to 100 mcg with a range of 50 to 250 mcg.

Continuous infusion: If BP is below target goal, begin a continuous infusion of 10 to 35 mcg/min, not to exceed 200 mcg/min.

A second manufacturer lists a rate of 0.5 to 1.4 mcg/kg/min. Titrate to blood pressure goal.

Septic or other vasodilatory shock *(no longer recommended for routine use for this indication)*: Do not administer a bolus. Begin with a continuous infusion of 0.5 to 6 mcg/kg/min. Titrate to blood pressure goal. Doses above 6 mcg/kg/min do not show a significant incremental increase in blood pressure.

Another source recommends:

Begin infusion at 100 to 180 mcg/min (0.1 to 0.18 mg/min) until BP is stabilized at a low normal for specific individual. Maintain with 40 to 60 mcg/min (0.04 to 0.06 mg/min). Titrate to desired effect.

DOSE ADJUSTMENTS

Patients with liver cirrhosis (Child-Pugh Class B and Class C) may have decreased responsiveness to phenylephrine. Higher-end doses may be required to achieve BP goal. ■ Patients with end-stage renal disease may have increased responsiveness to phenylephrine. Initiate dosing at lower end of dosing range.

DILUTION

IV injection: Dilute 10 mg (1 mL of a 10 mg/mL solution) with 99 mL of NS or D5W to provide a final concentration of 100 mcg/mL. Withdraw an appropriate dose from this solution prior to bolus administration.

Infusion: Dilute 10 mg in 500 mL of NS or D5W to provide a final concentration of 20 mcg/mL.

Storage: Store unopened vials at CRT in carton. Protect from light. Diluted solution should not be held for more than 4 hours at RT or for more than 24 hours under refrigeration. Discard any unused portion.

COMPATIBILITY

Compatibility information not available from manufacturer. Other source suggests specific **compatibilities** dependent on concentration and manufacturer; consult a pharmacist.

RATE OF ADMINISTRATION

IV injection: Administer by injection over 20 to 30 seconds.

Infusion: See Usual Dose. Titrate to maintain individual's low-normal BP. Use an infusion pump or microdrip (60 gtt/mL) to administer. Central line preferred.

ACTIONS

An alpha-1 adrenergic receptor agonist. Interacts with the receptors on the vascular smooth muscle cells, resulting in vasoconstriction. Increases in systolic blood pressure, diastolic blood pressure, mean arterial blood pressure, and total peripheral vascular resistance are observed within minutes of administration. As blood pressure increases, vagal activity also increases, resulting in a reflex bradycardia. Active on most vascular beds, including renal, pulmonary, and splanchnic arteries. Duration of effect is 15 to 20 minutes. Terminal half-life is 2.5 hours. Metabolized primarily by monoamine oxidase and sulfotransferase. Excreted in urine, primarily as inactive metabolites.

INDICATIONS AND USES

Treatment of clinically important hypotension resulting primarily from vasodilation in settings such as septic shock or anesthesia. *(No longer recommended for routine use in treatment of hypotension related to septic shock.)*

CONTRAINDICATIONS

Hypersensitivity to phenylephrine or any of its components.

PRECAUTIONS

Intravascular volume depletion should be corrected. ▪ Correct acidosis. Acidosis may reduce effectiveness of phenylephrine. ▪ Because of its pressor effects, phenylephrine can precipitate angina in patients with severe arteriosclerosis or history of angina, exacerbate underlying heart failure, and increase pulmonary arterial pressure. ▪ Avoid extravasation. Can cause necrosis or sloughing of tissue. ▪ Can cause peripheral and visceral vasoconstriction and ischemia to vital organs, particularly in patients with extensive peripheral vascular disease. ▪ Can cause severe bradycardia and decreased cardiac output. ▪ Can increase the need for renal replacement therapy in patients with septic shock. ▪ The pressor response to adrenergic drugs, including phenylephrine, can be increased in patients with autonomic dysfunction, such as may occur with spinal cord injuries. ▪ Contains bisulfites; use caution in allergic individuals. ▪ See Drug/Lab Interactions.

Monitor: Monitor vital signs. ▪ Check infusion site for free flow. Discontinue IV administration if vein infiltrates or is thrombosed. ▪ Monitor renal function. ▪ See Precautions, Drug/Lab Interactions.

Maternal/Child: Category C: safety for use in pregnancy or breast-feeding not established. ▪ Safety and effectiveness for use in pediatric patients not established.

Elderly: See Precautions; may have increased sensitivity to effects.

DRUG/LAB INTERACTIONS

Oxytocic drugs (e.g., oxytocin) potentiate the increasing blood pressure effects of sympathomimetic pressor amines, including phenylephrine, with the potential for hemorrhagic stroke. ▪ The pressor effect of phenylephrine is also increased in patients receiving **MAO inhibitors, tricyclic antidepressants, angiotensin, aldosterone, atropine, steroids, norepinephrine**

transporter inhibitors (e.g., atomoxetine), **or ergot alkaloids**. ■ The pressor effect of phenylephrine is decreased in patients receiving **alpha-adrenergic antagonists, phosphodiesterase type 5 inhibitors, mixed alpha- and beta-receptor antagonists** (e.g., labetalol, carvedilol), **calcium channel blockers, benzodiazepines, ACE inhibitors, or centrally acting sympatholytic agents**.

SIDE EFFECTS
The most common side effects are headache, nausea, and vomiting. Other reported side effects include arrhythmias, blurred vision, chest pain, diaphoresis, dyspnea, epigastric pain, extravasation, fullness of head, hypersensitivity (sulfite sensitivity), hypertension, hypertensive crisis, hypertensive induced bradycardia, ischemia, lower cardiac output, neck pain, nervousness, paresthesia, pruritus, pulmonary edema, rales, reflexive bradycardia, skin blanching, skin necrosis with extravasation, and tremor.

ANTIDOTE
To prevent sloughing and necrosis in areas of extravasation, with a fine hypodermic needle inject 5 to 10 mg of phentolamine diluted in 10 to 15 mL of NS liberally throughout the tissue in the extravasated area. Treatment should be started as soon as extravasation is recognized. Notify the physician of all side effects. IM injection may be preferable. Treat hypertension with phentolamine. Treat cardiac arrhythmias as indicated. Treat bradycardia with atropine. Resuscitate as necessary.

PHENYTOIN SODIUM BBW
(**FEN**-ih-toyn **SO**-dee-um)

Hydantoin
Anticonvulsant

Dilantin   pH 12

USUAL DOSE
Pretreatment: See Maternal/Child.

In all situations, transfer to oral therapy as soon as practical. See Precautions and Monitor. Treatment with phenytoin can be initiated either with a loading dose or an infusion. **Status epilepticus, anticonvulsant:** A *loading dose* of 10 to 15 mg/kg. One source recommends not exceeding a total dose of 1.5 Gm in 24 hours. Lethal dose estimated at 2 to 5 Gm. Another source suggests that 15 to 20 mg/kg is generally recommended. Follow with *maintenance doses* of 100 mg every 6 to 8 hours. Adjust dose based on phenytoin levels; see Monitor. Other measures, including concomitant administration of an IV benzodiazepine (such as diazepam) or an IV short-acting barbiturate, will usually be necessary for rapid control of seizures because of the required slow rate of administration of phenytoin. If seizure is not terminated, consider other anticonvulsants, barbiturates, or anesthesia. **Nonemergent loading and maintenance dosing:** 10 to 15 mg/kg as a *loading dose* followed by a *maintenance dose* of oral or IV phenytoin every 6 to 8 hours.

PEDIATRIC DOSE
Status epilepticus, anticonvulsant: 15 to 20 mg/kg as a *loading dose.* Follow with a *maintenance dose for age* (listed below):
Neonates: Begin with 5 mg/kg/24 hr in equally divided doses every 12 hours. Range is 4 to 8 mg/kg/24 hr in divided doses every 8 or 12 hours (2 to 4 mg/kg every 12 hours or 1.33 to 2.67 mg/kg every 8 hours).
Infants and other pediatric patients: Begin with 5 mg/kg/24 hr in equally divided doses every 8 to 12 hours (2.5 mg/kg every 12 hours or 1.67 mg/kg every 8 hours). Range varies according to age:
   6 months to 3 years: 8 to 10 mg/kg/24 hr (4 to 5 mg/kg every 12 hours or 2.67 to 3.33 mg/kg every 8 hours).
   4 to 6 years: 7.5 to 9 mg/kg/24 hr (3.75 to 4.5 mg/kg every 12 hours or 2.5 to 3 mg/kg every 8 hours).

7 to 9 years: 7 to 8 mg/kg/24 hr (3.5 to 4 mg/kg every 12 hours or 2.3 to 2.6 mg/kg every 8 hours).

10 to 16 years: 6 to 7 mg/kg/24 hr (3 to 3.5 mg/kg every 12 hours or 2 to 2.3 mg/kg every 8 hours).

DOSE ADJUSTMENTS

After the initial maintenance dose, subsequent maintenance doses should be individualized by monitoring serum levels of phenytoin to achieve a target therapeutic concentration. ■ Lower or less frequent dosing and a slower rate of administration may be required in elderly patients. ■ Use caution, lower dose, and slower rate of administration in seriously ill patients and cachectic patients. ■ Lower doses may also be required in patients with renal or hepatic disease or in those with hypoalbuminemia. Monitoring of unbound (free) phenytoin concentrations may be a better dosing guide. ■ Dose adjustment may be needed when switching between the sodium salt formulations (e.g., injection and capsules) and the free acid forms (e.g., suspension and infatabs). The free acid form contains approximately 8% more drug than the sodium salt form. ■ See Drug/Lab Interactions.

DILUTION

Available in 100- or 250-mg single-dose ampules or vials and in 100-mg single-dose syringes. After verifying patency, may be administered directly into a large peripheral or central vein through a large-gauge catheter. Alternately, may be further diluted in NS to a concentration of no less than 5 mg/mL and administered as an infusion. Use solution only when completely dissolved and clear.

Filters: Manufacturer recommends use of an in-line filter (0.22 to 0.55 microns) when administered as an infusion.

Storage: Store between 15° and 30° C (59° and 86° F). Infusion solutions should be administered immediately after preparation and must be completed within 1 to 4 hours. Do not refrigerate infusion solutions.

COMPATIBILITY

Manufacturer recommends not adding to IV solutions other than NS or mixing with other medications and states that "the addition of phenytoin to dextrose or dextrose-containing solutions will result in precipitation." Always flush line with NS before and after administration of any other drug through the same IV line. See Dilution.

Other sources suggest a few specific **compatibilities** dependent on concentration and manufacturer; consult a pharmacist.

RATE OF ADMINISTRATION

Because of the risk of local toxicity, IV phenytoin should be administered directly into a large peripheral or central vein through a large-gauge catheter. Before administration, the patency of the IV should be tested with a sterile saline flush. Follow the administration of phenytoin with a saline flush to avoid local venous irritation due to the alkalinity of the solution. In nonemergent situations, slower rates of administration should be used.

Adults: Administer slowly at a rate of 25 to 50 mg or fraction thereof over 1 minute. Do not exceed 50 mg/min.

Pediatric patients: Do not exceed 1 to 3 mg/kg/min (or 50 mg/min, whichever is slower). Another source suggests 0.5 mg/kg/min in neonates or 1 mg/kg/min in infants and other pediatric patients not to exceed 50 mg/min.

Elderly: Limit rate to 25 mg/min.

Infusion: Should be completed within 1 to 4 hours. Do not exceed 25 to 50 mg/min rate. Best if piggybacked to a **compatible** primary IV so phenytoin can be discontinued if side effects occur, but IV can be kept open.

ACTIONS

An anticonvulsant, chemically related to barbiturates. Selectively stabilizes seizure threshold and depresses seizure activity in the motor cortex. Mechanism of action may be due to increasing efflux or decreasing influx of sodium ions across the cell membrane during generation of the action potential. Effective control in emergency treatment of seizures may take 15 to 20 minutes because of rate of injection required. Highly protein bound. Metabolized by cytochrome P_{450} enzymes CYP2C9 and CYP2C19. Most of the drug is excreted in the bile as inactive metabolites. Urinary excretion of phenytoin and its metabolites occurs by glomerular filtration and tubular secretion. Half-life ranges from 10 to 15 hours. Crosses the placental barrier. Secreted in breast milk.

INDICATIONS AND USES

Treatment of generalized tonic-clonic status epilepticus and prevention and treatment of seizures during neurosurgery. Parenteral phenytoin should be used only when oral phenytoin administration is not possible.

CONTRAINDICATIONS

Known hypersensitivity to phenytoin or other hydantoin products. ▪ Bradycardia; sinoatrial, second-, or third-degree AV heart block; Adams-Stokes syndrome. ▪ A history of prior acute hepatotoxicity attributable to phenytoin. ▪ Coadministration with delavirdine (Rescriptor); see Drug/Lab Interactions.

PRECAUTIONS

Discontinue immediately for hypersensitivity reactions; with caution, substitute a nonhydantoin anticonvulsant. When substituting a new anticonvulsant, consideration should be given to avoiding structurally related drugs such as carboxamides (e.g., carbamazepine), barbiturates, succinimides, and oxazolidinediones (e.g., trimethadione). ▪ Angioedema has been reported. ▪ Abrupt withdrawal may cause increased seizure activity. Gradually reduce dose, discontinue, or substitute alternative antiepileptic agents if possible. ▪ Severe hypotension and cardiac arrhythmias have occurred with rapid infusion. Risk increases with increased rates, but adverse cardiac events have been reported at or below the recommended infusion rates. Cardiac arrhythmias have included bradycardia, heart block, ventricular tachycardia, and ventricular fibrillation and have resulted in asystole, cardiac arrest, and death. Severe complications are most commonly encountered in critically ill patients, elderly patients, and patients with hypotension and severe myocardial insufficiency. Careful cardiac monitoring is required during and after IV administration. Because of the risks of cardiac and local toxicity associated with IV phenytoin, oral phenytoin should be used whenever possible. ▪ Use caution with low serum albumin level, and adjust dose as indicated. Phenytoin is highly bound to serum protein (approximately 80% to 90% or more), and a reduced albumin causes an increase in free drug availability. ▪ Drug reaction with eosinophilia and systemic symptoms (DRESS), also known as multiorgan hypersensitivity, has been reported. Usually presents with fever, rash, lymphadenopathy, and/or facial swelling in association with other organ system involvement such as hepatitis, nephritis, hematologic abnormalities, myocarditis, or myositis. Eosinophilia is often present. Deaths have been reported. Discontinue therapy if an alternative etiology for S/S cannot be established. ▪ Severe cutaneous adverse reactions (SCARs) have been reported, including toxic epidermal necrolysis (TEN), Stevens-Johnson syndrome (SJS), acute generalized exanthematous pustulosis (AGEP), and DRESS. Deaths have occurred. Onset of symptoms is usually within 28 days but may occur later. Discontinue phenytoin at the first sign of a rash unless the rash is clearly not drug related. If a rash develops, the patient should be evaluated for S/S of SCARs. ▪ Selected patients of Asian ancestry with a specific human leukocyte antigen allele (HLA-B*1502) may have an increased risk of serious skin reactions (e.g., Stevens-Johnson syndrome, toxic epidermal necrolysis) from phenytoin therapy. ▪ Cases of acute hepatotoxicity, including hepatic failure, have been reported. These events may be part of the spectrum of DRESS or may occur in isolation. Reactions have included elevated liver function tests, eosinophilia, hepatomegaly, jaundice, and leukocytosis. Discontinue immediately and substitute alternative anticonvulsant therapy. ▪ Hematopoietic complications, some fatal, have been reported (e.g., agranulocytosis, granulocytopenia, leukopenia, thrombocytopenia, or pancytopenia with or without bone marrow suppression). ▪ Some reports suggest a relationship between phenytoin and the development of lymphadenopathy (local or generalized), including benign lymph node hyperplasia, pseudolymphoma, lymphoma, and Hodgkin disease. Lymph node involvement may occur with or without S/S resembling DRESS; see Monitor. ▪ Local toxicity, including purple glove syndrome (edema, discoloration, and pain distal to the injection site), has occurred and may or may not be associated with extravasation.

Irritation may range from slight tenderness to extensive necrosis and sloughing. ▪ Inhibits insulin release and may increase serum glucose; monitoring indicated in patients with diabetes. ▪ A small percentage of patients may be slow metabolizers of phenytoin. This appears to be genetically determined. If early signs of dose-related CNS toxicity develop, obtain serum levels immediately. ▪ Not effective for absence seizures; combined therapy is required if both conditions are present. ▪ Not indicated for seizures due to hypoglycemia or other metabolic causes. ▪ Use with caution in patients with porphyria. Phenytoin may exacerbate this disease. ▪ Antiepileptic drugs (AEDs) increase the risk of suicidal thoughts or behavior in patients taking these drugs for any indication. Patients treated with any AED for any indication should be monitored for the emergence or worsening of depression, suicidal thoughts or behavior, and/or any unusual changes in mood or behavior. Some psychotic symptoms and/or behavioral changes resolved without intervention. Others required dose reduction or discontinuation of the antiepileptic agent.

Monitor: Narrow margin of error between therapeutic and toxic dose. Plasma levels above 10 mcg/mL usually control seizure activity. The acceptable range is 10 to 20 mcg/mL. ▪ Consider monitoring free phenytoin levels in patients with hypoalbuminemia or renal or hepatic insufficiency (therapeutic range is 1 to 2 mcg/mL); fraction of unbound phenytoin is increased. ▪ Toxicity usually begins with nystagmus and may be seen at levels less than 20 mcg/mL. Serum levels sustained above the optimum range may produce confusional states referred to as delirium, psychosis, encephalopathy or, rarely, irreversible cerebellar dysfunction and/or cerebellar atrophy. Observe patient closely for signs of CNS side effects. At the first sign of acute toxicity, plasma levels are recommended. Reduce dose if levels are elevated. If symptoms persist, discontinuation of therapy is recommended. ▪ Periodic monitoring of CBC, platelets, albumin, urinalysis, and hepatic and renal function is recommended. ▪ Monitor ECG, BP, and respiratory status carefully during and after administration. ▪ Closely monitor patients who are gravely ill, have impaired liver function, or are elderly. May show early signs of toxicity. ▪ In all cases of lymphadenopathy, follow-up observation for an extended period is indicated, and alternative anticonvulsant therapy should be strongly considered. ▪ Observation of patient symptoms and evaluation of effectiveness of all medications is imperative. ▪ Monitor for S/S of hypersensitivity reactions. ▪ Observe for rash and discontinue if one appears; see Precautions. ▪ Monitor for symptoms of angioedema (e.g., facial, perioral or upper airway swelling). ▪ Determine absolute patency of vein. Avoid extravasation. Very alkaline; follow each injection with sterile NS to reduce local venous irritation; see Rate of Administration. ▪ Patients maintained with phenytoin should be given a dose the morning of surgery to maintain adequate serum levels. ▪ See Precautions and Drug/Lab Interactions.

Patient Education: May increase the risk of suicidal thoughts and behavior. Promptly report emergence or worsening of S/S of depression, any unusual changes in mood or behavior, or thoughts about self-harm. ▪ Effective birth control required for females of childbearing potential who are not planning a pregnancy. Hormonal contraceptive efficacy may be decreased; see Maternal/Child. ▪ Females who are pregnant or who become pregnant should be encouraged to enroll in the North American Antiepileptic Drug (NAAED) Pregnancy Registry. ▪ Do not discontinue phenytoin without consulting healthcare provider. ▪ Report S/S of dermatologic, hematologic, hepatic, or hypersensitivity reactions (e.g., anorexia, easy bruising, facial swelling, fever, jaundice, lymphadenopathy, mouth ulcers, nausea and vomiting, petechial or purpuric hemorrhage, rash, sore throat) or angioedema (e.g., facial, perioral, or upper airway swelling). ▪ Numerous drug interactions possible. Review all medications and alcohol use with provider. ▪ May cause increase in blood sugar. ▪ Good dental hygiene required to minimize development of gingival hyperplasia. ▪ May cause decreased coordination, dizziness, gait disturbance, and somnolence. Use caution when performing tasks that require alertness.

Maternal/Child: Avoid pregnancy. May cause fetal harm when administered to a pregnant woman. Prenatal exposure to phenytoin may increase the risk for congenital malformations and other adverse developmental outcomes; see manufacturer's prescribing information. Consider risks versus benefit. ▪ An increase in seizure frequency may occur because of alterations in phenytoin kinetics and decreased serum concentrations in pregnant females; may necessitate periodic monitoring of serum levels. Because of potential changes in protein binding, monitoring of phenytoin serum levels should be based on the unbound fraction. ▪ Newborns whose mothers received phenytoin during pregnancy may develop a life-threatening bleeding disorder that can be prevented by giving vitamin K to the mother before delivery and to the neonate after birth. ▪ Phenytoin is secreted in breast milk. Consider risk of infant exposure versus benefit of breast-feeding to the infant and benefit of treatment to the mother.

Elderly: See Dose Adjustments and Rate of Administration. ▪ Clearance tends to decrease with increasing age; lower or less frequent dosing may be required. ▪ Low serum albumin causing a decrease in protein binding may result in increased sensitivity to phenytoin.

DRUG/LAB INTERACTIONS

Interactions are numerous and potentially life threatening. Review of drug profile by pharmacist imperative. ▪ Phenytoin is highly protein bound and is prone to competitive displacement. ▪ Phenytoin is metabolized by CYP2C9 and CYP2C19 and is particularly susceptible to inhibitory drug interactions because it is subject to saturable metabolism. Inhibition of metabolism may produce significant increases in circulating phenytoin concentrations, increasing the risk of toxicity. ▪ Coadministration with **delavirdine** is contraindicated. Has potential for loss of virologic response and possible resistance to delavirdine or to the class of nonnucleoside reverse transcriptase inhibitors. ▪ Serum levels may be increased by **alcohol** (acute ingestion), **amiodarone, antiepileptic agents, azole antifungals, capecitabine, chloramphenicol, chlordiazepoxide, disulfiram, estrogens, fluorouracil, fluoxetine, fluvastatin, fluvoxamine, H₂ antagonists, isoniazid, methylphenidate, omeprazole, phenothiazines, salicylates, sertraline, sulfonamides, trazodone, and warfarin.** ▪ Serum levels and effectiveness may be decreased by **antineoplastics, carbamazepine, chronic alcohol abuse, diazepam, diazoxide, folic acid, fosamprenavir, nelfinavir, reserpine, rifampin, ritonavir, St. John's wort, theophylline, and vigabatrin.** ▪ Phenytoin serum levels may be increased or decreased by **phenobarbital, valproate sodium, and valproic acid.** Similarly, phenytoin may unpredictably affect the levels and efficacy of these drugs. ▪ The addition of withdrawal of drugs while patients are undergoing phenytoin therapy may require an adjustment of the phenytoin dose. ▪ Phenytoin will inhibit the effects of **azole antifungals, corticosteroids, doxycycline, estrogens, furosemide, irinotecan, oral contraceptives, paclitaxel, paroxetine, quinidine, rifampin, sertraline, teniposide, theophylline, and vitamin D.** Dose adjustment of these agents may be indicated. ▪ Because phenytoin is a potent enzyme inducer, it decreases plasma concentrations of **albendazole, HIV antivirals, antiepileptic agents, atorvastatin, chlorpropamide, clozapine, cyclosporine, digoxin, disopyramide, fluvastatin, folic acid, methadone, mexiletine, nifedipine, nimodipine, nisoldipine, praziquantel, quetiapine, simvastatin, and verapamil.** Adjust doses of these agents as indicated. ▪ Phenytoin when given with **fosamprenavir** alone may decrease the concentration of **amprenavir,** the active metabolite. Phenytoin when given with the combination of **fosamprenavir and ritonavir** may increase the concentration of **amprenavir.** ▪ May increase or decrease PT/INR responses when coadministered with **warfarin.** ▪ Alters **some clinical laboratory tests** (e.g., may decrease T_3 and T_4; may increase glucose, alkaline phosphatase, GGT, and TSH; and may produce low results in dexamethasone or metyrapone tests).

SIDE EFFECTS

The most common adverse reactions are nervous system reactions, including ataxia, decreased coordination, mental confusion, nystagmus, slurred speech, and somnolence. Other reported reactions include altered taste sensation, constipation, dizziness, drowsiness, dyskinesias, fever, headache, hyperplasia of gums, insomnia, local irritation/toxicity, nausea, nervousness, paresthesia, skin eruptions, tremors, vertigo, visual disturbances, and vomiting.

Serious adverse reactions, including acute hepatic failure, bradycardia, cardiac arrest, cardiovascular collapse, CNS depression, dermatologic reactions (including local toxicity, Stevens-Johnson syndrome, and toxic epidermal necrolysis), DRESS, heart block, hematopoietic complications, hypersensitivity reactions (including anaphylaxis [rare]), hypotension, lymphadenopathy, Peyronie's disease, respiratory arrest, tonic seizures, toxic hepatitis, and ventricular fibrillation, have been reported. Psychotic symptoms, including aggression, agitation, anger, anxiety, apathy, depersonalization, depression, emotional lability, hallucinations, hostility, irritability, and suicidal tendencies, have occurred with antiepileptic agents. Cerebellar atrophy has been reported and appears more likely in settings of elevated phenytoin levels and/or long-term phenytoin use.

Overdose: Ataxia, blurred vision, coma, dysarthria, hyperreflexia, hypotension, irreversible cerebellar dysfunction and atrophy, lethargy, nausea, nystagmus, slurred speech, tremor, and vomiting. Death is caused by respiratory and circulatory depression.

ANTIDOTE

Notify the physician of any side effects. If minor symptoms progress or any major side effect occurs, discontinue the drug and notify the physician; see Precautions. Obtain serum plasma levels at first signs of toxicity. If serum levels are excessive, symptoms persist, or major side effects appear, discontinue phenytoin and notify physician. Treat symptomatically, maintain a patent airway, and resuscitate as necessary. Discontinue phenytoin at the first sign of a rash unless the rash is clearly not drug related. If TEN or SJS is suspected, do not rechallenge; consider alternate therapy. Discontinue immediately if symptoms of angioedema develop. Evaluate for multiorgan hypersensitivity reactions (DRESS). Cardiovascular toxicity, including hypotension or cardiac arrhythmias, may respond to a decrease in infusion rate. Decrease rate or discontinue infusion for severe hypotension or cardiac arrhythmias. Local toxicity (purple glove syndrome) may resolve spontaneously. Hemodialysis may be useful in overdose.

PHOSPHATE
(**FOS**-fayt)

Electrolyte replenisher
Antihypophosphatemic

Potassium Phosphate, Sodium Phosphate

pH 5 to 7.8

USUAL DOSE

Dependent on individual needs of the patient.

TPN, adults and pediatric patients: 10 to 15 mM (310 to 465 mg) of phosphorus/liter of TPN solution should maintain normal serum phosphate. Larger amounts may be required. 1 mM equals 31 mg.

Acute hypophosphatemia: Adults and pediatric patients: 0.08 to 0.32 mM/kg of body weight as a *loading dose* equally distributed over 6 hours. *Maintain pediatric patients* with 0.5 to 1.5 mM/kg/24 hr. *Maintain adults* with 48.4 to 64.5 mM/24 hr.

INFANT DOSE

Infants receiving TPN: 1.5 to 2 mM/kg of body weight/day.

DOSE ADJUSTMENTS

Lower-end initial doses may be indicated in the elderly based on the potential for decreased organ function and concomitant disease or drug therapy.

DILUTION

Must be diluted in a larger volume of suitable IV solution and given as an infusion. Soluble in most commonly used IV solutions (see chart on inside back cover) except protein hydrolysate. Mix thoroughly. See Compatibility.

COMPATIBILITY

ALL FORMULATIONS

Mix thoroughly after each addition of supposedly **compatible** drugs or solutions. TPN solutions requiring the addition of phosphates and calcium salts must be mixed by the pharmacist to avoid a precipitate of calcium phosphate. Specific amounts, calculations, order, and temperature (precipitate forms more readily at room temperature) are required. Deaths have been reported.

POTASSIUM PHOSPHATE

Other sources suggest specific **compatibilities** dependent on concentration and manufacturer; consult a pharmacist.

SODIUM PHOSPHATE

Other sources suggest a few specific **compatibilities** dependent on concentration and manufacturer; consult a pharmacist.

RATE OF ADMINISTRATION

A usual dose is usually equally distributed over 6 hours. Other sources suggest administering up to 15 mM over 2 hours, up to 30 mM over 4 hours, and up to 45 mM over 6 hours. Potassium phosphate will be further limited by the maximum rate for potassium. Consider sodium/potassium content. Infuse slowly. Rapid infusion may cause phosphate or potassium intoxication. Serum calcium may be reduced rapidly, causing hypocalcemic tetany.

ACTIONS

Involved in bone deposition. Helps to maintain calcium levels, has a buffering effect on acid-base equilibrium, and influences renal excretion of the hydrogen ion. Normal levels in adults, 3 to 4.5 mg/dL of serum; in pediatric patients, 4 to 7 mg/dL. Excreted in urine.

INDICATIONS AND USES

To prevent or correct hypophosphatemia in patients with restricted or no oral intake.

CONTRAINDICATIONS

Any disease with high phosphate or low calcium levels, hyperkalemia (potassium phosphate), hypernatremia (sodium phosphate).

PRECAUTIONS

Rapid infusion may cause phosphate, sodium, or potassium intoxication. Serum calcium may be reduced, rapidly causing hypocalcemic tetany. ▪ Use sodium phosphate with caution in renal impairment, cirrhosis, cardiac failure, or any edematous, sodium-retaining state. ▪ Use potassium phosphate with caution in cardiac disease, renal disease, and digitalized patients. ▪ See Compatibility.

Monitor: Monitor serum calcium, potassium, phosphate, chlorides, and sodium. Discontinue when serum phosphate exceeds 2 mg/dL. ▪ See Drug/Lab Interactions.

Maternal/Child: Category C: safety for use in pregnancy not established.

Elderly: Differences in response between elderly and younger patients have not been identified. Lower-end initial doses may be appropriate in the elderly; see Dose Adjustments.

DRUG/LAB INTERACTIONS

May cause hyperkalemia with **potassium-sparing diuretics** (e.g., amiloride) **or angiotensin-converting enzyme inhibitors**.

SIDE EFFECTS

Elevated phosphates, reduced calcium levels and hypocalcemic tetany, elevated potassium levels causing cardiac arrhythmias, flaccid paralysis, heaviness of the legs, hypotension, listlessness, mental confusion, paresthesia of the extremities.

ANTIDOTE

For any side effect, discontinue the drug and notify the physician. Restore serum calcium with calcium gluconate or chloride. Shift potassium from serum to cells with 150 mL of 10% to 20% dextrose with 10 units regular insulin for each 20 Gm dextrose at 300 to 500 mL/hr. Correct acidosis with sodium bicarbonate. Reduce sodium by restriction, diuretics, or hemodialysis. Resuscitate as necessary.

PHYSOSTIGMINE SALICYLATE
(fye-zoh-**STIG**-meen sah-**LIS**-ah-layt)

USUAL DOSE
Postanesthesia: 0.5 to 1 mg initially. Repeat at 10- to 30-minute intervals until desired results obtained.

Anticholinergic toxicity: 0.5 to 2 mg initially. 1 to 4 mg may be repeated as necessary as life-threatening signs recur (arrhythmias, convulsions, deep coma). Maximum dose is 4 mg in 30 minutes.

PEDIATRIC DOSE
To be used in life-threatening situations only. 0.02 mg/kg/dose. May be repeated at 5- to 10-minute intervals only if toxic effects persist and there is no sign of cholinergic effects. Maximum total dose is 2 mg. See Maternal/Child.

DILUTION
May be given undiluted. Do not add to IV solutions. May be given through Y-tube of infusion set.

COMPATIBILITY
Compatibility information not available from manufacturer; consult a pharmacist.

RATE OF ADMINISTRATION
Rapid IV administration may cause bradycardia, hypersalivation, respiratory distress, and convulsions.

1 mg or fraction thereof over 1 to 3 minutes.

Pediatric rate: 0.5 mg or fraction thereof over at least 1 minute.

ACTIONS
An extract of *Physostigma venenosum* seeds. It inhibits the destructive action of acetylcholinesterase and prolongs and exaggerates the effects of acetylcholine. Stimulates parasympathetic nerve stimulation (pupil contraction, increased intestinal musculature tonus, bronchial constriction, salivary and sweat gland stimulation). Does enter the CNS. Onset of action occurs in 5 minutes and lasts about 1 hour. Rapidly hydrolyzed by cholinesterases.

INDICATIONS AND USES
To reverse CNS toxic effects caused by drugs capable of producing anticholinergic poisoning (e.g., atropine), other anticholinergic/antispasmodic agents, anticholinergic antiparkinson agents, and tricyclic antidepressants.

Unlabeled uses: Treatment of delirium tremens.

CONTRAINDICATIONS
Asthma, cardiovascular disease, diabetes, gangrene, mechanical obstruction of the intestines or urogenital tract, vagotonic states, patients receiving choline esters, depolarizing neuromuscular blocking agents (succinylcholine), or tricyclic antidepressants.

PRECAUTIONS
Rapid IV administration may cause bradycardia, hypersalivation, respiratory distress, and convulsions. ■ Contains bisulfites; use caution in allergic individuals.

Monitor: Atropine must always be available. ■ Monitor vital signs. ■ See Drug/Lab Interactions.

Maternal/Child: Safety for use in pregnancy and breast-feeding not established. ■ Has caused muscular weakness in neonates of mothers treated with other cholinesterase inhibitors for myasthenia gravis. ■ May contain benzyl alcohol; do not use in neonates.

DRUG/LAB INTERACTIONS

Potentiates **succinylcholine** and **other choline esters** (e.g., bethanechol). ▪ May antagonize CNS depressant effects of **diazepam**. ▪ May cause serious complications, including death, with **tricyclic antidepressants**.

SIDE EFFECTS

Anxiety, bradycardia, cholinergic crisis (overdose), coma, convulsions, defecation, delirium, disorientation, emesis, hallucinations, hyperactivity, hypersalivation, hypersensitivity, nausea, respiratory distress, salivation, seizures, sweating, urination.

ANTIDOTE

Keep physician informed of side effects. For excessive nausea or sweating, reduce dose. Discontinue drug for bradycardia; convulsions; excessive defecation, emesis, salivation, or urination; or respiratory distress. Treat cholinergic side effects (e.g., arrhythmias, bronchoconstriction) or hypersensitivity with the specific antagonist atropine sulfate in doses of 0.6 mg IV. May be repeated every 3 to 10 minutes. Endotracheal intubation or tracheostomy are considered prophylactic in anesthesia or crisis. Artificial ventilation, oxygen therapy, cardiac monitoring, adequate suctioning, and treatment of shock or convulsions must be instituted and maintained as necessary.

PHYTONADIONE BBW
(fye-toe-nah-**DYE**-ohn)

Vitamin (prothrombinogenic)
Antidote
Antihemorrhagic

Vitamin K$_1$

pH 5 to 7

USUAL DOSE

Should be given by the SC or oral route whenever possible; IM or IV administration has caused severe reactions and death; see Precautions.

Vitamin K deficiency: 2.5 to 10 mg/dose times 1 dose.

Anticoagulant-induced (warfarin or dicumarol) hypoprothrombinemia: 2.5 to 10 mg or more. Doses up to 25 mg and, rarely, 50 mg may be needed. May repeat in 6 to 8 hours if initial response is not adequate. Doses as low as 1 to 2 mg may be effective. Use the smallest dose that achieves effective results to prevent clotting hazards. Dosing recommendations based on INR and the presence or absence of bleeding are available in the medical literature.

Hypoprothrombinemia from other causes: 2.5 to 25 mg or more (rarely 50 mg) depending on the severity of the deficiency and the response obtained. Modify subsequent dosage (amount and frequency) based on the INR or clinical condition.

PEDIATRIC DOSE

See Usual Dose, Precautions, and Maternal/Child.

Vitamin K deficiency: 1 to 2 mg/dose times 1 dose.

Reversal of vitamin K antagonists (e.g., warfarin): Limited data available. One source suggests 0.03 mg/kg/dose IV for excessively prolonged INR (usually INR >8, no evidence of bleeding) due to vitamin K antagonist.

NEWBORN DOSE

See Usual Dose, Precautions, and Maternal/Child. Rarely given IV in the newborn.

Prophylaxis of vitamin K–deficiency bleeding in neonates: 0.5 to 1 mg IM within 1 hour of birth.

Treatment of vitamin K–deficiency bleeding in neonates: 1 mg SC or IM. Higher doses may be necessary if the mother has been receiving oral anticoagulants (e.g., warfarin [Coumadin]) or anticonvulsants (e.g., phenytoin [Dilantin]).

DOSE ADJUSTMENTS

See Drug/Lab Interactions.

DILUTION

Dilute with NS, D5NS, or D5W. Avoid use of other diluents that may contain benzyl alcohol. Dilution with at least 50 mL of diluent is recommended to facilitate prescribed rate of administration. Photosensitive; protect from light in all dilutions. Use immediately after preparation.

Filters: Not required by manufacturer; however, there should be no significant loss of potency with the use of a 0.22-micron filter.

Storage: Photosensitive; protect from light before use and in all dilutions. Store unopened ampules below 40° C (104° F), preferably between 15° and 30° C (59° and 86° F) in original carton. Protect from light and freezing. Discard diluted solution and drug remaining in ampule after single use.

COMPATIBILITY

Compatibility information not available from manufacturer. Other sources suggest a few specific **compatibilities** dependent on concentration and manufacturer; consult a pharmacist.

RATE OF ADMINISTRATION

Generally diluted in 50 mL of **compatible** solution and given over 15 to 20 minutes; not to exceed 1 mg/min. Too-rapid injection has caused severe reactions, including fatalities.

ACTIONS

Vitamin K, a fat-soluble vitamin, is essential for hepatic production of four blood coagulation factors (II [prothrombin], VII, IX, X). These are required for normal blood clotting. Onset of action is within 1 to 2 hours. Usually controls hemorrhage in 3 to 6 hours; normal INR should be obtained in 12 to 14 hours. Metabolized by the liver and eliminated in urine and feces. Crosses the placenta and is present in breast milk.

INDICATIONS AND USES

Treatment of the following coagulation disorders due to faulty formation of factors II, VII, IX, and X when caused by vitamin K deficiency or interference with vitamin K activity:

* Anticoagulant-induced hypoprothrombinemia caused by warfarin or indanedione derivatives
* Hypoprothrombinemia due to antibacterial therapy
* Hypoprothrombinemia secondary to factors limiting the absorption or synthesis of vitamin K (e.g., obstructive jaundice, biliary fistula, sprue, ulcerative colitis, celiac disease, intestinal resection, cystic fibrosis of the pancreas, and regional enteritis)
* Other drug-induced hypoprothrombinemia in which it is definitively shown that the result is due to interference with vitamin K metabolism (e.g., salicylates).
* Prophylaxis and treatment of vitamin K–deficiency bleeding in neonates.

CONTRAINDICATIONS

Hypersensitivity to phytonadione or any components of this medication.

PRECAUTIONS

Fatal and severe hypersensitivity reactions, including anaphylaxis, have occurred during and immediately after IV and IM injection. Reactions have occurred despite dilution to avoid rapid IV infusion and upon first dose. IV and/or IM is not the route of choice; used only when SC or oral route cannot be used.

■ As an alternative to administering phytonadione, discontinuation or reduction of the doses of drugs interfering with coagulation mechanisms (e.g., antibiotics, salicylates) should be considered. The severity of the coagulation disorder should determine whether phytonadione is required in addition to discontinuing or reducing the doses of interfering drugs. To correct excess anticoagulation after the use of warfarin (e.g., returning an increased INR to the desired range), consider the degree of elevation of the INR and the presence of clinically significant bleeding. ■ Coagulant effects of phytonadione are not immediate; improvement of INR may take 1 to 8 hours. Consider supplementation with whole blood transfusion or blood components if bleeding is severe. ■ When phytonadione is used to correct excessive anticoagulant-induced hypoprothrombinemia in a patient for whom anticoagulant therapy is indicated, the same clotting hazards that existed before beginning anticoagulant therapy will recur. Use the smallest dose of phytonadione possible and monitor INR. ▪ Cutaneous reactions, including eczematous reactions, scleroderma-like patches, urticaria, and delayed-type hypersensitivity reactions, have occurred with parenteral administration of phytonadione. Time of onset ranged from 1 day to 1 year after parenteral administration. Discontinue phytonadione for skin reactions and institute medical management.

Monitor: See Neonatal Dose, Precautions, and Drug/Lab Interactions. ▪ Monitor PT/INR regularly and as clinical conditions indicate. Coagulant effects of phytonadione are not immediate; improvement of INR may take 1 to 8 hours. Repeat PT/INR 6 to 8 hours after a dose. Subsequent dose(s) will be based on INR and clinical condition. ▪ Monitor for S/S of a hypersensitivity reaction (e.g., cardiorespiratory arrest, chest pain, cyanosis, diaphoresis, dyspnea, flushing, shock, tachycardia, and weakness). ▪ Monitor for cutaneous reactions.

Patient Education: Read the FDA-approved patient labeling. ▪ Promptly report signs of hypersensitivity. ▪ Gasping syndrome has occurred after administration of products containing benzyl alcohol to neonates and infants and pregnant females. ▪ Report the occurrence of new rashes. Cutaneous reactions may be delayed for up to 1 year after administration of phytonadione.

Maternal/Child: Safety for use during pregnancy not established. ▪ Pregnant females with vitamin K–deficiency hypoprothrombinemia may be at increased risk for bleeding diatheses during pregnancy and for hemorrhagic events at delivery. Subclinical maternal vitamin K deficiency during pregnancy has been implicated in rare cases of fetal intracranial hemorrhage. ▪ Use caution during breast-feeding. ▪ Safety and effectiveness for prophylaxis and treatment of vitamin K deficiency have been established in neonates. ▪ Use extreme caution in premature infants and neonates. Hemolysis, jaundice, and hyperbilirubinemia in newborns may result from an overdose of phytonadione. ▪ Neonates with vitamin K–deficiency bleeding should respond to administration of phytonadione with a shortening of the INR within 2 to 4 hours. If shortening of the INR is not seen, consider another diagnosis or coagulation disorder. ▪ May contain benzyl alcohol. Serious and fatal adverse reactions including "gasping syndrome" (characterized by CNS depression, gasping respirations, and metabolic acidosis) can occur in neonates and infants treated with benzyl alcohol–preserved medications, including phytonadione. Whenever possible, administer benzyl alcohol–free formulations in pediatric patients, pregnant females, and breast-feeding females. When used as recommended, there is no evidence to suggest that this small amount is associated with toxicity.

DRUG/LAB INTERACTIONS

Discontinue drugs **adversely affecting the coagulation mechanism** if possible (e.g., salicylates, antibiotics). ▪ May cause temporary resistance to **prothrombin-depressing oral anticoagulants**. When resuming anticoagulant therapy, a higher dose of anticoagulant or a change in therapy to a different class of anticoagulant (e.g., heparin) may be necessary. ▪ Phytonadione does not affect the anticoagulant action of heparin.

SIDE EFFECTS

The most common adverse reactions include cyanosis, diaphoresis, dizziness, dysgeusia, dyspnea, flushing, hypotension, and tachycardia. Other reported reactions include erythema, erythema perstans, hyperbilirubinemia, injection site reactions, pruritic plaques, and scleroderma-like lesions. Hypersensitivity reactions (including anaphylaxis), cardiac and/or respiratory arrest, shock, and death have occurred with parenteral route.

ANTIDOTE

Should not be necessary if dosage is accurately calculated before administration. Notify the physician of any side effects. Discontinue administration in the event of a severe hypersensitivity reaction. Treat hypersensitivity reactions as necessary.

PIPERACILLIN SODIUM AND TAZOBACTAM SODIUM

(pie-**PER**-ah-sill-in **SO**-dee-um and
tay-zoh-**BAC**-tam **SO**-dee-um)

Zosyn

**Antibacterial
(extended-spectrum penicillin
and beta-lactamase inhibitor)**

pH 5.5 to 6.8

USUAL DOSE

Measurement of both drugs is included in the total dose; for every 1 Gm of piperacillin there is 0.125 Gm of tazobactam (8:1 ratio).

12 Gm piperacillin/1.5 Gm tazobactam/24 hours given as 3.375 (3 Gm piperacillin/0.375 Gm tazobactam) every 6 hours. Usual duration of therapy is 7 to 10 days, based on severity of infection and patient progress.

Nosocomial pneumonia: 3.375 to 4.5 Gm every 6 hours. Also use an aminoglycoside. Continue aminoglycoside if *Pseudomonas aeruginosa* is isolated; may be discontinued if it is not isolated. Usual duration of therapy is 7 to 14 days.

PEDIATRIC DOSE

2 months to 9 months of age: 80 mg piperacillin/10 mg tazobactam per kg of body weight every 8 hours.

Over 9 months of age weighing up to 40 kg: 100 mg piperacillin/12.5 mg tazobactam per kg of body weight every 8 hours.

Pediatric patients over 40 kg: See Usual Dose.

DOSE ADJUSTMENTS

No dose adjustment needed in impaired liver function. ▪ Dose reduction may be required in the elderly. ▪ Adjust dose in adult patients with impaired renal function based on the following chart. ▪ Dose recommendations for pediatric patients with impaired renal function are not available.

Piperacillin/Tazobactam Dose Guidelines in Adults With Impaired Renal Function		
Renal Function (Creatinine Clearance, mL/min)	**All Indications (Except Nosocomial Pneumonia)**	**Nosocomial Pneumonia**
>40 mL/min	3.375 Gm q 6 hr	4.5 Gm q 6 hr
20-40 mL/min[a]	2.25 Gm q 6 hr	3.375 Gm q 6 hr
<20 mL/min[a]	2.25 Gm q 8 hr	2.25 Gm q 6 hr
Hemodialysis[b]	2.25 Gm q 12 hr	2.25 Gm q 8 hr
CAPD	2.25 Gm q 12 hr	2.25 Gm q 8 hr

[a]Creatinine clearance for patients not receiving hemodialysis.
[b]Hemodialysis removes 30% to 40% of piperacillin/tazobactam. Give an additional dose of 0.75 Gm following each dialysis session. No additional dose is necessary for CAPD patients.

DILUTION

Available in two different formulations: one with EDTA (edetate disodium dihydrate) and one without. **Compatibility** information differs; consult pharmacist. See Compatibility.

Reconstitute 2.25 Gm, 3.375 Gm, and 4.5 Gm with 10 mL, 15 mL, and 20 mL, respectively, with SWFI or NS (with or without preservatives) or D5W. Swirl until dissolved. Should be further diluted to desired volume (50 to 150 mL) with **compatible** infusion solutions (NS, SWFI, Dextran 6% in Saline, or D5W). *EDTA-containing formulation of Zosyn is compatible with all of the previously listed solutions plus LR.* If further diluted with SWFI, maximum recommended volume of SWFI per dose is 50 mL. May be reconstituted and instilled into an ambulatory IV infusion pump. Considered stable at RT for 12 hours when reconstituted and diluted to a final volume of 25 or 37.5 mL. See manufacturer's literature for additional information. Also available premixed in ADD-Vantage vials for use with ADD-Vantage infusion containers and as a frozen premixed solution.

Storage: Store unopened vials at RT. Use single-dose vials immediately after reconstitution; discard any unused portion after 24 hours at room temperature or 48 hours if refrigerated. Do not freeze vials after reconstitution. Stable for 24 hours at RT or for up to 7 days after dilution if refrigerated. Store frozen solution at $-20°$ C ($-4°$ F). Frozen solutions should be thawed at RT or under refrigeration. Do not force thaw. Thawed solutions are stable for 24 hours at RT or for 14 days if refrigerated. Do not refreeze.

COMPATIBILITY

Manufacturer states, "Should not be mixed with other drugs in a syringe or infusion bottle. Not chemically stable in solutions containing only sodium bicarbonate and/or solutions that significantly alter the pH. **Incompatible** with LR *(the EDTA-free formulation of Zosyn only)* and should not be added to blood products or albumin hydrolysates." Manufacturer recommends temporarily discontinuing other solutions infusing at the same site to avoid compatibility problems. Piperacillin may inactivate aminoglycosides (e.g., amikacin, gentamicin). Do not mix in the same solution. Separate administration required. Formulation containing EDTA **may be compatible** at the **Y-site** with amikacin or gentamicin. Selected doses, specific diluents, and amounts of diluent are required. Consult pharmacist or manufacturer's literature. See Drug/Lab Interactions.

Other sources suggest specific **compatibilities** dependent on concentration and manufacturer; consult a pharmacist.

RATE OF ADMINISTRATION

A single dose over 30 minutes as an intermittent infusion. Discontinue primary IV infusion during administration. Current data show that giving IV push over 2 to 3 minutes has been generally safe and tolerable when reconstituted with SWI 20 mL. Monitor for phlebitis and other infusion-related reactions.

Extended infusion method (unlabeled dosing): 3.375 to 4.5 Gm IV over 4 hours every 8 hours.

ACTIONS

An antimicrobial agent that combines the extended-spectrum penicillin piperacillin with the potent beta-lactamase inhibitor tazobactam. May be used in suspected polymicrobial infections due to its broad spectrum of activity. Acts by inhibiting septum formation and cell wall synthesis of susceptible bacteria. Bactericidal against gram-positive aerobes, gram-negative aerobes, and anaerobes that may be resistant to other antibiotics. Widely distributed into most body fluids and tissues. Mean tissue concentrations are 50% to 100% of plasma concentrations. Peak levels are achieved immediately at the completion of an infusion. Plasma half-life ranges from 0.7 to 1.2 hours. Metabolized and excreted in urine and, to a small extent, in bile. Crosses the placental barrier. Secreted in breast milk.

INDICATIONS AND USES

Treatment of patients with moderate to severe infections caused by piperacillin/tazobactam–susceptible strains of specific microorganisms in the following conditions: intra-abdominal (e.g., appendicitis complicated by rupture or abscess and peritonitis), gynecologic (e.g., postpartum endometritis and pelvic inflammatory disease), skin and skin structure (complicated and uncomplicated [e.g., cellulitis, cutaneous abscesses, and ischemic/diabetic foot infection]), community-acquired pneumonia (moderate severity only), and nosocomial pneumonia (moderate to severe severity). ■ Used in combination with aminoglycosides for nosocomial pneumonia caused by *Pseudomonas aeruginosa*.

Unlabeled uses: Treatment of septicemia.

CONTRAINDICATIONS

History of hypersensitivity reaction to any penicillin, cephalosporin, or beta-lactamase inhibitors (not absolute; see Precautions).

PRECAUTIONS

Serious and occasionally fatal hypersensitivity reactions have been reported in patients receiving piperacillin sodium and tazobactam; most likely to occur in patients with a history of penicillin, cephalosporin, or carbapenem hypersensitivity or sensitivity to multiple allergens.

There have been reports of individuals with a history of penicillin hypersensitivity experiencing severe reactions when treated with cephalosporins. Check history of previous hypersensitivity reactions to penicillins, cephalosporins, or other allergens. Actual incidence of cross-allergenicity not established but may be more common with first-generation cephalosporins. ▪ Serious skin reactions such as Stevens-Johnson syndrome, toxic epidermal necrolysis, drug reaction with eosinophilia and systemic symptoms (DRESS), and generalized exanthematous pustulosis have been reported. ▪ To reduce the development of drug-resistant bacteria and maintain its effectiveness, piperacillin/tazobactam should be used to treat or prevent only those infections proven or strongly suspected to be caused by bacteria. ▪ Sensitivity studies indicated to determine susceptibility of the causative organism to piperacillin. ▪ Avoid prolonged use of drug; superinfection caused by overgrowth of nonsusceptible organisms may result. ▪ Bleeding manifestations have been reported and may be associated with abnormal coagulation tests (e.g., clotting time, platelet aggregation, and PT). Patients with impaired renal function may be at increased risk for bleeding tendencies. If bleeding occurs, discontinue therapy and institute appropriate measures ▪ Leukopenia/neutropenia has been reported. Reaction appears to be reversible and is most common with prolonged therapy. ▪ Use caution in patients with CHF or those with a history of bleeding disorders or GI disease (e.g., colitis). ▪ *Clostridium difficile*–associated diarrhea (CDAD) has been reported. May range from mild diarrhea to fatal colitis. Consider in patients who present with diarrhea during or after treatment with piperacillin/tazobactam. ▪ Incidence of side effects (e.g., fever and rash) may be increased in patients with cystic fibrosis. ▪ Administration of higher than recommended doses has resulted in neuromuscular excitability and convulsions. Patients with renal impairment are at increased risk. ▪ In critically ill patients, the use of piperacillin sodium and tazobactam was found to be an independent risk factor for renal failure and was associated with delayed recovery of renal function compared with other beta-lactam antibacterial drugs. Consider alternative treatment options in critically ill patients. ▪ See Drug/Lab Interactions.

Monitor: Watch for early symptoms of a hypersensitivity reaction. ▪ Closely monitor patients who develop a skin rash. Discontinue therapy if lesions progress. ▪ Periodic evaluation of renal, hepatic, and hematopoietic systems and electrolytes recommended, especially with prolonged therapy. May cause hypokalemia; monitor closely. ▪ Contains 2.84 mEq (65 mg) of sodium/Gm. At the usual recommended doses, patients would receive 34.1 to 45.5 mEq (780 to 1,040 mg) per day. Observe for electrolyte imbalance and cardiac irregularities. May aggravate CHF, especially in the elderly. ▪ May cause thrombophlebitis; observe carefully and rotate infusion sites. ▪ Observe for increased bleeding tendencies in all patients, especially those with impaired renal function. ▪ See Drug/Lab Interactions.

Patient Education: Report promptly: fever, rash, sore throat, unusual bleeding or bruising, or seizures. ▪ May require alternate birth control. ▪ Promptly report diarrhea or bloody stools that occur during treatment or up to several months after an antibiotic has been discontinued; may indicate CDAD and require treatment.

Maternal/Child: Use during pregnancy only if clearly needed; data are insufficient. ▪ Use caution in breast-feeding. No information is available on the effects of use on the breast-fed infant or on milk production. ▪ Safety and effectiveness for use in pediatric patients under 2 months of age not established.

Elderly: No problems documented. Consider age-related organ function and concomitant disease or drug therapy. Elderly patients may respond with a blunted natriuresis to salt loading, which can be clinically important with regard to diseases such as CHF.

DRUG/LAB INTERACTIONS

Synergistic when used in combination with **aminoglycosides**. Synergism may be inconsistent; see Compatibility. ▪ Piperacillin may inactivate **aminoglycosides** by converting them to microbiologically inert amides. Coadministration with aminoglycosides in patients with end-stage renal disease requiring hemodialysis may result in significant reduction of aminoglycoside concentrations. Monitor closely. ▪ Concomitant administration with **vancomycin** may increase the incidence of acute kidney injury. Monitor renal function if concomitant use is required. No pharmacokinetic interactions have been noted between piperacillin/tazobactam and vancomycin. ▪ Concomitant administration with **probenecid** decreases rate of elimination of piperacillin/tazobactam, resulting in higher and more prolonged blood levels. Avoid coadministration unless benefit outweighs risk. ▪ Use caution with **anticoagulants** (e.g., heparin, warfarin) or **medications that affect platelet aggregation** (e.g., NSAIDs). Risk of bleeding may be increased. Monitoring of coagulation tests may be indicated. ▪ May be antagonized by **bacteriostatic antibiotics** (e.g., chloramphenicol, erythromycin, and tetracyclines); may interfere with bactericidal action. ▪ May decrease clearance and increase toxicity of **methotrexate;** monitor methotrexate levels. ▪ May prolong neuromuscular blockade with **vecuronium** or other nondepolarizing muscle relaxants. ▪ May cause **false-positive glucose** with Clinitest. ▪ **False-positive test results** using the Bio-Rad Laboratories Platelia Aspergillus EIA test in patients receiving piperacillin/tazobactam have been reported. ▪ See Side Effects.

SIDE EFFECTS
The most common side effects include constipation, diarrhea, headache, insomnia, and nausea. Abdominal pain; abnormal coagulation tests (e.g., increased bleeding time, prolonged PT and PTT); abnormal LFTs; arthralgia; candidiasis; CDAD; dyspepsia; electrolyte abnormalities, including hypokalemia; epistaxis; fever; flushing; hematologic abnormalities (anemia, thrombocythemia, thrombocytopenia); hypoglycemia; hypotension; increased AST, BUN, and serum creatinine; local reactions; myalgia; phlebitis; positive Coombs' test; pruritus; pseudomembranous colitis; rash (e.g., bullous, maculopapular, urticarial); renal failure; rhinitis; rigors; seizures; sinusitis; thrombophlebitis; and vomiting have been reported. Anaphylaxis can occur. Transient leukopenia, neutropenia, and eosinophilia can occur with prolonged therapy.

Post-Marketing: Agranulocytosis, dermatologic reactions (including acute generalized exanthematous pustulosis, exfoliative dermatitis, erythema multiforme, DRESS, Stevens-Johnson syndrome, and toxic epidermal necrolysis), eosinophilic pneumonia, hemolytic anemia, hepatitis, hypersensitivity reactions (including anaphylactic/anaphylactoid reactions), interstitial nephritis, jaundice, and pancytopenia.

ANTIDOTE
Notify physician immediately of any adverse symptoms. For severe symptoms, discontinue drug, treat hypersensitivity reactions (antihistamines, epinephrine, corticosteroids, airway management, oxygen), and resuscitate as necessary. Use anticonvulsants for seizures. Treat CDAD with fluids, electrolytes, protein supplements, and appropriate antibiotics (e.g., oral vancomycin) as indicated. In severe cases, surgical evaluation may be indicated. Mild cases may respond to drug discontinuation alone. Hemodialysis is effective in overdose.

POLATUZUMAB VEDOTIN-piiq

(**POOL**-a-**TOOZ**-ue-mab ve-**DOE**-tin)

Antineoplastic
Anti-CD79b-directed antineoplastic
Antibody-drug conjugate (ADC)

Polivy pH 5.3

USUAL DOSE

Pretreatment: Verify pregnancy status. Baseline studies indicated; see Monitor.

Premedication: If not already premedicated for the rituximab product, administer an anti-histamine (e.g., diphenhydramine) and an antipyretic (e.g., acetaminophen) at least 30 minutes before polatuzumab dose to prevent or attenuate infusion reactions.

Prophylaxis: Administer **prophylaxis** for *Pneumocystis jiroveci* pneumonia and herpesvirus throughout treatment with polatuzumab.

Polatuzumab vedotin-piiq: 1.8 mg/kg as an IV infusion every 21 days for 6 cycles in combination with bendamustine and a rituximab product. Administer polatuzumab, benda-mustine, and the rituximab product in any order on Day 1 of each cycle.

Bendamustine: 90 mg/M^2/day as an IV infusion on Day 1 and Day 2 of each cycle when given with polatuzumab and a rituximab product.

Rituximab product: 375 mg/M^2 as an IV infusion on Day 1 of each cycle when given with polatuzumab and bendamustine.

See prescribing information for chemotherapy drugs used in combination with polatuzumab vedotin-piiq.

DOSE ADJUSTMENTS

If a planned dose of polatuzumab is missed, administer as soon as possible. Adjust the schedule of administration to maintain a 21-day interval between doses. ▪ No starting dose adjustment is required in patients with mild hepatic impairment; see Precautions. ▪ Dose modifications for adverse reactions are outlined in the following chart.

Dose Modifications for Polatuzumab Vedotin-piiq Based on Adverse Reactions	
Event	**Dose Modification**
Grade 2–3 peripheral neuropathy	Hold polatuzumab dosing until improvement to Grade 1 or lower. If recovered to Grade 1 or lower on or before Day 14, restart polatuzumab with the next cycle at a permanently reduced dose of 1.4 mg/kg. If a prior dose reduction to 1.4 mg/kg has occurred, discontinue polatuzumab. If not recovered to Grade 1 or lower on or before Day 14, discontinue polatuzumab.
Grade 4 peripheral neuropathy	Discontinue polatuzumab.
Grade 1–3 infusion-related reaction	Interrupt polatuzumab infusion and give supportive treatment. For the first instance of Grade 3 bronchospasm, generalized urticaria, or wheezing, permanently discontinue polatuzumab. For recurrent Grade 2 urticaria, wheezing, or recurrence of any Grade 3 symptoms, permanently discontinue polatuzumab. Otherwise, upon complete resolution of symptoms, infusion may be resumed at 50% of the rate achieved before the interruption. In the absence of infusion-related symptoms, the rate of infusion may be escalated in increments of 50 mg/hr every 30 minutes. For the next cycle, infuse polatuzumab over 90 minutes. If no infusion-related reaction occurs, subsequent infusions may be administered over 30 minutes. Administer premedication for all cycles.
Grade 4 infusion-related reaction	Stop polatuzumab infusion immediately. Give supportive treatment. Permanently discontinue polatuzumab.

Dose Modifications for Polatuzumab Vedotin-piiq Based on Adverse Reactions—cont'd	
Event	**Dose Modification**
Grade 3–4 neutropenia[a,b]	Hold all treatment until ANC recovers to greater than 1,000/mcL. If ANC recovers to greater than 1,000/mcL on or before Day 7, resume all treatment without any additional dose reductions. Consider granulocyte colony-stimulating factor prophylaxis for subsequent cycles if not previously given. If ANC recovers to greater than 1,000/mcL after Day 7: • Restart all treatment. Consider granulocyte colony-stimulating factor prophylaxis for subsequent cycles, if not previously given. If prophylaxis was given, consider dose reduction of bendamustine. • If dose reduction of bendamustine has already occurred, consider dose reduction of polatuzumab to 1.4 mg/kg.
Grade 3–4 thrombocytopenia[a,b]	Hold all treatment until platelets recover to greater than 75,000/mcL. If platelets recover to greater than 75,000/mcL on or before Day 7, resume all treatment without any additional dose reductions. If platelets recover to greater than 75,000/mcL after Day 7: • Restart all treatment, with dose reduction of bendamustine. • If dose reduction of bendamustine has already occurred, consider dose reduction of polatuzumab to 1.4 mg/kg.

[a]Severity on Day 1 of any cycle.
[b]If primary cause is due to lymphoma, dose delay or reduction may not be needed.

DILUTION

Specific techniques required; see Precautions. Available as a lyophilized powder in a single-dose vial containing 140 mg. Reconstitute immediately before dilution. Calculate the number of vials required. For example, in a 70-kg patient:

$$1.8 \text{ mg/kg} \times 70 \text{ kg} = 126 \text{ mg}$$

$$126 \text{ mg} \div 140 \text{ mg/vial} = 0.9 \text{ vials; so 1 vial would be needed}$$

Reconstitute each vial with 7.2 mL of SWFI to yield 20 mg/mL. Direct the stream of diluent toward the side of the vial. Gently swirl to aid dissolution. *Do not shake.* Solution should be clear to slightly opalescent, colorless to slightly brown, and free of visible particulates. *Do not freeze or expose to direct sunlight.* Withdraw the calculated dose from the vial (126 mg [from the previous example] ÷ 20 mg/mL = 6.3 mL). This calculated dose must be further diluted in a minimum of 50 mL of NS, $1/2$NS, or D5W to achieve a final concentration of 0.72 to 2.7 mg/mL. Gently invert to mix the solution. *Do not shake. Do not freeze or expose to direct sunlight.*
Filters: Use of a sterile, nonpyrogenic, low–protein-binding in-line or add-on filter (0.2- or 0.22-micron pore size) is required.
Storage: Refrigerate vials at 2° to 8° C (36° to 46° F) in original carton to protect from light. Do not use beyond expiration date. *Do not freeze. Do not shake.* Reconstituted solution may be refrigerated for up to 48 hours or stored at RT up to a maximum of 8 hours before dilution. Discard vial when cumulative storage time before further dilution exceeds 48 hours. If not used immediately, store the fully diluted solutions depending on diluent according to the following chart.

Diluted Polatuzumab Vedotin-piiq Solution Storage Conditions[a]	
Diluent Used to Prepare Solution for Infusion	Diluted Polatuzumab Vedotin-piiq Solution Storage Conditions
NS	Up to 24 hours refrigerated at 2° to 8° C (36° to 46° F) **OR** Up to 4 hours at RT (9° to 25° C [47° to 77° F)
½NS	Up to 18 hours refrigerated at 2° to 8° C (36° to 46°F) **OR** Up to 4 hours at RT (9° to 25°C [47° to 77°F)
D5W	Up to 36 hours refrigerated at 2° to 8°C (36° to 46°F) **OR** Up to 6 hours at RT (9° to 25°C [47° to 77°F)

[a]To ensure product stability, do not exceed specified storage durations.

Limit transportation time (included in storage time) to 30 minutes at RT or 12 hours if refrigerated. Limit agitation of diluted product during preparation and transportation to administration site. Do not transport through an automated system (e.g., pneumatic tube or automated cart); agitation stress can result in aggregation. If transporting to a separate facility, remove air from the infusion bag to prevent aggregation. If air is removed, an infusion set with a vented spike is required to ensure accurate dosing during the infusion.

COMPATIBILITY

Manufacturer states, "Do not mix with or administer as an infusion with other drugs."

RATE OF ADMINISTRATION

Must be administered using a dedicated infusion line equipped with a sterile, nonpyrogenic, low–protein-binding, in-line or add-on filter (0.2- or 0.22-micron pore size) and catheter.

Initial dose: Administer polatuzumab as an IV infusion over 90 minutes. Monitor for infusion-related reactions during the infusion and for a minimum of 90 minutes after completion of the initial dose. If an infusion reaction occurs, interrupt the infusion and institute appropriate medical management.

Subsequent doses: If the initial infusion was well tolerated, administer polatuzumab over 30 minutes and monitor during the infusion and for at least 30 minutes after completion of the infusion.

ACTIONS

A CD79b-directed antibody-drug conjugate (ADC) with activity against dividing B-cells. It consists of three components: (1) the humanized immunoglobulin G1 (IgG1) monoclonal antibody specific for human CD79b, (2) the small molecule antimitotic agent monomethyl auristatin E (MMAE), and (3) a protease-cleavable linker maleimidocaproyl-valine-citrulline-p-amino-benzyloxycarbonyl (mc-vc-PAB) that covalently attaches MMAE to the polatuzumab antibody. It binds to CD79b, a B-cell–specific surface protein, which is a component of the B-cell receptor. Upon binding CD79b, polatuzumab vedotin-piiq is internalized and enables intracellular delivery of MMAE. MMAE binds to microtubules and kills dividing cells by inhibiting cell division and inducing apoptosis. MMAE protein binding is 71% to 77%. Terminal half-life of the antibody-conjugated MMAE is approximately 12 days. Terminal half-life of unconjugated MMAE is approximately 4 days. Metabolism has not been studied in humans, but it is expected to undergo catabolism to small peptides, amino acids, unconjugated MMAE, and unconjugated MMAE-related catabolites. MMAE is a substrate for CYP3A4.

INDICATIONS AND USES

Used in combination with bendamustine (Treanda, Bendeka) and a rituximab product for the treatment of adult patients with relapsed or refractory diffuse large B-cell lymphoma (DLBCL), not otherwise specified, after at least two prior therapies. This indication was granted accelerated approval based on complete response rate. Continued approval may be contingent on verification and description of clinical benefit in a confirmatory trial.

CONTRAINDICATIONS

Manufacturer states, "None."

PRECAUTIONS

Follow guidelines for handling cytotoxic agents. See Appendix A, p. 1308. ▪ For IV infusion only; *do not administer as an IV push or bolus*. ▪ Has been known to cause peripheral neuropathy, including severe cases. Peripheral neuropathy is predominantly sensory; however, motor and sensorimotor peripheral neuropathy also occur. May occur as early as the first cycle of treatment and has a cumulative effect. Polatuzumab may also exacerbate pre-existing peripheral neuropathy. ▪ Infusion-related reactions, including severe cases, have occurred. Delayed infusion reactions (as late as 24 hours after polatuzumab administration) have occurred. ▪ Can cause serious or severe myelosuppression, including anemia, neutropenia, and thrombocytopenia. ▪ Fatal and/or serious infections, including opportunistic infections such as sepsis, pneumonia (including *Pneumocystis jiroveci* and other fungal pneumonia), herpesvirus infection, and cytomegalovirus infection have occurred. ▪ Progressive multifocal leukoencephalopathy (PML) has been reported. ▪ May cause tumor lysis syndrome. Patients with a high tumor burden and rapidly proliferative tumor may be at increased risk. ▪ Serious cases of hepatotoxicity consistent with hepatocellular injury, including elevations of transaminases and/or bilirubin, have occurred. Pre-existing liver disease, elevated baseline liver enzymes, and concomitant medications may increase the risk of hepatotoxicity. ▪ Avoid administration in patients with moderate or severe hepatic impairment (bilirubin greater than 1.5 times the ULN); these patients are likely to have increased exposure to MMAE, which may increase the risk of adverse reactions. Has not been studied in these patients. ▪ Has not been studied in patients with severe renal impairment or in patients with ESRD. ▪ As with all therapeutic proteins, there is a potential for immunogenicity.

Monitor: Obtain baseline and periodic CBC, including platelet count, liver enzyme studies, and bilirubin. ▪ Cytopenias may require a delay, dose reduction, or discontinuation of therapy. Consider prophylactic granulocyte colony-stimulating factor administration; see Dose Adjustments. ▪ Monitor for symptoms of peripheral neuropathy (e.g., burning sensation, dysesthesia, gait disturbance, hyperesthesia, hypoesthesia, neuropathic pain, paresthesia, and weakness). May require delay, dose reduction, or discontinuation of therapy; see Dose Adjustments. ▪ Administer premedication and monitor for S/S of an infusion reaction (e.g., chills, dyspnea, fever, flushing, hypotension, and urticaria) during and after the infusion; see Rate of Administration. ▪ Closely monitor for S/S of infection. ▪ Monitor for new or worsening neurologic, cognitive, or behavioral changes. If PML is suspected, withhold therapy and any concomitant chemotherapy, and permanently discontinue if the diagnosis is confirmed. ▪ Monitor for early S/S of tumor lysis syndrome (e.g., flank pain, hematuria, hyperuricemia, hyperkalemia, hyperphosphatemia, hypocalcemia). Maintain hydration. Uric acid–lowering drugs (e.g., allopurinol [Aloprim]) may be indicated.

Patient Education: Verify pregnancy status of females of reproductive potential before initiating polatuzumab vedotin-piiq therapy. ▪ Avoid pregnancy. Females of reproductive potential should use effective birth control during treatment and for at least 3 months after the final dose. Report a suspected pregnancy immediately. ▪ Males with female sexual partners of reproductive potential should use effective contraception during treatment and for at least 5 months after the final dose. ▪ May impair male fertility. ▪ Promptly report S/S of infection (e.g., chills, cough, fever of 100.5° F or greater, pain with urination). ▪ Promptly report S/S of peripheral neuropathy (e.g., muscle weakness, numbness or tingling of the hands or feet). ▪ Promptly report S/S of an infusion reaction (e.g., breathing problems, chills, fever, or rash within 24 hours of an infusion). ▪ Promptly report changes in mood or unusual behavior; confusion; thinking problems; loss of memory; changes in vision, speech, or walking; and decreased strength or weakness on one side of the body. ▪ Promptly report symptoms of hepatotoxicity (abdominal pain, anorexia, dark urine, fatigue, jaundice). ▪ Promptly report any bleeding/bruising. ▪ Promptly report S/S of TLS (e.g., diarrhea, lethargy, nausea, vomiting). Periodic laboratory monitoring required. ▪ See Appendix D, p. 1311.

Maternal/Child: Avoid pregnancy; based on its mechanism of action, it can cause fetal harm. ■ Discontinue breast-feeding during treatment and for at least 2 months after the final dose. ■ Safety and effectiveness for use in pediatric patients not established.

Elderly: Numbers in clinical studies insufficient to determine whether elderly patients respond differently than younger subjects. Patients over 65 years of age had a higher incidence of serious adverse reactions.

DRUG/LAB INTERACTIONS

No clinical studies evaluating the drug-drug interaction potential of polatuzumab vedotin-piiq have been conducted. Another ADC drug that contains MMAE has the following drug interactions, and these interactions would likely result in similar effects on free MMAE and ADC. ■ Concomitant use with **a strong CYP3A4 inhibitor** (e.g., ketoconazole [Nizoral]) may increase free MMAE exposure, which may increase the incidence or severity of polatuzumab vedotin-piiq toxicities; monitor patients receiving ketoconazole or **other potent CYP3A4 inhibitors** (e.g., clarithromycin, itraconazole, nefazodone, saquinavir) closely for adverse reactions. ■ Concomitant use with rifampin, **a strong CYP3A4 inducer,** decreased MMAE and AUC and may reduce its effectiveness.

SIDE EFFECTS

The most common side effects reported include anemia, decreased appetite, diarrhea, fatigue, fever, neutropenia, peripheral neuropathy, pneumonia, and thrombocytopenia. Arthralgia; decreased phosphorus and potassium; dizziness; febrile neutropenia; hypoalbuminemia; hypocalcemia; hypokalemia; increased amylase, creatinine, ALT, AST, and lipase; leukopenia; lymphopenia; pancytopenia; sepsis; upper respiratory infections; vomiting; and decreased weight have also been reported. Serious adverse reactions include infusion-related reactions, hepatotoxicity, myelosuppression, peripheral neuropathy, progressive multifocal leukoencephalopathy, serious and opportunistic infections, and tumor lysis syndrome.

ANTIDOTE

Notify physician of all side effects. Treatment of most reactions will be supportive. Dose delay, dose modification, or discontinuation of therapy may be required in patients with severe or prolonged neutropenia, thrombocytopenia, peripheral neuropathy, or hepatotoxicity; see Dose Adjustments. G-CSF prophylaxis may be considered in patients with Grade 3 or Grade 4 neutropenia. If PML is suspected, hold polatuzumab vedotin-piiq. If PML is confirmed, discontinue polatuzumab vedotin-piiq. Interrupt or discontinue the infusion for an infusion-related reaction and institute appropriate medical management; see Dose Adjustments. Resuscitate as necessary.

PORFIMER SODIUM
(**POOR**-fih-mer **SO**-dee-um)

Photosensitizing agent
Antineoplastic

Photofrin

pH 7 to 8

USUAL DOSE

Pretreatment: Verify pregnancy status. Baseline studies indicated; see Monitor.

A course is a two-stage process requiring administration of both drug and light.

Stage one: Administration of porfimer: A single IV injection of 2 mg/kg. No further injection of porfimer sodium should be given in any one course of therapy.

Stage two: Illumination: Illumination with nonthermal laser light at 40 to 50 hours post-injection.

ESOPHAGEAL AND ENDOBRONCHIAL CANCER

2 mg/kg of porfimer sodium as an IV injection. Approximately 40 to 50 hours after the injection, standard endoscopic techniques are used for light administration and débridement. The laser system must be approved for delivery of a stable power output at a wavelength of 630 ± 3 nm. Light is delivered to the tumor by cylindrical OPTIGUIDE fiber-optic diffusers passed through the operating channel of an endoscope/bronchoscope. The choice of diffuser tip length depends on the length of the tumor. Diffuser length should be sized to avoid exposure of nonmalignant tissue to light and to prevent overlapping of previously treated malignant tissue. A second laser light application may be given 96 to 120 hours after injection. Before providing a second laser light treatment, the residual tumor should be gently débrided. Vigorous débridement may cause esophageal tumor bleeding; see Precautions.

Up to three courses may be given, but each must be separated by at least 30 days. Evaluate patients with esophageal cancer for the presence of a tracheoesophageal or bronchoesophageal fistula before each course. Evaluate all patients for possible erosion of the tumor into a major blood vessel.

Esophageal cancer: 2 mg/kg of porfimer sodium as an IV injection. A light dose of 300 joules/cm of diffuser length should be delivered by the specific process outlined previously. Light exposure time is set to 12 minutes and 30 seconds. Débridement of tumor may be performed 2 to 3 days later; see Precautions.

Endobronchial non–small-cell lung cancer: 2 mg/kg of porfimer sodium as an IV injection. A light dose of 200 joules/cm of diffuser length should be delivered by the specific process outlined previously. Light exposure time is set to 8 minutes and 20 seconds. Débridement of tumor should be performed 2 to 3 days later; see Precautions.

HIGH-GRADE DYSPLASIA (HGD IN BARRETT'S ESOPHAGUS [BE])

2 mg/kg of porfimer sodium as an IV injection. Approximately 40 to 50 hours after the injection, administration of light should be delivered by an X-cell Photodynamic Therapy (PDT) balloon with a fiber-optic diffuser. The choice of fiber-optic/balloon diffuser combination will depend on the length of Barrett's mucosa to be treated (see manufacturer's information). The objective of therapy is to expose and treat all areas of HGD and the entire length of Barrett's esophagus. The light dose administered is 130 joules/cm of diffuser length. Acceptable light intensity for the balloon/diffuser combinations ranges from 200 to 270 mW/cm of diffuser. Treatment time is dependent on the fiber-optic/balloon diffuser combination used (see manufacturer's information). A maximum of 7 cm of esophageal mucosa may be treated at the first light session. If possible, the area treated should include normal tissue margins of a few millimeters at both the proximal and distal ends. Nodules are pretreated at a light dose of 50 joules/cm of diffuser length with a short (2.5 cm) fiber-optic diffuser placed directly against the nodule. A second laser light application may be given to a previously treated segment that shows a "skip" area using a 2.5-cm fiber-optic diffuser at a light dose of 50 joules/cm of the diffuser length. Patients

Continued

with Barrett's esophagus greater than 7 cm should have the remaining untreated length of Barrett's epithelium treated with a second PDT course at least 90 days later. See Precautions.

Up to 3 courses (each separated by 90 days) may be given to a previously treated segment that still shows high-grade dysplasia, low-grade dysplasia, or Barrett's metaplasia, or to a new segment if the initial Barrett's segment was greater than 7 cm in length.

DOSE ADJUSTMENTS
No adjustments required.

DILUTION
Specific techniques required; see Precautions. Prepare immediately before use. Each vial of porfimer sodium must be reconstituted with 31.8 mL of D5W or NS. Concentration will be 2.5 mg/mL. Shake well until dissolved. An opaque solution; detection of particulate matter by visual inspection is difficult. Withdraw desired dose. Must be protected from bright light and used immediately.

Storage: Store unopened vials at CRT in carton to protect from light.

COMPATIBILITY
Manufacturer states, "Do not mix porfimer sodium with other drugs in the same solution."

RATE OF ADMINISTRATION
A single dose equally distributed over 3 to 5 minutes.

ACTIONS
The first light-activated drug (photosensitizing agent) for use in photodynamic therapy (PDT) to be approved in the United States. Treatment consists of a two-step process involving administration of drug and light. Cytotoxic and antitumor actions are light dependent and oxygen dependent and are the result of the propagation of radical reactions. PDT with porfimer causes direct intracellular damage by initiating radical chain reactions that damage intracellular membranes and mitochondria. After IV infusion of drug, it is allowed to circulate. It accumulates and is retained in tumors, skin, and organs of the reticuloendothelial system (e.g., liver, spleen) while largely clearing from other tissues. Has no apparent effect on tumors until it is activated by selective delivery of light (usually 40 to 50 hours postinfusion). Light activation induces a photochemical, not a thermal, effect that produces an active form of oxygen and releases thromboxane A_2. This process causes vasoconstriction, activation and aggregation of platelets, and increased clotting that contribute to ischemic necrosis leading to tissue and tumor death. The necrotic reaction and associated inflammatory response may evolve over several days. In patients with esophageal cancer, ability to swallow is improved, as is quality of life. Elimination half-life is very prolonged, up to several weeks. Highly protein bound.

INDICATIONS AND USES
Palliative treatment of patients with completely obstructing esophageal cancer or partially obstructing esophageal cancers that are unsuitable for treatment with thermal laser therapy. ▪ Treatment of microinvasive endobronchial non–small-cell lung cancer (NSCLC) in patients for whom surgery and radiotherapy are not indicated. ▪ Reduction of obstruction and palliation of symptoms in patients with completely or partially obstructing endobronchial non–small-cell lung cancer. ▪ Ablation of high-grade dysplasia (HGD) of Barrett's esophagus patients who do not undergo esophagectomy.

Unlabeled uses: Treatment of AIDS-related cutaneous Kaposi's sarcoma, primary or recurrent basal cell carcinoma, and squamous cell carcinoma.

CONTRAINDICATIONS
Known allergies to porphyrins, an existing tracheoesophageal or bronchoesophageal fistula, porphyria, or tumors eroding into a major blood vessel. ▪ Photodynamic therapy (PDT) is not suitable for emergency treatment of patients with severe acute respiratory distress caused by an obstructing endobronchial lesion because 40 to 50 hours are required between injection with porfimer sodium and laser light treatment. ▪ PDT is not suitable for patients with esophageal or gastric varices or for patients with esophageal ulcers greater than 1 cm in diameter.

PRECAUTIONS

Use rubber gloves and eye protection during preparation and administration. Avoid any skin or eye contact since that area will become photosensitive. Wipe up spills with a damp cloth. Dispose of all contaminated materials in a polyethylene bag to avoid accidental contact by others. Protection from light will be necessary if accidental exposure or overexposure occurs. See process in Patient Education. ■ Administered by or under the direction of the physician specialist with appropriate knowledge of the selected laser system. Facilities for monitoring the patient and responding to any medical emergency must be available. ■ Requires laser systems and a fiber-optic diffuser to activate. The FDA has approved several photodynamic lasers and the OPTIGUIDE fiber-optic diffuser for use with porfimer sodium. ■ Avoid exposure of skin and eyes to direct sunlight or bright indoor light; see Patient Education. ■ Porfimer elimination may be prolonged in patients with hepatic or renal impairment, and they may require longer precautionary measures for photosensitivity. ■ In the original studies for esophageal tumors, some experienced investigators indicated that natural sloughing action in the esophagus might be sufficient and débridement could needlessly traumatize the area. However, débridement may be performed after each light activation to minimize the potential for obstruction caused by necrotic debris. ■ A minimum of 4 weeks after completion of radiation therapy is recommended before treatment with PDT. This allows the acute inflammation produced by radiotherapy to subside. ■ 2 to 4 weeks should be allowed after PDT is complete before beginning any radiotherapy. ■ Thromboembolic events can occur following PDT with porfimer. More common in patients with other risk factors for thromboembolism (e.g., advanced cancer, cardiovascular disease, after a major surgery, or prolonged immobilization).

Esophageal tumors: Not recommended if the esophageal tumor is eroding into the trachea or bronchial tree; tracheoesophageal or bronchoesophageal fistula may result from treatment. Serious and sometimes fatal gastrointestinal and esophageal necrosis and perforation can occur after treatment. ■ Use extreme caution in patients with esophageal varices. Light should not be given directly to the variceal area because of the high risk of bleeding.

Endobronchial cancer: Interstitial fiber placement is preferred to intraluminal activation in noncircumferential endobronchial tumors that are soft enough to penetrate. Results in less exposure of the normal bronchial mucosa to light. ■ Patients with obstructing lung cancer who have received prior radiation therapy or who have tumors that are large, centrally located, cavitating, or extensive and extrinsic to the bronchus have a higher incidence of fatal hemoptysis. ■ An endobronchial tumor that invades deeply into the bronchial wall may create a fistula as the tumor resolves. ■ Use with extreme caution in endobronchial tumors located where treatment-induced inflammation could obstruct the airway (e.g., long or circumferential tumors of the trachea, tumors of the carina that involve both mainstem bronchi circumferentially, or circumferential tumors in the mainstem bronchus in patients with prior pneumonectomy).

HGD in Barrett's esophagus: Before initiating treatment with porfimer PDT, a diagnosis of HGD in Barrett's esophagus should be confirmed by a GI pathologist. ■ Long-term effect of PDT on HGD in Barrett's esophagus is unknown. There may be a risk of leaving cancerous cells behind or of leaving residual abnormal epithelium beneath the new squamous cell epithelium. ■ Esophageal strictures are a common adverse effect seen in patients treated with PDT for HGD in Barrett's esophagus. Nodule pretreatment and retreatment of the same mucosal segment more than once may influence the risk of developing an esophageal stricture. Usually occur within 6 months following PDT. May be managed with esophageal dilation; several dilations may be required.

Monitor: Obtain baseline CBC and monitor for anemia due to tumor bleeding. ■ Prevent extravasation at the injection site. Should extravasation occur, area must be protected from light. ■ Opiates may be required to control pain. ■ Observe patients carefully; most are critically ill, and many complications could occur. Monitor patients with **endobronchial tumors** closely between the laser light therapy and the mandatory débridement bronchoscopy for any evidence of respiratory distress, inflammation, mucositis, or necrotic debris that may cause obstruction of the airway. Immediate bronchoscopy may be required to remove secretions and debris to open the airway. ▪ Monitor for hemoptysis; may be a sign of progressive disease, or may result from resolution of a tumor that has eroded into a pulmonary artery. ▪ In patients who have received PDT for **HGD in Barrett's esophagus,** endoscopic biopsy surveillance should be conducted every 3 months until 4 consecutive negative evaluations for HGD have been recorded. Further follow-up should be performed every 6 to 12 months. ▪ Photosensitivity not transferable through skin to caregivers. ▪ See Precautions, Patient Education, and Drug/Lab Interactions.

Patient Education: Must observe precautions to avoid exposure of skin and eyes to direct sunlight or bright indoor light for at least 30 days. Some patients may remain photosensitive for up to 90 or more days. Photosensitivity is due to residual drug, which is present in all parts of the skin. Ambient indoor light is beneficial as it gradually inactivates the remaining drug through a photobleaching reaction. Do not remain in a darkened room. Do expose skin to ambient indoor light. Avoid bright indoor light from examination lamps, dental lamps, operating room lamps, and unshaded light bulbs. Limit time outdoors to necessary excursions, and completely cover body with clothing and shade face before going out. Conventional ultraviolet sunscreens are of no value because photoactivation is caused by visible light, not UV rays. Eyes will be sensitive to sun, bright lights, and car headlights; wear dark sunglasses with an average white light transmittance of less than 4%. After several weeks and before exposing any area of skin to direct sunlight or bright indoor light, test a small area of skin (not the face) for residual photosensitivity. Expose the small area of skin for 10 minutes. If no photosensitivity reaction (redness, swelling, or blistering) occurs within 24 hours, gradually resume normal outdoor activities. Exercise caution and increase skin exposure gradually. If some photosensitivity reaction occurs, continue precautions for 2 more weeks and then retest. Retest level of photosensitivity if traveling to a different geographic area with greater sunshine. ▪ Report chest pain (caused by inflammatory response within the area of treatment); may require prescription pain medication. ▪ Avoid pregnancy. Effective contraception necessary for females of reproductive potential during treatment and for 5 months after the last dose. Males with female partners of reproductive potential should use condoms during treatment and for 5 months after the last dose.

Maternal/Child: Based on animal studies, porfimer sodium can cause fetal harm. Effective contraception necessary. Has caused maternal and fetal toxicity in rats and rabbits (increased resorptions, decreased litter size, and reduced fetal body weight). ▪ Discontinue breast-feeding during treatment and for 5 months after the last dose. Serious reactions could occur in the infant. ▪ Safety and effectiveness for use in pediatric patients not established.

Elderly: Dose modification based on age is not required.

DRUG/LAB INTERACTIONS

No specific studies have been completed, but the following interactions are likely to occur. ▪ Use with **other photosensitizing agents** (e.g., griseofulvin, fluoroquinolones [e.g., ciprofloxacin], phenothiazines [e.g., prochlorperazine], sulfonamides [sulfisoxazole], ophthalmic solutions (AK-Sulf)], sulfonylurea hypoglycemic agents [tolbutamide], tetracyclines [doxycycline], thiazide diuretics [chlorothiazide]) could increase the photosensitivity reaction. ▪ Antitumor activity may be decreased by **dimethyl sulfoxide, beta-carotene, ethanol, formate, mannitol.** ▪ Antitumor activity may also be decreased by **allopurinol, calcium channel blockers** (e.g., diltiazem), **prostaglandin synthesis inhibitors** (NSAIDs [e.g., ibuprofen, naproxen]), **and tissue ischemia.** ▪ Effectiveness may be reduced by **drugs that decrease clotting, vasoconstriction** (e.g., nicardipine), **or platelet aggregation** (e.g., dipyridamole). ▪ **Glucocorticoid hormones** (e.g., dexamethasone) given before or with PDT may reduce the effectiveness of porfimer by inhibiting the production of thromboxane A_2.

SIDE EFFECTS

All diagnoses: May cause constipation. Most toxicities are local effects in the region of illumination and occasionally in surrounding tissues. Usually an inflammatory response induced by the photodynamic effects. Photosensitivity reactions occurred in 20% of patients in clinical studies. Reactions were usually mild to moderate erythema, but also included blisters, burning sensation, itching, and swelling. Less common skin manifestations included increased hair growth, skin discoloration, skin nodules, increased wrinkles, and skin fragility. Cases of fluid imbalance and thromboembolic events have been reported. Cataracts have been reported in one man with a family history of cataracts. Relationship to porfimer sodium unknown.

Post-Marketing: Infusion reactions (bradycardia, dizziness, hypertension, hypotension, urticaria).

Esophageal tumors: Bronchoesophageal or tracheoesophageal fistula can occur as a result of the disease or treatment, including débridement. Abdominal pain, anemia (more prevalent if tumor is located in the lower third of the esophagus), anorexia, arrhythmias (atrial fibrillation [more prevalent if tumor is located in the middle third of the esophagus], tachycardia), candidiasis, chest pain, coughing, dyspepsia, dysphagia, dyspnea, edema, eructation, esophageal edema (more prevalent if tumor is located in the upper third of the esophagus), esophageal tumor bleeding, esophageal stricture, esophagitis, fever, hematemesis, hypertension, hypotension, insomnia, nausea, pleural effusion, and vomiting may occur, as well as numerous others.

Endobronchial tumors: Coughing, dysphagia, dyspnea (may be life threatening), mucositis reaction (e.g., edema, exudate, and mucous plug obstruction), stricture, ulceration. Fatal hemoptysis has occurred (higher incidence in patients who have received radiation therapy).

High-grade dysplasia (HGD in Barrett's esophagus [BE]): Esophageal narrowing and esophageal stricture are common side effects and may require multiple dilations. Other side effects may include abdominal pain, anorexia, anxiety, arthralgia, back pain, chest discomfort or pain, dehydration, depression, diarrhea, dyspepsia, dysphagia, dyspnea, eructation, esophageal pain, fatigue, fever, headache, hiccups, hypertension, infections (bronchitis, sinusitis), insomnia, nausea and vomiting, odynophagia (pain on swallowing), pleural effusion.

ANTIDOTE

If an overdose of porfimer sodium is given, do not give the laser light treatment. Porfimer sodium is not dialyzable. Increased side effects and damage to normal tissue can be expected if an overdose of light is given. Keep physician informed of all side effects; most will be treated symptomatically. Some may be life threatening. Respiratory obstruction may require immediate bronchoscopy and removal of the obstruction with suction or forceps. Stent placement may be required in endobronchial stricture. Chest pain may require the use of opiates.

POSACONAZOLE
(**POE**-sa-**KON**-a-zole)

Antifungal
(azole derivative)

Noxafil

pH 2.6

USUAL DOSE

Pretreatment: Should be administered via a central venous line (e.g., central venous catheter or peripherally inserted central catheter [PICC]); see Precautions. Correct calcium, magnesium, and potassium deficiencies before initiating posaconazole. Baseline studies indicated; see Monitor.

Posaconazole dose: 300 mg as an IV infusion twice a day on the first day. Beginning on the second day, administer 300 mg once each day. Duration of treatment is based on recovery from immunosuppression or neutropenia and on clinical response.

Oral formulations may be substituted when appropriate.

DOSE ADJUSTMENTS

No dose adjustment is required in patients with an estimated glomerular filtration rate (eGFR) of 50 mL/min or greater; however, the intravenous vehicle Betadex Sulfobutyl Ether Sodium (SBECD) accumulates in patients with an eGFR of less than 50 mL/min. Use of oral posaconazole is recommended in these patients; see Precautions and Monitor. ■ No dose adjustment recommended in patients with mild to severe hepatic impairment (Child-Pugh Class A, B, or C); however, specific studies have not been conducted. ■ No dose adjustment indicated based on age, race, or gender. ■ Patients weighing more than 120 kg may have lower posaconazole levels. Monitor for breakthrough fungal infections.

DILUTION

Bring the 300-mg vial of posaconazole solution to RT. Aseptically transfer the contents of the vial (16.7 mL [18 mg/mL]) to a bag or bottle of ½NS, NS, D5W, D5½NS, D5NS, or D5W with 20 mEq KCl. Final concentration should be 1 to 2 mg/mL. Solution will be colorless to yellow.

Filters: Must be administered through a 0.22-micron polyethersulfone (PES) or polyvinylidene difluoride (PVDF) filter.

Storage: Refrigerate unopened vials at 2° to 8° C (36° to 46° F). Contains no preservatives; immediate use of the admixed product is preferred, but it may be refrigerated for up to 24 hours. Discard any unused solution.

COMPATIBILITY

Posaconazole should be prepared only in the solutions listed under Dilution. Use of other infusion solutions may result in particulate formation. Do not coadminister any products or diluents that are not listed by the manufacturer.

Manufacturer states that posaconazole is **compatible** with and can be infused at the same time through the same IV line **(Y-site)** as solutions listed under Dilution and the following products prepared in D5W or NS: amikacin, caspofungin, ciprofloxacin, daptomycin, dobutamine, famotidine, filgrastim, gentamicin, hydromorphone, levofloxacin, lorazepam, meropenem, micafungin, morphine, norepinephrine, potassium chloride, and vancomycin.

Manufacturer states that posaconazole is **incompatible** with and must not be diluted with LR, D5LR, and 4.2% sodium bicarbonate.

Other sources suggest a few specific **compatibilities** dependent on concentration and manufacturer; consult a pharmacist.

RATE OF ADMINISTRATION

Do not administer as an IV bolus. Administer through a 0.22-micron polyethersulfone (PES) or polyvinylidene difluoride (PVDF) filter.

Central venous catheter: Each dose as an IV infusion equally distributed over 90 minutes.

Single or initial dose (if a central venous catheter is not available): A single dose as an IV infusion equally distributed over 30 minutes.

ACTIONS

An azole antifungal agent. It blocks the synthesis of ergosterol, a key component of the fungal cell membrane, by inhibiting the cytochrome P_{450}–dependent enzyme lanosterol 14α-demethylase, which is responsible for the conversion of lanosterol to ergosterol. The depletion of ergosterol results in weakening of the structure and function of the fungal cell membrane (antifungal activity). Primarily circulates as the parent compound in plasma. Highly bound to human plasma proteins, predominantly albumin. Primarily metabolized via UDP glucuronidation and is a substrate for P-glycoprotein (P-gp) efflux. Mean terminal half-life is 27 hours. Primarily eliminated in feces as parent compound. Some minor excretion of metabolites occurs in urine and feces.

INDICATIONS AND USES

Prophylaxis of invasive *Aspergillus* and *Candida* infections in patients 18 years of age and older who are at high risk for developing these infections due to being severely immunocompromised, such as hematopoietic stem cell transplant (HSCT) recipients with graft-versus-host disease (GVHD) or patients with hematologic malignancies with prolonged neutropenia from chemotherapy.

CONTRAINDICATIONS

Known hypersensitivity to posaconazole or other azole antifungal agents. ▪ Concomitant administration with sirolimus. ▪ Concomitant administration with CYP3A4 substrates that prolong the QT interval (e.g., pimozide, quinidine). ▪ Coadministration with HMG-CoA reductase inhibitors primarily metabolized through CYP3A4 (e.g., atorvastatin, simvastatin). ▪ Coadministration with ergot alkaloids. ▪ See Drug/Lab Interactions.

PRECAUTIONS

Should be administered via a central venous line (e.g., central venous catheter or peripherally inserted central catheter [PICC]). If necessary, the initial dose may be administered through a peripheral IV line in advance of central venous line placement or to bridge the period during which a central venous line is replaced or is in use for other treatment. In clinical trials, multiple peripheral infusions resulted in infusion site reactions. **Do not administer as an IV bolus.** ▪ Avoid use of the IV formulation in patients with moderate or severe renal impairment (eGFR less than 50 mL/min) unless an assessment of the benefit versus risk to the patient justifies use; see Dose Adjustments. ▪ Concomitant administration with cyclosporine or tacrolimus increases the whole blood trough concentrations of these calcineurin inhibitors; see Drug/Lab Interactions. Nephrotoxicity and leukoencephalopathy (including deaths) have been reported in patients with elevated cyclosporine or tacrolimus concentrations. ▪ Has been associated with prolongation of the QT interval. Torsades de pointes has been reported. Use with caution in patients with potentially proarrhythmic conditions. Do not administer with drugs that are known to prolong the QTc interval and are metabolized through CYP3A4. Correct electrolyte abnormalities before administration. ▪ Hepatic toxicity (e.g., mild to moderate elevations in ALT, AST, alkaline phosphatase, total bilirubin, and/or clinical hepatitis) has been reported. Cases of more severe hepatic reactions, including cholestasis or hepatic failure (including deaths), have been reported in patients with serious underlying medical conditions (e.g., hematologic malignancy). Consider discontinuing posaconazole in patients who develop S/S of hepatic toxicity. ▪ Use with midazolam may prolong hypnotic and sedative effects of midazolam; see Drug/Lab Interactions. Benzodiazepine receptor antagonists should be available (e.g., flumazenil). ▪ Concomitant administration with vincristine has been associated with neurotoxicity and other serious adverse reactions, including seizures, peripheral neuropathy, syndrome of inappropriate antidiuretic hormone secretion, and paralytic ileus. Reserve azole antifungals (including posaconazole) for patients receiving a vinca alkaloid (including vincristine) who have no alternative antifungal treatment options; see Drug/Lab Interactions. ▪ Hypersensitivity reactions have been reported. ▪ Cross-resistance between azoles may occur; clinical significance unknown.

Monitor: Obtain baseline CBC, platelets, serum creatinine, and electrolytes. Monitor as indicated during therapy. ▪ Electrolyte disturbances, especially those involving potassium, magnesium, or calcium levels, should be monitored and corrected as necessary before and during therapy. ▪ Obtain baseline liver function tests and monitor throughout treatment. If elevations in ALT, AST, alkaline phosphatase, or total bilirubin occur, monitor for S/S of more severe hepatic injury. Consider discontinuation of posaconazole with the development of clinical S/S consistent with liver disease that may be attributable to posaconazole. ▪ Monitor serum creatinine levels closely in patients with moderate or severe renal impairment who receive posaconazole. ▪ Monitor for S/S of hypersensitivity reactions (e.g., chest pain, dizziness, dyspnea, fever, flushing, hypotension, nausea, pruritus, rash, rigors, urticaria). ▪ Closely monitor patients weighing more than 120 kg for breakthrough fungal infections; they may have lower posaconazole plasma drug exposure. ▪ See Drug/Lab Interactions.

Patient Education: Review of health history and complete medication profile, including over-the-counter medicines, vitamins, and herbal supplements, is imperative. ▪ Do not start a new medicine without consulting your healthcare provider. ▪ Review FDA-approved Patient Information. ▪ Use of effective birth control may be indicated. ▪ Promptly report S/S of a hypersensitivity reaction (e.g., itching, hives, shortness of breath). ▪ Promptly report S/S of liver toxicity (e.g., feeling very tired, flu-like symptoms, itchy skin, nausea or vomiting, yellowing of the eyes). ▪ Report a change in heart rate or rhythm. ▪ Additional precautions may be required with transfer to oral posaconazole.

Maternal/Child: May cause fetal harm when administered to pregnant females. ▪ There are no data on the presence of posaconazole in human milk, the effects on the breast-fed infant, or the effects on milk production. ▪ Safety and effectiveness for use in pediatric patients under 18 years of age not established.

Elderly: Safety profile similar to younger adults; dose adjustment not indicated.

DRUG/LAB INTERACTIONS

Interactions are numerous. Review of drug profile by pharmacist imperative.

Primarily metabolized via **UDP glucuronosyltransferase** and is a **substrate of P-glycoprotein (P-gp) efflux. Inhibitors or inducers** of these clearance pathways may affect posaconazole plasma concentrations. ▪ A strong **inhibitor of CYP3A4.** May increase plasma concentrations of drugs predominantly metabolized by CYP3A4. ▪ Concomitant administration with **sirolimus** is *contraindicated.* Blood concentrations of sirolimus may be increased approximately ninefold and result in sirolimus toxicity. ▪ Concomitant administration with **CYP3A4 substrates that prolong the QT interval** (e.g., pimozide, quinidine) is *contraindicated.* May result in increased plasma concentrations of the CYP3A4 substrates, leading to QTc prolongation and torsades de pointes. ▪ Coadministration with **HMG-CoA reductase inhibitors primarily metabolized through CYP3A4** (e.g., atorvastatin, lovastatin, simvastatin) is *contraindicated.* Increased plasma concentrations of these drugs can lead to rhabdomyolysis. ▪ Coadministration with **ergot alkaloids** is *contraindicated.* Increased plasma concentration of ergot alkaloids may lead to ergotism. ▪ Concomitant administration with **cyclosporine** or **tacrolimus** increases the whole blood trough concentrations of these calcineurin inhibitors. Reduce dose of cyclosporine to approximately three-fourths of the original dose and reduce the dose of tacrolimus to approximately one-third of the original dose. Monitor concentrations frequently during coadministration and after discontinuation of posaconazole. ▪ Concomitant use with **midazolam** increases midazolam plasma concentrations by approximately fivefold and prolongs the hypnotic and sedative effects of midazolam. Concurrent use with **other benzodiazepines** metabolized by CYP3A4 (e.g., alprazolam) could also result in increased plasma concentrations. If concomitant administration of these drugs with posaconazole is indicated, monitor patients closely, and a benzodiazepine receptor antagonist (e.g., flumazenil) should be available. ▪ **Efavirenz, rifabutin,** and **phenytoin** induce

UDP-glucuronidase and significantly decrease posaconazole plasma concentrations. Avoid concomitant use unless benefit outweighs risks. Monitor patients for breakthrough fungal infections. ■ **Rifabutin** is metabolized by CYP3A4; coadministration with posaconazole increases rifabutin plasma concentrations. If concomitant administration is indicated, monitor closely for breakthrough fungal infections and monitor full blood counts to avoid side effects (e.g., uveitis, leukopenia) from increased rifabutin plasma concentrations. ■ **Phenytoin** is metabolized by CYP3A4; coadministration with posaconazole increases phenytoin plasma concentrations. If concomitant administration is indicated, monitor closely for breakthrough fungal infections and monitor phenytoin concentrations frequently. Consider dose reduction of phenytoin. ■ **Atazanavir** and **ritonavir** are metabolized by CYP3A4, and posaconazole increases their plasma concentrations. Monitor frequently for adverse effects and toxicity of atazanavir and ritonavir if coadministration is indicated. ■ Concomitant administration with **fosamprenavir** may decrease posaconazole plasma concentrations; monitoring for breakthrough fungal infections is recommended. ■ **Vinca alkaloids** (e.g., vincristine, vinblastine) are substrates of CYP3A4; posaconazole may increase their plasma concentrations, leading to neurotoxicity and other adverse drug reactions. Reserve posaconazole for patients receiving a vinca alkaloid who have no alternative antifungal treatment options; see Precautions. ■ Posaconazole may increase the plasma concentrations of **calcium channel blockers** metabolized by CYP3A4. If coadministration is indicated, monitor frequently for side effects associated with calcium channel blockers. Dose reduction of the calcium channel blocker may be indicated. ■ May increase plasma concentrations of **digoxin**.

SIDE EFFECTS
Diarrhea, fever, hypokalemia, and nausea and vomiting are most common. The most serious side effects include arrhythmias and QT prolongation, hepatic toxicity, and hypersensitivity (including anaphylaxis). Abdominal pain, anemia, chills, constipation, cough, decreased appetite, dyspnea, epistaxis, fatigue, headache, hypertension, hypomagnesemia, peripheral edema, petechiae, rash, and thrombocytopenia have also been reported. Several other clinically significant adverse reactions were reported in less than 5% of patients during clinical trials.

Post-Marketing: Pseudoaldosteronism.

ANTIDOTE
Notify physician of all side effects; most will be treated symptomatically. If a hypersensitivity reaction occurs, discontinue the infusion and treat with oxygen, epinephrine, antihistamines, corticosteroids, or bronchodilators as indicated. Consider discontinuation of posaconazole if liver function tests are elevated and/or clinical S/S of liver disease attributable to posaconazole develop. No known specific antidote. Not removed by hemodialysis. Resuscitate as indicated.

POTASSIUM ACETATE AND POTASSIUM CHLORIDE

(po-**TASS**-ee-um **AS**-ah-tayt,
po-**TASS**-ee-um **KLOR**-eyed)

Electrolyte replenisher

pH 4 to 8

USUAL DOSE

Concentrated potassium solutions must be diluted before administration; direct injection of any concentrated solution can be instantly fatal. Maintenance potassium requirements should be incorporated into maintenance IV fluids. Intermittent IV potassium administration should be reserved for treatment of hypokalemia when the oral route is not feasible. Dose and rate of administration are dependent on specific patient condition. Starting dose based on losses, desired replacement, or maintenance.

Normal daily requirements: *Adults:* 40 to 80 mEq/24 hr.

Serum potassium level greater than 2.5 mEq/L: Rate should usually not exceed 10 mEq/hr or 200 mEq over a 24-hour period.

Serum potassium level less than 2 mEq/L and hypokalemia is a threat (e.g., potassium level less than 2 mEq/L and ECG changes and/or muscle paralysis): Rates up to 40 mEq/hr or 400 mEq over a 24-hour period can be administered. Continuous monitoring of ECG and frequent serum potassium determinations are required to prevent hyperkalemia and cardiac arrest.

PEDIATRIC DOSE

See comments under Usual Dose.

Normal daily requirements: *Newborn:* 2 to 6 mEq/kg/24 hr. ***Other pediatric patients:*** 2 to 3 mEq/kg/24 hr.

Another source recommends:

Maintenance: 2 to 4 mEq/kg/day.

Treatment of hypokalemia: 0.5 to 1 mEq/kg/dose infused at a rate of 0.5 mEq/kg/hr or less (maximum recommended single dose is 40 mEq). ECG and serum potassium monitoring recommended. Rates of 1 mEq/kg/hr have been used in critical care settings or critical care situations.

Potassium concentrate products may contain aluminum; see Precautions and Maternal/Child.

DOSE ADJUSTMENTS

Careful dose selection and adjustment is required in high-risk patients; see Precautions.
■ Reduce dose in impaired renal function. ■ Lower-end initial doses may be appropriate in the elderly based on potential for decreased organ function and concomitant disease or drug therapy.

DILUTION

Available in multiple forms. *Direct injection of any concentrated solution can be instantly fatal. Potassium chloride or acetate concentrate (2 mEq/mL) must be diluted in a larger volume of suitable IV solution and given as an infusion.* Compatible in most commonly used IV solutions; see chart on inside back cover. 40 mEq/L is the preferred dilution. 80 mEq/L is the usual maximum concentration and must be administered with caution. Avoid layering of potassium by thoroughly agitating the prepared IV solution. Also available as premixed concentrated solutions for administration via a peripheral or central line (route is dependent on concentration) and as premixed large volume solutions. In replacement therapy more concentrated solutions may be used and must be administered with caution. 40 mEq/100 mL is commonly used and must be controlled by an infusion pump and administered via a central line. In severe hypokalemia, solutions without dextrose are preferred (dextrose might decrease serum potassium level). Use only clear solutions. Check labels for aluminum content; see Precautions.

Storage: Most products may be stored at RT or CRT. See specific manufacturer requirements.

COMPATIBILITY

One manufacturer of premixed, highly concentrated solutions says, "Do not add supplementary medication."

Other sources suggest specific **compatibilities** dependent on concentration and manufacturer; consult a pharmacist.

RATE OF ADMINISTRATION

Because pain associated with peripheral infusion of potassium has been reported, administration via a central route is recommended whenever possible. Higher concentrations (40 mEq/100 mL) should be exclusively administered via a central line.

In general, a maximum of 10 mEq/hr of potassium chloride in any given amount of infusion fluid should not be exceeded. With serious potassium depletion (serum potassium under 2 mEq/L), 20 to 40 mEq/hr has been given with extreme caution, and patient must be on cardiac monitor and given via central line. Use of an infusion pump is recommended in all situations. Too-rapid infusion of hypertonic solutions may cause local pain and, rarely, vein irritation. Adjust rate of administration according to patient tolerance.

Pediatric rate: Usual rate is 0.5 mEq/kg/hr (up to 10 to 20 mEq/hr) or less. Infusion rates of up to 1 mEq/kg/hr (up to 40 mEq/hr) have been used in critical care settings.

ACTIONS

Potassium: Principal cation of intracellular fluid. Important for maintenance of body fluid composition and electrolyte balance. Participates in carbohydrate utilization and protein synthesis. Critical in the regulation of nerve conduction and muscle contraction, particularly in the heart. The normal serum potassium range is 3.5 to 5 mEq/L. The kidney normally regulates potassium balance but does not conserve potassium balance as well as or as promptly as it conserves sodium. Excreted in urine.

Chloride: The major extracellular anion. Closely follows the metabolism of sodium. Changes in the acid-base balance of the body are reflected by the changes in chloride concentration.

Acetate: An alternate source of bicarbonate by metabolic conversion in the liver.

INDICATIONS AND USES

Prevention or treatment of potassium deficiency when oral replacement is not feasible.
- Potassium chloride in dextrose solutions is indicated as a source of water, electrolytes, and calories.

CONTRAINDICATIONS

Hyperkalemia, renal failure, and any condition in which potassium retention is present.

Potassium chloride: Known hypersensitivity to potassium chloride.

Potassium acetate: Adrenal insufficiency.

PRECAUTIONS

Highly concentrated, ready-to-use potassium chloride injection is intended for the maintenance of serum potassium levels and for potassium supplementation in fluid-restricted patients who cannot accommodate additional volumes of fluid associated with potassium solutions of lower concentration. ■ To avoid potassium intoxication, do not infuse potassium infusions rapidly. ■ Administer with extreme caution, if at all, to patients with conditions predisposing to hyperkalemia and/or associated with increased sensitivity to potassium (e.g., acute dehydration, certain cardiac disorders such as CHF or AV block, extensive tissue injury or burns, severe renal impairment, potassium-aggravated skeletal muscle channelopathies [e.g., hyperkalemic periodic paralysis, paramyotonia congenita, and potassium-aggravated myotonia/paramyotonia]). ■ Administer with caution to patients who are at risk for experiencing hyperosmolality or acidosis, patients who are undergoing correction of alkalosis (conditions associated with a shift of potassium from intracellular to extracellular space), and patients treated concurrently or recently with agents or products that can cause hyperkalemia; see Drug/Lab Interactions. ■ Use solutions containing potassium with caution in patients with cardiac disease, particularly in the presence of renal disease. Cardiac monitoring is recommended. ■ Administration of concentrated potassium solutions can cause cardiac conduction disorders (including complete heart block) and other cardiac arrhythmias at any time during infusion.

Continuous cardiac monitoring is performed to aid in the detection of cardiac arrhythmias. Mild or moderate hyperkalemia may be asymptomatic and may be manifested only by increased serum potassium concentrations and, possibly, characteristic ECG changes. However, fatal arrhythmias can develop at any time during hyperkalemia. ▪ Potassium chloride may cause hyponatremia. Risk is increased in pediatric patients, elderly patients, postoperative patients, patients with psychogenic polydipsia, and patients treated with medications that increase the risk of hyponatremia; see Drug/Lab Interactions. Acute hyponatremia can lead to acute hyponatremic encephalopathy. Avoid potassium chloride injection in patients with or at risk for hyponatremia. If use cannot be avoided, monitor serum sodium concentrations. ▪ Solutions containing dextrose should be used with caution in patients with diabetes mellitus. ▪ Use potassium acetate with caution; excess administration may result in metabolic alkalosis. ▪ Use potassium acetate with caution in patients with metabolic or respiratory alkalosis and in patients with severe hepatic insufficiency. ▪ Administration of IV solutions can cause fluid and/or solute overload, resulting in dilution of serum electrolyte concentrations, overhydration, congested states, or pulmonary edema. The risk of dilutional states is inversely proportional to the electrolyte concentration. The risk of solute overload causing congested states with peripheral and pulmonary edema is directly proportional to the electrolyte concentration. ▪ Some solutions of potassium may contain aluminum. In impaired kidney function, aluminum may reach toxic levels. Premature neonates are particularly at risk because of their immature kidneys and requirement for calcium and phosphate, which also contain aluminum. Research indicates that patients with impaired renal function who receive more than 4 to 5 mcg/kg/day of parenteral aluminum are at risk for developing CNS or bone toxicity associated with aluminum accumulation.

Monitor: Patients requiring highly concentrated solutions should be kept on continuous cardiac monitoring and undergo frequent testing for serum potassium and acid-base balance. ▪ Potassium replacement should be guided primarily by ECG monitoring and secondarily by serum potassium levels, especially in patients taking digoxin. Serum potassium levels are not necessarily dependable indicators of tissue potassium levels. ▪ Continuous cardiac monitoring is preferable for infusions of over 10 mEq of potassium in 1 hour. ▪ Monitor changes in fluid balance, electrolyte concentration, and acid-base balance (e.g., serum potassium, sodium, chloride, bicarbonate, urinary output, pH). Only extracellular potassium can be measured; intracellular potassium equals 98% of total body potassium. Entire clinical picture must be considered. ▪ Confirm absolute patency of vein. Extravasation will cause severe tissue or nerve damage. Local pain and phlebitis may occur with concentrations greater than 40 mEq/L. ▪ See Drug/Lab Interactions.

Patient Education: Report burning or stinging at IV site promptly.

Maternal/Child: Effect unknown; use caution and only if clearly needed in pregnancy and breast-feeding. ▪ Safety and effectiveness for use of KCl in pediatric patients not established. However, use for treatment of potassium deficiency when oral therapy is not feasible is referenced in medical literature. Safety and effectiveness of potassium acetate for use in pediatric patients have been established.

Elderly: See Dose Adjustments. Monitoring of renal function suggested. ▪ Increased risk of hyperkalemia.

DRUG/LAB INTERACTIONS

Risk of hyperkalemia may be increased with concurrent administration of **angiotensin-converting enzyme inhibitors, angiotensin receptor blockers, tacrolimus,** and **cyclosporine**. ▪ Concurrent administration with **potassium-sparing diuretics** may cause hyperkalemia. ▪ Concurrent use with **medications associated with hyponatremia** (e.g., certain diuretics, antiepileptic and psychotropic medications) may increase the risk of hyponatremia. If concomitant use cannot be avoided, monitor serum sodium levels carefully.

SIDE EFFECTS

Abdominal pain, diarrhea, nausea, and vomiting are common side effects of potassium administration and may progress to potassium intoxication. Asystole,[a] bradycardia, cardiac arrest,[a] chest pain, dyspnea, extravasation, fever, hyperkalemia, hypersensitivity (manifested by rash and angioedema), hypervolemia, hyponatremia, hyponatremic encephalopathy, infection or pain at the site of injection, phlebitis, venous thrombosis, or ventricular fibrillation[a] may occur.

Potassium intoxication: Areflexia (absence of reflexes), cardiac arrest, cardiac arrhythmias (e.g., asystole, bradycardia, heart block, ventricular tachycardia or fibrillation), ECG abnormalities (including increased amplitude of T wave, disappearing P wave, QRS widening), hypotension, mental confusion, muscle weakness up to and including muscular and respiratory paralysis, paresthesias of the extremities, weakness. Progression of side effects may cause death.

Potassium deficit: Disruption of neuromuscular function, intestinal ileus, and dilatation.

ANTIDOTE

For any side effect, notify the physician. In the event of hyperkalemia, discontinue the infusion immediately and eliminate potassium-containing foods and medicines. Institute close ECG, laboratory, and other monitoring and, as necessary, corrective therapy to reduce serum potassium levels. For severe hyperkalemia (over 6.5 mEq/L plasma), insulin and dextrose may be administered to shift potassium into cells. Several regimens are described in the literature. One regimen recommends a bolus injection of 10 units of regular insulin followed by 50 mL of 50% dextrose. One manufacturer recommends IV dextrose, 10% to 25%, containing 10 units of regular insulin per 20 Gm of dextrose infused at 300 to 500 mL per hour. If P waves are absent, give calcium gluconate or chloride 0.5 to 1 Gm over 2 to 3 minutes (exceeds usual rate of administration). Do not use calcium, or use with extreme caution, if patient is receiving digoxin. All of these measures cause a shift of potassium into the cells and may be used simultaneously. Sodium polystyrene sulfonate (Kayexalate) orally or as retention enema is used to actually remove potassium from the body. Hemodialysis or peritoneal dialysis may be useful. Use caution in the digitalized patient; too-rapid removal of potassium may cause digoxin toxicity. Resuscitate as necessary. For extravasation, apply warm, moist compresses.

---

[a] Seen as a manifestation of rapid IV administration and/or hyperkalemia.

PRALATREXATE

(pral-a-**TREX**-ate)

Folotyn

Antineoplastic
(Antifolate)

pH 7.5 to 8.5

USUAL DOSE

Pretreatment: Verify pregnancy status. Vitamin supplementation required. 10 days before starting pralatrexate, begin folic acid 1 to 1.25 mg PO daily. Continue daily throughout the full course of therapy and for 30 days after the last dose of pralatrexate. Administer vitamin B_{12} (1 mg) IM within the 10 weeks before starting pralatrexate and every 8 to 10 weeks thereafter. Subsequent vitamin B_{12} injections may be given the same day as pralatrexate. Baseline studies indicated; see Monitor.

Pralatrexate: 30 mg/M^2 by IV push over 3 to 5 minutes via the side port of a free-flowing infusion of NS. Administer once weekly for 6 weeks in 7-week cycles until progressive disease or unacceptable toxicity occurs. Management of severe or intolerable side effects may require dose omission or reduction or interruption of therapy; see Dose Adjustments.

DOSE ADJUSTMENTS

Decrease initial dose to 15 mg/M^2 for patients with severe renal impairment (estimated glomerular filtration rate [eGFR] 15 to <30 mL/min/1.73 M^2). ■ Before administering any dose of pralatrexate, mucositis should be equal to or less than Grade 1, platelet count should be equal to or more than 100,000 cells/mm^3 for the first dose and equal to or greater than 50,000 cells/mm^3 for all subsequent doses, and the absolute neutrophil count (ANC) should be equal to or greater than 1,000 cells/mm^3. ■ Doses may be omitted or reduced based on patient tolerance. Do not make up omitted doses at the end of the cycle, and do not re-escalate once a dose reduction occurs for toxicity. See the following three charts for dose modifications based on patient symptoms.

Guidelines for Pralatrexate Dose Modifications for Mucositis			
Mucositis Grade[a] on Day of Treatment	**Action**	**Dose Upon Recovery to ≤ Grade 1**	**Dose Upon Recovery in Patients With Severe Renal Impairment**
Grade 2	Omit dose	Continue prior dose	Continue prior dose
Grade 2 recurrence	Omit dose	20 mg/M^2	10 mg/M^2
Grade 3	Omit dose	20 mg/M^2	10 mg/M^2
Grade 4	Stop therapy		

[a]Per National Cancer Institute Common Terminology Criteria for Adverse Events (NCI CTCAE), Version 4.0.

Guidelines for Pralatrexate Dose Modifications for Hematologic Toxicities				
Blood Count on Day of Treatment	**Duration of Toxicity**	**Action**	**Dose on Restart**	**Dose Upon Recovery in Patients With Severe Renal Impairment**
Platelets <50,000/mm³	1 week	Omit dose	Continue prior dose	Continue prior dose
	2 weeks	Omit dose	20 mg/M²	10 mg/M²
	3 weeks	Stop therapy		
ANC 500 to 1,000/ mm³ and no fever	1 week	Omit dose	Continue prior dose	Continue prior dose
ANC 500 to 1,000/ mm³ with fever or ANC <500/mm³	1 week	Omit dose, give G-CSF or GM-CSF support	Continue prior dose with G-CSF or GM-CSF support	Continue prior dose with G-CSF or GM-CSF support
	2 weeks or recurrence	Omit dose, give G-CSF or GM-CSF support	20 mg/M² with G-CSF or GM-CSF support	10 mg/M² with G-CSF or GM-CSF support
	3 weeks or 2nd recurrence	Stop therapy		

G-CSF, Granulocyte colony-stimulating factor; *GM-CSF,* granulocyte macrophage colony-stimulating factor.

Guidelines for Pralatrexate Dose Modifications for All Other Treatment-Related Toxicities			
Toxicity Grade[a] on Day of Treatment	**Action**	**Dose Upon Recovery to ≤ Grade 2**	**Dose Upon Recovery in Patients With Severe Renal Impairment**
Grade 3	Omit dose	20 mg/M²	10 mg/M²
Grade 4	Stop therapy		

[a]Per National Cancer Institute Common Terminology Criteria for Adverse Events (NCI CTCAE), Version 4.0.

DILUTION

Specific techniques for handling required; see Precautions. A clear yellow solution. ***Do Not Dilute.*** Aseptically withdraw the calculated dose directly into a syringe for immediate use. Available in single-dose vials containing 20 mg/mL or 40 mg/2 mL.

Filters: Specific information not available.

Storage: Refrigerate vials at 2° to 8° C (36° to 46° F) in original carton to protect from light until use. Unopened vial(s) are stable in original carton at RT for up to 72 hours. Discard if left at RT for more than 72 hours. Discard any unused portion of vial.

COMPATIBILITY

Manufacturer recommends administration via the side port of a free-flowing infusion of NS.

RATE OF ADMINISTRATION

A single dose by IV push over 3 to 5 minutes via the side port of a free-flowing infusion of NS.

ACTIONS

A folate analog metabolic inhibitor. It interferes with the growth of and leads to the destruction of cancer cells by inhibiting DNA, RNA, and protein synthesis. It competitively inhibits dihydrofolate reductase and folylpolyglutamyl synthetase. This inhibition results in the depletion of thymidine and other biologic molecules. May also affect healthy cells. Approximately 67% bound to plasma proteins. Half-life is 12 to 18 hours. Excreted as unchanged in urine (approximately 39%) and as unchanged drug and metabolites in feces.

INDICATIONS AND USES

Treatment of patients with relapsed or refractory peripheral T-cell lymphoma (PTCL). This indication is based on overall response rate. Clinical benefit such as improvement in progression-free survival or overall survival has not been demonstrated.

CONTRAINDICATIONS

Manufacturer states, "None."

PRECAUTIONS

Follow guidelines for handling cytotoxic agents; see Appendix A, p. 1308. ▪ Administered under the direction of a physician knowledgeable in its use and in a facility with adequate diagnostic and treatment facilities to monitor the patients and respond to any medical emergency. ▪ Bone marrow suppression can occur (e.g., anemia, neutropenia, and thrombocytopenia). Dose modification based on ANC and platelet count is required before each dose; see Dose Adjustments. ▪ May cause mucositis; see Dose Adjustments. ▪ To potentially reduce treatment-related hematologic toxicity and mucositis, folic acid and vitamin B_{12} supplementation is required. ▪ Severe dermatologic reactions, including skin exfoliation, toxic epidermal necrolysis, and ulceration, have been reported. May increase in severity with continued treatment, may involve skin and subcutaneous sites of known lymphoma, and may result in death. ▪ Tumor lysis syndrome has been reported. ▪ Serious adverse drug reactions, including toxic epidermal necrolysis and mucositis, were reported in patients with ESRD undergoing dialysis. ▪ Avoid pralatrexate use in patients with ESRD, including those undergoing dialysis, unless the potential benefit justifies the potential risk. ▪ Can cause hepatic toxicity and liver function abnormalities. Persistent liver function test abnormalities may be indicators of liver toxicity. ▪ Has not been studied in patients with hepatic impairment, and patients with selected liver test elevations were excluded from clinical trials.

Monitor: Obtain baseline CBC and platelets and serum chemistry tests, including renal and hepatic function. ▪ Monitor CBC and platelets and severity of mucositis weekly before each dose. ▪ Repeat serum chemistry tests, including renal and hepatic function, before the start of the first and fourth dose of a given cycle. ▪ Monitor patients with moderate to severe renal function closely. Adjust dose accordingly; see Dose Adjustments. ▪ Monitor patients with elevated liver enzymes closely (e.g., AST, ALT, transaminases). If liver function test abnormalities are greater than or equal to Grade 3, omit or modify dose; see Dose Adjustments. ▪ Observe for S/S of skin reactions (e.g., blisters, peeling and loss of skin, rash, sores); see Antidote. ▪ Monitor closely for S/S of tumor lysis syndrome (e.g., flank pain, hematuria, hyperkalemia, hyperphosphatemia, hyperuricemia, hypocalcemia, metabolic acidosis, urate crystalluria, and renal failure) and treat as appropriate. Allopurinol and hydration may be indicated for prevention and/or treatment of hyperuricemia. ▪ Monitor for thrombocytopenia (platelet count less than $50,000/mm^3$). Initiate precautions to prevent excessive bleeding (e.g., inspect IV sites, skin, and mucous membranes; use extreme care during invasive procedures; test urine, emesis, stool, and secretions for occult blood). ▪ Use prophylactic antiemetics to reduce nausea and/or vomiting and increase patient comfort. ▪ Observe closely for signs of infection. Prophylactic antibiotics may be indicated pending results of C/S in a febrile neutropenic patient.

Patient Education: A patient information guide is available from the manufacturer. ▪ Avoid pregnancy; effective birth control is recommended. ▪ Blood counts will be required at regular intervals. ▪ Take folic acid and vitamin B_{12} as prescribed to help reduce side effects. ▪ Report soreness in the mouth, redness of mucous membranes, difficulty swallowing, or ulcerations in the mouth. Discuss ways to avoid and/or manage mucositis with a healthcare professional. ▪ Promptly report S/S of infection (e.g., fever), S/S of bleeding (e.g., anemia, bruising), and S/S of tumor lysis syndrome (e.g., flank pain, hematuria). ▪ Promptly report S/S of skin reactions (e.g., blisters, peeling and loss of skin, rash, sores). ▪ Discuss medications (prescription and nonprescription) with a healthcare professional; see Drug/Lab Interactions. ▪ Avoid vaccination with live virus vaccines. ▪ See Appendix D, p. 1311.

Maternal/Child: Category D: avoid pregnancy. Can cause fetal harm. ■ Discontinue breast-feeding. ■ Safety and effectiveness for use in pediatric patients not established.
Elderly: No overall differences in effectiveness or safety based on age. ■ No dose adjustment required in elderly patients with normal renal function; however, dose selection should be cautious. Consider age-related organ impairment (e.g., bone marrow reserve, renal, hepatic) and monitor closely.

DRUG/LAB INTERACTIONS

Coadministration with **probenecid** (an inhibitor of multiple transporter systems, including the multidrug resistance–associated protein 2 [MRP2] efflux transporter) resulted in delayed renal clearance and an increase in pralatrexate exposure. ■ Concomitant administration of drugs that are substantially cleared by the renal system (e.g., **NSAIDs and sulfamethoxazole/trimethoprim**) may result in delayed clearance of pralatrexate. ■ Do not administer **live virus vaccines** to patients receiving antineoplastic drugs. ■ Not a substrate, inhibitor, or inducer of CYP_{450} isoenzymes and has a low potential for drug-drug interactions with drugs metabolized by these isoenzymes.

SIDE EFFECTS

The most common side effects are fatigue, mucositis, nausea, and thrombocytopenia. The most common serious side effects are dehydration, dyspnea, febrile neutropenia, fever, mucositis (stomatitis or mucosal inflammation of the GI and GU tracts), sepsis, and thrombocytopenia. Mucositis and thrombocytopenia were the most common reasons for discontinuing treatment. Other reported side effects include abdominal pain, abnormal liver function tests (e.g., AST, ALT, transaminases), anemia, anorexia, asthenia, back pain, constipation, cough, diarrhea, edema, epistaxis, hypokalemia, leukopenia, neutropenia, night sweats, pain in extremities, pharyngolaryngeal pain, pruritus, rash, tachycardia, tumor lysis syndrome, upper respiratory infection, vomiting.
Post-Marketing: Dermatologic reactions (e.g., skin exfoliation, toxic epidermal necrolysis, and ulceration).

ANTIDOTE

Treatment of most side effects will be supportive and may require dose adjustment or discontinuation. Discontinue pralatrexate if toxicity from side effects occurs (e.g., dermatologic reactions, Grade 4 treatment-related toxicities [e.g., mucositis], hematologic toxicities [persisting for 3 weeks], uncontrolled tumor lysis syndrome) and notify the physician; see Dose Adjustments. Administration of blood products and/or blood modifiers (e.g., darbepoetin, epoetin alfa, filgrastim, pegfilgrastim, sargramostim) may be indicated to treat bone marrow toxicity. Treat hypersensitivity reactions with epinephrine, antihistamines, and corticosteroids as needed. In addition to initiating supportive measures, leucovorin calcium (citrovorum factor, folinic acid) may be given PO, IM, or IV promptly to counteract inadvertent overdose. Resuscitate as indicated.

PROCAINAMIDE HYDROCHLORIDE

(proh-**KAYN**-ah-myd hy-droh-**KLOR**-eyed)

Antiarrhythmic

pH 4 to 6

USUAL DOSE

Loading dose: 0.2 to 1 Gm (100 mg/mL). 100 mg every 5 minutes or 20 mg every 1 minute may be given as an infusion until arrhythmia is suppressed or 500 mg is administered. Wait 10 minutes to allow adequate distribution, then resume dosing until arrhythmia is suppressed, maximum initial dose of 1 Gm is reached, or side effects appear (e.g., hypotension, QRS complex widening by 50%). Dose cautiously to avoid a hypotensive response. AHA recommends 20 mg/min as an infusion to a maximum total dose of 17 mg/kg. **Maintenance dose:** After arrhythmia is suppressed or maximum dose is reached, follow initial dose with an infusion of 1 to 4 mg/min (may require up to 6 mg/min). Titrate to control arrhythmias. Maintain with oral procainamide as soon as possible but at least 4 hours after last IV dose.

PEDIATRIC DOSE

See Maternal/Child; pediatric doses are unlabeled.

2 to 5 mg/kg of body weight. Do not exceed 100 mg/dose. Repeat as indicated every 10 to 30 minutes. Maximum dose in 24 hours is 30 mg/kg or 2 Gm. An alternate dose regimen is 2 to 6 mg/kg as a **loading dose** given over 5 minutes; follow with a **maintenance infusion** of 20 to 80 mcg/kg/min to control arrhythmias.

DOSE ADJUSTMENTS

Maintenance dose may be reduced in impaired or reduced renal function and in individuals over 50 years of age. ▪ See Drug/Lab Interactions.

DILUTION

IV injection: Dilute each 100 mg with 5 mL of D5W.

Infusion: Add 1 Gm of procainamide to 50, 250, or 500 mL of D5W. Yields 20 mg/mL, 4 mg/mL, or 2 mg/mL, respectively. 20 mg/mL should be used only as a loading dose. 2 and 4 mg/mL dilutions may be used for loading or maintenance based on fluid restrictions. Solution should be clear; may be light yellow. Discard if darker than light amber.

Pediatric infusion: Loading dose: Add a calculated loading dose (2 to 5 mg/kg) to a minimum of 10 mL D5W for each 100 mg or fraction thereof. More diluent may be used based on size of child and fluid restriction.

Maintenance infusion: See chart under Rate of Administration (Pediatric).

Storage: Photosensitive; protect from light. Store at CRT.

COMPATIBILITY

Compatibility information not available from manufacturer. Other sources suggest specific **compatibilities** dependent on concentration and manufacturer; consult a pharmacist.

RATE OF ADMINISTRATION

Administer loading dose at a rate of 20 to 50 mg/min. Use an infusion pump or a microdrip (60 gtt/mL) for infusion to deliver a constant rate. Up to 50 mg may be given by IV injection over 1 minute with extreme caution. After stabilized with loading dose, follow with a maintenance infusion at 1 to 4 mg/min.

Procainamide Infusion Rate (Adult)							
Desired Dose	**1 Gm in 500 mL D5W 2 mg/mL**				**1 Gm in 250 mL D5W 4 mg/mL**		
mg/min	**mg/hr**	**mL/min**	**mL/hr**	**mg/hr**	**mL/min**	**mL/hr**
1 mg/min	60	0.5	30	60	0.25	15
2 mg/min	120	1	60	120	0.5	30
3 mg/min	180	1.5	90	180	0.75	45
4 mg/min	240	2	120	240	1	60
5 mg/min	300	2.5	150	300	1.25	75
6 mg/min	360	3	180	360	1.5	90

Procainamide Infusion Rate (Pediatric)		
Desired Dose	**200 mg in 500 mL D5W 400 mcg/mL**	**200 mg in 125 mL D5W 1,600 mcg/mL**
mcg/kg/min	**mL/kg/min × kg = mL/min**	**mL/kg/min × kg = mL/min**
20 mcg/kg/min	0.05 × wt in kg	0.0125 × wt in kg
30 mcg/kg/min	0.075 × wt in kg	0.01875 × wt in kg
40 mcg/kg/min	0.1 × wt in kg	0.025 × wt in kg
50 mcg/kg/min	0.125 × wt in kg	0.03125 × wt in kg
60 mcg/kg/min	0.15 × wt in kg	0.0375 × wt in kg
70 mcg/kg/min	0.175 × wt in kg	0.04375 × wt in kg
80 mcg/kg/min	0.2 × wt in kg	0.05 × wt in kg

Example: To deliver 30 mcg/kg/min of a 400 mg/mL solution to a child weighing 20 kg, multiply 0.075 (mL/kg/min) × 20 (wt in kg) = an infusion rate of 1.5 mL/min.

ACTIONS

A procaine derivative. Exerts a depressing antiarrhythmic action on the heart, slowing the rate, slowing conduction, reducing myocardial irritability, and prolonging the refractory period. Decreases membrane permeability of the cell and prevents loss of sodium and potassium ions. Onset of action should occur in 2 to 3 minutes. Half-life is 3 to 4 hours. Crosses the placental barrier. Plasma levels decrease slowly; partially metabolized to the active metabolite NAPA; remaining drug excreted in the urine.

INDICATIONS AND USES

Suppress PVCs and recurrent ventricular tachycardia when lidocaine is contraindicated or has not suppressed ventricular arrhythmias. ▪ Treat wide-complex tachycardias difficult to distinguish from VT (lidocaine preferred). ▪ Rarely used ·in atrial fibrillation, paroxysmal atrial tachycardia, or arrhythmias caused by anesthesia. Safer drugs (e.g., verapamil, diltiazem) are readily available.

CONTRAINDICATIONS

Complete atrioventricular heart block, second- and third-degree AV block unless an electrical pacemaker is operative, pre-existing QT prolongation, torsades de pointes, known sensitivity to procainamide or any other local anesthetic of the ester type, myasthenia gravis, systemic lupus erythematosus.

PRECAUTIONS

Oral or IM administration is the route of choice; IV route for emergencies only. ▪ Use extreme caution in first- or second-degree blocks, ventricular tachycardia after a myocardial infarction, digoxin intoxication, CHF, any structural heart disease, and impaired liver or reduced kidney function. ▪ Predigitalize or cardiovert patients with atrial flutter or fibrillation to reduce incidence of sudden increase in ventricular rate as atrial rate is slowed. Use caution if used concurrently with other drugs that prolong QT interval (e.g., amiodarone). ■ Some clinicians recommend giving a dose the night before surgery and then discontinuing until after surgery. If an arrhythmia occurs, use lidocaine for ventricular arrhythmias and calcium channel blockers (e.g., diltiazem, verapamil) or beta-blockers (e.g., atenolol, propranolol) for supraventricular arrhythmias. Resume dosing after surgery and utilize oral dosing as soon as possible.

Monitor: Monitor the patient's ECG and BP continuously. Keep patient in a supine position. Hypotension can occur with rapid administration. ■ Discontinue IV use when the cardiac arrhythmia is interrupted or when the ventricular rate slows without regular atrioventricular conduction. ■ Small emboli may be dislodged when atrial fibrillation is corrected. ■ Monitor blood levels of procainamide and NAPA (active metabolite) in patients with renal impairment and in any patient receiving a constant infusion over 3 mg/min for more than 24 hours. ■ Monitor CBC, including WBC, differential, and platelets, with continued use; fatal blood dyscrasias have occurred with usual doses. ■ See Drug/Lab Interactions.

Maternal/Child: Category C: safety for use in pregnancy and breast-feeding and in pediatric patients not established. Consider quinidine as an alternate for use during pregnancy.

Elderly: Half-life of parent drug and active metabolite is prolonged; renal excretion reduced about 25% at age 50 and 50% at age 75. ■ Increased risk of hypotension.

DRUG/LAB INTERACTIONS

Potentiates or is potentiated by **neuromuscular blocking antibiotics** (e.g., kanamycin), **anticholinergics** (e.g., atropine), **thiazide diuretics, antihypertensive agents, muscle relaxants, succinylcholine, cimetidine, and others**. ■ May cause serious arrhythmias (e.g., prolongation of QT interval or other additive effects) with **other antiarrhythmic agents** (e.g., amiodarone, digoxin, disopyramide, lidocaine, quinidine). Lower doses of both drugs may be required. ■ Antagonizes **anticholinesterases** (e.g., neostigmine). ■ **Alcohol** may increase hepatic metabolism. ■ May **elevate AST levels.**

SIDE EFFECTS

Anorexia, bleeding, bruising, chills, dizziness, fever, flushing, giddiness, hallucinations, joint swelling or pain, mental confusion, nausea, skin rash, tremor, vomiting, weakness. May indicate onset of more serious side effects.

Major: Blood dyscrasias (e.g., agranulocytosis, bone marrow suppression, hypoplastic anemia, neutropenia, thrombocytopenia), hypotension with a BP drop over 15 mm Hg, lupus erythematosus-like symptoms, PR interval prolongation, QRS complex widening, QT interval prolongation, ventricular asystole, ventricular fibrillation, ventricular tachycardia.

ANTIDOTE

Notify the physician of any side effect. If minor symptoms progress or any major side effect appears, discontinue the drug immediately and notify the physician. Use dopamine or phenylephrine hydrochloride to correct hypotension. Treatment of toxicity is symptomatic and supportive. Infusion of $1/6$ M sodium lactate injection may reduce cardiotoxic effects. Hemodialysis may be indicated or urinary acidifiers may increase renal clearance. Resuscitate as necessary. Depending on arrhythmia, quinidine or lidocaine is an effective alternate. Consider insertion of a ventricular pacing electrode as a precautionary measure in case serious AV block develops.

PROCHLORPERAZINE EDISYLATE
(proh-klor-**PAIR**-ah-zeen eh-**DIS**-ah-layt)

Compazine

Phenothiazine
Antiemetic
Antipsychotic

pH 4.2 to 6.2

USUAL DOSE
A single IV dose should not exceed 10 mg. The maximum daily IV dose should not exceed 40 mg.

Control of severe nausea and vomiting: 2.5 to 10 mg; may be repeated one time in 1 to 2 hours if indicated.

Control of severe nausea and vomiting in adult surgical patients: 5 to 10 mg 15 to 30 minutes before induction of anesthesia or to control symptoms during or after surgery. Repeat once if necessary. Another source suggests 20 mg diluted in 1 L solution (see Dilution) during and/or after surgery.

Management of nausea and vomiting in emetic-inducing chemotherapy (unlabeled): One source suggests 10 to 20 mg 30 minutes before and 3 hours after treatment. Another source suggests 30 to 40 mg 30 minutes before and 3 hours after treatment. A third source suggests 0.8 mg/kg 30 minutes before and 3 hours after treatment and cites precipitous hypotension with larger doses; but another source suggests 2 mg/kg for highly emetogenic agents (e.g., cisplatin, dacarbazine) and 1 mg/kg for less emetogenic agents. Begin 30 minutes before chemotherapy, repeat every 2 hours for 2 doses, then every 3 hours for 3 doses. Treat extrapyramidal symptoms with diphenhydramine IM. These doses have not been recommended by the manufacturer and exceed the recommended maximum daily IV dose of 40 mg/24 hr.

Control of severe vascular and tension headaches (unlabeled): 10 mg given as an injection over 2 minutes. Sometimes given concurrently with dihydroergotamine 1 mg as an infusion over 30 minutes. Another regimen administers 3.5 mg of prochlorperazine over 5 minutes followed by dexamethasone 20 mg over 10 minutes.

PEDIATRIC DOSE
IV route not recommended for pediatric patients; safety has not been established; see Contraindications, Precautions, and Maternal/Child.

DOSE ADJUSTMENTS
Lower-end initial doses and more gradual adjustments may be indicated in the elderly and in debilitated or emaciated patients. ▪ See Drug/Lab Interactions.

DILUTION
May be given undiluted or each 5 mg (1 mL) may be diluted with 9 mL of NS. 1 mL will equal 0.5 mg. Larger amounts of NS may be used. May add doses over 10 mg to 50 mL to 1 liter of commonly used IV solution (e.g., D5W, NS, D5/$\frac{1}{2}$NS, Ringer's, or LR), and give as an intermittent or prolonged infusion. Handle carefully; may cause contact dermatitis. Slightly yellow color does not affect potency. Discard if markedly discolored.

Storage: Store below 40° C and protect from light and freezing.

COMPATIBILITY
Manufacturer recommends not mixing with other agents in a syringe.

Other sources suggest a few specific **compatibilities** dependent on concentration and manufacturer; consult a pharmacist.

RATE OF ADMINISTRATION
IV injection: Each 5 mg or fraction thereof over 1 minute.

Infusion: May be given at ordered rate, or rate may be increased or decreased as symptoms indicate. Use an infusion pump for infusion.

Management of nausea and vomiting associated with emetic-inducing chemotherapy: A single dose over 15 to 20 minutes as an *intermittent IV.*

ACTIONS

A phenothiazine derivative approximately six times more potent than chlorpromazine, with effects on the central, autonomic, and peripheral nervous systems. Has weak anticholinergic effects, moderate sedative effects, and strong extrapyramidal effects. A potent antiemetic, acting both centrally at the chemoreceptor trigger zone and peripherally by blocking the vagus nerve in the GI tract. Onset of action is prompt and lasting. Metabolized in the liver and excreted in urine and feces. Crosses placental barrier. Secreted in breast milk.

INDICATIONS AND USES

Control of severe nausea and vomiting. ▪ Used IM or PO in the treatment of schizophrenia and nonpsychotic anxiety.

Unlabeled uses: Use of higher doses to control nausea and vomiting associated with emetic-inducing chemotherapy. ▪ Treatment of severe vascular and tension headaches.

CONTRAINDICATIONS

Pediatric patients under 2 years or 10 kg (22 lb); pediatric patients with conditions that do not have an established dose; comatose or severely depressed states or in the presence of large amounts of CNS depressants (e.g., alcohol, barbiturates, narcotics); hypersensitivity to phenothiazines; breast-feeding and pregnancy, except labor and delivery; do not use in pediatric surgery.

PRECAUTIONS

Use IV only when absolutely necessary. IV not recommended for pediatric patients. ▪ Extrapyramidal symptoms caused by prochlorperazine may be confused with undiagnosed disease (e.g., Reye's syndrome, encephalopathy). ▪ May mask diagnosis of other conditions, including Reye's syndrome, brain tumor, drug intoxication, and intestinal obstruction. ▪ May produce ECG changes (e.g., prolonged QT interval, changes in T waves). ▪ Use caution in coronary disease, glaucoma, severe hypertension or hypotension, and in patients with bone marrow suppression. ▪ Use caution in patients with epilepsy. May lower the seizure threshold. ▪ Neuroleptic malignant syndrome (NMS), characterized by hyperpyrexia, muscle rigidity, autonomic instability, and altered mental status, has been reported with phenothiazine use. ▪ Tardive dyskinesia (potentially irreversible involuntary dyskinetic movements) may develop. Use the smallest doses and shortest duration of therapy to minimize risk. ▪ Anticholinergic and cardiac effects may be troublesome during anesthesia. For patients receiving phenothiazines, taper and discontinue preoperatively if they will not be continued after surgery. ▪ May discolor urine pink to reddish brown. ▪ Photosensitivity of skin is possible. ▪ May cause paradoxical excitation in pediatric patients and the elderly. ▪ Do not re-expose patients who have experienced jaundice, skin reactions, or blood dyscrasias in reaction to a phenothiazine. Cross-sensitivity may occur. ▪ May contain sulfites; use caution in patients with allergies.

Monitor: Keep patient in supine position and monitor BP and pulse before administration and between doses. ▪ Cough reflex may be suppressed. Monitor closely if nauseated or vomiting to prevent aspiration. ▪ See Drug/Lab Interactions.

Patient Education: Avoid use of alcohol or other CNS depressants (e.g., antihistamines, barbiturates). ▪ Request assistance for ambulation; may cause dizziness or fainting. ▪ Use caution performing tasks that require alertness. ▪ May cause skin and eye photosensitivity. Avoid unprotected exposure to sun.

Maternal/Child: Safety for use in pregnancy, breast-feeding, and pediatric patients not established; see Contraindications. ▪ Has been used during pregnancy for intractable nausea and vomiting; physician must decide if benefit outweighs risk. ▪ Use near term may cause maternal hypotension and adverse neonatal effects (e.g., extrapyramidal syndrome, hyperreflexia, hyporeflexia, jaundice). ▪ Fetuses and infants have a reduced capacity to metabolize and eliminate. ▪ Pediatric patients may metabolize antipsychotic agents more rapidly than adults. ■ Incidence of extrapyramidal reactions is relatively high in pediatric patients, especially in the presence of acute illness (e.g., measles, chickenpox, gastroenteritis).

Elderly: See Dose Adjustments and Precautions. ■ Have a reduced capacity to metabolize and eliminate and may have increased sensitivity to postural hypotension, anticholinergic and sedative effects. ■ Increased risk of extrapyramidal side effects (e.g., tardive dyskinesia, parkinsonism).

DRUG/LAB INTERACTIONS

Use with **epinephrine** not recommended; may cause precipitous hypotension. ■ Increased CNS respiratory depression and hypotensive effects with **narcotics, alcohol, anesthetics, barbiturates;** reduced doses of these agents usually indicated. ■ Additive effects with **MAO inhibitors, anticholinergics, antihistamines, antihypertensives, hypnotics, muscle relaxants, phenytoin, propranolol, rauwolfia alkaloids, and thiazide diuretics;** dose adjustment may be necessary. ■ Risk of cardiotoxicity increased with **pimozide**; concurrent use not recommended. ■ Risk of additive QT interval prolongation, cardiac depressant effects, and cardiac arrhythmias increased with **amiodarone, disopyramide, erythromycin, probucol, procainamide, and quinidine**. ■ Concurrent use with **antidepressants** or **MAO inhibitors** may increase effects of both drugs; risk of neuroleptic malignant syndrome may be increased. ■ Encephalopathic syndrome has been reported with concurrent use of **lithium;** monitor for S/S of neurologic toxicity. ■ May diminish effects of **oral anticoagulants.** ■ May lower seizure threshold. Dose adjustment of **anticonvulsants** may be necessary. ■ Use with **metrizamide** may lower seizure threshold; discontinue prochlorperazine 48 hours before **myelography,** and do not resume for 24 hours after test is completed. ■ Use caution during anesthesia with **barbiturates** (e.g., methohexital, thiopental); may increase frequency and severity of hypotension and neuromuscular excitation. ■ Capable of innumerable other interactions.

SIDE EFFECTS

Usually transient if drug discontinued but may require treatment if severe: anaphylaxis, blurring of vision, cardiac arrest, dermatitis, dizziness, drowsiness, dryness of mouth, dysphagia, elevated BP, extrapyramidal symptoms (e.g., abnormal positioning, extreme restlessness, pseudoparkinsonism, weakness of extremities), excitement, fever without etiology, hematologic toxicities (e.g., agranulocytosis, aplastic anemia, leukopenia, thrombocytopenia), hypersensitivity reactions, hypotension, photosensitivity, slurred speech, spastic movements (especially about the face), tachycardia, tardive dyskinesia, tightness of the throat, tongue discoloration, tongue protrusion, and many others. Overdose can cause convulsions, hallucinations, and death.

ANTIDOTE

Discontinue the drug at onset of any side effect and notify the physician. Discontinue prochlorperazine and all drugs not essential to concurrent therapy immediately if NMS occurs. Will require intensive symptomatic treatment, medical monitoring, and management of concomitant medical problems. Counteract hypotension with IV fluids and norepinephrine or phenylephrine; counteract extrapyramidal symptoms with benztropine mesylate or diphenhydramine. Maintain a clear airway and adequate hydration. *Epinephrine is contraindicated for hypotension.* Further hypotension will occur. Use diazepam for convulsions or hyperactivity. Follow with phenytoin. Phenytoin may be helpful in ventricular arrhythmias. In treating respiratory depression and unconsciousness, avoid analeptics such as doxapram; they may cause convulsions. Not removed by dialysis. Resuscitate as necessary.

PROMETHAZINE HYDROCHLORIDE BBW

(proh-**METH**-ah-zeen hy-droh-**KLOR**-eyed)

Phenothiazine
Antiemetic
Histamine H₁ antagonist

Phenergan

pH 4 to 5.5

USUAL DOSE

A vesicant; see Dilution, Rate of Administration, Contraindications, Precautions, Monitor, and Antidote. Deep IM injection is the preferred route of administration.

All uses: The Institute for Safe Medication Practices (ISMP) recommends 6.25 to 12.5 mg as a starting IV dose and limiting the concentration available to the 25 mg/mL product.

Nausea and vomiting: 12.5 to 25 mg every 4 to 6 hours as needed.

Allergic conditions: 25 mg. May repeat in 2 hours if necessary. Change to oral therapy as soon as possible.

Sedation, nighttime: 25 to 50 mg.

Sedation, perioperative: 25 to 50 mg. May combine with a reduced dose of narcotic analgesic and an anticholinergic drug (e.g., atropine).

Sedation, labor and delivery: 50 mg during early stage of labor. When labor fully established, may administer 25 to 75 mg with a reduced dose of a narcotic analgesic. May repeat every 4 hours to a maximum dose of 100 mg in a 24-hour period.

PEDIATRIC DOSE

IV use is rare and is limited to pediatric patients 2 years of age or older; see Contraindications and Maternal/Child. Adjust dose to the age, weight, and severity of condition. Use the minimum effective dose and avoid concomitant administration with other drugs with respiratory depressant effects. Do not exceed one-half of adult dose.

Adjunct to premedication: 1.1 mg/kg/dose.

DOSE ADJUSTMENTS

Reduced dose may be indicated in the elderly. See Drug/Lab Interactions.

DILUTION

Concentration should never exceed 25 mg/mL and IV push no faster than 12.5 mg/min if allowed by hospital protocol. Many hospitals now send promethazine diluted in 25 to 50 mL from the pharmacy. 1 mL (25 to 50 mg) diluted with 9 mL of NS equals 2.5 to 5 mg/mL. **The ISMP recommends further dilution with an additional 10 to 20 mL of NS.** Administer through Y-tube of a free-flowing IV.

Storage: Store at CRT. Protect from light. Do not use if solution has developed color or contains a precipitate.

COMPATIBILITY

May form a precipitate with heparin; flush heparinized infusion sets with SWFI or NS before and after administration.

Other sources suggest specific **compatibilities** dependent on concentration and manufacturer; consult a pharmacist.

RATE OF ADMINISTRATION

If allowed by local protocols, 12.5 mg may be given IV push over 1 minute; however, most hospitals require it to be diluted in 25 to 50 mL of fluid. Any doses greater than 12.5 mg must be given diluted.

ACTIONS

A phenothiazine derivative with effects on the central, autonomic, and peripheral nervous systems. It has antihistaminic, antiemetic, anticholinergic, anti–motion-sickness, and sedative effects. Promethazine is a competitive H₁ histamine receptor antagonist but does not block the release of histamine. Clinical effects are generally apparent within 5 minutes after an IV dose. Duration of action is 4 to 6 hours, but effects may persist up to 12 hours. Half-life ranges from 9 to 16 hours. Primarily metabolized in the liver and excreted in the urine.

INDICATIONS AND USES

Amelioration of allergic reactions to blood or plasma. ▪ An adjunct to the treatment of anaphylaxis after acute symptoms have been controlled with epinephrine and other standard measures. ▪ Treatment of other uncomplicated hypersensitivity reactions when oral therapy is impossible or contraindicated. ▪ Treatment of motion sickness. ▪ Preoperative, postoperative, and obstetric (during labor) sedation. ▪ Adjunct to analgesics for control of postoperative pain. ▪ Sedation and relief of apprehension; production of a light sleep from which a patient can be easily aroused. ▪ Prevention and control of nausea and vomiting associated with certain types of anesthesia and surgery. ▪ An adjunct to anesthesia and analgesia in selected surgical situations (e.g., repeated bronchoscopy, ophthalmologic surgery, and poor-risk patients). Given in conjunction with reduced amounts of narcotic analgesics.

CONTRAINDICATIONS

Comatose or severely depressed states. ▪ Hypersensitivity or an idiosyncratic reaction to phenothiazines. ▪ Pediatric patients under 2 years of age. ▪ Injection into an artery; may cause arteriospasm resulting in gangrene. ▪ SC administration; chemical irritation may result in necrotic lesions.

PRECAUTIONS

Ampule must state "for IV use." Deep IM injection preferred. ▪ Use with extreme caution in pediatric patients and the elderly; see Maternal/Child and Elderly. ▪ Can cause severe chemical irritation and tissue damage regardless of route of administration. Irritation and damage can result from perivascular extravasation, unintentional intra-arterial injection, and intraneuronal or perineuronal infiltration. Adverse event reports include abscesses, burning, erythema, gangrene, pain, palsies, paralysis, sensory loss, severe spasm of the distal vessels, swelling, thrombophlebitis, tissue necrosis, and venous thrombosis. ▪ Use should be avoided in patients with compromised respiratory function or in patients at risk for respiratory failure (e.g., COPD, sleep apnea); risk of potentially fatal respiratory depression is increased. ▪ May cause paradoxical excitation in pediatric patients and the elderly. ▪ Use with caution in patients with bladder neck obstruction, cardiovascular disease, narrow-angle glaucoma, liver dysfunction, prostatic hypertrophy, pyloroduodenal obstruction, or stenosing peptic ulcer. ▪ May produce ECG changes (e.g., prolonged QT interval, changes in T waves). ▪ May lower seizure threshold; use extreme caution in patients with known seizure disorders and with narcotics or local anesthetics that also lower seizure threshold. ▪ May contain sulfites; use caution in patients with allergies. ▪ Neuroleptic malignant syndrome (NMS), a rare syndrome manifested by hyperpyrexia, muscle rigidity, altered mental status, and autonomic instability (irregular BP and HR, tachycardia, diaphoresis, and cardiac dysrhythmias) has been reported in association with promethazine alone or in combination with antipsychotic drugs. ▪ Cholestatic jaundice has been reported.

Monitor: A vesicant; determine absolute patency of vein; extravasation will cause necrosis; see Contraindications and Precautions. ISMP suggests administering through large-bore veins. Administration through hand or wrist veins is strongly discouraged. ▪ Monitor frequently for S/S of extravasation (e.g., burning, erythema, pain, palsies, sensory loss, and swelling along IV site), especially along peripheral sites. ▪ Monitor for CNS effects (e.g., extrapyramidal effects, sedation). ▪ Sedative effect may require ambulation to be monitored. ▪ See Drug/Lab Interactions.

Patient Education: Avoid use of alcohol or other CNS depressants (e.g., antihistamines, barbiturates). ▪ Request assistance for ambulation; may cause dizziness or fainting. ▪ Use caution performing tasks that require alertness. ▪ May cause skin and eye photosensitivity. Avoid unprotected exposure to sun. ▪ Report stinging or burning at IV site promptly. ▪ Report any involuntary muscle movements.

Maternal/Child: Category C: safety for use in pregnancy and pediatric patients not established. Use only when clearly needed. ▪ Discontinue breast-feeding. ▪ Contraindicated in pediatric patients under 2 years of age. Post-marketing cases of respiratory depression and death have been reported. Concomitant administration with other respiratory depressants increases this risk. ▪ Use caution in pediatric patients 2 years of age or older. Use the minimum effective dose. ▪ Do not use for vomiting of unknown etiology in pediatric patients. Antiemetics are not recommended for treatment of uncomplicated vomiting in pediatric patients. Use should be limited to prolonged vomiting of known etiology. ▪ Extrapyramidal symptoms that can occur secondary to promethazine administration may be confused with CNS signs of an undiagnosed primary disease (e.g., encephalopathy or Reye's syndrome). Avoid use in pediatric patients with S/S suggestive of Reye's syndrome or other hepatic diseases. ▪ Excessively large doses of antihistamines in pediatric patients have caused sudden death. Hallucinations and convulsions have occurred with therapeutic doses and overdoses. Incidence of extrapyramidal reactions is increased in pediatric patients, especially in the presence of acute illness (e.g., measles, chickenpox, gastroenteritis). ▪ See Precautions and Contraindications.

Elderly: See Dose Adjustments and Precautions. ▪ May exhibit increased sensitivity to adverse effects, including anticholinergic (e.g., dry mouth, urinary retention), CNS, and extrapyramidal (e.g., tardive dyskinesia, parkinsonism) side effects.

DRUG/LAB INTERACTIONS

Promethazine may increase, prolong, or intensify the sedative action of **CNS depressants**. Avoid concurrent use or administer CNS depressants in reduced dosage. The dose of barbiturates should be reduced by at least one-half, and the dose of narcotics should be reduced by one-fourth to one-half. Dosage must be individualized. ▪ Additive effects with **MAO inhibitors, anticholinergics, antihistamines, antihypertensives, hypnotics,** and **muscle relaxants**; monitor for adverse effects. ▪ Use with epinephrine not recommended; may cause precipitous hypotension. ▪ Concurrent use with **other neuroleptic agents** (e.g., haloperidol) may increase the risk of NMS. ▪ Capable of innumerable other interactions. ▪ Selected **pregnancy tests** may show a false-negative or false-positive result. ▪ May cause an increase in blood glucose; consider when a **glucose tolerance test** is indicated.

SIDE EFFECTS

Angioneurotic edema, apnea, asthma, blurred vision, bradycardia, confusion, dermatitis, disorientation, dizziness, drowsiness, dryness of mouth, extrapyramidal symptoms, faintness, hallucinations, hematologic side effects (e.g., agranulocytosis, leukopenia, thrombocytopenia, thrombocytopenic purpura), hypersensitivity reactions, hypertension, halypotension, jaundice, nasal stuffiness, nausea, neuroleptic malignant syndrome, paradoxical reactions (e.g., abnormal movements, agitated behavior, delirium, hyperexcitability, nightmares), photosensitivity, respiratory depression, sedation, severe tissue injury (including gangrene), somnolence, tachycardia, urticaria, vomiting.

Overdose: Ataxia, athetosis, atropine-like S/S (e.g., dry mouth; fixed, dilated pupils; flushing), Babinski reflex, convulsions, deep sedation, GI symptoms, hyperreflexia, hypertonia, profound hypotension, respiratory depression, unconsciousness, and sudden death.

ANTIDOTE

Discontinue the drug immediately at onset of any side effect and notify the physician. Sympathetic block and heparinization have been used during acute management of promethazine extravasation (unintentional intra-arterial injection or perivascular extravasation). In some cases surgical intervention, including fasciotomy, skin graft, and/or amputation, has been required. Treatment of overdose is essentially symptomatic and supportive. Counteract hypotension with IV fluids, Trendelenburg position, norepinephrine, or phenylephrine; counteract extrapyramidal symptoms with benztropine mesylate or diphenhydramine. Epinephrine is contraindicated for hypotension; further hypotension will occur. Use diazepam or phenobarbital for convulsions or hyperactivity. Treatment of NMS includes discontinuation of all unnecessary drugs and intensive symptomatic treatment and monitoring. Dialysis does not appear to be helpful in overdose situations. Resuscitate as necessary.

PROPOFOL INJECTION
(**PROH**-poh-fohl in-**JEK**-shun)

General anesthetic
Anesthesia adjunct
Sedative

Diprivan

pH 7 to 8.5

USUAL DOSE

Pretreatment: Fluid correction required; see Monitor.

Lidocaine may be administered to minimize pain on injection of propofol. Administer before propofol injection or add to propofol immediately before administration. Do not exceed more than 20 mg lidocaine to 200 mg propofol.

SEDATION OF INTUBATED, MECHANICALLY VENTILATED ICU PATIENTS

Must be individualized and titrated to desired response. Given as a continuous infusion. Begin with an initial dose of 5 mcg/kg/min (0.3 mg/kg/hr) for 5 minutes. Allow at least 5 minutes between adjustments to reach peak drug effect and to avoid hypotension. Increase slowly over 5 to 10 minutes by 5 to 10 mcg/kg/min (0.3 to 0.6 mg/kg/hr) to desired level of sedation. Individualize to patient condition, response, blood lipid profile, and vital signs. Administration should not exceed 4 mg/kg/hr unless the benefits outweigh the risks. Some clinicians recommend reducing dose by approximately one-half for elderly (over 55 years) and debilitated. Check urinalysis and urine sediment before administration of propofol in patients at risk for renal failure; see Precautions and Monitor.

MAINTENANCE OF SEDATION IN MECHANICALLY VENTILATED OR RESPIRATORY-CONTROLLED ICU PATIENTS

5 to 50 mcg/kg/min (0.3 to 3 mg/kg/hr) or higher as a continuous infusion slowly titrated to desired level of sedation. Use caution with doses higher than 50 mcg/kg/min; may increase risk of hypotension. Bolus doses of 10 to 20 mg may be used to rapidly increase the depth of sedation in patients in whom hypotension is not likely to occur. Temporarily reduce dose once each day to assess neurologic and respiratory function and to determine minimum dose required for desired level of sedation. Average maintenance dose **under 55 years** is 38 mcg/kg/min; **over 55 years,** 20 mcg/kg/min. Average maintenance dose for **post–coronary artery bypass graft (CABG) patients** is usually low (median of 11 mcg/kg/min) because of high intraoperative opiates.

RELIEF OF PRURITUS ASSOCIATED WITH USE OF SPINAL OPIATES OR CHOLESTASIS (UNLABELED)

Subhypnotic doses of 10 to 15 mg as an IV injection or 0.5 to 1.5 mg/kg/hr as an infusion.

MANAGEMENT OF REFRACTORY STATUS EPILEPTICUS (UNLABELED)

Administer doses of 1 to 2 mg/kg as an IV injection over 5 minutes; may be repeated if seizure activity recurs. If indicated, follow with a maintenance infusion of 2 to 10 mg/hr. Adjust to achieve the lowest rate needed to suppress seizure activity. Decrease gradually to prevent withdrawal seizures.

Rapid sequence intubation (RSI): 1.5 to 2 mg/kg once (usual range 1 to 3 mg/kg) if permitted in your state/institution.

PEDIATRIC DOSE

To minimize pain on injection of propofol in pediatric patients, administer through larger veins or pretreat smaller veins with lidocaine. See Maternal/Child.

DOSE ADJUSTMENTS

All situations: Reduced dose required in presence of other CNS depressants. See Drug/Lab Interactions. ■ No dose adjustment required for gender, chronic hepatic cirrhosis, or chronic renal failure.

ICU sedation: Adjust infusion to maintain a light level of sedation through the wake-up assessment or weaning process.

DILUTION

Supplied in ready-to-use vials containing 10 mg/mL. Shake well before use. Do not use if there is evidence of excessive creaming or aggregation, if large droplets are visible, or if there are other forms of phase separation. Slight creaming, which should disappear after shaking, may be visible with prolonged standing. May be further diluted only with D5W. Do not dilute to a concentration less than 2 mg/mL (4 mL diluent to 1 mL propofol yields 2 mg/mL). More stable in glass than in plastic. Strict aseptic technique imperative; emulsion supports rapid growth of microorganisms. Failure to use strict aseptic technique has been associated with microbial contamination of the product with resultant fever, infection, sepsis, other life-threatening illnesses, and/or death. Prepare immediately before each use. Vials are never to be accessed more than once or used on more than one person because of the possible transmission of bloodborne pathogens (e.g., hepatitis B, hepatitis C, and HIV). Flush IV line at end of every 6 hours in extended procedures to remove residual propofol.

Filters: Use filters with caution. The pore size should be equal to or greater than 5 microns. Filters with a pore size less than 5 microns may impede the flow of propofol and/or cause a breakdown of the emulsion.

Storage: Protect from light and store below 22° C (72° F) but do not refrigerate. Discard infusion and tubing every 12 hours or every 6 hours if propofol has been transferred from the original container.

COMPATIBILITY

Manufacturer states, "Should not be mixed with other therapeutic agents prior to administration. **Compatibility** with blood/serum/plasma has not been established."

Other sources suggest specific **compatibilities** dependent on concentration and manufacturer; consult a pharmacist.

RATE OF ADMINISTRATION

Use of a syringe pump or volumetric pump recommended to provide controlled infusion rates. See Usual Dose for specific rates for specific age and/or indication. Decrease rate based on age, debilitation, or calculated risk. Must be individualized and titrated to desired level of sedation and changes in vital signs. Monitor respiratory function continuously. Continuous administration preferable to intermittent to avoid periods of undersedation or oversedation. Too-rapid administration (bolus dosing, too-rapid increase in infusion rate, overdose) can cause severe cardiorespiratory complications, especially in pediatric patients, adults over 55 years, debilitated or ASA III or IV risk patients. In all anesthesia, higher rates are generally required for the first 15 minutes, then appropriate responses can usually be maintained with a decrease of 30% to 50%. Control increased response to surgical stimulation or lightening of anesthesia (increased pulse rate, BP, sweating and/or tearing) with bolus injections of 25 to 50 mg **(adults under 55 years of age only),** slow injection of reduced doses, or by increasing the infusion rate **(adults under or over 55 years of age)** or by increasing the infusion rate **(pediatric patients).** If control not effective within 5 minutes, consider use of an opioid, barbiturate, or inhalation agent.

ACTIONS

A potent emulsified IV general anesthetic and sedation drug. Mechanism of action is poorly understood. Propofol is thought to produce its sedative/anesthetic effects by the positive modulation of the inhibitory function of the neurotransmitter GABA through the ligand-gated $GABA_A$ receptors. Can provide conscious (verbal contact maintained) or unconscious sedation depending on dose. Induces anesthesia rapidly and smoothly with minimal excitation, usually within 40 seconds. Depth of sedation easily and rapidly controlled by adjusting rate of infusion. Rapid onset of action facilitates accurate titration and minimizes oversedation. Due to extensive redistribution from the central nervous system to other tissues and high metabolic clearance, recovery from anesthesia or sedation is rapid. Time to awakening is dependent on duration of infusion. Discontinuation of an infusion after maintenance of anesthesia for 1 hour or sedation in the ICU for 1 day will result in rapid awakening. Prolonged infusions (e.g., 10 days in ICU) will result in drug accumulation and an increased time to awakening. By daily titration of the propofol dose to achieve only the minimum effective therapeutic concentration, rapid awakening within 10 to 15 minutes can occur even after long-term administration. Terminal half-life is

4 to 7 hours but may be up to 1 to 3 days after a 10-day infusion. Metabolized in the liver and excreted as metabolites in urine. Crosses placental barrier. Secreted in breast milk.

INDICATIONS AND USES

Adults: Induce and/or maintain anesthesia as part of a balanced anesthetic technique for inpatient and outpatient surgery. ▪ Initiate and maintain monitored anesthesia care (MAC) during diagnostic procedures (e.g., colonoscopy, dental procedures) and in conjunction with local/regional anesthesia during surgical procedures. ▪ Continuous sedation and control of stress responses in intubated, mechanically ventilated ICU patients (e.g., post-CABG, postsurgical, neuro/head trauma, ARDS, COPD, asthma, status epilepticus, tetanus). Continuous infusion of low doses allows controlled recovery of consciousness when required and for assessment.

Pediatric patients: Induction of anesthesia as a part of a balanced anesthetic technique for inpatient and outpatient surgery in pediatric patients over 3 years of age. ▪ Maintenance of anesthesia as part of a balanced anesthetic technique for inpatient and outpatient surgery in pediatric patients over 2 months of age. ▪ Not recommended for induction of anesthesia for pediatric patients under 3 years of age or for maintenance of anesthesia under 2 months of age. ▪ Not indicated for use in pediatric patients for ICU sedation or for MAC sedation for surgical, nonsurgical, or diagnostic procedures.

Unlabeled uses: Subhypnotic doses used for relief of pruritus associated with use of spinal opiates or cholestasis; treatment of status epilepticus refractory to standard anticonvulsant therapy.

CONTRAINDICATIONS

Known hypersensitivity to propofol or its components (e.g., soybean oil, glycerol, egg lecithin, sodium hydroxide) or any time general anesthesia or sedation is contraindicated.

PRECAUTIONS

All situations: For IV use only. ▪ Administered by or under the direct observation of the anesthesiologist. Must have responsibility only for anesthesia during surgery and/or procedures. In the ICU setting, may be administered to intubated, mechanically ventilated patients by persons skilled in medical management of critically ill patients and trained in cardiovascular resuscitation and airway management. Both life-threatening and fatal anaphylactoid and anaphylactic reactions have been reported. ▪ Strict aseptic technique required; see Dilution. ▪ Use caution in patients with compromised myocardial function, intravascular volume depletion, or abnormally low vascular tone (e.g., sepsis); may be more susceptible to hypotension. ▪ Avoid rapid bolus administration in the elderly, debilitated, or ASA-PS III or IV patients. May cause undesirable cardiopulmonary depression, including apnea, airway obstruction, hypotension, and oxygen desaturation. ▪ An emulsion; use caution in patients with lipid metabolism disorders (e.g., diabetic hyperlipidemia, pancreatitis, and primary hyperlipoproteinemia). ▪ May cause convulsions during recovery phase in patients with epilepsy. ▪ Use caution in patients with increased intracranial pressure or impaired cerebral circulation. Decrease in mean arterial pressure may cause decreases in cerebral perfusion. ▪ Propofol infusion syndrome has been reported and is characterized by severe metabolic acidosis, hyperkalemia, lipemia, rhabdomyolysis, hepatomegaly, renal failure, and ECG changes and/or cardiac failure. Major risk factors for the development of these events include decreased oxygen delivery to tissues; serious neurologic injury and/or sepsis; high dosages of one or more of the following pharmacologic agents: vasoconstrictors, steroids, or inotropes; and/or prolonged, high-dose infusions of propofol (greater than 5 mg/kg/hr for more than 48 hours). Deaths have occurred. Consider alternative means of sedation when there is a prolonged need for sedation, when large doses of propofol are required to maintain a desired level of sedation, or if a patient develops metabolic acidosis. ▪ Has no analgesic properties; provide pain relief or local anesthetic as indicated. Has been used successfully with midazolam (Versed), 1 to 3 mg, for initial induction. Midazolam provides better amnesia and causes less pain on injection, whereas propofol sustains sedation and allows more rapid recovery. ▪ May contain sulfites; use caution in patients with allergies. ▪ Abuse of propofol for recreational and other improper purposes has resulted in fatalities and other injuries. ▪ See Maternal/Child.

Monitor: *All situations:* Monitor for apnea if not intubated. Correct fluid volume deficiencies before administration. ▪ Will cause transient local pain during IV injection; minimize by using larger veins and lidocaine previous to injection. Use with midazolam reduces awareness of this pain. ▪ Apnea may occur during induction and last for more than 60 seconds. Intubation equipment, controlled ventilation equipment, oxygen, and facilities for resuscitation and life support must be available. Maintain a patent airway and ascertain adequate ventilation at all times. ▪ All vital signs must be monitored continuously. Use of a respiratory monitor required. ▪ Hypotension common during first 60 minutes; monitor closely. Significant hypotension or cardiovascular depression can be profound. ▪ To prevent profound bradycardia, anticholinergic agents (e.g., atropine, glycopyrrolate) may be required to modify increases in vagal tone due to concomitant agents (e.g., succinylcholine) or surgical stimulation. ▪ Bed rest required for a minimum of 3 hours after IV injection, or satisfy specific hospital rules for discharge. ▪ See Precautions and Drug/Lab Interactions.

ICU sedation: Observe for signs and symptoms of pain; may indicate need for opioids or analgesia, not an increase in propofol dose. ▪ Benzodiazepines (e.g., diazepam) and/or neuromuscular blocking agents (e.g., atracurium, succinylcholine) may also be used. ▪ Monitor triglycerides with long-term use (ICU sedation). Adjust if fat is inadequately cleared from body, and reduce other lipid administration. 1 mL of propofol contains approximately 0.1 Gm of fat (1.1 kcal). ▪ Dose may be reduced carefully to allow patient to awaken to a lighter level of sedation, allowing neurologic and respiratory assessment daily. Avoid rapid awakening; will cause anxiety, agitation, and resistance to mechanical ventilation. ▪ Monitor urinalysis and urine sediment on alternate days in patients at risk for renal impairment. ▪ Some formulations contain EDTA, a trace metal chelator. Formulations containing EDTA should not be infused for longer than 5 days without providing a drug holiday to safely replace estimated or measured zinc losses. Consider zinc supplementation in patients who may be predisposed (e.g., patients with burns, diarrhea, or major sepsis). ▪ Discontinue opioids and paralytic agents and optimize respiratory function before weaning from mechanical ventilation. ▪ Maintain light sedation until 15 minutes before extubation.

Patient Education: Avoid alcohol or other CNS depressants (e.g., antihistamines, benzodiazepines) for 24 hours following anesthesia. ▪ Do not perform tasks requiring mental alertness (e.g., driving, operating hazardous machinery, or signing legal documents) until the day after surgery or longer. All effects must have subsided. ▪ Discuss with parents or caregivers the risks, benefits, timing, and duration of surgery or procedures requiring anesthetic and sedation drugs; see Maternal/Child.

Maternal/Child: Use during pregnancy only if clearly needed. ▪ Not recommended for use in obstetric procedures, including cesarean section; no assurance of safety for fetus. ▪ Not recommended for use during breast-feeding. ▪ Has been approved for induction of anesthesia in pediatric patients 3 years to 16 years of age. Has been approved for maintenance of anesthesia in pediatric patients 2 months to 16 years of age. ▪ Distribution and clearance in pediatric patients 3 years to 12 years of age is similar to that seen in adults. ▪ Published studies suggest that repeated or prolonged exposures to anesthetic agents in utero (third trimester) and early in life (up to 3 years of age) may have negative effects on the developing brain, resulting in adverse cognitive or behavioral effects; see prescribing information for further discussion. Balance the benefits of appropriate anesthesia in pregnant females, neonates, and young children who require procedures with the potential risks described. ▪ Serious bradycardia may result with concomitant administration of fentanyl. ▪ Serious adverse effects (e.g., metabolic acidosis) occurred during ICU sedation in pediatric patients with respiratory infections and/or with doses in excess of recommendations for adults. Fatalities have occurred. ▪ A recent study identified an increase in deaths with propofol versus standard sedative agents. Manufacturer has issued a warning letter stating that propofol should not be used for sedation of pediatric patients in ICU. ▪ See Side Effects.

Elderly: Dose requirements decrease after age 55 due to reduced clearance and volume distribution and higher blood levels. Minimize undesirable cardiorespiratory depression (hypotension, apnea, airway obstruction, and/or oxygen desaturation) by using reduced doses and rates of administration. Avoid rapid single or repeated bolus doses; see Precautions. See Usual Dose and Dose Adjustments.

DRUG/LAB INTERACTIONS

Potentiated by **inhalational anesthetics, narcotics,** and **sedatives**. Anesthetic and sedative effects increased; systolic, diastolic, mean arterial pressure, and cardiac output are decreased. Dose adjustment may be indicated with concomitant use. ▪ Competition for chemoreceptor binding sites may occur if used in combination with **droperidol;** use of propofol as a single agent is suggested to control nausea and vomiting. ▪ In pediatric patients, serious bradycardia may result with concomitant administration of **fentanyl.** ▪ Concomitant use with **valproate** may lead to increased blood levels of propofol. Reduce the dose of propofol when coadministering with valproate. Monitor for signs of increased sedation or cardiorespiratory depression.

SIDE EFFECTS

Adults and pediatric patients: More likely to occur during loading boluses, with supplemental boluses, or during higher rate of administration. Apnea; bradycardia (profound); cough; dyspnea; headache; hypotension; hypoventilation; injection site burning, pain, stinging; nausea; and upper airway obstruction are most common. Urine may be green. Abdominal cramping, anaphylaxis (including bronchospasm, erythema, and hypotension), bucking/jerking/thrashing, clonic/myoclonic movement (rarely including convulsions and opisthotonos), dizziness, fever, flushing, hiccups, hypertension, tingling/numbness/coldness at injection site, twitching, and vomiting may occur.

Pediatric patients: Increased incidences of agitation, bradycardia, and jitteriness have occurred; apnea has been observed frequently. Abrupt discontinuation following prolonged infusion may result in agitation, flushing of the hands and feet, hyperirritability, and tremulousness.

Overdose: Cardiorespiratory depression (hypotension, apnea, airway obstruction, and/or oxygen desaturation).

ANTIDOTE

Keep physician informed of all side effects. Reduction of dose may be required or will be treated symptomatically. Discontinue the drug for major side effects, paradoxical reactions, or accidental overdose. A short-acting drug, a patent airway, and continuous controlled ventilation with oxygen until normal function assured should be adequate. Treat bradycardia and/or hypotension with increased rate of IV fluids, Trendelenburg position, vasopressors. Anticholinergic agents (e.g., atropine or glycopyrrolate) may be required. Treat hypersensitivity reactions and resuscitate as necessary.

PROPRANOLOL HYDROCHLORIDE

(proh-**PRAN**-oh-lohl hy-droh-**KLOR**-eyed)

Beta-adrenergic blocking agent
Antiarrhythmic

pH 2.8 to 3.5

USUAL DOSE

Acute heart rate control (atrial fibrillation/flutter, SVT) 1 mg over 1 minute, repeat every 2 minutes to a max of 3 doses. Ventricular tachycardia: 1 to 3 mg every 5 minutes up to a total of 5 g with other antiarrhythmic; see Monitor and Rate of Administration. Do not give additional propranolol if desired change in rate or rhythm is achieved. If there is no change in rhythm for at least 2 minutes after initial dose, cycle may be repeated one time. (AHA recommends 0.5 to 1 mg over 1 minute, repeated as needed up to a total dose of 0.1 mg/kg.) *No further propranolol may be given by any route for at least 4 hours.* Best results achieved if administered within 2 to 4 hours of symptom onset or thrombolytic therapy. Transfer to oral therapy as soon as possible.

PEDIATRIC DOSE (UNLABELED)

Tetrology: 0.15 to 0.25 mg/kg/dose IVPB over 10 minutes (maximum dose 1 mg), may repeat 1 time. Thyroid storm in adolescents: 0.5 to 1 mg slow IV push over 10 minutes. Tachyarrhythmias: 0.01 to 0.15 mg/kg/dose IVPB over 10 minutes, may repeat every 6 to 8 hours PRN. Max dose is age dependent: infant 1 mg/dose, children and adolescent 3 mg/dose.

DOSE ADJUSTMENTS

Lower-end initial doses may be indicated in the elderly based on potential for decreased organ function and concomitant disease or drug therapy. ▪ Consider dose reduction in patients with impaired hepatic function. ▪ See Drug/Lab Interactions. ▪ Reduce dose gradually to avoid rebound angina, myocardial infarction, or ventricular arrhythmias.

DILUTION

May be given undiluted; however, further dilution of each 1 mg in 10 mL D5W or NS. May be diluted in 50 mL of D5W, D5/$\frac{1}{2}$NS, D5NS, or NS for infusion.

Storage: Store at CRT. Protect from freezing or excessive heat.

COMPATIBILITY

Compatibility information not available from manufacturer. Other sources suggest specific **compatibilities** dependent on concentration and manufacturer; consult a pharmacist.

RATE OF ADMINISTRATION

1 mg/minute to avoid excessive hypotension and/or cardiac standstill. A single dose may be given as an infusion over 10 to 15 minutes. Allow adequate time for distribution; consider slow circulation time. Observe monitor and discontinue propranolol as soon as rhythm change occurs.

Pediatric rate: Extend rate of administration of a single dose by injection to a minimum of 5 minutes in pediatric patients.

ACTIONS

Propranolol is a nonselective beta-adrenergic blocker with antiarrhythmic effects. Cardiac response to sympathetic nerve stimulation is inhibited, slowing the HR (especially ventricular rate) by inhibiting atrioventricular conduction. Decreases the force of cardiac contractility and decreases arterial pressure and cardiac output. Blockade of beta$_2$-adrenergic receptors found predominantly in smooth muscle (e.g., vascular, bronchial, gastrointestinal, and genitourinary); leads to constriction in these tissues. Well distributed throughout the body, the onset of action occurs within 1 to 2 minutes and lasts about 4 hours. Half-life is 2 to 5.5 hours. Metabolized in the liver. Excreted primarily in the urine. Secreted in breast milk.

INDICATIONS AND USES

Reserve IV use for life-threatening situations or for those occurring under anesthesia. ▪ Short-term treatment to decrease ventricular rate in supraventricular tachycardia, including Wolff-Parkinson-White syndrome and thyrotoxicosis. ▪ Treatment of persistent and symptomatic PVCs that do not respond to conventional measures. ▪ Use in patients with atrial flutter or atrial fibrillation should be reserved for arrhythmias unresponsive to standard therapy or when more prolonged control is required. ▪ Control of ventricular rate in life-threatening, digoxin-induced arrhythmias (severe bradycardia may occur). ▪ Treatment of tachyarrhythmias due to excessive catecholamine action during anesthesia when other measures fail. ▪ Not the drug of first choice for treatment of ventricular arrhythmias unless arrhythmia is induced by catecholamines or digoxin. In critical situations, when cardioversion or other drugs are not indicated or effective, propranolol may be used with caution. (Use a low dose and administer very slowly so the failing heart maintains some sympathetic drive to maintain myocardial tone. May respond with NSR, but a reduction in ventricular rate is more likely.) ▪ Numerous other uses PO.

Unlabeled uses: Other beta-blockers (e.g., atenolol, esmolol) have been used in the perioperative period to reduce cardiac morbidity and mortality in patients at risk; propranolol was not used in these studies. ▪ Has been used for adjunctive treatment of pheochromocytoma following primary treatment with an alpha-adrenergic blocking agent (e.g., phenoxybenzamine, phentolamine) and for treatment of other refractory arrhythmias when benefit outweighs risk.

CONTRAINDICATIONS
Cardiogenic shock, sinus bradycardia, greater than first-degree heart block, bronchial asthma, known hypersensitivity to propranolol.

PRECAUTIONS
Oral administration is preferred. Use IV administration only when necessary. ▪ Not considered the drug of choice for arrhythmias in myocardial infarction. ▪ Used concurrently with digoxin or alpha-adrenergic blockers as indicated. ▪ Use with caution in overt CHF. May precipitate more severe failure. ▪ Use with extreme caution in asthmatics or in patients with lung disease or bronchospasm; can block bronchodilation produced by endogenous and exogenous catecholamine stimulation of beta receptors. ▪ Use with caution in patients with diabetes or in patients with a history of hypoglycemia. May cause hypoglycemia and mask the symptoms. ▪ Beta-blockade can mask symptoms of hyperthyroidism. Abrupt withdrawal of propranolol may be followed by exacerbation of symptoms, including thyroid storm. ▪ Use caution in patients with hepatic or renal impairment. ▪ May cause arrhythmia, angina, MI, or death if stopped abruptly. ▪ Beta-adrenergic receptor blockade can cause a reduction in intraocular pressure. Withdrawal of propranolol may lead to a return of elevated intraocular pressure. May also interfere with the screening test for glaucoma. ▪ IV dose used during surgery to replace an oral dose should be one-tenth of the oral dose. ▪ May cause severe bradycardia in patients with Wolff-Parkinson-White syndrome. See Drug/Lab Interactions.

Monitor: Continuous ECG and BP monitoring is mandatory during administration of IV propranolol. Monitoring of pulmonary wedge pressure or central venous pressure is recommended. Discontinue the drug when a rhythm change is noted and wait to note full effect before giving additional medication if indicated. ▪ See Precautions and Drug/Lab Interactions.

Patient Education: Report any breathing difficulty promptly.

Maternal/Child: Category C: safety for use in pregnancy and breast-feeding and in pediatric patients not established. Use only when clearly indicated. ▪ Bradycardia, hypoglycemia, and respiratory depression have been seen in neonates whose mothers received propranolol during labor or delivery.

Elderly: Lower-end initial doses may be indicated; see Dose Adjustments. ▪ Response of elderly versus younger patients not documented. ▪ Use with caution in age-related peripheral vascular disease; risk of hypothermia increased. ▪ May exacerbate mental impairment.

DRUG/LAB INTERACTIONS
Metabolism involves multiple pathways in the **cytochrome P$_{450}$ system.** Interactions with inhibitors, inducers, or substrates of this system are documented. ▪ Blood levels of

propranolol **increased** when administered concurrently **with substrates or inhibitors** such as amiodarone, cimetidine, ciprofloxacin, delavirdine, fluconazole, fluoxetine, fluvoxamine, imipramine, isoniazid, paroxetine, quinidine, ritonavir, rizatriptan, teniposide, theophylline, tolbutamide, zileuton, zolmitriptan. ■ Blood levels of propranolol **decreased** when administered concurrently with **inducers** such as cigarette smoke, ethanol, and rifampin. ■ Concurrent use with **propafenone** may produce additive negative inotropic and beta-blocking effects. ■ Concurrent administration with **quinidine** results in additive negative inotropic effects and beta-blockade and postural hypotension. ■ Concurrent use with **disopyramide** has been associated with additive hypotension, severe bradycardia, asystole, and heart failure. ■ Concurrent use with **amiodarone** results in additive negative chronotropic properties. ■ Decreases **lidocaine** clearance; lidocaine toxicity has been reported with concurrent use. ■ Effects additive when given with **other agents that slow A-V nodal conduction** (e.g., digoxin, lidocaine). ■ Concurrent use with **calcium channel blockers** that have negative inotropic and/or chronotropic activity (e.g., diltiazem, verapamil) may further depress myocardial contractility and A-V nodal conduction. Bradycardia, heart failure, and cardiovascular collapse have been reported with verapamil and beta-blockers. Bradycardia, hypotension, heart block, and heart failure have been reported with coadministration of diltiazem and beta-blockers. ■ Antihypertensive effects of **clonidine** may be antagonized by propranolol. Use with clonidine may precipitate acute hypertension or aggravate rebound hypertension if clonidine is stopped abruptly; discontinue propranolol several days before gradual withdrawal of clonidine. Monitor BP with concurrent use. ■ First-dose hypotension may be prolonged with **prazosin**. Postural hypotension has been reported when used concurrently with **doxazosin and terazosin**. ■ Coadministration with **reserpine** (a catecholamine-depleting drug) may result in hypotension, bradycardia, vertigo, syncope, or orthostatic hypotension. ■ Avoid concurrent use with **epinephrine.** Beta-blockade may lead to unopposed alpha-receptor stimulation, resulting in uncontrolled hypertension. ■ **Dobutamine or isoproterenol** may be administered to reverse the effects of propranolol. However, patients may experience protracted, severe hypotension. ■ **ACE inhibitors** (enalapril, lisinopril) may increase bronchial hyperactivity when given concurrently with propranolol. ■ Hypotension and cardiac arrest have been reported with concurrent use of **haloperidol** and propranolol. ■ Propranolol may increase serum levels of **theophylline and diazepam.** ■ Potentiates **ergot alkaloids**; monitor for peripheral ischemia; reduce ergot dose or discontinue beta-blocker. ■ Added hypotensive effect with **diuretics** (e.g., furosemide), **other antihypertensive agents** (e.g., enalapril, nitroglycerin), some **phenothiazines** (e.g., chlorpromazine), **and reserpine.** Reduced dose of one or both drugs may be indicated. ■ May prolong effects of **nondepolarizing muscle relaxants** (e.g., pancuronium). ■ May increase anticoagulant effects of **warfarin.** ■ May mask symptoms of hypoglycemia with **insulin and sulfonylureas** and result in prolonged hypoglycemia. ■ Can interfere with **numerous diagnostic and physiologic tests.** Consult literature. ■ May alter **thyroid function tests** and cause **elevations in BUN, serum potassium, triglycerides, serum transaminases, and alkaline phosphatase.** ■ Metabolism and release of catecholamines increased in **smokers;** increased doses may be required. May also interfere with therapeutic effects in **treatment of angina.** ■ Patients taking beta-blockers who are exposed to a potential allergen may be unresponsive to the usual dose of **epinephrine** used to treat a hypersensitivity reaction.

SIDE EFFECTS

AV conduction delays, bradyarrhythmias, bronchospasm, cardiac failure, cardiac standstill, erythematous rash, hallucination, hypotension, laryngospasm, nausea, paresthesia of the hands, respiratory distress, syncopal attacks, vertigo, visual disturbances. Many other side effects have been reported with oral propranolol and could be seen with the IV route; see manufacturer's literature.

ANTIDOTE

For any side effect or excessive dosage, discontinue the drug and notify the physician immediately. Treat bradycardia with atropine 0.25 to 1 mg. Isoproterenol may be used with caution if no response to vagal blockade. Serious bradycardia may require pacing.

Treat cardiac failure with digitalization and diuretics. Treat hypotension or depressed myocardial function with glucagon. Administer 50 to 150 mcg/kg IV followed by an infusion of 1 to 5 mg/hr (see glucagon monograph for correct dilution). Isoproterenol (Isuprel) and dopamine may also be useful; see Drug/Lab Interactions. Treat bronchospasm with isoproterenol and aminophylline. Treat other side effects symptomatically. Monitor ECG, HR, neurobehavioral status, and intake and output until stable. Not significantly removed by hemodialysis or peritoneal dialysis. Resuscitate as necessary.

PROTAMINE SULFATE BBW

(**PROH**-tah-meen **SUL**-fayt)

Antidote
(heparin antagonist)

pH 6 to 7

USUAL DOSE

Following a serious heparin overdose, discontinue heparin and administer protamine immediately.

Pretreatment: Corticosteroids and antihistamines can be used for patients at risk for protamine hypersensitivity.

IV heparin overdose: 1 mg of IV protamine neutralizes approximately 100 USP units of heparin. May be repeated if needed in 10 to 15 minutes. Never exceed 50 mg in any 10-minute period. Dose adjusted as indicated by coagulation studies. Any dose over 100 mg in 2 hours should be justified by coagulation studies (has its own anticoagulant effect). Because heparin disappears rapidly from the circulation, the dose of protamine required decreases rapidly with the time elapsed after heparin injection (e.g., 30 minutes after IV heparin, 0.5 mg [or one-half of the dose] of protamine may be sufficient to neutralize 100 USP units of heparin).

Subcutaneous heparin overdose: 1 to 1.5 mg IV protamine per 100 units of heparin. Some clinicians recommend a loading dose of 25 to 50 mg given slowly over 10 minutes followed by administration of the remainder of the calculated dose as a continuous infusion over 8 to 16 hours (the continuous infusion covers the absorption time seen with administration of SC heparin). See comments under IV heparin overdose.

Low-molecular-weight heparin overdose (unlabeled): 1 mg IV protamine for every 100 anti-factor Xa units of LMWH. If PTT remains prolonged 2 to 4 hours after the first dose, or if bleeding continues, consider administration of a second dose of 0.5 mg protamine for every 100 anti-factor Xa units. Only 60% to 75% of anti-factor Xa activity is neutralized. Excessive protamine doses can worsen bleeding potential. See comments under IV heparin overdose.

DOSE ADJUSTMENTS

Because heparin disappears rapidly from the system, reduce dose of protamine based on length of time elapsed since heparin dose (up to one-half if 30 minutes has elapsed).

■ Prompt administration of protamine may also decrease dose requirements.

DILUTION

May be given undiluted or may be further diluted with NS or D5W.

Storage: Store at CRT. Do not freeze. Discard remaining medication or diluted solution.

COMPATIBILITY

Manufacturer recommends not mixing with other drugs unless **compatibility** is known, and lists as **incompatible** with some antibiotics, including several cephalosporins and penicillins. Consider individualized rate adjustment necessary to produce desired effects.

Other sources suggest a few specific **compatibilities** dependent on concentration and manufacturer; consult a pharmacist.

RATE OF ADMINISTRATION

50 mg (5 mL) or fraction thereof over 10 minutes. Do not exceed 50 mg in 10 minutes. As an infusion, may be given over 2 to 3 hours with dosage titrated according to coagulation studies. Increase duration of infusion to 8 to 16 hours for treatment of SC heparin overdose. Use infusion pump or microdrip (60 gtt/mL) to administer. Too-rapid administration, high doses, or repeated doses can cause anaphylaxis, bradycardia, cardiovascular collapse, catastrophic pulmonary vasoconstriction, pulmonary hypertension, dyspnea, flushing, noncardiogenic pulmonary edema, sensation of warmth, or severe hypotension. Hypertension has also occurred.

ACTIONS

An anticoagulant if administered alone. In the presence of heparin, protamine forms a stable salt, neutralizing the anticoagulant effect of both drugs. Does not bind to low-molecular-weight fragments of LMWH preparations, leading to incomplete neutralization of anti-factor Xa. Each 1 mg of protamine can neutralize approximately 100 USP units of heparin. Onset of action is within 0.5 to 1 minute. Neutralization of heparin occurs within 5 minutes. Duration of action is about 2 hours.

INDICATIONS AND USES

To neutralize the anticoagulant activity of heparin in severe heparin overdosage.

Unlabeled uses: Neutralization of heparin administered during extracorporeal circulation in arterial and cardiac surgery or dialysis procedures. ▪ Heparin neutralization in pregnant females near delivery. ▪ Treatment of overdose of low-molecular-weight heparin (e.g., dalteparin, enoxaparin, tinzaparin). Neutralization of LMWH is not complete.

CONTRAINDICATIONS

Known hypersensitivity to protamine. ▪ Do not use for bleeding that occurs without prior exposure to heparin.

PRECAUTIONS

For IV use only. Can cause severe hypotension, cardiovascular collapse, noncardiogenic pulmonary edema, catastrophic pulmonary vasoconstriction, and pulmonary hypertension. Risk factors include high dose or overdose, rapid administration, repeated doses, previous administration of protamine, and current or previous use of protamine-containing drugs (e.g., NPH insulin, protamine zinc insulin, and certain beta-blockers). Allergy to fish, previous vasectomy (may have antiprotamine antibodies), severe left ventricular dysfunction, and abnormal preoperative pulmonary hemodynamics also may be risk factors. In patients with any of these risk factors, the risk versus benefit of protamine sulfate administration should be carefully considered. See Rate of Administration and Usual Dose. ▪ Must be administered in a facility equipped to monitor the patient and respond to any medical emergency. ▪ Pulmonary edema and/or circulatory collapse may occur in patients undergoing cardiac bypass surgery; etiology unknown. ▪ Protamine sulfate should not be given when bleeding occurs without prior heparin use.

Monitor: Coagulation studies (e.g., aPTT, ACT, heparin titration test with protamine, plasma thrombin time) may be indicated to monitor therapeutic response. ▪ Facilities to treat shock must be available; see Precautions. ▪ After cardiac surgery or dialysis procedures, even with adequate neutralization, further bleeding may occur any time within 24 hours (heparin "rebound"). Observe the patient continuously. Additional protamine sulfate may be indicated.

Maternal/Child: Category C: safety for use in pregnancy, breast-feeding, or pediatric patients not established.

DRUG/LAB INTERACTIONS

Specific information not available.

SIDE EFFECTS

Occur more frequently with too-rapid injection; anaphylaxis, back pain, bradycardia, dyspnea, feeling of warmth, flushing, lethargy, nausea, vomiting, severe hypertension or hypotension. Acute pulmonary hypertension, noncardiogenic pulmonary edema, catastrophic pulmonary vasoconstriction, circulatory collapse, capillary leak, or pulmonary edema may occur.

ANTIDOTE

Discontinue the drug and notify the physician, who may recommend a decrease in rate of administration or, if side effects are severe, symptomatic treatment such as administration of whole blood, vasopressors for hypotension, atropine for bradycardia, and oxygen for dyspnea. Resuscitate as necessary.

PROTEIN AMINO ACIDS, DEXTROSE, FAT EMULSION, AND ELECTROLYTES BBW

Nutritional therapy

(**PROH**-teen ah-**MEE**-noh **AS**-ids)

Kabiven ▪ Perikabiven

USUAL DOSE

Pretreatment: Obtain baseline labs; see Monitor. Correct severe fluid, electrolyte, and acid-base disorders before initiating therapy.

Kabiven: 19 to 38 mL/kg/day. Do not exceed 40 mL/kg/day.

Perikabiven: 27 to 40 mL/kg/day. Do not exceed 40 mL/kg/day.

Maximum infusion rate is based on the dextrose component. Individualize dose based on patient's clinical condition (ability to adequately metabolize amino acids, dextrose, and lipids), on patient's body weight and nutritional/fluid requirements, as well as on additional energy given orally/enterally to the patient. Dosage selection is based on fluid requirements, which can be used in conjunction with the nutritional requirements to determine final dosage. Products meet total nutritional requirements for protein, dextrose, and lipids in stable patients and can be individualized to meet specific needs with the addition of nutrients. Treatment may be continued for as long as is required by the patient's condition.

The recommended daily nutritional requirements for protein, dextrose, and lipids compared to the amount of nutrition provided by each product are shown in the following chart. See Rate of Administration for additional dosing instructions.

Nutritional Comparison				
	Nutrition Provided by Kabiven Recommended Dosage	Nutrition Provided by Perikabiven Recommended Dosage	Recommended Nutritional Requirements	
			Stable Patients	Critically Ill Patients[a]
Fluid (mL/kg/day)	19 to 38	27 to 40	30 to 40	Minimum needed to deliver adequate macronutrients
Protein[b] (Gm/kg/day)	0.6 to 1.3	0.64 to 0.94	0.8 to 1	1.5 to 2
Nitrogen (Gm/kg/day)	0.1 to 0.2	0.1 to 0.15	0.13 to 0.16	0.24 to 0.3
Dextrose (Gm/kg/day)	1.9 to 3.7	1.8 to 2.7	≤10	≤5.8
Lipids (Gm/kg/day)	0.7 to 1.5	0.95 to 1.4	1	≤1
Total energy requirement (kcal/kg/day)	16 to 32	18 to 27	20 to 30	25 to 30

[a]Do not use in patients with conditions that are contraindicated; see Contraindications.
[b]Protein provided as amino acids. When infused IV, amino acids are metabolized and utilized as the building blocks of protein.

Continued

DOSE ADJUSTMENTS

Stop infusion in patients with a serum triglyceride concentration above 400 mg/dL. Monitor levels. Once serum triglycerides are less than 400 mg/dL, restart infusion at a reduced rate. Advance rate in smaller increments toward target dosage, checking the triglyceride levels before each adjustment. ▪ Administer the recommended dosage in patients with renal impairment. Renal patients not needing dialysis require 0.6 to 0.8 Gm of protein/kg/day. Patients undergoing hemodialysis or continuous renal replacement therapy should receive 1.2 to 1.8 Gm of protein/kg/day up to a maximum of 2.5 Gm of protein/kg/day based on nutritional status and estimated protein losses. Dosage may require adjustment based on fluid, protein, and electrolyte requirements in these patients. Adjust dosage based on treatment for renal impairment, supplementing protein as indicated. If required, additional amino acids may be added to the Kabiven or Perikabiven bag or infused separately; see Compatibility. ▪ Lower-end initial dosing may be appropriate in the elderly based on the potential for decreased hepatic, renal, or cardiac function and on concomitant disease or drug therapy.

DILUTION

Kabiven and Perikabiven are sterile, hypertonic emulsions in a three-chamber container. The individual chambers contain one of the following, respectively: amino acids and electrolytes, dextrose, or lipid injectable emulsion. Available in multiple volumes. Process of activation is extensive. See manufacturer's prescribing information for **contents** of Kabiven and Perikabiven when mixed and for *Preparation Instructions* and *Instructions for Use.* An instructional video is available at www.KabivenUSA.com.

Inspect the bag before activation and discard if any of the following conditions exists: there is evidence of damage to the bag, more than one chamber is white, the solution is yellow, or any seal is already broken. *After activating the bag*, add any **compatible** additives (e.g., MVI and trace elements) via the additive port (white port) using an 18- to 23-gauge needle with a maximum length of 1.5 inches (40 mm). Mix thoroughly after each addition by inverting the bag to ensure a homogenous admixture. Visually inspect for particulate matter and discoloration before administration. Ensure that precipitates have not formed and that the emulsion has not separated. (Separation of the emulsion can be visibly identified by a yellowish streaking or the accumulation of yellowish droplets in the mixed emulsion.)

Filters: Use of a 1.2-micron in-line filter required.

Storage: *Kabiven and Perikabiven:* Before use, store at CRT. Avoid excessive heat and protect from freezing. If accidentally frozen, discard. Do not remove container from the overpouch until intended for use. Product should be used immediately after mixing and the introduction of additives. If not used immediately, the storage time and conditions before use should not be longer than 24 hours refrigerated at 2° to 8° C (36° to 46° F). After removal from refrigeration, the admixture should be infused within 24 hours. Any mixture remaining must be discarded.

Kabiven: In the absence of additives, once activated, the product remains stable for 48 hours at 25° C (77° F). If not used immediately, the activated bag can be stored for up to 7 days under refrigeration. After removal from refrigeration, the activated bag should be used within 48 hours.

COMPATIBILITY

Manufacturer states, "Ceftriaxone *must not be administered* simultaneously with calcium-containing intravenous solutions such as Kabiven or Perikabiven via a **Y-site** due to precipitation. However, may be administered sequentially if the infusion lines are thoroughly flushed between infusions with a **compatible** fluid. *Do not use administration sets and lines that contain DEHP.* Administration sets that contain polyvinyl chloride (PCV) components have DEHP as a plasticizer."

RATE OF ADMINISTRATION

For IV infusion only. Use a dedicated line without any connections. Multiple connections could result in air embolism. Use a 1.2-micron in-line filter. Use a nonvented infusion set or close the air inlet on a vented set. (Use of a vented intravenous administration set with a vent in the open position could result in air embolism.)

Kabiven: Maximum infusion rate is 2.6 mL/kg/hr via a **central vein**.

Perikabiven: Maximum infusion rate is 3.7 mL/kg/hr via a **central or peripheral vein**.

The maximum infusion rates listed correspond to 0.09 Gm/kg/hr of amino acids, 0.25 Gm/kg/hr of dextrose (the rate-limiting factor), and 0.1 Gm/kg/hr of lipids. The recommended duration of infusion is between 12 and 24 hours, depending on the clinical situation.

Dosing Instructions: 1. After determining the fluid requirements to be delivered (see preceding chart in Usual Dose), select the corresponding bag that will supply the correct volume of solution. 2. Determine the preferred duration of infusion (12 to 24 hours). 3. Ensure that the rate of infusion in mL/kg/day divided by the preferred duration of infusion in hours does not exceed the maximum infusion rate for the patient (i.e., 2.6 mL/kg/hr for **Kabiven** and 3.7 mL/kg/hr for **Perikabiven**). The infusion rate may need to be reduced and the duration of infusion increased in order not to exceed the maximum infusion rate. 4. Once the infusion rate in mL/kg/hr has been selected, calculate the infusion rate (mL/hr) using the patient's weight. 5. Compare the patient's nutrient requirements with the amount supplied by Kabiven or Perikabiven. Discuss any additions that may be required with a pharmacist or dietitian.

Example:

1. A stable, ambulatory 50-kg patient is to receive Kabiven at a rate of 30 mL/kg/day.

   30 mL/kg/day $\times$ 50 kg = 1,500 mL/day. A 1,540 mL bag is chosen.

2. To accommodate different therapies, an infusion duration of 12 hours is chosen.
3. Verify that the maximum rate has not been exceeded: 30 mL/kg/day $\div$ 12 = 2.5 mL/kg/hr.
4. 2.5 mL/kg/hr $\times$ 50 kg = 125 mL/hr.

ACTIONS

Kabiven and Perikabiven are used as a supplement or as the sole source of nutrition in patients, providing macronutrients (amino acids, dextrose, and lipids) and micronutrients (electrolytes) parenterally. The amino acids provide the structural units that make up proteins and are used to synthesize proteins and other biomolecules or are oxidized to urea and carbon dioxide as a source of energy. Dextrose is oxidized to carbon dioxide and water, yielding energy. Lipids provide biologically utilizable sources of calories and essential fatty acids. Fatty acids serve as an important substrate for energy production. Fatty acids are important for membrane structure and function, as precursors for bioactive molecules (such as prostaglandins), and as regulators of gene expression. The disposition of amino acids, dextrose, and electrolytes is essentially the same as those supplied by ordinary food. The elimination and oxidation rates of infused lipids depend on the patient's clinical condition. Elimination is faster and utilization is increased in postoperative patients and with sepsis, burns, and trauma, whereas patients with renal impairment and hypertriglyceridemia may show lower utilization of exogenous lipid emulsions.

INDICATIONS AND USES

Indicated as a source of calories, protein, electrolytes, and essential fatty acids for adult patients requiring parenteral nutrition when oral or enteral nutrition is not possible, is insufficient, or is contraindicated. May be used to prevent essential fatty acid deficiency or to treat negative nitrogen balance.

Limitation of use: Not recommended for use in pediatric patients under 2 years of age, including preterm infants, because the fixed content of the formulation does not meet the nutritional requirements of this age-group; see Maternal/Child.

CONTRAINDICATIONS

Known hypersensitivity to egg, soybean proteins, peanut proteins, corn or corn products, or any of the active substances or excipients. ▪ Severe hyperlipidemia or severe disorders of lipid metabolism characterized by hypertriglyceridemia (serum triglyceride concentration greater than 1,000 Gm/dL). ▪ Inborn error of amino acid metabolism. ▪ Cardiopulmonary instability (including pulmonary edema, cardiac insufficiency, myocardial infarction, acidosis, and hemodynamic instability requiring significant vasopressor support). ▪ Hemophagocytic syndrome.

PRECAUTIONS

For intravenous infusion only. **Kabiven** is indicated for administration into a *central vein* only (e.g., superior vena cava). Infusion of hypertonic nutrient injections into a peripheral vein may result in vein irritation, vein damage, and/or thrombosis. **Perikabiven** may be administered into a *peripheral or central vein*. Peripheral catheters should not be used for solutions with osmolarity of 900 mOsm/L or greater. The primary complication of peripheral access is venous thrombophlebitis. ▪ Not recommended for pediatric patients under 2 years of age, including preterm infants; see Maternal/Child. ▪ Stop infusion immediately for S/S of hypersensitivity reaction. ▪ Patients who require parenteral nutrition are at high risk for infections due to malnutrition and their underlying disease state. Decrease risk of septic complications with a heightened emphasis on aseptic technique in catheter placement and maintenance, as well as with aseptic technique in the preparation of the nutritional formula. ▪ A reduced or limited ability to metabolize the lipid contained in Kabiven and Perikabiven accompanied by prolonged plasma clearance may result in fat overload syndrome. Syndrome is characterized by a sudden deterioration in the patient's condition accompanied by fever, anemia, leukopenia, thrombocytopenia, coagulation disorders, hyperlipidemia, liver fatty infiltrations (hepatomegaly), deteriorating liver function, and central nervous system manifestations (e.g., coma). Cause of fat overload syndrome is unclear but is usually reversible with discontinuation of the lipid emulsion. ▪ Refeeding syndrome, characterized by the intracellular shift of potassium, phosphorus, and magnesium, may occur when refeeding severely undernourished patients with parenteral nutrition. Thiamine deficiency and fluid retention may also develop. Increase intake gradually to avoid overfeeding and to prevent these complications. ▪ Use with caution in patients with diabetes mellitus or hyperglycemia. Hyperglycemia or hyperosmolar syndrome may develop. Administration of dextrose at a rate exceeding the patient's utilization rate may lead to hyperglycemia, coma, and death; see Rate of Administration. ▪ Hepatobiliary disorders, including cholecystitis, cholelithiasis, cholestasis, hepatic steatosis, fibrosis, and cirrhosis, possibly leading to hepatic failure, have developed in patients without pre-existing liver disease who receive parenteral nutrition. Increase of blood ammonia levels and hyperammonemia may occur in patients receiving amino acid solutions. May indicate hepatic insufficiency or the presence of an inborn error of amino acid metabolism. A clinician knowledgeable in liver diseases should assess patients developing signs of hepatobiliary disorders. ▪ Parenteral nutrition–associated liver disease (PNALD) has been reported in patients receiving parenteral nutrition for extended periods. Exact etiology is unknown; see Antidote. ▪ Use with caution in patients with impaired liver function. ▪ Use with caution in patients with renal impairment, such as prerenal azotemia, renal obstruction, and protein-losing nephropathy. May be at increased risk for electrolyte and fluid volume imbalance. Patients developing signs of renal impairment should be assessed by a clinician knowledgeable in renal disease. ▪ Close monitoring of triglyceride levels is required to avoid consequences associated with hypertriglyceridemia. Serum triglyceride levels above 1,000 mg/dL have been associated with an increased risk of pancreatitis. ▪ Impaired lipid metabolism with hypertriglyceridemia may occur with conditions such as inherited lipid disorders, obesity, diabetes mellitus, and metabolic syndrome. In these cases, increased triglycerides can also be increased by dextrose and/or overfeeding; see Monitor and Dose Adjustments. ▪ Kabiven and Perikabiven contain no more than 25 mcg/L of aluminum. In impaired kidney function, aluminum may reach toxic levels. Research indicates that patients with impaired renal function who receive greater than 4 to 5 mcg/kg/day of parenteral aluminum are at risk for developing CNS or bone toxicity associated with aluminum accumulation. Tissue loading may occur at even lower rates of administration of total parenteral nutrition products.

Monitor: Frequent clinical evaluation and laboratory determinations are necessary for proper monitoring during administration. ▪ Obtain baseline labs, including electrolytes, serum triglycerides, blood glucose, liver/kidney function (BUN, SCr, liver function tests, ammonia), serum osmolarity, and CBC, including platelet and coagulation parameters. Repeat frequently as indicated by clinical condition. ▪ Monitor fluid status closely in patients with heart failure, pulmonary edema, or renal impairment. ▪ Evaluate patient's ability to eliminate and metabolize infused lipid emulsion by measuring serum triglyceride levels at baseline, with each increase in dosage, and regularly throughout treatment. ▪ Monitor patients for S/S of essential fatty acid deficiency. Laboratory tests are available to determine serum fatty acid levels. ▪ Monitor for S/S of a hypersensitivity reaction (e.g., altered mentation, bronchospasm, chills, cyanosis, dizziness, dyspnea, erythema, fever, flushing, headache, hypotension, hypoxia, nausea, rash, sweating, tachycardia, tachypnea, urticaria, vomiting). ▪ Monitor for S/S of early infection (e.g., fever, chills, hyperglycemia, leukocytosis). Check parenteral access device frequently. ▪ Monitor for S/S of fat overload syndrome. ▪ Monitor severely undernourished patients for S/S of refeeding syndrome. ▪ Monitor blood glucose levels and treat hyperglycemia to maintain optimum levels while infusing parenteral nutrition. Insulin may be administered or adjusted to maintain optimum blood glucose levels during parenteral nutrition administration. ▪ Monitor for thrombophlebitis, which may manifest as erythema, pain, tenderness, or a palpable cord. ▪ Monitor for S/S of hepatobiliary disorders (e.g., elevated LFTs/ammonia, jaundice). ▪ Monitor overall energy intake and other sources of lipid and dextrose, as well as drugs that may interfere with lipid and dextrose metabolism.

Patient Education: Report S/S of hyperglycemia, hypersensitivity reaction (e.g., bronchospasm, itching, rash, wheezing), hypoglycemia, infection (e.g., fever), nausea, vomiting, or fluid retention. ▪ Periodic laboratory tests and routine follow-up with healthcare provider required. ▪ Report any changes in prescription or nonprescription medications and supplements.

Maternal/Child: Category C: use during pregnancy only if clearly needed. Parenteral nutrition should be considered in cases of severe maternal malnutrition in which nutritional requirements cannot be fulfilled by enteral route because of the risks to the fetus associated with severe malnutrition, such as preterm delivery, low birth weight, intrauterine growth restriction, congenital malformations, and perinatal mortality. ▪ Use caution during breast-feeding. ▪ Safety and effectiveness in pediatric patients have not been established. Deaths in preterm infants after infusion of IV lipid emulsions have been reported. Autopsy findings included intravascular fat accumulation in the lungs. Preterm infants and low-birth-weight infants have poor clearance of IV lipid emulsion and increased free fatty acid plasma levels following lipid emulsion infusion. ▪ Not recommended for use in pediatric patients under 2 years of age, including preterm infants, because the fixed content of the formulation does not meet the nutritional requirements of this age-group.

Elderly: Differences in response between the elderly and younger patients have not been identified. Dose selection should be cautious; see Dose Adjustment.

DRUG/LAB INTERACTIONS

High levels of lipid in plasma may interfere with **some laboratory blood tests,** such as hemoglobin, triglycerides, bilirubin, LDH, and oxygen saturation, if blood is sampled before lipid has been cleared from the bloodstream. Lipids are normally cleared after a lipid-free interval of 5 to 6 hours in most patients. ▪ Kabiven and Perikabiven contain vitamin K, which can reverse coumarin and coumarin derivatives, including **warfarin**. Monitor laboratory parameters for anticoagulant activity in patients who are taking both Kabiven or Perikabiven and warfarin.

SIDE EFFECTS

Kabiven: The most common adverse reactions are decreased hemoglobin, decreased total protein, fever, hypertension, hypokalemia, increased gamma glutamyltransferase (GGT), nausea, vomiting. Less frequently reported reactions include decreased blood calcium, hyperglycemia, increased blood alkaline phosphatase, prolonged PT, pruritus, tachycardia. **Perikabiven:** The most common adverse reactions are fever, hyperglycemia, hypokalemia, and increased blood triglycerides. Less frequently reported reactions include hypoalbuminemia, increased alanine aminotransferase (ALT), increased blood alkaline phosphatase, increased BUN, increased C-reactive protein, increased GGT, nausea, phlebitis, and pruritus. A number of other reactions occurred in 1% or fewer of patients. See Precautions for serious adverse reactions that have been reported with Kabiven or Perikabiven. **Post-Marketing:** *Kabiven:* Cholestasis, hypersensitivity reaction (including anaphylaxis), infection, subependymal hemorrhage.

Perikabiven: Abdominal distension, abdominal pain, chest tightness, cholestasis, flushed face, infection.

ANTIDOTE

Notify the physician immediately of any adverse symptoms. Stop infusion for severely elevated electrolyte levels or triglyceride levels above 400 mg/dL. Monitor electrolytes and triglycerides. Re-initiate infusion at a reduced rate when laboratory values are within normal limits. Consider discontinuation or dosage reduction in patients who develop liver test abnormalities. Stop infusion immediately at the first sign of a hypersensitivity reaction and treat as indicated (antihistamines, epinephrine, corticosteroids, airway management, oxygen). Resuscitate as necessary. In the event of an overdose, fat overload syndrome may result. Stop infusion and allow lipids to clear from serum. Effects are usually reversible after the lipid infusion is stopped. The lipid administered and the fatty acids produced are not dialyzable.

PROTHROMBIN COMPLEX CONCENTRATE (HUMAN) BBW

Antihemorrhagic

(**PRO**-throm-bin **KOM**-plex **KAN**-sen-trayt [**HUE**-man])

Kcentra

USUAL DOSE

(International Units [IU])

Pretreatment: Dosing should be individualized based on the patient's baseline International Normalized Ratio (INR) value and body weight.

Vitamin K: Administer vitamin K (phytonadione) concurrently to maintain vitamin K–dependent factor levels once the effects of the prothrombin complex concentrate (human) have diminished.

Prothrombin complex concentrate (human): Coagulation factor levels may be unstable in patients with acute major bleeding who are receiving vitamin K. Obtain baseline INR (close to time of dosing). Using this INR and the patient's weight, individualize dose as shown in the following chart.

Prothrombin Complex Concentrate (Human) Dosing Guidelines			
	Pretreatment INR		
	2 to Less Than 4	4 to 6	Greater Than 6
Dose of prothrombin complex concentrate [human][a] (units[b] of factor IX/kg body weight)	25 IU/kg	35 IU/kg	50 IU/kg
Maximum dose (units of factor IX)[c]	Not to exceed 2,500 IU	Not to exceed 3,500 IU	Not to exceed 5,000 IU

[a]Dose is based on body weight. Dose is also based on actual potency as stated on the carton, which will vary from 20 to 31 factor IX units/mL.
[b]Units refer to international units.
[c]Dose is based on body weight up to but not exceeding 100 kg. For patients weighing more than 100 kg, maximum dose should not be exceeded.

Example dosing calculation for an 80-kg patient with a baseline INR of 5:

$$35 \text{ units of factor IX/kg} \times 80 \text{ kg} = 2,800 \text{ units of factor IX required}$$

For a vial with an actual potency of 30 units/mL factor IX, 93 mL would be given:

$$2,800 \text{ units} \div 30 \text{ units/mL} = 93 \text{ mL}$$

Repeat dosing with prothrombin complex concentrate is not supported by clinical data and is not recommended.

DILUTION   **(International units [IU])**

Available in a kit that contains 500 units of prothrombin complex concentrate in a single-use vial, a 20-mL vial of SWFI, a Mix2Vial filter transfer set, and an alcohol swab. The actual potency per vial of factors II, VII, IX, and X and of proteins C and S is stated on the carton (potency in IU is defined by factor IX content). When reconstituted, the final concentration of drug product in factor IX units will range from 20 to 31 units/mL (400 to 620 units/vial) depending on actual potency, which is listed on the carton. Nominal potency is 500 units per vial, which is approximately 25 units/mL after reconstitution. Record the lot number of the product in the patient's medical record when prothrombin complex concentrate is administered.

Begin the reconstitution process by bringing prothrombin complex concentrate and diluent vial to room temperature. Use of aseptic technique required. Remove vial tops and wipe stoppers with the alcohol swab. Open the Mix2Vial transfer set package, leaving transfer set in the clear package. Place **diluent vial** on a flat surface and hold vial tightly. Grip the Mix2Vial transfer set together with the clear package and push the plastic spike at the **blue end of the transfer set** firmly through the center of the diluent vial stopper. Carefully remove the clear package from the Mix2Vial transfer set. With the **prothrombin complex concentrate vial** firmly on a flat surface, invert the diluent vial with the transfer set attached and push the plastic spike of the **transparent adapter** firmly through the center of the stopper of the prothrombin complex concentrate vial. The diluent will automatically transfer into the prothrombin complex concentrate vial. With both vials still attached to the transfer set, gently swirl the prothrombin complex concentrate vial to ensure complete dissolution. **Do not shake.** Solution should be colorless, clear to slightly opalescent, and free from visible particles. With one hand, grasp the prothrombin complex concentrate side of the Mix2Vial transfer set, and with the other hand grasp the blue diluent side of the Mix2Vial transfer set, and unscrew the set into two pieces. Draw air into an empty, sterile syringe. While the prothrombin complex concentrate vial is upright, screw the syringe to the Mix2Vial transfer set. Inject air into the vial. While keeping the syringe plunger pressed, invert the system upside down and draw the concentrate into the syringe by pulling the plunger back slowly. Unscrew the syringe from the transfer set and attach to a suitable intravenous administration set. If the same patient is to receive more than one vial, contents of multiple vials may be pooled. Use a separate, unused Mix2Vial transfer set for each product vial.

Storage: Store lyophilized powder in carton at 2° to 25° C (36° to 77° F); protect from light and freezing. Stable for 36 months from date of manufacture. Do not use beyond the expiration date on the carton and vial labels. Product must be used within 4 hours following reconstitution. Reconstituted product can be stored at 2° to 25° C. If cooled, the solution should be warmed to 20° to 25° C (68° to 77° F, approximate room temperature) before administration. Do not freeze reconstituted product. Discard partially used vials.

COMPATIBILITY

Manufacturer states, "Do not mix with other medicinal products; administer through a separate infusion line. No blood should enter the syringe, as there is a possibility of fibrin clot formation."

RATE OF ADMINISTRATION

Administer at room temperature at a rate of 3 unit/kg/min up to 8.4 mL/min = 25 mL over about 3 minutes

ACTIONS

A purified, heat-treated, nanofiltered, and lyophilized nonactivated four-factor prothrombin complex concentrate prepared from human U.S. Source Plasma. Contains the vitamin K–dependent coagulation factors II, VII, IX, and X (together known as the prothrombin complex) and the antithrombotic proteins C and S. Factor IX is the lead factor for the potency of the preparation. (Human antithrombin III, heparin and human albumin, sodium chloride, and sodium citrate are listed as excipients.) A dose-dependent acquired deficiency of the vitamin K–dependent coagulation factors occurs during vitamin K antagonist (VKA) treatment. Vitamin K antagonists exert anticoagulant effects by lowering both factor synthesis and function. Administration of prothrombin complex concentrate rapidly increases plasma levels of the vitamin K–dependent coagulation factors II, VII, IX, and X as well as the antithrombotic proteins C and S. In clinical trials, prothrombin complex concentrate restored the decreased vitamin K–dependent clotting factors significantly faster than plasma in patients on warfarin. A single dose of prothrombin complex concentrate produced a rapid and sustained increase in plasma levels of factors II, VII, IX, and X within 30 minutes posttreatment with 87% less volume than with plasma. In addition, infusion time with prothrombin complex concentrate was seven times faster than with plasma. In most subjects, prothrombin complex concentrate decreased INR to less than or equal to 1.3 within 30 minutes. The relationship between this or other INR values and clinical hemostasis in patients has not been established.

INDICATIONS AND USES

Indicated for the urgent reversal of acquired coagulation factor deficiency induced by vitamin K antagonists (e.g., warfarin) therapy in adult patients with acute major bleeding. Not indicated for urgent reversal of vitamin K antagonist anticoagulation in patients without acute major bleeding.

CONTRAINDICATIONS

Patients with known anaphylactic or severe systemic reactions to prothrombin complex concentrate or any of its components, including heparin; factors II, VII, IX, and X; proteins C and S; antithrombin III; and human albumin. ■ Patients with disseminated intravascular coagulation (DIC). ■ Patients with known heparin-induced thrombocytopenia (HIT). Prothrombin complex concentrate contains heparin.

PRECAUTIONS

For IV use only. ■ Hypersensitivity reactions have been reported. ■ Both fatal and nonfatal arterial and venous thromboembolic complications have been reported. Patients being treated with VKA therapy have underlying disease states that predispose them to thromboembolic events. The potential benefits of reversing VKA should be weighed against the potential risks of thromboembolic events, especially in patients with a history of a thromboembolic event. Resumption of anticoagulation should be carefully considered as soon as the risk of thromboembolic events outweighs the risk of acute bleeding. ■ Prothrombin complex concentrate has not been studied in subjects who have had a thromboembolic event, myocardial infarction, disseminated intravascular coagulation, cerebrovascular accident, transient ischemic attack, unstable angina pectoris, or severe peripheral vascular disease within the previous 3 months. Prothrombin complex concentrate may not be suitable in patients who have had a thromboembolic event in the previous 3 months. ▪ Made from human blood and may contain infectious agents (e.g., HIV, Creutzfeldt-Jakob disease, hepatitis B, hepatitis C). Numerous steps in the manufacturing process are used to make the potential for transmission of infectious agents extremely remote. ▪ Prothrombin complex concentrate has not been studied in patients with congenital factor deficiencies.

Monitor: Monitor INR and clinical response during and after treatment. ▪ Standard clinical assessments (e.g., VS, hemoglobin measurements, CT assessments relevant to the type of bleeding [e.g., GI, cerebral]) may be used to evaluate effective hemostasis. ▪ Monitor for S/S of hypersensitivity reactions (e.g., angioedema, anxiety, bronchospasm, dyspnea, flushing, hypotension, nausea, pulmonary edema, tachycardia, urticaria, wheezing, vomiting). ▪ Monitor for signs and symptoms of thromboembolic events (e.g., deep venous thrombosis, pulmonary embolism, stroke) during and after administration of prothrombin complex concentrate.

Patient Education: Report any S/S of hypersensitivity promptly (e.g., hives, rash, tightness of chest, wheezing). ▪ Report S/S of thrombosis (e.g., limb or abdominal swelling and/or pain, chest pain or pressure, shortness of breath, loss of sensation or motor power, altered consciousness, vision, or speech). ▪ Prothrombin complex concentrate is made from human blood and may carry a remote risk of transmitting infectious agents. See Precautions.

Maternal/Child: Category C: safety for use during pregnancy, labor and delivery, and during breast-feeding not established; use only if clearly indicated. ▪ Safety and effectiveness for use in pediatric patients not established.

Elderly: Response similar to other age-groups.

DRUG/LAB INTERACTIONS

Specific information not available.

SIDE EFFECTS

The most common side effects observed were arthralgia, headache, hypotension, nausea, and vomiting. The most serious side effects were thromboembolic events, including deep vein thrombosis, pulmonary embolism, and stroke. Other side effects included abnormal breath sounds, chest pain, constipation, dyspnea, fluid overload, hypertension, hypokalemia, hypoxia, insomnia, intracranial hemorrhage, mental status changes, myocardial infarction, myocardial ischemia, pulmonary edema, respiratory distress, and tachycardia.

Post-Marketing: Hypersensitivity or allergic reactions (e.g., angioedema, anxiety, bronchospasm, dyspnea, flushing, hypotension, nausea, pulmonary edema, tachycardia, urticaria, vomiting, wheezing) and thromboembolic complications (arterial thromboembolic events [arterial thrombosis, acute MI], venous thromboembolic events [pulmonary embolism and venous thrombosis], and DIC).

ANTIDOTE

Notify physician of any side effect. If a severe hypersensitivity or anaphylactic-type reaction occurs, immediately discontinue administration and institute appropriate treatment (e.g., oxygen, hydrocortisone, epinephrine, diphenhydramine, famotidine).

RASBURICASE BBW
(ras-**BYOUR**-ih-kase)

Antihyperuricemic
Enzyme, urate-oxidase
(recombinant)

Elitek

USUAL DOSE
Pretreatment: Prehydration and baseline studies required; see Monitor.

0.2 mg/kg as a single daily dose each day for up to 5 days. Dosing beyond 5 days and/or administration of more than one course of rasburicase is not recommended. Safety and effectiveness of other schedules have not been evaluated. Alternate unlabeled single- and multiple-dose regimens have been used; see literature.

PEDIATRIC DOSE
Same as adult dose; see Maternal/Child.

DOSE ADJUSTMENTS
No dose adjustments recommended.

DILUTION
Available in 1.5- and 7.5-mg single-dose vials with manufacturer-supplied diluent (SWFI and Poloxamer 188). Determine the vial size and/or number of vials needed to provide the calculated dose. Reconstitute each 1.5-mg vial with 1 mL of diluent and each 7.5-mg vial with 5 mL of diluent. Final concentration is 1.5 mg/mL. Mix by swirling gently. *Do not shake.* Withdraw the calculated dose of reconstituted solution and inject into an infusion bag containing the appropriate volume of NS to achieve a final total volume of 50 mL. (For example a 20-kg child would receive a dose of 4 mg [20 kg × 0.2 mg/kg = 4 mg]. Reconstitute 3 vials, each with 1 mL of the diluent provided. Withdraw 2.7 mL of reconstituted solution and add to an infusion bag containing 47.3 mL of NS.)

Filters: *No filter should be used during reconstitution or infusion of rasburicase.*

Storage: Refrigerate unopened lyophilized drug product and diluent. Do not freeze; protect from light. Both the reconstituted and diluted product may be stored for 24 hours if refrigerated. Discard any unused product.

COMPATIBILITY
Manufacturer states, "Should be infused through a different line than that used for the infusion of other concomitant medications. If use of a separate line is not possible, the line should be flushed with at least 15 mL of NS prior to and after infusion with rasburicase."

RATE OF ADMINISTRATION
A single dose as an infusion equally distributed over 30 minutes. *Do not administer as a bolus infusion. Do not filter infusion.*

ACTIONS
A recombinant urate-oxidase enzyme produced by genetic engineering. Catalyzes enzymatic oxidation of uric acid into an inactive and soluble metabolite (allantoin). Onset of action is 4 hours. Mean terminal half-life is similar between pediatric and adult patients and ranges from 15.7 to 22.5 hours.

INDICATIONS AND USES
Initial management of plasma uric acid levels in pediatric and adult patients with leukemia, lymphoma, and solid tumor malignancies who are receiving anticancer therapy that is expected to result in tumor lysis and subsequent elevation of plasma uric acid.

Limitation of use: Indicated only for a single course of treatment.

CONTRAINDICATIONS
Glucose-6-phosphate dehydrogenase (G6PD) deficiency. ▪ History of anaphylaxis or severe hypersensitivity to rasburicase. ▪ History of development of hemolytic reactions or methemoglobinemia with rasburicase.

PRECAUTIONS
May cause serious and fatal hypersensitivity reactions, including anaphylaxis. Reactions may occur at any time during treatment, including with the first dose; see Monitor and Antidote.

■ Has caused severe hemolytic reactions in patients with G6PD deficiency. It is recommended that patients at higher risk for G6PD deficiency (e.g., patients of African or Mediterranean descent) be screened for G6PD deficiency before starting rasburicase therapy. See Contraindications and Antidote. ■ Methemoglobinemia has been reported. Patients developed serious hypoxemia, requiring intervention. See Antidote. ■ As with all therapeutic proteins, there is the potential for immunogenicity. May elicit antibodies that inhibit the activity of rasburicase.

Monitor: Monitor serum uric acid levels, electrolytes, and renal function before and during therapy. ■ Patients should be hydrated intravenously according to standard medical practice for the management of plasma uric acid in patients at risk for tumor lysis syndrome (TLS). ■ Observe for signs of TLS (e.g., hyperuricemia, hyperkalemia, hyperphosphatemia, and hypocalcemia). If untreated, may develop acute uric acid nephropathy, leading to renal failure. ■ Monitor for S/S of a hypersensitivity reaction (e.g., anaphylaxis, bronchospasm, chest pain and tightness, dyspnea, hypotension, hypoxia, shock, urticaria). ■ Screen patients at risk for hemolysis; see Contraindications and Precautions. Monitor for S/S of hemolysis (e.g., anemia, jaundice with increased indirect bilirubin and LDH, pallor, reduced haptoglobin). In studies, severe hemolytic reactions occurred within 2 to 4 days of the start of therapy. ■ Monitor for S/S of methemoglobinemia (e.g., cyanosis, dyspnea, headache, hypoxemia, lethargy, methemoglobin). ■ Will cause enzymatic degradation of uric acid within blood samples left at room temperature, resulting in falsely low uric acid levels. To ensure accurate measurement, blood must be collected into prechilled tubes containing heparin anticoagulant and immediately *immersed and maintained* in an ice water bath. Plasma samples must be prepared by centrifugation in a precooled centrifuge (4° C [39° F]). Plasma samples must be analyzed within 4 hours of sample collection.

Patient Education: Report blood in urine, painful urination, or signs of a hypersensitivity reaction promptly. ■ See Maternal/Child.

Maternal/Child: Based on animal studies, may cause fetal harm. Potential benefits must justify potential risks to fetus. ■ Breastfeeding is not recommended during treatment and for 2 weeks after the last dose. ■ Studied in pediatric patients from 1 month to 17 years of age. Pediatric patients under 2 years of age had a higher mean uric acid AUC and a lower rate of success at achieving normal uric acid concentrations by 48 hours than did older pediatric patients.

Elderly: No overall differences in pharmacokinetics, safety, and effectiveness were observed between elderly and younger patients.

DRUG/LAB INTERACTIONS

Studies have not been conducted. ■ Will cause enzymatic degradation of uric acid within blood samples left at room temperature, resulting in **falsely low uric acid levels;** see Monitor.

SIDE EFFECTS

The most common adverse reactions are abdominal pain, anxiety, constipation, diarrhea, fever, headache, hypophosphatemia, increased ALT, nausea, peripheral edema, pharyngolaryngeal pain, and vomiting. Serious adverse reactions observed are hemolysis, hypersensitivity reactions (e.g., anaphylaxis, arthralgia, chest pain, dyspnea, hypotension, injection site irritation, peripheral edema, rash, urticaria), methemoglobinemia, and severe rash. Other observed reactions include abdominal and GI infections, acute renal failure, fluid overload, hyperbilirubinemia, hyperphosphatemia, ischemic coronary artery disorders, mucositis, pulmonary hemorrhage, rash, respiratory distress/failure, sepsis, and supraventricular arrhythmias.

Post-Marketing: Anaphylaxis with potential fatal outcome, convulsions, muscle contractions (involuntary).

ANTIDOTE

Notify physician of all side effects. Should be immediately and permanently discontinued in patients who experience severe hypersensitivity reactions, hemolysis, or methemoglobinemia. Do not rechallenge. Treat anaphylaxis with epinephrine, corticosteroids (e.g., dexamethasone), oxygen, and antihistamines (diphenhydramine). Hemolysis or methemoglobinemia may require transfusion support. Methylene blue may be required for treatment of methemoglobinemia. There is no specific antidote. Resuscitate as indicated.

RAVULIZUMAB-cwvz BBW

(**RAV**-ue-**LIZ**-ue-mab)

Monoclonal antibody

Ultomiris

pH 7

USUAL DOSE

Pretreatment: Vaccinate patients for meningococcal disease according to current Advisory Committee on Immunization Practices (ACIP) recommendations for meningococcal vaccination in patients with complement deficiencies.

Premedication: Provide 2 weeks of antibacterial drug prophylaxis to patients if ravulizumab-cwvz must be initiated immediately and vaccines are administered less than 2 weeks before starting ravulizumab-cwvz therapy.

Paroxysmal nocturnal hemoglobinuria (PNH): Weight-based dosing for adults weighing 40 kg or greater consists of a loading dose followed 2 weeks later by a maintenance dose. Repeat maintenance doses every 8 weeks. Administer doses based on body weight as outlined in the following chart.

Ravulizumab-cwvz Weight-Based Dosing Regimen (PNH)			
Body Weight Range (kg)	**Loading Dose (mg)**	**Maintenance Dose (mg)**	
≥40 to <60 kg	2,400 mg	3,000 mg	
≥60 kg to <100 kg	2,700 mg	3,300 mg	Every 8 weeks
≥100 kg	3,000 mg	3,600 mg	

Atypical hemolytic uremic syndrome (aHUS): Weight-based dosing for adult and pediatric patients 1 month of age and older weighing 5 kg or greater consists of a loading dose followed 2 weeks later by a maintenance dose. Repeat maintenance doses every 4 or 8 weeks based on body weight as outlined in the following chart.

Ravulizumab-cwvz Weight-Based Dosing Regimen (aHUS)			
Body Weight Range (kg)	**Loading Dose (mg)**	**Maintenance Dose (mg) and Dosing Interval**	
≥5 to <10 kg	600 mg	300 mg	
≥10 to <20 kg	600 mg	600 mg	Every 4 weeks
≥20 to <30 kg	900 mg	2,100 mg	
≥30 to <40 kg	1,200 mg	2,700 mg	
≥40 to <60 kg	2,400 mg	3,000 mg	Every 8 weeks
≥60 to <100 kg	2,700 mg	3,300 mg	
≥100 kg	3,000 mg	3,600 mg	

For either indication, the dosing schedule is allowed to occasionally vary within 7 days of the scheduled infusion day (except for the first maintenance dose), but the subsequent dose should be administered according to the original schedule. For patients switching from eculizumab to ravulizumab-cwvz, administer the loading dose of ravulizumab-cwvz 2 weeks after the last eculizumab infusion, and then administer maintenance doses once every 8 weeks or every 4 weeks (depending on body weight) starting 2 weeks after loading dose administration.

DOSE ADJUSTMENTS

Age (18 to 83 years), sex, race, hepatic impairment, or any degree of renal impairment do not appear to influence the pharmacokinetics of ravulizumab-cwvz. ▪ Administration of PE/PI (plasmapheresis or plasma exchange or fresh-frozen plasma infusion) may reduce ravulizumab-cwvz serum levels. There is no experience with administration of supplemental doses of ravulizumab-cwvz.

DILUTION

Available in 300 mg/30 mL (10 mg/mL) single-dose vials. A clear to translucent, slight whitish color solution. The number of vials to be diluted is determined based on the individual patient's weight and the prescribed dose. Withdraw the calculated volume of ravulizumab-cwvz from the appropriate number of vials and dilute in an infusion bag using NS to a final concentration of 5 mg/mL. Mix gently. Do not shake. **Protect from light. Do not freeze.** Refer to the following administration reference charts. Allow the diluted solution to reach room temperature before infusion. Do not use an artificial heat source (e.g., microwave). Contains no preservatives. Administer the prepared solution immediately after preparation.

Ravulizumab-cwvz Loading Dose Administration Reference Table						
Body Weight Range (kg)[a]	Loading Dose (mg)	Ravulizumab-cwvz Volume (mL)	Volume of NaCl Diluent[b] (mL)	Total Volume (mL)	Minimum Infusion Time (hr)	Maximum Infusion Rate (mL/hr)
≥5 to <10 kg	600 mg	60 mL	60 mL	120 mL	3.8 hr	31 mL/hr
≥10 to <20 kg	600 mg	60 mL	60 mL	120 mL	1.9 hr	63 mL/hr
≥20 to <30 kg	900 mg	90 mL	90 mL	180 mL	1.5 hr	120 mL/hr
≥30 to <40 kg	1,200 mg	120 mL	120 mL	240 mL	1.3 hr	184 mL/hr
≥40 to <60 kg	2,400 mg	240 mL	240 mL	480 mL	1.9 hr	252 mL/hr
≥60 to <100 kg	2,700 mg	270 mL	270 mL	540 mL	1.7 hr	317 mL/hr
≥100 kg	3,000 mg	300 mL	300 mL	600 mL	1.8 hr	333 mL/hr

[a]Body weight at time of treatment.
[b]Dilute ravulizumab-cwvz using only 0.9% sodium chloride injection, USP.

Ravulizumab-cwvz Maintenance Dose Administration Reference Table						
Body Weight Range (kg)[a]	Maintenance Dose (mg)	Ravulizumab-cwvz Volume (mL)	Volume of NaCl Diluent[b] (mL)	Total Volume (mL)	Minimum Infusion Time (hr)	Maximum Infusion Rate (mL/hr)
≥5 to <10 kg	300 mg	30 mL	30 mL	60 mL	1.9 hr	31 mL/hr
≥10 to <20 kg	600 mg	60 mL	60 mL	120 mL	1.9 hr	63 mL/hr
≥20 to <30 kg	2,100 mg	210 mL	210 mL	420 mL	3.3 hr	127 mL/hr
≥30 to <40 kg	2,700 mg	270 mL	270 mL	540 mL	2.8 hr	192 mL/hr
≥40 to <60 kg	3,000 mg	300 mL	300 mL	600 mL	2.3 hr	257 mL/hr
≥60 to <100 kg	3,300 mg	330 mL	330 mL	660 mL	2 hr	330 mL/hr
≥100 kg	3,600 mg	360 mL	360 mL	720 mL	2.2 hr	327 mL/hr

[a]Body weight at time of treatment.
[b]Dilute ravulizumab-cwvz using only 0.9% sodium chloride injection, USP.

Filters: Administer only through a 0.2- or a 0.22-micron filter.

Storage: Store ravulizumab-cwvz vials refrigerated at 2° to 8° C (36° to 46° F) in original carton and protect from light. Do not freeze. Do not shake. If diluted solution is not used immediately, storage under refrigeration at 2° to 8° C (36° to 46° F) must not exceed 24 hours, taking into account the expected infusion time. Once removed from refrigeration, administer the diluted ravulizumab-cwvz infusion solution within 6 hours. Protect from light. Do not freeze or shake.

COMPATIBILITY

Compatibility information not available from manufacturer; consult a pharmacist.

RATE OF ADMINISTRATION

Administer through a 0.2- or a 0.22-micron filter. Administer as an IV infusion as outlined in the reference charts in Dilution.

ACTIONS

Ravulizumab-cwvz is a terminal complement inhibitor that specifically binds to the complement protein C5 with high affinity, thereby inhibiting its cleavage to C5a (the proinflammatory anaphylatoxin) and C5b (the initiating subunit of the terminal complement complex [C5b-9]) and preventing the generation of the terminal complement complex C5b-9. Ravulizumab-cwvz inhibits terminal complement-mediated intravascular hemolysis in patients with paroxysmal nocturnal hemoglobinuria (PNH) and complement-mediated thrombotic microangiopathy (TMA) in patients with atypical hemolytic uremic syndrome (aHUS). The mean terminal elimination half-lives in patients with PNH and aHUS are 49.7 and 51.8 days, respectively.

INDICATIONS AND USES

Treatment of adult patients with PNH. ▪ Treatment of adult and pediatric patients 1 month of age and older with aHUS to inhibit complement-mediated TMA.

Limitation of Use: Ravulizumab-cwvz is not indicated for the treatment of patients with Shiga toxin *Escherichia coli*–related hemolytic uremic syndrome (STEC-HUS).

CONTRAINDICATIONS

Patients with unresolved *Neisseria meningitidis* infection. ▪ Patients who are not currently vaccinated against *N. meningitidis* unless the risks of delaying ravulizumab-cwvz treatment outweigh the risks of developing a meningococcal infection.

PRECAUTIONS

For IV infusion only. ▪ Life-threatening meningococcal infection/sepsis has occurred. Meningococcal infection may become rapidly life-threatening or fatal if not recognized and treated early. ▪ Comply with the most current ACIP recommendations for meningococcal vaccination in patients with complement deficiencies. Revaccinate according to current medical guidelines, considering the duration of ravulizumab-cwvz therapy. ▪ A meningococcal vaccine must be administered at least 2 weeks before administering the first dose of ravulizumab-cwvz unless the risk of delaying ravulizumab-cwvz therapy outweighs the risk of developing a meningococcal infection. Vaccination reduces, but does not eliminate, the risk of meningococcal infections. ▪ Ravulizumab-cwvz blocks terminal complement activation; therefore there is an increased susceptibility to encapsulated bacterial infections, especially infections caused by *N. meningitidis* but also *Streptococcus pneumoniae, Hemophilus influenzae,* and, to a lesser extent, *Neisseria gonorrhoeae.* Administer vaccinations for the prevention of *S. pneumoniae* and *H. influenzae* type b (Hib) according to ACIP guidelines. ▪ Infusion reactions have occurred. However, in clinical trials these reactions did not require discontinuation of therapy. ▪ Continue established anticoagulant therapy during ravulizumab-cwvz treatment; the effect of withdrawal of anticoagulant therapy during ravulizumab-cwvz therapy has not been established. ▪ Ravulizumab-cwvz is available only through a restricted program under a Risk Evaluation and Mitigation Strategy (REMS). Under the ravulizumab-cwvz REMS, prescribers must enroll in the program. ▪ Treatment of aHUS should be a minimum duration of 6 months. Treatment duration beyond the initial 6 months should be individualized. ▪ As with all therapeutic proteins, there is a risk of immunogenicity.

Monitor: Closely monitor for early S/S of meningococcal infection (moderate to severe headache with nausea or vomiting, fever, or a stiff neck or stiff back; fever of 39.4° C [103° F] or higher; fever and a rash; confusion; and/or severe muscle aches with flu-like symptoms and light sensitivity) and evaluate patients immediately if infection is suspected. Consider discontinuation in patients who are undergoing treatment for serious meningococcal infection. ▪ Monitor for other types of infections or S/S of a worsening infection. ▪ Monitor for S/S of an infusion or hypersensitivity reaction (drop in blood pressure, infusion-related pain, and lower back pain) during infusion and for at least 1 hour after infusion. Slow or discontinue the infusion at the discretion of the physician. ▪ Monitor PNH patients who discontinue ravulizumab-cwvz for a minimum of 16 weeks to detect hemolysis identified by elevated LDH along with sudden decrease in PNH clone size or hemoglobin and to detect reappearance of symptoms such as fatigue, hemoglobinuria, abdominal pain, shortness of breath, major adverse vascular event (including thrombosis), dysphagia, or erectile dysfunction. If S/S of hemolysis occur after discontinuation, consider restarting therapy. ▪ Monitor aHUS patients who discontinue ravulizumab-cwvz therapy for a minimum of 12 months for TMA complications. TMA complications may be identified by clinical symptoms (e.g., angina, changes in mental status, dyspnea, increasing BP, seizure, or thrombosis) in addition to at least two of the following laboratory values observed concurrently (and confirmed by a second measurement 28 days apart): a decrease in platelet count of 25% or more compared with baseline or peak platelet count during treatment, an increase in SCr of 25% or more as compared with baseline or to nadir during treatment, or an increase in serum LDH of 25% or more as compared with baseline or to nadir during treatment. If S/S of TMA complications occur after discontinuation, consider restarting therapy. ▪ See Antidote.

Patient Education: Read the patient medication guide before initiating ravulizumab-cwvz. ▪ Meningococcal vaccination is required 2 weeks before initiating therapy if not previously vaccinated. Vaccination may not prevent meningococcal infection. Seek immediate medical attention if confusion, eyes sensitive to light, fever with or without a rash, headache associated with fever, nausea, vomiting, stiff back or neck, or muscle aches with flu-like symptoms occur. ▪ Carry ravulizumab-cwvz patient safety card at all times. ▪ Promptly report other S/S of an infection. Prevent gonorrheal infections; patients at risk should be tested regularly. ▪ Promptly report chills, dyspnea, and/or itching during or soon after an infusion. ▪ Patients with PNH or aHUS may develop hemolysis or TMA, respectively, when ravulizumab-cwvz therapy is discontinued. Prolonged monitoring (at least 16 weeks for patients with PNH and at least 12 months for patients with aHUS) is required. If ravulizumab-cwvz therapy is discontinued, keep Ultomiris Patient Safety Card on self for 8 months after the last dose.

Maternal/Child: There are no available data on ravulizumab-cwvz use in pregnant females. However, PNH in pregnancy is associated with adverse maternal outcomes, including worsening cytopenias, thrombotic events, infections, bleeding, miscarriages, and increased maternal mortality, as well as adverse fetal outcomes, including fetal death and premature delivery. aHUS is associated with adverse maternal outcomes, including pre-eclampsia and preterm delivery, and adverse fetal/neonatal outcomes, including intrauterine growth restriction, fetal death, and low birth weight. ▪ Discontinue breastfeeding during treatment and for 8 months after the final dose. ▪ The safety and efficacy of ravulizumab-cwvz for the treatment of PNH in pediatric patients have not been established. The safety and efficacy of ravulizumab-cwvz for the treatment of aHUS in pediatric patients 1 month of age and older have been established.

Elderly: Clinical studies of ravulizumab-cwvz did not include sufficient numbers of subjects 65 years of age and older to determine whether they respond differently from younger subjects.

DRUG/LAB INTERACTIONS

Continue established anticoagulant therapy during ravulizumab-cwvz treatment; the effect of withdrawal of anticoagulant therapy during ravulizumab-cwvz therapy has not been established.

SIDE EFFECTS

PNH: The most frequent side effects (>10%) were headache and upper respiratory tract infection. Serious side effects reported included fever and hyperthermia. Fatal sepsis has also occurred. Other side effects included abdominal pain, arthralgia, diarrhea, dizziness, nausea, and pain in extremity.

aHUS: The most frequent side effects (>20%) were diarrhea, fever, headache, hypertension, nausea, upper respiratory tract infections, and vomiting. Serious side effects reported included abdominal pain, hypertension, and pneumonia. Fatal sepsis has also occurred. Other side effects included alopecia, anemia, anxiety, arthralgia, back pain, constipation, cough, decreased appetite, decreased vitamin D, dry skin, dyspnea, edema, fatigue, GI infection, hypokalemia, hypotension, iron deficiency, lymphadenopathy, myalgia, pain in extremities, rash, tonsillitis, and urinary tract infection.

ANTIDOTE

Keep physician informed of all side effects. If an adverse reaction occurs during administration, slow or discontinue the infusion at the discretion of the physician. Interrupt ravulizumab-cwvz infusion and institute appropriate supportive measurements if signs of cardiovascular instability or respiratory compromise occur.

REMDESIVIR Antiviral
(rem-**DE**-si-vir)

Veklury

USUAL DOSE
200 mg IV on Day 1 followed by 100 mg once daily. Duration varies; generally 5 to 10 days based on specific patient needs and parameters.

PEDIATRIC DOSE
Weight 3.5 kg to less than 40 kg: 5 mg/kg/dose on Day 1 followed by 2.5 mg/kg/dose once daily.
Weight greater than 40 kg: 200 mg IV on Day 1 followed by 100 mg IV once daily.

DOSE ADJUSTMENTS
Renal: No dosage adjustment is required; however, no formal safety or pharmacokinetic data are available. The manufacturer does not recommend use for patients with eGFR less than 30 mL/min; however, short-term use is unlikely to result in significant toxicity.
Hepatic: No dosage adjustments are provided by the manufacturer. Studies suggest that if ALT is greater than 10 times the ULN; consider discontinuation. The drug should be discontinued if patient also exhibits signs of liver inflammation along with ALT elevation.

DILUTION
Preparation should occur on the day of administration. Diluted preparations in IV bags can be stored for 24 hours at room temperature or for 48 hours under refrigeration.
Injection solution concentrate (5 mg/mL) for adults and pediatric patients 40 kg or greater: Prior to dilution, allow injection solution vial to warm to room temperature. Withdraw and discard the required volume of NS from the infusion bag (40 mL for a 200-mg dose; 20 mL for a 100-mg dose). Transfer required volume of remdesivir, based on dose, to a 250-mL infusion bag and gently invert 20 times to mix the solution; *do not shake*. Discard unused portion.
Pediatric patients 3.5 kg to less than 40 kg:
Prefilled NS bag: From a bag of NS, withdraw a volume equal to the volume of the reconstituted remdesivir dose, plus additional volume as needed to result in a final concentration of 1.25 mg/mL. Withdraw the required volume of the reconstituted remdesivir solution for the patient-specific dose and add to the NS infusion bag. Gently invert the bag 20 times to mix the solution in the bag. *Do not shake*.

COMPATIBILITY
Do not administer simultaneously with any other medication or IV solutions other than normal saline.

RATE OF ADMINISTRATION
Administer as an IV infusion over 30 to 120 minutes.

ACTIONS
Remdesivir inhibits the SARS-CoV-2 RNA-dependent RNA polymerase (RdRp), which is necessary for viral replication. Remdesivir is a prodrug that is metabolized to the active nucleoside triphosphate metabolite, which then competes for incorporation into RNA chains, resulting in delayed chain termination during viral RNA replication. Remdesivir triphosphate can also inhibit viral RNA synthesis due to incorporation into the viral RNA template.

INDICATIONS AND USES
Remdesivir is FDA-approved for treatment of COVID-19 in hospitalized patients. Remdesivir should be used only in hospitalized patients.

CONTRAINDICATIONS
Hypersensitivity to remdesivir or any component of the formulation.

PRECAUTIONS
Hypersensitivity and infusion-related reactions: Hypersensitivity reactions, including anaphylactic and infusion-related reactions, have been reported during and after administration.

Hepatic effects: Elevated transaminases. Consider discontinuation in patients who develop ALT greater than 10 times the ULN, and discontinue if symptoms of liver inflammation appear.

Renal function impairment: Although the manufacturer recommends against use in patients with eGFR less than 30 mL/min, significant toxicity with a short duration of therapy (5 to 10 days) is unlikely.

Injectable dosage Form: Remdesivir contains cyclodextrin (sulfobutylether-beta-cyclodextrin; 6 g per 100 mg remdesivir [injection solution] or 3 g per 100 mg remdesivir [lyophilized powder]) as an excipient, which may accumulate in patients with renal impairment. The manufacturer recommends use of only the lyophilized powder in pediatric patients under 12 years of age or weighing less than 40 kg.

Monitor: Monitor for signs and symptoms of hypersensitivity reactions, including anaphylaxis, and for signs of liver inflammation. As clinically appropriate, monitor liver function and renal function tests.

Patient Education: Promptly report any signs of hypersensitivity (e.g., difficulty breathing, hives, itching, rash) or liver problems (e.g., dark urine, stomach pain, light-colored stools, or yellow skin or eyes) or infusion-related reactions (nausea, vomiting, sweating, shivering, dizziness).

Maternal/Child: Based on preliminary data, use in pregnant females should not be withheld if it is clinically needed. It is not known if remdesivir passes into breast milk.

Elderly: Refer to Usual Dose and Precautions.

DRUG/LAB INTERACTIONS
Choloroquine, hydroxychloroquine, and strong CYP-3A4 inducers may decrease the effectiveness of remdesivir.

SIDE EFFECTS
Skin rash, nausea, prolonged PT, elevated transaminases, hypersensitivity, seizures.

ANTIDOTE
Discontinue infusion and treat appropriately for severe hypersensitivity reactions. Stop treatment if ALTs are greater than 10 times the ULN.

RESLIZUMAB BBW
(res-**LIZ**-ue-mab)

Cinqair

Interleukin-5 antagonist
Monoclonal antibody (IgG4$_K$)

pH 5.5

USUAL DOSE
Pretreatment: Testing for eosinophilic phenotype indicated. See Maternal/Child.

Reslizumab: 3 mg/kg once every 4 weeks as an infusion over 20 to 50 minutes.

DOSE ADJUSTMENTS
No dose adjustments required based on age, gender, or race. Clinical studies have not been conducted to assess the effect of hepatic or renal impairment on the pharmacokinetics of reslizumab.

DILUTION
Supplied as a clear to slightly hazy/opalescent, colorless to slightly yellow solution in single-use vials containing 100 mg/10 mL (10 mg/mL). May contain a few translucent to white amorphous particulates. **Do not shake.** Aseptic technique required. Allow solution to reach room temperature. Withdraw the proper volume of reslizumab from the vial(s) based on the recommended weight-based dose and slowly add to a 50-mL infusion bag of NS. Gently invert to mix the solution. **Do not shake.**

Filters: Use of an infusion set with an in-line, low–protein-binding, 0.2-micron filter is required. **Compatible** with polyethersulfone (PES), polyvinylidene fluoride (PVDF), nylon, and cellulose acetate in-line infusion filters.

Storage: Before use, refrigerate at 2° to 8° C (36° to 46° F) in original carton to protect from light. Do not freeze. *Do not shake.* Administer diluted solution immediately after preparation or may be refrigerated or kept at RT (up to 25° C [77° F]), protected from light, for up to 16 hours. Time between preparation and administration should not exceed 16 hours. If refrigerated before administration, allow the diluted solution to reach RT. Discard unused portion.

COMPATIBILITY

Manufacturer states, "Do not mix or dilute with other drugs. Do not infuse concomitantly in the same IV line with other agents." **Compatible** with polyvinylchloride (PVC) or polyolefin infusion bags and with polyethersulfone (PES), polyvinylidene fluoride (PVDF), nylon, and cellulose acetate in-line infusion filters.

RATE OF ADMINISTRATION

For IV infusion only. Do not administer as an IV push or bolus. Use of an infusion set with an in-line, low–protein-binding, 0.2-micron filter is required.

Administer a single dose as an infusion over 20 to 50 minutes. Infusion time varies depending on total volume to be infused based on weight-based dosing. After administration, flush the IV line with NS to ensure that all of the reslizumab has been administered.

ACTIONS

Inflammation is an important component in the pathogenesis of asthma. Multiple cell types and mediators are involved in inflammation. Reslizumab is a humanized interleukin-5 antagonist monoclonal antibody (IgG4, kappa). IL-5 is the major cytokine responsible for the growth and differentiation, recruitment, activation, and survival of eosinophils. Reslizumab binds to IL-5, inhibiting the bioactivity of IL-5. By inhibiting IL-5 signaling, reslizumab reduces the production and survival of eosinophils, one of the cell types implicated in the inflammation seen with asthma. Specific mechanism of action not definitively established. Following administration of reslizumab, reductions in blood eosinophil counts were observed and maintained through 52 weeks of treatment. There is minimal distribution into the extravascular tissues. Reslizumab is degraded by enzymatic proteolysis into small peptides and amino acids. Half-life is approximately 24 days.

INDICATIONS AND USES

Add-on maintenance treatment of patients with severe asthma who have an eosinophilic phenotype and are 18 years of age or older. **Limitations of use:** Not indicated for the treatment of other eosinophilic conditions. ▪ Not indicated for the relief of acute bronchospasm or status asthmaticus.

CONTRAINDICATIONS

Known hypersensitivity to reslizumab or any of its excipients.

PRECAUTIONS

For IV use only. ▪ Administered by or under the direction of a physician knowledgeable in its use and in a facility equipped to monitor the patient and respond to any medical emergency. ▪ Hypersensitivity reactions, including anaphylaxis, have been reported. ▪ Should not be used to treat acute asthma symptoms or acute exacerbations. Do not use to treat acute bronchospasm or status asthmaticus. ▪ Malignant neoplasms have been reported. The majority were diagnosed within less than 6 months of exposure to reslizumab. The observed malignancies were diverse in nature and without clustering of any particular tissue type. ▪ No clinical studies have been conducted to assess the reduction of maintenance corticosteroid doses following administration of reslizumab. Do not discontinue systemic or inhaled corticosteroids abruptly upon initiation of reslizumab therapy. Reductions in corticosteroid dose, if appropriate, should be gradual and under physician supervision. ▪ Eosinophils may be involved in the immunologic response to some helminth infections. The effects of reslizumab on the immune response against parasitic infections are unknown. Patients with known parasitic infections were excluded from clinical studies. ▪ A therapeutic protein, there is a potential for immunogenicity. ▪ See Monitor.

Monitor: Monitor for S/S of a hypersensitivity reaction during and following completion of the infusion. In clinical trials, anaphylaxis was observed during or within 20 minutes after completion of the infusion and was reported as early as the second dose of reslizumab. Manifestations included decreased oxygen saturation, dyspnea, skin and mucosal involvement (including urticaria), vomiting, and wheezing. ■ If a taper in the maintenance steroid dose is initiated, monitor for systemic withdrawal symptoms and/or conditions previously suppressed by systemic corticosteroid therapy. ■ Treat pre-existing helminth infections before initiating reslizumab. Discontinue treatment until infection resolves in patients who become infected during therapy and do not respond to anti-helminth treatment.

Patient Education: Immediately report any S/S of a hypersensitivity reaction (e.g., chest discomfort, cough, dyspnea, postural dizziness, pruritus, rash, throat irritation, urticaria, wheezing) occurring during or after administration. ■ Does not treat acute asthma symptoms or acute exacerbations. Seek medical advice if asthma remains uncontrolled or worsens after initiation of treatment with reslizumab. ■ Malignancies have been reported. ■ Do not discontinue or reduce the dose of maintenance systemic or inhaled corticosteroids except under the direct supervision of a physician.

Maternal/Child: Use during pregnancy only if clearly needed. In females with poorly or moderately controlled asthma, evidence demonstrates an increased risk of pre-eclampsia in the mother and an increased risk of prematurity, low birth weight, and smaller for gestational age in the neonate. The level of asthma control should be closely monitored in pregnant females and treatment adjusted as necessary to maintain optimal control. Monoclonal antibodies such as reslizumab cross the placental barrier. The potential effects on a fetus are likely to be greater during the second and third trimester of pregnancy. Consider the long half-life of reslizumab. ■ Use caution during breastfeeding; effects unknown. ■ Safety and effectiveness for use in pediatric patients 17 years of age or younger not established.

Elderly: No overall differences in safety or effectiveness observed between younger patients and patients 65 years of age and older. No dose adjustment is necessary.

DRUG/LAB INTERACTIONS

No formal drug interaction studies have been performed. Population pharmacokinetics analyses indicate that concomitant use of either leukotriene antagonists (e.g., montelukast) or corticosteroids does not affect the pharmacokinetics of reslizumab.

SIDE EFFECTS

Oropharyngeal pain is the most common side effect. Less commonly reported adverse reactions include myalgia and transient creatine phosphokinase (CPK) elevations. Hypersensitivity reactions (including anaphylaxis) and malignancy are the most serious side effects.

ANTIDOTE

Keep the physician informed of all side effects. Most will be treated symptomatically. If a hypersensitivity reaction occurs, discontinue the infusion immediately and treat with oxygen, epinephrine, antihistamines (e.g., IV diphenhydramine), corticosteroids, albuterol, vasopressors (e.g., dopamine), and ventilation equipment as indicated. Symptoms of overdose were not noted in clinical trials. If overdose occurs, monitor patients for S/S of adverse effects. Resuscitate as necessary.

RETEPLASE RECOMBINANT
(**REE**-teh-place re-**KOM**-buh-nant)

Thrombolytic agent
(recombinant)

pH 7 to 7.4

USUAL DOSE
Pretreatment: Baseline assessment and studies indicated; see Monitor.

Administered concomitantly with heparin. Give a 5,000-unit IV bolus of heparin before the initial injection of reteplase, then give 10 units (10 mL) of reteplase as an IV injection. Follow with a 1,000 unit/hr continuous IV infusion of heparin for at least 24 hours. Give a second 10-unit bolus of reteplase 30 minutes after the first. See Dilution, Compatibility, and Rate of Administration. Aspirin is also used either during or following heparin treatment; an initial dose of 160 to 350 mg is followed by doses of 75 to 350 mg.

DOSE ADJUSTMENTS
The second bolus should not be given if serious bleeding in a critical location (e.g., intracranial, gastrointestinal, retroperitoneal, pericardial) occurs before it is due to be given.

DILUTION
Supplied in a kit with all components for reconstitution. Each kit contains a package insert and two of each of the following: single-use reteplase vials (10.8 units each), single-use diluent vials of SWFI (10 mL each), sterile 10-mL syringes with 20-gauge needles attached, sterile dispensing pins, sterile 20-gauge needles for administration, and alcohol swabs. Withdraw diluent with 20-gauge needle. Discard needle and put dispensing pin on syringe of diluent. Transfer diluent to vial of reteplase. Pin and syringe should remain in place while vial is swirled to dissolve reteplase. *Do not shake.* When completely dissolved, withdraw 10 mL reconstituted solution into the syringe (vials are 0.7 mL overfilled). Remove dispensing pin and replace with a 20-gauge needle for administration.

Storage: Kit should remain sealed to protect contents from light. Store at 2° to 25° C (36° to 77° F). Do not use beyond expiration date. Contains no preservatives; should be reconstituted immediately before use but may be stored at room temperature if used within 4 hours. Discard all unused solution and supplies.

COMPATIBILITY
Manufacturer states, "Should be given via an IV line in which no other medication is being simultaneously injected or infused. No other medication should be added to the injection solution containing reteplase. **Incompatible** with heparin; do not administer heparin in the same IV line unless the line is flushed through with NS or D5W before and after reteplase."

RATE OF ADMINISTRATION
Heparin: First 1,000 units over 1 minute. After this test dose, the balance of 4,000 units may be given over 1 minute. Follow with an infusion of 1,000 units/hr.

Reteplase: A single dose evenly distributed over 2 minutes. To avoid **incompatibilities** and ensure delivery of both doses, be sure to flush line with a minimum of 30 to 50 mL NS or D5W before and after each injection.

ACTIONS
A recombinant plasminogen activator. Exerts its thrombolytic action by generating plasmin from plasminogen through a specific process. Plasmin then degrades the fibrin matrix of the thrombus. Potency is expressed in units that are specific to reteplase. With therapeutic doses, a decrease in circulating fibrinogen makes the patient susceptible to bleeding. Onset of action is prompt, effecting patency of the vessel within 90 minutes in most patients. The FDA has allowed the manufacturer to claim superiority over alteplase at achieving patency within 90 minutes. Prompt opening of arteries increases probability of improved cardiac function. Half-life is 13 to 16 minutes. Cleared from the plasma

by the liver and kidneys. Mean fibrinogen level should return to baseline value within 48 hours.

INDICATIONS AND USES

Management of acute myocardial infarction (AMI) in adults for the improvement of ventricular function following AMI, the reduction of the incidence of congestive failure, and the reduction of mortality associated with AMI. Treatment should begin as soon as possible after the onset of symptoms of AMI. ▪ Current AHA and JAMA recommendations identify thrombolytic agents as Class I therapy in patients younger than 70 years with recent onset of chest pain (within 6 hours) consistent with AMI and at least 0.1 mV of ST-segment elevation in at least two ECG leads. Use in all other patients based on age, accurate diagnosis, and time from onset of chest pain.

CONTRAINDICATIONS

Active internal bleeding, arteriovenous malformation or aneurysm, bleeding diathesis, history of cerebral vascular accident, intracranial or intraspinal surgery or trauma within 2 months, intracranial neoplasm, severe uncontrolled hypertension.

PRECAUTIONS

Administered under the direction of a physician knowledgeable in its use and with appropriate emergency drugs and diagnostic and laboratory facilities available. ▪ Reperfusion arrhythmias occur frequently (e.g., sinus bradycardia, accelerated idioventricular rhythm, PVCs, ventricular tachycardia); have antiarrhythmic medications available at bedside. ▪ A greater alteration of hemostatic status than with heparin. Strict bed rest indicated to reduce risk of bleeding. Use extreme care with the patient; avoid any excessive or rough handling or pressure (including too-frequent BPs); avoid invasive procedures (e.g., arterial puncture, venipuncture, IM injection). If these procedures are absolutely necessary, use extreme precautionary methods (use radial artery instead of femoral, small-gauge catheters and needles, and sites that are easily observed and compressible where bleeding can be controlled; avoid handling of catheter sites; and use extended pressure application of up to 30 minutes). Minor bleeding occurs often at catheter insertion sites. Avoid use of razors and toothbrushes. ▪ Use extreme caution and weigh risks against anticipated benefits in the following situations: recent major surgery (e.g., coronary artery bypass graft, obstetric delivery, organ biopsy), previous puncture of noncompressible vessels (e.g., jugular, subclavian), cerebrovascular disease, recent GI or GU bleeding, recent trauma, hypertension (e.g., systolic BP equal to or greater than 180 mm Hg and/or diastolic BP equal to or greater than 110 mm Hg), high likelihood of left heart thrombus (e.g., mitral stenosis with atrial fibrillation), acute pericarditis, subacute bacterial endocarditis, hemostatic defects including those secondary to severe hepatic or renal disease, severe hepatic or renal dysfunction, pregnancy, diabetic hemorrhagic retinopathy or other hemorrhagic ophthalmic conditions, septic thrombophlebitis or occluded AV cannula at a seriously infected site, advanced age, patients currently receiving oral anticoagulants (e.g., warfarin [Coumadin]), or any other condition in which bleeding constitutes a significant hazard or would be particularly difficult to manage because of its location. ▪ Simultaneous therapy with continuous infusion of heparin is used to reduce the risk of rethrombosis. Markedly increases risk of bleeding. ▪ Standard treatment for myocardial infarction continues simultaneously with reteplase therapy except if temporarily contraindicated (e.g., arterial blood gases unless absolutely necessary). ▪ No experience with patients receiving repeat courses of reteplase. ▪ Cholesterol embolization has been reported and may be fatal.

Monitor: Best to establish separate IV lines for reteplase and heparin. If not appropriate, be sure to flush the IV line before and after each injection of reteplase. ▪ Baseline ECG, CPK, and clotting studies (TT, PTT, CBC, fibrinogen level, platelets) and baseline assessment (patient condition, pain, hematomas, petechiae, or recent wounds) should be completed before administration. Type and cross-match may also be ordered. ▪ Monitor ECG continuously, and record strips with greatest ST-segment elevation initially and every 15 minutes for at least 4 hours. A 12-lead ECG is indicated when therapy is complete. ▪ Maintain strict bed rest; monitor the patient carefully and frequently for anginal pain and signs of bleeding; observe catheter sites at least every 15 minutes and apply pressure dressings to any recently invaded site; watch for hematuria, hematemesis, bloody stool, petechiae, hematoma, flank pain, muscle weakness; do neuro checks every hour. Continue until normal clotting function returns. ▪ Watch for extravasation. ▪ See Precautions and Drug/Lab Interactions.

Patient Education: Compliance with all measures to minimize bleeding (e.g., strict bed rest) is very important. ▪ Avoid use of razors, toothbrushes, and other sharp items. ▪ Use caution while moving to avoid excessive bumping. ▪ Report all episodes of bleeding and apply local pressure if indicated. Expect oozing from IV sites.

Maternal/Child: Category C: has resulted in hemorrhage leading to spontaneous abortions in rabbits. Safety for use in pregnancy, breastfeeding, and pediatric patients not established.

Elderly: See Indications and Precautions. ▪ May have poorer prognosis following AMI or with pre-existing conditions that may increase the risk of intracranial bleeding. Select patients carefully to maximize benefits.

DRUG/LAB INTERACTIONS

Interaction of reteplase with other cardioactive drugs has not been studied. Risk of bleeding may be increased by **any medicine that affects blood clotting,** including anticoagulants (e.g., heparin, warfarin); **any medication that may cause hypoprothrombinemia, thrombocytopenia, or GI ulceration or bleeding** (e.g., selected antibiotics [e.g., cefotetan], aspirin, NSAIDs); **and/or any other medication that inhibits platelet aggregation** (e.g., clopidogrel, dipyridamole, glycoprotein GPIIb/IIIa receptor antagonists, valproic acid). Concurrent use not recommended with the exception of heparin and aspirin (in AMI) to reduce the risk of rethrombosis. If concurrent or subsequent use is indicated (e.g., management of acute coronary syndrome, percutaneous coronary intervention), monitor PT and aPTT closely. ▪ **Coagulation tests will be unreliable;** specific procedures can be used; notify the lab of reteplase use.

SIDE EFFECTS

Bleeding is most common: internal (GI tract, GU tract, intracranial, respiratory, or retroperitoneal sites), epistaxis, gingival, and superficial or surface bleeding (venous cutdowns, arterial punctures, sites of recent surgical intervention). Reperfusion arrhythmias are common; other serious arrhythmias may occur. A few hypersensitivity reactions, as well as fever, hypotension, nausea, and vomiting, have occurred. Cholesterol embolism has been reported and may be fatal. Clinical S/S may include acute renal failure, gangrenous digits, hypertension, infarctions (e.g., bowel, cerebral, myocardial, or spinal cord), pancreatitis, "purple toe" syndrome, renal artery occlusion.

ANTIDOTE

Notify physician of all side effects. Note even the most minute bleeding tendency. Oozing at IV sites is expected. Control minor bleeding by local pressure. For severe bleeding in a critical location, discontinue second dose of reteplase if it has not been given and any heparin therapy immediately. Whole blood, packed RBCs, cryoprecipitate, fresh-frozen plasma, platelets, desmopressin, tranexamic acid, and aminocaproic acid may all be indicated. Topical preparations of aminocaproic acid may stop minor bleeding. Consider protamine if heparin has been used. Treat bradycardia with atropine, reperfusion arrhythmias with lidocaine or procainamide; VT or VF may require cardioversion. Treat minor hypersensitivity reactions symptomatically. Discontinue drug and treat anaphylaxis as indicated; resuscitate as necessary. Discontinue therapy if any symptoms of cholesterol embolism occur.

Rh$_o$(D) IMMUNE GLOBULIN INTRAVENOUS (HUMAN) BBW
(ih-**MUNE GLAW**-byoo-lin **IN**-trah-ve-nes)

Rh$_o$(D)-IGIV, Rhophylac, WinRho SDF

Immunizing agent (passive)
Platelet count stimulator

pH 6.5 to 7.6

USUAL DOSE
(International units [IU])

Pregnancy, predelivery: *Rhophylac and WinRho SDF:* Confirm Rh$_o$(D)-negative status of patient. May be given IV or IM. 1500 IU (300 mcg) at 28 weeks' gestation. If *WinRho SDF* is administered early in the pregnancy, it should be repeated at 12-week intervals to maintain an adequate level of passively acquired anti-Rh.

Pregnancy, postdelivery: Confirm Rh$_o$(D)-negative status of patient. May be given IV or IM. Administer as soon as possible after delivery of a confirmed Rh$_o$(D)-positive baby. Usually given no later than 72 hours postdelivery. If the Rh status of the infant is unknown at 72 hours, administer to the mother at that time. Should be given as soon as possible up to 28 days after delivery. This second dose postdelivery (first dose given predelivery; see above) can reduce treatment failure.

Rhophylac: 1500 IU (300 mcg).

WinRho SDF: 600 IU (120 mcg).

Postabortion, amniocentesis (after 34 weeks' gestation), or any other manipulation late in pregnancy (after 34 weeks' gestation): Confirm Rh$_o$(D)-negative status of patient. May be given IV or IM. Administer immediately after abortion or procedure associated with increased risk of Rh isoimmunization. Must be given within 72 hours. One-half of a dose (a mini-dose [IM product]) may be given if a pregnancy terminates before 13 weeks' gestation; administration within 3 hours is preferred. According to the literature, this mini-dose can provide 100% effectiveness in preventing Rh immunization.

Rhophylac: 1500 IU (300 mcg).

WinRho SDF: 600 IU (120 mcg).

Postamniocentesis before 34 weeks' gestation or after chorionic villus sampling: Confirm Rh$_o$(D)-negative status of patient. May be given IV or IM. *Rhophylac or WinRho SDF:* 1500 IU (300 mcg) immediately after the procedure. Repeat *WinRho SDF* every 12 weeks during the pregnancy.

Threatened abortion: Confirm Rh$_o$(D)-negative status of patient. May be given IV or IM. *Rhophylac or WinRho SDF:* 1500 IU (300 mcg) as soon as possible.

Transfusion or fetal hemorrhage: Confirm Rh$_o$(D)-negative status of patient. May be given IV or IM. Administer within 72 hours of an incompatible event involving Rh$_o$(D)-positive blood such as exposure to incompatible blood transfusions (Rh+ whole blood or Rh+ red blood cells) or massive fetal hemorrhage.

Rhophylac: Give 100 IU (20 mcg) per each 2 mL transfused blood or per 1 mL erythrocyte concentrate. In cases of known or suspected excessive feto-maternal hemorrhage, the number of fetal red blood cells in the maternal circulation should be determined. If testing is not feasible and excessive feto-maternal hemorrhage cannot be excluded, administer a dose of 1500 IU (300 mcg).

WinRho SDF: Give up to 3000 IU (600 mcg) every 8 hours IV or 6000 IU (1,200 mcg) every 12 hours IM until the total dose is administered. Total IV dose is 45 IU (9 mcg) for every milliliter of Rh+ whole blood exposure or 90 IU (18 mcg) for every milliliter of Rh+ red blood cell exposure. Total IM dose is 60 IU (12 mcg) for every milliliter of Rh+ whole blood exposure or 120 IU (24 mcg) for every milliliter of Rh+ red blood cell exposure.

Treatment of immune thrombocytopenic purpura (ITP); adults and pediatric patients: *WinRho SDF:* Confirm Rh$_o$(D)-positive status of patient. Must be given IV. Hemoglobin should be greater than 10 Gm/dL. Give 250 IU/kg (50 mcg/kg) of body weight as the initial dose. May be given as a single dose or divided in half and given on 2 consecutive days. If response to the initial dose is adequate, maintenance doses of 125 to 300 IU/kg (25 to 60 mcg/kg) may be given. If response to the initial dose is inadequate, see Dose Adjustments. Dose and frequency based on patient's clinical response (e.g., RBC, hemoglobin, reticulocyte levels, and platelet counts); see Dose Adjustments.

PEDIATRIC DOSE
Treatment of ITP: *WinRho SDF:* See Usual Dose and Dose Adjustments.

DOSE ADJUSTMENTS   (International units [IU])
Pregnancy and obstetrical conditions: *WinRho SDF* suggests protection must be maintained throughout pregnancy once Rh$_o$(D) immune globulin is administered. Level of passively acquired anti-Rh$_o$(D) should not fall below levels required to prevent an immune response to Rh$_o$(D)-positive blood. Additional doses should be given every 12 weeks during pregnancy and at delivery unless the previous dose was administered within 3 weeks and there is less than 15 mL of fetomaternal red blood cell hemorrhage during delivery.

Suppression of Rh isoimmunization: *Rhophylac and WinRho SDF:* A large fetomaternal hemorrhage may cause an incorrect evaluation by standard tests of the amount of Rh$_o$(D) IGIV required. Assess the amount of hemorrhage and adjust dose accordingly.

Treatment of ITP: Adults and pediatric patients: *WinRho SDF:* If the hemoglobin level is less than 10 Gm/dL before or after the initial dose, reduce the initial dose and/or maintenance doses to 125 to 200 IU (25 to 40 mcg)/kg to minimize the risk of increasing the severity of anemia in the patient. ▪ In patients with adequate platelet response to the initial dose, adjust maintenance doses based on platelet and hemoglobin levels. ▪ If response to the initial dose is inadequate, adjust subsequent doses as follows:

Hemoglobin above 10 Gm/dL: redose with 250 to 300 IU (50 to 60 mcg)/kg.
Hemoglobin is 8 to 10 Gm/dL: redose with 125 to 200 IU (25 to 40 mcg)/kg.
Hemoglobin below 8 Gm/dL: use with caution; may increase severity of anemia.

DILUTION   (International units [IU])
Rhophylac: Available in a prefilled 2-mL syringe containing 1500 IU (300 mcg) for single-dose use. Bring to room or body temperature before use.
WinRho SDF: Available as a ready-to-use liquid. 5 IU equals 1 mcg. Withdraw the entire contents of the vial to obtain the labeled dose. If indicated, calculate a partial dose, then discard the excess from the syringe. The target fill volume of each vial is included in the following chart.

WinRho SDF Target Fill Volumes/Vial	
Vial Size	**Target Fill Volume**
600 IU (120 mcg)	0.5 mL
1,500 IU (300 mcg)	1.3 mL
2,500 IU (500 mcg)	2.2 mL
5,000 IU (1,000 mcg)	4.4 mL
15,000 IU (3,000 mcg)	13 mL

Storage: *Rhophylac:* Refrigerate syringes before use. Protect from light. Should not be used after expiration date. Discard unused product in syringe. ***WinRho SDF:*** Store unopened vials in refrigerator. Note expiration date. Do not freeze. Discard unused portion.

COMPATIBILITY
Rhophylac: Compatibility information not available from manufacturer; consult a pharmacist.

WinRho SDF: Manufacturer states, "Should be administered separately from other drugs." Dilute only with NS.

RATE OF ADMINISTRATION
Rhophylac: A single dose as a slow IV injection.

WinRho SDF: A single dose as an IV injection over 3 to 5 minutes.

ACTIONS   (International units [IU])
Rhophylac and WinRho SDF: Specialty immunoglobulins. A gamma globulin (IgG) fraction containing antibodies to the Rh$_o$(D) antigen (D Antigen). Reduces the incidence of Rh immunization of an Rh$_o$(D)-negative mother by an Rh$_o$(D)-positive infant before, during, and after delivery; reduces the likelihood of hemolytic disease in an Rh$_o$(D)-positive infant in present and future pregnancies. Has also been shown to increase platelet counts in nonsplenectomized Rh$_o$(D)-positive patients with immune thrombocytopenic purpura (ITP). A 1500-IU vial or syringe contains 300 mcg of anti-Rh$_o$(D), which can effectively suppress the immunizing potential of approximately 15 to 17 mL of Rh$_o$(D)-positive blood cells and, in addition, contains 25 to 40 mg of nonspecific gammaglobulin. Pooled from source plasma selected for high titers of Rh$_o$(D) antibody. Purified and standardized by several methods (e.g., solvent-detergent viral inactivation process to decrease the possibility of transmission of blood-borne pathogens [e.g., HIV, hepatitis]). Similar to native IgG that normally circulates in human plasma.

Rhophylac: Is thimerosal free, mercury free, and latex free. Contains albumin as a stabilizer. Half-life is 12 to 20 days. Anti-D IgG titers were measurable up to 9 weeks after injection.

WinRho SDF: Has also been shown to increase platelet counts in nonsplenectomized Rh$_o$(D)-positive patients with immune thrombocytopenic purpura (ITP). Platelet counts usually begin to rise in 1 to 2 days with peak effect in 7 to 14 days. Some effects last about 30 days. Contains 25 to 40 mg of nonspecific gammaglobulin. The liquid form contains maltose as a stabilizer; the lyophilized powder is stabilized with glycine, NaCl, and polysorbate 80. Half-life is 24 days. Crosses the blood-brain barrier.

INDICATIONS AND USES
Rhophylac and WinRho SDF: Suppression of Rh isoimmunization in nonsensitized Rh$_o$(D)-negative females during the normal course of pregnancy, within 72 hours after spontaneous or induced abortions, amniocentesis, chorionic villus sampling, ruptured tubal pregnancy, abdominal trauma or transplacental hemorrhage, unless the blood type of the fetus or father is known to be Rh$_o$(D)-negative. ▪ Suppression of Rh isoimmunization in Rh$_o$(D)-negative female pediatric patients and female adults in their childbearing years transfused with Rh$_o$(D)-positive red blood cells or blood components containing Rh$_o$(D)-positive RBCs.

WinRho SDF: Treatment of nonsplenectomized Rh$_o$(D)-positive pediatric patients with acute or chronic immune thrombocytopenic purpura (ITP), adults with chronic ITP, or pediatric patients and adults with ITP secondary to HIV infection in clinical situations requiring an increase in platelet counts to prevent excessive hemorrhage.

CONTRAINDICATIONS
Rhophylac and WinRho SDF: *All uses:* History of a prior severe hypersensitivity reaction to human immune globulin preparations or their components (*Rhophylac* contains albumin, *WinRho SDF* may contain thimerosal); patients with isolated IgA deficiency or pre-existing IgA antibodies (benefits must outweigh risks; risk of anaphylaxis is greater).

Suppression of Rh isoimmunization in pregnancy: For suppression of Rh isoimmunization in the mother. *Do not administer to the infant.* Not recommended for use in Rh$_o$(D)-negative individuals shown to be Rh immunized by standard screening tests.

WinRho SDF: *Treatment of ITP:* Not recommended for use in Rh$_o$(D)-negative or splenectomized individuals.

PRECAUTIONS

All uses: Confirm vial or syringe label—must state for IV or IV/IM use; several similar products are for IM use only (e.g., RhoGam). ▪ May risk transmission of infectious agents (e.g., hepatitis, HIV, possibly the Creutzfeldt-Jakob disease [CJD] agent); see Actions. ▪ May contain trace amounts of anti-A, anti-B, anti-C, and anti-E blood group antibodies. ▪ Use caution and weigh benefit versus risk in patients with known hypogammaglobulinemia or selective IgA deficiency; risk of severe hypersensitivity reactions or anaphylaxis is increased. ▪ Not intended for use in Rh+ individuals (with the exception of *WinRho SDF* in the treatment of ITP). ▪ Use with caution and monitor renal function in patients at risk for renal insufficiency. IGIV products have been reported to produce renal dysfunction in patients who are predisposed to acute renal failure or in those who have renal insufficiency. Most reports involve products that contain sucrose as a stabilizer. WinRho SDF does not contain sucrose.

Suppression of Rh isoimmunization in pregnancy: More than 1 dose of Rh₀(D) immune globulin may be required. A fetal RBC count can be done on maternal blood to determine the required dose. ▪ If a large fetomaternal hemorrhage occurs late in pregnancy or after delivery, Rh₀(D) IGIV should be administered in sufficient doses if there is any doubt about the mother's blood type (e.g., presence of passively administered anti-Rh₀(D) in maternal or fetal blood [positive Coombs' test]). ▪ See Monitor. ▪ Manufacturer recommends IM or IV use. Another source recommends IM injection when Rh₀(D) is used as an immunizing agent. ▪ Not effective in Rh₀(D)-negative females who have already been sensitized to the Rh₀(D) erythrocyte factor; however, if administered, the risk of side effects is not increased.

Treatment of ITP: IV route required for ITP. ▪ Rare cases of intravascular hemolysis have been reported. Usually occurs within 4 hours of administration. Complications may include clinically compromising anemia and multisystem organ failure, including ARDS. Fatalities have occurred. Serious complications, including severe anemia, acute renal insufficiency, renal failure, and DIC, have also been reported. Even if previous infusions have been uneventful, intravascular hemolysis and its complications may occur with subsequent infusions. ▪ If the hemoglobin level is less than 8 Gm/dL, use with extreme caution; may increase severity of anemia.

Monitor: *All uses:* See Precautions. ▪ Observe patient for at least 20 to 30 minutes after injection.

Suppression of Rh isoimmunization in pregnancy: Maintain accurate records of Rh factor and Rh₀(D)-IGIV. ▪ Obtain CBC and other appropriate lab work based on procedure or situation. ▪ Monitor vital signs if indicated.

Treatment of ITP: Obtain baseline RBC, hemoglobin, reticulocyte levels, and platelet counts. Monitor during therapy to determine clinical response. ▪ Given to Rh₀(D)-positive patients in this situation, interaction with RBC usually causes some degree of RBC hemolysis; observe carefully. Monitor for S/S of intravascular hemolysis (back pain, chills, fever, hemoglobinuria) for at least 8 hours after infusion. Perform a dipstick urinalysis at baseline, at 2 and 4 hours, and before the end of the monitoring period. ▪ Monitor for complications of intravascular hemolysis (IVH), including clinically compromising anemia (decreased hemoglobin, hypotension, pallor, and tachycardia), acute renal insufficiency (anuria, dyspnea, edema, or oliguria), or DIC (increased bruising and prolongation of bleeding or clotting time). ▪ If S/S of IVH or its complications occur, lab tests should be performed to confirm the diagnosis. Tests include but are not limited to CBC with platelets, haptoglobin, plasma hemoglobin, urine dipstick, BUN, SCr, LDH, direct and indirect bilirubin, and DIC-specific tests (e.g., D-dimer, fibrin degradation products [FDPs], fibrin split products [FSPs]). ▪ If transfusion is required, use Rh₀(D)-negative RBCs to avoid exacerbating ongoing IVH. Platelet products may contain RBCs; use caution if platelets from an Rh₀(D)-positive donor are used.

Patient Education: Report S/S of a hypersensitivity reaction (e.g., feeling of fainting, hives, itching, tightness in the chest, wheezing). ▪ Report feelings of dizziness, tiredness, weakness. *ITP:* May cause a considerable drop in hemoglobin; follow-up testing important. ■ Immediately report symptoms of back pain, chills, decreased urine output, discolored urine or hematuria, fever, sudden weight gain, fluid retention/edema, and/or shortness of breath. May indicate onset of intravascular hemolysis (IVH).

Maternal/Child: Category C: use only if clearly needed. ■ Rhophylac is not secreted in breast milk. Specific information is not available for WinRho SDF on safety during breastfeeding. ■ For the suppression of Rh isoimmunization in the mother; do not administer to the infant.

Elderly: When used for treatment of ITP, fatal outcomes associated with IVH and its complications occurred most frequently in patients over 65 years of age with comorbid conditions.

DRUG/LAB INTERACTIONS

Interaction with other drugs has not been evaluated. ■ Antibodies contained in $Rh_o(D)$ immune globulin may interfere with the body's immune response to certain **live virus vaccines.** Do not administer live virus vaccines (e.g., measles, mumps, polio, or rubella) for at least 3 months after $Rh_o(D)$ administration. ■ Trace amounts of anti-A, anti-B, anti-C, and anti-E blood group antibodies may be detectable in **direct and indirect antiglobulin (Coombs') tests** following treatment with $Rh_o(D)$. ■ May affect outcomes of **blood typing and antibody testing** in neonates. ■ The liquid formulation of WinRho SDF contains maltose, which may give **falsely high blood glucose levels** with certain types of blood glucose testing systems. Only testing systems that are glucose specific should be used to monitor blood glucose levels in patients receiving maltose-containing parenteral products such as WinRho SDF.

SIDE EFFECTS

All uses: Abdominal or back pain, arthralgias, asthenia, chills, diarrhea, dizziness, fever, headache, hyperkinesia, hypertension, hypotension, increased LDH, pruritus, rash, somnolence, and sweating. Hypersensitivity reactions, including anaphylaxis, have been reported rarely. Made from human plasma donors; transmission of selected diseases possible but not probable; see Precautions.

Suppression of Rh isoimmunization in pregnancy: Side effects are infrequent in $Rh_o(D)$-negative individuals. Only a few females have had treatment failures resulting in development of $Rh_o(D)$ antibodies.

ITP: Destruction of $Rh_o(D)$ red cells resulting in decreased hemoglobin (range was 0.4 to 6.1 Gm/dL). IVH (back pain, shaking chills, hemoglobinuria), acute onset and exacerbation of anemia, and renal insufficiency have been reported in $Rh_o(D)$-positive patients. Has rarely resulted in death.

ANTIDOTE

Keep physician informed of side effects; may require symptomatic treatment. Discontinue immediately if a hypersensitivity reaction occurs; treat as indicated (e.g., maintain airway, administer fluids, oxygen, epinephrine, diphenhydramine, corticosteroids [e.g., dexamethasone (Decadron)]). *ITP:* Treatment may have to be discontinued if drop in hemoglobin is too severe. Transfusion may be required.

RIFAMPIN
(rih-**FAM**-pin)

Antibacterial
(Rifamycin)
Antitubercular agent

Rifadin — pH 7.8 to 8.8

USUAL DOSE
Pretreatment: Baseline studies indicated; see Precautions and Monitor.

Dose and schedule may vary depending on treatment regimen selected. IV doses are the same as oral. Use oral dose form as soon as practical.

Tuberculosis (adults and pediatric patients 15 years of age or older): 10 mg/kg once a day when used in conjunction with other antitubercular agents in a daily regimen, or 10 mg/kg not to exceed 600 mg/dose two or three times a week when used in an intermittent multiple-drug regimen. Do not exceed 600 mg/day. Prescribed concurrently with other antitubercular drugs (e.g., ethambutol [Myambutol], isoniazid [INH], pyrazinamide, or streptomycin). Consult current CDC guidelines for suggested treatment regimens.

Meningococcal carriers: 600 mg every 12 hours for 2 days.

PEDIATRIC DOSE
Tuberculosis: 10 to 20 mg/kg of body weight once a day when used in conjunction with other antitubercular agents in a daily regimen or two or three times a week when used in an intermittent multiple-drug regimen. Do not exceed 600 mg/day. Prescribed concurrently with other antitubercular drugs (e.g., ethambutol [Myambutol], isoniazid [INH], pyrazinamide, or streptomycin).

Meningococcal carriers: *Under 1 month of age:* 5 mg/kg every 12 hours for 2 days. *Over 1 month of age:* 10 mg/kg every 12 hours for 2 days. Do not exceed 600 mg/dose.

DOSE ADJUSTMENTS
There are no dose adjustments provided in the manufacturer's prescribing information for patients with impaired hepatic function; use caution. ▪ No dose adjustment is necessary in impaired renal function; serum concentrations do not change. ▪ See Drug/Lab Interactions.

DILUTION
Each 600-mg vial must be initially diluted in 10 mL of SWFI (60 mg/mL). Swirl gently to dissolve. Withdraw desired dose and further dilute in 500 mL or 100 mL of D5W or NS; see Storage.

Storage: Store vials at CRT. Avoid excessive heat (temperatures above 40° C [104° F]). Protect from light. Reconstituted solution stable at RT for 30 hours. Use solution diluted in D5W within 8 hours; solution diluted in NS stable for 6 hours.

COMPATIBILITY
Manufacturer states, "May form a precipitate with diltiazem at the **Y-site.**" Infusion solutions other than D5W or NS are not recommended.

RATE OF ADMINISTRATION
A single dose diluted in 500 mL equally distributed as an infusion over 3 hours. In selected situations a single dose diluted in 100 mL may be administered over 30 minutes.

ACTIONS
A semi-synthetic antibiotic derivative of rifamycin. Has bactericidal activity in vitro against slow and intermittently growing *Mycobacterium tuberculosis* organisms and has been shown to be active against most strains of *Neisseria meningitidis* and *M. tuberculosis*. Inhibits bacterial DNA-dependent RNA polymerase activity in susceptible *M. tuberculosis* organisms but does not inhibit the mammalian enzyme. Rapidly distributed throughout the body and present in many organs and body fluids, including CSF. 80% protein bound. Metabolized in the liver. Undergoes enterohepatic circulation. Excreted in bile and urine. Half-life following repeated dosing is 3 to 4 hours. Crosses the placental barrier. Secreted in breast milk.

INDICATIONS AND USES

Treatment or retreatment of all forms of tuberculosis when the drug cannot be taken by mouth. ▪ Treatment of asymptomatic carriers of *Neisseria* meningitis. Not indicated for treatment of meningococcal infection because of rapid emergence of resistant meningococci.

Unlabeled uses: Used in combination with other agents in the treatment of certain atypical mycobacterial infections (e.g., *Mycobacterium avium*). ▪ Used in combination with other antistaphylococcal agents to treat serious staphylococcal infections.

CONTRAINDICATIONS

Hypersensitivity to rifampin or any of its components or to any rifamycins. ▪ Contraindicated in patients receiving ritonavir-boosted saquinavir; risk for severe hepatocellular toxicity is increased. ▪ Concomitant use with atazanavir, darunavir, fosamprenavir, saquinavir, and tipranavir; see Drug/Lab Interactions. ▪ Contraindicated in patients receiving praziquantel because therapeutically effective blood levels of praziquantel may not be achieved. In patients receiving rifampin who need immediate treatment with praziquantel, alternative agents should be considered. If treatment with praziquantel is necessary, rifampin should be discontinued 4 weeks before administration of praziquantel. Treatment with rifampin can then be restarted 1 day after completion of praziquantel treatment.

PRECAUTIONS

For IV use only. Do not administer IM or SC. ▪ Obtain cultures and susceptibility studies before starting therapy to confirm susceptibility of the organism to rifampin. Repeat studies periodically during therapy to monitor for the emergence of resistance. ▪ Resistance can emerge rapidly; appropriate susceptibility tests should be performed in the event of persistent positive cultures. ▪ Susceptibility tests also required before use as treatment for asymptomatic carriers of *Neisseria* meningitis. ▪ To reduce the development of drug-resistant bacteria and maintain its effectiveness, rifampin should be used to treat or prevent only those infections proven or strongly suspected to be caused by bacteria. ▪ Organisms resistant to rifampin are likely to be resistant to other rifamycins. ▪ Hepatoxicity of hepatocellular, cholestatic, and mixed patterns has occurred. Severity ranged from asymptomatic elevations in liver enzymes, isolated jaundice/hyperbilirubinemia, and symptomatic self-limited hepatitis to fulminant liver failure and death. Risk of liver damage is markedly increased if impaired liver function is present and when rifampin is given with other hepatotoxic agents (e.g., isoniazid [INH], halothane). Discontinue rifampin if hepatic damage occurs or worsens. ▪ Systemic hypersensitivity reactions may occur in patients taking rifampin. Manifestations of hypersensitivity (fever, laboratory abnormalities [including eosinophilia and liver abnormalities], and lymphadenopathy) may be present even without rash. If S/S occur, discontinue rifampin and administer supportive measures. ▪ Cases of severe cutaneous adverse reactions (SCAR) such as Stevens-Johnson syndrome (SJS), toxic epidermal necrolysis (TEN), acute generalized exanthematous pustulosis (AGEP), and drug reaction with eosinophilia and systemic symptoms (DRESS) syndrome have occurred. Discontinue rifampin immediately and institute appropriate therapy if S/S of severe cutaneous adverse reactions develop. ▪ May cause vitamin K–dependent coagulation disorders and bleeding. Consider discontinuation if abnormal coagulation tests and/or bleeding occur. Supplemental vitamin K administration should be considered when appropriate. ▪ May exacerbate porphyria. ▪ Use with caution in patients with diabetes; diabetes management may be more difficult. ▪ Not recommended for intermittent therapy; interruption of daily dosage regimen has resulted in rare renal hypersensitivity reactions when therapy was resumed. ▪ Urine, feces, sputum, sweat, teeth, and tears may be colored redorange. Soft contact lenses may be permanently stained. CSF may be light yellow. ▪ Pseudomembranous colitis has been reported. May range from mild to life-threatening. Consider in patients who present with diarrhea during or after treatment with rifampin.

Monitor: Obtain baseline measurements of hepatic enzymes (e.g., ALT and AST), bilirubin, SCr, CBC, and platelet count. Routine lab monitoring in patients with normal baseline labs is generally not necessary. However, patients should be seen monthly and questioned about symptoms that may indicate adverse reactions. ▪ Monitor liver function every 2 to 4 weeks in patients with pre-existing liver impairment. ▪ Monitor for S/S and clinical/laboratory signs of liver injury, especially if treatment is prolonged or given with other hepatotoxic drugs. ▪ Monitor coagulation tests during treatment (prothrombin time and other coagulation tests) in patients at risk for vitamin K deficiency (e.g., those with chronic liver disease, poor nutritional status, taking prolonged antibacterial drugs or anticoagulants). ▪ Monitor blood glucose closely in patients with diabetes. ▪ Notify physician immediately if flu-like symptoms develop; may be due to hepatotoxicity. ▪ Monitor for S/S of hypersensitivity reaction (e.g., acute bronchospasm, angioedema, conjunctivitis, DRESS, elevated liver transaminases, fever, flu-like syndrome [aches, chills, chest pain, cough, dizziness, fatigue, headache, itching, muscle pain, nausea, palpitations, shortness of breath, sweats, syncope, vomiting, weakness], hypotension, neutropenia, rash, thrombocytopenia, urticaria). ▪ Monitor for S/S of severe cutaneous adverse reactions. ▪ Thrombocytopenia has occurred. Reversible if rifampin is discontinued as soon as purpura occurs. Cerebral hemorrhage has occurred when rifampin has been continued or resumed after the appearance of purpura. Contact physician immediately if purpura occurs. ▪ Confirm patency of IV; avoid extravasation. Restart IV at a new site for any signs of inflammation or irritation. ▪ Do all lab tests and affected radiology studies before daily dose of medication. ▪ See Drug/Lab Interactions.

Patient Education: Reliability of hormonal contraceptives may be affected; use of nonhormonal contraceptives recommended. ▪ Do not take any other medication without medical advice. ▪ Avoid use of alcohol, other hepatotoxic agents (e.g., acetaminophen, NSAIDs, phenothiazines, some antineoplastic agents, sulfonamides), or herbal products. ▪ Review side effects with health care professional and promptly report abdominal pain, cough, darkened urine, itching, light-colored bowel movements, loss of appetite, malaise, nausea and vomiting, pain or swelling of the joints, rash with fever or blisters with or without peeling skin, shortness of breath, swollen lymph nodes, wheezing, or yellowish discoloration of the skin and eyes. ▪ May cause discoloration (yellow, orange, red, brown) of feces, sputum, sweat, urine, tears, and teeth. ▪ May permanently stain soft contact lenses. ▪ Do not interrupt daily dosage regimen.

Maternal/Child: Has teratogenic potential. Safety for use during pregnancy not established. Benefit must outweigh risk. See literature for best combinations with least known risk. ▪ Administration during the last few weeks of pregnancy may cause postnatal hemorrhages in mother and infant; treatment with vitamin K may be required. ▪ Closely monitor neonates of rifampin-treated mothers for adverse effects. ▪ Discontinue breastfeeding if mother requires treatment. ▪ Has been used in pediatric patients.

Elderly: Differences in response between elderly and younger patients have not been identified. ▪ See Dose Adjustments.

DRUG/LAB INTERACTIONS

Interactions are numerous and potentially life-threatening. Review of drug profile by pharmacist imperative. ▪ Hepatotoxicity, hepatic encephalopathy, and death associated with jaundice have occurred when rifampin is given with **other hepatotoxic agents** (e.g., alcohol, isoniazid). Discontinue one or both drugs for signs of hepatocellular damage. ▪ Concurrent use of rifampin with **saquinavir/ritonavir** (ritonavir-boosted saquinavir) is *contraindicated;* significant hepatocellular toxicity with markedly increased transaminase elevations has been reported. ▪ Concurrent use with praziquantel is *contraindicated;* see Contraindications. ▪ Concurrent administration with **atazanavir, darunavir, fosamprenavir, saquinavir,** and **tipranavir** is *contraindicated;* rifampin may substantially decrease plasma concentrations of these antiviral agents. Loss of antiviral effectiveness and/or development of viral resistance may result. ▪ Rifampin increases metabolism and clearance and decreases serum levels and effectiveness of numerous drugs. Manufacturer lists **antiarrhythmics, anticonvulsants, antiestrogens, antifungals, benzodiazepine-related drugs, beta-blockers, calcium channel blockers, chloramphenicol, clarithromycin, corticosteroids, cyclosporine, dapsone, diazepam, digoxin, doxycycline, efavirenz, fluoroquinolones, haloperidol, hepatitis C antivirals, indinavir, irinotecan, levothyroxine, methadone, narcotic analgesics, oral anticoagulants, oral hypoglycemic agents, oral or other systemic hormonal contraceptives, progestins, quinine, simvastatin, tacrolimus, theophylline, tricyclic antidepressants, and zidovudine.** Other sources add **amiodarone, benzodiazepines, buspirone, estrogens, lamotrigine, losartan,** and **ondansetron.** Increased doses of these drugs may be required. Monitor carefully. ▪ Increases requirements of **warfarin**; monitor PT/INR to establish and maintain required anticoagulant dose. ▪ Increases metabolism and decreases effectiveness of **oral or other systemic hormonal contraceptives**; use of effective nonhormonal contraception recommended. **Diabetes** may be more difficult to control. ▪ May reduce analgesic effects of **morphine and methadone.** Monitor carefully; an alternate analgesic may be required (see earlier statement). ▪ Concurrent use of **ketoconazole and rifampin** has resulted in decreased serum concentrations of both drugs. Treatment failure may occur when given concomitantly. ▪ Concomitant use of rifampin and **macrolide antibiotics** may decrease the metabolism of rifampin and increase the metabolism of the macrolide antibiotic. ▪ **Probenecid and co-trimoxazole** increase blood levels of rifampin. ▪ May decrease concentrations of enalaprilat, the active metabolite of **enalapril**, resulting in hypertension. Adjust dose as required. ▪ When taken concomitantly, decreased concentrations of **atovaquone** and increased concentration of rifampin have been observed. ▪ May induce metabolism of endogenous substrates including **adrenal hormones, thyroid hormones, and vitamin D.** Reduced levels of vitamin D may be accompanied by decreased serum calcium and phosphate and increased parathyroid hormone. ▪ Avoid concomitant administration with **cefazolin** in patients at increased risk of bleeding. ▪ Cross-reactivity and false-positive urine screening **tests for opiates** have been reported when using certain assays. Gas chromatography or mass spectrometry will distinguish rifampin from opiates. ▪ Therapeutic levels inhibit microbiologic assays of **serum folate and vitamin B$_{12}$.**

SIDE EFFECTS

Abnormal liver function tests, acute generalized exanthematous pustulosis, adrenal insufficiency, agranulocytosis, anorexia, ataxia, behavioral changes, bleeding, cholestasis, conjunctivitis (exudative), cramps, cutaneous reactions (e.g., flushing and itching with or without a rash), decreased hemoglobin, diarrhea, DIC, dizziness, drowsiness, edema of face and extremities, elevated BUN and serum uric acid, epigastric distress, eosinophilia, fatigue, flu-like symptoms (e.g., chills, fever, headache, malaise, muscle and bone pain), gamma-glutamyl transferase, gas, heartburn, hematuria, hemolytic anemia, hepatitis or a shock-like syndrome and abnormal liver function tests, hepatoxicity, hypersensitivity reactions (which may include anaphylaxis, conjunctivitis, DRESS syndrome, eosinophilia, erythema multiforme, pemphigoid reaction, pruritus, rash, sore mouth, sore tongue, Stevens-Johnson syndrome, toxic epidermal necrolysis, urticaria, vasculitis), hypotension, inability to concentrate, jaundice, leukopenia, menstrual disturbances, mental confusion, muscle weakness, myopathy (rare), nausea, numbness (generalized), pain in extremities, pseudomembranous colitis, psychosis, purpura, renal failure (acute), shortness of breath, thrombocytopenia, tooth discoloration (which may be permanent), visual disturbances, vitamin K–dependent coagulation disorders (abnormal prolongation of prothrombin time or low vitamin K–dependent coagulation factors), vomiting, wheezing.

Overdose: Abdominal pain; bilirubin levels and/or liver enzymes may increase rapidly; brown-red discoloration of feces, saliva, skin, sweat, tears, and urine is proportional to amount of overdose; headache, lethargy, nausea, and vomiting are immediate; pruritus; unconsciousness. Liver enlargement, possibly with tenderness, can develop within a few hours after severe overdose; bilirubin levels may increase and jaundice may develop rapidly. Arrhythmias, cardiac arrest, hypotension, and seizures have been reported in fatal overdoses.

ANTIDOTE

With increasing severity of any side effect, alterations in liver function tests, flu-like symptoms, purpura, thrombocytopenia, or symptoms of overdose, discontinue the drug and notify the physician immediately. Antiemetics (e.g., ondansetron, prochlorperazine) may be required to control nausea and vomiting. Forced diuresis will promote excretion. Hemodialysis may be indicated. If hemodialysis is not available, peritoneal dialysis can be used along with forced diuresis. In severe overdose or acute toxicity, maintain an adequate airway and confirm adequate respiratory exchange. Treat anaphylaxis and resuscitate as necessary.

RITUXIMAB BBW ▪
RITUXIMAB-abbs[a] BBW ▪
RITUXIMAB-pvvr[a] BBW ▪
RITUXIMAB-arrx[a] BBW

(rih-**TUK**-sih-mab)

Rituxan ▪ Truxima[a] ▪ Ruxience[a] ▪ Riabni[a]

Recombinant monoclonal antibody
Antineoplastic (anti-CD20)
Antirheumatic

pH 6.5

USUAL DOSE

Rituximab-abbs (Truxima)[a], rituximab-pvvr (Ruxience)[a], and rituximab-arrx (Riabni)[a] are biosimilar drugs of Rituxan (rituximab). Unless specifically stated otherwise, the information in the monograph applies to all formulations.

Pretreatment: Verify pregnancy status. Pretesting required and baseline studies indicated; see Precautions and Monitor.

Premedication: *Use recommended for all indications.* Acetaminophen and diphenhydramine are recommended before each dose to prevent or attenuate severe hypersensitivity and/or infusion reactions.

Rituximab (Rituxan and Truxima): Additional premedication (e.g., methylprednisolone 100 mg IV or equivalent) 30 minutes before each infusion is required for patients with rheumatoid arthritis (RA) and (for **Rituxan**) pemphigus vulgaris (PV).

Rituximab products: Patients with granulomatosis with polyangiitis (GPA [Wegener granulomatosis (WG)]) and microscopic polyangiitis (MPA) require additional premedication with methylprednisolone IV 1000 mg. Patients receiving the 90-minute infusion should receive the glucocorticoid component of their chemotherapy regimen before the rituximab infusion. PCP prophylaxis and/or antiherpetic viral prophylaxis required in specific indications; see Precautions. When administered for oncology-related indications, hydration and antihyperuricemic therapy are recommended for patients at risk for tumor lysis syndrome.

RITUXIMAB PRODUCTS

Relapsed or refractory, low-grade or follicular, CD20-positive, B-cell non-Hodgkin lymphoma (NHL):
Single agent: *Initial therapy:* 375 mg/M^2 as an infusion once a week for 4 or 8 doses. See Drug/Lab Interactions. ***Retreatment therapy:*** Patients who subsequently develop progressive disease may be retreated with 375 mg/M^2 as an IV infusion once each week for 4 doses.

Previously untreated follicular, CD20-positive, B-cell NHL: 375 mg/M^2 as an infusion, given on Day 1 of each cycle of chemotherapy for up to 8 doses. In patients with complete or partial response, initiate rituximab maintenance 8 weeks after completion of rituximab in combination with chemotherapy. Administer rituximab as a single agent every 8 weeks for 12 doses.

Nonprogressing, low-grade, CD20-positive, B-cell NHL (after first-line CVP chemotherapy): In patients who have not progressed following 6 to 8 cycles of CVP chemotherapy (stable disease), 375 mg/M^2 may be administered as an infusion once a week for 4 doses every 6 months for up to 16 doses.

Diffuse large B-cell, CD20-positive NHL: 375 mg/M^2 as an infusion on Day 1 of each cycle of chemotherapy for up to 8 doses.

Chronic lymphocytic leukemia (CLL): 375 mg/M^2 the day before the initiation of FC chemotherapy (fludarabine [Fludara] and cyclophosphamide [Cytoxan]) in the first cycle, then 500 mg/M^2 on Day 1 of Cycles 2 through 6 (every 28 days); see Precautions.

Granulomatosis with polyangiitis (GPA [WG]) and microscopic polyangiitis (MPA):
Induction treatment of patients with active GPA/MPA: Methylprednisolone: 1000 mg/day IV for 1 to 3 days followed by oral prednisone 1 mg/kg/day (not to exceed 80 mg/day and tapered per clinical practice) is recommended to treat severe vasculitis symptoms. This

---

[a]Please see p. xi for more information on biosimilars.

regimen should begin within 14 days before or with the initiation of rituximab and may continue during and after the 4-week course of treatment.

Rituximab: 375 mg/M^2 as an infusion once weekly for 4 weeks.

Follow-up treatment (for patients with GPA/MPA who have achieved disease control with induction treatment): Methylprednisolone: 100 mg IV. Complete 30 minutes before each rituximab infusion. ***Rituximab:*** Two 500-mg infusions separated by 2 weeks, followed by a 500-mg infusion every 6 months thereafter based on clinical evaluation. If induction treatment of active disease was with rituximab, follow-up treatment should be initiated within 24 weeks after the last rituximab induction infusion or based on clinical evaluation but no sooner than 16 weeks after the last induction dose. If induction treatment was with other standard immunosuppressants, rituximab follow-up treatment should be initiated within the 4-week period after achievement of disease control.

Therapeutic regimen with ibritumomab tiuxetan for treatment of NHL: *Rituximab:* 250 mg/M^2 as an IV infusion. Given in a specific protocol in combination with the radiotherapeutic antibody ibritumomab tiuxetan (Zevalin); see ibritumomab prescribing information.

RITUXAN AND TRUXIMA

Rheumatoid arthritis: Administer ***glucocorticoids*** (e.g., methylprednisolone [Solu-Medrol] 100 mg IV or equivalent) 30 minutes before each infusion of rituximab to reduce the incidence and severity of infusion reactions. Follow with a rituximab infusion of 1,000 mg. Repeat entire sequence one time in 2 weeks. Given in combination with methotrexate. Subsequent courses should be administered every 24 weeks or based on clinical evaluation but not sooner than every 16 weeks.

RITUXAN

Component of the therapeutic regimen with ibritumomab tiuxetan (Zevalin) for treatment of NHL: *Rituximab:* 250 mg/M^2 as an IV infusion. Given in a specific protocol in combination with the radiotherapeutic antibody ibritumomab tiuxetan; see ibritumomab prescribing information.

Pemphigus vulgaris: Additional premedication (e.g., methylprednisolone 100 mg IV or equivalent) 30 minutes before each infusion is required. Administer rituximab as two 1000-mg infusions separated by 2 weeks in combination with a tapering course of glucocorticoids. ***Maintenance treatment:*** 500 mg as an infusion at month 12 and every 6 months thereafter based on clinical evaluation. ***Treatment of relapse:*** 1,000 mg as an infusion. In addition, consider resuming or increasing the glucocorticoid dose based on clinical evaluation. Subsequent rituximab infusions may be administered no sooner than 16 weeks after the previous infusion.

PEDIATRIC DOSE

RITUXAN

Induction treatment of pediatric patients with active GPA/MPA: Administer Rituxan 375 mg/M^2 as an intravenous infusion once weekly for 4 weeks. Before the first Rituxan infusion, administer IV methylprednisolone 30 mg/kg (not to exceed 1 Gm/day) daily for 3 days. Continue with oral steroids per clinical practice.

Follow-up treatment (for pediatric patients with GPA/MPA who have achieved disease control with induction treatment): Administer Rituxan as two 250 mg/M^2 IV infusions separated by 2 weeks, followed by 250 mg/M^2 IV infusion every 6 months thereafter based on clinical evaluation. If induction treatment of active disease was with a rituximab product, initiate follow-up treatment with Rituxan within 24 weeks after the last induction infusion with a rituximab product or based on clinical evaluation but no sooner than 16 weeks after the last induction infusion with a rituximab product. If induction treatment of active disease was with other standard of care immunosuppressants, initiate Rituxan follow-up treatment with the 4-week period after achievement of disease control.

DOSE ADJUSTMENTS

No dose adjustments recommended. Has not been formally studied in patients with renal or hepatic impairment. See Rate of Administration. ■ Interrupt or slow infusion rate for infusion-related reactions. Continue the infusion at one-half the previous rate when symptoms subside.

DILUTION

Available in 100 mg/10 mL and 500 mg/50 mL (10 mg/mL) single-dose vials. Each single dose must be further diluted to a final concentration of 1 to 4 mg/mL with NS or D5W. 500 mg (50 mL) in 450 mL will yield 1 mg/mL; 500 mg (50 mL) in 75 mL will yield 4 mg/mL. Gently invert to mix solution. Contains no preservatives; discard any unused portion left in vial.

Storage: Refrigerate vials at 2° to 8° C (36° to 46° F); protect from light and freezing. Do not shake. Do not use beyond expiration date. Diluted solutions may be refrigerated for 24 hours and are stable at room temperature for an additional 24 hours (refrigeration preferred to RT).

COMPATIBILITY

Manufacturer states, "Rituximab should not be mixed or diluted with other drugs." No **incompatibilities** with polyvinylchloride or polyethylene bags have been observed.

RATE OF ADMINISTRATION

Must be given as an infusion. ***Do not administer as an IV push or bolus.*** Infusion reactions are a common occurrence and may be prevented or lessened with premedication and a reduced rate of infusion.

First infusion: Begin with an initial rate of 50 mg/hr (at this rate a 500-mg dose would be infused over 10 hours). If no discomfort or adverse effects occur, may be gradually increased by 50-mg/hr increments at 30-minute intervals to a maximum rate of 400 mg/hr. At any time that discomfort or adverse effects occur, interrupt or reduce the rate of infusion. When symptoms have completely resolved, the infusion can be restarted at half the previous rate. Discontinue the infusion for severe reactions and treat as indicated; see Antidote.

Subsequent infusions: If the patient did not tolerate the first infusion well, follow instructions under first infusion. If no discomfort or adverse effects occurred with the first infusion, use the following guidelines:

Standard infusion: Subsequent infusions may begin with an initial rate of 100 mg/hr and increased by 100-mg/hr increments at 30-minute intervals to a maximum rate of 400 mg/hr. See all precautionary measures under First Infusion (see above).

Previously untreated follicular NHL and diffuse large B-cell lymphoma (DLBCL) patients: If a Grade 3 or 4 infusion-related reaction did not occur during the first infusion, a subsequent 90-minute infusion can be administered with a glucocorticoid-containing chemotherapy regimen. Administer the corticosteroid, acetaminophen, and diphenhydramine; follow with rituximab. Administer 20% of rituximab dose equally distributed over the first 30 minutes and the remaining 80% of the dose equally distributed over 60 minutes. If this initial subsequent 90-minute infusion is tolerated, it can be repeated in the remaining infusions of the protocol. ▪ Patients who have clinically significant cardiovascular disease or who have a circulating lymphocyte count equal to or greater than 5,000/mm^3 before Cycle 2 should not be administered the 90-minute infusion.

ACTIONS

An antineoplastic agent. A humanized (Ig)G$_1$ monoclonal antibody produced by recombinant DNA technology. A CD20-directed cytolytic antibody designed to bind to the CD20 antigen found on the surface of normal (pre-B-lymphocytes and mature B-lymphocytes) and malignant B-lymphocytes. Upon binding to CD20, rituximab mediates B-cell lysis. Results in a rapid and sustained depletion of circulating and tissue-based B-cells. Cell lysis may be the result of complement-dependent cytotoxicity and antibody-dependent, cell-mediated toxicity. In oncology patients, rituximab may sensitize drug-resistant human B-cell lymphoma cell lines to cytotoxic chemotherapy. Detected in serum for 3 to 6 months after completion of therapy. B-cell depletion was sustained for 6 to 9 months posttreatment in 83% of patients. B-cell recovery begins at approximately 6 months, and most levels return to normal by 12 months following completion of treatment. B-cells are believed to play a role in the pathogenesis of rheumatoid arthritis (RA) and associated chronic synovitis. In this setting, B-cells may act at multiple sites in the autoimmune/inflammatory process, including through production of rheumatoid factor and other autoantibodies, antigen presentation, T-cell activation, and/ or proinflammatory cytokine production. In RA it induces depletion of peripheral B-lymphocytes, with near-complete depletion occurring in most patients within 2 weeks of the first dose. This B-lymphocyte depletion lasted for at least 6 months, followed by a gradual recovery. Treatment with rituximab in patients with RA was associated with a reduction of certain biologic markers for inflammation. A few patients had prolonged peripheral B-cell depletion lasting more than 3 years after a single course of treatment. Median half-life ranged from 18 to 32 days depending on diagnosis. Crosses the placental barrier. May be secreted in breast milk.

INDICATIONS AND USES

RITUXIMAB PRODUCTS: As a single agent in the treatment of patients with relapsed or refractory low-grade or follicular CD20-positive, B-cell NHL. ▪ In combination with CHOP (cyclophosphamide, doxorubicin, vincristine, and prednisone) or other anthracycline-based chemotherapy regimens for treatment in previously untreated diffuse large B-cell, CD20-positive NHL. ▪ Treatment of previously untreated follicular, CD20-positive, B-cell NHL in combination with first-line chemotherapy and as a single-agent maintenance therapy in patients achieving a complete or partial response to rituximab in combination with chemotherapy. ▪ Treatment of nonprogressing (including stable disease), low-grade, CD20-positive, B-cell NHL as a single agent after first-line cyclophosphamide, vincristine, and prednisone (CVP) chemotherapy. ▪ Treatment of patients with previously untreated and previously treated CD20-positive CLL. Used in combination with FC chemotherapy (fludarabine and cyclophosphamide). ▪ In combination with glucocorticoids for the treatment of adult patients with granulomatosis with polyangiitis (GPA [Wegener's granulomatosis (WG)]) and microscopic polyangiitis (MPA). ▪ In combination with ibritumomab tiuxetan as part of a therapeutic regimen for the treatment of patients with relapsed or refractory low-grade or follicular B-cell NHL or for the treatment of previously untreated follicular NHL in patients who have achieved a partial or complete response to first-line chemotherapy. *Rituxan and Truxima:* In combination with methotrexate to reduce S/S and to slow the progression of structural damage in adult patients with moderate to severe RA who have had an inadequate response to one or more TNF (tumor necrosis factor) antagonist therapies. *Rituxan:* Treatment of patients with moderate to severe pemphigus vulgaris. *Rituxan:* In combination with glucocorticoids for the treatment of pediatric patients 2 years of age and older with GPA Wegener's granulomatosis (WG) and MPA.

CONTRAINDICATIONS

Manufacturer states, "None."

PRECAUTIONS

For IV infusion only. Do not administer as an IV push or bolus. ▪ Has been given on an outpatient basis; however, rituximab should be administered by or under the direction of the physician specialist in facilities equipped to monitor the patient and respond to any medical emergency. ▪ Severe infusion-related reactions have occurred with rituximab infusions, and some have been fatal. Most severe reactions occur within 30 minutes to 2 hours of beginning the first infusion. Deaths within 24 hours of rituximab infusion have occurred. S/S of severe reactions may include hypotension, angioedema, hypoxia, urticaria, or bronchospasm. More severe manifestations may include anaphylactic and anaphylactoid events, pulmonary infiltrates, acute respiratory distress syndrome, myocardial infarction, ventricular fibrillation, and cardiogenic shock. ▪ Tumor lysis syndrome (TLS) has been reported within 12 to 24 hours after the first rituximab infusion in patients with NHL. S/S include renal insufficiency, hyperkalemia, hypocalcemia, hyperuricemia, or hyperphosphatemia. May cause acute renal failure requiring dialysis and has been fatal. ▪ TLS occurs more often in patients with high numbers of circulating malignant cells or high tumor burden. Consider prophylactic measures; see Monitor. ▪ Renal toxicity occurs more frequently in patients with high numbers of circulating malignant cells, high tumor burden, and/or TLS. Severe, including fatal, renal toxicity has occurred in patients with NHL. ▪ Safety of immunization with vaccines, particularly live virus vaccines, following rituximab therapy has not been studied. Review vaccination status. Administration of live virus vaccines is not recommended. Weigh benefit versus risk in NHL patients if a delay in treatment may occur for vaccination. ▪ Administer any CDC-recommended, non–live virus vaccinations to patients treated with rituximab at least 4 weeks before initiating treatment with rituximab. ▪ In CLL patients, *Pneumocystis jiroveci* pneumonia (PCP) and antiherpetic viral prophylaxis is recommended during treatment and for up to 12 months following treatment. ▪ In GPA (WG) and MPA patients, PCP prophylaxis is recommended during treatment and for at least 6 months following the last rituximab infusion. ▪ In PV patients, PCP prophylaxis is recommended during and after rituximab treatment. ▪ Mucocutaneous reactions (including lichenoid dermatitis, paraneoplastic pemphigus, Stevens-Johnson syndrome, toxic epidermal necrolysis, and vesiculobullous dermatitis), some with fatal outcomes, have been reported. Onset of reaction has been variable and includes reports of onset on the first day of rituximab exposure. ▪ Hepatitis B virus reactivation with fulminant hepatitis, hepatic failure, and death has been reported. For patients who show evidence of prior hepatitis B infection, consult physician with expertise in managing hepatitis regarding monitoring and consideration for HBV antiviral therapy; see Monitor. ▪ Not recommended for use in patients with severe active infections. ▪ Serious (including fatal) bacterial, fungal, and new or reactivated viral infections can occur during and following rituximab therapy. Infections have been reported in some patients with prolonged hypogammaglobulinemia (defined as hypogammaglobulinemia more than 11 months after rituximab exposure). New or reactivated viral infections have included JC virus (progressive multifocal leukoencephalopathy [PML], cytomegalovirus, herpes simplex virus, parvovirus B19, varicella zoster virus, West Nile virus, and hepatitis B and C). Deaths have occurred. ▪ JC virus infection resulting in PML and death can occur in rituximab-treated patients who have hematologic malignancies or autoimmune diseases. PML is a rare, progressive, demyelinating disease of the CNS. Usually leads to death or severe disability, and there is no effective treatment. Most patients with hematologic malignancies diagnosed with PML received rituximab in combination with chemotherapy or as part of a hematopoietic stem cell transplant. Patients with autoimmune diseases had prior or concurrent immunosuppressive therapy. Most cases of PML were diagnosed within 12 months of the last rituximab infusion. ▪ Cardiac adverse reactions, including ventricular fibrillation, myocardial infarction, and cardiogenic shock, have occurred. RA patients may have an increased risk of cardiovascular events. ▪ Not indicated for use in patients with RA who have responded to treatment with TNF antagonists (e.g., adalimumab [Humira], etanercept [Enbrel]). ▪ Abdominal pain, bowel obstruction, and perforation have been reported in patients receiving rituximab in combination with chemotherapy. Death has occurred. Mean time to GI perforation was 6 days (range 1 to 77 days) in patients with NHL. ▪ Use of concomitant immunosuppressants other than corticosteroids has not been studied in GPA (WG), MPA, or PV patients exhibiting peripheral B-cell depletion after treatment with rituximab. ▪ As with all therapeutic proteins, there is a potential for immunogenicity. ▪ See Rate of Administration, Drug/Lab Interactions, and Antidote.

Monitor: In patients with lymphoid malignancies who are receiving rituximab monotherapy, obtain a baseline CBC and platelet count and repeat before each course of therapy. In patients treated with rituximab and chemotherapy, obtain baseline CBC and platelet count at weekly to monthly intervals. Repeat more frequently in patients who develop cytopenias (e.g., leukopenia, neutropenia, thrombocytopenia). In RA, GPA (WG), or MPA patients, obtain a baseline CBC and platelet count and repeat at 2- to 4-month intervals during therapy. Duration of cytopenias may extend months beyond the treatment period. ▪ Screen all patients for HBV infection before treatment initiation. Monitor patients with evidence of current or prior HBV for clinical and laboratory signs of hepatitis or HBV reactivation during and for several months after treatment with rituximab. HBV reactivation has been reported up to 24 months after completion of rituximab therapy. ▪ Observe patient continuously for symptoms of infusion reactions, which are more common during the first infusion but can occur at any time; see Antidote. ▪ Monitor HR and BP frequently. ▪ ECG and pulmonary monitoring required during and in the immediate posttreatment period in patients with pre-existing cardiac or pulmonary conditions, in any patient who develops or has previously developed a clinically significant cardiopulmonary adverse event during treatment, and in patients with RA. ▪ Monitor patients with high numbers of circulating malignant cells (greater than or equal to 25,000/mm^3) with or without other evidence of high tumor burden for infusion reaction and tumor lysis syndrome. Monitoring of serum electrolytes, uric acid, and renal function indicated. ▪ Prevention and treatment of hyperuricemia due to TLS may be accomplished with adequate hydration and, if necessary, antihyperuricemia agents (e.g., allopurinol [Aloprim]); see Drug/Lab Interactions. ▪ Prevention and/or treatment of hyperphosphatemia, hyperkalemia, and hypocalcemia due to TLS is also indicated. ▪ Monitor closely for signs of renal failure, and discontinue rituximab in patients with a rising SCr or oliguria. ▪ Assess neurologic status frequently. Consider PML in patients with new-onset neurologic manifestations; consultation with a neurologist, brain MRI, and lumbar puncture may be required for diagnosis. ▪ Observe closely for signs of infection. Prophylactic antibiotics may be indicated pending results of C/S in a febrile neutropenic patient. ▪ Monitor for signs of mucocutaneous reactions. ▪ Use prophylactic antiemetics to reduce nausea and vomiting and increase patient comfort. ▪ Monitor for thrombocytopenia (platelet count less than 50,000/mm^3). Initiate precautions to prevent excessive bleeding (e.g., inspect IV sites, skin, and mucous membranes; use extreme care during invasive procedures; test urine, emesis, stool, and secretions for occult blood). ▪ Monitor patients closely for abdominal pain and repeated vomiting, especially early in the course of treatment. A thorough diagnostic evaluation is indicated; treat appropriately to prevent bowel obstruction and perforation. ▪ See Premedication in Usual Dose, Rate of Administration, Precautions, Drug/Lab Interactions, and Antidote.

Patient Education: Avoid pregnancy. Effective contraception recommended for females of reproductive potential during and for 12 months after rituximab therapy. See Maternal/Child. ▪ Read manufacturer's patient information sheet before each infusion. ▪ Discuss health history (e.g., presence of an infection, carrier of or had a previous hepatitis B virus infection, heart or lung problems, recent or scheduled vaccinations, scheduled surgeries) and prescription and nonprescription medications with the health care provider administering the rituximab. ▪ Review monitoring requirements and potential side effects before therapy. ▪ Promptly report any adverse reactions, including S/S of infection (e.g., cold or flu symptoms, dysuria, fever), infusion reactions (e.g., angioedema, breathing problems, chest pain, cough, dizziness, hypotension, palpitations, urticaria), severe mucocutaneous reactions (e.g., blisters, chest pain, painful sores or ulcers on the mouth, peeling skin, rash, and pustules), hepatitis (e.g., abdominal pain, yellow discoloration of the skin or eyes, worsening fatigue), tumor lysis syndrome (e.g., diarrhea, lethargy, nausea, vomiting), cardiovascular complications (e.g., chest pain, irregular heartbeats), or bowel obstruction/perforation (e.g., severe abdominal pain, repeated vomiting); immediate medical treatment may be indicated. ▪ New neurologic S/S (e.g., changes in vision, loss of balance or coordination, disorientation, or confusion) could be warning signs of PML. Report them promptly. ▪ Laboratory monitoring (e.g., CBC, renal function) required. ▪ See Appendix D, p. 1311.

Maternal/Child: Avoid pregnancy; effective contraception required; see Patient Education. Based on human data, can cause fetal harm due to B-cell lymphocytopenia in infants exposed to rituximab in utero. B-cell lymphocytopenia generally lasting less than 6 months has occurred in infants exposed to rituximab in utero. Use only if clearly needed. Monitor newborns and infants for signs of infection and manage accordingly. ▪ Do not breastfeed during treatment and for at least 6 months after the last dose of rituximab. ▪ The safety and effectiveness of **rituximab products** have not been established in pediatric patients; however, the safety and effectiveness for use of **Rituxan** in pediatric patients 2 years of age and older has been established for the treatment of GPA and MPA. Hypogammaglobulinemia has been observed in pediatric patients treated with rituximab.

Elderly: No overall differences in effectiveness were observed between different age groups of patients treated for diffuse large B-cell NHL. Cardiac and pulmonary adverse reactions (e.g., supraventricular arrhythmia, pneumonia, pneumonitis) occurred more frequently in the elderly. ▪ The numbers of elderly treated for low-grade or follicular NHL were insufficient to determine differences in response to therapy, but differences in safety or effectiveness were not identified. ▪ The incidence of Grade 3 and 4 adverse reactions was higher in patients over 70 years of age treated for CLL with R-FC. No observed benefit was seen with the addition of rituximab to FC in patients over 65 to 70 years of age. ▪ In older patients being treated for RA, GPA, or MPA, the incidence of side effects was similar to younger adults; however, the rate of serious side effects, including serious infection, malignancies, and cardiovascular events, was higher. ▪ The numbers of elderly patients treated for PV were insufficient to determine differences in response to therapy.

DRUG/LAB INTERACTIONS
Formal drug interaction studies have not been performed. ▪ Rituximab may lessen the therapeutic effect of **inactivated vaccines** and may enhance the adverse/toxic effects of **live vaccines**; see Precautions. ▪ Risk of renal toxicity increased in patients receiving concomitant therapy with **cisplatin** (the combination of cisplatin and rituximab is not an approved treatment regimen). ▪ Data on the safety of the use of biologic agents or **disease-modifying antirheumatic drugs** (DMARDs) other than methotrexate in RA patients are limited. Monitor patients closely for signs of infection with concurrent use of biologic agents or DMARDs other than methotrexate. ▪ In patients with CLL, rituximab did not alter the systemic exposure to fludarabine or cyclophosphamide. ▪ In patients with RA, concomitant administration of methotrexate or cyclophosphamide did not alter the pharmacokinetics of rituximab.

SIDE EFFECTS
Lymphoid malignancies: *CD20-positive, B-cell NHL:* The most common side effects are asthenia, chills, fever, infection, infusion-related reactions, and lymphopenia.
CLL: The most common side effects during clinical trials were infusion reactions and neutropenia.

Other reported reactions for NHL and CLL included abdominal pain, angioedema, anxiety, arthralgia, back pain, bronchospasm, chest tightness, cough, cytopenias (anemia, leukopenia, lymphopenia, neutropenia, thrombocytopenia), diarrhea, dizziness, dyspnea, flushing, headache, hepato-biliary toxicity, hyperglycemia, hypertension, hypotension, increased LDH, myalgia, nausea, night sweats, pain, peripheral edema, peripheral sensory neuropathy, pruritus, pulmonary toxicity, rash, rhinitis, rigors, sinusitis, throat irritation, urticaria, vomiting, weight gain.

Rheumatoid arthritis: Common side effects include infusion reactions, cardiac events, and infections (e.g., bronchitis, nasopharyngitis, sinusitis, URI, UTI). Other reported side effects include abdominal pain (upper), anxiety, arthralgia, asthenia, chills, dyspepsia, fever, hypercholesterolemia hypertension, migraine headache, nausea, paresthesia, pruritus, rhinitis, throat irritation, urticaria.

GPA (WG) and MPA: The most common side effects reported include anemia, diarrhea, headache, infections, infusion reactions, muscle spasm, nausea, and peripheral edema. Other commonly reported side effects include arthralgia, cough, dyspnea, epistaxis, fatigue, hypertension, hypogammaglobulinemia, increased ALT, insomnia, leukopenia, and rash. All major side effects associated with rituximab (e.g., infusion reactions, infections) may occur.

PV: The most common side effects reported include depression, infections, and infusion reactions. Other reported adverse reactions include abdominal pain (upper), alopecia, conjunctivitis, dizziness, fatigue, fever, headache, herpes simplex, herpes zoster, irritability, musculoskeletal pain, pruritus, skin disorders, tachycardia, and urticaria.

Serious but less frequently reported adverse reactions associated with rituximab therapy include angina, bowel obstruction and perforation, cardiac arrhythmias (e.g., supraventricular and ventricular tachycardia, ventricular fibrillation), hepatitis B reactivation with fulminant hepatitis and other viral infections (including JC virus infection resulting in PML), infusion reactions, mucocutaneous reactions (e.g., lichenoid dermatitis, paraneoplastic pemphigus, Stevens-Johnson syndrome, toxic epidermal necrolysis, and vesiculobullous dermatitis), renal failure, and tumor lysis syndrome (may occur within 12 to 24 hours). Infusion-related side reactions generally occur within 30 minutes to 2 hours of beginning of first infusion and may include any of the following S/S: angioedema, bronchospasm, chills/rigors, dizziness, fever, hypertension, hypotension, myalgia, pruritus, rash, urticaria, or vomiting.

Several other adverse reactions have been reported in fewer than 5% of study patients receiving rituximab.

Post-Marketing: Bowel obstruction and perforation, bronchiolitis obliterans (fatal), cardiac failure (fatal), disease progression of Kaposi's sarcoma, Grade 3 to 4 prolonged or late-onset neutropenia, hyperviscosity syndrome in Waldenström's macroglobulinemia, hypogammaglobulinemia (prolonged), increase in fatal infections in HIV-associated lymphoma and a reported increased incidence of Grade 3 and 4 infections in patients with previously treated lymphoma without known HIV infection, interstitial lung disease (fatal), lupus-like syndrome, marrow hyperplasia, mucocutaneous reactions (severe) including pyoderma gangrenosum (including genital presentation), optic neuritis, pancytopenia (prolonged), pleuritis, polyarticular arthritis, PRES, RPLS, serum sickness, systemic vasculitis, uveitis, vasculitis with rash, and viral infections, including PML.

ANTIDOTE

Keep physician informed of all side effects. May constitute a medical emergency or will be treated symptomatically as indicated. Infusion-related side effects generally resolve with slowing or interruption of the rituximab infusion and with supportive care (IV saline, diphenhydramine, bronchodilators such as albuterol or aminophylline, and acetaminophen). Most patients who have had non–life-threatening reactions have been able to complete the full course of therapy. Restart the infusion at half the previous rate after symptoms have resolved completely. Discontinue the infusion immediately for any life-threatening side effect (e.g., clinically significant bronchospasm, cardiac arrhythmias, Grade 3 or 4 infusion reactions, hypersensitivity reactions, hypotension, tumor lysis syndrome, or severe mucocutaneous reaction). Discontinue rituximab in any patient who develops a serious infection or experiences HBV reactivation. Initiate appropriate antiviral/anti-infective therapy as indicated. Discontinue treatment in patients who develop severe mucocutaneous reactions. Skin biopsy may be required to diagnose mucocutaneous reaction and guide treatment. Safety of readministration of rituximab to patients with severe mucocutaneous reactions has not been determined. Discontinue treatment in patients who develop PML; consider reduction or discontinuation of concomitant chemotherapy or immunosuppressive therapy. Discontinue treatment in patients with a rising SCr or oliguria. Treat severe infusion reactions/anaphylaxis with oxygen, antihistamines (diphenhydramine), epinephrine, and corticosteroids as indicated. Maintain a patent airway. Discontinue rituximab for serious or life-threatening cardiac arrhythmias and treat as indicated. Treat hypotension with IV fluids, Trendelenburg position, and, if necessary, vasopressors (e.g., norepinephrine, dopamine). Blood modifiers (e.g., darbepoetin alfa, epoetin alfa, filgrastim, pegfilgrastim, sargramostim) may be indicated to treat bone marrow toxicity. Tumor lysis syndrome requires correction of electrolyte abnormalities and monitoring of renal function and fluid balance. Supportive care, including dialysis, may be required. Resuscitate if indicated.

ROMIDEPSIN
(ROE-mi-DEP-sin)

Istodax

Antineoplastic
(histone deacetylase
[HDAC] inhibitor)

USUAL DOSE

Pretreatment: Verify pregnancy status. Baseline studies indicated; see Monitor.

Romidepsin: 14 mg/M^2 as an infusion over 4 hours. Administer on Days 1, 8, and 15 of a 28-day cycle; see Monitor. Cycles may be repeated every 28 days provided the patient continues to benefit from and tolerates the drug.

DOSE ADJUSTMENTS

Discontinuation or interruption with or without dose reduction to 10 mg/M^2 may be needed to manage adverse drug reactions as outlined in the following charts.

Romidepsin Dose Modification for Nonhematologic Toxicities Except Alopecia		
CTCAE[a] Grade on Day of Treatment	Action	Dose on Recovery
Grade 2 or 3 toxicity	Delay dose until toxicity returns to ≤Grade 1 or baseline	14 mg/M^2
Grade 3 toxicity recurrence	Delay dose until toxicity returns to ≤Grade 1 or baseline	Permanently reduce dose to 10 mg/M^2
Grade 4 toxicity	Delay dose until toxicity returns to ≤Grade 1 or baseline	Permanently reduce dose to 10 mg/M^2
Grade 3 or 4 toxicities recur after dose reduction	Discontinue therapy	

[a]Per Common Terminology Criteria for Adverse Events (CTCAE), Version 4.0.

Romidepsin Dose Modification for Hematologic Toxicities		
CTCAE[a] Grade on Day of Treatment	Action	Dose on Recovery
Grade 3 or 4 neutropenia or thrombocytopenia	Delay dose until ANC ≥1,500/mm^3 and/or platelet count ≥75,000/mm^3 or baseline	14 mg/M^2
Grade 4 febrile (≥38.5° C) neutropenia or thrombocytopenia that requires platelet transfusion	Delay dose until the specific cytopenia returns to ≤Grade 1 or baseline	Permanently reduce dose to 10 mg/M^2

[a]Per Common Terminology Criteria for Adverse Events (CTCAE), Version 4.0.

▪ No dose adjustments required based on age; gender; race; mild, moderate, or severe renal impairment; or mild hepatic impairment. ▪ Adjust starting dose for patients with moderate or severe hepatic impairment as shown in the following chart; see Monitor.

Recommendations for Starting Dose in Patients With Moderate and Severe Hepatic Impairment		
Hepatic Impairment	Bilirubin Levels	Romidepsin Dose
Moderate	>1.5 × ULN to ≤3 × ULN	7 mg/M^2
Severe	>3 × ULN	5 mg/M^2

ULN, Upper limit of normal.

DILUTION
Special techniques required; see Precautions: Romidepsin and diluent vials contain an overfill to ensure that the recommended volume can be withdrawn at a concentration of 5 mg/mL. Reconstitute each 10-mg single-dose vial with 2.2 mL of the supplied diluent. Inject diluent slowly into the vial of romidepsin and swirl contents until there are no visible particles. Concentration equals 5 mg/mL. Withdraw the calculated dose and further dilute in 500 mL NS.

Filters: Specific information not available.

Storage: Store vials in carton at CRT. Reconstituted solution is stable for up to 8 hours at RT. Diluted solutions are stable at RT for 24 hours, but use soon after dilution is recommended.

COMPATIBILITY
Manufacturer states, "The diluted solution is **compatible** with polyvinyl chloride (PVC), ethylene vinyl acetate (EVA), polyethylene (PE) infusion bags as well as glass bottles." No additional information available; consult a pharmacist.

RATE OF ADMINISTRATION
A single dose as an infusion equally distributed over 4 hours.

ACTIONS
A histone deacetylase (HDAC) inhibitor. HDACs catalyze the removal of acetyl groups from acetylated lysine residues in histones, resulting in the modulation of gene expression. Induces cell cycle arrest and apoptosis of some cancer cell lines. Mechanism of antineoplastic effect not fully characterized. Highly protein bound. It undergoes extensive metabolism in vitro by CYP3A4 with minor contributions from other cytochrome P_{450} isoenzymes. Half-life is approximately 3 hours. No accumulation of plasma concentration observed after repeated dosing.

INDICATIONS AND USES
Treatment of cutaneous T-cell lymphoma (CTCL) in adult patients who have received at least one prior systemic therapy. ▪ Treatment of peripheral T-cell lymphoma (PTCL) in adult patients who have received at least one prior therapy. This indication is approved under accelerated approval based on response rate. Continued approval for this indication may be contingent on verification and description of clinical benefit in confirmatory trials.

CONTRAINDICATIONS
Manufacturer states, "None."

PRECAUTIONS
Follow guidelines for handling cytotoxic agents. See Appendix A, p. 1308. ▪ Administered under the direction of a physician knowledgeable in its use in a facility with adequate diagnostic and treatment facilities to monitor the patients and respond to any medical emergency. ▪ Myelosuppression can occur (e.g., anemia, lymphopenia, neutropenia, and thrombocytopenia). Dose modification based on ANC, and platelet count is required; see Dose Adjustments. ▪ Serious and sometimes fatal infections, including pneumonia, sepsis, and viral reactivation (including Epstein-Barr and hepatitis B viruses), have been reported during or within 30 days of therapy. Patients with a history of prior treatment with monoclonal antibodies directed against lymphocyte antigens and patients with disease involvement of the bone marrow may be at increased risk for developing a life-threatening infection. ▪ Reactivation of Epstein-Barr viral infection leading to liver failure has occurred. In one case, ganciclovir prophylaxis failed to prevent Epstein-Barr viral reactivation. ▪ Several treatment-emergent ECG changes have been reported (e.g., T-wave and ST-segment changes, QT prolongation); clinical significance is unknown. Use caution in patients with congenital long QT syndrome or a history of significant CV disease or in patients taking antiarrhythmic or other medicines that can lead to significant QT prolongation; see Drug/Lab Interactions. ▪ Tumor lysis syndrome has been reported. Patients with advanced disease and/or high tumor burden are at greater risk. ▪ Use with caution in patients with moderate or severe hepatic impairment; see Dose Adjustments and Monitor. ▪ Renal impairment is not expected to influence ro-

midepsin exposure. Effect on end-stage renal disease (ESRD) has not been studied; use with caution in patients with ESRD.

Monitor: Due to the risk of QT prolongation, potassium and magnesium should be within the normal range before administration of romidepsin. ▪ Obtain baseline CBC, platelets, electrolytes, and liver function tests. Baseline CrCl or SCr may be indicated. ▪ Monitor CBC, platelets, and electrolytes during treatment and modify dose as indicated; see Dose Adjustments. ▪ Consider ECG monitoring and more frequent monitoring of electrolytes in at-risk cardiac patients; see Precautions. ▪ Monitor for signs of tumor lysis syndrome. Prevention and treatment of hyperuricemia may be accomplished with adequate hydration and, if necessary, antihyperuricemia agents (e.g., allopurinol). ▪ Monitor patients with hepatic impairment more frequently for toxicity, especially during the first cycle. ▪ Monitor for thrombocytopenia (platelet count less than 50,000/mm³). Initiate precautions to prevent excessive bleeding (e.g., inspect IV sites, skin, and mucous membranes; use extreme care during invasive procedures; test urine, emesis, stool, and secretions for occult blood). ▪ Use prophylactic antiemetics to reduce nausea and/or vomiting and increase patient comfort. ▪ Observe closely for signs of infection. Prophylactic antibiotics may be indicated pending results of C/S in a febrile neutropenic patient. ▪ Monitoring for hepatitis B reactivation and administration of antiviral prophylaxis should be considered in patients with evidence of prior hepatitis B infection.

Patient Education: Read patient insert carefully. ▪ Verify pregnancy status within 7 days of initiating romidepsin therapy. ▪ Avoid pregnancy; use of effective contraception is recommended for females of reproductive potential and for males with female partners of reproductive potential during treatment and for at least 1 month after the final dose. Because romidepsin may reduce the effectiveness of estrogen-containing contraceptives, alternative methods with non–estrogen-containing contraceptives (e.g., condoms, intrauterine device) should be used. ▪ May cause male and female infertility. ▪ Blood counts will be required at regular intervals. ▪ Report any history of hepatitis B before starting therapy. ▪ Maintain high fluid intake for at least 72 hours after each dose to decrease the risks associated with tumor lysis syndrome. ▪ Promptly report unusual bleeding, abnormal heartbeat, chest pain, or shortness of breath. ▪ Report burning on urination, cough, fever, flu-like symptoms, muscle aches, or worsening of skin problems. ▪ Nausea and vomiting are common. Prophylactic antiemetics are recommended. ▪ Discuss medications (prescription, nonprescription, and herbal) with a health care professional; see Drug/Lab Interactions. ▪ See Appendix D, p. 1311.

Maternal/Child: Based on its mechanism of action and findings from animal studies, romidepsin can cause fetal harm when administered to a pregnant female. ▪ Do not breastfeed during treatment and for at least 1 week after the last dose. ▪ Safety and effectiveness for use in pediatric patients not established.

Elderly: No differences in safety and effectiveness compared with younger patients were noted; however; greater sensitivity of some older patients cannot be ruled out.

DRUG/LAB INTERACTIONS

Concurrent use with **warfarin** may prolong PT and elevate INR. Monitoring of PT and INR recommended. ▪ **Strong CYP3A4 inhibitors** (e.g., atazanavir, clarithromycin, indinavir, itraconazole, ketoconazole, nefazodone, nelfinavir, ritonavir, saquinavir, and voriconazole) may increase concentrations of romidepsin; monitor for toxicity and follow dose modifications for toxicity; see Dose Adjustments. Use caution with concomitant use of **moderate CYP3A4** inhibitors (aprepitant, verapamil). ▪ Avoid coadministration with **rifampin (a strong CYP3A4 inducer).** In a pharmacokinetic drug interaction trial, romidepsin exposure was *increased* when coadministered with rifampin. Typically, coadministration of CYP3A4 inducers decreases concentrations of drugs metabolized by CYP3A4. The increase in exposure seen after coadministration with rifampin is likely due to rifampin's inhibition of an undetermined hepatic uptake process that is predominantly responsible for the disposition of romidepsin. It is unknown whether other **potent CYP3A4 inducers** (e.g., carbamazepine, phenobarbital, phenytoin, rifabutin, rifapentine, and St. John's wort) would alter the exposure of romidepsin. Avoid coadministration with other potent CYP3A4 inducers if possible. ■ Use caution with **drugs that inhibit the efflux transporter P-glycoprotein**; may increase concentrations of romidepsin. ■ Do not administer **live virus vaccines** to patients receiving antineoplastic drugs. ■ Concurrent use with other **drugs that prolong the QT interval** (e.g., antiarrhythmics [e.g., amiodarone, disopyramide, ibutilide, mexiletine, procainamide, quinidine], antihistamines, azole antifungals, fluoroquinolones, phenothiazines, and tricyclic antidepressants) may cause torsades de pointes and could be fatal.

SIDE EFFECTS

The most common side effects are anorexia, ECG T-wave changes, fatigue, infections, myelosuppression (e.g., anemia, lymphopenia, neutropenia, thrombocytopenia), nausea, and vomiting. Anemia, dyspnea, elevated AST, fatigue, hypomagnesemia, infection, pneumonia, QT prolongation, and thrombocytopenia were the most common reasons for discontinuing therapy. Adverse reactions categorized as severe included abdominal pain, acute renal failure, cardiopulmonary failure, cellulitis, central line infection, chest pain, deep venous thrombosis, dehydration, dyspnea, edema, elevated ALT and AST, fatigue, febrile neutropenia, fever, hyperbilirubinemia, hypersensitivity, hyperuricemia, hypoalbuminemia, hypocalcemia, hypophosphatemia, hypotension, hypoxia, infection, leukopenia, lymphopenia, nausea, neutropenia, pneumonitis, pulmonary embolism, reactivation of hepatitis B infection, sepsis, supraventricular arrhythmia, syncope, thrombocytopenia, ventricular arrhythmia, and vomiting. Other side effects reported include asthenia, constipation, dermatitis, diarrhea, dysgeusia, exfoliative dermatitis, hyperglycemia, hypermagnesemia, hypokalemia, hyponatremia, and pruritus.

ANTIDOTE

Treatment of most side effects will be supportive and may require dose delay, dose adjustment, or discontinuation; see Dose Adjustments. Discontinue if Grade 3 or 4 toxicities recur after dose reduction. Keep physician informed. Administration of blood products and/or blood modifiers (e.g., darbepoetin, epoetin alfa, filgrastim, pegfilgrastim, sargramostim) may be indicated to treat bone marrow toxicity. Treat hypersensitivity reactions with epinephrine, antihistamines, and corticosteroids as needed. No known antidote. Discontinue romidepsin and provide supportive therapy in overdose. Not known if romidepsin is dialyzable. Resuscitate if indicated.

SACITUZUMAB GOVITECAN
(**SAK**-i-**TOOZ** ue-mab **GOE**-vi-**TEE**-kan)

Antineoplastic agent
Topoisomerase I inhibitor

Trodelvy

USUAL DOSE
10 mg/kg IV on Days 1 and 8 of a 21-day treatment cycle. Continue until unacceptable toxicity or disease progression.

PEDIATRIC DOSE
Safety and efficacy have not been established.

DOSE ADJUSTMENTS
Renal: No dosage adjustments provided by manufacturer.
Hepatic: No dosage adjustments provided by manufacturer.
Hematologic: See manufacturer product information for specifics.

DILUTION
Allow vials to warm to room temperature. Reconstitute each vial with 20 mL of NS to a concentration of 10 mg/mL. Gently swirl vial for dissolution; may take up to 15 minutes; *do not shake*. Solution should be yellow and clear. After complete dissolution, immediately transfer the prescribed dose to a PVC, polypropylene, or ethylene/propylene copolymer infusion bag slowly to avoid foaming. Adjust volume in the infusion bag with NS as needed to a concentration of 1.1 to 3.4 mg/mL. Total volume per bag should not exceed 500 mL. If dose requires more than one 500-mL bag, divide and infuse sequentially.

COMPATIBILITY
Do not administer simultaneously with any other medication or IV solutions other than NS.

RATE OF ADMINISTRATION
Administer initial dose as an IV infusion over 3 hours; subsequent doses can be given over 1 to 2 hours if tolerated. Flush infusion line with 20 mL of NS. Do not give as an IV push or bolus. Administer infusion within 4 hours of administration (including infusion time).

ACTIONS
Sacituzumab govitecan is a topoisomerase 1 inhibitor, which leads to DNA damage, apoptosis, and cell death.

INDICATIONS AND USES
Breast cancer, urothelial cancer.

CONTRAINDICATIONS
Severe hypersensitivity to drug or any component of the formulation.

PRECAUTIONS
Bone marrow suppression, gastrointestinal (GI) toxicity, reduced UGT1A1 activity, polysorbate allergy, hypersensitivity.

Monitor: Blood counts prior to dose on Days 1 and 8 of each cycle and as clinically necessary. Hepatitis B virus screen prior to starting.

Patient Education: Advise patients to call physician if they experience infection, severe diarrhea, black or blood stools, dehydration or inability to take fluids by mouth, high blood sugar (confusion, increased thirst, hunger, frequent urination, fruity-smelling breath), electrolyte problems (mood changes, confusion, muscle weakness or pain, irregular heartbeat, vomiting), swelling, unexplained bruising or bleeding, numbness, not passing urine.

Maternal/Child: Check pregnancy status prior to use. Advise patient to use effective contraception during therapy and at least 6 months after last dose. May cause fetal harm. Breast-feeding is not recommended.

Elderly: Refer to adult dosing and precautions.

DRUG/LAB INTERACTIONS
5-ASA, bacille Calmette-Guérin (BCG) vaccine, baricitnib, brincidofovir, chloramphenicol ophthalmic, cladribine, clozapine, COVID-19 vaccines (may decrease effectiveness), moderate and strong CYP3A4 inducers (may decrease effectiveness of sacituzumab govitecan; avoid), strong CYP3A4 inhibitors (may increase serum concentration of sacituzumab govitecan; avoid), deferiprone, denosumab, dipyrone, echinacea, fexinidazole, fingolimod, inebilzumab, leflunomide, lenograstim, lipegfilgrastim, MMR vaccine (avoid), natalizumab, ocrelizumab, ofatumumab, ozanimod, pidotimod, pimecrolimus (avoid), ponesimod, promazine, rabies vaccine, roflumilast, spionimod, sipuleucel-T, smallpox and monkey pox vaccine, tacrolimus topical (avoid), talimogene laherparepvec (avoid), tertomotide, tofacitinib, UGT1A1 inducers and inhibitors (avoid), upadacitinib (avoid), live vaccines (avoid), varicella virus vaccine (avoid). Inactivated vaccines may have reduced response; give prior to start of therapy. Refer to package insert for further information.

SIDE EFFECTS
Alopecia; decreased albumin, calcium, glucose, phosphate, potassium, sodium, dehydration; edema; hyperglycemia; increased magnesium; pruritus; skin rash; xeroderma.

ANTIDOTE
Discontinue infusion and treat appropriately for severe hypersensitivity reactions.

SARGRAMOSTIM
(sar-**GRAM**-oh-stim)

Colony-stimulating factor
Hematopoietic agent

Leukine

pH 7.1 to 7.7

USUAL DOSE

Pretreatment: Baseline studies indicated; see Monitor.

Neutrophil recovery after induction chemotherapy in acute myelogenous leukemia (AML): 250 mcg/M²/day as an infusion over 4 hours. Begin on Day 11 or 4 days after induction chemotherapy is complete. Day 10 bone marrow should be hypoplastic with fewer than 5% blasts. Repeat sargramostim daily until absolute neutrophil count (ANC) is greater than 1,500/mm³ for 3 consecutive days or for a maximum of 42 days. Use same criteria if a second cycle of induction chemotherapy is indicated.

Autologous peripheral blood progenitor cell mobilization and collection: 250 mcg/M²/day as a 24-hour continuous infusion (or give SQ once daily). Continue at the same dose until adequate numbers of progenitor stem cells are collected. Collection of progenitor cells (apheresis) usually begins about Day 5 and is repeated daily. All cells are stored until predetermined targets are achieved. Consider other mobilization therapy if adequate numbers of progenitor cells are not collected.

Autologous peripheral blood progenitor cell transplantation: 250 mcg/M²/day as a 24-hour continuous infusion (or give SQ once daily). Begin immediately after infusion of harvested progenitor cells and continue until ANC is greater than 1,500/mm³ for 3 consecutive days.

Allogeneic or autologous bone marrow transplantation: 250 mcg/M²/day as a 2-hour infusion daily. Begin 2 to 4 hours after bone marrow infusion and not less than 24 hours after the last dose of chemotherapy or radiation therapy. Do not administer sargramostim until the post–marrow infusion ANC is less than 500 cells/mm³. Continue until ANC is greater than 1,500/mm³ for 3 consecutive days.

Allogeneic or autologous bone marrow transplantation: Treatment of delayed neutrophil recovery or graft failure: 250 mcg/M²/day as a 2-hour infusion daily for 14 days. Dose can be repeated after 7 days off therapy if neutrophil recovery has not occurred. If neutrophil recovery has still not occurred, give a third 14-day course of 500 mcg/M²/day after another 7 days off therapy. If there is still no improvement, it is unlikely that further dose escalation will be beneficial.

PEDIATRIC DOSE

Autologous peripheral blood progenitor cell transplantation, allogeneic or autologous bone marrow transplantation, allogeneic or autologous bone marrow transplantation (treatment of delayed neutrophil recovery or graft failure): See Usual Dose.

DOSE ADJUSTMENTS

For ANC above 20,000 cells/mm³ or WBC above 50,000 cells/mm³, interrupt sargramostim treatment or reduce dose by one-half. ■ For Grade 3 or 4 adverse reactions, reduce dose by 50% or interrupt dosing until the reaction abates. ■ See Antidote.

DILUTION

Available as a liquid formulation preserved with benzyl alcohol (500-mcg multiple-dose vial) or as a lyophilized powder (250-mcg single-dose vial). Reconstitute each 250-mcg vial with 1 mL SWFI with or without preservative. Direct diluent to the side of the vial and swirl gently. Avoid foaming or vigorous agitation. Do not shake. Do not mix together the contents of vials reconstituted with different diluents. Either product must be further diluted in NS for infusion. If the final concentration of sargramostim will be below 10 mcg/mL, albumin (human) must be added to the NS before addition of the sargramostim (1 mL of 5% albumin to each 50 mL NS). This will prevent adsorption of the drug into the components of the IV delivery system. Solution should be clear and colorless.

Filters: Manufacturer states, *"Do not use an in-line membrane filter for IV infusion of sargramostim."*

Storage: Must be refrigerated in all forms. Store in original carton to protect from light. Do not freeze or shake. Reconstituted product or any diluted solution should be used within 6 hours. Do not re-enter or reuse 250-mcg single-dose vial. Discard any unused portion. Liquid formulation can be refrigerated for up to 20 days after initial entry into vial.

COMPATIBILITY

Manufacturer recommends that no medication other than albumin be added to the infusion solution and that only NS be used to prepare IV solutions until specific **compatibility** data are available.

Other sources suggest specific **compatibilities** dependent on concentration and manufacturer; consult a pharmacist.

RATE OF ADMINISTRATION

See Usual Dose. Each single dose must be evenly distributed over 2, 4, or 24 hours. Do not use an in-line membrane filter. Reduce rate or temporarily discontinue for onset of any side effects that cause concern (e.g., hypersensitivity or infusion-related reactions).

ACTIONS

A human granulocyte-macrophage colony stimulating factor (rhu GM-CSF) produced by recombinant DNA technology. Induces partially committed progenitor cells to divide and differentiate in the granulocyte-macrophage pathways, which include neutrophils, monocytes/macrophages, and myeloid-derived dendritic cells. Is also capable of activating mature granulocytes and macrophages. Increases neutrophil, eosinophil, megakaryocyte, macrophage, and dendritic cell production. Reduces the duration of severe neutropenia. Mean terminal elimination half-life is approximately 3.84 hours.

INDICATIONS AND USES

To shorten time to neutrophil recovery and to reduce the incidence of severe, life-threatening, or fatal infections following induction chemotherapy in adult patients 55 years of age and older with acute myeloid leukemia (AML). ▪ For the mobilization of hematopoietic progenitor cells into peripheral blood for collection by leukapheresis in adult patients with cancer undergoing autologous hematopoietic stem cell transplantation. ▪ For the acceleration of myeloid reconstitution following autologous PBPC or bone marrow transplantation in adult and pediatric patients 2 years of age and older with non-Hodgkin lymphoma (NHL), acute lymphoblastic leukemia (ALL), and Hodgkin lymphoma (HL). ▪ For the acceleration of myeloid reconstitution in adult and pediatric patients 2 years of age and older undergoing allogeneic bone marrow transplantation from HLA-matched related donors. ▪ Treatment of adult and pediatric patients 2 years of age and older who have undergone allogeneic or autologous bone marrow transplantation in whom neutrophil recovery is delayed or failed. ▪ To increase survival in adult and pediatric patients from birth to 17 years of age acutely exposed to myelosuppressive doses of radiation (hematopoietic syndrome of acute radiation syndrome [H-ARS]). Administered as a subcutaneous injection.

Unlabeled uses: Primary prophylaxis of neutropenia in patients receiving chemotherapy (in settings other than transplant and AML) or who are at high risk for febrile neutropenia.

CONTRAINDICATIONS

History of serious hypersensitivity reactions, including anaphylaxis, to rhu GM-CSF such as sargramostim or to any components of sargramostim or yeast-derived products.

PRECAUTIONS

Should be administered under the direction of a physician knowledgeable about appropriate use in a facility equipped to monitor the patient and respond to any medical emergency. ▪ Due to the potential sensitivity of rapidly dividing hematopoietic progenitor cells, sargramostim should not be administered simultaneously with or within 24 hours preceding cytotoxic **chemotherapy** or **radiotherapy** or within 24 hours after chemotherapy. In one controlled trial, a higher incidence of adverse reactions, including higher mortality and a higher incidence of Grade 3 and 4 infections and Grade 3 and 4 thrombocytopenia, was observed. ▪ Serious hypersensitivity reactions, including anaphylactic reactions, have been reported. ▪ Sargramostim may cause infusion-related reactions, which usually occur after the first infusion in a particular cycle. These reactions may resolve with symptomatic treatment and usually do not recur with subsequent doses in the same cycle. ▪ Edema, capillary leak syndrome, and pleural and/or pericardial effusions have been reported. Use with caution in patients with pre-existing fluid retention, pulmonary infiltrates, or congestive heart failure. Sargramostim may aggravate fluid retention in patients with pre-existing pleural and pericardial effusions. Fluid retention may be reversible after interruption or dose reduction with or without diuretic therapy. ▪ Use with caution in patients with pre-existing cardiac disease. Supraventricular arrhythmias have been reported, particularly in patients with a previous history of cardiac arrhythmia. ▪ Use caution if considered for use in any malignancy with myeloid characteristics. Can act as a growth factor for any tumor type, particularly myeloid malignancies. ▪ Neutralizing antibodies may form after receiving sargramostim and may inhibit therapeutic effect. Incidence may be related to duration of exposure. Use sargramostim for the shortest duration required.

Monitor: Obtain a CBC with differential before administration and twice weekly thereafter to monitor for excessive leukocytosis (WBC above 50,000 cells/mm^3; or an ANC above 20,000 cells/mm^3). ▪ If blast cells appear or disease progression occurs, treatment should be discontinued. ▪ Anemia, leukocytopenia, and thrombocytopenia occur as side effects of various procedures; monitor carefully. ▪ Monitor for S/S of a hypersensitivity reaction (e.g., anaphylaxis, generalized erythema, flushing, rash, urticaria). ▪ Monitor for S/S of infusion-related reactions, particularly in patients with pre-existing lung disease. S/S may include dyspnea, flushing, hypotension, hypoxia, respiratory distress, syncope, and/or tachycardia. ▪ Observe for fluid retention; may cause peripheral edema, pleural effusion, and/or pericardial effusion. Monitor body weight and hydration status.

Patient Education: Read approved patient information guide. ▪ Review medical history with healthcare provider. ▪ Promptly report any signs or symptoms of infection (e.g., fever), infusion-related reactions, or hypersensitivity reactions (e.g., itching, swelling, redness at the injection site). ▪ Promptly report weight gain, fluid retention, irregular heartbeat, pain, or other adverse reactions.

Maternal/Child: Safety for use in pregnancy not established; use only if clearly needed. Use Leukine for injection (lyophilized product) reconstituted with SWFI without preservatives if use during pregnancy is required. ▪ Avoid breast-feeding during treatment and for at least 2 weeks after the last dose of sargramostim. ▪ Safety and effectiveness of sargramostim have been established in pediatric patients 2 years of age and older for autologous PBPCs and bone marrow transplantation, allogeneic bone marrow transplantation, and treatment of delayed neutrophil recovery or graft failure. ▪ Safety and effectiveness for these indications have not been established in pediatric patients under 2 years of age. ▪ Safety and effectiveness for use in pediatric patients have not been established in AML or for autologous PBPC mobilization and collection. ▪ Liquefied product contains benzyl alcohol. Exposure to benzyl alcohol has resulted in fatal adverse reactions, including "gasping syndrome" in neonates and low-birth-weight infants. Syndrome is characterized by CNS depression, metabolic acidosis, and gasping respirations. Leukine for injection (lyophilized product) reconstituted with SWFI without preservatives should be used for neonates and infants.

DRUG/LAB INTERACTIONS

Do not administer simultaneously with or within 24 hours preceding cytotoxic **chemotherapy** or **radiotherapy** or within 24 hours following chemotherapy. Rapidly dividing cells and the success of the treatment would be adversely affected by chemotherapy and radiation. ▪ Myeloproliferative effects may be potentiated by **lithium or corticosteroids;** avoid use if possible. If concurrent use cannot be avoided, monitor for clinical and laboratory signs of myeloproliferative effects.

SIDE EFFECTS

Autologous BMT: The most commonly reported adverse reactions include alopecia, anorexia, asthenia, diarrhea, edema, fever, GI disorder, malaise, mucous membrane disorder, nausea, rash, and vomiting. Other reported reactions include GI hemorrhage, liver damage, sepsis, and stomatitis.

Allogeneic BMT: The most commonly reported adverse reactions include abdominal pain, alopecia, anorexia, diarrhea, fever, headache, high glucose, hypertension, low albumin, nausea, rash, stomatitis, and vomiting. Other reported reactions include asthenia, chest pain, chills, dyspepsia, and pain.

AML: The most commonly reported adverse reactions include alopecia, diarrhea, fever, genitourinary abnormalities, infections, liver toxicity, metabolic laboratory abnormalities, nausea, neurotoxicity, pulmonary toxicity, skin reactions, stomatitis, vomiting, and weight loss. Other reported reactions include anorexia, chills, hypersensitivity reactions, and neuromotor and neuropsychiatric reactions.

Post-Marketing: Capillary leak syndrome, effusions, hypersensitivity reactions, immunogenicity, infusion-related reactions, injection site reactions, leukocytosis (including eosinophilia), pain (including abdominal, back, chest, and joint pain), supraventricular arrhythmias, and thromboembolic events.

Overdose: Chills, dyspnea, fever, headache, leukocytosis, malaise, nausea, rash, sinus tachycardia.

ANTIDOTE

Keep physician informed of all side effects. Most may be treated symptomatically, with temporary interruption of therapy or with a dose or rate reduction; see Dose Adjustments. Discontinue sargramostim for leukemic regrowth, if blast cells appear, or if there is progression of underlying disease. A maximum dose limit has not been determined; for accidental overdose, discontinue and monitor for WBC increase and respiratory symptoms. For ANC above 20,000 cells/mm^3 or WBC above 50,000 cells/mm^3, reduce dose by one-half or temporarily discontinue. Blood cell count should return to baseline level in 3 to 7 days. For any side effect that causes concern, reduce dose or temporarily discontinue. Dose reduction or interruption, with or without diuretic therapy, may reverse fluid retention. Infusion-related reactions may resolve with symptomatic treatment or by decreasing the rate of the infusion by 50%. If symptoms persist or worsen despite rate reduction, discontinue the infusion. May be able to administer subsequent infusions following the standard dose schedule with careful monitoring. Discontinue sargramostim permanently for serious hypersensitivity reactions. Treat as indicated and resuscitate as necessary.

SILDENAFIL BBW*
(sil-**DEN**-a-fil)

Revatio

**Vasodilating agent
Antihypertensive (pulmonary)**

*This drug is on the Black Box Warning list; however, a BBW is not provided in the parenteral prescribing information.

USUAL DOSE

Pretreatment: Baseline studies indicated; see Monitor.

Sildenafil: 2.5 mg (3.125 mL) or 10 mg (12.5 mL) as an IV bolus 3 times daily. Administer doses 4 to 6 hours apart. A 10-mg IV dose of sildenafil is equivalent to a 20-mg oral dose. Resume oral therapy as soon as tolerated. Treatment with doses higher than 10 mg IV (20 mg PO) three times a day is not recommended.

DOSE ADJUSTMENTS

No dose adjustments required for age, gender, race, weight, renal impairment (mild, moderate, or severe), or hepatic impairment (mild or moderate). Has not been studied in patients with severe hepatic impairment.

DILUTION

May be given undiluted. Aseptically withdraw the dose directly into a syringe for immediate use.

Filters: Specific information not available.

Storage: Store vials at CRT.

COMPATIBILITY

Compatibility information not available from manufacturer; consult a pharmacist.

RATE OF ADMINISTRATION

A single dose as an IV bolus.

ACTIONS

An inhibitor of cGMP-specific phosphodiesterase type 5 (PDE5) in the smooth muscle of the pulmonary vasculature where PDE5 is responsible for degradation of cGMP. Sildenafil increases cGMP within pulmonary vascular smooth muscle cells, resulting in relaxation. In patients with pulmonary arterial hypertension (PAH), this can lead to vasodilation of the pulmonary vascular bed and, to a lesser degree, vasodilation in the systemic circulation. PDE5 is also found in other tissues, including vascular and visceral smooth muscle, and in platelets. Sildenafil and its major metabolite are approximately 96% protein bound. Metabolized in the liver predominantly by CYP3A4 and other hepatic microsomal isoenzymes. Terminal half-life is about 4 hours. Findings suggest a lower clearance and/or a higher bioavailability of sildenafil in patients with PAH compared with healthy volunteers. Primarily excreted in feces and approximately 13% in urine.

INDICATIONS AND USES

Treatment of PAH (WHO Group 1) in patients who are currently prescribed oral sildenafil and are temporarily unable to take oral medications. Intended to improve exercise ability and delay clinical worsening. Delay in clinical worsening demonstrated with concurrent use of epoprostenol (Flolan). Studies establishing effectiveness included predominantly patients with NYHA Functional Class II-III symptoms and idiopathic etiology or etiology associated with connective tissue disease (CTD).

CONTRAINDICATIONS

Known hypersensitivity to sildenafil or any component of the product. ▪ Concomitant use of organic nitrates in any form, either regularly or intermittently, because of the greater risk of hypotension. ▪ Concomitant use of riociguat, a guanylate cyclase stimulator. PDE5 inhibitors, including sildenafil, may potentiate the hypotensive effects of riociguat.

PRECAUTIONS

Has vasodilatory properties, resulting in mild and transient decreases in BP. Use with caution in patients with resting hypotension (BP less than 90/50 mm Hg), fluid depletion, severe left ventricular outflow obstruction, autonomic dysfunction, and in patients undergoing antihypertensive therapy. ▪ Increase in mortality with increasing dose noted in pediatric patients; see Maternal/Child. ▪ Not recommended for use in patients with pulmonary veno-occlusive disease (PVOD); it may significantly worsen their cardiac status. Consider the possibility of associated PVOD if signs of pulmonary edema occur. ▪ Epistaxis has been reported in patients with PAH secondary to CTD and in patients treated with concomitant warfarin. ▪ Safety for use in patients with bleeding disorders or active peptic ulceration is unknown. ▪ Sudden loss of vision in one or both eyes has been reported. Nonarteritic anterior ischemic optic neuropathy (NAION), a cause of decreased vision (including permanent loss of vision), has been reported in temporal association with PDE5 inhibitors. Most, but not all, of these patients had underlying anatomic or vascular risk factors for developing NAION. A causal relationship between PDE5 inhibitor use and NAION has not been fully substantiated. ▪ Use with caution in patients with retinitis pigmentosa. ▪ Sudden decrease or loss of hearing has been reported; may be accompanied by dizziness and tinnitus. ▪ Use with caution in patients with an anatomic deformation of the penis (e.g., angulation, cavernosal fibrosis, or Peyronie's disease) or in patients with conditions that may predispose them to priapism (e.g., sickle cell anemia, multiple myeloma, or leukemia). Penile tissue damage and permanent loss of potency can result from priapism lasting more than 6 hours. ▪ Effectiveness and safety of sildenafil in PAH secondary to sickle cell anemia have not been established. Increased incidence of vaso-occlusive crisis requiring hospitalization has been reported in this patient population. ▪ See Drug/Lab Interactions.

Monitor: Obtain baseline studies as indicated by specific patient history. ▪ Monitor VS closely to note unsafe drops in BP. Monitoring of BP is especially important when sildenafil is coadministered with other BP-lowering drugs. ▪ Monitor for vision and/or hearing loss. ▪ See Precautions, Patient Education, and Drug/Lab Interactions.

Patient Education: Read manufacturer's patient education booklet carefully. ▪ Never take sildenafil with nitrate medicines or guanylate cyclase stimulators (e.g., riociguat [Adempas]); may cause a sudden and unsafe drop in BP. ▪ Do not take Viagra or other similar medications for erectile dysfunction with sildenafil. ▪ Seek immediate medical attention with a sudden loss of vision in one or both eyes. ▪ Seek prompt medical attention in the event of a sudden decrease or loss of hearing. ▪ Seek emergency help if an erection lasts for more than 4 hours. ▪ Discuss medications (prescription, nonprescription, and herbal) with a health care professional; see Drug/Lab Interactions.

Maternal/Child: Limited data show no clear association between sildenafil and major birth defects, miscarriage, or adverse maternal or fetal outcomes when used during pregnancy. ▪ Pregnant females with untreated PAH are at risk for heart failure, stroke, preterm delivery, and maternal and fetal death. ▪ Insufficient information about the effects of sildenafil on the breast-fed infant and no information on the effects of sildenafil on milk production. ▪ Use in pediatric patients, particularly chronic use, is not recommended. In a long-term study, mortality increased; deaths were first observed after about 1 year.

Elderly: Major differences in response compared with younger adults have not been identified; however, healthy elderly volunteers had a reduced clearance resulting in higher plasma concentrations. Dosing should be cautious. Consider age-related organ impairment and concomitant disease or drug therapy.

DRUG/LAB INTERACTIONS

Sildenafil is also marketed as Viagra. Do not take **Viagra or other PDE5 inhibitors** (e.g., tadalafil, vardenafil) concurrently with sildenafil. ▪ Potentiates the hypotensive effects of nitrates. Concurrent use with **nitrates** in any form is *contraindicated* (e.g., nitroglycerin in any form, isosorbide mononitrate, isosorbide dinitrate, street drugs called "poppers" [amyl nitrate or nitrite]). May result in an unsafe drop in BP. ▪ Concurrent use with **riociguat** is ***contraindicated***. ▪ Concurrent use with **alpha-adrenergic blocking agents** can lower BP significantly and lead to symptomatic hypotension. BP may be lowered further with this combined use of vasodilators by other variables, including intravascular volume depletion and concomitant use of other **antihypertensive drugs.** Monitor BP when coadministering BP–lowering drugs with sildenafil. ▪ Concomitant use of sildenafil with **ritonavir and other potent CYP3A4 inhibitors** (e.g., atazanavir, clarithromycin, indinavir, itraconazole, ketoconazole, nefazodone, nelfinavir, saquinavir, and voriconazole) *is not recommended.* ▪ **Cimetidine** and **erythromycin** may cause an increase in sildenafil plasma concentrations. ▪ **Potent CYP3A4 inducers** (e.g., carbamazepine, dexamethasone, phenytoin, phenobarbital, rifabutin, rifapentine, rifampin, and St. John's wort) may increase sildenafil clearance and reduce its effectiveness. ▪ **Bosentan** may increase sildenafil clearance; see Limitation of Use.

SIDE EFFECTS

The most common side effects are dyspepsia, dyspnea, epistaxis, erythema, flushing, headache, insomnia, and rhinitis. Serious side effects include hearing loss, hypotension, priapism, vaso-occlusive crisis, and vision loss. Other side effects reported include diarrhea, fever, gastritis, myalgia, paresthesia, and sinusitis. Additional adverse effects seen when sildenafil is administered in combination with epoprostenol (Flolan) include edema (including peripheral edema), nasal congestion, nausea, and pain in extremities. Retinal hemorrhage occurred in patients with risk factors for hemorrhage, including concurrent anticoagulant therapy.

Post-Marketing: Serious cardiovascular, cerebrovascular, and vascular events, including MI, cerebrovascular hemorrhage, hypertension, pulmonary hemorrhage, subarachnoid and intracerebral hemorrhages, TIA, ventricular arrhythmia, and sudden cardiac death have occurred at doses indicated for erectile dysfunction. NAION (with decreased vision, including permanent vision loss); sudden decrease or loss of hearing; seizure; and seizure recurrence.

ANTIDOTE

Treatment of most side effects will be supportive. Notify physician immediately if a serious side effect occurs (e.g., hearing loss, hypersensitivity, hypotension, priapism, vision loss). Treat hypersensitivity reactions with epinephrine, antihistamines, and corticosteroids as needed. Hemodialysis is not expected to be effective in overdose.

SODIUM ACETATE

(**SO**-dee-um **AS**-ah-tayt)

Electrolyte replenisher
Antihyponatremic
Alkalizing agent

pH 6 to 7

USUAL DOSE

Determined by nutritional needs, evaluation of electrolytes, and degree of hyponatremia. Some solutions may contain aluminum; see Precautions. Available in 2 mEq and 4 mEq/mL concentrations. Each mL provides 2 or 4 mEq each of sodium and acetate.

DOSE ADJUSTMENTS

Lower-end initial doses may be appropriate in the elderly based on the potential for decreased organ function and concomitant disease or drug therapy.

DILUTION

Must be added to larger volumes of IV infusion solutions including total parenteral nutrition. Use only clear solutions. Check labels for aluminum content; see Precautions.

Storage: Store at RT. Discard unused portion.

COMPATIBILITY

Compatibility information not available from manufacturer. Other sources suggest a few specific **compatibilities** dependent on concentration and manufacturer; consult a pharmacist.

RATE OF ADMINISTRATION

Administer at prescribed rate for infusion solutions. Rapid or excessive administration may produce sodium overload, water retention, alkalosis, or hypokalemia.

ACTIONS

An alkalizing agent and sodium salt. Sodium is the predominant cation of extracellular fluid. It controls water distribution throughout the body. Hypothalamus osmoreceptors, sensitive to osmolarity changes in the blood, control serum sodium concentration (142 mEq/L). Body fluid is lost when sodium content decreases and retained when sodium content increases. Sodium is excreted by the kidney. The acetate ion is metabolized to bicarbonate, thus providing a source of bicarbonate. It also acts as a hydrogen ion receptor.

INDICATIONS AND USES

To prevent or correct hyponatremia in patients with restricted intake, especially in individualized IV formulations when basic needs are not met by standard solutions. ▪ Treatment of mild to moderate acidotic states. ▪ Source of sodium ions in hemodialysis and peritoneal dialysis.

CONTRAINDICATIONS

Patients with hypernatremia or water retention.

PRECAUTIONS

Use with caution in impaired renal function, congestive heart failure, hypertension, peripheral or pulmonary edema, any condition resulting in salt retention, and in patients receiving corticosteroids. ▪ Use acetate-containing solutions with extreme caution in patients with metabolic or respiratory alkalosis and/or impaired hepatic function. ▪ Temporary therapy in acidosis. Treatment of primary condition must be instituted. ▪ Sodium bicarbonate is the drug of choice for use in severe acidosis that requires immediate correction. ▪ Some solutions of sodium acetate contain aluminum. In impaired kidney function, aluminum may reach toxic levels. Premature neonates are particularly at risk because of their immature kidneys and requirement for calcium and phosphate, which also contain aluminum. Research indicates that patients with impaired renal function who receive more than 4 to 5 mcg/kg/day of parenteral aluminum are at risk for developing CNS or bone toxicity associated with aluminum accumulation.

Monitor: Evaluate electrolytes frequently during treatment. ■ Evaluate fluid balance. ■ Rapid or excessive administration may produce alkalosis or hypokalemia. Cardiac arrhythmias may result from an intracellular shift of potassium. Many other complications may arise from electrolyte imbalance.

Maternal/Child: Category C: safety not established; use only if clearly needed.

Elderly: Differences in response between elderly and younger patients have not been identified. Lower-end initial doses may be appropriate in the elderly; see Dose Adjustments.

DRUG/LAB INTERACTIONS

Alkalinization of urine may increase the renal elimination and decrease the effects of many drugs, including **tetracyclines, lithium, methotrexate, and salicylates,** and may decrease the renal elimination and prolong the effects of others, including **anorexiants, flecainide, mecamylamine, quinidine, and sympathomimetics**.

SIDE EFFECTS

Hypernatremia, sodium level over 147 mEq/L, is most common (congestive heart failure, delirium, dizziness, edema, fever, flushing, headache, hypotension, oliguria, pulmonary edema, reduced salivation and lacrimation, respiratory arrest, restlessness, swollen tongue, tachycardia, thirst, weakness). Alkalosis and fluid or solute overload can occur.

ANTIDOTE

Notify the physician of any side effect. Reduce rate and notify physician at first sign of congestion or fluid overload. May be treated by sodium restriction and/or use of diuretics or dialysis. Resuscitate as necessary.

SODIUM BICARBONATE
(**SO**-dee-um bye-**KAR**-bon-ayt)

Electrolyte replenisher
Alkalizing agent

pH 7 to 8.5

USUAL DOSE

Adjusted according to pH, $Paco_2$, calculated base deficit, clinical response, and fluid limitations of the patient. In the presence of a low CO_2 content, adjust gradually to avoid unrecognized alkalosis. Correction to a CO_2 of 20 mEq/L within 24 hours will most likely result in a normal pH if the cause of acidosis is controlled and normal kidney function is present. Average dose for most indications is 2 to 5 mEq/kg/24 hr in adults and pediatric patients.

Cardiac arrest: 1 mEq/kg of body weight, only when appropriate (see Precautions; evidence supports little benefit and use may be detrimental). Repeat half dose in 10 minutes if indicated by blood pH and $Paco_2$.

PEDIATRIC DOSE

0.5 to 1 mEq/kg. For neonates and children up to 2 years of age, dose must never exceed 8 mEq/kg/24 hr of a 4.2% or more dilute solution; see Usual Dose, Monitor, and Maternal/Child.

DILUTION

May be diluted to a maximum concentration of 0.5 mEq/mL in dextrose solution and infuse over at least 2 hours.

COMPATIBILITY

Will form a precipitate with many drugs, including epinephrine. *If coadministration with epinephrine is indicated, give at separate sites.*

Other sources suggest specific **compatibilities** dependent on concentration and manufacturer; consult a pharmacist.

RATE OF ADMINISTRATION

Flush IV line thoroughly before and after administration. For infusion, dilute to a maximum concentration of 0.5 mEq/mL in dextrose solution and infuse over at least 2 hours. Maximum rate of administration if 1 mEq/kg/hour. See Pediatric Dose. Rapid or excessive administration may produce alkalosis, hypernatremia, hypocalcemia, and hypokalemia. Cardiac arrhythmias may result from an intracellular shift of potassium. Will also produce pain and irritation along injection site.

Cardiac arrest: Up to 1 mEq/kg over 1 to 3 minutes.

ACTIONS

An alkalizing agent and sodium salt. Helps to maintain osmotic pressure and ion balance. It is the buffering agent in blood. Bicarbonate ion elevates blood pH promptly. 99% reabsorbed with normal kidney function. Only 1% is excreted in the urine.

INDICATIONS AND USES

Metabolic acidosis (blood pH below 7.2 or plasma bicarbonate of 8 mEq/L or less) caused by circulatory insufficiency resulting from shock or severe dehydration, extracorporeal circulation of blood, severe renal disease, cardiac arrest (see Precautions), uncontrolled diabetes with ketoacidosis (low-dose insulin preferred), and primary lactic acidosis. ▪ Hyperkalemia. ▪ Hemolytic reactions requiring alkalinization of urine to reduce nephrotoxicity. ▪ Severe diarrhea. ▪ Barbiturate, methyl alcohol, or salicylate intoxication. ▪ Buffering solution to raise pH of IV fluids and medications.

CONTRAINDICATIONS

Diuretics known to produce hypochloremic alkalosis (e.g., thiazides), edema, hypertension, hypocalcemia (alkalosis may produce CHF, convulsions, hypertension, and tetany), hypochloremia (from vomiting, GI suction, or diuretics), hypernatremia, impaired renal function, metabolic alkalosis, respiratory alkalosis or acidosis, and any situation in which the administration of sodium could be clinically detrimental.

PRECAUTIONS

Temporary therapy in metabolic acidosis. Treatment of primary condition must be instituted. Best to partially correct acidosis and allow compensatory mechanisms to complete the correction. ▪ Use with caution in cardiac, liver, or renal disease; CHF; fluid/solute overload; elderly and postoperative patients with renal or cardiovascular insufficiency; and in patients receiving corticosteroids. ▪ Use in cardiac arrest indicated only in cases of prolonged resuscitation with effective ventilation or after return of spontaneous circulation after a long arrest interval. ▪ Adequate alveolar ventilation should control acid-base balance in most arrest situations except prolonged cardiac arrest, arrested patients with pre-existing metabolic acidosis, hyperkalemia, or tricyclic or barbiturate overdose.

Monitor: Confirm absolute patency of vein. Extravasation may cause chemical cellulitis, necrosis, ulceration, or sloughing. ▪ Flush IV line thoroughly before and after administration; many **incompatibilities**. ▪ Rapid or excessive administration may produce alkalosis, hypokalemia, and hypocalcemia. Cardiac arrhythmias may result from an intracellular shift of potassium. Many other complications may arise from electrolyte imbalance. ▪ Use only 50-mL ampules in cardiac arrest to prevent accidental overdose. Recent practice indicates smaller doses may be appropriate when indicated in cardiac arrest and may prevent secondary alkalosis. Adequate alveolar ventilation is imperative. Evaluate patient response and blood gases.

Maternal/Child: Category C: safety for use in pregnancy not established; use only if clearly needed. ▪ Use caution in breast-feeding. ▪ Doses in excess of 8 mEq/kg/24 hr and/or given too rapidly (10 mL/min) may cause intracranial hemorrhage, hypernatremia, and decrease in cerebrospinal fluid pressure in neonates and children under 2 years.

Elderly: Contains sodium; use caution in the elderly with renal or cardiovascular insufficiency with or without CHF; see Precautions.

DRUG/LAB INTERACTIONS

Alkalinization of urine may increase the renal elimination and decrease the effects of many drugs, including **tetracyclines, chlorpropamide, lithium carbonate, methotrexate,** salicylates, and may decrease the renal elimination and prolong the effects of others, including **anorexiants** (e.g., amphetamines), **flecainide, mecamylamine, quinidine, sympathomimetics** (e.g., dopamine, ephedrine).

SIDE EFFECTS

Rare when used with caution: alkalosis (hyperirritability and tetany), hypernatremia (edema, CHF), hypokalemia, local site venous irritation.

ANTIDOTE

Discontinue the drug and notify the physician of any side effect. Hypokalemia usually occurs with alkalosis. Sodium and potassium chloride must be supplemented as indicated for correction. Treatment of alkalosis often results in more alkalosis. Rebreathing expired air from a paper bag may help to control beginning symptoms of alkalosis. Calcium gluconate may help in severe alkalosis. Administration of a balanced hypotonic electrolyte solution (Isolyte H, Normosol-M, Plasma-lyte 56) with sodium and potassium chloride added may help to excrete the bicarbonate ion in the urine. Ammonium chloride may be indicated. Treat tetany as indicated (calcium gluconate). For extravasation, discontinue infusion; aspirate fluid, drug, and/or 3 to 5 mL of blood through the in-place needle, then remove the needle. Elevate the extremity and apply warm, moist compresses. Resuscitate as necessary.

SODIUM CHLORIDE
(**SO**-dee-um **KLOR**-eyed)

Electrolyte replenisher
Antihyponatremic

pH 4.5 to 7

USUAL DOSE

Highly individualized and dependent on age, weight, clinical condition of patient, concentration of salts in the plasma, and/or loss of body fluids.

Isotonic: (0.9% [NS], 9 Gm of sodium chloride/L or 154 mEq of sodium and 154 mEq of chloride [approximately 310 mOsm/L]) 1.5 to 3 L/24 hr.

Bacteriostatic isotonic NS contains benzyl alcohol as a preservative. It is used in small amounts (usually 1 to 2 mL) as a diluent for injectable drugs (IV, IM, SQ) or to flush IV lines. One study suggests that up to 30 mL/dose may be used in adults. However, the amount of benzyl alcohol that is tolerated within 24 hours in adults without toxic effects has not been determined. *Use only preservative-free sodium chloride in newborns for all indications.*

Hypertonic: Calculate sodium deficit. Total body water (TBW) is 45% to 50% in females and 50% to 60% in males.

$$\text{Na deficit in mEq} = \text{TBW [desired} - \text{observed plasma Na]}$$

Hypertonic (3%, 30 Gm of sodium chloride/L or 513 mEq of sodium and 513 mEq of chloride [approximately 1,030 mOsm/L] or 5%, 50 Gm of sodium chloride/L or 855 mEq of sodium and 855 mEq of chloride [approximately 1,710 mOsm/L]), 200 to

400 mL/24 hr. To correct *acute serious hyponatremia,* hypertonic sodium chloride is used to correct the serum sodium in 5 mEq/L/dose increments at a rate of no more than 0.5 mEq/hr until serum sodium is 125 mEq/L or neurologic symptoms improve. In the first 3 to 4 hours, an increase of plasma sodium at rates up to 1 mEq/L/hr may be tolerated in patients with distressing symptoms. **To prevent an overly rapid correction, an increase in plasma sodium of less than 10 mEq/L in the first 24 hours and an increase of less than 18 mEq/L in the first 48 hours is desired.** See Precautions.

Concentrated: To be used only as an additive in parenteral fluid therapy (14.6% contains 2.5 mEq of sodium and chloride/mL; 23.4% contains 4 mEq of sodium and chloride/mL).

DOSE ADJUSTMENTS

Dose selection should be cautious in the elderly, especially with hypertonic or concentrated solutions. Start at the lower end of the desired dosing range; consider the greater frequency of decreased organ function and of concomitant disease or drug therapy.

DILUTION

Isotonic and hypotonic sodium chloride are frequently combined with 5% or 10% dextrose. *Concentrated* must be diluted before use. Used only as an additive in parenteral fluids. Permits specific mEq for mEq replacement of sodium and chloride without contributing to fluid overload. Available in 14.6% strength in 20 mL, 40 mL, and 200 mL; 23.4% strength in 30 mL, 50 mL, 100 mL, and 200 mL.

Bacteriostatic isotonic available in 2-mL, 10-mL, and 30-mL vials ready for use as a diluent. Never use in neonates.

Storage: Store at CRT. Do not freeze.

COMPATIBILITY

Compatibility information not available from manufacturer; consult a pharmacist.

RATE OF ADMINISTRATION

IV infusions in flexible plastic containers: Do not hang in series connection, do not pressurize to increase flow rates without first fully evacuating residual air from the container, and do not use vented IV administration sets. All may result in air embolism.

Isotonic: A single daily dose equally distributed over 24 hours. Rate is dependent on age, weight, and clinical condition of the patient.

Hypertonic: One-half the calculated dose over at least 8 hours. Do not exceed 100 mL over 1 hour. Too-rapid infusion may cause local pain and venous irritation; reduce rate for tolerance; see Usual Dose.

Concentrated: Properly diluted in parenteral fluids and equally distributed over 24 hours. Never exceed hypertonic rate (see above) based on actual mEq of sodium chloride.

ACTIONS

Sodium: The predominant cation of extracellular fluid. It controls water distribution throughout the body. Hypothalamus osmoreceptors, sensitive to osmolarity changes in the blood, control serum sodium concentration (142 mEq/L). Body fluid is lost when sodium content decreases and retained when sodium content increases.

Chloride: The major extracellular anion. Closely follows the metabolism of sodium. Changes in the acid-base balance of the body are reflected by the changes in chloride concentration.

Distribution and excretion of sodium and chloride are largely under control of the kidney, which maintains a balance between intake and output.

INDICATIONS AND USES

Replace lost fluid or sodium and chloride ions in the body (e.g., hyponatremia, low salt syndrome, dehydration). ▪ Maintain fluid and electrolyte balance.

Hypotonic: Water replacement without increase of osmotic pressure or serum sodium levels; treatment of hyperosmolar diabetes requiring considerable fluid without excess sodium.

Isotonic: To replace sodium and chloride lost from vomiting because of obstructions and/or aspiration of GI fluids; treatment of metabolic alkalosis with fluid loss and sodium depletion. ▪ Diluent in parenteral preparations. ▪ To initiate and terminate blood transfusions without hemolyzing RBCs. ▪ Maintain patency and perform routine irrigations of many types of intravascular devices (e.g., catheters, implanted ports). ▪ Antidote for drug-induced hypercalcemia. Given concurrently with furosemide (Lasix). ▪ Priming solution in hemodialysis procedures.

Hypertonic: Used only when high sodium and/or chloride content without large amounts of fluid is required (e.g., electrolyte and fluid loss replaced with sodium-free fluids, excessive water intake resulting in drastic dilution of body water, emergency treatment of severe salt depletion, Addisonian crisis, diabetic coma). Caution: rapid correction of hyponatremia with concentrated NaCl may cause osmotic demyelination syndrome.

Concentrated: Used to meet the specific requirements of patients with unusual fluid and electrolyte needs (e.g., special problems of sodium electrolyte intake or excretion).

CONTRAINDICATIONS
Hypernatremia; fluid retention; situations in which sodium or chloride could be detrimental. 3% and 5% sodium chloride solutions are contraindicated with elevated, normal, or slightly decreased serum sodium and chloride levels. Bacteriostatic sodium chloride is contraindicated in newborns.

PRECAUTIONS
Use caution in circulatory insufficiency, congestive heart failure, edema with sodium retention, kidney dysfunction, hepatic disease, hypoproteinemia, in the elderly or debilitated individuals, and in patients receiving corticosteroids. ▪ Use with caution in surgical patients; see Monitor. ▪ More than 1 liter of NS may cause hypernatremia, which can result in loss of bicarbonate ions and acidosis. ▪ All uses require preservative-free solutions except the limited use of bacteriostatic NS as a diluent or flushing agent. ▪ Inadvertent direct injection or absorption of concentrated sodium chloride may cause sudden hypernatremia, cardiovascular shock, CNS disorders, extensive hemolysis, cortical necrosis of the kidneys, and severe local tissue necrosis with extravasation. Use extreme caution; see Dilution. ▪ Administration of IV solutions can cause fluid and/or solute overload, resulting in dilution of serum electrolyte concentrations, overhydration, congested states, or pulmonary edema. The risk of dilutional states is inversely proportional to the electrolyte concentration (increased fluids may dilute electrolyte concentration). The risk of solute overload causing congested states with peripheral and pulmonary edema is directly proportional to the electrolyte concentration (higher electrolytes pull in fluid, leading to fluid overload). ▪ Overly rapid correction of severe hyponatremia may lead to a neurologic disorder (osmotic demyelination syndrome [central pontine myelinolysis]), which may be irreversible; see Usual Dose.

Monitor: Maintain accurate intake and output; monitor electrolytes and acid-base balance, especially in prolonged therapy. ▪ Monitor vital signs as indicated. ▪ Monitor for signs of hyponatremia (sodium less than 135 mEq/L [e.g., disorientation, headache, lethargy, nausea, weakness]). May progress to coma and seizures. ▪ Excessive administration of potassium-free solutions may cause hypokalemia. ▪ Before and during use of hypertonic or concentrated sodium chloride, determine osmolar concentrations and chloride and bicarbonate content of the serum. Observe patient continuously to prevent pulmonary edema. ▪ Hypertonic solutions can cause vein damage; use a small needle and a large vein to reduce venous irritation and avoid extravasation; see Precautions.

Maternal/Child: Category C: safety for use during pregnancy not established; use only if clearly needed. ▪ Use caution in breast-feeding. ▪ Benzyl alcohol preservative in bacteriostatic sodium chloride has caused toxicity in newborns. Do not use. ▪ Is used in pediatric patients. Safety and effectiveness based on similarity of clinical conditions of pediatric and adult populations. Use caution in neonates or very small infants; the volume of fluid may affect fluid and electrolyte balance.

Elderly: Lower-end initial doses may be indicated in the elderly; see Dose Adjustments. ▪ Incidence of adverse reactions may be increased; monitor carefully, especially with renal or cardiac insufficiency with or without CHF. ▪ See Precautions.

DRUG/LAB INTERACTIONS
High sodium intake may reduce serum **lithium** concentrations.

SIDE EFFECTS
Fever, hypovolemia, and injection site reactions may occur.

Osmotic demyelination syndrome (central pontine myelinolysis) secondary to too-rapid correction with hypertonic solutions.

Due to sodium excess: Aggravation of existing acidosis, anorexia, cellular dehydration, deep respiration, disorientation, distension, edema, hydrogen loss, hyperchloremic acidosis, hypertension, increased BUN, nausea, oliguria, potassium loss, pulmonary edema, water retention, weakness. Excessive excretion of crystalloids to maintain normal osmotic pressure will increase excretion of potassium and bicarbonate and further increase acidosis. Other salts (e.g., iodide and bromide) used for therapy will also be excreted rapidly.

ANTIDOTE
Discontinue or decrease rate of infusion; notify the physician of side effects. Sodium excess can be treated by sodium restriction and/or use of diuretics or hemodialysis to remove excessive amounts. Observe patient carefully and treat symptomatically. Save balance of fluid for examination.

SODIUM FERRIC GLUCONATE COMPLEX
(**SO**-dee-um **FAIR**-ick **GLUE**-koh-nayt **KOM**-pleks)

Antianemic
Iron supplement

Ferrlecit

pH 7.7 to 9.7

USUAL DOSE
Dose is represented in terms of mg of elemental iron. Given as an infusion and may be administered during the dialysis session.

Treatment of iron deficiency in hemodialysis patients: 125 mg (10 mL)/dose. Doses above 125 mg may be associated with a higher incidence and/or severity of adverse events; see Side Effects. A minimum cumulative dose of 1 Gm of elemental iron is required by most patients. May be administered over eight sessions at sequential dialysis treatments to achieve a favorable hemoglobin or hematocrit response. Additional doses as necessary are indicated to maintain target levels of hemoglobin, hematocrit, and laboratory parameters of iron storage within acceptable limits. Use the lowest dose that achieves this goal.

PEDIATRIC DOSE
1.5 mg/kg (0.12 mL/kg) of elemental iron as a 1-hour infusion. Do not exceed 125-mg dose. Administer at 8 sequential dialysis sessions. See Maternal/Child.

DOSE ADJUSTMENTS
Begin at the low end of the dosing range in elderly patients. Consider decreased cardiac, hepatic, or renal function, and concomitant disease or other drug therapy.

DILUTION
Available in ampules or vials containing 62.5 mg/5 mL (12.5 mg/mL) of elemental iron.
Therapeutic dose: 125-mg (10-mL) dose may be diluted in 100 mL NS or may be given undiluted; see Rate of Administration.
Pediatric therapeutic dose: Dilute calculated dose in 25 mL of NS.

Filters: Specific studies not available from manufacturer. Filter needle not required by FDA for drug approval; however, use of a filter needle to withdraw it from an ampule should not have an adverse effect.

Storage: Store ampules at CRT. Do not freeze. Use immediately after dilution in NS.

COMPATIBILITY

Manufacturer states, "Do not mix with other medications or add to parenteral nutrition solutions." Known to be **compatible** only with NS.

RATE OF ADMINISTRATION

Too-rapid administration may cause hypotension associated with fatigue; light-headedness; malaise; severe pain in the chest, back, flanks, or groin; and weakness.

Infusion (adults and pediatric patients): A single dose as an infusion properly diluted and equally distributed over 60 minutes.

ACTIONS

A stable macromolecular complex in sucrose injection. Contains elemental iron as the sodium salt of a ferric ion carbohydrate complex. Used to replete the total body content of iron. Iron is critical for normal hemoglobin synthesis to maintain oxygen transport and necessary for metabolism and synthesis of DNA and various other processes. Half-life is approximately 1 hour. Doses of 1 mg/day are adequate to replenish losses in healthy non-menstruating adults. Iron complex is not dialyzable.

INDICATIONS AND USES

Treatment of iron-deficiency anemia in adult patients and pediatric patients 6 years of age or older with chronic kidney disease who are receiving hemodialysis and supplemental erythropoietin therapy; see Maternal/Child.

CONTRAINDICATIONS

All anemias not associated with iron deficiency. Hypersensitivity to sodium ferric gluconate complex or any of its components.

PRECAUTIONS

Use only when truly indicated to avoid excess storage of iron. Not recommended for use in patients with iron overload. ▪ Too-rapid administration may cause clinically significant hypotension; see Rate of Administration and Side Effects. ▪ Studies have included patients who have had prior iron dextran exposure with hypersensitivity reactions to at least one form of iron dextran. The majority of these patients tolerated Ferrlecit therapy without a subsequent hypersensitivity reaction. ▪ There have been rare occurrences of severe hypersensitivity reactions, including anaphylactic-type reactions, some of which have been life threatening and fatal. Administer in a facility equipped to monitor the patient and respond to any medical emergency. ▪ Serum iron levels greater than 300 mcg/dL combined with transferrin oversaturation may indicate iron poisoning; see Side Effects.

Monitor: Recumbent position during and after injection may help to prevent postural hypotension. Hypotensive effects may be additive to transient hypotension during dialysis and/or from too-rapid rate of infusion; monitor closely. Hypotensive reactions associated with fatigue; light-headedness; malaise; severe pain in the back, chest, flanks, or groin; and weakness may occur with IV iron. These symptoms may or may not be indicative of a hypersensitivity reaction and usually resolve within 1 or 2 hours. ▪ Observe continuously for a hypersensitivity reaction during an infusion and after administration for at least 30 minutes and until clinically stable. Monitor vital signs. ▪ Periodic monitoring of hemoglobin and hematocrit and iron storage levels recommended. Doses in excess of iron needs may lead to accumulation of iron in iron storage sites and iatrogenic hemosiderosis.

Patient Education: Report S/S of a hypersensitivity reaction (e.g., difficulty breathing, rash, shortness of breath) promptly. Report pain at injection site.

Maternal/Child: Category B: use during pregnancy only if potential benefit justifies potential risk to fetus. ▪ Safety for use during breast-feeding and in pediatric patients under 6 years of age not established. ▪ Contains benzyl alcohol; should not be used in neonates. Benzyl alcohol present in maternal serum may cross into human milk and may be orally absorbed by a breast-feeding infant.

Elderly: No age differences identified. Caution in the elderly suggested; see Dose Adjustments.

DRUG/LAB INTERACTIONS

May reduce absorption of concomitantly administered **oral iron preparations.** ▪ Concurrent administration of iron therapy with **dimercaprol** will result in the formation of a toxic complex. Either postpone iron therapy to at least 24 hours after dimercaprol or consider transfusions.

SIDE EFFECTS

Hypotension associated with fatigue; light-headedness; malaise; severe pain in the chest, back, flanks, or groin; and weakness may be caused by too-rapid infusion. Severe hypersensitivity reactions (e.g., angioedema, bronchospasm, cardiac arrest, cardiovascular collapse, dyspnea, edema [oral or pharyngeal], muscle spasm, pain [back or chest], pruritus, urticaria) have been reported rarely. The most commonly reported side effects include abdominal pain, back pain, chest pain, cramps, diarrhea, dizziness, dyspnea, fever, headache, hypersensitivity reactions, hypertension, hypotension, infection, injection site reactions, nausea and vomiting, pain, pharyngitis, pruritus, rhinitis, tachycardia, and thrombosis. Many other side effects occurred in less than 1% of patients and may or may not be attributable to sodium ferric gluconate complex.

Post-Marketing: Anaphylaxis, convulsions, dysgeusia, hypoesthesia, loss of consciousness, pallor, phlebitis, shock, and skin discoloration have been identified. In addition, post-marketing reports have identified that individual doses exceeding 125 mg may result in a higher incidence and/or severity of side effects, including abdominal pain, chest pain, diarrhea, dizziness, dyspnea, hypotension, nausea, paresthesia, peripheral swelling, and urticaria.

Overdose: Serum iron levels greater than 300 mcg/dL may indicate iron poisoning. May result in hemosiderosis, and excess iron may increase susceptibility to infection. If acute toxicity is seen, it may present as abdominal pain, diarrhea, or vomiting progressing to pallor or cyanosis, lassitude, drowsiness, hyperventilation due to acidosis, iatrogenic hemosiderosis, and cardiovascular collapse.

ANTIDOTE

Reduce rate or temporarily discontinue infusion for hypotension; volume expanders (e.g., albumin, hetastarch) may be indicated. Restart when resolved. Discontinue drug and treat hypersensitivity reactions or resuscitate as necessary; notify physician. Epinephrine and diphenhydramine should always be available. In overdose, monitor CBC, iron studies, vital signs, blood gases, and glucose and electrolytes. Maintain fluid and electrolyte balance. Correct acidosis with sodium bicarbonate. Iron complex is not dialyzable.

SODIUM THIOSULFATE

(**SOW**-dee-um thye-oh-**SUL**-fate)

Antidote

Pedmark

USUAL DOSE

Weight less than 5 kg = 10 Gm/m^2; weight 5–10 kg = 15 Gm/m^2; weight greater than 10 kg = 20 Gm/m^2

PEDIATRIC DOSE

See above.

DOSE ADJUSTMENTS

Renal: No dosage adjustments are provided by the manufacturer.

Hepatic: No dosage adjustments are provided by the manufacturer.

DILUTION

Calculate the dose (grams) and determine number of vials needed. Withdraw the calculated dose from the vial into the syringe or empty infusion bag. *Note:* Pedmark comes as 12.5-Gm/100 mL single-dose vial.

COMPATIBILITY

Do not administer simultaneously with any other medication or IV solutions other than normal saline.

RATE OF ADMINISTRATION

Administer as IV infusion over 15 minutes following cisplatin infusions.

ACTIONS

Sodium thiosulfate interacts directly with cisplatin to produce an inactive platinum species to help prevent ototoxicity.

INDICATIONS AND USES

Cyanide poisoning (alternative agent); to reduce ototoxicity associated with cisplatin in pediatric patients greater than 1 month of age

CONTRAINDICATIONS

History of severe hypersensitivity to sodium thiosulfate or any components

PRECAUTIONS

Hypersensitivity: Immediately discontinue infusion with any signs of allergic reaction and institute appropriate care.

Hypernatremia and hypokalemia: Monitor serum sodium and potassium levels at baseline and as clinically indicated. Withhold infusion if serum sodium is greater than 145 mmol/L.

Nausea and vomiting: Administer antiemetics prior to each infusion.

Monitor: Hypersensitivity/anaphylaxis during and after the infusion; sodium and potassium at baseline and as clinically indicated; nausea and vomiting. See package insert for dosage modifications based on adverse reactions.

Patient education: Notify provider of or any signs of allergic reaction or nausea.

Maternal/child: No information is available, as it is indicated only for pediatric patients. Refer to cisplatin monograph for information.

Elderly: No specific recommendations; refer to adult dosing.

DRUG/LAB INTERACTIONS

None is listed by the manufacturer.

SIDE EFFECTS

Hypersensitivity, nausea and vomiting, hypernatremia, and hypokalemia

ANTIDOTE

There is no antidote; stop infusion for hypersensitivity reactions and treat appropriately.

SOTALOL HYDROCHLORIDE BBW

(**SO**-tuh-lol hy-droh-**KLOR**-eyed)

Beta-adrenergic blocking agent
Antiarrhythmic

pH 6 to 7

USUAL DOSE

Pretreatment: Baseline ECG indicated; see Monitor.

To minimize the risk of induced arrhythmia, patients initiated or re-initiated on sotalol and patients who are converted from IV to oral administration should be hospitalized in a facility that can provide cardiac resuscitation and continuous ECG monitoring. CrCl must be greater than 60 mL/min. Baseline studies and correction of electrolyte abnormalities required before initiating therapy; see Precautions, Monitor, and Dose Adjustments.

Initial dose: 75 mg twice daily. If symptomatic arrhythmia is not controlled and dose is tolerated without excessive QTc prolongation (i.e., greater than 500 msec), may increase dose to 112.5 mg twice daily after 3 days. Continuous ECG monitoring required during dose escalation.

Dose for ventricular arrhythmias: 75 mg twice daily. Dose may be increased in increments of 75 mg/day every 3 days. Usual therapeutic effect is seen with doses of 75 to 150 mg twice daily. However, doses as high as 225 to 300 mg have been required in patients with refractory life-threatening arrhythmias.

Dose for symptomatic atrial fibrillation/atrial flutter (AFIB/AFL): 112.5 mg twice daily was found to be the most effective dose in studies. If symptomatic arrhythmia is not controlled and this dose is tolerated without excessive QTc prolongation (i.e., greater than 520 msec), increase dose to 150 mg twice daily.

Conversion from oral to IV Sotalol: Patients who have been stabilized on oral sotalol and are unable to take oral medications may be converted to IV sotalol using the following conversion chart.

Conversion From Oral Sotalol to IV Sotalol	
Oral Dose	**Intravenous Dose**
80 mg	75 mg (5 mL sotalol injection)
120 mg	112.5 mg (7.5 mL sotalol injection)
160 mg	150 mg (10 mL sotalol injection)

DOSE ADJUSTMENTS

Increase dosing interval to every 24 hours in patients with a CrCl between 40 and 60 mL/min. Sotalol is not recommended in patients with a CrCl less than 40 mL/min. ■ Titrate dose upward or downward as needed based on clinical effect, QT interval, or adverse reactions as described in Usual Dose.

DILUTION

Available in vials containing 150 mg/10 mL. Dilute required dose with NS, D5W, or LR as described in the following chart.

Sotalol Infusion Preparation to Compensate for Dead Space in the Infusion Set				
Target Dose	Sotalol Injection	Diluent	Volume Prepared	Volume to Infuse
75 mg	6 mL	114 mL	120 mL	100 mL
112.5 mg	9 mL	111 mL		
150 mg	12 mL	108 mL		
75 mg	6 mL	294 mL	300 mL	250 mL
112.5 mg	9 mL	291 mL		
150 mg	12 mL	288 mL		

Storage: Store at CRT. Protect from light and freezing.

COMPATIBILITY

Compatibility information not available from manufacturer; consult a pharmacist.

RATE OF ADMINISTRATION

A single dose equally distributed over 5 hours. Use of an infusion pump recommended.

ACTIONS

An antiarrhythmic with Class II (beta-adrenoreceptor blocking) and Class III (cardiac action potential duration prolongation) properties. The beta-blocking effect is noncardioselective. Slows heart rate, decreases AV nodal conduction, and increases AV nodal refractoriness. ECG shows dose-related increase in QT and QTc. Produces a reduction in systolic and diastolic BP and cardiac index and an increase in pulmonary capillary wedge pressure. Does not bind to plasma proteins and is not metabolized. Half-life is 12 hours. Excreted predominantly via the kidney in unchanged form. Crosses the placenta. Secreted in breast milk.

INDICATIONS AND USES

A substitute for oral sotalol in patients who are unable to take oral medications. ▪ Maintenance of normal sinus rhythm in patients with a history of highly symptomatic AFIB/AFL. ▪ Treatment of documented life-threatening ventricular arrhythmias.

CONTRAINDICATIONS

Bradycardia (HR below 50 beats/min), sick sinus syndrome, or second- or third-degree AV block unless a functioning pacemaker is present. ▪ Congenital or acquired long QT syndromes, QT interval greater than 450 msec. ▪ Cardiogenic shock, uncontrolled heart failure. ▪ CrCl less than 40 mL/min. ▪ Serum potassium less than 4 mEq/L. ▪ Bronchial asthma or related bronchospastic conditions. ▪ Known hypersensitivity to sotalol.

PRECAUTIONS

To minimize the risk of induced arrhythmia, patients initiated or re-initiated on sotalol and patients who are converted from IV to oral administration should be hospitalized for at least 3 days (or until steady-state drug levels are reached) in a facility that can provide cardiac resuscitation and continuous ECG monitoring. Personnel trained in the management of serious ventricular arrhythmias must be present. ▪ Can cause serious ventricular arrhythmias, primarily torsades de pointes (TdP), a polymorphic ventricular tachycardia associated with QTc prolongation. QTc prolongation is directly related to the concentration of sotalol. Factors that may increase the risk of TdP include a reduced CrCl, larger doses, female gender, sustained VT, and a history of cardiomegaly or CHF. ▪ The use of sotalol in conjunction with other drugs that prolong the QT interval has not been studied and is not recommended; see Drug/Lab Interactions. ▪ May cause bradycardia, which increases risk of TdP. ▪ Increased risk of TdP in patients with AFIB and sinus node dysfunction, especially after cardioversion. Sotalol increases bradycardia and QTc following cardioversion. ▪ Produces significant reductions in both systolic and diastolic BP. May cause deterioration in cardiac performance in patients with marginal cardiac compensation. ▪ Use caution in CHF. Beta blockade may depress myocardial contractility and precipitate or exacerbate heart failure. ▪ Use caution in the presence of heart failure controlled by digoxin. Both drugs slow AV conduction.

- Experience with use following acute MI is limited. Use caution, titrate dose carefully, and monitor patient closely. ▪ May cause angina, arrhythmia, or MI if discontinued abruptly; gradually reduce over 1 to 2 weeks if possible. ▪ May mask tachycardia occurring with hypoglycemia in diabetes and tachycardia of hyperthyroidism. ▪ In general, patients with bronchospastic disease should not receive beta-blockers. If sotalol is to be administered, use the smallest effective dose; see Contraindications. ▪ Use caution in patients with renal impairment; see Dose Adjustments. ▪ Patients with atrial fibrillation should be anticoagulated according to usual medical practice.

Monitor: Obtain baseline ECG to determine the QT interval. If baseline QT interval is greater than 450 msec, sotalol is not recommended. Monitor QT interval after the completion of each infusion. ▪ Measure and normalize serum potassium and magnesium levels before initiating therapy and as required during therapy. Pay special attention to electrolytes and acid-base status in patients with prolonged diarrhea or in patients receiving concomitant diuretics. ▪ Obtain baseline SCr and calculate CrCl to establish dosing interval. ▪ Monitor HR and BP. Monitor hemodynamics in patients with marginal cardiac compensation. ▪ In patients with life-threatening ventricular arrhythmias, the response to treatment should be evaluated by a suitable method (e.g., programmed electrical stimulation [PES] or Holter monitoring) at steady-state blood levels of the drug before continuing the patient on chronic therapy.

Patient Education: Do not discontinue therapy abruptly. ▪ Promptly report any breathing difficulty, syncope, or pain at injection site.

Maternal/Child: Category B: use during pregnancy only if clearly needed. ▪ Discontinue breast-feeding. ▪ Safety for use in pediatric patients not established. See prescribing information for unlabeled suggested oral doses for use in pediatric patients.

Elderly: Age-related differences in safety and effectiveness not identified; however, greater sensitivity of some elderly cannot be ruled out. Dose with caution, taking into account decreased renal function; see Dose Adjustments.

DRUG/LAB INTERACTIONS

Proarrhythmic events were more common in sotalol-treated patients also receiving **digoxin.** Unclear as to whether this is a drug interaction or is related to the presence of heart failure, which is a known risk factor for arrhythmias. ▪ Concurrent use with **calcium channel blockers** is expected to have additive effects on AV conduction, ventricular function, and BP. ▪ ▪ Beta-adrenergic blocking agents may be continued during the perioperative period in most patients; however, use caution with **selected anesthetic agents** that may depress the myocardium. Protracted severe hypotension and difficulty in restoring and maintaining normal cardiac rhythm after anesthesia have been reported. ▪ Concurrent use with **clonidine** may precipitate acute hypertension if one or both agents are stopped abruptly. ▪ Coadministration with **catecholamine-depleting drugs** (e.g., reserpine and guanethidine) may result in hypotension, bradycardia, vertigo, syncope, or orthostatic hypotension. ▪ Hyperglycemia may occur. Dosage of **insulin and other antidiabetic drugs** may require adjustment. ▪ Symptoms of **hypoglycemia may be masked.** ▪ Increased doses of **beta-agonists** such as albuterol, terbutaline, and isoproterenol may be required when administered concomitantly with sotalol. ▪ Patients taking **beta-blockers** who are exposed to a potential allergen may be unresponsive to the usual dose of epinephrine used to treat a hypersensitivity reaction. ▪ The use of sotalol in conjunction with other **drugs that prolong the QT interval** has not been studied and is not recommended. Such drugs include some phenothiazines, tricyclic antidepressants, oral macrolide antibiotics, Class I antiarrhythmics (e.g., disopyramide, procainamide, quinidine), and Class III antiarrhythmics (e.g., amiodarone). **Class I and III antiarrhythmic agents** should be withheld for at least three half-lives before dosing with sotalol. ▪ The presence of sotalol in the urine may result in **falsely elevated levels of urinary metanephrine** by certain methods.

SIDE EFFECTS

There is no clinical experience with IV sotalol. Side effects should be similar to those seen with oral sotalol therapy. The most common side effects (dose related) are asthenia, bradycardia, chest pain, dizziness, dyspnea, fatigue, headache, light-headedness, nausea, palpitations, and QT prolongation. Ventricular arrhythmia, primarily TdP, is the most common serious side effect. Other reported side effects include abdominal distension and pain, abnormal ECG, angina, bradycardia, cough, decreased appetite, diarrhea, dyspepsia, edema, fever, heart failure, hyperhidrosis, hypotension, infection, insomnia, musculoskeletal pain, tracheobronchitis, upper respiratory infection, visual disturbance, vomiting, and weakness. Other reactions have been reported.

Overdose: Bradycardia, bronchospasm, cardiac asystole, CHF, hypoglycemia, hypotension, premature ventricular complexes, prolongation of the QT interval, TdP, and ventricular arrhythmia.

ANTIDOTE

Notify physician of any side effects. If the QT interval increases to 500 msec or greater, reduce the dose, decrease the infusion rate, or discontinue therapy. Atropine, another anticholinergic drug, a beta-adrenergic agonist, or transvenous cardiac pacing may be used to treat bradycardia or cardiac asystole. A transvenous cardiac pacemaker may be required for second- or third-degree heart block. Epinephrine may be useful for treatment of hypotension. Aminophylline or aerosol beta-2–receptor stimulants (e.g., albuterol) may be useful for treatment of bronchospasm. DC cardioversion, magnesium sulfate, and potassium replacement may be required for treatment of TdP. Once TdP is terminated, transvenous cardiac pacing or an isoproterenol infusion may be used to increase heart rate.

SUGAMMADEX
(soo-**GAM**-ma-dex)

Antidote
Selective relaxant binding agent

Bridion pH 7 to 8

USUAL DOSE

Pretreatment: Baseline studies indicated; see Monitor.

A peripheral nerve stimulator should be used to determine when sugammadex should be initiated. Doses and timing of sugammadex administration should be based on monitoring for twitch responses and the extent of spontaneous recovery that has occurred. Before sugammadex administration and up until complete recovery of neuromuscular function, the patient should be well ventilated and a patent airway maintained. The recommended dose of sugammadex does not depend on the anesthetic regimen. Sugammadex can be used to reverse different levels of rocuronium-induced or vecuronium-induced neuromuscular blockade. Base dose on actual body weight.

For rocuronium and vecuronium: Deep blockade: 4 mg/kg as a single IV bolus injection is recommended if spontaneous recovery of the twitch response has reached 1 to 2 posttetanic counts (PTCs) and there are no twitch responses to train-of-four (TOF) stimulation following neuromuscular blockade.

Moderate blockade: 2 mg/kg as a single IV bolus injection is recommended if spontaneous recovery has reached the reappearance of the second twitch (T_2) in response to TOF stimulation following neuromuscular blockade.

Immediate reversal of rocuronium only: 16 mg/kg as a single IV bolus injection is recommended if there is a clinical need to reverse neuromuscular blockade soon (approximately 3 minutes) after administration of a single dose of 1.2 mg/kg rocuronium. The efficacy of the 16 mg/kg dose following administration of vecuronium has not been studied.

DOSE ADJUSTMENTS

Individualize dose based on extent of spontaneous recovery at time of administration (rocuronium and vecuronium) and whether there is a need to rapidly reverse the neuromuscular blocking agent (rocuronium only). ▪ Use of lower than recommended doses of sugammadex may lead to an increased risk of recurrence of neuromuscular blockade after initial reversal and is not recommended. ▪ No dose adjustment is recommended in patients with mild to moderate renal impairment. Sugammadex is not recommended for use in patients with severe renal impairment. ▪ No dose adjustment is recommended in patients with hepatic impairment, pulmonary complications, or cardiac disease (e.g., patients with ischemic heart disease, chronic heart failure, cardiac arrhythmias); see Precautions.

DILUTION

Available as a 100 mg/mL solution in a 2- or 5-mL single-dose vial. Solution is clear and colorless to slightly yellow-brown. Withdraw the calculated dose and inject into the IV line of a running infusion.

Filters: No data available from the manufacturer.

Storage: Store at CRT. Protect from light. If not protected from light, the vial must be used within 5 days.

COMPATIBILITY

May inject into the IV line of a running infusion with the following IV solutions: NS, D5W, D2.5/¼NS, D5NS, Isolyte P in D5W, RL, and Ringer's solution. Flush line with a **compatible** solution (e.g., NS) before and after administration of sugammadex. Manufacturer states that sugammadex should not be administered with other products and that it is physically **incompatible** with ondansetron and verapamil.

RATE OF ADMINISTRATION

Administer intravenously as a single bolus injection over 10 seconds. May administer into an existing IV line. Flush line with a **compatible** solution before and after administration.

ACTIONS

A modified gamma-cyclodextrin. Sugammadex forms a complex with rocuronium and vecuronium, thereby reducing the amount of neuromuscular blocking agent (NMBA) available to bind to nicotinic cholinergic receptors in the neuromuscular junction. This results in the reversal of neuromuscular blockade induced by rocuronium and vecuronium. Neither sugammadex nor the complex of sugammadex and the NMBA binds to plasma proteins or erythrocytes. Sugammadex is not metabolized by the liver. No metabolites of sugammadex have been observed, and the only route of elimination observed is renal excretion of the unchanged product. Elimination half-life is about 2 hours.

INDICATIONS AND USES

Reversal of the neuromuscular blockade induced by rocuronium bromide and vecuronium bromide in adults undergoing surgery.

Limitations of use: Sugammadex has not been studied for reversal following rocuronium or vecuronium administration in the ICU. ▪ Sugammadex should not be used to reverse neuromuscular blockade induced by <u>nonsteroidal</u> NMBAs such as succinylcholine or benzylisoquinolinium compounds (e.g., atracurium, cisatracurium, mivacurium) or to reverse neuromuscular blockade induced by <u>steroidal</u> NMBAs other than rocuronium or vecuronium.

CONTRAINDICATIONS

Known hypersensitivity to sugammadex or any of its components.

PRECAUTIONS

For IV administration only. ▪ Should be administered by a trained healthcare provider familiar with the use, actions, characteristics, and complications of NMBAs and NMB reversal agents. ▪ Ventilatory support is mandatory for patients until adequate spontaneous respiration is restored and the ability to maintain a patent airway is ensured. Should neuromuscular blockade persist after sugammadex administration or recur following extubation, appropriate steps should be taken to provide adequate ventilation. ▪ Hypersensitivity reactions have occurred in patients treated with sugammadex and can range from isolated skin reactions to serious systemic reactions (i.e., anaphylaxis, anaphylactic shock). ▪ Cases of marked bradycardia, some of which have resulted in cardiac arrest, have been observed within minutes after the administration of sugammadex. ▪ Delayed or minimal response to sugammadex has been reported in a small number of patients. ▪ A minimum waiting time is necessary before administration of a steroidal NMBA after the administration of sugammadex. ▪ Has been associated with increases in aPTT and PT/INR of up to 25% for up to 1 hour. ▪ Use with caution in patients with hepatic impairment accompanied by coagulopathy or severe edema. ▪ Sugammadex is not recommended for use in patients with severe renal impairment, including those requiring dialysis. ▪ See Drug/Lab Interactions.

Monitor: Obtain baseline SCr. ▪ Monitor the patient to ensure adequate ventilation and maintenance of a patent airway. Even if recovery from neuromuscular blockade is complete, other drugs used in the perioperative and postoperative period could depress respiratory function and necessitate the need for continued ventilator support. ▪ A peripheral nerve stimulation device capable of delivering a TOF stimulus is required. ▪ TOF monitoring alone should not be relied on to determine the adequacy of NMB reversal as related to a patient's ability to adequately ventilate and maintain a patent airway following tracheal extubation. Satisfactory recovery should be determined through the assessment of skeletal muscle tone and respiratory measurements in addition to the response to the peripheral nerve stimulator. ▪ Monitor for S/S of a hypersensitivity reaction. The most commonly reported hypersensitivity reactions were nausea, pruritus, and urticaria. Other reported hypersensitivity reactions have included bronchospasm, conjunctival edema, dermatologic reactions (erythema, flushing, rash, skin eruption), reduction in peak expiratory flow, and swelling of the pharynx, tongue, and/or uvula. ▪ Monitor for hemodynamic changes during and after reversal of neuromuscular blockade; see Antidote. ▪ Monitor coagulation parameters (e.g., aPTT, PT/INR) in patients with known coagulopathies, patients being treated with therapeutic anticoagulation, patients receiving thromboprophylaxis drugs other than heparin or LMWH, or patients receiving any thromboprophylaxis drugs and sugammadex at a dose of 16 mg/kg.

Patient Education: May reduce the efficacy of hormonal contraceptives. Females of reproductive potential who are using hormonal contraceptives should use an additional, non-hormonal contraceptive (e.g., condom, spermicide) for 7 days following sugammadex administration.

Maternal/Child: Use during pregnancy only if clearly needed. ▪ Use caution during breast-feeding. ▪ Safety and efficacy for use in pediatric patients have not been established.

Elderly: Dose adjustment is not generally needed in elderly patients with normal organ function, but an extended monitoring period to ensure complete reversal may be warranted. Risk of adverse events may be greater in patients with renal impairment. May be useful to monitor renal function.

DRUG/LAB INTERACTIONS

Toremifene has a high binding affinity for sugammadex. May cause displacement of vecuronium and rocuronium from the complex with sugammadex, thereby decreasing the effectiveness of sugammadex. Monitor for recurrence of NMB. Risk of displacement will be highest in the time period equivalent to 3 times the half-life of sugammadex. ▪ Sugammadex may bind to **progestogen**, thereby decreasing progestogen exposure and effectiveness. Patients using **hormonal forms of contraception** (oral and nonoral) who receive sugammadex must use an additional, nonhormonal contraceptive method or backup method of contraception for the next 7 days. ▪ Administration of **medications that can potentiate NMB** in the postoperative period (e.g., aminoglycosides, magnesium, vancomycin) may increase the possibility of recurrence of NMB. Monitor patients closely for recurrence if these medications must be administered. ▪ Sugammadex may interfere with the **serum progesterone assay**.

SIDE EFFECTS

The most common side effects are headache, hypotension, nausea, pain, and vomiting. Other side effects include abnormal QT interval, airway complication of anesthesia, anesthetic complication, anxiety, bradycardia, chills, cough, decreased RBC count, depression, dizziness, dry mouth, erythema, fever, flatulence, hypersensitivity reactions (including anaphylaxis), hypertension, hypocalcemia, hypoesthesia, increased blood creatine phosphokinase, insomnia, myalgia, procedural complications, pruritus, recurrence of prolonged NMB, restlessness, tachycardia, and wound hemorrhage.

Post-Marketing: Bradycardia, cardiac arrest, cardiac arrhythmias, dyspnea, hypersensitivity reactions (including anaphylaxis), laryngospasm, pulmonary edema, respiratory arrest, and wheezing.

ANTIDOTE

Treat anaphylaxis immediately with oxygen, epinephrine, antihistamines, vasopressors, corticosteroids, albuterol, IV fluids, and ventilation equipment as indicated. Treatment with an anticholinergic such as atropine should be administered if clinically significant bradycardia is observed. Sugammadex can be removed using hemodialysis with a high-flux filter but not a low-flux filter. Resuscitate as necessary.

SULFAMETHOXAZOLE AND TRIMETHOPRIM

(sul-fah-meh-**THOX**-ah-zohl and try-**METH**-oh-prim)

Antibacterial
Antiprotozoal

SMZ-TMP, TMP-SMZ

pH 9.5 to 10.5

USUAL DOSE

Pretreatment: Baseline studies and adequate hydration indicated; see Monitor and Maternal/Child.

Doses listed are based on the trimethoprim component of the drug. Maximum recommended dose is 960 mg trimethoprim and 4,800 mg sulfamethoxazole/24 hr (60 mL/24 hr).

Severe urinary tract infections and shigellosis in adults and pediatric patients over 2 months of age: 8 to 10 mg/kg/24 hr in equally divided doses every 6, 8, or 12 hours (2 to 2.5 mg/kg every 6 hours, 2.67 to 3.33 mg/kg every 8 hours, or 4 to 5 mg/kg every 12 hours). Administer for 14 days (urinary tract infections) or 5 days (shigellosis).

Pneumocystis jiroveci pneumonitis in adults and pediatric patients over 2 months of age: 15 to 20 mg/kg/24 hr in equally divided doses every 6 or 8 hours (3.75 to 5 mg/kg every 6 hours or 5 to 6.67 mg/kg every 8 hours) for up to 14 days.

DOSE ADJUSTMENTS

Reduce dose by one-half for CrCl between 15 and 30 mL/min. Use is not recommended in patients with a CrCl less than 15 mL/min. ▪ Reduced dose may be indicated in the elderly. ▪ See Monitor and Drug/Lab Interactions.

DILUTION

Each 5-mL ampule (16 mg trimethoprim/mL [80 mg/5 mL], 80 mg sulfamethoxazole/mL [400 mg/5 mL]) must be diluted in 125 mL D5W and given as an infusion. Reduce D5W to 75 mL for each 5-mL ampule if fluid restriction is required. Standard dilution must be used within 6 hours; fluid restriction dilution must be used within 2 hours. 5 mL may also be mixed in 100 mL of D5W and used within 4 hours. Available in 5-, 10-, and 30-mL vials. Concentration per mL same as 5-mL ampule. Discard if cloudiness or crystallization is present.

Storage: Store at RT; do not refrigerate. 10-mL and 30-mL vials may be multiple-dose containers. After entry into a multiple-dose vial, the remaining contents must be used within 48 hours.

COMPATIBILITY

Manufacturer states, "Do not mix with other drugs or solutions."

Other sources suggest specific **compatibilities** dependent on concentration and manufacturer; consult a pharmacist.

RATE OF ADMINISTRATION

A single dose must be infused over 60 to 90 minutes. Avoid rapid infusion or bolus injection.

ACTIONS

A broad-spectrum antibacterial and antiprotozoal combination agent with bactericidal action effective against gram-positive and gram-negative organisms. Blocks sequential steps in the biosynthesis of nucleic acids and proteins essential to many bacteria. Combination contains 400 mg sulfamethoxazole (a sulfonamide antimicrobial) and 80 mg trimethoprim (a dihydrofolate reductase inhibitor antibacterial) per each 5 mL. Metabolized in the liver and excreted in urine as metabolites and unchanged drug. Crosses placental barrier. Secreted in breast milk.

INDICATIONS AND USES

For use in adults and pediatric patients 2 months of age and older for the following indications: Treatment of severe or complicated urinary tract infections due to susceptible strains of designated organisms when oral therapy is not feasible and when the organism is not susceptible to single-agent antibacterials effective in the urinary tract (see prescribing information). ▪ Treatment of *Pneumocystis jiroveci* pneumonia. ▪ Treatment of enteritis caused by susceptible strains of *Shigella flexneri* and *Shigella sonnei*.

CONTRAINDICATIONS

Hypersensitivity to trimethoprim or sulfonamides. ▪ History of drug-induced immune thrombocytopenia with the use of trimethoprim and/or sulfonamides. ▪ Patients with documented megaloblastic anemia due to folate deficiency. ▪ Marked hepatic damage. ▪ Severe renal insufficiency when renal function status cannot be monitored. ▪ Pediatric patients under 2 months of age. ▪ Concomitant administration with dofetilide (Tikosyn).

PRECAUTIONS

To reduce the development of drug-resistant bacteria and maintain its effectiveness, sulfamethoxazole/trimethoprim should be used to treat or prevent only those infections proven or strongly suspected to be caused by bacteria. ▪ Sensitivity studies indicated to determine susceptibility of the causative organism to sulfamethoxazole/trimethoprim. ▪ Not for IM use. ▪ Fatalities associated with the administration of sulfonamides have occurred due to severe reactions, including Stevens-Johnson syndrome, toxic epidermal necrolysis, fulminant hepatic necrosis, agranulocytosis, aplastic anemia, and other blood dyscrasias. Discontinue therapy at the first appearance of a skin rash or any sign of adverse reaction. A skin rash may be followed by more severe reactions such as those listed previously. ▪ Hypersensitivity reactions of the respiratory tract have been reported with sulfonamide treatment. ▪ Severe cases of thrombocytopenia that are fatal or life-threatening have been reported and may be immune-mediated. ▪ Avoid use in treatment of streptococcal pharyngitis. Studies show that patients with group A beta-hemolytic streptococcal tonsillopharyngitis who are treated with sulfamethoxazole/trimethoprim have a greater incidence of bacteriologic failure than do those treated with penicillin. Failure to eradicate the organism may predispose the patient to sequelae such as rheumatic fever. ▪ Avoid use in patients with impaired liver or renal function, in patients with possible folate deficiency (e.g., elderly patients, patients with chronic alcohol use disorder, patients receiving anticonvulsant therapy, patients with malabsorption syndrome, and patients in malnutrition states), and in patients with severe allergies or bronchial asthma. Hematologic changes indicative of folic acid deficiency may occur in patients with pre-existing folic acid deficiency or kidney failure. These effects are reversible with folinic acid therapy. ▪ Use caution in patients with glucose 6-phosphate dehydrogenase (G-6PD) deficiency. Hemolysis may occur and is often dose related. ▪ Cases of hypoglycemia in nondiabetic patients has been reported and usually occurs after a few days of therapy. Patients with renal dysfunction, liver disease, or malnutrition, or patients receiving high doses of sulfamethoxazole/trimethoprim, are particularly at risk. ▪ Avoid use in patients with porphyria or thyroid dysfunction. Can precipitate porphyria crisis and hypothyroidism. ▪ Electrolyte abnormalities (including hyperkalemia and severe and symptomatic hyponatremia) can occur, particularly with higher doses. Patients with underlying disorders of potassium metabolism, patients with renal insufficiency, or patients who are taking drugs known to induce hyperkalemia may experience hyperkalemia at the lower recommended doses. ▪ Some products contain bisulfites; use caution in patients with allergies. ▪ Incidence of side effects markedly increased in AIDS patients. May not tolerate or respond to this drug. ▪ *Clostridium difficile*–associated diarrhea (CDAD) has been reported. May range from mild diarrhea to fatal colitis. Consider in patients who present with diarrhea during or after treatment with sulfamethoxazole/trimethoprim.

Monitor: Maintain adequate hydration to prevent crystalluria and stone formation. Monitor fluid intake and urinary output. ▪ Obtain baseline and periodic CBC with platelets. Monitor for any hematologic toxicity. Discontinue for any significant reduction in a blood-forming element. Thrombocytopenia usually resolves within a week after discontinuing sulfamethoxazole/trimethoprim. ▪ Urinalysis and renal function tests are also indicated. ▪ Monitor serum potassium, sodium, and glucose. ▪ Monitor closely for any signs of adverse reactions. Clinical signs such as arthralgia, cough, fever, jaundice, pallor, purpura, rash, shortness of breath, or sore throat may be early indications of serious reactions. ▪ Monitor for S/S of hypersensitivity reactions of the respiratory tract (e.g., cough, pulmonary infiltrates, shortness of breath). ▪ If extravasation occurs, discontinue and restart at a new site. May cause phlebitis. ▪ See Precautions and Drug/Lab Interactions.

Patient Education: Maintain adequate hydration. ▪ Report bruising or bleeding, fever, rash, or sore throat promptly. ▪ Possible skin photosensitivity. Avoid unprotected exposure to sunlight. ▪ Promptly report diarrhea or bloody stools that occur during treatment or up to several months after an antibiotic has been discontinued; may indicate CDAD and require treatment.

Maternal/Child: May cause fetal harm. Some epidemiologic studies suggest that exposure to sulfamethoxazole/trimethoprim during pregnancy may be associated with an increased risk of congenital malformations, particularly neural tube defects, cardiovascular malformations, urinary tract defects, oral clefts, and club foot. Benefits must outweigh risks. ▪ May contain benzyl alcohol, which has been associated with a fatal "gasping syndrome" in neonates. ▪ See Contraindications. ▪ Discontinue breast-feeding because of the potential risk for bilirubin displacement and kernicterus in the breast-fed infant. ▪ Contraindicated in pediatric patients under 2 years of age because of the potential risk of bilirubin displacement and kernicterus.

Elderly: See Dose Adjustments. ▪ Increased risk of severe side effects (e.g., bone marrow suppression, decrease in platelets with or without purpura, hyperkalemia, skin reactions), especially in impaired renal or liver function or with other drugs (e.g., diuretics).

DRUG/LAB INTERACTIONS

May enhance the nephrotoxicity of **cyclosporine**; avoid concurrent use. ▪ May potentiate **warfarin**; monitor PT/INR. ▪ May inhibit the hepatic metabolism of **phenytoin**; monitor phenytoin levels. ▪ May potentiate the effects of **oral hypoglycemics that are metabolized by CYP2C8** (e.g., pioglitazone, repaglinide) **or CYP2C9** (e.g., glipizide and glyburide) **or are eliminated renally via OCT2** (e.g., metformin). Careful monitoring of blood glucose may be warranted. ▪ Trimethoprim may increase serum concentrations of **dapsone**; monitor for toxic effects of dapsone (specifically methemoglobinemia). ▪ Potential for additive myelotoxicity when coadministered with **zidovudine**; monitor for hematologic toxicity. ▪ The sulfa component may displace **methotrexate** from its binding sites and competes with the renal transport of methotrexate, increasing free fraction of methotrexate and its potential for toxicity; avoid concurrent use. ▪ May decrease effectiveness of **tricyclic antidepressants**. ▪ Concurrent use with **leucovorin calcium** may cause treatment failure and increased mortality in HIV-infected patients being treated for *Pneumocystis jiroveci* pneumonia. ▪ Serum levels of **digoxin** may be increased with concurrent use; monitor digoxin levels. ▪ Increased sulfamethoxazole blood levels may occur in patients receiving **indomethacin**; avoid concurrent use. ▪ Patients receiving **pyrimethamine** as malaria prophylaxis and sulfamethoxazole/trimethoprim concurrently may develop megaloblastic anemia; avoid concurrent use. ▪ May form an insoluble precipitate in acid urine or cause crystalluria with **methenamine**; concurrent use not recommended. ▪ May decrease clearance and increase serum concentrations of **N-acetylprocainamide** (NAPA) **and procainamide**, resulting in prolongation of the QT_c interval. Monitor for clinical and ECG signs of procainamide toxicity and/or procainamide plasma concentrations. ▪ Trimethoprim may increase **dofetilide** plasma concentrations, increasing the risk for serious ventricular arrhythmias associated with QT interval prolongation, including torsades de pointes. Concurrent use is ***contraindicated***. ▪ Concurrent use with **rifampin** will increase elimination, reduce serum concentrations, and shorten half-life of trimethoprim. ▪ Concurrent use with **thiazide diuretics** in elderly patients may result in an increased incidence of thrombocytopenia with purpura; avoid concurrent use. ▪ Concurrent use with **angiotensin-converting enzyme inhibitors** may increase the risk of hyperkalemia; avoid concurrent use.

- Toxic delirium has been reported after concurrent use with **amantadine**; avoid concurrent use. ■ May interfere with **serum methotrexate assay and Jaffe assay for creatinine.**
- See Precautions.

SIDE EFFECTS

The most common adverse effects are anorexia, nausea, rash, urticaria, and vomiting. Serious side effects include CDAD, electrolyte abnormalities, embryo-fetal toxicity, hypersensitivity and other fatal reactions, hypoglycemia, infusion reactions, risk associated with concurrent use of leucovorin, sulfite sensitivity, and thrombocytopenia. Other reported reactions include abdominal pain; agranulocytosis; allergic myocarditis; angioedema; apathy; aplastic anemia; arthralgia; aseptic meningitis; ataxia; chills; conjunctival and scleral injection; convulsions; cough; crystalluria; depression; diarrhea; diuresis; drug fever; elevation of BUN, serum creatinine, serum transaminase, and bilirubin; eosinophilia; erythema multiforme; exfoliative dermatitis; fatigue; glossitis; hallucinations; headache; hemolytic anemia; Henoch-Schönlein purpura; hepatitis (including cholestatic jaundice and hepatic necrosis); hyperkalemia; hyponatremia; hypoprothrombinemia; insomnia; interstitial nephritis; leukopenia; local reactions (pain and irritation); megaloblastic anemia; methemoglobinemia; myalgia; nervousness; neutropenia; pancreatitis; periarteritis nodosa; peripheral neuritis; photosensitivity; pruritus; pseudomembranous enterocolitis; pulmonary infiltrates; renal failure; rhabdomyolysis; serum sickness–like syndrome; shortness of breath; Stevens-Johnson syndrome; stomatitis; systemic lupus erythematosus; thrombophlebitis; tinnitus; toxic epidermal necrolysis; toxic nephrosis with oliguria and anuria; uveitis; vertigo; and weakness.

Post-Marketing: Idiopathic thrombocytopenic purpura, QT prolongation resulting in ventricular tachycardia and torsades de pointes, thrombotic thrombocytopenia purpura.

ANTIDOTE

Notify the physician of any side effect. Discontinue the drug at any sign of major toxicity or bone marrow suppression. Some sources recommend leucovorin calcium 5 to 15 mg daily for treatment of bone marrow suppression. Peritoneal dialysis is not effective in toxicity; hemodialysis may be moderately effective in reducing serum levels. Acidification of urine may increase excretion. Hematologic changes indicative of folic acid deficiency may be reversed with folinic acid therapy. Evaluate hyponatremia; appropriate correction is necessary in symptomatic patients to prevent life-threatening complications. Treat anaphylaxis with epinephrine, corticosteroids, antihistamines, and vasopressors. Treat CDAD with fluids, electrolytes, protein supplements, and appropriate antibiotics (e.g., oral vancomycin) as indicated. In severe cases, surgical evaluation may be indicated.

TACROLIMUS BBW
(tah-**KROH**-lih-mus)

Immunosuppressant
Calcineurin inhibitor

Prograf

USUAL DOSE

Pretreatment: Verify pregnancy status; baseline studies indicated; see Monitor.

See Precautions. IV route used for patients unable to take oral medications; risk of anaphylaxis increased with IV administration. Transfer to oral therapy as soon as tolerated.

Whenever possible, administer the complete complement of vaccines before transplantation and treatment with tacrolimus.

For all indications: Dose regimens vary among transplant centers and approved or investigational use (range 0.01 to 0.05 mg/kg/day). Begin no sooner than 6 hours after transplantation in liver and heart transplant patients. In kidney transplant patients, initial dose may be administered within 24 hours of transplantation but should be delayed until renal function has recovered. Adults usually receive doses at the lower end of the range. Pediatric patients may require doses at the upper end of the range. Individualized adjustment based on clinical assessment of rejection or patients' tolerance is imperative and may be required on a daily basis. Adjunctive adrenal corticosteroid therapy early posttransplant is recommended. Initiate oral tacrolimus therapy as soon as feasible. Oral doses vary with specific organ transplant and in adults and pediatric patients (see literature). Total dose in mg/kg/day is given in equally divided doses every 12 hours. Begin 8 to 12 hours after IV tacrolimus is discontinued. Lower doses may be sufficient for maintenance therapy.

Prophylaxis of organ rejection in heart transplant: The recommended starting dose is 0.01 mg/kg/day as a continuous infusion. Used in combination with azathioprine or mycophenolate in addition to adrenal corticosteroids. Other immunosuppressants have also been used. See literature. See all comments and protocol under For All Indications above.

Prophylaxis of organ rejection in kidney transplant: The recommended starting dose is 0.03 to 0.05 mg/kg/day as a continuous infusion. Used in combination with azathioprine or mycophenolate in addition to adrenal corticosteroids. See all comments and protocol under For All Indications above.

Prophylaxis of organ rejection in liver transplant: The recommended starting dose is 0.03 to 0.05 mg/kg/day as a continuous infusion. Used in combination with adrenal corticosteroids. See all comments and protocol under For All Indications above.

PEDIATRIC DOSE

Has been used successfully in pediatric patients up to 16 years of age in liver transplants. See Usual Dose for mg/kg/day dose recommendations. Studies indicate that higher doses may be required to maintain blood trough concentrations similar to adults. Experience in pediatric heart and kidney transplant patients is limited but has been used. Consult literature. See Dilution and Maternal/Child.

DOSE ADJUSTMENTS

Dosing should be titrated based on clinical assessments of rejection and tolerability. ▪ Use lower end of the dosing range initially for patients with impaired renal or hepatic function (pretransplant or posttransplant). Renal impairment does not affect clearance of tacrolimus, but tacrolimus may cause nephrotoxicity, requiring a reduction in dose. ▪ Half-life is prolonged and clearance decreased in patients with severe hepatic impairment (Child-Pugh greater than or equal to 10). Higher levels resulting from decreased clearance can increase the risk of renal insufficiency. Dose reduction may be required. ▪ In kidney

Continued

transplant patients with postoperative oliguria, the initial dose of tacrolimus should be administered no sooner than 6 hours and within 24 hours of transplantation, but it may be delayed until renal function shows evidence of recovery. ■ Lower doses may be appropriate for maintenance. ■ Studies in kidney transplant patients indicate that African-American patients may require a higher dose to obtain trough concentrations comparable to those seen in White patients. ■ See Monitor and Drug/Lab Interactions.

DILUTION
Specific techniques required; see Precautions. Available as a 5-mg/mL solution in a 1-mL ampule. A 24-hour dose must be diluted with an appropriate amount of NS or D5W. Desired concentration is between 4 and 20 mcg/mL. May leach phthalate from polyvinylchloride containers; mix in glass or polyethylene infusion bottles. Use PVC-free IV tubing in pediatric patients.
Storage: Store between 20° and 25° C (68° and 77° F) before dilution. Discard diluted solution after 24 hours.

COMPATIBILITY
Manufacturer states, "Should not be mixed with solutions of pH 9 or greater." See Dilution.
Other sources suggest specific **compatibilities** dependent on concentration and manufacturer; consult a pharmacist.

RATE OF ADMINISTRATION
A single dose properly diluted and equally distributed over 24 hours as a continuous infusion. Use of a metriset (60 gtt/min) or infusion pump suggested.

ACTIONS
A potent immunosuppressive agent. Prolongs survival of allogeneic heart, kidney, and liver transplants. Inhibition of T-lymphocyte activation and proliferation results in immunosuppression. Highly protein bound. Metabolized primarily by the P450 enzyme system (CYP3A). Half-life ranges from 32 to 55 hours. Primarily excreted in feces. Minimal excretion in urine. Crosses the placental barrier. Secreted in breast milk.

INDICATIONS AND USES
Prophylaxis of organ rejection in adult and pediatric patients receiving allogeneic heart, kidney, and liver transplants in conjunction with other immunosuppressants.
Unlabeled uses: Treatment of autoimmune diseases (i.e., refractory rheumatoid arthritis). ■ Prevention and treatment of acute graft-versus-host disease.

CONTRAINDICATIONS
Hypersensitivity to tacrolimus or polyoxyl 60 hydrogenated castor oil.

PRECAUTIONS
Follow guidelines for handling hazardous agents. See Appendix A, p. 1308. ■ For IV use only. ■ Oral dosing preferred; begin as soon as feasible. Risk of anaphylaxis is increased by IV route versus oral route; use caution. *Reserve for patients unable to take oral medication.* ■ Usually administered in the hospital by or under the direction of a physician experienced in immunosuppressive therapy and management of organ transplant patients. ■ Adequate laboratory and supportive medical resources must be available. ■ Patients receiving immunosuppressants, including tacrolimus, are at increased risk of developing lymphomas and other malignancies (especially of skin). Risk appears to be related to intensity and duration of immunosuppression. ■ Has also been associated with a posttransplant lymphoproliferative disorder (PTLD), usually related to Epstein-Barr virus (EBV) infection. Risk of PTLD appears greatest in patients who are EBV-seronegative, which includes many young children. ■ Immunosuppressed patients are at increased risk for bacterial, viral, fungal, and protozoal infections, including opportunistic infections. May result in serious and fatal outcomes. ■ Opportunistic infections may include latent viral infections such as polyoma virus infections. Polyoma virus infections may result in polyoma virus–associated nephropathy (PVAN) and JC virus–associated progressive multifocal leukoencephalopathy (PML). PVAN is associated with serious outcomes, including deteriorating renal function

and kidney graft loss. PML is a serious progressive neurologic disorder caused by infection of the CNS by the JC virus. It typically occurs in immunocompromised patients. PML is rare but may result in irreversible neurologic deterioration and death, and there is no known effective treatment. Hemiparesis, apathy, confusion, cognitive deficiencies, and ataxia are the most commonly observed clinical signs. ▪ Patients receiving immunosuppression are at increased risk for developing cytomegalovirus (CMV), viremia, and CMV disease. ▪ Tacrolimus can cause acute or chronic nephrotoxicity. Use caution in impaired renal function; increases in SCr may require dose reduction or use of an alternate immunosuppressant; see Dose Adjustments, Monitor, and Drug/Lab Interactions. ▪ Use caution in severe hepatic dysfunction (mean Pugh score: greater than 10); clearance decreased; see Dose Adjustments. ▪ Post–liver transplant patients experiencing hepatic impairment may be at increased risk of developing renal insufficiency related to elevated tacrolimus concentrations. ▪ Can cause neurotoxicity, particularly at higher doses. The most severe neurotoxicities include posterior reversible encephalopathy syndrome (PRES), delirium, seizures, and coma; see Monitor. ▪ Hyperkalemia has been reported. ▪ Hypertension is a common adverse effect and may require hypertensive therapy; see Drug/Lab Interactions. ▪ Concurrent use with sirolimus is not recommended in liver or heart transplant patients. Regimen is associated with an increased risk of wound healing complications, renal function impairment, and insulin-dependent, posttransplant diabetes mellitus in heart transplant patients; regimen is associated with excess mortality, graft loss, and hepatic artery thrombosis in liver transplant patients. The safety and efficacy of tacrolimus and sirolimus have not been established in kidney transplant patients. ▪ New-onset diabetes mellitus has been reported in tacrolimus-treated heart, kidney, and liver transplant patients. May be reversible in some patients. African-American and Hispanic kidney transplant patients may be at an increased risk; see Monitor. ▪ Myocardial hypertrophy has been reported in pediatric patients and adults, particularly in those with high tacrolimus trough concentrations. Reversible in most cases with dose reduction or discontinuation of tacrolimus. ▪ May prolong the QT/QTc interval and cause torsades de pointes. Avoid use in patients with congenital long QT syndrome. Patients with CHF, bradyarrhythmias, or electrolyte abnormalities (e.g., hypokalemia, hypocalcemia, hypomagnesemia) and patients taking medicinal products that may lead to QT prolongation may be at increased risk; see Monitor and Drug/Lab Interactions. ▪ Pure red cell aplasia (PRCA) has been reported. ▪ See Drug/Lab Interactions.

Monitor: Obtain baseline CBC, differential, platelets, electrolytes, fasting glucose, BUN, SCr, and liver function tests. Monitor regularly during therapy. ▪ Contains a castor oil derivative; observe continuously for signs of a hypersensitivity reaction (e.g., acute respiratory distress syndrome [ARDS], dyspnea, pruritus, rash) for the first 30 minutes of the infusion and frequently thereafter. A source of oxygen and epinephrine must always be available. ▪ Monitor EBV serology during treatment. ▪ Observe for signs of infection (e.g., fever, sore throat, tiredness) or unusual bleeding or bruising. Adjust the immunosuppressive regimen to balance the risk of rejection with the risk of infection. ▪ Monitor urine output and SCr carefully. Overt nephrotoxicity occurs more frequently early after transplant. Acute nephrotoxicity is characterized by increasing SCr, hyperkalemia, and/or a decrease in urine output and is usually reversible. Chronic nephrotoxicity is usually progressive and is associated with increased SCr, decreased life of kidney graft, and characteristic histologic changes on renal biopsy. Consider changing to another immunosuppressive therapy in patients with persistent elevations of SCr who are unresponsive to dose adjustments. ▪ Monitor for S/S of neurotoxicity (e.g., changes in motor or sensory function, changes in mental status, coma, delirium, headache, paresthesias, tremors, seizures). ▪ Monitor for S/S of PRES (e.g., altered mental status, headache, hypertension, seizures, and visual disturbances). Diagnosis may be confirmed by MRI. Stabilize BP and consider dose reduction. Symptoms have reversed when immunosuppression is reduced or discontinued. ▪ Monitor for S/S of PML; apathy, ataxia, cognitive deficiencies, confusion, and hemiparesis are the most commonly observed clinical signs. Consultation with a neurologist may be indicated. ▪ Tacrolimus whole blood trough concentrations in conjunction with other laboratory and clinical parameters are used to evaluate rejection, toxicity, need for dose adjustment, and patient compliance. Risk of toxicity (e.g., nephrotoxicity, neurotoxicity, posttransplant diabetes mellitus) is increased with higher trough concentrations. Whole blood median trough concentrations may vary considerably during the first week but then stabilize. Most patients are stable when trough whole blood concentrations are between 5 and 20 ng/mL depending on indication and length of time since the transplant. The trough concentrations described above and in the manufacturer's prescribing information pertain only to oral administration of tacrolimus. Monitoring tacrolimus concentrations during a continuous IV infusion of tacrolimus may have some utility; however, the observed concentrations will not represent exposures comparable to those estimated by the trough concentrations observed in patients on oral therapy. ▪ Different methods are available for the assay of tacrolimus blood levels. Specific collection techniques and storage requirements are required. Contact the Clinical Laboratory for guidance. ▪ Blood concentration monitoring is not a replacement for renal and liver function monitoring and tissue biopsies. Monitor all parameters to evaluate efficacy, toxicity, and the possibility of organ rejection. ▪ Monitor BP; antihypertensives may be indicated; see Drug/Lab Interactions. ▪ Monitor electrolyte concentrations. May cause hyperkalemia or hypomagnesemia; see Drug/Lab Interactions. ▪ In patients with CHF, bradyarrhythmias, or electrolyte abnormalities (e.g., hypokalemia, hypocalcemia, hypomagnesemia) and in patients taking certain antiarrhythmics or other medicinal products that may lead to QT prolongation, consider obtaining an electrocardiogram and monitoring electrolytes periodically during treatment. ▪ May cause hyperglycemia. Monitor carefully; treatment may be required. ▪ Consider echocardiographic evaluation in patients who develop renal failure or clinical manifestations of ventricular dysfunction. Consider dose reduction or discontinuation of tacrolimus if myocardial hypertrophy is diagnosed. ▪ See Precautions and Drug/Lab Interactions.

Patient Education: Review manufacturer's medication guide. ▪ Female and male patients of reproductive potential should discuss family planning options, including effective contraception, with a health care provider before starting treatment with tacrolimus. ▪ Encourage female transplant patients who become pregnant and male patients who father a child and have been exposed to immunosuppressants, including tacrolimus, to enroll in the voluntary Transplantation Pregnancy Registry International. ▪ May compromise male and female fertility. ▪ Emphasize need for frequent routine lab work; compliance imperative. ▪ Interacts with many medications. Discuss any changes in drug regimen (prescription or nonprescription) with doctor or pharmacist. ▪ Promptly report any side effects (e.g., hypertension, nephrotoxicity, neurotoxicity, S/S of infection, heart failure). ▪ Review S/S of diabetes mellitus. ▪ Inform patient of increased risk of neoplasia, including malignant skin changes. Limit exposure to sunlight and ultraviolet light by wearing protective clothing and a broad-spectrum sunscreen with a high protection factor. Promptly report any skin changes. ▪ See Appendix D, p. 1311.

Maternal/Child: Data from post-marketing surveillance and an international pregnancy registry suggest that tacrolimus can cause fetal harm when administered to pregnant females. Infants exposed to tacrolimus in utero are at risk for prematurity, birth defects/congenital anomalies, low birth weight, and fetal distress. ▪ Has been associated with hyperkalemia and renal dysfunction in the fetus. ▪ May increase hyperglycemia in pregnant females with diabetes (including gestational diabetes); monitor maternal blood glucose levels regularly. ▪ May exacerbate hypertension in pregnant females and increase pre-eclampsia. Monitor and control blood pressure. ▪ Effects of tacrolimus on the breast-fed infant or on milk production have not been assessed. Use caution and consider risk versus benefit. ▪ Manufacturer has a general statement that safety and effectiveness have been established for use in pediatric liver, kidney, and heart transplant patients. However, data are limited on use of the IV formulation in pediatric kidney and heart transplant patients. Consult literature for suggested dosage regimens. ▪ Appears to be an increased risk for posttransplant lymphoproliferative disorder (PLPD) and primary EBV infection in immunosuppressed pediatric patients.

Elderly: Clinical trials did not include sufficient numbers of subjects 65 years of age and over to determine whether they respond differently from younger subjects. Clinical experience has not identified differences in response. In general, dose selection for an elderly patient should be cautious, starting at the lower end of the dosing range and taking into account age-related organ impairment and concomitant disease or drug therapy.

DRUG/LAB INTERACTIONS

Used concurrently with **adrenocorticosteroids and azathioprine or mycophenolate (CellCept).** ▪ Concomitant use of tacrolimus with **mycophenolic acid** (MPA) will increase MPA exposure more than exposure seen with concurrent use of MPA and cyclosporine. Monitor for MPA-associated toxicity and reduce MPA dose if needed. ▪ *Do not use simultaneously with cyclosporine.* If a change of immunosuppressants is indicated (tacrolimus to cyclosporine or cyclosporine to tacrolimus), avoid additive nephrotoxicity by waiting for at least 24 hours before starting the alternate drug. If elevated blood concentrations are present, further extend the interval between the two drugs. ▪ Concurrent use with **sirolimus** is not recommended; see Precautions. ▪ Coadministration with **strong CYP3A4 inhibitors** (e.g., azole antifungal agents, boceprevir, clarithromycin, letermovir, ritonavir, telaprevir) **and strong inducers** (e.g., rifampin), **including those that prolong the QT interval** (e.g., azole antifungals, clarithromycin), is not recommended without adjustments in tacrolimus dosing and close monitoring of tacrolimus whole blood trough concentration and associated side effects. ▪ Concurrent use with **other drugs that prolong the QT interval** may require dose adjustment and monitoring of the QT interval and trough concentrations. **Amiodarone** has been reported to increase tacrolimus whole blood concentration with or without concurrent QT prolongation. ▪ Use extreme caution with **other nephrotoxic agents** (e.g., aminoglycosides, amphotericin B, cisplatin, ganciclovir, nucleotide reverse transcriptase inhibitors [e.g., tenofovir], and protease inhibitors [e.g., ritonavir, indinavir]); risk of nephrotoxicity increased. ▪ Do not use **potassium-sparing diuretics** (e.g., spironolactone); increases risk of hyperkalemia. Other agents associated with hyperkalemia (e.g., **ACE inhibitors** and **angiotensin receptor blockers**) should be used with caution. ▪ **Calcium channel blockers, chloramphenicol, cimetidine, clotrimazole, danazol, erythromycin, estradiol, fluconazole, herbal products containing schisandra sphenanthera extracts, lansoprazole, metoclopramide, metronidazole, omeprazole, protease inhibitors** (e.g., ritonavir, saquinavir), **and troleandomycin** may inhibit the P450 enzyme system and increase tacrolimus blood levels, increasing toxicity potential. Tacrolimus toxicity may also be increased if given concurrently with **nefazodone.** ▪ Avoid concomitant use with **nelfinavir** unless benefits outweigh risks. ▪ When initiating therapy with **posaconazole or voriconazole** in patients already receiving tacrolimus, decrease tacrolimus dose to one-third of the original dose. Adjust subsequent tacrolimus doses based on tacrolimus whole blood concentrations. ▪ **Anticonvulsants, caspofungin, methylprednisone, rifamycins** (e.g., rifabutin, rifampin), **and St. John's wort** may induce the P450 enzyme system, decreasing effectiveness and leading to decreased tacrolimus blood levels and organ rejection. ▪ Tacrolimus may increase serum concentrations of **phenytoin.** ▪ **Grapefruit and grapefruit juice** may affect certain enzymes of the P450 system and should be avoided. ▪ **Do not use live virus vaccines** in patients receiving tacrolimus. Inactivated vaccines noted to be safe for administration after transplantation may not be sufficiently immunogenic during treatment with tacrolimus.

SIDE EFFECTS

The most common adverse reactions were abdominal pain, abnormal renal function, anemia, bronchitis, CMV infection, constipation, diabetes mellitus, diarrhea, fever, headache, hyperglycemia, hyperkalemia, hyperlipidemia, hypertension, hypomagnesemia, infection, insomnia, leukopenia, nausea, paresthesia, pericardial effusion, peripheral edema, tremor, and urinary tract infection. Additional adverse reactions reported in the different studies are listed below.

Heart transplant: Similar to above.

Kidney transplant: Other commonly reported reactions included arthralgia, asthenia, back pain, chest pain, cough, dizziness, dyspepsia, dyspnea, graft dysfunction, hypokalemia, hypophosphatemia, nephrotoxicity, pain, pruritus, rash, and vomiting.

Liver transplant: Abnormal LFTs, acidosis, anorexia, ascites, asthenia, atelectasis, back pain, bile duct disorder, dyspnea, EBV infection, gastroenteritis, GI hemorrhage, leukocytosis, nephrotoxicity, pain, peripheral edema, peritonitis, pleural effusion, pruritus, rash, sepsis, thrombocytopenia, vomiting.

Nephrotoxicity (abnormal renal function with increased SCr and BUN, oliguria) and neurotoxicity (delirium, headache, insomnia, paresthesia, tremor, seizures) may be dose limiting. Many other side effects have been reported; see Precautions and manufacturer's prescribing information.

Post-Marketing: Acute respiratory distress syndrome, agranulocytosis, cardiac arrhythmia, cerebral infarction, DIC, enterocolitis, febrile neutropenia, gastroesophageal reflux disease, GI perforation, hemolytic anemia, hepatotoxicity, interstitial lung disease, optic neuropathy, pain in extremity (including calcineurin-inhibitor–induced pain syndrome [CIPS]), PRES, PRCA, primary graft dysfunction, PML, and PVAN nephropathy are some of the many additional side effects reported.

ANTIDOTE

Notify the physician of all side effects. Most will be treated symptomatically. Tacrolimus dose may be decreased or discontinued or alternate immunosuppressive agents substituted. Nephrotoxicity, neurotoxicity, or hematopoietic depression may require temporary reduction of dose or discontinuation of therapy. Reduction in immunosuppression should be considered for patients who develop evidence of PVAN, PML, or CMV viremia and/or CMV disease. However, the risk that reduced immunosuppression represents to the functioning allograft must also be considered. If S/S of PRES occur, stabilize BP, and consider an immediate decrease of immunosuppression. Consider discontinuing tacrolimus if PRCA is diagnosed. Dialysis is not effective in overdose. Discontinue immediately if anaphylaxis occurs and treat with oxygen, epinephrine, corticosteroids, and/or antihistamines (e.g., diphenhydramine). Resuscitate as necessary.

TEDIZOLID PHOSPHATE

(te-**DIZ**-oh-lid **FOS**-fayt)

Sivextro

Antibacterial

(oxazolidinone)

USUAL DOSE

Pretreatment: Baseline studies indicated; see Monitor.

Tedizolid: 200 mg once daily for 6 days as an infusion over 1 hour. Alternately, may be given orally (with or without food).

DOSE ADJUSTMENTS

No dose adjustment necessary when changing from IV to oral doses. ▪ If a dose is missed or delayed, it should be administered as soon as possible any time up to 8 hours before the next scheduled dose. If less than 8 hours remain before the next dose, wait until the next scheduled dose. ▪ No dose adjustments indicated based on age, gender, weight, race, or any degree of hepatic or renal impairment.

DILUTION

Available in single-use vials containing 200 mg of tedizolid as a lyophilized powder. Reconstitute the 200-mg vial with 4 mL of SWFI. Gently swirl the contents and let the vial stand until completely dissolved and any foam disperses. Solution should be clear and colorless to pale yellow. Tilt the upright vial and insert a needle attached to a syringe to the bottom corner of the vial. Withdraw 4 mL of the reconstituted solution. *Do not invert the vial during extraction* of its contents. Further dilute by slowly injecting the 4 mL into a 250-mL bag of NS. Invert the bag gently to mix. *Do NOT shake*; may cause foaming.

Filters: Specific information not available.

Storage: Before use, vials may be stored at CRT. Total time from reconstitution to dilution to completion of administration of both reconstituted vials and/or fully diluted solutions should not exceed 24 hours at RT or under refrigeration at 2° to 8° C (36° to 46° F).

COMPATIBILITY

Tedizolid is **compatible** only with NS. Manufacturer states, "Other IV substances, additives, or other medications should not be added to tedizolid single-use vials or infused simultaneously through the same IV line or through a common IV port. If the same IV line is used for sequential infusion of additional medications, the line should be flushed before and after infusion of tedizolid with NS." It is **incompatible** with any solution containing divalent cations (e.g., calcium, magnesium), including LR injection and Hartmann's solution.

RATE OF ADMINISTRATION

A single dose as an infusion equally distributed over 1 hour. **Do not administer as an IV push or bolus.** If a common IV line is used to administer other drugs in addition to tedizolid, flush the IV line before and after each tedizolid infusion with NS.

ACTIONS

Tedizolid phosphate belongs to the oxazolidinone class of antibacterial drugs. It is a phosphate prodrug and is converted to tedizolid by phosphatases. Its antibacterial activity is mediated by binding to the 50S subunit of the bacterial ribosome, resulting in inhibition of protein synthesis. This mechanism of action is different from that of other non–oxazodidinone class antibacterial drugs; therefore cross-resistance between tedizolid and other classes of antibacterial drugs is unlikely. Bacteriostatic against designated strains of *Staphylococcus*, *Streptococcus,* and *Enterococcus*; see Indications. Peak plasma concentrations are achieved at the end of the 1-hour infusion. Penetrates into the interstitial space fluid of adipose and skeletal muscle tissue with exposure similar to free-drug exposure in plasma. Approximately 70% to 90% bound to human plasma proteins. Half-life is approximately 12 hours. The majority of elimination occurs via the liver. Primarily excreted as a microbiologically inactive sulfate conjugate in feces with some excretion in urine.

INDICATIONS AND USES

Treatment of adult patients with acute bacterial skin and skin structure infections (ABSSSI) caused by susceptible isolates of designated gram-positive microorganisms, including *Staphylococcus aureus* (both methicillin-susceptible [MSSA] and methicillin-resistant [MRSA] strains).

CONTRAINDICATIONS

Manufacturer states, "None."

PRECAUTIONS

For IV use only. ▪ Safety and efficacy for use in patients with neutropenia (neutrophil counts less than 1,000 cells/mm^3) have not been adequately evaluated. In an animal model of infection, the antibacterial activity of tedizolid was reduced in the absence of granulocytes. Consider alternative therapy when treating patients with neutropenia and ABSSSI. ▪ Specific sensitivity studies are indicated to determine susceptibility of the causative organism to tedizolid. ▪ To reduce the development of drug-resistant bacteria and maintain its effectiveness, tedizolid should be used to treat only those infections proven or strongly suspected to be caused by bacteria. ▪ *Clostridium difficile*–associated diarrhea (CDAD) has been reported for nearly all systemic antibacterial agents and may range in severity from mild diarrhea to fatal colitis. Consider in patients who present with diarrhea during or after treatment with tedizolid.

Monitor: Obtain baseline CBC with differential and platelets. ▪ Monitor for S/S of hypersensitivity (e.g., hypotension, rash, urticaria, tightness of the chest, wheezing).

Patient Education: Review FDA-approved patient information. ▪ Advise pregnant females and females of reproductive potential about possible risk to the fetus. ▪ Promptly report S/S of a hypersensitivity reaction (e.g., hives, rash, shortness of breath, wheezing). ▪ Promptly report diarrhea or bloody stools that occur during treatment or up to several months after an antibiotic has been discontinued; may indicate CDAD and require treatment.

Maternal/Child: Based on animal studies, tedizolid may cause fetal harm when administered to pregnant females. Use during pregnancy only if the potential benefit outweighs the possible risk to the fetus. ▪ Use caution during breast-feeding. ▪ Safety and effectiveness for use in pediatric patients not established.

Elderly: Numbers in clinical studies insufficient to determine whether the elderly respond differently than do younger subjects. No overall differences in pharmacokinetics were observed between elderly subjects and younger subjects.

DRUG/LAB INTERACTIONS

Tedizolid did not detectably inhibit or induce the metabolism of **cytochrome P450 enzyme substrates.** There was no degradation of tedizolid in human liver microsomes, indicating that tedizolid is unlikely to be a substrate for hepatic CYP450 enzymes. ▪ A reversible inhibitor of monoamine oxidase. Not evaluated because subjects taking MAO inhibitors were excluded from trials.

SIDE EFFECTS

The most common adverse reactions are diarrhea, dizziness, headache, infusion- or injection-related adverse reactions, nausea, and vomiting. CDAD, decreased WBC, dermatitis, eye disorders (e.g., asthenopia, blurred vision, visual impairment, vitreous floaters), flushing, hypersensitivity reactions, hypertension, hypoesthesia, increased hepatic transaminases, insomnia, myelosuppression (anemia, neutropenia, thrombocytopenia), oral candidiasis, palpitations, paresthesia, pruritus, seventh nerve paralysis, tachycardia, urticaria, and vulvovaginal mycotic infection have been reported. Peripheral and optic neuropathy have been described in patients treated with another member of the oxazolidinone class (e.g., linezolid) for longer than 28 days.

ANTIDOTE

Notify physician of any side effects. Discontinue the drug if indicated. Treat hypersensitivity reactions as indicated (e.g., diphenhydramine, epinephrine, albuterol) and resuscitate as necessary. Mild cases of CDAD may respond to discontinuation of tedizolid. Treat CDAD with fluids, electrolytes, protein supplements, and appropriate antibiotics (e.g., oral vancomycin) as indicated. In severe cases, surgical evaluation may be indicated. In the event of an overdose, discontinue tedizolid and provide supportive treatment as needed. Is not effectively removed from the circulation by hemodialysis.

TELAVANCIN BBW

(tel-a-**VAN**-sin)

Vibativ

Antibacterial
(lipoglycopeptide)

pH 4 to 5

USUAL DOSE

Pretreatment: Baseline studies indicated; see Monitor.

Complicated skin and skin structure infections (cSSSI): 10 mg/kg as an infusion once every 24 hours for 7 to 14 days. Duration of therapy is dependent on severity and site of infection and on the patient's clinical progress.

Hospital-acquired and ventilator-associated bacterial pneumonia (HABP/VABP): 10 mg/kg as an infusion once every 24 hours for 7 to 21 days. Duration of therapy is dependent on severity and site of infection and on the patient's clinical progress.

DOSE ADJUSTMENTS

Dose adjustment required in renal impairment as outlined in the following chart.

Telavancin Dosage Adjustment in Adult Patients With Renal Impairment	
Creatinine Clearance[a] (mL/min)	**Telavancin Dosage Regimen**
>50 mL/min	10 mg/kg every 24 hours
30 to 50 mL/min	7.5 mg/kg every 24 hours
10 to <30 mL/min	10 mg/kg every 48 hours

[a]Calculate using Cockcroft-Gault formula and ideal body weight. Use actual body weight if it is less than ideal body weight.

There is insufficient information to make specific dose recommendations for patients with end-stage renal disease (CrCl <10 mL/min), including patients undergoing hemodialysis. ■ Reduced doses may be indicated in the elderly based on age-related renal impairment. ■ No dose adjustment is recommended based on gender or in patients with mild or moderate hepatic impairment. Has not been studied in patients with severe hepatic impairment.

DILUTION

Reconstitute each 250-mg vial with 15 mL of D5W, SWFI, or NS (45 mL for a 750-mg vial). Resultant solution has a final concentration of 15 mg/mL. To minimize foaming during reconstitution, allow the vacuum of the vial to pull the diluent from the syringe into the vial. Do not forcefully inject the diluent into the vial. Do not forcefully shake the vial. Reconstitution time is generally under 2 minutes but can occasionally take as long as 20 minutes. Mix thoroughly to dissolve contents completely. Discard vial if vacuum does not pull diluent into vial. Doses of 150 to 800 mg must be further diluted in 100 to 250 mL of D5W, NS, or LR. Doses less than 150 mg or greater than 800 mg must be diluted in a sufficient volume to provide a final concentration of 0.6 to 8 mg/mL. Do not shake the final infusion solution.

Storage: Store unopened vials in refrigerator at 2° to 8° C (36° to 46° F). Excursions up to 25° C (77° F) are acceptable. Reconstituted and diluted solutions are stable for 12 hours at RT and for 7 days refrigerated. Total time in the vial plus the time in the infusion bag should not exceed 12 hours at RT and 7 days under refrigeration. The diluted solution can also be stored at −30° to −10° C (−22° to −14° F) for up to 32 days.

COMPATIBILITY

Manufacturer states, "Additives or other medications should not be added to telavancin single-use vials or infused simultaneously through the same IV line. If the same IV line is used for sequential infusion of additional medications, the line should be flushed before and after infusions of telavancin with D5W, NS, or LR."

Other sources suggest specific **compatibilities** dependent on concentration and manufacturer; consult a pharmacist.

RATE OF ADMINISTRATION

A single dose equally distributed as an infusion over 60 minutes. Rapid IV infusions can cause "red man syndrome"–like infusion-related reactions, including flushing of the upper body, urticaria, pruritus, or rash. Stopping or slowing the infusion may result in cessation of these reactions. If the same IV line is used for sequential infusion of additional medications, the line should be flushed before and after infusions of telavancin with D5W, NS, or LR.

ACTIONS

A lipoglycopeptide antibacterial that is a synthetic derivative of vancomycin. Bactericidal against gram-positive organisms, including susceptible strains of staphylococci, streptococci, and vancomycin-susceptible enterococci. Exerts bactericidal action through inhibition of cell wall synthesis. Highly protein bound, primarily to albumin. The metabolic pathway for telavancin has not been identified. Half-life is 6.6 to 9.6 hours. Primarily excreted by the kidney.

INDICATIONS AND USES

Treatment of adult patients with complicated skin and skin structure infections (cSSSIs) caused by susceptible isolates of gram-positive microorganisms, including *Staphylococcus aureus* (including methicillin-susceptible and methicillin-resistant isolates), *Streptococcus pyogenes, Streptococcus agalactiae, Streptococcus anginosus* group, or *Enterococcus faecalis* (vancomycin-susceptible isolates only). ▪ Treatment of adult patients with HABP/VABP caused by susceptible isolates of *S. aureus* (including methicillin-susceptible and methicillin-resistant isolates). Reserve use for when alternative treatments are not suitable.

CONTRAINDICATIONS

Known hypersensitivity to telavancin. ▪ Use of IV unfractionated heparin sodium is contraindicated; see Drug/Lab Interactions.

PRECAUTIONS

To reduce the development of drug-resistant bacteria and maintain its effectiveness, telavancin should be used to treat or prevent only those infections proven or strongly suspected to be caused by bacteria. ▪ Sensitivity studies are necessary to determine susceptibility of the causative organism to telavancin. ▪ Combination therapy may be clinically indicated if the documented or presumed pathogens include gram-negative organisms. ▪ Prolonged use of drug may result in superinfection caused by overgrowth of nonsusceptible organisms. ▪ New-onset or worsening renal impairment has been reported. Patients with underlying renal dysfunction or risk factors for renal dysfunction (diabetes mellitus, CHF, or hypertension) may be at increased risk. Patients who received concomitant medications known to affect kidney function (e.g., NSAIDs, ACE inhibitors, and loop diuretics) may also be at higher risk; see Drug Interactions. ▪ Patients with pre-existing moderate to severe renal impairment (CrCl less than or equal to 50 mL/min) who were treated with telavancin for HABP/VABP had increased mortality observed versus vancomycin. Use of telavancin in patients with pre-existing moderate to severe renal impairment should be considered only when the anticipated benefit outweighs the potential risk. ▪ Data from cSSSI trials suggest that clinical cure rates were lower in patients with baseline CrCl less than or equal to 50 mL/min. The same decrease in clinical cure rates was not seen in vancomycin-treated patients. These data should be considered when selecting antibacterial therapy for use in patients with baseline moderate/severe renal impairment. ■ Serious and sometimes fatal hypersensitivity reactions, including anaphylactic reactions, may occur after the first dose or subsequent doses. Telavancin is a semi-synthetic derivative of vancomycin; it is unknown whether patients with hypersensitivity reactions to vancomycin will experience cross-reactivity to telavancin. Use with caution in patients with known hypersensitivity to vancomycin. ■ *Clostridium difficile*–associated diarrhea (CDAD) has been reported. May range from mild diarrhea to fatal colitis. Consider in patients who present with diarrhea during or after treatment with telavancin. ■ Infusion-related reactions have been reported; see Rate of Administration and Monitor. ■ Has caused prolongation of the QTc interval. Use with caution in patients who are taking drugs known to prolong the QTc interval. Avoid use in patients with congenital long QT syndrome, known prolongation of the QTc interval, uncompensated heart failure, or severe left ventricular hypertrophy. ■ Does not interfere with coagulation. Increased risk of bleeding and effects on platelet aggregation have not been observed. However, has been shown to affect certain anticoagulation tests; see Drug/Lab Interactions. ■ There is no known cross-resistance between telavancin and other classes of antibiotics. Some vancomycin-resistant enterococci have a reduced susceptibility to telavancin. ■ See Maternal/Child.

Monitor: Obtain baseline CBC with differential and SCr. Monitor SCr every 48 to 72 hours, or more frequently if indicated, and at the end of therapy. If renal function deteriorates, the risk versus benefit of continuing therapy should be assessed. ■ Monitor for possible infusion-related reactions. ■ Monitor for S/S of hypersensitivity reactions.

Patient Education: Review manufacturer-supplied medication guide. ■ Females of child-bearing potential should have a pregnancy test before initiating therapy. Effective birth control should be used throughout therapy. A pregnancy registry has been established to monitor the outcomes of females who become pregnant while receiving telavancin. ■ Report all side effects promptly. ■ Promptly report diarrhea or bloody stools that occur during treatment or up to several months after telavancin has been discontinued; may indicate CDAD and require treatment.

Maternal/Child: Category C: adverse developmental outcomes in three animal species at clinically relevant doses raise concerns about potential adverse developmental outcomes in humans. Avoid use during pregnancy unless potential benefit justifies potential risk. ■ Females with childbearing potential should have a serum pregnancy test before receiving telavancin. A pregnancy registry has been established to monitor pregnancy outcomes in females exposed to telavancin during pregnancy. ■ Safety for use in breast-feeding not established and effects unknown; use caution. ■ Safety and effectiveness for use in pediatric patients have not been studied.

Elderly: In cSSSI trials, lower clinical cure rates were seen in patients over 65 years of age. Overall, treatment-emergent adverse events occurred with similar frequencies in patients of all age-groups studied. However, adverse events indicative of renal impairment occurred more frequently in the elderly. In HABP/VABP trials, treatment-emergent adverse events, deaths, and other serious adverse events occurred more often in patients 65 years of age or older. Consider age-related renal impairment; see Dose Adjustments.

DRUG/LAB INTERACTIONS

Use with caution in patients taking **medications known to prolong the QTc interval** (e.g., amiodarone and other antiarrhythmics, diphenhydramine, fosphenytoin, furosemide, itraconazole). Effects may be additive. ■ Concomitant use with **other agents that can affect renal function** (e.g., NSAIDs, diuretics, and ACE inhibitors) may increase the risk of renal toxicity. ■ May affect **certain anticoagulation tests.** Increases in PT, INR, aPTT, ACT, and coagulation-based factor X activity assays have been observed. Effects dissipate over time. Interference seen when using samples drawn between 0 and 18 hours after telavancin administration. Collect blood samples for these coagulation tests immediately before a patient's next telavancin dose to minimize interaction. Because aPPT test results are expected to be artificially prolonged after telavancin administration, concurrent use of intravenous unfractionated **heparin** is contraindicated. For patients who require aPTT monitoring while being treated with telavancin, a non–phospholipid-dependent coagulation test such as a factor Xa (chromogenic) assay or an alternative anticoagulant not requiring aPTT monitoring should be considered. ▪ Interferes with **urine qualitative dipstick protein assays** and **quantitative dye methods** (e.g., pyrogallol red-molybdate). However, microalbumin assays are not affected and can be used to monitor urinary protein excretion.

SIDE EFFECTS

The most common side effects include diarrhea, foamy urine, nausea, taste disturbances, and vomiting. The most serious side effects include cardiac events, CDAD, infusion-related reactions, nephrotoxicity (increased SCr, renal insufficiency, renal failure), and respiratory events. The most common events leading to discontinuation of therapy were acute renal failure, nausea, QTc prolongation, and rash. Other reported side effects include abdominal pain, decreased appetite, dizziness, infusion site pain and erythema, pruritus, and rigors.

Post-Marketing: Hypersensitivity reactions, including anaphylaxis.

ANTIDOTE

Notify the physician of all side effects. Initiate supportive care as indicated. Infusion-related reactions may respond to temporarily discontinuing or slowing the rate of infusion. Consider alternative antimicrobial therapy in patients who develop renal toxicity. Discontinue telavancin at the first sign of skin rash or other sign of hypersensitivity. Treat CDAD with fluids, electrolytes, protein supplements, and appropriate antibiotics (e.g., oral vancomycin) as indicated. In severe cases, surgical evaluation may be indicated. There is no information on the use of hemodialysis or continuous venovenous hemofiltration in toxicity.

TEMOZOLOMIDE

(te-moe-**ZOE**-loe-mide)

Antineoplastic
(alkylating agent)

Temodar

USUAL DOSE

Pretreatment: Verify pregnancy status. Baseline studies indicated; see Monitor.

IV and oral doses are therapeutically equivalent if the IV dose is administered equally distributed over 90 minutes. The oral form should be used as soon as tolerated by the patient.

Newly diagnosed glioblastoma multiforme (GBM [high-grade glioma]): Concomitant phase:75 mg/M^2 daily for 42 days. Given concomitantly with focal radiotherapy. No dose reductions are recommended during the concomitant phase; however, dose interruptions or discontinuation may occur based on toxicity. The temozolomide dose should be continued throughout the 42-day concomitant period up to 49 days if all of the following conditions are met:

- Absolute neutrophil count must be equal to or greater than 1.5 × 10^9/L (1,500/mm³).
- Platelet count must be equal to or greater than 100 × 10^9/L (100,000/mm³).
- Nonhematologic toxicity must be equal to or less than Grade 1 (except for alopecia, nausea, and vomiting).
- CBC and platelet count should be obtained weekly.
- Interrupt or discontinue temozolomide dosing based on the hematologic and nonhematologic criteria in the following chart. *Continued*

Temozolomide Dosing Interruption or Discontinuation During Concomitant Radiotherapy		
Toxicity	**TMZ Interruption[a]**	**TMZ Discontinuation**
Absolute neutrophil count	≥ 0.5 and $< 1.5 \times 10^9/L$	$< 0.5 \times 10^9/L$
Platelet count	≥ 10 and $< 100 \times 10^9/L$	$< 10 \times 10^9/L$
CTCAE nonhematologic toxicity (except for alopecia, nausea, vomiting)	CTCAE Grade 2	CTCAE Grade 3 or 4

TMZ, Temozolomide; *CTCAE*, Common Terminology Criteria for Adverse Events.
[a]Treatment with concomitant TMZ could be continued when all of the following conditions are met: ANC $\geq 1.5 \times 10^9/L$, platelet count $\geq 100 \times 10^9/L$, CTC nonhematologic toxicity Grade ≤ 1 (except for alopecia, nausea, vomiting).

Prophylaxis against *Pneumocystis jiroveci* pneumonia (PCP): Required for all patients during this concomitant therapy. PCP prophylaxis should be continued in patients who develop lymphocytopenia until they recover from lymphocytopenia (CTCAE Grade ≤ 1).

Newly diagnosed GBM (high-grade glioma]): *Maintenance phase:* 4 weeks after completing the temozolomide plus focal radiotherapy phase, temozolomide is administered for an additional 6 cycles of maintenance.

Cycle 1: The initial dose is 150 mg/M^2 once daily for 5 days followed by 23 days without treatment (a 28-day cycle); see Dose Adjustments.

Cycles 2 through 6: The dose can be increased to 200 mg/M^2 if the following conditions are met:

- Absolute neutrophil count is equal to or greater than $1.5 \times 10^9/L$ (1,500/mm^3)
- Platelet count is equal to or greater than $100 \times 10^9/L$ (100,000/mm^3)
- Nonhematologic toxicity is equal to or less than Grade 2 (except for alopecia, nausea, and vomiting).

The dose remains at 200 mg/M^2 per day for the first 5 days of each subsequent cycle except if toxicity occurs. If the dose was not increased at Cycle 2, it should not be increased for subsequent cycles. See Dose Adjustments for dose reduction or discontinuation during maintenance.

Refractory anaplastic astrocytoma: 150 mg/M^2 once daily for 5 consecutive days for each 28-day treatment cycle. This dose may be increased to 200 mg/M^2/day if both the nadir and day of dosing (Day 29, Day 1 of next cycle) ANC are equal to or greater than $1.5 \times 10^9/L$ (1,500/mm^3) and the nadir and day of dosing (Day 29, Day 1 of next cycle) platelet count are equal to or greater than $100 \times 10^9/L$ (100,000/mm^3). During treatment, a CBC should be obtained on Day 22 (21 days after the Day 1 dose of temozolomide) or within 48 hours of that day for each cycle. Repeat weekly until the ANC is above $1.5 \times 10^9/L$ (1,500/mm^3) and the platelet count exceeds $100 \times 10^9/L$ (100,000/mm^3). The next cycle of temozolomide should not be started until the ANC and platelet count exceed these levels. If the ANC falls to $< 1 \times 10^9/L$ (1,000/mm^3) or the platelet count is $< 50 \times 10^9/L$ (50,000/mm^3) during any cycle, reduce the next cycle by 50 mg/M^2 but not below 100 mg/M^2 (the lowest recommended dose). Therapy can be continued until disease progression. See the flowchart in Dose Adjustments.

DOSE ADJUSTMENTS

Newly diagnosed glioblastoma multiforme: Temozolomide dose must be adjusted according to the nadir ANC and platelet counts in the previous cycle and the ANC and platelet counts at the time of initiating the next cycle. Obtain a CBC and platelet count weekly during the concomitant phase and as indicated during the 4-week interim before beginning the maintenance phase. Obtain a baseline CBC and platelet count before beginning a cycle and repeat on Day 22 (21 days after the first dose of temozolomide in the cycle or within 48 hours of that day). Repeat weekly until the ANC is above $1.5 \times 10^9/L$ (1,500/mm^3) and the platelet count exceeds $100 \times 10^9/L$ (100,000/mm^3). The next cycle of temozolomide should not be started until the ANC and platelet count exceed these levels. This sequence is repeated for Cycles 1 through 6 of maintenance dosing. Base dose reductions during the next cycle on the lowest blood counts and worst nonhematologic toxicity during the previous cycle. Dose reductions or discontinuations during maintenance should be applied according to the following two charts.

Temozolomide Dose Levels for Maintenance Treatment		
Dose Level	**Dose (mg/M²/day)**	**Remarks**
−1	100 mg/M²/day	Reduction for prior toxicity
0	150 mg/M²/day	Dose during Cycle 1
1	200 mg/M²/day	Dose during Cycles 2 through 6 in absence of toxicity

Temozolomide Dose Reduction or Discontinuation During Maintenance Treatment		
Toxicity	**Reduce TMZ by 1 Dose Level[a]**	**Discontinue TMZ**
ANC	$<1 \times 10^9$/L	See [b]in footnote
Platelet count	$<50 \times 10^9$/L	See [b]in footnote
CTC nonhematologic toxicity (except for alopecia, nausea, vomiting)	CTC Grade 3	CTC Grade 4

TMZ, Temozolomide; *CTC*, Common Terminology Criteria.
[a]See preceding chart for temozolomide dose levels for maintenance treatment.
[b]TMZ is to be discontinued if a dose reduction to <100 mg/M² is required or if the same Grade 3 nonhematologic toxicity (except for alopecia, nausea, vomiting) recurs after dose reduction.

See the next page for temozolomide dose modifications for refractory anaplastic astrocytoma.

Temozolomide Dose Modification Table for Refractory Anaplastic Astrocytoma:

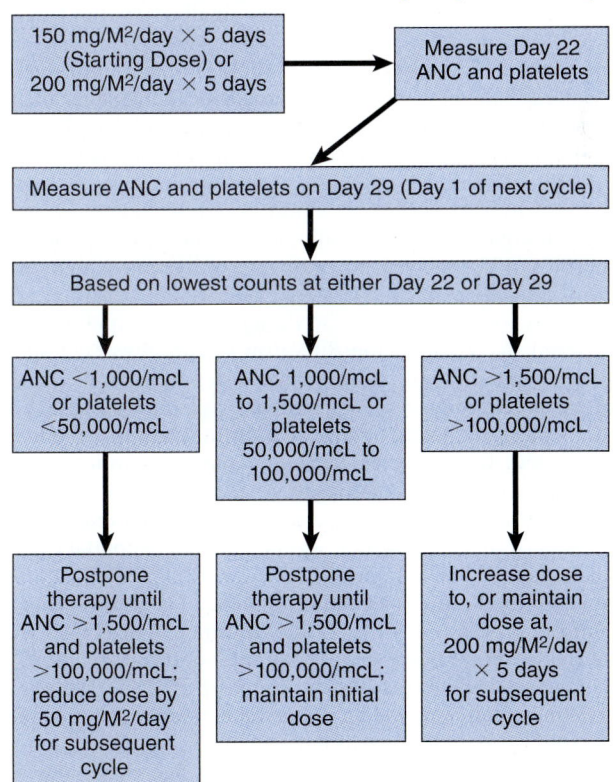

DILUTION

Specific techniques required; see Precautions. Bring vial(s) to room temperature before reconstitution. Reconstitute each 100-mg vial with 41 mL of SWFI. Swirl gently to dissolve; *do not shake;* will yield a concentration of 2.5 mg/mL of temozolomide. *Do not further dilute* the reconstituted solution. Withdraw up to 40 mL from each vial and transfer into an empty 250-mL PVC infusion bag for delivery with an infusion pump.

Filters: Specific information not available.

Storage: Refrigerate single-use vials at 2° to 8° C (36° to 46° F). Store reconstituted product at RT. Reconstituted solution must be used within 14 hours, including infusion time.

COMPATIBILITY

Manufacturer states, "Other medications should not be infused simultaneously through the same IV line." May be administered only in the same infusion line as NS.

RATE OF ADMINISTRATION

A single dose equally distributed over 90 minutes. Use of an infusion pump is recommended. Bioequivalence was established only with the 90-minute infusion. Infusion over a longer or shorter period may result in suboptimal dosing. In addition, the possibility of an increase in infusion-related adverse reactions cannot be ruled out. Flush IV lines before and after temozolomide infusion. Infusion must be complete within 14 hours of reconstitution.

ACTIONS

An imidazotetrazine derivative and alkylating agent. It is not directly active but undergoes rapid nonenzymatic conversion, as dacarbazine does, to the reactive compound 5-(3-methyl triazen-1-yl)-imidazole-4-carboxamide (MTIC) and to temozolomide acid metabolite. Cytotoxicity is thought to be due primarily to alkylation of DNA. Weakly bound to plasma proteins. Rapidly eliminated with a mean elimination half-life of 1.8 hours. Some excretion in urine and a very small amount in feces.

INDICATIONS AND USES

Treatment of adults with newly diagnosed glioblastoma multiforme. Initially given concomitantly with radiotherapy and then continued as maintenance treatment. ▪ Treatment of adults with refractory anaplastic astrocytoma (i.e., adults who have experienced disease progression on a drug regimen containing nitrosourea and procarbazine).

CONTRAINDICATIONS

Known history of hypersensitivity reaction to temozolomide or any of its components (e.g., urticaria, allergic reaction including anaphylaxis, toxic epidermal necrolysis, and Stevens-Johnson syndrome). ▪ Known history of hypersensitivity to dacarbazine.

PRECAUTIONS

Follow guidelines for handling cytotoxic agents. See Appendix A, p. 1308. ▪ Usually administered by or under the direction of the physician specialist in a facility with adequate diagnostic and treatment facilities to monitor the patient and respond to any medical emergency. ▪ Myelosuppression may be severe and dose limiting. May include prolonged pancytopenia, which may result in aplastic anemia. Deaths have been reported. Risk may be increased with concomitant use of other medications associated with aplastic anemia (e.g., carbamazepine, phenytoin, sulfamethoxazole/trimethoprim). ▪ Risk of myelosuppression increased in females and the elderly. ▪ Cases of myelodysplastic syndrome and secondary malignancies, including myeloid leukemia, have been observed. ▪ Prophylaxis against PCP is required for all patients being treated for newly diagnosed GBM receiving concomitant temozolomide and radiotherapy for the 42-day regimen. The longer dosing regimen may increase the risk of PCP; however, all patients, particularly those receiving steroids, should be monitored closely for symptoms of PCP regardless of the regimen. ▪ Severe, sometimes fatal hepatotoxicity have been reported. ▪ Use caution in patients with severe renal or hepatic impairment.

Monitor: Obtain a baseline CBC and platelet count. See Usual Dose for minimum levels required before administration of temozolomide. ▪ Obtain baseline liver function tests.

Repeat midway through the first cycle, before each subsequent cycle, and approximately 2 to 4 weeks after the last dose of temozolomide.

Patients with newly diagnosed GBM: Obtain a CBC and platelet count weekly during the concomitant phase and as indicated during the 4-week interim before beginning the maintenance phase. Obtain a baseline CBC and platelet count before beginning a maintenance dose (28-day cycles) and repeat on Day 22 (21 days after the first maintenance dose of temozolomide or within 48 hours of that day). Repeat weekly until the ANC is above 1.5 $\times$ 10⁹/L (1,500/mm³) and the platelet count exceeds 100 $\times$ 10⁹/L (100,000/mm³). This sequence is repeated for Cycles 1 through 6 of maintenance dosing.

Patients with refractory anaplastic astrocytoma: Obtain a CBC and platelet count on Day 1 of each cycle. During treatment (28-day cycles), a CBC should be obtained on Day 22 (21 days after the Day 1 dose of temozolomide or within 48 hours of that day for each cycle). Repeat weekly until the ANC is above 1.5 $\times$ 10⁹/L (1,500/mm³) and the platelet count exceeds 100 $\times$ 10⁹/L (100,000/mm³). Myelosuppression usually occurred within the first few cycles of therapy and was not cumulative. It occurred late in the treatment cycle and returned to normal, on average, within 14 days of nadir counts. (The median nadirs occurred at 26 days for platelets and 28 days for neutrophils.)

All indications: Nausea and vomiting may be significant. Prophylactic antiemetics may reduce nausea and vomiting and increase patient comfort. ▪ Observe closely for signs of infection. Prophylactic antibiotics may be indicated pending results of C/S in a febrile neutropenic patient. ▪ Monitor for thrombocytopenia (platelet count less than 50,000/mm³). Initiate precautions to prevent excessive bleeding (e.g., inspect IV sites, skin, and mucous membranes; use extreme care during invasive procedures; test urine, emesis, stool, and secretions for occult blood). ▪ Regardless of the regimen, monitor all patients, particularly those receiving steroids, for symptoms of PCP (dyspnea; fever; dry, nonproductive cough; characteristic x-ray).

Patient Education: Read the FDA-approved patient information. ▪ Avoid pregnancy; use of effective contraception recommended for females of reproductive potential during treatment with temozolomide and for at least 6 months after the final dose. Because of the potential for embryo-fetal toxicity and genotoxic effects on sperm cells, advise male patients with pregnant partners or female partners of reproductive potential to use condoms during treatment with temozolomide and for at least 3 months after the final dose. ▪ May impair male fertility. ▪ Male patients should not donate semen during treatment and for at least 3 months after the final dose. ▪ Promptly report a rash; swelling of the face, throat, or tongue; severe skin reaction; or troubled breathing. ▪ Report IV site burning or stinging promptly. ▪ Secondary malignancies have been reported. ▪ See Maternal/Child. ▪ See Appendix D, p. 1311. ▪ Additional precautions are required with the capsule form.

Maternal/Child: Based on its mechanism of action and findings from animal studies, temozolomide can cause fetal harm. Spontaneous abortions and congenital malformations, including polymalformations with central nervous system, facial, cardiac, skeletal, and genitourinary system anomalies, have been reported. ▪ Discontinue breast-feeding. ▪ Safety and effectiveness for use in pediatric patients not established. A 5-day regimen every 28 days using the oral formulation has been studied in selected pediatric patients from 3 to 18 years of age. Toxicity profile was similar to that seen in adults.

Elderly: Numbers in clinical studies are insufficient to determine whether the elderly respond differently than younger subjects. Dose selection should be cautious based on the potential for decreased organ function and concomitant disease or drug therapy. **In newly diagnosed patients with glioblastoma multiforme,** side effects were similar to those seen in younger patients. In the **anaplastic astrocytoma study,** patients 70 years or older had a higher incidence of Grade 4 neutropenia and Grade 4 thrombocytopenia in the first cycle of therapy.

DRUG/LAB INTERACTIONS

Valproic acid decreases the oral clearance of temozolomide by about 5%; clinical significance is not known. ▪ Administration of **live attenuated viral or bacterial vaccines** should be avoided.

SIDE EFFECTS

Newly diagnosed GBM: Myelosuppression may be severe and dose limiting. May include prolonged pancytopenia, which may result in aplastic anemia; deaths have been reported. Alopecia, anorexia, constipation, headache, nausea and vomiting, and thrombocytopenia were the most frequently reported side effects. The most commonly reported severe or life-threatening reactions were convulsions, fatigue, headache, and thrombocytopenia. Abdominal pain, arthralgia, blurred vision, confusion, coughing, diarrhea, dizziness, dry skin, dyspnea, erythema, hypersensitivity reactions (including anaphylaxis), insomnia, memory impairment, pruritus, radiation injury, rash, stomatitis, taste perversion, and weakness have also been reported.

Refractory anaplastic astrocytoma: Fatigue, headache, and nausea and vomiting were the most frequently reported side effects. Myelosuppression (neutropenia and thrombocytopenia) was the dose-limiting adverse reaction. Abdominal pain, abnormal coordination, abnormal gait, abnormal vision (blurred vision, vision changes, visual deficit), adrenal hypercorticism, amnesia, anemia, anorexia, anxiety, asthenia, ataxia, back pain, breast pain (female), confusion, constipation, convulsions (local and general), coughing, depression, diarrhea, diplopia, dizziness, dysphasia, fever, hemiparesis, insomnia, lymphopenia, myalgia, paresis, paresthesia, peripheral edema, pharyngitis, pruritus, rash, sinusitis, somnolence, URI, urinary incontinence, UTI, viral infection, and weight increase have been reported.

Injection site reactions: Erythema, irritation, pain, pruritus, swelling, and warmth at the infusion site; hematoma; and petechiae.

Post-Marketing: Alveolitis, cholestasis, diabetes insipidus, elevation of liver enzymes, erythema multiforme, hepatitis, hepatotoxicity (severe and sometimes fatal), hyperbilirubinemia, hypersensitivity reactions (including anaphylaxis), serious opportunistic infections with bacterial, viral (primary and reactivated), fungal, and protozoan organisms, interstitial pneumonitis, pneumonitis, prolonged pancytopenia that may result in aplastic anemia with fatal outcomes, pulmonary fibrosis, Stevens-Johnson syndrome, and toxic epidermal necrolysis.

ANTIDOTE

Keep physician informed of all side effects and CBC results. Temozolomide may need to be reduced or discontinued. Symptomatic and supportive treatment is indicated. Administration of whole blood products (e.g., packed RBCs, platelets, leukocytes) and/or blood modifiers (e.g., darbepoetin alfa, epoetin alfa, filgrastim, pegfilgrastim, sargramostim) may be indicated to treat bone marrow toxicity. Precautions are indicated for cancer patients with erythropoietin-stimulating agents (ESAs); see darbepoetin alfa and epoetin alfa monographs. Treat hypersensitivity reactions and/or anaphylaxis as indicated (e.g., epinephrine, corticosteroids, oxygen, and antihistamines [diphenhydramine]). There is no specific antidote. In the event of an overdose, hematologic evaluation is needed, and supportive measures should be provided as necessary. Resuscitate as indicated.

TEMSIROLIMUS

(**TEM**-sir-**OH**-li-mus)

Torisel

Antineoplastic
(kinase inhibitor)

USUAL DOSE

Pretreatment: Verify pregnancy status. Baseline studies indicated; see Monitor.

Premedication: To minimize the incidence of hypersensitivity reactions, administer diphenhydramine 25 to 50 mg IV 30 minutes before the start of each dose of temsirolimus; see Precautions and Monitor.

Temsirolimus: 25 mg as an infusion once a week until disease progression or unacceptable toxicity.

DOSE ADJUSTMENTS

Hold for absolute neutrophil count (ANC) less than 1,000/mm³, platelet count less than 75,000/mm³, or CTCAE Grade 3 or greater adverse reactions. Once toxicities have resolved to Grade 2 or less, restart therapy with the dose reduced by 5 mg/week to a dose no lower than 15 mg/week. ■ Consider dose reduction to 12.5 mg/week when coadministered with a strong CYP3A4 inhibitor; see Drug/Lab Interactions. If the strong inhibitor is discontinued, wait approximately 1 week before adjusting the temsirolimus dose upward to the indicated dose. ■ Consider a dose increase to 50 mg/week when coadministered with a strong CYP3A4 inducer; see Drug/Lab Interactions. If the strong inducer is discontinued, the temsirolimus dose should be returned to the dose used prior to initiation of the strong CYP3A4 inducer. ■ Decrease dose to 15 mg/week in patients with mild hepatic impairment (bilirubin >1 to 1.5 times the ULN or AST greater than ULN but bilirubin ≤ ULN); see Contraindications. ■ No dose adjustment indicated based on age, race, gender, or renal status. Not studied in hemodialysis patients.

DILUTION

Specific techniques required; see Precautions and Compatibility. Available as a kit containing a vial of temsirolimus and a vial of a manufacturer-supplied diluent. Temsirolimus and diluent vials contain overfill. A two-step dilution process is required. Reconstitute the temsirolimus vial with 1.8 mL of the provided diluent. Invert the vial several times to mix thoroughly. Allow time for foam to subside. Final concentration in temsirolimus vial is 10 mg/mL. Solution will be clear to slightly turbid and colorless to light-yellow. Withdraw the required amount of reconstituted temsirolimus and inject into a 250-mL container *(glass, polyolefin, or polypropylene)* of NS. Invert bag to mix; **see Compatibility.** Avoid excessive shaking. Use of non-DEHP, non-polyvinyl chloride (PVC) tubing (polyethylene-lined administration set is recommended) with appropriate filter is recommended. If a PVC administration set must be used, it should not contain DEHP. Temsirolimus contains polysorbate 80 when diluted, which increases the rate of DEHP extraction from PVC.

Filter: Use of an in-line polyethersulfone filter with a pore size not greater than 5 microns is recommended. If an administration set with an in-line filter is not available, a polyethersulfone end-filter should be used. The use of both an in-line and end-filter is not recommended.

Storage: Store unopened vials at 2° to 8° C (36° to 46° F). Protect from light. During handling and preparation, protect from excessive room light or sunlight. The temsirolimus/diluent mixture (10 mg/mL) is stable for up to 24 hours below 25° C (77° F) in the temsirolimus vial. Administration of the final product diluted in NS should be completed within 6 hours of adding the temsirolimus/diluent mixture to the NS.

COMPATIBILITY

Manufacturer states, "Final dilution for infusion should be stored in bottles (glass, polypropylene) or plastic bags (polypropylene, polyolefin) and administered through polyethylene-lined administration sets." Non–DEHP-containing materials must be used for administration. Manufacturer also states that undiluted temsirolimus should not be added directly to aqueous infusion solutions. A precipitate will form. In addition, "The stability of temsirolimus in other infusion solutions has not been evaluated. Addition of other drugs or nutritional agents to admixtures of temsirolimus in NS has not been evaluated and should be avoided. Temsirolimus is degraded by both acids and bases, and thus combinations of temsirolimus with agents capable of modifying solution pH should be avoided."

RATE OF ADMINISTRATION

A single dose as an infusion equally distributed over 30 to 60 minutes. Use of an infusion pump is recommended. Increase duration of infusion to 60 minutes in patients who experience a hypersensitivity reaction.

ACTIONS

An inhibitor of mTOR (mammalian target of rapamycin). Binds to an intracellular protein (FKBP-12); this protein-drug complex inhibits the activity of mTOR that controls cell division. Results in a cell cycle–specific (G1) growth arrest in treated tumor cells. In in vitro studies, temsirolimus inhibited the activity of mTOR and resulted in reduced levels of hypoxia-inducible factors HIF-1α and HIF-2α and the vascular endothelial growth factor. Both temsirolimus and sirolimus are extensively partitioned into formed blood elements. Extensively metabolized, primarily by C P450 3A4. Sirolimus is the principal metabolite and is active. Elimination is primarily via the feces and to a small extent via urine. Mean half-lives of temsirolimus and sirolimus were 17.3 and 54.6 hours, respectively.

INDICATIONS AND USES

Treatment of advanced renal cell carcinoma.

CONTRAINDICATIONS

Bilirubin greater than 1.5 times the ULN; see Dose Adjustments and Precautions.

PRECAUTIONS

Follow guidelines for handling cytotoxic agents. See Appendix A, p. 1308. ▪ Should be administered by or under the direction of the physician specialist in facilities equipped to monitor the patient and respond to any medical emergency. ▪ Hypersensitivity/infusion reactions have been reported. May occur early in the first infusion but may also occur with subsequent infusions. Premedication required to minimize the chance of a reaction; see Usual Dose. Use with caution in patients with known hypersensitivity to temsirolimus, its metabolites (including sirolimus), polysorbate 80, or any other components of the product. Use caution in patients who have known hypersensitivity to an antihistamine or who cannot receive prophylactic treatment with an antihistamine for medical reasons; see Monitor. ▪ Patients with moderate and severe hepatic impairment had increased rates of adverse reactions and deaths. Use caution when treating patients with mild hepatic impairment; see Dose Adjustments and Contraindications. ▪ Hyperglycemia/glucose intolerance is common. Initiation of or an increase in the dose of insulin and/or oral hypoglycemic agent therapy may be required. ▪ Elevated cholesterol and triglycerides are common. Initiation or adjustment of existing therapy may be required. ▪ May cause immunosuppression, thus increasing the risk of infections, including opportunistic infections. *Pneumocystis jiroveci* pneumonia (PJP), including fatalities, has been reported. May be associated with concomitant use of corticosteroids or other immunosuppressants. Consider prophylaxis of PJP when concomitant use of corticosteroids or other immunosuppressive agents is required. ▪ Cases of interstitial lung disease, some resulting in death, have been reported. ▪ Cases of fatal bowel perforation have been reported. ▪ Rapidly progressive and sometimes fatal acute renal failure has occurred. ▪ Has been associated with abnormal wound healing. Exercise caution when temsirolimus is used in the perioperative period. ▪ Patients who have CNS tumors and/or are receiving anticoagulation therapy may be at increased risk of intracerebral bleeding. ▪ Proteinuria (including cases of nephrotic syndrome) has occurred. ▪ The use of live virus vaccines and close contact with those who have received live virus vaccines should be avoided. See Drug Interactions.

Monitor: Obtain baseline and weekly CBC with differential and platelet count. Obtain a baseline chemistry panel, including bilirubin and liver function tests (ALT, AST), and repeat every 2 weeks. Monitor urine protein before the start of temsirolimus therapy and periodically thereafter. Obtain baseline radiographic assessment by lung CT or chest x-ray. Repeat assessments periodically. ▪ Monitor for S/S of a hypersensitivity/infusion reaction (e.g., anaphylaxis, apnea, bronchospasm, chest pain, dyspnea, flushing, hypotension, loss of consciousness, rash). If a reaction occurs, the infusion should be stopped and the patient should be observed for at least 30 to 60 minutes (depending on the severity of the reaction). At the discretion of the physician, and after a benefit-risk assessment, treatment may be resumed with the administration of an H_1-receptor antagonist (such as diphenhydramine) if not previously administered and/or an H_2-receptor antagonist (e.g., famotidine 20 mg IV) approximately 30 minutes before restarting the temsirolimus infusion. The infusion may be resumed at a slower rate; see Rate of Administration. ▪ Monitor for S/S of angioedema when temsirolimus is given concomitantly with ACE inhibitors or calcium channel blockers. ▪ Monitor serum glucose, cholesterol, and triglycerides before and during therapy. ▪ Monitor for S/S of infection. ▪ Monitor respiratory status. Patients may present with symptoms such as dyspnea, cough, hypoxia, and fever or may be asymptomatic. If clinically significant respiratory symptoms develop, consider withholding temsirolimus until after recovery of symptoms and improvement of radiographic findings related to pneumonitis. Opportunistic infections such as PJP should be considered in the differential diagnosis. Empiric treatment with corticosteroids and/or antibiotics may be considered. ▪ Monitor for S/S of bowel perforation (abdominal pain, acute abdomen, bloody stools, diarrhea, fever, metabolic acidosis). ▪ Monitor for thrombocytopenia (platelet count less than 50,000/mm^3); see Dose Adjustments and Contraindications. Initiate precautions to prevent excessive bleeding (e.g., inspect IV sites, skin, and mucous membranes; use extreme care during invasive procedures; test urine, emesis, stool, and secretions for occult blood).

Patient Education: Review medical history with health care provider. Temsirolimus may affect existing medical conditions (e.g., diabetes, high cholesterol, hyperlipidemia). Therapy may need to be adjusted. ▪ Review medication list (prescription, over-the-counter, and herbal [including past or present use of corticosteroids or immunosuppressants]) with health care provider. Interactions are possible. ▪ Promptly report any S/S of a hypersensitivity reaction (chest tightness, dyspnea, facial swelling, flushing, pruritus, rash, urticaria). ▪ Avoid pregnancy. Use effective contraception during treatment and for 3 months after completion of therapy. Males with partners of childbearing potential should use reliable contraception during treatment and for 3 months after completion of therapy. ▪ Male and female fertility may be compromised. ▪ Report excessive thirst or any increase in volume or frequency of urination. ▪ Promptly report S/S of nephrotic syndrome (e.g., fatigue; loss of appetite; swelling around the eyes, ankles, and feet; and weight gain). Acute renal failure may occur. ▪ Promptly report S/S of infection, new or worsening respiratory symptoms, new or worsening abdominal pain, or blood in stools. ▪ Wound healing complications may occur while on therapy. ▪ The use of live virus vaccines and close contact with those who have received live virus vaccines should be avoided. ▪ Increased risk of intracerebral bleed in patients who have CNS tumors and/or are receiving anticoagulants.

Maternal/Child: Avoid pregnancy; may cause fetal harm. ▪ Do not breast-feed during treatment with temsirolimus and for 3 weeks after the final dose. ▪ Safety and effectiveness for use in pediatric patients not established.

Elderly: Elderly patients may be more likely to experience certain side effects, including diarrhea, edema, and pneumonia.

DRUG/LAB INTERACTIONS

Concomitant use of **strong CYP3A4 inhibitors** (e.g., atazanavir, clarithromycin, indinavir, itraconazole, ketoconazole, nefazodone, nelfinavir, ritonavir, saquinavir, or voriconazole) may increase plasma concentrations of the active metabolite sirolimus. Avoid concomitant use if possible. If required, consider a dose reduction of temsirolimus to 12.5 mg/week and monitor closely for acute toxicity. If the strong inhibitor is discontinued, a washout period of approximately 1 week should be allowed before adjusting the temsirolimus dose upward to the indicated dose; see Dose Adjustments. ■ **Grapefruit juice** may increase plasma concentrations of sirolimus (a major metabolite of temsirolimus) and should be avoided. ■ **CYP3A4/5 inducers** (e.g., carbamazepine, dexamethasone, phenobarbital, phenytoin, rifabutin, rifampin) may decrease plasma concentrations of the active metabolite sirolimus, thus decreasing effectiveness. Avoid concomitant use if possible. If required, consider a dose increase to 50 mg/week. If the strong inducer is discontinued, the temsirolimus dose should be returned to the dose used before initiating the strong CYP3A4 inducer; see Dose Adjustments. ■ **Angioedema** has been reported in patients taking **mTOR inhibitors** such as temsirolimus in combination with **ACE inhibitors** (e.g., ramipril) or **calcium channel blockers** (e.g., amlodipine). ■ **St. John's wort** may decrease temsirolimus plasma concentrations, decreasing effectiveness. Avoid use. ■ Use caution with other **drugs that inhibit the efflux transporter P-glycoprotein (P-gp, ABCB1)** (e.g., protease inhibitors [e.g., nelfinavir]); may increase concentrations of temsirolimus. ■ Temsirolimus inhibits P-gp in vitro. Coadministration with drugs that are substrates of P-gp may result in increased concentration of substrates. No clinically significant effect is anticipated when coadministered with agents that are metabolized with CYP2D6 or CYP3A. ■ The combination of **sunitinib** (Sutent) and temsirolimus resulted in dose-limiting toxicity. ■ Do not administer **live virus vaccines** to patients receiving temsirolimus, and avoid close contact with those who have received live virus vaccines. ■ No clinically significant effect is anticipated when temsirolimus is coadministered with agents that are metabolized by CYP2D6 or CYP3A4.

SIDE EFFECTS

The most common side effects include anemia, anorexia, asthenia, edema, elevated alkaline phosphatase and AST, elevated SCr, hyperglycemia, hyperlipidemia, hypertriglyceridemia, hypophosphatemia, leukopenia, lymphopenia, mucositis, nausea, rash, and thrombocytopenia. Other reported side effects include abdominal pain, acne, angioneurotic edema–type reactions, arthralgia, back pain, chest pain, chills, conjunctivitis (including lacrimation disorder), constipation, convulsions, cough, depression, diarrhea, diabetes mellitus, dry skin, dysgeusia, dyspnea, edema, epistaxis, fever, headache, hemorrhage (GI, rectal), hypokalemia, increased bilirubin, increased total cholesterol, increased triglycerides, insomnia, myalgia, nail disorder, neutropenia, pain, pericardial effusion, pharyngitis, pleural effusion, pneumonitis, pruritus, rash, rhinitis, thrombophlebitis, urinary tract infections, vomiting, and weight loss. The most serious side effects include bowel perforation, hyperglycemia/glucose intolerance, hyperlipemia, hypersensitivity reactions, hypertension, infection (pneumonia, URI, wound [including postoperative] sepsis), interstitial lung disease, intracerebral hemorrhage, renal failure, venous thromboembolism (including DVT and pulmonary embolus [including fatal outcomes]), and wound healing complications.

Post-Marketing: Angioedema, cholecystitis, cholelithiasis, complex regional pain syndrome (reflex sympathetic dystrophy); extravasation with erythema, pain, pancreatitis, swelling, and warmth; injection site reactions; rhabdomyolysis; Stevens-Johnson syndrome.

ANTIDOTE

Keep physician informed of all side effects. Most minor side effects will be treated symptomatically. Monitor patient closely. Discontinue temsirolimus at the first sign of a hypersensitivity reaction. Monitor patient for 30 to 60 minutes. Treatment may be resumed at the discretion of the physician; see Monitor. Treat severe hypersensitivity reactions as indicated; may require epinephrine, airway management, oxygen, IV fluids, antihistamines (e.g., diphenhydramine), corticosteroids (e.g., hydrocortisone sodium succinate), and pressor amines (e.g., dopamine). Treat the development of interstitial lung disease as indicated. May require discontinuation of temsirolimus and/or treatment with corticosteroids and/or antibiotics. Some patients have been able to continue therapy without additional intervention. Discontinue in patients who develop nephrotic syndrome.

TENECTEPLASE
(teh-**NECK**-teh-plays)

Thrombolytic agent
(recombinant)

TNKase

pH 7.3

USUAL DOSE
Pretreatment: Baseline studies indicated; see Monitor.

Initiate therapy as soon as possible after the onset of acute myocardial infarction (AMI) symptoms. Total dose is based on patient weight and should not exceed 50 mg. See the following chart.

Tenecteplase Dosing Guidelines		
Patient Weight (kg)	Tenecteplase (mg)	Volume of Tenecteplase[a] to Be Administered (mL)
<60 kg	30 mg	6 mL
≥60 to <70 kg	35 mg	7 mL
≥70 to <80 kg	40 mg	8 mL
≥80 to <90 kg	45 mg	9 mL
≥90 kg	50 mg	10 mL

[a] From one vial of tenecteplase reconstituted with 10 mL of SWFI.

Concurrent administration of heparin and aspirin has been used in MI patients receiving tenecteplase therapy.

See most current guidelines for recommended doses of heparin and aspirin.

DOSE ADJUSTMENTS
None noted.

DILUTION
Remove the shield assembly from the manufacturer-supplied B-D® 10-mL syringe with TwinPak™ dual Cannula Device. Aseptically withdraw 10 mL of SWFI from the supplied diluent vial using the red hub cannula syringe filling device. Do not use bacteriostatic water for injection. Do not discard the shield assembly. Inject the 10 mL of SWFI into the tenecteplase vial, directing the diluent stream into the powder. Slight foaming may occur. Allow product to stand for several minutes. Gently swirl until contents are completely dissolved. Do not shake. The reconstituted preparation is colorless to pale yellow and contains tenecteplase 50 mg/10 mL. Withdraw the desired dose from the vial using the syringe. Once the appropriate dose is drawn into the syringe, stand the shield vertically on a flat surface with the green side down and passively recap the red hub cannula. Remove the entire shield assembly, including the red hub cannula, by twisting counterclockwise. **Note:** The shield assembly also contains the clear-ended blunt plastic cannula; retain for split septum IV access. The supplied syringe is **compatible** with a conventional needle and with needleless IV systems. See package insert for complete instructions for administration.

Storage: Store unopened vial at CRT or under refrigeration (at 2° to 8° C [(36° to 46° F]). Reconstitution immediately before use preferred, or may be refrigerated for up to 8 hours.

COMPATIBILITY
Manufacturer states, "Precipitation may occur when tenecteplase is administered in an IV line containing dextrose. Dextrose-containing lines should be flushed with a saline-containing solution prior to and following single bolus administration of tenecteplase."

RATE OF ADMINISTRATION

A single bolus dose over 5 seconds. Flush line with saline-containing solution to ensure delivery of entire dose.

ACTIONS

A tissue plasminogen activator and enzyme produced by recombinant DNA technology. Binds to fibrin in a thrombus and converts plasminogen to plasmin. This initiates local fibrinolysis and dissolution of the clot. Onset of action is prompt. Cleared via hepatic metabolism. Terminal half-life is 90 to 130 minutes.

INDICATIONS AND USES

For use in the reduction of mortality associated with AMI. Treatment should be initiated as soon as possible after the onset of AMI symptoms.

CONTRAINDICATIONS

Active internal bleeding, history of cerebrovascular accident, intracranial or intraspinal surgery or trauma within the past 2 months, intracranial neoplasm, arteriovenous malformation or aneurysm, known bleeding diathesis, and severe uncontrolled hypertension.

PRECAUTIONS

Administered under the direction of a physician knowledgeable in its use and with appropriate emergency drugs and diagnostic and laboratory facilities available. ▪ The most common complication is bleeding. Bleeding may be internal (involving intracranial or retroperitoneal sites or the GI, GU, or respiratory tracts) or external bleeding, especially at arterial and venous puncture sites. Use extreme care with the patient; avoid IM injections and any trauma to the patient. Avoid invasive procedures (e.g., arterial puncture and venipuncture). If these procedures are absolutely necessary, use precautionary methods. To minimize bleeding from noncompressible sites, avoid internal jugular and subclavian venous punctures. If an arterial puncture is necessary, use an upper extremity vessel that is accessible to manual compression, apply pressure for at least 30 minutes, and monitor the puncture site closely. ▪ Use extreme caution in the following situations: recent major surgery (e.g., CABG, organ biopsy, previous puncture of noncompressible vessels), recent trauma, cerebrovascular disease, recent GI or GU bleeding, hypertension (systolic BP at or above 180 and/or diastolic BP at or above 110), high likelihood of left heart thrombus (e.g., mitral stenosis with atrial fibrillation), acute pericarditis, subacute bacterial endocarditis, hemostatic defects (including those secondary to severe hepatic or renal disease), severe hepatic dysfunction, pregnancy or obstetric delivery, diabetic hemorrhagic retinopathy or other hemorrhagic ophthalmic conditions, septic thrombophlebitis or occluded AV cannula at a seriously infected site, advanced age, patients currently receiving oral anticoagulants (e.g., warfarin), recent administration of GP IIb/IIIa inhibitors (e.g., eptifibatide), or any other condition in which bleeding constitutes a significant hazard or would be particularly difficult to manage because of its location. In the presence of any of these situations, the risk versus benefit of tenecteplase therapy must be evaluated. ▪ The use of thrombolytics can increase the risk of thromboembolic events in patients with high likelihood of left heart thrombus, such as patients with mitral stenosis or atrial fibrillation. ▪ Cholesterol embolism has been reported rarely in patients treated with all types of thrombolytic agents. See Side Effects. ▪ Reperfusion arrhythmias (e.g., sinus bradycardia, accelerated idioventricular rhythm, ventricular premature depolarization, ventricular tachycardia) may occur following coronary thrombolysis. Manage with standard antiarrhythmic measures. Have antiarrhythmic medications readily available. ▪ Physicians should choose either thrombolysis or PCI as the primary treatment strategy for reperfusion in patients with large ST-segment elevation myocardial infarctions. Rescue PCI or subsequent elective PCI may be performed after administration of thrombolytic therapies if medically appropriate; however, the optimal use of adjunctive antithrombotic and antiplatelet therapies in this setting is unknown. ▪ Standard management of MI should be implemented concomitantly with tenecteplase therapy. Simultaneous therapy with heparin and aspirin is used to reduce the risk of rethrombosis. Increases risk of bleeding; see Usual Dose. ▪ Readministration of tenecteplase to patients who have received prior plasminogen activator therapy has not been studied. Use caution if deemed necessary, and monitor for signs of hypersensitivity or anaphylactic reactions. ▪ Hypersensitivity reactions have been reported.

Monitor: Obtain appropriate clotting studies (e.g., PT, PTT, aPTT, fibrinogen levels), CBC, and platelet count. ▪ Diagnosis-specific baseline studies (e.g., ECG, troponin) are indicated. Baseline assessment (patient condition, pain, hematomas, petechiae, or recent wounds) should be completed before administration. ▪ Type and cross-match may also be ordered. ▪ Maintain strict bed rest; monitor the patient carefully and frequently for pain and signs of bleeding; observe catheter sites and apply pressure dressings to any recently invaded site; watch for hematuria, hematemesis, bloody stool, petechiae, hematoma, flank pain, muscle weakness; and perform frequent neuro checks. Continue until normal clotting function returns. ▪ Monitor vital signs and ECG. ▪ Monitor for S/S of a hypersensitivity reaction during and for several hours after administration (e.g., anaphylaxis, angioedema, laryngeal edema, rash, and urticaria). ▪ See Precautions and Drug/Lab Interactions.

Patient Education: Compliance with all measures to minimize bleeding (e.g., strict bed rest) is very important. ▪ Avoid use of razors, toothbrushes, and other sharp items. Use caution while moving to avoid excessive bumping. ▪ Report all episodes of bleeding and apply local pressure if indicated. Expect oozing from IV sites.

Maternal/Child: Safety for use in pregnancy, breast-feeding and pediatric patients not established. Use in pregnancy only if the potential benefits justify the potential risk to the fetus.

Elderly: In clinical studies, 30-day mortality rates and incidence of adverse events (e.g., intracranial hemorrhage, stroke, major bleeds) were higher in elderly patients. In elderly patients, the benefits of tenecteplase on mortality should be weighed against the risk of increased adverse events, including bleeding.

DRUG/LAB INTERACTIONS

Formal studies have not been performed. ▪ Risk of bleeding may be increased by **any medicine that affects blood clotting,** including anticoagulants (e.g., heparin, warfarin); **and/ or any other medication that inhibits platelet aggregation** (e.g., clopidogrel, dipyridamole, glycoprotein GPIIb/IIIa receptor antagonists [e.g., eptifibatide, tirofiban]). Concurrent use not recommended with the exception of heparin and aspirin to reduce the risk of rethrombosis. If concurrent or subsequent use indicated (e.g., management of acute coronary syndrome, percutaneous coronary intervention), monitor coagulation studies closely. ▪ Use caution with **any medication that may cause hypoprothrombinemia, thrombocytopenia, or GI ulceration or bleeding** (e.g., selected antibiotics [e.g., cefotetan], aspirin, NSAIDs, valproic acid). ▪ **Coagulation test and/or measures of fibrinolytic activity** may be unreliable unless specific procedures are used to prevent in vitro artifacts; notify the lab of tenecteplase use.

SIDE EFFECTS

Bleeding is the most common adverse reaction: internal (GI tract, GU tract, retroperitoneal, or intracranial), epistaxis, gingival bleeding, hematoma, and superficial or surface bleeding (venous cutdowns, arterial punctures, sites of recent surgical intervention). Hypersensitivity reactions (e.g., anaphylaxis, angioedema, laryngeal edema, rash, and urticaria) have been reported rarely. Fever, hypotension, nausea and vomiting, and reperfusion arrhythmias have occurred. Cholesterol embolization can occur with thrombolytic therapy, but has been reported rarely. Clinical features may include livedo reticularis; "purple toe" syndrome; acute renal failure; gangrenous digits; hypertension; pancreatitis; MI; cerebral, spinal cord, or bowel infarction; retinal artery occlusion; and rhabdomyolysis. Several other adverse events have been reported. These reactions are frequently sequelae of the underlying disease, and the effect of tenecteplase on the incidence of these events is unknown.

ANTIDOTE

Notify physician of all side effects. Note even the most minute bleeding tendency. Oozing at IV sites is expected. Control minor bleeding by local pressure. For severe bleeding in a critical location or suspected intracranial bleeding, discontinue any heparin or antiplatelet therapy immediately. Draw blood for type and cross-match and transfuse as indicated. Consider administration of protamine if heparin has been used. Treat reperfusion arrhythmias with standard antiarrhythmic therapy. Treat minor hypersensitivity reactions symptomatically. Discontinue drug and treat anaphylaxis as indicated; resuscitate as necessary.

TENIPOSIDE BBW
(teh-**NIP**-ah-side)

Antineoplastic
(mitotic inhibitor)

VM-26, Vumon

pH 5

USUAL DOSE

Pretreatment: Verify pregnancy status. Baseline studies indicated; see Monitor.
Adults: *All indications and doses are unlabeled.*
Acute lymphoblastic leukemia: 165 mg/M^2 by IV infusion on Days 1, 4, 8, and 11 during consolidation on the "Linker" regimen.
Refractory non-Hodgkin lymphoma: Given as an IV infusion. Dosage schedules include 30 mg/M^2 for 10 days or 50 to 100 mg/M^2 weekly as a single agent; or 60 to 70 mg/M^2 weekly in combination with other chemotherapy agents.

PEDIATRIC DOSE

See Precautions and Maternal/Child. Optimum dose not established.
Acute lymphocytic leukemia (ALL): 165 mg/M^2 in combination with cytarabine 300 mg/M^2. Both drugs are given twice weekly for 8 to 9 doses. An alternate regimen includes teniposide 250 mg/M^2 and vincristine 1.5 mg/M^2 once each week for 4 to 8 weeks plus prednisone 40 mg/M^2 PO daily for 28 days.

DOSE ADJUSTMENTS

Reduce dose by one-half in patients with Down's syndrome and leukemia (increased sensitivity to myelosuppressive chemotherapy). Higher doses may be used in subsequent courses based on degree of myelosuppression and mucositis. Must be individualized. ■ Reduced dose may be necessary in severe renal or hepatic impairment.

DILUTION

Specific techniques required; see Precautions. Must be diluted and given as an infusion. May leach the toxic plasticizer DEHP from PVC infusion bags or sets; prepare and store in bottles (glass, polypropylene) or plastic bags (polypropylene, polyolefin) and administer through polyethylene-lined administration sets (e.g., lipid administration sets or low DEHP–containing nitroglycerin IV sets). Undiluted teniposide has caused acrylic or ABS plastic devices to crack and leak; handle carefully during dilution process. **Compatible** with NS or D5W. Final concentration of 0.1, 0.2, 0.4, or 1 mg/mL desired. Contains 10 mg/mL. 100 mg (10 mL) in 990 mL yields 0.1 mg/mL, in 490 mL yields 0.2 mg/mL, in 240 mL yields 0.4 mg/mL, in 90 mL yields 1 mg/mL. Precipitation may occur at recommended concentrations, especially with excessive agitation. Avoid contact of diluted solution with any other drugs or fluids; flush IV line with D5W or NS before and after administration.
Storage: Refrigerate unopened ampules in original packaging. Do not refrigerate diluted solutions; 1 mg/mL should be administered within 4 hours; all other dilutions are stable at RT for up to 24 hours.

COMPATIBILITY

Manufacturer states, "Heparin solution can cause precipitation of teniposide; flush IV line thoroughly with D5W or NS before and after administration of teniposide. Because of potential for precipitation, **compatibility** with other drugs, infusion materials, or IV pumps cannot be ensured." See Dilution, Rate of Administration, and Precautions/Monitor.

Other sources suggest specific **compatibilities** dependent on concentration and manufacturer; consult a pharmacist.

RATE OF ADMINISTRATION

Total desired dose, properly diluted and evenly distributed over at least 30 to 60 minutes. Infusion time may be extended. Flush IV line with D5W or NS before and after administration to avoid precipitation of teniposide in IV catheter. Rapid infusion may cause marked hypotension or increased nausea and vomiting.

ACTIONS

An antineoplastic agent. A semi-synthetic derivative of podophyllotoxin related to etoposide. Cell cycle–specific for the late S or early G_2 phase, thus preventing cells from entering mitosis. Cytotoxic effects are related to the relative number of single- and double-strand DNA breaks produced in cells. Has a broad spectrum of in vivo antitumor activity against murine tumors, including hematologic malignancies and various solid tumors. Active against certain murine leukemias with acquired resistance to cisplatin, doxorubicin, amsacrine, daunorubicin, mitoxantrone, or vincristine. Highly protein bound; limits distribution within the body (a beneficial effect). Plasma levels increase with dose. Terminal half-life is 5 hours. Metabolized primarily in the liver. Only about 10% excreted as unchanged drug in urine.

INDICATIONS AND USES

Induction therapy in refractory childhood acute lymphoblastic leukemia. Used in combination with other antineoplastic agents.

Unlabeled uses: Has been used as an unlabeled agent in several adult protocols (e.g., refractory non-Hodgkin lymphoma and neuroblastoma).

CONTRAINDICATIONS

Hypersensitivity to teniposide, etoposide (no cross-sensitivity to date), or a history of prior severe hypersensitivity reactions to other drugs formulated in Cremophor EL (e.g., cyclosporine, paclitaxel).

PRECAUTIONS

Follow guidelines for handling cytotoxic agents. See Appendix A, p. 1308. Always wear impervious gloves when handling ampules containing teniposide. After contact with skin, wash immediately and thoroughly with soap and water; after contact with mucous membranes, flush immediately and thoroughly with water. ▪ Usually administered by or under the direction of the physician specialist. ▪ Adequate diagnostic and treatment facilities must be readily available. ▪ May cause severe myelosuppression with resulting infection or bleeding. ▪ Causes severe myelosuppression when used in combination with other chemotherapeutic agents. Sepsis, sometimes fatal, may result. ▪ Use caution in patients with impaired hepatic or renal function; may reduce plasma clearance and increase toxicity. ▪ Hypersensitivity reactions, including anaphylaxis, may occur with initial dosing or with repeated exposure. ▪ Incidence of hypersensitivity may be increased in patients with brain tumors or neuroblastoma. ▪ Acute CNS depression, hypotension, and metabolic acidosis occurred in patients receiving high-dose teniposide pretreated with antiemetic drugs; use caution. ▪ Pediatric patients with ALL in remission on teniposide maintenance therapy have shown an increased risk of developing secondary acute nonlymphocytic leukemia (ANLL). ▪ Reduce dose in patients with Down syndrome. ▪ See Drug/Lab Interactions.

Monitor: Bone marrow suppression; occurs early with indicated doses and can be profound. Obtain baseline hemoglobin, WBC count with differential, and platelet count. Monitor frequently during therapy, before each dose, and after therapy. See Dose Adjustments. ▪ Severe hypersensitivity reactions can occur with teniposide and may be life threatening. Epinephrine, oxygen, and other emergency supplies must be at the bedside. Monitor patient continuously and take vital signs very frequently during the first hour and at intervals thereafter. ■ Monitor renal and hepatic function tests before and during therapy. ■ Determine absolute patency and quality of vein and adequate circulation of extremity. Avoid extravasation; can cause local tissue necrosis and thrombophlebitis. ■ Precipitation sufficient to occlude central venous access catheters has occurred; monitor infusion closely, and flush thoroughly before and after administration. ■ Use prophylactic antiemetics to increase patient comfort. ■ Steady-state volume of distribution increases with a decrease in plasma albumin levels; monitor pediatric patients with hypoalbuminemia carefully. ■ If severe myelosuppression occurs, bone marrow examination should be repeated before a decision to continue therapy is made. ■ Monitor for thrombocytopenia (platelet count less than 50,000/mm³). Initiate precautions to prevent excessive bleeding (e.g., inspect IV sites, skin, and mucous membranes; use extreme care during invasive procedures; test urine, emesis, stool, and secretions for occult blood). ■ Observe closely for signs of infection. Prophylactic antibiotics may be indicated pending results of C/S in a febrile neutropenic patient.

Patient Education: Report IV site burning or stinging promptly. ■ Avoid pregnancy; effective birth control recommended for males and females. ■ Males should consider the possibility of storing sperm for future artificial insemination. ■ Report any signs of hypersensitivity promptly (e.g., chills, difficult breathing, fever, flushing, rapid heartbeat, rash). ■ Secondary acute nonlymphocytic leukemia (ANLL) has been reported (see Precautions). ■ Interacts with many medications. Discuss all drugs (prescription or non-prescription) with doctor or pharmacist. ■ See Appendix D, p. 1311.

Maternal/Child: Category D: avoid pregnancy. May cause fetal harm; see Patient Education. ■ Potential for serious adverse reactions in nursing infants; discontinue breast-feeding. ■ Contains benzyl alcohol; not recommended for use in premature infants. ■ Intended for use in pediatric patients, but see Precautions/Monitor. ■ When used as a single agent, side effects in pediatric patients from 2 weeks to 20 years of age are similar to other age-groups.

Elderly: Monitor renal, hepatic, and hematologic function closely.

DRUG/LAB INTERACTIONS

Concomitant use with **vincristine sulfate** has resulted in neurotoxicity, including severe cases of neuropathy. ■ **Sodium salicylate, sulfamethizole, and tolbutamide** displace teniposide from protein-binding sites. Can cause substantial increases in free drug levels and increase toxicity of teniposide. ■ May result in clinically significant drug interactions with **other drugs highly bound to protein** (e.g., buprenorphine, calcium channel blocking agents, phenothiazines). ■ May increase plasma clearance and increase intracellular levels of **methotrexate.** ■ **Phenobarbital, fosphenytoin, and phenytoin** increase clearance of teniposide; may reduce effectiveness. ■ Depressant and hypotensive effects of **antiemetics** may be additive with alcohol in teniposide. ■ May cause additive effects with **bone marrow–suppressing agents or agents that cause blood dyscrasias** (e.g., amphotericin B, antithyroid agents [methimazole], azathioprine, chloramphenicol, ganciclovir, interferon, plicamycin, zidovudine) **and radiation therapy.** ■ Do not administer **live virus vaccines.**

SIDE EFFECTS

Most are reversible if detected early. Hypersensitivity reactions (e.g., bronchospasm, chills, confusion, dyspnea, facial flushing, fever, headache, hypertension, hypotension, tachycardia, urticaria) have occurred and can be fatal if not treated promptly. Myelosuppression (anemia, leukopenia, neutropenia, thrombocytopenia) occurs early, can be profound, and recovery can be delayed. Alopecia, asthenia, bleeding, diarrhea, fever, hypotension/cardiovascular, infection, mucositis, nausea and vomiting, rash, thrombophlebitis. Hepatic dysfunctions, metabolic abnormalities, neurotoxicity, and renal dysfunction have occurred in fewer than 1% of patients.

Overdose: Acute CNS depression, hypotension, and metabolic acidosis.

ANTIDOTE

Keep physician informed of all side effects. Symptomatic treatment is often indicated. Discontinue teniposide and treat hypersensitivity reactions immediately (epinephrine, antihistamines [e.g., diphenhydramine], cimetidine, corticosteroids [e.g., dexamethasone], bronchodilators [e.g., theophylline], IV fluids). Consider risk/benefit before rechallenging any patient who has had a severe hypersensitivity reaction. Pretreatment with corticosteroids and antihistamines and constant observation are imperative. Administration of whole blood products (e.g., packed RBCs, platelets, leukocytes) and/or blood modifiers (e.g., darbepoetin alfa, epoetin alfa, filgrastim, pegfilgrastim, sargramostim) may be indicated to treat bone marrow toxicity. Consider diazepam or phenytoin for seizures. Hypotension is usually due to a rapid infusion rate; discontinue temporarily. Trendelenburg position and IV fluids should reverse the hypotension; vasopressors (e.g., dopamine) may be required. In addition to antiemetics (e.g., ondansetron), rate reduction may reduce nausea and vomiting. For extravasation, discontinue the drug immediately and administer into another site. Resuscitate as necessary.

TERLIPRESSIN

(ter-li-**PRES**-sin)

Terlivaz

Antidiuretic hormone analog; hormone, posterior pituitary

USUAL DOSE

Initial dose: 0.85 mg IV every 6 hours for 3 days

Maintenance dose: Beginning on day 4, adjust dose based on serum creatinine (SeCr) as follows:

- If SeCr has decreased by greater than or equal to 30% from baseline, continue 0.85 mg IV every 6 hours until 24 hours after patient achieves two consecutive SeCr values of less than or equal to 1.5 mg/dL or for a maximum of 14 days.
- If SeCr has decreased less than 30% from baseline, give 1.7 mg IV every 6 hours; continue until 24 hours after two consecutive SeCr values of less than or equal to 1.5 mg/dL or for a maximum of 14 days
- If SeCr is greater than or equal to baseline, discontinue terlipressin.

PEDIATRIC DOSE

Not established

DOSE ADJUSTMENTS

Renal: No dosage adjustments are necessary for the initial dosage; subsequent dose adjustments should be determined based on SeCr response starting on day 4 (see dosing above). Patients with SeCr greater than 5 at the time of initiation are unlikely to experience benefit.

Hepatic: No dosage adjustments are provided by the manufacturer.

Other dosage adjustments:

Fluid overload—Along with reducing fluid administration and judicious use of diuretics, temporarily interrupt, reduce, or stop terlipressin until the patient volume status improves.

Ischemic signs or symptoms—Stop terlipressin with signs of ischemia.

Respiratory effects—Stop terlipressin if patient develops hypoxia or increase in respiratory symptoms.

DILUTION
IV bolus: Reconstitute each vial with 5 mL normal saline.

COMPATIBILITY
Do not administer simultaneously with any other medication or IV solutions other than normal saline.

RATE OF ADMINISTRATION
Give via IV bolus slowly over 2 minutes through a peripheral or central line. Flush line after administration.

ACTIONS
Terlipressin is a synthetic vasopressin analog; a majority of activity results from conversion to lysine–vasopressin via slow enzymatic cleavage, producing an extended duration of systemic vasoconstriction. Terlipressin reduces portal pressure and blood flow into portal vessels, increasing effective arterial blood volume and mean arterial pressure, thus increasing blood flow to the kidneys.

INDICATIONS AND USES
Hepatorenal syndrome, to improve kidney function in adults with hepatorenal syndrome with rapid reduction in kidney function

CONTRAINDICATIONS
Patients with ongoing coronary, peripheral, or mesenteric ischemia; hypoxia; or worsening respiratory symptoms.

PRECAUTIONS
Black Box Warning: Terlipressin may cause serious or fatal respiratory failure. Patients with volume overload or with acute or chronic liver failure grade 3 are at increased risk. Assess oxygenation saturation before beginning. Do not start terlipressin if patient is experiencing hypoxia (SpO_2 less than 90%) until oxygenation levels improve. Monitor patients for hypoxia using continuous pulse oximetry during treatment, and stop terlipressin if SpO_2 decreases below 90%.

Monitor: Serum creatinine, oxygen saturation (baseline and continuous during therapy); Acute-on Chronic Liver Failure Grade and volume status (baseline and periodically during treatment); signs and symptoms of fluid overload or ischemia.

Patient education: Notify provider of swelling (fluid overload), any difficulty breathing, chest pain, or any signs of allergic reaction.

Maternal/child: Terlipressin causes uterine contractions and endometrial ischemia. Based on its mechanism of action and animal data, in utero exposure may cause fetal harm. It is not know if terlipressin is present in breast milk. According to the manufacturer, the decision to breastfeed during therapy should consider risks to infant, the benefits of breastfeeding, and the benefits to treatment for the mother.

Elderly: No specific recommendations; refer to adult dosing.

DRUG/LAB INTERACTIONS
Drugs that cause bradycardia; certinib, desmopressin, fexinidazole (avoid), fingolimod, ivabradine, lacosamide, midodrine, ozanimod, ponesimod (avoid), siponimod, tofacitinib

SIDE EFFECTS
Abdominal pain, diarrhea, nausea, dyspnea, respiratory failure, bradycardia, ischemia, hypervolemia, sepsis, pleural effusion, gangrene, hyponatremia, headache

ANTIDOTE
There is no antidote; stop terlipressin and treat supportively based on symptoms.

THIAMINE HYDROCHLORIDE
(**THIGH**-ah-min hy-droh-**KLOR**-eyed)

Vitamin B$_1$

USUAL DOSE

Transfer to PO doses when practical; see Precautions. Administer before dextrose solutions in the poorly nourished to avoid the development of acute symptoms of thiamine deficiency.

Thiamine deficiency (prophylaxis): Administered as part of a TPN program and based on individual patient needs (average daily requirement in a normal healthy adult is 1 mg). Average supplementation in TPN is 6 mg/day; may be increased to 25 to 50 mg/day in patients with a history of alcohol abuse. In critically ill adults, an initial dose of up to 100 mg has been used. May be followed with 50 to 100 mg daily until a regular balanced diet can be eaten. IV dextrose solutions or high carbohydrate diets increase thiamine requirements and may worsen symptoms in patients who are thiamine deficient.

Beriberi: 5 to 30 mg IV or IM 3 times daily for up to 2 weeks. Continue PO for 1 month.

Alcohol withdrawal syndrome: 100 mg IV or IM daily for several days. Administer concurrently with IV glucose. Follow with 50 to 100 mg/day PO.

Wernicke's encephalopathy: An initial dose of 100 mg IV. Larger doses may be required in the first 24 hours with extreme caution. Follow with 50 to 100 mg daily until a normal diet is resumed.

PEDIATRIC DOSE

Thiamine deficiency (prophylaxis and/or treatment): Administered as part of a TPN program and based on individual patient needs (average daily requirement in a normal healthy infant or child ranges from 0.2 mg in infants to 0.9 mg in 9- to 13-year-olds). Up to 10 to 25 mg/24 hr may be used in critically ill pediatric patients. See comments under Usual Dose.

Beriberi: 10 to 25 mg/24 hr. Follow with 10 to 50 mg PO daily for 2 weeks, then 5 to 10 mg PO daily for 1 month.

DILUTION

May be given by IV injection or added to most IV solutions and given as an infusion. See chart on inside back cover.

Storage: Can be refrigerated; protect from freezing and from light.

COMPATIBILITY

Unstable in neutral or alkaline solutions. Do not use in combination with alkaline solutions (e.g., acetates, barbiturates, carbonates, citrates, copper ions). **Incompatible** with solutions containing sulfites and other oxidizing and reducing agents.

RATE OF ADMINISTRATION

100 mg or fraction thereof over 5 minutes. For 100 mg or larger doses, equal distribution over an extended time as an infusion is preferred.

ACTIONS

A water-soluble vitamin, thiamine is necessary to most metabolic processes in humans, especially carbohydrate metabolism. Widely distributed in all body tissues, metabolized in the liver, and excreted in urine.

INDICATIONS AND USES

Prophylaxis or treatment of thiamine deficiency syndromes including beriberi (wet or dry), Wernicke's encephalopathy, or peripheral neuritis.

CONTRAINDICATIONS

Known hypersensitivity to thiamine hydrochloride.

PRECAUTIONS

Not commonly administered IV; PO or IM is preferred. ▪ Rarely used alone, it is more often administered as a multiple B vitamin. ▪ In thiamine deficiency, administer thiamine before giving any glucose load to prevent the sudden onset of Wernicke's encephalopathy or add 100 mg to each of the first few liters of IV fluid to avoid precipitating heart failure. ▪ Requirements may be increased in certain conditions (e.g., alcoholism, burns, GI disease, or malabsorption). ▪ Supplementation is necessary in patients receiving total parenteral nutrition (usually administered as a multivitamin). ▪ S/S of thiamine deficiency (e.g., ataxia, edema, heart failure, neuritis, ocular signs) may respond within hours of thiamine administration and disappear within days. Confusion and psychosis may be slower to respond and may not improve if nerve damage has occurred.

Patient Education: Dietary consultation indicated to prevent relapse.

Maternal/Child: Category A: use only if clearly needed. ▪ Use caution in breast-feeding.

SIDE EFFECTS

Anaphylaxis and death caused by hypersensitivity reaction can occur with IV administration. Recent studies have shown that hypersensitivity reactions can occur with equal frequency by any route. Incidence after IV administration is less than 0.1%. May increase in frequency with repeat injections. Other reactions include feeling of warmth, nausea, pain, pruritus, sweating, urticaria, and weakness.

ANTIDOTE

Discontinue the drug, treat hypersensitivity reactions or resuscitate as necessary, and notify the physician.

THIOTEPA BBW
(thigh-oh-**TEP**-ah)

Antineoplastic
(alkylating agent/nitrosurea)

Tepadina

pH 5.5 to 7.5

USUAL DOSE
Pretreatment: Verify pregnancy status. Baseline studies indicated; see Monitor.
Adenocarcinoma of the breast or ovary (thiotepa and Tepadina): 0.3 to 0.4 mg/kg every 1 to 4 weeks. Dose must be carefully individualized. A slow response does not necessarily indicate a lack of response. Increasing the frequency of dosing may only increase toxicity. Initially the higher dose in the given range is commonly administered. After maximum benefit is obtained by initial therapy, it is necessary to continue the patient on maintenance therapy (1- to 4-week intervals). The maintenance dose should be adjusted weekly on the basis of pretreatment control blood counts and subsequent blood counts. Maintenance doses should not be administered more frequently than weekly.

PEDIATRIC DOSE
Class 3 beta-thalassemia: *Tepadina:* Two administrations of 5 mg/kg IV approximately 12 hours apart on Day −6 before allogeneic hematopoietic progenitor (stem) cell transplantation (HSCT) in conjunction with high-dose busulfan and cyclophosphamide as outlined in the following chart. See busulfan and cyclophosphamide monographs.

Dosage Regimen for Allogeneic HSCT in Pediatric Patients With Class 3 Beta-Thalassemia											
	Day Before Transplantation										
Treatment	Day −10	Day −9	Day −8	Day −7	Day −6	Day −5	Day −4	Day −3	Day −2	Day −1	Day 0
Busulfan IV weight-based dose q 6 hr[a]	X X X X	X X X X	X X X X	X X X X							
Tepadina IV 5 mg/kg twice (approximately 12 hours apart)					X X						
Cyclophosphamide IV 40 mg/kg/day						X	X	X	X		
Stem cell infusion											X

[a]**Busulfan IV weight-based dose:** 1 mg/kg q 6 hr for patients less than 9 kg; 1.2 mg/kg q 6 hr for patients 9 to 16 kg; 1.1 mg/kg q 6 hr for patients 16.1 kg to 23 kg; 0.95 mg/kg q 6 hr for patients 23.1 to 34 kg; 0.8 mg/kg q 6 hr for patients more than 34 kg.

DOSE ADJUSTMENTS
Reduce dose or discontinue if WBC or platelet count falls rapidly. ■ To continue optimal effect and to preserve correlation between dose and blood counts, maintenance doses should not be administered more frequently than weekly. ■ *Thiotepa:* Usually contraindicated but can be used with extreme caution and in low doses in patients with existing hepatic, renal, or bone marrow damage if benefits outweigh risks and are accompanied by hepatic, renal, and hematopoietic function tests.

DILUTION
Specific techniques required; see Precautions. Each 15-mg vial is reconstituted with 1.5 mL of SWFI (10 mg/mL). Each 100-mg vial is reconstituted with 10 mL of SWFI (10 mg/mL). Mix manually by repeated inversions. A hypotonic solution; further dilute with NS before administration. Must be filtered through a 0.22-micron filter before

administration. Final solution should be clear; may occasionally show opalescence. Do not use if hazy or opaque or if a precipitate is present.

Thiotepa: May then be given through a Y-tube or three-way stopcock of a free-flowing IV infusion.

Tepadina: Dilute to a final concentration between 0.5 and 1 mg/mL. Use of a central venous catheter is required when used for **class 3 beta-thalassemia**.

Filters: Filter through a 0.22-micron filter before administration. See Dilution.

Storage: **Thiotepa:** Must be refrigerated before and after reconstitution. Protect from light at all times. Use reconstituted solution within 8 hours. Use diluted solution immediately. **Tepadina:** Refrigerate before and after reconstitution; do not freeze. Use reconstituted solution within 8 hours. After dilution, **Tepadina** is stable for 24 hours refrigerated and for 4 hours at RT. Immediate use is preferred.

COMPATIBILITY

Compatibility information not available from manufacturer. Other sources suggest specific **compatibilities** dependent on concentration and manufacturer; consult a pharmacist.

RATE OF ADMINISTRATION

Thiotepa and Tepadina: Use of a 0.22-micron filter required.

Adenocarcinoma of the breast or ovary (thiotepa and Tepadina): A single dose of 0.3 to 0.4 mg/kg by rapid IV administration.

Class 3 beta-thalassemia: **Tepadina:** A single dose in a concentration of 0.5 to 1 mg/mL. Administer through a central venous catheter over 3 hours. Flush catheter with 5 mL of NS before and after infusion.

ACTIONS

An alkylating agent chemically and pharmacologically related to nitrogen mustard. Has antitumor activity and is cell-cycle phase–nonspecific. The radiomimetic action is thought to occur through the release of ethylenimine radicals which, like irradiation, disrupt DNA bonds. Results in inhibition of protein, RNA, and DNA synthesis. It is metabolized extensively in the liver and has one major active metabolite (TEPA). Half-life is 1.4 to 3.7 hours in adults. Some urinary excretion of drug and metabolite.

INDICATIONS AND USES

Tepadina: To reduce the risk of graft rejection when used in conjunction with high-dose busulfan and cyclophosphamide as a preparative regimen for allogeneic hematopoietic progenitor (stem) cell transplantation (HPSCT) for pediatric patients with class 3 beta-thalassemia.

Thiotepa and Tepadina: Treatment of adenocarcinoma of the breast and ovary. ■ For controlling intracavitary effusions secondary to diffuse or localized neoplastic diseases of various serosal cavities. ■ Treatment of superficial papillary carcinoma of the urinary bladder.

Thiotepa: Although now largely superseded by other treatments, thiotepa has been effective against other lymphomas, such as lymphosarcoma and Hodgkin disease.

CONTRAINDICATIONS

Thiotepa and Tepadina: Known hypersensitivity to thiotepa.

Tepadina: Concomitant use with live or attenuated vaccines.

Thiotepa: Hepatic, renal, or bone marrow damage unless need is greater than the risk.

PRECAUTIONS

Thiotepa and Tepadina: Follow guidelines for handling cytotoxic agents. See Appendix A, p. 1308. ■ Administered by or under the direction of the physician specialist. ■ Can cause fetal harm; see Maternal/Child and Patient Education. ■ Hypersensitivity reactions (including anaphylaxis), laryngeal edema, rash, urticaria, and wheezing have been reported. ■ Some evidence of carcinogenicity; risk of secondary malignancy is increased.

Thiotepa: Highly toxic to the hematopoietic system. Death from septicemia and hemorrhage has occurred as a direct result of hematopoietic depression. ■ Death has occurred after intravesical administration, caused by bone marrow depression from the systematically absorbed drug. ■ See Dose Adjustments and Side Effects.

Tepadina: Risk of myelosuppression may be increased during treatment of breast and ovarian cancer if bone marrow is compromised by prior irradiation or chemotherapy.

Tepadina high-dose therapy: Myelosuppression is profound and occurs in all patients treated with high doses of Tepadina together with other chemotherapy in the preparative regimen for class 3 beta-thalassemia. May cause bone marrow ablation with resulting infection or bleeding. Do not begin the preparative regimen if a stem cell donor is not available. ■ Tepadina or its active metabolites may be excreted in the skin of patients undergoing high-dose therapy. May cause blistering, desquamation, pruritus, skin discoloration, and peeling that may be more severe in the axillae, groin, neck area, skin folds, and under dressings. Skin reactions from accidental exposure may also occur. Wash skin thoroughly with soap and water. Flush mucous membranes. ■ Hepatic veno-occlusive disease may occur with high-dose therapy in conjunction with busulfan and cyclophosphamide. ■ Fatal encephalopathy has occurred in patients treated with high doses of thiotepa. Other CNS toxicities (e.g., amnesia, apathy, coma, confusion, disorientation, drowsiness, forgetfulness, hallucinations, headache, inappropriate behavior, psychomotor retardation, seizures, and somnolence) have occurred.

Monitor: *Thiotepa and Tepadina:* Obtain baseline and weekly CBC and platelet counts during therapy and for at least 3 weeks after therapy has been discontinued. ■ Obtain baseline SCr, BUN, and/or liver function tests in patients with renal or hepatic impairment and monitor during treatment. Patients with CrCl less than 30 mL/min and/or a bilirubin level greater than 1.5 to 3 times the ULN (with any AST) may be at increased risk for toxicity due to accumulation of drug and metabolite. ■ Be alert for signs of bone marrow suppression or infection. Use of prophylactic antibiotics may be indicated pending results of C/S in a febrile neutropenic patient. ■ Prophylactic antiemetics may increase patient comfort. ■ Monitor for thrombocytopenia (platelet count less than 50,000/mm³). Initiate precautions to prevent excessive bleeding (e.g., inspect IV sites, skin, and mucous membranes; use extreme care during invasive procedures; test urine, emesis, stool, and secretions for occult blood). ■ Monitor for S/S of hypersensitivity reactions. ■ See Drug/Lab Interactions.

Tepadina high-dose therapy: Monitor CBC and platelets and provide supportive care until hematopoietic recovery. Monitor for cutaneous toxicity. Change occlusive dressings and clean the covered skin at least twice daily through 48 hours after administration of Tepadina. Change bed sheets daily. ■ Monitor for hepatic veno-occlusive disease by physical examination, serum transaminases, and bilirubin daily through BMT Day +28. ■ Monitor for S/S of CNS toxicity, including intracranial hemorrhage and seizures.

Patient Education: Verify pregnancy status before initiating therapy. Effective contraception should be used by females during therapy and for 6 months after the final dose. ■ Males should use effective contraception during therapy and for 1 year after the final dose. ■ Male and female fertility may be compromised. May damage spermatozoa and testicular tissue, resulting in possible genetic abnormalities; consider sperm conservation before therapy begins. ■ Promptly report S/S of bleeding (e.g., black stools, bruising, change in urine color, epistaxis), infection (e.g., fever, chills), or suspected pregnancy. ■ Promptly report S/S of hypersensitivity reaction (anaphylaxis, laryngeal edema, rash, urticaria, and wheezing). ■ Pediatric patients receiving high-dose therapy should shower or bathe with water at least twice daily through 48 hours after Tepadina administration. ■ See Appendix D, p. 1311.

Maternal/Child: Avoid pregnancy. Can cause fetal harm; see Patient Education. Has a mutagenic potential. ■ Discontinue breast-feeding. ■ Safety and effectiveness for use in pediatric patients not established except *Tepadina* for prevention of graft rejection in pediatric patients undergoing allogeneic HSCT. Safety and effectiveness of Tepadina in neonates have not been established.

Elderly: Safety and effectiveness of Tepadina as a preparative regimen before HSCT for patients with class 3 beta-thalassemia have not been established in elderly patients. Clinical studies for this indication did not include subjects 65 years of age and older. For all other indications, studies did not include sufficient numbers of subjects over age 65 years to determine whether elderly subjects respond differently than younger subjects. Differences have not been seen. Dose selection should be cautious, taking into account age-related organ impairment and concomitant disease states or drug therapy.

DRUG/LAB INTERACTIONS

Thiotepa and Tepadina: Possible pharmacokinetic interactions with any concomitantly administered medications have not been formally investigated. ▪ **Other drugs that cause bone marrow suppression** (e.g., amphotericin B [all formulations], ganciclovir [Cytovene]) should be avoided. ▪ In vitro studies suggest that thiotepa is metabolized by CYP3A4 and CYP2B6 to its active metabolite TEPA. Avoid coadministration of **strong CYP3A4 inhibitors** (e.g., itraconazole, clarithromycin, ritonavir) and **strong CYP3A4 inducers** (e.g., rifampin, phenytoin). May increase toxicity or reduce efficacy. Consider alternative medications with no or minimal potential to inhibit or induce CYP3A4. If use cannot be avoided, monitor closely for adverse drug reactions. ▪ In vitro studies also suggest that thiotepa inhibits CYP2B6; clinical relevance unknown. Inhibition of CYP2B6 may reduce the conversion of **cyclophosphamide** to its active metabolite. Reduction in conversion appears to be sequence dependent, with a greater reduction in the conversion to the active metabolite when thiotepa is administered 1.5 hours before the IV administration of cyclophosphamide compared with administration of thiotepa after IV cyclophosphamide. ▪ May potentiate **succinylcholine.** May cause prolonged apnea. ▪ Do not administer **live virus vaccines** to patients receiving antineoplastic drugs.

Thiotepa: Avoid combination, either simultaneously or sequentially, with **cancer chemotherapeutic agents or therapeutic modalities** (e.g., nitrogen mustard, cyclophosphamide, radiation therapy) that have the same mechanism of action. Will increase toxicity without increasing therapeutic benefit. Allow complete recovery verified by WBC count before using a second agent.

SIDE EFFECTS

Thiotepa and Tepadina for treatment of adenocarcinoma of the breast and ovary: Abdominal pain, alopecia, amenorrhea, anaphylactic shock, anorexia, asthma, blurred vision, conjunctivitis, dermatitis, dizziness, dysuria, fatigue, fever, headache, interference with spermatogenesis, laryngeal edema, nausea, pain at injection site, rash, urinary retention, vomiting, and wheezing. Bone marrow suppression (anemia, leukopenia, thrombocytopenia) may be life threatening, is dose related, and can occur with usual doses.

Tepadina as part of the preparative regimen for class 3 beta-thalassemia: Anemia; cytomegalovirus infection; diarrhea; elevated ALT, AST, and bilirubin; hematuria; hemorrhage; mucositis; neutropenia; thrombocytopenia; and rash are most common. Serious reactions include acute graft-versus-host disease, CNS toxicity (e.g., seizures), cutaneous toxicity (e.g., blistering, desquamation, peeling, pruritus, skin discoloration), hemorrhage (e.g., GI, intracranial, subarachnoid), hepatic veno-occlusive disease, hypersensitivity (e.g., anaphylaxis, asthma, laryngeal edema, rash, urticaria, wheezing), and infection (pneumonia, pseudomonas).

ANTIDOTE

Minor side effects will be treated symptomatically if necessary. Notify the physician of serious side effects. If platelet count falls below 150,000/mm³ or WBCs fall below 3,000/mm³, discontinue use and notify physician. Provide supportive care as needed for myelosuppression (e.g., bleeding, infections, symptomatic anemia, thrombocytopenia) until adequate hematopoietic recovery. Administration of whole blood products (e.g., packed RBCs, platelets, or leukocytes) and/or blood modifiers (e.g., darbepoetin alfa, epoetin alfa, filgrastim, pegfilgrastim, sargramostim) may be indicated to treat bone marrow toxicity. Discontinue the drug for severe or life-threatening CNS toxicity and provide supportive care. Discontinue the drug and treat hypersensitivity reactions as indicated.

TIGECYCLINE FOR INJECTION BBW
(tye-ge-**SYE**-kleen)

Antibacterial
(glycylcycline)

Tygacil

pH 7.8

USUAL DOSE
Pretreatment: Verify pregnancy status. Baseline studies indicated; see Precautions and Monitor.

Tigecycline: 100 mg as an initial dose. Follow with 50 mg every 12 hours. Recommended duration of treatment is 5 to 14 days for complicated skin and skin structure infections and complicated intra-abdominal infections and 7 to 14 days for community-acquired bacterial pneumonia. Duration of treatment is based on the severity and site of the infection and the patient's clinical and bacteriologic progress.

PEDIATRIC DOSE
See Maternal/Child.

DOSE ADJUSTMENTS
In patients with severe impaired liver function (Child-Pugh Class C), the initial dose remains the same, but subsequent doses should be reduced to 25 mg every 12 hours. ▪ No dose adjustment is indicated for impaired renal function, for mild to moderate impaired liver function (Child-Pugh Class A and Child-Pugh Class B), or in patients undergoing hemodialysis. ▪ No dose adjustment is indicated based on age, gender, or race. ▪ There are no data to provide dosing recommendations in pediatric patients with hepatic impairment; see Maternal/Child.

DILUTION
Reconstitute each 50-mg vial with 5.3 mL of NS, D5W, or LR (yields 10 mg/mL). Use 2 vials for the 100-mg dose. Swirl gently until lyophilized powder is dissolved. Reconstituted solution should be yellow to orange in color. Immediately withdraw 5 mL from each of two vials for the 100-mg dose (vials have overfill) or from one vial for the 50-mg dose and add to a 100-mL IV bag of D5W, NS, or LR for infusion. Maximum concentration should be 1 mg/mL.

Filters: No data available from manufacturer.

Storage: Store unopened vials at CRT. Reconstituted solution may be stored at RT for up to 6 hours. Fully diluted solution in the IV bag may be stored at RT for up to 24 hours or for 6 hours in the vial and the remaining time in the IV bag, or the fully diluted solution in either D5W or NS may be refrigerated at 2° to 8° C (36° to 46° F) for up to 48 hours following immediate transfer of the reconstituted solution into the IV bag.

COMPATIBILITY
The following drugs **should not** be administered simultaneously through the same **Y-site** as tigecycline: amphotericin B (conventional), amphotericin B lipid complex, diazepam, esomeprazole, and omeprazole.

Y-site: Compatible at the **Y-site** when used with NS or D5W: amikacin, aminophylline, dobutamine, dopamine, gentamicin, LR solution, lidocaine, metoclopramide, morphine, norepinephrine, piperacillin/tazobactam, potassium chloride, propofol, and tobramycin.

Other sources suggest specific **compatibilities** dependent on concentration and manufacturer; consult a pharmacist.

RATE OF ADMINISTRATION
Flush IV line with D5W, NS, or LR before and after infusion of tigecycline if other drugs are administered through the same line; see Compatibility. Consider **compatibility** of other drugs when flushing the line.

A single dose as an infusion over 30 to 60 minutes.

ACTIONS

A broad-spectrum tetracycline class antibacterial agent that is bacteriostatic against specific aerobic gram-positive and gram-negative microorganisms and specific anaerobic microorganisms; see prescribing information. Inhibits protein translation in bacteria by binding to a specific ribosomal subunit and blocking entry of specific molecules into the A site of the ribosome, thereby inhibiting protein synthesis. Plasma protein binding is approximately 71% to 89%. Extensively distributed beyond the plasma volume and into tissues. For example, concentrations have been identified in the bone, colon, gallbladder, synovial fluid, and lung. Mean half-life is 42.4 hours. Not extensively metabolized. 59% of a dose is excreted in bile and feces, and 33% is excreted in urine.

INDICATIONS AND USES

Treatment of patients 18 years of age and older with infections caused by susceptible strains of designated microorganisms in complicated skin and skin structure infections, complicated intra-abdominal infections, and community-acquired bacterial pneumonia. **Limitations of use:** Tigecycline is not indicated for treatment of diabetic foot infections. ▪ Tigecycline is not indicated for treatment of hospital-acquired or ventilator-associated pneumonia. In a comparator clinical trial, greater mortality and decreased efficacy were reported in the patients treated with tigecycline.

CONTRAINDICATIONS

Known hypersensitivity to tigecycline. Contains no excipients or preservatives.

PRECAUTIONS

An increase in all-cause mortality has been observed in a meta-analysis of Phase 3 and 4 clinical trials in tigecycline-treated patients versus comparator-treated patients. The cause of this increase has not been established. Tigecycline should be reserved for use in situations in which alternative treatments are not suitable. ▪ A trial of patients with hospital-acquired (including ventilator-associated) pneumonia failed to demonstrate the efficacy of tigecycline; see Limitations of Use. ▪ Sensitivity studies are indicated to determine susceptibility of the causative organism to tigecycline. Treatment may begin after culture and sensitivity studies are drawn. Re-evaluate after results are known. ▪ To reduce the development of drug-resistant bacteria and maintain its effectiveness, tigecycline should be used to treat only those infections proven or strongly suspected to be caused by bacteria. ▪ Cross-resistance and/or antagonism between tigecycline and other antibiotics have not been observed. ▪ Not affected by resistance mechanisms seen with other antibiotics (e.g., β-lactamases or ribosomal protection and efflux seen with other tetracyclines). However, some ESBL-producing isolates may confer resistance to tigecycline via other resistance mechanisms. ▪ Structurally similar to the tetracycline class of antibiotics; may have similar side effects (e.g., antianabolic action [which has led to acidosis, azotemia, hyperphosphatemia, and increased BUN], photosensitivity, and pseudotumor cerebri). ▪ Anaphylactic reactions have been reported. Should be avoided in patients with a history of hypersensitivity to tetracyclines; may have cross-sensitivity. ▪ Acute pancreatitis, including fatalities, has been reported. ▪ Monotherapy with tigecycline should be avoided in patients with complicated intra-abdominal infections secondary to clinically apparent intestinal perforation; sepsis/septic shock has occurred. ▪ Abnormalities in total bilirubin, PT, and transaminases have been seen in patients treated with tigecycline. Isolated cases of significant hepatic dysfunction and hepatic failure have also been reported; see Monitor. ▪ May cause permanent discoloration of the teeth during tooth development; see Maternal/Child. ▪ Avoid prolonged use of drug; superinfection caused by overgrowth of nonsusceptible organisms may result. ▪ Use caution in patients with severe liver impairment. Reduced dose and monitoring for treatment response are indicated; see Dose Adjustments. ▪ *Clostridium difficile*–associated diarrhea (CDAD) has been reported. May range from mild diarrhea to fatal colitis. Consider in patients who present with diarrhea during or after treatment with tigecycline.

Monitor: Monitor vital signs carefully. ▪ Obtain baseline CBC with differential, and monitor as indicated. ▪ Monitor liver function. If abnormal liver function tests develop, monitor closely for worsening hepatic function and evaluate for risk/benefit of continuing therapy. Hepatic dysfunction may occur after tigecycline is discontinued. ▪ Monitor patients with severe hepatic impairment for treatment response; see Precautions and Dose Adjustments. ▪ Monitor for S/S or laboratory abnormalities suggestive of acute pancreatitis. ▪ Observe for signs of hypersensitivity reactions (e.g., chills, fever, hives, rash, shortness of breath). ▪ See Precautions and Drug/Lab Interactions.

Patient Education: Avoid pregnancy; use effective contraceptive measures; see Drug/Lab Interactions. Should pregnancy occur, notify physician immediately and discuss potential hazards. ▪ Promptly report diarrhea or bloody stools that occur during treatment or up to several months after an antibiotic has been discontinued; may indicate CDAD and require treatment. ▪ Promptly report S/S of hypersensitivity (e.g., chills, fever, hives, rash, shortness of breath) and/or S/S of liver dysfunction (e.g., jaundice or yellow sclera).

Maternal/Child: Use during the second and third trimester of pregnancy may cause permanent discoloration of deciduous teeth and reversible inhibition of bone growth. Use of effective contraception required; see Drug/Lab Interactions. ▪ Use during tooth development (the last half of pregnancy, infancy, and childhood to the age of 8 years) may cause permanent discoloration of the teeth and is not recommended. ▪ Because of the risk of dental discoloration and inhibition of bone growth, avoid breast-feeding if taking tigecycline for longer than 3 weeks. Consider interrupting breast-feeding and pumping and discarding breast milk during treatment and for 9 days after the last dose to minimize drug exposure to breast-fed infant. ▪ Safety and effectiveness for use in pediatric patients under 18 years of age have not been evaluated due to the observed increase in mortality associated with tigecycline in adult patients. Tigecycline should not be used in pediatric patients unless no alternative antibacterial drugs are available. Under these circumstances, the following doses are suggested: *Pediatric patients 8 to 11 years of age* should receive 1.2 mg/kg every 12 hours (not to exceed 50 mg every 12 hours). *Pediatric patients 12 to 17 years of age* should receive 50 mg every 12 hours.

Elderly: Response similar to that seen in younger adults; however, the potential for greater sensitivity to side effects cannot be disregarded.

DRUG/LAB INTERACTIONS

May decrease clearance of warfarin. INR should be monitored if tigecycline is administered with warfarin. ▪ May render **oral contraceptives** less effective, resulting in pregnancy or breakthrough bleeding. ▪ Tigecycline is a substrate of P-glycoprotein (P-gp). Clinical relevance is not known. Coadministration of **P-gp inhibitors** (e.g., ketoconazole or cyclosporine) or **P-gp inducers** (e.g., rifampin) could affect the pharmacokinetics of tigecycline. ▪ No reported interactions with lab tests.

SIDE EFFECTS

Nausea and vomiting are the most common side effects and are the primary reason for discontinuing therapy. Other commonly reported side effects include abdominal pain, diarrhea, headache, and increased ALT. Less commonly reported side effects include abnormal healing; abscess; anemia; asthenia; bilirubinemia; CDAD; dizziness; dyspepsia; hyponatremia; hypoproteinemia; increased alkaline phosphatase, amylase, AST, and BUN; infection; phlebitis; pneumonia; rash. Sepsis/septic shock and death occurred in a few patients with complicated infections.

Post-Marketing: Acute pancreatitis, anaphylactic reactions, hepatic cholestasis, jaundice, severe skin reactions (including Stevens-Johnson syndrome), and symptomatic hypoglycemia in patients with and without diabetes.

Overdose: Increased incidence of nausea and vomiting.

ANTIDOTE

Keep physician informed of all side effects. Most minor side effects will be treated symptomatically; monitor closely. If minor side effects are progressive or if any major side effect occurs, discontinue the drug, treat hypersensitivity reactions, or resuscitate as necessary. Mild cases of CDAD may respond to discontinuation of tigecycline. Treat CDAD with fluids, electrolytes, protein supplements, and appropriate antibiotics (e.g., oral vancomycin) as indicated. In severe cases, surgical evaluation may be indicated. Not removed by hemodialysis.

TIROFIBAN HYDROCHLORIDE

Antiplatelet agent

(ty-roh-**FYE**-ban hy-droh-**KLOR**-eyed)

Aggrastat   pH 5.5 to 6.5

USUAL DOSE

Pretreatment: Baseline studies indicated; see Monitor.

Tirofiban: A *loading infusion* of 25 mcg/kg administered within 5 minutes followed by a *maintenance infusion (CrCl over 60 mL/min)* of 0.15 mcg/kg/min for up to 18 hours; see Dose Adjustments for dosing in patients with a CrCl equal to or less than 60 mL/min. See Rate of Administration for additional administration information. Has been used in combination with aspirin, clopidogrel (Plavix), and heparin or bivalirudin (Angiomax).

DOSE ADJUSTMENTS

After loading dose of 25 mcg/kg administered within 5 minutes, reduce maintenance dose to 0.075 mcg/kg/min for up to 18 hours in patients with a CrCl equal to or less than 60 mL/min. ▪ No dose adjustment indicated based on age, race, gender, or hepatic impairment.

DILUTION

Multiple forms and strengths available. Available as an infusion solution in a 5 mg/100 mL vial or a 12.5 mg/250 mL bag (50 mcg/mL) or as a bolus vial containing 3.75 mg/15 mL (250 mcg/mL). Remove overwrap of the infusion bag. Plastic may be somewhat opaque due to sterilization process. Opacity should diminish. Squeeze inner container to check for leak. Discard if leakage noted; sterility is impaired.

Bolus dose: Withdraw bolus dose of tirofiban from the 15-mL premixed bolus vial into a syringe. Alternatively, the bolus dose may be administered from the 100-mL premixed vial or from the 250-mL premixed bag. Do not dilute. Refer to the following equations to calculate bolus volume.

The recommended bolus volume using the 15-mL premixed bolus vial:

$$\frac{\text{Bolus Volume}}{\text{(mL)}} = \frac{25 \text{ mcg/kg} \times \text{body weight (kg)}}{250 \text{ mcg/mL}}$$

The recommended bolus volume using the 100-mL premixed vial or 250-mL premixed bag:

$$\frac{\text{Bolus Volume}}{\text{(mL)}} = \frac{25 \text{ mcg/kg} \times \text{body weight (kg)}}{50 \text{ mcg/mL}}$$

Storage: Store unopened containers at 25° C (77° F). Variations from 15° to 30° C (59° to 86° F) are acceptable (CRT). Protect from light during storage. Do not freeze. Discard unused solution.

COMPATIBILITY

Do not add other drugs or remove solution directly from the bag with a syringe. Should not be administered in the same IV line as diazepam.

Compatibile at the **Y-site** with amiodarone, argatroban, atropine, bivalirudin, dobutamine, dopamine, epinephrine, famotidine, furosemide, heparin, lidocaine, midazolam, morphine, nitroglycerin IV, potassium chloride, propranolol.

RATE OF ADMINISTRATION

Loading infusion: 25 mcg/kg administered within 5 minutes via a syringe or IV pump. For patients weighing 167 kg or more, it is recommended that the bolus dose be administered via syringe from the 15-mL premixed bolus vial to ensure delivery time does not exceed 5 minutes.

Maintenance infusion: *CrCl greater than 60 mL/min:* 0.15 mcg/kg/min for up to 18 hours. *CrCl equal to or less than 60 mL/min:* 0.075 mcg/kg/min for up to 18 hours.

Administer the maintenance infusion from the 100-mL premixed vial or 250-mL premixed bag via an IV pump immediately following the bolus dose.

Infusion rate for CrCl greater than 60 mL/min using the 100-mL premixed vial or 250-mL premixed bag can be calculated as follows:

$$\text{Infusion Rate for CrCl} > 60 \text{ mL/min (mL/hr)} = \frac{0.15 \text{ mcg/kg/min} \times \text{Body weight (kg)} \times 60 \text{ min/hr}}{50 \text{ mcg/mL}}$$

Example calculation of infusion rate for 60-kg patient with CrCl greater than 60 mL/min using the 100-mL premixed vial or 250-mL premixed bag:

$$\text{Infusion Rate for CrCl} > 60 \text{ mL/min (mL/hr)} = \frac{0.15 \text{ mcg/kg/min} \times 60 \text{ kg} \times 60 \text{ min/hr}}{50 \text{ mcg/mL}} = 10.8 \text{ min/hr}$$

Infusion rate for CrCl 60 mL/min or less using the 100-mL premixed vial or 250-mL premixed bag can be calculated as follows:

$$\text{Infusion Rate for CrCl} \leq 60 \text{ mL/min (mL/hr)} = \frac{0.075 \text{ mcg/kg/min} \times \text{Body weight (kg)} \times 60 \text{ min/hr}}{50 \text{ mcg/mL}}$$

ACTIONS

A nonpeptide antagonist of the platelet glycoprotein GPIIb/IIIa receptor. It inhibits platelet aggregation by preventing the binding of fibrinogen to the receptor site on activated platelets. Inhibits platelet aggregation in a dose- and concentration-dependent manner. When given according to the recommended regimen, greater than 90% inhibition is attained within 10 minutes. Bleeding time is prolonged. Inhibition is reversible, with aggregation returning to baseline in more than 90% of patients within 4 to 8 hours following cessation of the infusion. Half-life is approximately 2 hours. Cleared from the plasma primarily by renal excretion, with about 65% of the unchanged drug appearing in the urine and about 25% appearing in feces. Metabolism is limited.

INDICATIONS AND USES

Indicated to reduce the rate of thrombotic cardiovascular events (combined end point of death, myocardial infarction, or refractory ischemia/repeat cardiac procedure) in patients with non–ST elevation acute coronary syndrome (NSTE-ACS).

CONTRAINDICATIONS

Severe hypersensitivity (e.g., anaphylaxis) to tirofiban. ▪ A history of thrombocytopenia following prior exposure to tirofiban. ▪ Active internal bleeding or a history of bleeding diathesis, major surgical procedure, or severe physical trauma within the previous month.

PRECAUTIONS

For intravenous use only. ▪ Bleeding is the most common complication encountered during therapy. Most bleeding associated with tirofiban occurs at the arterial access site for cardiac catheterization; see Monitor. Fatal bleeding events have been reported.

- Concomitant use of fibrinolytics, oral anticoagulants, and antiplatelet drugs increases the risk of bleeding; see Drug/Lab Interactions. ▪ Profound thrombocytopenia has been reported. Previous exposure to GPIIb/IIIa receptor antagonists (e.g., eptifibatide, tirofiban) may increase the risk of developing thrombocytopenia. ▪ Patients treated with tirofiban plus heparin were more likely to experience decreases in platelet counts than were patients on heparin alone. ▪ Plasma clearance is decreased in patients with moderate to severe renal insufficiency; see Dose Adjustments. Safety and effectiveness not established for use in patients on hemodialysis. ▪ Hypersensitivity reactions, including anaphylaxis, have been reported in post-marketing. They have occurred during initial infusion and during readministration.

Monitor: Obtain platelet count, hemoglobin, and hematocrit before therapy, within 6 hours following the loading infusion, and at least daily thereafter. More frequent monitoring may be indicated. ▪ If platelet count drops to below 90,000/mm³, additional platelet counts should be performed to exclude pseudothrombocytopenia. If thrombocytopenia is confirmed, heparin and tirofiban should be discontinued and appropriate therapy initiated. ▪ Obtain an aPTT before treatment and carefully monitor the anticoagulant effects of heparin by repeated determinations of aPTT; adjust heparin dose accordingly. ▪ Monitor for S/S of hypersensitivity or infusion-related reactions (e.g., anaphylaxis, hypotension, pruritus, rash, urticaria, or wheezing). ▪ Monitor the patient for signs of bleeding; take vital signs (avoiding automatic BP cuffs); observe any invaded sites at least every 15 minutes (e.g., sheaths, IV sites, cutdowns, punctures, epidural sites, Foleys, NGs); watch for hematuria, hematemesis, bloody stool, petechiae, hematoma, flank pain, muscle weakness. Perform neuro checks frequently. If during therapy bleeding cannot be controlled with pressure, tirofiban and heparin infusions should be discontinued. ▪ Use care in handling patient; minimize use of urinary catheters, nasotracheal intubation, and nasogastric tubes. Avoid arterial puncture, venipuncture, epidural procedures, and IM injection. Use extreme precautionary methods and only compressible sites if these procedures are absolutely necessary (i.e., avoid subclavian or jugular veins). Apply pressure for 30 minutes to any invaded site and then apply pressure dressings. Saline or heparin locks suggested to facilitate blood draws.

Patient Education: Compliance with all measures to minimize bleeding (e.g., strict bed rest, positioning) is imperative. ▪ Avoid use of razors, toothbrushes, and other sharp items. ▪ Use caution while moving to avoid excessive bumping. ▪ Promptly report S/S of a hypersensitivity reaction (e.g., hives, rash, shortness of breath or troubled breathing, swelling of eyelids, lips, or face) and all episodes of bleeding, and apply local pressure if indicated. ▪ Expect oozing from IV sites.

Maternal/Child: Although published data cannot definitively establish the absence of risk, available case reports have not established an association between tirofiban use during pregnancy and major birth defects, miscarriage, or adverse maternal or fetal outcomes. Myocardial infarction is a medical emergency in pregnancy and can be fatal to the pregnant woman and fetus if left untreated. ▪ No data on the presence of tirofiban in human milk, the effects of the drug on the breast-fed infant, or the effects of the drug on human milk production. Consider risk versus benefit. ▪ Safety and efficacy for use in pediatric patients not established.

Elderly: Effectiveness similar to that seen in younger patients. ▪ Dose adjustment based solely on age is not necessary. Consider age-related renal impairment; see Dose Adjustments.

DRUG/LAB INTERACTIONS
Use caution when given with drugs that affect hemostasis (e.g., **anticoagulants** [e.g., apixaban, heparin, rivaroxaban, warfarin], **NSAIDs**, **platelet aggregation inhibitors** [e.g., clopidogrel, dipyridamole], or **thrombolytic agents** [e.g., alteplase, reteplase, streptokinase]). Risk of bleeding is increased.

SIDE EFFECTS
Bleeding is the most frequent adverse event. Laboratory findings related to bleeding include decrease in hemoglobin, hematocrit, and platelet count and occult blood in urine and feces. Other side effects that occur at an incidence of greater than 1%, regardless of drug relationship, are bradycardia, dissection of the coronary artery, dizziness, edema, hypersensitivity reactions (e.g., hives, rash), leg pain, nausea, pelvic pain, sweating, thrombocytopenia, and vasovagal reflex.

Post-Marketing: Hypersensitivity reactions (including anaphylaxis), severe thrombocytopenia. Fatal bleeding events have been reported.

ANTIDOTE
Keep physician informed of laboratory values and side effects. Discontinue the infusion of tirofiban and heparin if any serious bleeding not controllable with pressure occurs. If platelet count drops to below 90,000 mm^3, obtain additional platelet counts to exclude pseudothrombocytopenia. If thrombocytopenia is confirmed, discontinue tirofiban and heparin. Platelet transfusion may be required. If a hypersensitivity reaction should occur, discontinue the infusion and treat as indicated by severity (e.g., epinephrine, dopamine, theophylline, antihistamines [e.g., diphenhydramine], and/or corticosteroids as necessary).

No specific antidote is available. Overdosage should be treated by assessment of the patient's clinical condition and cessation or adjustment of the drug infusion as appropriate. Hemodialysis may be useful in an overdose situation.

TOBRAMYCIN SULFATE BBW
(toe-brah-**MY**-sin **SUL**-fayt)

**Antibacterial
(aminoglycoside)**

pH 3 to 6.5

USUAL DOSE
Pretreatment: See Maternal/Child.

Tobramycin: 3 mg/kg of body weight/24 hr equally divided into 3 doses and given every 8 hours (1 mg/kg every 8 hours). Up to 5 mg/kg equally divided into 3 or 4 doses may be given in life-threatening infections (1.25 mg/kg every 6 hours or 1.67 mg/kg every 8 hours). Reduce to usual dose as soon as feasible. For obese patients, the dosing weight used to calculate the mg/kg dose is achieved by adding the ideal or lean body weight (IBW) to 40% of the excess over IBW.

$$\text{Dosing weight} = \text{IBW} + 0.4 \, (\text{Total body weight} - \text{IBW})$$

Do not exceed 5 mg/kg/day unless serum levels are monitored.

Studies suggest that in certain populations a single daily dose of 5 to 7 mg/kg (instead of divided into 2 to 3 doses) may provide higher peak levels and enhance drug effectiveness while actually reducing or having no adverse effects on risk of toxicity. Various procedures for monitoring blood levels are in use. Some health facilities are monitoring with trough levels; others may draw levels at predetermined times and plot the concentration on nomograms. Depending on the protocol in place, doses or intervals may be adjusted. See Dose Adjustments and Precautions.

Patients with cystic fibrosis: One source suggests 7.5 to 10.5 mg/kg/24 hr equally divided into 3 doses and given every 8 hours for 7 to 21 days (2.5 to 3.5 mg/kg every 8 hours).

PEDIATRIC DOSE
In pediatric and neonatal patients, monitor serum levels. Wide interpatient variability; see Monitor and Maternal/Child.

Over 1 week of age: 6 to 7.5 mg/kg of body weight/24 hr in 3 or 4 equally divided doses (1.5 to 1.89 mg/kg every 6 hours or 2 to 2.5 mg/kg every 8 hours). Another source suggests the same as adult dose.

A single daily dose is also being used in pediatric patients. See comments under Usual Dose.

Severe cystic fibrosis: 10 mg/kg/day in equally divided doses every 6 hours (2.5 mg/kg every 6 hours).

NEONATAL DOSE
1 week of age or less: Up to 4 mg/kg of body weight/24 hr in two equal doses every 12 hours (up to 2 mg/kg every 12 hours). Lower doses may be safer because of immature kidney function. 2.5 mg/kg every 18 hours or 3 mg/kg every 24 hours may provide acceptable peak and trough levels in neonates weighing less than 2,000 Gm. See Maternal/Child.

DOSE ADJUSTMENTS
Reduce daily dose commensurate with amount of renal impairment and/or increase intervals between injections. Measurement of serum concentrations following a loading dose of 1 mg/kg is suggested. Adjust subsequent doses accordingly. ▪ Once-daily dosing is not usually used in patients with ascites, burns covering more than 20% of the total body surface area, CrCl less than 40 mL/min (including patients requiring dialysis), CrCl greater than 120 mL/min, cystic fibrosis, endocarditis, mycobacterium infections, or in infants or during pregnancy. ▪ Reduced doses or extended intervals may be required in the elderly. ▪ See Drug/Lab Interactions.

DILUTION
Prepared solutions equal 10 or 40 mg/mL. Further dilute each single dose in 50 to 100 mL of NS or D5W and administer through an additive tubing. Also available in ADD-Vantage vials for use with ADD-Vantage infusion containers. Reduce volume of diluent proportionately for pediatric patients.

Storage: Store at CRT.

COMPATIBILITY
Manufacturer states, "Do not physically premix with other drugs; administer separately." Inactivated in solution with beta-lactam antibiotics (e.g., cephalosporins, penicillins) and vancomycin; do not mix in the same solution. Appropriate spacing required because of physical **incompatibilities.** See Drug/Lab Interactions.

Other sources suggest specific **compatibilities** dependent on concentration and manufacturer; consult a pharmacist.

RATE OF ADMINISTRATION
Each single dose, properly diluted, over a minimum of 20 and a maximum of 60 minutes.

ACTIONS
An aminoglycoside antibiotic with potential neuromuscular blocking action. Inhibits protein synthesis in bacterial cells. Bactericidal against specific gram-negative bacilli, including *Escherichia coli, Klebsiella, Proteus,* and *Pseudomonas.* Well distributed through all body fluids. Usual half-life is 2 to 2.5 hours. Half-life is prolonged in infants, postpartum females, fever, liver disease and ascites, spinal cord injury, cystic fibrosis, and the elderly; shorter in severe burns. Crosses the placental barrier. Excreted in the kidneys.

INDICATIONS AND USES
Short-term treatment of serious infections caused by susceptible organisms. Indicated infections include septicemia; lower respiratory tract infections; CNS infections (meningitis); intra-abdominal infections (including peritonitis); skin, bone, and skin structure infections; and complicated and recurrent urinary tract infections. ▪ Primarily used when penicillin and other less toxic antibiotics are ineffective or contraindicated. ▪ Concurrent therapy with a penicillin or cephalosporin sometimes indicated.

CONTRAINDICATIONS
Known tobramycin or aminoglycoside sensitivity. Sulfite sensitivity may be a contraindication.

PRECAUTIONS
Use extreme caution if therapy is required over 7 to 10 days. ▪ Sensitivity studies necessary to determine susceptibility of causative organism to tobramycin. ▪ To reduce the development of drug-resistant bacteria and maintain its effectiveness, tobramycin should be used to treat or prevent only those infections proven or strongly suspected to be caused by bacteria. ▪ Superinfection may occur from overgrowth of nonsusceptible organisms. ▪ Use caution in infants, children, the elderly, and patients with congestive heart failure, extensive burns, or muscular disorders. ▪ May contain sulfites; use caution in patients with asthma. ▪ Potentially nephrotoxic, ototoxic, and neurotoxic. Risk for neurotoxicity (e.g., auditory and vestibular ototoxicity) increased in patients with pre-existing renal damage or in normal renal function with prolonged use. Partial or total irreversible deafness may continue to develop after tobramycin is discontinued. ▪ Aminoglycosides are nephrotoxic; risk for nephrotoxicity increased in patients with impaired renal function and in patients who receive high doses or prolonged therapy. ▪ Single daily dosing has been used effectively in abdominal, pelvic inflammatory, and GU infections in patients with normal renal function. Not recommended in bacteremia caused by *Pseudomonas aeruginosa,* endocarditis, meningitis, during pregnancy, or in patients less than 6 weeks postpartum. Limited data available for use in all other situations (e.g., burns, pediatric patients or the elderly, cystic fibrosis, renal impairment). ▪ *Clostridium difficile*–associated diarrhea (CDAD) has been reported. May range from mild diarrhea to fatal colitis. Consider in patients who present with diarrhea during or after treatment with tobramycin.

Monitor: Watch for decrease in urine output, rising BUN and SCr, and declining CrCl levels. Dose may need to be reduced. ▪ Closely monitor renal and eighth cranial nerve function, especially in patients with known or suspected reduced renal function at onset of therapy and in patients who develop signs of renal dysfunction during therapy. Monitor urine for decreased specific gravity, increased protein, and the presence of cells or casts. Serial audiograms are recommended, particularly in high-risk patients. ▪ Closely monitor patients with impaired renal function for nephrotoxicity and neurotoxicity (e.g., auditory and vestibular ototoxicity, convulsions, muscle twitching, numbness, tingling); nephrotoxicity may be reversible. ▪ Routine evaluation of hearing is recommended. ▪ Narrow range between toxic and therapeutic levels. Periodically monitor peak and trough concentrations to avoid peak serum concentrations above 12 mcg/mL and trough concentrations above 2 mcg/mL (indicates accumulation). With traditional dosing, therapeutic levels are between 4 and 8 mcg/mL depending on site and severity of infection. Accumulation, excessive peak concentrations, advanced age, cumulative doses, and dehydration may contribute to ototoxicity and nephrotoxicity. ▪ Maintain good hydration. ▪ Monitor serum calcium, magnesium, potassium, and sodium; levels may decline. ▪ In extended treatment, monitoring of serum levels, electrolytes, renal, auditory, and vestibular functions daily is recommended. ▪ See Drug/Lab Interactions.

Patient Education: Report promptly dizziness, hearing loss, weakness, or any changes in balance. ▪ Effective birth control required. Avoid pregnancy. ▪ Promptly report diarrhea or bloody stools that occur during treatment or up to several months after an antibiotic has been discontinued; may indicate CDAD and require treatment.

Maternal/Child: Category D: avoid pregnancy; use during pregnancy and breast-feeding only when absolutely necessary. Potential hazard to fetus. ▪ Peak concentrations are generally lower in infants and young children. ▪ Use extreme caution in premature infants and neonates; immature kidney function will result in prolonged half-life. ▪ See Precautions.

Elderly: Consider less toxic alternatives. ▪ Monitor renal function and drug levels carefully. Measurement of CrCl more useful than BUN or SCr to assess renal function. ▪ Half-life prolonged; longer intervals between doses may be more important than reduced doses. ▪ See Precautions, Dose Adjustments, and Side Effects.

DRUG/LAB INTERACTIONS

Synergistic when used in combination with **beta-lactam antibiotics** (e.g., cephalosporins, penicillins) **and vancomycin.** Synergism may be inconsistent; see Compatibility.

▪ Concurrent and/or sequential use topically or systemically with any other neurotoxic, ototoxic, or nephrotoxic agents should be avoided. May have dangerous additive effects with **anesthetics and other neuromuscular blocking antibiotics** (e.g., other aminoglycosides). ▪ **Neuromuscular blocking muscle relaxants** (e.g., atracurium, succinylcholine) are potentiated by aminoglycosides. *Apnea can occur.* ▪ May be antagonized by **bacteriostatic antibiotics** (e.g., chloramphenicol, erythromycin, and tetracycline); bactericidal action may be affected. ▪ **Magnesium sulfate** may reduce the antibiotic activity of tobramycin. ▪ Aminoglycosides are potentiated by **anticholinesterases** (e.g., edrophonium), **antineoplastics** (e.g., nitrogen mustard, cisplatin). ▪ See Side Effects.

SIDE EFFECTS

Occur more frequently with impaired renal function, higher doses, prolonged administration, dehydration, in the elderly, and in patients receiving other ototoxic or nephrotoxic drugs.

Dizziness; fever; headache; increased AST, ALT, and serum bilirubin; itching; lethargy; rash; roaring in the ears; seizures; urticaria; vomiting.

Major: Apnea; blood dyscrasias; CDAD; cylindruria; elevated BUN, nonprotein nitrogen (NPN), and creatinine; hearing loss; leukocytosis; neuromuscular blockade; oliguria; proteinuria; seizures (large doses); tinnitus; vertigo.

ANTIDOTE

Notify the physician of all side effects. If minor side effects persist or any major symptom appears, discontinue the drug and notify the physician. Evidence of impaired renal, vestibular, or auditory function requires discontinuation of tobramycin or a dose adjustment. Treatment is symptomatic or a reduction in dose may be required. Mild cases of CDAD may respond to discontinuation of drug. Treat CDAD with fluids, electrolytes, protein supplements, and appropriate antibiotics (e.g., oral vancomycin) as indicated. In severe cases, surgical evaluation may be indicated. In overdose hemodialysis may be indicated. Monitor fluid balance, CrCl, and plasma levels carefully. Complexation with ticarcillin may be as effective as hemodialysis. Consider exchange transfusion in the newborn. Calcium salts or neostigmine may reverse neuromuscular blockade. Resuscitate as necessary.

TOCILIZUMAB BBW
(**TOE**-si-**LIZ**-oo-mab)

Antirheumatic; disease-modifying
anti-rheumatic drug (DMARD)
Monoclonal antibody

Actemra

pH 6.5

USUAL DOSE

Pretreatment: Pretesting and baseline studies required and prescreening may be indicated; see Monitor.

Before initial use, the absolute neutrophil count (ANC) should be equal to or greater than 2,000/mm³, platelet count should be equal to or greater than 100,000/mm³, and ALT and AST should be no more than 1.5 times the ULN.

Rheumatoid arthritis (RA): Initial adult dose in rheumatoid arthritis: 4 mg/kg as an IV infusion once every 4 weeks. Increase dose to 8 mg/kg every 4 weeks based on clinical response. May be used as monotherapy or in combination with methotrexate or other nonbiologic DMARDs as an IV infusion or SC injection. Doses above 800 mg per infusion are not recommended. See prescribing information for SC dosing, intervals, and dose adjustments. When transitioning from IV to SC administration, administer the first SC dose instead of the next scheduled IV dose.

Polyarticular juvenile idiopathic arthritis (PJIA): *Weight less than 30 kg:* 10 mg/kg.

Weight at or above 30 kg: 8 mg/kg. Administer as an IV infusion once every 4 weeks. May be used alone or in combination with methotrexate. Do not adjust dose based on a single-visit body weight; weight may fluctuate. See prescribing information for SC dosing and intervals. When transitioning from IV to SC administration, administer the first SC dose instead of the next scheduled IV dose

Systemic juvenile idiopathic arthritis (SJIA): *Weight less than 30 kg:* 12 mg/kg.

Weight equal to or more than 30 kg: 8 mg/kg. Administer as an IV infusion once every 2 weeks. May be used as an IV infusion or as a SC injection alone or in combination with methotrexate. Do not adjust dose based on a single-visit body weight; weight may fluctuate. See prescribing information for SC dosing and intervals. When transitioning from IV to SC administration, administer the first SC dose instead of the next scheduled IV dose

Cytokine release syndrome (CRS): *Weight less than 30 kg:* 12 mg/kg.

Weight 30 kg or more: 8 mg/kg. Administer as an IV infusion over 60 minutes. May be used alone or in combination with corticosteroids. If no clinical improvements in the S/S of CRS occur after the first dose, up to 3 additional doses may be administered. The interval between consecutive doses should be at least 8 hours. Doses exceeding 800 mg per infusion are not recommended. For IV administration only; SC administration is not approved for CRS.

DOSE ADJUSTMENTS

When given IV on a mg/kg basis, patients with a body weight 100 kg or greater are predicted to have a mean steady-state exposure higher than mean values for the patient population. Therefore doses exceeding 800 mg are not recommended; see Usual Dose. No specific dose adjustments required based on age, gender, race, or mild or moderate renal impairment. ▪ Hold therapy in patients with severe infections until infection is controlled. ▪ Dose reduction has not been studied in PJIA or SJIA. Dose interruptions are recommended for liver enzyme abnormalities, low neutrophil counts, and low platelet counts in patients with PJIA or SJIA at levels similar to those outlined in the following charts for patients with rheumatoid arthritis (RA). May require interruption or discontinuation of tocilizumab and/or dose modification, interruption, or discontinuation of other concomitant medications (e.g., methotrexate) until evaluation of the clinical situation. The decision to discontinue tocilizumab for a lab abnormality should be based on medical assessment of the individual. ▪ The effects of severe renal impairment or hepatic impairment have not been studied. ■ The following charts outline dose adjustments for adults with RA based on ANC, platelets, and liver function tests.

Tocilizumab Dose Recommendations for Adults With RA With a Low Absolute Neutrophil Count (ANC)	
Lab Value (cells/mm³)	**Recommendation**
ANC >1,000/mm³	Maintain dose.
ANC 500 to 1,000/mm³	Hold tocilizumab dosing. When ANC >1,000/mm³, resume tocilizumab at 4 mg/kg and increase to 8 mg/kg as clinically appropriate.
ANC <500/mm³	Discontinue tocilizumab.

Tocilizumab Dose Recommendations for Adults With RA With a Low Platelet Count	
Lab Value (cells/mm³)	**Recommendation**
Platelet count 50,000 to 100,000/mm³	Hold tocilizumab dosing. When platelet count is >100,000/mm³, resume tocilizumab at 4 mg/kg and increase to 8 mg/kg as clinically appropriate.
Platelet count <50,000/mm³	Discontinue tocilizumab.

Tocilizumab Dose Recommendations for Adults With RA With Liver Enzyme Abnormalities	
Lab Value	**Recommendation**
>1 to 3 × ULN	Dose modify concomitant DMARDs (RA) or immunomodulatory agents (GCA) if appropriate. For persistent increases in this range, reduce tocilizumab dose to 4 mg/kg or hold dosing until ALT and/or AST have normalized.
>3 to 5 × ULN (confirmed by repeat testing)	Hold tocilizumab dosing until <3 × ULN, and follow recommendations above for >1 to 3 × ULN. For persistent increases >3 × ULN, discontinue tocilizumab.
>5 × ULN	Discontinue tocilizumab.

ULN, Upper limit of normal.

DILUTION

Available as a solution for single use (20 mg/mL). For patients weighing 30 kg or more, the solution must be further diluted to 100 mL in NS or 0.45 NS. For patients weighing less than 30 kg, dilute to 50 mL in NS or 0.45 NS. From a 100-mL (or 50-mL) infusion bag or bottle, withdraw a volume of NS or 0.45 NS equal to the volume of solution required for the calculated dose. Slowly add tocilizumab and avoid foaming by gently inverting the bag or bottle. Bring fully diluted solution to RT before administration.

For Intravenous Use: Volume of Tocilizumab Injection per kg of Body Weight		
Dose	**Indication**	**Volume of Tocilizumab Injection per kg of Body Weight**
4 mg/kg	Adult RA	0.2 mL/kg
8 mg/kg	Adult RA PJIA, SJIA, and CRS (≥30 kg of body weight)	0.4 mL/kg
10 mg/kg	PJIA (<30 kg of body weight)	0.5 mL/kg
12 mg/kg	SJIA and CRS (<30 kg of body weight)	0.6 mL/kg

Filters: Specific information not available.
Storage: Refrigerate unopened vials in original carton at 2° to 8° C (36° to 46° F). Do not use beyond expiration date. Protect from light. Do not freeze. Fully diluted solutions for

infusion using NS may be refrigerated at 2° to 8° C (36° to 46° F) or stored at RT for up to 24 hours. Fully diluted solutions for infusion using 0.45 NS may be refrigerated at 2° to 8° C (36° to 46° F) for up to 24 hours or stored at RT for up to 4 hours. Protect from light. Discard unused solution.

COMPATIBILITY
Manufacturer states, "Fully diluted solutions are **compatible** with polypropylene, polyethylene, and polyvinyl chloride infusion bags and with polypropylene, polyethylene, and glass infusion bottles. Tocilizumab should not be infused concomitantly in the same intravenous line with other drugs."

RATE OF ADMINISTRATION
A single dose as an infusion equally distributed over 60 minutes. Do not administer as an IV push or bolus.

ACTIONS
A recombinant humanized antihuman interleukin 6 (IL-6) receptor monoclonal antibody. Binds specifically to both soluble and membrane-bound IL-6 receptors. Inhibits IL-6–mediated signaling through these receptors. IL-6 is a pro-inflammatory cytokine produced by a variety of cell types. IL-6 is also produced by synovial and endothelial cells leading to local production of IL-6 in joints affected by inflammatory processes such as rheumatoid arthritis. IL-6 has been shown to be involved in diverse physiologic processes such as T-cell activation, induction of immunoglobulin secretion, initiation of hepatic acute-phase protein synthesis, and stimulation of hematopoietic precursor cell proliferation and differentiation. Following administration, increases in hemoglobin and decreases in C-reactive protein, rheumatoid factor, erythrocyte sedimentation rate, and serum amyloid A were observed. ANC counts decreased to the nadir 3 to 5 days after administration, and neutrophils recovered toward baseline in a dose-dependent manner. Half-life is concentration dependent and ranges from 11 to 13 days in adults depending on the dose administered. Half-life in pediatric patients ranges from 16 to 17 days.

INDICATIONS AND USES
Treatment of adults with moderately to severely active rheumatoid arthritis who have had an inadequate response to one or more disease-modifying antirheumatic drugs (DMARDs), such as methotrexate, and biologics (e.g., adalimumab, etanercept, infliximab, rituximab). ■ Treatment of patients 2 years of age and older with active polyarticular juvenile idiopathic arthritis (PJIA). ■ Treatment of patients 2 years of age and older with active systemic juvenile idiopathic arthritis (SJIA). ■ Treatment of adult and pediatric patients 2 years of age and older with chimeric antigen receptor (CAR), T-cell–induced, severe or life-threatening cytokine release syndrome. ■ Subcutaneous administration is approved for treatment of adult patients with giant cell arteritis (GCA).

CONTRAINDICATIONS
Known hypersensitivity to tocilizumab.

PRECAUTIONS
Administered under the direction of a physician knowledgeable in its use in a facility with adequate diagnostic and treatment facilities to monitor the patients and respond to any medical emergency. ■ Patients treated with tocilizumab are at increased risk for serious and sometimes fatal infections. Patients were often taking concomitant immunosuppressants such as methotrexate or corticosteroids, which may have predisposed them to infection. The most common serious infections included bacterial arthritis, cellulitis, diverticulitis, gastroenteritis, herpes zoster, pneumonia, sepsis, and UTIs. Reported infections include active tuberculosis (which may present with pulmonary or extrapulmonary disease), invasive fungal infections (e.g., aspergillosis, candidiasis, cryptococcus, pneumocystosis, which may present with disseminated rather than localized disease), and bacterial, viral, and other infections caused by opportunistic pathogens. ■ Do not administer tocilizumab to patients with an active infection, including localized infections. Assess the risks and benefits of tocilizumab before initiating in patients with chronic or recurrent infection, patients who have been exposed to tuberculosis, patients with a history of a serious or an opportunistic infection, patients who have resided or traveled in areas of

endemic tuberculosis or endemic mycoses, or patients with underlying conditions that may predispose them to infection. ▪ Evaluate patients for TB risk factors and latent TB before initiating therapy; see Monitor. ▪ Viral reactivation has been reported with immunosuppressive biologic therapies. Cases of herpes zoster exacerbation have been reported with tocilizumab. Cases of hepatitis B reactivation have not been reported, but patients who screened positive for hepatitis were excluded from studies. ▪ Serious cases of hepatic injury have been observed. Some of these cases have resulted in liver transplant and death. Time to onset ranged from months to years after treatment initiation. ▪ Has not been studied in patients with active hepatic disease or hepatic impairment, including patients with positive HBV (hepatitis B virus) or HCV (hepatitis C virus) serology. Use is not recommended. ▪ Has not been studied in patients with severe renal impairment. ▪ Use caution in patients who may be at risk for GI perforation (e.g., diverticulitis) and in patients with pre-existing or recent-onset demyelinating disorders (e.g., multiple sclerosis, chronic inflammatory demyelinating polyneuropathy). ▪ Hypersensitivity reactions, including anaphylaxis and death, have been reported. Emergency medical equipment and medications for treating these reactions must be readily available. ▪ Tocilizumab is associated with a higher incidence of neutropenia and elevated transaminases, a reduction in platelet counts, and increases in lipids; see Monitor and Dose Adjustments. ▪ Infusion-related reactions have occurred; see Side Effects. ▪ As with all therapeutic proteins, there is the potential for immunogenicity. ▪ Treatment may result in an increased risk of malignancy. ▪ Do not administer live virus vaccines. All patients, especially PJIA and SJIA patients and elderly patients, should be brought up-to-date with immunizations before beginning therapy. ▪ Patients with severe or life-threatening CRS often have cytopenias or elevated ALT or AST resulting from lymphodepleting chemotherapy or the CRS. The decision to administer should take into account the potential benefit of treating the CRS versus the risk of short-term treatment; see Usual Dose/Pretreatment.

Monitor: Evaluate patients for TB risk factors and latent TB with a TB skin test before tocilizumab use and during therapy. Patients testing positive in TB screening should be treated with a standard TB regimen before initiating therapy with tocilizumab. Consider treatment in patients with a history of latent or active TB when an adequate course of treatment cannot be confirmed and in patients who have a negative test for latent TB but have risk factors for TB. Consultation with a specialist in TB diagnosis and treatment is encouraged. Closely monitor all patients for S/S of tuberculosis. May present with pulmonary or extrapulmonary disease. ▪ Screening for viral hepatitis may be indicated. ▪ In RA patients, obtain baseline CBC, platelets, and liver function tests (e.g., ALT, AST, alkaline phosphatase, total bilirubin). ▪ Monitor neutrophils and platelets 4 to 8 weeks after start of therapy and then every 3 months thereafter; see Dose Adjustments. ▪ Monitor liver function tests every 4 to 8 weeks after start of therapy for the first 6 months and then every 3 months thereafter. Initiating therapy in patients with elevated transaminases ALT or AST greater than 1.5 times the ULN is not recommended; see Dose Adjustment. ▪ Measure liver function tests promptly in patients who report symptoms that may indicate liver injury (e.g., anorexia, dark urine, fatigue, jaundice, right upper abdominal discomfort). Interrupt therapy if liver function tests are abnormal. Tocilizumab should be restarted only in patients with another explanation for liver test abnormalities and after normalization of liver tests. ▪ In PJIA and SJIA patients, obtain baseline CBC, platelets, and liver function tests. Monitor neutrophils, platelets, ALT, and AST before the second infusion and every 4 to 8 weeks for PJIA and every 2 to 4 weeks for SJIA. ▪ In RA, PJIA, and SJIA patients, obtain baseline lipid studies (e.g., cholesterol [HDL, LDL, and total], triglycerides). Repeat in 4 to 8 weeks. Manage patients according to clinical guidelines for management of hyperlipidemia. ▪ Closely monitor for S/S of infection during and after treatment with tocilizumab; S/S may be lessened due to suppression of the acute-phase reactants. Hold tocilizumab if a serious infection, an opportunistic infection, or sepsis develops, and appropriate evaluation and treatment should be initiated promptly. ▪ Monitor for S/S of hypersensitivity or infusion-related reactions (e.g., anaphylaxis, generalized erythema, hypotension, pruritus, rash, urticaria, or wheezing); most hypersensitivity reactions have occurred between the second and fourth infusion but can occur at any time, even if they have not occurred with earlier infusions. Have occurred in patients who received premedication; see Side Effects. ▪ Monitor for S/S of GI perforation (e.g., new-onset abdominal pain). ▪ Monitor for S/S potentially indicative of demyelinating disorders. ▪ See Precautions and Drug/Lab Interactions.

Patient Education: Read FDA-approved medication guide before starting therapy. ▪ Promptly report S/S of an allergic reaction (e.g., rash, itching, wheezing), infusion reaction (e.g., dizziness, headache), or infection (e.g., chill, cough, with or without a fever). Report severe, persistent abdominal pain promptly. ▪ Discuss previous infections, current infections, or exposure to TB. ▪ May cause fetal harm. Report suspected or known pregnancy. Pregnancy registry has been established. ▪ Routine laboratory monitoring required. ▪ All vaccinations should be brought up-to-date before starting tocilizumab.

Maternal/Child: Use during pregnancy only if the potential benefit justifies the potential risk to the fetus. Monoclonal antibodies are increasingly transported across the placenta as pregnancy progresses, with the largest amount transferred during the third trimester. ▪ A pregnancy registry has been established; contact manufacturer. ▪ Consider risk versus benefit with breast-feeding. ▪ Safety and effectiveness have been established for use only in pediatric patients 2 years of age or older with SJIA, PJIA, and CRS. ▪ Risks and benefits should be considered before administering live or live-attenuated vaccines to infants exposed to tocilizumab in utero.

Elderly: Incidence of infection is higher in elderly patients. Clinical studies for CRS did not include sufficient numbers of patients 65 years of age and older to determine whether they respond differently from younger patients. Use caution; see Precautions.

DRUG/LAB INTERACTIONS

Formal drug interaction studies have not been conducted. ▪ Avoid concurrent use with **biological DMARDS** such as TNF antagonists (e.g., adalimumab, etanercept, infliximab), IL-1R antagonists, anti-CD20 monoclonal antibodies, and selective costimulation modulators; may increase immunosuppression and risk of infection. ▪ Increased frequency and magnitude of LFT elevations may be seen when tocilizumab is coadministered with other potentially **hepatotoxic medications** (e.g., methotrexate). ▪ Inhibition of IL-6 signaling in patients treated with tocilizumab may restore CYP450 activities to higher levels, resulting in an increased metabolism of drugs that are CYP450 substrates. Concurrent use showed an increase in metabolism and lower serum concentrations of **omeprazole** and **simvastatin**. This effect may be clinically relevant with CYP450 substrates with a narrow therapeutic index, in which the dose is individually adjusted (e.g., **warfarin, cyclosporine, theophylline**). Therapeutic monitoring of effect (INR) and/or serum concentrations is indicated to adjust the dose of these drugs with initiation or termination of tocilizumab. Use caution with CYP3A4 substrate drugs in which a decrease in effectiveness is undesirable (e.g., **atorvastatin, oral contraceptives**). The effect of tocilizumab on CYP450 enzyme activity may persist for several weeks after therapy is discontinued. ▪ Do not administer **live virus vaccines**.

SIDE EFFECTS

RA: The most common adverse reactions include headache, hypertension, increased ALT, injection site reactions, nasopharyngitis, and upper respiratory tract infections. The most common serious infections include bacterial arthritis, cellulitis, diverticulitis, gastroenteritis, herpes zoster, pneumonia, sepsis, and UTIs. The most common side effects that required discontinuation of therapy were increased hepatic transaminase values and serious infections. Infusion-related reactions have been reported. Hypertension frequently occurred during infusion, and headache and skin reactions (e.g., pruritus, rash, urticaria) were reported within the next 24 hours. Hypersensitivity reactions (e.g., anaphylactoid and anaphylactic) did occur in a few patients. Other side effects reported include bronchitis, conjunctivitis, cough, dizziness, dyspnea, elevated lipids, gastric ulcer, gastritis, GI perforation (seen primarily in patients taking concomitant NSAIDs, corticosteroids, or methotrexate), hypothyroidism, increased total bilirubin, increased weight, leukopenia, mouth ulceration, nephrolithiasis, neutropenia, oral herpes simplex, peripheral edema, stomatitis, thrombocytopenia, and upper abdominal pain.

PJIA: Side effects consistent with those seen in RA and SJIA patients.

SJIA: The most common adverse reactions included diarrhea, headache, nasopharyngitis, and upper respiratory tract infections. Anaphylaxis, decreased platelet count, development of anti-tocilizumab antibodies, increased liver function tests and lipids, infections, infusion reactions, macrophage activation syndrome (MAS), and neutropenia have been reported.

CRS: No adverse reactions related to tocilizumab were reported in a retrospective analysis.

Post-Marketing: Drug-induced liver injury, fatal anaphylaxis, hepatitis, hepatic failure, jaundice, pancreatitis, Stevens-Johnson syndrome.

ANTIDOTE

Notify physician of any side effects; most will be treated symptomatically. During clinical studies, most infusion-related reactions were mild to moderate. Interrupt therapy for decreases in ANC and platelets and increases in liver function studies as outlined in Dose Adjustments. Therapy may need to be interrupted in patients who develop infections. Discontinue tocilizumab for any serious reaction or infection. Treat infusion and hypersensitivity reactions as indicated (e.g., oxygen, diphenhydramine, epinephrine, corticosteroids, vasopressors, and/or fluids). Resuscitate as necessary.

TOPOTECAN HYDROCHLORIDE BBW

(toh-poh-**TEE**-kan hy-droh-**KLOR**-eyed)

Hycamtin

Antineoplastic
(topoisomerase I inhibitor)

pH 2.5 to 3.5

USUAL DOSE

Pretreatment: Verify pregnancy status. Baseline studies indicated; see Monitor.

Verify dose using body surface area before dispensing. Recommended dose should generally not exceed 4 mg IV. Before giving the initial dose, the baseline neutrophil count must be at least 1,500/mm^3 and baseline platelet count must be at least 100,000/mm^3.

Ovarian cancer and small-cell lung cancer: 1.5 mg/M^2 as an infusion each day for 5 consecutive days (Days 1 through 5 of a 21-day course). Begin the second course on Day 22. See Dose Adjustments.

Cervical cancer: 0.75 mg/M^2 as an infusion on Days 1, 2, and 3. On Day 1 follow with cisplatin 50 mg/M^2. Repeat every 21 days. See cisplatin monograph for prehydration requirements.

Non–small-cell lung cancer (unlabeled): 1.5 mg/M^2 as an infusion each day for 5 consecutive days. Repeat every 21 days.

DOSE ADJUSTMENTS

Do not begin subsequent courses of topotecan until neutrophils recover to more than 1,000/mm^3, platelets recover to 100,000/mm^3, and hemoglobin recovers to 9 mg/dL (with transfusion if necessary). ■ **For single-agent use,** reduce dose to 1.25 mg/M^2 for (1) neutrophil counts less than 500 cells/mm^3, or administer granulocyte-colony stimulating factor (G-CSF) starting no sooner than 24 hours after the last dose of topotecan; or (2) platelet counts less than 25,000 cells/mm^3 during the previous cycle. ■ **For combination use with cisplatin,** reduce dose to 0.6 mg/M^2 (and further to 0.45 mg/M^2 if necessary) for (1) febrile neutropenia (defined as neutrophil counts less than 1,000 cells/mm^3 with temperature greater than or equal to 38° C [100.4° F]), or administer G-CSF starting no sooner than 24 hours after the last dose of topotecan; or (2) platelet counts less than 25,000 cells/mm^3 during the previous cycle. See cisplatin monograph for specific dose adjustments. ■ **For single-agent use,** reduce dose to 0.75 mg/M^2 in patients with moderate impaired renal function (CrCl 20 to 39 mL/min). There are inadequate data at this time to recommend a dose in severe renal impairment. ■ Dose adjustment may be required in the elderly because of age-related renal impairment.

DILUTION

Specific techniques required; see Precautions. Available as a 4-mg lyophilized powder in a single-dose vial. Reconstitute each 4-mg vial with 4 mL of SWFI (1 mg/mL). Also available as a generic in a 4 mg/4 mL solution in a single-use vial. Withdraw the calculated dose and further dilute in NS or D5W.

Filters: No data available from manufacturer.

Storage: *Hycamtin:* Store unopened vials in cartons protected from light between 20° and 25° C (68° and 77° F). Reconstituted solutions contain no preservative; use immediately. Solutions diluted for infusion are stable at room temperature in soft light for 24 hours. *Generic:* Store unopened vials in cartons protected from light and refrigerated between 2° and 8° C (36° and 46° F). Solutions diluted for infusion are stable for no more than 4 hours at RT or for 12 hours if refrigerated.

COMPATIBILITY

Compatibility information not available from manufacturer. Other sources suggest specific **compatibilities** dependent on concentration and manufacturer; consult a pharmacist.

RATE OF ADMINISTRATION

A single dose as an infusion evenly distributed over 30 minutes.

ACTIONS

A class of antineoplastic agent that inhibits the enzyme topoisomerase I required for DNA replication. It is a semi-synthetic derivative of camptothecin. Causes cell death by damaging DNA produced during the S-phase of the cell cycle. Undergoes pH-dependent hydrolysis in plasma, and minor additional metabolism occurs in the liver. Terminal half-life is 2 to 3 hours. Moderately bound to plasma protein (35%). Excreted in urine and, to a lesser extent, in feces.

INDICATIONS AND USES

As a single agent for treatment of patients with metastatic carcinoma of the ovary after disease progression on or after initial or subsequent chemotherapy. ▪ As a single agent for treatment of patients with small-cell lung cancer with platinum-sensitive disease who progressed at least 60 days after initiation of first-line chemotherapy. ▪ In combination with cisplatin for treatment of patients with stage IV-B, recurrent, or persistent carcinoma of the cervix not amenable to curative treatment.

Unlabeled uses: Treatment of non–small-cell lung cancer.

CONTRAINDICATIONS

History of severe hypersensitivity reactions to topotecan.

PRECAUTIONS

Follow guidelines for handling cytotoxic agents. See Appendix A, p. 1308. ▪ Administered by or under the direction of the physician specialist. ▪ Adequate diagnostic and treatment facilities must be available to meet any medical emergency. ▪ May cause severe myelosuppression. Bone marrow suppression (primarily neutropenia) is the dose-limiting toxicity. Severe myelotoxicity has been reported when topotecan is administered in combination with cisplatin. Anemia, neutropenia, febrile neutropenia, pancytopenia, and thrombocytopenia have been reported; see Monitor. ▪ Use with caution in impaired renal function; clearance decreased. ▪ Neutropenic enterocolitis (typhlitis) has been reported. Fatalities have occurred; see Monitor. ▪ Interstitial lung disease (ILD), including fatalities, has occurred; risk increased in patients with a history of ILD, lung cancer, pulmonary fibrosis, thoracic irradiation, and the use of pneumotoxic drugs and/or colony-stimulating factors; see Monitor.

Monitor: Baseline neutrophil count must be at least 1,500/mm³ and platelets at least 100,000/mm³ before the initial dose. ▪ Obtain a baseline CBC with differential and platelets. ▪ Monitor before each course and frequently during treatment. Platelet count must be 100,000/mm³, neutrophils 1,000/mm³, and hemoglobin 9 mg/dL before a course of therapy can be repeated. Anemia is frequent and transfusion is often indicated. ▪ Baseline CrCl and BUN suggested. ▪ Monitor vital signs. ▪ Maintain adequate hydration. ▪ Nausea and vomiting can be frequent and may be severe; use prophylactic administration of antiemetics to increase patient comfort. ▪ Observe closely for S/S of infection. Prophylactic antibiotics may be indicated pending results of C/S in a febrile neutropenic patient. ▪ Not a vesicant, but monitor injection site for inflammation and/or extravasation. Severe cases have been reported. If S/S of extravasation occur, discontinue infusion and manage as indicated. ▪ Monitor for S/S of ILD (e.g., cough, dyspnea, fever, and/or hypoxia). ▪ Monitor for signs of neutropenic colitis (e.g., fever, neutropenia, and abdominal pain). ▪ Monitor for thrombocytopenia (platelet count less than 50,000/mm³). Platelet transfusions may be required. Initiate precautions to prevent excessive bleeding (e.g., inspect IV sites, skin, and mucous membranes; use extreme care during invasive procedures; test urine, emesis, stool, and secretions for occult blood).

Patient Education: Females should use effective contraception during treatment and for at least 1 month after the last dose of topotecan. ▪ May damage spermatozoa. Males with a female sexual partner of reproductive potential should use effective contraception during and for 3 months after treatment with topotecan. ▪ Potential risk for impaired fertility in both male and female patients. Discuss family planning options if appropriate. ▪ Report any unusual or unexpected symptoms or side effects as soon as possible (e.g., signs of infection [e.g., chills, fever, night sweats] or signs of bleeding [e.g., bruising, black tarry stools]). ▪ May cause loss of strength or fatigue. Use caution when driving or operating machinery. ▪ See Appendix D, p. 1311.

Maternal/Child: Avoid pregnancy; can cause fetal harm; see Patient Education. ▪ Discontinue breast-feeding. ▪ Safety and effectiveness for use in pediatric patients not established.

Elderly: Safety and effectiveness similar to younger adults. ▪ Consider age-related renal impairment; see Dose Adjustments. Monitoring of renal function may be useful.

DRUG/LAB INTERACTIONS

May cause severe prolonged myelosuppression and Grade 3 or 4 nonhematologic effects (e.g., diarrhea, lethargy, nausea, vomiting) with **cisplatin.** ▪ Concurrent administration of **G-CSF (filgrastim)** can prolong the duration of neutropenia. If used, do not administer until at least 24 hours after the final dose of topotecan. ▪ Concurrent or consecutive administration of **other bone marrow suppressants** (e.g., cyclophosphamide, paclitaxel) **or radiation therapy** may produce additive bone marrow suppression. Dose reduction may be required based on blood cell counts. ▪ Concurrent use with **hydantoins** (e.g., phenytoin) may decrease plasma concentrations of topotecan. Specific guidelines for topotecan dose adjustment are not available. Consider alternatives to phenytoin when possible. ▪ Do not administer **palifermin** within 24 hours before or after topotecan; coadministration may increase the severity and duration of oral mucositis. ▪ Do not administer **live virus vaccines.**

SIDE EFFECTS

Bone marrow suppression, primarily neutropenia, is the dose-limiting toxicity of topotecan.

Ovarian cancer: The most common hematologic adverse reactions were anemia (Grade 3 and 4), febrile neutropenia, neutropenia (Grade 4), and thrombocytopenia (Grade 4). The most common nonhematologic adverse reactions were diarrhea, dyspnea, fatigue, nausea, and vomiting. Other reported reactions included abdominal pain, asthenia, constipation, elevated bilirubin and hepatic enzymes, intestinal obstruction, pain, and sepsis.

Small-cell lung cancer: The most common hematologic adverse reactions were anemia (Grade 3 and 4), febrile neutropenia, neutropenia (Grade 4), and thrombocytopenia (Grade 4). The most common nonhematologic adverse reactions were abdominal pain, asthenia, dyspnea, fatigue, nausea, and pneumonia. Other reported reactions included elevated bilirubin and hepatic enzymes, pain, and sepsis.

Cervical cancer: The most common hematologic adverse reactions were anemia (Grade 3 and 4), neutropenia (Grade 3 and 4), and thrombocytopenia (Grade 3 and 4). The most common nonhematologic adverse reactions were infection/febrile neutropenia, pain, and vomiting. Other reported reactions included asthenia, chills, fatigue, fever, lethargy, malaise, rigors, stomatitis-pharyngitis, sweating, and weight gain or loss.

Post-Marketing: Abdominal pain associated with neutropenic enterocolitis, extravasation, hypersensitivity reactions (including anaphylaxis), interstitial lung disease, severe bleeding, skin and subcutaneous tissue disorders (e.g., angioedema, severe dermatitis, severe pruritus).

ANTIDOTE

Keep physician informed of all side effects. Withhold topotecan until myelosuppression has improved to minimum requirements. Neutropenia recovery may be aided by G-CSF (filgrastim, pegfilgrastim) under specific conditions; see Dose Adjustments or Drug/Lab Interactions. Anemia often required RBC or whole blood transfusions. Thrombocytopenia may require platelet transfusion. Death can result from the progression of many side effects. Discontinue topotecan if a new diagnosis of ILD is confirmed. No known antidote for overdose. If an overdose is suspected, monitor for bone marrow suppression and institute supportive care measures (e.g., prophylactic G-CSF and antibiotic therapy) as appropriate. Treat hypersensitivity reactions with oxygen, epinephrine, corticosteroids, and antihistamines.

TRANEXAMIC ACID
(**TRAN**-eks-am-ik **AS**-id)

Cyklokapron

Antifibrinolytic
Antihemorrhagic

pH 6.5 to 8

USUAL DOSE
Dental extraction in adults and pediatric patients with hemophilia: *Preoperative:* Normal renal function required. 10 mg/kg IV immediately before surgery. *Postoperative:* 10 mg/kg IV every 6 to 8 hours for 2 to 8 days.

Trauma-associated hemorrhage (unlabeled): A loading dose of 1,000 mg IV over 10 minutes followed by an infusion of 1,000 mg over 8 hours. Treatment should begin within 8 hours of injury.

Surgery, blood loss reduction (unlabeled): Several regimens have been studied and include: 10-30 mg/kg depending on type of surgery. mg/kg IV over 30 minutes

DOSE ADJUSTMENTS
Lower-end initial and/or reduced doses may be indicated in the elderly based on the potential for decreased organ function and concomitant disease or drug therapy.
- Reduce dose in impaired renal function according to the following chart.

Tranexamic Dose Guidelines in Impaired Renal Function	
Serum Creatinine (mg/dL)	**Dose**
1.36-2.83 mg/dL	10 mg/kg two times per day
2.83-5.66 mg/dL	10 mg/kg once per day
>5.66 mg/dL	10 mg/kg every 48 hours or 5 mg/kg every 24 hours

DILUTION
100 mg equals 1 mL of prepared solution. Further dilute a single dose with at least 50 mL **compatible** infusion solutions (e.g., NS, dextrose solutions in water or various concentrations of NS); see Compatibility. Prepare solution immediately before use; discard any unused solution.

Storage: Store ampules at CRT. Prepare the same day it is to be administered.

COMPATIBILITY
Do not mix with blood and do not mix with solutions containing penicillins. See Drug/Lab Interactions.

Solutions: May be mixed with IV solutions, including solutions containing electrolytes, carbohydrates, amino acids, or dextran.

Additive: Compatible with heparin.

RATE OF ADMINISTRATION
100 mg/min over 5 minutes. Too-rapid infusion may cause hypotension.

ACTIONS
An inhibitor of fibrinolysis. Inhibits plasminogen activation and, at higher concentrations, inhibits plasmin. About 10 times more potent than aminocaproic acid. Onset of

action is prompt. Half-life approximately 2 hours. Excreted in urine primarily as unchanged drug. Crosses the placental barrier. Secreted in breast milk.

INDICATIONS AND USES

Reduce or prevent hemorrhage and reduce the need for replacement therapy in hemophilia patients during and following tooth extraction.

Unlabeled uses: Trauma-associated hemorrhage, prevention of perioperative bleeding associated with cardiac surgery and spinal surgery, reduction of blood loss associated with orthopedic surgery or cesarean section.

CONTRAINDICATIONS

Acquired defective color vision, active intravascular clotting, subarachnoid hemorrhage, and hypersensitivity to tranexamic acid or its ingredients.

PRECAUTIONS

For short-term use only (2 to 8 days). ▪ Focal areas of retinal degeneration have been seen in animals, and visual abnormalities have been noted in post-marketing reports; see Monitor. ▪ Rapid administration in any form may cause hypotension. ▪ Whole blood transfusions may be given if necessary but must be given through a second infusion site. ▪ In patients with upper urinary tract bleeding, ureteral obstruction due to clot formation has been reported. ▪ Risk of venous or arterial thrombosis increased in patients with a previous history of thromboembolic disease. ▪ Thromboembolic events (e.g., central retinal artery and vein obstruction, cerebral thrombosis, deep vein thrombosis, pulmonary embolism) have been reported rarely in patients receiving tranexamic acid for indications other than hemorrhage prevention in patients with hemophilia. ▪ Patients with DIC being treated with tranexamic acid require the strict supervision of a physician specialist. ▪ Convulsions have been reported with tranexamic acid treatment. ▪ See Compatibility and Drug/Lab Interactions.

Monitor: Use only in conjunction with general and specific tests to determine the amount of fibrinolysis present. ▪ In repeated treatment or if treatment will last more than several (2 to 3) days, a complete ophthalmologic examination (visual acuity, color vision, eyeground, visual fields) should be done before and at regular intervals during treatment. Discontinue use if changes are found.

Patient Education: May produce dizziness; request assistance with ambulation and use caution performing tasks that require alertness (e.g., driving or operating machinery).

Maternal/Child: Category B: use caution and only if clearly needed in pregnancy and breast-feeding. ▪ Use in pediatric patients has been limited. Available data suggest that the mg/kg dose for adults can be used.

Elderly: Lower-end initial or reduced doses may be indicated; see Dose Adjustments. ▪ Monitoring of renal function suggested.

DRUG/LAB INTERACTIONS

No formal Drug Interaction studies between tranexamic acid and other drugs have been conducted. ▪ Concomitant use with **factor IX complex** (e.g., AlphaNine SD, Mononine, Konyne) or **anti-inhibitor coagulant concentrates** (e.g., Feiba) is not recommended; may increase the risk for venous or arterial thrombosis.

SIDE EFFECTS

Allergic dermatitis, diarrhea, giddiness, hypotension, nausea and vomiting. Thromboembolic events (e.g., central retinal artery and vein obstruction, cerebral thrombosis, deep vein thrombosis, pulmonary embolism) have been reported rarely.

Post-Marketing: Chromatopsia and visual impairment, convulsions, and thromboembolic events as above have been reported.

ANTIDOTE

All side effects may subside with reduced dosage or rate of administration. Discontinue use of drug if any changes are found during follow-up ophthalmologic examinations. Resuscitate as necessary.

TRASTUZUMAB BBW ▪
TRASTUZUMAB-dkst[a] BBW ▪
TRASTUZUMAB-dttb[a] BBW ▪
TRASTUZUMAB-pkrb[a] BBW ▪
TRASTUZUMAB-anns[a] BBW ▪
TRASTUZUMAB-qyyp[a] BBW

(traz-**TOO**-zah-mab)

Monoclonal antibody
Antineoplastic

Herceptin, Ogivri[a], Ontruzant[a], Herzuma[a], Kanjinti[a], Trazimera[a]

pH 6

USUAL DOSE

Trastuzumab-dkst (Ogivri)[a], trastuzumab-pkrb (Herzuma)[a], trastuzumab-dttb (Ontruzant)[a], trastuzumab-anns (Kanjinti)[a], and trastuzumab-qyyp (Trazimera)[a] are biosimilar drugs of trastuzumab (Herceptin). Unless specifically stated otherwise, monograph information and the use of the name *trastuzumab* or *trastuzumab product(s)* applies to all six formulations.

DO NOT substitute trastuzumab products for or with ado-trastuzumab emtansine.

Pretreatment: Verify pregnancy status. Preassessment required to determine appropriate patient selection, and baseline studies indicated; see Precautions and Monitor.

Premedication: Pretreatment with antihistamines (e.g., diphenhydramine) and/or corticosteroids (e.g., dexamethasone) may be indicated and is suggested for patients being retreated after a hypersensitivity reaction or a severe infusion reaction; see Precautions. Pretreatment may not be successful; hypersensitivity reaction and/or infusion reaction may recur. Combination therapies may require additional premedication; refer to product monographs.

Adjuvant treatment of breast cancer: Administer according to one of the following dose regimens and schedules for a total of 52 weeks of trastuzumab therapy (extending adjuvant treatment beyond 1 year is not recommended):

1. *During and following paclitaxel, docetaxel, or docetaxel/carboplatin:* Administer an initial dose of *trastuzumab* 4 mg/kg as an infusion over 90 minutes. Follow with a dose of 2 mg/kg as an infusion over 30 minutes at weekly intervals for the first 12 weeks when given in combination with *paclitaxel or docetaxel* or for 18 weeks when given in combination with *docetaxel/carboplatin.* Beginning 1 week after the last 2-mg/kg weekly dose of *trastuzumab,* administer *trastuzumab* 6 mg/kg as an infusion over 30 to 90 minutes every 3 weeks.

2. *As a single agent within 3 weeks of completion of multimodality, anthracycline-based chemotherapy regimens,* administer an initial dose of *trastuzumab* 8 mg/kg as an infusion over 90 minutes. Follow with a dose of 6 mg/kg as an infusion over 30 to 90 minutes every 3 weeks.

3. See clinical studies in prescribing information for different treatment regimens used. In all studies, *trastuzumab* was initiated *after completion of the doxorubicin and cyclophosphamide treatment cycles.*

Metastatic breast cancer: *Initial dose:* 4 mg/kg as an infusion over 90 minutes. Follow with a *maintenance dose* of 2 mg/kg as an infusion over 30 minutes at weekly intervals. Trastuzumab is administered until tumor progression.

Metastatic breast cancer in combination therapy with paclitaxel: *Trastuzumab* dose as above. *Paclitaxel dose:* 175 mg/M^2 over 3 hours every 21 days for at least 6 cycles. See paclitaxel monograph.

Metastatic gastric cancer in combination with cisplatin and capecitabine or 5-fluorouracil: *Initial dose:* 8 mg/kg as an infusion over 90 minutes. Follow with a dose of 6 mg/kg as an

---

[a]Please see p. xi for more information on biosimilars.

infusion over 30 to 90 minutes every 3 weeks until disease progression. See individual monographs and/or prescribing information and specific protocol for doses of cisplatin andcapecitabine or 5-fluorouracil.

DOSE ADJUSTMENTS

Withhold trastuzumab dose for at least 4 weeks for either (1) equal to or greater than a 16% absolute decrease in left ventricular ejection fraction (LVEF) from baseline assessment, or (2) LVEF below institutional limits of normal and equal to or greater than 10% absolute decrease in LVEF from baseline assessment.

May resume trastuzumab if within 4 to 8 weeks the LVEF returns to normal limits and the absolute decrease from baseline is equal to or less than 15%. Discontinue permanently for a persistent (more than 8 weeks) LVEF decline or for suspension of trastuzumab dosing on more than three occasions for cardiomyopathy. ▪ See prescribing information for recommended actions if a dose is missed by either 1 week or less or by more than 1 week.

DILUTION

Check vial labels to ensure use of trastuzumab and **not** ado-trastuzumab emtansine.

420-mg multiple-dose vial (Herceptin, Ogivri, Herzuma, Kanjinti, and Trazimera): Manufacturers with the exception of Kanjinti supply a vial of bacteriostatic water for injection (BWFI) for dilution. Confirm content of vial; 20 mL is required to obtain the correct concentration. Inject diluent slowly directed at the lyophilized cake. Swirl gently; ***do not shake***. Allow vial to stand for 5 minutes; slight foaming is permissible. Will yield a multidose solution containing 21 mg/mL. Label vial immediately with a "do not use after" date 28 days from date of reconstitution. SWFI may be used to reconstitute trastuzumab for patients with a known hypersensitivity to benzyl alcohol, but the calculated dose must be withdrawn, used immediately, and the balance of the reconstituted solution discarded. Reconstituted solution must be further diluted and given as an infusion. Withdraw the calculated dose from the reconstituted vial (21 mg/mL) and add it to an infusion bag containing 250 mL of NS. Gently invert to mix the solution.

150-mg single-dose vial (Herceptin, Herzuma, Ogivri, and Ontruzant): Reconstitute each vial with 7.4 mL of SWFI (SWFI not supplied). Inject diluent slowly at the lyophilized cake. Swirl gently; ***do not shake***. Allow vial to stand for 5 minutes; slight foaming is permissible. Will yield a single-dose solution containing 21 mg/mL. Use immediately after reconstitution.

Filters: In-line filters are not necessary but may be used (0.2-micron filters were evaluated with ***Herceptin***).

Storage: Refrigerate unopened and reconstituted vials at 2° to 8° C (36° to 46° F). Vials reconstituted with supplied diluent are stable for 28 days after reconstitution. Discard remaining diluent. Discard reconstituted trastuzumab product after expiration date written or stamped on vial. Immediate use preferred if reconstituted with SWFI. However, it may be stored for up to 24 hours refrigerated at 2° to 8° C (36° to 46° F). Discard unused portion whether used immediately or refrigerated for up to 24 hours. Solutions diluted in NS, including those diluted in polyvinyl chloride or polyethylene bags, may be refrigerated for no more than 24 hours before use. This storage time is in addition to the time allowed for the reconstituted vials. Do not freeze reconstituted or diluted trastuzumab products. If needed, refrigerated and unopened 420 mg vials of Trazimera may be removed from the refrigerator and stored at RT up to 30° C (86° F) for a single period of up to 3 months in the original carton to protect from light. Once removed, do not return to the refrigerator, and discard after 3 months or by the expiration date stamped on the vial, whichever occurs first. Write the revised expiration date in the space provided on the carton labeling.

COMPATIBILITY

Manufacturer states, "Do not reconstitute with drugs other than BWFI or SWFI. Further dilute infusion with NS. *Infusions should not be administered or mixed with dextrose solutions. Do not mix trastuzumab products with other drugs.*" Is **compatible** with polyethylene and polyvinylchloride infusion bags and tubing.

RATE OF ADMINISTRATION

For infusion only; do not administer as an IV push or bolus. Use of a microdrip (60 gtt/min) or other IV controller suggested. Decrease rate of infusion for mild or moderate infusion reactions.

Initial dose: A single dose as an infusion over a minimum of 90 minutes. Observe for chills, fever, or other infusion-associated symptoms; see Precautions/Monitor.

Maintenance dose: If the initial dose was well tolerated, administer a single dose as an infusion over 30 to 90 minutes (based on regimen; see Usual Dose).

ACTIONS

A recombinant DNA–derived humanized monoclonal antibody that selectively binds with high affinity to the extracellular domain of the human epidermal growth factor receptor 2 (HER2) protein. Inhibits proliferation and mediates an antibody-dependent cellular toxicity in cancer cells that overexpress the HER2 protein. Half-life increases and clearance decreases with increasing doses. May cross the placental barrier. May be secreted in breast milk.

INDICATIONS AND USES

Indicated for adjuvant treatment of breast cancer that is HER2-overexpressing, node-positive or node-negative (ER/PR-negative or with one high-risk feature). May be used as part of a treatment regimen that may consist of (1) doxorubicin (Adriamycin), cyclo-phosphamide (Cytoxan), and either paclitaxel (Taxol) or docetaxel (Taxotere); (2) part of a treatment regimen with docetaxel and carboplatin; or (3) a single agent following multimodal anthracycline-based therapy *(Herceptin, Ogivri, and Ontruzant only)*. ▪ As a single agent for treatment of patients with metastatic breast cancer whose tumors over-express the HER2 protein and who have received one or more chemotherapy regimens for their metastatic disease. ▪ In combination with paclitaxel (Taxol) for the first-line treatment of patients with metastatic breast cancer whose tumors overexpress the HER2 protein and who have not received chemotherapy for their metastatic disease. ▪ In com-bination with cisplatin and capecitabine (Xeloda) or 5-fluorouracil (5-FU) for treatment of patients with HER2-overexpressing metastatic gastric or gastroesophageal junction adenocarcinoma who have not received prior treatment for metastatic disease *(Herceptin, Ogivri, and Ontruzant only)*. ▪ Select patients for therapy based on an FDA-approved companion diagnostic for trastuzumab.

CONTRAINDICATIONS

None known when used as indicated; see Precautions.

PRECAUTIONS

Do not administer as an IV push or bolus. ▪ Trastuzumab should be used only in patients whose tumors have HER2 overexpression or HER2 gene amplification in tumor speci-mens. Tumor histology differs; use FDA-approved tests for specific tumor type (breast or gastric cancers) to assess HER2 overexpression and HER2 gene amplification. Must be performed in laboratories with demonstrated proficiency in the specific technology. ▪ Ad-ministered by or under the direction of the physician specialist. May be given on an out-patient basis. ▪ Adequate laboratory and supportive medical resources must be available. ▪ Emergency equipment and drugs for treatment of left ventricular dysfunction and/or infusion reactions must be immediately available; see Antidote. ▪ Use with caution in patients with known hypersensitivity to trastuzumab, Chinese hamster ovary cell proteins, benzyl alcohol, or any component of this product. ▪ Serious and fatal infusion reactions and pulmonary toxicity have been reported. Retreatment after full recovery from an infusion reac-tion has been tried following pretreatment with antihistamines and/or corticosteroids. Some tolerated treatment; others had another severe reaction. ▪ Can cause subclinical and clinical cardiac failure. Incidence of cardiac dysfunction was highest in patients who received trastuzumab with an anthracycline-containing chemotherapy regimen (e.g., doxorubicin [Adriamycin]) and in elderly patients; see Drug/Lab Interactions. ▪ Can cause left ventricular cardiac dysfunction, ar-rhythmias, hypertension, disabling cardiac failure, cardiomyopathy, and cardiac death. May also cause asymptomatic decline in left ventricular ejection fraction (LVEF). ▪ Use extreme caution in treating patients with pre-existing cardiac dysfunction or pulmonary compromise. Pre-existing cardiac disease or prior cardiotoxic therapy (e.g., anthracyclines), radiation therapy to the chest, or pre-existing pulmonary compromise secondary to intrinsic lung disease and/or malignant pulmonary involvement may decrease ability to tolerate trastuzumab. ■ May exacerbate chemotherapy-induced neutropenia.

Monitor: Select patients based on HER2 protein overexpression or HER2 gene amplification in tumor specimens. Assessment of HER2 protein overexpression and HER2 gene amplification should be performed using FDA-approved tests specific for breast or gastric cancers. Improper assay performance can lead to unreliable results. ■ Obtain baseline CBC with differential and platelet count and repeat as needed. ■ Monitor all vital signs before and during therapy. ■ Treatment with trastuzumab can result in the development of ventricular dysfunction and CHF. Evaluate left ventricular function before and during treatment. For all treatment regimens (monotherapy and/or combination therapies), patients should have a thorough baseline cardiac assessment, including a history and physical exam and determination of LVEF by an echocardiogram or a MUGA scan. Monitoring and assessment may not identify all patients at risk for developing cardiotoxicity. ■ Monitor closely throughout treatment for S/S of deteriorating cardiac function (e.g., cough, dyspnea, paroxysmal nocturnal dyspnea, peripheral edema, S_3 gallop, or reduced ejection fraction [symptomatic or asymptomatic]). Suggested monitoring schedule includes a repeat evaluation of left ventricular function (echocardiogram or MUGA scan) every 3 months during treatment with trastuzumab and at least every 6 months for 2 years after completion of treatment if trastuzumab was used as a component of adjuvant therapy. More frequent monitoring should be used for patients with pre-existing cardiac dysfunction and/or if S/S of deteriorating cardiac function develop; see Dose Adjustments. ■ Onset and clinical course of infusion reactions are variable. Most occur during or immediately following the infusion or within 24 hours. Monitor patient until symptoms completely resolve. Chills and/or fever occur in 40% of patients during the first infusion. May be treated with acetaminophen, diphenhydramine, and meperidine with or without reduction in the rate of infusion. During infusion, monitor closely; asthenia, bronchospasm, dizziness, dyspnea, headache, hypotension (may be severe), hypoxia, nausea, pain (may be at tumor site), rash, rigors, and vomiting have also occurred. ■ Monitor closely; in addition to the symptoms of infusion reaction previously noted, severe and sometimes fatal hypersensitivity reactions (e.g., anaphylaxis, angioedema, bronchospasm, hypotension, urticaria) and pulmonary reactions (e.g., dyspnea, interstitial pneumonitis, pulmonary infiltrates, pleural effusions, noncardiogenic pulmonary edema, pulmonary fibrosis, pulmonary insufficiency, hypoxia, and ARDS) have occurred during and after the infusion. ■ Monitor for thrombocytopenia (platelet count less than 50,000/mm³). Initiate precautions to prevent excessive bleeding (e.g., inspect IV sites, skin, and mucous membranes; use extreme care during invasive procedures; test urine, emesis, stool, and secretions for occult blood). ■ Not a vesicant; if extravasation occurs, discontinue infusion and restart using another vein.

Patient Education: During infusion, promptly report chills and/or fever and other S/S of infusion reaction. ■ Promptly report cough, difficulty breathing, weight gain, and swelling of extremities. ■ Avoid pregnancy; use effective contraception during treatment and for at least 7 months after the last dose of trastuzumab. ■ See Appendix D, p. 1311.

Maternal/Child: Avoid pregnancy. Verify pregnancy status of females of reproductive potential before initiating trastuzumab. Can cause fetal harm. Increases the risk for oligohydramnios and oligohydramnios sequence manifesting as pulmonary hypoplasia, skeletal abnormalities, and neonatal death. Pregnant females who receive *Herceptin* are encouraged to enroll in the MotHER Pregnancy Registry and to report the trastuzumab exposure to the manufacturer (Genentech). ■ There is no information on the presence of trastuzumab in human milk, the effects on the breast-fed infant, or the effects on milk production. Consider the developmental and health benefits of breast-feeding along with the mother's clinical need for trastuzumab treatment and any potential adverse effects on the breast-fed child from trastuzumab or from the underlying maternal condition. This consideration should also take into account the trastuzumab washout period of 7 months. ■ Safety and effectiveness for use in pediatric patients not established.

Elderly: Advanced age may increase the risk of cardiac dysfunction.

DRUG/LAB INTERACTIONS

No formal drug interaction studies have been done. Use with **paclitaxel** may decrease trastuzumab clearance and increase serum levels. Paclitaxel concentration is not affected. ■ The plasma concentration of capecitabine, carboplatin, cisplatin, docetaxel, doxorubicin, and paclitaxel was not altered when used in combination with trastuzumab. ■ Risk of cardiotoxicity increased with concurrent use or previous use of **anthracyclines** (e.g., doxorubicin). Patients who receive anthracycline after stopping trastuzumab may also be at increased risk for cardiac dysfunction. If possible, physicians should avoid anthracycline-based therapy for up to 7 months after stopping trastuzumab. If anthracyclines are used, carefully monitor the patient's cardiac function. ■ Bone marrow toxicity may be additive with **other antineoplastic agents** (e.g., anthracyclines, cyclophosphamide).

SIDE EFFECTS

Cardiomyopathy, pulmonary toxicity, infusion reactions, and exacerbation of chemotherapy-induced neutropenia are the most serious side effects. Anemia, chills, cough, diarrhea, dysgeusia, dyspnea, fatigue, fever, headache, infections, infusion reactions, insomnia, mucosal inflammation, myalgia, nasopharyngitis, nausea, neutropenia, rash, stomatitis, thrombocytopenia, upper respiratory tract infections, vomiting, and weight loss are most common. Side effects that cause interruption or discontinuation of therapy include severe infusion reactions, pulmonary toxicity, congestive heart failure, and a decline in left ventricular cardiac function. Abdominal pain, accidental injury, acne, anorexia, arthralgia, asthenia, back pain, bone pain, depression, dizziness, edema, flu syndrome, headache, herpes simplex, hypersensitivity reactions, hypotension, neuropathy, pain (may be at tumor site), paresthesia, peripheral edema, peripheral neuritis, pharyngitis, rash, rhinitis, sinusitis, and tachycardia have been reported in more than 5% of patients. Many other serious side effects have been reported in some patients (e.g., cardiac arrest, coagulation disorder, death, hypersensitivity reactions [e.g., angioedema, bronchospasm, dyspnea, urticaria, wheezing], hypertension, hypotension, noncardiogenic pulmonary edema, pancytopenia, pericardial or pleural effusion, pulmonary infiltrates, pulmonary insufficiency and hypoxemia requiring O_2 and/or ventilatory support, shock arrhythmia, syncope, vascular thrombosis).

Post-Marketing: Serious adverse events including hypersensitivity reactions and infusion reactions, including some with a fatal outcome; and pulmonary events including ARDS and death. Symptoms occurred most commonly during the infusion, but some occurred 24 hours or more after the infusion. Renal toxicity (glomerulopathy) and immune thrombocytopenia have also been reported. Cases of possible tumor lysis syndrome have been reported. Cases of oligohydramnios and oligohydramnios sequence manifesting as pulmonary hypoplasia, skeletal abnormalities, and neonatal death have been reported when trastuzumab has been administered to pregnant females.

ANTIDOTE

Notify physician of all side effects. Most will be treated symptomatically. Decrease rate of infusion for mild or moderate infusion reactions. Interrupt infusion if dyspnea or clinically significant hypotension occurs. Discontinue trastuzumab for severe or life-threatening infusion reactions. Discontinue infusion in patients who develop anaphylaxis, angioedema, ARDS, and interstitial pneumonitis. Discontinue trastuzumab in patients receiving adjuvant therapy, and withhold therapy in patients with metastatic disease for clinically significant decrease in left ventricular function; see Dose Adjustments. Safety of continuation or resumption of therapy has not been studied. Treatment may include diuretics, ACE inhibitors, inotropic agents, beta-blockers, and/or supplemental oxygen. Infusion reaction is treated with acetaminophen, diphenhydramine, and meperidine. Administration of whole blood products (e.g., packed RBCs, platelets, leukocytes) and/or blood modifiers (e.g., darbepoetin alfa, epoetin alfa, filgrastim, pegfilgrastim, sargramostim) may be indicated to treat bone marrow toxicity from concurrent antineoplastics. Treat hypersensitivity reactions (may be more frequent with coadministration of paclitaxel) with epinephrine, antihistamines, corticosteroids, bronchodilators, and oxygen. To treat extravasation, apply cold compresses and elevate extremity. Resuscitate as indicated.

TRILACICLIB
(**TRY**-la-**SYE**-klib)

Cosela

Antineoplastic
Cyclin-dependent kinase inhibitor

USUAL DOSE
240 mg/M^2/dose IV. Given prior to a platinum/etoposide or topotecan-based chemotherapy; should be completed within 4 hours before the start of chemotherapy.

PEDIATRIC DOSE
Safety and efficacy have not been established.

DOSE ADJUSTMENTS
Renal: No dosage adjustments provided by manufacturer.

Hepatic: Do not use in moderate or severe impairment (total bilirubin >1.5 times the ULN).

See prescribing information for dose modifications based on side effects.

DILUTION
Reconstitute each vial with 19.5 mL of D5W or NS to a concentration of 15 mg/mL. Swirl the vial gently for up to 3 minutes until completely dissolved; ***do not shake***. Reconstituted solution should be yellow or clear; do not use if solution is cloudy, discolored, or contains particulates. Withdraw appropriate dose volume and dilute in infusion bag of NS or D5W. Final concentration of diluted solution should be 0.5 to 3 mg/mL. Invert infusion bag gently; ***do not shake***.

COMPATIBILITY
Do not administer simultaneously with any other medication or IV solutions other than NS or D5W.

RATE OF ADMINISTRATION
Administer as an IV infusion over 30 minutes and complete infusion within 4 hours before start of chemotherapy. Flush the infusion line with at least 20 mL of D5W or NS after completing infusion. Give with an infusion set that has an in-line 0.2- or 0.22-micron filter.

ACTIONS
Selective and reversible cyclin-dependent kinase 4 and 6 inhibitor (CDK4/6). Through this inhibition, it prevents cells from proliferating in the presence of chemotherapy, thus leading to myelopreservation.

INDICATIONS AND USES
Chemotherapy-induced myelosuppression.

CONTRAINDICATIONS
Hypersensitivity (anaphylaxis) to trilaciclib or any component of the formulation.

PRECAUTIONS
Infusion-related reactions: Infusion-site reactions, including thrombophlebitis and phlebitis, have been reported.

Pulmonary toxicity: Severe, life-threatening, or fatal interstitial lung disease/pneumonitis have been reported.

Hypersensitivity: Acute hypersensitivity reactions, including anaphylaxis, facial edema, and urticaria, have been reported.

Monitor: Monitor for S/S of infusion site reactions, thrombophlebitis, phlebitis, and signs of acute drug hypersensitivity reactions (edema of face, eye, tongue; urticaria; pruritus; anaphylaxis) and pulmonary symptoms.

Patient Education: Advise patients to call physician if they experience headache, stomachache, or weakness that gets worse. Educate patients on signs of hypersensitivity reactions (rash; hives; red, blistered, swollen skin; chest tightness; wheezing; trouble breathing or swallowing; hoarseness; swelling of face, lips, mouth, tongue, or throat).

Maternal/Child: Check pregnancy status prior to use. Advise patient to use effective contraception during therapy and for at least 3 weeks after last dose. May cause fetal harm. Breast-feeding is not recommended.

Elderly: See Usual Dose and Precautions.

DRUG/LAB INTERACTIONS
Cisplatin, dalfampridine, dofetilide, metformin.

SIDE EFFECTS
Fatigue, headache, hyperglycemia, hypocalcemia, hypokalemia, hypophosphatemia, increased AST, infusion-related reaction, injection site reaction, peripheral edema, skin rash, thrombosis.

ANTIDOTE
Discontinue infusion and treat appropriately for severe hypersensitivity reactions.

VALPROATE SODIUM BBW
(val-**PROH**-ayt **SO**-dee-um)

Depacon

Anticonvulsant

pH 7.6

USUAL DOSE
Pretreatment: Verify pregnancy status. Baseline studies indicated; see Precautions and Monitor.

Adults and pediatric patients 10 years of age or older: For all indications optimal clinical response is usually achieved with doses less than 60 mg/kg/24 hr. Usual therapeutic range of plasma levels is 50 to 100 mcg/mL. A total daily dose exceeding 250 mg should be given in divided doses. Oral and IV doses are considered to be equivalent and should be given at previously established intervals (e.g., every 6 or 8 hours). However, the equivalence shown between the IV and oral formulations at steady state was evaluated only in an every-6-hour regimen. If the IV formulation is given two or three times a day, close monitoring of trough plasma levels may be needed. See Precautions, Monitor, and Drug/Lab Interactions. Use of IV formulation for more than 14 days has not been studied. Transfer to oral dosing as soon as practical.

Complex partial seizures (monotherapy [initial]): Begin with an initial dose of 10 to 15 mg/kg/24 hr. May be increased by 5 to 10 mg/kg/week until desired clinical response achieved or until side effects are dose limiting.

Complex partial seizures (conversion to monotherapy): Begin with an initial dose of 10 to 15 mg/kg/24 hr. May be increased by 5 to 10 mg/kg/week until desired clinical response achieved or until side effects are dose limiting. Concomitant antiepilepsy drug (AED) dosage can usually be reduced by 25% every 2 weeks. Dose of AEDs may be decreased at the beginning of valproate therapy or decrease may be delayed for 1 to 2 weeks to avoid unwanted seizures.

Complex partial seizures (adjunctive therapy): Begin with an initial dose of 10 to 15 mg/kg/24 hr. May be increased by 5 to 10 mg/kg/week until desired clinical response achieved. Has been used in combination with either carbamazepine or phenytoin. Dose adjustment of these drugs is not usually needed; however, drug interactions may occur; monitor plasma concentrations, especially during early therapy.

Simple and complex absence seizures: Begin with an initial dose of 15 mg/kg/24 hr. May be increased by 5 to 10 mg/kg/week until seizures are controlled or side effects are dose limiting.

PEDIATRIC DOSE
No IV dose recommendations are available from the manufacturer for pediatric patients under 10 years of age. See Maternal/Child.

DOSE ADJUSTMENTS
Monitor plasma concentrations when transferring from oral to IV or IV to oral; dose increases or decreases may be indicated. ■ Reduce initial dose in the elderly; base subsequent

doses on clinical response and/or development of side effects. ■ Reduced dose or discontinuation of therapy may be indicated if there is evidence of decreased food or fluid intake or excessive somnolence in the elderly. ■ Reduced dose or discontinuation of therapy may be indicated if there is evidence of bruising, hemorrhage, or a disorder of hemostasis/coagulation. ■ No dose adjustments required for impaired renal function, gender, or race. ■ See Maternal/Child and Drug/Lab Interactions.

DILUTION

Available as a clear, colorless solution in a 500 mg/5 mL single-dose vial. Each single dose should be diluted with at least 50 mL of D5W, NS, or LR.

Storage: Store vials at CRT. Diluted solutions stable at CRT for 24 hours. No preservative added; discard unused contents of vial.

COMPATIBILITY

Compatibility information not available from manufacturer. Other sources suggest a few specific **compatibilities** dependent on concentration and manufacturer; consult a pharmacist.

RATE OF ADMINISTRATION

A single dose as an infusion over 60 minutes. Manufacturer has recommended that a rate of 20 mg/min not be exceeded; however, results of a single study suggest that selected patients tolerated rates from 1.5 to 3 mg/kg/min, allowing administration of up to 15 mg/kg/dose over 5 to 10 minutes. Incidence of side effects may be increased with too-rapid infusion.

ACTIONS

An anticonvulsant. A sodium salt of valproic acid. Therapeutic effect in epilepsy may result from increased brain concentrations of gamma-aminobutyric acid (GABA). Peak effect occurs at the end of a 60-minute infusion or 4 hours after an oral dose. Plasma protein binding is high and is concentration dependent. Concentration in CSF is similar to unbound concentrations in plasma (10%). Half-life range is 13 to 19 hours. The half-life will be in the lower part of the range in patients receiving other enzyme-inducing antiepileptic agents (e.g., carbamazepine, phenobarbital, phenytoin). Metabolized in the liver. 30% to 50% excreted in changed form in urine. Crosses placental barrier. Secreted in breast milk.

INDICATIONS AND USES

Use of IV product indicated in the following specific conditions when oral administration of valproate products (e.g., divalproex sodium) is temporarily not feasible. ■ Treatment of complex partial seizures occurring in isolation or with other seizures (monotherapy or adjunctive therapy). ■ Treatment of simple and complex absence seizures (monotherapy or adjunctive therapy). ■ Adjunctive treatment of multiple seizure types that include absence seizures.

Unlabeled uses: Used alone or in combination with other antiepileptic drugs for treatment of patients with status epilepticus (refractory) who have not responded to other therapies.

Limitation of use: Because of the risk to the fetus of decreased IQ, neural tube defects, and other major congenital malformations, which may occur very early in pregnancy, valproate products should not be used to treat females with epilepsy or bipolar disorder who are pregnant or who plan to become pregnant unless other medications have failed to provide adequate symptom control or are otherwise unacceptable. Valproate should not be administered to a woman of childbearing potential unless other medications have failed to provide adequate symptom control or are otherwise unacceptable.

CONTRAINDICATIONS

Known hypersensitivity to valproate products. ■ Patients with hepatic disease or significant hepatic dysfunction. ■ Patients known to have mitochondrial disorders caused by mutations in mitochondrial DNA polymerase γ (POLG) gene (e.g., Alpers-Huttenlocher syndrome), and pediatric patients under 2 years of age who are suspected of having a POLG-related disorder. ■ Patients with known urea cycle disorders. ■ Prophylaxis of migraine headaches in pregnant females and in females of childbearing potential who are not using effective contraception.

PRECAUTIONS

Use of IV valproate for more than 14 days has not been studied. ■ Safety of doses above 60 mg/kg/day is not known. ■ Has caused fatal hepatic failure. Incidents usually occur during the first 6 months of treatment. Patients with a history of hepatic disease, patients taking multiple anticonvulsants, pediatric patients, patients with congenital metabolic disorders, patients with severe seizure disorders accompanied by cognitive impairment, and patients with organic brain disease may be at particular risk.

Pediatric patients under 2 years of age are at the greatest risk. If valproate is used in pediatric patients under 2 years of age with or without these increased risk factors, benefits must outweigh risks; use only as a sole agent and with extreme caution. Incidence of fatal hepatotoxicity decreases in progressively older patient groups. ■ Cases of life-threatening pancreatitis have been reported in both pediatric patients and adults receiving valproate. Some of the cases have been described as hemorrhagic with rapid progression from initial symptoms to death. May occur at any time from shortly after initiation of therapy to years later. If pancreatitis is diagnosed, valproate should be discontinued. ■ Patients with hereditary neurometabolic syndromes caused by DNA mutations of the mitochondrial DNA polymerase γ (POLG) gene (e.g., Alpers-Huttenlocher syndrome) have an increased risk of valproate-induced liver failure and death; see Contraindications and Monitor. ■ Hyperammonemic encephalopathy, sometimes fatal, has been reported in patients with urea cycle disorders (UCD). Before starting valproate, consider a possible diagnosis of UCD in patients with a history of unexplained encephalopathy or coma, encephalopathy associated with a protein load, pregnancy-related or postpartum encephalopathy, unexplained cognitive impairment, a history of elevated plasma ammonia or glutamine, cyclical vomiting or lethargy, episodic extreme irritability, ataxia, low BUN, protein avoidance, a family history of UCD or unexplained infant deaths, or any other S/S of UCD. ■ Hyperammonemia may be present even with normal liver function tests. Hyperammonemic encephalopathy should be considered in patients who present with lethargy and vomiting or altered mental status. Hyperammonemia should also be considered in patients who present with hypothermia (unintentional drop in body temperature to less than 35° C [95° F]). Elevation of ammonia may also be asymptomatic. ■ Hyperammonemia with or without encephalopathy has been reported with concomitant administration of valproic acid and topiramate (Topamax). Has occurred in patients who have tolerated either drug alone. S/S in most cases abated with discontinuation of either drug. ■ Hypothermia has occurred with valproate therapy both in conjunction with and in the absence of hyperammonemia. Can also occur in patients using concomitant topiramate with valproate after starting topiramate therapy or after increasing the dose of topiramate. ■ Hypothermia may be manifested by a variety of clinical abnormalities, including lethargy, confusion, coma, and significant alterations in other major organ systems such as the cardiovascular and respiratory systems. ■ Antiepileptic drugs (AEDs) increase the risk of suicidal thoughts or behavior in patients taking these drugs for any indication. Patients treated with any AED for any indication should be monitored for the emergence or worsening of depression, suicidal thoughts or behavior, and/or any unusual changes in mood or behavior. Some behavioral changes resolved without intervention. Others required dose reduction or discontinuation of valproate. ■ The frequency of adverse events (particularly elevated liver enzymes and thrombocytopenia) may be dose-related. The benefit of improved therapeutic effect with higher doses should be weighed against the possibility of a greater incidence of adverse reactions. ■ Incidence of thrombocytopenia increases at total trough concentrations greater than 110 mcg/mL in females and greater than 135 mcg/mL in males. ■ Valproate use has also been associated with decreases in other cell lines and myelodysplasia. ■ Drug reaction with eosinophilia and systemic symptoms (DRESS), also known as multiorgan hypersensitivity, has been reported in patients receiving valproate therapy. May be fatal or life threatening. Initial S/S include fever, rash, and/or lymphadenopathy associated with other organ system involvement (e.g., arthralgia, hematologic abnormalities, hepatitis, myocarditis, myositis, nephritis). Eosinophilia is often present. Discontinue valproate and use alternative therapy. ■ Plasma protein binding is decreased and free fraction is increased in the elderly, in hyperlipidemic patients, in chronic hepatic disease, in impaired renal function, and in the presence of other drugs; see Drug/Lab Interactions. Total plasma concentrations may be normal, but free concentrations may be substantially elevated in these patients. ■ Antiepilepsy drugs should not be abruptly discontinued in patients being treated for major seizure activity. Reduce AED doses gradually to prevent status epilepticus. ■ Can cause major congenital malformations, particularly neural tube defects (e.g., spina bifida). In addition, valproate can cause decreased IQ scores and neurodevelopmental disorders after in utero exposure. Do not administer to a woman of childbearing potential unless other medications have failed to provide adequate symptom control or are otherwise unacceptable. In such situations, effective contraception should be used. Do not use to treat non–life-threatening conditions (e.g., migraine) or in females of childbearing age who are not using effective contraception. See Contraindications and Maternal/Child. ▪ In vitro studies suggest that valproate may stimulate the replication of the HIV and CMV viruses under certain experimental conditions. The clinical significance of this is unknown but should be kept in mind when evaluating patients with HIV or CMV who are receiving valproate. ▪ Not recommended for use in patients with acute head trauma for the prophylaxis of posttraumatic seizures.

Monitor: Obtain baseline CBC with platelet counts and coagulation tests and monitor during therapy. Repeat before planned surgery and during pregnancy. Thrombocytopenia, inhibition of the secondary phase of platelet aggregation, and abnormal coagulation parameters (e.g., low fibrinogen, coagulation factor deficiencies, acquired von Willebrand disease) have been reported. ▪ Obtain baseline serum liver testing and monitor frequently during therapy, especially during the first 6 months. ▪ Observe closely for nonspecific symptoms that may precede serious or fatal hepatotoxicity (e.g., anorexia, facial edema, lethargy, loss of seizure control, malaise, weakness, vomiting). ▪ Abdominal pain, anorexia, nausea, and vomiting may be symptoms of pancreatitis and should be evaluated promptly. ▪ Valproate products should be used only after other anticonvulsants have failed in patients over 2 years of age who are clinically suspected of having a hereditary mitochondrial disease. Closely monitor during treatment for the development of acute liver injury with regular clinical assessments and serum liver testing. Perform POLG mutation testing and screening as indicated (e.g., family history, unexplained encephalopathy, refractory epilepsy [focal, myoclonic], status epilepticus at presentation, developmental delays, psychomotor regression, axonal sensorimotor neuropathy, myopathy cerebellar ataxia, ophthalmoplegia, or complicated migraine with occipital aura). ▪ Therapeutic serum levels for most patients will range from 50 to 100 mcg/mL; however, a good correlation has not been established between daily dose, serum levels, and therapeutic effect. Some patients may be controlled with lower or higher serum concentrations. One contributing factor is the nonlinear, concentration-dependent protein binding of valproate, which affects the clearance of the drug. ▪ Total serum valproic acid concentration is affected by variable free-fractions of drug; consider hepatic metabolism and protein binding when interpreting valproic acid concentrations. ▪ Monitor antiepileptic concentrations more frequently whenever concomitant AEDs are being introduced or withdrawn, and observe closely for seizure activity. ▪ Monitor serum concentrations more frequently if any of the risk factors listed in Dose Adjustments or Precautions are present, and when any drugs that affect hepatic enzymes are introduced or discontinued; see Drug/Lab Interactions. ▪ When used as replacement therapy, the equivalence shown between the IV and oral formulations was evaluated only in an every-6-hour regimen. If valproate sodium is given two or three times daily, close monitoring of trough plasma levels may be needed to ensure therapeutic levels are being maintained. ▪ Evaluate for S/S of UCD; see Precautions and Antidote. ▪ Consider hyperammonemia encephalopathy in patients who develop unexplained lethargy and vomiting or changes in mental status. Consider hyperammonemia in patients who present with hypothermia. Elevations of ammonia may also be asymptomatic; monitor plasma ammonia levels closely; see Antidote. Treat hyperammonemia and assess for underlying UCD. ▪ Observe patient closely for signs of CNS side effects; see Precautions. ▪ Monitor for S/S of DRESS. ▪ See Dose Adjustments, Precautions, and Drug/Lab Interactions for additional monitoring requirements.

Patient Education: May cause drowsiness; determine effects before driving or operating any machinery. ▪ Avoid pregnancy; use effective contraception; see Maternal/Child. ▪ Read the patient information leaflet provided by manufacturer, and discuss your medical history and concurrent prescription and nonprescription medications with your healthcare provider. ▪ Promptly report symptoms such as changes in mental state, fever, jaundice, lethargy, lymphadenopathy, rash, unexplained lethargy, unintentional drop in body temperature to less than 35° C (95° F); may be symptoms of serious side effects (e.g., hepatotoxicity, hyperammonemia, hypersensitivity) and require prompt evaluation and treatment. ▪ Promptly report abdominal pain, anorexia, nausea, and/or vomiting. May indicate pancreatitis; medical evaluation may be required. ▪ May increase the risk of suicidal thoughts and behavior. Promptly report emergence or worsening of the S/S of depression, any unusual changes in mood or behavior, or thoughts about self-harm. ▪ There have been reports of male infertility coincident with valproate therapy. ▪ Females who are pregnant or who become pregnant should be encouraged to enroll in the North American Antiepileptic Drug (NAAED) Pregnancy Registry. ▪ See Maternal/Child.

Maternal/Child: Valproate can cause fetal harm when administered to a pregnant woman. Avoid pregnancy; see Contraindications. Valproate should not be used to treat females with epilepsy or bipolar disorder who are pregnant or who plan to become pregnant unless other medications have failed to provide adequate symptom control or are otherwise unacceptable. There is an increased risk for major congenital malformations, particularly neural tube defects (e.g., spina bifida) and other birth defects such as craniofacial defects, cardiovascular malformation, hypospadias, and limb malformations. In addition, valproate can cause decreased IQ scores and neurodevelopmental disorders (including autism spectrum disorders) following in utero exposure. In utero exposure to valproate may also result in hearing impairment or hearing loss. The incidence of congenital malformations associated with the use of valproate by females with seizure disorders during pregnancy is higher than in females with seizure disorders who use other AEDs. The increased teratogenic risk from valproate in females with epilepsy is expected to be reflected in an increased risk in other indications (e.g., bipolar disorder, migraine). ▪ Evidence suggests that folic acid supplementation before conception and during the first trimester decreases the risk for congenital neural tube defects in the general population. It is not known whether the risk of neural tube defects or decreased IQ in the offspring of females receiving valproate is reduced by folic acid supplementation. Dietary folic acid supplementation before conception and during pregnancy is recommended. Tests to detect neural tube and other defects should be considered as part of routine prenatal care in pregnant females receiving valproate. ▪ To prevent major seizures, do not discontinue valproate abruptly in these patients; can precipitate status epilepticus, resulting in maternal and fetal hypoxia and a threat to life. ▪ When used during pregnancy, valproate has caused hepatic failure or clotting abnormalities in the mother that may result in hemorrhagic complications in the neonate. Deaths have been reported. If clotting parameters are abnormal in the mother, then these parameters should also be monitored in the neonate; see Monitor. ▪ Has caused hepatic failure in infants exposed to valproate in utero. ▪ Has caused hypoglycemia in infants exposed to valproate in utero. ▪ Use with caution during breast-feeding; is excreted in human milk. Monitor the breast-fed infant for signs of liver damage, including jaundice and unusual bruising or bleeding. ▪ Neonates under 2 months of age have a markedly decreased ability to eliminate valproate compared with older pediatric patients and adults. ▪ Pediatric patients 3 months to 10 years of age have 50% higher clearance rates based on weight compared to adults. ▪ Younger pediatric patients, especially those receiving enzyme-inducing drugs (e.g., carbamazepine, phenobarbital, phenytoin) will require larger maintenance doses to achieve therapeutic valproic acid concentrations. ▪ IV product has not been studied in pediatric patients under 2 years of age. If used, use as a sole agent with extreme caution. ▪ Pediatric patients under 2 years of age are at an increased risk for developing fatal hepatotoxicity. ▪ See Precautions and Monitor.

Elderly: May be more prone to adverse events. Initial dose should be lower, and dosage should be increased slowly. Rate of clearance decreased, free fraction increased; see Dose Adjustments. ▪ Monitor for fluid and nutritional intake, dehydration, somnolence, and other adverse events. Dose reduction or discontinuation of valproate should be considered in patients with decreased food or fluid intake and in patients with excessive somnolence. ▪ A higher percentage of patients over 65 years of age reported accidental injury, infection, pain, somnolence, and tremor.

DRUG/LAB INTERACTIONS

Clearance increased and effectiveness reduced by **drugs that induce hepatic enzymes** (e.g., phenytoin, carbamazepine, phenobarbital, primidone, ritonavir); increased monitoring of valproate and concomitant drug concentrations indicated. ▪ **Aspirin** decreases protein binding, inhibits metabolism, and increases free concentration of valproate; use caution and monitor valproate concentrations if administered concomitantly. ▪ Peak concentrations increased if coadministered with **felbamate**; reduced dose of valproate indicated. ▪ Metabolism may be decreased and serum levels increased when given concurrently with **erythromycin.** ▪ **Carbapenem antibiotics** (e.g., ertapenem, meropenem) may reduce serum valproic acid concentrations to subtherapeutic levels, resulting in loss of seizure control. Monitor valproic acid levels. Consider alternative antibacterial or anticonvulsant therapy if serum valproate concentrations drop significantly or seizure control deteriorates. ▪ **Estrogen-containing contraceptives** may increase the clearance of valproate, decreasing valproate concentration and potentially increasing seizure frequency; monitor serum valproate concentrations and clinical response when adding or discontinuing estrogen-containing products. ▪ **Rifampin** may increase clearance of valproate and require dose adjustment. ▪ Inhibits metabolism of **barbiturates** (e.g., phenobarbital) **and primidone,** increasing their effects. Monitor for neurologic toxicity; obtain barbiturate serum levels and reduce barbiturate dose as indicated. ▪ May decrease serum levels of carbamazepine. **Carbamazepine** decreases plasma concentrations of valproate, and a loss of seizure control may occur; monitor carefully and increase valproate dose if indicated. ▪ Concomitant use with **clonazepam** may induce absence status in patients with a history of absence-type seizures. ▪ **Displaces some protein-bound drugs** (e.g., carbamazepine, diazepam, phenytoin, tolbutamide, warfarin). In addition to decreasing protein binding, may also decrease the metabolism of diazepam and phenytoin. Dose adjustments and serum concentrations may be indicated. ▪ **Phenytoin** with valproate has caused breakthrough seizures in patients with epilepsy; adjust dose of phenytoin as indicated by serum concentrations. ▪ Hyperammonemia with or without encephalopathy, as well as hypothermia, has been reported with concomitant administration of valproic acid and **topiramate**; see Precautions. ▪ Monitor coagulation tests if administered with **anticoagulants** (e.g., warfarin). ▪ CNS effects may be increased when given concurrently with **CNS depressants** (e.g., **benzodiazepines and tricyclic antidepressants**). ▪ May decrease clearance and increase effects of **amitriptyline and nortriptyline**. Dose reduction of these drugs may be required. ▪ Inhibits metabolism of **ethosuximide**; monitor serum concentrations of both drugs with concomitant administration. ▪ Concurrent administration of **lamotrigine** and valproate may increase lamotrigine levels. Dose of lamotrigine should be reduced. ▪ Serious skin reactions have been reported with concurrent use of **lamotrigine** and valproic acid. ▪ Decreases clearance and may increase toxicity of **zidovudine**. ▪ **Rufinamide** (Banzel) clearance is decreased by valproate. Concentrations were increased by less than 16% to 70% depending on the concentration of valproate. Patients stabilized on rufinamide before initiating valproate therapy should begin valproate at a low dose and titrate to a clinically effective dose. Similarly, patients on valproate should begin rufinamide at a dose lower than 10 mg/kg/day (pediatric patients) or 400 mg/day (adults). ▪ Concomitant use with **propofol** may lead to increased blood levels of propofol. Reduce dose of propofol and monitor patients closely for signs of increased sedation or cardiorespiratory depression. ▪ See package insert for additional information about many drugs that do not present significant clinical interactions. ▪ May alter **thyroid function tests.** ▪ May cause **false-positive urine ketone test.**

SIDE EFFECTS
Abdominal pain, alopecia, amblyopia/blurred vision, amnesia, anorexia with weight loss, asthenia, ataxia, bronchitis, constipation, depression, diarrhea, diplopia, dizziness, dyspepsia, dyspnea, ecchymosis, emotional lability, fever, flu syndrome, headache, increased appetite with weight gain, infection, insomnia, nausea, nervousness, nystagmus, peripheral edema, pharyngitis, rhinitis, somnolence, thinking abnormally, thrombocytopenia, tinnitus, tremor, and vomiting are most common. Accidental injury, back pain, chest pain, euphoria, hypesthesia, injection site inflammation, injection site pain, rash, sweating, taste perversion, and vasodilation were the next most commonly reported side effects. Psychiatric symptoms, including aggression, agitation, anger, anxiety, apathy, depersonalization, depression, emotional lability, hallucinations, hostility, irritability, and suicidal tendencies, have also been reported. Frequency of elevated liver enzymes and thrombocytopenia may be dose related. Fatal hepatotoxicity (anorexia, facial edema, lethargy, loss of seizure control, malaise, sweating, vasodilation, vomiting, weakness) has occurred. See Precautions for other reported serious adverse events.
Overdose: Somnolence, deep coma, heart block, and hypernatremia. Some fatalities have been reported.

Post-Marketing: Many adverse reactions have been reported during post-approval use of valproate sodium. The frequency of reactions and/or causal relationship to valproate may be difficult to determine. Some of the reported reactions have included dermatologic reactions (e.g., erythema multiforme, nail and nail bed disorders, photosensitivity, Stevens-Johnson syndrome, toxic epidermal necrolysis), endocrine abnormalities (e.g., elevated testosterone, hirsutism, hyperandrogenism, secondary amenorrhea), enuresis, Fanconi's syndrome, hair color and texture changes, hematologic reactions (e.g., anemia including macrocytic with or without folate deficiency, aplastic anemia, bone marrow suppression), hypersensitivity reactions (including anaphylaxis), neurologic reactions (e.g., parkinsonism, acute or subacute cognitive decline and behavioral changes [apathy or irritability] with cerebral pseudoatrophy on imaging, acute or subacute encephalopathy in the absence of elevated ammonia levels, elevated valproate levels, or neuroimaging changes), osteopenia, osteoporosis, reproductive reactions (e.g., aspermia, azoospermia, male infertility), and weight gain.

ANTIDOTE

Keep physician informed of all side effects. Some may respond to a decrease in the rate of administration. Discontinue immediately if signs of suspected or apparent significant hepatic dysfunction appear (e.g., hyperammonemia, elevated liver function tests) or S/S of underlying UCD. Hepatic dysfunction may progress after valproate is discontinued. Discontinue if S/S of DRESS occur. Initiate alternate therapy. Reduce dose or discontinue if bruising, hemorrhage, or abnormal coagulation parameters occur (e.g., thrombocytopenia). Discontinue if S/S of pancreatitis occur. All of the above situations may be life threatening and will require immediate symptomatic treatment. Consideration should be given to discontinuing valproate in patients who develop hypothermia. Maintain a patent airway and resuscitate as indicated. Support patient as required in treatment of overdose; monitor and maintain adequate urine output. Hemodialysis is effective in overdose. Naloxone may reverse CNS depressant effects in overdose but may also reverse antiepilepsy effects of valproate. Psychotic symptoms may require dose reduction or discontinuation of valproate.

VANCOMYCIN HYDROCHLORIDE
(van-koh-**MY**-sin hy-droh-**KLOR**-eyed)

Antibacterial
(tricylic-glycopeptide)

pH 2.5 to 5

USUAL DOSE
500 mg every 6 hours or 1 Gm every 12 hours. Administer each dose at a rate of 10 mg/min or over 60 minutes, whichever is longer. Normal renal function required.

Other sources recommend 15 to 20 mg/kg/dose (with a usual maximum of 2 Gm/dose) every 8 to 12 hours. In seriously ill patients with complicated infections, a loading dose of 25 to 30 mg/kg (actual body weight) may be administered.

Prevention of enterococcal endocarditis in selected penicillin-allergic patients having GI, biliary, or GU surgery or instrumentation (unlabeled): *Adults and adolescents:* AHA recommends 1 Gm IV before the procedure. Give gentamicin 1.5 mg/kg IV concurrently in high-risk patients (not to exceed 120 mg). Infusion must be administered over at least 60 minutes and should be completed within 30 minutes of starting the procedure. Gentamicin may not be necessary in moderate-risk patients. Vancomycin alone may be indicated in selected patients having dental procedures or upper respiratory tract surgery or instrumentation. Consult recent recommendations of the American Heart Association or the American Dental Association.

Treatment of patients with oxacillin-resistant staphylococcal endocarditis who have a native cardiac valve: 30 mg/kg/24 hr (not to exceed 2 Gm/day unless serum concentrations are inappropriately low) equally divided into 2 doses (15 mg/kg every 12 hours) for 6 weeks.

Treatment of patients with oxacillin-resistant endocarditis who have a prosthetic valve or other prosthetic material: 30 mg/kg/24 hr (not to exceed 2 Gm/day unless serum concentrations are inappropriately low) equally divided into 2 doses (15 mg/kg every 12 hours) for 6 weeks or longer. Given in conjunction with oral or IV rifampin 300 mg every 8 hours for 6 weeks or longer and IM or IV gentamicin 3 mg/kg/day equally divided into 2 to 3 doses (1 mg/kg every 8 hours or 1.5 mg/kg every 12 hours) during the first 2 weeks of vancomycin therapy.

Treatment of endocarditis caused by viridans streptococci or *Streptococcus bovis* in patients unable to take a beta-lactam antibiotic: 30 mg/kg/24 hr (not to exceed 2 Gm/day unless serum concentrations are inappropriately low) equally divided into 2 doses (15 mg/kg every 12 hours) for 4 weeks (native valve endocarditis) to 6 weeks (prosthetic valve endocarditis).

Treatment of enterococcal endocarditis when penicillin G or ampicillin cannot be used: 30 mg/kg/24 hr equally divided into 2 doses (15 mg/kg every 12 hours) for 6 weeks. Given in conjunction with IM or IV gentamicin 1 mg/kg every 8 hours for 6 weeks.

Perioperative prophylaxis in selected surgeries (e.g., cardiac, prosthetic valve, coronary artery bypass, joint replacement, craniotomy) when a cephalosporin cannot be used or there is a high incidence of methicillin-resistant staphylococci at the institution (unlabeled use): 15 mg/kg within 120 minutes before surgery; should be completed within 30 minutes before the start of surgery. May be repeated one or more times if surgery is prolonged or major blood loss occurs. Postoperative doses are considered generally unnecessary and are not recommended.

Prevention of neonatal Group B streptococcal disease: Used for females with penicillin hypersensitivity who should not receive β-lactam anti-infectives or if resistance to clindamycin or erythromycin is known or suspected. 1 Gm every 12 hours until delivery. Initiate at the beginning of labor or rupture of membranes. Another source recommends 20 mg/kg/dose (maximum of 2 Gm/dose) every 8 hours from onset of labor until delivery.

PEDIATRIC DOSE
Pediatric patients 1 month of age or older: 10 mg/kg IV infused over at least 60 minutes every 6 hours. Another source recommends: *Mild to moderate infections:* 40 to 45 mg/kg/24 hr equally divided and given every 6 or 8 hours (10 to 11.25 mg/kg every 6 hours or 13.33 to

15 mg/kg every 8 hours). *Severe infections:* 45 to 60 mg/kg/24 hr equally divided and given every 6 or 8 hours (11.25 to 15 mg/kg every 6 hours or 15 to 20 mg/kg every 8 hours). 60 mg/kg/24 hr given in divided doses every 6 hours (15 mg/kg/dose) has been recommended for treatment of meningitis. Do not exceed 2 Gm in 24 hours.

Prevention of enterococcal endocarditis in selected penicillin-allergic patients having GI, biliary, or GU surgery or instrumentation: 20 mg/kg before the procedure. Give gentamicin 1.5 mg/kg concurrently in high-risk patients (not to exceed 120 mg). Gentamicin may not be necessary in moderate-risk patients. Infusion of vancomycin must be administered over at least 60 minutes and should be complete within 30 minutes of starting the procedure. Note comments about dental and upper respiratory surgery or instrumentation under Usual Dose.

NEONATAL DOSE
15 mg/kg as an initial dose. See Maternal/Child. Follow with 10 mg/kg. Adjust interval based on age and/or weight as follows:

Infants up to 1 week of age: Give every 12 hours.

Infants 1 week to 1 month of age: Give every 8 hours.

The American Academy of Pediatrics recommends 10 to 15 mg/kg. Adjust dose and interval based on weight and/or age as follows:

Postnatal Weight and Age	Dose and Interval
Less than 1.2 kg and under 7 days of age	15 mg/kg/dose every 18 to 24 hours
Less than 1.2 kg and 7 days of age or older	15 mg/kg/dose every 18 to 24 hours
1.2 to 2 kg and under 7 days of age	10 to 15 mg/kg/dose every 12 to 18 hours
1.2 to 2 kg and 7 days of age or older	10 to 15 mg/kg/dose every 8 to 12 hours
Over 2 kg and under 7 days of age	10 to 15 mg/kg/dose every 8 to 12 hours
Over 2 kg and 7 days of age or older	10 to 15 mg/kg/dose every 6 to 8 hours

DOSE ADJUSTMENTS
Reduce total daily dose in premature infants and elderly patients. Greater dose reductions than expected may be necessary in these patients because of impaired renal function.
■ Dose reduction required in impaired renal function. In all renally impaired patients (including functionally anephric and anuric patients), the initial dose should be no less than 15 mg/kg. After the initial dose, subsequent doses are reduced based on CrCl; *see prescribing information.* In patients with marked renal impairment, it may be more convenient to give a maintenance dose of 250 to 1,000 mg every several days rather than administering the drug on a daily basis. For anuria, subsequent doses of 1,000 mg every 7 to 10 days have been suggested. Monitoring of serum levels is recommended.

DILUTION
Available premixed and frozen, or reconstitute each 500-mg vial with 10 mL of SWFI. Each 500 mg must be further diluted with 100 mL of NS or D5W and given as an intermittent infusion. Also **compatible** in D5NS, LR, D5LR, D5 Normosol-M, Isolyte E, and acetated Ringer's injection. Concentrations greater than 5 mg/mL are not recommended. Also available in ADD-Vantage vials for use with ADD-Vantage infusion containers.

Storage: Store vials at CRT. After reconstitution, vials may be stored in a refrigerator for 96 hours. Maintains potency for 2 weeks in D5W or NS. Solutions prepared from ADD-Vantage vials are stable for 24 hours at room temperature and for 14 days if refrigerated. However, good professional practice suggests that compounded admixtures should be administered as soon after preparation as possible. Frozen premixed containers should be stored at or below −20° C (−4° F). Thaw at RT or under refrigeration. Do not force thaw. Once thawed, product is stable for 72 hours at RT or for 30 days if refrigerated.

COMPATIBILITY

Several sources recommend not admixing with other drugs. They suggest it is **incompatible** with alkaline solutions (e.g., aminophylline, aztreonam, barbiturates, chloramphenicol, dexamethasone, sodium bicarbonate) and may form a precipitate with heavy metals. May inactivate aminoglycosides; should also not be combined in the same solution with albumin, selected cephalosporins, foscarnet, or selected penicillins; if administered concurrently, administer at separate sites or separate intervals (flush IV line with a **compatible** solution before and after administration).

Other sources suggest specific **compatibilities** dependent on concentration and manufacturer; consult a pharmacist.

RATE OF ADMINISTRATION

Severe hypotension, with or without flushing of the face, neck, chest, and extremities, and cardiac arrest can occur with too-rapid injection.

A single dose properly diluted (concentration of no more than 5 mg/mL) at a rate not to exceed 10 mg/min or 60 minutes, whichever is longer. Another reference suggests each 500-mg increment over a minimum of 30 minutes. This intermittent infusion is the preferred route of administration because of high incidence of thrombophlebitis.

Pediatric rate: A single dose over a minimum of 60 minutes.

ACTIONS

A tricyclic glycopeptide antibiotic, it is bactericidal against gram-positive organisms. Bactericidal action results from the inhibition of cell wall synthesis. Also alters bacterial cell-membrane permeability and RNA synthesis. Well distributed in most body tissues and fluids, including pleural, pericardial, ascitic, and synovial fluids; in urine; in peritoneal dialysis fluid; and in atrial appendage tissue. Penetration into the CSF occurs when the meninges are inflamed. Half-life is 4 to 6 hours in patients with normal renal function. Vancomycin is excreted in biologically active form in the urine. Crosses the placental barrier. Secreted in breast milk.

INDICATIONS AND USES

Treatment of serious or severe infections caused by susceptible strains of methicillin-resistant (beta-lactam–resistant) *Staphylococcus aureus* (MRSA). ▪ Treatment of gram-positive infections in penicillin-allergic patients; for patients who cannot receive or who have failed to respond to other drugs, including the penicillins or cephalosporins; and for infections caused by vancomycin-susceptible organisms that are resistant to other antimicrobial drugs. ▪ Empiric therapy when MRSA is suspected. ▪ Treatment of staphylococcal endocarditis and other infections due to staphylococci, including septicemia, bone, lower respiratory tract, and skin and skin structure infections that do not respond or are resistant to other antibiotics. ▪ Treatment of endocarditis caused by other gram-positive organisms. Depending on the causative organism, vancomycin may be used alone or in combination with other antimicrobial agents. ▪ Parenteral form may be used orally for pseudomembranous colitis/staphylococcal enterocolitis caused by *C. difficile*.

Unlabeled uses: Prophylaxis against enterococcal endocarditis in moderate or high-risk (prosthetic heart valves, congenital or rheumatic heart disease) penicillin-allergic patients undergoing GI, biliary, or GU surgery or instrumentation.

CONTRAINDICATIONS

Known hypersensitivity to vancomycin. Solutions containing dextrose may be contraindicated in patients with allergies to corn or corn products.

PRECAUTIONS

To reduce the development of drug-resistant bacteria and maintain its effectiveness, vancomycin should be used only to treat or prevent infections proven or strongly suspected to be caused by bacteria. ▪ Sensitivity studies necessary to determine susceptibility of the causative organism to vancomycin. ▪ Prolonged use of drug may result in superinfection caused by overgrowth of nonsusceptible organisms. ▪ Nephrotoxicity has occurred. Systemic vancomycin has resulted in acute kidney injury (AKI). Risk increases as serum levels increase and in patients with underlying renal impairment, patients with comorbidities, and patients receiving concomitant therapy with a drug known to be nephrotoxic. ▪ Ototoxicity has been reported with vancomycin, mostly in patients receiving excessive doses, who have an underlying hearing loss, or who are receiving concomitant therapy with another ototoxic agent such as an aminoglycoside. It may be transient or permanent. Use with caution in patients with renal impairment. Risk of ototoxicity is increased by high, prolonged blood concentrations. ▪ *Clostridium difficile*–associated diarrhea (CDAD) has been reported. May range from mild diarrhea to fatal colitis. Consider in patients who present with diarrhea during or after treatment with vancomycin. ▪ Risk of high sodium load with Vancomycin Injection, USP with Sodium Chloride, USP. Each 100 mL contains 0.9 Gm of sodium chloride. Avoid use of this formulation in patients with CHF, elderly patients, and patients requiring restricted sodium intake. ▪ Oral vancomycin has a local effect only (e.g., in the bowel); not for systemic use. ▪ Reversible neutropenia has been reported; see Monitor.

Monitor: Monitor renal function in all patients receiving vancomycin; see Precautions. ▪ Monitoring of serum levels may be indicated in patients at increased risk for developing nephrotoxicity and/or ototoxicity (e.g., patients with underlying renal dysfunction or changing renal function, patients receiving concomitant aminoglycosides [e.g., gentamicin]) or in patients receiving prolonged courses of therapy (e.g., treatment of endocarditis); see Drug/Lab Interactions. ▪ Determine absolute patency of vein. Necrosis and sloughing will result from extravasation. The frequency and severity of thrombophlebitis may be minimized by slow infusion of vancomycin and by rotation of venous access sites. ▪ Monitor BP during infusion. ▪ Severe hypotension (with or without flushing of the face, neck, chest, and extremities) and cardiac arrest can occur with too-rapid injection (red man or red neck syndrome). ▪ Auditory testing indicated with prolonged use. ▪ Periodic monitoring of leukocyte count recommended in prolonged therapy. ▪ See Drug/Lab Interactions.

Patient Education: Report all side effects promptly. ▪ Promptly report diarrhea or bloody stools that occur during treatment or up to several months after an antibiotic has been discontinued; may indicate CDAD and require treatment.

Maternal/Child: Use during pregnancy only if clearly needed. ▪ Safety for use in breast-feeding not established; discontinue breast-feeding. ▪ Confirmation of desired serum concentrations suggested in pediatric patients. Neonates have immature renal function; blood levels may be excessive. In premature infants, vancomycin clearance decreases as postconceptional age decreases. Longer dosing intervals may be necessary, and close monitoring of vancomycin serum concentrations is recommended.

Elderly: Clearance may be reduced; dosage reduction and monitoring required.

DRUG/LAB INTERACTIONS

Synergistic with **aminoglycosides** against many strains of *Staphylococcus aureus* and streptococci; see package insert. Combined use may increase risk of ototoxicity and nephrotoxicity. ▪ Additive toxicities may occur with *systemic or topical* use of **other nephrotoxic, neurotoxic, or ototoxic drugs** (e.g., aminoglycosides, amphotericin B, bacitracin, cisplatin, colistin, ethacrynic acid, furosemide, polymyxin B). Use with caution in combination with vancomycin; serial monitoring of renal and auditory function indicated. ▪ May enhance neuromuscular blockade with **nondepolarizing muscle relaxants** (e.g., pancuronium). ▪ Frequency of infusion-related reactions, including erythema, flushing, hypotension, pruritus, and urticaria, increases with concomitant administration of **anesthetic agents**. This infusion-related reaction may be minimized by administering vancomycin as a 60-minute infusion before anesthetic induction. Concomitant administration of vancomycin and anesthetic agents has been associated with erythema and histamine-like flushing in pediatric patients.

SIDE EFFECTS

Agranulocytosis, anaphylaxis, cardiac arrest, CDAD, chills, drug fever, dyspnea, eosinophilia, infusion-related events (anaphylactoid reactions, dyspnea, flushing of the upper body, hypotension, pain and muscle spasm of the chest and back, pruritus, urticaria, wheezing), interstitial nephritis, nausea, nephrotoxicity, neutropenia, ototoxicity (e.g., dizziness, hearing loss, tinnitus, vertigo), pain or inflammation at the injection site, pruritus, pseudomembranous colitis, rash (including exfoliative dermatitis, Stevens-Johnson syndrome, and vasculitis), red neck or red man syndrome, thrombocytopenia, and thrombophlebitis.

Post-Marketing: Drug rash with eosinophilia and systemic symptoms (DRESS).

ANTIDOTE

Notify the physician of all side effects. Hearing loss may progress even if drug is discontinued. If minor side effects are progressive or any major side effect occurs, discontinue the drug, treat hypersensitivity reaction, or resuscitate as necessary. Temporarily discontinue or slow rate of infusion for an infusion-related reaction. Fluids, antihistamines, corticosteroids, and vasopressors (e.g., dopamine) may be required. Mild cases of CDAD may respond to discontinuation of drug. Treat CDAD with fluids, electrolytes, protein supplements, and appropriate antibiotics (e.g., oral vancomycin) as indicated. In severe cases, surgical evaluation may be indicated. Hemodialysis or CAPD will not decrease blood levels in toxicity.

VASOPRESSIN INJECTION
(vay-so-**PRESS**-in in-**JEK**-shun)

Vasostrict

Hormone
Antidiuretic

pH 2.5 to 4.5

USUAL DOSE

Vasodilatory shock: *Postcardiotomy shock:* Initiate therapy at 0.03 units/min. Titrate to target BP as outlined in Dose Adjustments. Maximum dose is 0.1 units/min.

Septic shock: Initiate therapy at 0.01 units/min. Titrate to target BP as outlined in Dose Adjustments. Maximum dose is 0.07 units/min.

GI variceal hemorrhage (unlabeled): 0.2 to 0.4 units/min as an infusion. Titrate as needed to a maximum dose of 0.8 units/min; maximum recommended duration is 24 hours at highest effective dose.

PEDIATRIC DOSE

All IV doses and uses are unlabeled; however, studies in pediatric patients have been conducted. See literature.

GI hemorrhage: 0.002 to 0.005 units/kg/min as an infusion. Gradually increase dose as needed to a maximum dose of 0.01 units/kg/min.

DOSE ADJUSTMENTS

Titrate up by 0.005 units/min at 10- to 15-minute intervals if needed until target BP response or maximum dose is reached. ▪ Goal of treatment is optimization of perfusion to critical organs, but aggressive treatment can compromise perfusion of organs, such as the gastrointestinal tract, whose function is difficult to monitor. Titrate to the lowest dose compatible with a clinically acceptable response. ▪ After target BP has been maintained for 8 hours without the use of catecholamines, taper vasopressin by 0.005 units/min every hour as tolerated to maintain target BP. ▪ Lower-end initial dosing may be appropriate in the elderly based on the potential for decreased organ function and concomitant disease or drug therapy.

DILUTION

Available as a 1-mL multiple-dose vial containing 20 units/mL. Dilute in NS or D5W as outlined in the following chart.

Preparation of Vasopressin Diluted Solution			
		Mix	
Fluid Restriction?	**Final Concentration**	**Vasopressin**	**Diluent**
No	0.1 units/mL	2.5 mL (50 units)	500 mL
Yes	1 unit/mL	5 mL (100 units)	100 mL

Storage: Refrigerate unopened vials between 2° and 8° C (36° and 46° F). Do not freeze. Storage conditions and expiration periods for vasopressin vials are summarized in the following chart. Mark revised 12-month expiration date on vials removed from refrigeration.

Storage Conditions and Expiration Periods for Vasopressin			
	Unopened/Refrigerated (2° to 8° C [36° to 46° F])	**Unopened/Room Temperature (20° to 25° C [68° to 77° F])**	**Opened (After First Puncture)**
1-mL vial	Until manufacturer expiration date	12 months or until manufacturer expiration date, whichever is earlier	48 hours

Diluted solution may be stored for 18 hours at RT or 24 hours under refrigeration.

COMPATIBILITY
Compatibility information not available from manufacturer. Other sources suggest specific **compatibilities** dependent on concentration and manufacturer; consult a pharmacist.

RATE OF ADMINISTRATION
Infusion: See Usual Dose for recommended rates for each diagnosis. Use of a central venous catheter is recommended. Titrate rate so that perfusion remains adequate while BP is optimized. Do not discontinue abruptly; see Dose Adjustments.

ACTIONS
A polypeptide hormone that causes contraction of vascular and other smooth muscles and antidiuresis. The vasoconstrictive effects of vasopressin are mediated by vascular V_1 receptors. The antidiuretic effects are mediated by vascular V_2 receptors. At therapeutic doses, exogenous vasopressin elicits a vasoconstrictive effect in most vascular beds, including the splanchnic, renal, and cutaneous circulation. It also triggers contractions of smooth muscles in the GI tract mediated by muscular V_1 receptors and by the release of prolactin and ACTH via V_3 receptors. At lower concentrations typical for the antidiuretic hormone, vasopressin inhibits water diuresis via renal V_2 receptors. In patients with vasodilatory shock, vasopressin increases systemic vascular resistance and mean arterial BP and reduces the dose requirements for norepinephrine. The pressor effect is proportional to the infusion rate. Vasopressin tends to decrease heart rate and cardiac output. Onset of action is rapid, with peak effects occurring in 15 minutes. Pressor effects fade within 20 minutes after stopping an infusion. There is no evidence of tachyphylaxis or tolerance to the pressor effect of vasopressin. Predominantly metabolized in the liver and kidney to inactive metabolites. Excreted in the urine, primarily as inactive metabolites.

INDICATIONS AND USES
To increase BP in adults with vasodilatory shock (e.g., postcardiotomy shock or septic shock) who remain hypotensive despite fluids and catecholamines.
Unlabeled uses: Gastroesophageal variceal hemorrhage; in-hospital cardiac arrest (in combination with epinephrine and methylprednisolone).

CONTRAINDICATIONS
Hypersensitivity to 8-L-arginine vasopressin or chlorobutanol.

PRECAUTIONS
Use in patients with impaired cardiac response may worsen cardiac output. ▪ Use with caution in patients with vascular disease, especially coronary artery disease; may cause cardiac ischemia. Small doses may precipitate anginal pain, and larger doses may cause

myocardial infarction. ▪ May cause ischemia of other organs (e.g., GI tract, kidneys); use lowest effective dose. ▪ May produce water intoxication; use with caution in patients with asthma, epilepsy, heart failure, migraine, renal impairment, or any condition in which a rapid addition to extracellular water could be hazardous.

Monitor: Monitor BP, HR, and ECG. ▪ Monitor fluid and electrolyte status, serum and urine sodium, urine specific gravity, urine and serum osmolality, and urine output. ▪ Monitor IV site very closely, especially if it is a peripheral site; a central venous catheter is preferred. Produces intense vasoconstriction. Avoid extravasation; vasoconstriction that may result in severe tissue necrosis and gangrene can occur. ▪ Use an indwelling urinary catheter to confirm urine output and monitor closely. ▪ Fluid restriction may be indicated; initial signs of water intoxication include drowsiness, listlessness, and headache and can rapidly progress to coma and convulsions. ▪ See Rate of Administration, Precautions, and Drug/Lab Interactions.

Maternal/Child: Category C: safety for use during pregnancy not established; use only if clearly needed. ▪ May produce tonic uterine contractions that could threaten the continuation of pregnancy. ▪ Increased clearance of vasopressin in the second and third trimesters of pregnancy may necessitate the use of higher doses for treatment of postcardiotomy or septic shock. ▪ Safety for use during breast-feeding not established. ▪ Safety and effectiveness for use in pediatric patients with vasodilatory shock not established.

Elderly: See Precautions; elderly patients may be more sensitive to adverse effects. ▪ Dose selection should be cautious in elderly patients; see Dose Adjustments.

DRUG/LAB INTERACTIONS
Vasodilators (e.g., nitroglycerin, nitroprusside sodium) counteract the vasoconstrictive effects of vasopressin. ▪ Concomitant use with **catecholamines** (e.g., epinephrine, norepinephrine) is expected to result in an additive effect on mean arterial BP and other hemodynamic parameters. ▪ **Indomethacin** may prolong the effect of vasopressin. ▪ Use with ganglionic blocking agents may increase the effect of vasopressin on mean arterial BP. ▪ **Furosemide** increases the effect of vasopressin on osmolar clearance and urine flow. ▪ Use with **drugs suspected of causing SIADH** (e.g., selective serotonin reuptake inhibitors, tricyclic antidepressants, haloperidol, chlorpropamide, enalapril, methyldopa, pentamidine, vincristine, cyclophosphamide, ifosfamide, felbamate) may increase the pressor effect in addition to the antidiuretic effect of vasopressin. ▪ Use with **drugs suspected of causing diabetes insipidus** (e.g., demeclocycline, lithium, foscarnet, clozapine) may decrease the pressor effect in addition to the antidiuretic effect of vasopressin.

SIDE EFFECTS
The most common adverse reactions include bradycardia, decreased cardiac output, hyponatremia, ischemia (coronary, digital, mesenteric, skin), and tachyarrhythmias. Other reported adverse reactions include acute renal insufficiency, angina, atrial fibrillation, decreased platelets, gangrene, headache, hemorrhagic shock, hypersensitivity reactions, increased bilirubin, intractable bleeding, ischemic lesions, and right heart failure.

Overdose: Hyponatremia, ischemia (coronary, mesenteric, peripheral), nonspecific GI symptoms, rhabdomyolysis, and ventricular tachyarrhythmias.

ANTIDOTE
Monitor patient carefully. Notify physician of any side effect. Monitor fluid intake and urine output to ensure adequate hydration. Extravasation and/or ischemia at the injection site should be reported immediately to prevent tissue necrosis and gangrene. If extravasation occurs, stop the infusion immediately and disconnect, leaving cannula in place. Gently aspirate extravasated solution. Elevate extremity and initiate treatment of extravasation with phentolamine. If water intoxication should occur, treat with water restriction and discontinue vasopressin. If possible, discontinue gradually as described in Rate of Administration to prevent a rapid fall in BP. Direct pressor effects will resolve within minutes of withdrawal of treatment.

VECURONIUM BROMIDE BBW
(veh-kyour-**OH**-nee-um **BRO**-myd)

Neuromuscular blocking agent
(nondepolarizing)
Anesthesia adjunct

Norcuron ✦

pH 3.5 to 4.5

USUAL DOSE

Adjunct to general anesthesia: Must be individualized, depending on previous drugs administered and degree and length of muscle relaxation required. To maximize clinical benefit and to minimize the possibility of overdose, the monitoring of muscle twitch response to peripheral nerve stimulation is advised.

Initial starting dose: 0.08 to 0.1 mg/kg (80 to 100 mcg/kg) of body weight initially as an IV bolus. Must be used with adequate anesthesia and/or sedation and after unconsciousness induced. One source suggests using IBW for obese patients (equal to or greater than 30% of IBW).

Maintenance dose: Determine need for *maintenance dose* based on beginning symptoms of neuromuscular blockade reversal determined by a peripheral nerve stimulator. *IV bolus injection:* 0.01 to 0.015 mg/kg (10 to 15 mcg/kg) will be required in approximately 25 to 40 minutes and every 12 to 20 minutes thereafter to maintain muscle relaxation. Higher doses (0.15 to 0.28 mg/kg) at longer intervals have been given with proper ventilation without causing adverse cardiac effects. *Continuous infusion:* 1 mcg/kg/min. Begin 20 to 40 minutes after initial bolus dose. Initiate infusion only after early evidence of spontaneous recovery from the bolus dose. Adjust infusion rate to maintain a 90% suppression of twitch response. (Average infusion rate: 0.8 to 1.2 mcg/kg/min.)

Support of intubated, mechanically ventilated, adult ICU patients (unlabeled): Initial IV bolus dose of 0.08 to 0.1 mg/kg (80 to 100 mcg/kg) followed by a continuous IV infusion of 0.8 to 1.7 mcg/kg/min (usual range: 0.8 to 1.2 mcg/kg/min). To reduce the possibility of prolonged neuromuscular blockade and other possible complications that might occur after long-term use in the ICU, vecuronium should be administered in carefully adjusted doses by or under the supervision of experienced clinicians who are familiar with appropriate peripheral nerve stimulator muscle monitoring techniques.

PEDIATRIC DOSE

Adjunct to general anesthesia: *10 to 16 years of age:* See Usual Dose.

1 to 10 years of age: May require an initial dose that is slightly higher than the initial adult dose, and maintenance doses may be required on a more frequent basis.

Under 1 year of age: See Dose Adjustments and Maternal/Child.

DOSE ADJUSTMENTS

Reduce initial dose by 15% (i.e., 0.06 to 0.085 mg/kg) if administered more than 5 minutes after inhalation general anesthetics. If a maintenance vecuronium infusion is initiated in the presence of steady-state concentrations of enflurane or isoflurane, it may be necessary to reduce the infusion rate 25% to 60% 45 to 60 minutes after the intubating dose. Under halothane anesthesia, a reduction in infusion rate may not be necessary. ■ If intubation is performed using succinylcholine, a reduction of the initial dose of vecuronium to 0.04 to 0.06 mg/kg with inhalation anesthesia and to 0.05 to 0.06 mg/kg with balanced anesthesia may be required. Succinylcholine must show signs of wearing off before vecuronium is given. Use caution. ■ Reduced dose may be required with numerous drugs; see Drug/Lab Interactions. ■ Reduced dose may be required in renal or hepatic impairment. Preparation by dialysis before surgery is recommended for patients with renal failure. In an emergency surgery when dialysis cannot be accomplished, consider a lower initial dose. ■ Infants between 7 weeks and 1 year may require a slightly lower dose, and recovery time will be extended.

DILUTION

Each 10 mg must be reconstituted to 10 (20) mL with a **compatible** IV solution (e.g., SWFI or BWFI). May be given by IV injection, or 10 (20) mg may be further diluted to a final volume of 100 mL with NS, D5W, D5NS, or LR and given as an infusion of 0.1 (0.2) mg/mL concentration. Concentrations of 1 mg/mL have been used in the ICU setting or in fluid-restricted patients.

Storage: Store dry powder in original carton at CRT and protect from light. When reconstituted with an IV solution without preservatives (e.g., SWFI), refrigerate, use within 24 hours, and discard unused product. When reconstituted with BWFI, store at RT or refrigerated and use within 5 days.

COMPATIBILITY

Manufacturer states, "Has an acid pH. Reconstituted vecuronium should not be mixed with alkaline solutions (e.g., barbiturates) in the same syringe or administered simultaneously during IV infusion through the same needle or the same IV line."

Other sources suggest specific **compatibilities** dependent on concentration and manufacturer; consult a pharmacist.

RATE OF ADMINISTRATION

Adjunct to general anesthesia: A single dose as an IV bolus over 30 to 60 seconds. If maintenance dose is given as an infusion, adjust rate to specific dose desired as outlined in Usual Dose.

Mechanical ventilation support in ICU: See Usual Dose for specific rates and criteria.

ACTIONS

A nondepolarizing neuromuscular blocking agent about one-third more potent than pancuronium with a shorter duration of neuromuscular blockade. Acts by competing for cholinergic receptors at the motor end plate. Onset of action is within 1 minute and is dose dependent. Vecuronium produces good or excellent intubation conditions within 2.5 to 3 minutes and maximum neuromuscular blockade (paralysis) within 3 to 5 minutes. Under balanced anesthesia, clinically required neuromuscular blockade lasts approximately 25 to 30 minutes. Time to recovery to 25% of control (clinical duration) is approximately 25 to 40 minutes, and recovery is usually 95% complete at approximately 45 to 65 minutes after injection of the intubating dose. Up to three times the therapeutic dose has been given without significant changes of hemodynamic parameters in good-risk surgical patients. Excreted as metabolites in bile and urine. Crosses the placental barrier.

INDICATIONS AND USES

Adjunctive to general anesthesia, to facilitate endotracheal intubation and to relax skeletal muscles during surgery or mechanical ventilation.

Unlabeled uses: To facilitate mechanical ventilation in ICU patients.

CONTRAINDICATIONS

Known hypersensitivity to vecuronium.

PRECAUTIONS

For IV use only. ▪ Administered by or under the supervision of experienced clinicians who are familiar with its actions and the possible complications that might occur after its use. ▪ Maintenance of an adequate airway and respiratory support is imperative. Appropriate emergency drugs and equipment for monitoring the patient and responding to any medical emergency must be readily available. ▪ Use extreme caution in elderly patients, obese patients, and patients with cirrhosis, cholestasis, edematous states, or circulatory insufficiency; delay in onset or prolonged recovery is possible. ▪ In patients with myasthenia gravis or Lambert-Eaton myasthenic syndrome, small doses may have profound effects; use of a small test dose and a peripheral nerve stimulator may be of value in monitoring the response to vecuronium. ▪ Severe anaphylactic reactions have been reported with neuromuscular blocking agents; some have been fatal. Use caution in patients who have had an anaphylactic reaction to another neuromuscular blocking agent (depolarizing or nondepolarizing); cross-reactivity has occurred. ▪ Long-term use in the ICU to facilitate mechanical ventilation may be associated with prolonged paralysis and/or skeletal muscle weakness. Symptoms consistent with disuse muscle atrophy can develop in patients immobilized for extended periods. In addition, ICU patients may experience acid-base and/or electrolyte imbalances, debilitation, hypoxic episodes, and/or the use of other drugs (e.g., broad-spectrum antibiotics, narcotics, steroids) that can prolong the effects of vecuronium. Careful monitoring with a peripheral nerve stimulator during administration and recovery is strongly recommended. ▪ Patients with severe obesity or neuromuscular disease may pose airway and/or ventilator problems requiring special care; use caution. ▪ Many drugs used in anesthetic practice have triggered malignant hyperthermia (MH). Data are insufficient to establish whether or not vecuronium is capable of triggering MH. ▪ Vecuronium has no known effect on consciousness, the pain threshold, or cerebration (i.e., no analgesic or sedative properties). Patient may be conscious and completely unable to communicate by any means. Vecuronium administration must be accompanied by adequate anesthesia or sedation. Administer analgesics as needed.

Monitor: This drug produces apnea. Continuous monitoring with controlled artificial ventilation with oxygen must be available at all times. Maintain a patent airway. ▪ Use a peripheral nerve stimulator to monitor response to vecuronium and avoid overdose. ▪ Have reversal agents available (e.g., edrophonium, neostigmine, pyridostigmine with atropine or glycopyrrolate); see Antidote. ▪ Action is altered by dehydration, electrolyte imbalance, and acid-base imbalance. ▪ Recovery time extended in infants 7 weeks to 1 year. ▪ See Drug/Lab Interactions. *Mechanical ventilation support in ICU:* Physical therapy is recommended to prevent muscular weakness, atrophy, and joint contracture. Muscular weakness may be first noticed during attempts to wean patients from the ventilator.

Maternal/Child: Category C: use in pregnancy only if use justifies potential risk to fetus. Has been used during cesarean section; monitor infant carefully. Action may be enhanced by magnesium administered for the management of toxemia of pregnancy. ▪ Use caution during breast-feeding. ▪ Safety for use in infants under 7 weeks of age has not been established. ▪ Some preparations contain benzyl alcohol; do not use in premature infants. ▪ See Dose Adjustments.

Elderly: Differences in response compared to younger adults not observed. Lower-end initial doses may be appropriate based on the potential for decreased organ function and concomitant disease or drug therapy. ▪ Duration of neuromuscular block may be prolonged.

DRUG/LAB INTERACTIONS
Potentiated by **acidosis, hypokalemia, calcium channel blockers, general anesthetics, many antibiotics** (e.g., clindamycin), **aminoglycosides, polypeptide antibiotics** (e.g., bacitracin, colistimethate), **tetracyclines, vancomycin, diuretics, diazepam and other muscle relaxants, magnesium sulfate, quinidine, and others.** May need to reduce dose of vecuronium. Use with caution. ▪ Effects may be decreased by **acetylcholine, alkalosis, anticholinesterases, azathioprine, carbamazepine, and phenytoin.** ▪ **Succinylcholine** may enhance the neuromuscular blocking effect and duration of action of vecuronium and must show signs of wearing off before vecuronium is given. Use caution.

SIDE EFFECTS
The most common adverse reaction consists of an extension of the drug's pharmacologic action and may range from skeletal muscle weakness to profound and prolonged skeletal muscle paralysis resulting in respiration insufficiency or apnea. Muscular weakness and atrophy may occur with long-term use (1 to 3 weeks).

Post-Marketing: Hypersensitivity reactions, including anaphylaxis, bronchospasm, erythema, hypotension, tachycardia, and urticaria.

ANTIDOTE
All side effects are medical emergencies. Treat symptomatically. Controlled artificial ventilation must be continuous until full muscle control returns. Edrophonium, pyridostigmine, or neostigmine given with atropine or glycopyrrolate will probably reverse the muscle relaxation. Resuscitate as necessary.

VEDOLIZUMAB

Integrin receptor antagonist
Monoclonal antibody

Entyvio

pH 6.3

USUAL DOSE

Pretreatment: Updating of immunizations required, and pre-screening for tuberculosis (TB) may be indicated; see Monitor.

Vedolizumab: 300 mg as an IV infusion over 30 minutes at 0, 2, and 6 weeks and then every 8 weeks thereafter. Discontinue in patients who show no evidence of therapeutic benefit by Week 14. Consider pretreatment with standard medical therapy in patients who experience mild to moderate infusion-related reactions or hypersensitivity reactions; see Antidote.

DOSE ADJUSTMENTS

No dose adjustments indicated. ▪ Pharmacokinetics in patients with renal or hepatic insufficiency has not been studied.

DILUTION

Available as a white to off-white lyophilized powder in a single-use vial containing 300 mg. Bring vial to room temperature before reconstitution. Reconstitute with 4.8 mL SWFI using a syringe with a 21- to 25-gauge needle. Direct the SWFI to the glass wall of the vial to avoid excessive foaming. Gently swirl the vial for at least 15 seconds to dissolve the powder. *Do not vigorously shake or invert.* Allow solution to sit for up to 20 minutes. May be gently swirled. If not fully dissolved, allow another 10 minutes. Do not use if not fully dissolved within 30 minutes. Solution should be clear or opalescent, colorless to light brownish yellow. Once dissolved, gently invert the vial 3 times. Using a syringe with a 21- to 25-gauge needle, immediately withdraw 5 mL (300 mg) from the vial and add to an infusion bag or bottle containing 250 mL of NS or LR. Mix gently.

Filters: Specific information not available.

Storage: Refrigerate unopened vials at 2° to 8° C (36° to 46° F). Retain in original package to protect from light. Use reconstituted solution immediately or refrigerate for 8 hours (SWFI). Solutions diluted in NS may be stored for 12 hours at RT or for 24 hours refrigerated. Solutions diluted in LR should be used immediately if at RT or may be stored for 6 hours if refrigerated. All storage times include initial reconstitution, dilution, and administration time. Do not freeze vials, reconstituted solutions, or diluted solutions. Discard any unused portion.

COMPATIBILITY

Manufacturer states, "Do not add other medicinal products to the prepared infusion solution or intravenous infusion set."

RATE OF ADMINISTRATION

Do not administer as an IV push or bolus; for IV infusion only.

Administer a single dose (300 mg) as an IV infusion equally distributed over 30 minutes.

Flush line before the infusion and after infusion is complete with 30 mL of NS or LR.

ACTIONS

A recombinant humanized monoclonal antibody, vedolizumab is an integrin receptor antagonist. It specifically binds to the α4β7 integrin and blocks the interaction of α4β7 integrin with mucosal addressin cell adhesion molecule-1 (MAdCAM-1) and inhibits the migration of memory T-lymphocytes across the endothelium into inflamed gastrointestinal parenchymal tissue. Does not bind to or inhibit function of the α4β1 and αEβ7 integrins and does not antagonize the interaction of α4 integrins with vascular cell adhesion molecule-1 (VCAM-1). The interaction of the α4β7 integrin with MAdCAM-1 has been implicated as an important contributor to the chronic inflammation that is a hallmark of ulcerative colitis and Crohn's disease. A reduction in GI inflammation has been observed in rectal biopsy specimens. Clearance depends on both linear and nonlinear pathways. Serum half-life is approximately 25 days.

INDICATIONS AND USES

Treatment of adults with moderately to severely active ulcerative colitis (UC) to induce and maintain clinical response and clinical remission, improve the endoscopic appearance of the mucosa, and achieve corticosteroid-free remission. ■ Treatment of adults with moderately to severely active Crohn's disease (CD) to achieve clinical response and clinical remission and corticosteroid-free remission. ■ Indicated in adults with UC and CD who have had an inadequate response to, lost response to, or were intolerant to a tumor necrosis factor (TNF) blocker or immunomodulator or who had an inadequate response with, were intolerant to, or demonstrated dependence on corticosteroids.

CONTRAINDICATIONS

Known serious or severe hypersensitivity reaction to vedolizumab or any of its excipients.

PRECAUTIONS

Do not administer as an IV push or bolus; for IV infusion only ■ Administered under the direction of a physician knowledgeable in its use in a facility with adequate diagnostic and treatment facilities to monitor the patient and respond to any medical emergency. ■ Has been associated with infusion-related reactions and hypersensitivity reactions, including anaphylaxis. Reactions may occur during or several hours after the infusion. ■ Effects on the immune system may increase the risk of infection, including opportunistic infection. ■ Not recommended for patients with active, severe infections until the infections are controlled. ■ Use caution in patients with a history of recurring severe infections. ■ Progressive multifocal leukoencephalopathy (PML) has been reported with another integrin receptor antagonist; see Monitor. ■ Elevations of transaminase and/or bilirubin have occurred. May be a predictor of severe liver injury that may lead to death or the need for a liver transplant; see Monitor. ■ Update all vaccinations before initiating treatment with vedolizumab. Non–live virus vaccines (e.g., influenza) may be administered if indicated. No data on the secondary transmission of infection by live virus vaccines. ■ As with all therapeutic proteins, there is the potential for immunogenicity. Anti-vedolizumab antibodies may develop and should be considered if there is an inadequate response or a reduced therapeutic effect to treatment.

Monitor: Consider screening for tuberculosis (TB). ■ Monitor for S/S of a hypersensitivity reaction (e.g., bronchospasm, dyspnea, flushing, hypertension, rash, tachycardia, urticaria) during the infusion and for several hours after completion. ■ Assess neurologic status frequently. S/S associated with PML are diverse and occur over days to weeks. May include progressive weakness on one side of the body, clumsiness of the limbs, disturbances of vision, or changes in thinking, memory, and orientation leading to confusion and personality changes. Progression of deficits usually leads to severe disability or death over weeks to months. Withhold vedolizumab if PML is suspected; consultation with a neurologist is indicated. If PML is confirmed, discontinue vedolizumab permanently. ■ Monitor for S/S of liver injury (e.g., elevated bilirubin, elevated liver function tests, jaundice). Discontinue vedolizumab in patients with jaundice or other evidence of significant liver injury. ■ Monitor for S/S of infection.

Patient Education: Read medication guide carefully. ■ Review medical conditions and medications with healthcare provider before beginning treatment. ■ Promptly report any new medical problems (e.g., new or sudden change in thinking, eyesight, balance, or strength). ■ Report infections. ■ Report any symptoms of infusion or hypersensitivity reactions immediately (e.g., difficulty breathing, dizziness, feeling faint, itching, nausea). ■ Discuss potential risks and benefits of treatment (e.g., risk of PML). ■ Report any symptoms that may indicate liver injury (e.g., anorexia, dark urine, fatigue, jaundice, right upper abdominal discomfort).

Maternal/Child: Use during pregnancy only if the benefits to the mother outweigh the risk to the fetus. Published data suggest that the risk of adverse pregnancy outcomes in females with inflammatory bowel disease is associated with increased disease activity. Adverse pregnancy outcomes include preterm delivery, low-birth-weight infants, and infants small for gestational age at birth. A pregnancy exposure registry has been created. Contact manufacturer for information. ▪ Data suggest that vedolizumab is secreted in human milk. Use caution if required during breast-feeding; effects on breast-fed infant and on milk production unknown. ▪ Administration of vedolizumab during pregnancy could affect immune responses in the newborns and infants exposed in utero. Safety of administering live or live-attenuated vaccines in exposed infants is unknown. ▪ Safety and effectiveness for use in pediatric patients not established.

Elderly: Safety and effectiveness similar to that seen in younger adults.

DRUG/LAB INTERACTIONS

Because of the potential for increased risk of PML and other infections, avoid the concomitant use of vedolizumab with **natalizumab**. ▪ Because of the increased risk of infections, avoid the concomitant use of vedolizumab with **TNF blockers** (e.g., infliximab). ▪ Benefits must outweigh risks if **live virus vaccines** are to be administered concurrently with vedolizumab; see Precautions. ▪ Prior treatment with **TNF blockers** (e.g., infliximab), coadministered **immunomodulators** (including azathioprine, 6-mercaptopurine, methotrexate), and coadministered **aminosalicylates** did not have a clinically meaningful effect on the pharmacokinetics of vedolizumab.

SIDE EFFECTS

Arthralgia, back pain, bronchitis, cough, fatigue, fever, headache, influenza, nasopharyngitis, nausea, oropharyngeal pain, pain in extremities, pruritus, rash, sinusitis, and upper respiratory tract infection are most common. Infusion-related reactions and hypersensitivity reactions, including anaphylaxis, have occurred. Other serious side effects include liver injury (e.g., hepatitis), malignancies, PML, and serious infections such as anal abscess, cytomegaloviral colitis, giardiasis, *Listeria* meningitis, salmonella sepsis, sepsis (some fatal), and tuberculosis.

ANTIDOTE

Keep physician informed of all side effects. Most will be treated symptomatically. Discontinue vedolizumab at the first sign of liver injury. Discontinue infusion if any S/S of a serious hypersensitivity or infusion reaction occur. Treat with epinephrine, corticosteroids, diphenhydramine, bronchodilators, and oxygen as indicated. In clinical trials, patients with mild to moderate infusion-related reactions or hypersensitivity reactions were pretreated with standard medical therapy (e.g., acetaminophen, antihistamines, and/or hydrocortisone) before the next infusion. Withhold vedolizumab if S/S suggestive of PML occur; if diagnosis is confirmed, discontinue permanently. Consider withholding vedolizumab if a severe infection occurs.

VERAPAMIL HYDROCHLORIDE
(ver-**AP**-ah-mil hy-droh-**KLOR**-eyed)

Calcium channel blocker
Antiarrhythmic

pH 4.1 to 6

USUAL DOSE
ECG and BP monitoring recommended.

Verapamil: 5 to 10 mg initially (0.075 to 0.15 mg/kg of body weight). May cause transient bradycardia or hypotension. 10 mg (0.15 mg/kg) may be repeated in 30 minutes if needed to achieve appropriate response. Maximum total dose is 20 mg. AHA recommendation is 2.5 to 5 mg as an initial dose. Repeat 5 to 10 mg if needed every 15 to 30 min. Maximum dose 20 mg. Alternately, give 5 mg every 15 min to a total dose of 30 mg.

PEDIATRIC DOSE
ECG and BP monitoring mandatory. See Maternal/Child.

Infants up to 1 year of age: 0.1 to 0.2 mg/kg of body weight (usually 0.75 to 2 mg). Repeat in 30 minutes if indicated.

1 to 15 years of age: 0.1 to 0.3 mg/kg (usually 2 to 5 mg). Do not exceed 5 mg. Repeat in 30 minutes if response not adequate. Repeat dose should not exceed 10 mg as a single dose.

DOSE ADJUSTMENTS
Reduced dose may be required in hepatic or renal disease, especially with repeat dosing. ■ Dose selection should be cautious in the elderly. Reduced doses may be indicated based on the potential for decreased organ function and concomitant disease or drug therapy. ■ See Drug/Lab Interactions.

DILUTION
IV injection: May be given undiluted through Y-tube of tubing containing D5W, NS, or Ringer's solution for infusion.

Filters: No data available from manufacturer.

Storage: Store between 15° and 30° C (59° and 86° F). Protect from light and freezing. Do not use if discolored or particulate matter present. Discard unused solution.

COMPATIBILITY
Manufacturer states, "Not recommended for dilution with sodium lactate in polyvinyl chloride bags. Will precipitate in any solution with a pH greater than 6." Lists as **incompatible** with albumin, amphotericin B (conventional), hydralazine, sulfamethoxazole/trimethoprim.

Other sources suggest specific **compatibilities** dependent on concentration and manufacturer; consult a pharmacist.

RATE OF ADMINISTRATION
IV injection: A single dose over a minimum of 2 minutes for adults and pediatric patients. Extend to 3 minutes in the elderly.

ACTIONS
A calcium antagonist. It inhibits calcium (and possibly sodium) ion influx through slow channels into conductile and contractile myocardial cells and vascular smooth muscle cells. Slows conduction through the AV node, prolongs effective refractory period within the AV node, and reduces ventricular rates in patients with atrial flutter and/or atrial fibrillation and a rapid ventricular response. Prevents re-entry phenomena through the AV node. Reduces myocardial contractility, afterload, arterial pressure, systemic vascular resistance, and oxygen demand. Effective within 3 to 5 minutes. Hemodynamic effects last about 20 minutes, but antiarrhythmic effects may last up to 6 hours. Does not alter total serum calcium levels. Metabolized in the liver. Half-life range is 2 to 5 hours. Crosses the placental barrier. Excreted in urine and feces. Secreted in breast milk.

INDICATIONS AND USES

Treatment of supraventricular tachyarrhythmias, including (1) conversion to normal sinus rhythm of paroxysmal supraventricular tachycardia, including those associated with accessory bypass tracts (Wolff-Parkinson-White [WPW] and Lown-Ganong-Levine [LGL] syndromes); and (2) temporary control of rapid ventricular rate in atrial flutter or atrial fibrillation (except when the atrial flutter and/or atrial fibrillation are associated with accessory bypass tracts [WPW and LGL syndromes]).

Unlabeled uses: Alternative drug after adenosine to terminate re-entry SVT with narrow QRS complex and adequate BP and preserved LV function (AHA guidelines).

CONTRAINDICATIONS

Patients with atrial fibrillation or flutter and an accessory bypass tract (e.g., Wolff-Parkinson-White or Lown-Ganong-Levine syndromes), cardiogenic shock, congestive heart failure (severe) unless secondary to supraventricular tachyarrhythmia treatable with verapamil, known hypersensitivity to verapamil, second- or third-degree AV block (unless functioning artificial pacemaker is in place), severe hypotension, sick sinus syndrome (unless functioning artificial pacemaker in place), patients receiving IV beta-adrenergic blocking drugs (e.g., propranolol) within a few hours, and ventricular tachycardia.

PRECAUTIONS

Administer in a facility with adequate personnel, equipment, and supplies to monitor the patient and respond to any medical emergency. A small fraction (less than 1%) of patients may respond with life-threatening adverse responses, including rapid ventricular rate in atrial flutter/fibrillation with an accessory bypass tract, marked hypotension, or extreme bradycardia/asystole. ▪ Valsalva maneuver is recommended before use of verapamil in paroxysmal supraventricular tachycardia if clinically appropriate. ▪ May produce hypotension. Usually transient and asymptomatic, but can cause dizziness. ▪ Has rarely caused second- and third-degree AV block and, in extreme cases, asystole. More common in patients with sick sinus syndrome (SA nodal disease); see Elderly. ▪ Caution required in hepatic and renal disease, especially if repeated dosing is required. ▪ Use extreme caution in patients with hypertrophic cardiomyopathy. ▪ May cause marked hemodynamic deterioration and ventricular fibrillation in patients with wide-complex ventricular tachycardia. ▪ When heart failure is not severe or rate related, it should be controlled with digoxin and diuretics before using verapamil. ▪ Patients with pulmonary wedge pressure above 20 mm Hg and/or ejection fraction below 30% may experience acute worsening of heart failure. ▪ May precipitate respiratory muscle failure in patients with muscular dystrophy. ▪ May increase intracranial pressure during anesthesia induction in patients with supratentorial tumors. Use caution and monitor closely. ▪ Reduction of myocardial contractility may worsen CHF in patients with severe left ventricular dysfunction.

Monitor: Continuous ECG and BP monitoring recommended. ▪ Emergency resuscitation drugs and equipment must always be available. ▪ Maintain bed rest until effects on HR, BP, and potential dizziness are evaluated. ▪ See Drug/Lab Interactions.

Maternal/Child: Category C: safety for use in pregnancy not yet established; use only when clearly indicated. ▪ Discontinue breast-feeding. ▪ Controlled studies have not been conducted in pediatric patients. Has been used in pediatric patients, including infants and newborns. Results of treatment were similar to those in adults. However, in rare instances severe hemodynamic side effects (e.g., bradycardia, hypotension, or a rapid ventricular rate in atrial flutter/fibrillation) have occurred in infants and neonates. Use caution and monitor closely.

Elderly: May have an increased hypotensive effect; see Rate of Administration. ▪ Half-life may be prolonged; see Dose Adjustments. ▪ Elderly patients are more likely to have sick sinus syndrome, which may increase the risk of second- or third-degree AV block, bradycardia and, in extreme cases, asystole.

DRUG/LAB INTERACTIONS

Potentiates **digoxin;** lower dose may be appropriate. Both drugs slow AV conduction. Monitor for AV block and bradycardia. ▪ Do not give concomitantly (within a few hours) with **IV beta-adrenergic blocking drugs**; see Contraindications. Both drugs depress myocardial contractility and AV node conduction; monitor patient closely. Use with extreme caution with **oral or ophthalmic beta-blockers.** ▪ Do not administer **disopyramide** within 48 hours before or 24 hours after verapamil. ▪ Use caution with **inhalation anesthetics.** Both depress cardiovascular activity. Titrate each carefully to avoid excessive cardiovascular depression. ▪ Coadministration with **amiodarone** may result in bradycardia, hypotension, and decreased cardiac output. Monitor closely. ▪ Potentiates **cyclosporine, carbamazepine, and theophyllines.** Monitor serum levels of these drugs and adjust dose as needed. ▪ Potentiates **nondepolarizing muscle relaxants** (e.g., vecuronium); dose reduction of either drug may be required. ▪ Metabolism may be decreased and serum concentrations may be increased by **itraconazole.** ▪ Verapamil may increase serum concentrations of **dofetilide.** One source says avoid use; another says concurrent use contraindicated. ▪ Avoid concomitant use of **ivabradine** and verapamil. Concurrent use increases serum concentrations of ivabradine, which may exacerbate bradycardia and conduction disturbances. ▪ Verapamil may increase serum concentrations of **HMG-CoA reductase inhibitors, imipramine, sirolimus, and tacrolimus.** Monitor serum levels and/or monitor for S/S of toxicity; adjust dose as needed. ▪ Concomitant use of **HMG-CoA reductase inhibitors** has been associated with reports of myopathy and rhabdomyolysis. In patients receiving verapamil, limit dose of simvastatin to 10 mg daily and limit lovastatin dose to 40 mg daily. Dose reductions for other HMG-CoA reductase inhibitors may also be required. ▪ May increase effects of certain **benzodiazepines** (e.g., midazolam, triazolam) and **buspirone**; monitor and adjust doses as indicated. ▪ May cause excessive hypotension with **other antihypertensive drugs** (vasodilators and diuretics). ▪ Serum concentrations and effectiveness of verapamil may be decreased by **barbiturates, calcium salts,** and **phenytoin**. ▪ Concomitant use with **IV dantrolene** may result in cardiovascular collapse. ▪ Use caution with **quinidine**; may cause hypotension. ▪ Highly protein bound; use with caution with **other highly protein-bound drugs** (e.g., oral hypoglycemics, warfarin). ▪ Variable effects when administered with **lithium.** Has caused decreased effectiveness of lithium and may cause neurotoxicity. ▪ Monitor heart rate with concurrent use of verapamil with **clonidine;** has resulted in sinus bradycardia requiring pacemaker insertion. ▪ **Grapefruit juice** may affect certain enzymes of the P_{450} enzyme system and increase the serum concentrations of verapamil and should be avoided.

SIDE EFFECTS
Abdominal discomfort, asystole, bradycardia, dizziness, headache, second- and third-degree heart block, heart failure, hypersensitivity reactions (including anaphylaxis, bronchospasm/laryngospasm, itch, urticaria), rapid ventricular rate (Wolff-Parkinson-White and Lown-Ganong-Levine syndromes), hypotension (symptomatic), increased ventricular response in atrial flutter, nausea, PVCs, skin eruptions (including rare reports of erythema multiforme), seizures (rare), tachycardia (severe).

ANTIDOTE
Discontinue verapamil and notify physician promptly if hypotension, bradycardia, or second- or third-degree heart block occurs. Keep physician informed of all side effects. Treatment will depend on clinical situation. Calcium chloride may reverse effects of verapamil and can be used in toxicity. Glucagon may also be used in toxicity; see glucagon monograph. Rapid ventricular response (due to antegrade conduction in atrial flutter/fibrillation with WPW or LGL syndromes) should respond to cardioversion, procainamide, and/or lidocaine. Treat bradycardia, AV block, and asystole with standard AHA protocol (atropine, pacing). Norepinephrine, calcium chloride, or dopamine will reverse hypotension. Treat hypersensitivity reactions or resuscitate as necessary. Not removed by hemodialysis.

VINBLASTINE SULFATE BBW
(vin-**BLAS**-teen **SUL**-fayt)

VLB

Antineoplastic
(mitotic inhibitor-vinca alkaloid)

pH 3.5 to 5

USUAL DOSE
Pretreatment: Baseline studies indicated; see Monitor. See Maternal/Child.
Auxiliary labeling required; see Precautions.

Vinblastine: 3.7 mg/M^2 initially. Administered once every 7 days, increasing the dose to specific amounts (5.5, 7.4, 9.25, 11.1 mg/M^2) by a single step each week until the WBC count is decreased to 3,000 cells/mm^3, remission is achieved, or a maximum dose of 18.5 mg/M^2 is reached. Maintenance dose is one step below any dose that causes leukopenia (3,000 cells/mm^3 or less), once every 7 to 14 days. Usually 5.5 to 7.4 mg/M^2. Continue treatment for 4 to 6 weeks. Up to 12 weeks often necessary.

PEDIATRIC DOSE
See Maternal/Child.

One source suggests 2.5 mg/M^2 initially. Use same procedure as for adult dose using steps to 3.75, 5, 6.25, and 7.5 mg/M^2. Maximum dose is 12.5 mg/M^2. Maintenance dose is calculated by same parameters as Usual Dose (above). Usually differs with each individual. Other sources suggest that initial doses vary depending on the schedule used, use of vinblastine as a single agent, or its use in a combination regimen. Some suggested doses are:

Letterer-Siwe disease (unlabeled): As a single agent, an initial dose of 6.5 mg/M^2.

Hodgkin disease: An initial dose of 6 mg/M^2 in combination with other chemotherapeutic agents.

Testicular cancer: An initial dose of 3 mg/M^2 in combination with other chemotherapeutic agents.

DOSE ADJUSTMENTS
Reduce dose by 50% if serum bilirubin above 3 mg/dL. ▪ Often used with other antineoplastic drugs and corticosteroids in reduced doses and/or extended intervals to achieve tumor remission.

DILUTION
Specific techniques required; see Precautions. Each 10 mg is diluted with 10 mL of NS for injection. 1 mg equals 1 mL. Also available in liquid form (1 mg/mL). May be given by IV injection or through Y-tube of a free-flowing IV infusion.

Storage: Store in refrigerator before and after dilution. Potency maintained for 28 days after dilution if reconstituted with bacteriostatic NS.

COMPATIBILITY
Manufacturer suggests that the pH not be altered from between 3.5 to 5 by an additive or a diluent, and it recommends NS as a diluent and not admixing with other drugs in the same container.

Other sources suggest specific **compatibilities** dependent on concentration and manufacturer; consult a pharmacist.

RATE OF ADMINISTRATION
IV injection: Total desired dose, properly diluted, over 1 minute.

ACTIONS
An alkaloid of the periwinkle plant with antitumor activity. Cell cycle–specific for M phase. Thought to interfere with the metabolic pathways of amino acids. Sometimes pharmacologically effective without any noticeable improvement in symptoms of malignancy. Cell energy production and synthesis of nucleic acid may also be inhibited. Half-life is 24.8 hours. Metabolism mediated by the hepatic cytochrome P$_{450}$ isoenzymes in the CYP 3A subfamily. Some excretion through bile and urine.

INDICATIONS AND USES

To suppress or retard neoplastic growth. Remission and probable cure have been achieved with bleomycin and cisplatin in testicular malignancies. Response has been noted in Hodgkin disease, non-Hodgkin lymphomas, choriocarcinoma, Kaposi's sarcoma, mycosis fungoides, breast and renal cell malignancies. ▪ Used to treat many other malignancies.

CONTRAINDICATIONS

Bacterial infection or leukopenia below 3,000 cells/mm^3.

PRECAUTIONS

Follow guidelines for handling cytotoxic agents. See Appendix A, p. 1308. ▪ Usually administered by or under the direction of the physician specialist. ▪ Manufacturer provides an auxiliary sticker labeled "Fatal if given intrathecally, for IV use only" and an overwrap labeled "Do not remove covering until moment of injection. Fatal if given intrathecally. For intravenous use only." Each and every syringe containing a specific dose and prepared in advance of actual administration must be labeled with the provided auxiliary sticker and packaged in this overwrap. If intrathecal injection should occur, immediate neurosurgical intervention is required; consult package insert for immediate steps to be taken. ▪ May cause corneal ulceration with accidental contact to the eye. ▪ Use caution in presence of ulcerated skin areas, cachexia, or impaired liver function. ▪ Leukocyte and platelet counts have fallen precipitously in patients with malignant-cell infiltration of the bone marrow following moderate doses of vinblastine. Further administration is not recommended. ▪ Acute pulmonary reactions including acute shortness of breath and severe bronchospasm have been reported in patients receiving vinca alkaloids. Occurs most frequently when given in combination with mitomycin-C. Onset of reaction may occur minutes to hours after vinca administration and up to 2 weeks following the mitomycin dose.

Monitor: WBC count must be checked before each dose. Must be above 4,000 cells/mm^3. ▪ Determine absolute patency, quality of vein, and adequate circulation of extremity. Severe cellulitis may result from extravasation. Rinse syringe and needle with venous blood before withdrawal from the vein; see Antidote. ▪ Leukopenia is dose-limiting toxicity. Nadir occurs 5 to 10 days after therapy. Recovery occurs within another 7 to 14 days. ▪ Be alert for signs of bone marrow suppression or infection. ▪ Prophylactic antibiotics may be indicated pending results of C/S in a febrile neutropenic patient. ▪ Thrombocytopenia is rare, but may occur in patients whose bone marrow has been impaired by prior radiation therapy or other bone marrow suppressants. If platelet count is less than 50,000/mm^3, initiate precautions to prevent excessive bleeding (e.g., inspect IV sites, skin, and mucous membranes; use extreme care during invasive procedures; test urine, emesis, stool, and secretions for occult blood). ▪ Observe for increased uric acid levels; may require increased doses of antigout agents; allopurinol (Aloprim) preferred. ▪ Maintain adequate hydration. ▪ Prophylactic antiemetics may increase patient comfort. ▪ See Drug/Lab Interactions.

Patient Education: Avoid pregnancy; effective birth control recommended. ▪ Report IV site burning or stinging promptly. ▪ Report chills, fever, sore mouth, or throat promptly. ▪ Maintain adequate hydration; avoid constipation. ▪ See Appendix D, p. 1311.

Maternal/Child: Category D: avoid pregnancy. May produce teratogenic effects on the fetus. Has a mutagenic potential. ▪ Discontinue breast-feeding. ▪ Do not use diluents containing benzyl alcohol in premature infants.

Elderly: Leukopenic response may be increased in malnutrition or with skin ulcers.

DRUG/LAB INTERACTIONS

Inhibited by **some amino acids, glutamic acid, and tryptophan.** ▪ Potentiated by **other bone marrow suppressants** (e.g., antineoplastics, radiation therapy). ▪ Do not administer **live virus vaccines** to patients receiving antineoplastic drugs. ▪ Acute pulmonary reactions can occur with **mitomycin-C;** see Precautions. ▪ May inhibit effects of **phenytoin;** increased doses of phenytoin may be needed. ▪ **Erythromycin** decreases metabolism and increases toxicity of vinblastine. ■ Use caution with **any drug that inhibits P₄₅₀ enzymes** (e.g., calcium channel blockers, antifungal agents, bromocriptine, cimetidine, clarithromycin, cyclosporine, danazol, metoclopramide); may increase vinblastine blood levels and increase toxicity. ■ Effect of **bleomycin** is significantly enhanced if vinblastine is administered 6 to 8 hours before bleomycin administration.

SIDE EFFECTS

Usually dose related and not always reversible: abdominal pain, alopecia, anorexia, cellulitis, constipation, convulsions, diarrhea, dizziness, extravasation, gonadal suppression, headache, hemorrhage, ileus, leukopenia (severe), malaise, mental depression, myelosuppression, nausea, numbness, oral lesions, paresthesias, peripheral neuritis, pharyngitis, Raynaud's syndrome, reflex depression (deep tendon), skin lesions, thrombophlebitis, tumor site pain, vomiting, weakness.

ANTIDOTE

For extravasation, discontinue the drug immediately and administer into another vein. Hyaluronidase should be injected locally into extravasated area. Use a fine hypodermic needle. Elevate extremity. Moist heat may be helpful. Notify the physician of all side effects; symptomatic treatment is often indicated. Administration of whole blood products (e.g., packed RBCs, platelets, leukocytes) and/or blood modifiers (e.g., darbepoetin alfa, epoetin alfa, filgrastim, pegfilgrastim, sargramostim) may be indicated to treat bone marrow toxicity. Glutamic acid blocks toxicity of vinblastine but also blocks its antineoplastic activity.

VINCRISTINE SULFATE BBW ▪
VINCRISTINE SULFATE LIPOSOME
INJECTION BBW

(vin-**KRIS**-teen **SUL**-fayt)
(vin-**KRIS**-teen **SUL**-fayt **LIP**-oh-sohm in-**JEK**-shun)

Antineoplastic
(mitotic inhibitor-vinca alkaloid)

VCR, Vincasar PFS ▪ Marqibo

pH 3.5 to 5.5 • pH not available

USUAL DOSE

Pretreatment: Verify pregnancy status. Baseline studies/assessment indicated; see Monitor.

CONVENTIONAL VINCRISTINE

Auxiliary labeling required; see Precautions.

Neurotoxicity appears to be dose related. Use extreme care in calculating and administering vincristine. Overdose may be fatal.

1.4 mg/M^2 administered once every 7 days. Various dosage schedules have been used with caution.

MARQIBO (LIPOSOMAL VINCRISTINE)

2.25 mg/M^2 as an IV infusion over 1 hour once every 7 days. Liposomal vincristine has different dosage recommendations than conventional vincristine. Verify drug name and dose before preparation and administration.

PEDIATRIC DOSE

CONVENTIONAL VINCRISTINE

Weight over 10 kg: 1.5 to 2 mg/M^2 once each week.
Weight 10 kg (22 lb) or less: 0.05 mg/kg of body weight once a week. See comments under Usual Dose.

MARQIBO (LIPOSOMAL VINCRISTINE)

Safety and effectiveness for use in pediatric patients not established.

DOSE ADJUSTMENTS

CONVENTIONAL VINCRISTINE: In impaired hepatic function, reduce initial doses by 50% if direct bilirubin above 3 mg/dL. May be increased gradually based on individual response.
▪ Usually given with other antineoplastic drugs and corticosteroids in reduced doses to achieve tumor remission. ▪ See Drug/Lab Interactions.

MARQIBO (LIPOSOMAL VINCRISTINE)

Recommended Dose Modifications for Marqibo-Related Peripheral Neuropathy	
Severity of Peripheral Neuropathy Signs/Symptoms[a]	**Modification of Marqibo Dose and Regimen**
Patient develops Grade 3 (severe symptoms, limiting self-care activities of daily living [ADL][b]) or persistent Grade 2 (moderate symptoms, limiting instrumental ADL[c]) peripheral neuropathy.	Interrupt Marqibo. If the peripheral neuropathy remains at Grade 3 or 4, discontinue Marqibo. If the peripheral neuropathy recovers to Grade 1 or 2, reduce the Marqibo dose to 2 mg/M^2.
Patient has persistent Grade 2 peripheral neuropathy after the first dose reduction to 2 mg/M^2.	Interrupt Marqibo for up to 7 days. If the peripheral neuropathy increases to Grade 3 or 4, discontinue Marqibo. If peripheral neuropathy recovers to Grade 1, reduce the Marqibo dose to 1.825 mg/M^2.
Patient has persistent Grade 2 peripheral neuropathy after the second dose reduction to 1.825 mg/M^2.	Interrupt Marqibo for up to 7 days. If the peripheral neuropathy increases to Grade 3 or 4, discontinue Marqibo. If the toxicity recovers to Grade 1, reduce the Marqibo dose to 1.5 mg/M^2.

[a]Grading based on the National Cancer Institute Common Terminology Criteria for Adverse Events (CTCAE), v4.0.
[b]Self-care ADL: Refers to bathing, dressing/undressing, feeding self, using the toilet, taking medications, not bedridden.
[c]Instrumental ADL: Refers to preparing meals, shopping for groceries and clothes, using telephone, managing money, etc.

DILUTION

CONVENTIONAL VINCRISTINE: *Specific techniques required; see Precautions.* Apply auxiliary label and package in manufacturer-supplied overwrap; see Precautions. Available in preservative-free solutions (1 mg/mL). May be given by IV injection or through Y-tube or of a free-flowing IV infusion. Occasionally further diluted in 50 mL or more NS or D5W and given as an infusion. To reduce the potential for fatal medication errors due to incorrect route of administration, vincristine should be diluted in a flexible plastic container and prominently labeled as indicated for intravenous use only.

MARQIBO (LIPOSOMAL VINCRISTINE): *Specific techniques required; see Precautions.* Marqibo will be prepared in the pharmacy by a very specific process that takes approximately 60 to 90 minutes. Dedicated, uninterrupted time is required due to extensive monitoring of temperature and time required for preparation. When prepared according to directions, each single-dose vial contains 5 mg/31 mL (0.16 mg/mL). Refer to manufacturer's literature for a detailed outline of the preparation procedure. Contact manufacturer if questions arise about preparation.

Items required by the pharmacy to prepare Marqibo include:
- Marqibo kit
- Water bath*
- Calibrated thermometer (0° to 100° C)*
- Calibrated electronic timer*
- Sterile venting needle or other suitable device equipped with a sterile 0.2-micron filter
- 1-mL or 3-mL sterile syringe with needle, and a 5-mL sterile syringe with needle

*Manufacturer will send the water bath, calibrated thermometer, and calibrated electronic timer to the medical facility at the initial order of Marqibo and will replace them every 2 years.

Filters: *Marqibo (liposomal vincristine):* 0.2-micron filter required during preparation; however, *do not use with in-line filters*.

Storage: *Conventional vincristine:* Store in refrigerator. Retain in carton to protect from light. Store upright. Solutions diluted with NS to a concentration of 0.0015 to 0.08 mg/mL are stable for 24 hours when protected from light or for 8 hours under normal light at 25° C (77° F).

Marqibo (liposomal vincristine): Store Marqibo kit in refrigerator at 2° to 8° C (36° to 46° F). *Do not freeze.* Once prepared, may be stored at CRT for no more than 12 hours.

COMPATIBILITY

CONVENTIONAL VINCRISTINE

Manufacturer suggests that the pH not be altered from between 3.5 to 5.5 by an additive or a diluent, and it recommends NS or D5W as a diluent and not admixing with other drugs in the same container.

Other sources suggest specific **compatibilities** dependent on concentration and manufacturer; consult a pharmacist.

MARQIBO (LIPOSOMAL VINCRISTINE)

Manufacturer states, "Do not mix with other drugs."

RATE OF ADMINISTRATION

CONVENTIONAL VINCRISTINE

"Fatal if given intrathecally; for IV use only."

IV injection: Total desired dose, properly diluted, over 1 minute.

Infusion: A single dose over 5 to 10 minutes or as a continuous infusion (based on specific protocols).

MARQIBO (LIPOSOMAL VINCRISTINE)

For IV use only; fatal if given by other routes. A single dose as an IV infusion equally distributed over 1 hour. Administer through a secure and free-flowing venous access line.

ACTIONS

CONVENTIONAL VINCRISTINE: An alkaloid of the periwinkle plant with antitumor activity. Cell cycle–specific for the M phase. It binds to tubulin, altering the tubulin polymerization equilibrium and resulting in altered microtubule structure and function. It stabilizes the spindle apparatus, preventing chromosome segregation and triggering metaphase arrest and inhibition of mitosis. Well distributed except in spinal fluid. Extensively metabolized with a half-life of 85 hours. Primarily excreted through feces.

MARQIBO (LIPOSOMAL VINCRISTINE): Vincristine encapsulated in sphingomyelin/cholesterol liposomes. Its mechanism of action, distribution, and elimination is similar to that of conventional vincristine.

INDICATIONS AND USES

CONVENTIONAL VINCRISTINE: Treatment of acute leukemia. ▪ Useful in combination with other oncolytic agents for Hodgkin disease, non-Hodgkin malignant lymphomas, rhabdomyosarcoma, neuroblastoma, and Wilms' tumor.

MARQIBO (LIPOSOMAL VINCRISTINE): Treatment of adults with Philadelphia chromosome-negative (Ph-) acute lymphoblastic leukemia (ALL) in second or greater relapse or adults whose disease has progressed following two or more antileukemia therapies. Indication based on overall response rate; clinical benefit such as improvement in overall survival not verified.

Unlabeled uses: **Conventional vincristine:** Treatment of idiopathic thrombocytopenic purpura; treatment of Kaposi's sarcoma, breast and bladder cancer.

CONTRAINDICATIONS

Both formulations: Demyelinating form of Charcot-Marie-Tooth syndrome.

Marqibo (liposomal vincristine): Hypersensitivity to vincristine sulfate or any of the components of Marqibo.

PRECAUTIONS

BOTH FORMULATIONS: Follow guidelines for handling cytotoxic agents. See Appendix A, p. 1308. ▪ Administered by or under the direction of the physician specialist. ▪ Sensory and motor neuropathies are common and cumulative. Risk of neurologic toxicity is greater in patients with pre-existing neuromuscular disorders or when other potentially neurotoxic drugs are coadministered; see Monitor. ▪ Myelosuppression may require dose adjustment. ▪ Tumor lysis syndrome leading to acute uric acid nephropathy has occurred; see Monitor.

CONVENTIONAL VINCRISTINE: Manufacturer provides an auxiliary sticker labeled "Fatal if given intrathecally, for IV use only" and an overwrap labeled "Do not remove covering until moment of injection. For intravenous use only. Fatal if given by other routes." Each and every infusion bag or syringe containing a specific dose and prepared in advance of actual administration must be labeled with the provided auxiliary sticker and packaged in this overwrap. If intrathecal injection should occur, immediate neurosurgical intervention is required; consult package insert for immediate steps to be taken. ▪ If central nervous system leukemia is diagnosed, additional agents may be required because vincristine does not appear to cross the blood-brain barrier in adequate amounts. ▪ Acute shortness of breath and severe bronchospasm have been reported following administration of vinca alkaloids. These reactions occur most frequently when the vinca alkaloid is administered in combination with mitomycin-C. Onset of these reactions may occur minutes to several hours after the vinca alkaloid is injected and may occur up to 2 weeks after the dose of mitomycin. Progressive dyspnea requiring chronic therapy may occur. Reaction may require aggressive treatment, especially if pre-existing pulmonary dysfunction is present. Vincristine should not be readministered. ▪ Use extreme caution in combination with radiation therapy. Should not be given to patients while they are receiving radiation therapy through radiation ports that include the liver. ▪ May cause corneal ulceration with accidental contact to the eye; flush eyes with water immediately. ▪ Use caution in pre-existing neuromuscular disease or impaired liver function. ▪ Not recommended for use in patients receiving radiation therapy that involves the liver.

MARQIBO (LIPOSOMAL VINCRISTINE): For IV use only; fatal if given by other routes. ▪ Death has occurred with intrathecal administration. ▪ Has different dose recommendations than conventional vincristine. Verify drug name and dose before preparation and administration to avoid overdose. ▪ Constipation and bowel obstruction have occurred. ▪ Can cause severe fatigue requiring dose delay, reduction, or discontinuation of therapy. ▪ Fatal liver toxicity and elevated AST have occurred. ▪ The influence of renal impairment and severe hepatic impairment has not been evaluated.

Monitor: *Both Formulations:* Monitor CBC and platelets, bilirubin, and liver function tests before therapy and at frequent intervals. ▪ Determine absolute patency and quality of vein and adequate circulation of extremity. Severe cellulitis may result from extravasation; see Antidote. ▪ Monitor neurologic status before therapy and at frequent intervals. Symptoms of neuropathy may include areflexia, arthralgia, burning sensation, cranial neuropathy, decreased vibratory sense, hyperesthesia, hypoesthesia, hyporeflexia, ileus, jaw pain, muscle spasm, myalgia, neuralgia, paresthesia, or weakness. ▪ Be alert for signs of bone marrow suppression or infection. Prophylactic antibiotics may be indicated pending results of C/S in a febrile neutropenic patient. ▪ Observe for increased uric acid levels; may require increased doses of antigout agents (allopurinol [Aloprim] preferred) and may require alkalinization of urine. Monitor for early signs of tumor lysis syndrome (e.g., flank pain and hematuria). ▪ Maintain adequate hydration. ▪ Prophylactic antiemetics may increase patient comfort. ▪ Monitor for hyponatremia and inappropriate secretion of antidiuretic hormone (ADH); may require fluid limitation. ▪ Institute a prophylactic bowel regimen to prevent potential constipation, bowel obstruction, and/or paralytic ileus. ▪ Monitor for thrombocytopenia (platelet count less than 50,000/mm³). Initiate precautions to prevent excessive bleeding (e.g., inspect IV sites, skin, and mucous membranes; use extreme care during invasive procedures; test urine, emesis, stool, and secretions for occult blood). ▪ See Drug/Lab Interactions.

Patient Education: *Both formulations:* Avoid pregnancy; nonhormonal birth control recommended. ▪ Report IV site burning or stinging promptly. ▪ See Appendix D, p. 1311. ▪ Use adequate dietary fiber, hydration, stool softeners and, if necessary, laxatives to avoid constipation.

Maternal/Child: *Both formulations:* Category D: avoid pregnancy. Can cause fetal harm. ▪ Discontinue breast-feeding.

Marqibo (liposomal vincristine): Safety and effectiveness for use in pediatric patients not established.

Elderly: *Both formulations:* Neurotoxicity may be more severe (observe closely for constipation, ileus, and urinary retention). Dose selection should be cautious.

DRUG/LAB INTERACTIONS

Studies have not been conducted for Marqibo, but it is expected to have interactions similar to conventional vincristine. ▪ Acute pulmonary reactions can occur with **mitomycin-C.** ▪ Do not administer **live virus vaccines** to patients receiving antineoplastic drugs. ▪ May decrease levels and effectiveness of **digoxin and phenytoin.** Monitor serum levels of digoxin and phenytoin; increased doses of these drugs may be required. ▪ A substrate for cytochrome P_{450} isoenzymes (CYP3A). Avoid concurrent use of **drugs known to inhibit cytochrome P_{450} isoenzymes** (e.g., atazanavir, clarithromycin, indinavir, itraconazole, ketoconazole, nefazodone, nelfinavir, ritonavir, saquinavir) and **inducers of cytochrome P_{450} enzymes** (e.g., carbamazepine, dexamethasone, phenobarbital, phenytoin, rifabutin, rifampin, St. John's wort). ▪ Although not yet studied, it is likely that there will be interactions, and concomitant use should be avoided with **inhibitors of P-gp** (e.g., amiodarone, clarithromycin, diltiazem, erythromycin, itraconazole, ketoconazole, protease inhibitors [e.g., nelfinavir, ritonavir], quinidine, sirolimus, tacrolimus) and **inducers of P-gp** (e.g., rifampin, St. John's wort).

SIDE EFFECTS

CONVENTIONAL VINCRISTINE: Frequently dose related and not always reversible: abdominal pain, alopecia, anemia (rare), ataxia, bronchospasm, cellulitis, constipation, convulsions, cranial nerve damage, diarrhea, dysuria, extravasation, fever, foot-drop, gonadal suppression, headache, hepatic veno-occlusive disease, hypersensitivity reactions (e.g., anaphylaxis, edema, rash), hypertension, hypotension, leukopenia (rare), muscle wasting, nausea, neuritic pain, oral lacerations, paralytic ileus, paresthesias, polyuria, reflex changes, sensory impairment, shortness of breath, SIADH, thrombocytopenia (rare), thrombophlebitis, tingling and numbness of extremities, upper colon impaction, uric acid nephropathy, vomiting, weakness, weight loss.

MARQIBO (LIPOSOMAL VINCRISTINE): Anemia, constipation, decreased appetite, diarrhea, fatigue, febrile neutropenia, fever, insomnia, nausea, and peripheral sensory and motor neuropathy are most common. Asthenia, bowel obstruction, cardiac arrest, hypotension, ileus, increased AST, mental status changes, muscle weakness, neutropenia, pain, pneumonia, renal disorders, respiratory distress and/or failure, septic shock, staphylococcal bacteremia, and thrombocytopenia have also been reported. Extravasation, hepatic toxicity, and tumor lysis syndrome have occurred.

ANTIDOTE

For extravasation, discontinue the drug immediately and administer into another vein. Hyaluronidase may be injected locally into extravasated area. Use a fine hypodermic needle. Elevate extremity; moist heat may be helpful. Notify the physician of all side effects; symptomatic treatment is often indicated. Will probably reduce dose at earliest signs of neurologic toxicity (tingling and numbness of extremities). Discontinue for inappropriate ADH secretion or hyponatremia. Treat with fluid restriction and diuretics. Phenobarbital may be needed for convulsions. Use enemas or cathartics to treat constipation or prevent ileus. Folinic acid, 100 mg IV every 3 hours for 24 hours and then every 6 hours for at least 48 hours, may be helpful in overdose. Supportive measures still required. Administration of whole blood products (e.g., packed RBCs, platelets, leukocytes) and/or blood modifiers (e.g., darbepoetin alfa, epoetin alfa, filgrastim, pegfilgrastim, sargramostim) may be indicated to treat bone marrow toxicity. Hemodialysis is not likely to be helpful in an overdose situation.

VINORELBINE BBW

(vin-**OR**-el-been)

Antineoplastic
(mitotic inhibitor-vinca alkaloid)

Navelbine

pH 3.5

USUAL DOSE

Pretreatment: Verify pregnancy status. Baseline studies indicated; see Monitor.

Single agent: 30 mg/M^2 administered IV over 6 to 10 minutes once each week until disease progression or dose-limiting toxicity.

In combination with cisplatin: 25 mg/M^2 administered as an IV injection or infusion over 6 to 10 minutes once weekly on Days 1, 8, 15, and 21 of a 28-day cycle in combination with cisplatin 100 mg/M^2 on Day 1 only of each 28-day cycle. **An alternative regimen** is vinorelbine 30 mg/M^2 as an IV injection or infusion over 6 to 10 minutes once a week in combination with cisplatin 120 mg/M^2 on Days 1 and 29, then every 6 weeks.

DOSE ADJUSTMENTS

Reduce or withhold dose based on hematologic toxicity or hepatic insufficiency (e.g., hyperbilirubinemia) on the day of treatment. For patients with both hematologic toxicity and hepatic insufficiency, administer the lower of the doses determined appropriate from the following charts.

Vinorelbine Dose Adjustments for Hematologic Toxicity	
Neutrophils (cells/mm^3) on Day of Treatment	**Dose of Vinorelbine**
≥1,500 cells/mm^3	100%
1,000 to 1,499 cells/mm^3	50%
<1,000 cells/mm^3	Do not administer. Repeat neutrophil count in 1 week. If 3 consecutive weekly doses are held because neutrophil count is <1,000 cells/mm^3, discontinue vinorelbine.
For patients who experience fever and/or sepsis while neutrophil count is <1,500 or have 2 consecutive weekly doses held due to neutropenia, subsequent doses of vinorelbine should be:	
≥1,500 cells/mm^3	75%
1,000 to 1,499 cells/mm^3	37.5%
<1,000 cells/mm^3	Do not administer vinorelbine. Repeat neutrophil count in 1 week.

Vinorelbine Dose Adjustments for Impaired Hepatic Function	
Total Bilirubin (mg/dL)	**Dose of Vinorelbine**
≤2 mg/dL	100%
2.1 to 3 mg/dL	50%
>3 mg/dL	25%

Appropriate dose reductions for cisplatin should be made when vinorelbine is used in combination. During one study, more than 50% of patients required a dose reduction of vinorelbine due to myelosuppression. ▪ No dose adjustment is required for impaired renal function. ▪ If Grade 2 or greater neurotoxicity develops, discontinue vinorelbine.

DILUTION

Specific techniques required; see Precautions.

Available as a colorless to pale-yellow solution in single-dose vials containing 10 mg/mL or 50 mg/5 mL. Each 10 mg (1 mL) must be further diluted with 4 to 19 mL

NS, D5W, ½NS, D5/½NS, R, or LR. Desired concentration is 0.5 to 2 mg/mL (4 mL diluent yields 2 mg/mL concentration, 19 mL yields 0.5 mg/mL concentration). Other references recommend diluting a single dose to a minimum total volume of 100 mL. Must be given into the side-arm port of a free-flowing IV infusion.

Storage: Refrigerate vials and protect from light. Do not freeze. Unopened vials are stable at room temperature for up to 72 hours. Diluted solution are stable for 24 hours under normal room light when stored at 5° to 30° C (41° to 86° F).

COMPATIBILITY

Manufacturer recommends mixing only with solutions listed under Dilution.

Other sources suggest specific **compatibilities** dependent on concentration and manufacturer; consult a pharmacist.

RATE OF ADMINISTRATION

A vesicant; ensure proper needle or catheter position before administration to avoid extravasation.

Total desired dose, properly diluted over 6 to 10 minutes through the side-arm port of a free-flowing IV. After administration, flush with at least 75 to 125 mL of diluent solution. Inadequate flushing of the vein after administration may increase the risk of phlebitis.

ACTIONS

An antineoplastic agent. A semi-synthetic vinca alkaloid that interferes with microtubule assembly. Antitumor activity is thought to be due primarily to inhibition of mitosis at metaphase through its interaction with tubulin. Demonstrates high binding to platelets and lymphocytes. Elimination half-life is 27 to 43 hours. Metabolized in the liver by hepatic cytochrome P_{450} isoenzymes in the CYP3A subfamily. Excreted in feces and, to a lesser extent, in urine.

INDICATIONS AND USES

In combination with cisplatin for first-line treatment of patients with locally advanced or metastatic non–small-cell lung cancer (NSCLC). ■ As a single agent for treatment of patients with metastatic NSCLC.

Unlabeled uses: Treatment of breast, cervical, and ovarian cancers.

CONTRAINDICATIONS

Manufacturer states "None." Do not administer to patients with pretreatment neutrophil counts less than 1,000 cells/mm³.

PRECAUTIONS

Follow guidelines for handling cytotoxic agents. See Appendix A, p. 1308. ■ *For IV administration only;* inadvertent intrathecal administration of other vinca alkaloids has resulted in death. Syringes containing vinorelbine should be labeled "For IV use only. Fatal if given by other routes." ■ Administered by or under the direction of the physician specialist. ■ Adequate diagnostic and treatment facilities must be readily available. ■ Severe myelosuppression manifested by neutropenia, anemia, and thrombocytopenia occurs with vinorelbine. Serious infection, septic shock, hospitalization, and death may occur. Neutropenia is the major dose-limiting toxicity. ■ Drug-induced liver toxicity (manifested by elevations of AST and bilirubin) can occur. ■ Severe and fatal paralytic ileus, constipation, intestinal obstruction, necrosis, and perforation have been reported. Initiate a prophylactic bowel regimen, including routine use of stool softeners, hydration, and adequate dietary fiber intake, to mitigate these side effects. ■ Extravasation of vinorelbine can result in severe irritation, local tissue necrosis, and/or thrombophlebitis. ■ Sensory and motor neuropathies, some severe, have been reported. ■ Pulmonary toxicity, including severe acute bronchospasm, interstitial pneumonitis, and ARDS has been reported. Deaths have occurred. ■ Use caution in patients with hepatic impairment. ■ See Monitor and Drug/Lab Interactions.

Monitor: Obtain baseline CBC, differential, platelets, and liver function tests. ■ Monitor CBC, differential, and platelets before each dose. Neutropenia is dose-limiting. Neutropenia nadirs occur between 7 and 10 days after the dose, and recovery should occur within the following 7 to 14 days; see Dose Adjustments. ▪ Monitor hepatic function periodically during treatment; see Dose Adjustments. ▪ Monitor for S/S of constipation/ileus (e.g., abdominal pain, bowel movements, bowel sounds). ▪ Promptly evaluate patients with alterations in their baseline pulmonary functions or with new onset of cough, dyspnea, hypoxia, or other symptoms. Onset of pulmonary toxicity has occurred in 3 to 8 days. ▪ Monitor for new or worsening S/S of neuropathy (e.g., hyperesthesia, hyporeflexia, muscle weakness, paresthesia). ▪ Determine absolute patency and quality of vein and adequate circulation of extremity; see Antidote. ▪ Be alert for any sign of infection. Infections must be brought under control before beginning therapy with vinorelbine. ▪ Use of prophylactic antibiotics may be indicated pending results of C/S in a febrile neutropenic patient. ▪ Maintain adequate hydration. ▪ Prophylactic antiemetics may increase patient comfort. ▪ Monitor for thrombocytopenia (platelet count less than 50,000/mm^3). Initiate precautions to prevent excessive bleeding (e.g., inspect IV sites, skin, and mucous membranes; use extreme care during invasive procedures; test urine, emesis, stool, and secretions for occult blood). ▪ See Precautions and Drug/Lab Interactions.

Patient Education: Report burning or stinging at IV site promptly. ▪ Report chills, fever, difficulty breathing, or shortness of breath promptly. ▪ Avoid pregnancy. Females of reproductive potential should use highly effective contraception during therapy and for 6 months after the final dose. Males with female sexual partners of reproductive potential should use highly effective contraception during and for 3 months after therapy. ▪ May damage spermatozoa and decrease fertility in male patients. ▪ Follow a diet rich in fiber, drink fluids liberally to stay hydrated, and use stool softeners to avoid constipation. ▪ Report new or worsening numbness, tingling or decreased sensation, or muscle weakness. ▪ See Appendix D, p. 1311.

Maternal/Child: Avoid pregnancy; based on its mechanism of action, vinorelbine can cause fetal harm. ▪ Discontinue breast-feeding during treatment and for 9 days after the final dose. ▪ Safety and effectiveness for use in pediatric patients have not been established but have been investigated. In one study, vinorelbine was considered to be ineffective when used in doses similar to those used in adults in a limited number of pediatric patients with recurrent solid malignant tumors (e.g., rhabdomyosarcoma/undifferentiated sarcoma, neuroblastoma, and CNS tumors). Toxicities were similar to those reported in adults.

Elderly: No overall difference in safety, efficacy, and pharmacokinetic parameters have been observed between the elderly and younger adult patients.

DRUG/LAB INTERACTIONS

Drugs that inhibit the cytochrome P$_{450}$ isoenzymes in the CYP3A subfamily (e.g., azole antifungals and macrolides) may inhibit the metabolism of vinorelbine and increase its toxicity. ▪ Neurotoxicity may be increased by **other neurotoxic drugs** (e.g., antineoplastics [such as cisplatin, paclitaxel]); may require discontinuation of vinorelbine. Vestibular and auditory deficits have been observed, usually when vinorelbine is used in combination with cisplatin. ▪ Do not administer **live virus vaccines** to patients receiving antineoplastic drugs. ▪ **Mitomycin-C** may cause or aggravate acute pulmonary reactions (e.g., acute shortness of breath, bronchospasm). ▪ Neutropenia is significantly higher when used in combination with **cisplatin.** ▪ Additive bone marrow suppression may occur with **radiation therapy and/or other bone marrow–suppressing agents** (e.g., azathioprine, chloramphenicol, melphalan); dose reductions may be required.

SIDE EFFECTS

Neutropenia is the major dose-limiting toxicity and may be significantly greater in combination regimens. Other commonly reported adverse reactions are anemia, asthenia, constipation, injection site reactions, leukopenia, liver enzyme elevation (AST and bilirubin), nausea, peripheral neuropathy, and vomiting. Additional adverse reactions occurring in at least 5% of patients receiving vinorelbine as a single agent include alopecia, chest pain, diarrhea, dyspnea, phlebitis, and thrombocytopenia. When used in combination with cisplatin, adverse reactions reported in at least 10% of patients included alopecia, arthralgia, constipation, decreased appetite, decreased weight, diarrhea, embolism, fatigue, fever, hematologic toxicity (anemia, leukopenia, neutropenia, febrile neutropenia, thrombocytopenia), impaired hearing, increased SCr, infection, injection site reactions, lethargy, malaise, myalgia, nausea, ototoxicity, paresthesia, peripheral numbness, phlebitis, taste alterations, thrombosis, vomiting, and weakness.

Post-Marketing: Abdominal pain, anaphylactic reaction, angioedema, back pain, blistering, deep venous thrombosis, dermatitis, dysphagia, electrolyte imbalance (including hyponatremia), esophagitis, flushing, gait disturbance, headache, hypertension, hypotension, jaw pain, loss of tendon reflex, mucosal inflammation, muscular weakness, palmarplantar erythrodysesthesia syndrome, pancreatitis, pneumonia, pruritus, pulmonary edema, pulmonary embolism, radiation recall phenomenon, rash, sloughing of skin, tachycardia, tumor pain, urticaria, vasodilation, vestibular disorder.

ANTIDOTE

Notify the physician of all side effects; symptomatic treatment is often indicated. For severe reactions, discontinue vinorelbine or reduce subsequent doses. Discontinue vinorelbine for development of Grade 2 or greater neurotoxicity, interstitial pneumonitis, or ARDS. See Dose Adjustments. For extravasation, discontinue the drug immediately and administer into another vein. Institute recommended management measures based on institutional policies. Elevation of the extremity, application of dry heat, and hyaluronidase administration have been used for treatment of extravasation. Bone marrow toxicity is reversible after discontinuing vinorelbine. Administration of whole blood products (e.g., packed RBCs, platelets, leukocytes) may be indicated. Darbepoetin alfa, epoetin alfa, filgrastim, pegfilgrastim, or sargramostim may be used to promote bone marrow recovery but may not be given within 24 hours of a dose of cytotoxic therapy or until 24 hours after a dose of cytotoxic therapy.

VON WILLEBRAND FACTOR/COAGULATION FACTOR VIII COMPLEX (HUMAN)

Antihemorrhagic

(von **WILL**-a-brand **FAK**-tor/koh-**AG**-yoo-**LAY**-shun **FAK**-tor VIII **KOM**-plex) (**HYOO**-man)

Wilate

USUAL DOSE

(International units [IU])

Pretreatment: Prophylactic vaccinations recommended; see Patient Education.

One IU of von Willebrand factor:Ristocetin Cofactor (VWF:RCo) is approximately equal to the level of VWF:RCo activity found in 1 mL of fresh human plasma. The ratio between VWF:RCo and FVIII activities in Wilate is approximately 1:1. When using a FVIII-containing VWF product, continued treatment may cause an excessive rise in FVIII activity; see Monitor.

Calculate the required dose using the following formula:

Required IU = Body weight (kg) × Desired VWF:RCo rise (%) (IU/dL) × 0.5 (IU/kg per IU/dL)

Adjust dose and frequency of administration according to the clinical effectiveness in each patient. The following chart provides estimated doses for minor and major hemorrhages.

Guide to Wilate Dosing for Treatment of Minor and Major Hemorrhages			
Type of Hemorrhage	**Loading Dose (IU VWF:RCo/kg)**	**Maintenance Dose (IU VWF:RCo/kg)**	**Therapeutic Goal**
Minor Hemorrhages	20 to 40 IU/kg	20 to 30 IU/kg every 12 to 24 hours[a]	VWF:RCo and FVIII activity trough levels of >30%
Major Hemorrhages	40 to 60 IU/kg	20 to 40 IU/kg every 12 to 24 hours[a]	VWF:RCo and FVIII activity trough levels of >50%

[a]Maintenance doses may need to be continued for up to 3 days for minor hemorrhages and 5 to 7 days for major hemorrhages. Repeat doses may be administered for as long as needed based on repeated monitoring of appropriate clinical and laboratory measures.

Recommendations for dosing in minor and major surgeries is provided in the following chart.

Guide to Wilate Dosing for Treatment in Minor and Major Surgeries in All vWD[a] Types						
Type of Surgery	**Loading Dose (IU VWF: RCo/kg) (Within 3 Hours Before Surgery)**	**VWF:RCo Peak Levels (% of Normal)**	**Maintenance Dose (IU VWF: RCo/kg)**	**VWF:RCo Trough Levels (% of Normal)**	**Frequency of Doses (hours)**	**Duration of Therapy (days)**
Minor (including tooth extraction)	30 to 60 IU/kg	50%	15 to 30 IU/kg or half the loading dose	Greater than 30%	12 to 24 hours	Until wound healing achieved, up to 3 days
Major	40 to 60 IU/kg	100%	20 to 40 IU/kg or half the loading dose	Greater than 50%	12 to 24 hours (at least 2 doses within the first 24 hours after the start of surgery)	Until wound healing achieved, up to 6 days or more

[a]vWD, von Willebrand disease.

See prescribing information for an alternate formula to determine loading dose based on patient's individual in vivo recovery (IVR) determined before surgery.

Performing appropriate lab tests once a day after surgery is recommended to ensure adequate VWF:RCo and FVIII activity levels are reached and maintained. To decrease the risk of perioperative thrombosis, FVIII activity levels should not exceed 250%.

PEDIATRIC DOSE
Follow the general recommendations for dosing and administration for adults. See Usual Dose and Maternal/Child.

DOSE ADJUSTMENTS
Adjust dose according to the extent and location of bleeding and the patient's clinical condition. ▪ vWD Type 3 patients with GI bleeding may require higher doses.

DILUTION   (International units [IU])
Available in 5-mL and 10-mL vials containing either 500 or 1,000 IU VWF:RCo and 500 or 1,000 IU FVIII activities. Provided as a kit containing a single-dose vial of powder, a vial of diluent, a Mix2Vial transfer device, a 10-mL syringe, an infusion set, and 2 alcohol swabs. Consult instructions for reconstitution and injection in the package insert. Warm to room temperature (25° C) before dilution and maintain throughout reconstitution. If a water bath is used for warming (temperature should not exceed 37° C [98° F]), do not allow water to come into contact with the latex-free rubber stopper or vial caps. The total number of IUs available is clearly marked on each vial. Record the batch number of each vial. Should be used immediately after reconstitution. Solution should be clear or slightly opalescent.

Filters: Incorporated into the Mix2Vial.

Storage: Store in original carton to protect from light. Stable for 36 months from date of manufacture when refrigerated at 2° to 8° C (36° to 46° F). Do not freeze. May be stored at RT (maximum of 25° C [77° F]) for up to 6 months. Label vial with date removed from refrigeration. Once stored at RT, do not return to refrigeration. Shelf life expires 6 months from date of removal from refrigeration or on the expiration date on the product vial, whichever is earlier. Administer immediately after reconstitution. Discard any unused solution.

COMPATIBILITY
Manufacturer states, "Must not be mixed with other medicinal products or administered simultaneously with other IV preparations in the same infusion set."

RATE OF ADMINISTRATION
A single dose as an infusion at 2 to 4 mL/min. Reduce rate of administration or interrupt the infusion if a marked increase in pulse occurs.

ACTIONS
A purified, lyophilized von Willebrand factor (VWF) and coagulation factor VIII complex that is obtained from pooled human plasma. VWF and FVIII are normal constituents of human plasma. Patients with VWD have a deficiency or abnormality of VWF; this results in low FVIII activity and an abnormal platelet function, which causes excessive bleeding. VWF promotes platelet aggregation and platelet adhesion on damaged vascular endothelium; it also serves as a stabilizing carrier protein for the procoagulant protein FVIII, an essential cofactor in the activation of factor X, leading to the formation of thrombin and fibrin. VWF activity is measured with an assay that uses an agglutinating cofactor called Ristocetin (RCo). The VWF:RCo assay provides a quantitative measurement of VWF function by determining how well VWF helps platelets adhere to one another. Reduced VWF:RCo activity indicates a deficiency of VWF. Half-life varies based on type of VWD (1, 2, or 3).

INDICATIONS AND USES
On-demand treatment and control of bleeding episodes and perioperative management of bleeding in pediatric patients and adults with von Willebrand disease.

Limitation of use: Not indicated for the treatment of hemophilia A.

CONTRAINDICATIONS
History of anaphylactic or severe systemic reactions to plasma-derived products, any ingredient in the formulation, or components of the container.

PRECAUTIONS

For IV use only. ▪ Administered under the direction of a physician knowledgeable in the treatment of coagulation disorders in a facility with adequate diagnostic and treatment facilities to monitor the patient and respond to any medical emergency. ▪ Hypersensitivity reactions, including anaphylaxis, have occurred; see Monitor. ▪ Manufactured from human plasma. Risk of transmitting infectious agents (e.g., HIV, hepatitis and, theoretically, Creutzfeldt-Jakob disease) has been greatly reduced by screening, testing, and manufacturing techniques. However, risk of transmission cannot be totally eliminated. ▪ Hepatitis A and B vaccines are recommended for patients receiving plasma derivatives. ▪ Thrombotic events have been reported. Use caution in patients with known risk factors for thrombosis. ▪ Inhibitors may develop with large or frequent doses; see Monitor.

Monitor: Monitor BP and pulse during infusion. If a marked increase in pulse occurs, either reduce rate of infusion or interrupt the infusion. ▪ Throughout the infusion, monitor for S/S of a hypersensitivity reaction (e.g., angioedema, burning and stinging at injection site, chills, fever, flushing, headache, hives, hypotension, nausea, tachycardia, tightness of the chest, urticaria, vomiting, wheezing). Evaluate for the presence of inhibitors if an anaphylactic reaction occurs. ▪ Appropriate laboratory tests should be performed on the patient's plasma at suitable intervals to ensure that adequate VWF:RCo and FVIII activity levels have been reached and are maintained. Monitoring is also required to avoid sustained excessive VWF and FVIII activity. When using a VWF product that contains FVIII, continued treatment may cause an excessive rise in FVIII activity. Excessive activity levels may increase the risk of thrombotic events. In the postsurgery period, monitoring should be done daily if possible, and FVIII levels should not exceed 250%. ▪ Monitor for development of VWF and FVIII inhibitors (neutralizing antibodies). Consider formation of inhibitors and perform assays if bleeding is not controlled with usual doses.

Patient Education: Review manufacturer's medication guide. ▪ Prophylactic hepatitis A and hepatitis B vaccines recommended. ▪ Promptly report S/S of a hypersensitivity reaction (e.g., dizziness, hives, itching, rash, tightness of the chest). ▪ Frequent blood tests (e.g., monitoring of VWF:RCo and FVIII activity) are required to ensure effectiveness and reduce the risk of thrombotic events. ▪ Inhibitors may develop if expected VWF activity plasma levels are not attained or if bleeding is not controlled with adequate or repeat dosing; notify treating physician. ▪ Report symptoms of possibly transmitted viral infections immediately. Symptoms may include anorexia, arthralgias, fatigue, jaundice, low-grade fever, nausea, or vomiting.

Maternal/Child: Use during pregnancy or labor and delivery only if clearly needed. ▪ Safety for use during breast-feeding is unknown; consider benefit versus risk. ▪ Approved for use in pediatric patients. No dose adjustment is required.

Elderly: Numbers insufficient to determine differences in response compared with younger adults.

DRUG/LAB INTERACTIONS

Specific information not available.

SIDE EFFECTS

The most common side effects reported are dizziness, hypersensitivity reactions, and urticaria. The most serious adverse reactions were hypersensitivity reactions.

Post-Marketing: Abdominal pain, anaphylactic reaction, chest discomfort, chills, cough, dyspnea, factor VIII inhibition, fever, flushing, headache, hypotension, nausea, paresthesia, rash, tachycardia, and vomiting.

ANTIDOTE

Keep the physician informed of side effects. Slow or interrupt infusion for a marked increase in pulse rate or mild hypersensitivity reaction. Discontinue the infusion immediately if a severe hypersensitivity reaction or thrombotic event (e.g., chest pain, dyspnea, leg pain, MI) occurs, and evaluate for the presence of inhibitors. Treat hypersensitivity as necessary (e.g., antihistamines, epinephrine, corticosteroids), and treat thrombotic events with appropriate measures. Resuscitate as necessary.

VON WILLEBRAND FACTOR (RECOMBINANT)
(von **WILL**-a-brand **FAK**-tor)

Antihemorrhagic

Vonvendi

USUAL DOSE
(International units [IU])

Each vial is labeled with the actual amount of recombinant von Willebrand factor (rVWF) activity in international units (IU) as measured with the Ristocetin cofactor assay (VWF:RCo). Hemostasis cannot be ensured until factor VIII coagulation activity (FVIII:C) level reaches 0.4 IU/mL (40% of normal activity).

If the patient's baseline plasma FVIII:C level is below 40% or unknown, it is necessary to administer an approved recombinant, non–VWF-containing factor VIII (e.g., Advate) with the first infusion of recombinant von Willebrand factor (rVWF) in order to achieve a hemostatic plasma level of FVIII:C.

If an immediate rise in FVIII:C is not necessary or if the baseline FVIII:C level is sufficient to ensure hemostasis, recombinant von Willebrand factor (rVWF) may be administered without recombinant factor VIII.

Initial dose: 40 to 80 IU/kg. For each bleeding episode, administer an approved recombinant, non–VWF-containing factor VIII (e.g., Advate) within 10 minutes of the initial dose of rVWF if factor VIII baseline levels are below 40% or unknown. A ratio of 1.3:1 (30% more) VWF to factor VIII is recommended. The following chart provides estimated doses for minor and major hemorrhages.

Vonvendi Dosing Guidelines for Treatment of Minor and Major Hemorrhages		
Hemorrhagic Event	**Initial Dose[a]**	**Subsequent Dose**
Minor (e.g., readily managed epistaxis, oral bleeding, menorrhagia)	40 to 50 IU/kg	40 to 50 IU/kg every 8 to 24 hours (as clinically required)
Major[b] (e.g., severe or refractory epistaxis, menorrhagia, GI bleeding, CNS trauma, hemarthrosis, or traumatic hemorrhage)	50 to 80 IU/kg	40 to 60 IU/kg every 8 to 24 hours for approximately 2 to 3 days (as clinically required). Maintain trough levels of VWF:RCo greater than 50% for as long as necessary.

[a]If recombinant factor VIII is administered, see its package insert for reconstitution and administration instructions.
[b]A bleed can be considered major if RBC transfusion is either required or potentially indicated or if bleeding occurs in a critical anatomic site (e.g., intracranial or GI hemorrhage).

The initial dose of rVWF should achieve greater than 60% VWF levels (based on VWF:RCo greater than 0.6 IU/mL), and an infusion of recombinant factor VIII should achieve factor VIII levels greater than 40% (FVIII:C greater than 0.4 IU/mL). To calculate specific doses using the correct ratio of 1.3:1, the following formula is recommended:

$$\text{Vonvendi dose (IU)} = \text{Dose in (IU/kg)} \times \text{Weight (kg)}$$
$$\text{Recombinant factor VIII dose (IU)} = \text{Vonvendi dose} \div 1.3$$

DOSE ADJUSTMENTS
Adjust dose according to the extent and location of bleeding. ▪ Administer subsequent doses as long as clinically required.

DILUTION
(International units [IU])

Provided as a kit containing a single-dose vial of powder, a vial of diluent, and a Mix2Vial reconstitution device. Consult instructions for reconstitution and administration in the package insert. Use of plastic syringes is recommended. Warm to room temperature (25° C) before dilution and maintain throughout reconstitution. The total number of IUs available is clearly marked on each vial (approximately 650 or 1,300 IU of

VWF:RCo). Record the batch number of each vial. Should be used immediately after reconstitution. Solution should be clear or slightly opalescent. Use a new Mix2Vial transfer set and syringe for each vial of drug.

If more than one vial is required, the contents of each vial must be drawn into individual syringes that should be left attached to the vial until ready to infuse to reduce the risk of contamination.

Filters: Incorporated into the Mix2Vial.

Storage: Store refrigerated at 2° to 8° C (36° to 46° F) in original carton to protect from light. Do not freeze. May be stored at RT (maximum of 30° C [86° F]) for up to 12 months. Label vial with date removed from refrigeration. Once stored at RT, do not return to refrigeration. Do not use beyond the expiration date on the product vial. Administer immediately after reconstitution, or store at RT not to exceed 27° C (81° F) for up to 3 hours. Do not refrigerate after reconstitution. Discard after 3 hours.

COMPATIBILITY

Manufacturer states, "Do not mix with other medicinal products. Use plastic syringes; proteins in the product tend to stick to the surface of glass syringes."

RATE OF ADMINISTRATION

A single dose may be administered as an infusion up to a maximum rate of 4 mL/min; consider patient comfort. Reduce rate of administration or interrupt the infusion if an increase in heart rate occurs.

ACTIONS

A purified, recombinant von Willebrand factor (rVWF) expressed in Chinese hamster ovary (CHO) cells. Patients with von Willebrand disease (vWD) have a deficiency or abnormality of VWF; this results in low factor VIII activity and an abnormal platelet function, which causes excessive bleeding. VWF re-establishes platelet adhesion at the site of vascular damage, providing primary hemostasis (shortening of bleeding time occurs immediately), and it stabilizes factor VIII by binding to it and preventing its rapid degradation. This latter action is slightly delayed. VWF activity is measured with an assay that uses an agglutinating cofactor called Ristocetin (RCo). The VWF:RCo assay provides a quantitative measurement of VWF function by determining how well VWF helps platelets adhere to one another. Reduced VWF:RCo activity indicates a deficiency of VWF. A sustained increase of factor VIII coagulation activity (FVIII:C) was observed 6 hours after a single infusion of rVWF. Half-life ranged from 19.1 to 21.9 hours depending on the dose administered.

INDICATIONS AND USES

On-demand treatment and control of bleeding episodes in adults (age 18 and older) diagnosed with von Willebrand disease.

CONTRAINDICATIONS

Life-threatening hypersensitivity reactions to von Willebrand factor (recombinant) or constituents of the product or to hamster or mouse proteins.

PRECAUTIONS

For IV use only. ■ Administered under the direction of a physician knowledgeable in the treatment of coagulation disorders in a facility with adequate diagnostic and treatment facilities to monitor patient and respond to any medical emergency. ■ Hypersensitivity reactions, including anaphylaxis, have occurred; see Monitor. ■ Thrombotic events, including disseminated intravascular coagulation (DIC), venous thrombosis, pulmonary embolism, MI, and stroke, can occur, particularly in patients with known risk factors for thrombosis. ■ Neutralizing antibodies (inhibitors) to VWF and/or factor VIII can occur; see Monitor.

Monitor: Monitor BP and heart rate during infusion. If an increase in heart rate occurs, either reduce rate of infusion or interrupt the infusion. ■ Throughout the infusion, monitor for S/S of a hypersensitivity reaction (e.g., acute respiratory distress, angioedema, chest tightness, hypotension, lethargy, nausea, paresthesia, pruritus, restlessness, urticaria, vomiting, wheezing). ■ Appropriate laboratory tests should be performed on the patient's plasma at suitable intervals. If expected VWF activity plasma levels are not attained or if bleeding episode is not controlled with an appropriate dose, perform an assay that measures the presence of VWF or factor VIII inhibitors. ▪ Monitor plasma levels of VWF:RCo and factor VIII activities to avoid sustained excessive VWF and/or factor VIII activity levels, which may increase the risk of thrombotic events. ▪ Monitor for early S/S of thrombotic events such as cough, discoloration, dyspnea, hemoptysis, pain, swelling, and syncope.

Patient Education: Review manufacturer's medication guide. ▪ Promptly report S/S of a hypersensitivity reaction (e.g., dizziness, hives, itching, rash, tightness of the chest). ▪ Frequent blood tests (e.g., monitoring of VWF:RCo and FVIII activity) are required to reduce the risk of thrombotic events. ▪ Report a lack of clinical response to therapy; may be a manifestation of an inhibitor. ▪ If traveling, bring an adequate supply of medication based on current treatment regimen.

Maternal/Child: Use during pregnancy or labor and delivery only if clearly needed. ▪ Safety for use during breast-feeding not known; consider benefit versus risk. ▪ Safety and effectiveness for use in pediatric patients under 18 years of age not established.

Elderly: Numbers insufficient to determine differences in response compared with younger adults.

DRUG/LAB INTERACTIONS
Specific information not available.

SIDE EFFECTS
The most common side effect is generalized pruritus. Chest discomfort, dizziness, dysgeusia, hot flush, hypertension, infusion site paresthesia, nausea, tachycardia, and tremor have occurred.

ANTIDOTE
Keep the physician informed of side effects. Slow or interrupt infusion for an increase in heart rate or mild hypersensitivity reaction. Discontinue the infusion immediately if a severe hypersensitivity reaction or thrombotic event (e.g., chest pain, dyspnea, leg pain, MI) occurs. Treat hypersensitivity as necessary (e.g., antihistamines, epinephrine, corticosteroids), and treat thrombotic events with appropriate measures. Resuscitate as necessary.

VORICONAZOLE
(**vor**-ih-**KOH**-nah-zohl)

Antifungal
(azole derivative)

VFEND IV

USUAL DOSE

Pretreatment: Verify pregnancy status. Pretesting required; see Precautions and Monitor. Obtain baseline electrolytes and correct calcium, magnesium, and potassium deficiencies before initiating voriconazole.

Duration of treatment is based on severity of the underlying disease, recovery from immunosuppression, and clinical response.

Voriconazole Dose Guidelines in Adults			
Infection	**Loading Dose**	**IV Maintenance Dose[a]**	**Oral Maintenance Dose[a]**
Invasive aspergillosis[b, c]	6 mg/kg q 12 hr for the first 24 hours	4 mg/kg q 12 hr	200 mg q 12 hr[d]
Candidemia in nonneutropenic patients and in other deep tissue *Candida* infections	6 mg/kg q 12 hr for the first 24 hours	3 to 4 mg/kg q 12 hr[e, f]	200 mg q 12 hr[d, e, f]
Esophageal candidiasis			200 mg q 12 hr[d, g]
Scedosporiosis and fusariosis[c]	6 mg/kg q 12 hr for the first 24 hours	4 mg/kg q 12 hr	200 mg q 12 hr[d]

[a]In healthy volunteer studies, a 200-mg oral dose every 12 hours provided an exposure (AUC) similar to a 3-mg/kg IV dose every 12 hours; a 300-mg oral dose every 12 hours provided an exposure (AUC) similar to a 4-mg/kg IV dose every 12 hours.

[b]In a clinical study of invasive aspergillosis, the median duration of IV voriconazole was 10 days (range 2 to 85 days). Median duration of oral therapy was 76 days (range 2 to 232 days).

[c]IV therapy should be continued for at least 7 days.

[d]Patients who weigh 40 kg or more should receive an oral maintenance dose of 200 mg q 12 hr. Adult patients who weigh less than 40 kg should receive an oral maintenance dose of 100 mg q 12 hr.

[e]In clinical trials, patients with candidemia received 3 mg/kg q 12 hr as primary therapy, and patients with other deep tissue *Candida* infections received 4 mg/kg as salvage therapy. Appropriate dose should be based on the severity and nature of the infection.

[f]Treat for at least 14 days following resolution of symptoms or following last positive culture, whichever is longer.

[g]Treat for a minimum of 14 days and for at least 7 days following the resolution of symptoms.

For all indications: A switch between IV and oral formulations is appropriate because of high bioavailability of oral formulations. Depending on diagnosis, may switch to oral formulation when a patient has shown clinical improvement and can tolerate oral therapy; see Patient Education.

PEDIATRIC DOSE

Initiate therapy with an IV infusion regimen. Consider an oral regimen only after there is a significant clinical improvement. Note that an 8 mg/kg IV dose will provide voriconazole exposure approximately twofold higher than a 9 mg/kg oral dose. Oral bioavailability may be limited in pediatric patients 2 to 12 years of age with malabsorption and very low body weight for age. IV voriconazole administration is recommended.

Voriconazole Dose Guidelines in Pediatric Patients 2 to 12 Years of Age and 12 to 14 Years of Age With Body Weight Less Than 50 kg			
Infection	**Loading Dose**	**IV Maintenance Dose**	**Oral Maintenance Dose**
Invasive aspergillosis[a] Candidemia in nonneutropenic patients and in other deep tissue *Candida* infections[b] Scedosporiosis and fusariosis	9 mg/kg q 12 hr for the first 24 hours	8 mg/kg q 12 hr after the first 24 hours	9 mg/kg q 12 hr (maximum dose of 350 mg q 12 hr)
Esophageal candidiasis[c]	Not evaluated	4 mg/kg q 12 hr	9 mg/kg q 12 hr (maximum dose of 350 mg q 12 hr)

[a]Based on a population pharmacokinetic analysis in 112 immunocompromised pediatric patients 2 years to less than 12 years of age and 26 immunocompromised pediatric patients 12 years to less than 17 years of age.
[b]In the phase 3 clinical trials, patients with invasive aspergillosis (IA) received IV treatment for at least 6 weeks and up to a maximum of 12 weeks. Patients received IV treatment for at least the first 7 days of therapy and then could be switched to oral therapy.
[c]Study treatment for primary or salvage invasive candidiasis and candidemia (ICC) or EC consisted of IV voriconazole, with an option to switch to oral therapy after at least 5 days of IV therapy based on subjects meeting switch criteria. For subjects with primary or salvage ICC, voriconazole was administered for at least 14 days after the last positive culture. A maximum of 42 days of treatment was permitted. Patients with primary or salvage EC were treated for at least 7 days after the resolution of clinical signs and symptoms. A maximum of 42 days of treatment was permitted.

DOSE ADJUSTMENTS

Adult patients with an inadequate response weighing 40 kg or more: Increase the oral maintenance dose from 200 mg every 12 hours (similar to 3 mg/kg IV every 12 hours) to 300 mg every 12 hours (similar to 4 mg/kg every 12 hours). If unable to tolerate the 300-mg oral dose, decrease it by 50-mg increments to a minimum of 200 mg orally every 12 hours.

Adult patients with an inadequate response weighing less than 40 kg: Increase the oral maintenance dose from 100 mg every 12 hours to 150 mg every 12 hours. If unable to tolerate the 150-mg dose, decrease it to 100 mg orally every 12 hours. ▪ Reduce the IV maintenance dose to 3 mg/kg every 12 hours in patients unable to tolerate treatment. ▪ If phenytoin is being administered concurrently, increase the IV maintenance dose of voriconazole to 5 mg/kg every 12 hours or from 200 to 400 mg orally every 12 hours (or 100 mg to 200 mg orally every 12 hours in patients weighing less than 40 kg); see Drug/Lab Interactions. ▪ When voriconazole is coadministered with efavirenz (Sustiva), increase voriconazole oral maintenance dose to 400 mg every 12 hours and decrease efavirenz dose to 300 mg every 24 hours. ▪ No dose adjustment is indicated based on age or gender or in patients with baseline liver function tests (ALT, AST) up to 5 times the ULN (see Precautions and Monitor). ▪ In patients with mild to moderate hepatic cirrhosis (Child-Pugh Class A and B), use the standard loading dose but reduce the maintenance dose by one-half. ▪ No dose adjustment is required in patients with a CrCl of 50 mL/min or greater; however, the intravenous vehicle, sulfobutyl ether beta-cyclodextrin sodium (SBECD), accumulates in patients with a CrCl of less than 50 mL/min. Use of oral voriconazole is recommended in these patients; see Precautions and Monitor. ▪ A 4-hour hemodialysis session does not remove a sufficient amount of voriconazole to warrant dose adjustment.

Pediatric patients 2 to 12 years of age and 12 to 14 years of age weighing less than 50 kg: If patient response is inadequate and the patient is able to tolerate the initial IV maintenance dose, the maintenance dose may be increased by 1 mg/kg steps. ▪ If patient response is inadequate and the patient is able to tolerate the oral maintenance dose, the dose may be increased by 1 mg/kg steps or 50 mg steps to a maximum of 350 mg every 12 hours. ▪ If patient is unable to tolerate the initial IV maintenance dose, reduce the dose by 1 mg/kg steps. ▪ If patient is unable to tolerate the oral maintenance dose, reduce the dose by 1 mg/kg or 50 mg steps.

Pediatric patients 12 to 14 years of age weighing 50 kg or more and pediatric patients 15 years of age and older regardless of body weight: Use the optimal method for titrating dose recommended for adults.

DILUTION

Reconstitute each vial with exactly 19 mL SWFI. Use of a standard 20-mL (nonautomated) syringe is recommended to facilitate exact measurement. Volume will be 20 mL (10 mg/mL). Discard the vial if a vacuum is not present to pull the diluent into the vial. Shake until all powder is dissolved. Calculate the required dose based on patient weight (see the following chart). Must be further diluted for infusion in D5W, D5LR, LR, NS, D5/½NS, D5NS, ½NS, or D5W with 20 mEq KCl. Withdraw a volume equal to the calculated dose of voriconazole from an infusion bag or bottle (30 mL in the following example). The volume of diluent left in the infusion bag or bottle should be enough to allow a final concentration of not less than 0.5 mg/mL or greater than 5 mg/mL after voriconazole is added. Withdraw the required volume of reconstituted drug and add to the infusion bag or bottle. For example, a patient weighing 50 kg will require a loading dose of 300 mg (6 mg/kg × 50 kg), which equals 30 mL of reconstituted drug (1½ vials). Withdraw and discard 30 mL of solution from a 100-mL infusion bag and add the 30 mL of reconstituted drug. Final concentration equals 3 mg/mL.

Required Volumes of 10 mg/mL Voriconazole Concentrate					
	Volume of Voriconazole Concentrate (10 mg/mL) Required for:				
Body Weight (kg)	3 mg/kg Dose (number of vials)	4 mg/kg Dose (number of vials)	6 mg/kg Dose (number of vials)	8 mg/kg Dose (number of vials)	9 mg/kg Dose (number of vials)
10 kg	—	4 mL (1 vial)	—	8 mL (1 vial)	9 mL (1 vial)
15 kg	—	6 mL (1 vial)	—	12 mL (1 vial)	13.5 mL (1 vial)
20 kg	—	8 mL (1 vial)	—	16 mL (1 vial)	18 mL (1 vial)
25 kg	—	10 mL (1 vial)	—	20 mL (1 vial)	22.5 mL (2 vials)
30 kg	9 mL (1 vial)	12 mL (1 vial)	18 mL (1 vial)	24 mL (2 vials)	27 mL (2 vials)
35 kg	10.5 mL (1 vial)	14 mL (1 vial)	21 mL (2 vials)	28 mL (2 vials)	31.5 mL (2 vials)
40 kg	12 mL (1 vial)	16 mL (1 vial)	24 mL (2 vials)	32 mL (2 vials)	36 mL (2 vials)
45 kg	13.5 mL (1 vial)	18 mL (1 vial)	27 mL (2 vials)	36 mL (2 vials)	40.5 mL (3 vials)
50 kg	15 mL (1 vial)	20 mL (1 vial)	30 mL (2 vials)	40 mL (2 vials)	45 mL (3 vials)
55 kg	16.5 mL (1 vial)	22 mL (2 vials)	33 mL (2 vials)	44 mL (3 vials)	49.5 mL (3 vials)
60 kg	18 mL (1 vial)	24 mL (2 vials)	36 mL (2 vials)	48 mL (3 vials)	54 mL (3 vials)
65 kg	19.5 mL (1 vial)	26 mL (2 vials)	39 mL (2 vials)	52 mL (3 vials)	58.5 mL (3 vials)
70 kg	21 mL (2 vials)	28 mL (2 vials)	42 mL (3 vials)	—	—
75 kg	22.5 mL (2 vials)	30 mL (2 vials)	45 mL (3 vials)	—	—
80 kg	24 mL (2 vials)	32 mL (2 vials)	48 mL (3 vials)	—	—
85 kg	25.5 mL (2 vials)	34 mL (2 vials)	51 mL (3 vials)	—	—
90 kg	27 mL (2 vials)	36 mL (2 vials)	54 mL (3 vials)	—	—
95 kg	28.5 mL (2 vials)	38 mL (2 vials)	57 mL (3 vials)	—	—
100 kg	30 mL (2 vials)	40 mL (2 vials)	60 mL (3 vials)	—	—

Filters: No data available from manufacturer.

Storage: Store unopened vials at CRT. Immediate use of reconstituted vials is preferred; however, they may be refrigerated up to 24 hours at 2° to 8° C (37° to 46° F). Discard partially used vials.

COMPATIBILITY

Must not be infused concomitantly with any blood product or short-term infusion of concentrated electrolytes, even if the two infusions are running in separate IV lines or cannulas. Electrolyte disturbances such as hypokalemia, hypomagnesemia, and hypocalcemia should be corrected before initiation of voriconazole; see Precautions. Voriconazole can be infused at the same time as other IV solutions containing (nonconcentrated) electrolytes but must be infused through a separate line. Voriconazole can be infused at the same time as total parenteral nutrition (TPN) but must be infused in a separate line. If infused through a multiple-lumen catheter, TPN needs to be administered using a different port from the one used for voriconazole. Manufacturer states that voriconazole should not be diluted with 4.2% sodium bicarbonate solution. **Compatibility** with other concentrations of sodium bicarbonate is unknown; do not use.

Other sources suggest a few specific **compatibilities** dependent on concentration and manufacturer; consult a pharmacist.

RATE OF ADMINISTRATION

A single dose as an infusion *over 1 to 2 hours*. Do not exceed a rate of 3 mg/kg/hr.

ACTIONS

A triazole antifungal agent. Inhibits a fungal cytochrome P_{450}-mediated essential step in fungal ergosterol biosynthesis. With a loading dose regimen, peak and trough plasma concentrations close to steady-state concentrations are achieved within the first 24 hours. Extensively distributed into tissues. Plasma protein binding (estimated at 58%) is not affected by varying degrees of hepatic and renal insufficiency. Metabolized by cytochrome P_{450} enzymes (CYP2C19 is significantly involved). Terminal half-life is dose dependent and is not useful in predicting accumulation or elimination. Eliminated via hepatic metabolism; less than 2% is excreted unchanged in urine.

INDICATIONS AND USES

For use in patients 2 years of age and older in treatment of the following infections: Treatment of invasive aspergillosis caused by *Aspergillus fumigatus* and other species of *Aspergillus*. ▪ Treatment of candidemia in nonneutropenic patients and the following *Candida* infections: disseminated infections in the skin and infections in the abdomen, kidney, bladder wall, and wounds. ▪ Treatment of serious fungal infections caused by *Scedosporium apiospermum* and *Fusarium* species, including *Fusarium solani,* in patients intolerant of or refractory to other therapy. ▪ Treatment of esophageal candidiasis.

CONTRAINDICATIONS

Hypersensitivity to voriconazole or any of its components. Use caution in patients exhibiting hypersensitivity to other azole antifungals (e.g., fluconazole, itraconazole, ketoconazole); see Precautions. ▪ Coadministration is specifically **contraindicated** with CYP3A4 substrates (e.g., pimozide, quinidine); increased plasma concentrations of these drugs may result in QT prolongation and torsades de pointes. ▪ Coadministration is **contraindicated** with the following drugs: barbiturates, carbamazepine, efavirenz (400 mg every 24 hours or higher with a *standard dose* of voriconazole), ergot alkaloids, rifabutin, rifampin, ritonavir, sirolimus, St. John's wort, and tolvaptan; see Drug/Lab Interactions.

PRECAUTIONS

Do not give as an IV bolus; for infusion over 1 to 2 hours only. ▪ Specimens for fungal culture, serologic testing, and histopathologic testing should be obtained before therapy to isolate and identify causative organisms. Therapy may begin as soon as all specimens are obtained and before results are known. Reassess after test results are known. ▪ Correct electrolyte disturbances such as hypokalemia, hypomagnesemia, and hypocalcemia before initiation of voriconazole. ▪ Infusion-related hypersensitivity reactions, including anaphylaxis, chest tightness, dyspnea, faintness, fever, flushing, nausea, pruritus, rash, sweating, and tachycardia have occurred. Usually appear at the beginning of the infusion. If a hypersensitivity reaction occurs, discontinue the infusion. ▪ Consider use in patients with severe hepatic insufficiency only if the benefit outweighs potential risk; monitor carefully for drug toxicity. ▪ Serious hepatic reactions (including clinical hepatitis, cholestasis, and fulminant hepatic failure, including fatalities) have occurred. Usually occur in patients with serious underlying medical conditions (e.g., hematologic malignancy); however, hepatic reactions, including hepatitis and jaundice, have occurred in patients with no other identifiable risk factors. If liver function tests become markedly elevated compared with baseline, voriconazole should be discontinued unless medical judgment of benefit versus risk justifies continued use. Liver function usually improves with discontinuation of voriconazole. ■ Pancreatitis has been reported; see Monitor. ■ Consider use of IV formulation in patients with a CrCl less than 50 mL/min only if the benefit outweighs potential risk. Accumulation of SBECD may occur with the IV formulation; use of the oral formulation is recommended. ■ Acute renal failure has been reported, usually in patients receiving concomitant nephrotoxic drugs or in patients who have concurrent medical conditions that may result in decreased renal function; see Drug/Lab Interactions. ■ May cause prolongation of the QT interval on ECG and, rarely, torsades de pointes. Use with caution in patients with proarrhythmic conditions (e.g., congenital or acquired QT prolongation, cardiotoxic chemotherapy, cardiomyopathy [in particular when heart failure is present], sinus bradycardia, existing symptomatic arrhythmias, hypokalemia, and concomitant medications that may also prolong the QT interval). ■ Because of the enzymes involved in metabolism, Asian populations may be poor metabolizers, and serum concentrations may be elevated from 2 to 4 times higher than normal metabolizers. Some Whites and Blacks are also poor metabolizers. ■ Blurred vision, color vision changes, and/or photophobia are common but may be associated with higher serum concentrations and/or doses. Usually resolves within 2 weeks of the end of voriconazole therapy. If therapy continues beyond 28 days, the effects of voriconazole therapy on visual function are not known. Prolonged visual adverse effects, including optic neuritis and papilledema, have been reported. ■ Serious exfoliative cutaneous reactions, such as Stevens-Johnson syndrome, have been reported. ■ Photosensitivity skin reactions have been reported. If a phototoxic reaction occurs, the patient should be referred to a dermatologist, and discontinuation should be considered. If therapy is continued despite the occurrence of phototoxicity-related skin lesions, dermatologic evaluation should be performed on a systematic and regular basis to allow for early detection and management of premalignant lesions. Squamous cell carcinoma and melanoma have been reported during long-term therapy. If skin lesions consistent with premalignant skin lesions, squamous cell carcinoma, or melanoma develop, therapy should be discontinued; see Patient Education and Maternal/Child. ■ Fluorosis (mottled enamel of human teeth caused by fluoride) and periostitis (inflammation of the periosteum) have been reported during long-term therapy. Discontinue treatment in patients who develop skeletal pain or radiographic findings consistent with either of these diagnoses. ■ Fungi with reduced susceptibility to one azole antifungal agent may also be less susceptible to other azole derivatives. Cross-resistance may occur and may require alternative antifungal therapy. ■ Oral maintenance doses adjusted based on weight (above or below 40 kg); see product literature.

Monitor: Obtain baseline electrolytes and make rigorous attempts to correct calcium, magnesium, and potassium before initiating voriconazole. Monitor electrolytes during therapy; may cause hypocalcemia, hypokalemia, and hypomagnesemia. ■ Obtain baseline liver function tests (e.g., alkaline phosphatase, ALT, AST, bilirubin), serum creatinine, and electrolytes in all patients. ■ Monitor liver function tests at least weekly for the first month of treatment. A higher incidence of liver enzyme elevations was observed in pediatric patients. May decrease monitoring to monthly during continued use if no clinically significant changes are noted. ■ Monitor pancreatic function (e.g., serum amylase) in adults and pediatric patients with risk factors for acute pancreatitis (e.g., recent chemotherapy, hematopoietic stem cell transplantation [HSCT]). ■ Monitor serum creatinine during therapy, more frequently in patients with a CrCl less than 50 mL/min. If an increase in serum creatinine occurs, consider changing to the oral formulation. ■ Monitor for S/S of hypersensitivity reactions; see Precautions and Antidote. ■ Monitor visual acuity, visual field, and color perception if treatment continues beyond 28 days. ▪ If a rash develops, serious cutaneous reactions (e.g., Stevens-Johnson syndrome) may develop; see Side Effects and monitor closely. Consider discontinuing voriconazole. ▪ See Precautions, Drug/Lab Interactions, and Antidote.

Patient Education: Review of health history and medication profile is imperative. ▪ Avoid pregnancy; effective contraception required; see Drug/Lab Interactions. Should pregnancy occur, notify physician immediately and discuss potential hazards. ▪ Do not drive at night; changes to vision, including blurring and/or photophobia, may occur. Ophthalmologic monitoring is required with prolonged use. ▪ If a change in vision occurs, avoid hazardous tasks, such as driving or operating machinery. ▪ Avoid strong, direct sunlight; protective clothing and sunscreen with a high SPF are recommended. ▪ Promptly report S/S of a hypersensitivity reaction (e.g., itching, hives, shortness of breath) or a serious skin reaction (e.g., severe sunburn, blistering or peeling of skin). ▪ Additional precautions required with transfer to oral voriconazole.

Maternal/Child: Avoid pregnancy; may cause fetal harm. Teratogenic in rats and embryotoxic in rabbits. Use of effective contraception is required in females of childbearing age. ▪ No data are available regarding the presence of voriconazole in human milk, the effects of voriconazole on the breast-fed infant, or the effects on milk production. ▪ Safety and effectiveness for use in pediatric patients under 2 years of age not established. ▪ Frequency of phototoxicity reactions is higher in pediatric patients. Stringent measures for photoprotection are warranted; see Patient Education. In pediatric patients experiencing photoaging injuries such as lentigines or ephelides, sun avoidance and dermatologic follow-up are recommended, even after discontinuation of therapy. ▪ A higher incidence of liver enzyme elevations was observed in pediatric patients.

Elderly: Safety profile similar to younger adults. ▪ Use caution; consider decreased cardiac, hepatic, or renal function and effects of concomitant disease or other drug therapy. ▪ Monitor liver and renal function closely.

DRUG/LAB INTERACTIONS

Interactions are numerous and potentially life threatening. Review of drug profile by pharmacist is imperative.

Contraindicated with **CYP3A4 substrates** (e.g., **pimozide, quinidine**); increased plasma concentrations of these drugs may result in QT prolongation and torsades de pointes. ▪ Contraindicated with **long-acting barbiturates, carbamazepine, rifampin, St. John's wort, and tolvaptan;** these drugs may significantly increase metabolism and decrease serum concentrations of voriconazole. ▪ **Contraindicated** with **high-dose (400 mg every 12 hours) ritonavir**; decreases serum concentrations of voriconazole. **Low-dose ritonavir (100 mg every 12 hours)** reduces voriconazole concentration to a lesser extent. Coadministration should be avoided unless assessment of the benefit versus risk to the patient justifies voriconazole use. ▪ **Contraindicated** with **sirolimus**; metabolism of sirolimus is decreased, and serum concentrations are significantly increased by voriconazole. ▪ **Contraindicated** with **rifabutin**; voriconazole significantly increases the serum concentrations of rifabutin, and rifabutin significantly decreases voriconazole serum concentrations. ▪ Coadministration of standard doses of voriconazole with **efavirenz** doses of 400 mg every 24 hours or higher is **contraindicated.** Voriconazole increases serum concentrations of efavirenz, and efavirenz decreases serum concentrations of voriconazole. If coadministration is required, dose adjustment of both drugs is indicated. Increase voriconazole oral maintenance dose to 400 mg every 12 hours and decrease efavirenz to 300 mg every 24 hours. Restore the initial dose of efavirenz when treatment with voriconazole is discontinued. ▪ **Contraindicated** with **ergot alkaloids**; serum concentrations of ergot alkaloids may be increased and may lead to ergotism. ▪ Avoid concomitant use with **fluconazole.** Potential for voriconazole toxicity remains if voriconazole is initiated within 24 hours of the last dose of fluconazole. ▪ May decrease the metabolism and increase serum levels of **cyclosporine.** If concurrent administration with voriconazole is indicated, reduce the dose of cyclosporine by one-half and monitor cyclosporine serum levels frequently. When voriconazole is discontinued, monitor cyclosporine levels frequently and increase the dose as necessary. ■ May decrease the metabolism and increase serum levels of **methadone** and increase risk of QT prolongation. If concurrent administration with voriconazole is indicated, monitor closely and decrease dose of methadone as necessary. ■ Increases concentration and half-life of **alfentanil, fentanyl, oxycodone, and sufentanil**. Dose reduction and extended monitoring recommended. ■ May decrease the metabolism and increase serum levels of **tacrolimus and tolvaptan**. If concurrent administration with voriconazole is indicated, reduce the dose of tacrolimus by one-third and monitor tacrolimus serum levels frequently. When voriconazole is discontinued, monitor tacrolimus levels frequently and increase the dose as necessary. ■ Concurrent use with **warfarin** may cause a significant increase in PT or INR. Monitor PT or INR closely and adjust warfarin dose as necessary. ■ May decrease the metabolism and increase serum concentrations of CYP3A4 substrates, such as selected **HMG-CoA reductase inhibitors, selected benzodiazepines** (e.g., alprazolam, midazolam, triazolam), **selected calcium channel blockers** (e.g., felodipine), **vinca alkaloids** (e.g., vinblastine, vincristine), and CYP2C9 substrates such as **sulfonylureas** (e.g., glipizide, glyburide, tolbutamide) and **NSAIDs**. In patients receiving a **vinca alkaloid**, reserve the use of azole antifungals, including voriconazole, for patients who have no alternative antifungal treatment options. To reduce the potential for toxic effects that may be caused by these drugs (e.g., rhabdomyolysis, prolonged sedative effect, cardiac toxicity, GI toxicity, neurotoxicity, hypoglycemia), close monitoring for toxic effects of all of these drugs is indicated, and in most cases dose reduction is indicated during concomitant administration of voriconazole. ■ Concomitant administration with **everolimus**, a CYP3A4 inhibitor and substrate and a P-pg substrate, is not recommended; plasma exposure of everolimus is likely to be increased. ■ Concurrent use with **phenytoin** may require dose adjustments of both drugs. Phenytoin increases metabolism and decreases serum concentrations of voriconazole. An increased dose of voriconazole is indicated; see Dose Adjustments. Voriconazole decreases the metabolism of phenytoin and increases serum concentrations. Monitor phenytoin serum concentrations and reduce dose as necessary to avoid toxicity. ■ May decrease the metabolism and increase serum levels of **selected HIV protease inhibitors** (e.g., amprenavir, nelfinavir, saquinavir). Selected HIV protease inhibitors (e.g., amprenavir, saquinavir) may decrease the metabolism of voriconazole and increase its serum levels. Monitor frequently for drug toxicity with coadministration of voriconazole and HIV protease inhibitors. ■ May decrease the metabolism and increase serum levels of **omeprazole**. If concurrent administration with voriconazole is indicated, reduce a dose of omeprazole of 40 mg or more by one-half. The metabolism of other selected proton pump inhibitors may react similarly. ■ **Nonnucleoside reverse transcriptase inhibitors** (NNRTIs) such as delavirdine may decrease the metabolism of voriconazole and increase its serum concentrations. Voriconazole may inhibit the metabolism of the same NNRTIs and increase their serum levels. Monitor frequently for drug toxicity with coadministration of voriconazole and NNRTIs. ■ Concurrent use with **other nephrotoxic drugs** (e.g., aminoglycosides, cyclosporine) may result in decreased renal function or acute renal failure. ■ Concurrent use with **oral contraceptives** may increase concentrations of both drugs. Monitor for adverse events related to each drug. Should not reduce the effectiveness of oral contraception.

SIDE EFFECTS

Adult: Abdominal pain, chills, diarrhea, dyspnea, fever, hallucinations, headache, hypokalemia, increases in liver function tests, nausea, peripheral edema, rash, respiratory disorders, sepsis, tachycardia, visual disturbances, and vomiting occur most frequently.

Pediatric patients: Abdominal distention, abdominal pain, abnormal ALT, abnormal LFT, constipation, cough, diarrhea, dizziness, dyspnea, epistaxis, fever, hallucinations, headache, hemoptysis, hyperglycemia, hypertension, hypoalbuminemia, hypocalcemia, hypokalemia, hypomagnesemia, hypophosphatemia, hypotension, mucosal inflammation, nausea, peripheral edema, photophobia, rash, renal impairment, tachycardia, thrombocytopenia, upper respiratory tract infections, visual disturbances, and vomiting are most common. Side effects that most often led to discontinuation of therapy include elevated liver function tests, rash, and visual disturbances. Blurred vision, color vision change, and/or photophobia are common but may be associated with higher serum concentrations and/or doses. Hypersensitivity reactions, including anaphylaxis, have been reported. Rarely, Stevens-Johnson syndrome and photosensitivity skin reactions have been reported. In patients with photosensitivity reactions, squamous cell cancer and melanoma have been reported. Numerous other side effects may occur, including QT prolongation and, rarely, torsades de pointes.

Post-Marketing: Pancreatitis in pediatric patients, prolonged visual adverse events, including optic neuritis and papilledema.

ANTIDOTE

Notify physician of all side effects; most will be treated symptomatically. If a hypersensitivity reaction (e.g., an infusion reaction) occurs, discontinue the infusion and treat with oxygen, epinephrine, antihistamines (e.g., diphenhydramine), corticosteroids (e.g., dexamethasone), or bronchodilators (e.g., albuterol) as indicated. Consider discontinuation of voriconazole if liver function tests are elevated and/or clinical S/S of liver disease attributable to voriconazole develop, if visual disturbances occur, if an increase in serum creatinine occurs, if a rash develops (may be the first sign of an exfoliative skin disorder), or if a phototoxic reaction occurs. No known specific antidote. Hemodialysis may assist in the removal of some voriconazole in accidental overdose and in the removal of SBECD. Resuscitate as indicated.

ZIDOVUDINE BBW
(zye-**DOH**-vyou-deen)

Antiviral

Azidothymidine, AZT, Retrovir

pH 5.5

USUAL DOSE
Pretreatment: Baseline studies indicated; see Monitor.

Treatment of HIV infection (symptomatic or asymptomatic): 1 mg/kg every 4 hours. Initiate oral therapy as soon as possible. (The recommended oral dose of zidovudine is 300 mg twice daily in combination with other antiretroviral agents.) Usually part of a multidrug regimen; see Drug/Lab Interactions.

Prevention of maternal-fetal HIV transmission: 2 mg/kg of total body weight over 1 hour when labor begins. Follow with an infusion of 1 mg/kg/hr (of total body weight) until umbilical cord is clamped.

PEDIATRIC DOSE
See Maternal/Child.

To avoid medication errors when preparing pediatric doses, use extra care to calculate the appropriate dose based on body weight (kg). Follow with oral therapy; see comments in Usual Dose.

Treatment of HIV infections in pediatric patients 4 weeks to less than 18 years of age, weight greater than 4 kg: Recommendations for pediatric oral dosing (capsules or syrup) can be found in the prescribing information. Should not exceed the recommended adult dose. See Dose Adjustments.

NEONATAL DOSE
See Maternal/Child.

Treatment of HIV infections (unlabeled): Oral dosing preferred but may be given IV.

Premature neonates (gestational age under 30 weeks) under 6 weeks of age: 1.5 mg/kg IV every 12 hours. Increase to 2.3 mg/kg every 12 hours at 4 weeks of age.

Premature neonates (gestational age 30 to 35 weeks) under 6 weeks of age: 1.5 mg/kg IV every 12 hours. Increase to 2.3 mg/kg IV every 12 hours at 15 days of age.

Full-term infants (gestational age 35 weeks or more) under 6 weeks of age: 3 mg/kg IV every 12 hours.

Prevention of maternal-fetal HIV transmission: Start neonatal dosing within 12 hours after birth and continue through 6 weeks of age. Oral dosing preferred but may be given IV. Consider impaired hepatic or renal function; see Precautions.

Recommended Neonatal Doses of Zidovudine		
Route	Total Daily Dose	Dose and Frequency
Oral	8 mg/kg/day	2 mg/kg every 6 hours
IV	6 mg/kg/day	1.5 mg/kg infused over 30 minutes every 6 hours

Use an appropriate-sized syringe with 0.1-mL graduation to ensure accurate dosing of the syrup formulation in neonates.

DOSE ADJUSTMENTS
Dose selection should be cautious in the elderly based on the potential for decreased organ function and concomitant disease or drug therapy. ■ Reduce dose to 1 mg/kg every 6 to 8 hours in patients with a CrCl less than 15 mL/min or in patients with ESRD who are being maintained on hemodialysis or peritoneal dialysis. ■ Data are insufficient to recommend dose adjustment in patients with hepatic impairment. Monitor for hematologic toxicity. ■ Dose interruption may be required in the presence of significant anemia and/or neutropenia. ■ Dose adjustment may be required in anemia and/or with other drugs. See Monitor, Drug/Lab Interactions, and Antidote.

DILUTION

Each vial of zidovudine contains 200 mg in 20 mL (10 mg/mL). Withdraw the calculated dose and add to a sufficient volume of D5W to achieve a final concentration no greater than 4 mg/mL. To avoid medication errors when preparing a pediatric dose, use extra care to calculate the appropriate dose based on body weight (kg).

Filters: Not required by manufacturer; no further data available from manufacturer.

Storage: Store undiluted vials at 15° to 25° C (59° to 77° F). Protect from light. Chemically and physically stable after dilution for 24 hours at RT or 48 hours refrigerated at 2° to 8° C (36° to 46° F). However, as an added precaution against microbial contamination, manufacturer recommends use within 8 hours if stored at 25° C (77° F) and 24 hours if refrigerated.

COMPATIBILITY

Manufacturer states, "Admixture in biologic or colloidal fluids (e.g., blood products, protein solutions) is not recommended."

Other sources suggest specific **compatibilities** dependent on concentration and manufacturer; consult a pharmacist.

RATE OF ADMINISTRATION

Intermittent infusion: Each single dose properly diluted must be delivered at a constant rate over 1 hour. Avoid rapid infusion or IV bolus.

Continuous infusion: Prevention of maternal-fetal HIV transmission: 2 mg/kg equally distributed over 1 hour, followed by 1 mg/kg/hr until umbilical cord clamped.

Neonates: A single dose infused over 30 minutes.

ACTIONS

A pyrimidine nucleoside analog active against HIV. Through a specific process this thymidine analog interferes with reverse transcriptase, thus inhibiting viral replication. Metabolized by glucuronidation in the liver and excreted through the kidneys. Oral dosing half-life is approximately 0.5 to 3 hours in adults. Crosses the placental barrier. Secreted in breast milk.

INDICATIONS AND USES

Treatment of HIV-1 infection in combination with other antiretroviral agents. ▪ Prevention of maternal-fetal HIV-1 transmission. In most cases, should be given in combination with other antiretroviral drugs. Protocol includes oral zidovudine beginning between week 14 and week 34 of gestation, continuing until labor begins, IV dosing during labor, and zidovudine syrup or IV dosing to the newborn; see Maternal/Child.

CONTRAINDICATIONS

Life-threatening hypersensitivity reactions to any of the components.

PRECAUTIONS

For IV use only. Do not give IM or SC. ▪ Incidence of adverse reactions appears to increase with disease progression. ▪ Has been associated with hematologic toxicity, including neutropenia and severe anemia, particularly in patients with advanced HIV. ▪ Use with caution in patients with bone marrow compromise as indicated by a granulocyte count of less than 1,000/mm³ or hemoglobin below 9.5 Gm/dL. Hematologic toxicities appear to be related to pretreatment bone marrow reserve and to dose and duration of therapy. ▪ Prolonged use of zidovudine has been associated with symptomatic myopathy and myositis with pathologic changes similar to those produced by HIV disease. ▪ Lactic acidosis and severe hepatomegaly with steatosis have been reported with the use of some nucleoside analogs, including zidovudine. Deaths have occurred. Female sex and obesity may increase risk. Suspend therapy in any patient who develops clinical or laboratory findings suggestive of lactic acidosis or pronounced hepatotoxicity (which may include hepatomegaly and steatosis, even in the absence of marked transaminase elevations). ▪ Use with caution in patients with severe hepatic impairment; may be at increased risk for hematologic toxicity. ▪ Hepatic decompensation has occurred in HIV/HCV co-infected patients receiving combination antiretroviral therapy for HIV and interferon alfa with or without ribavirin for HCV. ▪ Use with caution in patients with severely impaired renal function (CrCl less than 15 mL/min); see Dose Adjustments. ▪ Immune reconstitution syndrome has been reported in patients treated with combination antiretroviral therapy, including zidovudine. Patients may develop an inflammatory response to indolent opportunistic infections (e.g., *Mycobacterium avium*, CMV, *Pneumocystis jiroveci* pneumonia [PCP], or tuberculosis). May require further evaluation and treatment. ▪ Autoimmune disorders (e.g., Graves' disease, polymyositis, and Guillain-Barré syndrome) have been reported in the setting of immune reconstitution; may occur months after initiation of therapy. ▪ Treatment has been associated with loss of subcutaneous fat. The incidence and severity of lipoatrophy are related to cumulative exposure. The fat loss (which is most evident in the face, limbs, and buttocks) may be only partially reversible, and improvement may take months to years after switching to a non–zidovudine-containing regimen. ▪ Vial stoppers contain dry natural rubber latex (a latex derivative); may cause hypersensitivity reactions in latex-sensitive individuals. ▪ See Drug/Lab Interactions.

Monitor: Obtain blood cell counts to monitor for hematologic toxicity, including neutropenia, severe anemia, and occasionally reversible pancytopenia. Anemia may occur as early as 2 to 4 weeks. Neutropenia usually occurs after 6 to 8 weeks of therapy; dosage adjustments and/or transfusions may be required. More frequent monitoring is required in patients with poor bone marrow reserve and advanced disease. ▪ Monitor liver function. ▪ Obtain baseline CD4 lymphocyte count and monitor as indicated. ▪ Regularly assess for signs of lipoatrophy during therapy. If feasible, therapy should be switched to an alternative regimen if there is suspicion of lipoatrophy. ▪ Closely monitor patients receiving zidovudine and interferon alfa, with or without ribavirin (Rebetol), for treatment-associated toxicities, especially hepatic decompensation, neutropenia, and anemia. Discontinuation of zidovudine and dose reduction or discontinuation of interferon, ribavirin, or both may be required if worsening clinical toxicities are seen (e.g., hepatic decompensation [e.g., Child-Pugh score greater than 6]). ▪ Observe closely; not a cure for HIV infections. Patients may acquire illnesses associated with AIDS or AIDS-related complex (ARC), including opportunistic infections. ▪ See Drug/Lab Interactions.

Patient Education: Zidovudine is not a cure. Remain under the care of a physician when using zidovudine, and avoid actions that can spread HIV-1 infection to others. ▪ Promptly report abdominal pain, decreased appetite, diarrhea, jaundice, muscle weakness, shortness of breath, rapid breathing, or unusual sleepiness; may indicate lactic acidosis or hepatoxicity. ▪ Major side effects are neutropenia and/or anemia. ▪ Requires frequent lab work and close follow-up with physician; keep all appointments. ▪ Inform health care provider of an allergy to latex. ▪ Promptly report S/S of infection, because inflammation from a previous infection may occur soon after combination antiretroviral therapy, including when zidovudine is started. ▪ Loss of subcutaneous fat may occur; regular assessments indicated. ▪ Manufacturer has a pregnancy exposure registry that monitors pregnancy outcomes in women exposed to zidovudine during pregnancy. ▪ Check with physician before taking any other medications.

Maternal/Child: Safety for use during pregnancy has been evaluated. Risk versus benefit appears justified only in HIV-infected mothers. Congenital deformities not increased in studies. Hyperlactatemia, which may be due to mitochondrial dysfunction, has been reported in infants with in utero exposure to zidovudine-containing products. Because the fetus is most susceptible to the potential teratogenic effects of drugs during the first 10 weeks of gestation and because the risks of therapy with zidovudine during this period are not fully known, women in the first trimester of pregnancy who do not require immediate initiation of antiretroviral therapy for their own health may consider delaying use. (Indication for prevention of maternal-fetal HIV-1 transmission is based on use after 14 weeks of gestation.) ▪ Discontinue breast-feeding because of the potential for HIV-1 transmission (in HIV-negative infants), development of viral resistance (in HIV-positive infants), and serious adverse reactions in breast-fed infants. ▪ Has been studied in HIV-infected pediatric patients over 6 weeks of age who have HIV-related symptoms or are asymptomatic with abnormal lab values, indicating significant HIV-related immunosuppression. Has also been studied in neonates perinatally exposed to HIV. ▪ To monitor maternal-fetal outcomes, an Antiretroviral Pregnancy Registry has been established. See prescribing information.

Elderly: Differences in response between elderly patients and younger patients have not been identified. Dose selection should be cautious; see Dose Adjustments. Consider impaired hepatic and renal function.

DRUG/LAB INTERACTIONS

Probenecid may inhibit glucuronidation or reduce renal excretion of zidovudine, increasing zidovudine toxicity. ▪ Use with **atovaquone, fluconazole, methadone,** or **valproic acid** may increase zidovudine serum concentrations; monitoring indicated; dose adjustment of zidovudine is not indicated. ▪ **Rifamycins** (e.g., rifampin) may increase clearance, reduce zidovudine serum levels, and reduce effectiveness. ▪ Antagonized by **doxorubicin, stavudine, and ribavirin.** Avoid concurrent use. ▪ Exacerbation of anemia due to ribavirin has been seen in patients co-infected with HIV/HCV when zidovudine is part of the HIV regimen; coadministration is not advised. ▪ Hematologic toxicity increased with **ganciclovir, interferons, or other bone marrow suppressants or cytotoxic agents.** Close clinical and laboratory monitoring indicated if coadministration is necessary. ▪ **Phenytoin** levels may increase or decrease; monitor carefully to ensure proper dosing. ▪ **Phenytoin** may also increase zidovudine levels by decreasing clearance. ▪ Use with **acyclovir** may cause neurotoxicity (drowsiness, lethargy). ▪ Combination therapy with zidovudine and **interferon alfa,** with or without **ribavirin,** may increase risk of hepatic decompensation, neutropenia, and anemia. Discontinuation of zidovudine and/or dose reduction or discontinuation of interferon alfa, ribavirin, or both should be considered if worsening clinical toxicities are observed. ▪ Prescribing information states that dose modification is also not warranted with coadministration of **clarithromycin, lamivudine, probenecid, or rifampin.** Other sources suggest drug adjustments with some adverse reactions.

SIDE EFFECTS

Frequency and severity of adverse events are greater in patients with more advanced infection at the time of initiation of treatment. Anorexia, headache, malaise, nausea, and vomiting are most common with oral and IV administration. Anemia and neutropenia were reported frequently with IV administration. Abdominal cramps, abdominal pain, anaphylaxis, arthralgia, asthenia, chills, constipation, dyspepsia, fatigue, granulocytopenia, hepatomegaly (severe), hyperbilirubinemia, increased liver function tests (e.g., ALT, AST, alkaline phosphatase), injection site reaction (e.g., pain, redness), insomnia, musculoskeletal pain, myalgia, neuropathy, pancytopenia (reversible), and thrombocytopenia have also been reported. Side effects most commonly reported in *pediatric patients* were anemia, cough, fever, and neutropenia.

ANTIDOTE

Notify physician of all side effects; most will be treated symptomatically. Moderate anemia or granulocytopenia may respond to a reduction in dose. Interrupt zidovudine therapy for significant anemia (hemoglobin less than 7.5 Gm/dL or a greater than 25% reduction from baseline) or significant neutropenia (granulocyte count less than 750/mm^3 or a greater than 50% reduction from baseline). Transfusions may be required. If marrow recovery occurs following dose interruption, resumption of therapy may be appropriate using adjunctive measures such as epoetin alfa (Epogen). Suspend treatment if clinical or laboratory findings suggestive of lactic acidosis or pronounced hepatotoxicity occur. Rash may be the first sign of a more serious reaction (e.g., anaphylaxis, Stevens-Johnson syndrome); notify physician and treat with diphenhydramine, epinephrine, and corticosteroids as indicated. Antimicrobial therapy may be indicated to treat opportunistic infections. Not removed by hemodialysis or peritoneal dialysis.

ZOLEDRONIC ACID
Bisphosphonate

(**ZOH**-leh-dron-ick **AS**-id)

Reclast ▪ Zometa
pH 6 to 7 ▪ pH 2

USUAL DOSE
RECLAST AND ZOMETA

Pretreatment: Verify pregnancy status. Baseline studies and an oral examination indicated before initiation of therapy; see Monitor and Precautions. Prehydration required. Always used with adequate hydration and appropriate monitoring. See Dose Adjustments, Precautions, and Monitor.

RECLAST

Administration of acetaminophen after Reclast administration may reduce the incidence of acute-phase reaction symptoms; see Side Effects. In clinical studies, a standard dose of acetaminophen was given with the infusion and for the next 72 hours as needed.

Treatment of Paget's disease: One dose of 5 mg as an infusion over no less than 15 minutes. Supplemental calcium and vitamin D are required, particularly during the 2 weeks following administration.

Treatment of osteoporosis in men and postmenopausal women and treatment and prevention of glucocorticoid-induced osteoporosis: A single dose of 5 mg given once a year as an infusion over at least 15 minutes.

Prevention of osteoporosis in postmenopausal women: A single dose of 5 mg given every 2 years as an infusion over at least 15 minutes.

ZOMETA

Hypercalcemia of malignancy (corrected serum calcium equal to or greater than 12 mg/dL [3 mmol/L]): One dose of 4 mg as an infusion over no less than 15 minutes.

Experience is limited, but retreatment with the same dose may be considered if serum calcium does not return to normal or remain normal after initial treatment. Wait at least 7 days from completion of the first infusion to allow full response.

Multiple myeloma and metastatic bone lesions from solid tumors: 4 mg as an infusion over no less than 15 minutes every 3 to 4 weeks. A CrCl greater than 60 mL is required; see Dose Adjustments. Optimal duration of therapy is unknown. Concurrent daily administration of PO calcium 500 mg and a multivitamin with 400 units vitamin D is recommended.

DOSE ADJUSTMENTS
RECLAST AND ZOMETA

Dose adjustment is not indicated based on age or race. Studies have not been conducted in patients with hepatic or severe renal impairment; see Dilution, Precautions, and Elderly.

RECLAST

No dose adjustment required in patients with a CrCl of 35 mL/min or greater.

ZOMETA

Hypercalcemia of malignancy: Dose adjustments are not necessary in patients with mild to moderate renal impairment before beginning treatment (SCr less than 4.5 mg/dL). If renal function deteriorates, consider if the potential benefit of continued treatment outweighs the possible risk.

Multiple myeloma and metastatic bone lesions from solid tumors: Reduce the initial and following doses in patients with mild to moderate renal impairment based on the following chart:

Zometa Dose Adjustments in Multiple Myeloma and Metastatic Bone Lesions	
Baseline Creatinine Clearance	**Zoledronic Acid Recommended Dose**
Greater than 60 mL/min	4 mg
50 to 60 mL/min	3.5 mg
40 to 49 mL/min	3.3 mg
30 to 39 mL/min	3 mg

Measure SCr before each Zometa dose and withhold if renal condition deteriorates. In clinical studies, renal deterioration was defined as an increase in SCr of 0.5 mg/dL in patients with a normal baseline SCr and an increase in SCr of 1 mg/dL in patients with an abnormal baseline SCr. When the CrCl has returned to within 10% of the baseline value, resume dosing at the same dose administered before treatment interruption.

DILUTION
RECLAST
A 5-mg dose is available in a 100-mL ready-to-infuse solution. If previously refrigerated, allow solution to reach room temperature before administration.
ZOMETA
Available in two formulations: (1) a single-use prediluted solution containing 4 mg in 100-mL solution, and (2) a concentrate containing 4 mg in 5 mL.
Single-use, ready-to-use-bottle: 100 mL of solution equals a 4-mg dose of zoledronic acid and may be administered without further dilution.

Single-Use, Ready-to-Use Bottle Zometa Dilution Recommendations for Reduced Doses in Patients With a CrCl Less Than or Equal to 60 mL/min		
Remove and discard the following Zometa ready-to-use solution (mL)	**Replace with the following volume of NS or D5W (mL)**	**Dose (mg)**
12 mL	12 mL	3.5 mg
18 mL	18 mL	3.3 mg
25 mL	25 mL	3 mg

Concentrate with 4 mg in 5 mL for single use: Vials contain overfill; measure accurately. Withdraw desired volume from vial as outlined in the following chart. Must be further diluted immediately in 100 mL of NS or D5W and given as an infusion.

4-mg Concentrate in 5 mL for Single Use Zometa Dilution Recommendations for Reduced Doses in Patients With a CrCl Less Than or Equal to 60 mL/min	
Recommended Dose (mg)	**Volume of Zometa (mL)**
4 mg	5 mL
3.5 mg	4.4 mL
3.3 mg	4.1 mL
3 mg	3.8 mL

Filters: Not required by manufacturer; however, use of a filter should not have an adverse effect.
Storage: *Reclast:* Store at CRT. Stable for 24 hours refrigerated at 2° to 8° C (36° to 46° F) after opening. *Zometa:* Store vials and ready-to-use container in carton at CRT. Use immediately after dilution or manipulation of ready-to-use container is preferred. Diluted

solution may be refrigerated but must be used and the infusion completed within 24 hours of mixing. If refrigerated, bring to RT before administration. Do not store undiluted solution in a syringe (to avoid inadvertent injection).

COMPATIBILITY
RECLAST AND ZOMETA
Must not be mixed with calcium or other divalent cation–containing infusion solutions (e.g., LR). Should be administered as a single IV solution in a line separate from all other drugs.

RATE OF ADMINISTRATION
A single dose equally distributed over no less than 15 minutes. After infusion is finished, flush IV line with 10 mL NS. An increase in renal toxicity that can progress to renal failure can result from shorter infusion times.
RECLAST
A vented IV set is required.

ACTIONS
ZOLEDRONIC ACID
A bisphosphonate that inhibits osteoclast-mediated bone resorption. Used as a bone resorption inhibitor in Paget's disease (Reclast) and as a hypocalcemic agent to reduce hypercalcemia in oncology patients (Zometa). After administration, it rapidly partitions to the bone and localizes preferentially at sites of high bone turnover. Inhibits osteoclastic (destructive to bone) activity and induces osteoclast apoptosis (fragmentation of a cell into particles for elimination). Blocks the osteoclastic resorption of mineralized bone and cartilage through its binding to bone. Inhibits the increased osteoclastic activity and skeletal calcium release induced by various tumors. Decreases serum calcium and phosphorus and increases urinary calcium and phosphorus excretion. Plasma protein binding of zoledronic acid is low. Not metabolized. Most bound to bone and slowly released back into the systemic circulation. Primarily excreted intact via the kidney. Half-life is triphasic with a terminal half-life of 146 hours.

RECLAST
In Paget's disease, it localizes preferentially at sites of high bone turnover and promotes bone of normal quality with no evidence of impaired bone remodeling or mineralization effect. Returns patients to normal levels of bone turnover; see Indications.

ZOMETA
In oncology patients with hypercalcemia, it reduces serum calcium concentrations by inhibiting bone resorption. Reduction in calcium levels is seen in 24 to 48 hours, but maximum response may take up to 7 days.

INDICATIONS AND USES
RECLAST
Treatment of Paget's disease of the bone in men and women. Treatment indicated to induce remission (normalization of serum alkaline phosphatase) in patients with elevations in serum alkaline phosphatase of two times or higher than the upper limit of the age-specific reference range and in patients who are symptomatic or are at risk for complications from their disease. Paget's disease of the bone is a chronic focal skeletal disorder characterized by greatly increased and disorderly bone remodeling. Excessive osteoclastic bone resorption is followed by irregular osteoblastic new bone formation, which leads to replacement of the normal bone architecture by disorganized, enlarged, and weakened bone structure. ▪ Prevention and treatment of osteoporosis in postmenopausal women. In osteoporosis diagnosed by a bone mineral density test or prevalent vertebral fractures, Reclast reduces the incidence of hip, vertebral, and nonvertebral osteoporosis-related fractures. In patients at high risk for fracture (defined as a recent low-trauma hip fracture), Reclast reduces the incidence of new clinical fractures. ▪ Treatment to increase bone mass in men with osteoporosis. ▪ Treatment and prevention of glucocorticoid-induced osteoporosis in men and women who are initiating or continuing systemic glucocorticoids in a daily dose that is equivalent to 7.5 mg or more of prednisone and who are expected to remain on glucocorticoids for at least 12 months.

Limitation of use: Safety and effectiveness for treatment of osteoporosis are based on 3 years of clinical data. Optimal duration of therapy is unknown. Re-evaluate the need for continued therapy on a periodic basis. Consider discontinuation of therapy after 3 to 5 years in patients at low risk for fracture. Patients who discontinue therapy should have their risk for fracture re-evaluated periodically.

ZOMETA

Treatment of hypercalcemia of malignancy (HCM), which is defined as an albumin-corrected calcium (cCa) greater than or equal to 12 mg/dL (3 mmol/L) using the following formula:

$$cCa \text{ in mg/dL} = Ca \text{ in mg/dL} + 0.8 [4 \text{ Gm/dL} - \text{Patient albumin (Gm/dL)}]$$

■ Treatment of patients with multiple myeloma and patients with documented bone metastases from solid tumors in conjunction with chemotherapy. Prostate cancer should have progressed after treatment with at least one hormonal therapy.

Limitation of use: Safety and efficacy for use in the treatment of hypercalcemia associated with hyperparathyroidism or with other non–tumor-related conditions has not been established.

CONTRAINDICATIONS

RECLAST AND ZOMETA

Hypersensitivity to zoledronic acid or any of its components.

RECLAST

Hypocalcemia in patients with a CrCl less than 35 mL/min, and in patients with evidence of acute renal impairment.

PRECAUTIONS   (International units [IU])

RECLAST AND ZOMETA

A patient being treated with Zometa should not be treated with Reclast or another bisphosphonate (e.g., ibandronate, pamidronate). ■ Bisphosphonates have been associated with deterioration of renal function and potential renal failure. Multiple cycles of zoledronic acid, doses over 4 or 5 mg, and/or a rate of administration less than 15 minutes increase this risk. Patients who are elderly, are dehydrated, are receiving diuretics or other nephrotoxic drugs, or have pre-existing renal impairment may also be at increased risk. In trials and post-marketing events, renal deterioration progressing to renal failure and dialysis has occurred in patients, including those treated with approved doses infused over 15 minutes. ■ Use with caution in patients with aspirin-sensitive asthma; although not seen in zoledronic acid trials, bronchoconstriction has been reported when other bisphosphonates have been given to these patients. ■ Osteonecrosis of the jaw (ONJ) has been reported in patients receiving bisphosphonates. The majority of cases have been in cancer patients undergoing dental procedures. However, some cases have been reported in patients with postmenopausal osteoporosis treated with either oral or IV bisphosphonates. Risk factors include cancer, concomitant therapy (e.g., chemotherapy, radiotherapy, corticosteroids, angiogenesis inhibitors), and comorbid conditions (e.g., anemia, coagulopathies, infection, pre-existing oral disease). Risk may also increase with duration of exposure to bisphosphonates. Post-marketing experience suggests a greater frequency of reports based on tumor type (advanced breast cancer or multiple myeloma); see Drug/Lab Interactions. ■ A routine oral exam is recommended before beginning therapy with bisphosphonates. Patients, especially cancer patients, should consider appropriate preventive dentistry and avoid invasive dental procedures during bisphosphonate therapy. Dental surgery may exacerbate ONJ in patients who develop ONJ while undergoing bisphosphonate therapy. ■ Severe and occasionally incapacitating bone, joint, and/or muscle pain has been reported. Onset of symptoms may be days to months after initiation of therapy. Symptoms usually resolve when zoledronic acid is discontinued. A subset of patients had a recurrence of symptoms when rechallenged with the same drug or another bisphosphonate. ■ Atypical subtrochanteric and diaphyseal femoral fractures have been reported in bisphosphonate-treated patients. May be bilateral. Many patients report prodromal pain in the affected area (usually presenting as dull, aching thigh pain) weeks to months before a complete fracture occurs. Patients presenting with thigh or groin pain in the absence of trauma should be evaluated to rule out an incomplete femur fracture. Patients presenting with an atypical fracture should also be assessed for S/S of fracture in the contralateral limb. Poor healing of these fractures has also been reported. ▪ Use with caution in patients with hepatic impairment; has not been adequately studied and data are limited. ▪ See Monitor.

Reclast

Hypocalcemia may occur. Pre-existing hypocalcemia and disturbances of mineral metabolism must be treated before initiating therapy. Concurrent dosing with calcium and vitamin D during therapy is required and is especially important in the 2 weeks following Reclast administration. ▪ Effectively treat disturbances of calcium and mineral metabolism (e.g., hypoparathyroidism, thyroid surgery, parathyroid surgery, malabsorption syndromes, excision of the small intestine) before initiating therapy with Reclast.

Zometa

Calcium is bound to serum protein; concentration fluctuates with changes in blood volume. Changes in serum calcium (especially during rehydration) may not reflect true plasma levels. Measurement with ionized calcium levels is preferred. If unavailable, all calcium measurement should be corrected for albumin to establish a basis for treatment and evaluation of treatment. ▪ Hypocalcemia has been reported. Cardiac arrhythmias and adverse neurologic events (numbness, seizures, tetany) have been reported secondary to severe hypocalcemia. Correct hypocalcemia before beginning Zometa therapy. Adequately supplement with calcium and vitamin D. ▪ Mild or asymptomatic hypercalcemia will be treated with conservative measures (e.g., saline hydration, with or without diuretics [after correcting hypovolemia]). Consider patient's cardiovascular status. ▪ Not recommended for patients with bone metastases with a SCr greater than 3 mg/dL (265 micromol/L) or for patients with hypercalcemia of malignancy with a SCr greater than 4.5 mg/dL (400 micromol/L). These patients were excluded from the studies. After considering other treatment options, use only if benefit outweighs risk of renal failure. ▪ Retreatment may increase potential for renal failure; before retreatment, consider other available treatment options and risk versus benefit; evaluate serum creatinine before each dose. ▪ May be used adjunctively with chemotherapy, radiation, or surgery.

Monitor: Reclast and Zometa: Serum phosphate levels may decrease (hypophosphatemia) and may require treatment. Short-term supplemental therapy may also be required for hypocalcemia or hypomagnesemia. ▪ See Precautions and Drug/Lab Interactions.

Reclast: S/S of Paget's disease range from no symptoms to severe morbidity due to bone pain, bone deformity, pathologic fractures, and neurologic and other complications. Serum alkaline phosphatase provides an objective measure of disease severity and response to therapy. Diagnosis can be confirmed by radiographic evidence. ▪ Obtain baseline measurement of serum alkaline phosphatase, serum calcium, electrolytes, phosphate, magnesium, and SCr. Monitor as indicated. Obtain serum creatinine and calculate CrCl before each dose. ▪ Supplemental calcium and vitamin D required; see Usual Dose. Very important in the 2 weeks following Reclast administration. ▪ Adequate hydration required; a minimum of two glasses of liquid is recommended before dosing on day of administration. Additional hydration is required in patients undergoing diuretic therapy. ▪ Monitor calcium and mineral levels (phosphate and magnesium) closely in patients with disturbances of calcium and mineral metabolism (e.g., hypoparathyroidism, thyroid surgery, parathyroid surgery, malabsorption syndromes, excision of the small intestine). ▪ Bone mineral density should be evaluated 1 to 2 years after initiation of therapy in patients being treated for osteoporosis.

Zometa: Obtain baseline measurements of serum calcium (corrected for serum albumin), electrolytes, phosphate, magnesium, SCr, and CBC with differential. Monitor all closely as indicated by baseline results. ▪ Monitor SCr before each dose to identify renal deterioration. During clinical studies, deterioration was considered as an increase of 0.5 mg/dL if the patient had a normal baseline; if the patient had an abnormal baseline, deterioration was considered as an increase of 1 mg/dL. ▪ Patients with cancer-related hypercalcemia are often dehydrated. Must be adequately hydrated orally and/or IV before treatment is initiated. Hydration with saline is preferred to facilitate the renal excretion of calcium and to correct dehydration. A pretreatment urine output of 2 L/day is recommended. Maintain adequate hydration and urine output throughout treatment. ■ Correct hypovolemia before using diuretics. ■ Avoid overhydration in patients with compromised cardiovascular status. Observe frequently for signs of fluid overload.

Patient Education: RECLAST AND ZOMETA: Review manufacturer's medication guide. ■ Avoid pregnancy; use of effective birth control recommended during and after treatment. Report a suspected pregnancy; may cause fetal harm. ■ Regular visits and assessment of lab tests imperative. ■ Take only prescribed medications. Discuss all medications, allergies (including aspirin sensitivity), and medical history with physician. ■ Adequate hydration required. Drink at least two glasses of fluid before infusion. ■ Report abdominal cramps, chills, confusion, fever, muscle spasms, sore throat, and/or any new medical problems promptly. ■ Flu-like symptoms may occur within the first 3 days of therapy. Usually resolve within 3 days of onset but may last for up to 7 to 14 days. Administration of acetaminophen may reduce incidence of symptoms. ■ Good dental hygiene and routine dental care required. Obtain a dental exam before initiating therapy, and avoid invasive dental procedures during therapy. Report any oral symptoms such as loosening of a tooth, pain, swelling or nonhealing of sores, or discharge. ■ Report development of bone, joint, or muscle pain promptly. Onset of pain is variable. ■ Report thigh, hip, or groin pain promptly.

RECLAST: Calcium and vitamin D supplementation required to maintain calcium levels. ■ Tell your physician if you have had surgery to remove some or all of the parathyroid glands in your neck, have had sections of your intestine removed, or are unable to take calcium supplements. ■ Promptly report muscle spasms and/or numbness or tingling sensations (especially around the mouth); may indicate hypocalcemia. ■ Patients being treated with Reclast should not be treated with Zometa or other bisphosphonates.

ZOMETA: Dietary restriction of calcium and vitamin D may be required in hypercalcemia of malignancy. ■ An oral calcium supplement of 500 mg and a multivitamin with 400 IU of vitamin D are recommended for patients with multiple myeloma and bone metastasis of solid tumors. ■ Patients being treated with Zometa should not be treated with Reclast or other bisphosphonates.

Maternal/Child: Category D: avoid pregnancy; may cause fetal harm. ■ Discontinue breast-feeding. ■ Not indicated for use in pediatric patients. Because of long-term retention in bone, zoledronic acid should be used in pediatric patients only when potential benefit outweighs potential risk. Has been used in pediatric patients with severe osteogenesis imperfecta; see manufacturer's prescribing information.

Elderly: Response similar to that seen in younger patients. ■ Use with caution based on age-related impaired organ function and concomitant disease or other drug therapy. Monitor renal function closely. Elderly patients are at increased risk for acute renal failure. ■ Monitor fluid and electrolyte status. ■ Acute-phase reactions occur less frequently in the elderly; see Side Effects.

DRUG/LAB INTERACTIONS
RECLAST AND ZOMETA

Concurrent use with **loop diuretics** may increase risk of hypocalcemia or nephrotoxicity. ■ Concurrent use with **aminoglycosides** or **calcitonin** may have an additive hypocalcemic effect that may persist for a prolonged period. ■ Use caution when administered with other potentially **nephrotoxic drugs** (e.g., aminoglycosides, cisplatin, NSAIDs); the risk of renal deterioration is increased. Consider monitoring of SCr. ■ Use with caution when administered with **renally eliminated drugs** (e.g., digoxin). Possible development of renal impairment may lead to increased exposure of these drugs. Use caution and consider monitoring of SCr. ■ In vitro studies indicate that it does not inhibit microsomal CYP_{450} enzymes. ■ Concomitant administration of **drugs associated with ONJ** (e.g., bevacizumab, denosumab, everolimus, pazopanib, sorafenib, sunitinib, or corticosteroids) may increase the risk of ONJ.

ZOMETA

Does not interfere with any known primary cancer therapy. ▪ Concurrent use with **thalidomide** does not result in a significant change in the pharmacokinetics of zoledronic acid or creatinine clearance; no dose adjustment indicated. ▪ Effects may be antagonized by **calcium-containing preparations or vitamin D;** avoid use.

SIDE EFFECTS

RECLAST AND **Z**OMETA

Abdominal pain, anorexia, atypical femur fracture, conjunctivitis, constipation, dehydration, diarrhea, dyspnea, episcleritis, flu-like syndrome (e.g., arthralgias and/or bone pain, chills, fever, flushing, and myalgias), headache, hypersensitivity reactions (including rare case of anaphylaxis, angioedema, and urticaria), hypocalcemia (abdominal cramps, confusion, muscle spasms), hypomagnesemia, hypophosphatemia, hypotension, injection site reactions, nausea, ocular inflammation (e.g., iritis, uveitis, scleritis, orbital inflammation and edema), osteonecrosis (primarily of the jaw), rash, renal impairment, and vomiting. In addition to the previously noted side effects, an acute-phase reaction (e.g., chills, fatigue, fever, headache, influenza-like illness, or muscle, bone, or joint pain) and nausea and vomiting were reported. Symptoms may be significant and lead to dehydration. This acute-phase reaction may occur within the first 3 days, is usually mild to moderate, and lasts only a few days. However, in some patients the resolution of symptoms may take 7 to 14 days or longer.

RECLAST

The most commonly reported side effects are arthralgia, fever, headache, myalgia, and pain in extremities. Other important side effects include diarrhea, eye inflammation, flu-like illness, nausea, and vomiting. In addition to the previously noted side effects, abdominal distension, anemia, asthenia, atrial fibrillation, back pain, dizziness, dyspepsia, fatigue, hypertension, lethargy, musculoskeletal stiffness, pain, paresthesia, peripheral edema, and vertigo have also been reported.

ZOMETA

The most commonly reported side effects are anemia, bone pain, constipation, dyspnea, fatigue, fever, nausea, and vomiting. In addition to the previously noted side effects, agitation, anxiety, bronchoconstriction, chest pain, confusion, cough, dysphagia, edema, granulocytopenia, hypokalemia, increased serum creatinine, pancytopenia, pleural effusion, pruritus, somnolence, thrombocytopenia, urinary tract infection, and weakness have occurred in 10% or more of patients. Fluid overload, hypokalemia, hypomagnesemia, and hypophosphatemia may occur more often with the use of concurrent fluid and diuretics.

Post-Marketing: Acquired Fanconi syndrome; acute renal failure; angioneurotic edema; asthma exacerbation; atypical subtrochanteric and diaphyseal femoral fractures; blurred vision; bradycardia; bronchospasm; dehydration secondary to diuretic therapy, fever, or GI losses; dry mouth; hematuria; hyperesthesia; hyperkalemia; hypernatremia; hypersensitivity reactions (including anaphylactic reaction/shock, angioedema, bronchoconstriction, Stevens-Johnson syndrome, toxic epidermal necrolysis, and urticaria); hypertension; hypocalcemia (cardiac arrhythmias, numbness, seizures, and tetany have occurred with severe hypocalcemia); hypophosphatemia; increased SCr; increased sweating; influenza-like illness (asthenia, fatigue or malaise, fever persisting for more than 30 days); interstitial lung disease (ILD) with positive rechallenge; musculoskeletal pain (severe); osteonecrosis (primarily of the jaw but also of other anatomic sites, including ankle, external auditory canal, femur, hip, humerus, knee, and wrist); proteinuria; and weight increase.

Overdose: Clinically significant hypocalcemia (e.g., abdominal cramps; confusion; irregular heartbeats; muscle cramps in the hands, arms, feet, legs, or face; numbness and tingling around the mouth, fingertips, or feet), hypophosphatemia (e.g., unusual tiredness or weakness), and hypomagnesemia (e.g., muscle trembling or twitching) may occur. Elevated SCr levels and renal tubular necrosis may occur with excessive dose or rate of administration.

ANTIDOTE

RECLAST AND ZOMETA

Keep physician informed of side effects. According to the manufacturer, no specific treatment was required in most cases of flu-like syndrome, GI symptoms, and infusion site reactions, and the symptoms subsided in 24 to 48 hours. Some side effects may respond to symptomatic treatment. IV fluids may be required for dehydration. Magnesium and phosphorus may require replacement if depletion is too severe. If mild, all will probably return toward normal in 7 to 10 days. For asymptomatic or mild to moderate hypocalcemia (6.5 to 8 mg/100 mL [1 dL] corrected for serum albumin), short-term calcium therapy (e.g., calcium gluconate) may be indicated. Discontinue drug for any symptoms of hypersensitivity or overdose. Discontinue for severe bone, joint, or muscle pain. Treat anaphylaxis and resuscitate as indicated.

ZOMETA

Monitor serum calcium and use vigorous IV hydration, with or without diuretics, for 2 to 3 days. Monitor intake and output to ensure adequacy and balance. Use short-term IV calcium therapy if indicated. Potassium phosphate and/or magnesium sulfate may be required to treat hypophosphatemia and hypomagnesemia.

APPENDIX A
Recommendations for the Safe Use and Handling of Cytotoxic Drugs

Numerous references are available on the topic of guidelines, recommendations, and regulations for handling antineoplastic and other hazardous agents.

The Department of Health and Human Services in the Centers for Disease Control and Prevention has publications and other references that cover all aspects of the topic at www.cdc.gov/niosh. Click on Hazards & Exposures, then click on Antineoplastic Agents, and finally on NIOSH Publications. Links to several informative documents can be found on this page, including *Preventing Occupational Exposure to Antineoplastic and Other Hazardous Drugs in Health Care Settings* and the *NIOSH List of Antineoplastic and Other Hazardous Drugs in Healthcare Settings, 2016.* The latter document discusses the criteria used to define hazardous drugs and places drugs into three different groups: (1) antineoplastic drugs, (2) nonantineoplastic drugs that meet one or more of the NIOSH criteria for a hazardous drug, and (3) drugs that primarily pose a reproductive risk to men and women who are actively trying to conceive and women who are pregnant or breast-feeding. This publication also provides general guidance on personal protective equipment and engineering controls when working with hazardous drugs in health care settings.

The United States Pharmacopeia published General Chapter <800> in the First Supplement to USP 39–NF 34. The purpose of this chapter is to describe practice and quality standards for handling hazardous drugs in health care settings and to help promote patient safety, worker safety, and environmental protection. The new general chapter defines processes intended to minimize the exposure to hazardous drugs in health care settings.

Other frequently cited guidelines on handling hazardous drugs are available from the American Society of Health-System Pharmacists, the Oncology Nursing Society, and the International Society of Oncology Pharmacy Practitioners.

Together these guidelines and regulations represent the recommendations of many diverse groups and have been established to promote not only patient safety but also worker safety and environmental protection.

APPENDIX B
FDA Pregnancy Categories

The FDA is no longer using these categories, but many drug monographs have not been updated in the prescribing information, so these categories will remain in the appendixes for now. The new categories include Reproductive Considerations, Pregnancy Considerations, and Breastfeeding Considerations. No drug should be used during pregnancy unless clearly needed and the risks to the fetus are outweighed by the benefits to the mother.

Category A   Adequate studies have not demonstrated a risk to the fetus in any trimester.

Category B   May have caused adverse effects in animals, but no adverse effects have been demonstrated in humans in any trimester, or no demonstrated risk in animals, but there are no adequate studies in pregnant women.

Category C   Animal studies have shown an adverse effect, but there are no adequate studies in pregnant women or no animal studies and no studies in pregnant women.

Category D   Definite fetal risks. May be given in spite of risks if needed in life-threatening conditions.

Category X   Will cause fetal abnormalities. Risk of use outweighs benefits. Not recommended for use at any time during pregnancy. Consider alternatives before treating a pregnant woman.

Consider all men and women capable of conception when any drug in Category D or Category X is to be administered. Discuss birth control options to avoid pregnancy if a specific drug in these categories must be administered. Some drugs require birth control for months after all dosing is complete. Research complete information and keep patient informed.

APPENDIX C
U.S. Department of Health and Human Services, National Institutes of Health, National Cancer Institute Common Terminology Criteria for Adverse Events (CTCAE)

In Appendix C we have in the past incorporated the Common Toxicity Criteria (CTC) provided by the U.S. Department of Health and Human Services, the National Institutes of Health, and the National Cancer Institute. It was referred to throughout the text as the National Cancer Institute Common Toxicity Grading Criteria (NCI CTGC). This listing has been expanded and updated by these organizations and is too expansive to be included in an appendix. Web access to this material is available at www.cancer.gov. Search for CTCAE (Common Terminology Criteria for Adverse Events Version 5.0). Printed copies are available free of charge; call 1-800-4-CANCER (1-800-422-6237).

APPENDIX D
Information for Patients Receiving Immunosuppressive Agents

- Report allergic or sensitivity reactions you may have had to drugs or food.
- Report other medical problems you may have (e.g., exposure to chickenpox; herpes zoster; infections; bone marrow, heart, kidney, or liver problems).
- Provide a complete list of all medications you take, prescription and nonprescription.
- In most situations birth control is essential and may be required for both patient and partner. Nonhormonal birth control reduces the possibility of drug interactions, but compliance is imperative. If there is any possibility you or your partner may be pregnant, inform your physician promptly.
- Discontinue breast-feeding.
- Take only prescribed medication(s) in the exact amounts prescribed and at the times prescribed. This will help to maintain correct blood levels and avoid drug interactions.
- Confirm procedure if you should miss a dose. If any questions, notify physician.
- Confirm procedure for correct storage of your medication(s).
- Close monitoring by your physician is very important; keep all appointments and have all required lab work done on schedule. Your medications may interfere with some test results. Discuss with your physician.
- Do not take any immunizations without your physician's approval. Polio vaccine is especially virulent in your condition; request family members to defer immunization, and either avoid friends who have been immunized or wear a protective mask covering your nose and mouth while visiting. Live vaccines should be avoided.
- Dental procedures may need to be completed before starting therapy or deferred until therapy is completed. Use caution with your toothbrush, toothpicks, or dental floss. Alternate methods of dental hygiene may be necessary should your gums become tender, inflamed, or bleed.
- Review all side effects with your physician. Confirm those that may be a special problem for you and discuss solutions and expectations.
- Avoid anyone with an infection or fever. Report symptoms such as chills, fever, cough, hoarseness, lower back or side pain, painful or difficult urination. Take precautions when in crowded areas indoors, and consider wearing a mask.
- Wash hands before touching your eyes or the inside of your nose.
- Report unusual bleeding, bruising, black tarry stools, blood in urine, or pinpoint red spots on your skin (petechiae).
- Report redness, swelling, or soreness in the mouth (symptoms of stomatitis).
- Report mild hair loss, nausea and vomiting, rash, tiredness, weakness.
- Avoid accidental cuts whenever possible (e.g., razors, fingernail and toenail clippers).
- Avoid contact sports in which you might be bruised or injured.
- Drink adequate amounts of fluids to prevent increases in serum uric acid concentrations. Allopurinol and/or alkalinization of urine may be required.
- Anesthesia during dental, surgical, or emergency treatment may be a problem. It is best to consult with your physician, but inform all health care professionals about the medications you are taking before they treat you in any way.

APPENDIX E
Recently Approved Drugs

- Imetelstat (Rytelo)
- Ceftobiprole medocaril (Zevtera)
- Cefepime plus enmetazobactam (Exblifep)
- Mosunetuzumab (Lunsumio)
- Axatilimab (Niktimvo)
- Donanemab (Kisunla)
- Atezolizumab (Tecentriq)

INDEX

Note: Page numbers followed by "f" indicate figures, "t" indicate tables, and "b" indicate boxes.

Color type indicates generic drug name.
*See http://evolve.elsevier.com/IVMeds for detailed information.

Color type indicates generic drug name.
*See http://evolve.elsevier.com/IVMeds for detailed information.

Color type indicates generic drug name.
*See http://evolve.elsevier.com/IVMeds for detailed information.

Color type indicates generic drug name.
*See http://evolve.elsevier.com/IVMeds for detailed information.

Color type indicates generic drug name.
*See http://evolve.elsevier.com/IVMeds for detailed information.

Color type indicates generic drug name.
*See http://evolve.elsevier.com/IVMeds for detailed information.

Direct anti-globulin (C$_{oo}$mbs') tests, Rh$_o$(D) immune globulin intravenous (human) with, 1076

Disease-modifying antirheumatic drugs
anifrolumab with, 83
rituximab with, 1088

Disoproxil fumarate, pantoprazole sodium with, 951–952

Disopyramide
chlorpromazine hydrochloride with, 284
ciprofloxacin with, 290
droperidol with, 446.e2–446.e3
erythromycin lactobionate with, 506
granisetron hydrochloride with, 622
ibutilide fumarate with, 660
insulin human aspart with, 701
insulin human injection with, 705
oxaliplatin with, 923
phenytoin sodium with, 997
procainamide hydrochloride with, 1032
propranolol hydrochloride with, 1045–1046
romidepsin with, 1092–1093
verapamil hydrochloride with, 1208–1209

Disseminated gonococcal infections
cefotaxime sodium for, 237
ceftriaxone sodium for, 263

Disseminated intravascular coagulation (DIC)
aminocaproic acid for, 53
heparin sodium for, 624

Disulfiram (Antabuse)
aminophylline with, 59
caffeine/sodium benzoate with, 198.e2
diazepam with, 390
fosphenytoin sodium with, 589–590
metronidazole hydrochloride with, 819–820

Disulfiram *(Continued)*
theophylline in D5W with, 1151.e6–1151.e7

Diuretics
alprostadil with, 42
amikacin sulfate with, 51
amphotericin B with, 73
buprenorphine hydrochloride with, 190–191
clofarabine with, 305–306
cosyntropin with, 320
dexamethasone sodium phosphate with, 376–377
diazepam with, 390
droperidol with, 446.e2–446.e3
enalaprilat with, 464–465
epinephrine hydrochloride with, 471–472
epoprostenol sodium with, 488
ethacrynic acid with, 516.e2–516.e3
foscarnet sodium with, 581
gentamicin sulfate with, 607
hydralazine hydrochloride with, 635
hydrocortisone sodium succinate with, 639
hydromorphone hydrochloride with, 643–644
ibuprofen lysine with, 658
inotuzumab ozogamicin with, 701.e5
insulin human aspart with, 701
insulin human injection with, 705
irinotecan hydrochloride with, 714
ketorolac tromethamine with, 735–736
mannitol with, 782
meperidine hydrochloride with, 786.e4
methadone hydrochloride with, 796.e5–796.e6
methylprednisolone sodium succinate with, 810
morphine sulfate with, 837–838
ondansetron hydrochloride with, 916
pantoprazole sodium with, 951–952

Color type indicates generic drug name.
*See http://evolve.elsevier.com/IVMeds for detailed information.

Color type indicates generic drug name.
*See http://evolve.elsevier.com/IVMeds for detailed information.

Color type indicates generic drug name.
*See http://evolve.elsevier.com/IVMeds for detailed information.

Color type indicates generic drug name.
*See http://evolve.elsevier.com/IVMeds for detailed information.

Color type indicates generic drug name.
*See http://evolve.elsevier.com/IVMeds for detailed information.

Color type indicates generic drug name.
*See http://evolve.elsevier.com/IVMeds for detailed information.

---

*See http://evolve.elsevier.com/IVMeds for detailed information.

Color type indicates generic drug name.
*See http://evolve.elsevier.com/IVMeds for detailed information.

Color type indicates generic drug name.
*See http://evolve.elsevier.com/IVMeds for detailed information.

Color type indicates generic drug name.
*See http://evolve.elsevier.com/IVMeds for detailed information.

Solution Compatibility Chart

Intravenous Medication	D2½W	D5W	D10W	D5/¼NS	D5/½NS	D5NS	NS	½NS	R	LR	D5R	D5LR	Dextran 6%/D5W/NS	Fruc 10%/W/NS	Invert sug 10%/W/NS
Acetazolamide	C	C	C	C	C	C	C	C	C	C	C	C	C	C	C
Acyclovir		C		C	C	C	C			C					
Aminophylline	C	C	C	C	C	C	C	C	C	C	C	C	C		
Antithymocyte Globulin	C	C	C	C	C	C	C	C							
Ascorbic Acid	C	C	C	C	C	C	C	C	C	C	C	C	C	C	C
Aztreonam		C	C	C	C	C	C			C	C		C		
Calcium Chloride		C	C	C	C	C	C			C	C	C	C		
Calcium Gluconate		C	C			C	C			C		C		W	
Cefazolin Na		C	C	C	C	C	C			C	C		C		W
Cefoperazone Na		C	C	C		C	C			C		C			
Cefotaxime Na		C	C	C	C	C	C				C				W
Cefotetan		C					C								
Cefoxitin Na		C	C	C	C	C	C			C	C		C		C
Ceftazidime		C	C	C	C	C	C			C	C				W
Ceftriaxone Na		C	C		C		C								W
Cefuroxime Na		C	C	C	C	C	C			C	C				W
Clindamycin		C	C		C	C	C			C	C				
Dexamethasone		C					C								
Dobutamine HCl		C	C		C	C	C	C		C		C			
Dopamine HCl		C	C		C	C	C			C		C			
Doxycycline		C					C		C						W
Epinephrine	C	C	C	C	C	C	C			C	C	C	C	C	C
Famotidine		C	C				C			C					
Fentanyl		C					C								
Folic Acid		C					C								
Furosemide		C	C			C	C			C		C			
Gentamicin		C	C				C		C	C					
Heparin Na	C	C[a]		C	C	C	C[a]	C	C		C	C	C	C	C
Hydrocortisone Phosphate		C	C				C	C							
Hydrocortisone Na Succinate	C	C	C	C	C	C	C	C	C	C	C	C	C	C	C
Hydromorphone HCl		C	C		C	C	C	C	C	C	C	C		W	
Imipenem-Cilastatin		C[4]	C[4]	C[4]	C[4]	C[4]	C[10]								
Insulin (Regular)		C[P]	C		C		C[P]			C	C				
Isoproterenol	C	C[P]	C	C	C	C	C[P]	C	C	C	C	C	C	C	C
Kanamycin		C	C			C	C				C				
Labetalol		C		C		C	C		C	C	C	C			
Lidocaine		C[P]			C	C	C	C		C		C			
Magnesium Sulfate		C					C			C					
Meperidine HCl	C	C	C	C	C	C	C	C	C	C	C	C	C	C	C
Meropenem		C[1]	C[1]	C[1]		C[1]	C[4]		C[4]	C[4]		C[1]			